S0-BAU-769

PHYSIOLOGIC BASIS OF MODERN SURGICAL CARE

Physiologic Basis of Modern Surgical Care

EDITOR

Thomas A. Miller, M.D.

Professor and Vice Chairman,
Department of Surgery,
University of Texas Medical School,
Houston, Texas

CONTRIBUTING EDITOR

Brian J. Rowlands, M.D., F.R.C.S.

Professor and Chairman,
Department of Surgery,
Queen's University,
Belfast, Ireland;
Formerly Associate Professor of Surgery,
Department of Surgery,
University of Texas Medical School,
Houston, Texas

With 741 illustrations

The C.V. Mosby Company

St. Louis · Washington, D.C. · Toronto 1988

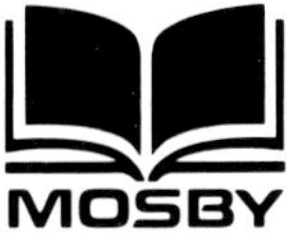

A TRADITION OF PUBLISHING EXCELLENCE

Editor: Terry Van Schaik
Assistant editor: Patricia Gregory
Project manager: Patricia Gayle May
Manuscript editors: Mary Cusick Drone
Marilyn Kinney Wynd
Susan McRoberts Hermance

Printed in the United States of America

The C.V. Mosby Company
11830 Westline Industrial Drive 63146

Library of Congress Cataloging-in-Publication Data

Physiologic basis of modern surgical care.

Includes bibliographies and index.
1. Physiology, Pathological. 2. Surgery. I. Miller, Thomas A. (Thomas Allen). II. Rowlands, Brian J. [DNLM: 1. Physiology. 2. Surgery. WO 102 P578]
RB113.P47 1988 616.07 87-24666
ISBN 0-8016-3421-0

C/MV/MV 9 8 7 6 5 4 3 2 1 01/B/014

Contributors

Joseph F. Amaral, M.D.
Assistant Clinical Instructor in Surgery,
Department of Surgery,
Brown University Medical School;
Haffenreffer Surgical Research Fellow,
Rhode Island Hospital,
Providence, Rhode Island

Stanley W. Ashley, M.D.
Research Fellow,
Department of Surgery,
Washington University School of Medicine,
St. Louis, Missouri

James L. Austin, M.D.
Assistant Professor of Surgery,
Department of Surgery,
University of Missouri Health Sciences Center;
Staff Surgeon,
Department of Surgical Services,
Harry S. Truman Memorial Veterans Administration Hospital,
Columbia, Missouri

Charles M. Balch, M.D.
Professor and Head, Division of General Surgery and Chairman,
Department of General Surgery,
University of Texas M.D. Anderson Hospital and Tumor Institute;
Professor and Associate Chairman, Department of Surgery,
University of Texas Medical School at Houston,
Houston, Texas

Dennis F. Bandyk, M.D.
Associate Professor of Surgery,
Department of Surgery,
Medical College of Wisconsin;
Chief, Vascular Surgery Service,
Department of Surgery,
Wood Veterans Administration Medical Center,
Milwaukee, Wisconsin

Giacoma Basadonna, M.D.
Assistant Professor,
Third Department of Surgery,
University of Milan,
Milan, Italy

Donald P. Becker, M.D.
Professor of Surgery/Neurosurgery,
Department of Surgery,
UCLA School of Medicine;
Chief of Neurosurgery,
Department of Surgery,
UCLA Medical Center,
Los Angeles, California

James M. Becker, M.D.
Associate Professor of Surgery,
Director of Gastrointestinal Surgery,
Department of Surgery,
Washington University School of Medicine,
St. Louis, Mo.

George S. Benson, M.D.
Professor of Surgery/Urology,
Department of Surgery,
Division of Urology,
University of Texas Medical School at Houston;
Urology Staff,
Department of Surgery/Urology,
Hermann Hospital;
Consultant Staff,
Shriners Hospital for Crippled Children,
Houston, Texas

Kirby I. Bland, M.D.
Professor and Associate Chairman,
Department of Surgery,
University of Florida College of Medicine;
Staff Surgeon,
Shands Hospital at the University of Florida,
Gainesville, Florida

Roger A. Bonau, M.D.
Resident, Department of Surgery,
Vanderbilt University Medical School,
Nashville, Tennessee

Edward L. Bove, M.D.
Associate Professor of Surgery;
Director, Pediatric Cardiac Surgery,
Department of Surgery,
University of Michigan Medical Center,
Ann Arbor, Michigan

John W. Brown, M.D.
Associate Professor of Surgery,
Section of Cardiothoracic Surgery,
Department of Surgery,
Indiana University School of Medicine;
Attending Cardiothoracic Surgeon,
Indiana University Hospitals and
Riley Children's Hospital,
Indianapolis, Indiana

Christopher W. Bryan-Brown, M.D.
Professor,
Departments of Surgery and Anesthesiology,
University of Texas Medical School at Houston;
Attending Anesthesiologist,
Hermann Hospital,
Houston, Texas

Juan A. Cabrera, M.D.
Instructor/Research Coordinator in Neurosurgery,
Division of Neurosurgery,
Department of Surgery,
University of Texas Medical School;
Staff Neurosurgeon,
Hermann Hospital,
Houston, Texas

Michael D. Caldwell, M.D., Ph.D.
Associate Professor of Surgery,
Department of Surgery,
Brown University Medical School;
Associate Surgeon,
Rhode Island Hospital,
Providence, Rhode Island

Laurence Y. Cheung, M.D.
Professor and Chairman,
Department of Surgery,
University of Kansas School of Medicine,
Kansas City, Kansas

G. Patrick Clagett, M.D.
Professor and Chief,
Division of Vascular Surgery,
Department of Surgery,
University of Texas Southwestern Medical School;
Dallas Veterans Administration Medical Center,
Parkland Memorial Hospital,
Dallas, Texas

Orlo H. Clark, M.D.
Professor of Surgery,
Department of Surgery,
University of California at San Francisco;
Staff Physician,
Department of Surgical Service,
Veterans Administration Medical Center,
San Francisco, California

Rolando Colon, M.D.
Research Fellow,
Cardiovascular Research Laboratory,
Texas Heart Institute;
Resident,
Department of Surgery,
University of Texas Medical School,
Houston, Texas

Edward M. Copeland, III, M.D.
Professor and Chairman,
Department of Surgery,
University of Florida College of Medicine;
Chief of Surgery,
Department of Surgery,
Shands Hospital at the University of Florida,
Gainesville, Florida

Joseph N. Corriere, Jr., M.D.
Professor of Surgery/Urology,
Director of the Division of Urology,
Department of Surgery,
University of Texas Medical School at Houston;
Chief of Urology,
Hermann Hospital,
Houston, Texas

John M. Daly, M.D.
Professor of Surgery,
University of Pennsylvania Medical School,
Philadelphia, Pennsylvania

David R. Dantzker, M.D.
Professor and Director,
Division of Pulmonary Medicine,
Department of Internal Medicine,
University of Texas Medical School at Houston;
Staff Physician,
Department of Pulmonary Services,
Hermann Hospital,
Houston, Texas

Haile T. Debas, M.D., F.R.C.S.(C)
Professor and Chairman,
Department of Surgery,
University of California at San Francisco;
Moffit-Long Hospitals,
San Francisco, California

Clifford W. Deveney, M.D.
Professor of Surgery,
Department of Surgery,
Oregon Health Sciences University;
Chief, Surgery,
Veterans Administration Hospital,
Portland, Oregon

Philip E. Donahue, M.D.
Professor of Surgery,
Department of Surgery,
University of Illinois at Chicago;
Chairman, Division of General Surgery,
Cook County Hospital,
Chicago, Illinois

Charles D. Ericsson, M.D.
Associate Professor of Medicine,
Program in Infectious Disease and Clinical Microbiology,
University of Texas Medical School at Houston;
Staff Physician,
Department of Medicine,
Hermann Hospital,
Houston, Texas

Peter J. Fabri, M.D.
Professor and Vice Chairman,
Department of Surgery,
University of South Florida College of Medicine,
Tampa, Florida

Ronald Fairman, M.D.
Assistant Clinical Professor,
Department of Surgery,
University of Pennsylvania Medical School,
Philadelphia, Pennsylvania

O. Howard Frazier, M.D.
Professor of Surgery,
Director, Division of Cardiovascular and Thoracic Surgery,
Department of Surgery,
University of Texas Medical School at Houston;
Director, Cardiac Transplant Program;
Director, Cardiovascular Surgical Research Laboratories,
Texas Heart Institute;
Chief, Cardiovascular Surgery,
Hermann Hospital,
Houston, Texas

Thomas R. Gadacz, M.D.
Associate Professor of Surgery,
Department of Surgery,
Johns Hopkins University School of Medicine;
Chief, Surgical Service,
Baltimore Veterans Administration Medical Center,
Baltimore, Maryland

Glenn W. Geelhoed, M.D.
Professor of Surgery,
Department of Surgery,
George Washington University Medical School;
Chief, Surgical Endocrinology,
Director, Surgical Research,
Attending Surgeon,
George Washington University Hospital,
Washington, D.C.;
Consultant, Surgery Branch, National Cancer Institute,
National Institutes of Health,
Bethesda, Maryland

Bruce L. Gewertz, M.D.
Associate Professor,
Department of Surgery,
University of Chicago Medical School;
Director, Surgical Education,
Pritzker School of Medicine at the University of Chicago,
Chicago, Illinois

Philip Gildenberg, M.D., Ph.D.
Clinical Professor of Surgery/Neurosurgery,
University of Texas Medical School,
Houston, Texas

Alan M. Graham, M.D.
Assistant Professor of Surgery,
Department of Surgery
McGill University Medical School,
Royal Victoria Hospital,
Montreal, P.Q., Canada

Linda M. Graham, M.D.
Associate Professor of Surgery,
Division of Peripheral Vascular Surgery,
Department of Surgery,
University of Michigan Medical School,
Ann Arbor, Michigan

A. Gerson Greenburg, M.D., Ph.D.
Professor of Surgery,
Program on Medicine,
Brown University Medical School;
Surgeon-in-Chief,
Miriam Hospital,
Providence, Rhode Island

Christine Idzikowski, OTR/L
Director,
Occupational Therapy Department,
University Hospitals of Cleveland,
Cleveland, Ohio

Larry W. Jenkins, Ph.D.
Associate Professor of Neurology,
Department of Neurology,
Medical College of Virginia,
Virginia Commonwealth University,
Richmond, Virginia

Barry D. Kahan, M.D., Ph.D.
Professor of Surgery,
Director, Division of Immunology and Organ Transplantation,
Department of Surgery,
University of Texas Medical School at Houston;
Surgeon Director, End Stage Renal Disease Center,
Department of End Stage Renal Disease,
Hermann Hospital,
Houston, Texas

Kenji Kakizaki, M.D.
Staff Surgeon,
Sendai National Hospital,
Sendai, Japan

Jeffrey Katz, M.D., Ch.B.
Assistant Professor,
Department of Anesthesiology,
University of Texas Medical School at Houston;
Attending Staff,
Department of Anesthesiology,
Hermann Hospital,
Houston, Texas

Gordon L. Kauffman, Jr., M.D.
Professor of Surgery and Physiology,
Chief, Division of General Surgery,
Department of Surgery,
Pennsylvania State University College of Medicine,
Milton S. Hershey Medical Center,
Hershey, Pennsylvania

Dennis R. Kopaniky, M.D., Ph.D.
Assistant Professor of Surgery,
Director, Spinal Cord Injury Service,
Division of Neurosurgery,
Department of Surgery,
University of Texas Medical School at Houston;
Staff Neurosurgeon,
Hermann Hospital,
Houston, Texas

Barry A. Levine, M.D.
Professor of Surgery,
Department of Surgery,
University of Texas Medical School at San Antonio;
Attending Surgeon,
Department of Surgery,
Medical Center Hospital and Audie Murphy Memorial Veterans Hospital,
San Antonio, Texas

Charles D. Livingston, M.D.
Surgical Practice;
Formerly Resident, Department of Surgery,
University of Texas Medical School at San Antonio,
San Antonio, Texas

Charles W. Lloyd, Pharm.D.
Assistant Professor,
Department of Pharmaceutics,
School of Pharmacy,
University of Michigan,
Ann Arbor, Michigan

Alan H. Lockwood, M.D.
Professor of Neurology,
Department of Neurology,
University of Texas Medical School at Houston;
Attending Physician,
Department of Neurology,
Hermann Hospital,
Houston, Texas

Marc I. Lorber, M.D.
Associate Professor of Surgery,
Director, Division of Organ Transplantation and Immunology,
Department of Surgery,
Yale University School of Medicine,
New Haven, Connecticut

Harold R. Mancusi-Ungaro, M.D.
Assistant Professor of Surgery,
Division of Plastic and Reconstructive Surgery,
Director, University Hospital Burn Unit,
Department of Surgery,
University of Colorado Health Sciences Center,
Denver, Colorado

Stephen J. Mathes, M.D.
Professor of Surgery,
Head, Division of Plastic Surgery,
Department of Surgery,
University of California at San Francisco,
San Francisco, California

David W. McFadden, M.D.
Instructor in Surgery,
Department of Surgery,
Johns Hopkins University Medical School,
Baltimore, Maryland

Irvin G. McQuarrie, M.D., Ph.D.
Associate Professor of Neurosurgery,
Department of Surgery,
Associate Professor of Developmental Genetics and Anatomy,
Case Western Reserve University School of Medicine,
Assistant Neurosurgeon,
University Hospitals of Cleveland;
Medical Investigator in Neurosurgery,
Veterans Administration Medical Center,
Cleveland, Ohio

Ronald C. Merrell, M.D.
Associate Professor of Surgery,
Department of Surgery,
University of Texas Medical School at Houston;
Chief, "Green" Surgery Service,
Hermann Hospital,
Houston, Texas

Thomas A. Miller, M.D.
Professor and Vice Chairman,
Department of Surgery,
University of Texas Medical School at Houston;
Chief, "Blue" Surgery Service,
Hermann Hospital,
Houston, Texas

Michael E. Miner, M.D., Ph.D.
Professor of Surgery,
Director, Division of Neurosurgery,
Department of Surgery,
University of Texas Medical School at Houston;
Director of Neurosurgery,
Hermann Hospital,
Houston, Texas

Elvira L. Muller, M.D.
Chief Resident in Surgery,
Department of Surgery,
UCLA School of Medicine,
Los Angeles, California

Stuart I. Myers, M.D.
Assistant Professor of Surgery,
Department of Surgery,
University of Texas Medical School at Houston;
Chief, Section of Vascular Surgery,
Hermann Hospital,
Houston, Texas

Heber H. Newsome, Jr., M.D.
Professor and Interim Chairman,
Department of Surgery,
Chairman, Division of General/Trauma Surgery,
Medical College at Virginia,
Virginia Commonwealth University,
Richmond, Virginia

John E. Niederhuber, M.D.
Professor of Surgery and Oncology,
Professor of Molecular Biology and Genetics,
Departments of Surgery, Oncology, and Molecular Biology and Genetics,
Johns Hopkins University School of Medicine,
Baltimore, Maryland

Philip R. Orlander, M.D.
Assistant Professor of Medicine,
Division of Endocrinology,
Department of Internal Medicine,
University of Texas Medical School at Houston;
Attending Physician,
Department of Internal Medicine,
Hermann Hospital,
Houston, Texas

Mark B. Orringer, M.D.
Professor of Surgery,
Head, Section of Thoracic Surgery,
Department of Surgery,
University of Michigan,
Ann Arbor, Michigan

Donald H. Parks, M.D.
Associate Professor of Surgery,
Chief, Division of Plastic Surgery,
Department of Surgery,
University of Texas Medical School at Houston;
Chief, Plastic Surgery,
Hermann Hospital,
Houston, Texas

Gary L. Pellom
Assistant Professor of Surgery,
Department of Surgery,
State University of New York at Buffalo School of Medicine;
Attending Surgeon,
Buffalo Children's Hospital,
Buffalo, New York

Henry A. Pitt, M.D.
Associate Professor of Surgery and Vice Chairman,
Department of Surgery,
Johns Hopkins University School of Medicine,
Baltimore, Maryland

Lennart Rabow, M.D.
Chief of Neurosurgery,
University Hospital,
Linkoping, Sweden

Daniel H. Raess, M.D.
Assistant Professor of Surgery,
Section of Cardiothoracic Surgery,
Indiana University School of Medicine,
Indianapolis, Indiana

Howard A. Reber, M.D.
Professor and Vice Chairman,
Department of Surgery,
University of California at Los Angeles,
Los Angeles, California;
Chief, Surgical Service,
Veterans Administration Medical Center—Sepulveda,
Sepulveda, California

J. David Richardson, M.D.
Professor of Surgery and Vice Chairman,
Department of Surgery,
University of Louisville School of Medicine,
Louisville, Kentucky

Layton F. Rikkers, M.D.
Professor and Chairman,
Department of Surgery,
University of Nebraska Medical Center,
Omaha, Nebraska

Joyce M. Rocko, M.D.
Associate Professor of Surgery,
Department of Surgery,
University of Medicine and Dentistry at New Jersey,
New Jersey Medical School;
Director, Emergency/Trauma Services,
University Hospital,
Newark, New Jersey

John L. Rombeau, M.D.
Associate Professor of Surgery,
University of Pennsylvania Medical School,
Philadelphia, Pennsylvania

Brian J. Rowlands, M.D., F.R.C.S.
Professor and Chairman,
Department of Surgery,
Queen's University,
Belfast, Ireland;
Formerly Associate Professor of Surgery,
Department of Surgery,
University of Texas Medical School at Houston,
Houston, Texas

Richard P. Saik, M.D.
Associate Professor of Surgery, Department of Surgery,
University of California at San Diego;
Medical Director of Surgery,
Scripps Clinic,
San Diego, California

Andrew M. Seal, M.D., M.S., F.R.C.S.(C)
Associate Professor of Surgery,
Department of Surgery, Faculty of Medicine,
University of British Columbia;
Active Staff,
Department of Surgery,
UBC Health Sciences Centre Hospital,
Vancouver, British Columbia, Canada

Joseph H. Sellin, M.D.
Associate Professor of Medicine and Physiology,
Division of Gastroenterology, Departments of Internal Medicine and Physiology,
University of Texas Medical School at Houston;
Staff Gastroenterologist,
Hermann Hospital,
Houston, Texas

David N. Shapiro, M.D.
Assistant Professor of Pediatrics,
Division of Hematology and Oncology,
Department of Pediatrics,
University of Michigan Medical Center;
Mott Children's Hospital,
Ann Arbor, Michigan

Kenneth R. Sirinek, M.D., Ph.D.
Professor of Surgery,
Department of Surgery,
University of Texas Medical School at San Antonio;
Attending Surgeon,
Medical Center Hospital,
San Antonio, Texas

James C. Stanley, M.D.
Professor of Surgery,
Head, Division of Vascular Surgery,
Department of Surgery,
University of Michigan Medical School,
Ann Arbor, Michigan

Alton L. Steiner, M.D.
Professor of Medicine,
Director of Endocrinology,
Department of Internal Medicine,
University of Texas Medical School at Houston;
Attending Physician,
Department of Internal Medicine,
Hermann Hospital,
Houston, Texas

Thomas R. Stevenson, M.D.
Assistant Professor of Surgery,
Section of Plastic Surgery,
University of Michigan Medical School,
Ann Arbor, Michigan

Harvey J. Sugerman, M.D.
David M. Hume Professor of Surgery,
Department of Surgery,
Medical College of Virginia,
Virginia Commonwealth University,
Richmond, Virginia

Kenneth G. Swan, M.D.
Professor of Surgery,
Chief, General Surgery,
Department of Surgery,
University of Medicine and Dentistry of New Jersey,
New Jersey Medical School,
Newark, New Jersey

Brian L. Thiele, M.D.
Professor of Surgery,
Department of Surgery,
Pennsylvania State University College of Medicine;
Chief, Vascular Surgery,
Milton S. Hershey Medical Center,
Hershey, Pennsylvania

Martin J. Tobin, M.D.
Assistant Professor of Medicine,
Division of Pulmonary Medicine,
Department of Internal Medicine,
University of Texas Medical School at Houston;
Attending Physician,
Hermann Hospital,
Houston, Texas

Alan S. Tonnesen, M.D.
Associate Professor of Anesthesiology,
Department of Anesthesiology,
University of Texas Medical School at Houston;
Medical Director, Surgical Intensive Care Unit,
Hermann Hospital,
Houston, Texas

David H. Van Buren, M.D.
Fellow, Division of Immunology and Organ Transplantation,
Department of Surgery,
University of Texas Medical School at Houston,
Houston, Texas

Gage Van Horn, M.D.
Professor of Neurology,
Department of Neurology,
University of Texas Medical School at Houston;
Attending Physician,
Department of Neurology,
Hermann Hospital,
Houston, Texas

David J. Wainwright, M.D.
Assistant Professor of Surgery,
Division of Plastic and Reconstructive Surgery,
University of Texas Medical School at Houston;
Attending Surgeon,
Plastic Surgery/Burn Unit,
Hermann Hospital,
Houston, Texas

William E. Walker, M.D., Ph.D.
Associate Professor of Surgery,
Division of Cardiothoracic Surgery,
Department of Surgery,
University of Texas Medical School at Houston;
Houston, Texas

Thonas R. Weber, M.D.
Professor of Surgery,
Departments of Surgery and Pediatrics,
St. Louis University School of Medicine;
Director, Department of Surgery,
Cardinal Glennon Children's Hospital,
St. Louis, Missouri

Andrew S. Wechsler, M.D.
Professor of General and Thoracic Surgery,
Assistant Professor of Physiology,
Department of Surgery,
Duke University Medical Center;
Attending Surgeon,
Duke Hospital,
Durham, North Carolina

Edward J. Weinman, M.D.
Professor and Director,
Division of Nephrology,
Department of Internal Medicine,
University of Texas Medical School at Houston;
Director of Nephrology,
Hermann Hospital,
Houston, Texas

Walter H. Whitehouse, Jr., M.D.
Associate Professor of Surgery,
Section of Peripheral Vascular Surgery,
Department of Surgery,
University of Michigan Medical School,
Ann Arbor, Michigan

Richard E. Wilson, M.D.
Professor of Surgery,
Department of Surgery,
Harvard Medical School;
Chief of Surgical Oncology,
Department of Surgery,
Brigham and Women's Hospital,
Dan Farber Cancer Institute,
Boston, Massachusetts

Christopher K. Zarins, M.D.
Professor of Surgery,
Chief, Vascular Surgery,
Department of Surgery,
University of Chicago Medical Center,
Chicago, Illinois

Frank G. Zavisca, M.D., Ph.D.
Associate Professor of Anesthesia,
Department of Anesthesiology,
Texas Tech University Health Sciences Center;
Attending Anesthesiologist,
Lubbock General Hospital,
Lubbock, Texas

Michael J. Zinner, M.D.
Associate Professor and Vice Chairman,
Department of Surgery,
Johns Hopkins School of Medicine,
Baltimore, Maryland

Preface

The past two decades have experienced unparalleled advances in the practice of surgery. The ability to aliment patients intravenously and maintain growth and development in the absence of normal gastrointestinal function, to transplant organs almost at will with the expectation of long-term survival, to support the multiply injured or critically ill patient with a variety of machines (often controlled by computers) until normal body function returns, and to replace blood vessels, various other tissues, and even hearts with artificial substitutes are just a few of the many strides that have been made in the field of surgery in recent years. These advances have placed a tremendous responsibility, not only on the contemporary medical student and the trainee in surgery, but also on the practicing surgeon to have a sound knowledge of current surgical physiology if optimum care of patients both diagnostically and in terms of prevention and treatment is to be rendered. Although a number of books have been published over the years to bring this physiologic information to the doorstep of the surgeon, most of this source material on surgical physiology is either a simple extension of basic science oriented without appropriate clinical application, or primarily a collection of clinical treatises in which important physiologic facts and concepts are only treated superficially, with very little emphasis on their importance in the management of surgical disorders. In our role as educators of medical students and surgical house officers, the contributors to this volume and I have been concerned with the tremendous gap that exists between the fund of information learned in physiology during the basic science courses in medical school and the inability to apply this information to clinical care. It is frightening to consider how wide this gap must be among practicing surgeons who may have failed to adequately keep abreast of updated physiologic information, modern advances in surgery, or a combination of the two.

The purpose of the present volume is to bridge this gap by attempting to approach surgical disease as derangements in normal physiology. Thus, in diagnosing surgical disorders, we have explained signs and symptoms in terms of physiologic dysfunction and correlated them with the use of laboratory and radiologic modalities where appropriate. This book is not meant to replace standard textbooks of surgery, nor is it a comprehensive discussion of all aspects of surgical disease. Rather, its purpose is to emphasize that surgical disease is basically a derangement in normal physiology and that the best way to diagnose and treat it is to understand thoroughly this deviation from normal.

No single individual is an expert on all aspects of surgical physiology. In selecting contributors for this book I have recruited individuals who have not only made substantial clinical contributions in their respective fields, but who are also fully current on the physiologic processes pertinent to the topics that they have been asked to address. In addition, each contributor has been made aware of the tremendous importance of critically assessing current knowledge of physiologic processes within his given discipline and applying that which is important to the given clinical situation. Each has admirably achieved this goal.

To cover the fundamental information necessary in a volume on surgical physiology, the book itself has been divided into nine sections. The first section concerns general information pertinent to the human body as a whole. The remaining eight sections focus specifically on the various organ systems, including the alimentary tract, the endocrine system, and the cardiothoracic system. The physiologic information addressed in this book is primarily focused on the needs of the general surgeon. Since the current practice of general surgery only rarely involves diseases affecting the reproductive organs, disorders of the head and neck other than the thyroid and parathyroid glands, and disorders of the musculoskeletal system, specific chapters dealing with these entities have not been included. On the other hand, the well-trained general surgeon does need a solid working knowledge of the physiology of the cardiovascular and urinary systems, as well as various components of the nervous system, including the evaluation of an unconscious patient, the initial management of the patients with head injuries, and the approach to management of nerve injuries. Further, in having a broad-based understanding of endocrinology, information relative to the normal physiology and pathophysiology of the pituitary gland is essential. For these reasons specific chapters involving these organ systems have been included. Although some overlap invariably occurs, every effort has been made to minimize this as much as possible through careful editing. To prevent as much redundancy as possible each author(s) has adapted his chapter to a specific format, and each chapter has been reviewed with great care to ensure that the author discusses physiologic principles and processes rather than delivering an extensive treatise on some disease, which can be readily obtained in most major textbooks of surgery. Each contributor has also been asked to include a current bibliography that comprises the most important references in each field of discussion to provide a basis for further reading by the student of surgery. Depending on the subject being considered, some chapters will have more reference material than others.

To publish a book of this nature demands the cooperation of many individuals. I am indeed appreciative of each of the authors, many of whom are active, busy clinical surgeons, for the important contribution that each has made. I am particularly grateful for the invaluable help provided by Dr. Brian Rowlands, who has served as Contributing Editor in this venture and who is responsible for careful editing of most of the chapters on metabolism, endocrinology, and nutrition. I am also aware that behind the scenes in the production of each chapter are multiple secretaries who assisted in typing, reading, rereading, and photocopying each manuscript. For these many unnamed individuals, I express a special word of gratitude. Finally, I am especially grateful to the representatives of The C.V. Mosby Co. who originally approached me about writing such a volume. Individuals associated with The C.V. Mosby Co. with whom I have worked during completion of the book and whose friendship I value include Terry Van Schaik and Mary Drone. For the publisher's patience, encouragement, and help along the way, I offer many thanks.

Thomas A. Miller

SPECIAL ACKNOWLEDGEMENT

The editor wishes to express a formal ''thank you'' and note of appreciation to Mrs. Inci Akkaya, his personal secretary, for the important role that she played in bringing this book to completion. The untold hours of typing and retyping of manuscript, as well as ensuring that the many details necessary to produce a book of this nature were attended to, are gratefully acknowledged.

Contents

This book is dedicated to my parents,
Marion R. and Joseph E. Miller, who made it all possible
and to my wife, Janet, and our children, David, Bill, and Laurie,
who made it all worthwhile.

PHYSIOLOGIC BASIS OF MODERN SURGICAL CARE

Part One GENERAL CONSIDERATIONS IN THE MANAGEMENT OF SURGICAL PATIENTS

1 Metabolic Response to Starvation, Stress, and Sepsis

Joseph F. Amaral and Michael D. Caldwell

The metabolic response to stress, starvation, and sepsis may be viewed as a complex series of neuroendocrine reflexes induced by these factors and resulting in an integrated attempt by the organism to mobilize energy substrates, to preserve oxygen and substrate delivery, and to maintain essential body functions.[69] These metabolic alterations involve changes in the distribution and use of water, proteins, fats, and carbohydrates. As such, an understanding of normal body composition is essential to make discussion of the metabolic response itself meaningful.

BODY COMPOSITION

Body composition has been defined by Moore[129] as "the study of the total mass and volume of body components in relation to body size, body configuration, age, sex, disease, and concentration changes." It may be considered from several aspects including tissue anatomy, chemical composition, or metabolic structure (Fig. 1-1), with the latter two the most important with regard to energy stores and intermediary metabolism.

Chemical Composition

All living organisms may be considered as complex and organized arrangements of fats, proteins, carbohydrates, minerals, and electrolytes in an aqueous environment. Although the percentage of each of these chemical groups varies among and within species, by far the largest component of all living organisms is water.

Water

Water is an important substance involved in virtually all physiologic processes. Its physiochemical properties result largely from its electron structure. The hydrogen ions have a slightly positive charge, whereas the oxygen molecule, with its lone pair of electrons, has a negative charge. This difference allows extensive hydrogen bonding and a relatively high dipole moment[121] that causes the water molecules to orient themselves in an external electric field in such a way that they act as an electric buffer. When ionic substances are placed in water, a hydrational shell forms around the individual ions, reducing their electrochemical attraction.[121] Thus water keeps electrolytes and other polar molecules in solution and allows them independent motion, which is important in nutrient transport.

The extensive hydrogen bonding capacity of water molecules causes them to orient themselves in a highly organized structure similar to ice. This structure accounts for the relatively high boiling point of water, its relatively high freezing point, and its high specific heat (the energy required to raise the temperature of 1 g of a substance 1° C). This latter property allows water to exert a major role in temperature regulation since a large amount of heat is lost as water evaporates (perspiration) and a large amount of heat is required to raise the temperature of water. The extensive hydrogen bonding of water also makes it important in establishing the tertiary structure of proteins and other molecules.

Total body water (TBW) is divisible into two components: intracellular water (ICW) and extracellular water (ECW). These two components are separated by cell membranes. Measurement of body fluid compartments uses dilution techniques (Fig. 1-2), which are based on the concept that a substance that distributes itself equally and exclusively throughout a given compartment (e.g., TBW) can be used to determine the volume of that compartment. This procedure is done by injecting a known amount of the substance and measuring its concentration at steady state as well as measuring the amount excreted during the period of time required to reach steady state. Thus:

$$\text{Volume} = \frac{\text{Amount injected} - \text{Amount excreted}}{\text{Steady state concentration}}$$

Since the amount lost is usually negligible, the convention is to use:

$$\text{Volume} = \frac{\text{Amount injected}}{\text{Steady state concentration}}$$

Numerous substances are available that allow measurement of various fluid compartments (Fig. 1-3), of which TBW is most accurately measured.

TBW varies with age, sex, body build, physical activity, disease, and state of hydration. TBW can be measured accurately using deuterium oxide or tritiated water. For a healthy adult male, TBW constitutes approximately 60% of total body weight, and for a healthy adult female, it constitutes approximately 50% (Table 1-1). The differences in the proportion of TBW reflect the quantity of

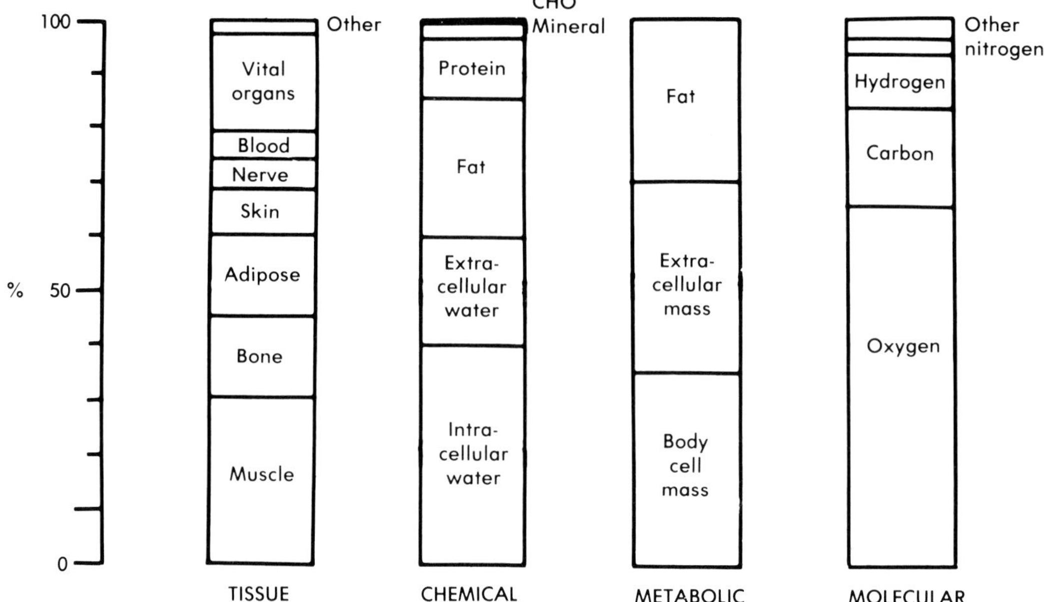

Fig. 1-1 Body composition in adult man. (From Shizgal, H.M. In Fischer, J.E., editor: Surgical nutrition, Boston, 1983, Little, Brown & Co.; Bell, G.H., Davidson, J.N., and Emslie-Smith, D.: Textbook of physiology and biochemistry, London, 1972, Churchill Livingstone, Inc.; and Mitchell, H.H., et al.: J. Biol. Chem. **158:**625, 1945.)

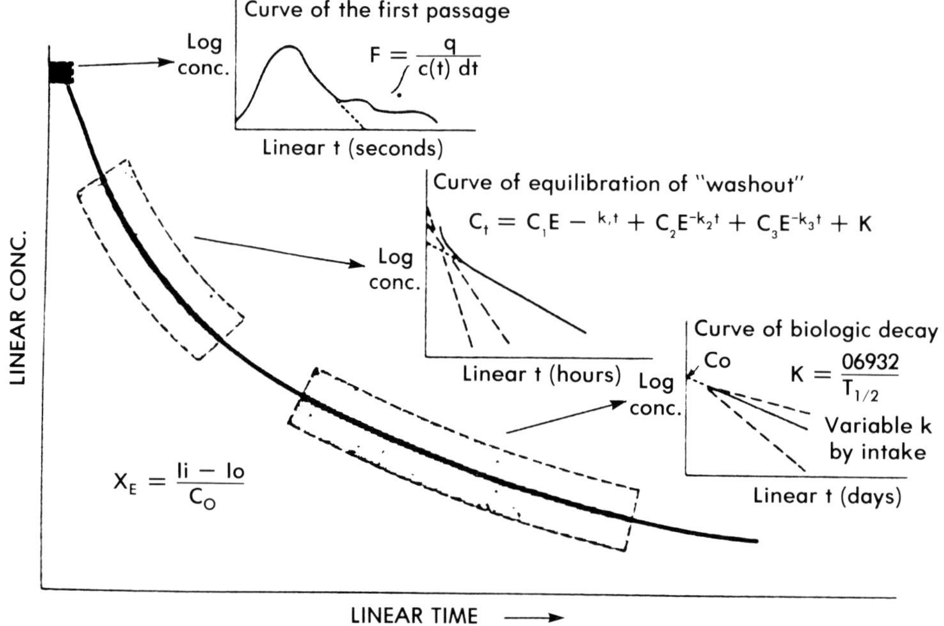

Fig. 1-2 Isotope dilution principle. A stylized curve, divided into three approximate portions, is shown for dilution of an ion in body water components followed over time. The first portion is the "first pass" through heart and lungs and represents the formulation used for cardiac output measurements. The second declining slope (of variable pitch according to the element) represents the sum of a series of slopes, determined by rate-limiting membranes and flux rates. The final portion of the curve is a single exponential representing the biologic halftime of the element in the body. Mathematic formulations are shown for each portion of the curve. (From Moore, F.D.: J.P.E.N. **4:**227, 1980.)

skeletal muscle and adipose tissue present in the two sexes. Adipose tissue contains little ICW, whereas skeletal muscle has one of the largest water contents of all tissues (Table 1-2). Women, with their larger adipose tissue stores and smaller skeletal muscle mass, have less TBW than males. Similarly, the TBW of young, lean athletes is greater than that of elderly, obese nonathletes.

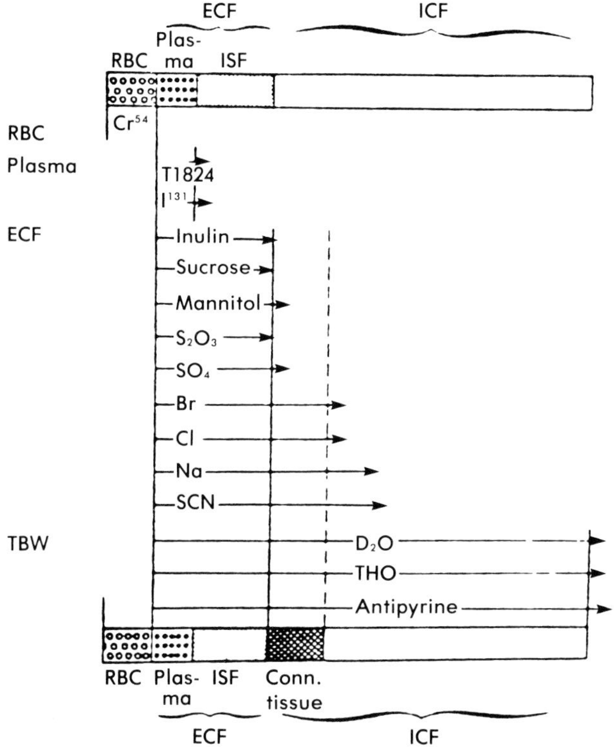

Fig. 1-3 Substances used to measure the body fluid compartments. (From Winters, R.W.: The body fluids in pediatrics, Boston, 1973, Little, Brown & Co., Inc.)

Table 1-1 **DISTRIBUTION OF TOTAL BODY WATER IN INFANTS, CHILDREN, AND ADULTS**

	Total Body Water (%)	
Age	Men	Women
0-1 day	79	79
1-10 days	74	74
1-3 months	72.3	72.3
3-6 months	70.1	70.1
6-12 months	60.4	60.4
1-2 years	58.7	58.7
2-3 years	63.5	63.5
3-5 years	62.2	62.2
5-10 years	61.5	61.5
10-16 years	58.9	57.3
17-39 years	60.6	50.2
40-59 years	54.7	46.7
60+ years	51.5	45.5

Modified from Maxwell, M.H., and Kleeman, C.R.: Clinical disorders of fluid and electrolyte balance, ed. 3, New York, 1979, McGraw-Hill Book Co.

TBW as a percentage of body weight decreases steadily with age (see Table 1-1). Newborn infants have the highest percentage, with 75% to 80% of body weight representing water. This percentage decreases during the first few months after birth to approximately 65% of the body weight, where it remains for the remainder of infancy and childhood. The reduction in TBW is primarily the result of reduction in ECW (Fig. 1-4). Until the age of 12, no difference in TBW is noted between males and females. With advancing age, TBW as a percentage of body weight decreases to a low of 52% and 47% in males and females, respectively.[129] This results primarily from a decrease in ICW since ECW remains unchanged.[121]

The size of the ECW space depends on the method used for determining it. Large molecules such as inulin, mannitol, or sucrose appear to underestimate the ECW compartment because of the slower diffusion of these larger molecules into noncellular spaces.[121] An ECW space of 15% to 16% of body weight is usually reported with these methods.[121] Assessment of the ECW with small molecules such as $^{35}SO_4$, ^{82}Br, and ^{24}Na appears to overestimate the extracellular fluid space because of the ability of these small ions to diffuse into cells. An ECW space of 21% to 27% of body weight is usually reported when these methods are used.[121]

The ECW occupies 20% of the body weight (and therefore 30% to 40% of TBW). It is divided into plasma (5% of body weight) and interstitial fluid (15% of body weight). The interstitial fluid occupies a rapidly equilibrating functional space between cells and a slowly equilibrating (or nonequilibrating) space composed of epithelial cell secretions, connective tissue, joint space, and cerebrospinal fluids, the so-called transcellular space.[49] The functional interstitial fluid accounts for 90%, and the transcellular space accounts for 10% of the total interstitial fluid.

The transcellular space should not be equated with the "third space." The transcellular fluids are a normal component of the ECW and do not affect the functional volume of the extracellular space. The third space results from abnormalities in the permeability of cells such as

Table 1-2 **DISTRIBUTION OF WATER IN THE VARIOUS TISSUES OF A 70-KG MAN**

Tissue	Water (%)	Body Weight (%)	Liters of Water per 70 kg
Skin	72	18	9.07
Muscle	75.6	41.7	22.1
Skeleton	22	15.9	2.45
Brain	74.8	2	1.05
Liver	68.3	2.3	1.03
Heart	79.2	0.5	0.28
Lungs	79	0.7	0.39
Kidneys	82.7	0.4	0.25
Spleen	75.8	0.2	0.1
Blood	83	8	4.65
Intestine	74.5	1.8	0.94
Adipose tissue	10	±10	0.7

From Skeleton, H.: Arch. Int. Med. **40**:140, 1927. Copyright 1927, American Medical Association.

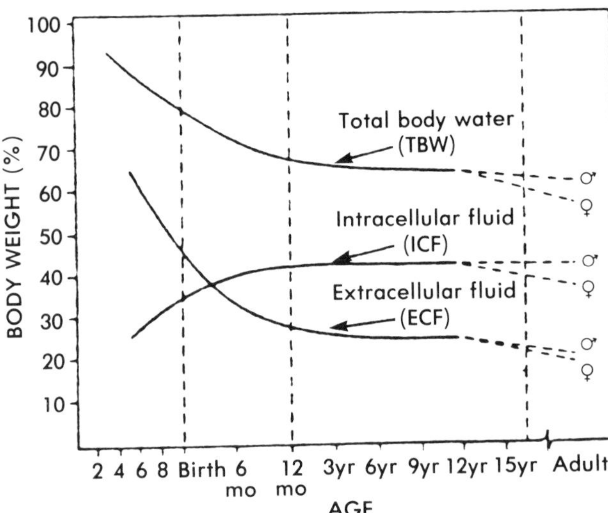

Fig. 1-4 Distribution of body fluids in children as a function of age and sex. (From Winters, R.W.: The body fluids in pediatrics, Boston, 1973, Little, Brown & Co., Inc. Reproduced by permission of Pediatrics **28:**169, 1961.)

Table 1-3 **ELECTROLYTE COMPOSITION OF THE BODY FLUID COMPARTMENTS**

Electrolytes	Serum (mEq/L)	Serum Water (mEq/L)	Interstitial Fluid (mEq/L)	Intracellular Fluid (Muscle) (mEq/kg of H_2O)
Cations				
Sodium (Na^+)	142	152.7	145	± 10
Potassium (K^+)	4	4.3	4	156
Calcium (Ca^{++})	5	5.4		3.3
Magnesium (Mg^{++})	2	2.2		26
Total cations	153	165	149	195
Anions				
Chloride (Cl^-)	102	109.7	114	± 2
Bicarbonate (HCO_3^{2-})	26	28	31	± 8
Phosphate (HPO_4^{2-})	2	2.2		95
Sulfate (SO_4^{2-})	1	1.1		20
Organic acids	6	6.5		
Protein	16	17.2		55
Total anions	153	165	145	180+

From Maxwell, M.H., and Kleeman, C.R.: Clinical Disorders of Fluid and Electrolyte Metabolism, ed. 3, New York, 1979, McGraw-Hill Book Co.

those abnormalities seen after ischemia and those seen with inflammation that increases the size of the extracellular space but not the volume of the ECW. Third-space size is proportional to the severity of the injury. Since fluid and electrolytes in the third space are derived from functional extracellular fluid, the increase in size of the extracellular space reduces the functional extracellular volume.

Direct measurement of the ICW compartment is extremely difficult since substances that equilibrate only in the intracellular space have not been defined. Consequently, the ICW space is estimated as the difference between TBW and ECW. The ICW space varies from individual to individual. In healthy normal adults it constitutes approximately 30% to 40% of body weight (55% of TBW). Since fat has little ICW and skeletal muscle has the highest percentage of ICW, athletic muscular individuals have a higher proportion of ICW; but females, the obese, and the elderly have a smaller muscle mass and therefore have a smaller percentage of their body weight as ICW.

The electrolyte composition of the various fluid compartments is noted in Table 1-3. The major cations are sodium and potassium, and the major anions are chloride and bicarbonate. The absolute amount of a particular ion can only be measured by cadaveric analyses, but the total exchangeable amount of an ion can be estimated by the dilution technique. The total exchangeable amount represents that portion of the total amount that is available for exchange and equilibration with a labeled form of the compound. Total exchangeable sodium is not equivalent to total body sodium. A large amount, approximately 1000 mEq, is present in a nonexchangeable form in bone.[130] The total exchangeable potassium is more closely equivalent to the total body potassium (less than 0.5% is nonexchangeable).[130]

Sodium is the major extracellular cation, and potassium is the major intracellular cation (Table 1-4). The ECW space is approximated by the total body sodium, the ICW space by the total body potassium, and the TBW by the sum of total body sodium and total body potassium. Moore[130] has used this relationship to estimate TBW from total exchangeable sodium (Na_e) and potassium (K_e) using the formula below:

$$TBW = \frac{(Na_e + K_e) + 70}{163} (\pm 2\ L)$$

The differing ionic compositions of the various fluid compartments are the result of variations in the permeabilities and active transport mechanisms present in the cell membranes separating these spaces. There is a great diversity among the transcellular fluids in this regard (Table 1-5).

Fat (Lipids)

Until the 1950s, lipids, the second largest chemical constituent of the body, were considered relatively inert substances that served as a source of protection and insulation. They now are recognized as essential components of energy metabolism providing 9.3 kcal/g, hormonal synthesis (steroids), hormonal regulation and action (prostaglandins), and neural transmission (sphingomyelins). In addition, they are required for general cellular integrity and stability (cell membrane phospholipids and cholesterol). Many of the functions of lipids require fatty acids that cannot be synthesized by human beings. The three major essential fatty acids are arachidonic acid, linoleic acid, and linolenic acid.

Total body fat varies inversely with total body water in normal individuals. During the first 4 months of life, there is a decrease in the percentage of total body fat—expressed as percent of total body weight (Table 1-6). After puberty the total body fat content increases, with increase greater in females than in males. In healthy adult males total body fat accounts for approximately 25% of body weight, and in healthy adult females fat accounts for ap-

Table 1-4 **TOTAL AND EXCHANGEABLE AMOUNTS OF ELECTROLYTES IN FLUID COMPARTMENTS OF ADULT MAN**

Compartment	Sodium	Potassium	Magnesium	Chloride	Bicarbonate
	(mEq/kg of Body Weight)				
Total extracellular	52.8	2.5	21.8	27.8	6.8
Total intracellular	5.2	51.3	8.2	5.2	5.9
Total body	58	53.8	30	33	12.7
Total exchangeable	41	52.8	3.4, 4.9, 10*	33	12.7
Total body intracellular concentration (mEq per liter intracellular water)	14.4	14.3	22.8	14.4	16.4

From Ruch, T.C., and Patton, H.D.: Physiology and biophysics, vol. 2, Philadelphia, 1974, W.B. Saunders Co.
*Equilibrated for 24, 48, and 89 hours respectively. Total exchangeable magnesium is a function of time of equilibration.

Table 1-5 **MEAN ELECTROLYTE COMPOSITION OF TRANSCELLULAR FLUIDS**

Fluid	Na^- meq/L	K^- meq/L	Cl^- meq/L	HCO_3^- meq/L	H^+ meq/L
Saliva	33	20	34	0	—
Gastric juice	60	10	130	0	90
Bile	149	5	101	45	—
Pancreatic juice	141	5	77	92	—
Ileal fluid	129	11	116	29	—
Cecal fluid	80	21	48	22	—
Cerebrospinal fluid	141	3	127	23	—
Sweat	45	5	58	0	—

Modified from Rose, B.D.: Clinical physiology of acid-base and electrolyte disorders, New York, 1977, McGraw-Hill Book Co.

Table 1-6 **BODY COMPOSITION OF INFANTS AND CHILDREN AS FUNCTION OF AGE**

Age (Months)	Body Weight (kg)	Whole Body (g/100 g)			
		Water	Protein	Lipid	Other
Birth	3.5	75.1	11.4	11	2.5
4	7	60.2	11.4	26.3	2.1
12	10.5	59	14.6	23.9	2.5
24	13	61	15.7	20.6	2.7
36	15	62	16.4	18.3	3.3

From Fomon, S.J.: Infant nutrition, ed. 2, Philadelphia, 1974, W.B. Saunders Co.

proximately 35% of body weight (Fig. 1-5). During advancing age, there is an increase in the percentage of body weight occupied by fat. However, it is of note that body weight often remains unchanged with age. Since total body weight equals body fat plus fat-free tissues, a decrease in fat-free tissue is thought to occur with aging.[77]

The percentage of body weight occupied by fat is also inversely related to the level of physical activity. Muscular athletic individuals have a greater muscle mass and smaller percentage of body fat than sedentary individuals of similar body weight.[12] These changes are somewhat adaptive, however. For example, a long-distance swimmer benefits from the buoyancy and insulation provided by fat and often has a greater amount of fat than a long-distance runner of equivalent body build.[12] This presumably results from a difference in caloric intake between these two groups.

Approximately 50% of the fat in human beings is located in the subcutaneous tissue, but the distribution of the subcutaneous tissue varies with age, sex, and physical activity.[77] Children have a large amount of subcutaneous tissue over their triceps but only a small amount of subcutaneous tissue in their abdominal walls. The distribution is reversed in adults. Changes in the body fat distribution, occurring as a result of weight gain, are not equally distributed.[77] For this reason, serial measurement of an isolated anthropometric index may not adequately reflect body composition changes in malnourished people who are being repleted. However, changes in the body fat distribution occurring as a result of weight loss are equally distributed. A 10% loss in triceps skin fold will be accompanied by a concomitant 10% loss in the size of the subcutaneous tissues of other areas such as the hips, abdomen, thighs, and breasts.[77]

Total body fat is defined as the difference between total body weight and fat-free mass (see the following equation). Fat contains very little water and virtually no potassium. On the other hand, the total water content of fat-free tissue averages 73.2% of total body water (TBW),[149] and the potassium content of fat-free tissues averages 68.1 mEq/kg.[77] Consequently, fat-free tissue may be approximated from either TBW or total exchangeable potassium (K_e) and the total body fat (TBF) estimated by inference. Equations for these calculations are:

For TBW: $TBF = BW - (TBW/0.732)$
and
$\%TBF = 1 - (\%TBW/0.732)$

For K_e: $TBF = BW - (K_e)/68.1$
and
$\%TBF = [BW - (K_e/68.1)]/BW$

where TB is body weight. It should be noted that these methods assume that the hydration and potassium content of that portion of the body that is fat free is constant. However, these assumptions are not always valid because the hydration of the fat-free tissue can vary considerably (e.g., greatest in edematous states and least in dehydrated states).

A third method used in calculating total body fat involves the measurement of the specific gravity of the individual by underwater weighing procedure.[11,12,20,77] This method is based on the finding that normal human fat has a density of 0.9 g/ml and nonfat tissue has an average density of 1.1 g/ml at 37° C. At 37° C, the density of an average reference male containing 15.3% body fat is 1.064 g/ml.[10] With the use of these values the percentage fat in an individual can be determined by measuring his density (D) in water as indicated by the equation:

$$\%\text{Fat} = [(4.570/D) - 4.142] \times 100^{20}$$

Although the density of human fat changes only with temperature, the density of fat-free tissue changes with age, degree of obesity, and degree of hydration.[77] Changes in weight are not simply the result of increases or decreases in body fat. Overweight or underweight as compared to the reference male is not equal to more or less fat. These changes involve tissue that is both fat and fat free. Tissue

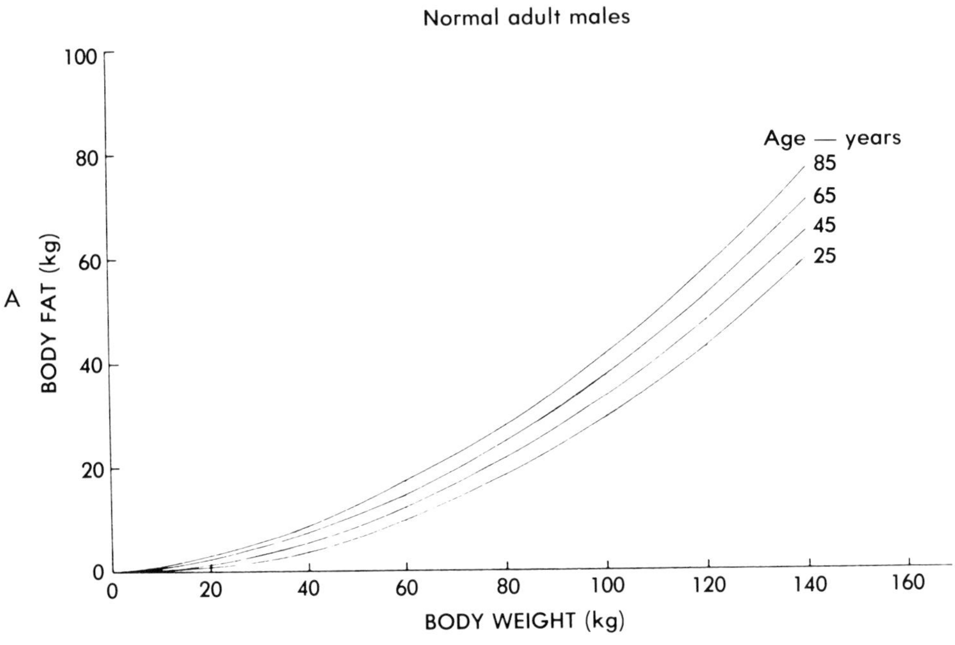

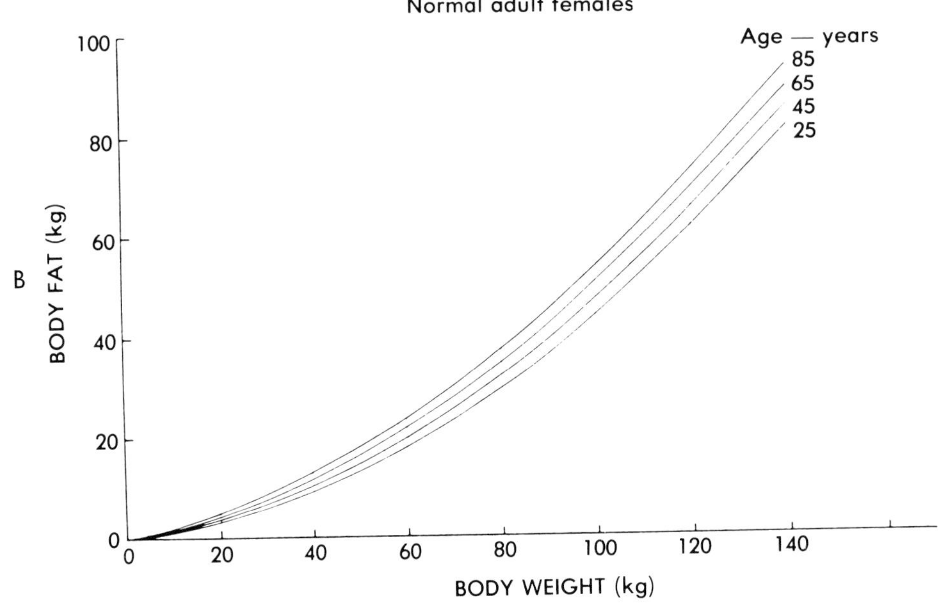

Fig. 1-5 Relationship of total body fat, **A,** in men, and **B,** in women as a function of total body weight and age. (From Moore, F.D.: The body cell mass and its supporting environment, Philadelphia, 1963, W.B. Saunders Co.)

termed obese tissue by Keys and Grande[77] has a density at 37° C of 0.9478 g/ml and is 73% fat. The proportion (in grams [g]) of the body made up by obese tissue can be determined as:

$$g = (1.064/D) - 1/(1.064/0.9478) - 1$$
$$g = 8.1566$$

The amount of obese tissue present is "g × BW," and the amount of nonobese tissue is "BW − obese tissue." Total body fat can then be calculated as:

$$\text{TBF} = (\text{Obese tissue} \times 0.73) + (\text{Nonobese tissue} \times 0.153)$$

where 0.73 and 0.153 are the proportion of fat in obese and nonobese tissues respectively. When estimates of total body fat made by densitometric methods are compared to calculations of total body fat made from TBW, the densitometric methods give a higher estimate of total body fat.[11,12] Densitometric methods give a lower estimate of total body fat when compared to calculations of total body fat made from total exchangeable potassium.[11,13]

A fourth method used to calculate total body fat involves the measurement of the uptake of an inert, highly fat-soluble gas such as cyclopropane or krypton.[109] The assumption made in this technique is that the gas will only go into fat cells. Thus it should yield a more accurate measurement of total body fat than the other methods noted. When compared to measurements made by TBW determination, similar results are obtained.[142] When compared to K_e measurements or densitometric measurements, lower values are obtained.[189] However, no data are available comparing the inert gas method with cadaver analyses.

Proteins

Proteins are essential components of all living cells and are involved in virtually all body functions. These molecules serve as enzymes, hormones, neurotransmitters, immunoglobins, and transport molecules. They are also essential components of all cell membranes as well as various cellular components including receptors, transport systems, and contractile elements. As such, they are necessary for the metabolism, growth, regulation, replication, protection, repair, communication, and motion of individual cells as well as the coordinated function of the entire organism. Consequently, it is somewhat remarkable that total body proteins account for only 15% of the body weight in a healthy adult male and that over 80% of the total body protein is present in skeletal muscle and connective tissue.

As a result of its numerous and varied functions, protein, unlike fat, undergoes considerable daily turnover. Approximately 2.5% of the total body protein (250 g in a 70-kg adult male) is broken down and resynthesized each day.[189] More than half of this turnover is accounted for by daily secretory processes, white cell turnover, hemoglobin turnover, muscle protein turnover, and plasma protein turnover. The total turnover rate of body protein diminishes progressively with age.[135] The protein synthesis rate per kilogram of body weight decreases from 25 g/kg/day in the neonate to 7 g in a 1-year-old infant. In the average adult male and female, protein synthesis is 3.2 and 2.6 g/kg of body weight per day, respectively, whereas in an elderly male and female, it is 2.6 and 1.9 g, respectively.

The synthesis rate of transport protein, such as albumin, remains unchanged with increasing age, but the breakdown rate (and presumably synthesis rate) of skeletal muscle decreases (Table 1-7). If the total turnover rate of protein is expressed per lean body mass rather than body weight, an increase in turnover is noted with aging. Since the lean body mass decreases with aging as a result of a reduction in skeletal muscle mass and the synthesis rate of albumin is unchanged, it is apparent that the changes in protein turnover per kilogram body weight are the result of a decrease in skeletal muscle mass.

Total body protein may be determined by one of two methods: (1) measurement of total exchangeable potassium; or (2) measurement of total body nitrogen by neutron activation. Total body nitrogen (TBN) is linearly related to total exchangeable potassium in both normal and decreased conditions.[83,183] The average exchangeable potassium to nitrogen ratio in tissue is 3 mEq/g nitrogen.[130] Thus:

$$\text{TBN} = K_e/3$$

Table 1-7 **COMPARISON OF WHOLE BODY PROTEIN BREAKDOWN WITH ESTIMATES OF MUSCLE PROTEIN BREAKDOWN AND ALBUMIN SYNTHESIS IN YOUNG AND OLD ADULT HUMAN BEINGS**

		Whole Body Protein Breakdown* (g/day)			Muscle Protein Breakdown† (g/day)			Albumin Synthesis‡ (g/day)		
Group	Mean Age (Years)	Per kg Body Weight	Per kg Body Cell Mass	Per gram Creatinine	Per kg Body Weight	Per kg Body Cell Mass	Per gram Creatinine	Per kg Body Weight	Per kg Body Cell Mass	Per gram Creatinine
Males										
Young	22	2.94	6.7	115	0.76	1.74	30	0.19	0.39	7
Old	70	2.64	7.5	163	0.53	1.50	32	0.15	0.40	8.4
Females										
Young	20	2.35	6.1	103	0.64	1.69	28			
Old	76	1.94	6.6	166	0.31	1.05	26			

From Valgeirsdòttir, K.V., and Munro, H.N.: © Am. J. Clin. Nutr. **31**:1608, 1978.
*Measured by administration of ^{15}N-glycine [92].
†Measured as 3-methylhistidine output in urine and computed as muscle protein [92].
‡Measured by administration of ^{15}N-glycine [31].

where K_e equals exchangeable potassium. Total body protein (TBP) is directly proportional to total body nitrogen (TBN) by a factor of approximately 6.25. Thus:

$$TBP = (6.25)(TBN) = (6.25)(K_e/3) = 2.08\ K_e$$

Total body nitrogen can also be measured using neutron activation analysis.[83,87] When tissues are irradiated with neutrons from either a cyclotron or a plutonium source, gamma rays specific for a substance capturing the neutron are emitted. For nitrogen, gamma rays of 10.83 Mev are emitted. Consequently, measurement of the gamma rays produced after neutron activation allows determination of total body nitrogen. In general the results obtained with either method correlate well with each other.

Carbohydrates

Carbohydrates serve as the energy source of the body when energy is rapidly required, providing 4 kcal/g. They also serve important roles in cell-membrane function and stability (glycoproteins and glycolipids), hormone function (glycoproteins), and as precursors of lipid and nonessential amino acid synthesis. In addition, the brain, red cells, white cells, and wounds are to a large extent glucose-dependent tissues. Of the three major sugars found in the human body (glucose, fructose, and galactose), glucose is the primary carbohydrate. In addition to ingested carbohydrates, glucose is readily available from pyruvate and lactate, gluconeogenic amino acids (alanine and glutamine), the glycerol moiety of lipids, and its storage form, glycogen.

Most of the body's glycogen is stored in the liver, skeletal muscle, and cardiac muscle. Muscle glycogen is used primarily by the muscle itself because muscle lacks glucose 6-phosphatase. In contrast, hepatic glycogen is primarily used in providing glucose to glucose-dependent tissues. Since little glycogen is stored in the liver, the hepatic stores of glycogen are rapidly depleted by an overnight fast. Cahill has estimated the total hepatic glycogen content of a 70-kg male to be 75 g and the total muscle glycogen content to be 150 g.[22]

The total carbohydrate content of the body is approximately 300 g.[99] Except by cadaver analysis, no method is available to measure total body carbohydrate. However, it is of note that the daily intake of carbohydrate approximates the total body stores.

Lean Body Mass and Body Cell Mass

Based on densitometric measurements, Behnke[11,12] proposed the division of total body weight into fat and lean body mass. The lean body mass was defined as that portion of the body mass with the least amount of essential body fat compatible with health. The essential body fat was thought to represent 2% to 10% of the total body weight. However, because the essential body fat cannot be differentiated from the nonessential body fat, most investigators have redefined lean body mass as the portion of body mass devoid of all fat, the so-called fat-free body.[77] Although "fat-free body" and "lean body mass" are often used interchangeably, there is a small (2% to 10%) difference between them (Table 1-8). This chapter subsequently

Table 1-8 **COMPARISON OF BODY CELL MASS, LEAN BODY MASS, AND FAT FREE BODY**

	Body Cell Mass (BCM)	Lean Body Mass (LBM)	Fat Free Body (FFB)
Anatomy	**All body cells** Protoplasm Nucleus Membrane $[ICK]_{AV} = 150 mE/L_{ICW}$	**All body cells} BCM** Plus: Plasma, ECF, TCF } ECF Tendon, Fascia, Collagen, Elastin, Dermis, Skeleton } ECS (ECF + ECS) } ECT "2% = 10% essential lipid"} Fat	Same as LBM But No Lipid at All
Function	**Cellular metabolism** Respiration Oxidation Synthesis Cretion Mitosis	**Cellular Metabolism** Support Transport Circulation Protection Integument	Same as LBM
Composition	$[K_e - ECK] \times f = BCM$ $f = 7.5$ to 10 *or* $K_e \times 8.33 = BCM$ 70-kg man $3200 \times 8.33 = 26.6$ kg Calories 2.7 to 3.6 $Cal/hr/kg_{BCM}$	**Density = 1100** $\% LBM = 100 - \frac{495}{d} - 450$ 70-kg man Approx 50 kg Calories 110 $Cal/hr/kg_{LBM}$	$FFB = \frac{TBW}{f}$ $f = 0.695 - 0.735$ 70-kg man $\frac{36.4}{0.732} = 49.7$ Calories (Same as LBM)

From Moore, F.D.: J.P.E.N. **4**:227, 1980.

refers only to the fat-free body, but it should be kept in mind that the same statements are generally true for lean body mass. Since the total body weight is equal to total body fat plus the fat-free body, the size of the fat-free body can be determined by the same methods used to determine the size of the total body fat.

The fat-free body mass is divisible into the extracellular mass, composed primarily of water, and the body cell mass, composed of all the metabolically active cells in the body.[129,130] The cells in the body cell mass are actively involved in energy exchange, protein synthesis, enzyme replication, and morphogenesis.[129] Therefore the body cell mass is composed of the skeletal muscle mass (60%), visceral cell mass (20%), and the peripheral cell mass (20%) (see Table 1-8).[130] The peripheral cell mass includes blood cells and connective tissue cells.

Although the body cell mass cannot be measured directly, it can be calculated from the exchangeable potassium, the exchangeable sodium, the total body nitrogen (TBN), or the intracellular water. Since over 98% of the total body potassium is intracellular, a linear relationship exists between body cell mass (BCM) and the total body potassium (TBP), total exchangeable potassium, and intracellular water. Histochemical analysis has demonstrated that approximately one fourth of the wet weight of cells is protein.[85] Consequently,

$$BCM = (TBP)\ (4) = (2.08\ K_e)\ (4) = 8.33\ K_e$$
$$BCM = (TBN)\ (6.25)\ (4) = 25\ (TBN)$$

Since the average cell has 150 mEq of intracellular potassium per liter[130] and since each cell is composed of 25.8% solids (74.2% water),[85] body cell mass is also equivalent to:

$$K_e\ (1000/0.732)/150 = (K_e)\ (9.10)$$

or

$$ICW/0.742$$

Each of these methods yields a different value for the body cell mass of a given individual. This is most obvious when the two methods presented for K_e are used. However, any of these methods provide accurate estimates of sequential changes in an individual or differences among populations if the same method is used throughout the study.

Measurements of total exchangeable potassium by whole body ^{40}K counting or of total body nitrogen by neutron activation are difficult to perform and require equipment that is expensive and not readily available. To avoid these practical problems, Shizgal and coworkers[174] developed a method to estimate total exchangeable potassium from isotope dilution measurements of total body water (TBW) and total exchangeable sodium. As noted previously, TBW is approximately equal to the sum of the total exchangeable sodium and potassium. Thus:

$$Na_e + K_e/TBW = R$$

where R is constant. Na_e and TBW can be easily measured by isotope dilution with deuterium oxide or tritiated water and ^{22}Na. The constant, R, can be approximated by measurement of the sodium, potassium, and water of whole blood. Thus:

$$K_e = [(R)\ (TBW)] - Na_e$$

and

$$BCM = 8.33\ K_e \text{ or } 9.10\ K_e$$

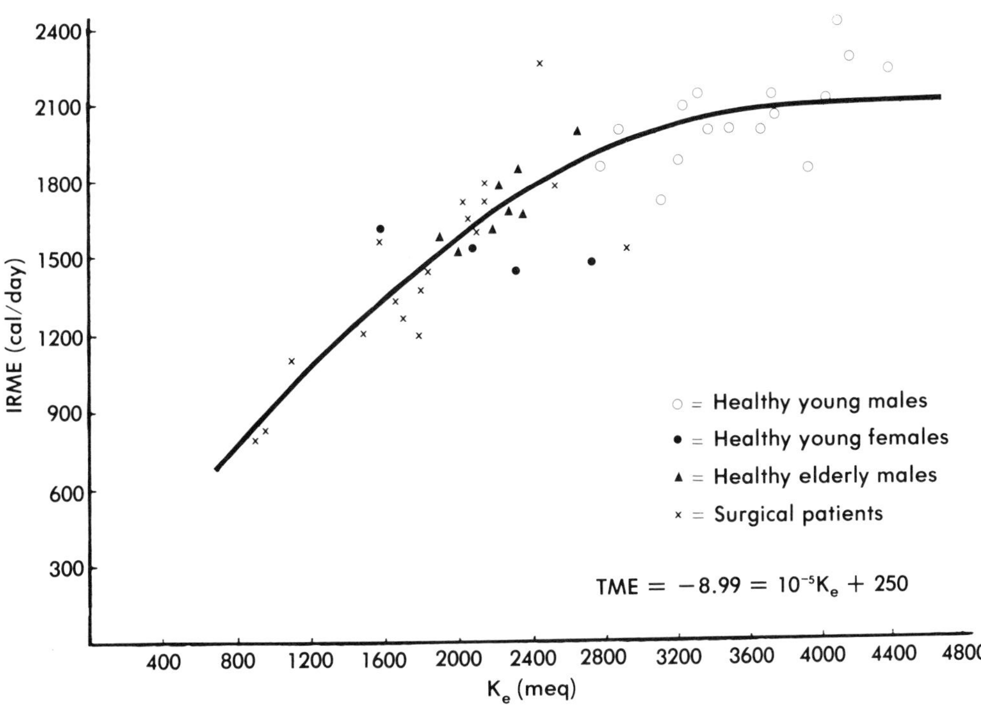

Fig. 1-6 Relationship of total body energy expenditure to the total exchangeable potassium (K_e). (From Kinney, J.M., Lister, J., and Moore, F.D.: Ann. N.Y. Acad. Sci. **110:**711, 1963.)

As might be expected, body cell mass increases with age until the middle years of life. With advancing age, the percentage of body weight composed of the body cell mass decreases as a result of a decrease in skeletal muscle mass. In addition, males generally have a greater percentage of body weight composed of body cell mass than females, athletic individuals greater than sedentary individuals, and lean individuals greater than obese individuals. Thus the body cell mass varies from 20% of body weight in morbidly obese people to 54% in lean athletic males.[157]

A direct correlation exists between total energy expenditure and body cell mass, whereas other measurements of body composition such as total body mass and fat-free body demonstrate a variable or poor correlation.[100] Kinney, Lister, and Moore[100] have demonstrated an oxygen consumption of 8 to 10 ml O_2/kg body cell mass and an energy expenditure of 2.7 to 3.6 kcal/kg/hour body cell mass. As noted in Fig. 1-6, total exchangeable potassium (and therefore body cell mass) is linearly related to the total metabolic energy expenditure in healthy adults and surgical patients until 1800 cal/day are expended. However, when measurements of total metabolic energy expenditure greater than this are included, the relationship is parabolic. This relationship is believed to reflect the lower resting metabolic rate of skeletal muscles per milliequivalent intracellular potassium when compared to visceral tissues. Skeletal muscle, which provides approximately 50% of the total body potassium, accounts for only 15% of the body's resting energy expenditure. On the other hand, visceral tissues, such as brain, heart, and kidneys, which provide only 10% of the total body potassium, account for 70% of the body's resting energy expenditure.[41] Consequently, individuals with a small body cell mass have less skeletal muscle mass and a good correlation of K_e with total metabolic energy expenditure. In contrast, individuals with a large body cell mass have a smaller increase in total metabolic energy expenditure when compared to K_e because skeletal muscle at rest contributes significantly to K_e but not to total metabolic energy expenditure.

ESTIMATION OF BODY COMPOSITION BY SEX AND BODY WEIGHT*

$TBW = 0.7945\,(BWt) - 0.0024\,(BWt)^2 - 0.0015\,(age)(BWt)$ (males)

$TBW = 0.6981\,(BWt) - 0.0026\,(BWt)^2 - 0.0012\,(age)(BWt)$ (females)

$ICW = 0.623\,(TBW) - 0.0016\,(age)\,(TBW)$ (males)

$ICW = 0.553\,(TBW) - 0.0007\,(age)\,(TBW)$ (females)

$Fat = BWt - TBW/0.732$

$ECW = TBW - ICW$

$K_e = 150\,(ICW) + 4\,(ECW)$

$Na_e = 163.2\,(TBW) - K_e - 69$

From Moore, F.D.: The body cell mass and its supporting environment, Philadelphia, 1963, W.B. Saunders Co.

*TBW, total body water; BWt, body weight; ICW, intracellular water; ECW, extracellular water; K_e, exchangeable potassium; Na_e, exchangeable sodium.

Table 1-9 **ESTIMATION OF TOTAL BODY WATER BY AGE, SEX, AND BODY WEIGHT**

Sex	Age (Years)	Total Body Water (Liters)	95% Conf. Limits (%)
Males	16-30	0.4 (BWt*) + 13	±16
	31-60	0.4 (BWt) + 11	±17
	61-90	0.34 (BWt) + 12	±16
Females	16-30	0.31 (BWt) + 11.6	±13
	31-90	0.33 (BWt) + 8.84	±21

From Moore, F.D.: J.P.E.N. **4**:227, 1980.

*BWt, body weight.

Changes in Body Composition with Stress, Sepsis, and Starvation

The body composition of a human being at any given moment is influenced significantly by the individual's age, sex, physical activity, and previous nutritional status as well as by concurrent infections, injuries, and disease processes. Changes produced by age, sex, and physical activity have been discussed at length. Tables 1-9 and 1-10, plus the boxed material at left provide a summary of the formulas derived from multiple body composition studies of normal individuals.[129,130] These formulas can be applied to any healthy adult under normal circumstances to estimate the components of body composition.

Ultimately, body composition is the net result of the total chemical constituents taken in minus the total chemical constituents used and excreted. Since carbohydrates and lipids primarily serve as a source of calories, this relationship can be simplistically stated as,

$$\Delta BC = [(C_{in} + N_{in} + WS_{in}) - (C_{out} + N_{out} + WS_{out})]$$

where Δ is change; BC is body composition; C is calories; N is nitrogen; W is water; and S is solutes (electrolytes and minerals). Under normal steady-state conditions, the quantities of these components taken in equal the quantities used or lost, and there is no net change in body composition (BC = 0). If the quantity of a component taken in is greater than the quantity used, this component either is stored (BC > 0), thus changing body composition, or is lost (BC < 0). For example, if caloric intake is greater than caloric loss or expenditure, energy will be stored in

Table 1-10 **ESTIMATION OF TOTAL EXCHANGEABLE POTASSIUM BY AGE, SEX, AND BODY WEIGHT**

Sex	Age (Years)	Exchangeable Potassium (mEq)	95% Conf. Limits (%)
Males	16-30	38 (BWt*) + 735	±23
	31-60	26 (BWt) + 1383	±20
	61-90	27 (BWt) + 723	±16
Females	16-30	18 (BWt) + 1250	±20
	31-60	17 (BWt) + 1176	±23
	61-90	18 (BWt) + 757	±29
By Total Body Water (TBW)			
Males and females	20-60	97.4 (TBW) − 409	±10
	61-84	2 + 77 (TBW)	±17

From Moore, F.D.: J.P.E.N. **4**:227, 1980.

*BWt, body weight.

the body in the form of lipids and carbohydrates. If water intake is greater than output, water will be retained (e.g., edema). Fortunately, regulatory mechanisms exist that protect against an increase in body water (see Chapter 2) as well as other nutrients. Consequently, for a net increase to be seen in total body water, there must be a neuroendocrine alteration present as well. Such is the case after trauma and surgery when elevated secretion rates of aldosterone and vasopressin promote the retention of salt and water. On the other hand, excess nitrogen intake is not stored, and, as already noted, maximum rates of protein synthesis exist in each individual. When the intake of nitrogen exceeds the need, the excess nitrogen is converted into urea and is excreted.

There are five basic situations in which intake does not equal output—dehydration and the four catabolic stresses defined by Moore as fasting, starvation, injury, and febrile illness.[129] In dehydration, the loss of water exceeds the intake resulting in a reduction in total body water that is distributed throughout the intracellular water and extracellular water. In fasting and in starvation (prolonged fasting), caloric and nitrogen expenditures are the same or less than those of a normal individual, but the intake of these substrates is markedly reduced or absent. As a result, there is a loss of total body lipids, carbohydrates, and nitrogen. In patients with injury or febrile illness, caloric and nitrogen expenditures are greater than those of the normal individual. The increase in energy expenditure produced by an injury or infection is in proportion to the severity of the insult. Burns are the most severe injury, and generalized sepsis is the most severe febrile illness (Fig. 1-7). A healthy adult undergoing an elective operation increases his resting energy expenditure by approximately 10%, but the same individual with a severe burn increases his resting energy expenditure by 40% to 120%, depending on the size and the degree of the burn injury.[98] A minor febrile illness or a minor febrile complication after an elective operation increases the resting energy expenditure by 13% for each degree Celcius of temperature elevation,[47] but generalized sepsis increases the resting energy expenditure by 15% to 50%.[98] The changes in body composition resulting from an increase in caloric and nitrogen expenditure during injury and febrile illness are frequently compounded by reductions in intake as a result of anorexia and ileus. However, if the increased measurements are adequately met by exogenous substrate sources (enteral or parenteral), little change in body composition will occur.[31,87,130,173]

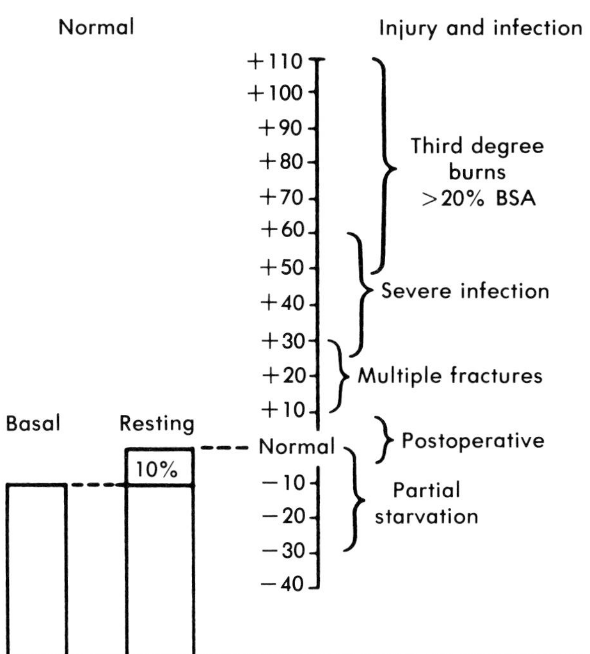

Fig. 1-7 Resting energy expenditure during injury and starvation in man. (From Kinney, J.M.: The application of indirect calorimetry to clinical studies. In Kinney, J.M., editor: Assessment of energy metabolism in health and disease, Columbus, Ohio, 1980, Ross Laboratories.)

NORMAL METABOLISM: INTERMEDIARY METABOLISM AND SUBSTRATE INTERACTIONS

Body composition remains in a steady state when four essential conditions are met: (1) energy is supplied in sufficient quantities to meet the metabolic demands of all the body's tissues; (2) carbohydrates are supplied in sufficient quantities to meet the requirements of glucose-dependent tissues, such as those of the brain, red cells, and white cells; (3) nitrogen is supplied in sufficient quantities to meet the obligatory synthesis of protein; and (4) water and solutes (electrolytes and minerals) are supplied in sufficient quantities to replace daily obligatory losses (water and electrolyte metabolism). In addition, these conditions must be met in the face of varying dietary intakes and varying daily energy requirements. This achievement is possible as a result of numerous substrate to substrate interactions (e.g., conversion of protein to carbohydrates) and the neuroendocrine regulation of intermediary metabolism.

Energy Metabolism

All metabolic processes in cells either produce energy (exergonic reactions) or use energy (endergonic reactions). The energy required for the operation of all biologic processes in nonphotosynthetic cells is derived from the inherent energy present in the structure of organic molecules.[108] The chemical energy produced by the processing of these organic molecules is transferred to the phosphate bonds of purine nucleotides as well as other molecules with phosphate bonds such as phosphagens. As noted in Table 1-11, the hydrolysis of the phosphate bonds of aden-

Table 1-11 **ENERGY RELEASED ($G^{O\prime}$) DURING HYDROLYSIS OF HIGH-ENERGY PHOSPHATE COMPOUNDS**

Reaction	$G^{o\prime}$ (Joules/Mol)
ATP + $H_2O \rightarrow$ ADP + Pi	−36,800
ADP + $H_2O \rightarrow$ AMP + Pi	−36,000
ATP + $H_2O \rightarrow$ AMP + PPi	−40,600
PPi + $H_2O \rightarrow$ 2Pi	−31,800
AMP + $H_2O \rightarrow$ A + Pi	−12,600

Based on data from Lehninger, A.L.: Biochemistry: the molecular basis of cell structure and function, ed. 2, Menlo Park, California, 1975, Worth Publishing, Inc.

osine 5′-triphosphate (ATP) or its precursors releases a considerable amount of energy that can be used to drive other biologic processes. The formation of these compounds with high energy phosphate group transfer potential is usually a result of the transfer of reducing equivalents from the substrate by reduction of NAD^+, flavoproteins, and other coenzymes followed by coupled oxidative phosphorylation of adenosine 5′-diphosphate (ADP) in the mitochondria.[107]

Although ATP serves as a carrier of chemical energy in all living cells, it is not a reservoir of energy.[108] The intracellular concentrations of ATP are small, highly regulated, and rapidly depleted. Reservoirs of energy (phosphagens), such as phosphocreatine, do exist in some cells.[108] These reservoirs accept high-energy phosphate bonds when the intracellular concentration of ATP is high and transfer a phosphate group to ADP nucleotides when the availability of ATP is low.[108]

The intracellular concentrations of adenine nucleotides also provide the cell with a sensitive control mechanism for regulating energy-producing and energy-using processes in cells. Atkinson[7] has introduced the concept of energy charge to explain this regulatory mechanism. Adenylate energy charge (EC) represents the balance between energy-using processes and energy-producing processes. It is defined by the equation:

$$EC = (ATP + 0.5\ ADP)/(ATP + ADP + AMP)$$

A normal energy charge signals that energy-producing processes and energy-using processes are in balance. If the energy charge is increased, energy-producing processes are exceeding energy-using processes, and a resultant reduction of energy-producing processes occurs. If the energy charge is decreased, energy-using processes are exceeding energy-producing processes, resulting in a decrease in energy-using processes that may jeopardize cell survival.

The major energy-producing processes include the catabolism of carbohydrates, proteins, and lipids. Each of these substrate groups can provide part of the energy present in their structure through cytoplasmic catabolic reactions (e.g., glycolysis). The remainder of the available energy present in these substrates is released during oxidation of the remaining carbon fragments in the intramitochondrial tricarboxylic acid cycle (TCA). The final common pathway into the TCA cycle for carbohydrates, proteins, and lipids is through the formation of acetyl coenzyme A (CoA) (Fig. 1-8). For each molecule of acetyl-CoA completely oxidized in the TCA cycle, two molecules of carbon dioxide, three molecules of nicotinamide adenine dinucleotide (reduced form) (NADH), one molecule of flavin adenine dinucleotide (FADH), and one molecule of guanosine 5′-triphosphate (GTP)[190] are produced. In total, 12 high-energy phosphates are formed. Unlike carbohydrates and lipids, amino acids may also directly enter the TCA cycle at one of the intermediate reactions (see Fig. 1-8).

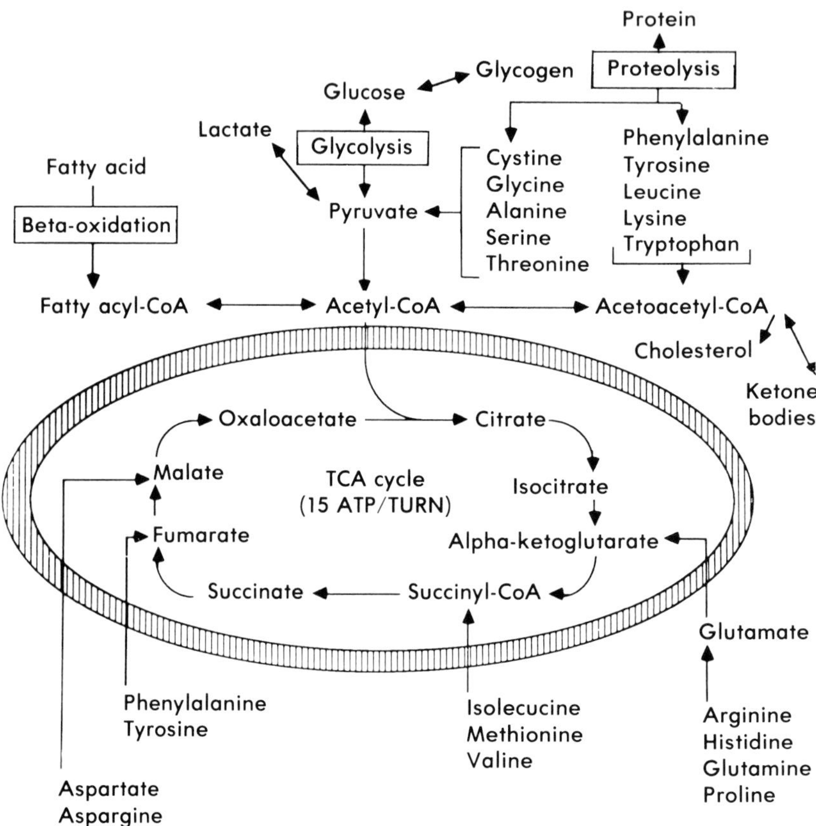

Fig. 1-8 Pathways for production and use of acetyl-CoA. (From Gann, D.S., Amaral, J.F., and Caldwell, M.D.: Metabolic response to injury, stress, and starvation. In Davis, J.H., et al.: Clinical surgery, St. Louis, 1987, The C.V. Mosby Co.)

Carbohydrate Metabolism

In the cytoplasm of all cells, one molecule of glucose is catabolized to pyruvate through the Embden-Meyerhoff pathway to yield two molecules of pyruvate, two molecules of ATP, and one molecule of NADH (Fig. 1-9). The completion of glycolysis (i.e., glucose to lactate) uses one molecule of NADH in the conversion of pyruvate to lactate. Conversely, the conversion of pyruvate to acetyl-CoA produces one molecule of NADH. Since the oxidation of acetyl-CoA in the TCA cycle produces 12 high-energy phosphates (HEP), the complete oxidation of one molecule of glucose to carbon dioxide and water produces 26 high-energy phosphates $[(2 \times 12) + 2]$ and four molecules of NADH. The latter molecules produce 12 high-energy phosphates (three high-energy phosphates per molecule of NADH) through coupled oxidative phosphorylation. Consequently, the total energy produced in the complete oxidation of one molecule of glucose to carbon dioxide and water is equivalent to 38 high-energy phosphates. This result is in contrast to glycolysis where only two high-energy phosphates are produced in the conversion of glucose to lactate. As noted in Fig. 1-9, there are three nonreversible reactions in glycolysis: (1) the conversion of glucose to glucose 6-phosphate, catalyzed by hexokinase; (2) the conversion of fructose 6-phosphate to fructose 1,6-biphosphate, catalyzed by 1-phosphofructokinase; and (3) the conversion of phospho*enol*pyruvate to pyruvate, catalyzed by pyruvate kinase. These reactions are irreversible because they lose a considerable amount of energy as heat. It is the presence of these three nonreversible reactions that drives glucose to pyruvate. In addition, phosphofructokinase and pyruvate kinase act as the major regulators of glycolysis.[141]

Once the catabolism of glucose has begun, it rapidly proceeds to pyruvate. Under aerobic conditions, most tissues oxidatively decarboxylate pyruvate to acetyl-CoA and

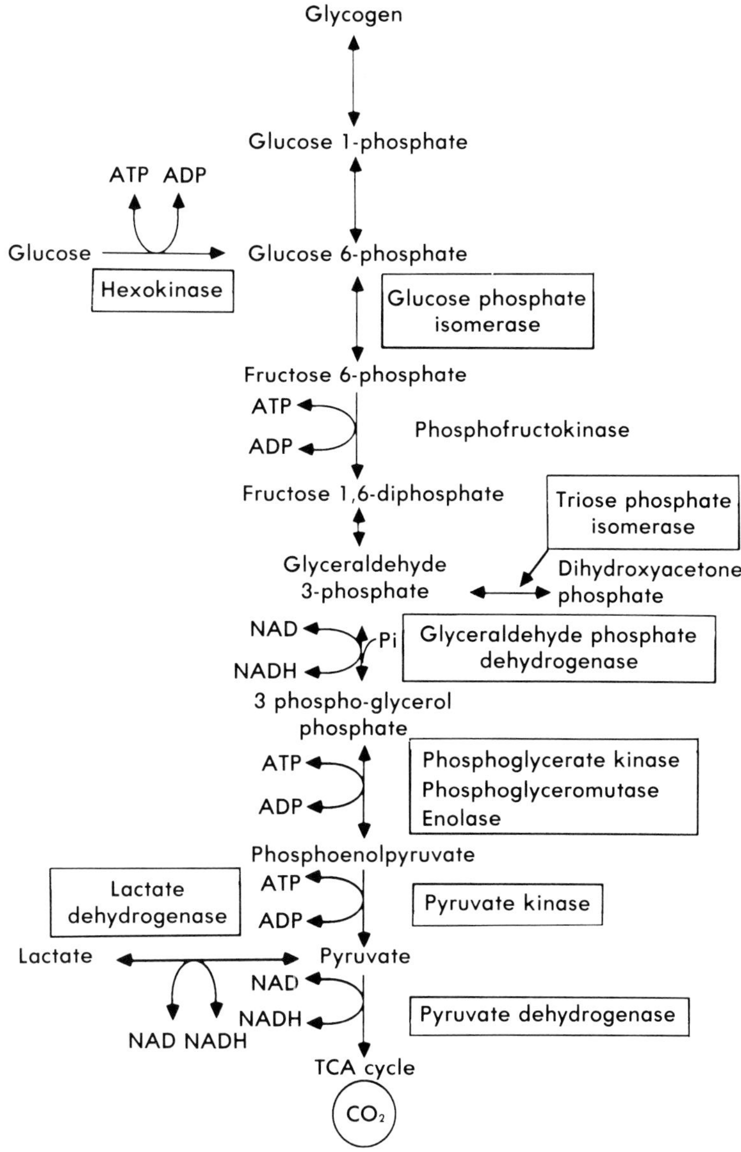

Fig. 1-9 Catabolism of glucose and major carbohydrate precursors. (From Gann, D.S., Amaral, J.F., and Caldwell, M.D.: Metabolic response to injury, stress, and starvation. In Davis, J.H., et al.: Clinical surgery, St. Louis, 1987, The C.V. Mosby Co.)

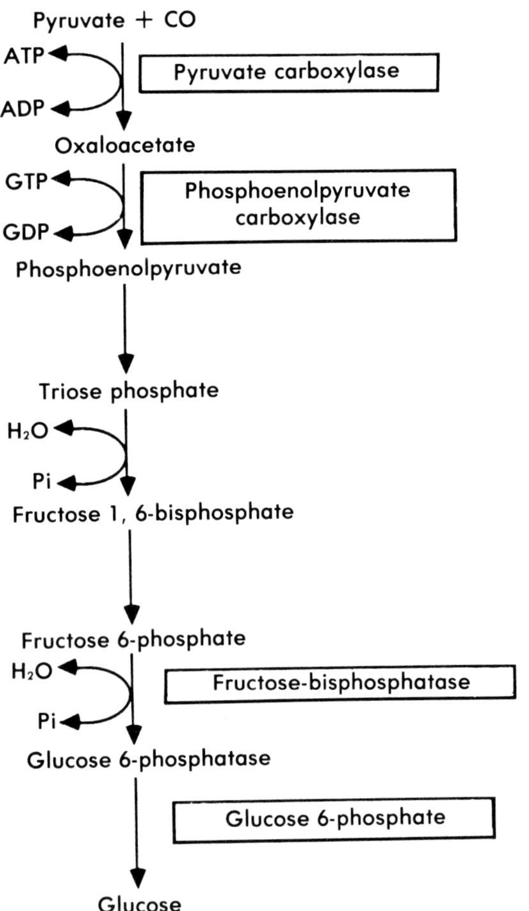

Fig. 1-10 Gluconeogenic pathway in the liver and the kidney. (From Gann, D.S., Amaral, J.F., and Caldwell, M.D.: Metabolic response to injury, stress, and starvation. In Davis, J.H., et al.: Clinical surgery, St. Louis, 1987, The C.V. Mosby Co.)

then oxidize the acetyl-CoA in the TCA cycle. Under anaerobic conditions, pyruvate cannot be decarboxylated, and it is converted instead to lactate. As a result, elevated tissue and plasma concentrations of lactate (and pyruvate) are characteristic of ischemia and anoxia. Some tissues, such as erythrocytes and leukocytes, are capable of glycolysis only. These cells lack the ability to oxidize pyruvate and acetyl-CoA even under aerobic conditions. Therefore they derive all their energy from conversion of glucose to pyruvate and lactate. Carbohydrates other than glucose can also be metabolized through glycolysis. For example, fructose, galactose, mannose, and triose sugars can enter glycolysis after modification by endergonic reactions. Similarly, pentose sugars may also enter the glycolytic pathway.

As noted earlier, the total carbohydrate stores of the human body are limited and are rapidly depleted.[22] In addition, red cells, white cells, and the brain are glucose-dependent tissues that are unable to use nonglucose energy substrates. Thus glucose must be made continuously available. The synthesis of glucose through a process called gluconeogenesis can proceed from lactate, pyruvate, and amino acids, but gluconeogenesis is not simply the reversal of glycolysis because the unidirectional reactions make glycolysis irreversible. However, gluconeogenic tissues, such as the liver and the kidney, contain four enzymes that essentially allow glycolysis to proceed in reverse fashion from pyruvate (and lactate) to glucose (Fig. 1-10). The first of these enzymes, pyruvate carboxylase, in the presence of ATP, carbon dioxide, and biotin, converts pyruvate to oxaloacetate in the mitochondria. (Although it does not act as a cofactor, acetyl-CoA must be present in excess for this reaction to proceed.[14]) Oxaloacetate is then converted to phospho*enol*pyruvate by the cytoplasmic enzyme

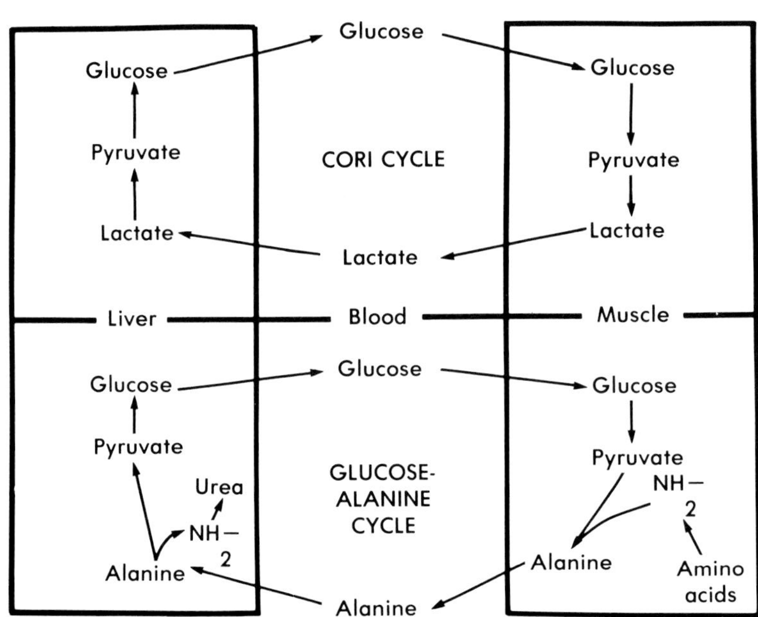

Fig. 1-11 Glucose-lactate (Cori) cycle and glucose-alanine cycle. (From Gann, D.S., and Amaral, J.F.: The pathophysiology of trauma and shock. In Zuidema, G.D., Rutherford, W.F., and Ballinger, W.F., editors: The management of trauma, Philadelphia, 1984, W.B. Saunders Co.)

phospho*enol*pyruvate carboxylase and guanosine 5′-triphosphate (GTP). Since the oxaloacetate is found in the mitochondria and phospho*enol*pyruvate carboxylase in the cytoplasm, oxaloacetate must cross the mitochondrial membranes into the cytoplasm. However, since the mitochondrial membranes are relatively impermeable to oxaloacetate, it is thought that oxaloacetate leaves the mitochondria as either malate or aspartate, which can be transported through the mitochondrial membranes and then reconverted to oxaloacetate in the cytoplasm.[124]

Once phospho*enol*pyruvate is formed, glycolysis can easily proceed in reverse fashion to fructose 1,6-biphosphate. The enzyme fructose 1,6-biphosphate is required to form fructose 6-phosphate. This enzyme is present in the liver and kidney and to a lesser extent in skeletal muscle. However, it is not present in adipose tissue, smooth muscle, or cardiac muscle.[81] Fructose 6-phosphate can then proceed to glucose 6-phosphate by the reversible glycolytic reaction catalyzed by glucosephosphate isomerase, but the conversion of glucose 6-phosphate to glucose requires the last of the gluconeogenic enzymes, glucose phosphatase. This enzyme is present in the liver and kidney but not skeletal, smooth, or cardiac muscle. Any glucose 6-phosphate that might be formed in skeletal muscle must either be converted to glycogen, be used in glycolysis, or be used in the hexose monophosphate shunt because skeletal muscle cannot release free glucose as a result of the absence of glucose 6-phosphatase. The glucose 6-phosphate formed in the liver and kidney can be converted to glucose and released into the circulation.

Since there is a constant production of lactate and pyruvate in aerobic glycolytic tissues and in all tissues during anaerobic conditions, a constant source of lactate and pyruvate is available to gluconeogenic tissues such as the liver and kidney. In the liver and kidney, these substrates can be converted back to glucose and released into the circulation. The newly formed glucose is then available to glucose-dependent tissues for reconversion to lactate in the so-called Cori cycle (Fig. 1-11). However, it should be noted that this reconversion does not result in a net increase in glucose carbon since lactate is itself derived from glucose.[55]

Protein and Amino Acid Metabolism

Energy and glucose can also be derived from the metabolism of amino acids. Although the partial catabolism and transformation of all alpha-amino acids to their alpha-keto acid derivatives can occur in most tissues, the complete oxidation of alpha-amino acids to urea and carbon dioxide occurs primarily in the liver and secondarily in the kidney.[106] In general the catabolism of all amino acids (except lysine) involves the removal of the alpha-amino acid group from the carbon skeleton to form ammonia and an alpha-keto acid. This is followed by the conversion of ammonia to urea and by the conversion of the alpha-keto acids to TCA-cycle intermediates or precursors.[134,136]

Removal of the alpha-amino group can occur by one of three processes: (1) transamination; (2) oxidative deamination; and (3) nonoxidative deamination.[81,124] The most common mechanism is transamination. Transaminases (aminotransferases) interconvert a pair of amino acids and a pair of alpha-keto acids (Fig. 1-12). This process requires the presence of pyridoxyl phosphate (vitamin B_6) for the transfer of the amino group. These reactions are freely reversible and function both in synthesis and in catabolism. At least 12 of the amino acids undergo transamination including the branched chain amino acids, valine, leucine, and isoleucine. The most notable transaminases are glutamic-oxaloacetic transaminase (GOT or aspartate transaminase) and glutamic-pyruvic transaminase (GPT or alanine transaminase). Through the collective action of all the transaminases, the alpha-amino groups are usually collected in the form of glutamate or alanine. Since alpha-ketoglutarate can accept the alpha-amino group of all the amino acids that are transaminated, including alanine, it serves as the final common amino group acceptor to form glutamate.

Mallette, Exton, and Park[119] have proposed and Felig[59] has expanded the concept of an alanine-glucose cycle similar to the Cori cycle (see Fig. 1-11). In peripheral tissues, amino acids are transaminated with pyruvate to form alanine and an alpha-keto acid. The alanine is then transported to the liver where it is transaminated with alpha-ketoglutarate to form pyruvate and glutamate. The pyruvate can then be converted back to glucose and released into the circulation where it may be taken up by peripheral tissues and converted to pyruvate and lactate.

The oxidative deamination of glutamate by glutamate dehydrogenase is an important mechanism in the liver for the removal of the amino group (see Fig. 1-12). Since alpha-ketoglutarate is the common acceptor for all transaminases, substantial amounts of glutamate are formed. Consequently, the oxidative deamination of glutamine allows for the regeneration of alpha-ketoglutarate and the removal of free ammonia. Oxidative deamination of other amino

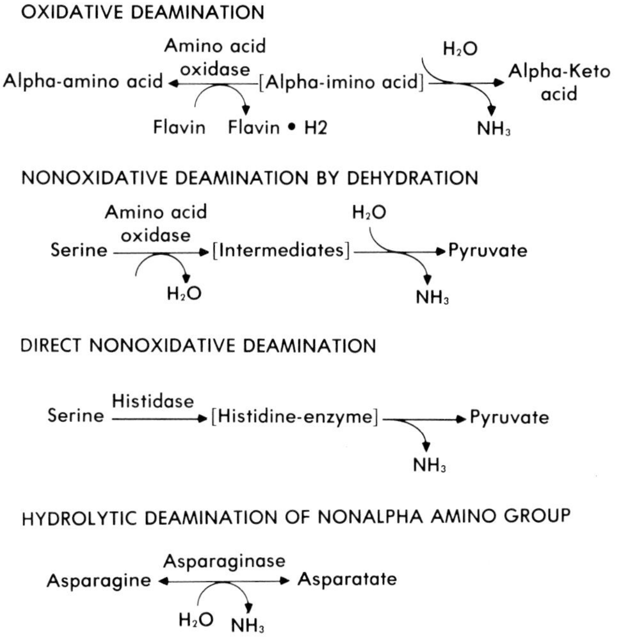

OXIDATIVE DEAMINATION

Alpha-amino acid ← Amino acid oxidase (Flavin → Flavin • H2) → [Alpha-imino acid] (+ H_2O → NH_3) → Alpha-Keto acid

NONOXIDATIVE DEAMINATION BY DEHYDRATION

Serine → Amino acid oxidase (→ H_2O) → [Intermediates] (+ H_2O → NH_3) → Pyruvate

DIRECT NONOXIDATIVE DEAMINATION

Serine → Histidase → [Histidine-enzyme] (→ NH_3) → Pyruvate

HYDROLYTIC DEAMINATION OF NONALPHA AMINO GROUP

Asparagine ← Asparaginase (H_2O → NH_3) → Asparatate

Fig. 1-12 Mechanisms for removal of the amino group. (From Gann, D.S., Amaral, J.F., and Caldwell, M.D.: Metabolic response to injury, stress, and starvation. In Davis, J.H., et al.: Clinical surgery, St. Louis, 1987, The C.V. Mosby Co.)

acids is also possible through the action of alpha-amino acid oxidases that are present in the liver and kidney. However, with the exception of glutamate dehydrogenase, these enzymes do not appear to exert a major physiologic role in humans.[106,136] Three amino acids, serine, threonine, and histidine, are primarily deaminated nonoxidatively (see Fig. 1-12).[124] The former two amino acids undergo nonoxidative deamination by dehydration, whereas histidine undergoes direct deamination. The nonalpha-amino groups of glutamine and aspargine are removed by hydrolytic deamination.[124]

Free ammonia, even in small concentrations, is poorly tolerated by cells. Four mechanisms exist to handle the free ammonia produced by oxidative or nonoxidative deamination, thereby keeping the intracellular (and extracellular) concentration of this substance low. Free ammonia can be added to glutamate by glutamine synthetase to form glutamine. This is the primary mechanism for the elimination of ammonia in brain cells and muscle cells. The free ammonia may also be added to alpha-ketoglutarate, forming glutamate in the freely reversible reaction catalyzed by glutamate dehydrogenase. The resulting glutamate may be used as an amino acid in protein, as a precursor in arginine and citrulline synthesis, or as an alpha-amino group donor in transaminase reactions. A third mechanism for ammonia elimination is through its excretion by the kidney. Two thirds of the ammonia excreted by the kidney is derived from the amide nitrogen of glutamine from renal arterial blood and one third from the alpha-amino nitrogen of renal arterial amino acids.[190]

Although these three mechanisms remove a substantial amount of the ammonia formed, most of it is cleared by the liver with subsequent entry into the urea cycle (Krebs-Henseleit cycle).[106] As noted in Fig. 1-13, the urea cycle essentially involves the cleavage of a molecule of urea from arginine. The ammonia is first combined with carbon dioxide in the presence of ATP to form carbamylphosphate. Carbamylphosphate then condenses with ornithine to form citrulline, which, through a series of reactions, forms arginine. The arginine is then cleaved into urea and ornithine by urease, thereby reestablishing the cycle. The net energy cost of this cycle is four high-energy phosphates derived from three molecules of ATP. Atkinson and Bourke have recently suggested an important role for ureagenesis in the maintenance of pH homeostasis.[8] Since the oxidation of amino acids yields both bicarbonate and ammonium ions, the urea cycle promotes the neutralization of the bicarbonate ion by the proton of the ammonium ion during the formation of carbonylphosphate.

The remaining carbon skeletons of amino acid deamination or transamination are converted either to intermediates of the TCA cycle or to precursors of acetyl-CoA, such as pyruvate and acetoacetate. Consequently, all the carbon skeletons of amino acids can be oxidized in the TCA cycle to carbon dioxide and water. The carbon skeletons of all the amino acids may also be converted to glucose or fat. As such, they may be classified as glucogenic, ketogenic, or glucogenic and ketogenic (Table 1-12). Seven (alanine, serine, glycine, cysteine, cystine, proline,

Table 1-12 **PATHWAYS FOR THE USE OF AMINO ACID CARBON FRAGMENTS**

Gluconeogenesis	Ketogenesis	Gluconeogenesis and Ketogenesis
Alanine	Leucine	Isoleucine
Arginine		Lysine
Aspartic Acid		Phenylalanine
Aspargine		Tyrosine
Cystine		Tryptophan
Glutamic Acid		
Glycine		
Histidine		
Hydroxyproline		
Methionine		
Proline		
Serine		
Threonine		
Valine		

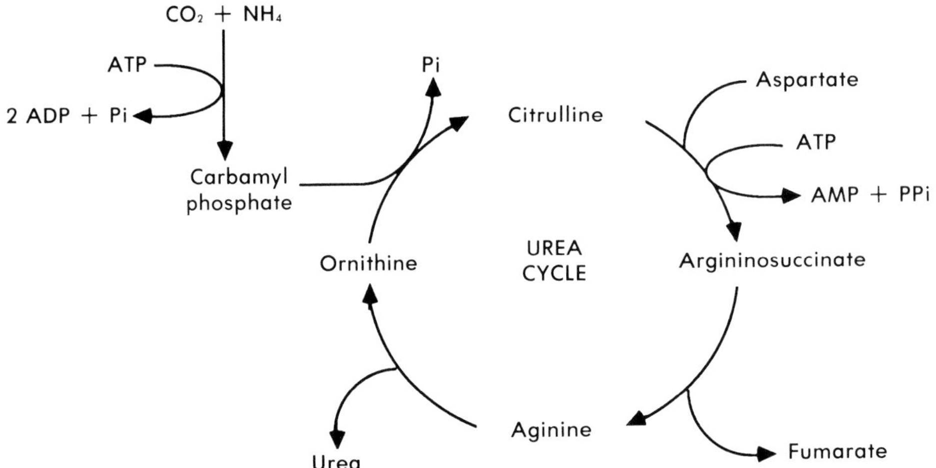

Fig. 1-13 Urea cycle. (From Gann, D.S., Amaral, J.F., and Caldwell, M.D.: Metabolic response to injury, stress, and starvation. In Davis, J.H., et al.: Clinical surgery, St. Louis, 1987, The C.V. Mosby Co.)

and hydroxyproline) of the 22 most common amino acids in proteins are converted to pyruvate. Depending on the redox state of the cell, the pyruvate can either be used for gluconeogenesis or converted to acetyl-CoA. Five amino acid carbon skeletons (phenylalanine, tyrosine, tryptophan, leucine, and lysine) form acetoacetate that may be converted to acetyl-CoA and either oxidized in the TCA cycle or used in fatty-acid synthesis. In addition, in the process of producing acetoacetate, phenylalanine and tyrosine are also cleaved to fumarate, and tryptophan is cleaved to alanine. Thus they may be used both in glucogenesis and in ketogenesis. Lysine may also be used both in glucogenesis and ketogenesis, but its precursor for gluconeogenesis is not known. In contrast, leucine forms one molecule of acetyl-CoA and one molecule of acetoacetate. Since neither acetyl-CoA nor acetoacetate can be converted to pyruvate, the carbon skeleton of leucine can only be used for ketogenesis or oxidation.

It should be apparent that any compound that enters the TCA cycle as acetyl-CoA cannot be used as a precursor of glucose. This relates to the fact that by the time it reaches malate, the acetyl-CoA that entered the TCA cycle has been completely oxidized. However, the carbon skeletons of amino acids that are TCA-cycle intermediates can be used for gluconeogenesis. In addition to phenylalanine and tyrosine, which enter the TCA cycle as fumarate, three amino acids enter as succinyl-CoA (isoleucine, methionine, and valine), and two other amino acids enter as oxaloacetate (aspartate and aspargine) and give amino acids that enter as alpha-ketoglutarate (glutamate, glutamine, proline, histidine, and arginine) (Fig. 1-14). Consequently, all of these amino acids may be used either in gluconeogenesis or oxidation. Quantitatively, in the isolated perfused liver, only alanine, serine, threonine, and glycine are used in significant amounts for gluconeogenesis.[165]

As noted previously, excess nitrogen cannot be stored. When the protein intake is excessive, the amino acids resulting from proteolysis are catabolized to nitrogen and a carbon skeleton. The nitrogen is converted to urea and the carbon skeleton to either glucose, lipid, or carbon dioxide depending on the needs of the cell and the redox state present. Similarly, when glucose is needed but unavailable, excess ingested proteins or existing body proteins are degraded. Although it may be imperceptible, the use of existing body protein for energy or gluconeogenesis always results in the loss of some cellular function.

Lipid Metabolism

The final and greatest source of energy in the body is lipid. Stored in adipose tissues as triglycerides, lipids can be released on demand and transported to most tissues for use as an energy source. Tissues capable of using lipids include the liver, kidney, heart, and skeletal muscle; such use, however, must occur under aerobic conditions. Nonlipid-using tissues include erythrocytes, leukocytes, and nerve cells.

Triglycerides are composed of three fatty-acid chains linked together by a glycerol molecule. During lipolysis, the fatty acids are sequentially cleaved off the glycerol moiety by lipases. The remaining glycerol moiety can then be used for glucose synthesis or converted to pyruvate (see Fig. 1-9). In contrast, fatty acids themselves cannot be used as substrate for gluconeogenesis since they are ultimately broken down to acetyl-CoA.

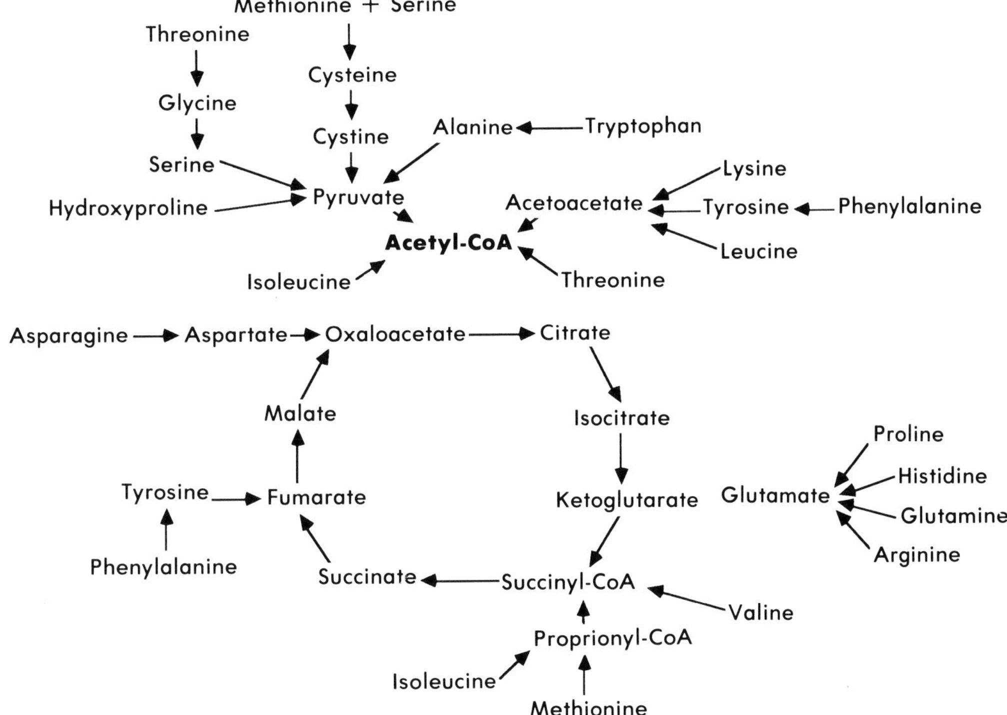

Fig. 1-14 Pathways through which the carbon skeletons of alpha-amino acids enter the TCA cycle.

The catabolism of fatty acids can be divided into two stages. These stages include beta oxidation in the outer mitochondrial membrane to produce molecules of acetyl-CoA and the processing of acetyl-CoA in the mitochondria to produce carbon dioxide and energy or ketone bodies (Fig. 1-15).[23,120] Only the first step in fatty-acid catabolism requires energy. In this step, the enzyme thiokinase adds CoA to a fatty acid producing a fatty acyl-CoA (Fig. 1-15). After a sequence of reactions, the final two carbons on the fatty acyl-CoA are cleaved off, resulting in the production of one molecule of acetyl-CoA and a new fatty acyl-CoA that is two carbon atoms shorter than the parent fatty acyl-CoA. This process of beta oxidation yields five high-energy phosphates per acetyl-CoA formed and, with even-numbered fatty-acid chains, continues until the entire fatty acid has been cleaved to acetyl-CoA. In the case of odd-numbered fatty-acid chains, beta oxidation continues until a three-carbon fatty acyl-CoA (propionyl-CoA) remains. The latter substance may then be converted to succinyl-CoA and enter the TCA cycle.

The acetyl-CoA that results from the oxidation of fatty acids can be used in one of three available pathways (see Fig. 1-15).[23,139] The first involves the intramitochondrial oxidation of acetyl-CoA through the TCA cycle to two molecules of carbon dioxide and 12 high-energy phosphates (HEP). Thus the total oxidation of a 20-carbon fatty acid, for example, yields

$$169 \text{ HEP} = [(10 \times 5) + (10 \times 12) - 1].$$

The second pathway involves the ketogenic pathway in the liver (Fig. 1-16). Through the action of the enzyme thiolase, two molecules of acetyl-CoA combine to form acetoacetyl-CoA in a freely reversible reaction. Acetoacetyl-CoA can then be converted to 3-hydroxy-3-methylglutaryl-CoA, the precursor in cholesterol synthesis and ketone body formation. The three ketone bodies, acetoacetate, beta-hydroxybutyrate, and acetone are normally produced and released by the liver. Under conditions in which there is an abundance of hepatic glycogen, beta-hydroxybutyrate predominates; under conditions in which the liver glycogen is low, acetoacetate predominates. The ketone bodies that are released by the liver can then be used by a variety of peripheral tissues, such as cardiac and skeletal muscle, as a source of energy by conversion back to acetyl-CoA.

The final pathway for use of acetyl-CoA is in the synthesis of fatty acids and triglycerides (see Fig. 1-15). This pathway is stimulated by neuroendocrine mechanisms and low cytoplasmic concentrations of fatty acids. Lipogenesis

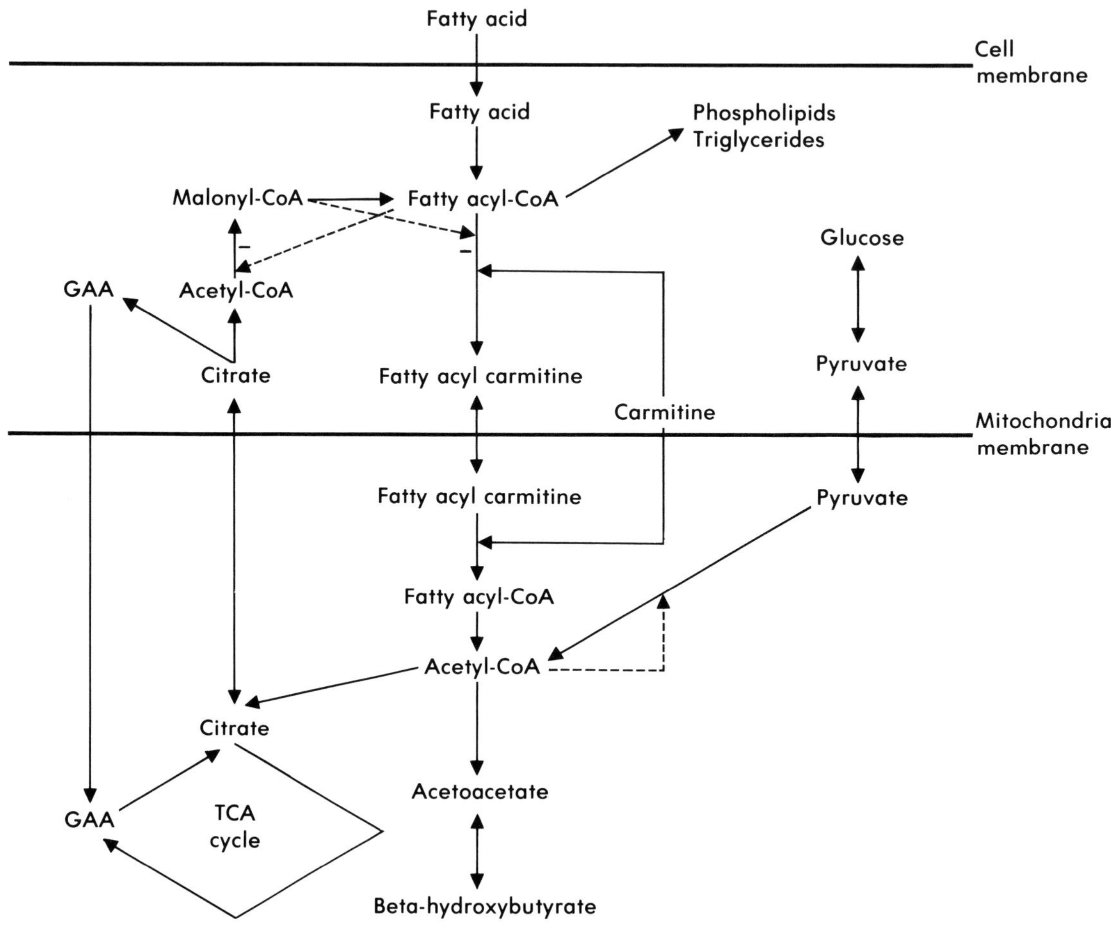

Fig. 1-15 Metabolic pathways of fatty-acid metabolism in the liver. (From Gann, D.S., and Amaral, J.F.: The pathophysiology of trauma and shock. In Zuidema, G.D., Rutherford, W.F., and Ballinger, W.F., editors: The management of trauma, Philadelphia, 1984, W.B. Saunders Co.)

is a cytoplasmic process that requires malonyl-CoA. Malonyl CoA is formed from acetyl-CoA by acetyl-CoA carboxylase. When fatty-acid levels are low, the rate-limiting enzyme in malonyl-CoA formation, acetyl-CoA carboxylase, is stimulated, leading to increased intracellular concentrations of malonyl-CoA.[103] In turn, the elevated concentrations of malonyl-CoA inhibit carnitine acetyltransferase, the enzyme necessary for transport of acetyl-CoA into the mitochondria,[123] resulting in an increased concentration of cytoplasmic acetyl-CoA that can then be used for malonyl-CoA synthesis and ultimately for the synthesis of triglycerides and other lipids. In contrast, when the intracellular concentrations of fatty acids are elevated, the rate-limiting enzyme in malonyl-CoA synthesis (acetyl-CoA carboxylase) is inhibited. Malonyl-CoA concentrations decrease, thereby stimulating carnitine acetyltransferase and increasing the transport of acetyl-CoA into the mitochondria for oxidation and ketogenesis.[123] The inhibition of acetyl-CoA carboxylase also results in the accumulation of cytoplasmic citrate that, in turn, inhibits glycolysis through inhibition of phosphofructokinase, the so-called Randle effect.[141]

NEUROENDOCRINE REGULATORY MECHANISMS

Stimuli and Mechanism of Action of the Neuroendocrine System

The pathways of intermediary metabolism and substrate to substrate interactions noted previously are under the local control of substrate availability, cellular redox potential, and cellular energy availability. The integration of this control is governed by the neuroendocrine system. This system may be thought of as a reflex physiologic network in which alterations in homeostasis are perceived by specialized receptors that are located both peripherally and centrally. The receptors transmit their information to the central nervous system where the afferent signals are processed and modulated, resulting in release or inhibition of numerous neuroendocrine effectors that produce physiologic changes aimed at correcting the alterations in homeostasis. In the absence of significant injury, sepsis, or starvation, alterations in homeostasis are small, and the responses of the neuroendocrine system to stimuli are directed at fine tuning and integrating the functioning of the organism. In the presence of significant injury, sepsis, or starvation, the stimuli are multiple and intensified, and the reflexes are directed at an integrated attempt by the organism to preserve oxygen delivery, mobilize energy substrates, and minimize pain (Fig. 1-17).[69] The major stimuli affecting neuroendocrine reflexes include: (1) changes in the circulating body fluids; (2) changes in the oxygen, hydrogen ion, and carbon dioxide concentrations in tissues and blood; (3) changes in ambient and core temperature; (4) changes in substrate availability; (5) emotional arousal; (6) pain; and (7) infection.

Critical to the initiation of the neuroendocrine response is the perception of the stimulus. Paraplegics do not respond to stimuli below the level of cord transection. This lack of response is thought to be the result of the absence of afferent impulses reaching the brain.[51] However, conscious perception of the stimulus is not required. An individual responds to a stimulus in the presence of anesthesia, but the response may not be the same had anesthesia been absent.

Changes in the circulating body fluids may result from the direct loss of blood (as in hemorrhage), from the loss of plasma volume (as in third-space losses and dehydration), or from the inability of the body fluids to circulate (as in cardiac failure or pulmonary embolism). The changes in circulating body fluids are sensed by high-pressure baroreceptors in the carotid arteries and aorta and by low-pressure stretch receptors in the right atrium. Under normal conditions, the afferent signals from these receptors exert a tonic inhibition of the release of many hormones and of the activities of the central and autonomic nervous systems.[72] When baroreceptor or stretch receptor activities decrease (e.g., a decrease in blood pressure or blood volume), the tonic inhibition is released, resulting in the increased secretion of adrenocorticotropic hormone

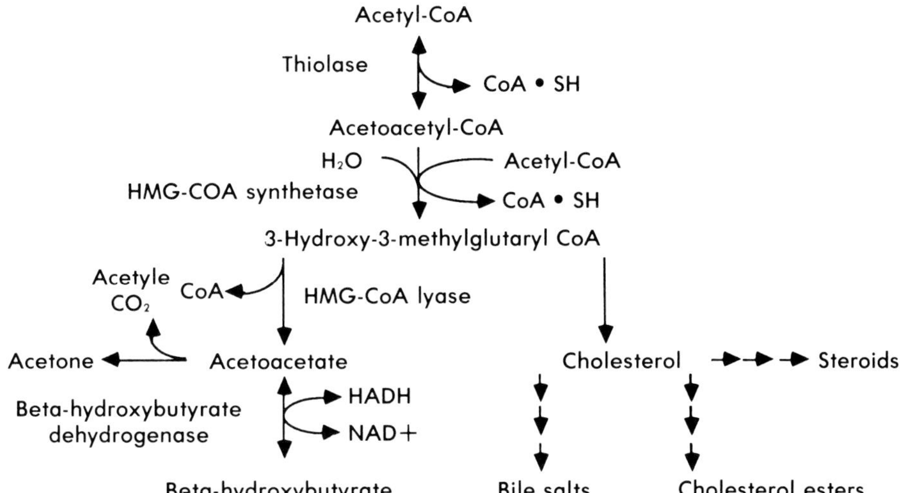

Fig. 1-16 Ketogenic pathway and cholesterol pathway in the liver. (From Gann, D.S., Amaral, J.F., and Caldwell, M.D.: Metabolic response to injury, stress, and starvation. In Davis, J.H., et al.: Clinical surgery, St. Louis, 1987, The C.V. Mosby Co.)

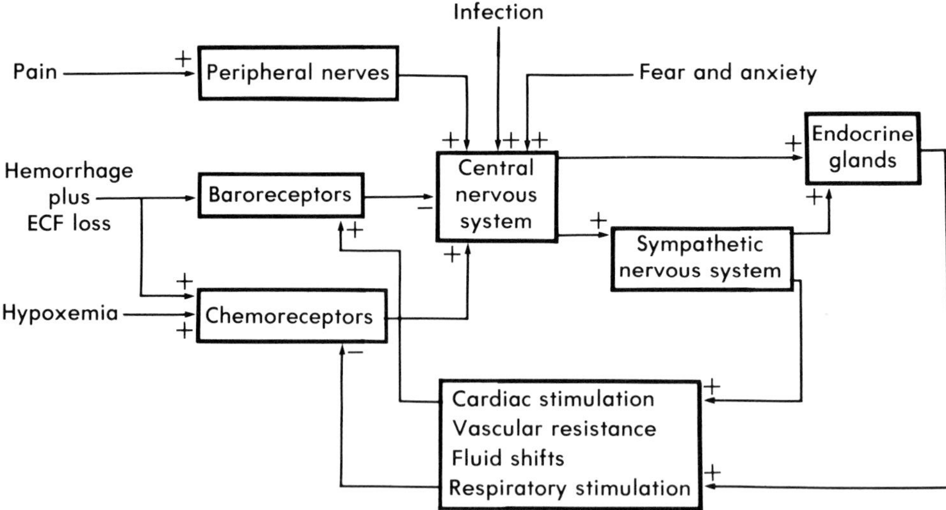

Fig. 1-17 Overview of the neuroendocrine reflexes induced by shock and trauma. (From Gann, D.S., and Amaral, J.F.: The pathophysiology of trauma and shock. In Zuidema, G.D., Rutherford, W.F., and Ballinger, W.F., editors: The management of trauma, Philadelphia, 1984, W.B. Saunders Co.)

(ACTH), vasopressin, beta-endorphin, and growth hormone through central pathways and resulting in the increased secretion of epinephrine, norepinephrine, renin, and glucagon through peripheral autonomic neural pathways. These responses bring about further neuroendocrine changes such as the inhibition of insulin secretion by epinephrine[163] and the stimulation of aldosterone secretion by renin and ACTH.[93]

Changes in blood concentrations of oxygen, hydrogen ion, and carbon dioxide initiate neuroendocrine responses through the activation of peripheral chemoreceptors. The chemoreceptors, which are located in the aortic and carotid bodies, have an extremely high blood-flow rate.[79] Under normal conditions, these receptors are not activated. However, changes primarily in oxygen and secondarily in carbon dioxide and in hydrogen ions are sensed by these receptors, which results in the activation of neuroendocrine pathways. Because of the high blood flow through the chemoreceptors, the partial pressure of oxygen (Po_2) of arterial blood, chemoreceptor tissue, and venous blood is nearly the same. However, a drop in blood flow will increase the oxygen extraction by the chemoreceptor tissue, decrease the venous Po_2, and through an unknown mechanism, activate the chemoreceptor.[79] Consequently, a decrease in circulating volume or pressure not only inhibits baroreceptors and stretch receptors but also activates chemoreceptors.

Pain and emotion also activate the neuroendocrine system. The former acts through the projections of peripheral nociceptive receptors to the central nervous system, and the latter through projections from the limbic areas of the brain to the hypothalamus and lower brainstem nuclei.[73] Through these pathways, pain and emotional arousal bring about increased hypothalamic, autonomic, adrenomedullary, and adrenocortical activities, the so-called flight or fight reaction of Cannon.[26]

Abnormalities in core and ambient temperatures, as well as infection, also stimulate neuroendocrine reflexes. Changes in the core temperature of the body are sensed in the preoptic area of the hypothalamus. These changes may result from alterations in ambient temperature, a loss of the normal insulating barrier of the skin (e.g., burns), a reduction in hepatic thermogenesis produced by inadequate blood flow or substrate supply, or in response to inadequate peripheral vasoconstriction or vasodilation. Infection may also decrease the core temperature through the action of endotoxin. Infection may further stimulate neuroendocrine reflexes through a direct action of endotoxin on the hypothalamus[50] or through secondary changes in blood volume, oxygen concentration, substrate concentrations, and pain.

The primary substrate alterations that activate the neuroendocrine system are those induced by changes in the plasma glucose concentration. Plasma glucose alterations are sensed by receptors in the hypothalamus and the pancreas. A decrease in plasma glucose concentration stimulates the release of catecholamines, cortisol, growth hormone, and vasopressin through central mechanisms and stimulates the release of glucagon both by central pathways (autonomic nervous system) and peripheral pathways (direct pancreatic activation).[48] In addition, the secretion of insulin is inhibited through central pathways (autonomic nervous system) and directly by the pancreas itself.[163]

All these stimuli are commonly produced by injury, sepsis, and starvation. Furthermore, these stimuli rarely occur singly. Generally the individual perceives multiple stimuli that occur both simultaneously and sequentially. Thus the neuroendocrine response is the summation of all the stimuli the individual perceives and processes. According to classic endocrine feedback mechanisms, the elevation of serum cortisol resulting from one set of stimuli would be expected to inhibit the release of ACTH by a new set of stimuli. Following most injuries, this is not true. The secretion of ACTH is unchanged or increased (potentiated), and the secretion of cortisol may also increase. The mechanism of action of this physiologic facilitation is unknown, but it appears to take 60 to 90 minutes to be of sufficient magnitude to offset the inhibition and lasts for at least 24 hours.[71] Physiologic facilitation and potentiation have been demonstrated with sequential hemorrhages,[115] repeated operations,[114] in response to hypoxia and surgery,[156] with pain and hemorrhage,[13] and with elevated core temperature and hemorrhage.[196] Consequently, the response to an injury or an alteration in homeostasis may be modified by previous stimuli, and the response to a second set of stimuli may be different than if they had occurred first.

The efferent limb of the neuroendocrine system arises from two primary areas—the hypothalamic-pituitary axis and the autonomic regions of the brainstem. The output from the former region involves the release of numerous pituitary hormones, and the output from the latter region involves changes in the neural activities of the sympathetic and parasympathetic nervous systems. Both sets of output either may cause direct changes in physiologic functions or may stimulate or inhibit the secretion of peripheral endocrine organs.

The hormones secreted by endocrine organs and the autacoids produced by tissues fall into one of five chemical classes. These include the fatty-acid derivatives of cholesterol (cortisol, aldosterone) or arachidonic acid (prostaglandins), proteins (insulin, glucagon), glycoproteins (thyroid-stimulating hormone, adrenocorticotropin), small polypeptides (vasopressin, enkephalin), and the amines (catecholamines, serotonin). All these agents act on cellular receptors that are either on the surface of cell membranes or in the cytoplasm of the cell. These cellular receptors are neither fixed nor unchangeable. Instead, they are in a dynamic state in which the number of receptors on cells can be increased (up regulation) or decreased (down regulation) according to need. Furthermore, the affinity of these receptors for their specific hormone can also be changed.[167]

Steroid hormones (and possibly thyroxine), which are freely permeable to cell membranes, bind to cytosolic receptors in target cells.[145,147] The hormone-receptor complex migrates to the cell nuclei where it interacts with DNA to modulate the transcription of messenger RNA and ultimately the synthesis of enzymatic, structural, and regulatory proteins (Fig. 1-18, *A*).[145] This may, in part, explain the 1- to 2-hour delay in the action of steroid hormones. In contrast, the action of most peptide and amine hormones, which generally bind to cell surface receptors, is faster and of shorter duration. In general, these hormones act either through alterations in the intracellular concentrations of cyclic adenosine monophosphate (cAMP) or calcium, the so-called second messengers,[160,181] or through other intermediates (growth hormone through somatomedins). The second messenger system of hormonal action operates primarily through the activation and inactivation of regulatory proteins and enzymes rather than through the synthesis of new proteins. This difference explains the faster onset of action and shorter duration of effect of hormones that operate through this system in contrast to those of steroid and other lipid-soluble hormones.

The adrenergic receptor system may be considered the prototype for examining the mechanisms of second messengers since all the second messenger pathways known are represented in the four adrenergic receptors ($alpha_1$, $alpha_2$, $beta_1$, and $beta_2$) (Fig. 1-18, *B*). $Beta_1$ and $beta_2$ receptors (differentiated on the basis of radioligand-binding affinity) both function through the activation of membrane-bound adenylate cyclase, which in turn leads to the production of cAMP.[160] The increased intracellular concentration of cAMP activates an inactive protein kinase by attaching to a binding protein on the protein kinase molecule. The attachment of cAMP to the regulatory subunit protein results in the release of an active protein kinase that in turn phosphorylates an inactive phosphorylase kinase to an active form. The active phosphorylase kinase then phosphorylates dephospho-regulatory enzymes, possibly resulting in the activation of the regulatory enzyme (e.g., glycogen phosphorylase) or in its inactivation (e.g., glycogen synthetase) (Fig. 1-19).[78] In addition, active protein kinase may directly act on dephosphoregulatory enzymes without the activation of phosphorylase kinase. In contrast, $alpha_2$ receptor activation inhibits membrane-bound adenylate cyclase thereby decreasing the concentration of cAMP and active protein kinase. Activation of $alpha_1$ adrenergic receptors results in an increase in phosphatidylinositol turnover that then mediates an increase in intracellular calcium from intracellular and extracellular sources.[56,160] The increase in intracellular calcium activates a calcium-binding protein kinase or phosphorylase kinase (see Fig. 1-18, *B*).

The actions of intracellular cAMP and calcium in the coupling of receptor activation with hormonal action (stimulus-response coupling) are not independent. Instead, there is a duality to this system in which the actions of calcium and cAMP are highly interrelated, termed synarchic control by Rasmusen.[160] As noted in Fig. 1-20 and the boxed material on p. 24, there are five basic patterns to the synarchic control of hormone-response coupling through cAMP and calcium. In coordinate control, a hormone activates both a calcium-activating receptor and a cAMP-activating receptor, either one of which may produce the response alone. In hierarchal control, separate stimuli activate independently the calcium and cAMP pathways that are both necessary for a given response. In sequential control, the activation of one of the two lines of the system leads to the activation of the other limb. Although the first limb can produce the response, activation of the second limb augments the response. In redundant control, two separate stimuli independently activate the two different limbs of the messenger system, either one of which can produce the response. Finally, in antagonist control, one stimulus activates one limb of the messenger system that leads to the response, and a second stimulus activates the second limb, which inhibits the ability of the first limb to produce the response. Although each of these control mechanisms can occasionally be found in cells in pure form, most of the presently known hormone-response–coupling mechanisms involve mixed patterns.[160]

Hormonal Regulation of Metabolism

The neuroendocrine system is able to regulate metabolic reactions through three basic processes. First, it may increase substrate availability so that by simple stoichiometry (mass action), reactions proceed in a desired direction. This process can be brought about either by an increase in the plasma concentration of a substrate or by alterations in blood flow and its distribution. Second, the neuroendocrine effectors can alter the membrane transport properties of cells for a given substrate so that more or less of the substrate enters or leaves the cell. Third, the neuroendocrine effectors can alter the activity or synthesis of key regulatory enzymes that are necessary for reactions to proceed.

Most hormones operate through more than one of these processes. For example, insulin stimulates both glycogen synthetase and the transport of glucose into cells. In this manner, insulin not only activates the enzymatic mechanisms necessary for glycogenesis, it also increases the availability of the necessary substrates. It would be futile

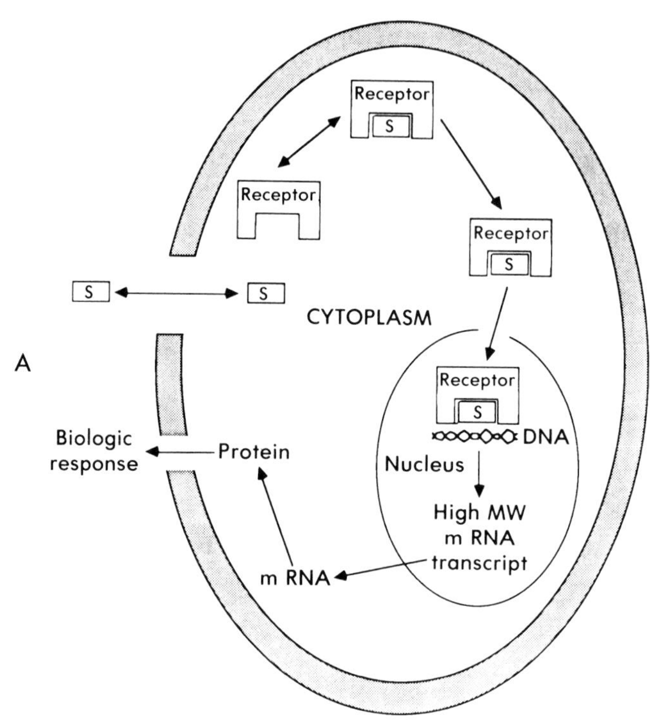

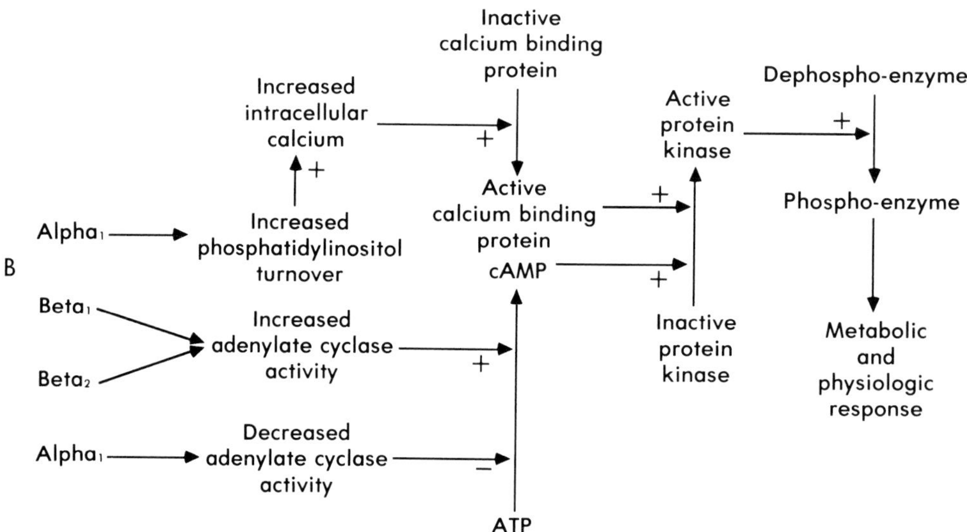

Fig. 1-18 **A,** Proposed mechanism of action of steroid hormones. **B,** Proposed mechanism of action of peptide hormones through the second messenger system. (**A,** From Gann, D.S., Amaral, J.F., and Caldwell, M.D.: Neuroendocrine response to injury, stress, and starvation. In Davis, J.H., et al.: Clinical surgery, St. Louis, 1987, The C.V. Mosby Co. **B,** From Gann, D.S., and Amaral, J.F.: The pathophysiology of trauma and shock. In Zuidema, G.D., Rutherford, W.F., and Ballinger, W.F., editors: The management of trauma, Philadelphia, 1984, W.B. Saunders Co.)

for a hormone to stimulate opposing processes in a given cell. If a hormone stimulated both glycogenesis and glycogenolysis, there would be no net effect. As a result, most hormones not only activate the enzymes necessary for one metabolic pathway, they also inhibit the enzymes necessary for the opposing process. Thus epinephrine, through an $alpha_1$ mechanism, activates glycogen phosphorylase and inactivates glycogen synthetase, whereas insulin inactivates glycogen phosphorylase and activates glycogen synthetase.

The coordinated control of metabolism also requires that a hormone not have opposing actions in different tissues. Thus by increasing amino acid uptake in skeletal muscle and decreasing amino acid degradation in the liver, insulin promotes the availability of an abundant substrate supply for the enzymes of protein synthesis it activates. Cortisol

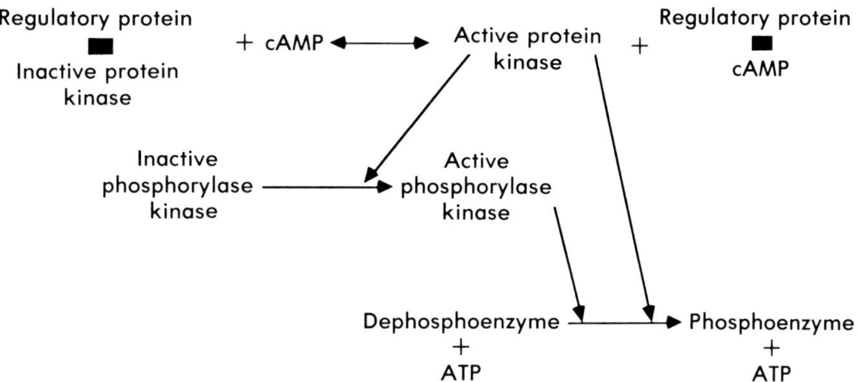

Fig. 1-19 Activation of protein kinase leading to enzymatic or physiologic response. Activation of the dephospho-enzyme by phosphorylation may be brought about either directly by the active protein kinase or indirectly through the activation of a phosphorylase kinase by the active protein kinase. (From Gann, D.S., Amaral, J.F., and Caldwell, M.D.: Neuroendocrine response to injury, stress, and starvation. In Davis, J.H., et al.: Clinical surgery, St. Louis, 1987, The C.V. Mosby Co.)

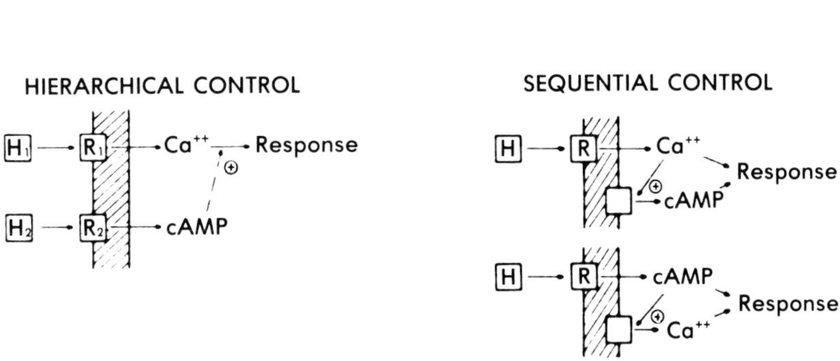

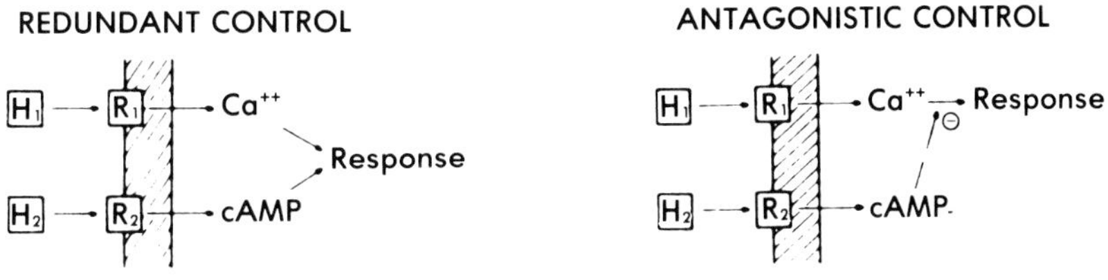

Fig. 1-20 Patterns of synarchic regulation by calcium and cAMP. (From Rasmusen, H.: Calcium and cAMP as synarchic messengers, New York, 1981, John Wiley & Sons, Inc.)

CALCIUM-CYCLIC AMP INTERACTIONS IN STIMULUS-RESPONSE COUPLING

1. Effects of calcium on cAMP messenger systems
   A. Stimulates cAMP production—brain, adrenal cortex, pancreatic islets, adrenal medulla, slime mold
   B. Stimulates cAMP hyrolysis—brain, heart, liver, kidney, fly salivary gland, many other tissues
   C. Activates phosphoprotein product of cAMP-dependent protein kinase, glycogenolysis in many tissues
2. Effects of cAMP on calcium messenger system
   A. Increases calcium entry across plasma membrane—heart, synapse
   B. Increases calcium release from mitochondria—kidney, liver, fly salivary gland, others
   C. Increases calcium uptake by microsomes—heart, uterus, liver, smooth muscles
   D. Increases calcium efflux across plasma membrane—smooth muscle, heart
   E. Decreases sensitivity of response elements to calcium—smooth muscle, heart
   F. Increases sensitivity of response element to calcium—phosphorylase beta kinase, liver, muscle
3. Interrelated activities
   A. cAMP-dependent and calcium-dependent protein kinases act upon same protein substrate—liver, brain, adrenal cortex
   B. Regulate sequential steps in metabolic or transport process—secretion in fly salivary gland, glycogenolysis

From Rasmusen, H.: Calcium and cAMP as synarchic messengers, New York, Copyright ©1981. Reprinted by permission of John Wiley & Sons, Inc.

produces an inhibition of amino acid uptake in skeletal muscle, increases amino acid uptake by the liver, and stimulates hepatic gluconeogenic enzymes. These processes ensure that an abundant supply of amino acids will be available to the liver for cortisol-stimulated gluconeogenesis.

The primary hormones involved in the regulation of metabolism include insulin, cortisol, epinephrine, glucagon, growth hormone, vasopressin, and somatostatin. Insulin is the primary anabolic hormone promoting the synthesis of glycogen, proteins, and lipids. Cortisol, epinephrine, glucagon, and vasopressin are the primary catabolic hormones promoting the breakdown of glycogen, proteins, and lipids as well as the synthesis of glucose from gluconeogenic amino acids, lactate, and pyruvate. In contrast, the actions of growth hormone initially are anabolic, but its late effects are primarily catabolic.

Insulin, Glucagon, and Somatostatin

Insulin, composed of two polypeptide chains, one containing 21 amino acids and the other 30 amino acids, and glucagon, a 29-amino acid polypeptide, are produced and secreted by the pancreatic B cells (Beta islets of Langerhans) and A cells (alpha islets of Langerhans), respectively. The secretion of both of these hormones is under the control of at least three mechanisms: circulating substrates (glucose, amino acids, and free fatty acids), the autonomic nervous system, and other circulating hormones.

Under normal physiologic conditions, glucose is the most important regulator of insulin and glucagon secretion. When the plasma concentration of glucose increases, the secretion of insulin increases, and the secretion of glucagon decreases. When the plasma concentration of glucose decreases, the secretion of insulin decreases, and the secretion of glucagon increases. These changes are probably the result of a direct action of glucose on pancreatic islet cells and not a result of neuroendocrine modulation of the pancreas by other neuroendocrine effectors.[188] The direct action of glucose on islet cell function may be mediated either through a glucoreceptor on the surface of the islet cell or through the intracellular metabolism of glucose in the islet cells.[60]

Elevations in the plasma concentration of amino acids stimulate the release of both insulin and glucagon. Most, if not all, of the amino acids increase insulin secretion, but the potency of amino acids in stimulating glucagon secretion is variable.[153] In general, the more gluconeogenic amino acids appear to stimulate glucagon secretion.[153]

High concentrations of fatty acids stimulate the secretion of insulin and inhibit the secretion of glucagon. Conversely, low concentrations of free fatty acids inhibit the secretion of insulin and stimulate the secretion of glucagon. The potency of fatty acids in regulating insulin and glucagon secretion is substantially less than that of glucose.[153]

The stimulation of insulin secretion and the inhibition of glucagon secretion after the administration of an oral glucose load is greater than that following the intravenous administration of glucose.[125] Similarly, the stimulation of both insulin and glucagon secretion is greater after an oral protein or amino acid load than it is after the intravenous administration of amino acids and protein.[159] This effect is thought to be the result of the higher concentrations of substrate in the pancreas, the potentiation by gastrointestinal hormones of the substrate effect on the pancreas, and the effect of neural input to the pancreas that has been stimulated by eating.[153] The gastrointestinal hormones, cholecystokinin, gastrin, vasoactive intestinal peptide (VIP), substance P, neurotensin, and gastric inhibitory peptide (GIP) all increase the secretion of both insulin and glucagon in pharmacologic concentrations.[153,161] Although gastrin does appear to potentiate the release of glucagon and insulin induced by amino acids and GIP in physiologic concentrations appears to augment the release of insulin by glucose,[153] the physiologic role of the gastrointestinal hormones is not certain.

The pancreatic A cells and B cells both have alpha- and beta-adrenergic receptors that alter the secretion of insulin and glucagon. Alpha adrenergic stimulation of the pancreas inhibits the secretion of both insulin and glucagon, whereas beta adrenergic stimulation of the pancreas stimulates the secretion of both insulin and glucagon.[92,154] However, the alpha and beta adrenergic receptor density of A cells and B cells is not the same. The beta adrenergic receptor density of A cells is greater than that of B cells.[154] As a result, increased sympathetic stimulation of the pancreas or increased circulating concentrations of epinephrine or norepinephrine increase the secretion of glucagon but decrease the secretion of insulin.[92,154] In contrast, isoproterenol infusion increases the secretion of both insulin and glucagon.[154] In addition to sympathetic stimulation, the parasympathetic limb of the autonomic nervous system alters pancreatic hormone secretion. Both acetylcholine infusion and direct parasympathetic stimulation of the pancreas increase the secretion of both insulin and glucagon.[153]

In addition to the gastrointestinal hormones and the autonomic nervous system, other hormones alter the secretion of insulin and glucagon. Beta endorphin appears to directly increase the secretion of insulin and glucagon,[63] insulin inhibits the release of insulin and stimulates the release of glucagon,[153] and glucagon inhibits the release of glucagon and stimulates the release of insulin.[61,153] Insulin and glucagon appear to exert their action both directly on islet cells and by the alterations they produce in circulating substrates.[153] Cortisol stimulates the release of insulin and glucagon, but it appears to have no direct activity on the secretory ability of A cells and B cells. Instead, cortisol is believed to increase glucagon secretion through an increase in plasma amino acids and to increase insulin secretion by an increase in plasma glucose. In this regard, both cortisol and epinephrine are able to inhibit the peripheral actions of insulin, and both are thought to exert a major role in insulin resistance.[52,62]

Somatostatin, a tetradecapeptide, is a potent inhibitor of both insulin and glucagon secretion.[161,188] In addition to its location in pancreatic D cells, somatostatin is found in the hypothalamus, limbic system, brainstem, spinal cord, other neural tissue, salivary glands, parafollicular thyroid cells, kidneys, and in gastrointestinal tissue.[161] Although somatostatin was originally named for its ability to inhibit growth hormone secretion, somatostatin is now recognized to inhibit the secretion of thyroid stimulating hormone (TSH), renin, calcitonin, gastrin, secretin, and cholecystokinin as well as insulin and glucagon.[161] In addition, somatostatinergic nerve fibers are involved in the projection of impulses from peripheral sensory organs to the neuroaxis.[161]

The role somatostatin exerts in the physiologic regulation of insulin and glucagon secretion is not known precisely. The A, B, and D cells all have somatostatin receptors that, when activated, inhibit the secretion of glucagon, insulin, and somatostatin respectively. Although the mechanism of action of somatostatin is thought to be mediated primarily by the local diffusion of somatostatin from D cells to A cells and B cells,[161,188] recent evidence suggests that somatostatin reaching the pancreas through the blood stream may be more important.[94] The effects of somatostatin on A cells are transient, but the effects on B cells are persistent.[188] This persistence may account for the relative hyperglycemia that occurs in patients with somatostatinomas or after the long-term administration of somatostatin.[188]

The physiologic actions of glucagon occur primarily in the liver and are mediated through an increase in intracellular cAMP. The activation of glycogen phosphorylase and the inhibition of glycogen synthetase by glucagon promotes the breakdown of glycogen to glucose (glycogenolysis).[141] In addition, glucagon stimulates gluconeogenesis through the stimulation of phospho*enol*pyruvate carboxykinase, amino acid transport, and amino acid transamination.[105,141] The net result is an increase in hepatic production and release of glucose that under basal conditions accounts for 75% of the glucose produced by the liver.[187]

Glucagon also exerts an important influence over hepatic lipid metabolism. In addition to stimulating lipolysis in adipose tissue and the liver, glucagon inhibits acetyl-CoA carboxylase, the enzyme that converts acetyl-CoA to malonyl-CoA.[153] In turn, the reduction in malonyl-CoA produces inhibition of triglyceride synthesis and activation of carnitine acyl transferase. The latter increases fatty acid transfer to the mitochondria and therefore increases the oxidation of acetyl-CoA and ketogenesis.[23,153]

Peripheral actions of glucagon include the stimulation of lipolysis in adipose tissue, of glycogenolysis in skeletal muscle, and of myocardial contractility.[152,155,187] However, these actions do not appear to be of physiologic significance in human beings.[152,155,187]

As a result of glucagon's ability to increase hepatic glucose production, mobilize fat, and increase ketogenesis, glucagon is important in normal metabolism and more so in the metabolism of altered states. However, the effects of glucagon are evanescent.[64] After 30 to 60 minutes, the activity assigned to glucagon decreases even if plasma glucagon concentrations remain elevated. Therefore it appears that an increase in glucagon concentration rather than the absolute amount of glucagon present is a key determinant of glucagon activity.[64] This effect also appears to be true of other cAMP-mediated hormones (the burst effect).

The physiologic activity of insulin is primarily in the liver, skeletal muscle, and adipose tissue, but it does affect many other peripheral tissues. Notable exceptions include erythrocytes and wounded tissue. Insulin promotes the entry of glucose into cells by stimulating the membrane transport of glucose. The increased intracellular concentrations of glucose are used in glycogen synthesis (stimulation of glycogen synthetase and inhibition of glycogen phosphorylase) and in glycolysis (stimulation of glucokinase, phosphofructokinase, and pyruvate kinase) to produce energy.[141] In addition, insulin inhibits gluconeogenesis through the inhibition of phospho*enol*pyruvate carboxylase and the stimulation of phosphofructokinase and pyruvate kinase.[141]

Insulin also increases the membrane transport of amino acids into the liver and peripheral tissues. The increased intracellular concentrations of amino acids are used in protein synthesis (stimulation of protein synthesis and inhibition of proteolysis). By inhibiting gluconeogenesis and amino acid oxidation, insulin further directs the intracellular amino acids to protein synthesis.[105]

In adipose tissue, insulin stimulates lipogenesis and inhibits lipolysis as it does in the liver. By stimulating lipoprotein lipase, insulin also makes triglycerides more available for uptake from the plasma by adipose tissue. Glycerol synthesis and the pentose-phosphate shunt also are increased by insulin in adipose tissue and the liver. Thus insulin is the primary anabolic hormone promoting the storage of lipid, glucose, and protein.

Although insulin and glucagon oppose each other in the metabolic processes each stimulates, a bihormonal response is necessary for maintenance of glucose homeostasis after a protein meal.[161] If insulin were secreted alone in response to a protein meal, the increase in protein synthesis and decrease in hepatic glucose production would result in hypoglycemia. Conversely, if glucagon were secreted alone, the decrease in protein synthesis and the increase in hepatic gluconeogenesis would result in hyperglycemia. However, when a rise in glucagon is accompanied by an increase in insulin, hepatic glucose production remains unchanged and euglycemia is maintained. In this regard, Unger[186] has proposed the insulin/glucagon (I/G) ratio as a quantitative measure of hepatic glucose balance. When the I/G ratio is greater than 5, anabolism and protein synthesis are favored. When the I/G ratio is less than 3, glycogenolysis, gluconeogenesis, and lipolysis are favored. However, the validity of this relationship has been questioned.[60]

ACTH, Cortisol, and Epinephrine

The primary hormones released in response to any physiologic or psychologic stress are the glucocorticoids and catecholamines. These hormones are in large part responsible for the "flight or fight reaction." The release of cortisol is under the control of adrenocorticotropic hormone (ACTH), a 39-amino acid polypeptide released from the chromophobe cells in the anterior pituitary. In turn, the release of ACTH is itself under the inhibitory influence of cortisol and the stimulatory influence of corticotropin–releasing factor (CRF) produced by the hypothalamus. The release of CRF (and ACTH-cortisol) is stimulated by all the stimuli noted previously and is potentiated by vasopressin, oxytocin, and angiotensin II.[75,118] ACTH acts directly on cells of the adrenal zona fasciculata, stimulating the production and release of cortisol through a cAMP–mediated conversion of cholesterol to pregnenolone.[198]

The catecholamines (epinephrine, norepinephrine, and dopamine) are the prototypical neuroendocrine effectors that act as neurotransmitters and hormones.[36] Epinephrine, produced almost exclusively by the adrenal medulla, functions primarily as a hormone, whereas norepinephrine and dopamine function primarily as neurotransmitters.[36] Although the adrenal medulla may be viewed as a collection of postganglionic sympathetic neurons without axons that release their neurotransmitters into the general circulation, the activation of the sympathetic nervous system does not occur in an all-or-none fashion, and it is not synonymous with adrenomedullary secretion.[70] Similarly, adrenomedullary stimulation is not synonymous with the complete activation of the sympathetic nervous system. Numerous stimuli have been identified that lead to increased secretion of catecholamines from the adrenal medulla (e.g., hypotension, hypoxia, hypoglycemia, pain, and fear), but the exact mechanisms involved in adrenomedullary control remain poorly understood.[70]

Both cortisol and epinephrine function as "counter-regulatory" hormones, mediating catabolic processes throughout the body. In the liver, cortisol inhibits several key glycolytic enzymes (glucokinase, phosphofructokinase, and pyruvate kinase), the pentose-phosphate shunt, and the actions of insulin.[141,198] In addition, cortisol stimulates the hepatic uptake of amino acids, transaminases, and several gluconeogenic enzymes (pyruvate carboxylase, phospho*enol*pyruvate carboxykinase, and glucose 6-phosphatase), as well as potentiating the actions of glucagon and epinephrine.[52,141,198] As a result, the production of glucose, lactate, and pyruvate by the liver is increased.

The metabolic effects of epinephrine are similar to those of glucagon but are more widespread, affecting peripheral tissues as well as the liver. In the liver, epinephrine stimulates glycogenolysis (alpha$_1$-mediated stimulation of glycogen phosphorylase and inhibition of glycogen synthetase),[160] lipolysis (beta$_1$-mediated activation of triacylglycerol lipase),[57] ketogenesis (beta$_1$-mediated inhibition of acetyl-CoA carboxylase leading to decreased malonyl-CoA and increased carnitine acyl transferase),[78] and gluconeogenesis (beta$_1$-mediated inhibition of phosphofructokinase and hexokinase by the products of glycolysis and glycogenolysis).[3] Thus epinephrine serves to increase hepatic glucose production and lipid breakdown.

Although both glucagon and epinephrine increase glucose production by the liver, glucose use by peripheral tissues is not the same in the presence of epinephrine as it is in the presence of glucagon.[105] Glucagon promotes the use of glucose by peripheral tissues through the stimulation of insulin secretion. In contrast, epinephrine inhibits both the release and the action of insulin, thereby decreasing glucose use in insulin-dependent peripheral tissues. However, epinephrine serves to increase glucose availability to insulin-insensitive tissues such as the brain, whereas glucagon does not shunt glucose to insulin-insensitive tissues.[105]

In adipose tissue, epinephrine increases lipolysis (beta$_1$-mediated activation of triacylglycerol lipase). In peripheral tissues, epinephrine stimulates glycogenolysis (alpha$_1$) and inhibits stimulated glucose uptake through a beta$_2$ and alpha$_1$ mechanism.[29,151] As a result of increased substrate availability, glycolysis is increased in skeletal muscle, and large amounts of lactate are produced and released into the circulation. The lactate can then be taken up by the liver for subsequent gluconeogenesis (Cori cycle). Therefore, during stressful conditions, epinephrine and cortisol both promote a rise in blood sugar and make glucose more available to glucose-dependent tissues. Both of these hormones also promote the breakdown of lipid and thereby its use as a source of fuel. Whereas the actions of epinephrine are direct, many of the actions of cortisol occur as a result of the potentiation or inhibition of other hormones—the so-called permissive action of cortisol.

Growth Hormone and Vasopressin

Growth hormone is a 191-amino acid polypeptide that is released from acidophilic cells in the anterior pituitary gland. Its secretion is under the control of a releasing factor (growth hormone–releasing factor) and by an inhibiting factor (somatostatin).[76] Elevation of blood glucose or free fatty acids stimulates the release of growth hormone.[76] In addition, the release of growth hormone is stimulated by vasopressin, ACTH, alpha melanocyte–stimulating hormone, and estrogen, and its release is inhibited by cortisol, thyroxine, and growth hormone itself.

In addition to its ability to promote protein synthesis and RNA synthesis and to increase in linear growth, growth hormone exhibits an important role in the regulation of metabolic processes. Its effects are biphasic, composed of early effects of 3- to 4-hours' duration and late effects of longer duration.[76] In muscle and liver, growth hormone increases amino acid uptake and protein synthesis.[67] In addition, growth hormone stimulates glucose uptake in skeletal muscle and antagonizes the lipolytic effects of catecholamines in adipose tissue while increasing protein synthesis.[67] Therefore the early effects of growth hormone are similar to insulin. In fact, growth hormone directly stimulates the secretion of insulin by pancreatic B cells during its early phase.[93] The late effects of growth hormone include an increased mobilization of fatty acids and ketone bodies by adipose tissue as a result of increased lipolysis. This action of growth hormone occurs only in the presence of cortisol.[34] In addition, it inhibits insulin-stimulated glucose uptake and use, thereby producing a profound stimulation of insulin release by hyperglycemia.[93]

Arginine vasopressin (antidiuretic hormone) is a nonapeptide that is released by the posterior pituitary. Although released primarily in response to an increase in plasma osmolality and to a reduction in effective circulating volume,[94,95] vasopressin release is also stimulated by hypoglycemia through nonosmotic pathways.[96] Vasopressin is a powerful stimulator of hepatic glycogenolysis (alpha-receptor) and also stimulates hepatic gluconeogenesis.[66,97] As such, it may exert an important role in elevating the blood glucose after injury and during hypoglycemia.

THE METABOLIC RESPONSE IN STARVATION, INJURY, AND SEPSIS

Fasting and Starvation

In the absence of food, fasting humans must supply the energy required for daily activities, glucose for glucose-dependent tissue, essential amino acids, and essential fatty acids from existing body stores. Cahill[22] has estimated that the average resting 70-kg male using 1800 kcal of energy per day requires 180 g of glucose daily—for the metabolism of nervous tissue (144 g) and for other glycolytic tissue (red blood cells [RBCs], white blood cells [WBCs,], and the renal medulla) (36 g) (Fig. 1-21). Since the available glycogen in the liver is only 75 g (Table 1-13), this amount will not suffice for either the energy requirements or the glucose needs of a fasting male. Although there are an additional 150 g of glucose in skeletal muscle as glycogen, as noted previously, it cannot be released from skeletal muscle as free glucose as a result of the absence of glucose 6-phosphatase. Therefore it is apparent that the energy requirements and glucose requirements of fasting human beings must be supplied from noncarbohydrate sources and by gluconeogenesis.

The daily energy requirements can be met by the mobilization of approximately 160 g of triglycerides from adipose tissue in the form of free fatty acids.[19] The free fatty acids, as well as ketone bodies produced by the liver, are used throughout the body by nonglycolytic tissues such as the heart, kidney, muscle, and liver. In the liver, energy

Table 1-13 **THE FUEL COMPOSITION OF NORMAL HUMANS**

Fuel	Weight (kg)	Calories
Tissues		
Fat (adipose triglyceride)	15	141,000
Protein (mainly muscle)	6	24,000
Glycogen (muscle)	0.15	600
Glycogen (liver)	0.075	300
TOTAL		165,900
Circulating Fuels		
Glucose (extracellular fluid)	0.02	80
Free fatty acids (plasma)	0.0003	3
Triglycerides (plasma)	0.003	30
TOTAL		113

From Cahill, G.F.: Reprinted by permission of N. Engl. J. Med. **282:**668, 1970.

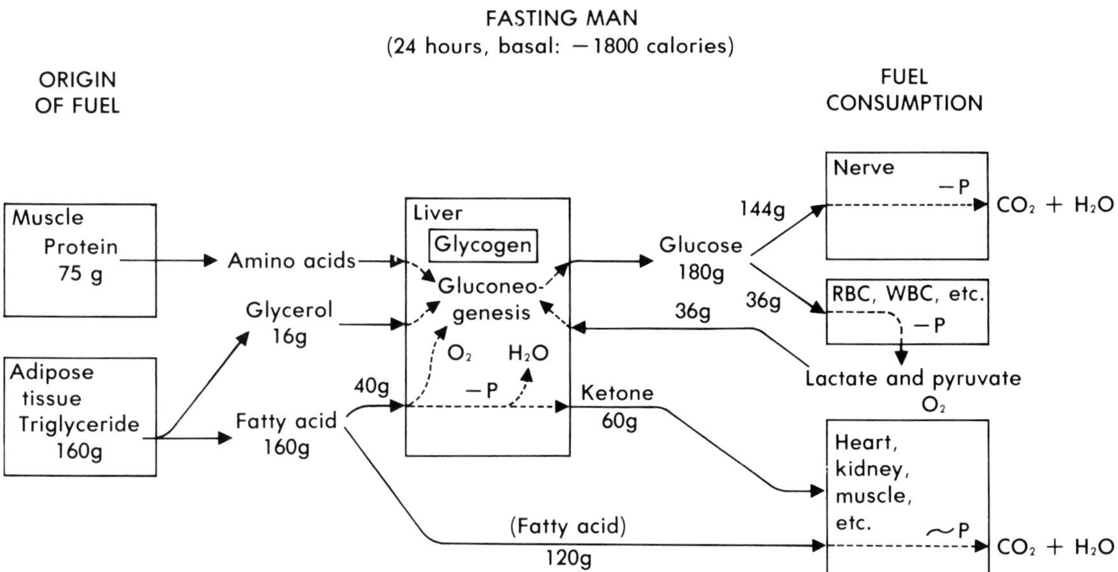

Fig. 1-21 Flow diagram of fuel metabolism in normal fasted man. (From Cahill, G.F.: Reprinted by permission of N. Engl. J. Med. **282:** 669, 1970.)

derived from beta oxidation of fat and from oxidation of acetyl-CoA is used to drive the necessary gluconeogenic processes. Gluconeogenic substrates are available from three sources (Table 1-14). First, the lipolysis of 160 g of triglycerides releases 16 g of glycerol that can be converted by the liver to glucose. Second, some glucose-dependent tissue (i.e., RBCs and WBCs) converts glucose to lactate and pyruvate that may then be reused in the liver by the Cori cycle to produce new glucose. In addition to the 36 g of lactate and pyruvate produced in this manner, skeletal muscle can also release lactate and pyruvate by the breakdown of glycogen and glucose. Third, approximately 75 g of skeletal muscle protein is degraded daily during starvation, and the resulting amino acids are used in the liver for gluconeogenesis. Consequently, the energy required during brief fasting is derived primarily from adipose tissue. In contrast, the glucose required is supplied from lactate, pyruvate, glycogen, and amino acids.

Table 1-14 **AMOUNT OF GLUCOSE PRODUCED FROM LACTATE, GLYCEROL, AND AMINO ACIDS DURING STARVATION**

Glucose Precursor	Grams of Glucose Produced per Day: 3 or 4 Days of Starvation	Grams of Glucose Produced per Day: Several Weeks of Starvation
Glycerol*	19	19
Lactate + pyruvate†	39	39
Amino acids‡	41	16
Total glucose produced from above precursors by liver and kidney cortex§	99	74
Maximum glucose available for oxidation by the brain (i.e., glycerol and amino acid as precursors)‖	60	35
Fuel requirement of brain (glucose equivalents)¶	120	120
Suggested alternative fuel to glucose for brain**	Ketone bodies	Ketone bodies

From Newsholme, E.A., and Start, C.: Regulation in metabolism, New York, 1975, Reprinted by permission of John Wiley & Sons, Inc.

*Amount of glucose produced from glycerol is estimated from the amount of triglyceride hydrolyzed per day. In starvation, 190 g of triglyceride is required to satisfy the caloric needs of the subject. Since glycerol represents 10% of triglyceride it can provide 19 g of glucose per day. This amount is confirmed by measurement of glycerol uptake by liver and kidney using catheterization techniques.

†Amount calculated from glucose 1-C turnover studies in man that gives values between 27 and 58 g/day, and this is *not* affected by the dietary state. Also the measurement of lactate and pyruvate uptake by the liver and kidney in man by catheterization techniques estimates glucose formation as 39 g/day.

‡Amount calculated from nitrogen excreted in urine (100 g protein produces 57 g glucose; 1 g nitrogen is equivalent to 6 to 25 g protein). In early stages of starvation approximately 12 g nitrogen is excreted per day, but this is decreased in prolonged starvation to 4 to 7 g/day. Catheterization studies in subjects undergoing prolonged starvation indicate an uptake of amino acids by liver and kidney that could theoretically produce 26 g glucose per day.

§In prolonged starvation the hepatic-renal glucose production as measured by catheterization techniques provides an estimate of 86 g glucose per day, which is in good agreement with the 74 g obtained in this calculation.

‖Catheterization techniques have been used to measure the A-V differences across the brain. In prolonged starvation, glucose oxidation by the brain (excluding glucose converted to lactate, which is converted back to glucose in the liver and kidney) is estimated as 24 g/day.

¶Oxygen uptake or total fuel use is measured by catheterization techniques.

**The rate of ketone body uptake by the brain has been estimated from A-V differences using catheterization techniques. These studies strongly suggest that ketone bodies are the alternative fuel to glucose during starvation.

During the first 2 to 4 days of fasting, there is a rapid increase in the urinary nitrogen excretion from 5 to 7 g per day to approximately 8 to 11 g per day.[131] This increase is associated with the previously noted breakdown of 50 to 75 g of protein per day. The rapid proteolysis of skeletal muscle protein does not continue during more prolonged fasting. During the next 20 to 40 days of fasting, the urinary nitrogen excretion begins gradually to decline and eventually reaches its nadir of 2 to 4 g of nitrogen per day.[131] This decline is the result of ketoadaptation to starvation. In this process, the brain, which does not normally use ketone bodies for fuel, adapts its metabolism and transport systems to use ketone bodies.[148] This adaptation results in a significant reduction in the amount of glucose needed by this glucose-dependent tissue and consequently in the amount of amino acid substrate necessary for gluconeogenesis (Fig. 1-22). Protein conservation follows with only 20 to 30 g of protein catabolized per day.[22]

Concurrent with these adaptations to starvation is a reduction in the resting energy expenditure by as much as 31%.[96] In part, the reduction in resting energy expenditure is the result of a reduction in body cell mass produced by the breakdown of muscle and other proteins. However, the reduction in body size is less than the reduction in resting energy expenditure.[35,96] Other factors that may contribute to the reduction in resting energy expenditure include a reduction in voluntary work, a decrease in body temperature, a decrease in cardiac work, a decrease in sympathetic nervous system activity, and a decrease in muscle activity.

The changes in metabolism accompanying fasting and starvation are primarily regulated by decreased concentrations of insulin and increased concentrations of glucagon in response to decreasing glucose concentrations.[22,23,131] The decreased insulin concentrations promote an increase in lipolysis in adipose tissue and a decrease in glucose uptake in insulin-dependent tissues. The increased concentrations of glucagon promote hepatic gluconeogenesis. These changes (including the decreased secretion of insulin and increased secretion of glucagon) may be further augmented by slight increases in the concentrations of epinephrine, ACTH, cortisol, and growth hormone.[150,187] However, an actual increase in these hormones is not necessary since basal concentrations of the counter regulatory hormones will be unopposed by the reduced secretion of insulin that is stimulated by hypoglycemia.

Thus through four major adaptive mechanisms, a reduction in resting energy expenditure, the use of protein for gluconeogenesis, the use of fat for energy, and keto-adaptation of the brain, a human being is able to survive for prolonged periods of time without food. As a result of the decreased excretion of urea and nitrogen during prolonged starvation, water intake is also reduced. However, it is apparent that this condition cannot be maintained indefinitely. In the average 70-kg male, there are approximately 170,000 calories and 6000 g of protein (see Table 1-13). If it could all be used, starvation for up to 100 days would be tolerated. However, this is not possible because of the loss of essential body functions as body protein is consumed and not replenished. In fact, acute weight losses of 30% to 40% of body weight are usually fatal and associated with a rapid increase in urinary nitrogen excretion and a rapid decline in plasma glucose.[110,131,180]

Injury and Sepsis

Cuthbertson,[38,39] in his classic studies of the metabolic response to long-bone fractures, defined two phases of the metabolic response to injury—an ebb or shock phase and a flow phase. Moore[128] subsequently divided the flow phase into catabolic and anabolic stages. The ebb phase, constituting the first several hours after injury, is characterized by hyperglycemia and the restoration of circulatory volume and tissue perfusion. Once perfusion is restored, the flow phase begins. It is characterized by generalized catabolism, negative nitrogen balance, hyperglycemia, and heat production. The flow phase is the best-studied phase and may last from days to weeks depending on the severity of the injury, the previous health of the individual, and medical intervention. Finally, once volume deficits have been corrected, pain has been eliminated, wounds have been closed, infection has been controlled, and complete oxygenation has been restored, the anabolic phase begins.[69] This phase can be divided into a slow but progressive reaccumulation of protein followed by the reaccumulation of body fat. Since protein synthesis cannot exceed 3 to 5 g of nitrogen per day, the protein repletion phase may be considerably longer than the catabolic phase in which protein is broken down.

The posttraumatic state is characterized by starvation, immobilization, and repair. Although starvation and immobilization are both associated with decreased energy requirements, reparative processes increase energy needs. As a result, the overall energy requirements of traumatized and septic individuals are increased. The increase in energy need varies directly with the severity of injury and the complications that develop. In this regard, the most severe injury is the burn, and the most severe complication is sepsis (see Fig. 1-7). Despite the use of protein and carbohydrate for calories, most of the energy used after trauma and after sepsis is derived from fat. This use is reflected in the low respiratory quotients noted after injury and sepsis. For example, Wilmore[195] found respiratory quotients of 0.70 to 0.76 after severe burns. In addition, septic injury appears to have a greater lipid dependence for energy than nonseptic injury.[6,137]

Increased lipolysis is seen in both the ebb phase and the flow phase of the metabolic response to injury. During the ebb phase, elevated concentrations of cortisol, catecholamines, glucagon, growth hormone, ACTH, increased sympathetic nervous system activity, and depressed concentrations of insulin favor lipolysis. The presence of cortisol appears to be necessary for the remainder of the hormonal agents to be effective.[58,171] Elevated concentrations of glycerol and free fatty acids during the ebb phase are well documented.[33,80,144] However, Kovach and associates[104] have noted that elevation of plasma free fatty acids may not occur after severe hemorrhage as a result of intense vasoconstriction in adipose tissue producing minimum blood flow.

During the flow phase, net lipolysis persists despite an increase in the concentration of insulin. Increased free fatty acids have been documented after trauma, burns, and

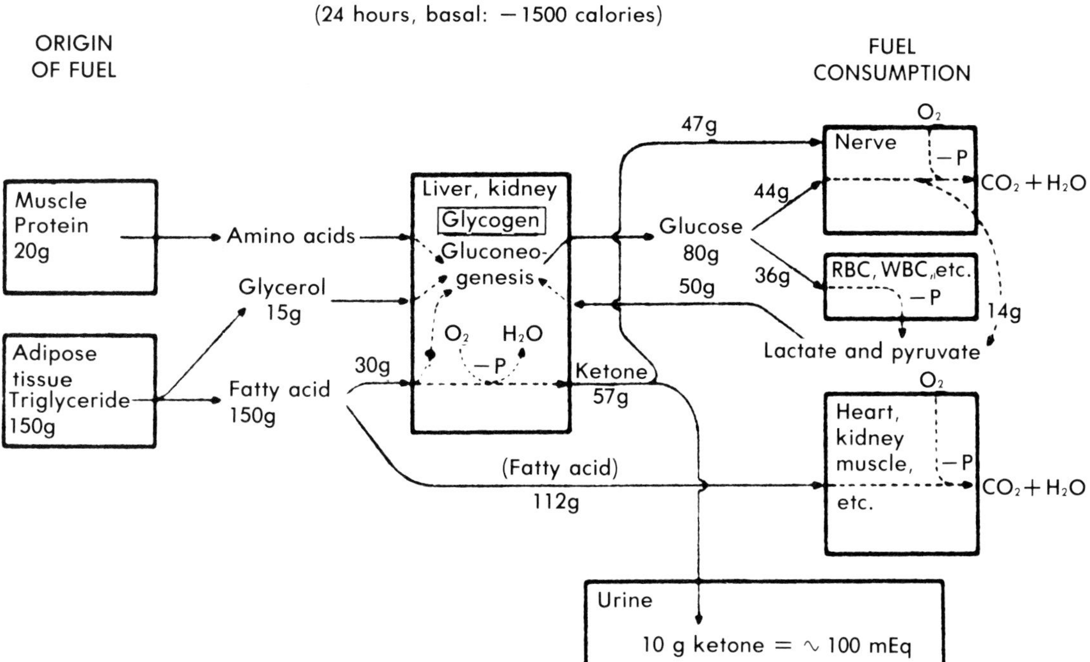

Fig. 1-22 Flow diagram of fuel metabolism in starved man after adaptation. (From Cahill, G.F.: N. Engl. J. Med. **282:**672, 1970.)

sepsis.* The fatty acids are used throughout the body for energy. In both the ebb and flow phase, the high concentration of intracellular fatty acids and the elevated concentration of glucagon inhibit acetyl-CoA carboxylase thereby decreasing malonyl-CoA concentrations and fatty-acid synthesis. In hepatocytes, the decreased conentration of malonyl-CoA also stimulates carnitine acyl transferase thereby increasing the transport of acetyl-CoA into the mitochondria for oxidation and ketogenesis. However, the activity of ketogenesis after shock, injury, and sepsis is variable and correlates with the severity of injury.[146,176,179] After major injury and sepsis, ketogenesis is low or absent, whereas after minor injury and sepsis, it is increased but to a lesser extent than is seen during nonstressed starvation.[17,127] During starvation, the inhibition of acetyl-CoA carboxylase also results in the accumulation of cytoplasmic citrate that in turn inhibits glycolysis through phosphofructokinase inhibition (Randle effect).[141] However, after shock and major injury, citrate does not accumulate.[44,132] This lack of accumulation may play a role in the persistence of glycolysis after injury.

Unlike fasting and starvation, hyperglycemia is a hallmark of the response to injury, sepsis, and stress. An increase in blood glucose occurs during both the ebb and flow phases and is proportional to the severity of the injury.[27,126] There is also an increased concentration of lactate, pyruvate, organic phosphates, total amino acids, glycerol, and free fatty acids. Changes in lactate, pyruvate, and alanine have also been found to correlate with the severity of injury.[146] The rise in the concentrations of glucose and other solutes contributes to an elevated plasma osmolality after hemorrhage and injury that is thought to be critical in the complete restitution of blood volume and plasma proteins.[21,43,68,74,95] The hyperosmolality appears to augment the transcapillary refill phase and the plasma protein restoration phase of blood volume restitution by mediating the movement of water from cells to the interstitium and ultimately to the plasma.[43,68,74]

The metabolic changes in carbohydrate metabolism arise primarily as the result of the actions and interactions of catecholamines, cortisol, glycogen, insulin, growth hormone, and somatostatin.† It is apparent that the elevated blood glucose concentration results from increased hepatic production and from impaired peripheral uptake that are under endocrine control. Both the ebb and the flow phases are associated with hyperglycemia, increased gluconeogenesis, and hepatic and peripheral insulin resistance. However, the mechanisms involved in these carbohydrate "abnormalities" are different. During the ebb phase, plasma insulin is clearly depressed in relationship to the degree of hyperglycemia.[27,37,133,193] This results from decreased B-cell sensitivity to glucose that is secondary to catecholamines, somatostatin, reduced pancreatic blood flow, and the increased activity of the sympathetic nervous system.‡ However, during the flow phase, B-cell sensitivity returns to normal, and insulin concentrations rise to more appropriate values. Nevertheless, hyperglycemia persists.[91,193]

In both the ebb and the flow phases, there is a delayed rate of assimilation of a glucose load, glucosuria, and a resistance to exogenously administered insulin.[2,18,28] Despite this "diabetes of injury," glucose uptake and use by peripheral tissues in both the ebb and the flow phases have been demonstrated consistently to be greater than under normal circumstances.* The resistance to insulin is manifested in a decreased glucose clearance. Consequently, the high plasma glucose concentration and the attendant increase in plasma-tissue glucose concentration gradient appear to overcome the resistance of peripheral tissues to glucose entry. The insulin resistance that develops appears to result from the action of catecholamines, cortisol, and other factors.[52,62,151,162,163]

Hepatic carbohydrate metabolism is also affected by insulin resistance. During the ebb phase, elevated concentrations of catecholamines, cortisol, and glucagon and a decreased concentration of insulin result in rapid glycogenolysis and an outpouring of glucose from the liver. In addition, these hormonal alterations stimulate gluconeogenesis from alanine, lactate, and pyruvate. Growth hormone also is involved in these processes by inhibiting glucose uptake through inhibition of glucokinase. During the flow phase, gluconeogenesis persists despite near-normal concentrations of insulin. This persistence appears to result from insulin resistance and produces a continued flow of glucose from the liver. Therefore the hyperglycemia that results after injury results from a combination of increased glucose production and glucose release and from a peripheral resistance to the entrance of glucose.

After injury and during sepsis, glucose must be provided not only to red cells, white cells, renal medulla, and neural tissues, but also to wounded tissue.[24,86,185] Glucose uptake in wounded tissue is increased by up to 100%. Wounds demonstrate a lack of insulin sensitivity and do not increase their glucose uptake or glycogenesis in response to insulin.[139,140,194] The accelerated glucose uptake in wounded tissue and possibly in septic tissue appears to correlate with the degree of inflammatory cellular infiltrate.[185] In addition, it has recently been demonstrated that the accelerated glycolysis of wounded tissue may be aerobic and not anaerobic as thought previously.[24] In aerobic glycolysis, glycolysis proceeds to lactate in the presence of adequate oxygen. Thus oxygen consumption and carbon dioxide production are normal, but lactate production is accelerated. Increased lactate production may be related to an inability of the NADH shuttle to transfer reducing equivalents from the cytoplasm to the mitochondrion.[89,138] Metabolic derangements suggestive of aerobic glycolysis have also been seen in septic tissue.[164] In this regard, it is of note that aerobic glycolysis is characteristic of the cellular infiltrate.[166]

As one might expect, negative nitrogen balance and net proteolysis are characteristic of the posttraumatic and the septic states.[1,175] However, only 20% of the protein broken down is used for calories.[48] The remainder is used in gluconeogenesis. As noted previously, the production of

*References 17, 122, 128, 137, 146, 176, 179.

†References 27, 28, 52, 62, 162, 163.

‡References 18, 45, 80, 86, 151, 154.

*References 42, 116, 158, 168, 182, 193.

lactate in the presence of oxygen primarily results from the actions of cortisol, glucagon, catecholamines, and the decreased effectiveness of insulin.

The rise in urinary nitrogen is associated with an increased excretion of urea, sulfur, phosphorous, potassium, magnesium, and creatinine, suggesting the breakdown of intracellular material.[38,65] Isotope dilution studies suggest that this loss of protein results from the loss of cell mass rather than cell number.[38] The nitrogen-to-sulfur and nitrogen-to-potassium ratios suggest that this loss occurs mainly from muscle.[38] The marked increase in the urinary excretion of 3-methylhistidine during trauma, sepsis, and burns also suggests the importance of skeletal muscle in this response.[15,117,192] Analysis of the protein content and the incorporation of radiolabeled amino acids in visceral tissues and skeletal muscle confirm that it is skeletal muscle that is depleted while visceral tissue (liver, kidney) is spared.[169] This is the opposite of nonstressed starvation in which visceral protein is used before muscle protein and has been termed visceral translocation of protein.[98,169]

The alterations in plasma amino acids are not well defined during the ebb and flow phases. During the ebb phase, little change in total amino acid concentrations were noted by Elwyn and associates[53] until the late phases of shock. In addition, it appears that these changes result primarily from a decreased hepatic uptake[53] and not an increased peripheral release as was thought previously.[54] During the flow phase, alterations in plasma amino acids appear to be related to the severity of injury and the specific type of injury.[30,40,66,197] Alanine, the major gluconeogenic amino acid, appears to be released from peripheral tissues and taken up by the liver for gluconeogenesis. Early in the flow phase, the concentration of alanine in plasma is increased, but as the injury persists, serum alanine decreases, presumably as a result of its lack of availability in peripheral tissues and its continued hepatic uptake. Branched-chain amino acids and aspartate and aspargine are transaminated in peripheral tissues, and their remaining carbon fragments are used in the TCA cycle. Nonetheless, muscle concentrations of amino acids generally reveal normal or elevated concentrations of all amino acids except alanine, glutamine, and arginine.[5]

The net catabolism of protein can result from either increased catabolism, decreased synthesis, or a combination of the two. Available data on total body protein turnover suggest that after injury, the net changes in catabolism and synthesis depend on the severity of the injury.[16] Elective operations and minor injury appear to result in a decreased rate of synthesis with a normal rate of protein catabolism.[34,144] Severe trauma, burns, and sepsis appear to be associated with increases in both synthesis and catabolism but with a greater increase in the latter, resulting in net catabolism.[16,97,117,177] In this regard, it is important to note that accelerated proteolysis and a high rate of gluconeogenesis persist after injury and during sepsis.[30,143] This persistence appears to result from an inhibition of ketoadaptation after injury and sepsis. Unlike starvation, ketogenesis is not prominent, and it does not fuel the brain in significant amounts. Therefore a high requirement for glucose and therefore gluconeogenesis persists. The mechanism for this inhibition of ketoadaptation is not understood presently. Clowes and associates[32] have recently presented evidence suggesting the involvement of a circulating peptide containing 33 amino acids in this response. In addition, Baracos and associates[9] have proposed that interleukin-1 (a human leukocyte pyrogen) may be responsible for the accelerated proteolysis that accompanies fever and sepsis.

The net catabolism of protein that occurs after any injury is dependent on the prior nutritional status and intake, sex, and age of the individual as well as the severity of the injury. Young healthy males lose more protein in response to an injury than do women or the elderly.[173] In addition, the urinary excretion of nitrogen is less after a second operation if it closely follows the first.[175,176] This decline is presumably the result of a reduction in available protein stores. Finally, negative nitrogen balance can be reduced or virtually eliminated by high caloric and nitrogen supplementation.[28,100,170,177,178] Together, these facts suggest that the loss of protein that occurs after injury is not entirely obligatory to the injury but is also a manifestation of acute starvation.[179]

Despite a negative nitrogen balance and energy balance after injury, most wounds heal.[101,180] Kinney, Lister, and Moore[100] have termed this ability of wound healing to proceed in the presence or absence of abundant substrate supply, the biologic priority of wound healing. However, the biologic priority of wound healing should not be taken to mean that wound healing is normal in the severely injured patient. As Levenson and associates[112] have noted, "Whereas the healing of a wound after injury appears satisfactory, it may be neither normal nor optimal." In examining the healing of laparotomy wounds in normal and burned (35%) rodents, Levenson and associates[112,113] noted a distinct delay in the wound healing of burned animals. Similarly, rodents with a fractured femur did not heal a skin incision as well as rodents with a skin incision alone.[35] The biologic priority of wound healing also does not mean that wound healing cannot be improved in severely injured patients. Large open wounds, such as burns, are associated with an inhibition of nitrogen anabolism of the host and may result in protein malnutrition and death if the substrate demands of the wounds are not met exogenously. It is not clear whether the administration of protein improves wound healing per se. However, it has been shown to reduce negative nitrogen balance. Some investigators have also noted an improvement in wound healing with protein supplementation,[82,102,191] but others have been unable to document any change.[4,25]

In summary, generalized catabolism, hyperglycemia, persistent gluconeogenesis, protein wasting, negative nitrogen balance, heat production, and loss of the body mass that parallel the severity of the injury are characteristic after trauma and during sepsis. Most of the energy necessary for biologic processes to proceed is derived from fat. The net catabolism of 300 to 500 g of lean body cell mass per day is apparently required as a source of amino acids for gluconeogenesis. The persistence of the injury, particularly sepsis, through unknown mechanisms produces inhibition of the usual adaptive mechanisms that occur in starvation, resulting in the persistence of a highly catabolic state. This state, in turn, leads to protein wasting and malnutrition and ultimately in multiple organ failure[84] and in death if the stimuli are not eliminated.

SUMMARY

Starvation, stress from injury or surgical procedures, and sepsis induce a series of metabolic changes that are regulated by neuroendocrine reflexes and result in mobilization of substrates from endogenous tissue stores. These metabolic changes ensure that energy is available for vital functions, that oxygen delivery is maintained, and that reparative processes take place. An understanding of these complex metabolic interactions depends on an appreciation of normal homeostasis and the distribution of body water, proteins, fat, and carbohydrates. The role of each component of body tissue is important in periods of starvation, stress, and sepsis, especially when the ability to replenish endogenous food stores is impaired as a result of either the inability to consume adequate nutrients or the excessive consumption of tissue stores. The mechanisms described in this chapter illustrate the complexity of the metabolic response to stress, the interrelationships between the neuroendocrine responses and substrate mobilization and use, and the importance of adequate energy and tissue stores for survival and repair of the organisms under conditions of nutrient deprivation.

REFERENCES

1. Abbott, W.E., and Anderson, K.: The effect of starvation, infection, and injury on the metabolic processes and body composition, Ann. N.Y. Acad. Sci. **110:**941, 1963.
2. Allison, S.P., Hinton, P., and Chamberlain, J.J.: Intravenous glucose tolerance insulin and free fatty acid levels in burn patients, Lancet **2:**1116, 1968.
3. Altszuler, N., et al.: Glucose metabolism and plasma insulin level during epinephrine infusion in the dog, Am. J. Physiol. **212:**677, 1967.
4. Andrews, R.P., Morgan, H.C., and Jurkiewicz, M.J.: Relationship of dietary protein to the healing of experimental burns, Surg. Forum **6:**72, 1955.
5. Askanazi, J., et al.: Muscle and plasma amino acids following injury, Ann. Surg. **192:**78, 1980.
6. Askanazi, J., et al.: Respiratory distress secondary to a high carbohydrate load, Surgery **86:**596, 1980.
7. Atkinson, D.E.: The energy charge of the adenylate pool as a regulator parameter interaction with feedback modifiers, Biochemistry **7:**4030, 1966.
8. Atkinson, D.E., and Bourke, E.: The role of ureagenesis in pH homeostasis, Trends Biochem. Sci. **9:**297, 1984.
9. Baracos, V., et al.: Stimulation of muscle protein degradation and prostaglandin E_2 release by leukocyte pyrogen (interleukin-1), N. Engl. J. Med. **308:**553, 1983.
10. Baylis, P.H., Zerbe, R.L., and Robertson, G.L.: Arginine vasopressin response to insulin-induced hypoglycemia in man, J. Clin. Endocrinol. Metab. **53:**935, 1981.
11. Behnke, A.R.: Physiologic studies pertaining to deep sea diving and aviation, especially in relation to the fat content and composition of the body, Harvey Lect. **37:**198, 1941.
12. Behnke, A.R., and Wilmore, J.H.: Evaluation and regulation of body build and composition, Englewood Cliffs, N.J., 1974, Prentice Hall, Inc.
13. Bereiter, D.A., Plotsky, P.M., and Gann, D.S.: Tooth pulp stimulation potentiates the ACTH response to hemorrhage in cats, Endocrinology **111:**1127, 1982.
14. Bie, P.: Osmoreceptors, vasopressin, and control of renal water excretion, Physiol. Rev. **60:**961, 1980.
15. Bilmazer, C., et al.: Quantitative contribution by skeletal muscle to elevated rates of whole-body protein breakdown in burned children as measured by 3-MEH output, Metabolism **27:**671, 1978.
16. Birkhain, R.H., et al.: Effects of major skeletal trauma on whole body protein turnover in man measured by L-[1,14_C] -leucine, Surgery **88:**294, 1980.
17. Birkhain, R.H., et al.: A comparison of the effects of skeletal trauma and surgery on the ketosis of starvation in man, J. Trauma **21:**513, 1981.
18. Black, P.R., et al.: Mechanisms of insulin resistance following injury, Ann. Surg. **196:**420, 1982.
19. Browne, J.S.L., and Schenker, V.: Conferences on metabolic aspects of convalescence including bone and wound healing: transactions of the third meeting, New York, 1943, Joshiah Macy Jr., Publications.
20. Brozek, J., et al.: Densitometric analysis of body composition: revision of some quantitative assumptions, Ann. N.Y. Acad. Sci. **110:**113, 1963.
21. Byrnes, G.J., Pirkle, J.C., Jr., and Gann, D.S.: Cardiovascular stabilization after hemorrhage depends upon restitution of blood volume, J. Trauma **18:**623, 1978.
22. Cahill, G.F.: Starvation in man, N. Engl. J. Med. **668:**282, 1970.
23. Cahill, G.F.: Ketosis, J.P.E.N. **5:**281, 1981.
24. Caldwell, M.D., et al.: Evidence for aerobic glycolysis in λ-carrageenan wounded skeletal muscle, J. Surg. Res. **37:**63, 1984.
25. Calloway, D.H., et al.: Effect of previous level of protein feeding on wound healing and on metabolic response to injury, Surgery **37:**935, 1955.
26. Cannon, W.B.: The wisdom of the body, New York, 1939, W.W. Norton and Co., Inc.
27. Carey, L.C., Lowery, B.D., and Cloutier, C.T.: Blood sugar and insulin response in human shock, Ann. Surg. **172:**342, 1970.
28. Carey, L.C., Cloutier, C.T., and Lowery, B.D.: Growth hormone and adrenal cortisol response to shock and trauma in the human, Ann. Surg. **174:**451, 1971.
29. Chaisson, J.L., et al.: Inhibitory effect of epinephrine on insulin-stimulated glucose uptake by rat skeletal muscle, J. Clin. Invest. **68:**706, 1981.
30. Clowes, G.H.A., Randall, H., and Cha, C.: Amino acid and energy metabolism in septic and traumatized patients, J.P.E.N. **4:**195, 1980.
31. Clowes, G.H.A., Randall, H., and Cha, C.: Effects of parenteral alimentation on metabolism in septic patients, Surgery **88:**531, 1980
32. Clowes, G.H.A., et al.: Muscle proteolysis induced by a circulating peptide in patients with sepsis or trauma, N. Engl. J. Med. **308:**545, 1983.
33. Coran, A.G., et al.: Fat and carbohydrate metabolism during hemorrhagic shock in the unanesthetized baboon, Surg. Forum **9:**10, 1971.
34. Crane, C.W., et al.: Protein turnover in patients before and after elective orthopedic operations, Br. J. Surg. **64:**129, 1977.
35. Crowley, C.V., et al.: Effects of environmental temperature and femoral fracture on wound healing in rats, J. Trauma **17:**436, 1977.
36. Cryer, P.E.: Physiology and pathophysiology of the human sympathoadrenal neuroendocrine system, N. Engl. J. Med. **303:**436, 1980.
37. Cryer, P.E., Herman, C.M., and Sode, J.: Carbohydrate metabolism in the baboon subjected to gram-negative septicemia. I. Hyperglycemia with depressed plasma insulin concentrations, J. Lab. Clin. Med. **79:**622, 1972.
38. Cuthbertson, D.P.: Observations on the disturbance of metabolism by injury to the limbs, Q. J. Med. **1:**233, 1932.
39. Cuthbertson, D.P.: Further observations on the disturbance of metabolism caused by injury, with particular reference to the dietary requirements of fracture cases, Br. J. Surg. **23:**505, 1936.
40. Dale, G., et al.: The effect of surgical operation on venous plasma free amino acids, Surgery **81:**295, 1977.
41. Drabkin, D.L.: The distribution of the chromoproteins, hemoglobin, myoglobin and cytochrome C, in the tissue of different species, and the relationship to the total content of each chromoprotein to body mass, J. Biol. Chem. **182:**317, 1950.
42. Drucker W.R., and Dekieweit, J.C.: Glucose uptake by diaphragms

from rats subjected to hemorrhagic shock, Am. J. Physiol. **206:**317, 1964.
43. Drucker, W.R., Chadwick, C.D.J., and Gann, D.S.: Transcapillary refill in hemorrhage and shock, Arch. Surg. **116:**1344, 1981.
44. Drucker, W.R., et al.: Citrate metabolism during surgery, Arch. Surg. **85:**557, 1962.
45. Drucker, W.R., et al.: The effect of persisting hypovolemic shock on pancreatic output of insulin. In Kovach, A.G.B., Stoner, H.B., and Spitzer, J.J., editors: Neurohumoral and metabolic response to injury, New York, 1978, Plenum Publishing Corp.
46. Reference deleted in galleys.
47. Dubois, E.F.: The mechanism of heat loss and temperature regulation, Lane Medical Lectures, 1937, Stanford University Press.
48. Duke, J.H., et al.: Contribution of protein to caloric expenditure following injury, Surgery **68:**168, 1970.
49. Edelman, I.S., and Leibman, J.: Anatomy of body water and electolytes, Am. J. Med. **27:**256, 1959.
50. Egdahl, R.H.: The differential response of the adrenal cortex and medulla to bacterial endotoxin, J. Clin. Invest. **38:**1120, 1959.
51. Egdahl, R.H.: Pituitary-adrenal response following trauma to the isolated leg, Surgery **46:**9, 1959.
52. Eigler, N., Sacca, L., and Sherwin, R.S.: Synergistic interactions of physiologic increments of glucagon, epinephrine, and cortisol in the dog, J. Clin. Invest. **63:**114, 1979.
53. Elwyn, D.H., et al.: Interorgan transport of amino acids in hemorrhagic shock, Am. J. Physiol. **231:**377, 1976.
54. Engel, F.L.: The significance of the metabolic changes during shock, Ann. N.Y. Acad. Sci. **55:**383, 1956.
55. Exton, J.H.: Gluconeogenesis, Metabolism **21:**945, 1972.
56. Fain, J.N.: Involvement of phosphatidylinositol breakdown in elevation of cytosol Ca^{2+} by hormones and relationship to prostaglandin formation. In Kohn, L.D., editor: Hormone receptors, vol. 6, New York, 1982, John Wiley & Sons, Inc.
57. Fain, J.N., and Garcia-Sainz, J.A.: Adrenergic regulation of adipocyte metabolism, J. Lipid Res. **24:**945, 1983.
58. Fain, J.N., Kovacev, V.P., and Scow, R.O.: Effect of growth hormone and dexamethasone on lipolysis and metabolism in isolated fat cells of the rat, J. Biol. Chem. **240:**3522, 1965.
59. Felig, P.: The glucose-alanine cycle, Metabolism **22:**179, 1973.
60. Felig, P.: The endocrine pancreas: diabetes mellitus. In Felig, P., et al., editors: Endocrinology and metabolism, New York, 1981, McGraw-Hill Book Co.
61. Felig, P., Wahren, J., and Hendler, R.: Influence of physiologic hyperglucagonemia on basal and insulin inhibited splanchnic glucose output in normal man, J. Clin. Invest. **58:**961, 1976.
62. Felig, P., et al.: Hormonal interactions in the regulation of blood glucose, Recent Prog. Horm. Res. **35:**501, 1979.
63. Feldman, M., et al.: Beta-endorphin and the endocrine pancreas, N. Engl. J. Med. **208:**350, 1983.
64. Fradkin, J., et al.: Evidence for an important role of changes in rather than absolute concentrations of glucagon in the regulation of glucose production in humans, J. Clin. Endocrinol. Metab. **50:**698, 1980.
65. Frawley, J.P., Artz, C.P., and Howard, J.M.: Muscle metabolism and catabolism in combat casualties, Arch. Surg. **71:**612, 1955.
66. Freund, H.R., Ryan, J.A., and Fischer, J.E.: Amino acid derangements in patients with sepsis: treatment with branched chain amino acid rich infusions, Ann. Surg. **188:**423, 1978.
67. Frohman, L.A.: Diseases of the anterior pituitary. In Felig, P., et al., editors: Endocrinology and metabolism, New York, 1981, McGraw-Hill Book Co.
68. Gann, D.S.: Endocrine control of plasma protein and volume, Surg. Clin. North Am. **56:**1135, 1976.
69. Gann, D.S., and Amaral, J.F.: The pathology of trauma and shock. In Fridema, G.D., Rutherford, W.F., and Bullinger, W.F., editors: The management of trauma, Philadelphia, 1984, W.B. Saunders Co.
70. Gann, D.S., and Lilly, M.P.: The neuroendocrine response to multiple trauma, World J. Surg. **7:**101, 1983.
71. Gann, D.S., Cryer, G.L., and Pirkle, J.C., Jr.: Physiological inhibition and facilitation of adrenocortical response to hemorrhage, Am. J. Physiol. **232:**R5, 1977.
72. Gann, D.S., Ward, D.G., and Carlson, D.E.: Neural control of ACTH: a hemostatic reflex, Recent Prog. Horm. Res. **35:**357, 1978.
73. Gann, D.S., Dallman, M.F., and Engeland, W.C.: Reflex control and modulation of ACTH and corticosteroids. In McCann, S.M., editor: Endocrinology physiology. III. International review of physiology, vol. 24, Baltimore, 1981, University Park Press.
74. Gann, D.S., et al.: Role of solute in the early restitution of blood volume after hemorrhage, Surgery **94:**439, 1983.
75. Gibbs, D.M.: Measurement of hypothalamic releasing factors in hypophyseal-portal blood, Regul. Pept. (In press.)
76. Goodman, H.M.: The pituitary gland. In Mountcastle, V.S., editor: Medical physiology, ed. 14, St. Louis, 1980, The C.V. Mosby Co.
77. Grande, F., and Keys, A.: Body weight, body composition, and calorie status. In Goodhart, R.S., and Shihs, M.E., editors: Modern nutrition in health and disease, Philadelphia, 1980, Lea & Febiger.
78. Greengard, P.: Phosphorylated proteins as physiological effectors, Science **199:**146, 1978.
79. Guyton, A.C.: Textbook of medical physiology, ed. 6, Philadelphia, 1981, W.B. Saunders Co.
80. Halmagyi, D.F.J., Irving, M.H., and Varga, D.: Effect of adrenergic blockade on the metabolic response to hemorrhagic shock, J. Appl. Physiol. **25:**384, 1968.
81. Harper, H.A., Rodwell, V.W., and Mayes, P.A.: Review of physiological chemistry, ed. 16, Los Altos, Calif., 1977, Lange Medical Publications.
82. Harvey, S.C., and Howes, E.L.: Effect of high protein diet on the velocity of growth of fibroblasts in the healing wound, Ann. Surg. **91:**641, 1930.
83. Harvey, T.C., et al.: Measurement of whole body nitrogen by neutron activation analysis, Lancet **2:**359, 1973.
84. Hassett, J., and Border, J.R.: The metabolic response to trauma and sepsis, World J. Surg. **7:**125, 1983.
85. Hastings, A.B.: The electrolytes of tissue and body fluids, Harvey Lect. **36:**91, 1940-1941.
86. Hiebert, J.M., et al.: Insulin response to hemorrhagic shock in the intact and adrenalectomized primate, Am. J. Surg. **125:**501, 1973.
87. Hill, G.L., et al.: Multi-element analysis of the living body by neutron activation analysis—application to critically ill patients receiving intravenous nutrition, Br. J. Surg. **66:**868, 1979.
88. Hinton, P., et al.: Insulin and glucose to reduce catabolic response to injury in burned patients, Lancet **1:**767, 1971.
89. Hochachka, P.N.: Living without oxygen, Cambridge, Mass., 1980, Harvard University Press.
90. Howard, J.E., Bingham, R.S., Jr., and Mason, R.E.: Studies on convalescence-Nitrogen and mineral balances during starvation and graduated feeding in healthy young males at bed rest, Trans. Assoc. Am. Physicians **59:**242, 1946.
91. Kahn, C.R.: Insulin resistance, insulin insensitivity and insulin unresponsiveness: a necessary definition, Metabolism **27:**1893, 1973.
92. Kaneto, A., Kajinuma, H., and Kosaka, K.: Effect of splanchnic nerve stimulation on glucagon and insulin output in the dog, Endocrinology **96:**143, 1975.
93. Kaplan, N.M., and Bartter, F.C.: The effect of ACTH, renin angiotensin II and various precursors on biosynthesis of aldosterone by adrenal slices, J. Clin. Invest. **41:**715, 1962.
94. Kawai, K., et al.: Circulating somatostatin acts on the islet of Langerhans by way of a somatostatin poor compartment, Science **218:**417, 1982.
95. Kenney, P.R., Allen-Rowlands, C.F., and Gann, D.S.: Glucose and osmolality as predictors of injury severity, J. Trauma **23:**712, 1983.
96. Keys, A., et al.: The biology of human starvation, Minneapolis, 1950, University of Minnesota Press.
97. Kien, C.L., et al.: Increased rates of whole body protein synthesis and breakdown in children recovering from burns, Ann. Surg. **187:**383, 1978.
98. Kinney, J.M.: Energy requirements in injury and sepsis, Acta Anaesthesiol. Scand. **55:**15, 1974.
99. Kinney, J.M., and Gump, F.E.: The metabolic response to injury. In American College of Surgeons, editors: Manual of pre and postoperative care, Philadelphia, 1983, W.B. Saunders Co.
100. Kinney, J.M., Lister, J., and Moore, F.D.: Relationship of energy

expenditure to total exchangeable potassium, Ann. N.Y. Acad. Sci. **110:**711, 1963.

101. Kinney, J.M., et al.: Tissue composition of weight loss in surgical patients. I. Elective operations, Ann. Surg. **168:**459, 1968.
102. Kobak, M.W., et al.: The relation of protein deficiency to experimental wound healing, Surg. Gynecol. Obstet. **85:**751, 1947.
103. Korchak, H.M., and Masoro, E.J.: Changes in the level of the fatty acids synthesizing enzymes during starvation, Biochem. Biophys. Acta **58:**354, 1962.
104. Kovach, A.G.B., et al.: Blood flow, oxygen consumption, and free fatty acid release in subcutaneous adipose tissue during hemorrhagic shock in control and phenoxybenzamine-treated dogs, Circ. Res. **26:**733, 1970.
105. Kraus-Friedmann, H.: Hormonal regulation of hepatic gluconeogenesis, Physiol. Rev. **64:**170, 1984.
106. Krebs, H.A.: The metabolic fate of amino acids. In Munroe, H.N., and Allison, J.B., editors: Mammalian protein metabolism, New York, 1964, Academic Press, Inc.
107. Lehninger, A.L.: Bioenergetics, ed. 2, Menlo Park, Calif., 1972, The Benjamin/Cummings Publishing Co.
108. Lehninger, A.L.: Biochemistry: the molecular basis of cell structure and function, ed. 2, New York, 1975, Worth Publishing, Inc.
109. Lesser, G.T., Deutsch, S., and Markofsy, T.: Use of independent measurement of body fat to evaluate overweight and underweight, Metabolism **20:**792, 1971.
110. Levenson, S.M., and Seifter, E.: Starvation. In Fischer, J.E., editor: Metabolic and physiologic responses, Boston, 1982, Little, Brown & Co., Inc.
111. Levenson, S.M., Seifter, E., and Van Winkle, W.: Nutrition. In Hunt, R.K., and Dunphy, J.W., editors: Fundamentals of wound management, New York, 1979, Appleton-Century-Crofts.
112. Levenson, S.M., et al.: The effect of thermal burns on wound healing, Surg. Gynecol. Obstet. **99:**74, 1954.
113. Levenson, S.M., et al.: Effect of thermal burns on wound healing, Ann. Surg. **146:**357, 1957.
114. Lilly, M.P., and Gann, D.S.: The effect of repeated operation on the response of the adrenal cortex to infused ACTH, Surg. Forum **33:**10, 1982.
115. Lilly, M.P., Engeland, W.C., and Gann, D.S.: Adrenal response to repeated hemorrhage: implications for studies of trauma, J. Trauma **22:**809, 1982.
116. Long, C.L., et al.: Carbohydrate metabolism in men: effect of elective operations and major injury, J. Appl. Physiol. **31:**110, 1971.
117. Long, C.L., et al.: Muscle protein catabolism in the septic patient as measured by 3-methyl histidine excretion, Am. J. Clin. Nutr. **30:**1349, 1977.
118. Makara, G.: Pathways by which stressful stimuli activate the pituitary-adrenal system. In Regulatory peptides. (In press.)
119. Mallette, L.E., Exton, J.H., and Park, C.R.: Control of gluconeogenesis from amino acids in the perfused rat liver, J. Biol. Chem. **244:**5713, 1969.
120. Masoro, E.J.: Lipids and lipid metabolism, Annu. Rev. Physiol. **39:**301, 1977.
121. Maxwell, M.H., and Kleeman, C.R.: Dynamics of body water and electrolytes. In Clinical disorders of fluid and electrolyte metabolism, ed. 4, New York, 1987, McGraw-Hill Book Co.
122. Mays, E.T.: The effect of surgical stress on plasma-free fatty acids, J. Surg. Res. **10:**315, 1970.
123. McGarry, J.D., and Foster, D.W.: Hormonal control of ketogenesis: biochemical considerations, Arch. Intern. Med. **137:**495, 1977.
124. McGilvery, R.W.: Biochemistry—a functional approach, Philadelphia, 1970, W.B. Saunders Co.
125. McIntyre, N., Holdsworth, C.D., and Turner, D.S.: Intestinal factors in the control of insulin secretion, J. Clin. Endocrinol. Metab. **25:**1317, 1965.
126. Meguid, M.M., et al.: Hormone-substrate interrelationships following trauma, Arch. Surg. **109:**776, 1974.
127. Miller, J.D.B., Bistran, B.R., and Blackburn, G.L.: Failure of postoperative infection to increase nitrogen excretion in patients maintained on peripheral amino acids, Am. J. Clin. Nutr. **30:**1523, 1977.
128. Moore, F.D.: Bodily changes in surgical convalescence, Ann. Surg. **137:**289, 1953.
129. Moore, F.D.: The body cell mass and its supporting environment, Philadelphia, 1963, W.B. Saunders Co.
130. Moore, F.D.: Energy and the maintenance of the body cell mass, J.P.E.N. **4:**228, 1980.
131. Moore, F.D., and Brennan, M.F.: Surgical injury: body composition, protein metabolism and neuroendocrinology. In Ballinger, W.F., et al., editors: Manual of surgical nutrition, Philadelphia, 1975, W.B. Saunders Co.
132. Morris, A.S., et al.: The role of effectors of phosphofructokinase on the regulation of aerobic glycolysis in a λ-carrageenan wounded muscle, Metabolism. (In press.)
133. Moss, G.S., et al.: Serum insulin response in hemorrhagic shock in baboons, Surgery **68:**34, 1970.
134. Munro, H.N.: Biochemical aspects of protein metabolism. In Munro, H.N., and Allison, J.B., editors: Mammalian protein metabolism, New York, 1964, Academic Press, Inc.
135. Munro, H.N., and Young, V.R.: Protein metabolism in the elderly: observations relating to dietary needs, Postgrad. Med. **63:**143, 1978.
136. Munro, H.N., and Crim, M.C.: The proteins and amino acids. In Goodhart, R.S., and Shils, M.E., editors: Modern nutrition in health and disease, Philadelphia, 1980, Lea & Febiger.
137. Nanni, G., et al.: Increased lipid fuel dependence in the critically ill septic patient, J. Trauma **24:**14, 1983.
138. Needham, A.E.: Regeneration of wound healing. In Albercrombie, M., editor: Methuen's monographs on geological subjects, New York, 1952, John Wiley & Sons, Inc.
139. Nelson, K.M., and Turinsky, J.: Analysis of postburn insulin unresponsiveness in skeletal muscle, J. Surg. Res. **31:**404, 1981.
140. Nelson, K.M., and Turinsky, J.: Local effect of burn on skeletal muscle insulin responsiveness, J. Surg. Res. **31:**288, 1981.
141. Newsholme, E.A., and Start, C.: Regulation in Metabolism, New York, 1973, John Wiley & Sons, Inc.
142. Norris, A.H., Lundry, T., and Shock, N.W.: Trends in selected indices of body composition in men between the ages 30 and 80 years, Ann. N.Y. Acad. Sci. **110:**623, 1963.
143. O'Donnell, T.F., et al.: Proteolysis associated with a deficit of peripheral energy fuel substrates in septic man, Surgery **80:**192, 1976.
144. O'Keefe, S.J.D., Sender, P.M., and James, W.P.T.: Catabolic loss of body nitrogen in response to surgery, Lancet **2:**1035, 1974.
145. O'Malley, B.W., and Schrader, W.T.: The receptors of steroid hormones, Sci. Am. **234:**32, 1976.
146. Oppenheim, W., Williamson, D., and Smith, R.: Early biochemical changes and severity of injury in man, J. Trauma **20:**135, 1980.
147. Oppenheimer, J.H.: Thyroid hormone action at the cellular level, Science **203:**971, 1979.
148. Owen, O.E., et al.: Brain metabolism during fasting, J. Clin. Invest. **46:**1589, 1967.
149. Pace, H., and Rathbun, E.N.: Studies in body composition. III. The body water and chemically combined nitrogen content in relation to fat content, J. Biol. Chem. **158:**685, 1945.
150. Palmblad, J., et al.: Effect of total energy withdrawal (fasting) on the levels of growth hormone, thyrotropin, cortisol, adrenaline, norepinephrine, T_4, T_3 and rT_3 in healthy males, Acta Med. Scand. **201:**15, 1977.
151. Palmer, B.Q., et al.: Epinephrine acutely mediates skeletal muscle insulin resistance, Surgery **94:**172, 1983.
152. Parmley, W.W., Glick, G., and Sonnenblick, E.H.: Cardiovascular effects of glucagon in man, N. Engl. J. Med. **12:**279, 1968.
153. Porte, D., Jr., and Halter, J.B.: The endocrine pancreas and diabetes mellitus. In Williams, R.H., editor: Textbook of endocrinology, Philadelphia, 1981, W.B. Saunders Co.
154. Porte, D., Jr., Smith, P.H., and Ensinick, J.W.: Neurohumoral regulation of the pancreatic islet A and B cells, Metabolism **25:**1453, 1976.
155. Posefsky, T., et al.: Metabolism of forearm tissues in man: studies with glucagon, Diabetes **25:**128, 1976.
156. Raff, H., Shinsako, J., and Dallman, M.F.: Surgery potentiates adrenocortical responses to hypoxia in dogs, Proc. Soc. Exp. Biol. Med. **172:**400, 1983.
157. Randall, H.T.: Water, electrolytes and acid base balance. In Goodhart, R.S., and Shils, M.E., editors: Modern nutrition in health and disease, Philadelphia, 1980, Lea & Febiger.

158. Randle, P.J., and Smith, G.H.: Regulation of glucose uptake by muscle. I. The effect of insulin, anaerobosis and cell poisons on the uptake of glucose and release of potassium by isolated rat diaphragm, Biochem. J. **70:**409, 1958.
159. Raptis, S., et al.: Differences in insulin, growth hormone, and pancreatic enzyme secretion after intravenous and intraduodenal administration of mixed amino acids in man, N. Engl. J. Med. **288:**1199, 1973.
160. Rasmusen, H.: Calcium and cAmp as synarchic messengers, New York, 1981, John Wiley & Sons, Inc.
161. Reichlin, S.: Somatostatin, N. Engl. J. Med. **309:**1495, 1983.
162. Rizza, R.A., Mandarino, L.J., and Gerich, J.E.: Cortisol-induced insulin resistance in man: impaired suppression of glucose production and stimulation of glucose utilization due to a postreceptor defect of insulin action, J. Clin. Endocrinol. Metab. **54:**131, 1982.
163. Rizza, R.A., et al.: Adrenergic mechanisms for the effect of epinephrine on glucose production and clearance in man, J. Clin. Invest. **65:**682, 1980.
164. Romanosky, A.J., et al.: Increased muscle glucose uptake and lactate release after endotoxin administration, Am. J. Physiol. **239:**E311, 1980.
165. Ross, B.D., Hems, R., and Krebs, H.A.: The rate of gluconeogenesis from various precursors in the perfused rat liver, Biochem. J. **102:**942, 1967.
166. Ross, R.: The fibroblast and wound repair, Biol. Rev. **43:**51, 1968.
167. Roth, T., and Grunfeld, C.: Endocrine systems: mechanisms of disease, target cells, and receptors. In William, R.H., editor: Textbook of endocrinology, Philadelphia, 1981, W.B. Saunders Co.
168. Russell, J.A., Long, C.N.H., and Engel, F.L.: Biochemical studies of shock: peripheral tissues on the metabolism of protein and carbohydrate during hemorrhagic shock in the rat, J. Exp. Med. **79:**1, 1944.
169. Ryan, N.T.: Metabolic adaptations for energy production during trauma and sepsis, Surg. Clin. North Am. **56:**1073, 1976.
170. Schrier, R.W., Berl, W.T., and Anderson, R.J.: Osmotic and nonosmotic control of vasopressin release, Am. J. Physiol. **236:**F321, 1979.
171. Shafrir, E., and Steinberg, D.: The essential role of the adrenal cortex in the response of plasma free fatty acids, cholesterol, and phospholipids to epinephrine injection, J. Clin. Invest. **39:**310, 1960.
172. Shearer, J., et al.: Effect of starvation on the local and systemic metabolic effects of the λ-carrageenan wound, Am. J. Surg. **147:**456, 1984.
173. Shizgal, H.M., Milne, C.A., and Spainer, H.A.: The effect of nitrogen-sparing intravenously administered fluids on postoperative body composition, Surgery **86:**60, 1979.
174. Shizgal, H.M., et al.: The indirect measurement of total exchangeable potassium, Am. J. Physiol. **233:**F253, 1977.
175. Siegel, J.H., et al.: Physiological and metabolic correlations in human sepsis, Surgery **86:**163, 1979.
176. Smith, R., et al.: Initial effect of injury on ketone bodies and other blood metabolites, Lancet **1:**1, 1975.
177. Stein, T.P., et al.: Changes in protein synthesis after trauma: importance of nutrition, Am. J. Physiol. **233:**E348, 1977.
178. Stephens, R.V., and Randall, H.T.: Use of a concentrated, balanced, liquid elemental diet for nutritional management of catabolic states, Ann. Surg. **170:**642, 1969.
179. Stoner, H.B., et al.: The relationships between plasma substrates and hormones and the severity of injury in 277 recently injured patients, Clin. Sci. **56:**563, 1979.
180. Studley, H.O.: Percentage of weight loss, a basic indicator of surgical risk, JAMA **106:**458, 1936.
181. Sutherland, E.W.: Studies on the mechanism of hormone action, Science **177:**401, 1972.
182. Swerlick, R.A., Drucker, N.A., and McCoy, S.: Insulin effectiveness in hypovolemic dogs, J. Trauma **21:**1013, 1981.
183. Tarso, P.J., Spafford, M.S., and Blaw, M.: The metabolism of water and electrolytes in congestive heart failure, J. Lab. Clin. Med. **41:**280, 1953.
184. Talvo, P.J., et al.: Exchangeable potassium as a parameter of body composition, Metabolism **9:**456, 1960.
185. Turinsky, J.: Glucose metabolism in the region recovering from burn injury, Endocrinology **113:**1370, 1983.
186. Unger, R.H.: Diabetes and the alpha cell, Diabetes **25:**136, 1976.
187. Unger, R.H., and Orci, L.: Glucagon and the A cell: physiology and pathophysiology, N. Engl. J. Med. **304:**1518, 1981.
188. Unger, R.H., Dobbs, R.E., and Orci, L.: Insulin, glucagon, and somatostatin secretion in the regulation of metabolism, Annu. Rev. Physiol. **40:**307, 1978.
189. Valgcirsdottir, K., and Munro, H.N.: Protein and amino acid metabolism. In Fischer, J.E., editor: Surgical nutrition, Boston, 1983, Little, Brown & Co., Inc.
190. White, A., Handler, P., and Smith, E.L.: Principles of biochemistry, New York, 1973, McGraw-Hill Book Co.
191. Williamson, M.B., McCarthy, T.H., and Fromm, H.J.: Relation of protein nutrition to the healing of experimental wounds, Proc. Soc. Exp. Biol. Med. **77:**302, 1951.
192. Williamson, O.H., et al.: Muscle-protein catabolism after injury in man, as measured by urinary excretion of 3-methyl histidine, Clin. Sci. Mol. Med. **52:**527, 1977.
193. Wilmore, D.W., Mason, A.D., and Pruitt, B.A.: Insulin response to glucose in hypermetabolic burn patients, Ann. Surg. **183:**314, 1976.
194. Wilmore, D.W., et al.: Influence of the burn wound on local and systemic responses to injury, Ann. Surg. **186:**444, 1977.
195. Wilmore, D.W., et al.: Effect of injury and infection on visceral metabolism and circulation, Ann. Surg. **192:**491, 1980.
196. Wood, C.E., et al.: Hormonal and hemodynamic responses to 15 ml/kg hemorrhage in conscious dogs: responses correlate to body temperature, Proc. Soc. Exp. Biol. Med. **167:**15, 1981.
197. Woolfe, L.I., Groves, A.C., and Moore, J.P.: Arterial plasma amino acids in patients with serious postoperative infections and in patients with major fractures, Surgery **79:**283, 1976.
198. Yates, F.E., Marsh, D.J., and Maran, J.W.: The adrenal cortex. In Mountcastle, U.B., editor: Medical physiology, ed. 14, St. Louis, 1980, The C.V. Mosby Co.

2 *Peter J. Fabri*

Fluid and Electrolyte Physiology and Pathophysiology

The human body can be likened to a sac of electrolyte-rich fluids in which is suspended or dissolved a complex network of solids known collectively as "organs." The common medium of these fluids is water; the electrolytes are a mixture of primarily monovalent and divalent ions. The total volume of water, known as total body water, accounts for approximately 60% of total body mass. Substances are continually added to and excreted from this aqueous environment, and only through a system of homeostatic, protective mechanisms is the composition and distribution of this fluid-based system maintained. Disease, pharmaceuticals, and medical interventions all have the potential to disrupt the balance of this fluid medium and result in clinically evident fluid and electrolyte disturbances. To achieve the desired goal of preventing or treating such disturbances, the nature, composition, and interrelationships of these fluids and the homeostatic mechanisms that maintain them must be clearly understood.

MAINTENANCE OF THE INTERNAL MILIEU: TOTAL BODY WATER

Water is the universal solvent of the human body. The total volume of this substance is subdivided into discrete parts known as intracellular, extracellular, and transcellular water. These parts are separated by semipermeable membranes equipped with energy-consuming, work-producing pumps that are usually based on an ATP-ase enzyme system. These pumps are able to maintain electrochemical and concentration gradients across membranes that result in a marked difference in composition of the intracellular and extracellular spaces. Water, on the other hand, passively follows the laws of osmotic and ionic equilibrium. It traverses these membranes freely in order to maintain an equal number of solute molecules (osmolality) and ionic particles (tonicity) per unit volume on each side of such semipermeable membranes. This difference between the control of solute/ions and that of water results in marked differences in volume and electrolyte composition of the two spaces. The normal balance can be disturbed by changing the number of solute molecules on either side of the membrane (e.g., hypoalbuminemia, hyperglycemia) or by disrupting its enzyme-based pumps (e.g., shock, digitalis).

The extracellular space can be considered an open system in that the alimentary tract serves as a mode of entrance (and occasionally exit) of water and solute and the lungs, kidneys, and skin serve as excretory conduits. Entrance and excretion of water and solute are controlled by active systems that are under homeostatic (nervous or hormonal) control. Thus the composition of this open, extracellular system can be maintained within relatively tight limits.[35] Nonstandard entrance routes such as the administration of fluids intravenously bypass the normal entry control mechanisms and directly add water and solute to the extracellular space. In this circumstance, the *intrinsic* ability of the excretory systems to maintain osmotic and ionic stability becomes the limiting factor in maintaining ionic stability and composition of the extracellular space. Failure of these excretory control mechanisms, either by inability to conserve or increase loss, threatens the chemical stability of the extracellular fluids.

Table 2-1 **NORMAL DISTRIBUTION OF BODY WATER AS PERCENT OF BODY WEIGHT**

	Men (percent)	Women* (percent)
Total body water	60	55
Extracellular water	15	15
Intracellular water	45	40

*Values are less than equivalent for men because women have a relatively greater amount of adipose tissue.

The intracellular space, on the other hand, is a closed space. The only route of entrance and exit is across the semipermeable cellular membrane and its contained enzyme systems. Therefore the extracellular space can be thought of as the conduit and the buffer zone of the intracellular space. Only by transfer from or to the extracellular space can intracellular composition be changed. This complex system, richly furnished with active transport mechanisms and buffer zones, rigidly protects the stability of the body fluids and maintains constancy of the internal milieu. Two thirds of the total body water (usually about 60% of total body weight) is intracellular, and one third is extracellular (Table 2-1).

Extracellular Water

The extracellular space is composed of the vascular space (blood cells plus plasma) and the extravascular space (interstitial fluid and lymph). Cerebrospinal fluid is a specialized subspace of extracellular fluid. The vascular and extravascular spaces are in relative continuity, separated only by the rather permeable basement membranes of the blood vessel walls. When these vessels are intact, the formed, cellular elements of the blood remain contained in the intravascular space, whereas the aqueous, noncellular plasma undergoes continuous "filtration" through the pores of the vessel walls into the extravascular space. The extravascular space, however, is continuously "drained" by a system of lymphatic channels that return protein-rich extracellular fluid to the vascular space through the lymphatic ducts. This continuous-cycle system results in moment-to-moment renewing of the interstitial, pericellular space, bringing fresh nutrients from and carrying waste products to the vascular space, which is in direct continuity with normal routes of incretion and excretion.

The volume of intravascular fluid (blood) is determined by the oncotic effect of blood cells and large molecules such as albumin, as well as the rate of return of lymph. The volume of the extravascular fluid space depends on the balance between "filtration" of plasma and "drainage" of lymph. Plasma is continuously filtered across the vascular pores, particularly at the capillary level. The rate of filtration is governed by Starling's law, which takes into account net hydrostatic pressure, net oncotic pressure, and pore size (reflectance). Fluid shifts across the vascular membrane are controlled by the summed effect of hydrostatic and oncotic pressures. Hydrostatic pressure exists in both the vessel (mean capillary pressure) and the tissue (mean tissue pressure). The difference results in a vector force that typically acts to drive fluid into the extravascular space. Simultaneously, this vector is offset by an oncotic pressure vector, which is the net difference between plasma oncotic pressure and tissue oncotic pressure adjusted for a permeability factor (reflectance) that varies as the "size" of the pores changes. Ordinarily these vectors, on the average, tend to cancel, and there is no net flux of fluid across the membrane. However, alteration in any of the main forces can lead to marked derangement in fluid distribution and the development of clinical edema. The balanced forces in Starling's equation result in the passage of fluid across the vascular membrane into the interstitial (extravascular) space. Not yet considered is the "drainage" effect of the lymphatic system that tends to remove filtered plasma from the interstitium. Obstruction of lymphatics by complications such as tumor and infection can further impair fluid clearance and result in localized edema or lymphedema.

Osmolality and Tonicity

The composition of extracellular water is reflected by the concentration of solutes. Ordinarily, extracellular composition is maintained within tight boundaries by renal control mechanisms (e.g., antidiuretic hormone and aldosterone). These control mechanisms, however, tend to respond to the concentration of a given substance rather than to the total amount of all substances. Concentration represents the combined effect of the amount of a given substance (numerator) dissolved in a given amount of water (denominator). Thus abnormalities in concentration may represent changes in the amount of solute, amount of water, or both. The concentration of total solute of a given substance is most easily measured by plasma osmolality (mOsm/kg). This value indicates the ratio of solute to water in the plasma and in the extravascular space. Since extracellular water is in equilibrium with intracellular water, shifts of membrane permeable water result in maintenance of osmotic equality throughout total body water. In other words, accumulation of intracellular solute is compensated by a shift in water from the extracellular space to the intracellular space until osmolality is equal. The concentration of total ions, indicating ionic strength, is approximated by assessing the concentration of the principal extracellular cation, sodium. Changes in sodium concentration represent changes in tonicity, a term related to but not synonymous with osmolality. Typically, tonicity and osmolality change together, and hyperosmolality usually includes hypertonicity.[29] However, any substance that has a low molecular weight and a sizable concentration will contribute to serum osmolality. Thus conditions such as hyperglycemia, azotemia, hyperlactatemia, and accumulation of ethanol will raise osmolality without a change in tonicity.

The contributing factors to osmolality can be understood more clearly by using the osmolal gradient. This represents the difference between calculated (Osm[c]) and measured (Osm[m]) osmolality. Calculated osmolality is estimated by the formula:

$$\text{Osm(c)} = 1.86(\text{Na}) + \text{Glu}/18 + \text{BUN}/2.8$$

where Na is serum sodium concentration in mEq/L, Glu is serum glucose in mg/100 ml, and BUN is blood urea nitrogen in mg/100 ml. Ordinarily the osmolal gradient is less than 10 mOsm/kg where:

$$\text{osmolal gradient} = \text{Osm(m)} - \text{Osm(c)}$$

A gradient greater than 10 mOsm/kg represents the accumulation of some unmeasured, osmotically active substance such as lactate, ethanol, and mannitol. A common error in clinical practice is to assume that a change in measured osmolality represents an increase or decrease in water. As might be anticipated, osmolality is a concentration term and therefore can be disrupted by a change in amount of solute (e.g., azotemia) or amount of water (e.g., dehydration) or both (e.g., hyperosmolar coma). Since measured osmolality equals the ratio of solute molecules to water:

$$\text{Osm} = \text{Solute/water}$$

total body solute must equal osmolality multiplied by total body water, which can be estimated as 60% of total body weight, as shown by the formula:

$$\text{Solute} = \text{Osm} \times 0.6 \times \text{wt}$$

Estimation of this compound variable allows assessment of changes in total body solute, and, by inference, permits an appraisal of changes in body water.

Electrolyte Composition

As previously indicated, intracellular and extracellular fluids vary in concentration of electrolytes. The total body content of each electrolyte[16] has been estimated by direct assay[12] and by radionuclide exchange (exchangeable ion).[6,31,32] The distribution of these electrolytes is unequal and results in marked concentration differences throughout the body (Table 2-2).

Most of the difference between total body content (gravi-

Table 2-2 **ELECTROLYTE COMPOSITION**

	Na	K	Cl	Ca	Mg
Total body content (mEq/kg)	67	58	42	940	32
Exchangeable content (mEq/kg)	41	44	30	—	—
Intracellular concentration (mEq/L)	10	160	3	2	26
Plasma water concentration (mEq/L)	152	5	110	5	3
Serum concentration (mEq/L)	142	5	103	5	—

metric) and exchangeable content is accounted for as substance in bone. As a glance at Table 2-2 will confirm, and contrary to the impression gained from evaluating serum electrolytes, the content of total exchangeable sodium (Na) is roughly equal to the content of total exchangeable potassium (K). The sum of these ions (exchangeable Na + K) validly estimates total body cations that are roughly equally divided between intracellular and extracellular water. Accordingly, the serum sodium concentration (or conversely the intracellular potassium concentration) represents the ratio of total body cations to total body water, as shown below:

$$\text{Na (Serum)} = (\text{Na} + \text{K}) / (0.6 \times \text{wt})$$

By a process analogous to osmolality, cross-multiplying serum sodium concentration by an estimate of total body water yields total body exchangeable cations. An estimate, therefore, of total body water, total body solute, and total body cations allows serial assessment of fluid and electrolyte balance.

HOMEOSTATIC CONTROL MECHANISMS

General Concepts

The kidney is the cornerstone of the homeostatic mechanisms controlling fluid and electrolyte balance. Although it is true that fluid losses from the skin, lungs, and gastrointestinal tract may be impressive, the kidney is the only part of the system that is able to "control" its output. Accepting that fact, it is helpful to think of renal homeostasis as "throwing the baby out with the bath water, and catching the baby before it goes down the drain." In other words, glomerular filtration, the frontline initiator of excretion, is relatively nonspecific. It only limits excretion of substances that are associated with large proteins. Glomerular filtrate, therefore, is an ultrafiltrate of plasma. This ultrafiltrate passes through the proximal tubule where approximately 95% of most solute and most of the water are reabsorbed. In effect, control of absorption to this point is really a question of "what isn't reabsorbed." Final modification of urinary composition takes place in the distal tubule and collecting duct[27] where sodium is exchanged for hydrogen or potassium[23] and the remaining water either is or is not reabsorbed, depending on the status of antidiuretic hormone.[18]

Sodium and Water Homeostasis

Intracellular water is in equilibrium with extracellular water through osmotic and ionic neutrality. A small gradient is accounted for by anion proteins, which results in a concentration inequality referred to as the Gibbs-Donnan distribution. Extracellular water is controlled largely by plasma volume and serum sodium concentration.

Sodium and water conservation must be considered together since their control mechanisms are inseparable. Water deficits or excesses are compensated by changes in antidiuretic hormone (ADH) release (from the pituitary) and effect (renal collecting duct).[3] Changes in sodium homeostasis are accompanied by both ADH and mineralocorticoid responses. A decrease in plasma volume stimulates baroreceptors located in sites such as the right atrium and carotid body, as well as in the juxtaglomerular apparatus and macula densa of the kidney.[7] The baroreceptor response results in an increase in ADH release from the posterior pituitary and causes decreased loss of solute free water in the collecting duct of the kidney. (As the serum sodium concentration falls, ADH release will be inhibited, and further water conservation will be blunted.) The simultaneous effect of decreased glomerular filtration leads to decreased sodium delivery to the juxtaglomerular apparatus of the kidney. Renin release is triggered, which causes cleavage of angiotensinogen into the decapeptide angiotensin I. This latter substance is converted in the lung to the octapeptide angiotensin II by the angiotensin-converting enzyme. Angiotensin II is a potent vasoconstrictor substance that also directly stimulates aldosterone release from the zona glomerulosa of the adrenal cortex. The resultant increase in aldosterone increases sodium reabsorption in the distal tubule of the kidney in exchange for potassium and/or hydrogen ions.

As serum sodium concentration changes, release of ADH from the posterior pituitary is altered by osmoreceptors in the hypothalamus. Very small changes (2 mOsm) can predictably result in a measurable change in plasma ADH levels. Corresponding changes in thirst perception and the permeability of the collecting duct of the kidney to water also occur. In the case of hypernatremia, thirst increases, and maximum concentration of solute-free water occurs in the kidney. This can be corroborated by a high measured urine osmolality (usually >500 mOsm). During hyponatremia, ADH release is inhibited, the stimulus for water conservation in the collecting duct ceases, and solute-free water ("free water") is excreted, resulting in a hypotonic (<280 mOsm/kg) urine and a return of serum sodium to normal. In addition, the zona glomerulosa of the adrenal appears to be sensitive to changes in serum sodium concentration, resulting in feedback control of aldosterone release.

Potassium Homeostasis

Control of serum potassium levels is quite unlike sodium. Potassium is primarily an intracellular ion, with concentration manifold greater than plasma. Yet the extracellular concentration is extremely important in maintaining electrochemical gradients across cell membranes that facilitate depolarization of electrically active cells such as cardiac muscle and specialized conduction cells. Therefore control of extracellular potassium is important. Typically mammalian diets contain large amounts of potassium, such that conservation of potassium is not usually a problem unless losses are excessive (diuretics, diarrhea) or renal mechanisms are abnormal (hyperaldosteronism).

Potassium conservation and excretion tend to be the mirror image of sodium. Potassium, for example, stimulates the release of aldosterone from the adrenal.[4] While the majority of potassium reabsorption (like sodium) occurs in the proximal tubule, at the distal tubule potassium is excreted in response to the aldosterone stimulus. Sodium can be reabsorbed almost entirely within the nephron, whereas potassium conservation is less complete until profound body deficits occur. Distal tubular flow rate is also a major factor in potassium homeostasis. As flow rates increase, potassium excretion becomes inappropriately high. Although total body potassium distribution is affected by renal mechanisms, it is also subject to exchange mechanisms at the cell surface of all cells such that, as sodium (or hydrogen) is transported out, potassium reenters the intracellular fluid (probably insulin-dependent). Likewise, in severe acidosis or alkalosis, plasma potassium levels may change as a result of the fluxes of potassium that are consequent to the hydrogen ion shifts.

Acid/Base Conservation

With the exception of several specialized body fluids, the pH of body water is very closely guarded. Normal plasma pH (7.4 ± 0.05) generally is representative of the pH of total body water, although the pH of fluids such as cerebrospinal fluid and intracellular fluid may transiently diverge from that of plasma because of differing controlling factors and influences. For practical purposes, however, the pH of all compartments of body water can be assumed to be equal.

In order to appreciate the intricacies of acid/base balance, a solid understanding of the basic chemical concepts of acids, bases, and dissociation is essential. Acids are substances that have the capability of donating protons (hydrogen ions; hydronium ions). Bases, conversely, are substances that have the ability to accept protons during chemical reactions. Both acids and bases are ionic compounds that, when dissolved in water, have the ability to dissociate into cationic and anionic species. This dissociation is rarely complete, and the ratio of dissociated to nondissociated chemicals is determined by the dissociation constant. Acids, when dissociated, contribute hydrogen ions (H^+) and a corresponding anion (An^-) to the total ionic composition of the solution. Bases typically contribute a cation and a hydroxyl (OH^-) ion.

A typical acid (or base) dissociation can be described by the chemical reaction:

$$HAn = H^+ + An^-$$

The dissociation constant is determined by the ratio of products to reactants; therefore:

$$K = [H^+]\,[An^-]\,/\,[HAn]$$

where the brackets represent concentration in solution. Taking the logarithm of both sides of this equation results in a useful and familiar form of the dissociation equation:

$$\log K = \log H^+ + \log([An^-]\,/\,[HAn])$$
$$pK = pH - \log([An^-]\,/\,[HAn])$$
$$pH = pK + \log([An^-]\,/\,[HAn])$$

The dissociation constant (and consequently the pK) takes into account the simultaneous equilibrium of water.

In the human, many acid/base pairs (buffer pairs) exist in simultaneous equilibrium. This means that the ambient pH of the body determines the ratio of anion to dissociated acid for a number of acids present in the body. Although substances such as phosphoric acid, proteins, and amino acids are all present in abundance and could be used as estimates of acid/base status, the carbonic acid/bicarbonate buffer system is most commonly used for this purpose. The reason for using this buffer system is clear. The major homeostatic mechanisms of acid/base control are pulmonary (the excretion of carbon dioxide) and renal (the conservation of bicarbonate and excretion of hydrogen ions). Consequently, this buffer pair reflects the efficacy of the homeostatic mechanisms that are operative in compensating for changes in acid or base gain or loss. In addition, bicarbonate and carbon dioxide (PCO_2) are easily measured in plasma.

The general dissociation equation, when applied to the bicarbonate/carbonic acid buffer system, is known as the Henderson-Hasselbalch equation:

$$pH = 6.1 + \log([HCO_3]\,/\,[H_2CO_3])$$

where $[HCO_3-]$ is the concentration of bicarbonate and $[H_2CO_3]$ is the concentration of carbonic acid. Since the concentration of carbonic acid is determined by the partial pressure of carbon dioxide and the solubility of carbon dioxide in water is 0.03:

$$pH = 6.1 + \log([HCO_3]\,/\,0.03\,PCO_2)$$

and

$$[H^+] = 24\,(PCO_2\,/\,[HCO_3])$$

Current technology allows the direct measurement of pH and PCO_2 in arterial (or venous) blood, enabling the estimation of bicarbonate concentration by the above equation. Alternatively, measurement of bicarbonate concentration and pH would enable calculation of PCO_2.

Other electrolytes enter the body pool only by ingestion (or injection), but acids (and bases) are rarely present in the diet. Acid is a product of metabolism and is added to total body water as a function of the rate of metabolism and the fractional use of acid-producing metabolites (Table 2-3).

In general, net acid production is approximately 1 mEq/kg/day (2 to 3 mEq/kg/day in infants) and is primarily caused by the production of sulfuric acid from metabolism of thiols; phosphoric acid from metabolism of organic phosphates; and other organic acids from the metabolism of proteins, carbohydrates, and fats. Any addition of base (e.g., antacids) or compounds that generate base (e.g., citrate, lactate) will tend to offset the daily endogenous acid load.

To maintain acid/base equilibrium, the body must ex-

Table 2-3 **PHYSIOLOGIC FACTORS AFFECTING PLASMA ACIDITY**

Through Plasma Bicarbonate Changes	Through Plasma P_{CO_2}
Rate of hydrogen ion input	Rate of carbon dioxide production
Rate of hydrogen ion or bicarbonate loss (Gastrointestinal)	Rate of alveolar ventilation
Availability of buffers	
Bicarbonate space of distribution	
Rate of net renal acid excretion	

crete a quantity of acid equal to endogenous production (plus any exogenous acid and minus any exogenous base). This is accomplished primarily by renal excretion of fixed acid in the form of phosphates and ammonia. Ammonia is produced by metabolism of glutamine in the kidney and excreted into the renal tubular lumen. Simultaneously, monohydrogen phosphate is filtered at the glomerulus. Hydrogen ions, filtered or secreted, are trapped by the buffering capability of these two proton acceptors and excreted. In addition, through a carbonic anhydrase-dependent system, the tubular epithelial cell is capable of generating a hydrogen and a bicarbonate ion from carbonic acid (dissolved carbon dioxide) and reabsorbing the bicarbonate while the hydrogen ion is excreted. This regenerates the bicarbonate pool and facilitates acid/base stability. If the bicarbonate pool becomes excessive, renal excretion of bicarbonate is increased by a complex mechanism dependent on the decreased hydrogen ion in the tubular fluid. In effect, the kidney is able to directly influence acid excretion by three mechanisms: excretion of phosphate (affected by glomerular filtration and parathyroid hormone), synthesis of ammonia, and control of the directional flow of bicarbonate.

The last of the three mechanisms just enumerated requires further comment. Because of the ready availability of carbon dioxide and water (and consequently carbonic acid), the kidney, through carbonic anhydrase, can control the abundance of hydrogen ions and bicarbonate. By directing the excretion of hydrogen ions into the tubular lumen and the return of bicarbonate to plasma, the kidney has a great capacity to excrete acid and control base. Only when the renal mechanisms responsible for reabsorption of base or excretion of acid are compromised does the renal contribution to acid/base balance become limited. In normal circumstances, the rate at which the kidney returns bicarbonate to the body is equivalent to the rate of sodium/hydrogen exchange in the distal tubule. Although the proximal tubule is quantitatively the most important site of bicarbonate reabsorption in the kidney, with a small contribution from the loop of Henle, the distal segment is capable of "fine tuning" the acid/base excretory balance.

As indicated, carbon dioxide (and its hydrated form, carbonic acid) plays a central role in maintenance of acid/base homeostasis. The major parameter of carbon dioxide concentration in the blood is its partial gas pressure (P_{CO_2}). The P_{CO_2} of arterial blood (venous blood has increased P_{CO_2} caused by addition of carbon dioxide from tissue metabolism) is determined by the balance between the amount of alveolar (effective) ventilation ($\dot{V}_A$) in the lung and the amount of carbon dioxide produced per minute (V_{CO_2}). Further stated, the arterial P_{CO_2} is actually proportional to the ratio of carbon dioxide production to alveolar ventilation. Normal metabolism consumes oxygen and a fuel substrate (carbohydrate, protein, fat), with the subsequent production of carbon dioxide to be excreted by ventilation. The amount of carbon dioxide produced per volume of oxygen consumed is determined by the "mix" of fuel and is known as the *respiratory quotient* (RQ). At a higher respiratory quotient (e.g., during pure carbohydrate metabolism when 1 mol of carbon dioxide is produced for each mole of oxygen consumed [RQ = 1]), even though metabolic rate is constant, more carbon dioxide is produced than during metabolism of pure fat (RQ = 0.7). Both an increase in metabolic rate and an increase in respiratory quotient will increase carbon dioxide production. Total minute ventilation is the sum of alveolar ventilation (effective breathing) and dead space ventilation (ineffective, wasted breathing). The product of the alveolar ventilation and respiratory rate is the minute alveolar ventilation and is the portion of breathing that is effective in eliminating carbon dioxide and absorbing oxygen. Conversely, dead space ventilation is air that must be moved into and out of the lungs but does not contribute to gas exchange. Dead space ventilation can be anatomic (trachea, large bronchi, cysts) or physiologic. Physiologic dead space commonly increases during diseases involving the lung and leads to a smaller percentage of each breath that contributes to gas exchange. The amount of alveolar ventilation determines the adequacy of carbon dioxide elimination. When alveolar ventilation increases without an increase in carbon dioxide production, P_{CO_2} falls, resulting in decreased H_2CO_3 and respiratory alkalosis. Alternatively, a decrease in alveolar ventilation relative to carbon dioxide production causes increased P_{CO_2} with resulting increased H_2CO_3 and respiratory acidosis.

PATHOPHYSIOLOGY AND TREATMENT OF SPECIFIC ELECTROLYTE AND ACID/BASE ABNORMALITIES

In order to understand abnormalities of electrolyte homeostasis, some attention must be given to normal daily requirements (Table 2-4). Although it is true that a state of electrolyte balance requires that intake is equal to losses (and losses can be minimized), realistically there will be daily excretion of electrolytes of a fairly predictable magnitude, allowing a range of estimated daily needs. Under normal conditions, losses are primarily through urinary excretion and those secondary to evaporation from the skin and water losses through the lungs. These latter two sources are referred to as insensible losses because they are not visible or readily measurable and amount to 500 to 800 ml of water daily with almost negligible amounts of sodium and chloride. Urine is the major sensible loss (one that is viable and measurable) and averages between 1200 and 1500 ml of water daily with 10 to 30 mEq of sodium and 20 to 60 mEq of potassium. Another sensible loss is water loss through the feces, which is usually quite mini-

Table 2-4 **ADULT DAILY REQUIREMENTS**

	Normal	Minimal
Water (total)	1500 ml/m^2	(870 ml/m^2)
Water (insensible)	500 ml/m^2	—
Sodium	0.7 - 3.6 mEq/kg	(0.3 mEq/kg)
Potassium	0.7 - 2.1 mEq/kg	(0.3 - 0.5 mEq/kg)
Chloride	0.7 - 3.6 mEq/kg	(0.3 mEq/kg)
Calcium	0.4 - 1.1 mEq/kg	(0.2 mEq/kg)
Magnesium	0.3 - 0.7 mEq/kg	(0.2 - 0.4 mEq/kg)

Modified from Goodenough, R.D., and Burke, J.F.: Fluid, electrolyte, and acid-base homeostasis in surgery. In Burke, J.F.: Surgical physiology, Philadelphia, 1983, W.B. Saunders Co.

mal. Losses greater than those routinely encountered (e.g., diarrhea) will result in corresponding increases in requirements; decreases in normal excretion rates (e.g., renal failure) will necessitate a reduction in intake.

Abnormalities of Water Balance

Disturbances in the amount of distribution of total body water are common in clinical practice. Since water distributes throughout the body, restricted in its movement only by osmotic and ionic barriers, abnormalities in amount with maintenance of normal electrolyte concentrations are frequent. An isotonic increase in total body water results in edema, whereas an isotonic decrease produces clinical dehydration. Since electrolyte conservatory mechanisms are extremely efficient, deviation from isotonicity is uncommon except at the extremes of age when compensatory mechanisms are less adequate or access to water or salt is restricted. In infants and elderly, therefore, hypertonic (sodium >145) and hypotonic (sodium <135 mEq/L) abnormalities are more commonly found and require attention to both the volume abnormality and the concentration problem. It is important, however, to realize that isotonic abnormalities in total body water are more prevalent in adults than other fluid derangements only because compensatory mechanisms maintain the concentration of important solutes. In circumstances in which a coexistent problem compromises these compensatory mechanisms (e.g., renal disease, inappropriate ADH secretion, diuretic use, adrenal insufficiency) a superimposed fluid loss or gain may very well not be isotonic.

Dehydration is an absolute decrease in total body water and usually represents a balanced loss between intracellular and extracellular volume. Dehydration can be assessed on clinical grounds alone, and in fact there is no readily available test that identifies it in the absence of a coexistent abnormality of concentration. Blood urea nitrogen and consequently osmolality are frequently elevated to a variable degree, however, and may be supportive of the diagnosis when the creatinine concentration is normal and the blood urea nitrogen/creatinine ratio >20. Up to 5% decrease in total body water can escape clinical detection without appropriate suspicion by history. Thirst is usually present, however, and is an accurate sign of water deficit. Losses greater than 5% usually lead to conditions such as sunken eyes, loss of skin turgor with tenting of presternal skin, and dry mucous membranes. Greater than 10% dehydration will commonly demonstrate hemodynamic changes with tachycardia and postural hypotension.

Treatment of dehydration requires an understanding of the composition of the fluid deficits. Isotonic dehydration reflects a loss of all fluid compartments (and their contained electrolytes) and is corrected by infusing intravenously a balanced salt solution such as Ringer's lactate solution (Table 2-5). Concomitant abnormalities in concentration or tonicity are best assessed by the serum sodium concentration; such electrolyte abnormalities should be treated simultaneously with management of the volume deficit. For example, in hypernatremic states water alone as 5% dextrose in water is used for replacement (Table 2-5). The appropriate intravenous fluid should be administered to correct one half of the estimated abnormality over 24 hours. This approach is used since most deficits develop over a period of days or weeks and the patient has usually adjusted to them. Rapid replacement of losses may actually impose a greater risk than the deficit itself.

Edema can be related to an underlying disease (cardiac, renal, hepatic) or, as is more common in modern practice, abundant or excessive intravenous fluid administration. Excesses in extracellular fluid typically are susceptible to gravity and hence are most pronounced in dependent areas. Conditions such as pretibial and ankle edemas are common in the upright patient. Presacral edema or pitting of the skin overlying the iliac spine is more likely in the recumbent patient.

Water intoxication represents a specific abnormality of water balance. Ordinarily, large amounts of ingested or administered water can be excreted quantitatively without resultant volume excess or ionic dilution. Very marked amounts, however, particularly in a setting of compromised homeostatic mechanisms, can result in edema, hyponatremia, and dilution of other electrolytes as well. (For a further discussion, refer to section on hyponatremia.)

Treatment of fluid excess requires an understanding of cause and an assessment of the integrity of homeostatic mechanisms, particularly renal, hepatic, and CNS function. In the setting of normal compensation, simple fluid restriction or decreased administration is likely to be effective. When simultaneous abnormalities in renal, hepatic, adrenal, or cardiac physiology exist, careful attention to intake and output (an "accountant" approach) is indicated. Only by specific accounting of all volumes, concentrations, and amounts can aggravation or creation of abnormalities be prevented.

Abnormalities of Sodium

Since sodium is the major cation of the fluid most commonly analyzed in the laboratory (serum or plasma), it is surprising that abnormalities in sodium concentration are not more frequent. Although hypernatremia and hyponatremia are seen, they are rigorously prevented by compensatory mechanisms at the renal level and under the control of antidiuretic hormone (ADH). In fact, very small changes in sodium concentration (and subsequently osmolality) result in a measurable change in ADH release in the

Table 2-5 **COMPOSITION OF COMMON SOLUTIONS USED FOR INTRAVENOUS THERAPY**

Solutions	Glucose (g/L)	Na (mEq/L)	Cl (mEq/L)	HCO_3 (mEq/L)	K (mEq/L)	Ca (mEq/L)
5% Dextrose and water	50	—	—	—	—	—
0.9% Sodium chloride (normal saline)	—	154	154	—	—	—
0.45% Sodium chloride (half-normal saline)	—	77	77	—	—	—
3% Sodium chloride (hypertonic saline)	—	513	513	—	—	—
Lactated Ringer's solution	—	130	109	28*	4	2.7

*Exists in solution as lactate and is ultimately metabolized to bicarbonate (HCO_3).

same direction. When renal concentrating mechanisms are defective[22] (e.g., washout of renal medullary concentration gradient as with diuretics, partial tubular dysfunction from incipient or resolving acute tubular necrosis, or massive sodium loss in interstitial nephritis), abnormalities in serum sodium are more common.

Hyponatremia

Virtually all acute, stressful situations (e.g., infection, anesthesia, and surgery) are accompanied by release of ADH and conservation of free water.[20] This homeostatic mechanism is very effective in preserving extracellular volume when combined with sodium conservation, which depends on a decrease in delivered sodium or perfusion pressure at the juxtaglomerular apparatus.[7] Consequently, hyponatremia in adult patients at the time of admission is distinctly uncommon. However, once a patient has received intravenous administration of hypotonic fluids (e.g., 0.45% saline), the inability to excrete the ''free'' water in the face of an obligatory ADH release frequently results in a decrease in serum sodium to some degree.

When hyponatremia is present, spurious causes must be excluded. This is accomplished most simply by evaluating the serum osmolality. Since osmolality measures the amount of solute per *mass* of water instead of volume, it is independent of the amount of water in a volume of serum. Normally, serum is 94% water. Increases in protein or lipid concentrations can, however, alter the amount of water and lead to an analytic error in sodium determination. Osmolality is not so affected. Consequently, hyponatremia with normal osmolality would raise the suspicion of paraproteinemia (e.g., multiple myeloma, macroglobulinemia) or hyperlipidemia.

Alternatively, an increase in an extracellular solute such as glucose (or mannitol) causes a shift in water from the intracellular to extracellular space to conserve osmotic equality. This results in a subsequent ''dilution'' of sodium but a maintained osmolality because of the presence of another osmotically active substance, mainly glucose. Confirmation of hyperglycemia in the setting of normal osmolality will justify a fall in sodium of approximately 1.6 mEq/L for each 100 mg/100 ml rise in blood sugar above normal.

When true hyponatremia does occur (low sodium plus low osmolality), evaluating how the kidney is behaving allows a rational interpretation of the probable pathophysiology. A careful assessment of overall fluid and electrolyte status (weight change, input and output summaries. presence or absence of edema) is essential.[33] Characterizing the patient as ahead or behind in volume allows appropriate interpretation of the renal response, which is best ascertained by measuring the urinary osmolality and sodium concentration.

During active sodium conservation, urinary sodium is typically low (<5 mEq/L). This indicates either that there is a true deficit in sodium or that the kidney ''thinks'' there is one. The latter occurs when circulating substances (e.g., aldosterone) are inappropriately present in edematous states such as cirrhosis and chronic congestive heart failure. In each of these settings, however, the patient is both edematous and has ascites. In the absence of either of these findings, true sodium depletion is probably present. Sodium administration should be guided by an estimate of the deficit, which must be considered independently of (added to) volume deficits that are isotonic (Na = 140 mEq/L). The sodium deficit approximates 0.6 mEq/kg per milliequivalent fall in serum sodium. Unless neurologic symptoms ensue, which would mandate urgent treatment, the sodium replacement should take 24 to 48 hours. After one half of the deficit has been replaced, serum electrolyte levels should be rechecked.

When urinary sodium is increased (>20 mEq/L), simple sodium depletion can be excluded. Sodium conservation either will not or cannot take place. This occurs in the setting of abnormal ADH release, adrenal insufficiency, recent use of diuretics, or intrinsic renal tubular dysfunction as in renal failure or interstitial nephritis. This can be clarified by measuring urinary osmolality.

Since the normal response to hyponatremia and hypoosmolality is excretion of solute-free water (and dilute urine), the finding of a urine osmolality above that of serum indicates an abnormal ADH response.[5,20] This implies a continued release of ADH in spite of a hypoosmolar state. If this is present at the time of admission or in the absence of intravenous fluids, it implies a CNS abnormality (e.g., head trauma, intracranial tumor) or an ectopic site of production (e.g., bronchogenic carcinoma). In the patient receiving hypotonic fluids, this finding more commonly reflects the release of ADH associated with a central ''acute phase response'' to stress or illness. In either event, fluid balance will be ''ahead'' as is the total amount of sodium in the body. The hyponatremia means that water is ''more ahead'' than sodium. This paradoxic increased sodium in the face of decreased serum sodium concentration results in a high urinary sodium excretion (>20 mEq/L) and a high salt excretion fraction (>5%).[9]

The finding of isosthenuria (urine osmolality equals serum osmolality) implies intrinsic renal dysfunction or pharmacologic dysfunction from diuretics. The finding of low urine osmolality and high urine sodium, however, suggests that ADH release is appropriately terminated but that sodium is not being conserved. This situation is seen in mineralocorticoid insufficiency.

Laboratory evaluation of the renal response to hyponatremia can be enlightening but does not replace clinical assessment. Since hyponatremia means either a decrease in sodium or an increase in water, appropriate interpretation of readily available data should allow discrimination. A decrease in sodium requires the presence of a route of loss and usually is associated with weight loss. Alternatively, an increase in water should be manifested by a gain in weight and excess fluid intake over output.

In the patient who is not receiving intravenous fluids, a serum sodium below 135 mEq/L constitutes hyponatremia and deserves investigation. In the patient who is receiving hypotonic fluids, however, mild hyponatremia is common enough to be almost expected. Although it is not normal, mild hyponatremia down to 130 mEq/L can be ignored. A sodium of 125 to 130 mEq/L justifies vigorous diagnostic efforts to identify the cause. A serum sodium level of 120 to 125 mEq/L necessitates vigorous institution of appropriate therapy. A sodium of <120 mEq/L is a medical emergency and frequently requires careful administration of hypertonic saline for correction. It is not the low sodium per se that is detrimental, but rather the increase in the intracellular fluid compartment that accompanies this circumstance. This intracellular volume increase is especially detrimental to brain cells since the brain is contained within a fixed space with little or no room for expansion. When brain cells swell, an increase in intracranial pressure ultimately develops and presents clinically by a variety of manifestations, including apathy, confusion, weakness, nausea, and occasionally vomiting. If this water intoxication is not corrected, it will ultimately lead to convulsions, stupor, and possibly even death.

Hypernatremia

The body rigorously defends itself against hyperosmolality. Even a small rise results in increased ADH release and subsequent free water retention by the kidney, unless, of course, ADH release cannot occur (diabetes insipidus), ADH is ineffective (nephrogenic diabetes insipidus), or the patient is prevented from access to water (infants, geriatric patients, unconscious or restrained patients). A simple review of the clinical situation will often identify the cause. Since hypernatremia implies either an increase in sodium or a decrease in water, both must be considered. An increase in sodium can result from vigorous administration of normal saline or sodium bicarbonate. A decrease in water can occur by renal or extrarenal mechanisms. Nonrenal causes should be clinically apparent and include such symptoms as diarrhea and excessive sweating. In addition to the forms of diabetes insipidus (pituitary dysfunction or nephrogenic), renal sources must include osmotic diuresis with obligatory "free" water loss. In all cases, treatment is simple. Administration of hypotonic solutions will restore sodium concentration; and, when sodium excess is a component, judicious diuretic use will hasten sodium excretion.

Care in treating hypernatremia must be exercised, however, since a rapid change in sodium concentration is of greater clinical importance than the actual sodium concentration. Too rapid correction of sodium abnormalities can result in dramatic CNS effects, including seizures. Accordingly, treatment should be planned to correct one half of the estimated deficit over 24 hours. In the case of hypernatremia, this usually translates into the administration of 2 ml of free water per kg over 24 hours for each milliequivalent of planned decrease in serum sodium concentration.

In the patient with head injury or recent neurosurgical intervention with accompanying diabetes insipidus, unless actual hypophysectomy has been performed, early administration of vasopressin should be discouraged. Careful replacement of losses will maintain fluid and electrolyte balance until the usually transient abnormality resolves. Accordingly, hypernatremia should be avoidable. If permanent diabetes insipidus is anticipated, however, administration of vasopressin or its synthetic analog, desmopressin acetate (DDAVP), should be instituted. Serious complications of diabetes insipidus (or inappropriate ADH secretion) are not a function of difficulty in treatment, but rather failure of recognition. Anticipation of such problems will greatly simplify their subsequent management.

Abnormalities of Potassium

Since mammals usually ingest large amounts of potassium, it is not surprising that most abnormalities in potassium balance are the result not of intake but of excretion. Further, the very narrow range of normal potassium concentration in plasma and the relatively massive adjacent intracellular pool[6] (with exchange influenced by variables such as pH and drugs) makes control of serum potassium both important and tenuous. This importance is underscored by the critical nature of severe potassium abnormalities on the cardiac, neural, and muscular systems and evidenced by the diligent monitoring of potassium concentrations that occurs in operating suites and intensive care units. An understanding of the common circumstances leading to potassium abnormalities will facilitate maintenance of normal homeostasis and simplify treatment of abnormalities.[26]

Hyperkalemia

Since the kidney is the major site of potassium excretion, compromised renal function is almost always a component of hyperkalemia.[14,38] Although increased potassium levels can occur from either excess intake or decreased excretion, the former is quite rare and is usually iatrogenic and occurs in the setting of administering massive intravenous doses of potassium (or potassium-containing drugs such as penicillin) or giving potassium to a patient receiving a drug that inhibits potassium excretion (spironolactone, triamterene). Abnormalities of excretion are common and can be caused by intrinsic abnormalities of renal function (acute, oliguric renal failure), disturbances in hormonal control of potassium exchange (hypoaldosteronism, adrenal insufficiency), or alterations in the potassium exchange mechanism per se (drugs, acidosis). Occasionally serum potassium factitiously is elevated (compared to plasma potassium) because of release of K^+ from platelets in thrombocytosis.[19]

Hyperkalemia produces predictable clinical consequences that affect neuromuscular function (weakness, irritability) and cardiac conduction (peaking of T waves, prolongation of PR and QT intervals, widening of QRS complexes, and heart block). Monitoring of the electrocardiogram provides a simple, noninvasive method of assessing change in the hyperkalemic or potentially hyperkalemic patient. Predictable changes, beginning with T-wave peaking, are the harbingers of subsequent complications, which are evidenced by alterations in the shape and duration of the major electrocardiogram complexes.

Since hyperkalemia poses a life-threatening problem, urgent and definitive correction is imperative. Transient decrease in serum potassium can be accomplished by translocating potassium back into cells with glucose and insulin, and the membrane effects of hyperkalemia can be offset by the administration of calcium. In the rare patient with reasonable renal function, potassium diuresis can be induced by use of loop-active diuretics. More commonly, potassium is removed from the body by the use of potassium-exchanging resins (sodium polystyrene sulfonate [Kayexalate]) that can be given by mouth or rectum and predictably lower potassium. This is accomplished, however, through exchange with sodium and may alter fluid and sodium balance. Institution of peritoneal or hemodialysis is clearly the most effective, long-term approach to potassium control in the patient with renal compromise. It is important to remember, however, that continued administration of hypertonic glucose, as in parenteral nutrition support, will result in a predictable and sustained fall in serum potassium as the egress of potassium associated with catabolism is prevented.

Hypokalemia

Hypokalemia is a common electrolyte abnormality in both hospitalized and ambulatory patients.[4,21] Although it may be precipitated by an underlying disease (mineralocorticoid excess as in Cushing's syndrome, potassium loss from colonic villous adenoma, potassium wasting in renal disease) or by decreased potassium intake (low-potassium diet), most hypokalemia is iatrogenic in that it is induced pharmacologically by agents having potassium wasting as a side effect.[25] Most notable are the diuretic agents currently used in the management of hypertension and fluid overload. The loop-acting agents in particular are associated with a substantial potassium loss in the urine. Other classes of drugs, however, also induce hypokalemia.[37,39] Recent increased use of amphotericin B in the treatment of immune-compromised patients has uncovered a profound and difficult-to-manage hypokalemia.[28] Use of newer synthetic penicillins in ultrahigh concentration is also associated with increased renal potassium loss and subsequent hypokalemia.

Hypokalemia may manifest itself in various ways (e.g., muscle weakness, paralysis). More frequently, however, hypokalemia produces myocardial irritability and subsequent arrhythmias such as frequent premature contractions, sustained tachycardias, and potentiation of digitalis toxicity. Although these complications are more feared than common, they are serious complications and justify both respect and careful monitoring. Treatment is simple. Administration of potassium as the chloride salt will correct the usual associated chloride-dependent alkalosis, decrease renal potassium loss, and correct the hypokalemia. However, the degree of hypokalemia is very poorly correlated to the magnitude of potassium deficit. Therefore strict guidelines for replacement are dangerous. Since the hazards of hypokalemia appear to be virtually eliminated by institution of treatment rather than total correction, the identification of the abnormality and institution of treatment are more important than the rapidity of treatment. Frequently, discontinuation of the offending drug or control of the underlying disease will be necessary for long-term potassium control.

Abnormalities of Chloride

Since chloride is the most abundant anion in plasma, it is not surprising that its range of variation is large and its mechanism of variation somewhat passive. The high concentration of chloride in gastric juice accounts for the hypochloremia that accompanies the metabolic alkalosis of conditions such as gastric outlet obstruction, repetitive vomiting, and pyloric stenosis. Chloride is absorbed in large quantities from the gut, and its level is controlled by urinary excretion. Most reabsorption of chloride occurs in the proximal tubule of the kidney in association with sodium absorption. A considerable component is also actively reabsorbed in Henle's limb.[36] Alterations in proximal tubule absorption (osmotic diuretics) or Henle's limb (loop-active diuretics) will lead to hypochloremia and metabolic alkalosis. In addition, in the presence of "hormone-dependent" (e.g., aldosterone) alkalosis, the fraction of chloride that is reabsorbed is decreased. This interaction of chloride and bicarbonate is important in the evaluation of the patient with metabolic alkalosis.

Chloride is present in abundance in gastrointestinal secretions. Substantial chloride loss can result from gastrointestinal fluid losses from the upper tract (e.g., gastric outlet obstruction) or lower tract (e.g., diarrhea). Assessment of the chloride deficit provides complementary information in the evaluation of volume depletion secondary to gastrointestinal losses.

Isolated Acid/Base Abnormalities

The availability of routine measurement of "arterial blood gases" has resulted in a much clearer understanding of the nature and treatment of acid/base disturbances in clinical practice. On the basis of the normal physiologic determinants previously described and the pathophysiologic mechanisms that will be enumerated, acid/base disturbances can be classified into acidosis or alkalosis; each of these categories can be further subdivided into metabolic and respiratory, as well as combined metabolic/respiratory. Tables, nomograms, and algorithms have been developed for the assessment of the excess or deficit of acid (or base) to assist the clinician in management. Unfortunately, all of these aids are of only limited practical value because of the concurrent and efficient efforts of the compensatory mechanisms of the body to correct the acid/base disturbance. In other words, the onset of a disturbance in pH (by change in either HCO_3 or PCO_2) results in very rapid initiation of respiratory and metabolic compensatory mechanisms to partially correct the pH. It is essential in planning treatment of acid/base disturbances to keep this compensation in mind, lest overaggressive management results in new, iatrogenic acid/base disturbances in the opposite direction.

Acidosis

As described previously, acidosis can occur by the absolute gain in acid or loss of base from the body. Since the buffering system of the body is "open" in the sense that the CO_2/HCO_3 system uses both respiratory and renal control systems, all but the most acute form of acidosis will be combined with compensatory adjustments. Consequently all respiratory disturbances will have a metabolic compensatory component, and metabolic imbalance will stimulate respiratory compensation. Frequently, the pH is remarkably well corrected, and only a careful review of the historical facts associated with the illness will allow a clear analysis of the inciting cause. Occasionally, the cause is so elusive that only disturbing the system with exogenous alkali and observing the respiratory response (or lack thereof) will determine the primary problem.

Respiratory Acidosis. Pure respiratory acidosis is the simplest of the acid/base disturbances conceptually because it results from a decrease in effective alveolar ventilation (relative to carbon dioxide production). Normal carbon dioxide production from metabolic processes is approximately 450 L/day (20,000 mmol). Whenever carbon dioxide elimination lags behind production, respiratory acidosis ensues. The consequent laboratory abnormalities include a decrease in pH and an increase in PCO_2. It is important to look at the pH first since compensatory hypercapnea in the setting of profound metabolic alkalosis is not uncommon, particularly in patients receiving mechanical ventilation by an intermittent (intermittent mandatory ventilation, intermittent demand ventilation) modality. Once respiratory acidosis is identified, a differential consideration of causes must include central respiratory depression (e.g., narcotics, intrinsic CNS disease), mechanical causes of decreased ventilation and/or increased dead space (e.g., tension pneumothorax, hemothorax, massive pleural effusions), or pathophysiologic causes of increased carbon dioxide production. The common causes of acute or chronic respiratory acidosis are summarized as follows:

- Airway obstruction
- Respiratory center depression
- Neuromuscular defects
- Restrictive lung diseases
- Smoke inhalation
- Inadequate mechanical ventilation

Appropriate treatment logically follows an identification of the underlying mechanism and may include ventilatory assistance to enhance alveolar ventilation to eliminate the retained carbon dioxide and thereby correct the acidic pH.

Metabolic Acidosis. In marked contradistinction to respiratory acidosis, metabolic acidosis can result from a variety of causes that include gain of metabolic acids above excretion rates and loss of bicarbonate greater than its rate of regeneration.[1,2,8,18] Again, clinical evaluation and elucidation of the underlying mechanism greatly simplifies the task of evaluating the data. Also, it is important to avoid jumping to a conclusion of acidosis on the basis of only a decrease in the bicarbonate concentration of the serum since this finding may also represent metabolic compensation for a respiratory alkalosis.

As is true with all biologic systems, electrical neutrality is maintained in all fluid compartments throughout the body by balancing the total number of cations with the total number of anions. In the extracellular compartment under normal conditions, the concentration of the cation sodium roughly equals the sum of the concentrations of the anions, chloride, and bicarbonate, except for a small anion gap of 8 ± 2 mEq/L. An increase in this gap can give an important clue concerning the cause of the acidosis. Thus it is helpful to subdivide metabolic acidosis into those categories that manifest an increase in unmeasured anions *(anion gap)* and those that do not and that subsequently have a normal anion gap and absolute or relative hyperchloremia. As a generality, metabolic acidosis associated with the accumulation of organic acid will have an associated anion gap, whereas that caused by a loss of bicarbonate will have a normal anion gap. The distinction is important. Although both causes may require replacement of bicarbonate to correct the acidosis, the former group will require correction of an associated metabolic abnormality, and the latter will require attention to the site of bicarbonate loss (e.g., fistula).

Anion Gap Acidosis. Any metabolic acidosis that is caused by the accumulation of organic (and therefore not measured by routine electrolytes) acid will have a calculated anion gap (uremia, diabetic ketoacidosis, lactic acidosis, and drug ingestion). In some circumstances, e.g., diabetic ketoacidosis, combined mechanisms are operative, and the component caused by ketoacids is proportional to the anion gap. The presence of an acidosis with an anion gap >14 mEq/L implies either an ingestion or an endogenous metabolic abnormality. Of the four commonly ingested substances (methanol, ethylene glycol, ethanol, and isopropanol), only methanol (formic acid) and ethylene glycol (oxalic acid) produce a metabolic acidosis. Ethylene glycol produces oxaluria, whereas methanol ingestion usually produces rapid retinal blindness. Acetylsalicylic acid (aspirin) and paraldehyde can also produce metabolic acidosis if ingested in large amounts.

Endogenous production of organic acid in excess of excretory capacity is seen in uremia, diabetic ketoacidosis, and lactic acidosis. (In addition, some inborn errors of metabolism can produce acidosis in neonates.) Each is usually identifiable by the company it keeps: acidosis caused by renal failure is associated with the clinical and metabolic abnormalities of uremia; diabetic ketoacidosis is usually seen in known diabetics and is associated with hyperglycemia, dehydration, and ketosis in urine and serum[11]; lactic acidosis can be caused by a variety of clinical states but usually represents hypoperfusion, sepsis, postictal or acute alcohol intoxication.[34] Lactic acidosis is associated with an increase in lactate in the blood (>4 mEq/L) and an altered ratio of lactate to pyruvate (>30:1) and other oxidation-reduction pairs (e.g., acetoacetate/betahydroxybutyrate,

NAD/NADH). It is important to recognize, in addition, that lactic acid may represent a component of the metabolic acidosis caused by diabetic ketoacidosis, methanol poisoning, and salicylate intoxication.

Treatment of all forms of anion gap acidosis is both supportive (restore circulation, correct acidosis with bicarbonate) and specific (correct underlying abnormality). Bicarbonate should be given in adequate quantities to keep the pH above 7.2 and/or the bicarbonate level above 15 mEq/L. Situations with ongoing tissue hypoxia may require substantial replacement, whereas transient problems such as postictal lactic acidosis usually correct themselves spontaneously. When bicarbonate is required, the bicarbonate deficit can be determined by a variety of formulas. An easy-to-remember fact is that the bicarbonate space corresponds roughly to one half of total body water (approximately 30% of total body weight in kilograms). Thus:

$$HCO_3 \text{ deficit} = 0.3 \times \text{wt} \times (24 - HCO_3)$$

Usually one half of the calculated deficit is replaced to avoid overcorrection following which blood gasses are repeated before infusing additional bicarbonate. In patients with compromised renal function and metabolic acidosis, it is important to remember that disorders of potassium, magnesium, and phosphate are commonly found and should be sought.

Nonanion Gap Acidosis (Hyperchloremic). Causes of metabolic acidosis with a normal anion gap include bicarbonate loss, inability to excrete hydrogen ion, or administration of exogenous HCl, NH_4Cl. Most commonly there is either a perceived source of bicarbonate loss or an abnormality in the kidney (or adrenal). Recognized bicarbonate loss is usually from the gastrointestinal tract distal to the pylorus and may include duodenal fistula, biliary drainage, pancreatic fistula, small intestinal fistula, ureterosigmoidostomy, and diarrhea. Intrinsic renal losses of bicarbonate include interstitial nephritis, renal tubular acidosis,[17,36,40] adrenal insufficiency, hypoaldosteronism,[43] and acetazolamide administration.

Treatment of nonanion gap acidosis requires correction of the existing acidosis plus routine administration of bicarbonate on a regular basis. The dosage of bicarbonate required will depend on the underlying disease, its magnitude, and the need for dialysis. Guidelines for acute correction are the same as for anion gap acidosis: calculate bicarbonate deficit (base deficit), estimate bicarbonate space, and administer only as much as should correct one half of the predicted deficit over a period of 24 hours.

As indicated previously, compensation for metabolic acidosis is usual and is manifested as hyperpnea, tachypnea, nasal flaring, or even Kussmaul's respiration. The degree of compensatory hyperventilation in a stable, chronic metabolic acidosis (as opposed to the acute changes seen in conditions such as sepsis and hypovolemia) can be predicted[1] by the following formula:

$$P_{CO_2} = 1.5\,(HCO_3) + \Delta$$

where HCO_3 is mEq of HCO_3^- and Δ is 8 ± 2 mEq/L. Recognition of this compensatory phenomenon will assist in preventing iatrogenic metabolic alkalosis from overtreatment with bicarbonate.

Alkalosis

As is the case with acidosis, alkalosis may be either respiratory or metabolic in origin. In contradistinction to acidosis, it is the metabolic component that is rather simple to define and correct, whereas respiratory alkalosis may have a myriad of causes.

Respiratory Alkalosis. Respiratory alkalosis is probably the most common acid/base disturbance in clinical medicine and can be induced by a multitude of underlying conditions. The pathophysiologic mechanism is excess alveolar ventilation above the requirements of carbon dioxide production. This abnormality typically represents some form of CNS overstimulation but may include as causes those factors summarized below:

Anxiety
Fever
Salicylate intoxication
CNS disorders
Intrathoracic processes
Hypoxemia
Hepatic insufficiency
Gram-negative septicemia
Pregnancy
Mechanical hyperventilation

Treatment of respiratory alkalosis must be directed at correcting the underlying cause (e.g., correct fever with antipyretics). In patients requiring assisted ventilation, use of intermittent demand systems will tend to minimize the typical overventilation that is seen with controlled or assist/controlled ventilation. Other attempts at increasing P_{CO_2} such as inspired carbon dioxide, rebreathing devices, and added mechanical dead space are relatively ineffective.

Metabolic Alkalosis. The fundamental abnormality in pure metabolic alkalosis is an absolute or relative excess of base (primarily bicarbonate) in extracellular fluid.[2,21,30] This excess tends to be offset by a compensatory decrease in minute alveolar ventilation with subsequent hypercarbia. The mechanisms underlying metabolic alkalosis are the loss of hydrogen (with chloride), gain of exogenous base, or extracellular fluid–volume contraction. Identification of the latter two mechanisms should be straightforward, although gain of exogenous base may be masked as in blood transfusions (citrate) or intravenous infusions of fresh frozen plasma (citrate) or lactated Ringer's solution.

The most common clinically important form of metabolic alkalosis is a result of loss of hydrogen ion and chloride from the stomach or the kidney. These two varieties can be separated by attention to the amount of urinary chloride. Low urinary chloride (<10 mEq/L) reflects a "chloride responsive" alkalosis that will correct itself by the appropriate administration of saline[24] (usually with some potassium). This variety is typically related to volume contraction, gastric losses, or base administration. High urinary chloride (>10 mEq/L) indicates a "chloride-resistant" alkalosis[13] (caused by hyperaldosteronism, increased plasma desoxycorticosterone, exogenous corticosteroids, licorice ingestion or carbenoxolone therapy, and chloruretic diuretics) and suggests a renal origin, more specifically a "hormone" or drug-related effect on tubular function causing a change in tubular resorption of bicarbonate and increased excretion of H^+ and K^+.[10,15] This latter variety is dependent on (although not initiated by) hypokalemia,[37,41] and correction of the potassium deficit is essential to restoration of acid/base balance.[4] Active reabsorption of potassium in the distal renal tubule in "exchange" for H^+ leads to the paradox of acid urine (paradoxic aciduria) associated with hypokalemic alkalosis. Occasionally, massive doses of potassium are required to achieve equilibrium. When clinically significant hypoventilation develops as compensation for metabolic alkalosis, more rapid treatment may be needed.[42] Two approaches are described, including administration of acid or inducing renal tubular acidosis with acetazolamide. Recent experience with 0.1 normal (N) HCl infusions (or as high as 0.2 N) has shown this form of treatment to be quite safe if administered through a central venous line. The dose of H^+ should be calculated by determining base excess (or increase in bicarbonate above 25 mEq/L), and multiplying it by one half of estimated total body water (0.3 × weight). One half of this calculated amount is then administered over 24 hours. Although anecdotal experience suggests that acetazolamide administration is effective, no controlled studies exist to confirm this contention.

Combined Acid/Base Disorders

It is crucial to realize that acid/base disorders are in no way limited to a single pathophysiologic mechanism. Consequently, combinations of abnormalities are common. In order to distinguish single from combined disturbances, an objective approach is essential. Most standard texts contain graphs that indicate the 95% probability range for single acid/base disorders; i.e., the laboratory values that are 95% likely to represent a single pathophysiologic abnormality. In addition, numerous empiric equations have been developed to identify compensatory changes as opposed to coexistent abnormalities. Characteristics of isolated acid/base disturbances are listed in Table 2-6.

Certain combinations of acid/base disturbances are encountered commonly enough clinically to also justify listing. The components of these combinations and the clinical settings in which they are likely to occur are summarized below:

1. *Respiratory acidosis and metabolic alkalosis* occur in patients with chronic respiratory acidosis with superimposed congestive heart failure requiring diuretics.
2. *Respiratory acidosis and metabolic acidosis* occur in patients with cardiopulmonary arrest, chronic lung disease in shock, and chronic renal failure with respiratory insufficiency.
3. *Respiratory alkalosis and metabolic acidosis* occur in hepatic failure caused by central hyperventilation plus hepatic or renal insufficiency.
4. *Respiratory alkalosis and metabolic alkalosis* occur in hepatic cirrhosis with hyperventilation associated with vomiting or in chronic respiratory failure following institution of vigorous mechanical ventilation.
5. *Metabolic acidosis and metabolic alkalosis* are actually sequential rather than simultaneous. It is identified when the anion gap is greater than the HCO_3 deficit and occurs with progressive contraction alkalosis caused by vomiting when hypotension develops.

Table 2-6 **IDENTIFICATION OF ISOLATED ACID/BASE DISTURBANCES**

Disturbance	Effect
Metabolic acidosis	P_{CO_2} should fall by 1 to 1.5 times the fall in HCO_3
Metabolic alkalosis	P_{CO_2} should rise by 0.5 to 1 times the rise in HCO_3
Respiratory acidosis (acute)	Plasma HCO_3 should be <30 mEq/L
Respiratory acidosis (chronic)	Plasma HCO_3 should rise by 4 mmol/10 mm Hg rise in P_{CO_2}
Respiratory alkalosis (acute)	Plasma HCO_3 should fall by 2.5 mmol/10 mm Hg fall in P_{CO_2} (usually >18 mEq/L)
Respiratory alkalosis (chronic)	Plasma HCO_3 should fall at least as much as acute but not <15 mEq/L

Modified from Schrier, R.W., editor: Renal and electrolyte disorders, Boston, 1980, Little, Brown, & Co., Inc.

PRINCIPLES OF FLUID THERAPY

In any patient requiring intravenous fluid therapy, three categories of fluid loss must be taken into consideration. These include losses related to normal body maintenance, losses resulting from the patient's underlying disease, and any existing fluid deficits. As indicated in an earlier section of this chapter, all patients have normal maintenance requirements related to daily sensible and insensible losses. These losses will vary somewhat depending on the person's age, body build, and sex but generally average between 2000 and 2500 ml of fluid every 24 hours. The major sensible loss is urine, and the major insensible loss is related to evaporative losses from the skin and water losses through the lungs. All of these losses are primarily water losses containing only minimal amounts of electrolytes. If an individual patient requires intravenous therapy for only short periods of time, replacement of electrolyte losses is generaly unnecessary, and maintenance volume losses can be replaced with solutions of 5% dextrose and water (see Table 2-5). If prolonged intravenous therapy is expected, consideration of the small but consistent daily electrolyte losses will need to be taken into account and can generally be managed by giving 1 mEq/kg of body weight of sodium, chloride, and potassium daily. Thus if a patient requires 2500 ml of fluid to meet normal maintenance needs, 1500 ml could be provided as dextrose and water, and the remaining 1000 ml could be given as half normal saline with the addition of appropriate amounts of potassium chloride (see Table 2-5).

Losses arising from the patient's underlying disease must also be replaced. In surgical patients, these losses are almost always from some portion of the gastrointestinal tract. As a general rule, intestinal secretions, bile, or pancreatic juice can be replaced on a volume-to-volume basis with a balanced salt solution such as Ringer's lactate or normal saline, whereas losses from an actively secreting stomach are replaced with half normal saline solution (see

Table 2-7 **COMPOSITION OF GASTROINTESTINAL SECRETIONS**

	Volume (ml/24 hr)	Na (mEq/L)	K (mEq/L)	Cl (mEq/L)	HCO_3^- (mEq/L)
Stomach	1000-2000	60-100	10-20	100-130	—
Pancreas	300-800	135-145	5-10	70-90	95-120
Bile	300-600	135-145	5-10	90-130	30-40
Intestine (primarily small)	2000-4000	120-140	5-10	90-140	30-40

Table 2-5). In addition, each of these secretions contains varying amounts of potassium. Generally, gastric secretions contain about twice the amount of potassium as exists in secretions from the small intestine, bile, or pancreas (Table 2-7). To prevent the development of problems with hypokalemia, 10 to 20 mEq of potassium for every liter of fluid loss from any of these sites should be administered. If long-term intravenous therapy is required, these requirements may increase and should be monitored by the determination of serum electrolyte values every 2 to 3 days.

Another source of abnormal losses in patients who are septic is an increased evaporative loss from the skin and respiratory tract. As much as 1000 ml daily may occur over and above normal insensible losses if the body temperature is markedly elevated. In patients with persistent temperature elevations above 101° F (38.4° C), 500 to 1000 ml of additional fluid may be required daily. Since such fluid loss is primarily water, it can generally be replaced with a dextrose and water intravenous solution.

Finally, existing solute or volume deficits must also be corrected. Again, such deficits generally arise from the gastrointestinal tract and are the result of such problems as vomiting, diarrhea, or sequestration of fluid as may occur in patients with bowel obstruction. A correct estimate of these losses is often difficult, but careful attention to physical findings and important historical information from the patient summarizing the duration of disease and the frequency and amount of fluid losses (e.g., through vomiting or diarrhea) are usually helpful in deriving an appropriate estimate of the magnitude of underlying deficits. As emphasized previously, only one half of this calculated estimate should be replaced in a given 24-hour period, and the patient reassessed clinically and with supporting laboratory data before attempting any further deficit replacement.

If the principles just enumerated are followed, the large majority of patients requiring intravenous therapy can be managed without difficulty. Especially pertinent in such management is frequent reassessment of the patient clinically and daily review of the patient's input and output records to ensure that the proper amount of fluid is being given. Daily weights are especially helpful in this regard and can give valuable clues as to whether abrupt changes in fluid balance (either fluid overload or fluid deficit) are occurring. Further, attention to such detail helps prevent the development of any major imbalances that may occur insidiously before they become clinically obvious.

SUMMARY

The plasma is a subset of the total fluid (extracellular fluid) that bathes the cells. As such it allows an indirect look at cellular events and the interaction between the cells and the extracellular fluid. Fluid and electrolyte disorders are legion and commonplace. The correct, critical interpretation of laboratory parameters to identify the pathophysiologic mechanisms underlying these abnormalities requires a willingness to go beyond the obvious. A logical, analytic approach to the meaning of the observed laboratory disturbances should lead to an insight into the significance of the observation. A cookbook approach to "correct" the abnormal test result may actually worsen the situation.

It is critical to appreciate that a concentration actually represents a ratio of the amount of a substance to the amount of fluid in which it is dissolved or suspended. Abnormalities in concentration can be caused by a change in either component. Attention to a variety of clinical factors (weight changes, vital signs, nursing notes, even history and physical examination) often provides the insight necessary to identify the true problem and chart its solution.

SUGGESTED READINGS

Brenner, B.M., and Stein, J.H., editors: Acid-base and potassium homeostasis, vol. 2 of Contemporary issues in nephrology, New York, 1978, Churchill Livingstone.

Diem, K., editor: Water and electrolyte balance. In Documenta Geigy, scientific tables, Ardsley, N.Y., 1962, Geigy Pharmaceuticals.

Goodenough, R.D., and Burke, J.F.: Fluid, electrolyte and acid-base homeostasis in surgery. In Burke, J.F., editor: Surgical physiology, Philadelphia, 1983, W.B. Saunders.

Maxwell, M.H., and Kleeman, C.R., editors: Clinical disorders of fluid and electrolyte metabolism, New York, 1980, McGraw-Hill Book Co.

Murphy, J.E., Preuss, H.G., and Henry, J.B.: Evaluation of renal function and water, electrolyte, and acid-base balance. In Henry, J.B., editor: Clinical diagnosis and management by laboratory methods, Philadelphia, 1984, W.B. Saunders.

Narins, R.G., et al.: Diagnostic strategies in disorders of fluid, electrolyte, and acid-base homeostasis, Am. J. Med. **72**:496, 1982.

Schrier, R.W., editor: Renal and electrolyte disorders, Boston, 1980, Little, Brown & Co.

Shoemaker, W.C.: Fluids and electrolytes in the adult. In: Shoemaker, W.C., and Thompson, W.L., editors: Critical care—state of the art, vol. 3, Fullerton, Calif., 1982, The Society of Critical Care Medicine.

Vanatta, J.C., and Gogelman, M.J.: Moyer's fluid balance, Chicago, 1976, Year Book Medical Publishers, Inc.

REFERENCES

1. Albert, M.D., Dell, R.B., and Winters, R.W.: Quantitative displacement of acid base equilibrium in metabolic acidosis, Ann. Intern. Med. **66**:312, 1967.
2. Arruda, J.A.L., and Kurtzman, N.A.: Metabolic acidosis and alkalosis, Clin. Nephrol. **7**:201, 1977.
3. Bie, P.: Osmoreceptors, vasopressin, and control of renal water excretion, Physiol. Rev. **60**:961, 1980.
4. Boyd, J.E., and Mulrow, T.J.: Further studies of the influence of potassium on aldosterone production in the rat, Endocrinol. **90**:299, 1972.
5. Cooke, C.R., Turin, M.D., and Walker, W.G.: The syndrome of inappropriate antidiuretic hormone secretion (SIADH): pathophysio-

logic mechanisms in solute and volume regulation, Medicine **58:**240, 1979.

6. Corsa, L., et al.: Measurement of exchangeable potassium in man by isotope dilution, J. Clin. Invest. **29:**1280, 1950.
7. Davis, J.O., and Freeman, R.H.: Mechanisms regulating renin release, Physiol. Rev. **56:**1, 1976.
8. Emmett, M., et al.: The pathophysiology of acid-base changes in chronically phosphate-depleted rats, J. Clin. Invest. **59:**291, 1977.
9. Espinel, C.H.: The FeNa test, JAMA **6:**579, 1976.
10. Fanestil, D.O., and Park, C.S.: Steroid hormones and the kidney, Annu. Rev. Physiol. **43:**637, 1981.
11. Felig, P.: Diabetic ketoacidosis, N. Engl. J. Med. **290:**1360, 1974.
12. Forbes, R.M., Mitchell, H.H., and Cooper, A.R.: Further studies on the gross composition and mineral elements of the adult human body, J. Biol. Chem. **223:**969, 1956.
13. Garella, S., Chazan, J.A., and Cohen, J.J.: Saline resistant metabolic alkalosis or "chloride-wasting nephropathy." Report of four cases with severe potassium depletion, Ann. Intern. Med. **73:**31, 1970.
14. Gennari, F.J., and Cohen, J.J.: Role of the kidney in potassium homeostasis: lessons from acid base disturbances (editorial), Kidney Int. **8:**1, 1975.
15. Gill, J.R., and Bartter, F.C.: Evidence for a prostaglandin-independent defect in chloride reabsorption in the loop of Henle as a proximal cause of Bartter's syndrome, Am. J. Med. **65:**766, 1978.
16. Gruber, U.F., and Allgower, M.: Water and electrolyte balance. In Diem, K., editor: Documenta Geigy, scientific tables, Ardsley, N.Y., 1970, Geigy Pharmaceuticals.
17. Halperin, M.L., et al.: Studies on the pathogenesis of type 1 (distal) renal tubular acidosis as revealed by the urinary P_{CO_2} tensions, J. Clin. Invest. **53:**669, 1974.
18. Handler, J.S., and Orloff, J.: Antidiuretic hormone, Annu. Rev. Physiol. **43:**611, 1981.
19. Harmann, R.C., and Mellinkoff, S.M.: The relationship of platelets to the serum potassium concentration, J. Clin. Invest. **34:**938, 1955.
20. Hays, R.M.: Antidiuretic hormone, N. Engl. J. Med. **295:**659, 1976.
21. Hodgkin, J.E., Soeprono, F.F., and Chan, D.M.: Incidence of metabolic alkalemia in hospitalized patients, Crit. Care Med. **8:**725, 1980.
22. Imai, M., and Kokko, J.: Sodium urea and water transport in the thin ascending limb of Henle: generation of osmotic gradients by passive diffusion of solutes, J. Clin. Invest. **53:**393, 1974.
23. Jorgensen, P.L.: Sodium and potassium ion pumps in kidney tubules, Physiol. Rev. **60:**864, 1980.
24. Kassirer, J.P., et al.: The critical role of chloride in the correction of hypokalemic alkalosis in man, Am. J. Med. **38:**172, 1965.
25. Knochel, J.P.: Role of glucoregulatory hormones in potassium homeostasis, Kidney Int. **11:**443, 1977.
26. Kunau, R.T., and Stein, J.H.: Disorders of hypo- and hyperkalemia, Clin. Nephrol. **7:**173, 1977.
27. Kunau, R.T., Webb, H.L., and Borman, S.C.: Characteristics of sodium reabsorption in the loop of Henle and distal tubule, Am. J. Physiol. **227:**1181, 1974.
28. Lipner, H.I., et al.: The behavior of carbenicillin as a non-reabsorbable anion, J. Lab. Clin. Med. **290:**1184, 1974.
29. Loeb, J.N.: The hyperosmolar state, N. Engl. J. Med. **290:**1184, 1984.
30. Madias, N.E., Ayus, J.C., and Adroque, H.J.: Increased anion gap in metabolic alkalosis: the role of plasma-protein equivalency, N. Engl. J. Med. **300:**1421, 1979.
31. Moore, F.D.: Determination of total body water and solids with isotopes, Science **104:**157, 1946.
32. Moore, F.D., et al.: Body composition: total body water and electrolytes: intravascular and extravascular phase volumes, Metabolism **5:**447, 1956.
33. Oh, M.S., and Carroll, H.J.: Decreased anion gap and hyponatremia, N. Engl. J. Med. **298:**111, 1978.
34. Oliva, P.B.: Lactic acidosis, Am. J. Med. **48:**209, 1970.
35. Pitts, R.F.: Physiology of the kidney and body fluids: volume and composition of the body fluids, Chicago, 1968, Year Book Medical Publishers, Inc.
36. Rocha, A.S., and Kokko, J.P.: Sodium chloride and water transport in the medullary thick ascending limb of Henle: evidence for active chloride transport, J. Clin. Invest. **52:**612, 1973.
37. Roscoe, J.M., et al.: Effect of amphotericin-B on urine acidification in rats: implications for the pathogenesis of distal renal tubular acidosis, J. Lab. Clin. Med. **89:**463, 1977.
38. Schultze, R.G.: Recent advances in the physiology and pathophysiology of potassium excretion, Arch. Intern. Med. **131:**885, 1973.
39. Sebastian, A., and Morris, R.C., Jr.,: Renal tubular acidosis, Clin. Nephrol. **7:**216, 1977.
40. Sebastian, A., McSherry, E., and Morris, R.C., Jr.: Renal potassium wasting in renal tubular acidosis, J. Clin. Invest. **50:**667, 1971.
41. Seldin, D.W., and Rector, R.C., Jr.: The generation and maintenance of metabolic alkalosis, Kidney Int. **1:**306, 1972.
42. Shear, L., and Brandman, I.S.: Hypoxia and hypercapnia caused by respiratory compensation for metabolic alkalosis, Am. Rev. Respir. Dis. **107:**836, 1973.
43. Szylman, P., et al.: Role of hyperkalemia in the metabolic acidosis of isolated hypoaldosteronism, N. Engl. J. Med. **294:**361, 1976.

3 Surgical Nutrition

Roger A. Bonau and John M. Daly

The provision of intravenous and enteral nutritional support to hospitalized patients has developed over the past 20 years and has stimulated investigation into related areas such as nutritional assessment, the provision of specialized formulas, and the application of nutritional principles to many clinical situations. These principles are founded on the complex interrelationships between endogenous and exogenous sources of proteins and energy and their modification by starvation and disease states. Protein-calorie malnutrition in hospitalized patients is being increasingly recognized. Biochemical indices and anthropometric studies have demonstrated that malnutrition occurs in up to 50% of surgical patients[7] and is associated with significantly increased morbidity and mortality. Several factors, e.g., disease process and treatment, influence the development of malnutrition, but absence of one of the warning signs detailed in the boxed material below does not exclude the presence of malnutrition or its subsequent development.[16]

Protein-calorie malnutrition occurs as one of three clinical entities: marasmus, kwashiorkor, and a mixture of the two. Marasmus is simple starvation resulting from prolonged inadequate intake of all nutrients. Cahill[17] described the adaptive processes to starvation, which includes use of available endogenous energy stores, predominately fat. The initial, relatively high urinary loss of protein decreases as the body adapts to a lipid source of calories. Prolonged starvation leads to continued reduction of protein stores. Clinically, patients with marasmus exhibit loss of subcutaneous fat, diminution of muscle mass, and weight loss. Biochemical markers of visceral protein status may be relatively normal. Kwashiorkor occurs as a result of diets lacking in protein but with sufficient calories. Patients with this entity exhibit signs of protein loss, including reduction of visceral mass and muscle bulk, edema, and hair loss. The degree of weight loss is variable because of adequate calorie intake. Laboratory biochemical markers are usually abnormal with low serum concentrations of albumin, transferrin, and prealbumin. Cellular immunity is depressed and may be demonstrated by anergy to skin test antigens and depression of the total lymphocyte count. The third kind of protein-calorie malnutrition, a mixed marasmus-kwashiorkor type, is most common in hospitalized patients. Underlying malnutrition is enhanced by stress resulting from a given disease, its treatment, or its complications. These patients are at high risk for increased morbidity and mortality.

NUTRITIONALLY HIGH-RISK PATIENT—FOR HOSPITAL-ASSOCIATED MORBIDITY AND MORTALITY

- Gross underweight: Weight-for-height below 80% of standard
- Gross overweight: Weight-for-height above 120% of standard
- Recent loss of 10% or more of usual body weight
- Alcoholism
- No oral intake for over 10 days on simple intravenous solutions
- Protracted nutrient losses
  - Malabsorption syndromes
  - Short-gut syndromes/fistulas
  - Renal dialysis
  - Draining abscesses, wounds
- Increased metabolic needs
  - Extensive burns, infection, trauma
  - Protracted fever
- Intake of drugs with antinutrient or catabolic properties: steroids, immunosuppressants, antitumor agents

Modified from Butterworth, C.E.: Malnutrition in hospital patients: assessment and treatment. In Goodhart, R.S., and Shils, M.E., editors: Modern nutrition in health and disease, Philadelphia, 1980, Lea & Febiger.

ENERGY STORAGE AND STARVATION

Starvation in humans results in a reliance on endogenous fuel reserves to satisfy energy and protein requirements. Endogenous stores are in three forms, including carbohydrate, protein, and fat. Carbohydrate, along with water, is stored as glycogen intracellularly. The amount of stored glycogen is limited, and it is a relatively inefficient fuel on a per weight basis. Total liver and muscle glycogen stores provide approximately 900 calories in healthy humans (Table 3-1).[17] Protein is stored predominantly in lean body mass intracellularly in an aqueous environment. Approximately 24,000 calories are potentially available in healthy humans from protein. In addition to its role as an energy source, protein also serves other essential functions in tissue repair and homeostasis. Fat is stored intracellularly in a nonaqueous environment[17] and constitutes the major fuel

Table 3-1 **TISSUE FUEL COMPOSITION OF NORMAL MAN**

Fuel*	Kg	Calories
Fat (adipose triglyceride)	15	141,000
Protein (mainly muscle)	6	24,000
Glycogen (muscle)	0.15	600
Glycogen (liver)	0.075	300
TOTAL		165,900

Modified from Cahill, G.F.: N. Engl. J. Med. **282:**668, 1970.
*Total available carbohydrate fuel is approximately 900 calories.

source with over 140,000 calories potentially available in healthy humans. Although fat stores also provide insulation, their major role is energy provision.

During brief starvation, body reserves are used for nutritional requirements. Following a 24-hour fast, resting energy expenditures, approximately 1800 calories in a healthy person, are derived from glycogen, protein, and fat. Glycogen stores are inadequate to meet these requirements, necessitating the use of other fuel reserves. Starvation initially results in increased production of urinary urea, reflecting mobilization of endogenous protein reserves to meet energy requirements. Increased urea production in the liver is a consequence of an increased release of $-NH_2$ moieties for gluconeogenesis from amino acid precursors. Alanine and glutamine are released from muscle breakdown, and additional alanine is released from the gut proportionate to glutamine uptake by the splanchnic bed. The resulting production of hepatic glucose is used by the brain and other glycolytic tissues such as red blood cells. Red blood cells convert glucose into lactate and pyruvate that are transported back to the liver and act as gluconeogenic precursors. This energy requiring activity is called the Cori cycle.

Energy for these activities is derived from the oxidation of fat.[65] The fall in plasma glucose concentrations during starvation is reflected by a corresponding fall in plasma insulin and a rise in plasma glucagon concentrations, resulting in an increase in lipolysis with corresponding increased free fatty acid levels. Fatty acids may be used for energy by certain tissues or may be oxidized to ketone bodies by the liver; they may then be used for energy by the liver and other tissues.

Prolonged starvation is characterized by the conversion from a glucose to a lipid system of energy use. Continued reliance on glucose would require continued skeletal muscle breakdown for gluconeogenesis precursors. This would severely compromise other important functions of proteins, including enzymatic, structural, and transport requirements. Continued use of fat for energy is characterized by a fall in urinary urea, reflecting decreased amino acid efflux from skeletal muscle, and by a corresponding increase in plasma concentrations of free fatty acids and ketone bodies. The brain converts to the use of ketone bodies for energy. Prolonged starvation may be tolerated for approximately 50 days because of the size of normal fat reserves in humans.

STRESSED STARVATION

The addition of some stress (e.g., sepsis, trauma, burns, or a major elective surgical procedure) complicates the picture of simple starvation. Stressed starvation is characterized by increased energy and protein requirements without the usual adaptive, protein-conserving mechanisms that are present in simple starvation. This is reflected by increased mobilization of muscle amino acids required for hepatic gluconeogenesis and for local functions, e.g., wound repair and immune responses. The Cori cycle activity is increased. As a result, lipolysis is enhanced without a corresponding fall in skeletal muscle breakdown. The magnitude of injury appears to be the major determinant of urinary urea nitrogen losses.

The goal of nutritional support in the setting of starvation, with or without stress, is to meet requirements of energy, proteins, minerals, and vitamins exogenously, using various routes of administration. The ability to preserve body mass and function by nutritional support will be discussed in the following sections.

NUTRITIONAL ASSESSMENT

In surgical patients, malnutrition is associated with delayed wound healing, decreased resistance to infection, and other potential complications.[68] Implementation of perioperative nutritional intervention results in the reversal of markers associated with malnutrition such as improvement in short half-life serum protein concentrations and reversal of skin test anergy, and in turn is associated with reduced postoperative morbidity and mortality.[71] Assessment of operative risk requires qualitative and quantitative methods of nutritional assessment. Nutritional assessment techniques correlate physiologic and body compositional aberrations with useful clinical markers that are associated with malnutrition. Standard methods for assessing nutritional status include a history and physical examination, anthropometric measurements, laboratory determinations, and measurement of immune competence.

Nutritional assessment should be undertaken in all patients under consideration for nutritional support and should be used as a guideline to quantitate the degree of malnutrition.

History and Physical Examination

Nutritional deficiencies may be generalized or may involve only specific nutrients. Certain clinical entities are associated with generalized nutritional deficiencies; e.g., alcoholism is associated with protein-calorie malnutrition and deficits of various vitamins and minerals, including niacin and zinc. Specific operative procedures may be responsible for individual vitamin and mineral deficiencies. Ileal resection or diversion may result in steatorrhea with deficiencies in fat-soluble vitamins and magnesium.

A complete dietary history may give clues to underlying deficiencies, including a history of recent weight loss or use of fad diets.[46] The medical history should evaluate prior operations or conditions that may have resulted in nutritional deficits (e.g., folate deficiency as a result of a prior gastrectomy or a history of chronic illness such as pancreatic insufficiency may indicate deficiencies of the fat-soluble vitamins). The social history may help explain underlying deficiencies. Poverty, alcoholism, and fad diets have all been implicated in malnutrition. Finally, a careful systems review should uncover symptoms associated with anorexia and weight loss. The presence of nausea and vomiting, diarrhea, melena, abdominal pain, dysphagia, peripheral edema, and fever are often present in disease states that are associated with protein-calorie malnutrition, as shown in Table 3-2.

A careful physical examination will identify most patients with malnutrition (see boxed material on p. 53). Overall patient appearance should be noted. Although most patients will not be obviously emaciated, the presence of pallor, edema, skin lesions, and muscle wasting are clinical determinants of malnutrition. The integument

Table 3-2 **NUTRITIONAL DEFICIENCIES COMMONLY ASSOCIATED WITH DISEASE STATES**

Nutrient	Clinical State
Protein	Burns, nephrosis, alcoholism, surgery, protein-losing enteropathy
Fat	Gluten enteropathy, blind loop syndrome, tropical sprue, pancreatic insufficiency, ileal resection, gastrectomy, short bowel syndrome
Potassium	Surgery, intestinal bypass
Calcium	Chronic renal failure, gastrectomy, intestinal bypass
Iron	Hemorrhage, gastrectomy
Magnesium	Alcoholism, intestinal bypass surgery, malabsorption syndromes, intestinal and biliary fistulas, acute pancreatitis, diabetes, parathyroid disease, renal disease, diuretic therapy
Zinc	Alcoholism, surgery
Vitamin A	Chronic obstructive lung disease, congestive heart failure, pancreatic insufficiency, fever, thyrotoxicosis, gastrectomy, bile salt depletion, sprue, cystic fibrosis
Vitamin D	Gastrectomy, cirrhosis, pancreatic insufficiency
Vitamin K	Pancreatic insufficiency, obstructive jaundice, cholestyramine ingestion, prolonged antibiotic therapy
Vitamin E	Pancreatitis, cystic fibrosis, steatorrhea, gastrectomy
Thiamine	Wernicke encephalopathy, beriberi, thyrotoxicosis, fever, diuresis, prolonged antacid therapy
Riboflavin	Alcoholism, fever
Niacin	Alcoholism
Pyridoxine	Thyrotoxicosis, alcoholism
Folate	Alcoholism, psoriasis, rheumatoid arthritis, fever, liver disease, sickle cell disease, leukemia, thyrotoxicosis, gastrectomy, macrocytic anemia, gluten-induced enteropathy, malignancy
Vitamin B_{12}	Ileal resection, pernicious anemia, regional enteritis, blind loop syndrome, thyrotoxicosis, alcoholism, gastrectomy
Vitamin C	Drug addiction, fever, rheumatoid arthritis, alcoholism, thyrotoxicosis, congestive heart failure, peptic ulcer disease

Modified from Grant, J.P., Custer, P.B., and Thurlow, J.: Surg. Clin. North Am. **61**:437, 1981.

often provides specific and general signs of nutritional deficiency states. Loss of hair is associated with protein deficiency. Loss of subcutaneous fat may be associated with calorie depletion. Iron deficiency may be the cause of spoon-shaped nails. Niacin deficiency, pellagra, may result in a symmetric, hyperpigmented skin rash over body parts exposed to sunlight.

The oral cavity is commonly affected in malnutrition. The absence of teeth or the presence of caries may contribute to the underlying deficiency. Glossitis is associated with vitamin B deficiency; and swollen, bleeding gums are associated with vitamin C deficiency.

Muscle wasting is the most recognizable sign of protein-calorie malnutrition. It may be associated with peripheral edema. All muscle groups may be affected, although signs may be more obvious in the small muscles of the hand and in the muscles of facial expression.

Anthropometric Measurements

Anthropometry is the science that deals with the measurement of the size, weight, and proportions of the human body. Body proportions or composition may be assessed using analytic methods to determine total body nitrogen, potassium, and water. For the most part, however, these methods are not clinically useful, and more simplified methods of determining body composition have been used. These standardized anthropometric measurements have been compared with direct body composition analyses; they may be helpful in determining nutritional status, although this appears to be more likely in groups rather than individuals.

The body can be divided into six compartments: fat, skin and skeleton, extracellular mass, plasma protein, visceral protein, and somatic protein mass.[46] Assessment of the various compartments is useful in quantifying the type and degree of deficits present (Fig. 3-1). Assessing compartment losses is important not only for determining nutrient needs but also for determining individual deficits.

Somatic Protein Mass

Anthropometric measurements of somatic protein mass (skeletal muscle) are body weight and mid-upper arm muscle circumference. Body weight should be measured at the time of hospital admission in all surgical patients and can be compared to ideal body weight as derived from the Metropolitan Life Insurance Co. tables. However, a comparison of actual to ideal body weight may have little clinical application because of the wide range of weights for any given frame size. In addition, obesity is prevalent in our society so that actual weight may be greater than ideal weight. Substantial recent weight loss may have occurred in a given patient, also obscuring the meaning of actual weight measurements. More useful is the comparison of body weight to previously known weight. Insufficient caloric intake results in increased use of endogenous fat and protein stores for caloric needs, resulting in weight loss. Extracellular sodium and water may be retained in protein-depleted patients, causing an underestimation of malnutrition when determined by body weight. However, loss of weight over a prolonged period (weeks) is usually specific for decreased energy intake in relation to energy needs.

The mid-upper arm circumference has been found to be a simple anthropometric estimate of skeletal muscle mass. The mid-upper arm is defined as the midpoint between the olecranon and the acromial process. The circumference of the arm muscle at this point calculated with the use of the triceps skinfold thickness is compared with results in standard tables. Less than 60% of standard is considered abnormal.

Body Fat Mass

Depletion of body fat is an indicator of inadequate caloric intake relative to energy needs. Body fat is also determined anthropometrically by measurement of skinfold thickness. This method is justified because subcutaneous fat accounts for approximately 50% of total body fat. Var-

PHYSICAL SIGNS ASSOCIATED WITH MALNUTRITION

Dietary Obesity
Excess weight
Excessive weight
Excessive skin folds
Excessive abdominal girth

Undernutrition
Lethargy, mental and physical
Low weight in relation to height
Diminished skin folds
Exaggerated skeletal prominences
Loss of elasticity of skin

Protein-Calorie Deficiency Disease
Edema
Muscle wasting
Low body weight
Psychomotor change
Dyspigmentation of the hair
Thin, sparse hair
Moon face
Flaky pain dermatosis
Areas of hyperpigmentation

Vitamin A Deficiency
Xerosis of skin
Follicular hyperkeratosis
Xerosis conjunctivae
Keratomalacia
Bitot's spots

Riboflavin Deficiency
Angular stomatitis
Cheilosis
Magenta tongue
Central atrophy of lingual papillae
Nasolabial dyssebacia
Angular palpebritis
Scrotal and vulval dermatosis
Corneal vascularization

Thiamin Deficiency
Loss of ankle jerks
Sensory loss and motor weakness
Calf-muscle tenderness
Cardiovascular dysfunction
Edema

Niacin Deficiency
Pellagrous dermatosis
Scarlet and raw tongue
Tongue fissuring
Atrophic lingual papillae
Malar and supraorbital pigmentation

Vitamin C Deficiency
Spongy and bleeding gums
Folliculosis
Petechiae
Ecchymoses
Intramuscular or subperiosteal hematoma
Epiphyseal enlargement (painful)

Vitamin D Deficiency
Active rickets (in children)
Epiphyseal enlargement (over 6 months of age, painless)
Beading of ribs
Craniotabes (under 1 year of age)
Muscular hypotonia
Healed rickets (in children or adults)
Frontal and parietal bossing
Knock-knees or bow legs
Deformities of thorax
Osteomalacia (in adults)
Local or generalized skeletal deformities

Iron Deficiency
Pallor of mucous membranes
Koilonychia
Atrophic lingual papillae

Modified from Scrimshaw, N.S.: Cecil textbook of medicine, Philadelphia, 1979, W.B. Saunders Co.

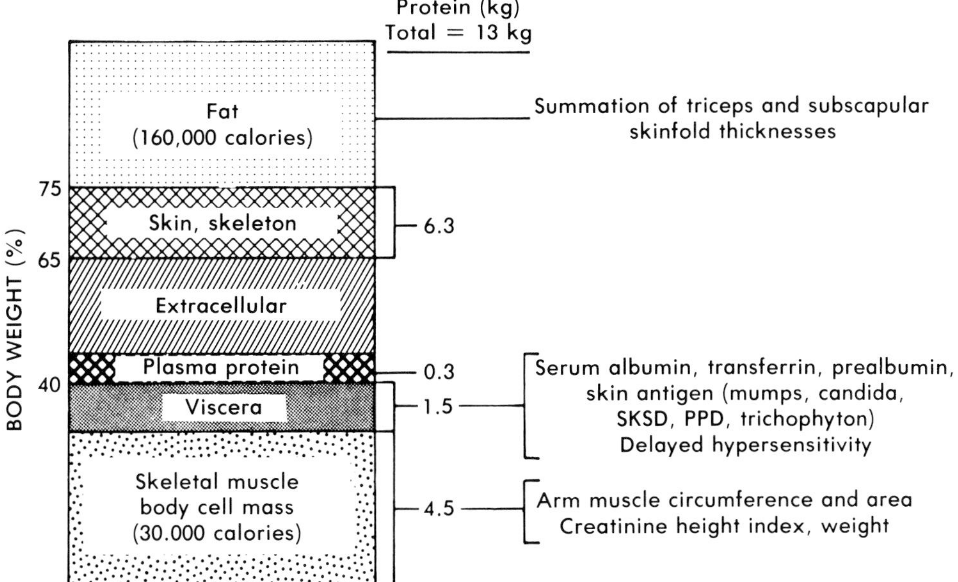

Fig. 3-1 Body composition components and corresponding nutritional assessment methods. (Modified from Blackburn, G.L., and Bothe, A.: Cancer Bulletin **30:**88, 1978.)

ious sites can be used for measurement of skinfold thickness, including thigh, calf, biceps, suprailiac, and chin. The summation of measurements taken at three or four different sites (Durnin's equation) may also be used. However, the most common method for assessing subcutaneous fat has been the use of triceps and subscapular skin folds. Triceps and subscapular skin folds are easier to measure, and the measurements tend to be more accurate than that of other skin folds in edematous patients.

Laboratory Determinations

Estimation of somatic and visceral protein mass can be obtained by laboratory tests. Depletion of somatic mass can be determined by measurement of 24-hour urinary creatinine excretion in the presence of normal renal function. Creatinine is the breakdown product of creatine, a liver-synthesized energy molecule that is stored in skeletal muscle. By measurement of the 24-hour urinary creatinine excretion in the absence of renal impairment, skeletal muscle mass is assessed indirectly. Known 24-hour urinary creatinine levels for normal adults of similar sex and height can be compared to an actual patient measurement. The ratio of the patient's 24-hour urinary creatinine excretion to normal values, expressed as a percentage, is called the creatinine-height index (CHI). A CHI of 100% indicates normal lean body mass. Depletion of lean body mass should result in a CHI of less than 80%.[8] Nevertheless, this methodology suffers from the use of "ideal" values found in tables and from the difficulties encountered in obtaining accurate 24-hour urine collections.

Visceral protein mass is estimated by measurement of plasma transport protein concentrations. The ideal measurable plasma protein should have a short half-life (high rate of synthesis and catabolism) with few factors altering catabolism.[36] Current laboratory methods measure plasma levels of albumin, transferrin, prealbumin, and retinol-binding protein.

Serum albumin concentration is not an ideal transport protein for estimation of visceral protein mass. Its metabolic half-life is approximately 20 days. Albumin is present to a great extent in the extravascular space, which affects its rate of catabolism. Albumin can be mobilized from this pool into the vascular space. In addition, hydrational changes may affect serum concentrations. Thus serum concentrations may not adequately assess visceral protein mass, particularly in the acute setting. Nevertheless, depressed serum albumin concentrations are associated with chronic visceral protein mass depletion when plasma levels fall below 3.0 g/ml.

Plasma transferrin concentration is a better estimate of visceral protein mass. It has a metabolic half-life of 8 days and has a smaller total body pool. Hepatic transferrin synthesis rates may be affected by different nutrient deficiencies (e.g., iron deficiency) that have marked underlying protein depletion.

Finally, short half-life proteins such as prealbumin and retinol-binding protein have also been used for estimation of visceral protein mass. Prealbumin is involved in the transport of thyroid hormone. It has a metabolic half-life of 2 days. However, it is rapidly depressed in nonmalnourished patients with traumatic injuries or sepsis.[46] Retinol-binding protein has a metabolic half-life of 12 hours. This serum protein is considered unreliable in patients with renal failure because it is cleared by the kidneys. In addition, it is very sensitive to other factors, including stress, which has limited its clinical use.

Immune Competence

Anergy to skin-test antigens has been shown to be a predictor of septic complications.[60] Although delayed cutaneous hypersensitivity is usually considered a test specifically for cell-mediated immunity, both cell-mediated and humoral immune responses are interrelated. Specifically, subsets of T lymphocytes, T-helper, and T-suppressor cells

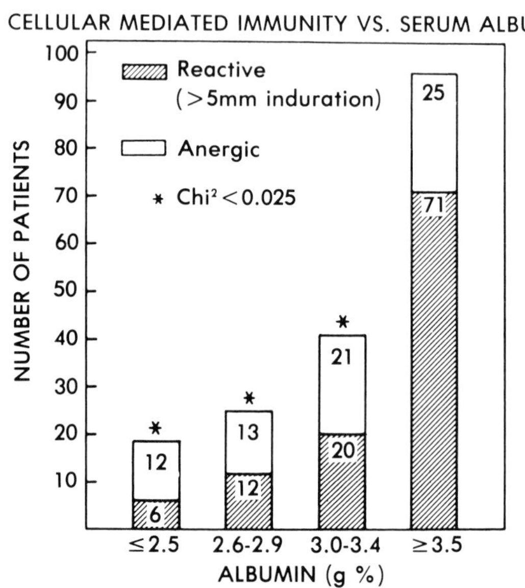

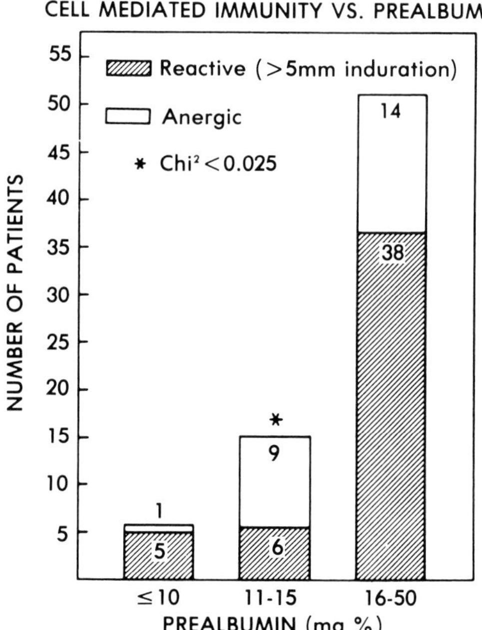

Fig. 3-2 Correlation of cell-mediated immunity with laboratory markers of nutritional status. (Modified from Grant, J.P., Custer, P.B., and Thurlow, J.: Surg. Clin. North Am. **61**:437, 1981.)

interact with B cells, allowing and controlling the ability of B cells to produce antibodies. Therefore depression of T-cell function as measured by anergy to skin-test antigens helps assess the ability of the patient to mount an immune response to injury and infection. Various skin-test antigens used include mumps, tuberculin, and *Candida* species. A positive response has a diameter of induration greater than 5 mm. A patient is considered anergic if induration fails to form to all skin-test antigens, although a graded system of immune responsiveness may be used.

The immune system may be depressed in old age and by trauma, inhalational anesthetic agents, drugs, malignancy, and oncologic therapy.[47,64] Malnutrition is also associated with impairment of the immune response.[57] Reversal of skin test anergy in malnourished patients has been demonstrated following nutritional repletion.[28] This supports the belief that nutritional intervention is useful in immune-suppressed patients. Nevertheless, because of the complexity of the immune system, as well as the ability of various factors to alter the immune response, delayed cutaneous hypersensitivity skin testing should be considered complementary to other means of assessing nutritional status (Fig. 3-2).

Accuracy of Nutritional Assessment

There is no complete agreement on the accuracy and usefulness of the various techniques used to determine nutritional status because of the lack of one specific, accurate test to which the other techniques of nutritional assessment may be compared. The prognostic nutritional index (PNI) is an attempt to correlate various methods of nutritional assessment with the occurrence of postoperative morbidity and mortality through stepwise regression analyses[69] as shown below:

$$\text{PNI}(\%) = 158 - 16.6(\text{ALB}) - 0.78(\text{TSF}) - 0.20(\text{TFN}) - 5.8(\text{DH})$$

where PNI is an estimate of the risk of a complication occurring in an individual patient; ALB is the serum albumin concentration (g/100 ml); TSF is the triceps skinfold thickness (mm); TFN is the serum transferrin concentration (mg/100 ml); and DH is delayed hypersensitivity reactivity to any of three recall antigens (0 = nonreactive, 1 = <5 mm induration, 2 = >5 mm induration). The prognostic nutritional index has been shown to be accurate in predicting which surgical patients were at a high risk for postoperative morbidity and mortality. Application of perioperative nutritional support to patients considered to be high risk reduced postoperative morbidity and mortality in a retrospective study.[71] However, other investigators have questioned the ability of preoperative nutritional assessment to predict postoperative morbidity and mortality.[80]

The history and physical examination have been prospectively compared to anthropometric data, laboratory data, delayed cutaneous hypersensitivity, and highly sophisticated direct body composition analyses as a method of nutritional assessment.[3] Two clinicians trained in nutritional assessment techniques independently examined 59 patients and categorized them into one of three groups: normal, mild malnutrition, and severe malnutrition. The two examiners agreed on the classification in 48 of the 59 patients (81%). Furthermore, the clinical evaluation of nutritional status was then compared to the objective measurements. There was a significant correlation in all tests with the clinical status, except for total lymphocyte count. The clinical status was also able to separate the patients into groups with significantly different mean values for six of the nine objective measurements.

Finally, the investigators demonstrated that the morbidity of these patients correlated with the clinical nutritional status. They concluded that

> general clinical assessment is a reproducible and valid technique for evaluating nutritional status before surgery. Unless further studies show that laboratory measurements of nutritional status are more accurate than clinical evaluation or provide better prognostic information, we suggest that carefully performed history-taking and physical examinations are sufficient for nutritional assessment.[3]

However, it should also be noted that objective evaluation of nutritional status also correlated with clinical outcome and allowed a means to quantitate nutritional status changes with supplementation. These evaluations, however, are adjuncts to and not replacements for a thorough medical history and a complete physical examination.

ENTERAL NUTRITION

Use of an intact gastrointestinal tract for nutritional support should be the initial step in alimentation. The concept of enteral alimentation is not new; in patients unable to eat, ancient Egyptians and Greeks attempted artificial alimentation through the use of nutrient enemas and clysters. The use of large bore tubes with bolus "home-style" feeding was used in past years but was not well accepted because of patient discomfort with this technique. Recent technical advances, however, have improved the quality of the equipment and the method of delivery and have increased the spectrum of available nutrient formulas.

An understanding of intestinal physiology is important to a discussion of enteral nutrition because of the variety of dietary formulas and gastrointestinal abnormalities encountered in clinical situations. The reader should refer to discussions elsewhere in this book on intestinal physiology, digestion, and absorption.

Indications for Enteral Nutrition

Malnourished patients with an intact gastrointestinal tract should initially be given enteral nutritional support. The specific disease processes affecting oral nutrition are diverse. In general, patients who are unable or unwilling to eat or unable or unwilling to eat enough should be considered for enteral nutritional support.

Patients with upper gastrointestinal or oral malignancies commonly develop problems resulting in an inability to eat. Many patients develop difficulty in chewing or swallowing as a result of their underlying disease process. In addition, radiation or chemotherapy treatment for various malignancies may result in stomatitis, mucositis, or nausea, which may affect oral intake. Finally, some patients may have a functional intestinal tract but be unable to eat

Table 3-3 **INDICATIONS AND ROUTE FOR NUTRITIONAL SUPPLEMENTATION WITH NORMAL GASTROINTESTINAL FUNCTION**

Oral	Nasoenteric	Gastrostomy or jejunostomy
Normal nutritional status with increased nutritional needs	Difficulties in swallowing	Oral or upper GI: Obstruction Dysfunction Fistula
Mild protein-calorie malnutrition with normal or increased nutritional requirements	Increased nutritional needs	Chronic enteral nutritional support
	Moderate-to-severe protein-calorie malnutrition	
	Anorexia	

Modified from Hearne, B.E., and Daly, J.M.: Enteral nutrition. In Kirkpatrick, J., editor: Nutritional metabolism in the surgical patient, Mt. Kisco, N.Y., 1983, Futura Publishing Co., Inc.

as a result of proximal atrophy, obstruction, or fistula. These patients may receive enteral support through various enteric catheters.

Patients may be able to eat but often are unwilling to do so either because of a lack of desire to eat or because of unwanted side effects from eating. Patients with anorexia nervosa and cancer are commonly encountered in this category. Unwillingness to eat is probably the single most important cause of malnutrition in cancer patients.

Patients with substantially increased energy expenditures and catabolism often are unable or unwilling to eat enough to meet their requirements. Patients with major skeletal trauma or sepsis may have a 40% increase in energy expenditures, whereas those with major burns may have increases of 60% to 100% above normal levels. Such patients commonly require nutritional support.

Finally, patients may have difficulty in digestion or absorption of various nutrients because of anatomic or physiologic lesions; e.g., following total pancreatectomy there may be impaired digestion of fats, even with supplemental oral pancreatic enzymes. Patients undergoing abdominal radiation commonly develop inadequate terminal digestion and absorption of various nutrients.

Selection of Enteral Nutrient Delivery

Patients who require enteral nutritional supplementation may be supported through various routes of administration. These are either oral, nasoenteric, or enteric (gastrostomy or jejunostomy) (Table 3-3). The selection of the route of administration should parallel the underlying indication for nutritional support. In general, patients with only moderately insufficient oral intake may be supplemented orally with aggressive dietary counseling. Patients with more severe deficiencies of higher nutrient needs commonly require tube feedings (Table 3-3).[48]

Use of silicone rubber or polyurethane small-bore feeding tubes has significantly reduced patient discomfort caused by older, large-bore, inflexible nasogastric tubes. Longer catheters with mercury-weighted ends may be used for nasoduodenal feedings. For patients who require long-term enteral support, surgically placed gastrostomy or jejunostomy catheters are more direct routes for feedings. These feeding enterostomies have been considered a routine part of complicated surgical procedures by some surgeons.[40]

Table 3-4 **JEJUNOSTOMY FEEDING SCHEDULE***

Day	Strength	Dosage (ml/hour)
1	¼	50
2	½	75
3	½	100
4	¾	100
5	Full	100

*Volume increase precedes concentration increase in jejunostomy feeding schedule.

Gastric feedings are advantageous in some patients. Osmolality of the feeding formula is rarely of significant consideration because of the ability of the stomach to dilute hyperosmolar solutions. In addition, bolus feedings may be used and thereby reduce patient care time. However, gastric outlet obstruction, obtundation, or laryngeal incompetence are contraindications for this mode of feedings because of the high incidence of aspiration.[76]

Jejunal feedings require continuous pump infusions. Diarrhea is more commonly encountered than in gastric feedings because of the delivery of hyperosmolar feedings into the small intestine. The presence of hyperosmolar solutions in the intestine results in diffusion of water into the intestinal lumen. In order to reduce the incidence of diarrhea, jejunal feedings should be started with dilute solutions, and the concentration of feedings increased only after the patient is tolerating adequate volumes (Table 3-4). If diarrhea persists, antiperistaltic agents may be added to the feeding formula, or the delivery rate may be decreased.

Dietary Formulations

Currently available dietary formulations may be divided among blenderized formulas, nutritionally complete commercial formulas, chemically defined formulas, and modular formulas.

Blenderized tube feedings may be composed of any food that can be blenderized. These may be prepared at home or may be commercial preparations. Caloric distribution of these formulas should parallel a normal diet. Blenderized

Table 3-5 **POTENTIAL COMPLICATIONS OF ENTERAL NUTRITION AND ASSOCIATED PREVENTIVE MEASURES**

Complication	Prevention
MECHANICAL	
Regurgitation and aspiration	Elevate patient to 30-degree angle
Tube or ostomy leak or malfunction	Use careful surgical technique and local care
Erosion of external nares	Tape tube to prevent contact with nares
Erosion of tube lumen	Use small diameter silicone rubber or polyurethane tubes
Clogging of tube lumen	Irrigate before and after feeding with 50 ml tepid water; use appropriate bore tube with formula and mode of administration
Otitis media	Use small bore, soft feeding tube
GASTROINTESTINAL	
Nausea, vomiting, or bloating	Reduce flow rate; increase time interval between intermittent feedings
Diarrhea or cramping	Reduce flow rate; reduce formula concentration; appropriate formula selection
METABOLIC	
Hyperglycemia and glycosuria, osmotic diuresis, and hyperosmotic dehydration	Monitor urine for glucose and acetone; blood glucose; serum electrolytes
Edema	Monitor body weight; fluid and salt requirements; intake and output
Prerenal azotemia	Monitor blood urea nitrogen and creatinine

Modified from Hearne, B.E., and Daly, J.M.: Enteral nutrition. In Kirkpatrick, J., editor: Nutritional metabolism in the surgical patient, Mt. Kisco, N.Y., 1983, Futura Publishing Co., Inc.

formulas are indicated most often in patients with feeding gastrostomies unable to eat by mouth.

Nutritionally complete commercial formulas vary in protein, carbohydrate, and fat composition. Several are flavored and are considered suitable for oral supplementation. Several formulas use sucrose or glucose as carbohydrate sources and are suitable for lactose-deficient patients. Commercial formulas are convenient, sterile, low cost; they are the most frequently used diet given to patients requiring tube feedings.

Chemically defined formulas are commonly called elemental diets. The nutrients are provided in a predigested and readily absorbed form. These diets are not often used in oral feedings since the presence of amino acids in the formula markedly reduces its palatability. They are useful in patients with digestive disturbances, e.g., in patients with radiation enteritis or pancreatic insufficiency. However, they are more expensive than nutritionally complete commercial formulas and are hyperosmolar, which may cause cramping and diarrhea.

Modular formulations include special formulas used for specific nutrient needs or because of organ dysfunction. Single-nutrient formulas are used to modify other enteral formulas, tailoring them for specific needs. Patients with renal or hepatic failure may require specialized modular formulas that take into account underlying fluid and amino acid abnormalities.

Complications of Enteral Nutrition

Complications of enteral nutrition may be considered mechanical, gastrointestinal, or metabolic (Table 3-5). Mechanical problems relate to the placement and care of tubes used for feedings. In general, placement of the tubes should be followed by radiologic verification of proper intraluminal positioning. Intraoperative placement of a jejunostomy can be verified by the installation of saline into the catheter while the jejunum is compressed immediately distal to the catheter. Placement of small-bore nasogastric tubes should always be verified radiologically before initiation of feedings, particularly if they are placed in obtunded patients or patients with a poor cough reflex. The presence of symptoms of peritoneal irritation in patients being fed through a jejunostomy tube warrants further evaluation to ensure that dislodgement of the catheter has not resulted in the intraperitoneal delivery of feedings. Attachment of the stomach or small bowel to the anterior abdominal wall reduces the chance of accidental intraperitoneal catheter dislodgement.

Gastrointestinal side effects of enteral feedings are common. These include abdominal distention, diarrhea, and vomiting. Gastric feedings usually are better tolerated by bolus infusion. However, the presence of 200 ml or more residual volume may indicate gastric atony or distal obstruction. Feedings should be stopped in patients with this quantity of residual volume. Proper monitoring of residual volume reduces the incidence of vomiting. Patients being fed intragastrically should be started on small amounts of full-strength formulas, with gradually increasing volumes as tolerated.

Patients being fed through a jejunostomy tube are more likely to develop diarrhea than when other delivery routes are used. The presence of the hyperosmolar feeding in the proximal small intestine results in a passive diffusion of water into the lumen to render the intraluminal contents isotonic. If the infusion rate is too rapid for a given osmolality, diarrhea occurs. Therefore patients with jejunostomies should be able to tolerate a sufficient volume of the infusate before the concentration is increased. If diarrhea occurs, either an antiperistaltic agent should be added to the infusate, or its rate of delivery decreased until symptoms abate. Finally, each patient should be matched to a defined formula. This should reduce the incidence of gastrointestinal side effects in patients with lactose intolerance caused by infusion of a lactose-based carbohydrate source. Additionally, patients not demonstrating a specific need for elemental diets could be fed other nutritionally balanced commercial formulas that may be less hyperosmolar and less expensive.

Metabolic complications can occur with enteral feedings. Glucose intolerance can result from the relative infusion of too much glucose. Patients receiving tube feedings, particularly those with constant infusions, should be monitored serially for blood and urine glucose levels. Diabetic patients may require exogenous insulin or a lower rate of nutrient delivery. Hypertonic dehydration can result from the intraluminal loss of free water. Free water can be given to reduce the chance of this occurring. Infusion rates can also be reduced if the problem develops.

Tube feedings may be contraindicated in situations of severe gastrointestinal dysfunction, upper gastrointestinal bleeding, and intractable vomiting and diarrhea. Nasogastric feedings are especially contraindicated in obtunded patients.

Clinical Trials of Enteral Nutrition

Enteral nutrition has been favorably compared to parenteral nutrition in several clinical trials. Rombeau and Barot[76] compared 10 seriously ill patients fed enterally with 10 similar patients given total parenteral nutrition and demonstrated that the patients given enteral nutrition achieved better nitrogen balances.[76] Other studies have consistently demonstrated that patients on enteral nutrition achieve at least similar nutritional gains when compared to patients on total parenteral nutrition.[2,14]

McArdle and associates[62] compared nutritional benefits in patients randomized to receive enteral or parenteral nutrition. Although the nitrogen balances from both groups were similar, the patients on parenteral nutrition demonstrated high levels of blood cortisol and plasma insulin concentrations compared to those patients on enteral nutrition. In addition, patients receiving parenteral alimentation also demonstrated a significant decrease in free fatty acid levels compared to the other group. This was presumably the result of decreased lipolysis as a result of increased circulating insulin levels present in the group receiving parenteral nutrition. Other benefits of enteral nutrition included decreased cost, ease of solution handling, and decreased septic complications.

PARENTERAL NUTRITION

The ability to provide complete, intravenous feedings to patients in a clinically practical manner has been appreciated since the late 1960s.[32] The application of total parenteral nutrition (TPN), as an adjunct or as primary therapy to a variety of clinical situations has resulted in its general acceptance as a safe, clinically useful technique. Although relatively few major advances in the delivery techniques of TPN have been made since 1968, widespread application of TPN has resulted in a greater understanding of underlying physiologic principles. In turn, this has allowed a standardization of methodology with a resultant decrease in complications associated with TPN.

Indications

The initial application of TPN was as supportive care in critically ill patients with severe nutritional deficiencies. The technique of feeding these patients parenterally was initially referred to as hyperalimentation. However, more recent studies demonstrated its usefulness in patients who were not nutritionally depleted but who required only maintenance of their nutritional state. Although the ability to improve clinical outcome through the judicious application of TPN has been demonstrated in several disease states such as in enterocutaneous fistulae, in other situations the evidence of improved clinical outcome has been indirect. For example, for a variety of reasons it has been difficult to demonstrate improved clinical outcome by the addition of TPN in patients with cancer undergoing chemotherapy, although cellular immunity and nutritional status may be improved. The greatest difficulty in conducting these clinical trials in a randomized prospective fashion is the ethical dilemma of not feeding patients who are severely malnourished. Therefore the evidence for improved clinical outcome in these situations may continue to be indirect.

TPN should be initiated in patients who fulfill the following three criteria: (1) patients who are malnourished or as a result of their medical care are unable to maintain their current nutritional state; (2) patients who cannot maintain an adequate enteral intake or who do not have a functional gastrointestinal tract; and (3) patients whose clinical outcome is improved by the application of TPN.

Techniques

The provision of hypertonic nutrient solutions necessitates the use of a large-bore, high-flow vein, to decrease the possibility of thrombophlebitis. These criteria are met by delivery of these solutions into the superior vena cava. Infraclavicular percutaneous subclavian venous catheterization has been a safe and effective method since its use for delivery of TPN was initiated by Dudrick and associates.[32] Although delivery of TPN into the superior vena cava may be accomplished by other methods of catheter introduction by way of the saphenous, basilic, or jugular (external and internal) veins, the higher incidence of infection and thrombophlebitis with these techniques precludes their use except when subclavian vein catheterization is contraindicated.[26]

After the patient has been reassured and the procedure explained, insertion of the subclavian catheter is best accomplished with the patient in a slight Trendelenburg position, with a sheet roll placed longitudinally under the spine. The skin of the shoulder, neck, and chest is shaved, defatted with acetone, and covered with a povidone-iodine solution. The infraclavicular area is draped, and local anesthesia is infiltrated into the skin and periosteum of the inferior portion of the clavicle at its midpoint. Venipuncture is accomplished by introduction of a large-bore needle attached to a syringe into the area anesthetized and advancement of the needle paralleled to the floor, aiming at the suprasternal notch. A flashback of venous blood signals successful venipuncture. The patient is asked to perform the Valsalva maneuver as the syringe is removed, and the catheter is introduced without forcing. The needle is withdrawn, the catheter at its entrance site anchored to the skin with a suture, and its end attached to the intravenous tubing. The bottle of intravenous fluid is lowered to ensure venous return into the tubing. A sterile, secure dressing is then placed over the introduction site, and a chest x-ray film is taken to ensure accurate placement of the catheter tip without pneumothorax.

TPN may be initiated after the chest x-ray film confirms correct positioning of the catheter. Although many patients will be able to tolerate their calculated caloric requirements initially, a gradual increase in caloric loads until requirement levels are reached is preferable. The solutions may be prepared with lower amounts of dextrose initially and increased gradually, with full amounts of nitrogen, trace minerals, vitamins, and fluids provided daily. Full-strength solutions may also be prepared initially but delivered at lower rates, which are gradually increased as tolerated by the patient. In either instance, similar guidelines for patient management should be followed. Body weight should be measured daily, vital signs should be taken at least every 4 hours, and fluid balance observed every 8 hours. Urinary sugar and acetone should be measured every 6 hours; whereas serum electrolyte concentrations, blood urea nitrogen, and blood glucose should be measured at least daily until stable and every 2 days thereafter. Liver function studies, serum albumin, calcium, and phosphorus should be determined weekly.

Complications

Potential complications of TPN may be divided into technical, infectious, and metabolic.

Although subclavian vein catheterization is widely used, it is not free of potential complications. These complications can be minimized by rigid adherence to the previously described techniques. If catheterization is performed by those who have performed few catheterizations, adequate supervision can further reduce the incidence of complications. A list of potential complications associated with catheterization of the superior vena cava is summarized in the boxed material at right. Arterial puncture during catheterization is indicated by the filling of a syringe with bright red blood. The needle should be withdrawn, and firm pressure applied for several minutes. Pneumothorax is the most common technical complication. This may be suggested if air is aspirated into the syringe during insertion. The needle should be withdrawn, and the patient observed for signs of respiratory distress. A chest x-ray film should be obtained to rule out pneumothorax and to check the catheter position after all insertions. TPN should not be initiated until the chest x-ray film is reviewed. This will reduce the incidence of hydrothorax. Catheter embolism is an iatrogenic complication that may occur when the catheter is withdrawn through the needle used for insertion, either for repositioning of the catheter or after a failed venipuncture. Joint withdrawal of the catheter and needle should eliminate this complication.

Infectious complications associated with TPN are potentially serious. Contamination may occur as a result of faulty techniques of catheter insertion or maintenance, infusion of contaminated solutions, or use of the subclavian catheter for other purposes such as infusion of medications. Most patients receiving TPN are predisposed to infectious complications because of the nature of the underlying disease, their nutritional state, and interference of host defense mechanisms from treatment.[82]

Management of patients who become febrile while receiving TPN requires a methodic approach because of the potential seriousness of catheter sepsis. A diligent examination and fever workup should be instituted to rule out other potential sources of the fever. Failure to demonstrate another cause requires removal of the nutrient solution and tubing. Cultures of the solution, peripheral blood, and central venous blood should be taken. Positive cultures, cardiovascular instability, or persistent fever require replacement of the indwelling catheter. To avoid complications

COMPLICATIONS OF CENTRAL VENOUS CATHETERIZATION

- Pleural space
  - Pneumothorax
  - Tension pneumothorax
  - Hemothorax
  - Hydrothorax (intrapleural infusion)
- Mediastinum
  - Hemomediastinum
  - Hydromediastinum
  - Superior vena cava syndrome
- Neck
  - Subcutaneous emphysema
  - Arterial injury (hematoma, arteriovenous malformation, false aneurysm, stenosis)
    - Subclavian artery
    - Carotid artery
    - Cervical and thoracic arteries
  - Nerve injury
    - Phrenic nerve
    - Vagus nerve
    - Recurrent laryngeal nerve
    - Brachial plexus
  - Lymphatic injury to the thoracic duct
  - Tracheal injury
- Veins
  - Laceration with hemorrhage
  - Air embolism
  - Catheter embolism (paradoxic embolism)
  - Cardiac arrhythmia
  - Myocardial perforation (hydropericardium, tamponade)
  - Coronary sinus block (tamponade)
  - Venobronchial fistula
  - Hepatic vein thrombosis
  - Superior vena cava thrombosis (pulmonary embolism)
  - Catheter sepsis

Modified from Ryan, J.A.: Complications of total parenteral nutrition. In Fischer, J.E., editor: Total parenteral nutrition, Boston, 1976, Little, Brown & Co., Inc.

Table 3-6 **METABOLIC COMPLICATIONS AND POSSIBLE CAUSES ASSOCIATED WITH TPN**

Complication	Possible Cause
Carbohydrate Metabolism	
Hyperglycemia	Excessive rate of infusion of glucose Insufficient endogenous insulin secretion Sepsis Glucocorticoids
Hyperosmolar nonketotic dehydration (hyperosmolar syndrome)	Persistent hyperglycemia Osmotic diuresis Dehydration
Hypoglycemia	Abrupt interruption of TPN infusion Excessive insulin
Amino Acid Metabolism	
Elevated blood urea nitrogen	Intrinsic renal disease Dehydration Excessive rate of infusion of amino acids Low caloric nitrogen ratio of TPN solution
Hyperammonemia	Intrinsic liver disease
Electrolyte and Mineral Metabolism	
Hypokalemia	Insufficient potassium intake relative to losses and anabolic requirements
Hypophosphatemia	Insufficient phosphate intake relative to losses and anabolic requirements
Hypomagnesemia	Insufficient magnesium intake relative to losses and anabolic requirements

Modified from Reinhardt, G.F.: Surg. Clin. North Am. **57**:1283, 1977.

associated with catheter reinsertion, the catheter may be changed over a guide wire. The tip of the removed catheter should be cultured, and broad spectrum antibiotics initiated if blood cultures continue to remain positive.

Table 3-6 reviews common potential metabolic complications of TPN. Infusions of hypercaloric solutions may result in glucose intolerance. A normal adult can use 0.5 g of glucose per kilogram per hour. For a 70-kg person, this extrapolates to the use of 3500 calories per day. Patients who are severely catabolic, as is often the case in burns, polytrauma, and severe sepsis, may use up to 6000 calories per day. However, glucose tolerance is often unpredictable. In addition, many patients will be either frankly diabetic or may have underlying disease that renders them relatively glucose intolerant, as may be the case in severe sepsis or trauma. Therefore these patients may exceed the glucose renal threshold with resultant hyperglycemia and glucosuria. Diligent monitoring of urinary sugar and blood glucose levels is necessary to prevent potentially severe complications from occurring.

The ability of patients to metabolize large glucose loads is directly related to their ability to mount an insulin response to the infused glucose. Studies conducted on the insulin response in nondiabetic patients receiving TPN have demonstrated several points: (1) abrupt initiation of hypercaloric feedings results in insulin levels four to six times basal levels by 6 hours; (2) continued infusion is associated with lowering of both the insulin and glucose levels; (3) the glucose tolerance test was normal during TPN, demonstrating the ability of the normal pancreas to increase insulin production if faced with increasing glucose load; and (4) cessation of TPN does not usually result in rebound hypoglycemia.[81] Diabetic patients cannot mount an insulin response, or their hormonal response may be inadequate. Other patients with severe sepsis or polytrauma may have diminished ability to produce sufficient insulin relative to the hyperglycemic state (Fig. 3-3). In addition, increased adrenal stimulation with resultant increased production of glucocorticoids also influences glucose tolerance in these patients. Finally, although rebound hypoglycemia is usually not a complication of TPN cessation in normal patients, a gradual reduction of TPN or use of a hypocaloric dextrose infusion after TPN is stopped is recommended.

To avoid osmotic diuresis, TPN is maintained at a rate that results in blood glucose levels below 225 mg/100 ml and urinary glucose levels below 2 g/100 ml. Patients with diabetes mellitus or persistent glycosuria will require exogenous administration of crystalline insulin, which may be added to the nutrient solution in dosages up to 60 U/1000 calories to achieve a reduction in blood glucose concentration. This protocol should prevent the development of nonketotic hyperosmolar coma that occurs when the rate of glucose infusion far exceeds the ability of the cells to metabolize glucose leading to hyperglycemia, glycosuria, and osmotic diuresis. Dehydration and coma may ensue and should be treated along the same lines as the management of diabetic coma by stopping the hypertonic carbohydrate infusion and giving intravenous fluids, electrolytes, and insulin to normalize hydration, acid-base balance, and blood glucose. Patients at risk include those with sepsis, burns, polytrauma, or diabetes mellitus. Treatment consists of infusion of dextrose solutions with isotonic or half-strength saline plus insulin. Measurement of serum electrolytes and blood glucose levels, as well as clinical assessment, will allow appropriate rehydration.

Infusion of amino acid solutions is also associated with potential complications. A rising blood urea nitrogen level

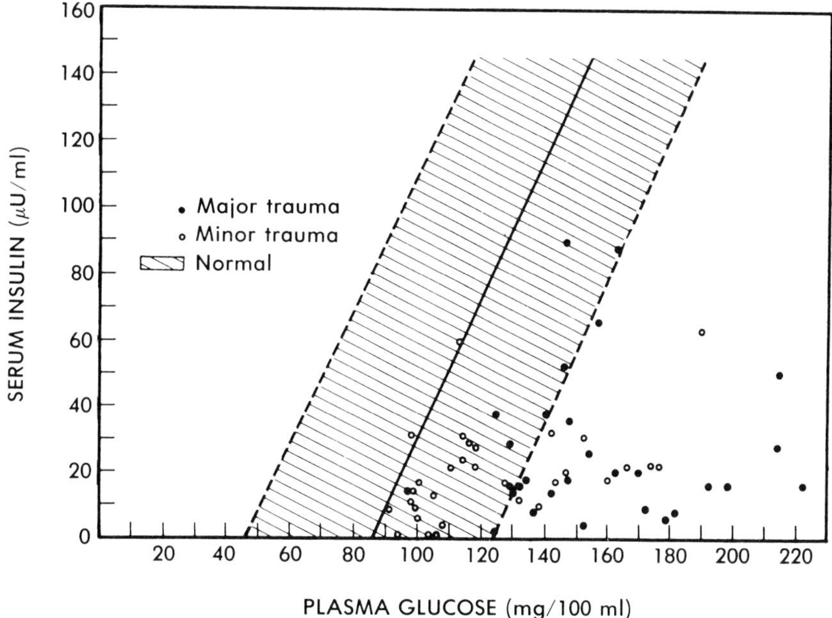

Fig. 3-3 Demonstration of elevated plasma glucose concentrations with inappropriately low insulin levels in patients with minor and major trauma. Normal levels are represented by the heavy line with two standard deviations. (Modified from Meguid, M.M., et al.: Arch. Surg. **109**:776, 1974. Copyright 1974, American Medical Association.)

may be indicative of excess provision of amino acids, prerenal azotemia, renal disease, or a combination of all three. Reduction of the amino acid load and appropriate hydration is the treatment of choice. Hyperammonemia primarily occurs in patients with hepatic disease. Although it may be related to free ammonia infused in protein hydrolysates, this entity can occur with infusions of crystalline amino acids that contain essentially no free ammonia.[49]

Hyperchloremic metabolic acidosis can occur with infusions of crystalline amino acids because of the liberation of hydrochloric acid as the amino acids are used. Reducing the chloride intake decreases the incidence of metabolic acidosis. This reduction may be accomplished by providing potassium and sodium as their acetate salts.[49]

Serum electrolyte and trace metal abnormalities are a common complication of TPN. These deficiencies can be the result of inadequate intake to compensate for losses or because of the increased requirements during continued anabolism. These ions include potassium, phosphorus, calcium, and magnesium. Potassium may be further depleted as a result of the intracellular influx of potassium secondary to the infusion of dextrose and increased serum insulin levels.

TPN can result in significant hypophosphatemia, characterized by malaise, lethargy, perioral paresthesias, tremors, and dysarthrias. Progression can lead to coma and death. Phosphorus is an essential intracellular anion involved in protein synthesis. Trapping of the ion in protein synthesis may result in hypophosphatemia. Phosphorus should be added to TPN in doses of 15 to 30 mEq/L in ordinary circumstances and 30 to 50 mEq/L in severely malnourished patients.

Calcium and magnesium are also required for the anabolic process. Calcium should be added to TPN in amounts of 4.5 to 9 mEq daily. In pediatric patients, 4 mEq/kg of body weight should be added daily. Approximately 24 mEq of magnesium daily are required for normal adults. These levels may be increased in severely malnourished patients who may also manifest evidence of zinc and selenium deficiencies. Renal function should be observed closely because requirements for electrolytes and minerals may be reduced.

Essential fatty acid deficiency may result in patients infused with fat-free dextrose and amino acid solutions. This is reflected in the lowered serum levels of linoleic and arachidonic acids and increased serum eicosatrienoic acid. The deficiency may be corrected by the infusion of a fat emulsion in amounts of about 10% of nonprotein calories. Currently, fat emulsions are available in concentrations of 10% or 20%.

Other metabolic complications, including fluid overload, vitamin abnormalities, and trace element deficiencies, are usually iatrogenic and may be easily corrected by provision of daily supplements of vitamin and mineral supplements to replenish deficiencies and replace ongoing losses (Table 3-7).

Glucose vs. Fat

The use of fat emulsions as a calorie source for parenteral feedings in patients has been investigated for many years. The ability to provide nitrogen parenterally by infusion of protein hydrolysates has been available since the 1930s but was not used clinically because of the absence of a feasible means to provide calories. In the late 1960s, Dudrick and associates[32] were able to demonstrate normal growth in puppies and infants through the use of amino acid solutions and hypertonic dextrose infused into the superior vena cava. Consequently, dextrose was the pre-

Table 3-7 **FLUID AND NUTRITIONAL DEFICIENCIES DURING TPN**

Deficiency	Supplemental Feeding Technique
Water	Decrease rate of TPN infusion Administer 5% dextrose in water intravenously Replace using enteric feedings; water or dilute nutritional solution
Iron	Use appropriate dosage of intramuscular iron preparation
Trace elements (copper, zinc, manganese, chromium, cobalt, fluoride)	Present in variable and usually insufficient amounts as contaminants in TPN solutions; present to some degree in blood and blood products Replace using enteric feedings; trace element concentrates, elemental diets, liquid or higher diets
Essential fatty acids	Replace using enteric feedings, intravenous fat preparations

Modified from Reinhardt, G.F.: Surg. Clin. North Am. **57:**1283, 1977.

ferred caloric source. Further modifications in preparation techniques of parenteral fat emulsions reduced many of the complications associated with their early use, including fever and infection.

Parenteral fat emulsions contain soybean oil as a source of fatty acids, an emulsifier (egg yolk phospholipid in Intralipid), and other agents to obtain isotonicity such as glycerol. Administration of a fat emulsion as a calorie source has theoretic advantages. Because of the higher caloric value of fats compared to glucose, more total calories can be provided by fat emulsions than by glucose if equal amounts are given. In addition, fat emulsions are isotonic and therefore may be delivered by way of peripheral veins. For these reasons, parenteral fat emulsions have distinct advantages in certain types of peripheral parenteral nutrition that will be discussed later.

The use of fat emulsions eliminates the potential complication of essential fatty acid deficiency that may result from fat-free TPN. Fatty acids are required for several important functions, including prostaglandin synthesis and cholesterol metabolism. The most important fatty acids appear to be linoleic, linolenic, and arachidonic acid, of which only linoleic is considered essential.

The absence of fatty acid intake in long-term TPN patients is associated with fatty acid deficiency.[63] Levels of linoleic and arachidonic acids are decreased. As the level of linoleic acid decreases, serum levels of oleic acid, an endogenous fatty acid, increase. In turn, elongation and desaturation of oleic acid lead to increases of eicosatrienoic acid, a fatty acid that is considered unique to essential fatty acid deficiency. Depletion of essential fatty acids may lead to an impaired immune response, impaired wound healing, and platelet dysfunction. Clinically, the presence of dry, scaly skin, hair loss, and delayed wound healing may be related to an essential fatty acid deficiency.

The use of fat emulsions has been investigated in several clinical trials. Jeejeebhoy and associates[53] compared nitrogen balances in two groups of patients with gastrointestinal disease. Both groups received equal amounts of amino acids, minerals, and vitamins daily. Nonprotein calories were provided as 100% dextrose in one group and by 17% dextrose/83% lipid in the other group. There was no significant difference in nitrogen balance between the two groups. In the lipid-based group, there was a rise in free fatty acids and ketone bodies with concomitant lower insulin levels, demonstrating that lipid had become the major energy source. Other investigators compared the effects of different levels of dextrose and lipid intake on protein metabolism and demonstrated no disadvantage as long as significant amounts of fat calories were provided.[4,59]

The infusion of lipid-based TPN to critically ill patients remains controversial. The use of lipid-based TPN eliminates the incidence of essential fatty acid deficiency, which may be more prevalent in patients with increased requirements for fatty acids. In addition, many of these patients have concurrent respiratory problems and may require ventilatory support. The use of hypercaloric dextrose infusions in these patients theoretically results in increased glucose oxidation with resultant increased carbon dioxide production. This may increase ventilatory demands and may result in respiratory and acid/base complications.[13] However, Long and co-workers[58] studied the use of fat emulsions in injured patients and demonstrated that nitrogen conservation is accomplished if dextose calories are infused at levels corresponding to the resting metabolic rate. The provision of fat calories did not correlate with nitrogen-sparing efficacy of TPN.

Because of the relatively cheaper costs associated with dextrose-based regimens compared to lipid-based regimens, the use of fat as the major caloric source may be justified only in patients with respiratory difficulties, glucose intolerance, and subclavian vein thrombosis (preventing infusion of hypercaloric dextrose infusions centrally). The clearest indication for the infusion of fat emulsions is in the prevention of essential fatty acid deficiency and as a supplemental source of parenteral calories.

Peripheral Parenteral Nutrition

The parenteral solution most widely used perioperatively to reduce protein catabolism is hypocaloric dextrose. A 1 L amount of a 5% dextrose solution yields 50 g of carbohydrate. This is obviously insufficient to meet the patient's energy requirements at an average level of total fluid intake. However, nitrogen balance is improved in patients receiving a hypocaloric dextrose solution when compared with patients receiving saline solutions without dextrose. Theoretically, the carbohydrate calorie intake in hypocaloric dextrose infusions is used for endogenous caloric needs. This in turn reduces the caloric requirements to be provided by gluconeogenesis. Substrates for hepatic gluconeogenesis are derived from the catabolism of peripheral muscle, providing amino acids (predominantly alanine) as a carbon skeleton source for the endogenous conversion to glucose. By providing at least some calories exogenously, the rate of gluconeogenesis and, in turn, protein catabolism is reduced. However, infusion of dextrose alone does not eliminate the requirements for amino acids other than as an energy source.

In order to reduce protein losses further, Blackburn and associates[9] proposed infusions of amino acid solutions to patients without a caloric source. They demonstrated that, in contrast to hypocaloric dextrose solutions, infusions of amino acids alone would result in nitrogen balance in surgical patients. It was theorized that the provision of amino acids reduced the requirements of endogenous protein as a calorie source (through hepatic gluconeogenesis) and as visceral and transport substrates. Caloric requirements would be met partially by the hepatic conversion of endogenous and exogenous amino acids to glucose. Most of the caloric requirements in other tissues were provided by endogenous fat stores that were mobilized as a result of decreased insulin levels. Increased lipolysis was reflected by increased serum levels of free fatty acids and ketone bodies.

Other investigators were also able to demonstrate improved nitrogen balance in patients receiving amino acid solutions compared to patients receiving only hypocaloric dextrose.[24] However, the advantage of infusing only amino acid solutions as opposed to amino acids plus hypocaloric dextrose has been disputed by others.[34] These latter investigators were able to demonstrate improvement in nitrogen balance when hypocaloric dextrose was added to the amino acid infusions. It was speculated that the advantages of low insulin and glucose levels were overstated and that infusions of hypocaloric glucose simply allow adjustments to be made of how much fat is actually mobilized to meet caloric requirements.[84]

The use of protein-sparing solutions has been compared to TPN and hypocaloric dextrose infusions in surgical patients.[24] Although nitrogen balance was improved when either TPN or amino acid solutions were infused postoperatively, there was no difference in clinical outcome between those patients receiving hypocaloric dextrose and those receiving amino acids. Indeed, only patients receiving TPN were able to demonstrate clinical improvement. It seems clear that TPN is preferable in patients who require more nutritional support than can be provided by hypocaloric dextrose.

Because of the increased costs of protein-sparing amino acid solutions and the inability to improve clinical outcome, their routine perioperative use is contraindicated. It appears that they can be best used in those patients (e.g., obese patients) who may benefit from only nitrogen-sparing without actual anabolism. Finally, this regimen is useful in those patients who require nutritional support but in whom subclavian vein catheterization is contraindicated. In the latter group of patients, caloric requirements may be met by peripheral infusions of isotonic fat emulsions.

Specialized Amino Acid Solutions

The ability to modify calorie sources, calorie and nitrogen quantities, trace minerals, vitamins, and fluid volumes allows the physician to tailor nutrients to suit the specific needs of the patient. Certain clinical situations may require different proportions or elimination of certain amino acids. Three specific clinical settings have created roles for specialized amino acid formulations.

Renal Insufficiency

Renal insufficiency, whether functional or organic, is a common complication in patients following multiple trauma or sepsis. Acute renal failure that occurs in this setting is often reversible and is characterized by increased protein catabolism combined with an inability to excrete protein breakdown products. The result is an increase in blood urea nitrogen with concurrent loss of body cell mass. Nutritional intervention in this setting is complicated by the patient's inability to tolerate normal nitrogen or fluid volumes in standard TPN regimens.

Patients with oliguric renal insufficiency should be given sufficient fluid to compensate for insensible and measurable losses. Additional fluid may be deleterious. Therefore protein and calorie administration must be tailored for these limitations. Guidelines for fluid intake may be liberalized in patients undergoing peritoneal dialysis and hemodialysis.

An obvious limiting factor in the provision of protein is the contribution of that protein to the underlying azotemia. Protein catabolism can be reduced by provision of adequate calories, as in other catabolic states. Nevertheless, positive nitrogen balance cannot be achieved by high calorie intake only; protein must be given concurrently. Protein catabolism results in amino acids entering into a metabolic pool from which the individual amino acids are either reused for protein synthesis or further deaminated with resultant urea production. The goal of nutritional intervention in patients with renal failure should be to provide sufficient protein to meet demands for protein synthesis with a reduction in protein catabolism.[52] Nutritional therapy with the use of high-calorie, low-protein diets in a setting of renal failure has resulted in improved nitrogen balance, weight gain, and reduction of blood urea nitrogen concentration.[44]

Provision of high-quality protein or essential amino acids alone allows use of available urea for production of nonessential amino acids, reduction of the nitrogen load and blood urea nitrogen levels, and achievement of positive nitrogen balance. Dietary therapy in the surgical patient with renal insufficiency is often hindered by gastrointestinal dysfunction resulting from the underlying pathology, operative treatment, hypermetabolic states, and renal insufficiency itself. The efficacy of parenteral administration of essential amino acids and hypertonic dextrose was demonstrated by Dudrick and associates,[31] who showed improvement of nitrogen balance and weight gain with concomitant maintenance or reduction in blood urea nitrogen levels.

Controversy exists as to the proper amino acid mixture to use in renal failure patients. Caloric intake should be high with concomitant fluid and nitrogen restriction.

Whether nitrogen sources of only essential amino acids or a combination of essential and nonessential amino acids are more efficacious remains debatable. Some investigators have reasoned that, since these patients are hypercatabolic, perhaps a mixture of essential and nonessential amino acids can more adequately provide nitrogen requirements.[5] Others have reasoned that, because of the catabolic nature of these patients, there is an increased requirement of essential amino acids.[41]

In a prospective controlled trial, Abel and associates[1] randomized 53 patients to receive either hypertonic dextrose or hypertonic dextrose plus essential amino acids. Both groups received similar quantities of nonprotein calories. They demonstrated a significantly higher recovery from renal failure in those patients receiving the essential amino acids plus hypertonic dextrose. The improved outcome was reflected by improvement in the underlying renal failure as a result of nutritional support (Fig. 3-4). Freund, Atamian, and Fischer[41] studied patients with renal insufficiency and infused a balanced amino acid solution containing both essential and nonessential amino acids plus hypertonic dextrose. They demonstrated significantly increased mortality in patients receiving the balanced amino acid solution when compared with patients treated with only essential amino acids plus the hypertonic dextrose previously studied.[1] However, studies by Leonard, Luke, and Sieger[56] and Feinstein and associates[35] demonstrated no significant improvement in renal failure patients given an essential amino acid solution compared with patients receiving essential and nonessential amino acids. Both groups included patients undergoing dialysis during the course of their treatment. Although nitrogen requirements are higher in patients undergoing dialysis, the use of dialysis allows more liberalization of fluid and nitrogen intake and may negate any advantage of a solution containing only essential amino acids. Further prospective, randomized clinical trials are required before the role of essential amino acid solutions in acute and chronic renal failure can be completely assessed.

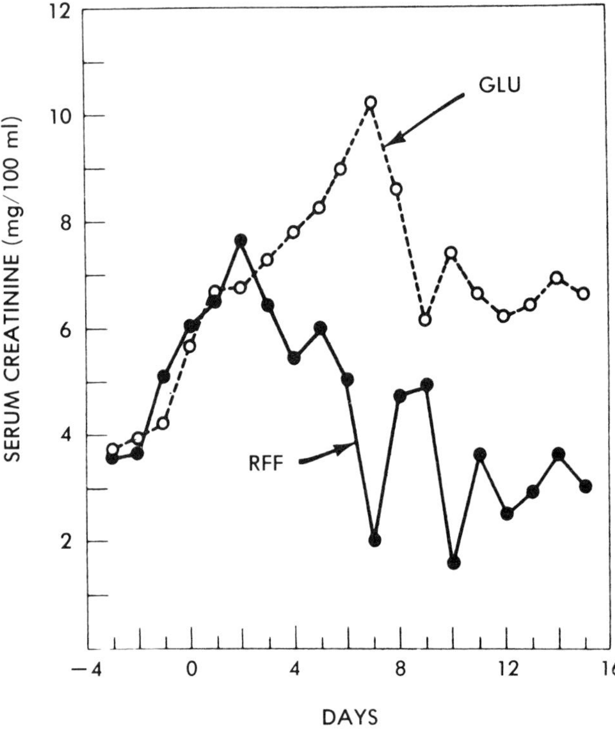

Fig. 3-4 Reduction of mean serum creatinine with infusion of renal failure formula *(RFF)* compared to patients receiving glucose *(GLU)*. (Modified from Abel, R.M., et al. Reprinted by permission of N. Engl. J. Med. **288:**695, 1973.)

Hepatic Encephalopathy

Numerous metabolic alterations occur in patients with hepatic failure. These alterations, singly or in combination, have been proposed as causative agents in hepatic encephalopathy, a condition consisting of various neuropsychiatric abnormalities that may be manifested in patients with hepatic failure. In recent years, attention has focused on neurotransmitted precursor concentrations and toxic metabolites as important causative agents in hepatic encephalopathy (Fig. 3-5).

Several investigators have reported plasma and urine amino acid abnormalities that occur in patients with encephalopathy.[18] Plasma aminograms in patients with encephalopathy typically demonstrate abnormally low levels of the branched chain amino acids with corresponding high levels of the aromatic amino acids, tyrosine, phenylalanine, and free tryptophan, as well as methionine.[38] Morgan, Milsom, and Sherlock[67] compared the levels of plasma leucine plus isoleucine plus valine to phenylalanine plus tyrosine and demonstrated a correlation between this ratio and the severity of liver disease. Branched chain amino acids are primarily metabolized in skeletal muscle, whereas aromatic amino acids and methionine are primarily metabolized in the liver. Severe hepatic dysfunction that occurs in the setting of hypercatabolism results in the typical plasma amino acid patterns of low branched chain amino acids (BCAAs)/aromatic amino acids (Fig. 3-6).

Transport of amino acids across the blood-brain barrier appears to be regulated by plasma amino acid concentrations. Several amino acids competitively share the same transport mechanisms. Increased plasma concentrations of aromatic amino acids with lowered BCAA concentrations allows greater entry of the aromatic amino acids into the brain.[75] Fischer and Baldessarini[37] proposed that abnormal plasma acid levels may alter brain amino acid patterns and, in turn, brain neurotransmitter levels, with resultant encephalopathy. Abnormal plasma ratios of BCAAs to aromatic amino acids would preferentially allow increased transportation of aromatic amino acids across the blood-brain barrier.

Increased plasma levels of phenylalanine will contribute to already elevated levels of brain tyrosine. Accumulation of phenylalanine and tyrosine in the brain results in increased levels of beta-hydroxylated phenyldothylamines including octopamine by way of increased levels of brain tyramine. Increased brain phenylalanine may also interfere with normal tyrosine metabolism. Elevated urinary and plasma levels of octopamine have been demonstrated in patients with hepatic encephalopathy.[61] Intestinal bacterial enzymes can directly metabolize dietary proteins, also resulting in increased levels of plasma tyramine. These substances are weak neurotransmitters, but with substantial brain accumulation they can replace normal neurotransmitters in neural synapses.

Elevated levels of plasma-free tryptophan readily cross the blood-brain barrier and are implicated in abnormal brain serotonin production.[55] Additionally, elevated plasma-free tryptophan levels have been implicated in sleep disorders.[51] Plasma and brain methionine have also been implicated in encephalopathy.

Patients with hepatic failure manifest unique biochemical and physiologic alterations. In addition, these patients are often malnourished, requiring nutritional intervention during treatment. Studies in animals with experimentally induced encephalopathy demonstrated that administration of amino acid solutions containing a greater proportion of the branched chain amino acids and a reduced proportion of methionine and the aromatic amino acids resulted in amelioration of encephalopathy and a normalization of the plasma amino acid patterns.[77]

Clinical studies have been conducted to evaluate solutions containing a greater proportion of branched chain amino acids and a reduced proportion of aromatic amino acids and methionine. A study of 63 patients by Freund

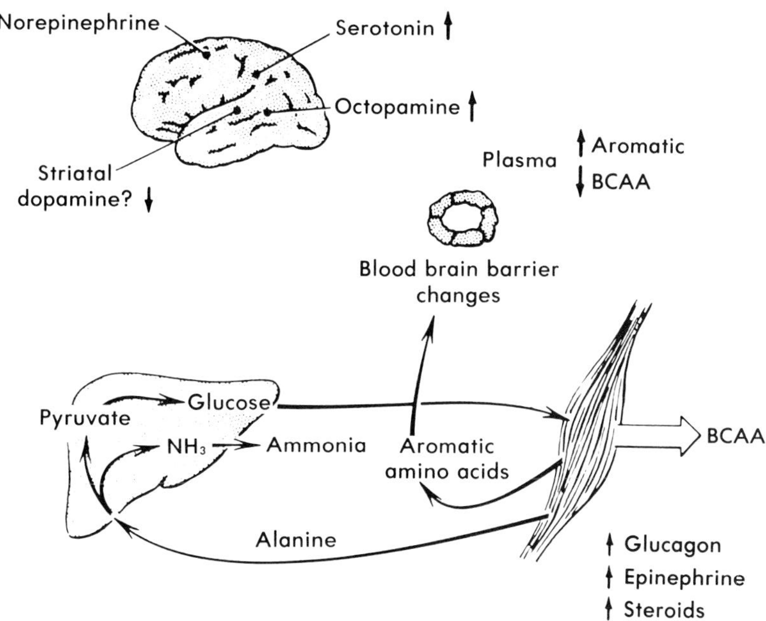

Fig. 3-5 Overall metabolic scheme leading to hepatic coma. (Modified from Fischer, J.E., and Bower, R.H.: Surg. Clin. North Am. **61:**653, 1981.)

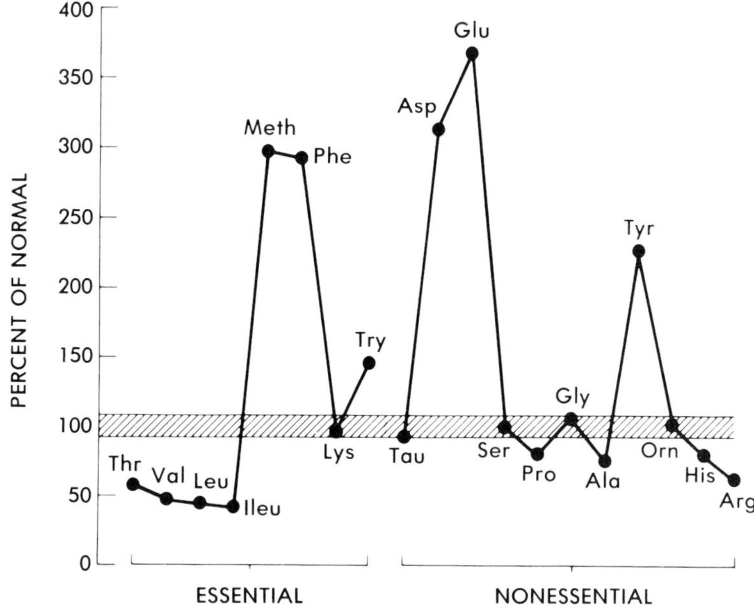

Fig. 3-6 Abnormal plasma amino acid pattern in patients with chronic liver disease expressed as percent of normal. (Reprinted with permission from Rosen, H.M., et al.: Gastroenterology **72:**483, 1972, © by Williams and Wilkins.)

and associates[42] demonstrated that improved nutritional support with positive nitrogen balance could be achieved by branched chain amino acid–enriched solutions in patients with hepatic insufficiency and protein intolerance. These patients maintained or improved their hepatic encephalopathy in response to increased nutritional intake. Other controlled studies comparing high branched chain amino acid solutions with standard types of therapy in hepatic encephalopathy demonstrated significant improvement in encephalopathy and concurrent improvement in nutritional status in patients receiving specialized amino acid formulas.[20,50,78]

Other studies have not demonstrated similar results in encephalopathic patients receiving specialized amino acid formulas.[66] Encephalopathy occurs as a combination of several metabolic disturbances, including increased levels of short-chain fatty acids and ammonia. Other concurrent complications such as hypovolemia, hepatorenal syndrome, or gastrointestinal bleeding, may prohibit improvement in mental status with nutritional supplementation. In addition, nutritional intervention with specialized formulas in hepatic failure of different causes other than alcoholic cirrhosis have not yet been adequately studied. Nevertheless, it would appear that specialized nutritional formulas may improve amino acid tolerance and nutritional status in patients with hepatic encephalopathy.

STRESS AND SEPSIS

Increased energy expenditure and skeletal muscle catabolism are characteristic features of sepsis and multiple trauma.[19] Energy- and nitrogen-conserving mechanisms used by the body in simple starvation are altered in this setting, leading to rapid depletion of lean body mass.

Skeletal muscle preferentially uses the branched chain amino acids (BCAA), leucine, isoleucine, and valine for energy production. The individual BCAA is deaminated to its individual keto acid and an amino group. The keto acids are further metabolized and decarboxylated, resulting in ATP production.[83] The donation of the amino group contributes to the production of alanine and glutamine by combining with pyruvate and glutamate, respectively.[79] In addition, the carbon skeletons of valine and isoleucine may be converted to glutamine by way of the tricarboxylic acid cycle.[45] Alanine and glutamine are released by skeletal muscle and are used by the liver for glucose production.[73]

The role of BCAAs in skeletal muscle protein turnover has been studied by various investigators. In vitro studies demonstrated that the BCAAs were able to promote protein synthesis and inhibit protein degradation.[15,43] It was postulated that the BCAAs may play important roles in the muscle protein-sparing effect of amino acid solutions.

Studies in catabolic patients paralleled these results. Plasma aminograms in septic patients demonstrated decreased concentrations of BCAAs and increased concentrations of other amino acids not catabolized by skeletal muscle.[83] Increased muscle proteolysis in traumatized patients are postulated as resulting directly in the increased glucose turnover and the amino acid abnormalities present in these patients.[23] Catabolic clinical settings have been demonstrated to cause increased protein catabolism and decreased protein synthesis (Fig. 3-7).[6,74]

As a result of these findings, it is hypothesized that amino acid solutions enriched with the BCAAs may be more nitrogen sparing in hypermetabolic patients than standard amino acid solutions. Studies in animals suggested that infusion of BCAAs may result in improved nitrogen sparing.[10] Studies in patients following surgery demonstrated that infusion of BCAA-enriched solutions

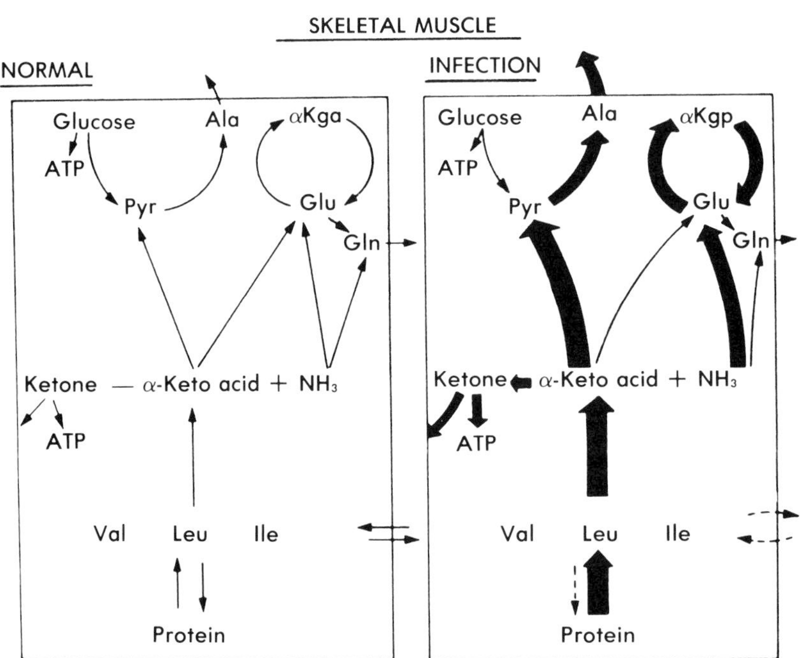

Fig. 3-7 The role of branched chain amino acids in response to infection. (Modified from Wannemacher, R.W.: Am. J. Clin. Nutr. [© American Society for Clinical Nutrition] **30:**1269, 1977.)

improved nitrogen balance on peak "stress" days.[54] These investigators further postulated that the nitrogen-sparing effect of BCAAs was related to the amount of BCAAs present in the solutions.[21] However, studies in patients following surgery demonstrated no improvement on nitrogen balance by BCAA-enriched solutions, although these solutions did result in increased uptake of BCAAs across skeletal muscle.[29] Subsequent clinical studies demonstrated that solutions enriched with BCAAs but relatively lower in leucine than standard amino acid solutions resulted in lower nitrogen balance and increased whole body protein catabolism in the postoperative patients receiving the BCAA-enriched solutions. Correction of the leucine imbalance improved nitrogen balance and decreased whole body protein catabolism but was not significantly different compared with the standard amino acid solution.[11]

Conclusive evidence of improved nitrogen sparing as a result of BCAA-enriched solutions in stressed patients has not been demonstrated. The level of the BCAAs present in standard amino acid solutions may be sufficient to optimize nitrogen-sparing mechanisms in a variety of stressed conditions. BCAA-enriched solutions may be more beneficial in a severely stressed population such as in severe, prolonged sepsis. The difficulty in conducting randomized, prospective studies in these patients has handicapped attempts at answering this important question. Additionally, the identification of the patient population that may benefit from BCAA-enriched solutions is unknown and may actually be relatively small. These important questions need to be answered by well conducted, prospective, randomized trials before the widespread use of BCAA-enriched solutions can be justified.

NUTRITION AND CANCER

The association between weight loss, malnutrition, and cancer has been well established. Nutritional support of cancer patients has gained increased acceptance as a valuable adjuvant for several reasons. The successful use of nutritional support has been demonstrated in clinical trials involving noncancer patients, suggesting that similar results may be possible in cancer patients. In addition, aggressive, multimodality treatment regimens that have been credited with improving survival rates for various types of malignancies are also associated with systemic, toxic effects that may impair the ability of the patient to maintain an adequate intake of nutrients. Often this occurs in patients with existing nutritional deficits. Finally, improvements in delivery and composition of nutritional support have resulted in a greater acceptance of this modality as a viable tool in the management of cancer patients.

Anorexia, a common symptom in malignancies, results in diminished nutrient intake and weight loss. Host and tumor requirements for energy and protein may be greater than nutrient intake in cancer patients with anorexia, which results in a greater use of endogenous fuel reserves. Patients with gastrointestinal malignancies may have reduced nutrient intake because of the mechanical obstruction of the tumor. Compounding the effects of the tumor on nutrient availability to the host are the nutritionally debilitating effects of surgery, radiation therapy, or chemotherapy. The resulting weight loss has been previously documented in various types of malignancies using different criteria.[30,72]

Malnutrition in cancer patients often is characterized as "cancer cachexia," which is a sign and symptom complex, including inanition, anorexia, weakness, wasting, and organ dysfunction. Cachexia may be present in patients with advanced metastatic or localized disease, demonstrating an inconsistent relationship between tumor burden, stage, and histologic characteristics of the malignancy. The true cause of cancer cachexia is often unclear. Nevertheless, a variety of etiologic factors, involving decreased nutrient intake and increased or deranged nutrient requirements, is usually present (Fig. 3-8), leading to altered substrate metabolism associated with cancer (see the boxed material on p. 68).

Cancer patients may have decreased nutrient intake for a variety of reasons and often do not demonstrate the nor-

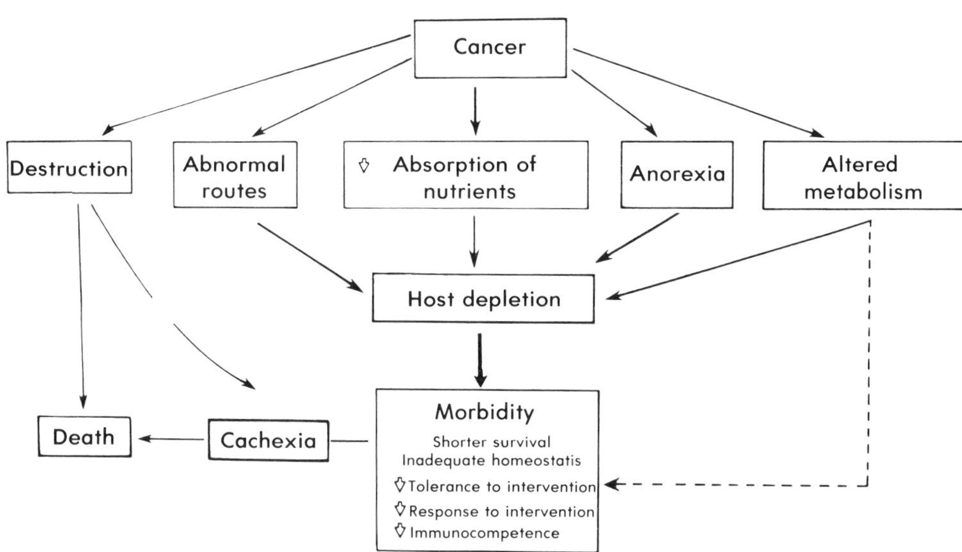

Fig. 3-8 Mechanisms leading to host depletion and morbidity in patients with cancer. (Modified from Costa, G.: Cancer Res. **37:**2327, 1977.)

ALTERED SUBSTRATE METABOLISM IN CANCER PATIENTS

Carbohydrate Metabolism
Abnormal response to glucose tolerance test
Increased insulin resistance (hepatic and peripheral)
Increased gluconeogenesis from alanine and lactate
Increased Cori cycle activity

Protein Metabolism
"Nitrogen trapping" by the tumor
Increased protein turnover
Impaired muscle protein synthesis

Fat Metabolism
Increased neutral fat breakdown and fatty acid use for energy

Energy Expenditure
Increased energy expenditure
Inefficient energy expenditure

mal response to starvation by the conservation of endogenous nutrient stores. Malnutrition in cancer patients may contribute to a number of severe sequelae. Protein-calorie malnutrition may result in weight loss and a compromise of visceral and somatic protein compartments that are vital to enzymatic, structural, and mechanical function. Immunocompetence may be compromised with resultant increased susceptibility to infection.[27] Treatment regimens involving radiation, chemotherapy, and surgery may also contribute to impaired immunity. In addition, poor wound healing, prolonged ileus, and increased morbidity and mortality following surgical procedures have been linked to poor nutritional status in cancer patients. Review of autopsy reports in cancer patients has demonstrated that malnutrition is implicated in at least 22% of cancer deaths.[70] Therefore patients with cancer who are malnourished and who are or will undergo treatment for their malignancy may benefit from nutritional support.

The selection of the route for administration of nutritional support in cancer patients does not differ from that in noncancer patients. If gastrointestinal function is adequate, oral supplementation should be the initial form of support. However, an unwillingness or an inability of the patient to tolerate oral feedings should be followed by an attempt at tube feeding. Nevertheless, patients with cancer often have inadequate gastrointestinal function. In these patients, parenteral feedings usually offer the best alternative for nutritional support.

The use of nutritional support in cancer patients previously was discouraged because of fear of enhanced tumor growth. Various animal studies have demonstrated that tumor growth may be enhanced by dietary manipulations. However, interpretations of animal studies should be tempered with caution. In rats, tumor burdens are disproportionately large, and tumor growth rates are very high in contrast to patients with cancer. In addition, in contrast to animals, patients with cancer receiving nutritional support usually receive concurrent antineoplastic therapy in these studies. Indeed, various investigators have been unable to demonstrate increased tumor growth in patients receiving antineoplastic therapy and nutritional support.[12,25]

The use of nutritional support in patients with cancer remains a controversial subject. Malnourished cancer patients receiving antineoplastic therapy usually receive nutritional support. The benefits of nutritional support in these patients were demonstrated by retrospective studies. Prospective, randomized trials involving malnourished patients with cancer are difficult to conduct, and most physicians are unwilling to withhold nutritional support in these patients if they are to receive concurrent treatment. Prospective randomized trials of TPN in cancer patients undergoing treatment have been conducted and recently reviewed.[12] The results of these studies are inconclusive and somewhat conflicting. The majority of these studies failed to demonstrate a significant increase in tumor response in patients receiving TPN. However, many of the series contained a limited number of patients, and most were not malnourished. In addition, benefits of TPN were demonstrated in several of the studies, particularly in patients undergoing surgery for gastrointestinal neoplasms.

Drawing solid conclusions from these trials is difficult. Trials in patients with malignancies that carry a dismal prognosis may fail to demonstrate statistical improvement when receiving TPN as a result of the low number of these patients that respond to any treatment. Nevertheless, retrospective data do indicate that an improvement in nutritional status in cancer patients may be advantageous. Ultimately, the implementation of nutritional support in these patients should be based on several principles. First, malnutrition should not be allowed to interfere with required cancer therapy by diminishing the ability of the patient to withstand therapeutic procedures. Second, no patient should be allowed to develop malnutrition as a result of necessary treatment. Finally, only those patients with a hope of a meaningful therapeutic response should be considered for nutritional support.

LONG-TERM NUTRITIONAL SUPPORT

Nutritional intervention has been found to be efficacious in a variety of clinical settings. Increased use of this treatment modality has resulted in a reduction of associated complications with associated greater efficiency of delivery systems. Technical advances have allowed application of nutritional support for nonhospitalized patients.[33] Patients who would otherwise have little hope for life because of refractory malnutrition, either from their underlying disease or its treatment, can maintain adequate nutrient intake from home parenteral and home enteral nutrition.

Home Parenteral and Enteral Nutrition

Home parenteral nutrition (HPN) is indicated in patients who are unable to eat and absorb enough nutrients for maintenance. The specific diseases and/or subsequent treatments that create a need for HPN in patients are varied. The majority of patients currently receiving HPN are patients with short-bowel syndromes. These patients usually suffer from extensive Crohn's disease, mesenteric infarction, or severe abdominal trauma.[39] Other reported cases include patients with severe intestinal obstruction, radiation enteritis, cancer, necrotizing enterocolitis, or congenital short-bowel syndrome.[85]

The majority of these patients cannot receive adequate

nutrition enterally, although compensatory mucosal growth with resultant increased efficiency of absorption can occur in some patients and may either reduce or remove the need for continued HPN. Other categories of patients requiring HPN include those with malabsorption syndromes, intestinal pseudo-obstruction, radiation enteritis, and severe anorexia nervosa.[85]

Complications of HPN parallel those of in-hospital total parenteral nutrition. Patients with proximal gastrointestinal tract obstruction or diversion may receive their nutrition at home enterally, by way of gastrostomy or jejunostomy. Debilitated patients have been fed for many years through nasoenteric feeding tubes, the more recently developed silastic tubes being considerably more comfortable than earlier examples. Advantages to home enteral nutrition parallel those of in-hospital programs: lower cost, ease of administration, and fewer complications.[22]

SUMMARY

Subclinical and clinical malnutrition have become increasingly recognized in hospitalized surgical patients and have been shown to be associated with increased morbidity and mortality. The metabolic response to starvation and surgical stress, e.g., trauma, operative procedures, and infection, leads to an erosion of lean body mass and endogenous fat stores, which, if allowed to persist, will ultimately lead to organ failure and death. The development of techniques of nutritional support by way of enteral or parenteral routes on the basis of sound physiologic principles has allowed the provision of optimal nutritional therapy to all patients at all times and has minimized the devastating effects that nutritional failure may have on patient outcome and survival.

REFERENCES

1. Abel, R.M., et al.: Improved survival from acute renal failure after treatment with intravenous essential L-amino acids and glucose, N. Engl. J. Med. **288:**695, 1973.
2. Allardyce, D.B., and Groves, A.C.: A comparison of nutritional gains resulting from intravenous and enteral feeding, Surg. Gynecol. Obstet. **139:**179, 1974.
3. Baker, J.P., et al.: Nutritional assessment: a comparison of clinical judgement and objective measurements, N. Engl. J. Med. **306:**969, 1982.
4. Baker, J.P., et al.: Randomized trial of total parenteral nutrition in critically ill patients: metabolic effects of varying glucose-lipid ratios as the energy source, Gastroenterology **87:**53, 1984.
5. Bergstrom, J., Furst, P., and Josephson, B.: Factors affecting the nitrogen balance in chronic uremic patients receiving essential amino acid intravenously or by mouth, Nutr. Metab. **14**(suppl.):162, 1972.
6. Birkhahn, R.H., et al.: Effects of major skeletal trauma on whole body protein turnover in man measured by L-(1,14C)-leucine, Surgery **88:**294, 1980.
7. Bistrian, B.R., et al.: Protein status of general surgical patients, JAMA **230:**858, 1974.
8. Bistrian, B.R., et al.: Therapeutic index of nutritional depletion in hospitalized patients, Surg. Gynecol. Obstet. **141:**512, 1975.
9. Blackburn, G.L., et al.: Protein sparing therapy during periods of starvation with sepsis or trauma, Ann. Surg. **177:**589, 1973.
10. Blackburn, G.L., et al.: Branched chain amino acid administration and metabolism during starvation, injury, and infection, Surgery **86:**307, 1979.
11. Bonau, R.A., et al.: High branched amino acid solutions: relationship of composition to efficacy, J.P.E.N. **8:**622, 1984.
12. Brennan, M.F.: Total parenteral nutrition in the cancer patient, N. Engl. J. Med. **305:**375, 1981.
13. Burke, J.F., et al.: Glucose requirements following burn injury, parameters of optimal glucose infusion and possible hepatic and respiratory abnormalities following excessive glucose intake, Ann. Surg. **190:**274, 1979.
14. Burt, M.E., Gorschboth, C.M., and Brennan, M.F.: A controlled, prospective, randomized trial evaluating the metabolic effects of enteral and parenteral nutrition in the cancer patient, Cancer **49:**1092, 1982.
15. Buse, M.G., and Reid, S.S.: Leucine: a possible regulator of protein turnover in muscle, J. Clin. Invest. **56:**1250, 1975.
16. Butterworth, C.E., and Weinsier, R.L.: Malnutrition in hospital patients: assessment and treatment. In Goodhart, R.S., and Shils, M.E., editors: Modern nutrition in health and disease, Philadelphia 1980, Lea & Febiger.
17. Cahill, G.F.: Starvation in man, N. Engl. J. Med. **282:**668, 1970.
18. Cascino, A., et al.: Plasma amino acids imbalance in patients with liver disease, Dig. Dis. Sci. **23:**591, 1978.
19. Cerra, F.B., et al.: Correlations between metabolic and cardiopulmonary measurements in patients after trauma, general surgery, and sepsis, J. Trauma **19:**621, 1979.
20. Cerra, F.B., et al.: Cirrhosis, encephalopathy, and improved results with metabolic support, Surgery **94:**612, 1983.
21. Cerra, F.B., et al.: Nitrogen retention in critically ill patients is proportional to the branched chain amino acid load, Crit. Care Med. **11:**775, 1983.
22. Chrysomilides, S.A., and Kaminski, M.V.: Home enteral and parenteral nutritional support: a comparison, Am. J. Clin. Nutr. **34:**2271, 1981.
23. Clowes, G.H.A., Randall, H.T., and Cha, C.J.: Amino acid and energy metabolism in septic and traumatized patients, J.P.E.N. **4:**195, 1980.
24. Collins, J.P., Oxby, C.B., and Hill, G.L.: Intravenous amino acids and intravenous hyperalimentation as protein-sparing therapy after major surgery: a controlled clinical trial, Lancet 1:788, 1978.
25. Copeland, E.M., III., Daly, J.M., and Dudrick, S.J.: Nutrition and Cancer, Int. Adv. Surg. Oncol. **4:**1, 1981.
26. Daly, J.M., and Long, J.M.: Intravenous hyperalimentation: techniques and potential complications, Surg. Clin. North Am. **61:**583, 1981.
27. Daly, J.M., Dudrick, S.J., and Copeland, E.M., III: Effects of protein depletion and repletion on cell-mediated immunity in experimental animals, Ann. Surg. **188:**791, 1978.
28. Daly, J.M., Dudrick, S.J., and Copeland, E.M., III: Intravenous hyperalimentation: effect on delayed cutaneous hypersensitivity in cancer patients, Ann. Surg. **192:**587, 1980.
29. Daly, J.M., et al.: Effects of postoperative infusion of branched chain amino acids on nitrogen balance and forearm muscle substrate flux, Surgery **94:**151, 1983.
30. DeWys, W.D., et al.: Prognostic effect of weight loss prior to chemotherapy in cancer patients, Am. J. Med. **69:**491, 1980.
31. Dudrick, S.J., Steiger, E., and Long, J.M.: Renal failure in surgical patients: treatment with intravenous essential amino acids and hypertonic glucose, Surgery **68:**180, 1970.
32. Dudrick, S.J., et al.: Long-term parenteral nutrition with growth, development, and positive nitrogen balance, Surgery **64:**134, 1968.
33. Dudrick, S.J., et al.: Update on ambulatory home hyperalimentation, Nutr. Sup. Ser. **1:**18, 1981.
34. Elwyn, D.J., et al.: Protein and energy sparing of glucose added in hypocaloric amounts to peripheral infusions of amino acids, Metabolism **27:**325, 1978.
35. Feinstein, E.I., et al.: Clinical and metabolic responses to parenteral nutrition in acute renal failure, Medicine **60:**124, 1981.
36. Fischer, J.E.: Nutritional assessment before surgery, Am. J. Clin. Nutr. **35:**1128, 1982.
37. Fischer, J.E., and Baldessarini, R.J.: False neurotransmitters and hepatic failure, Lancet **2:**75, 1971.
38. Fischer, J.E., et al.: The role of plasma amino acids in hepatic encephalopathy, Surgery **78:**276, 1975.
39. Fleming, C.R., et al.: Home parenteral nutrition for management of the severely malnourished adult patient, Gastroenterology **79:**18, 1980.
40. Freeman, J.B., and Fairfull-Smith, R.J.: Current concepts of enteral feeding, Adv. Surg. **16:**75, 1983.

41. Freund, H., Atamian, S., and Fischer, J.E.: Comparative study of parenteral nutrition in renal failure using essential and nonessential amino acid containing solutions, Surg. Gynecol. Obstet. **151**:652, 1980.
42. Freund, H., et al.: Infusion of branched chain enriched amino acid solution in patient with hepatic encephalopathy, Ann. Surg. **196**:209, 1982.
43. Fulks, R.M., Li, J.B., and Goldberg, A.L.: Effects of insulin, glucose, and amino acids on protein turnover in rat diaphragm, J. Biochem. **250**:290, 1975.
44. Giovannetti, S., and Maggiore, Q.: A low-nitrogen diet with proteins of high biologic value for severe chronic uraemia, Lancet **1**:1000, 1964.
45. Goldberg, A.L., and Chang, T.W.: Regulation and significance of amino acid metabolism in skeletal muscle, Fed. Proc. **37**:2301, 1978.
46. Grant, J.P., Custer, P.B., and Thurlow, J.: Current techniques of nutritional assessment, Surg. Clin. North Am. **61**:437, 1981.
47. Haffejee, A.A., and Angorn, I.B.: Nutritional status and the nonspecific cellular and humoral immune response in esophageal carcinoma, Ann. Surg. **189**:475, 1979.
48. Hearne, B.E., and Daly, J.M.: Enteral nutrition. In Kirkpatrick, J., editor: Nutrition and metabolism in the surgical patient, Mt. Kisco, N.Y., 1983, Futura Publishing Co., Inc.
49. Heird, W.C., et al.: Hyperammonemia resulting from intravenous alimentation using a mixture of synthetic L-amino acids, J. Pediatr. **81**:162, 1972.
50. Horst, D., et al.: Comparison of dietary protein with an oral, branched chain enriched amino acid supplement in chronic portal-systemic encephalopathy: a randomized controlled trial, Hepatology **4**:279, 1984.
51. James, J.H., et al.: Brain tryptophan, plasma free tryptophan and distribution of plasma neutral amino acids, Metabolism **25**:471, 1976.
52. Jeejeebhoy, K.N.: Nutritional support of the azotemic patient, Urol. Clin. North Am. **1**:345, 1974.
53. Jeejeebhoy, K.N., et al.: Metabolic studies in total parenteral nutrition with lipid in man: comparison with glucose, J. Clin. Invest. **57**:125, 1976.
54. Kern, K.A., et al.: The effect of a new branched chain enriched amino acid solution on postoperative catabolism, Surgery **92**:780, 1982.
55. Knell, A.J., et al.: Dopamine and serotonin metabolism in hepatic encephalopathy, Br. Med. J. **23**:549, 1974.
56. Leonard, C.D., Luke, R.G., and Sieger, R.R.: Parenteral essential amino acids in acute renal failure, Urology **6**:154, 1975.
57. Lloyd, A.V.C.: Tuberculin test in children with malnutrition, Br. Med. J. **3**:529, 1968.
58. Long, J.M., et al.: Effect of carbohydrate and fat intake on nitrogen excretion during total intravenous feeding, Ann. Surg. **185**:417, 1977.
59. Macfie, J., Smith, R.C., and Hill, G.L.: Glucose or fat as a nonprotein source? A controlled clinical trial in gastroenterological patients requiring intravenous nutrition, Gastroenterology **80**:103, 1981.
60. MacLean, L.D., et al.: Host resistance in sepsis and trauma, Ann. Surg. **182**:207, 1975.
61. Manghani, K.K., et al.: Urinary and serum octopamine in patients with portal-systemic encephalopathy, Lancet **2**:943, 1975.
62. McArdle, A.H., et al.: A rationale for enteral feeding as the preferable route for hyperalimentation, Surgery **90**:616, 1981.
63. McCarthy, M.C., Cottam, G.L., and Turner, W.W.: Essential fatty acid deficiency in critically ill surgical patients, Am. J. Surg. **142**:747, 1981.
64. McIrvine, A.J., and Mannick, J.A.: Lymphocyte function in the critically ill surgical patient, Surg. Clin. North Am. **63**:245, 1983.
65. Meguid, M.M., Collier, M.D., and Howard, L.J.: Uncomplicated and stressed starvation, Surg. Clin. North Am. **61**:529, 1981.
66. Millikan, W.J., et al.: Total parenteral nutrition with F080 in cirrhotics with subclinical encephalopathy, Ann. Surg. **197**:294, 1983.
67. Morgan, M.Y., Milsom, J.P., and Sherlock, S.: Plasma ration of valine, leucine, and isoleucine to phenulalanine and tyrosine in liver disease, Gut **19**:1068, 1978.
68. Mullen, J.L., et al.: Implications of malnutrition in the surgical patient, Arch. Surg. **114**:121, 1979.
69. Mullen, J.L., et al.: Prediction of operative morbidity and mortality by preoperative nutritional assessment, Surg. Forum **30**:80, 1979.
70. Mullen, J.L., et al.: Protein synthesis dynamics in human gastrointestinal malignancies, Surgery **87**:331, 1980.
71. Mullen, J.L., et al.: Reduction of operative morbidity and mortality by combined preoperative and postoperative nutritional support, Ann. Surg. **192**:604, 1980.
72. Nixon, D.W., et al.: Protein calorie undernutrition in hospitalized cancer patients, Am. J. Med. **68**:683, 1980.
73. Odessy, R., Khairallah, E.A., and Goldberg, A.L.: Origin and possible significance of alanine production by skeletal muscle, J. Biochem. **249**:7323, 1974.
74. O'Keefe, S.J.D., Sender, P.M., and James, W.P.T.: "Catabolic" loss of body nitrogen in response to surgery, Lancet **2**:1035, 1974.
75. Oldendorf, W.H., and Szabo, J.: Amino acid assignment to one of three blood-brain barrier amino acid carriers, Am. J. Physiol. **230**:94, 1976.
76. Rombeau, J.L., and Barot, L.R.: Enteral nutritional therapy, Surg. Clin. North Am. **61**:605, 1981.
77. Rosen, H.M., et al.: Influences of exogenous intake and nitrogen balance on plasma and brain aromatic amino acid concentrations, Metabolism **27**:393, 1978.
78. Rossi-Fanelli, F., et al.: Branched chain amino acids vs. lactulose in the treatment of hepatic coma, Dig. Dis. Sci. **27**:929, 1982.
79. Ruderman, N.B., and Berger, M.: The formation of glutamine and alanine in skeletal muscle, J. Biochem. **249**:5500, 1974.
80. Ryan, J.A., and Taft, D.A.: Preoperative nutritional assessment does not predict morbidity and mortality in abdominal operations, Surg. Forum **31**:96, 1980.
81. Sanderson, I.: Insulin response in patients receiving concentrated infusions of glucose and casein hydrolysates for complete parenteral nutrition, Ann. Surg. **179**:387, 1974.
82. Sanderson, I., and Deitel, M.: Intravenous hyperalimentation without sepsis, Surg. Gynecol. Obstet. **136**:577, 1973.
83. Wannemacher, R.W.: Key role of various individual amino acids in host response to infection, J. Biochem. **249**:5500, 1974.
84. Watters, J.M., and Freeman, J.B.: Parenteral nutrition by peripheral vein, Surg. Clin. North Am. **61**:593, 1981.
85. Wolfe, B.M., et al.: Experience with home parenteral nutrition, Am. J. Surg. **146**:7, 1983.

4

Charles M. Balch and Richard E. Wilson

Immunity and the Immunocompromised Surgical Patient

The function of the immune system is to protect the body's internal environment from foreign proteins, cells, microorganisms, and other substances. Alterations in the immune system are important components in the evaluation of the surgical patient, both in the setting where a surgical disease such as cancer or infection adversely affects it and where the surgical procedure itself such as the transplant of an organ induces alterations in immunity.

The immune system is a highly integrated, complex homeostatic system whose primary function is to discriminate between substances that are its own (''self'') and those that are foreign (''not self''). After recognizing a foreign substance, the immune system must be able to eliminate the invader. Its capability of doing so represents a dynamic interplay between the presentation of the antigen and the response by the cellular constituents of this system and their products. The diverse roles of these different cellular participants in the immunologic repertoire are being identified with increasing precision. It is clear that the types of responding cells and the effectiveness of antigen elimination are influenced by how the antigen is presented (i.e., route, dose, and timing), the immune competence of the patient, and the patient's genetic background. Abnormal or defective immunity results from imbalances between antigen presentation and the corresponding host immunologic responses. Increasingly, the surgeon should be able to identify abnormalities in immunologic responses, to assess the impact of surgical treatment (both favorable and adverse) on the immunologic system, and to assess the impact of postoperative treatments that may be immunosuppressive.

AN OVERVIEW OF THE HUMAN IMMUNE SYSTEM

A basic understanding of the immune system is facilitated by categorizing lymphoid cells into functional components. The most extensively studied cell is the lymphocyte. Despite their uniform microscopic appearance, there are actually two categories of lymphocytes, which are designated as T cells and B cells. Both types of cells originate from stem cells in the bone marrow, but the maturation and differentiation of T cells is dependent on the thymus gland. Thus thymus-dependent (T) lymphocytes mediate cellular immunity, and bone-marrow derived (B) lymphocytes mediate humoral (antibody) immunity (Fig. 4-1). In recent years, T lymphocytes have been further subdivided into functional categories such as suppressor and helper cells. Natural killer and killer cells have been defined as a special group of granular lymphocytes with characteristics distinctive from both T and B lymphocytes. Macrophages, monocytes, and granulocytes have usually been described as nonspecific ''scavenger'' cells. However, more recent evidence suggests that macrophages have an important role in antigen presentation and in influencing the types of immunologic responses that result.

Cellular Components

B Lymphocytes

The B-lymphocyte system is concerned with the manufacture of an enormous variety of antibodies with specificity for virtually all foreign antigens. B lymphocytes, which generally reside in the spleen and lymph nodes, are committed to becoming antibody-producing plasma cells when stimulated by the presence of particular antigens (Fig. 4-2). Plasma cells can synthesize and secrete approximately 2000 identical antibody molecules per second. They usually die within a few days after reaching maturity. It is estimated that mature individuals have developed the genes necessary to code for the production of 1,000,000 to 100,000,000 antibodies that have different specificities.

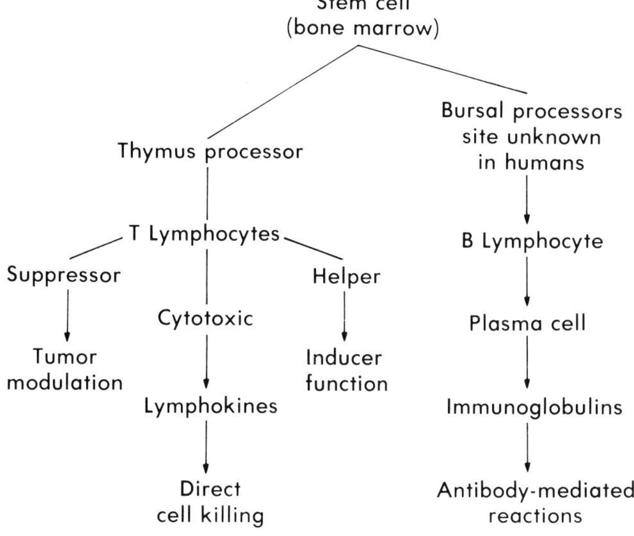

Fig. 4-1 Sequence of lymphocyte maturation for T and B lymphocytes. Precursor stem cells are derived from bone marrow. T lymphocytes are activated by thymic hormones and differentiate into cytotoxic, suppressor, and helper cells. These functions overlap and affect the B lymphocytes in the production of antibodies. (From Wilson, R.E.: Surgical problems in immunodepressed patients, Philadelphia, 1984, W.B. Saunders Co.)

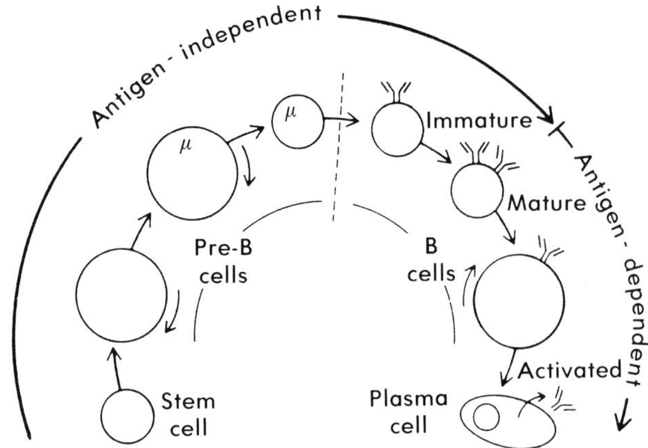

Fig. 4-2 Hypothetical model of the life history of a B lymphocyte. Changes in expression of the immunoglobulin genes may reflect different stages of differentiation. Cells at stages of B-cell differentiation that are involved in considerable proliferative activity are represented by large circles with accompanying arrows. (From Cooper, M.D., Kearney, J., and Scher, I.: B Lymphocytes. In Paul, W.E., editor: Fundamental immunology, New York, 1984, Raven Press.)

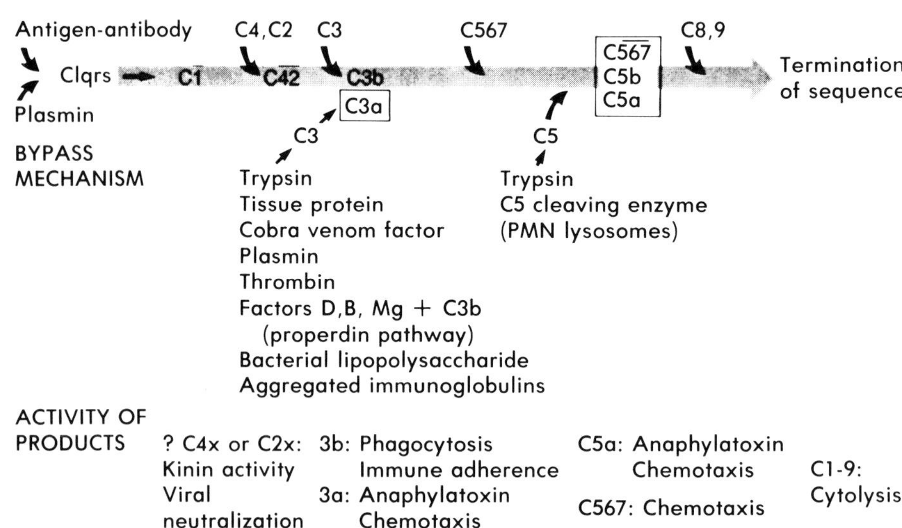

Fig. 4-3 Cascade of complement activation. Full cytolytic activity occurs only when all components (C1-C9) are activated in sequence. The alternate complement pathway permits activation to proceed at the C3a level, bypassing the need for C1, C4, and C2. (From Bellanti, J.A.: Immunology II, Philadelphia, 1985, W.B. Saunders Co.)

The system is thus well-designed to deal with unpredictable and unforeseen microbial and toxic agents. In fact, most types of bacterial infections involve B-lymphocyte immune responses.

Once an antibody has combined with an antigen, an amplification system is triggered that involves the activation of complement[16] (Fig. 4-3) and the infiltration of granulocytes. The complement system comprises at least 20 different serum glycoproteins. These proteins generally circulate as inactive precursor forms that elicit proteolytic activity once they are activated. Nine major components of this system (i.e., C1 to C9) have been recognized, several of which exist in various subunits (i.e., C1q, r, and s). The major biologic functions that result from activation of complement include enhancement of phagocytosis (opsonization) and viral neutralization, mediation of inflammation, cell lysis (e.g., antibody-coated bacteria or cells), and modulation of immune responses.

The products of antibody-secreting cells are immunoglobulin molecules (Fig. 4-4). Some of their characteristics are shown in Table 4-1. This group of proteins has several structural features in common. They are constructed of one or several units, each of which consists of two heavy polypeptide chains and two light polypeptide chains. Each unit possesses two combining sites for the antigen. The antigen-combining site of an individual antibody molecule is created by contributions from specialized regions of both the heavy and the light chains and is termed the *variable* region of the molecule. The *constant* region of the antibody molecule is responsible for the distinct biologic functions of each class of antibody. For example, IgM antibodies can activate the complement system; IgA antibodies are secreted into a variety of bodily fluids and provide secretory immunity; IgE antibodies are fixed as specific receptors on mass cells and basophils; IgD antibodies act almost exclusively as membrane receptors for antigen; and IgG antibodies mediate a variety of functions, including the ability to be transferred across the placenta.

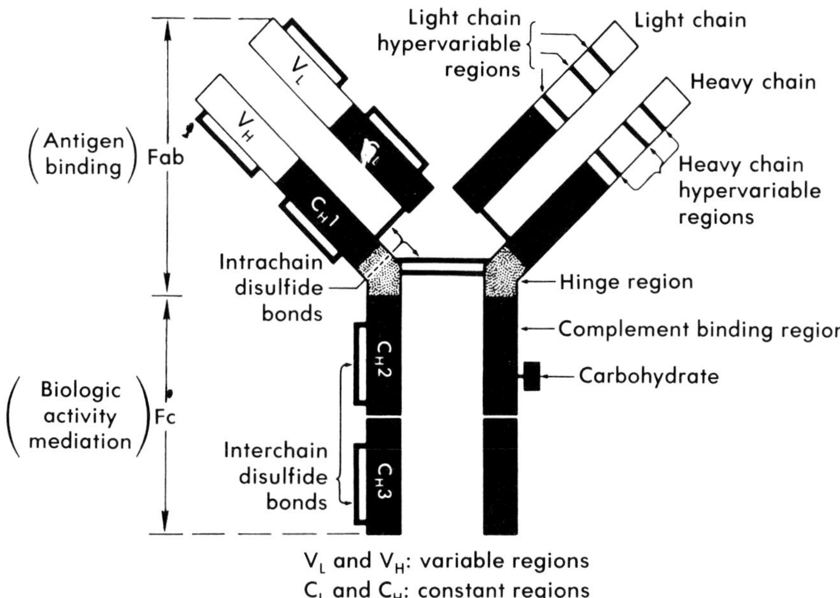

Fig. 4-4 Structure of an immunoglobulin molecule. Representation of an IgG molecule indicates the chain and domain structure molecule and the existence of hypervariable regions with variable regions of both H and L chains. (From Wasserman, R.L., and Capra, J.D. In Horawitz, M.I., and Pigman, W., editors: Immunoglobulins in the glycoconjugates, New York, 1977, Academic Press, Inc.)

Table 4-1 **TYPES OF IMMUNOGLOBULINS AND THEIR FUNCTIONS**

Characteristic	IgG	IgM	IgA	IgD	IgE
Serum Ig	75%-85%	5%-10%	7%-15%	0.3%	0.003%
Biologic property	2° antibody response	1° antibody response	Mucous secretions	B-lymphocyte surface molecule	Anaphalaxis allergy
Binding to cells	K cells, macrophages, granulocytes	K cells	—	—	Mast cells
Complement binding	C, A*	C	A	A	—
Molecular weight	150,000	950,000	160,000	175,000	190,000

*C, classic; A, alternate.

T Lymphocytes

T lymphocytes have a different range of functional capabilities. Their influence appears to rely more on cell to cell interactions and recognition of particular cell surface components. T-cell–mediated destruction of cells or microorganisms is independent of both antibody and the complement system. T-cell–mediated cytolysis requires intimate contact between a viable effector cell and its target (Fig. 4-5). The cytolytic event itself is independent of protein synthesis, DNA synthesis, and RNA synthesis. A variety of mediators (lymphokines) is released from sensitized lymphocytes after they have been exposed to a specific antigen that facilitates this cellular immunologic event (Fig. 4-6).

T cells are the predominant lymphocyte type that circulates in the blood and in lymph; they are also found in the thymus, lymph nodes, and spleen. Important subgroups of T cells can be classified by their functional properties and include cytotoxic, helper, and suppressor T cells. More recent evidence suggests that even these subsets of cells can be refined into precursor cells, inducer cells, and activated cells (see boxed material on p. 75).

The interactions among these cells are considerable. Macrophages and monocytes may also play an important role as accessory cells in these cytolytic events, both during the inductive phase and, as scavenger cells, after immune cytolysis has occurred.

Cytotoxic T cells can kill cells or microorganisms by direct contact after reacting with particular surface antigens, including products of genes encoded in the major histocompatibility complex. Thus they are important participants in immune responses directed against certain viruses, tumors, and transplanted tissues since their antigens are exposed at the cell surface. Considerable information is now available about the T-cell receptor for antigen, including its molecular structure.[1] Once the cytotoxic T cell has engaged cells or microbes bearing antigen, there are multiple steps in the lytic event that include: (1) cell to cell contact (requiring calcium and/or magnesium); (2) the lytic event; and (3) rupture of the membrane with loss of its cytoplasmic contents. The target cell serves only to display antigen and does not even have to be viable to be subject to lytic attack. The effector cell, in contrast, survives the interaction that destroys the target cell and can go on to kill other targets.

Another subpopulation is the *helper (or inducer) T cells,* so named because they interact with B cells in the production of antibodies and with other T cells in the development of mature cytotoxic T cells. Helper T cells, therefore, have a positive or amplifying influence on many types of immune responses. The initial activation of the helper T cell depends on its corecognition of antigen and a particular type of histocompatibility antigen (HLA-DR), which is usually expressed on the surface of a specialized antigen-presenting cell. The precise function of the antigen-presenting cell in this activation process has not been fully clarified, but an important element is its production of interleukin-1.

Suppressor T cells constitute a very important subpopulation that can exert a negative regulatory effect on both antibody responses and T-cell effector responses. This is an important conceptual advance in immunology, for it is increasingly evident that a weak or absent immune response may be the result of active suppression rather than passive unresponsiveness. This regulatory system may be responsible for the maintenance of tolerance to "self" antigens as well. Several different subgroups of human T cells have been shown to have suppressor activity, and macrophages are also capable of functioning as suppressor cells. The regulation of immune responses by suppressor cells may occur by several different mechanisms.

Granular Lymphocytes with Natural Killer and Killer Cell Function

In the past, natural killer (NK) cells and killer (K) cells have been classified as "null" cells that had lymphocyte characteristics but lacked classic T- and B-cell markers. NK cells and K cells are functional definitions; therefore it

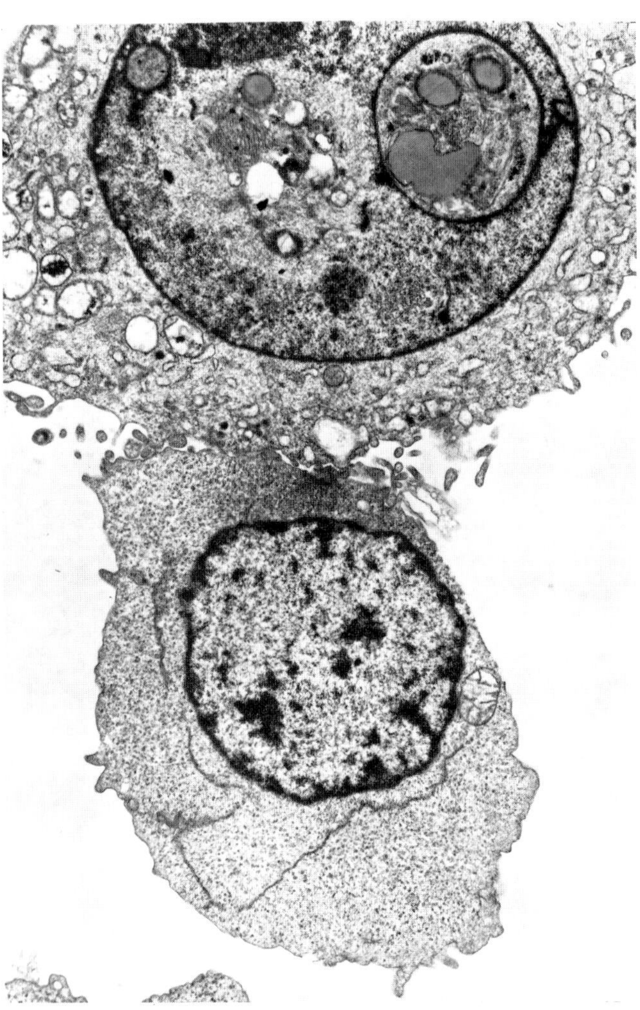

Fig. 4-5 Electron photomicrograph of a cytotoxic T lymphocyte in process of killing an autologous melanoma tumor cell. The cytolytic event is independent of antibody and complement.

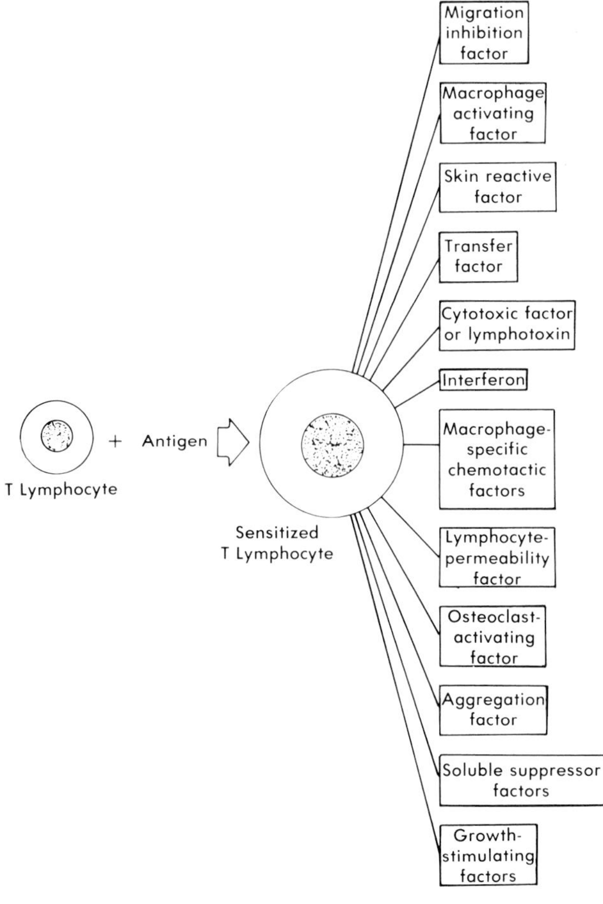

Fig. 4-6 Partial list of lymphokines produced by sensitized lymphocytes. Many of the cellular products have valuable biologic functions in the cellular immune reactions mediated by T lymphocytes. (From Wilson, R.E.: Surgical problems in immunodepressed patients; Philadelphia, 1984, W.B. Saunders Co.)

is preferable to describe this group of cells as granular lymphocytes because of the abundant azurophilic granules in their cytoplasm (Fig. 4-7).

In contrast to T lymphocytes, granular lymphocytes with NK- and K-cell function lack immunologic specificity and can kill cells across organ, strain, and even species barriers. Thus the cytotoxicity of these cells is not restricted to products of the major histocompatibility gene complex. One common feature of these cells is the display of a membrane receptor for the Fc portion of immunoglobulin (especially the IgG isotype) (see Fig. 4-4), but a number of cell-surface antigens identified by monoclonal antibodies have recently been described on NK cells as well. The NK-cell–mediated cytotoxicity can be accomplished totally in the absence of antibody, whereas K-cell function requires the presence of antibody to ''bridge'' the effector and the target cell causing contact and lysis.

Macrophages

Phagocytes have traditionally been viewed as scavenger cells that engulf particulate debris. However, it is becoming increasingly evident that the mononuclear phagocytes—monocytes and macrophages—have an important role in initiating and regulating the immune responses to a number of antigens.[10] These cells have been studied less extensively than lymphocytes, primarily because of the difficulty in obtaining relatively pure populations for analysis. Nevertheless, experiments to date in both animals and humans indicate that monocytes and macrophages have important regulatory influences on lymphocyte responsiveness. In addition to their cellular interactions, these phagocytes exert their influences by elaborating

FUNCTIONAL T-CELL POPULATIONS DEFINED IN MICE

Helper T cells
Ig-recognizing helper T cells
Lymphokine-secreting T cells
Inducer of suppression
First-order suppressor cells (Ts1)
Second-order suppressor cell (Ts2)
Antigen-specific suppressor cells
Suppressor effector T cells
Third-order suppressor cell (Ts3)
Ia-recognizing suppressor
Idiotype-recognizing suppressor cells
Cytotoxic effector T cells
Contrasuppressor effector T cells
Ly12 T cells

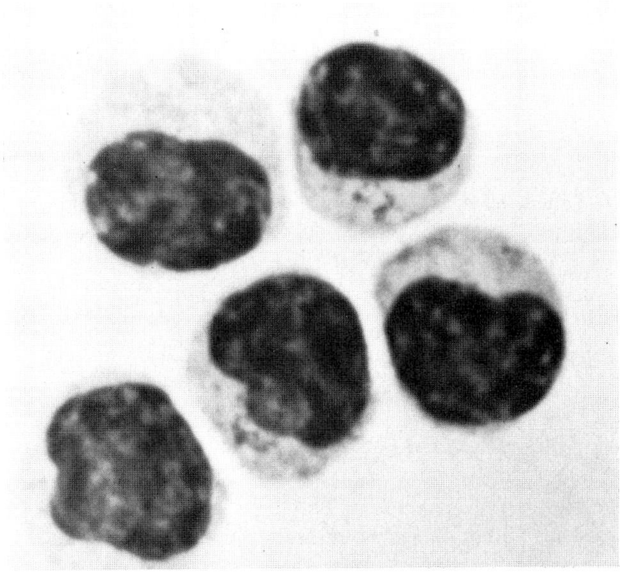

Fig. 4-7 Granular lymphocytes with abundant cytoplasm containing azurophilic granules. They have been termed ''null cells'' in the past because they do not express the classic surface markers for T and B lymphocytes. They do express Fc receptors for immunoglobulin. Granular lymphocytes function as natural killer (NK) cells, and as antibody-dependent cytotoxic cells (ADCC) and are probably the precursors of IL-2–activated killer (LAK) cells.

SECRETORY PRODUCTS OF MACROPHAGES

ENZYMES
Lysozyme
Neutral proteases
- Plasminogen activator
- Collagenase
- Elastase
- Angiotensin-convertase

Acid hydrolases
- Proteases
- Lipases
- Ribonucleases
- Phosphatases
- Glycosidases
- Sulfatases

COMPLEMENT COMPONENTS
C1, C2, C3, C4, C5
Factor B
Factor D
Properdin
C3b inactivator
β1H

ENZYME INHIBITORS
α_2-Macroglobulin
Plasmin inhibitors

BINDING PROTEINS
Transferrin
Transcobalamin II
Fibronectin

ENDOGENOUS PYROGENS

REACTIVE METABOLITES OF OXYGEN
Superoxide
Hydrogen peroxide
Hydroxyl radical

BIOACTIVE LIPIDS
Arachidonate metabolites
- Prostaglandin E_2
- 6-Keto-prostaglandin $F_{1\alpha}$
- Thromboxane
- Leukotriene
- Hydroxy-eicosa-tetraeneoic acids
- Platelet-activating factors

FACTORS CHEMOTACTIC FOR NEUTROPHILS

FACTORS REGULATING SYNTHESIS OF
Proteins by other cells

FACTORS PROMOTING REPLICATION OF
Lymphocytes-IL-1
Myeloid precursors-CSF
Fibroblasts

FACTORS INHIBITING REPLICATION OF
Lymphocytes
Tumor cells

From Shevach, E.M.: Macrophages and other accessory cells. In Paul, W.E., editor: Fundamental immunology, New York, 1984, Raven Press. Modified from Nathan, C.F., Murray, H.W., and Cohn, Z.A.: N. Engl. J. Med. **303:**622, 1980.

many substances, including complement components, lysosome, interferon, plasminogen activators, chemotactic factor, and numerous enzymes (see the boxed material on p. 75). Recently an important group of suppressor macrophages has been characterized that exerts influence by elaborating prostaglandin E_2 and suppressing various aspects of cellular immune function.

Activation of macrophages occurs after antigen exposure and is also under the influence of T-cell products. A consequence of this macrophage activation is the development of its capacity to destroy certain types of bacteria that have been phagocytosed. Macrophages also play an important role as "accessory cells" that are required in the amplification of certain T-cell functions by stimulating them to divide and proliferate.

Granulocytes

Granulocytes engulf foreign material in three well-defined steps: (1) chemotaxis; (2) ingestion; and (3) killing. Clarification of these steps is essential to identify specific cellular defects in surgical patients at risk for the development of infections.

Chemotaxis refers to the directed migration of phagocytic cells out of capillaries toward the source of chemotactic factors that are generated at the site of inflammation. Their precise mechanism is unclear, but these factors can activate a local site on the plasma membrane and direct previous random movement of a cell toward the site of chemotactic factor. Two principal chemotactic factors in humans are believed to be polypeptide portions of the third and fifth components of complement. T lymphocytes also secrete a lymphokine that serves as a chemotactic factor for monocytes and macrophages.

Phagocytosis, or the ingestion step, has two components—attachment of the organism to the phagocytic cell wall and engulfment. The first process (attachment) is augmented by opsonization, the coating of microbes with antibody. In recent years the nature of opsonization has been defined more clearly. For example, it is now known that more efficient phagocytosis of microorganisms requires activation and fixation of the third component of complement to the surface of the organism, which may occur through the interaction of the organism with specific antibodies of the IgG or IgM class.

The final step is the killing process. Intracellular enzymes are activated, and a complex series of oxidative and other metabolic processes is initiated to kill the microorganism or target cell.

Immune Regulation

Amplifying Systems

Among the most important regulatory functions of the T-lymphocyte population is the capacity of *helper T cells* to cooperate with B lymphocytes in the stimulation of the latter to proliferate and to differentiate into antibody-secreting plasma cells. B-cell responses to most protein antigens are absolutely dependent on T-cell help. Such antigens are generally designated thymus-dependent antigens since they fail to stimulate responses in mice that congenitally lack a thymus. Although other types of antigens such as soluble polysaccharides and bacterial lipopolysaccharides have been thought capable of stimulating antibody responses without the need for T cells or their products, recent work indicates that even these responses are dependent on T-cell influences, at least in certain circumstances.

T-cell help can be delivered in at least two distinct ways. One way, often referred to as "cognate help," requires the direct interaction of the helper T cell and the responding B cell. The T cell appears to recognize determinants on antigenic molecules already bound to the B cell. These T cells also recognize a histocompatibility gene product on the B-cell surfaces; the product is referred to as a Class II MHC molecule or DR antigen. The second mechanism by which T cells can participate in B-cell activation is through the release of soluble, nonspecific helper factors referred to as lymphokines. Among the lymphokines are *growth factors,* principally B-cell growth factor, which regulates B-cell proliferation and response to antigenic stimulation, and *differentiation factors,* which cause proliferating B cells to develop into antibody-secreting cells.

Recent evidence has also demonstrated that macrophages can function as helper or *accessory macrophages* involving T-cell proliferation. For example, macrophages are 10 to 80 times more effective as stimulators of allogeneic T-cell proliferation than purified lymphocytes. One possible reason for the ability of macrophages to function as stimulators is that they are the only population in the cell pool that bears the appropriate cell-surface histocompatibility antigens. Another explanation is that macrophages produce essential mediators (such as interleukin-1) required for T-cell proliferation.

Suppressor Systems

An important regulatory function of T cells is their capacity to suppress immune responses. Current research indicates that the activation of *suppressor T cells* to mediate their function actually requires the participation of other cells, which act as part of a suppressor circuit. They include inducer cells, suppressor-precursor cells, and suppressor-effector cells. Thus suppression of immune responses by T cells is a multistep process in which different subsets of T cells are involved. Both internal feedback and amplification loops involving the process of suppression have been demonstrated, and they constitute a highly complicated regulatory system. Some of the effects have been shown to be mediated by soluble factors with or without antigen specificity and genetic restriction.

Recently it has been demonstrated that macrophages and monocytes also have an important regulatory role in many types of immune responses and can act efficiently as suppressor cells. One mechanism of action is the elaboration of prostaglandin E_2 by suppressor macrophages. Prostaglandin E_2 is a potent inhibitor of lymphocyte proliferation, possibly by interfering with the elaboration and binding of interleukin-2. Abnormal levels of suppressor macrophage function have been demonstrated in patients with Hodgkin's lymphoma, head and neck carcinoma, and colon carcinoma.[2] A third group of suppressor cells is identified by a monoclonal antibody (Leu. 7 antibody).[13] These cells can regulate both the differentiation of B lymphocytes and the proliferative responses of T lymphocytes. This suppressor cell activity requires an immune complex activation.

Mediators

Lymphokines function to regulate the proliferation and differentiation of lymphocytes (see Fig. 4-6). Thus lymphocytes communicate among themselves by producing polypeptides with characteristics similar to hormones and neurotransmitters. They exert their effect in a microenvironment (e.g., an inflammatory site) but usually do not have a generalized or systemic effect on other organs. These molecules or factors are nonantibody products affecting lymphocyte clonal expansion.

The literature is confusing about the different types and functions of lymphokines because many were studied with impure preparations and relatively crude separations of the cells they influence. But with the advent of recombinant DNA technology, monoclonal antibodies, and cell-sorting methodologies, exciting and important data are emerging. The major classes of molecules include the following.

INTERLEUKIN-1 (FORMERLY LYMPHOCYTE-ACTIVATING FACTOR). Interleukin-1 (IL-1) functions to activate T cells and is probably an important process in the amplification of T-cell functions. It may also be important in the regulation of body temperature because it is associated with the febrile response. IL-1 is produced by macrophages, and it may mediate some of the accessory functions of macrophage influence on T-cell proliferation. One of its activities is to stimulate the production of IL-2 (see following paragraph); the production of IL-1 is suppressed by glucocorticoids. This interrelationship may be one explanation of why patients receiving steroids have infection with an inappropriately low-febrile response.

INTERLEUKIN-2 (FORMERLY T-CELL GROWTH FACTOR). Interleukin-2 (IL-2) triggers T cells, natural killer cells, and activated killer cells of the granular lymphocyte series. In fact, T lymphocytes will not undergo DNA synthesis in the absence of IL-2. This observation may explain why glucocorticoids inhibit antigen and lectin-induced T-cell mitosis since steroids inhibit IL-2 production in a reversible, concentration-dependent manner. It is not known whether IL-2 affects all T-cell subsets—cytotoxic, helper, and suppressor cells—or whether it has a more selective effect. Recently a functional subclass of cells called lymphokine-activated killer cells has been shown to acquire the ability to kill a wide spectrum of human and murine cancer cells after incubation with IL-2 (Fig. 4-8).[7,9]

PROSTAGLANDIN E_2. Prostaglandin E_2 (PGE_2) and other metabolites of arachidonic acid represent an important group of regulatory molecules whose action in the control of immune function is only beginning to be understood. One primary effect of PGE_2 is to decrease mitogen response and mitosis by T lymphocytes. The sources of PGE_2 are macrophages, monocytes, and, to some extent, neutrophils. PGE_2 production is increased in cancer patients. Prostaglandins represent an important mediator in inflammatory reactions, and their action may be blocked by indomethacin or aspirin. Lymphokines produced by sensitized lymphocytes are capable of stimulating prostaglandin production by macrophages. Since prostaglandin in turn inhibits lymphokine formation and T-cell mitogenesis, this PGE_2 response by macrophages can serve as an important form of negative feedback control.

The effects of prostaglandins are limited to the microenvironment where they are produced. It is not surprising, therefore, that prostaglandins may actually have diametric effects by stimulating T cells as a positive feedback me-

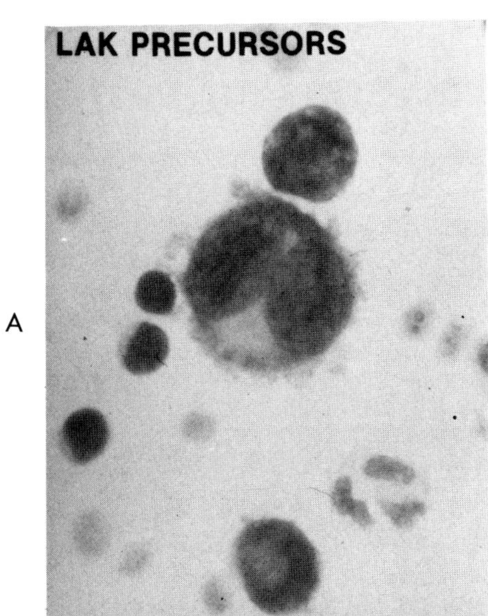

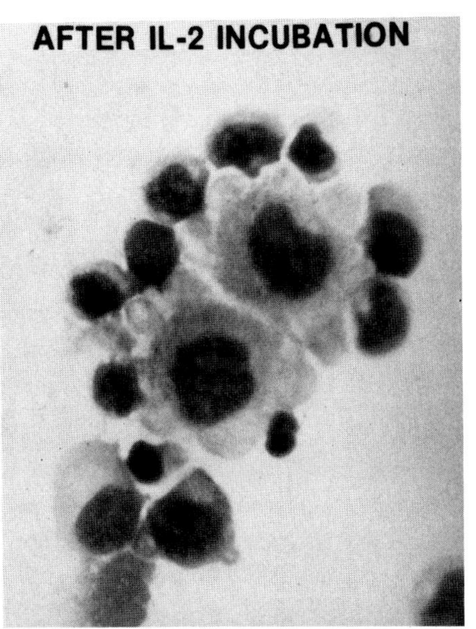

Fig. 4-8 Photomicrographs of IL-2–activated killer (LAK) cell precursors **(A)** and LAK effector cells **(B)** binding to autologous metastatic melanoma targets. LAK precursors from peripheral blood were not capable of binding or killing autologous melanoma tumor cells from the same patient. After a 3-day incubation period with IL-2, the lymphocytes were capable of binding and killing the patient's own metastatic melanoma. (From Balch, C.M., Itoh, K., and Tilden, A.B.: Cellular immune defects in patients with melanoma involving interleukin-2–activated lymphocyte cytotoxicity and a serum suppressor factor, Surgery **98**(2):151, 1985.)

diator. Thus PGE_2 induces immature thymocytes, B lymphocytes, and hematopoietic cell precursors to differentiate and acquire the functional, morphologic, and immunologic characteristics of mature lymphocytes or blood-forming cells. Once cells have matured, PGE_2 is primarily inhibitory, exerting a variety of effects on leukocyte functions. Thus PGE_2 inhibits: (1) T- and B-cell proliferation; (2) leukocyte chemotaxis, aggregation, spread, and oxidative metabolism; (3) cell-mediated cytotoxicity either by natural killer cells or cytotoxic T cells; and (4) release of inflammatory mediators, monokines, or lymphokines from mass cells, basophils, neutrophils, monocytes, or lymphocytes. In addition, PGE_2 and PGD_2 both inhibit platelet aggregation.

Prostaglandins are capable of playing pro-inflammatory as well as anti-inflammatory roles. Exogenously added prostaglandins induce fever, erythema, increased vascular permeability, and vasodilation. PGE_2 is particularly active as a vasodilator and appears to exert its physiologic effects through changes in intracellular cAMP.

INTERFERON. Interferon is a lymphokine that is not a single substance but is a family of proteins produced by many types of animal cells in response to viral infection and other stimuli. In the human, interferons are produced primarily by leukocytes, fibroblasts, and lymphocytes and are classified as alpha, beta, and gamma depending on from which of these cells they originate. Macrophages can also produce interferon. Interferon has been shown experimentally to possess a number of immunologic effects, including enhancement of macrophage activity and augmentation of the cytotoxic activities of lymphocytes with natural killer activity. Its most important role appears to be in the inhibition of the growth of viruses. Pure preparations of interferon are now available. Although some studies suggest that interferon may be of use in the treatment of those tumors suspected of being associated with viruses (e.g., benign juvenile laryngeal papillomatosis), its therapeutic value in the treatment of human cancer remains to be established.

B-CELL FACTORS. B-cell factors are only in a preliminary stage of characterization. They are known to be distinct moieties from interleukin-2 and may play a role in B-cell mitosis and differentiation. T lymphocytes produce at least two such factors: (1) a B-cell growth factor, which induces the proliferation of B lymphocytes; and (2) a B-cell differentiation factor, which induces the differentiation of B cells into plasma cells. Some reports suggest that T cells may produce factors that determine the immunoglobulin heavy-chain class and subclass that an activated B cell will ultimately express.

IDIOTYPES (ANTIANTIBODIES). The amino acid determinants on the heavy and light chains of immunoglobulins can themselves act as antigens because of their structural uniqueness. Such immunoglobulin Region V antigenic determinants are designated idiotopes, and the collection of idiotopes on an antibody molecule is its idiotype. T cells and antibodies specific for idiotypes may play an important role in the regulation of the immune system.

LYMPHOCYTE SURFACE MARKERS. The lymphocyte membrane is a complex biologic structure. Many membrane proteins are concerned with structural and metabolic integrity, whereas other proteins (such as differentiation antigens and histocompatibility antigens) expressed at the membrane surface reflect the cell's specialized function(s). Biologically, these latter surface constituents are important for cell to cell or cell to antigen interaction in their microenvironment and as receptors for activation (or deactivation) of cell function as part of an immune response that takes place in concert with other lymphoid cells. Experimentally, these diverse surface constituents are extremely valuable as biologic markers or fingerprints for characterizing lymphocyte traits. Some of these proteins are designated as *cell surface antigens* because they elicit antibodies when injected into another host (e.g., monoclonal antibodies), and they are to be distinguished from naturally incurring foreign antigens (e.g., those on microorganisms). Other markers have been termed *cell surface receptors* because they spontaneously bind certain indicator cells or molecules (e.g., viral, complement, or immunoglobulin receptors).

Table 4-2 **DIFFERENT WAYS OF CHARACTERIZING HUMAN T AND B LYMPHOCYTES**

Category	B Cells	T Cells
By stages of maturation	Pre-B cell Immature B cell Mature B cell Plasma cell	Pre-T cell Immature T cell Mature T cell
By surface markers	Surface immunoglobulin	T-cell antigen
By function	Antibody-producing cell (IgM, IgG, IgE, IgA, IgD)	Cytotoxic cell Helper cell Suppressor cell

Immunologic reagents that detect surface membrane markers have become valuable probes to detect different patterns of marker expression (called the surface phenotype) on specialized subpopulations of lymphocytes. As a result, the actual cellular participants in different immune responses can now be discerned more precisely from a crowd of bystander lymphoid cells in blood and lymphoid tissues. Much progress in this regard has been made in human immunology to the extent that several dozen distinct surface markers have been cataloged, as well as the myriad of antigenic specificities that represent products in the major histocompatibility complex present on all cells (Table 4-2).

MONITORING THE IMMUNE SYSTEM

Clinical Assessment of Immune Function

Correlation of either in vitro or in vivo assays for immune function with observed immune reactivity in humans is far from ideal. The techniques for measuring immune function are crude, and the results are frequently confused by the presence of sepsis or other associated problems in immunodepressed surgical patients. Nevertheless, the rapid development of sophisticated technology has permitted more quantitative and precise assays of immune function at the cellular and even the molecular level. Without question, the availability of monoclonal antibodies (Fig. 4-

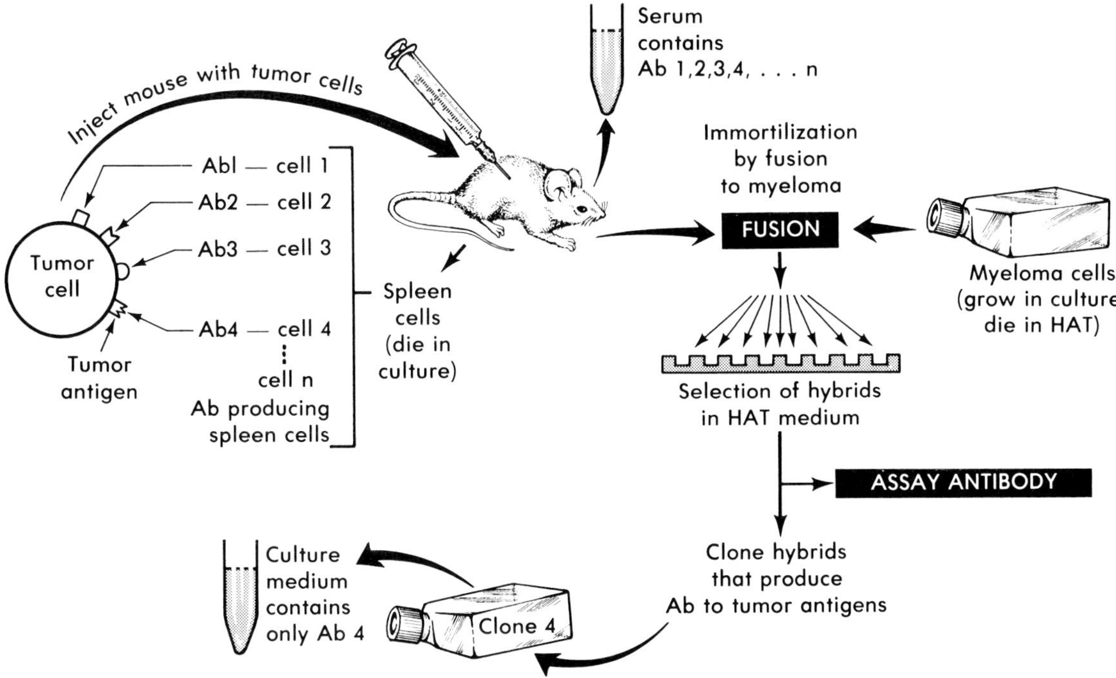

Fig. 4-9 Monoclonal antibody production. Tumor cells contain multiple tumor antigens, each of which elicits a separate type of antibody when the tumor is injected into a mouse. B lymphocytes are harvested from the spleen of the immunized mouse and are fused to myeloma cells. Myeloma cells fused to lymphocytes are able to grow in HAT medium, whereas nonfused myeloma cells and lymphocytes from the spleen die. Subclones of the hybridomas can then be isolated to produce antibody to a single tumor antigen. (From Kearney, J.F.: Hybridomas and monoclonal antibodies. In Paul, W.E., editor: Fundamental immunology, New York, 1984, Raven Press.)

9) and genetically engineered biologics are the two most important technical advances of this decade.[4]

Monoclonal antibodies are made from cloned hybridomas that can produce large quantities of pure antibodies. This technique has already had an enormous impact because it can provide reagents with a purity and potency not previously obtainable by other means. Although cultured myeloma cells can be adapted to grow indefinitely in tissue culture, they manufacture irrelevant immunoglobulins, whereas plasma cells producing a specific antibody will not grow for more than a few days in tissue culture. In the hybridization technique, plasma cells from immunized mice can be fused with the myeloma cells to form a hybrid cell line, and subclones of antibody-producing hybridomas can then be isolated. Thus the genetic machinery directing the production of antibodies is taken over by the plasma cell while the genes from the cultured myeloma cell allow the hybridoma to grow in tissue culture indefinitely.

Gene cloning is another remarkable advance wherein a specific gene fragment can be inserted into a bacteriophage and grown in susceptible bacteria on an indefinite basis. As shown in Fig. 4-10, a gene of interest can be digested by sequence-specific restriction enzymes into gene fragments. These fragments are introduced into bacteriophage vectors and then plated into susceptible bacteria. The clones of bacteria that contain the gene of interest can be identified using specific DNA probes. Further subcloning is then used to isolate the bacteria containing the cloned gene. The genetically engineered bacteria are then cultured indefinitely; any products produced by the bacteria under direction of the cloned gene can be harvested in the supernatant fluid. Examples of cloned gene products include many types of hormones and biologics (e.g., IL-2 and interferon).

In Vitro Assays

In vitro assays are used either to define the presence of specific components of the immune system or to test the activity of these components, once identified.

Some advantages of cloned DNA or hybridoma products include the following: (1) an inexhaustible and specific product is established; (2) cloning separates molecular elements at the genetic level before their actual synthesis by isolating unique DNA sequences or gene products; (3) sensitivity and specificity of a cloned reagent are controlled by the user rather than being limited by the supply or purity of the reagent itself; and (4) reproducibility is possible because the reactivities of monoclonal antibodies, gene probes, and cloned antigens are predetermined, specific, and consistent.[4] Some uses of monoclonal antibodies are listed in the boxed material on p. 81. Examples of DNA hybridization to monitor certain disease states are shown in Table 4-3. Cytofluorimetry using labeled monoclonal antibodies can now define various subsets of lymphocytes with considerable precision.[12] Thus it is possible to determine whether or not there are mature circulating T cells,

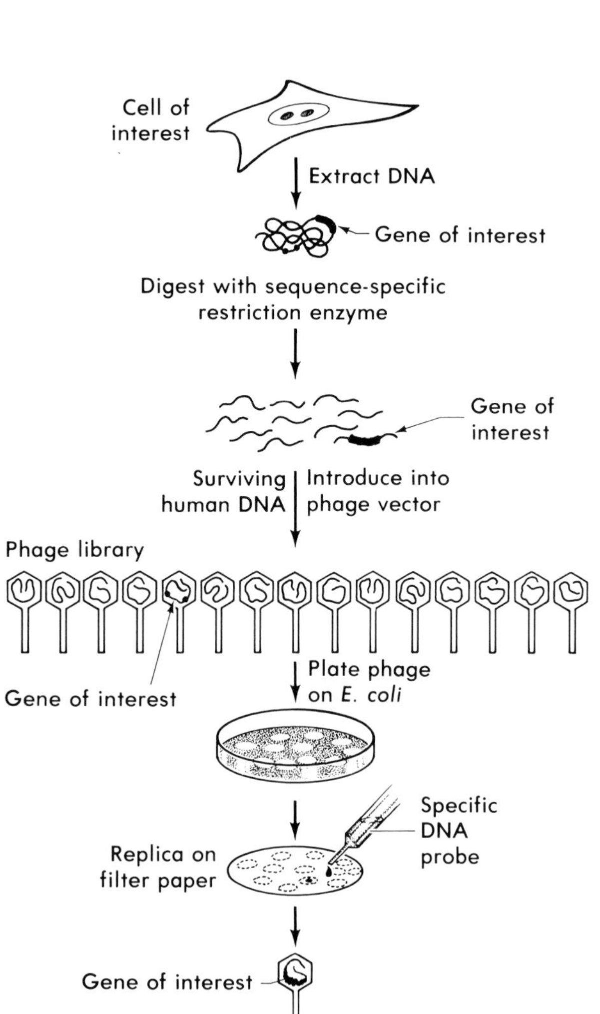

Fig. 4-10 One method of gene cloning. DNA molecules can be reconstructed by joining gene sequences from one source to other sequences of different origins. The product is often described as recombinant DNA. A key to this technique is the ability of restriction enzymes to cleave DNA at particular, short nucleotide sequences and to rejoin them in hybrid form while retaining their function. (From Balch, C.M.: Immune responses to tumor antigens and their clinical applications, Surgery **100:**562, 1986.)

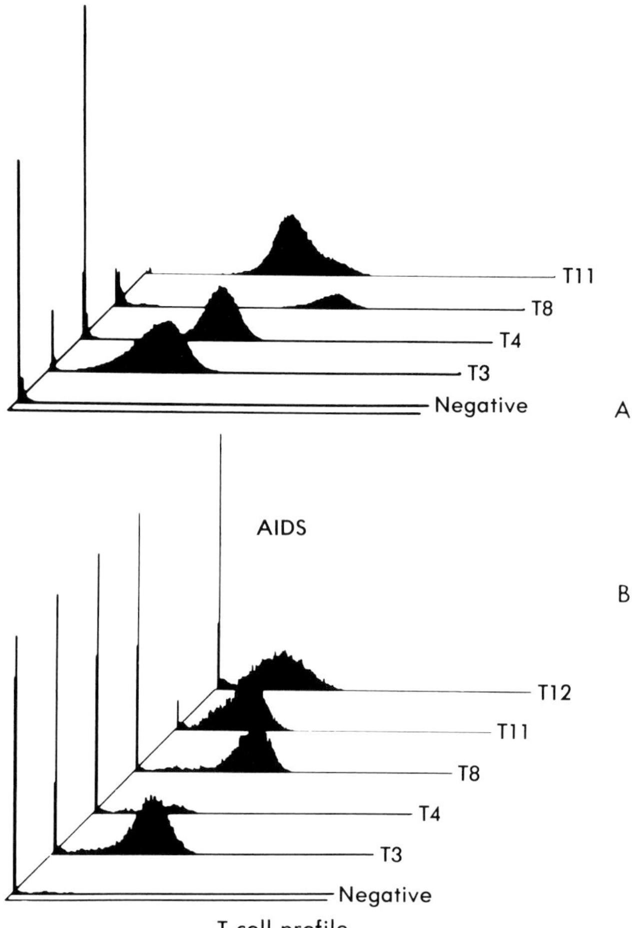

Fig. 4-11 Monoclonal antibody characterization of human T cell subpopulations. **A,** Normal. **B,** Patient with acquired immune deficiency syndrome (AIDS). Reactivity of T-cell–specific monoclonal antibody as defined on a cell sorter by direct immunofluorescence. For this technique, 50,000 cells were quantitated with anti-T_3 (defining a constant subunit of T-cell receptor on all mature T cells), anti-T_4 (inducer T cells equal 66% of T cells), anti-T_8 (suppressor T cells equal 33% of T cells), anti-T (sheep erythrocyte receptor on all T cells), and anti-T_{11} (mature T cells). There is a reversal of T_4/T_8 ratio in the AIDS patient as compared with the normal individual. (From Wilson, R.E.: Surgical problems in immunodepressed patients, Philadelphia, 1984, W.B. Saunders Co.)

Table 4-3 **EXAMPLES OF USE OF DNA HYBRIDIZATION TO DETECT VIRAL NUCLEIC ACID IN HOSTS WITH CHRONIC INFECTIONS OR NONINFECTIOUS DISEASES**

Disease	Viral Probe
Chronic hepatitis	Hepatitis B virus
Latent central nervous system herpes simplex virus	Herpes simplex virus–1 DNA
Latent varicella-zoster virus in sensory ganglia	Varicella-zoster–virus DNA fragments
Acquired immunodeficiency syndrome	Human T-cell leukemia virus
Laryngeal papilloma (active, inactive, and adjacent tissue)	Cloned papilloma–virus DNA
Atherosclerosis	Herpes simplex virus 1 or 2
Nasopharyngeal carcinoma and Burkitt's lymphoma	Cloned Epstein-Barr–virus DNA
Central nervous system lymphoma	Cloned Epstein-Barr–virus DNA
Hepatocellular carcinoma in alcoholic liver disease	Hepatitis B–virus DNA
Kaposi's sarcoma	Hepatitis B–virus DNA
Various human malignant processes	Various retrovirus genes

From Engleberg, N.C., and Eisenstein, B.I.: Reprinted by permission of N. Engl. J. Med. **311:**892, 1984.

USES OF MONOCLONAL ANTIBODIES

DIAGNOSTIC AND TECHNICAL USES

1. Identification and characterization of cell-surface molecules (e.g., differentiation antigens on lymphocytes, hormone receptors, histocompatibility antigens, and tumor antigens)
2. Detection of protein antigens by radioimmunoassay (RIA) (e.g., CEA and hormones)
3. Standardization of tissue typing reagents
4. Large-scale purification of biologically active substances (e.g., interferon)

THERAPEUTIC USES

1. Delivery of radioisotopes or drugs to tumor cells
   a. To detect micrometastases
   b. To destruct tumor cells
2. Manipulation of the immune system
   a. To eliminate specific effector cells
   b. To kill suppressor cells
   c. To passively immunize against tumors

helper T cells, suppressor-cytotoxic T cells, normal thymocytes, and precursor T cells in the early stages of differentiation and whether or not activated and mature suppressor-cytotoxic T cells are present. Ratio analysis of different subsets may be used to define immunologically abnormal states such as that in the acquired immune deficiency syndrome (AIDS) patient population (Fig. 4-11). In patients with AIDS there is a reversal of the normal helper–suppressor cell ratio (normally 2:1) so that the suppressor cells greatly outnumber the helper lymphocytes.

B-cell function can be quantitated by enumerating those lymphocytes with immunoglobulin isotopes on their surface membrane as well as by measuring serum immunoglobulin levels. It is possible to measure an antigen-antibody complex by measuring its binding with protein A of staphylococcus or the binding of the C1q component of complement. In addition, blocking of Fc receptors in a reaction such as the antibody-dependent cell cytotoxicity assay can reflect the presence of antigen-antibody complexes. Polyethylene glycol precipitation of immune complexes can be simply defined by differences in light absorption. Complement components can be accurately measured, and deficiencies involving the pathway of complement activation cascade can be identified.

In addition to the use of the flow cytometry evaluation of lymphocyte subsets (using a fluorescence-activated cell sorter), five areas of lymphocyte function can be evaluated by other types of in vitro analysis: (1) proliferation; (2) lymphokine production; (3) cytotoxic activity; (4) helper cell function; and (5) macrophage suppression. These assays use certain lectins to stimulate subsets of lymphocytes and macrophages while the rate of proliferation, cytotoxicity, or soluble products so produced are measured. These soluble products such as interferon and interleukins are becoming increasingly more important as biologic response modifiers.

Usually the identification of the immunologic status of a given surgical patient is fairly straightforward. Screening for basic functions identifies most patients with either profound B- or T-lymphocyte abnormalities. Bone marrow deficiency can quickly be identified from a complete blood count. More sophisticated screening requires expert assistance because of the complexities of the instrumentation and the reagents involved.

In Vivo Assays

To date in vivo assays of immune function are not sufficiently reproducible or reliable to use in a clinical setting. The most representative in vivo measure of cellular immune function is the dinitrochlorobenzene (DNCB) assay. After an initial skin contact with DNCB, a challenge with the same substance is made on the skin 14 days later. Since this antigen represents a new contact for delayed hypersensitivity, the induced response can be quantitated by the degree of skin reactivity and provides an index of T-cell immune responsiveness. Skin testing with other substances such as *Candida,* mumps virus, tuberculous bacteria, streptokinase, and streptodornase represents measurement of recall antigens. The maximum response occurs within 48 to 72 hours, measuring erythema and induration as the end point.

TYPES OF SURGICAL PATIENTS WITH IMMUNODEPRESSION

It can no longer be considered a rarity for hospitalized surgical patients to have some level of immune depression. Alterations in immune function occur so broadly, although frequently only to a minimum degree, that the majority of surgical patients may be expected to have some altered component of the immune system.[16] All practicing surgeons must recognize the problems and the consequences of immune depression to diagnose and to treat surgical disease more effectively. Alterations in immune function can be classified as either random (unintentional) or medically induced.

Random Immunodepression

The category of random immunodepressed patients includes those born with congenital defects of immune function as well as patients in the older age group who have a spontaneous reduction in immune reactivity. Acquired causes of immune deficiency include those resulting from infections, trauma, primary malignancy, nutritional deficiency, and disease states associated with autoimmunity. Many alterations in immune function can occur in this broad spectrum of unintentional immune deficiency depending on the degree of host responsiveness. Quantitative defects range from the profound immunodeficiency diseases resulting from hematopoietic stem-cell defects with reduced T-cell, B-cell, and phagocytic activity to the mild senescence of the immune system in many older patients.

The congenital deficiencies are very heterogenous, and each must be accurately defined to determine prognosis and potential therapy.[3] The severe combined immunodeficiency group is associated with both T- and B-cell disorders. This group includes four subtypes: (1) reticular dysgenesis with a hematopoietic stem-cell defect (reduced T-cell, B-cell, and phagocytic activity); (2) "Swiss" type with lymphocytic stem-cell defect (reduced T-cell and B-cell activity); (3) severe combined immunodeficiency with adenosine deaminase deficiency (reduced T-cell activity and variable B-cell alteration); and (4) severe combined immunodeficiency with B cells (T-cell abnormality alone). Primary T-cell deficiencies include purine/nucleotide phosphorylase deficiency and thymic maldevelopment as is seen in patients with the DiGeorge syndrome.

There is a wide diversity of disorders of B-cell function resulting in hypogammaglobulinemia or agammaglobulinemia. The Wiskott-Aldrich syndrome is associated with an abnormality in one or more of the interacting cells in the afferent limb of the immune arc even though the effector limb is intact. It is associated with severe thrombocytopenia, frequent episodes of bleeding, and recurrent infections. Finally there is a group of immunodeficiency diseases associated with the inability of effective immunologic components to survive in the circulation. Some of these disorders involve the catabolic pathways for such molecules or result from circulating anti-lymphocyte antibodies. One such disorder—intestinal lymphagiectasia—is associated with a loss of both lymphocytes and immunoglobulin into the bowel as a result of dilated lymphatics of the small intestine.

An anticipated alteration in immune function occurs with aging. Older patients have an increased susceptibility to infection and also have an increased incidence of autoimmunity. One of the most definable immunologic alterations that occurs with aging is thymic involution. By age 50, there is 15% or less of the original thymic capability. This alteration has been well-defined by studies of transplantation in aging mice.[15] It may be that loss of suppressor cell function regulated by thymic function may increase the risk for autoimmune disorders. Other flaws in immune regulation may be more clearly defined as newer techniques become available.

Heading the list of acquired forms of unintentional immunosuppression are those diseases associated with viral infections. Although infections with the Epstein-Barr virus are the most common, most notably mononucleosis, certainly the AIDS patient population associated with human T-cell leukemia virus Type III (HTLV-3) is the most spectacular.[5] The resultant reversal of the helper/suppressor cell ratios makes the patients susceptible to opportunistic infections with organisms such as *Pneumocystis carinii* and to the induction of rare malignancies such as Kaposi's sarcoma. Other important viral infections associated with alterations in suppressor T-cell function and immunoglobulins are those with cytomegalovirus and hepatitis B virus. Careful evaluation of patients with a broad variety of viral illnesses is certain to delineate even a greater number of immunodepressed states associated with these agents.

Traumatic injuries, especially thermal burns, are associated with the activation of suppressor T cells.[8] It is possible that immune complex formations from damaged tissue play an important role in the altered immune function in traumatized patients for both suppressor factors in serum and cells have been identified in these circumstances. The thymus becomes atrophic, particularly in youngsters with burns, and responses to T-dependent antigens are depressed. Most of the alterations in T-cell function appear to be related to the induction of suppressor cell activity, but indirectly, antibody production is also markedly reduced.

Patients with the immune complex diseases such as systemic lupus erythematosus (SLE), Sjögren's syndrome, polymyositis, rheumatoid arthritis, scleroderma, and the various vasculitidies demonstrate progressive alteration in immune function with circulating and tissue-fixed autoantibodies, and many are associated with a much higher incidence of lymphoid malignancies. When corticosteroid and other immunodepressive agents are used for therapy in this patient population, the patients present a dual problem in altered immune function for the surgeon. Likewise, patients with granulomatous disease of the intestine have a significantly higher level of immune complexes in the circulating blood that interfere with all cells expressing Fc receptors such as macrophages and granular lymphocytes.

The common denominator for many patients with chronic sepsis, malnutrition, and wasting illness is the chronicity of their protein-calorie deficiency and the continued catabolism that accompanies this defect. The reversal of such a deficiency by hyperalimentation has had a dramatic effect on immune function in these patients. The usual consequence in the depleted and malnourished patient is an increased risk for sepsis, decreased antibody production, and inefficient wound healing.

Although it is widely accepted that cancer induction may result from some alteration in immune surveillance on the part of the host and that there may be a failure of natural immunity to eradicate genetically dissimilar cancer cells, attempts to reliably detect abnormalities of immune capability at the time that tumors are found have been uniformly unrevealing. More sophisticated identification of specific antibodies and variations involving subsets of lymphoid cells may help to elucidate abnormalities in immune response in cancer patients in the future. Once the patient becomes cachectic in association with widespread metastatic malignancy and malnutrition, there is little question that a broad reduction in immune function takes place. However, only in such primary tumors as Hodgkin's disease and multiple myeloma have alterations in immune response been defined.

Correlations have been made between the level of dinitrochlorobenzene (DNCB) reactivity and the prognosis for patients with head and neck cancers, malignant melanoma, bladder cancers, and some lung cancers. The anergic state of Hodgkin's disease patients relates to cellular immunity with a well-recognized reduction in delayed cutaneous hypersensitivity to both primary and secondary antigens. However, there does not appear to be any correlation between immune depression and outcome in patients with Hodgkin's disease, and it is not a part of the staging system. Recently Hodgkin's disease patients have been shown to contain circulating phagocytic cells that can release prostaglandins (PGE_2) that can specifically inhibit T-cell proliferation. Patients with nonHodgkin's lymphoma often have abnormalities in antibody production with monoclonal gammopathies. Cell-mediated immunity varies according to the type of lymphoma found. Again, evaluation of immune function in cancer patients depends not only on the underlying disease but on the treatment that has been instituted for the cancer patient. Both must be taken into account when defining the state of immune reactivity.

Induced Abnormalities of Immune Function

For surgical patients, anesthesia per se is often responsible for a reduction in T-cell function. The extent of both the surgery and the underlying surgical disease affects this phenomenon. Sepsis, trauma, cancer, or immunologic diseases modify the primary anesthetic effect. Spinal anesthesia is less likely to be associated with altered immune response than is general anesthesia.

The most dramatic demonstration of induced immune response is that achieved in the transplant recipient. The requirement for major alterations in T-cell and B-cell function by a variety of techniques produces a profound effect on immune function. It is now recognized that the induction of immunologic enhancement, again by a reversal of the helper/suppressor ratio, is associated with the best long-term preservation of transplanted organs. In the renal allograft system, protection from antibody attack and from immune complex destruction of vascular structures and minimization of cellular infiltrates preserve long-term function of transplanted kidneys. Obviously the goal of the transplant immunologist is to provide the most specific form of immune nonreactivity possible to permit protection of the host from viral and bacterial infections, cancer induction, and immune-complex diseases. Maintaining a minimum level of immune suppression, with bursts of increased therapy when acute rejection episodes occur, is the strategy now widely adopted by transplant centers. Unfortunately, most immunosuppressive therapy is still nonspecific in nature and depends on gross alteration in T-cell and B-cell responsiveness.

The attack on the immune system takes place at all three points in the immune arc—the afferent arc, the central zone, and the efferent arc. Antigen processing by macrophages and dendritic cells is most crucial. The central site may be defined as the entire host response mechanism subsequent to antigen processing, and it involves the central lymphoid tissue. The efferent arc is that portion of the system that takes place within the grafted tissue itself. The major effect of clinical suppression is to alter T-cell responses with drugs such as azathioprine, corticosteroids, anti-lymphocyte serum, and cyclosporin A. This latter substance seems to have a propensity for permitting suppressor cells to survive, thus inducing a more efficient form of enhancement.[14] In general, there is a sparing of B-cell function so that immediate-type hypersensitivity reactions and antibody production are much less affected than delayed-type reactions. Thus bacterial infections are much less serious for transplant recipients because their ability to produce antibodies is intact, while viral and fungal diseases are more prevalent because T-cell immunity is depressed. Cancer induction, autoimmune diseases, and vasculitis are common sequelae in patients who undergo long-term immunosuppression for allograft survival. Although most transplant recipients can be maintained at a level of reasonable homeostasis, many of their body functions are unusually brittle, and their "immune reserve" is greatly reduced. The potential for unusual complications of surgical disease and therapy is great, but when proper steps are taken, surgical risks can be significantly reduced in this patient population.

Corticosteroids affect immune function in a variety of ways. They are probably the drugs most frequently used in transplant recipients, and the requirement for high doses of a drug like prednisone during rejection episodes in allografted patients is associated with the greatest incidence of complications. Most of these complications are infectious in nature, but the effects on the gastrointestinal tract, the skeletal system, the metabolic activity of all cells, and acid-base balance are equally dramatic. Many other patients besides transplant recipients receive corticosteroids, however, so it is essential for the surgeon to identify a history of steroid administration in all patients. Corticosteroid actions on lymphocytes include decreased DNA synthesis, decreased RNA synthesis, membrane destabilization, and decreased interleukin-2 and interferon production. Steroids have direct actions on macrophages as well, including stabilization of lysosomal and cellular membranes, loss of phagocytic activity, and decreased function of dendritic cells. Complement production is decreased since macrophages serve as a major source of complement in the body. A general reduction in inflammatory reactions, depression of protein synthesis resulting from a catabolic effect, and changes in membrane transport are also net effects of corticosteroid activity. Most actions of corticosteroid therapy are dose related; for patients receiving chronic steroid therapy, alternate-day treatment may frequently be associated with fewer complications and aberrations of immune response.

Chemotherapeutic agents for the management of malignancy may also have very specific actions that affect protein synthesis and cellular proliferative processes. Patients receive chemotherapeutic agents either for the primary treatment of lymphoproliferative disorders or when those patients with solid tumors are at high risk for recurrence or have known metastatic disease. Adjuvant therapeutic protocols are becoming more aggressive but of shorter duration so that effects on immune responses may be less noticeable over the long-term in those patients treated with such agents. However, the net effect of chemotherapeutic agents on the immune response system must be considered for each drug as well as for the underlying malignant disease process. With each class of drugs, marked differences in the potential for altering immune responses exist.

All alkylating chemotherapy agents (e.g., L-Phenylalanine mustard and cyclophosphamide [Cytoxan]) are associated with some degree of bone marrow depression and have a propensity for leukemia induction. Pancytopenia is common during the nadir from chemotherapy, but bone marrow function at other times is usually adequate. Specific suppression of antibody production and suppressor cell activity has been identified with cyclophosphamide, and synergy with radiation therapy is common with this class of drugs. Cyclophosphamide has actually been used as an alternative agent to azathioprine (an antimetabolite drug) for immune suppression in transplant recipients. The antimetabolites act primarily during the DNA-synthetic phase of the cell cycle. Both T- and B-lymphocyte function can be reduced during chemotherapy with these drugs. For example, 5-fluorouracil, another antimetabolite, specifically blocks DNA synthesis through its effect on thymidylate synthetase, while methotrexate blocks the enzyme dihydrofolate reductase and its role in purine synthesis. Most of the antitumor antibiotics (e.g., doxorubicin [Adriamycin]), plant alkyloids (e.g., vincristine), and enzymes (e.g., L-asparaginase) also interfere with DNA production. They either intercolate, thus interfering with DNA replication, alter spindle proteins during mitosis, or otherwise compromise reparative processes and lymphocyte production that are so necessary for the immune response to proceed. Most of the synthetic chemotherapeutic agents such as hydroxyurea and platinum-containing compounds behave like alkylating agents, with the production of free radicals and the subsequent cross-linking of complementary DNA strands within the cell. These effects are primarily on rapidly proliferating cell populations, but they include lymphoid and bone marrow cells along with malignant ones.

Patients undergoing splenectomy may have reduced immune responsiveness. The most serious component of this immunodepressed state is the inability to handle overwhelming bacterial infection, primarily with encapsulated organisms such as pneumococcus, meningococcus, and influenza.[16] Associated with this postsplenectomy syndrome is disseminated intravascular coagulation, adult respiratory distress syndrome, and shock. The rapidity with which this syndrome may be lethal (12 to 24 hours) has produced the greatest cause for concern. In general, the risk for occurrence in patients undergoing splenectomy without hematologic disorders and not receiving other immunosuppressive agents is considered minimum. However, immunizing patients undergoing splenectomy with polyvalent vaccine (Pneumovax) directed against pneumococcal capsular polysaccharides is now accepted surgical practice.

Most of the functional abnormalities in immune response that occur following splenectomy are short-term, but alteration in T- and B-cell numbers probably persists. There is no evidence of skin test anergy or alteration in delayed hypersensitivity, but IgM production can be reduced following splenectomy, at least transiently. Unquestionably, because of these immune disturbances, there has been a reduction in the incidence of splenectomy following trauma and as a part of other surgical procedures, with attempts being made to preserve the spleen whenever feasible and safe.

Finally, radiation therapy also influences immune function.[16] Cells that require reproduction for their function are most sensitive to irradiation. T lymphocytes are especially susceptible to ionizing radiation. This response forms the basis for the use of x-ray therapy of renal allografts that has been common practice in many transplant centers, particularly when cadaver donor grafts are involved. Current knowledge indicates that the mechanism of radiation therapy is through induction of breaks (usually single) in the deoxyriboside backbone of the DNA double helix. In addition, the production of free radicals within radiated cells as well as various hydroperoxides induce an alkylating effect. The net result of these reactions is interference with cell reproduction in the S phase of cell division. Fully differentiated cells do not seem to be harmed by radiation. Thus antibody production is much less affected by radiation than is cell-mediated reactivity, resulting in radiation's major effect being on the ability of the host to respond to a new antigen.

In view of these effects, it is not surprising that radiation has been associated with the development of a number of malignancies including leukemias, lymphomas, sarcomas of bone and soft tissue, various skin malignancies, thyroid cancer, bladder cancer, and liver tumors.[16] The latency period between exposure to radiation and the induction of cancer is generally long. For example, the latency period for the development of the induction of thyroid cancer following neck irradiation for swollen lymph nodes in children, a not uncommon practice several decades ago, has often been as long as 20 to 30 years. Thus when a particular malignancy is treated with radiotherapy, the potential for the delayed development of a radio-induced malignancy must always be considered.

ASSOCIATED PROBLEMS IN IMMUNOCOMPROMISED PATIENTS

Patients with either acquired or induced immunologic abnormalities are at greater risk for a wide variety of medical problems even without subjection to a surgical procedure. The underlying disease state responsible for the immunodepression, the therapy the patient is receiving, and the documented abnormality in immune function must be considered when evaluating the overall immune potential of a given individual. Deficits in immune responsiveness may make the surgical patient more susceptible to a variety of serious complications, either common or unique, with the severity generally related to the degree of immunosuppression achieved.[16] The five major problems in immunodepressed patients are sepsis, gastrointestinal disease, metabolic derangement, cardiopulmonary dysfunction, and growth of malignant cells.

Sepsis. Septic complications are usually the most frequent and certainly the most likely to be lethal of all of the associated problems with which immunodepressed patients must deal. Bacterial, fungal, viral, and protozoan agents may all be responsible for infections. Many of the pathogens are unusual and frequently are saprophytic and opportunistic. Often little immunity is developed against these organisms, or the immunity that had been present is no longer active. The most frequent bacterial infections result from *Mycobacterium tuberculosis* and species of *Pseudomonas, Listeria, Legionella, Serratia,* or other nosocomial sources. Since neutrophil function is usually active, most patients do not manifest standard staphylococcal or streptococcal infections, and coliform organisms produce sepsis only in certain settings, such as bowel perforation. Viral infections are usually caused by cytomegaloviruses, hepatitis B virus, or Epstein-Barr virus.

Fungal infections can be extremely difficult to manage. The most common fungal conditions are aspergillosis, mucormycosis, blastomycosis, coccidioidomycosis, or actinomycosis. *Candida albicans* is probably the most frequent of all hyphal forms. These agents are particularly aggressive and difficult to eradicate because immune defenses are usually severely depressed when these infections appear. Protozoan and other organisms are by no means rare in this patient population. They include *Pneumocystis carinii, Mycoplasma* spp., and *Nocardia* spp.

Fevers of unknown origin are common in immunocompromised patients and demand intensive and carefully planned evaluation. The most common portals of entry for pathogenic organisms are through the respiratory and gastrointestinal tracts, but spread to the central nervous system, the liver, and the kidney is not uncommon. Common presenting diagnoses are pneumonia, lung abscess, meningitis, hepatitis, urinary sepsis, and wound infections.

Gastrointestinal Disease. Preexisting gastrointestinal disease often flares when immunosuppression becomes apparent. Such problems include acid-peptic disease, diverticulitis, perianal sepsis, hepatitis, cholecystitis, and esophagitis. Thus it is important to be aware of any underlying gastrointestinal abnormalities and to take whatever prophylactic steps are possible to avoid complications from them. The type of therapy patients are receiving plays an important role in stimulating further gastrointestinal disease, particularly gastritis, esophagitis, and duodenal ulcer. Most of the chemotherapeutic agents produce gastrointestinal or mucosal ulceration and mucositis; many of the complications of steroid therapy have to do with esophagitis, gastritis, and duodenal ulcer disease. Fluid restriction and constipation resulting from inactivity and dietary restriction may be responsible for diverticulitis, and cholestatic disease in the liver can occur with the use of a variety of drugs. Prolonged nasogastric intubation as well as radiation or oral drug administration can produce severe esophagitis. Gastrointestinal symptoms, particularly relating to duodenal ulcer disease, may be muted and much less painful when patients are on corticosteroids, yet perforation and gastrointestinal bleeding can occur despite minimum symptomatology.

Metabolic Derangements. Protein-calorie malnutrition is one of the major metabolic derangements in patients with immunocompromised function. Patients on corticoids are susceptible to steroid-induced diabetes mellitus, particularly if they have a family history of diabetes. The diabetes results in further muscle wasting and a higher risk for sepsis unless appropriate treatment is instituted. Cataract development, aseptic necrosis of the hip, and the neurologic complications of diabetes may all ensue. Postoperative problems involving wound healing, such as gastrointestinal fistulas and perforation of otherwise contained gastrointestinal lesions, also produce their own serious metabolic complications. Hyponatremia is frequent in this patient population, and metabolic alkalosis may occur with vomiting or with other abnormalities of the gastrointestinal tract. Hypokalemia is seen in patients receiving corticosteroids as well as in those patients with diarrhea, fistula formation, and vomiting. On the other hand, if renal failure and renal insufficiency take place, hyperkalemia is the most serious complication, accompanied by metabolic acidosis. Calcium and magnesium metabolism may be markedly disturbed either in the form of hypocalcemia with renal failure or in the secondary hyperparathyroidism resulting from renal failure. The risk of hypercalcemia from enteral tube feedings is also a possibility.

Cardiopulmonary Disease. Many immunodepressed patients have evidence of vascular disease, with or without hypertension and cardiovascular complications. Certainly all renal failure patients have premature arteriosclerosis as do patients with immune complex diseases. Chronic anemia worsens cardiac function, and many of the septic complications can, in fact, involve the myocardium. Therefore fluid and metabolic management should include careful evaluation of cardiac performance status. Certain chemotherapeutic agents such as doxorubicin (Adriamycin) have a substantial risk for myocardial toxicity if they exceed recommended dosages. The combination of doxorubicin with mediastinal radiation therapy greatly increases the risk of cardiomyopathy. Bleomycin presents a complicating problem with respiratory insufficiency, especially if oxygen levels in the inspired air are maintained above 30% during anesthesia. This is particularly the case if surgery is performed within 3 weeks of the last dose of bleomycin therapy.

Pulmonary insufficiency accompanying pulmonary sepsis must be searched for and corrected if present. Pericarditis can occur with malignant tumor involvement of the pericardium or can result from tuberculosis or uremia. Endocarditis from central venous catheters can be avoided by using meticulous aseptic technique in catheter placement and maintenance. Pleural effusions occur frequently, and they may be a septic focus as well. Thrombophlebitis and phlebothrombosis are more frequent in immunocompromised patients even in the face of thrombocytopenia or abnormalities involving production of clotting factors.

Development of Malignancies. There is a clear increase in the incidence of certain forms of primary malignancy in patients who are immunosuppressed. Those patients with congenital abnormalities and many patients with immune complex disease have a higher incidence of lymphoma and leukemia. Renal transplant recipients and patients with AIDS are also at increased risk to develop nonHodgkin's lymphomas and Kaposi's sarcomas. In general, immunosuppressed patients have a higher incidence of epithelial cancers, particularly those of the uterine cervix and basal cell and squamous cell carcinoma of the skin. Their incidence of lymphoma is approximately one-hundredfold greater than in the normal population. The most common form in the transplant recipient is diffuse histiocytic lymphoma.[11] Interestingly, half of the lymphomas identified in transplant recipients have involved the central nervous system, a privileged site since it is lacking in lymphocytes. There is likewise a risk of leukemia induction from chemotherapy, particularly with alkylating agents.[6] Radiation-induced malignancy is usually in the form of sarcomas, most frequently after treatment of breast cancer and pelvic tumors, or epithelial tumors such as thyroid cancers following head and neck irradiation. Recognition of this greater risk for the induction of malignancies makes it important for physicians to screen for them in this at-risk population.

SURGICAL MANAGEMENT OF THE IMMUNOCOMPROMISED SURGICAL PATIENT

Nutrition

Whenever possible, nutrition should be optimized in the immunocompromised patient population. If the gastrointestinal tract is functional, oral nutrition is best and should be encouraged with frequent, appetizing, high-caloric intake supported by appropriate vitamins and minerals. Before any surgical procedure, every attempt should be made to achieve an anabolic state. If oral intake is not possible or is inadequate, intravenous therapy should be instituted, either as peripheral venous alimentation or central venous alimentation. It is possible to administer 1500 to 3000 calories per day by these techniques. Various central venous administration solutions can be selected for patients with differing needs and circumstances. Patients in renal failure or those with requirements for low potassium or low sodium may be selectively treated with proper solutions. The surgeon should work closely with dietary and metabolic consultants to speed the preparation of patients preoperatively and to help restore the nutritional status of patients postoperatively.

Biologic Treatments

Appropriate biologic therapy requires identification and definition of immunologic deficiencies. Blood and blood products are the most frequent forms of biologic treatments effectively used in this patient population. Platelets, white cells, and red cells can all be valuable in selected circumstances. Potential therapy for T-cell deficiency includes thymosin and levamisole but they are still investigational treatments. Both agents appear to restore immune function in individuals whose T-cell function is depressed. With genetic engineering techniques, lymphokines such as interferon and interleukin can be produced in large quantities. It may be possible in the future to stimulate macrophage production of interferon and interleukin-1 or T-cell production and interleukin-2 to help correct an immunologic deficiency. Exciting investigational work by Mule and associates[9] with interleukin therapy to tumor-bearing animals indicates that lymphokine-activated killer cells (LAK) may play a role in reducing metastases in experimental tumor models, and Phase I trials are in progress in patients with malignant diseases. Development of these types of specific passive immune therapy may have very important implications in management of all forms of immunosuppressed individuals.

Pharmacologic Agents

Pharmacologic agents include antibiotics, corticosteroids, chemotherapeutic agents for cancer therapy, insulin and other hormones, and potentially anabolic agents. Once again diagnosis of a specific abnormality permits more specific pharmacologic therapy. Antibiotics should be used prophylactically in this patient population for surgical procedures, preferably in short, high-dose bursts of treatment during the time of the operative procedure. Careful bowel preparation before any intra-abdominal operation with nonabsorbable antibiotics is also advisable. Any infection, draining sinus, or catheter drainage should be cultured so that if sepsis should arise, sensitivities are known, and immediate therapy can be instituted. Constant antibiotic therapy should be avoided since it leads to a greater incidence of superinfections, fungal overgrowth, and secondary complications. Corticosteroids must be given during and immediately after any operative procedure in a patient who has had steroids in the previous year even if he is not receiving these agents at the time of operation. Patients on corticosteroid therapy should be carefully monitored for steroid-induced diabetes. Appropriate insulin therapy should be administered as necessary when hyperalimentation is given. Pain medicine should be used sparingly but effectively, and patients should be encouraged to be mobile both before and after operative procedures. This mobility will reduce the risk of thrombophlebitis, pressure sores, and pneumonia, as well as increase a sense of patient "well being."

It may be possible in the future to use specific subset deletion of selected lymphoid cell populations should this be desired to alter immunologic reactivity. For instance, an overabundance of suppressor cells might be treated with anti-suppressor monoclonal antibodies, or cytotoxic T cells might be eliminated in autoimmune reactivity. Corticosteroids also block autoimmune damage because of their general effect on T-cell lymphocyte populations.

Modification of Standard Surgical Approaches

There are two major admonitions for the surgeon dealing with the immunosuppressed patient population: (1) diagnosis of disease is more difficult in the immunosuppressed patient and requires more dependence on objective measurements; and (2) surgical approaches may have to be modified when treating abdominal disease, requiring more gastrointestinal decompression, diversion, and drainage, and more staging of operative procedures.[16] Naturally, wound closure and tissue repair is greatly altered, and special efforts must be made to avoid infection and wound dehiscence. More diligence must be exercised to prevent wound complications, thrombophlebitis, postoperative pneumonia, and pressure ulcers. Whenever possible, prophylactic correction of potentially complicating lesions should be performed before induced immunodepression is begun. For instance, duodenal ulcer disease is best treated by surgical correction, gallstones should be removed by cholecystectomy, diverticulitis should be treated by resection of the involved colon, secondary hyperparathyroidism should be treated surgically, and gingivitis should be treated with careful periodontal surgery. These types of procedures are much more easily and safely performed in the subject who is free of the additional complications related to immune depression.

Management of abdominal disease is the area that surgeons often have to deal with in immunodepressed patients. Acute abdominal problems occur more frequently in these patients, and there are many confusing aspects to the differential diagnosis of abdominal pain. Patients on chemotherapy at the time of their lowest blood counts (i.e., maximum marrow depression) often are seen with a neutropenic enteropathy, which must be distinguished from perforated duodenal ulcer, acute appendicitis, acute cholecystitis, or diverticulitis. As already mentioned, gastritis—with or without bleeding—is common in these patients, and decisions for or against surgery must often be made. In general, conservative management should be applied to gastrointestinal bleeding, particularly secondary to gastritis, but radical subtotal gastrectomy may be required if bleeding cannot be controlled with vasopressin, antacids, and anti-H_2 receptor therapy. The use of feeding tubes at the time of any abdominal surgery to permit better alimentation postoperatively is a worthwhile concept. This route is safer and more efficient than using central hyperalimentation by the venous route. On rare occasions, exploratory laparotomy is necessary in the absence of a clear-cut indication should silent perforation be suspected that cannot be adequately demonstrated by the usual techniques. This is true for both the upper and lower intestinal tracts.

Perforated diverticulitis is one of the most serious and insidious complications in this entire population group. The constipation and dehydration that go with the chronically ill, bedridden, and often diet-restricted patient increase the risk for diverticulitis abscesses, which often fail to be walled off by omentum and frequently are seen with diffuse peritonitis. They are best diagnosed by using a limited barium enema, even in the face of minimum symptoms. Any patient with lower abdominal discomfort, a change in bowel habits, left-lower quadrant or suprapubic tenderness, or fever of unknown origin should be considered for a barium study. Surgical treatment should consist of resecting the infected, perforated colonic segment, exteriorizing the proximal bowel as an end colostomy, and performing either a mucous fistula or Hartmann turn-in of the distal segment, depending on the ease with which the former could be brought to the anterior abdominal wall. No attempt at anastomosis is appropriate, nor is simple drainage sufficient.

Pseudomembranous colitis secondary to *Clostridium difficile* toxin is not rare in this patient population and is best treated with intensive antibiotic therapy. This lesion may involve the entire colon and can be lethal because of both blood and protein loss or invasive sepsis if not adequately managed. Vancomycin is the most efficient form of therapy, although subtotal colectomy may be required for emergency control. Radiation colitis can also be seen in some of these patients; it is an insidious problem seen months or years after the original radiation therapy and results in progressive vasculitis and fibrosis of the gut wall. In patients with this problem, it is best to consider bowel bypass if resection is not feasible. Conservative management short of an operative procedure is usually unwarranted since a combination of obstruction and perforation may coexist in these patients.

There is a higher incidence of intra-abdominal postoperative complications in immunodepressed patients, including acute cholecystitis, acute pancreatitis, mesenteric vascular thrombosis, and acute duodenal ulcer. In addition, pulmonary emboli or pneumonia involving the diaphragmatic surface of the lung may mimic epigastric abdominal disease. Postoperative pancreatitis is far more lethal than the standard forms of pancreatitis and should be treated more aggressively. Hemorrhagic pancreatitis has been documented to occur more frequently in this population. Operative intervention in pancreatitis should be reserved for its complications—namely, pancreatic abscess, fistula, or persistent pseudocyst. Cholecystostomy or common duct exploration may be required for stones that have induced pancreatitis; the extent of any such operative procedure depends on the operative status of the patient. Anastomotic leaks are more likely to occur in bowel surgery with intra-abdominal abscess formation and peritonitis frequently resulting. Therefore diversion and decompression should be planned in a more comprehensive manner. Proper wound closure should be performed to avoid dehiscence and evisceration. Through-and-through sutures are generally necessary in these patients. Any infected abdominal wound requires open packing and skin-to-peritoneal layer retention sutures without any attempt at individual layered closure.

Consultation with colleagues who specialize in infectious disease, cardiology, pulmonary medicine, hematology-oncology, and nephrology should be used liberally for the management of these patients where needed, because these individuals are more prone to cardiopulmonary problems, vascular complications, and sepsis. The usual surgical management of "nonsurgical" aspects of the patient may not suffice for these individuals. They need the most expert and intensive type of care to survive any requisite surgical procedures.

SUMMARY

The immune system is a highly integrated, complex, and homeostatic system whose primary function is to discriminate between substances that are its own ("self") and those that are foreign ("not self"). Its ability to accomplish this feat is dependent on the dynamic interplay between the presentation of an antigen to a host and the response by cellular constituents of this system and their products. The types of responding cells and the effectiveness of antigen elimination are influenced by the route, dose, and timing of antigen presentation, the immune competence of the host, and his genetic makeup.

An imbalance between antigen presentation and the corresponding host immunologic response may have direct effects on surgical disease as well as postoperative convalescence following its treatment. Patients with either acquired or induced immunologic abnormalities are at a greater risk for a wide variety of medical problems even in the absence of being subjected to a surgical procedure. Thus one must consider the underlying disease state responsible for the immunodepression, the therapy the patient is receiving, and the documented abnormality in immune function when evaluating the overall immune potential of a given patient. By identifying abnormalities in immune response and their impact on surgical treatment and correcting them if possible or preventing their further deterioration, surgical care will be optimized and the risk of complications following an operation greatly minimized.

REFERENCES

1. Acuto, O., and Reinherz, E.L.: The human T-cell receptor—structure and function, N. Engl. J. Med. **312:**1100, 1985.
2. Balch, C.M., et al.: Prostaglandin E_2-mediated suppression of cellular immunity in colon cancer patients, Surgery **95:**71, 1984.
3. Blaese, R.M.: T and B cell immunodeficiency diseases. In Parker, C.W., editor: Clinical immunology, vol. 1, Philadelphia, 1980, W.B. Saunders Co.
4. Engleberg, N.C., and Eisenstein, B.I.: The impact of new cloning techniques on the diagnosis and treatment of infectious diseases, N. Engl. J. Med. **311:**892, 1984.

5. Gallo, R.C.: Human T-cell leukemia (lymphotropic) retroviruses and their causative role in T-cell malignancies and acquired immune deficiency syndrome, Cancer **55:**2317, 1985.
6. Green, M.H., et al.: Acute nonlymphocytic leukemia after therapy with alkylating agents for ovarian cancer: a study of five randomized clinical trials, N. Engl. J. Med. **307:**1416, 1982.
7. Grimm, E.A., et al.: Lymphokine-activated killer cell phenomenon: lysis of natural killer-resistant fresh solid tumor cells by interleukin-2 activated autologous human peripheral blood lymphocytes, Surgery **98:**151, 1985.
8. McIrvine, A.J., et al.: Depressed immune response in burn patients: use of monoclonal antibodies and functional assays to define the role of suppressor cells, Ann. Surg. **196:**297, 1982.
9. Mule, J.J., et al.: Adoptive immunotherapy of established pulmonary metastases with LAK cells and recombinant interleukin-2, Science **225:**1487, 1984.
10. Nathan, C.F., Murray, H.W., and Cohn, Z.A.: The macrophage as an effector cell, N. Engl. J. Med. **303:**622, 1980.
11. Penn, I.: Malignant lymphomas in organ transplant recipients, Transplant. Proc. **7:**1047, 1979.
12. Reinherz, E.L., and Schlossman, S.F.: Regulation of the immune response—inducer and suppressor T-lymphocyte subsets in human beings, N. Engl. J. Med. **303:**370, 1980.
13. Tilden, A.B., Abo, T., and Balch, C.M.: Suppressor cell function of human granular lymphocytes identified by the HNK-1 (Leu 7) monoclonal antibody, J. Immunol. **130:**1171, 1983.
14. VanBuren, C.T., et al.: The cellular target of cyclosporin A action in humans, Surgery **92:**167, 1982.
15. Weksler, M.C., Innes, J.D., and Goldstein, G.: Immunological studies of aging. IV. The contribution of thymic involution to the immune deficiencies of aging mice and reversal with thymopoietin 32-36, J. Exp. Med. **148:**996, 1978.
16. Wilson, R.E., editor: Surgical problems in immune-depressed patients, Philadelphia, 1984, W.B. Saunders Co.

5 David H. Van Buren and Barry D. Kahan

Physiologic Basis of Transplantation

Successful clinical transplantation is limited not by technical pitfalls but rather by the immune process that mediates rejection of the transplanted tissue or organ. Thus the physiologic basis of transplantation rests on understanding the immunologic rejection process. The goal of the transplant surgeon is to manipulate either the host (i.e., the recipient of the transplanted organ or tissue) or the allograft (i.e., the organ or tissue being transplanted from a donor within the same species) to avert, minimize, or reduce this physiologic process. Immunologic events leading to allograft rejection are classified as afferent, central, and efferent limbs[144]: the afferent limb includes presentation and T-lymphocyte recognition of foreign histocompatibility antigens; the central includes proliferation, differentiation, and production of lymphokines by T cells and of humoral antibody by B cells; and the efferent limb includes the action of the immune mediators to destroy the graft. For a discussion of the basic concepts of immunity and the immune response, see Chapter 4.

ALLOGRAFT REJECTION

Afferent Limb: Presentation and Recognition of Antigens

Histocompatibility Antigens

Early experiments in the development of clinical transplantation revealed the presence of a single, strong antigenic system controlling the outcome of transplantation in every species studied. Antigen (Ag) disparity between the host and the graft initiates the immune response and ultimately the rejection process. The presence of preformed antibodies directed against donor Ags because of presensitization of the recipient results in accelerated rejection. In the case of humans, the major histocompatibility complex (MHC) Ags[3-5] include Class I and II molecules, encoded by sites on the sixth autosomal chromsome. Class I Ags, which are present on the cell surface of almost all nucleated cells, represent gene products of the HLA-A, B, and C loci within the major histocompatibility complex. These membrane-bound glycoproteins consist of a 44,000-dalton heavy chain noncovalently bonded to a 11,500-dalton beta-microglobulin light chain (Fig. 5-1, *A*). HLA-A, B, and C Ags are serologically defined histocompatibility Ags because they are identified on lymphocytes using a microcytotoxicity assay in which antibodies of known specificity cause complement-dependent lysis of antigen-bearing cells[93,171]; hence the abbreviation HLA for human lymphocyte antigen.

The Class II Ag, structurally composed of a 34,000-dalton heavy chain covalently linked to a 29,000-dalton light chain (Fig. 5-1, *B*), is limited in distribution to vascular endothelium and cells of lymphoreticular origin, specifically B lymphocytes, activated T lymphocytes, monocytes, and dendritic cells.[5,53,199,213] Within the human major histocompatibility complex the HLA-D Ag is a Class II Ag. In practice, HLA-D disparity is detected by the proliferative response of normal peripheral blood lymphocytes on allogeneic stimulation (i.e., stimulation resulting from recipient cells responding to the nonidentity of cells from a donor within the same species) in the mixed lymphocyte culture (MLC) reaction (Fig. 5-2). In unrelated donor renal transplants, Class II Ag identity may correlate better with renal allograft survival than Class I iden-

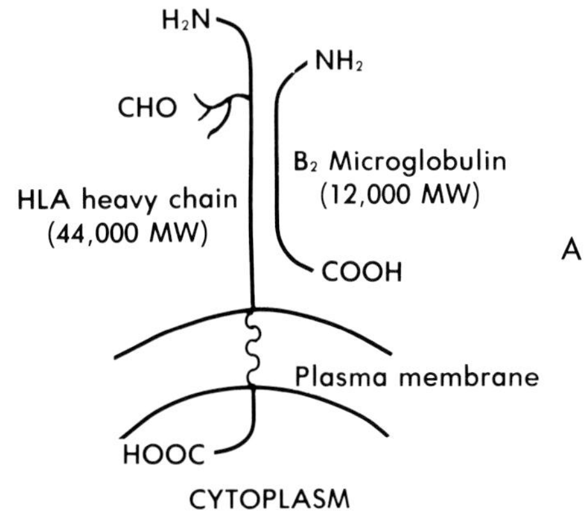

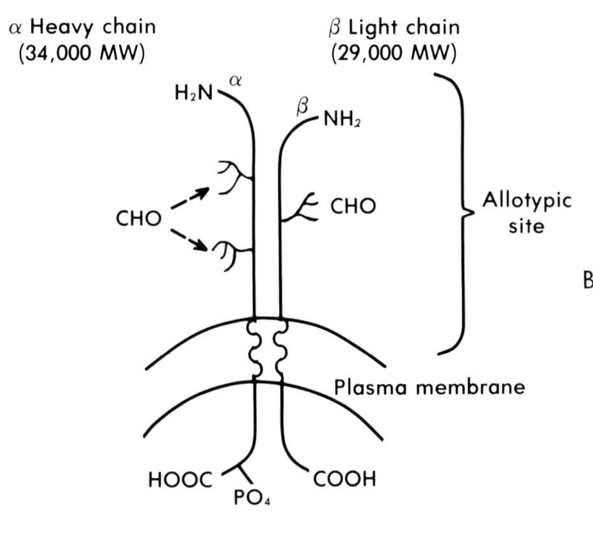

Fig. 5-1 **A**, Class I antigen molecular structure. **B**, Class II antigen molecular structure.

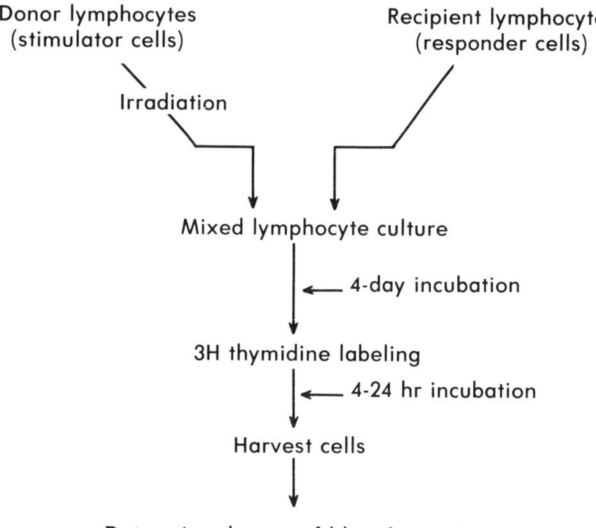

Fig. 5-2 Mixed lymphocyte reaction, which is an in vitro determination of histocompatibility. Proliferative response is determined by incorporation of ^{3}H-thymidine.

tity: graft survival across donor-recipient combinations causing high MLC stimulation indicative of a significant Class II Ag mismatch was 18% in contrast to 88% survival with weak Class II Ag differences.[6] A "D-related" or DR-Ag system, which appears to be closely linked to the HLA-D region, has been serologically defined by the reaction of specific antibodies against purified B cells. Dendritic cells, which include the epidermal Langerhans cell, the follicular dendritic cell, and the interdigitating reticulum cell, all express Class II Ags,[199] which are potent stimulators of the MLC reaction.[213] Dendritic cells are widely distributed throughout connective tissue and thus have a potent effect to enhance organ immunogenicity.

As previously indicated, Class II Ags have also been demonstrated on the surface of vascular endothelial cells. Paul, van Es, and Baldwin[172] reported a renal distribution of Class II Ags limited to the intertubular capillaries and veins. Umbilical vein endothelium also expresses Class II Ags.[93] Thus Class II Ags residing on the surface of vascular endothelium may cause allosensitization of peripheral lymphocytes as they circulate through the graft.

The ABO system of blood typing is the only non-HLA histocompatibility system that has been identified to mediate rejection in humans.[3,5] Renal transplantation across an ABO incompatibility is almost always unsuccessful.[179,197] The recipient responds as a presensitized host, because he bears circulating isoantibodies toward foreign blood group antigens, thereby resulting in hyperacute rejection (see below). Renal function ceases within minutes to hours. Lewis Ags, which are gene products of the ABO, Rh, secretor, and Lewis loci[206] may also influence renal allograft survival. Oriol and co-workers[166] implicated incompatible Lewis Ags as the cause of renal allograft failure. Both Lewis and HLA-Ag disparities display negative additive effects on transplant survival; however, HLA identity cannot override the deleterious influence of a Lewis mismatch.[234] Lewis Ags are expressed on lymphocytes and on epithelial cells of both the distal convoluted tubules and collecting ducts. Spitalnik and associates[206] reported that eight Lewis-negative individuals with circulating anti-Lewis antibodies who received Lewis-incompatible grafts all displayed allograft rejection. Unlike the incompatibility of the Lewis system, Rh incompatibility is relatively unimportant, except possibly in a presensitized Rh(−) recipient.[67] Currently ABO incompatibility between donor and recipient is routinely avoided by blood grouping, but Lewis mismatches are only sought if there has been an extensive recipient transfusion history.

Presensitization resulting in donor Ag–specific antibodies and strong major histocompatibility complex disparity, especially with regard to the Class II antigen system, preclude allograft longevity. Tissue typing techniques identify these circumstances so they might be avoided. With the use of humoral and cellular immune techniques, tissue typing identifies the transplantation Ags of the potential recipient and donor. Lymphocytotoxic antibodies specific for the various HLA antigens detect antigens present on peripheral lymphocytes. Lymphocytic death indicates that the patient bears the distinctive HLA Ag. Histocompatibility matching of the HLA-A and HLA-B loci are performed clinically. The degree of MLC response between donor and recipient correlates with the compatibility of the allograft and recipient. Because the MLC requires a 5-day in vitro incubation, serologic techniques have been developed to recognize Ags that provoke this cellular response. These Ags are identified with the use of cytotoxic antibodies directed against B lymphocytes.

Antigen Recognition

Sensitization of host lymphocytes by histocompatibility Ags on the cell surface of transplanted cells represents the initial step in allograft rejection. Bretscher and Cohn[25] proposed a two-signal theory of antigen recognition (Fig. 5-3). The first signal results from the binding of Ag to a receptor on Ag-sensitive cells. This interaction, inducing a conformation change in the receptor site, produces a second signal to the cell that results in activation.

Lafferty and Cunningham[125] proposed that Ag recognition alone activated T lymphocytes and emphasized the importance of the Class II Ags. According to their hypothesis, the induction of T lymphocytes, a two-step process, requires the introduction of a foreign antigen bound to membrane receptors of the responsive cell. The stimulator cell, which presents the Ag to the responsive cell, expresses Class II Ags.[68,134,239] The first signal is transmitted to the responsive cell by Ag binding. Simultaneously an induction stimulus, the second signal, is generated by the stimulator cell after it is bound to the responsive T cell by an Ag bridge (Fig. 5-4, *A*).

Bach, Bach, and Sondel[6] proposed an alternative model to explain alloimmune induction (Fig. 5-4, *B*). This

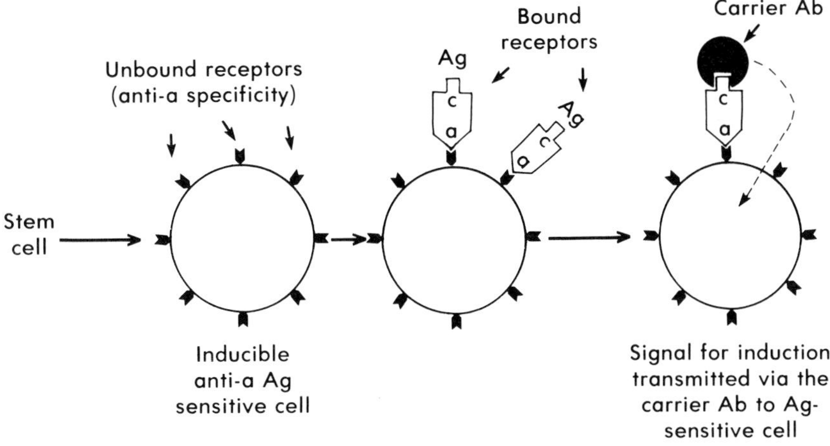

Fig. 5-3 Two-signal theory of antigen recognition proposed by Bretscher and Cohn.[25]

theory, also a two-signal process, requires the interaction of the T helper (T_H) and cytotoxic T lymphocyte (CTL) populations in response to antigenic stimulation. The stimulator cell expresses both a lymphocyte-defined (LD) Ag, which is a Class II Ag; and a serologically defined Ag, which represents a Class I HLA-A, B, and C Ag. The LD Ag is difficult to define serologically. LD Ag disparity is associated with a significant MLC response. The second signal is generated by the proliferating helper T cell population stimulated by LD Ags. The two subpopulations of T lymphocytes, proliferating helper and cytotoxic T lymphocytes, respond to LD and serologically defined Ag disparities, respectively. The serologically defined Ags are both stimulators and targets for the cytotoxic T cells, whereas the LD Ag stimulus results in MLC proliferation and augmentation of cytotoxic T-cell generation.

Although Bach and associates' model is generally accepted as a reasonable explanation for Ag recognition, the major weakness of this model has been the inability to explain cytotoxic T-cell activation when Class II Ag disparity did not exist.[156,190,191] In contrast, Lafferty and Cunningham's hypothesis[125] stressed the importance of a stimulator cell expressing Class II Ags to function as the Ag-presenting cell when interacting with the responsive T-cell population. A unification of these two theories is commonly accepted (Fig. 5-4, *C*); i.e., that alloimmune induction requires MHC antigen presentation to responsive T lymphocytes by Ag-presenting cells expressing Class II Ag.[177] The necessity of cell-to-cell cooperation for alloantigenic sensitization has been demonstrated by the inability of killed cells to stimulate cytotoxic T-cell populations although they bear the appropriate histocompatibility Ag.

Monoclonal antibodies, homogenous antibodies resulting from the hybridization of myeloma and B-lymphocyte cell lines, have been used to elucidate the cellular events of Ag recognition. Cell surface markers distinctive for human T lymphocytes at various stages of differentiation are recognized by murine monoclonal antibodies.[182] The helper T-cell subpopulation (T4 positive), which expresses cell surface markers T1, T3, T12, and T4, comprises 55% to 60% of the circulating T-cell population. The T4 population generally acts physiologically as an inducer for the maturation of cytotoxic T cells and as a helper for the maturation of antibody-producing B cells. When in vitro techniques are used to expand and clone T4 populations, some of the T4 clones display cytotoxic activity directed against Class II Ags. The stimuli for cell-mediated lympholysis (Fig. 5-5) (i.e., the specific destruction of target cells after presensitization) determines the subset of T cell involved. T4 clones direct a cytotoxic response to Class II Ags, whereas cytotoxic T8 clones kill cells with Class I Ags identical to those of the initial sensitizing cell. Thus the T4 and T8 cells appear to have different receptors specific for Class II and Class I Ags, respectively. The T4 population also provides inducer activity for T-to-T interactions. The cytotoxic/suppressor T-cell subset (T8), bearing T1, T3, T12, and T8 cell surface markers, accounts for 20% to 30% of the peripheral lymphocytes and mediates suppressor functions and Class I Ag CTL activity.[183] Maximum T8 cytotoxicity directed toward Class I MHC surface Ags requires T4 cells. In a primary MLC (see Fig. 5-2), the T8 cells are the major cytotoxic effector population, and the cells induce the proliferative response and stimulate the T8 subset to achieve maximal cytotoxicity.[3-5,183]

These receptors for Class I and II Ags present on T8 and T4 cells, respectively, function in Ag recognition. In addition, the T3 cell surface marker appears to be required for Ag recognition by both lymphoid subpopulations. Monoclonal antibodies directed against T3 molecules prevent recognition and thus cytotoxic activity. The clonal cytotoxic activity is directly related to the cell surface density of the T3 Ags. Both the T3 Ags and the T4 or T8 Ags are required for Ag recognition and subsequent clonal cell-mediated lympholysis. Reinherz and associates[183] proposed that the T3 region binds to the polymorphic region of the MHC molecule, whereas the T8 and T4 region binds to the constant region of the Class I or Class II molecule.

Immune induction requires the presentation of graft Ags by an Ag-presenting cell to the T lymphocytes. Ag-presenting cells that lack Class II Ags are unable to elicit a

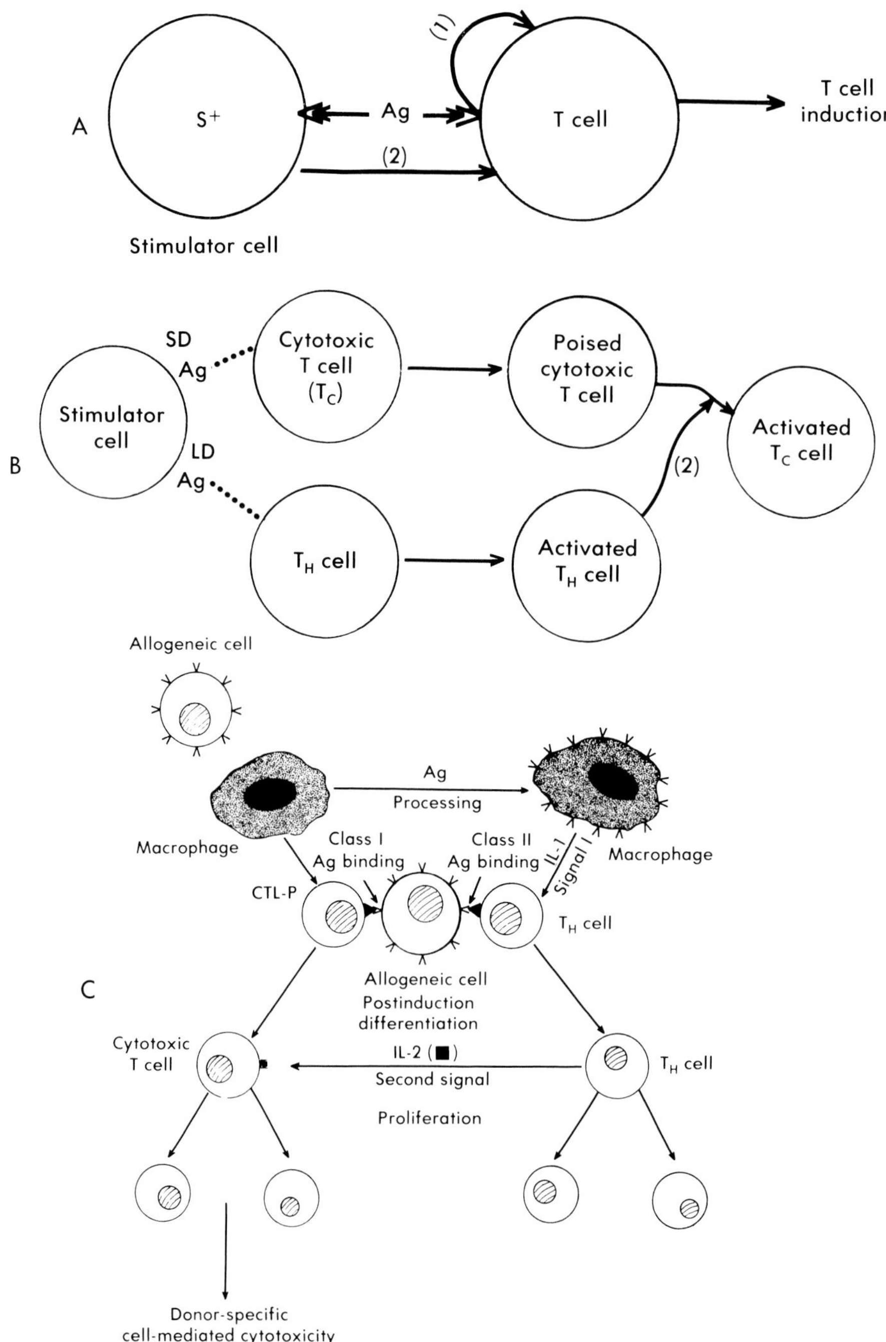

Fig. 5-4 **A,** T-cell induction proposed by Lafferty and Cunningham.[125] Signal 1: Responsive T cell binds antigen to its surface receptor. Signal 2: Inductive stimulus from stimulator cell *(S^+)*, which also binds antigen. Both signals are required for T-cell induction. **B,** T-cell induction theory proposed by Bach, Bach, and Sondel.[6] Cytotoxic T cell *(T_C)* is converted to poised Tc upon binding of serologically defined antigen present on stimulator cell. Final differentiation of T_C occurs after T_H cell binds lymphocyte-defined (LD) antigen on stimulator cell and delivers signal 2 from activated T_H cell. **C,** Alloimmune induction initiated by presentation and recognition of histocompatibility antigen. First signal, mediated by IL-1, occurs with antigen recognition and binding. Second signal, mediated by IL-2, is generated by T_H cells after activation. *CTL-P,* precursor cytotoxic T cell; *T_H,* T-helper cell; *IL-1,* interleukin 1; *IL-2,* interleukin 2.

primary MLC reaction.[177] Thus Class II Ag expression, not necessarily disparity, is essential for sensitization. The expression of both Class I and Class II Ags leads to T4 and T8 subset stimulation and maximum cell-mediated lympholysis.

Central Limb: Proliferation and Differentiation of T Cells and Production of Lymphokines

The two-signal theory of Ag recognition and response hypothesizes that the first signal results from Ag binding and presentation. The first signal is mediated by the lymphokine interleukin-1 (IL-1), a 31–amino acid peptide of molecular weight 12,000-14,000,[151,152] which is released from macrophages, a subset of which expresses Class II Ags and functions as Ag-presenting cells. When the supernatant of mitogen-stimulated spleen cells[126] containing IL-1 is added to cultures of allogeneic lymphocytes and Ag-bearing cells lacking Class II Ags, there is induction of specific cytotoxic activity. Although IL-1 is a nonspecific molecule, it causes maturation of precursor T4 lymphocytes to respond in the presence of alloantigen presentation.[152] The most significant biologic effect of IL-1 is the induction of conditions under which T4 cells can produce the second signal, the lymphokine interleukin-2 (IL-2). Although IL-2 production can take place in an IL-1–deficient medium, the presence of IL-1 amplifies IL-2 synthesis.[170] The second signal, IL-2, plays a crucial role in alloimmune induction by converting precursor cytotoxic T8 lymphocytes into cytotoxic effectors capable of destroying allogeneic targets.

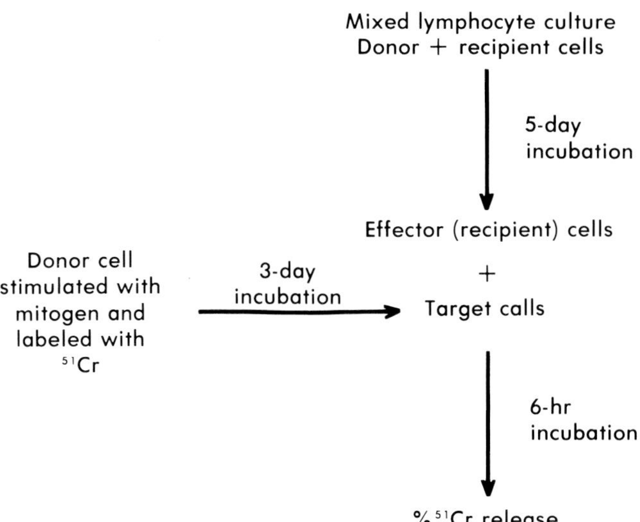

Fig. 5-5 Cell-mediated lympholysis test. Percentage of ^{51}Cr release is proportional to major histocompatibility complex disparity and killing of target cells by effector cells.

T4 cells produce IL-2 after interacting with alloantigen-presenting cells in the presence of IL-1. Ag-stimulated T-helper and cytotoxic T lymphocytes express IL-2 receptors on activation, therefore becoming responsive to IL-2.[170] Thus IL-2 stimulation causes proliferation of cytotoxic T cells and facilitates expression of cytotoxic capacities.[56] IL-2 also augments natural killer cell activity,[80] and may have a role in B-cell maturation.[56] In addition to producing IL-2, stimulated T4 cells also synthesize a variety of other lymphokines, including lymphocyte mitogenic factors, macrophage-activating factors, and gamma interferon, which recruit lymphoid cells, stimulate their proliferation, and engender cytotoxic activity.[56]

Efferent Limb: Action of the Immune Mediators to Destroy the Graft

The rejection process (Table 5-1), which is initiated by Ag recognition and lymphocyte activation, is ultimately effected by: (1) cytotoxic T cells reacting specifically with

Table 5-1 **THE REJECTION PROCESS**

Rejection	Time Course	Clinical Signs and Symptoms	Mechanism	Pathology	Response to Antirejection Therapy
Hyperacute	Sudden onset, min/hr after revascularization	Abrupt loss of graft function; no perfusion	Humoral with preformed anti-HLA antibodies	Fibrin thrombi within arterioles Endothelial cell sloughing, platelet aggregation	(−) Irreversible process
Accelerated	Rapid loss of graft function 72-100 hr after transplant	Abrupt loss of graft function; tender, swollen allograft	Cellular presensitization: destruction by specific Tc or antibody-dependent killer cell-mediated cytotoxicity	Interstitial hemorrhage Fibrinoid necrosis of small arterial vessels	(±)
Acute rejection	First 4 months after transplant	Graft swelling and fever, oliguria	Cellular; delayed-type hypersensitivity mechanism	Prominent interstitial and perivascular mononuclear infiltration and interstitial edema	(+)
Chronic rejection	Gradual decline in graft function	Progressive loss of graft function Hypertension Glomerulopathy	Humoral	Obliterative vascular changes Interstitial fibrosis	(−)

Class I Ag-bearing cells; (2) nonspecific effector cells activated by a lymphokine mechanism; and/or (3) humoral antibodies, including a variety of complement-dependent and lymphocyte-dependent moieties.[29] Clinically, graft rejection is classified on the basis of its timing as hyperacute, accelerated, acute, or chronic. Hyperacute rejection is characterized by a sudden, irreversible cessation of graft function minutes to hours after revascularization. This form of rejection is thought to be secondary to host presensitization, i.e., to the presence of preformed antidonor antibodies. Further, it is not amenable to any of the pharmacologic immunosuppressive agents. A classic setting for hyperacute rejection is ABO incompatibility wherein circulating antidonor hemagglutinins rapidly thrombose the graft after binding to endothelial cells and through their Fc tails, attracting platelet deposition and granulocyte activation. Preformed anti-HLA antibodies, the usual cause of hyperacute rejection, may be induced by prior transplants, transfusions, or pregnancy.[117,178,232,233] Both Jeannet and associates[103] and Pierce[174] demonstrated a correlation between a positive pretransplant microcytotoxicity crossmatch and the occurrence of hyperacute rejection.

Microscopically the hyperacutely rejected transplant shows fibrin thrombi within small arteries and arterioles, capillary dilation, endothelial cell sloughing, platelet aggregation, and adhesion of polymorphonuclear leukocytes. Both animal and human renal allograft studies[27,28,158] suggest that rejection is initiated by a primary immune injury to the vascular endothelium. The circulating antibodies bind together with complement specifically to the histocompatibility Ags exposed on the vascular endothelial cell surface. Platelet aggregation and subsequent release of platelet factors and vasoactive substances occur at the site of injury. Vasoconstriction progresses to thrombosis after aggregation of platelets, red blood cells, and polymorphonuclear leukocytes produce thrombus formation, organization, and fibrin deposition as terminal events in the ischemic cascade. The ultimate result is a lack of perfusion to the transplant organ. Sometimes the reaction is not immediate but rather occurs 24 to 48 hours after transplantation, in which case it is denoted delayed hyperacute rejection. Lucas and associates[143] demonstrated the occurrence of antibodies specifically binding histocompatibility Ags in renal transplant patients with this syndrome. There was a dose-response relationship between the pretransplant antibody titer and the severity of postoperative renal failure. Delayed rejection appeared to be the result of a weaker immune response than that which caused hyperacute rejection.

Accelerated rejection frequently produces rapid loss of graft function; in many cases it is refractory to antirejection therapy. The graft usually functions satisfactorily for 72 to 100 hours, but then graft function declines precipitously. Histologically there are vascular lesions of capillary disruption with interstitial hemorrhage, hemorrhagic infarcts, and fibrinoid necrosis of small arterial vessels. Two pathogenetic mechanisms appear to mediate the response: cellular presensitization with rapid graft destruction by specific T-cytotoxic cells, or a secondary antibody production of a moiety that depends on lymphocytes to execute cytotoxicity.[1]

Acute rejection, unlike the accelerated or hyperacute mechanisms, tends to be reversible with therapy. Acute rejection episodes are the most common type, affecting 65% to 85% of renal allografts and usually occurring during the first 4 months following surgery with a peak incidence at 5 weeks.[7] The clinical features of cell-mediated renal allograft rejection include graft swelling and tenderness, fever, oliguria, and hypertension. Laboratory assessment reveals an increased serum creatinine, and the diagnosis may be confirmed by percutaneous needle biopsy. The histologic features include prominent interstitial and perivascular mononuclear infiltrates with interstitial edema. Macrophages and T lymphocytes, specifically cytotoxic T cells, are the predominant infiltrating cell types. In addition, T4 helper cells mediating delayed-type hypersensitivity mechanisms are important contributors. In mild-to-moderate cellular rejection, two cell types predominate within the interstitial cellular infiltrates[80]: macrophages comprising 40% to 50%, and T lymphocytes, 30% to 40%. Microscopically, infiltrating T cells include cytotoxic T cells (Tc) bearing the T8 cell surface marker and helper T4 cells. In severe cellular rejection the cellular infiltrate is composed of 60% macrophages, 20% to 30% polymorphonuclear leukocytes, and 15% T lymphocytes, the majority of which are Tc cells.[85,180,214]

After the activation of T4 and T8 lymphocytes, circulating immune cells recognize the allograft at the periphery. The T4 cells play a critical role by releasing lymphokines that recruit and activate immunologically incompetent lymphocytes and macrophages toward the allograft[97] through a delayed-type hypersensitivity mechanism. This mechanism is specific, although the target cytotoxic cell activated by lymphokines is not.[161] On the one hand, the delayed-type hypersensitivity effector T4 cell does not directly mediate allograft damage but secretes lymphocytotoxins responsible for cellular destruction and lymphokines that attract and activate macrophages, lymphocytes, and natural killer cells to mediate cellular necrosis.[146] On the other hand, the cytotoxic T8 lymphocyte displays specific activity against Class I alloantigen on the graft, thereby participating in the tissue destruction. Although the Tc cell is the predominant specific lymphocyte involved in cellular rejection, the T4 helper cell is an important component of the process because of its ability to magnify the cellular response by recruitment of other immune elements. In sum, cytotoxic T cells specifically react with the Class I alloantigen disparity, whereas the delayed-type hypersensitivity mechanism of T4 helper cells causes a nonspecific response in recognition of the Class II alloantigen disparity.

Acute rejection episodes may be precipitated by viral syndromes[42,140] that are caused by the following:

1. Direct viral damage, e.g., as in mumps or influenza viral syndromes, releases increased amounts of histocompatibility Ags from the graft.
2. Viral Ags expressed during a clinical infection may cross-react with donor histocompatibility Ags. Thus the immune response directed against the virus can potentially result in graft rejection.
3. The virus may augment the host's immune system by acting as an adjuvant, making him more susceptible

to an acute rejection episode; although in most cases, particularly with cytomegalovirus, the infection tends to induce immunodepression.

4. Nonspecific immune augmentation may occur because of the presence of circulating Ag antibody complexes.[42]

From the opposite standpoint, allograft rejection sometimes produces activation of a latent viral infection, caused either by lymphocyte transformation or by release of virus from damaged donor kidney cells.[140]

Chronic rejection is characterized by a gradual decline in graft function and tends to be unresponsive to steroid antirejection therapy and to eventuate in transplant failure. The clinical syndrome of progressive deterioration of graft function following renal transplantation includes hypertension and glomerulopathy with hematuria and/or proteinuria. Graft damage has been ascribed to a humoral process based on detection of donor-specific circulating antibodies in recipient sera.[99,173,175,232] Deposition of immunoglobulins and complement on glomerular capillary walls and low serum complement levels[173] suggest that the humoral antibodies mediate a glomerular lesion. The immunoglobulin deposits appear to produce obliterative vascular changes eventuating in interstitial fibrosis.[7] Chronic rejection tends to be a separate pathologic and clinical entity reflecting an alloantibody response rather than the result of recurrent acute rejection episodes.

Overview of Rejection Process

The immunologic events leading to allograft rejection include afferent, central, and efferent limbs. The *afferent limb,* which involves the presentation and recognition of the histocompatibility Ags, is initiated by sensitization of host lymphocytes by histocompatibility Ags. Alloimmune induction requires the presentation of histocompatibility Ags to responding populations of T lymphocytes by an Ag-presenting cell expressing Class II Ags. The T4 receptor of the T_H cell and the T8 receptor of the Tc cell bind to the constant region of Class II and Class I Ags, respectively. Simultaneously the T3 region of the T_H and Tc cells binds to the polymorphic region of histocompatibility Ags. The expression and binding of both Class I and Class II Ags results in the stimulation of both T8 and T4 subpopulations.

Lymphocyte induction, the *central limb* of the immune response, has been hypothesized as being a two-signal process: the first signal occurring with Ag recognition and binding, and the second signal being generated by the T_H cell following its activation. The first signal is mediated by IL-1, a peptide released from the Ag-presenting macrophage following binding of histocompatibility Ags. IL-1 induces the maturation of precursor T_H lymphocytes and amplifies IL-2 synthesis by the T_H cell. T_H cells produce IL-2 following cell-cell interaction with the Ag-presenting cell bearing Class II Ag. The second signal, IL-2, induces maturation of the precursor cytotoxic T8 lymphocytes into cytotoxic effector cells and also stimulates their proliferation. In addition, IL-2 stimulates natural killer cell activity and B-cell maturation. Other lymphokines produced by the T4 cells nonspecifically stimulate the recruitment, proliferation, and cytotoxic activity of lymphoid cells.

These varied cell populations participate in the *efferent limb*. The clinical manifestation of this process is the rejection of the transplanted allograft. Allograft rejection is classified as hyperacute, accelerated, acute, or chronic. Hyperacute rejection occurs abruptly following revascularization. Presentation and the subsequent presence of preformed antibodies are responsible for this irreversible process. Accelerated rejection characterized by rapid loss in graft function 3 to 5 days following transplantation also results from presensitization. Graft destruction by specific cytotoxic T8 cells following cellular presensitization is pathognomonic for this type of rejection. Acute rejection, the most frequently encountered rejection process, occurs typically during the first 4 months following transplantation and is partially mediated by a delayed-type hypersensitivity mechanism. Following activation of the T4 and T8 lymphocyte subpopulation, the delayed-type hypersensitivity effector T4 cell indirectly mediates allograft destruction by the secretion of lymphocytotoxins and lymphokines. The lymphokines result in the recruitment and activation of lymphoid cells, which cause nonspecific cellular destruction of the allograft. Specific cytotoxicity is mediated by mature T8 lymphocytes when Class I disparity exists. The T4 cell amplifies the specific cytotoxic response and induces the nonspecific response through the delayed-type hypersensitivity mechanism. Chronic rejection, characterized by a gradual decline in graft function, is caused by a humoral process. Donor-specific circulating antibodies have been found in recipient sera, and Ag-antibody complexes have been implicated in graft destruction.

IMMUNOLOGIC STRATEGIES TO PREVENT REJECTION

The ultimate goal in organ transplantation is to achieve immunologic tolerance of the host for his graft, thereby obviating any rejection process. This end result might be obtained either by alteration of the allograft antigens to abrogate immunogenicity or by immunosuppression of the host. Although there have been important experimental leads toward the goal of decreasing graft immunogenicity either by in vitro cultivation or by ultraviolet exposure, only the second, recipient immunosuppressive approach has proven clinical efficacy. The ideal immunosuppressive regimen that would specifically dampen host responses toward donor, but not toward third-party, antigens represents a nirvana toward which there has been intensive inquiry. For the present, the immunosuppressive modalities used currently for organ transplantation are nonspecific, altering host responses not only toward histocompatibility but also toward an array of other antigens. In general, three types of agents are used: physical irradiation, chemical agents exemplified by corticosteroids and antiproliferative agents, and biologic agents such as antilymphocyte sera and monoclonal antibodies.

Immunosuppressive Modalities

Irradiation

Dempster, Lennox, and Boag[46] demonstrated the immunosuppressive potential of irradiation in alloimmunity when they showed that irradiation of rabbit hosts before skin allografting resulted in graft prolongation. Hamburger and associates[79] and Murray and co-workers[155] each used total body irradiation in renal transplant recipients with limited but unequivocal success. Hume and associates[98] abandoned total body irradiation because of its associated toxicity in favor of local graft radiotherapy because total body irradiation of four renal recipients resulted in severe bone marrow depression and fatal infections in two patients. Kaufman and co-workers[112] showed that 90% of irradiated renal allografts receiving six doses of 150 R over 12 to 15 days survived significantly longer than control grafts and that this treatment reversed acute rejection episodes. Subsequent clinical trials tend to support the effectiveness of local graft radiation in human renal transplant recipients. Uncontrolled trials by Levitt and colleagues[136] and Birtch and associates[20] noted improved immunosuppression by graft radiation used in conjunction with other immunosuppressive agents. Fidler and co-workers[60] demonstrated the benefit of graft irradiation in instances when other immunosuppressive agents could not be used because of life-threatening infections.

Despite these observations, the efficacy of graft irradiation used in conjunction with standard immunosuppressive agents, specifically corticosteroids, was questioned by Godfrey and Salaman.[69,70] In a controlled study, patients were randomized to treatment with methylprednisolone alone or in conjunction with radiotherapy. Patients treated with combination therapy demonstrated a 58% incidence of early rejection reversal compared to a 50% incidence of reversal in those receiving steroids only. However, the combined therapy decreased the longevity of the allograft. Combination therapy yielded a 26% graft survival at 1 year compared with a 50% survival in the control group. Thus local graft irradiation increased the rate of reversal of allograft rejection but adversely affected the ultimate fate of the graft. A prospective randomized study by Pilepich and associates[176] investigating the clinical effect of graft irradiation in conjunction with corticosteroids yielded similar conclusions. The control group, receiving only methylprednisolone as acute rejection therapy, had an 84.5% incidence of acute rejection reversal and a 54% graft survival. In the experimental group treated with local graft irradiation and steroid pulse therapy, recurrent rejection episodes were significantly increased (i.e., there was a 75% rejection reversal rate and a 22% graft survival). Those treated with corticosteroids only had an improved prognosis with respect to graft longevity and ease of acute rejection reversal. Thus the clinical studies of Godfrey and Salaman[69,70] and Pilepich and co-workers[176] have clearly shown consistently inferior results of local graft irradiation on long-term graft survival when used in conjunction with steroids. These findings, coupled with the superiority of other immunologic strategies in managing graft rejection, underscore the very limited clinical application of local graft irradiation; and, as suggested by Fidler and colleagues,[60] this modality should be reserved only for those patients who have life-threatening infections requiring the cessation of other therapeutic options.

Because of the potent immunodepressive effect of radiotherapy and the need to minimize other organ toxicity, a regimen called total lymphoid irradiation (TLI) to focus on cervical, axillary, mediastinal, para-aortic, splenic, and ilioinguinal nodes, was devised by Kaplan[110] and first applied for treatment of Hodgkin's disease. After therapy, hosts displayed a state of immunosuppression characterized by T lymphocytopenia, decreased alloreactivity, and induction of nonspecific T suppressor cells.[142] A decreased number and function of T cells were documented for years after therapy.[63] Decreased alloreactivity after TLI was ascribed to induction of T suppressor cells capable of inhibiting MLC reactions[115] and graft vs. host responses, in which donor T lymphocytes recognize nonidentity of the recipient and respond to lymphohematopoietic alloantigens. Although TLI decreases cell-mediated immunity and prolongs allograft survival in mice,[202] success in large mammal models has not been consistent.[142] Even if the logistic issue that TLI must be performed before transplantation is ignored, the complications associated with its administration (i.e., nausea, vomiting, possible increased incidence of lymphoma, and opportunistic infections)[159] have limited its application in the clinical arena.

Chemical Agents

CORTICOSTEROIDS. Corticosteroids cause a multitude of effects on the immune system.[50] Steroids act at the cellular level by entering the cell and binding to specific cytoplasmic receptors, forming a complex that is transported to the nucleus, where it is bound and affects cellular function by inhibiting DNA transcription. Steroids cause generalized lymphopenia[57] secondary to a redistribution of lymphocytes, particularly T4 cells, to the extravascular pool.[83] In humans the lymphopenia is not secondary to a corticosteroid-sensitive lytic effect as it is in rodents.[203] Human lymphocytes are corticoresistant.[32] The nonspecific lymphopenia is a beneficial effect of steroids in organ transplantation, because the cellular sequestration diminishes the potential of lymphocytes, particularly cytotoxic T lymphocytes, to infiltrate the allograft.[50]

Steroids also affect antigen recognition and subsequent immune induction by inhibiting Class Ia antigen expression[13,14,160,204] by interrupting the interaction between antigen-presenting cells and T cells and by decreasing interleukin production (Fig. 5-6), which dampens lymphocyte proliferation.[65,111,131] In addition, corticosteroids lessen the inflammatory response of rejection because of decreased monocyte and macrophage cytolytic activity[185,186] and impaired accumulation of monocytes at an inflammatory site.[41] All of these effects probably contribute to the generalized global and profound immunosuppression caused by corticosteroids.

ANTIPROLIFERATIVE AGENTS. The antiproliferative agents used for immunosuppression in transplantation are cyclosporine (CsA) and azathioprine (Aza). CsA, a cyclic endecapeptide fungal metabolite, acts selectively on T cells. Both the activation of T helper cells and the induction of cytotoxic T lymphocytes are decreased, but suppressor cell activity is less affected.[87] In contrast, Aza, an analog of 6-mercaptopurine, competitively inhibits de novo purine synthesis by all cells and consequently interferes with the proliferation of all rapidly dividing cells, including lymphocytes. Both of these pharmacologic agents tend to be

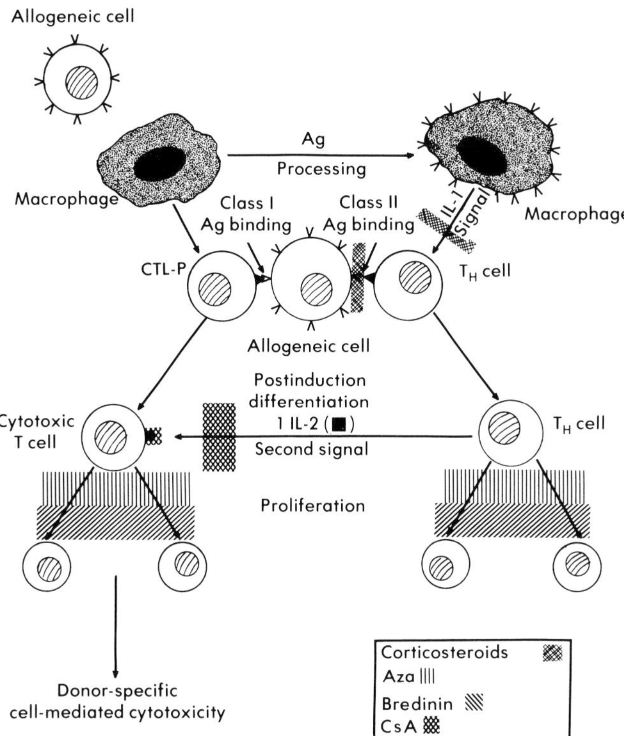

Fig. 5-6 Sites of action of various immunosuppressive agents attempting to interrupt lymphocyte induction and proliferation. *CTL-P,* precursor cytotoxic T cell; T_H, T-helper cell; *IL-1,* interleukin 1; *IL-2,* interleukin 2; *CsA,* cyclosporine; *AZA,* azathioprine.

used in conjunction with corticosteroids to obtain adequate immunosuppression for transplantation.

Azathioprine. The demonstration by Schwartz and Dameshek[193] that rabbits treated with 6-mercaptopurine were unable to synthesize humoral antibody on challenge with bovine serum albumin provided the foundation for the era of chemical immunosuppression. Azathioprine is an imidazole derivative of 6-mercaptopurine that is more consistently absorbed from the gastrointestinal tract. Azathioprine competitively inhibits the de novo synthesis of purines by blocking the conversion of inosine monophosphate to adenosine and guanidine monophosphates. This immunosuppressive agent has its effect on T lymphocytes during early phases of proliferation (see Fig. 5-6). Because it also competes with purine incorporation in a variety of tissues, its side effects are pleiotropic: granulocytopenia, thrombocytopenia, and alopecia. Additional therapeutic complications include pancreatitis, hepatic dysfunction, and febrile idiosyncratic responses. The most severe complication resulting from its use is bone marrow depression evidenced by leukocytopenia, thrombocytopenia, and reticulocytopenia, placing patients at increased risk for life-threatening opportunistic infections. Because the antiproliferative effects on the marrow occur at a lower dose than the immunosuppressive dose for most patients, Azathioprine displays a low therapeutic index and is only a weak immunosuppressant. Azathioprine toxicity is treated by drug withdrawal. After 5 days clonal proliferation occurs with return of bone marrow elements and the threat of allograft rejection.

Bredinin. Bredinin, an imidazole nucleoside, has been used experimentally and to a limited extent clinically in Japan as an immunosuppressive agent. Uchida, Yokota, and Akiyama[223] demonstrated prolonged survival of canine renal allografts with this agent. Its mode of action appears to be twofold: to competitively inhibit the conversion of inosinic monophosphate to guanylic monophosphate and to interfere with intracellular cyclic AMP levels.[188] Its immunosuppressive capacity is estimated to be comparable to that of Azathioprine (see Fig. 5-6), whereas associated marrow depression is less prominent.[164] The drug is not metabolized in the liver and demonstrates no significant hepatotoxicity.[109,164] Its use has been associated with significant anorexia and subsequent weight loss in the canine model.[223] This experimental immunosuppressant may have potential benefits in appropriate clinical circumstances.

Cyclosporine. Cyclosporine (CsA), a cyclic endecapeptide fungal metabolite, was shown in animal studies by Borel[22] and Borel and associates[23] to inhibit T-cell responses, thus preventing the development of cell-mediated cytotoxicity and inhibiting the induction of delayed-type hypersensitivity reactions. CsA did not suppress antibody production to lipopolysaccharide antigens in nude mice, suggesting that the drug had no direct effect on B cells. Further, CsA displays little myelotoxicity even at high doses. Thus hosts treated with CsA display a relatively low incidence of serious bacterial infections. Inhibition of humoral responses dependent on helper T cell functions[95,231] results in suppression of the response toward allografts. This specificity of CsA for T lymphocytes makes it particularly effective for the prevention of infection in transplantation.

The effect of CsA is reversible,[47,133] suggesting that this agent does not act by clonal deletion of uncommitted immunocompetent cells. Rather, CsA acts on the immune system by affecting the immunoregulatory T cell. On T-lymphocyte stimulation, the binding of antigen or mitogen results in the activation of the T cell.[2] Co-stimulator activity can be provided by both IL-1 and IL-2.[130] IL-2 provides the co-stimulatory activity for precursor cytotoxic T cells,[225,226], and IL-1 supplies the inductive signal for helper T cells.[227] When activated T cells are cultured in the presence of antigen or mitogen, T-lymphocyte growth factor, IL-2, is produced by the helper T cell population. Activated T lymphocytes proliferate when exposed to this growth factor. In vitro models have shown that CsA inhibits the activation of resting T lymphocytes through disruption of IL-2 and, to a lesser extent, IL-1 production (see Fig. 5-6). The CsA inhibition is both dose-[87,88,231] and time-dependent.[231] When added to mixed lymphocyte cultures at the initiation of the incubation, CsA inhibits T-cell proliferation, IL-2 production, and T-cell responsiveness to exogenous IL-2. However, when added at 48 or 72 hours after stimulation, CsA has little effect on proliferation. Further, the drug only inhibits the activity of mature cytotoxic T lymphocytes at high concentrations, indicating an early effect on immune cell generation at the usual therapeutic doses.

The arrest of in vitro antigen-induced proliferation by CsA occurs with both cloned helper T and cytotoxic T cell populations. CsA inhibits alloantigen-driven proliferation to a greater extent than lymphokine-induced stimulation.[167] In addition to inhibiting resting T-cell activation as evidenced by depressed proliferation on alloantigen stimulation, CsA also inhibits the production of IL-2 by T4 cells.[89,91] This effect occurs early in lymphocyte activation before gene transcription since cell lines that constitutively produce IL-2 are unaffected by CsA. Pharmacologic doses of CsA in mice inhibit the production and release of IL-1.[26] These effects hinder T-cell activation by limiting the availability of the second signal. Thus CsA inhibits the proliferation and function of cytolytic T lymphocytes by: (1) suppressing helper T cell secretion of mitogenic lymphokines, and (2) prohibiting antigen-induced clonal expansion of activated T cells.[226]

Hess[86] recently demonstrated that the immunosuppressive effect of CsA on the MLC can be partially overridden by addition of exogenous IL-2. When CsA is initially added to a mixed lymphocyte reaction, it prevents precursor cytotoxic T cells from acquiring responsiveness to IL-2. However, when IL-2 is added soon thereafter, the suppression of cytotoxic T-cell activity caused by CsA is reversed. The effect of CsA appears to be limited to the inhibition of both IL-2 production and responsiveness of precursor cytotoxic T lymphocytes to IL-2. Once this responsiveness has been acquired, Tc cells become sensitized and able to clonally expand in the presence of IL-2.

The ability to respond to IL-2 appears to depend on the presence of a receptor for this growth factor,[86,130,169,171] referred to as the Tac marker, found on cells stimulated with mitogens and alloantigens.[150] This marker is recognized by a monoclonal antibody. Prebinding of this antibody prevents the binding of IL-2 to mitogen-stimulated T lymphocytes and abrogates IL-2–dependent proliferation. Palacios and Moller[171] suggested that CsA blockade of receptors to stimulatory cell HLA-DR antigens resulted in the lack of responsiveness to IL-2 and inhibition of T-cell growth factor production. They proposed that the expression of IL-2 receptors was induced by the signals from HLA-DR antigens on stimulator cells. Thus, by blocking receptors for DR antigens on T cells, CsA would inhibit expression of IL-2 receptors. However, it is now clear from experiments both in the mouse and in humans that CsA blocks neither histocompatibility antigen reception nor IL-2 receptor expression.

The expression of the IL-2 receptor is thought to occur as the activated T cell moves from the G_0 to late G_1 phase of the cell cycle.[129,150,207,228] IL-2 production occurs predominantly during the late G_1 phase following expression of the IL-2 receptor.[129] After cultured T lymphocytes are incubated with CsA, they accumulate in the early phase of the G_1 stage of the cell cycle.[119] Consequently CsA appears to arrest the progression of the cell cycle at a stage before the expression of the IL-2 receptor and the production of T-cell growth factor.

The exact mechanism by which the proposed cellular events occur is unknown. CsA possibly acts at the membrane or in the cytoplasm to alter generation of a derepressor gene or at the nucleus to affect gene regulation. A cytoplasmic mechanism was recently advanced when Colombani, Robb, and Hess[33] demonstrated competitive inhibition of CsA binding to T lymphocytes by calmodulin inhibitors and interruption of calmodulin-dependent enzyme activity with CsA binding, indicating that CsA binds to T-lymphocyte–associated calmodulin. Calmodulin, a 16,000- to 18,000-dalton cytoplasmic protein, is involved in the early events of cell activation through calmodulin-dependent phosphodiesterase activity. The inhibition of this enzyme system prevents the activation of cyclic nucleotides, protein kinases, and phosphorylases and ultimately precludes synthesis of protein, prostaglandins, messenger RNA, and DNA. CsA-calmodulin binding is a possible mechanism accounting for the interruption in T-lymphocyte activation and the abrogation of the normal immune response.

The inability to acquire IL-2 sensitivity after CsA treatment seems to be limited to precursor cytotoxic T lymphocytes. Alloantigen activation of suppressor T lymphocytes is sensitive to IL-2 stimulation and less affected by CsA. Although CsA preferentially inhibits precursor cytotoxic T lymphocyte induction, it passively permits suppressor T-cell activation.[87] When they are exposed to CsA during rechallenge with alloantigen, primed lymphocytes proliferate, generating an increase in suppressor cell population size and activity.[88,90,91] In addition, CsA-treated lymphocytes cultured with IL-2 demonstrate a selective suppressor cell expansion. Both alloantigen activation and stimulation with exogenous IL-2 result in suppressor cell proliferation even in the presence of CsA. The mechanism by which IL-2 induces suppressor cell proliferation is unknown. The possible mechanisms include direct stimulation of the suppressor population by IL-2, an IL-2–sensitive amplifying population, or an IL-2–responsive suppressor precursor population.[59]

Suppressor cells do not prevent the cytoxic effector cells from responding to IL-2, but they inhibit precursor cytotoxic T lymphocytes from acquiring this responsiveness.[89,91] Removal of adherent suppressor cells by nylon-wool fractionation restores the ability of primed lymphocytes to generate a cytotoxic response toward a sensitizing alloantigen. Suppressor cells may prevent the production of IL-2[123] or inhibit the recruitment of competent precursor cells.[77,187] CsA appears to augment suppressor cell activity passively more than actively because of a relative insensitivity of this population to CsA.

The disequilibrium between the cytotoxic and suppressor arms of the cellular immune response is the basis for the use of CsA in transplantation. Such disequilibrium results in immunosuppression and alloantigen-specific, CsA-induced tolerance. This specific immunologic unresponsiveness is mediated by the effect of suppressor cells and not by clonal deletion.[87,88] Because of this parallel, CsA-induced immunosuppression is synergistic with maneuvers to produce unresponsiveness.[107,222,236] The administration of oral CsA in combination with extracted donor antigens prolonged rat renal allograft survival greater than a comparable dose of CsA alone. Treatment of recipients with a single dose of extracted histocompatibility antigens the day before transplantation and a 3- or 5-day course of CsA beginning at that time led to allograft prolongation. Cyclic CsA therapy in conjunction with a single dose or multiple doses of extracted donor-soluble antigen prolonged graft survival compared with hosts receiving only the initial administration of antigens and CsA. The specific suppressor cell-mediated immunosuppression initiated by administration of CsA and extracted antigens can be maintained with cyclic CsA.[237] In a less clinically relevant model, Homan and associates[96] prolonged rat renal allograft survival by pretreatment of the recipients with a 2-week course of CsA and intraperitoneal injection of 10^8 intact donor spleen cells for 2 weeks before transplantation. In these models, temporary unresponsiveness was achieved in spite of limited immunosuppressive therapy by the emergency of donor-specific suppressor elements.

Biologic Agents

Antilymphocyte Sera. Potent, nonspecific, immunosuppressive antibodies can be produced by immunizing a xenogeneic host, i.e., a species-divergent host, toward human lymphocytes. These sera opsonize the corresponding peripheral blood cellular elements leading to their auto-destruction. In addition, antibody binding onto lymphocytes may "blind" them to antigenic stimuli or, alternatively, nonspecifically stimulate them into a pathway not destructive to the graft. Immunosuppression with antilymphocyte sera (ALS) or purified globulin fractions (ALGs) has been demonstrated in experimental animal trials to prevent skin allograft rejection in mice,[75] rats,[235] and primates[9] and to prevent rejection of vascularized allografts in experimental canine renal[132,149,210] and hepatic[210] transplantation. Starzl and associates[210] reported that clinical use of ALG in renal transplantation, with the use of prophylactic therapy during the first week after transplantation, reduced the frequency and severity of early rejection episodes. However, subsequent clinical studies have not yielded unequivocal evidence supporting the use of ALS prophylactically. In a nonrandomized study Sheil and co-workers[198] demonstrated that prophylactic ALG decreased by 7% to 21% the incidence of acute rejection episodes. Taylor, Ackman, and Horowitz[218] and Novick and associates[162] in randomized controlled studies demonstrated improved graft survival and fewer rejection episodes, with a relative absence of reported side effects of serum sickness, anaphylactoid reactions, vascular thrombosis, or infection. On the other hand, well-controlled studies by other groups[12,229] suggest no therapeutic benefit from the *prophylactic use* of ALG, but rather a significant risk of fatal infections.

Alternatively, ALG can be used for the *therapy* of acute renal allograft rejection episodes. Glass and colleagues[66] found insignificant differences in renal allograft survival rates (i.e., 53%, 61%, and 49%) between groups randomized for high-dose steroids or ALG in combination with either low-dose or high-dose steroids. They recommended sequential rather than simultaneous use of ALG and high-dose steroids for rejection therapy. Simonian and co-workers[200] reported a 13% increased incidence of viral sepsis and a 13% incidence of serum sickness when antithymocyte globulin was used in conjunction with high-dose steroids to reverse acute renal allograft rejection episodes but an improved 1-year allograft survival from 38% to 100%. The prophylactic and acute therapeutic benefits of ALG in clinical transplantation remain controversial, in view of the increased risks of patient morbidity and mortality. Indeed there is no consensus that ALS provides a steroid-sparing effect.

The methods of production of ALS are varied. The most common method immunizes heterologous equine or rabbit hosts with either thymic T or cultured B-blastoid lymphocytes to yield a polyclonal product containing a heterogenous array of antibodies reactive with T cells, as well as a range of other normal lymphoid elements.[36] There are several disadvantages of the product. First, only 5% to 10% of the total antithymocyte globulin (ATG) dose is responsible for the therapeutic effect.[37] Second, there is appreciable batch-to-batch variability. Third, side effects, including serum sickness and increased cytomegalovirus infections, are prominent.

Monoclonal Antibodies. Monoclonal antibodies may provide an immunosuppressive agent, which obviates some of the disadvantages of polyclonal antilymphocyte sera. Kohler and Milstein[118] demonstrated that monoclonal antibodies with specificity for T-lymphocyte membrane determinants can be produced by alloimmune B cell–plasma cytoma cell hybrids. On this basis Kung and associates[122] generated a panel of monoclonal antibodies specific for T-lymphocyte subpopulations. These monoclonal anti-T cell antibodies have been used both for immunologic monitoring of immunosuppressed patients and for treatment of allograft rejection.

Two primary types of reagents are of interest: one recognizes helper-inducer (T4) and the other suppressor-cytotoxic (T8) T-lymphocyte subpopulations. An elevation of the ratio of T4/T8 has been associated with acute rejection episodes.[38,51,52] Chatenoud and co-workers[31] found this association in 71% of renal transplant recipients undergoing an acute rejection episode. Of the patients followed longitudinally, 22% had elevations in this ratio not associated with allograft rejection; however, in these cases the change in T-cell subset dynamics was transient. Colvin and associates[34] also noted an association between the helper-inducer to suppressor-cytotoxic cell ratio and renal allograft rejection in 80% of his patients. Other investigators[153,195] have been unable to demonstrate this correlation. On the other hand, it is consistent that a reversal in ratio in renal transplant recipients is associated with viral, specifically herpes, and cytomegalovirus infections.[192,195] Schooley and colleagues[192] noted that all patients who had primary or reactivated herpes virus infections displayed a reversal in the T-cell subset ratio. Initial observations suggest that the ratio affords a barometer of the immune state that is useful to differentiate renal allograft rejection from viral infections when renal dysfunction occurs in the period following transplant.

Therapeutic use of monoclonal antibodies induces immunosuppression by T-lymphocyte depletion. In vitro treatment of harvested bone marrow cells with monoclonal antibodies that react specifically with peripheral T lymphocytes has been claimed to lyse mature T cells, as evidenced by the reduction of rosette formation with sheep red blood cells by 89% and completely inhibited responses to T-cell mitogens, concanavalin A, and phytohemagglutinin.[196] After monoclonal antibody therapy. Michaelides, Hogarth, and McKenzie[148] decreased T-cell responsiveness in in vitro assays with prolongation of murine skin and tumor allograft survival. In subhuman primates, injection of OKT4 monoclonal antibodies resulted in the disappearance of T4 lymphocytes from the peripheral circulation,[104,106] but the ratio of T-cell subsets was not altered, suggesting that the T4 antigen had been removed from the surface by modulation. There was an associated prolonged skin allograft survival. On the other hand, administration of monoclonal antibodies specific for cytotoxic T cells had no beneficial effect on skin allograft longevity.[104-106] Monoclonal antibodies reactive with all T cells induced modulation that resulted in decreased immunologic function and prolonged skin allograft survival in rhesus monkeys.[105]

These promising experimental results led to clinical trials with the use of monoclonal antibodies. Although the goal of monoclonal antibody therapy is specific T-cell subset immunosuppression, the initial clinical trials evaluated the efficacy of an OKT3 monoclonal antibody reactive with all mature T cells because of their easier production and thus clinical availability.[37] The treatment of cadaveric renal transplant recipients with biopsy-proven acute allograft rejection resulted in an immediate depletion of T3 reactive T cells within minutes of administration. All rejection episodes were reversed within 2 to 7 days. Within the 3 to 12 month follow-up period, five patients had subsequent rejection episodes, two of which were unresponsive to conventional therapy. After 5 to 7 days of monoclonal antibody therapy, there was a gradual return of T lymphocytes reactive with other T-cell markers but not with OKT3 monoclonal antibodies, indicating that antigenic modulation had occurred but had not interfered with the immunosuppressive effect of the monoclonal reagent.[36] One patient developed antibodies to the monoclonal reagent and subsequently underwent irreversible allograft rejection. The occurrence of OKT3 reactive peripheral T lymphocytes corresponded with the initial clinical signs and symptoms of rejection. However, this was unusual, provided only a single course was used. A recent multicenter randomized clinical trial comparing the administration of OKT3 monoclonal antibodies and high-dose steroids for acute renal allograft rejection confirms the efficacy of this immunosuppressive modality.[71] A 2-week course of monoclonal antibodies resulted in significantly improved rejection reversal and 1-year graft survival when compared to steroid therapy. Additionally, monoclonal antibody therapy allowed for a concomitant lowering of the dosage of the other immunosuppressive drugs. The majority of patients developed antibodies to OKT3 monoclonal antibodies; however, their presence did not affect the therapeutic outcome. Another monoclonal antibody, which apparently recognizes the E-rosette–forming cell receptor or a surface structure closely related to it, did not affect allograft rejection[221] in 19 renal allograft recipients. A third monoclonal antibody, denoted anti-T12, which reacts with a T-cell surface marker on thymic T lymphocytes, was moderately effective in reversing acute cellular, but not humoral, rejection mechanisms.[116]

Significant in vivo toxicity associated with the administration of monoclonal antibodies has not been noted.[37] The clinical efficacy, the duration of administration, and the ability to repeatedly administer the reagent are all limited by the frequent immune responses to murine immunoglobulin.[101] The therapeutic use of monoclonal antibodies results neither in specific unresponsiveness nor in durable graft function since second rejection episodes occur frequently. These findings probably relate to the fact that monoclonal antibodies only deplete select subsets of T lymphocytes involved in the rejection process.

Induction of Immunologic Unresponsiveness

In addition to methods for preventing graft rejection directly by various immunosuppressive agents, methods have also been developed to halt the rejection process through the establishment of a state of immunologic unresponsiveness (see boxed material below). One such approach is through the induction of anti-idiotypic antibodies, which are substances that enhance antibodies directed against histocompatibility antigen, antigen-antibody complexes, and suppressor cell activity.[78] The classic model of antibody-mediated unresponsiveness uses enhancing antibodies raised by immunization of hosts with lyophilized tissue extracts. Experimentally, long-term survival of skin allografts,[35,208] heterotopic cardiac allografts,[43] and renal allografts[216] was achieved by passive transfer of enhancing antibodies directed against either Class I or Class II antigens. Antibodies directed against Class II antigens inhibit in vitro mixed lymphocyte culture reactions[49,194] and theoretically prevent the recognition stage of the allograft response. Antibodies directed against Class I antigens probably inhibit the effector mechanism of antigen response by inhibiting induction of cytolytic T lymphocytes. Antibodies specific for Class I or II antigens might mediate passive enhancement by acting at any of the three stages of the transplant response. Enhancing antibodies could mask donor alloantigens on the graft,[208] thereby preventing induction of cell-mediated cytotoxicity and antigen recognition. A second possibility is the formation of antigen-antibody complexes[208] that cause immunosuppression by specific binding to antigen-reactive cells.[10] This opsonization would cause these cells to be phagocytized by the reticuloendothelial system of the host. In addition, passively transferred antibodies may have a central effect to promote suppressor cell differentiation. The third possibility is that

MECHANISMS OF IMMUNOLOGIC UNRESPONSIVENESS

Antigenic Deletion
In vitro culture

Host Response Modification
Cellular: Suppressor T-cell activation
Humoral: Anti-idiotypic antibodies
Enhancing antibodies
Antigen-antibody complex formation

the antibodies coat graft antigens, making them inaccessible to effector mechanisms.

The clinical use of passive enhancement for specific immunosuppression has been limited because of the possibility of transferred antibody-mediated damage to the grafted organ. Stuart, Fitch, and McKearn[216] demonstrated enhanced renal allograft survival but severe graft injury with monoclonal alloantibodies directed against both Class I and Class II antigens. Hart and Fabre[81] suggested that the efficacy of this regimen could be increased by using non-complement-fixing monoclonal xenoantibodies directed against Class I and Class II histocompatibility antigens. Mouse monoclonal antibodies directed against human histocompatibility antigens have failed to provide transplantation enhancement in large mammal models.

Anti-idiotypic antibodies are moieties directed against the specific receptor sites present on the surface of immunocompetent cells reactive to donor histocompatibility antigens. Deletion of these cell clones would produce specific tolerance toward histocompatibility antigens. In animal models immunization with T lymphoblasts, which have been sensitized toward donor histocompatibility antigens and carry on their surface specific antidonor idiotypic receptors, results in the production of anti-idiotypic antibodies specific for the recognition site. Deletion of cells bearing the idiotype would ultimately produce tolerance toward the lymphoid cells used to prime the T lymphoblasts. The recognition site or idiotype would act as an immunogen, because its structure is not native to the lymphoid cell.[97] Some individuals believe that the idiotypic determinant of the T-cell receptor is similar or identical to the antigen-binding idiotype of B-lymphocyte surface immunoglobulins, in the case of a single alloantigen.[16,17,19] The presence of idiotypic binding sites on immunoglobulin molecules has been demonstrated by the capacity of B lymphocytes to absorb the specific activity of an anti-idiotypic antiserum raised against T-cell receptors sensitized to the same alloantigen.[16] There is no evidence that the T-lymphocyte receptors express any idiotypes not present on corresponding alloantibody molecules, although the converse is not true.[19] Anti-idiotypic antibodies that interact with both T-cell receptor sites and alloantibodies directed against the same antigen can specifically coat idiotype-positive B and T lymphocytes.

The T-cell idiotype structure is a two-chain (alpha and beta) complex having a molecular weight of 150,000 daltons with each chain weighing 70,000 daltons.[18] It has been hypothesized that each chain is the product of a gene locus, one of which is linked to the major histocompatibility complex and the other to the region coding for the immunoglobulin heavy chain.[230] Since the T-cell idiotype is coded for by genes linked to those determining the variable regions of the immunoglobulin heavy chain,[17,121,230] fine specificity is determined by immunoglobulin structure.[120,230] The T-cell receptor is associated on the surface with the OKT3 T-cell marker.

Anti-idiotypic antibodies induce specific transplantation tolerance in rodent models. Binz and Wigzell[19] demonstrated that anti-idiotypic antibodies cause selective inhibition of T-cell responses in rats and mice. Elimination of T cells involved in allograft rejection responses (mixed lymphocyte culture reactions, cell-mediated lympholysis, and graft vs. host reactions) occurred without affecting third-party reactions. Efforts to duplicate these results of anti-idiotypic antibodies in the primate[215] succeeded in causing mixed lymphocyte culture inhibition but failed to create in vivo unresponsiveness.

Although the clinical use of anti-idiotypic antibodies for selective immunosuppression has not been tested, it has been hypothesized that anti-idiotypic antibodies may mediate the immunologic unresponsiveness resulting from blood transfusions. Sera from transfused patients who had successfully undergone renal allotransplantation inhibited mixed lymphocyte culture reactions, wherein the stimulating HLA alloantigen corresponded to the disparate donor specificity.[201] Sera from patients who had rejected renal allografts either did not inhibit the mixed lymphocyte response; or if inhibition was present, it did not correlate with the appropriate histocompatibility specificity. Anti-idiotypic antibodies demonstrated in the sera of transfused renal transplant recipients using indirect immunofluorescence[55] reacted only with T lymphocytes, bearing the very donor mismatched HLA-B antigen specificity. In an experimental model with three to four transfusions,[157] murine sera inhibited mixed lymphocyte culture responses specifically toward stimulator cells of donor type but not toward a third party. The inhibitory effect appeared to be mediated by antibodies directed against the T-cell recognition site rather than the surface antigens of the stimulator cells. Thus clinical and experimental studies suggest that blood transfusions may generate anti-idiotypic antibodies that specifically inhibit the immune response.

Specific tolerance toward foreign transplantation antigens is the ultimate goal of immunosuppressive therapy. Renal transplant recipients bearing long-term allografts may display donor-specific unresponsiveness that in at least some instances seems to be mediated by suppressor T cells.[137] Peripheral blood lymphocytes from unresponsive patients suppress the in vitro induction of cell-mediated lympholysis activity toward the donor cells. In vitro mixed lymphocyte cultures induce the proliferation of suppressor T cells, which either directly[61,92,224] or through soluble noncytotoxic factors[184,189] inhibit the primary differentiation proliferation of cytotoxic T cells reactive with the specific transplantation antigens. Since allosensitization toward a renal allograft results not only in generation of cytotoxic T cells but also in the development of suppressor cells bearing the T8 phenotype[30] and in the inhibition of donor-specific cell-mediated lympholysis activity, patients without rejection or with well-controlled responses may display only suppressor activity.

The classic model of unresponsiveness is the induction of neonatal transplantation tolerance by the intravenous administration of allogeneic splenic cells into newborn mice, resulting in permanent acceptance of donor allografts.[94] Cytotoxic activity cannot be expressed by hosts toward cells bearing the specific tolerated donor antigens. This antigen-specific tolerance appears to result from the generation of suppressor T cells.

Gorczynski and MacRae[72,73] have proposed that two

separate populations of suppressor cells induce tolerance by means of different mechanisms. Suppressor population A induces neonatal tolerance by inhibiting the development of precursor cytotoxic T cells from stem cells. Thus suppressor A causes clonal deletion to achieve tolerance. Suppressor population B inhibits the final differentiation of precursor cytotoxic T cells into the cytotoxic effector cell. In this setting the tolerance maintained by the active cellular process of peripheral inhibition can be adoptively transferred. Neonatally induced tolerance can be reversed by the infusion of syngeneic immunocompetent cells only across a Class I antigen disparity. Class II antigen tolerance cannot be abrogated by this mechanism.[76]

When Class II antigen incompatibility exists, induction of unresponsiveness in adult animals occurs secondary to suppressor cell induction acting through an active cellular process. Tolerance to a Class I antigen disparity induced in the neonatal model can be reversed by the administration of immunocompetent cells that replace those removed by clonal deletion. Transplantation tolerance through the induction of suppressor cells has not been achieved clinically.

An alternative approach to the generation of unresponsiveness is manipulation of the allograft. The passenger leukocyte concept introduced by Snell[203] and supported by Billingham[15] postulates that donor leukocytes passively transferred in the allograft are critical to the induction of immunity. Because passenger leukocytes are stimulator cells bearing histocompatibility antigens, they may serve as the primary sensitizing agents.[40] This hypothesis suggests that immunogenicity may be reduced by eliminating the passenger leukocyte. Two techniques have been proposed to accomplish this: (1) through incubation of the allograft with complement and antigen-specific (Ia) monoclonal antibodies, and (2) through in vitro cell culture.

In vitro cultivation of an allograft before transplantation was successfully used for endocrine tissue by Lafferty and associates,[127] who prolonged the survival of thyroid tissue in an allogeneic host after in vitro cell culture under an atmosphere of 95% oxygen and 5% carbon dioxide, since passenger leukocytes are sensitive to high oxygen tension and extended periods of culture. The success of this allogeneic transplant was not the result of a deficient host immune system. When the host received a second, uncultured allograft from the same donor strain, both allografts were rejected. In addition, successful transplantation of allogeneic cultured thyroid cells followed by injection of donor peritoneal exudate cells caused subsequent graft loss.[128] The findings suggest that during the process of cultivation thyroid cells lose their contaminating passenger leukocytes, leading to an afferent blockade and failure of sensitization. However, injection of peritoneal exudate cells or subsequent transplantation of uncultured thyroid cells bearing passenger leukocyte stimulator cells introduces the structures necessary for histocompatibility antigen recognition and causes rejection by cytotoxic lymphocyte induction. Similar principles have been applied to transplantation of isolated pancreatic islet cells, leading to reversal of chemically induced diabetes in the rodent.[24,113,124] Furthermore, canine islet cells cultured for 1 week may be depleted of dendritic cells expressing Ia antigens, which serve as allogeneic stimulators.[64] Burn wounds grafted with cultured human epidermal cells,[84] which have lost their ability to stimulate allogeneic lymphocytes in epidermal cell-lymphocyte reactions, are free of the Ia positive Langerhans cells.[199] Thus in vitro maintenance of tissues in a controlled environment results in a loss of immunogenicity secondary to a decrease in antigen-specific, positive stimulator cells.

In support of the theory that culture techniques decrease graft alloreactivity is the observation that Class II histocompatibility antigens are present on passenger leukocytes but not on parenchymal endocrine cells of pancreatic islet cells, thyroid follicular cells, and adrenal cortical cells. Class II antigen expression is limited to interstitial dendritic cells.[82] Indeed, incubation of an allograft with complement and monoclonal antibody specific for Class II antigens prolongs graft survival without the need for pretransplantation in vitro cultivation.[58] Thus both in vitro culturing and pretreatment with antibodies directed to Class II antigens achieve the same ultimate result, i.e., depletion of Ia positive, immunogenic cells. Allograft rejection does not require that there be Class II antigen differences[154] but only that there be the ability to present a Class I antigenic disparity in an immunogenic manner.

Overview of Therapy to Prevent Rejection

Immunosuppressive therapy has been directed toward the allograft to decrease graft immunogenicity and toward the host to depress the response to the immunogenetic allograft. Clinical application has been demonstrated only with the latter approach. Total body irradiation has been used historically as an immunosuppressive modality, but it has been abandoned because of the high incidence of severe bone marrow depression and subsequent infectious complications. Local graft irradiation, which avoids the systemic side effects of radiation when used in conjunction with corticosteroids, has detrimental effects on the rate of rejection reversal and graft survival. Total lymphoid irradiation, which uses the immunodepressive effect of radiotherapy while minimizing systemic toxicity, results in an immunosuppressive state characterized by T-cell lymphopenia and decreased alloreactivity secondary to induction of T-suppressor cells. The inconsistent experimental results and the complications associated with this modality, specifically nausea, vomiting, and the possible increased incidence of lymphoma, have limited its application.

The chemical agents for transplant immunosuppression include corticosteroids and antiproliferative agents. Corticosteroids create an immunosuppressive state by decreasing the number of circulating lymphocytes, affecting antigen recognition, and decreasing the inflammatory response of rejection. The generalized lymphopenia resulting from steroid administration is caused by a redistribution of lymphocytes, particularly T4 cells to the extravascular pool. The second mechanism of steroid immunosuppression is through an alteration in the antigen recognition process. Corticosteroids both inhibit the expression of Class II antigens and decrease interleukin production. The third known immunosuppressive mechanism attributed to steroids is decreased inflammatory response at the rejection site through interference with the recruitment and cytotoxic activation of macrophages.

Azathioprine, an analog of 6-mercaptopurine, and bredinin, an imidazole nucleoside, both competitively inhibit de novo synthesis and consequently inhibit the early phase of T-lymphocyte proliferation. The immunosuppressive capability of these two agents is comparable; however, bredinin has less bone marrow and hepatic toxicity.

Cyclosporine (CsA), an endecapeptide and fungal metabolite, inhibits the induction of cell-mediated cytotoxicity and the delayed-type hypersensitivity reaction by inhibiting T-cell activation. CsA inhibits the production of IL-2 by T4 cells and antigen-induced proliferation of activated T cells. CsA arrests the progression of activated T cells during the cell cycle before the expression of the IL-2 receptor. IL-2 sensitivity, a prerequisite for cytotoxic T-cell proliferation, is dependent on the presence of this receptor. CsA administration not only results in immunosuppression but also induces alloantigen-specific tolerance. This unresponsiveness is mediated by the passive expansion of suppressor T cells.

Biologic agents used for immunosuppression include antilymphocyte sera and monoclonal antibodies. Antilymphocyte sera results in nonspecific immunosuppression by producing opsonization of peripheral lymphoid cells and by antibody binding to lymphocytes, thus "blinding" them to antigenic stimuli. The prophylactic and therapeutic use of antilymphocyte sera to prevent or reverse rejection episodes is not generally accepted because of equivocal clinical results and significant associated morbidity. Monoclonal antibodies have been used in experimental and clinical transplantation to avoid the disadvantage of polyclonal antilymphocyte sera. Monoclonal antibodies have been used for both immunologic monitoring and for the treatment of allograft rejection. Although not a pathognomic indicator, an elevation in the T4/T8 ratio has been associated with acute rejection episodes. The ratio is more often used to differentiate between renal allograft rejection and a viral infection when renal dysfunction occurs in the period following transplant. Monoclonal antibodies are used therapeutically to decrease the T-lymphocyte responsiveness by specific T-cell subset immunosuppression. Recent clinical trials have demonstrated the efficacy of OKT3 monoclonal antibody therapy in reversing allograft rejection and in prolonging graft survival.

Methods to prevent the side effects of nonspecific immunosuppression through the establishment of immunologic unresponsiveness include the development of anti-idiotypic antibodies, enhancing antibodies directed against histocompatibility antigens, antigen-antibody complexes and suppressor cell activity. Enhancing antibodies directed against Class I and Class II antigens and antigen-antibody complex formulation have created unresponsiveness in experimental models, but the development of antibody-mediated damage to the graft has limited their clinical use. Anti-idiotypic antibodies that are directed against the specific T-cell receptor site produce alloantigen-specific tolerance by clonal deletion of these immunocompetent cells. Anti-idiotypic antibodies have induced unresponsiveness in rodent models, but experimentation in primates has been unsuccessful. It has been hypothesized that immunologic unresponsiveness resulting from blood transfusion is associated with this mechanism. Suppressor cell-mediated unresponsiveness through either the inhibition of precursor cytotoxic T-cell development or differentiation yields transplantation tolerance, although induction of suppressor cells has not been advanced clinically. The ultimate goal is to achieve successful transplantation through the establishment of specific tolerance to the allograft. Experimental attempts to achieve this goal through immunologic manipulation of the graft or host have had limited success. Currently, nonspecific means are used to preclude the effector mechanism of the allograft response and prevent graft destruction.

CLINICAL TRANSPLANTATION

The modern era of organ transplantation began with the first successful grafting of a kidney between identical twins in 1954.[147] Subsequent advances in knowledge concerning the pathogenesis of rejection and the ability to manipulate this immune response by various therapeutic strategies have allowed transplantation to proceed to a point where many diseased organs can now be replaced with a minimum of difficulty. Kidney transplantation is relatively commonplace throughout the United States and many other countries, and organs such as the liver and heart are now being transplanted with increasing frequency. Although allograft rejection continues to be an important problem, cyclosporine has done much to improve graft survival rates. Thus for many organs the availability of donors has posed more of a problem than the potential difficulties surrounding the rejection process. To gain insight into the advances that have been made in organ transplantation over the last three decades, this section will briefly review the current status of organs that are transplantable. For purposes of discussion, three types of donor grafts should be recognized. These include: (1) grafting between twins in which the immunologic match is identical between host and donor, (2) living-related grafts in which there is considerable immunologic similarity between the host and donor, but not to the same degree as with twins, and (3) cadaveric grafts obtained from unrelated individuals (i.e., subjects who are brain dead, but in whom function of the organ to be potentially transplanted is normal) in which immunologic matching between host and donor may be quite dissimilar, even though every attempt is made before transplantation to optimize this match as much as possible. For renal transplantation, all three types of grafts have been used. For transplantation of organs such as the liver and heart, it is obvious that only cadaver grafts can be used.

Renal Transplantation

Approximately 6000 to 10,000 new patients annually develop end-stage renal disease in the United States, requiring treatment with either chronic dialysis or renal transplantation. For patients 55 years old or less, renal transplantation has emerged as the treatment of choice. This relates to the recent advances in immunosuppression, particularly the discovery of cyclosporine, which has drastically improved both renal allograft and patient survival. Before the availability of cyclosporine, survival rates for patients receiving cadaveric allografts approached 90%, whereas graft survivals approximated 50%. With the advent of cyclosporine, graft and patient 1-year survival rates of 80% and 95%, respectively,[108] have been achieved in cadaveric transplantation. Similar results have been obtained in patients receiving living-related donor kidneys. With HLA-identical grafts, graft survival has approached 90% to 95%, and for all other living-related grafts 75% to 85% graft survival has been obtained.[108]

Historically, patient survival following renal transplantation with a kidney from a living-related donor always exceeded that achieved when hemodialysis was the renal replacement therapy used. In contrast, patient survival after cadaveric transplantation generally paralleled that associated with hemodialysis.[100] With the use of cyclosporine, however, a clear improvement in patient survival following cadaveric transplantation has been observed when compared with hemodialysis. In addition, such renal transplantation patients have also demonstrated a significantly improved rehabilitation rate when compared to those treated with hemodialysis.[54] Without question, both the longevity and quality of life have been clearly improved when this therapeutic modality has been used.

In patients receiving renal transplantation, the transplanted kidney is usually placed in the iliac fossa through a lower abdominal incision in a retroperitoneal fashion. Generally, the blood supply is assured by anastomosing the renal artery to the hypogastric artery in an end-to-end fashion. The renal vein is anastomosed to the iliac vein end-to-side. Urinary tract continuity is usually established by a ureteroneocystostomy by placing the ureter through a submucosal tunnel to prevent the subsequent development of reflux. The success of this surgical approach has been clearly demonstrated in the thousands of kidneys that have been transplanted over the last 30 years.

Heart Transplantation

Since the performance of the first human cardiac transplant by Dr. Christiaan Barnard in December 1967,[11] several hundred heart transplants have been performed to prolong the life expectancy of patients with end-stage cardiac disease. Although enthusiasm for cardiac transplantation has waxed and waned over the last two decades, the use of cyclosporine to treat rejection has clearly improved the clinical outcome and rejuvenated the interest and excitement associated with this procedure.

Patients considered suitable candidates for cardiac transplantation are generally limited to those with a life expectancy of several weeks because of functional Class IV cardiac disease refractory to medical or surgical therapy.[168] Generally, candidates for cardiac transplantation should be under the age of 50, and without an underlying malignant disease, insulin-dependent diabetes mellitus, severe peripheral vascular disease, morbid obesity, or an active infectious process. In addition, a high fixed pulmonary vascular resistance is generally considered a contraindication for this procedure.

Cardiac allotransplantation is usually performed orthotopically; the recipient heart is removed, leaving a remnant of the right and left atria posteriorly.[141] The atria, pulmonary artery, and aorta from the donor heart are then anastomosed primarily. Heterotopic cardiac transplantation has also been performed in which the allograft is connected in parallel with the native heart.[163] The theoretic advantage of this latter procedure is the maintenance of the native myocardium to sustain the recipient for reimplantation, if the donor organ undergoes acute irreversible rejection.

The current overall survival rate at 1 and 2 years for cardiac allotransplantation is 80% and 75%, respectively.[62] Regularly scheduled right endocardial biopsies in conjunction with cardiac catheterization with the use of coronary angiography are used to evaluate the status of the transplanted heart. Although fever, hemodynamic instability, signs of congested heart failure, arrhythmias, and electrocardiographic alterations are clinical indices suggesting a rejection, histologic evaluation of the endocardium is usually necessary to rule out a rejection episode. Although rejection may occur at any time following transplantation, late graft failure is often associated with atherosclerotic coronary artery disease of the transplanted heart. To minimize the likelihood of this problem, most patients at present are treated prophylactically with antithrombogenic agents.

Liver Transplantation

Liver transplantation is now considered an accepted therapeutic modality for a number of hepatic disorders and in certain conditions the treatment of choice. As with heart transplantation, the general acceptance of this procedure has paralleled the significant improvement in survival resulting from the use of cyclosporine. Before the use of cyclosporine, Starzl and co-workers,[211] pioneers in clinical hepatic transplantation, reported a 1- and 5-year survival rate of 32.9% and 20%, respectively, between 1963 and 1980. Immunosuppression with cyclosporine has drastically improved these results, with the actuarial survival rates at 1 and 5 years now being 69.7% and 62.8%, respectively.[212]

Indications for liver transplantation are only now becoming clearly defined. In the pediatric population, biliary atresia is the most common clinical condition in which this procedure is used. The 1- and 5-year actuarial survival rates for this population of patients is 76.2% and 73.7%, respectively.[74] Because clinical success with hepatic transplantation has exceeded that of the Kasai procedure for biliary atresia, it is now considered the treatment of choice for this pediatric disease. Other pediatric conditions in which hepatic transplantation offers a therapeutic alternative include various inborne errors of metabolism such as Wilson's disease, tyrosinemia, glycogen storage disease, and the alpha$_1$-antitrypsin deficiency.

In the adult population the most common indications for liver transplantation include end-stage, primary, biliary cirrhosis; sclerosing cholangitis; and chronic active hepatitis. Those patients with a positive antigen for hepatitis B are usually not accepted as suitable candidates for transplantation because of the significant risk of recurrence of hepatitis. Similarly, those patients older than 60 years of age and/or those individuals with significant cardiopulmonary disease, advanced alcoholic disease, sepsis, or those deemed psychologically unfit for transplantation because of potential difficulty with immunologic drug compliance are also eliminated as acceptable transplant candidates. The role of hepatic transplantation in malignant disease remains uncertain. Although the literature is replete with examples of transplantation in patients with a variety of malignant disorders, including hepatocellular carcinoma, cholangiocarcinoma, and hemangioendothelioma, the relatively high recurrence rate in patients with neoplastic disease has questioned the value of this procedure in this patient population. As a general rule, patients with hepatic malignancy secondary to an extrahepatic source are no longer considered acceptable candidates for liver transplantation. If the malignancy is primary and confined to the liver parenchyma, hepatic transplantation is still considered an acceptable therapeutic modality in selected patients.

Despite the increasing use of liver transplantation in the treatment of various hepatic diseases, even when performed by the most skilled surgeon, this operation is a formidable procedure. Not only is the donor hepatectomy technically demanding, but the recipient operation involves a number of anastomoses requiring the utmost in surgical skill, including those involving the biliary tract, the inferior vena cava above and below the liver, the portal vein, and the hepatic artery.

In deciding whether a patient is a suitable candidate for hepatic transplantation, the most important determinants are clearly the extent to which the patient's underlying disease is interfering with quality of life and how transplantation will ultimately influence the long-term prognosis of this disease.

Lung Transplantation

Transplantation of the lung can be performed either by itself or as an en bloc heart-lung combination. Clinical experience with solitary lung transplants has been fraught with considerable problems, including infection, hemorrhagic consolidation, and severe rejection, although this latter problem appears to be less noteworthy with the availability of cyclosporine. Most centers in which solitary transplants have been performed have had few survivors beyond 1 month. For this reason the heart-lung combination transplant has gained in popularity. Not only does the combined transplant ensure a better blood supply to the transplanted bronchus, which has historically been a major problem with solitary pulmonary transplants in which anastomotic dehiscence of the bronchus has frequently occurred, but the operation is also technically more feasible than the solitary transplant and provides a maximum amount of lung parenchyma to optimize function of the allograft.[102] Currently, heart-lung grafting boasts 1- and 2-year survival rates approaching 70% and 60%, respectively.[44] As with other transplants, the use of cyclosporine has contributed greatly to this success.

Although clinical experience with lung transplantation has been limited when compared with kidney, heart, or liver transplantation, potential recipients include those individuals with irreversible and terminal pulmonary failure. Among individuals who have received lung transplants have been patients with end-stage pulmonary vascular disease such as primary pulmonary hypertension, and those with severe parenchymal disease, including chronic obstructive pulmonary disease, respiratory burns, pulmonary fibrosis, toxic pneumonitis, and bronchiectasis.

Pancreas Transplantation

More than 1 million patients currently exist in the United States with insulin-dependent diabetes mellitus. An additional 10,000 to 15,000 new cases can be expected each year. Despite exacting control of the serum glucose by exogenously administered insulin, the complications associated with this disease continue to be plaguing problems. These are primarily associated with the microangioplastic lesions that result from the aberrant diabetic carbohydrate metabolism, giving rise to a severe retinopathy that may ultimately lead to blindness, nephropathy eventuating in renal failure and uremia, and peripheral vascular disease that is commonly associated with neuropathy and limb loss. Pancreatic transplantation in rodent models has successfully prevented and in some cases halted the progression of these microangiopathic lesions;[8,181] thus it is not surprising that enormous efforts have been made to develop a successful means of transplanting pancreatic tissue in humans.

Since 1966 over 500 human pancreatic transplants have been attempted with varying degrees of success, the outcome being influenced greatly by the magnitude of the rejection process. With the advent of cyclosporine, a renewed interest has emerged in the feasibility of both segmental and whole organ transplantation of the pancreas. Of the two approaches, segmental pancreatic grafting is technically less complex. It encompasses transplantation of the body and tail of the pancreas with the use of the splenic artery and vein to reestablish vascularization. Control of pancreatic duct drainage has been the major technical difficulty encountered with this procedure. Although attempts at intraperitoneal transplantation with intraabdominal pancreatic drainage have proven successful in large animal models, this procedure has been abandoned clinically because of the high complication rate encountered in patient trials.[217] Other approaches have included duct ligation[114] or duct obliteration by the intraductal injection of synthetic polymers[48] in an attempt to manage the pancreatic exocrine secretion. Unfortunately, blockage of exocrine function ultimately led to sclerosis of the pancreas and the eventual failure of its endocrine function.[21]

Because of these difficulties, current interest has focused on the use of whole organ pancreatic transplants. With this procedure the pancreas and a portion of duodenum surrounding the papilla of Vater are transplanted en bloc.[139,209] The approach most commonly used is to anastomose the duodenum to the urinary bladder in order to provide a means of exocrine drainage.[205] The splenic artery and vein are then anastomosed to the hypogastric artery and external iliac vein, respectively, to reestablish blood supply. The ultimate future of this technique remains to be determined, but results to date have been quite encouraging and have demonstrated not only long-term functional survival (up to 4 years) but also normalization of the glucose intolerance.

In addition to the vascularized pancreatic allograft, treatment of diabetes has also been attempted with transplantation of isolated pancreatic islet cells. For this procedure, the pancreas is mechanically and enzymatically disrupted to harvest the islet cells. These cells are then transferred to the donor. A variety of donor sites have been used, including the testes, the peritoneal cavity, the spleen, and the portal vein, the latter being the most often used. Although this technique has been quite successful experimentally in preventing or halting the metabolic consequences of diabetes in various animal models,[8,181] clinical trials to date in diabetic human subjects have failed to abrogate the need for insulin. Thus, at present, whole organ transplantation appears to show the most promise if the transplanted pancreas is ever to be used in the treatment of diabetes mellitus.

Small Bowel Transplantation

Annually thousands of patients become victims of the short gut syndrome, usually secondary to thrombosis or embolization of the superior mesenteric artery, necessitating massive intestinal resection. The minimal digestive absorptive capacity with which these patients is left is often inadequate to maintain a normal nutritional status, requiring the use of long-term parenteral alimentation for survival. Obviously, replacement of this missing intestine with a small bowel transplant would be highly desirable.

Experimentally, small bowel transplantation has been successfully performed in animals since 1959. Lillehei, Goott, and Miller[138] were the first to describe this technique with a canine model. Continuing experimental refinements have made the technique of small bowel transplantation quite feasible from a technical standpoint. As with other organ transplants, the major problem in making small bowel transplantation a clinically useful modality concerns the control of rejection. The magnitude of this problem directly relates to the length of intestine transplanted. Large segments of small intestine have resulted experimentally in a graft vs. host reaction because of the large amount of intestinal mesenteric lymphoid tissue also transplanted.[45] When small segments of intestine are transplanted, this is less of a problem, but the allograft still undergoes the standard rejection process. Immunosuppression regimens that have recently been successful in preventing the rejection process and graft vs. host disease in various experimental models include cyclosporine administration,[39] donor organ irradiation,[135] and microsurgical excision of mesenteric lymph nodes.[220] Although several attempts have been made clinically to transplant human intestine, all patients have died because of technical difficulties associated with the operation, sepsis, graft rejection, or a combination of these factors. Until these problems are more effectively managed, human intestinal transplantation must be viewed at present as an experimental procedure.

Bone Marrow Transplantation

The indications for bone marrow transplantation include severe inherited immune deficiency disorders, bone marrow failure, and certain malignancies.[219] The potentially fatal inherited diseases for which bone marrow transplantation has been used include various hemoglobinopathies such as thalassemia and sickle cell disease; immunodeficiency states; and certain enzymatic disorders such as mucopolysaccharoidosis, osteopetrosis, chronic granulomatous disease, adenosine deaminase deficiency, and Diamond-Blackfan anemia. Acquired disorders of marrow failure responding to bone marrow transplantation have included aplastic anemia and various malignancies such as acute lymphocytic leukemia, acute nonlymphocytic leukemia, chronic myelogenous leukemia, hairy cell leukemia, Hodgkin's disease, non-Hodgkin's lymphoma, neuroblastoma, multiple myeloma, and acute myelofibrosis. Marrow transplantation has also been used in selected cases of marrow failure secondary to toxic chemotherapeutic agents.

Bone marrow for transplantation has been obtained from syngeneic, allogeneic, and autologous sources. Whereas syngeneic marrow transplantation refers to a transfer of bone marrow between genetically identical twins, allogeneic marrow transplantation requires the donor and recipient to be HLA-identical siblings. Recipients of allogeneic or syngeneic marrow are pretreated with immunosuppressive agents and myeloablative drugs if the underlying cause of marrow failure is a malignancy. In autologous transplantation, marrow is harvested during remission and cryopreserved. The marrow is then replanted following myeloablative antineoplastic therapy to eliminate residual malignant cells. Of interest, autologous transplantation has been as effective in treating acute nonlymphocytic and chronic myelogenous leukemia as has allogeneic or syngeneic marrow transplantation.[238]

The major complications associated with bone marrow transplantation have included rejection of the grafted marrow, graft vs. host disease, and potentially lethal infections. If the transplanted marrow functions only briefly and a marrow biopsy reveals the absence of marrow elements, this indicates that the recipient has rejected the donor marrow because of presensitization, usually resulting from prior blood transfusions. Graft vs. host disease results from the transplanted T cells reacting to the genetically different host cells. The lymphohematopoietic system, including the skin, liver, and gastrointestinal tract, are primarily affected by the graft vs. host response, which is manifest clinically as dermatitis, diarrhea, alterations in liver function, weight loss, and a high susceptibility to infection. Graft vs. host disease occurs in 30% to 70% of allogeneic marrow transplant recipients and results in death in 20% to 40% of those individuals affected.[165]

The infectious complications following bone marrow transplantation usually occur within the first several weeks before the production of granulocytes by the grafted marrow. The recipient is susceptible to all types of infections, including bacterial, fungal, and herpes simplex infections. After the first month following grafting, the increase in the peripheral white blood cell count suggests the engraftment of the donor marrow. Subsequent infections include cytomegalovirus and *Pneumocystis carinii* infections, both of which are usually manifested as interstitial pneumonias. The use of prophylactic trimethoprim-sulfamethoxazole has greatly reduced the incidence of interstitial pneumonia secondary to *Pneumocystis*. Those patients having cytomegalovirus as the offending organism are much less fortunate, and many of these individuals will die because no current effective treatment exists. Thus, to prevent cytomegalovirus infections, hyperimmune globulin is usually administered prophylactically early after transplantation.

Corneal Transplantation

Corneal transplantation, also referred to as corneal grafting or penetrating keratoplasty, is performed in the United States at a rate of approximately 10,000 operations per year. The success of this procedure is limited only by the technical skills of the surgeon and not by the immune response. This is because the cornea is an immunologically privileged structure in which oxygen is derived from the oxygen content of the internal aqueous humor rather than from specific blood vessels. Consequently, circulating antibodies are isolated from the transplanted cornea. When they occur, rejection episodes are usually mild and develop at a rate of only 10% to 12%. If rejection becomes a problem, it is usually ablated by the use of topical steroids. In over 90% of operations performed, corneal transplantation proves to be successful. Currently, corneal transplantation is the procedure of choice for all patients suffering from opaque corneas. It is limited only by the availability of donor corneas.

The persistence of the immunologically privileged status of the transplanted cornea depends on the vascularity of the graft. Scarring of the cornea results in an increased vascularity and consequently an increased risk of rejection. Under this circumstance the cornea has a 25% incidence of irreversible rejection. Maumenee[145] first attributed graft failure to immunologic rejection. Rejection occurs primarily through a cellular immune response. Previous corneal grafting resulting in corneal scarring and increased vascularity have been associated with graft failure. Histocompatibility matching is not routinely necessary, but is beneficial in the presence of heavily vascularized corneas.

SUMMARY

Successful transplantation of organs or tissues rests on an understanding of the immunologic rejection process. The events leading to allograft rejection consist of afferent, central, and efferent limbs. The presentation and recognition of foreign antigens are manifestations of the afferent limb. The central limb encompasses the proliferation, differentiation, and production of lymphokines by T cells and of humoral antibody by B cells, whereas the efferent limb represents the activation of various cell populations that ultimately lead to the rejection of the transplanted tissue or organ. Clinically, allograft rejection is classified as hyperacute, accelerated, acute, or chronic.

A variety of immunologic strategies have been used to avert, minimize, or reduce the rejection response of the host or the immunogenicity of the allograft. The latter approach has only had limited success experimentally with nonvascularized grafts. Host immunosuppression by means of physical agents (i.e., total body, graft, or lymphoid irradiation) or various chemical substances (i.e., corticosteroids, cyclosporine, azathioprine, or bredinin) nonspecifically diminish the immune response. Biologic agents (i.e., antilymphocyte sera and monoclonal antibodies) provide both generalized and specific immunosuppressive effects. Antilymphocyte sera nonspecifically depletes the host of lymphoid cells, whereas monoclonal antibodies delete a specific T-cell subset. Anti-idiotypic antibodies, enhancing antibodies, antigen-antibody complexes, and stimulation of suppressor cell activity have also been used to create a state of specific immunologic unresponsiveness; but these strategies have been limited primarily to various experimental models. To date, immunologic manipulation to achieve transplantation tolerance has not progressed to a level satisfactory for clinical use. Consequently, nonspecific means to repress the effector mechanism of the allograft rejection response still remain necessary.

Knowledge currently available concerning the rejection process and the ability to minimize it with various immunosuppressive modalities, particularly cyclosporine, has made clinical transplantation a reality. Kidney transplantation, for example, is currently the procedure of choice in the management of patients with end-stage renal disease and clearly improves the quality of life when compared with chronic dialysis. Other organs that are being transplanted with increasing frequency include the liver and the heart. No longer is successful clinical transplantation of these organs limited by technical pitfalls but rather by the immune process mediating rejection of the transplanted organ or tissue. As further strategies are developed to avert this process, it is anticipated that other organs that can be technically transplanted such as the lung, pancreas, and small intestine will become treatment options for patients suffering from such devastating disorders as end-stage lung disease, insulin-dependent diabetes, and the short bowel syndrome, respectively.

REFERENCES

1. Anderson, C.B., and Newton, W.T.: Accelerated human renal allograft rejection, Arch. Surg. **110:**1230, 1975.
2. Andrus, L., and Lafferty, K.J.: Inhibition of T-cell activity by cyclosporin A, Scand. J. Immunol. **15:**449, 1982.
3. Bach, F.H., and van Rood, J.J.: The major histocompatibility complex—genetics and biology, Part I, N. Engl. J. Med. **295**(15):806, 1976.
4. Bach, F.H., and van Rood, J.J.: The major histocompatibility complex—genetics and biology, Part II, N. Engl. J. Med. **295**(15):872, 1976.
5. Bach, F.H., and van Rood, J.J.: The major histocompatibility complex—genetics and biology, Part III, N. Engl. J. Med. **295**(15)927, 1976.
6. Bach, F.H., Bach, M.L., and Sondel, P.M.: Differential function of major histocompatibility complex antigens in T lymphocyte activation, Nature **259:**273, 1976.
7. Balch, C.M., and Diethelm, A.G.: The pathophysiology of renal allograft rejection: a collective review, J. Surg. Res. **12**(5):350, 1972.
8. Ballinger, W.F., and Lacy, P.E.: Transplantation of intact pancreatic islets in rats, Surgery **72:**175, 1972.

9. Balner, H., Dersjant, H., and van Bekkum, D.W.: Testing of antihuman lymphocyte sera in chimpanzees and low primates, Transplantation **8:**281, 1969.
10. Barber, W.H., Hutchinson, I.V., and Morris, P.J.: Enhancement of rat kidney allografts using haptenated alloantigens and antihapten antibody, Transplantation **36:**475, 1983.
11. Barnard, C.N.: A human cardiac transplant, S. Afr. Med. J. **41:**1271, 1967.
12. Bell, P.R.F., et al.: Medical research council trial of antilymphocyte globulin in renal transplantation, a multicenter randomized double-blind placebo controlled clinical investigation, Transplantation **35:**539, 1983.
13. Belsito, D.V., et al.: Effect of glucocorticosteroids on epidermal Langerhans cells, J. Exp. Med. **155:**291, 1982.
14. Berman B., et al.: Modulation of expression of epidermal Langerhans cell properties following in situ exposure to glucocorticoids, J. Invest. Dermatol. **80:**168, 1983.
15. Billingham, R.E.: The passenger cell concept in transplantation immunology, Cell. Immunol. **2:**1, 1971.
16. Binz, H., and Wigzell, H.: Shared idiotypic determinants on B and T lymphocytes reactive against the same antigenic determinants. I. Demonstration of similar or identical idiotypes on IgG molecules and T-cell receptors with specificity for the same alloantigens, J. Exp. Med. **142:**197, 1975.
17. Binz, H., and Wigzell, H.: Antigen binding idiotypic receptors from T lymphocytes: an analysis of their biochemistry, genetics, and use as immunogens to produce specific immune tolerance, Cold Spring Harbor Symp. Quant. Biol. **41:**275, 1976.
18. Binz, H., and Wigzell, H.: Shared idiotypic determinants on B and T lymphocytes reactive against the same antigenic determinants, Scand. J. Immunol. **5:**559, 1976.
19. Binz, H., and Wigzell, H.: Idiotypic, alloantigen-reactive T lymphocyte receptors and their use to induce specific transplantation tolerance, Prog. Allergy **23:**154, 1977.
20. Birtch, A.G., et al.: Controlled clinical trial of antilymphocyte globulin in human renal allografts, Transplant. Proc. **3:**762, 1971.
21. Blanc-Brunat, N., et al.: Pathology of the pancreas after intraductal neoprene injection in dogs and diabetic patients treated by pancreatic transplantation, Diabetologia **25:**97, 1983.
22. Borel, J.F.: Comparative study of in vitro and in vivo drug effects on cell-mediated cytotoxicity, Immunology **31:**631, 1976.
23. Borel, J.F., et al.: Effects of the new antilymphocyte peptide cyclosporin A in animals, Immunology **32:**1017, 1977.
24. Bowen, K.M., Andrus, L., and Lafferty, K.J.: Successful allotransplantation of mouse pancreatic islets to nonimmunosuppressed recipients, Diabetes **29**(suppl. 1):98, 1980.
25. Bretscher, P., and Cohn, M.: A theory of self-nonself discrimination, Science **169:**1042, 1970.
26. Bunjes, D., et al.: Cyclosporin A mediates immunosuppression of primary cytotoxic T cell responses by impairing the release of interleukin 1 and interleukin 2, Eur. J. Immunol. **11:**657, 1981.
27. Busch, G.J., et al.: Human renal allografts: the role of vascular injury in early graft failure, Medicine **59**(1):29, 1971.
28. Busch, G.J., et al.: A primate model of hyperacute renal allograft rejection, Am. J. Pathol. **79:**31, 1975.
29. Carpenter, B.: Mechanisms of rejection: update 1982, Transplant. Proc. **15:**259, 1983.
30. Charpentier, B.M., et al.: Expression of OKT8 antigen and Fc and receptors by suppressor cells mediating specific unresponsiveness between recipient and donor in renal-allograft-tolerant patients, Transplantation **36:**495, 1983.
31. Chatenoud, L., et al.: Interest in and limitations of monoclonal anti-T cell antibodies for the follow-up of renal transplant patients, Transplantation **36:**45, 1983.
32. Claman, H.N.: Corticosteroids and lymphoid cells, N. Engl. J. Med. **291:**1154, 1974.
33. Colombani, P.M., Robb, A, and Hess, A.D.: Cyclosporin A binding to calmodulin: a possible site of action on T lymphocytes, Science **228:**337, 1985.
34. Colvin, R.B., et al.: Circulating T-cell subsets in 72 human renal allograft recipients: the OKT4+/OKT8+ cell ratio correlates with reversibility of graft injury and glomerulonephropathy, Transplant. Proc. **15:**1166, 1983.
35. Corson, J.: Active inhibition of the allograft response in H-2 incompatible mice, Transplantation **10:**484, 1970.
36. Cosimi, A.B.: The clinical usefulness of antilymphocyte antibodies, Transplant. Proc. **15:**583, 1983.
37. Cosimi, A.B., et al.: Treatment of acute renal allograft rejection with OKT3 monoclonal antibody, Transplantation **32:**535, 1981.
38. Cosimi, A.B., et al.: Monoclonal antibodies for immunologic monitoring and treatment in recipients of renal allografts, N. Engl. J. Med. **305:**308, 1981.
39. Craddock, G.H., et al.: Small bowel transplantation in the dog using cyclosporine, Transplantation **35:**284, 1983.
40. Cunningham, A.J., and Lafferty, K.J.: A simple, conservative explanation of the H-2 restriction of interactions between lymphocytes (editorial), Scand. J. Immunol. **6:**1, 1977.
41. Dale, D.C., Fauci, A.S., and Wolff, S.M.: Alternate-day prednisone: leukocyte kinetics and susceptibility to infections, N. Engl. J. Med. **291:**1154, 1974.
42. David, D.S., et al.: Viral syndromes and renal homograft rejection, Ann. Surg. **175**(2):257, 1972.
43. Davies, D.A.L., and Alkins, B.J.: What abrogates heart transplant rejection in immunological enhancement? Nature **247:**294, 1974.
44. Dawkins, K.D., et al.: Long-term results, hemodynamics, and complications after combined heart and lung transplantation, Circulation **71:**919, 1985.
45. Deltz, E., et al.: Development of graft-versus-host reaction in various target organs after small intestine transplantation, Transplant. Proc. **13:**1215, 1981.
46. Dempster, W.J., Lennox, B., and Boag, J.W.: Prolongation of survival of skin homotransplants in the rabbit by irradiation of the host, Br. J. Exp. Pathol. **31:**670, 1950.
47. Denham, S., et al.: Reversible suppression of allo-antibody production by cyclosporin, Int. Arch. Allergy Appl. Immunol. **62:**453, 1980.
48. Dubenard, J.M., et al.: A new method of preparation of segmental pancreatic grafts for transplantation: trials in dogs and in man, Surgery **84:**633, 1978.
49. Duc, H.T., Kinsky, R.G., and Voisin, G.A.: Ia versus K/D antigens in immunological enhancement of tumor allografts, Transplantation **25:**182, 1978.
50. Dupont, E., Wybran, J., and Toussant, C.: Glucocorticosteroids and organ transplantation, Transplantation **37**(4):331, 1984.
51. Ellis, T.M., et al.: Alterations in human regulatory T lymphocyte subpopulations after renal allografting, J. Immunol. **127:**2199, 1981.
52. Ellis, T.M., et al.: Immunological monitoring of renal allograft recipients using monoclonal antibodies to human T lymphocyte subpopulations, Transplantation **33:**317, 1982.
53. Evans, R.L., et al.: Peripheral human T cell sensitized in mixed leukocyte culture synthesize and express Ia-like antigens, J. Exp. Med. **148:**1440, 1978.
54. Evans, R.W., et al.: The quality of life of patients with end-stage renal disease, N. Engl. J. Med. **312:**553, 1985.
55. Fagnilli, L., and Singal, D.P.: Blood transfusions may induce anti-T cell receptor antibodies in renal patients, Transplant. Proc. **14:**319, 1982.
56. Farrar, J.J., et al.: The biochemistry, biology, and role of IL-2 in the induction of cytotoxic T cell and Ab-forming B cell responses, Immunol. Rev. **63:**129, 1982.
57. Fauci, A.S., and Dale, D.C.: The effect of in vivo hydrocortisone on subpopulations of human lymphocytes, J. Clin. Invest. **53:**240, 1974.
58. Faustman, D., et al.: Prolongation of murine islet allograft survival by pretreatment of islets with antibody directed to Ia determinants, Proc. Natl. Acad. Sci. (USA) **78**(8):5156, 1981.
59. Feldman, M., et al.: T-T interactions in induction of suppressor and helper T cells—analysis of membrane phenotype of precursor and amplifier cells, J. Exp. Med. **145:**793, 1977.
60. Fidler, J.P., et al.: Radiation reversal of acute rejection in patients with life-threatening infections, Arch. Surg. **107:**256, 1973.
61. Folch, H., and Waksman, B.H.: The splenic suppressor cell. II. Suppression of the mixed lymphocyte reaction by thymus-dependent adherent cells, J. Immunol. **113:**140, 1974.

62. Frazier, O.H., and Cooley, D.A.: Cardiac transplantation, Surg. Clin. North Am. **66**(3):477, 1986.
63. Fuks, Z., et al.: Long-term effects of radiation on T and B lymphocytes in peripheral blood of patients with Hodgkin's disease, J. Clin. Invest. **58:**803, 1976.
64. Gebel, H.M., et al.: Ia-bearing cells within isolated canine islets, Transplantation **36**(3):346, 1983.
65. Gillis, S., Crabtree, G.R., and Smith, K.A.: Glucocorticoid-induced inhibition of T cell growth factor production, J. Immunol. **123:**1624, 1979.
66. Glass, N.R., et al.: A comparative study of steroids and heterologous antiserum in the treatment of renal allograft rejection, Transplant. Proc. **15:**617, 1983.
67. Gleason, R.E., and Murray, J.E.: Report from kidney transplant registry, Transplantation **5:**343, 1967.
68. Glimcher, L.H., et al.: Ia antigen-bearing B cell tumor lines can present protein antigen and alloantigen in major histocompatibility complex-restricted fashion to antigen-reactive T cells, J. Exp. Med. **155:**445, 1982.
69. Godfrey, A.M., and Salaman, J.R.: Radiotherapy in treatment of acute rejection of human renal allografts, Lancet **1:**938, 1976.
70. Godfrey, A.M., and Salaman, J.R.: Is graft irradiation of value in renal transplant rejection? Transplant. Proc. **9:**1005, 1977.
71. Goldstein, G., et al.: A randomized clinical trial of OKT3 monoclonal antibody for acute rejection of cadaveric renal transplants, N. Engl. J. Med. **313:**337, 1985.
72. Gorczynski, R.M., and MacRae, S.: Suppression of cytotoxic response to histocompatible cells. I. Evidence for two types of T lymphocyte-derived suppressors acting at different stages in the induction of a cytotoxic response, J. Immunol. **122:**737, 1979.
73. Gorczynski, R.M., and MacRae, S.: Suppression of cytotoxic response to histocompatible cells. II. Analysis of the role of two independent T suppressor pools in maintenance of neonatally induced allograft tolerance in mice, J. Immunol. **122:**747, 1979.
74. Gordon, R.D., et al.: Indications for liver transplantation in the cyclosporine era, Surg. Clin. North Am. **66**(3):541, 1986.
75. Gray, J.G., Monaco, A.P., and Russell, P.S.: Heterologous mouse antilymphocyte serum to prolong skin homografts, Surg. Forum **15:**142, 1964.
76. Gruchalla, R.S., Strome, P.G., and Streilein, J.W.: Analysis of neonatally induced tolerance of H_2 alloantigens. III. Ease of abolition of tolerance of Class I but not Class II antigens with infusions of syngeneic immunocompetent cells, Transplantation **36:**318, 1983.
77. Gulberg, M., and Larsson, E.L.: Studies on induction and effector function of concanavain A-induced suppressor cells that limit TCGF production, J. Immunol. **128:**746, 1982.
78. Halle-Pannenko, O., Pritchard, L.L., and Rappaport, H.: Alloimmunization activated suppressor cells, Transplantation **36:**60, 1983.
79. Hamburger, J., et al.: Renal homotransplantation in man after radiation of the recipient, Am. J. Med. **32:**854, 1962.
80. Hancock, W.W.: Analysis of intragraft effector mechanisms associated with human renal allograft rejection: immunohistological studies with monoclonal Abs, Immunol. Rev. **77:**61, 1984.
81. Hart, D.N.J., and Fabre, J.W.: Passive enhancement of rat renal allografts using mouse monoclonal xenoantibodies, Transplantation **32:**431, 1981.
82. Hart, D.N.J., et al.: Major histocompatibility complex antigens in the rat pancreas, isolated pancreatic islets, thyroid, and adrenal, Transplantation **36**(4):431, 1983.
83. Haynes, F., and Fauci, A.S.: The differential effect of in vivo hydrocortixone on the kinetics of subpopulations of human peripheral blood thymus-derived lymphocytes, J. Clin. Invest. **61:**703, 1978.
84. Hefton, J.M., et al.: Grafting of burn patients with allografts of cultured epidermal cells, Lancet **2:**428, 1983.
85. Hersh, E.M., et al.: Lymphocyte activation during allograft rejection, Transplant. Proc. **3**(1):457, 1971.
86. Hess, A.D.: Effect of interleukin 2 on the immunosuppressive action of cyclosporine, Transplantation **39**(2):62, 1985.
87. Hess, A.D., and Tutschka, P.J.: Effect of cyclosporin A on human lymphocyte responses in vitro. I. CsA allows for the expression of alloantigen-activated suppressor cells while preferentially inhibiting the induction of cytolytic effector lymphocytes in MLR, J. Immunol. **124**(6):2601, 1980.
88. Hess, A.D., Tutschka, P.J., and Santos, G.W.: Effect of cyclosporin A on human lymphocyte responses in vitro. II. Induction of specific alloantigen unresponsiveness mediated by a nylon wool-adherent suppressor cell, J. Immunol. **126:**961, 1981.
89. Hess, A.D., Tutschka, P.J., and Santos, G.W.: Effect of cyclosporin A on human lymphocyte responses in vitro. III. CsA inhibits the production of T-lymphocyte growth factors in secondary mixed lymphocyte responses but does not inhibit the response of primed lymphocyte to TCGF, J. Immunol. **128:**355, 1982.
90. Hess, A.D., Tutschka, P.J., and Santos, G.W.: Effect of cyclosporine on the induction of cytotoxic T lymphocytes: role of interleukin 1 and interleukin 2, Transplant. Proc. **15:**2248, 1983.
91. Hess, A.D., et al.: Effect of cyclosporin A on human lymphocyte responses in vitro. IV. Production of T cell stimulator growth factors and development of responsiveness to these growth factors in CsA-treated primary MLR cultures, J. Immunol. **128:**360, 1982.
92. Hirano, T., and Norden, A.A.: Cell-mediated immune response in vitro. I. The development of suppressor cells and cytotoxic lymphocytes in mixed lymphocyte cultures, J. Immunol. **116:**1115, 1976.
93. Hirschberg, H., Braathen, L.R., and Thorsby, E.: Ag presentation by vascular endothelial cells and epidermal Langerhans cells: the role of HLA-DR, Immunol. Rev. **66:**57, 1982.
94. Holan, V., Chutna, J., and Hasek, M.: Specific suppression of antigen-reactive cells in neonated transplantation tolerance, Nature **274:**895, 1978.
95. Homan, W.P., et al.: Studies on the immunosuppressive properties of cyclosporin A in rats receiving renal allografts, Transplantation **29:**361, 1980.
96. Homan, W.P., et al.: Prolongation of renal allograft survival in the rat by pretreatment with donor antigen and cyclosporin A, Transplantation **31:**423, 1981.
97. Hopt, U.T., et al.: Lymphocyte recruiting capacity of cells infiltrating rejecting sponge matrix allografts in vivo, Transplant. Proc. **15:**367, 1983.
98. Hume, D.M., and Wolf, J.S.: Abrogation of the immune response: irradiation therapy and lymphocyte depletion, Transplantation **5:**1174, 1967.
99. Hume, D., et al.: Glomerulonephritis in human renal homotransplants, Transplant. Proc. **2**(3):361, 1970.
100. Hutchinson, T.A., et al.: Prognostically controlled comparison of dialysis and renal transplantation, Kidney Int. **26:**44, 1984.
101. Jaffers, G.J., et al.: The human immune response to murine OKT3 monoclonal antibody, Transplant. Proc. **15:**646, 1983.
102. Jamieson, S.W., et al.: Operative technique for heart-lung transplantation, J. Thorac. Cardiovasc. Surg. **87:**930, 1984.
103. Jeannet, M., et al.: Humoral antibodies in renal allotransplantation in man, N. Engl. J. Med. **282**(3):111, 1970.
104. Jonker, M., Goldstein, G., and Balner, H.: Effects of in vivo administration of monoclonal antibodies specific for human T cell subpopulations on the immune system in a rhesus monkey model, Transplantation **35:**521, 1983.
105. Jonker, M., Malissen, B., and Mawas, C.: The effect of in vivo application of monoclonal antibodies specific for human cytotoxic T cells in rhesus monkeys, Transplantation **35:**374, 1983.
106. Jonker, M., et al.: In vivo application of monoclonal antibodies specific for human T cell subsets permits the modification of immune responsiveness in rhesus monkeys, Transplant. Proc. **15:**235, 1983.
107. Kahan, B.D., Yoshimura, N., and Yasumura, T.: Induction of donor-specific unresponsiveness in rat kidney transplantation with donor antigen and three cycles of cyclosporine, Transplant Proc. **17:**1387, 1985.
108. Kahan, B.D., et al.: Clinical and experimental studies with cyclosporin in renal transplantation, Surgery **97:**125, 1985.
109. Kamata, K., et al.: Immunosuppressive effect of bredinin on cell-mediated and humoral immune reactions in experimental animals, Transplantation **35:**144, 1983.
110. Kaplan, H.S.: Hodgkin's disease, Cambridge, Mass., 1972, Harvard University Press.

111. Kaplan, M.P., et al.: Suppression of interleukin-2 production by methylprednisolone, Transplant. Proc. **15**:407, 1983.
112. Kaufman, H.M., et al.: Prolongation of renal homograft function by local graft radiation, Surg. Gynecol. Obstet. **120**:49, 1965.
113. Kedinger, M., et al.: In vitro culture reduces immunogenicity of pancreatic endocrine islets, Nature **270**:736, 1977.
114. Kelly, W.D., et al.: Allotransplantation of the pancreas and duodenum along with the kidney in diabetic nephropathy, Surgery **61**:827, 1967.
115. King, D.P., Strober, S., and Kaplan, H.S.: Suppression of mixed leukocyte response and of graft versus host diseases by spleen cells following total lymphoid irradiation, J. Immunol. **126**:1140, 1981.
116. Kirkman, R.L., et al.: Treatment of acute renal allograft rejection with monoclonal anti-T12 antibody, Transplantation **36**:620, 1983.
117. Kissmeyer-Nielsen, F., et al.: Hyperacute rejection of kidney allografts associated with preexisting humoral antibodies against donor cells, Lancet **2**:662, 1966.
118. Kohler, G., and Milstein, C.: Continuous cultures of fused cells secreting antibody of predefined specificity, Nature **256**:495, 1975.
119. Koponen, M., Geider, A., and Loor, F.: The effects of cyclosporins on the cell cycle of T lymphoid cell lines, Exp. Cell Res. **140**:237, 1982.
120. Krammer, P.H., and Eichmann, K.: T-cell receptor idiotypes are controlled by genes in the heavy chain linkage group and the major histocompatibility complex, Nature **270**:733, 1977.
121. Krawinkel, V., et al.: On the structure of the T cell receptor for antigen, Cold Spring Harbor Symp. Quant. Biol. **41**:285, 1976.
122. Kung, P.C., et al.: Strategies for generating monoclonal antibodies defining human T lymphocyte differentiation antigens, Transplant. Proc. **12**:141, 1980.
123. Kupiec-Weglinski, J.W., et al.: Population of cyclophosphamide-sensitive T suppressor cells maintain cyclosporin-induced allograft survival, Transplant. Proc. **15**(suppl.):2357, 1983.
124. Lacy, P.E., Davie, J.M., and Finke, E.H.: Effect of organ culture on islet rejection, Diabetes **29**(suppl):93, 1980.
125. Lafferty, K.J., and Cunningham, A.J.: A new analysis of allogeneic interactions, Aust. J. Exp. Biol. Med. Sci. **53**(1):27, 1975.
126. Lafferty, K.J., Andrus, L., and Prowse, S.J.: Role of lymphokine and antigen in the control of specific T cell responses, Immunol. Rev. **51**:279, 1980.
127. Lafferty, K.J., et al.: Thyroid allograft immunogenicity is reduced after a period in organ culture, Science **188**:259, 1975.
128. Lafferty, K.J., et al.: Effect of organ culture on the survival of thyroid allografts in mice, Transplantation **22**:138, 1976.
129. Lalande, M.E., et al.: Quantitative studies on the precursors of cytotoxic lymphocytes. VI. Second signal requirements of specifically activated precursors isolated 12 hours after stimulation, J. Exp. Med. **151**:12, 1980.
130. Larsson, E.L.: Cyclosporin A and dexamethasone suppress T cell responses by selectively acting at distinct sites of the triggering process, J. Immunol. **124**(6):2828, 1980.
131. Larsson, E.L., Iscove, N.N., and Coutinno, A.: Two different factors are required for induction of T-cell growth, Nature **283**:664, 1980.
132. Lavson, R.K., et al.: The prolongation of canine renal homograft function using antilymphocyte sera as an immunosuppressive agent, Transplantation **5**:169, 1967.
133. Leapman, S.B., et al.: Cyclosporin A prevents the appearance of cell surface "activation" antigens, Transplantation **34**:94, 1982.
134. Lechler, R.F., and Batchelor, J.R.: Restoration of immunogencity to passenger cell-depleted kidney allografts by the addition of donor strain dendritic cells, J. Exp. Med. **155**:31, 1982.
135. Lee, K.K.W., and Schraut, W.H.: In vitro allograft irradiation prevents graft vs. host disease in small bowel transplantation, J. Surg. Res. **38**:364, 1985.
136. Levitt, S.H., et al.: Radiation for immunosuppression in human organ transplantation, Acta Radiol. (Ther.) **10**:329, 1971.
137. Liburd, E.M., et al.: Evidence of suppressor cells and reduced CML induction, Transplant. Proc. **10**:557, 1978.
138. Lillehei, R.C., Goott, B., and Miller, F.A.: The physiological response of the small bowel of the dog to ischemia including prolonged in vitro presentation of the bowel with successful replacement and survival, Ann. Surg. **150**:543, 1959.
139. Lillehei, R.C., et al.: Pancreaticoduodenal allotransplantation: experimental and clinical experience, Ann. Surg. **172**:405, 1970.
140. Lopez, C., et al.: Association of renal allograft rejection with viral infections, Am. J. Med. **56**:280, 1974.
141. Lower, R.R., and Shumway, N.E.: Studies on orthotopic homotransplantation of the canine heart, Surg. Forum **11**:18, 1960.
142. Lowry, R.P., et al.: Bone marrow transplantation following total lymphoid irradiation, Transplantation **36**:16, 1983.
143. Lucas, Z.J., et al.: Early renal transplant failure associated with subluminal sensitization, Transplantation **10**(6):522, 1970.
144. Mason, D.W.: The mechanism of allograft rejection—progress and problems, Transplant. Proc. **15**:264, 1983.
145. Maumenee, A.E.: The influence of donor-recipient sensitization on corneal grafts, Am. J. Ophthalmol. **34**:142, 1951.
146. McKenzie, I.F.C.: Alloaggression, Transplant. Proc. **15**:269, 1983.
147. Merrill, J.P., et al.: Successful homotransplantation of human kidney between identical twins, JAMA **160**:277, 1956.
148. Michaelides, M., Hogarth, P.M., and McKenzie, I.F.C.: The immunosuppressive effect of monoclonal anti-Lyt-1.1 antibodies in vivo, Eur. J. Immunol. **11**:1005, 1981.
149. Mitchell, R.M., et al.: The effect of heterologous immune serum on canine renal homografts, Transplantation **4**:323, 1966.
150. Miyawaki, T., et al.: Cyclosporine A does not prevent expression of Tac antigen, a probable TCGF receptor molecule on mitogen-stimulated human T cell, J. Immunol. **130**:2727, 1983.
151. Mizel, S.B.: Physiochemical characterization of lymphocyte activity factor, J. Immunol. **122**:2167, 1979.
152. Mizel, S.B.: Interleukin 1 and T cell activation, Immunol. Rev. **63**:51, 1982.
153. Morris, P.J., et al.: Role of T-cell subset monitoring in renal allograft recipients, N. Engl. J. Med. **306**:1110, 1982.
154. Morrows, C.E., et al.: Lack of donor-specific tolerance in mice with established anti-Ia-treated islet allografts, Transplantation **36**(6):691, 1983.
155. Murray, J.E., et al.: Study on transplantation immunity after total body irradiation: clinical and experimental investigation, Surgery **48**:272, 1960.
156. Nabholtz, M., et al.: Cell-mediated cell lysis in vitro: control of killer cell production and target specificities in the mouse, Eur. J. Immunol. **4**:378, 1974.
157. Nagarkatti, P.S., Joseph, S., and Singal, D.P.: Induction of antibodies by blood transfusions capable of inhibiting responses in MLC, Transplantation **36**:695, 1983.
158. Najarian, J.S., and Perpes, R.J.: Participation of humoral antibody in allogeneic organ transplantation rejection, Surgery **62**:213, 1967.
159. Najarian, J.S., et al.: Total lymhoid irradiation and kidney transplantation: a clinical experience, Transplant. Proc. **13**:417, 1981.
160. Norlung, J.J., Acles, A.E., and Lerner, A.B.: The effect of ultraviolet light and certain drugs on Ia bearing Langerhans cells in murine epidermis, Cell. Immunol. **60**:50, 1981.
161. North, R.J.: The concept of the activated macrophage, J. Immunol. **121**:806, 1978.
162. Novick, A.C., et al.: A controlled randomized double-blind study of antilymphoblast globulin in cadaver renal transplantation, Transplantation **35**:175, 1983.
163. Novitzky, D., Cooper, D.K.C., and Barnard, C.N.: The surgical technique of heterotopic heart transplantation, Ann. Thorac. Surg. **36**:176, 1983.
164. Okubo, M., Kamata, K., and Yokota, K.: Effect of bredinin on cellular and humoral immunity responses and on canine kidney allograft survival, Transplant. Proc. **12**:515, 1980.
165. O'Reilly, R.J.: Allogeneic bone marrow transplantation: current status and future directions, Blood **62**:941, 1983.
166. Oriol, R., et al.: The Lewis system: new histocompatibility antigens in renal transplantation, Lancet **1**(2):574, 1978.
167. Orosz, C.G., et al.: Analysis of cloned T cell function. I. Dissection of cloned T cell proliferative responses using cyclosporin A, J. Immunol. **129**:1865, 1982.
168. Oyer, P.E., Stinson, E.B., and Reitz, B.A.: Cardiac transplantation: 1980, Transplant. Proc. **13**:199, 1981.
169. Palacios, R.: Cyclosporin A inhibits the proliferative response and the generation of helper, suppressor, and cytotoxic T-cell functions, Cell. Immunol. **61**:453, 1981.

170. Palacios, R.: Mechanisms of T cell activation: role and functional relationships of HLA-DR Ags and interleukins, Immunol. Rev. **63:**73, 1982.
171. Palacios, R., and Moller, G.: Cyclosporin A blocks receptors for HLA-DR antigens on T cells, Nature **290:**792, 1981.
172. Paul, L.C., van Es, L.A., and Baldwin, W.M.: Antigens in human renal allografts, Clin. Immunopathol. **19:**206, 1981.
173. Petersen, V.P., et al.: Late failure of human renal transplants, Medicine **54**(1):45, 1975.
174. Pierce, J.C.: Crossmatching for organ transplantation II, Transplant. Proc. **4**(4):447, 1972.
175. Pierce, J.C., Kay, S., and Lee, H.M.: Donor-specific IgG antibody and the chronic rejection of human renal allografts, Surgery **78**(1):14, 1975.
176. Pilepich, M.V., et al.: Renal graft irradiation in acute rejection, Transplantation **35:**208, 1983.
177. Pimsler, M., Treal, J., and Forman, J.: Ag-presenting cells in T cell responses, Immunogenetics **12:**297, 1981.
178. Porter, K.A.: Morphological aspects of renal homograft rejection, Br. Med. Bull. **21**(2):171, 1965.
179. Porter, K.A.: Histopathology in clinical renal transplantation, Transplant. Proc. **6**(4):79, 1974.
180. Porter, K.A., et al.: The role of lymphocytes in the rejection of canine renal homotransplants, Lab. Invest. **13**(9):1080, 1964.
181. Reckard, C.R., and Barker, C.F.: Transplantation of isolated pancreatic islets across strong and weak histocompatibility barriers, Transplant. Proc. **5:**761, 1973.
182. Reinherz, E.L., and Schlossman, S.F.: The differentiation and function of human T lymphocytes, Cell **19:**821, 1980.
183. Reinherz, E.L., Meuer, S.C., and Schlossman, S.F.: The human T cell receptor: analysis with cytotoxic T cell clones, Immunol. Rev. **74:**83, 1983.
184. Rich, S.S., and Rich, R.R.: Regulatory mechanisms in cell-mediated immune responses. II. A genetically restricted suppressor of mixed lymphocyte reactions released by alloantigen-activated spleen cells, J. Exp. Med. **142:**1391, 1975.
185. Rinehart, J.J., et al.: Effect of corticosteroids on human monocyte function, J. Clin. Invest. **54:**1337, 1974.
186. Rinehart, J.J., et al.: Effect of corticosteroid therapy on human monocyte function, N. Engl. J. Med. **292:**236, 1975.
187. Rode, H.N., Uotila, M., and Gordon, J.: Regulation of mixed leukocyte culture reaction by suppressor cells, Eur. J. Immunol. **8:**213, 1978.
188. Sakaguchi, K., et al.: Mode of action of bredinin with guanylic acid on L5278Y mouse leukemia cells, J. Antibiot. **29:**1320, 1976.
189. Sasportes, M., et al.: Suppression of the human allogeneic response in vitro with primed lymphocytes and suppressive supernates, J. Exp. Med. **152:**2705, 1980.
190. Schendel, D.J., and Bach, F.H.: Genetic control of cell-mediated lympholysis in mouse, J. Exp. Med. **140:**1534, 1974.
191. Schendel, D.J., Alter, B.J., and Bach, F.H.: The involvement of LD and SD-region differences in MLC and CML: a three-cell experiment, Transplant. Proc. **5:**1651, 1973.
192. Schooley, R.T., et al.: Association of herpes virus infections with T-lymphocyte subset alterations, glomerulopathy, and opportunistic infections after renal transplantation, N. Engl. J. Med. **308:**507, 1983.
193. Schwartz, R., and Dameshek, W.: Drug-induced immunological tolerance, Nature **183:**1682, 1959.
194. Schwartz, R.H., Fathman, C.G., and Sachs, D.H.: Inhibition of stimulation of murine mixed lymphocyte cultures with an alloantiserum directed against a shared Ia determinant, J. Immunol. **116:**929, 1976.
195. Severyn, W., et al.: The role of immunological monitoring in transplantation, Heart Transplant. **1:**222, 1982.
196. Sharp, T.G., et al.: T-cell depletion of human bone marrow using monoclonal antibody and complement-mediated lysis, Transplantation **35:**112, 1983.
197. Sheil, A.G.R., et al.: ABO blood group incompatibility in renal transplantation, Transplantation **8**(3):299, 1969.
198. Sheil, A.G.R., et al.: Antilymphocyte globulin in patients with renal allografts from cadaveric donors, Lancet **2:**227, 1973.
199. Silberber-Sinakin, I., et al.: Langerhans cells: role in contact hypersensitivity and relationship to lymphoid dendritic cells and to macrophages, Immunol. Rev. **53:**203, 1980.
200. Simonian, S.J., et al.: Reversal of acute cadaveric renal allograft rejection with added ATG treatment, Transplant Proc. **15:**604, 1983.
201. Singal, D.P., Joseph, S., and Szewczuk, M.K.: Possible mechanisms of beneficial effect of pretransplant blood transfusions on renal allograft survival in man, Transplant. Proc. **14:**316, 1982.
202. Slavin, S., et al.: Use of total lymphoid irradiation in tissue transplantation in mice, Transplant. Proc. **9:**1001, 1977.
203. Snell, G.D.: The homograft reaction, Annu. Rev. Microbiol. **11:**439, 1957.
204. Snyder, D.S., and Unanue, K.R.: Corticosteroids inhibit murine macrophage Ia expression and interleukin 1 production, J. Immunol. **129**(5):1803, 1982.
205. Sollinger, H.W., et al.: Clinical and experimental experience with pancreatico-cystostomy for exocrine pancreatic drainage in pancreas transplantation, Transplant. Proc. **16:**749, 1984.
206. Spitalnik, S., et al.: Correlation of humoral immunity to Lewis blood group antigens with renal transplant rejection, Transplantation **37**(3):265, 1984.
207. Stadler, B.M., et al.: Relationship of cell cycle to recovery of IL-2 activity from human mononuclear cells, human and mouse T cell lines, J. Immunol. **127:**1936, 1981.
208. Staines, N.A., Guy, K., and Davies, D.A.L.: The dominant role of Ia antibodies in the passive enhancement of H-2 incompatible skin grafts, Eur. J. Immunol. **5**(11):782, 1975.
209. Starzl, T.E., Iwatsuki, S., and Shaw, B.W.: Pancreaticoduodenal transplantation in humans, Surg. Gynecol. Obstet. **159:**265, 1984.
210. Starzl, T.E., et al.: The use of heterologous antilymphoid agents in canine renal and liver homotransplantation and in human renal homotransplantation, Surg. Gynecol. Obstet. **124:**301, 1967.
211. Starzl, T.E., et al.: Evolution of liver transplantation, Hepatology **2:**614, 1982.
212. Starzl, T.E., et al.: Orthotopic liver transplantation in 1984, Transplant. Proc. **17:**250, 1985.
213. Steinman, R.M., et al.: Studies with a monoclonal antibody to mouse dendritic cells, Transplant. Proc. **15:**299, 1983.
214. Strom, T.B., et al.: Cellular components of allograft rejection: identity, specificity, and cytotoxic function of cells infiltrating acutely rejecting allografts, J. Immunol. **118:**2020, 1977.
215. Strong, D.M., et al.: Anti-idiotypic antibody in the primate. I. Characterization specificity against cells primed for histocompatibility determinants, Transplantation **29:**367, 1980.
216. Stuart, F.P., Fitch, F.W., and McKearn, T.J.: Enhancement of renal allografts with idiotypic and anti-idiotypic monoclonal alloantibodies, Transplant. Proc. **14:**313, 1982.
217. Sutherland, D.E.R., et al.: Segmental pancreas transplantation from living related and cadaver donors, Surgery **90:**159, 1981.
218. Taylor, H.E., Ackman, C.F.D., and Horowitz, I.: Canadian clinical trial of antilymphocyte globulin in human cadaver renal transplantation, Can. Med. Assoc. J. **115:**1205, 1976.
219. Thompson, C.B., and Thomas, G.D.: Bone marrow transplantation, Surg. Clin. North Am. **66:**589, 1986.
220. Theide, A., et al.: Successful manipulation of GVH-reaction in semi-allogeneic intestinal transplantation in rat by treatment of the donor recipient (abstract), Lyon, 1982, Seventh International Congress in Microsurgery.
221. Thurlow, P.J., et al.: A monoclonal anti-pan T-cell antibody, Transplantation **36:**293, 1983.
222. Tsuda, T., and Kahan, B.D.: A potential synergistic effect of donor antigenic extracts and cyclosporine on the prolongation of rat renal allografts, Transplantation **35**(5):483, 1983.
223. Uchida, H., Yokota, K., and Akiyama, N.: Effectiveness of a new drug bredinin, on canine kidney allotransplant survival, Transplant. Proc. **11:**865, 1979.
224. Wagner, H., et al.: Regulation of T cell-mediated cytotoxic allograft responses. I. Evidence for antigen-specific suppressor T cells, Eur. J. Immunol. **6:**873, 1976.
225. Wagner, H., et al.: T-T cell interactions during in vitro cytotoxic T lymphocyte response, J. Immunol. **124:**1058, 1980.

226. Wagner, H., et al.: Intrathymic differentiation of cytotoxic T lymphocyte precursors, J. Immunol. **125:**2532, 1980.
227. Wagner, H., et al.: T-T cell interactions during cytotoxic T lymphocyte responses: T cell–derived helper factor (interleukin 2) as a probe to analyze CTL responsiveness and thymic maturation of CTL progenitors, Immunol. Rev. **51:**215, 1980.
228. Wagner, H., et al.: Dissection of the proliferative and differentiative signals controlling murine cytotoxic T lymphocyte responses, J. Exp. Med. **155:**1876, 1982.
229. Wechter, W.J., et al.: Antithymocyte globulin (ATGAM) in renal allograft recipients, Transplantation **28:**294, 1979.
230. Weinberger, J.Z., et al.: Hapten-specific T-cell responses to 4-hydroxy-3-nitrophenyl acetyl. I. Genetic control of delayed-type hypersensitivity by VH and I-A region genes, J. Exp. Med. **149:**1336, 1979.
231. White, D.J., et al.: Cyclosporin A: an immunosuppressive agent preferentially active against proliferating T cells, Transplantation **27:**55, 1979.
232. Williams, G.M., et al.: Studies in hyperacute and chronic renal homograft rejection in man, Surgery **62**(1):204, 1967.
233. Williams, G.M., et al.: Hyperacute renal homograft rejection in man, N. Engl. J. Med. **299**(12):611, 1968.
234. Williams, G., Pegrum, G.D., and Evans, C.A.: Lewis Ags in renal transplantation, Lancet **1**(2):878, 1978.
235. Woodruff, M.F.A., and Anderson, N.A.: Effect of lymphocyte depletion by thoracic duct fistula and administration of antilymphocyte serum on the survival of skin homografts in rats, Nature **200:**702, 1963.
236. Yasumura, T., and Kahan, B.D.: Prolongation of rat kidney allografts by pretransplant administration of donor antigen extract or whole blood transfusion combined with a short course of cyclosporine, Transplantation **36:**603, 1983.
237. Yasumura, T., and Kahan, B.D.: Prolongation of allograft survival by repeated cycles of donor antigen and cyclosporine in rat kidney transplantation, Transplantation **38:**418, 1984.
238. Yeager, A.M., et al.: Autologous bone marrow transplantation in patients with acute nonlymphocytic leukemia, using ex vivo marrow treatment with 4-hydroperoxycylcophosphamide, N. Engl. J. Med. **315:**141, 1986.
239. Zitron, I.M., et al.: The cellular stimuli for the rejection of established islet allografts, Diabetes **30:**242, 1981.

6

Charles D. Ericsson and Brian J. Rowlands

Surgical Infection: Principles of Management and Antibiotic Usage

Although the antibiotic era of medicine, which began nearly 50 years ago, has revolutionized the treatment of surgical infection, problems of an infectious nature, particularly when developing during the postoperative period, continue to complicate clinical management of surgical patients, often lengthening the hospital stay and increasing the cost of providing medical care. The explanation for this continuing problem with infection is obviously multifactorial, but the widespread use of antibiotics has frequently resulted in an unrealistic overdependence on their effectiveness in treating disease, with a consequent violation of established surgical principles and the breakdown of isolation procedures. In the face of this antibiotic overusage, a reservoir of antibiotic-resistant microorganisms has emerged in the hospital environment.

These trends have been further accentuated by the technologic developments in surgical diagnosis and the sophisticated anesthetic techniques currently available that allow the performance of more complex surgical procedures. In addition, the ability to successfully resuscitate and manage severely traumatized patients who would have died as recently as a decade ago, the growing use of more toxic immunosuppressive drugs in transplant and oncologic patients, and the more aggressive treatment of surgical disease in the aged and debilitated patient all favor the development of hospital-acquired infections. Thus the surgeon must have a clear understanding of those factors that are responsible for the development of infection as well as a knowledge of the microorganisms likely to be implicated if the morbidity and mortality associated with this problem are to be reduced.

THE BIOLOGY OF SURGICAL INFECTION

Under normal circumstances the wide range of microorganisms, all with the potential for causing infection, to which the human body is continually exposed is held in abeyance by a variety of local and systemic host-defense mechanisms. This balance, which maintains normal health, may be disrupted by a variety of factors. They include the number and the virulence of microorganisms attempting to gain access to the host tissues and/or alterations in host resistance that limit the capacity to prevent infection. Surgical management perioperatively is directed at ensuring a favorable balance between the patient and the bacteria to which he is exposed.

A certain quantitative level of bacteria must be present for infection to develop.[19] The greater the virulence of a bacterium, the fewer the number of microorganisms that will be needed to initiate an infection. For example, an individual who would be resistant to infection from most organisms may need to inhale only a few bacteria of a virulent strain such as the plague bacilla to become dangerously ill. Furthermore, the way inoculated pathogens gain nourishment also influences the likelihood of infection. Traumatized tissue and collections of blood or blood products are all forms of pabulum from which pathogens may gain nourishment. As a generalization, a bacterial count exceeding 1000 organisms per gram of tissue or per milliliter of biologic fluid represents a population of bacteria in which mere colonization can no longer be considered to exist. If this figure exceeds 100,000 organisms (i.e., 10^5) per similar unit of measurement, significant bacterial contamination is present and may result in a severe life-threatening infection.[19] On occasion, when considerable bacterial contamination has occurred, measures can be taken to lessen its potentially deleterious effects. An example would be the case in which traumatic disruption of the large intestine (from either blunt or penetrating injury) results in significant fecal soilage and exposure of the peritoneal cavity to a large bacterial load. By repeated saline lavage of the exposed abdominal contents, this load can be considerably decreased, greatly lessening the degree of such contamination.

In addition to the quantity and virulence of pathogens, the adequacy of host-defense mechanisms will also determine whether an infection ultimately develops. Thus an organism may be highly virulent but have little opportunity to cause an infection if the host resistance is great and an adequate environment for bacterial growth is lacking. This endogenous host resistance is comprised of both cellular and humoral components as well as a series of chemical and mechanical barriers.[16] These barriers represent the first level of resistance and include keratinized skin that prevents the penetration of bacteria, various skin-derived lipids with antimicrobial activity, and the bacterial flora that normally reside in sweat glands and hair follicles and compete with pathogenic bacteria for an ecologic niche. The various epithelial mucous membranes lining the gastrointestinal tract, vagina, and respiratory tract are also important barriers through their ability to maintain a pH nonconducive to colonization of certain bacteria and through the production of immunoglobulins, such as IgA, which occurs in the gut. These chemical and mechanical barriers are also responsible for the distinctive organisms that normally inhabit various tissues such as the gram-positive bacteria, which are normally present in the upper respiratory tract, and the gram-negative bacteria, which normally reside in the anus and the rectum.

Once these barrier mechanisms are altered, local defense mechanisms are triggered as bacteria gain access to the damaged tissue.[16,19] An increase in local vascular permeability is observed in injured cells secondary to the release of various vasoactive substances from the kallikrein-kinin system. This increased permeability results in the influx of plasma immunoglobulins, complement, components of the phagocytic system, and various clotting factors. A complex interplay among these substances results in confinement of the infection and limitation of its spread. Clotting factors attempt to wall off the process by platelet aggregation and fibrin deposition at the same time that the immunoglobulins (particularly IgG and IgM) interact with antigenic components on the bacterial wall. This latter reaction activates the complement system, leading to direct bacterial injury, neutrophil chemotaxis, and opsonization of the bacterial wall.

These humoral reactants also trigger the third line of defense—the cellular mechanisms of the host defense.[16,19] They include phagocytic cells and the reticuloendothelial system. The humoral events just enumerated direct the movement of phagocytes to the site of tissue injury where phagocytosis of both opsonized bacteria and other particulate debris is accomplished. These ingested substances are then digested enzymatically and ultimately absorbed into the phagocytes' cytoplasm, with the predominant cell being the polymorphonuclear leukocyte.

The reticuloendothelial system is composed of both fixed and wandering components. The fixed components consist of phagocytes that line vascular channels and serve to eliminate pathogens and other foreign debris that have reached the bloodstream when bacteremia develops. These phagocytes are located in the hepatosplenic circulation and lymphatic system. The wandering components include nonthymic-dependent lymphocytes (i.e., B lymphocytes) and thymic-dependent lymphocytes (i.e., T lymphocytes). The B lymphocytes function primarily through the production of circulating antibodies that are instrumental in killing bacteria. In contrast, the immunity effected by T lymphocytes is cell-mediated and occurs primarily through the induction of mononuclear macrophages to ingest and destroy pathogens to which they have been sensitized. T lymphocytes are active primarily against viruses and fungi and certain intracellular bacteria. In the majority of infections, however, the major mechanism of immunity is through B lymphocytes.

FACTORS PREDISPOSING FOR SURGICAL INFECTION

Existent or incubating infections at the time of admission to a hospital are difficult to prevent and may require surgery to effect adequate treatment, but the incidence of hospital-associated infections can often be reduced by attention to detail and by the administration of appropriate measures perioperatively to improve host resistance to infection. Knowledge of these measures is crucial to optimum patient care. Some important principles that reduce postoperative infection in surgical patients are listed in the boxed material at above right.

A wide variety of factors may compromise an individual's host-defense mechanisms to deal adequately with bacterial contamination at the time of surgery. A detailed discussion of operating room hygiene and the principles to be followed to ensure the maintenance of a safe operating room environment is beyond the scope of this chapter and has been adequately addressed elsewhere.[1,16,19] Nevertheless, the single most important factor contributing to the development of infection at the time of surgery is *faulty aseptic technique*. The degree of bacterial contamination (as well as the type, number, and virulence of the contaminating bacteria) and the adequacy of the underlying local and systemic host-defense mechanisms are important determinants of whether a bacterial inoculum subsequently gives rise to infection. Furthermore, the presence of devitalized, unhealthy, and traumatized tissue within a wound clearly decreases local resistance to bacterial invasion and growth. Thus every effort should be made to handle tissues gently, remove devitalized and/or necrotic tissues and foreign bodies, and carefully obliterate any potential dead space. In addition, undue pressure from retractors, ligatures, large bites of tissue that impair local blood flow, inopportune spillage of visceral contents (e.g., stomach and intestine), inadequate hemostasis resulting in hematoma formation, and excessive use of diathermy coagulation are to be avoided.

PRINCIPLES LEADING TO A REDUCTION OF POSTOPERATIVE INFECTION IN SURGICAL PATIENTS

1. Short preoperative stay
2. Hexachlorophene shower before surgery
3. Minimum shaving of operative site
4. Exemplary surgical technique (short, safe procedure with minimum contamination)
5. Greater care in operations performed on the elderly, obese, malnourished, and diabetic patients
6. Meticulous attention to hemostasis
7. No drains brought to surface through the operative wound
8. Frequent audit of each surgeon's wound infection rate

The extent to which these principles are followed will not only influence the outcome of a surgical repair (e.g., an intestinal anastomosis) but will also have a direct bearing on the subsequent development of a wound infection. In a series of 40,662 wounds studied over a 7-year period, the incidence of wound infection postoperatively was directly related to adherence to these principles and the resulting wound type (Table 6-1).[9] For a *clean* wound in which the respiratory, digestive, or genitourinary tract was not entered during surgery and the wound was primarily closed and undrained, the incidence of infection was 1.8%. For a *clean-contaminated* wound in which any of these organ systems was entered but without unusual contamination, the infection rate was 9.1%. If the wound was *contaminated,* which indicates an open, fresh, traumatic wound (e.g., gunshot wound to the colon) or a major break in sterile technique, the incidence of infection averaged 18.4%. Finally, in a *dirty* wound, which includes old traumatic wounds and those involving clinical infection or perforated viscera, the infection rate was 41.8%. In this study, the duration of operation, its complexity, and the

Table 6-1 **INDICATIONS FOR USE OF ANTIBIOTIC PROPHYLAXIS IN SURGICAL PATIENTS**

Wound Classification	Rate of Infection Without Antibiotics	Indication for Prophylaxis or Short-Term Therapy	Examples	Selected Exceptions
Clean—digestive, respiratory, genitourinary (GU) tract not entered	1%	Usually none	Herniorrhaphy	Implantation of prosthetic devices; obese patient; diabetic patient with *Clostridium perfringens* colonization
Clean-contaminated—digestive, respiratory or GU tract entered without visible, gross contamination	5%-10%	Generally high	Elective colonic surgery; vaginal hysterectomy	Elective appendectomy, cholecystectomy (surgical technique renders procedures "clean") unless obstructive jaundice present; esophagogastroduodenal operations "clean" unless malignancy, hydrogen-hemorrhage, perforation, obstruction, or prolonged antagonist therapy present
Contaminated—visible contamination from hollow viscus or fresh traumatic wound with contamination less than 3 hr old; major break in sterile technique	10%-20%	Generally high	Colonic operations secondary to high-risk gunshot or knife wounds	Elderly patient, undebrided necrotic material, and difficulty with hemostasis may require a 7- to 10- day course of antibiotic therapy
Dirty—old traumatic wound, clinically infected or abscessed tissue	>20%*	None†	Perforated appendix; colonic diverticular abscess	None†

*Pertains to old traumatic wounds that did not initially appear infected.
†Presently all dirty wounds should be treated with a *long-term* course of antibiotic therapy, usually 7 to 10 days.

experience and meticulousness of the surgeon performing the procedure were also important determinants in the subsequent development of wound infection. Of equal note, for all types of wounds, the use of diathermy coagulation doubled the infection rate.

A number of preoperative factors may also predispose the surgical patient to the development of infection. In a prospective study over a 5-year period involving over 23,649 surgical wounds, important risk factors found to be associated with the subsequent development of wound infections included old age, diabetes, obesity, malnutrition, and a perioperative hospital stay in excess of 2 weeks.[10] In another study analyzing 917 surgical patients retrospectively, risk factors found to be associated with the development of postoperative infection (wound infections as well as other infections) were obvious weight loss, malnutrition, malignancy, diabetes, alcoholism, and the previous use of steroids or cytotoxic drugs.[20] If none of these risk factors was present, the incidence of infective complications postoperatively was only 5.8%. With one risk factor, this incidence increased to 17%; with four risk factors present, a 39% postoperative infection rate was noted. The mortality rate was 7.2% if one or more risk factors was present, in contrast to 0.6% with no clinical risk factor. Other factors that have been shown to be predictive of serious postoperative infection include anemia, hypoalbuminemia, lymphopenia, abnormal immunoglobulins, and abnormal delayed hypersensitivity skin testing indicating the presence of anergy, an index of malnutrition that was discussed in Chapter 3.* Since so many of these risk factors are directly related to the patient's underlying nutritional status, every effort should be made to establish nutritional and metabolic normalcy before surgery (see Chapter 3) if surgery can be deferred. Finally, there is increasing evidence that a patient with an active infection at the time of surgery is at increased risk for developing a second remote focus of infection postoperatively. For this reason, active infections, such as those involving the urinary tract or the upper respiratory tract, should be eliminated before surgery is performed.

In addition to the preoperative and intra-operative measures already discussed, a number of other factors may also contribute to postoperative infection. Exogenous infections acquired during surgery from the operating room environment, the patient's nasopharynx, or the surgical team or after surgery secondary to cross infection may also occur. Such infections are caused mainly by staphylococcal organisms and fortunately account for only 5% of the total incidence of surgical infection. Factors related to the development of such an infection include the density of bacterial contamination in the operating room, the amount of personnel movement during the operation, the number of persons on the surgical team, the adequacy of hemostasis, the type of skin preparation, and the use of closed

*References 7, 15, 21, 24, 26, 33.

suction drainage.[6,8] Staphylococcal organisms may also be introduced into a patient's body as a contaminant during intravenous catheter placement. Meticulous attention to sterile technique during insertion and management of such catheters will usually obviate this problem. The insertion of other foreign substances such as urinary catheters and endotracheal tubes may also result in bacterial contamination and/or violation of normal host-defense mechanisms.

The extent to which a given individual's host defenses are compromised varies considerably and is dependent on the type and number of underlying risk factors. This compromise may be as simple as a transiently avascular wound that was inadvertently colonized at the time of wound closure. Some patients are compromised through the use of invasive procedures including tracheal intubation, urinary bladder catheterization, and arterial and central venous line placement. Other patients have a generalized depression of their immune system such as those patients with diabetes who are more susceptible to certain types of infections (e.g., *Clostridium perfringens*) or the cancer patient who receives chemotherapy, becomes neutropenic, and requires a surgical procedure, which places him at high risk for postoperative infection. In this latter example, not only are general host defenses compromised, but frequently the operative site can act as a local breeding ground when, for technical reasons, necrotic malignant tissue cannot be adequately debrided. Most of the commonly recognized factors that predispose to surgical infection are related to impaired host defenses and to increases in the number of potentially infecting flora (Table 6-2).

CLASSIFICATION OF SURGICAL INFECTION

Approximately 30% of surgical patients will either enter the hospital with an infection or subsequently develop one during the course of their postoperative care. Surgical infection may be classified according to its mode of presentation or its causative organism. A practical approach to classification is offered in the boxed material below.

CLASSIFICATION OF SURGICAL INFECTION

INFECTION PRESENT WHEN ADMITTED TO HOSPITAL

1. *Underlying surgical disease*—responsible for admission (e.g., appendicitis, cholecystitis)
2. *After injury*—related to delayed recognition or treatment (e.g., peritonitis following blunt trauma)
3. *Nonsurgical*—unrelated to surgical problem or injury (e.g., pneumonia)
4. *Incubating*—incubating at admission and manifesting later (e.g., community-acquired hepatitis)

POSTOPERATIVE INFECTION (USUALLY NOSOCOMIAL)

Regional

1. *Surgical*—related to the operative procedure (e.g., wound, intra-abdominal infection)
2. *Surgical care*—related to breeches in local defenses (e.g., urinary tract infection, phlebitis, pneumonia)
3. *After injury*—unrecognized or uncontrolled by surgery (e.g., lymphadenitis, peritonitis)

Systemic

1. *Nosocomial bacteremia*—usually related to underlying infection that is frequently localized (e.g., infected catheter site, pelvic abscess)

Table 6-2 **RELATIONSHIP OF FACTORS THAT PREDISPOSE TO SURGICAL INFECTION AND THE VARIABLES THAT RELATE TO INFECTION**

Factors	Increased Virulence of Organisms or Flora	Increased Number of Potentially Infecting Organisms	Decreased Host Resistance
Patient-related	Prolonged hospital stay (increased colonization with aerobic gram-negative bacilli)	Diabetes (*Clostridia* colonization of skin); poor hygiene; patient preparation for surgical procedures (failure to decrease number of stool, skin, or other flora)	Malnutrition and decreased albumin; malignancy; diabetes; alcoholism; obesity; jaundice; extremes of age; leukopenia; abnormal immunoglobulins; abnormal skin testing; bypassing local defenses— Tracheal intubation; Urinary bladder catheterization; Intravenous catheterization
Drugs	—	Prophylactic antibiotics (decrease in protective normal flora with overgrowth of other potentially infecting flora)	Corticosteroids; cytotoxic agents
Technical and/or perioperative	—	Faulty technique (bacterial contamination); complexity and duration of operation; hygiene of surgeon and supporting personnel	Lack of hemostasis; devitalized tissue; foreign body
Environmental	—	Defective air and traffic control in operating room; defective sterilization techniques	—

In patients who are admitted to surgical services with evidence of infection, operative intervention is usually required to effect adequate treatment. Infectious diseases of this nature include appendicitis, cholecystitis, diverticular abscess, and gangrene of the leg as well as other conditions. Although a period of antibiotic coverage before surgery is usually indicated to improve outcome, antibiotics by themselves are usually not efficacious in controlling the infectious process.

Of the types of infectious processes coming to the attention of a surgeon, the most frequent is postoperative, and, in general, this classification implies a hospital-acquired infection, commonly referred to as a *nosocomial infection*. Basically, this type of infection is caused by the patient's own endogenous normal flora; if he has resided in the hospital for as little as 2 or 3 days, this flora may include what are generally considered hospital isolates (e.g., species of *Pseudomonas* and *Serratia*). An example is the burn patient whose burn eschar becomes heavily colonized with an organism such as *Pseudomonas aeruginosa* before the wound infection and its systemic spread become clinical problems. This example underscores a generalization about infections in postoperative surgical patients—the majority of the infections are caused by relatively avirulent organ-

Table 6-3 **SELECTED VIRULENCE PROPERTIES OF MICROORGANISMS AND THEIR IMPORTANCE TO SURGICAL PATIENT MANAGEMENT**

Organism	Property	Management Problem
AEROBIC BACTERIA		
Gram-positive		
Staphylococcus aureus	Methicillin resistance	Drug of choice—vancomycin—more toxic than nafcillin
	Intracellular survival	Must drain abscesses and treat over a long period of time to avoid infectious complications
Streptococcus pyogenes (Group A beta-hemolytic streptococcus)	Exotoxin production	May cause devastating sepsis even in young adults
Enterococcus *(Streptococcus faecalis)*	Antibiotic resistance	Must be treated with correct synergistic combination of antibiotics
Gram-negative		
Pseudomonas aeruginosa	Exotoxin production	Must use beta-lactam and an aminoglycoside antibiotic for optimum control of exotoxin production
	Perivascular infiltration causing coagulation necrosis	Must treat with adequate dosages of antibiotics to penetrate necrotic areas and over a long period of time to avoid relapse
Species of *Serratia, Providencia,* and many other gram-negative organisms	Antibiotic resistance	In large institutions in which antibiotic resistance often occurs, must use newer, more expensive antibiotics
ANAEROBIC BACTERIA		
Gram-positive		
Clostridium perfringens	Alpha toxin production	Sometimes must remove focus of infection to control hemolysis and sepsis (e.g., hysterectomy)
Clostridium difficile	Cytotoxin production	Often must treat antibiotic-associated enterocolitis with expensive oral vancomycin
Gram-negative		
Bacteroides fragilis	Endotoxin	Must recognize as a potential cause of septic shock
	Heparinase	Local thrombosis may complicate infection (e.g., pelvic septic thrombophlebitis)
	Penicillin resistance	Must treat with appropriate antianaerobic antibiotics
Fungi		
Candida albicans	Pseudohyphae formation under certain conditions	Presence of pseudohyphae in clinical specimen is not necessary to invoke a pathogenic role for the organism
Mucor	Tendency to invade blood vessels and extend along adipoidal planes	Must debride widely beyond apparent line of demarcation using frozen section as a guide
VIRUSES		
Influenza virus	Mutagenic drift of neuraminidase	Must change vaccines to maintain protection
Herpes simplex	Latency	Reactivation of herpes infections may complicate postoperative care
PROTOZOA		
Toxoplasmosis	Potential reactivation of infection	Reactivation of latent infection may complicate AIDS; patients may require brain biopsy for diagnosis

isms. Although normal endogenous flora account for most surgical infections and the microorganisms are in and of themselves relatively avirulent, this by no means indicates that the ensuing infections will be trivial. These normal flora, once they do establish infection, often have virulence properties that are important to understanding the extent of the infection that subsequently develops and the design of the therapeutic intervention. Hospital flora such as *Pseudomonas aeruginosa* may become part of the colonizing flora of the patient and later cause or contribute to the development of a hospital-acquired infection that may be resistant to treatment with even multiple antibiotic regimens. Selected organisms and their special virulence properties or antibiotic-resistance problems are listed in Table 6-3. This table does not include the microbiology of all surgical infections but does underscore that certain microbial properties dictate an approach to therapeutic management and that relatively avirulent organisms may still cause infections that can be difficult to treat.

Finally, nosocomial infection caused by organisms acquired directly from the environment do occur, but they comprise a minority of these infections. Examples include infections derived from contaminated respiratory equipment resulting in pneumonia, intravenous fluid contaminants resulting in sepsis, and the infrequent situation in which a surgeon himself may be a nasal carrier of an organism such as *Staphylococcus*, resulting in direct inoculation of a wound or prosthesis. Most postoperative infections, however, are a consequence of breaches in the patient's host defenses that result from the surgical procedure itself or secondary to the relatively invasive techniques of modern surgical care.

A more difficult and insidious problem occurring postoperatively is the patient who develops signs and symptoms of an infection that seem totally unrelated to the previously performed surgical procedure. In these instances in which a typical postoperative infection has been excluded, the surgeon is well advised to retake carefully a history from the patient who may now reveal complaints that were present before surgery but were forgotten or overshadowed in the patient's mind because of the original acute or worrisome circumstances that precipitated the surgery. Careful reexamination of the patient to identify the source of a perplexing fever may reveal localizing, but subtle, clues missed earlier (e.g., lymphadenopathy, splenomegaly, or heart murmur).

Diagnosing an infection that was incubating before surgery but that does not manifest itself until after surgery taxes the genius of even the most astute physician. Under these circumstances, consultation with an expert in infectious diseases is clearly warranted. Such a patient may prove to have hepatitis, an enigmatic viral syndrome like mononucleosis, or a more insidious disease such as tuberculosis or bacterial endocarditis. Although a true fever of unknown origin (implying a continuing fever for 3 weeks and an unrevealing, in-hospital investigation spanning at least 2 weeks) may not be present, localizing or diagnostic signs or symptoms that indicate the source of infection are usually existent even though they may be extremely subtle and quite elusive.

Another approach to classifying surgical infection relates to its clinical manifestations. Infections that arise in tissues begin as a *cellulitis*. It is manifested clinically by local tenderness, heat, swelling, redness, and pain. Because this type of infection has no localized areas of pus formation, it does not lend itself to drainage and can often be managed by rest, application of local heat, adjunctive antibiotic therapy, and elevation if an extremity is involved. If left untreated, cellulitis may spread through adjacent tissue planes (as occurs with a beta-hemolytic streptococcus) or remain localized to form an abscess (as may occur with staphylococcus).

In contrast to cellulitis, an *abscess* denotes a local collection of necrotic tissue, white cells, and bacteria designated clinically as pus. The increased osmotic pressure that exists within a walled-off abscess can result in considerable movement of water into the area from adjacent tissues resulting in pronounced pressure that is seen clinically as severe pain and tenderness. Not only to provide symptomatic relief but also to prevent the risk of bacterial spread along adjacent tissue planes or through the blood or lymphatic vessels, all abscesses should be drained or excised. Adjunctive antibiotic therapy is usually indicated to control adequately any bacteria that may have entered the lymph or blood during the drainage process.

Not uncommonly, products of infection from areas of cellulitis or abscess formation gain access to the blood and lymph systems. Occasionally during the spread of infection, lymph channels may become infected and are seen clinically as hyperemic streaks. This condition is acute *lymphangitis*, colloquially referred to as blood poisoning. If this infection is not controlled, the involved lymph nodes may later abscess and progress to a more severe state of infection known as *suppurative lymphangitis*. Invasion of vascular channels by bacteria is referred to as *bacteremia*. When the bacteremia involves dissemination throughout the body, *septicemia* exists. Because of the dire consequences that may result from bacterial spread both lymphatically and throughout the vascular system, aggressive treatment is always indicated and includes appropriate antibiotic therapy and local management of the source of infection with abscess drainage if present.

POSTOPERATIVE INFECTIONS

Normal body temperature is maintained by the thermoregulatory center in the hypothalamus within very narrow limits (98.6° ± 0.9° F) and varies only slightly throughout a given 24-hour period. It is highest in the early evening and lowest in the early morning hours. Thus an elevation in temperature above normal daily fluctuations represents the presence of fever, which should be assumed to be infectious in origin until proven otherwise.

It is not uncommon during the postoperative period for a patient to become febrile. Although the infectious process responsible for this event can vary considerably, an understanding of the types of infection that develop postoperatively and their clinical manifestations assists greatly in expediting diagnosis and in instituting appropriate treatment. In approaching the problem of postoperative fever, attention should be focused on infections related to the sur-

CAUSES OF POSTOPERATIVE FEVER

- Respiratory tract infections
  - Atelectasis
  - Pneumonia
- Urinary tract infections
- Wound infections
  - Early wound infections
    - *Streptococcus* species
    - *Clostridium* species
  - Late wound infections
    - *Staphylococcus* species
    - Mixed aerobic-anaerobic organisms
- Thrombophlebitis
  - Upper extremity (almost always catheter-related infections)
  - Lower extremity (usually related to venous stasis and not infected)
- Intra-abdominal causes
  - Peritonitis
  - Abscess
- Miscellaneous causes (considerably less common)
  - Gastrointestinal infections
  - Blood transfusion reaction
  - Allergies
  - Dehydration
  - Undrained sterile fluids (e.g., pleural fluid, hematoma)
  - Pancreatitis
  - Blood transfusion–related infections (e.g., non-A hepatitis, non-B hepatitis, cytomegalovirus)

gical procedure itself and other iatrogenic maneuvers (e.g., placement of a urinary catheter) that may alter host defenses (see boxed material above).

The timing of the onset of fever is a classic aid in determining the possible etiology of these infections. A temperature elevation in the first day or two following surgery is usually related to atelectasis involving one or both lungs. In the next 24 to 48 hours, urinary tract manifestations may become apparent. Under most conditions, wound infections do not cause fever until 3 to 5 days postoperatively, although streptococcal and clostridial wound infections can be seen as early as 48 hours after surgery. Thrombophlebitis almost never occurs before the third postoperative day and usually does not become apparent until a week to 10 days following surgery. A mnemonic to assist in remembering this sequence of fever onset is *wind* (pulmonary), *water* (urinary), *wound,* and *walking* (phlebitis), although venous disorders involving the lower extremities as a cause of postoperative fever are generally less commonly encountered than those associated with phlebitis secondary to upper-extremity venous catheter placement (i.e., intravenous lines). Despite the convenience of these guidelines, they should not preclude careful examination of other potential sources for infection. Furthermore, exceptions to the timing of these guidelines and fever patterns are legion so that the rational assessment of postoperative fever should begin with an organized approach to diagnosis (Fig. 6-1).

In addition to careful elicitation of the patient's history, which may give clues to the source of infection (e.g., shortness of breath that may signify pulmonary atelectasis or inordinate incisional pain that may indicate a wound infection), during the physical examination stress should be given to "high pay-off" areas. Wounds and drain sites must be inspected carefully. Patients with urinary bladder catheters should be examined for signs of urinary tract infection (e.g., flank pain and cloudy urine). Intravenous catheter sites may be a source of serious infection even though the evidence for inflammation at the catheter site may be subtle. Swelling in the arm distal to a subclavian catheter might indicate septic thrombophlebitis. This diagnosis is important not only because it dictates the need for antibiotic therapy but also because embolic disease to the lungs does occur and is probably underdiagnosed; adjunctive heparin therapy should be more strongly considered in this situation than has been recommended in the past.[14]

In any evaluation of postoperative fever, examination of the skin throughout the body is also appropriate. Rashes indicative of allergic reactions can generate an entirely different therapeutic intervention from that for pustular lesions consistent with metastatic-embolic lesions in an apparently septic patient in whom antibiotic therapy will be needed. These latter lesions can be uncapped, and the pustular contents can be Gram stained. Yeast forms may be seen on such stains suggesting the diagnosis of systemic candidiasis, which should be confirmed by punch biopsy of an isolated pustule to demonstrate yeast forms deep in the corium, which would imply hematogenous spread. In contrast, intertriginous yeast infections are common, can be managed with local creams, and are not usually confused with the pustular lesions of systemic candidiasis. Finally, infected decubitus ulcers are usually evident if the skin is carefully evaluated.

Careful assessment of the lungs and chest tube sites, if present, is mandatory to exclude pneumonitis and other pulmonary infections such as empyema. In the workup of any postoperative fever, a chest radiogram should be considered a routine part of the examination. Evaluation of the abdomen may disclose peritonitis or a suspected subphrenic or other deep abscess. The rectal and pelvic examinations must not be excluded; otherwise, perirectal and pelvic abscesses might be missed.

The laboratory can be useful in assessing postoperative fever; however, its use is all too frequently substituted for a proper clinical evaluation of the patient. Routine culturing of the patient need not include a sputum sample if there is no realistic concern for pulmonary infection (i.e., no cough, no rales during pulmonary auscultation, and a normal chest radiogram). As a rule, however, the blood and urine should be cultured. Other sites (e.g., cerebrospinal fluid, pleural fluid, and peritoneal fluid) should also be cultured when appropriate. All specimens should be Gram stained; this information should then be evaluated before embarking on therapy. Generally, empiric use of antibiotics for postoperative fever is discouraged. Only when an established source of infection has been defined or is strongly suspected should antibiotic coverage be rendered. Obviously, in life-threatening conditions such as meningitis, sepsis, or any infection where bacteremia is presumed,

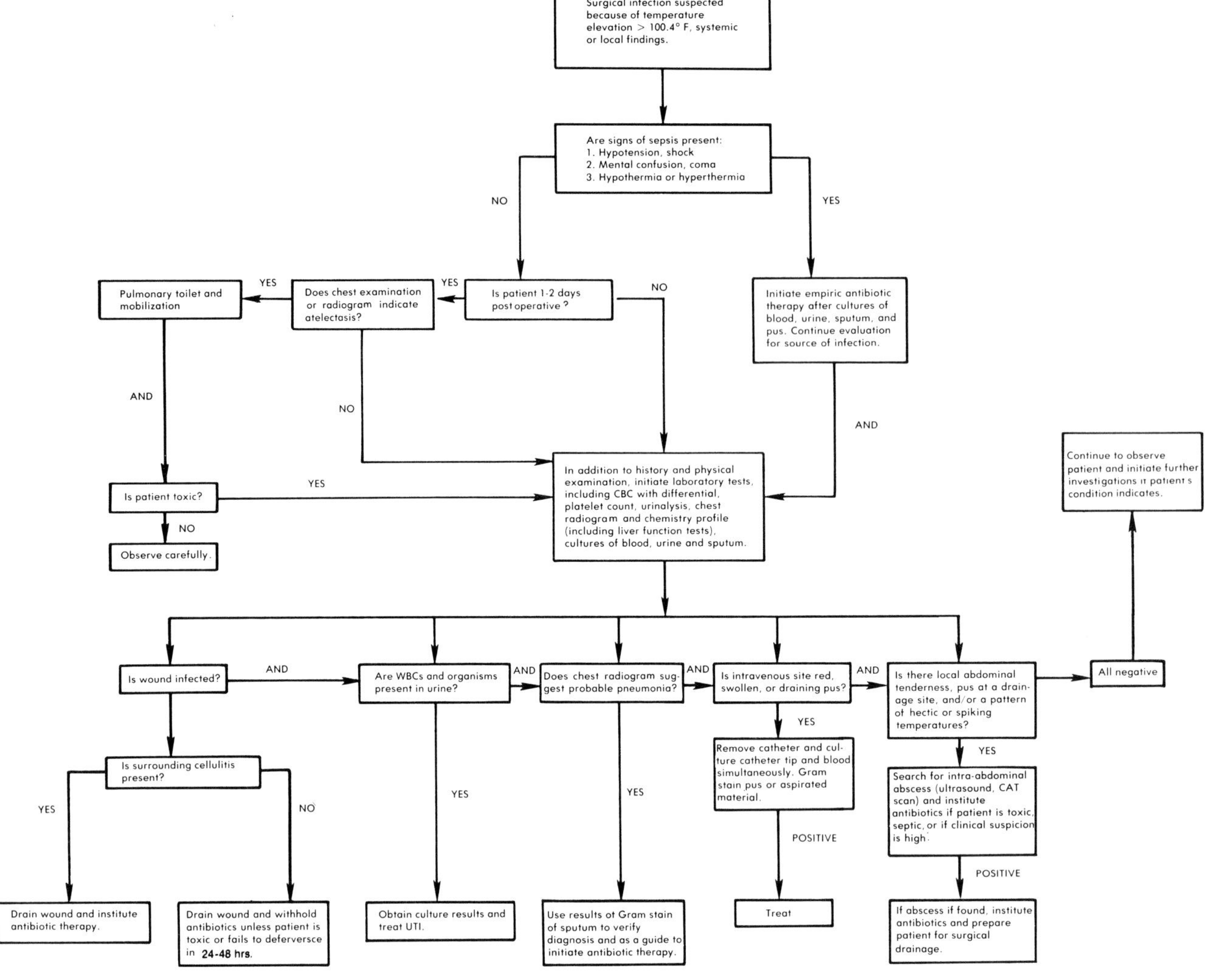

Fig. 6-1 Approach to the clinical management of the surgical patient with postoperative fever.

empiric antibiotic therapy logically precedes even examination of a Gram-stained specimen. Once Gram's stain and/or culture results are available, the antibiotic regimen can be altered as appropriate.

Types of Postoperative Infections

Respiratory Infections

The most common cause of fever in the immediate 24 hours after surgery is pulmonary atelectasis. This condition represents the collapse of alveoli as a result of inadequate postoperative tidal volumes and bronchiolar constriction. These areas of collapse result in retention of bronchial secretions and the entrapment of bacteria. As alveolar macrophages and systemically recruited neutrophils attempt to eradicate these bacteria, fever ensues. Atelectasis is commonly related to the immediate adverse postoperative effects of anesthesia and systemic analgesia on pulmonary expansion, which limit the efficiency of both inspiration and expiration as well as the tidal volume. Splinting painful upper-abdominal incisions may have similar adverse effects. Any surgical patient may develop atelectasis postoperatively, but patients at particular risk include the elderly, those with chronic obstructive lung disease, and those who are chronic cigarette smokers. Since atelectasis is the inciting event in the development of postoperative pneumonia, every effort should be employed to ensure its prevention as well as its treatment when it occurs. Both prevention and treatment go hand-in-hand and are directed at preventing or reexpanding collapsed alveoli. This goal can be accomplished in patients through early ambulation, frequent coughing and deep breathing, frequent changes in position when in bed, and the use of blow-bottles or balloons to improve pulmonary expansion.

When management of atelectasis is ineffective, pneumonia results. Patients requiring ventilatory assistance in the early postoperative period are also at risk for this problem. Overall, pneumonia occurs on surgery services with a frequency of approximately 5.1 cases per 1000 hospital discharges and is associated with a greater morbidity and mortality than other infections.[13] The rate of this infection is highest among intensive care unit patients. In addition to its frequency in patients with retained bronchial secretions and atelectasis, pneumonia commonly arises as a result of the aspiration of oropharyngeal contents or because of a breach of normal host defenses by the presence of tracheal intubation, which allows the introduction of various hospital pathogens into the tracheobronchial tree during assisted ventilation. Characteristically the diagnosis of pneumonia is made by the demonstration of an infiltrate on a chest x-ray film and the identification of purulent tracheobronchial secretions.

Because of the life-threatening potential of pulmonary infections, every effort should be made to prevent their development. As already stated, in patients not requiring ventilator assistance, vigorous attempts to prevent atelectasis and to enhance expectoration of any retained bronchial secretions should be used. If mechanical ventilation is required, frequent suctioning of the tracheal tube should be administered, and attempts should be made to wean the patient from the ventilator as soon as possible.

Efforts to minimize the likelihood of aspiration of oropharyngeal and gastric contents are equally important in the prevention of postoperative pneumonia. Thus removal of tubes that alter the normal function of the gastroesophageal (i.e., a nasogastric tube) and pharyngoesophageal sphincters (i.e., an endotracheal tube) and discontinuation of drugs that depress the central nervous system should be effected as early as can be done safely. Prevention of aspiration becomes particularly problematic in the patient who requires a nasogastric tube to receive intensive antacid or hydrogen-antagonist therapy to prevent stress ulcer formation; the stomach thereby becomes a reservoir for the overgrowth of hospital-acquired organisms. By an ascending route these organisms may heavily colonize the oropharynx, and, if aspirated, they may correspondingly cause respiratory tract infection.[12] There is no adequate solution to this risk except to remove the nasogastric tube as soon as the patient's status permits. Some patients may aspirate acid stomach contents as opposed to organism-containing oropharyngeal secretions. If samples of the aspirate can be obtained, acid aspiration can be recognized by assessing the pH of bronchial secretions.[41] After acid aspiration, a chemical pneumonitis may evolve, but it often does not become infected and is resolved without antibiotic therapy.

Any episode of aspiration should be treated as though oropharyngeal contents have been aspirated and infection might ensue. Although steroids have no therapeutic role in its management,[40] antibiotics should be started as soon as aspiration is observed or suspected and should be continued for approximately 3 days if the chest radiogram does not indicate a developing pneumonia. If an infiltrate is present on the radiogram taken on day 3 and the patient is afebrile, antibiotics should be continued for a 7- to 10-day course. If the patient has an infiltrate and is febrile, the possibility of pneumonia should be reevaluated by obtaining a culture and Gram's stain of the sputum to be certain the correct antimicrobial agent is being administered.

The choice of antibiotics for the treatment of aspiration pneumonia is controversial.[22] Penicillin G was once the mainstay of therapy for aspiration of oropharyngeal contents that had not yet become colonized with hospital flora. Recently concern has been expressed about the failure of penicillin G to treat necrotizing pneumonias and lung abscesses caused by oral anaerobes that produce beta-lactamases and inactivate penicillin. Although this point has not been studied specifically in the use of antibiotics in the immediate postaspiration period, probably a beta-lactamase–stable, antianaerobic antibiotic such as clindamycin should be used in place of penicillin G. When hospital flora have been aspirated, an aminoglycoside such as tobramycin should be added to the regimen. In many hospitals the new, anti-*Pseudomonas* cephalosporins such as ceftazidime may successfully supplant aminoglycoside usage. If antibiotics cannot be instituted within several hours after the aspiration, it is reasonable to observe the patient, if he is stable, and to treat him appropriately only if a pneumonia develops.

Another source of postoperative pneumonia that is indirectly hospital-acquired is secondary to bacteremic spread of infection. These pneumonias should be suspected when the chest x-ray film reveals widespread patchy involvement, particularly if it appears nodular. As a rule, any surgical patient who develops pneumonia without a clearly identifiable cause might have a distant focus of infection that has seeded the lungs. This possibility is best assessed by obtaining a careful history and performing a physical examination. For a further discussion of pneumonia, see Chapter 35.

Urinary Tract Infections

The largest percentage of infections that occur on surgery services arise in the urinary tract (approximately 13.3 cases per 1000 hospital discharges).[13] This circumstance is a simple consequence of the placement of urinary bladder catheters. Although serious infectious problems may ensue from the catheterization of the elderly male with an unrecognized prostate infection or obstruction, most urinary tract problems occur because closed urinary drainage systems eventually become colonized by enteric bacteria such as *Escherichia* from which the patient may become infected. No measure is particularly effective in preventing these catheter-related infections, although a number of approaches have been tried including the administration of antibiotics (both systemic and local), the use of special tubes with irrigants, and various regimens of catheter care.[36] Use of prophylactic antibiotics encourages infection by resistant bacteria or the fungus *Candida* (especially in diabetics). Frequent catheter care with cleansing of the urethral meatus leads to an increased frequency of urinary tract infections so that only daily (rather than more frequent) catheter care has become standard practice. The best prevention of urinary tract infections is to avoid prolonged catheterization and to use alternatives such as intermittent catheterization or, in the case of men, condom catheters whenever possible. Regardless of the technique of drainage, patients should be kept well hydrated so that the bladder is constantly flushed, thereby decreasing the number of potentially infecting bacteria.

Many physicians overreact to the presence of more than 10^5 organisms in the patient's urine without first obtaining a urinalysis to prove the presence (or absence) of pyuria. Colonization without pyuria can usually be resolved without the use of antibiotics simply by removing the patient's catheter and maintaining adequate hydration. In the patient with significant bacteriuria and pyuria in combination and a high temperature elevation in the range of 103° to 104° F, a source of infection other than the bladder should be sought. Pyelonephritis with its attendant high frequency of bacteremia may be present under these circumstances and require aggressive antibiotic therapy; simple cystitis rarely causes high fever. The majority of catheterized patients with bacteriuria and pyuria have a low-grade fever secondary to a simple catheter-related cystitis. The principles of management in this latter circumstance include removal of the catheter, if possible, and in most instances a single dose of an antimicrobial agent that is excreted in the urine. For those patients in whom catheter placement must remain in the presence of pyuria, the use of a brief course of an antibiotic is warranted to prevent the bladder from becoming a nidus for systemic infection. This latter condition is most likely to occur if the catheter becomes obstructed.

Although most postoperative urinary tract infections occur in association with indwelling urethral catheters, occasionally such infections develop in the early postoperative period secondary to urinary stasis and necessitate catheter placement as a therapeutic measure. Patients at risk for this problem include those with prostatic hypertrophy, various neuromuscular disorders such as multiple sclerosis, and previous anorectal procedures that have resulted in ineffective postoperative voiding, and those individuals in whom a spinal anesthetic was used. Under most circumstances, a urinary catheter should be prophylactically placed in such patients before surgery to prevent these stasis problems and should be removed as soon as normal voiding can be ensured. If a catheter-associated infection develops, the principles of treatment outlined previously should be followed.

Wound and Soft-Tissue Infection

Another common postoperative infection is the wound or soft-tissue infection that occurs at a rate of 8.9 cases per 1000 hospital discharges.[13] The concept underlying this infection is that skin flora or the flora involved with a mucous membrane have contaminated a surgical wound that, when closed, allows these organisms to become invaders along the opposing fascial planes of the wound that do not possess adequate host defenses until revascularization occurs. The best prevention of a wound infection is careful surgical technique that includes leaving skin wounds open when they are known to be contaminated and decreasing the concentration of potentially infecting organisms by maneuvers such as wound irrigation and, in the case of abdominal incisions, lavaging the peritoneal cavity with normal saline or antimicrobial-containing solutions before wound closure.

Phlebitis

Although phlebitis of the lower extremities may develop in any patient following surgery (see Chapter 53 about venous disorders) and result in postoperative fever, it seldom has a bacterial cause. In contrast, the phlebitis that is catheter-related is a true infection not uncommonly observed in surgical patients and may result in bacteremia and sepsis. As discussed previously, bacteremia denotes the presence of bacteria in the bloodstream, but septicemia denotes not only bacteremia but also the physiologic consequences of release of mediators of inflammation (notably caused by endotoxemia) with the resultant risks of cardiovascular shock. Often the surgical literature uses the term "surgical sepsis" to mean surgical infection; this term can be misleading and should be reserved for situations in which true sepsis is present.

An intravenous (I.V.) catheter breaches local skin defenses and allows a portal of entry for skin flora (e.g., *Staphylococcus aureus,* but also, with increasing recognition, *Staphylococcus epidermidis*). As the patient resides longer in the hospital, gram-negative bacilli may also cause catheter-related bacteremia. Careful studies have implicated the I.V. catheter as the source of bacteremia by semiquantitative culture of the skin surrounding the catheter and by culture of the catheter tip by rolling it onto an agar plate upon its removal.[25] By convention, the catheter site is a nidus of infection only when the tip culture count exceeds the skin count or when frank pus can be expressed from an intravenous catheter site and organisms are shown by Gram's stain or culture. A common mistake in performing a tip culture count is to withdraw the catheter tip, sterilely snip off the tip, and drop it into a culture broth. Then when the culture is positive, a catheter site infection is assumed. However, unless visible pus was present at the catheter site, acceptable alternative explanations include contaminating skin colonizers that grew to large numbers in the liquid media or bacteremia from another focus that seeded the catheter. The more relevant culture to obtain when catheter-related bacteremia or sepsis is suspected is a blood culture. If the site is inflamed, pus from the site should be cultured. Differential therapeutic decisions cannot and should not be made from unquantified cultures of catheter tips.

Three therapeutic decisions involving I.V. catheters are particularly controversial. The first is bacteremia caused by *Staphylococcus aureus,* often secondary to infected I.V. catheters. *Staphylococcus aureus* is notorious for persisting within leukocytes and disseminating widely throughout the body.[27] It cannot be treated with a short course of antibiotics without risking subsequent serious infections such as osteomyelitis or infective endocarditis. A body of data has suggested that if the focus of infection is removable (e.g., an I.V. catheter that can be removed or a furuncle that can be rapidly drained), then the patient can be treated with a relatively short course of antibiotics, specifically, 2 weeks.[37] The qualifier is that during the 2 weeks of therapy, the patient should not develop circulating teichoic acid antibodies, which indicate an immunologic reaction to the cell wall teichoic acid in a staphylococcus. The presence of such antibodies suggests an intravascular or deep-seated staphylococcal infection that needs long-term therapy. Conflicting evidence reveals the occasional case of endocarditis that develops despite adherence to appropriate principles of short-course anti-staphylococcal therapy.[39] Furthermore, the focus of infection is too frequently not removed quickly, and the patient's problem then is sustained *Staphylococcus* bacteremia, which is all too likely to have caused seeding of distant foci. Many infectious disease specialists recommend a conservatively long (4 to 6 weeks) course of antibiotics for all but the most clearly defined cases of staphylococcal bacteremia resulting from a removable focus. Depending on the circumstances, a portion of the long-term therapy may be administered orally, but most infectious disease experts insist on at least 2 weeks of intravenous therapy.

A second and relatively common therapeutic dilemma is the approach to *Candida albicans* fungemia related to an infected I.V. catheter site. Until recently the usual approach was to remove the catheter and, because *C. albicans* is an avirulent pathogen, to rely on host defenses to clear the infection. The status of the host is the operative variable. In patients with obvious host deficits (e.g., underlying cancer, lowered defenses as a result of chemotherapy, and poor nutritional status), fungemia treated only with catheter removal has led to a small proportion of patients developing deep-seated *Candida* infections.[4] The current recommendation is a short course (7 to 10 days) of amphotericin B for fungemic hosts whose defense status is questionable. This recommendation for the use of amphotericin B is still controversial and is probably best effected in consultation with an infectious disease expert.

The third difficulty in the treatment of infected I.V. catheter sites arises when thrombophlebitis supervenes. If a central vein is thrombosed and infected, high-dose antimicrobial therapy often suffices. The incidence of pulmonary embolism in this setting is probably higher than previously thought, and the use of heparin may be appropriate for selected patients.[14] A difficult problem is documented bacteremia believed to be secondary to an infected I.V. catheter site—the catheter has been removed, an antibiotic has been started, the patient's temperature has not subsided in a timely fashion, and a palpable venous cord is present. Efforts to aspirate the vein are usually unrevealing but worth attempting. The judgment that needs to be made is whether or not to excise a possibly infected vein, to hope that a long course of antibiotics will eventually control the infection, or to treat the patient with a conventional course of antibiotics for approximately 10 days and, when the antibiotics are stopped, discover if the vein itself was infected based on whether or not the patient becomes bacteremic again. The right decision simply must be individualized. Veins that appear grossly normal at the time of surgery may in fact contain multiple microabscesses in their walls when they are sectioned and examined microscopically.[29] These veins might not have been suspected as the source of bacteremia or sepsis because typical indications of inflammation such as erythema or warmth may have been lacking.

Intraabdominal Infections

The majority of infections that occur in the abdominal cavity postoperatively are related to bacterial contamination from operations involving the biliary tract or the intestine. Occasionally, spontaneous gastrointestinal perforations may be responsible for postoperative intraadominal infection. The subset of patients in which this circumstance may arise includes the individual with multisystem organ failure in whom a stress ulcer penetrates the full thickness of the gastric wall and those individuals requiring chronic immunosuppression with corticosteroids or other toxic agents. An even less common cause of intraabdominal infection is primary peritonitis caused by peritoneal contamination from hematogenous or lymphatic sources, which may occur in a patient with end-stage liver disease and portal hypertension.

Since the vast majority of intraabdominal infections are related to previous abdominal surgeries, the circumstances surrounding this type of surgery bear directly on the likelihood of developing a postoperative infection and its clinical presentation. For example, if a patient has an elective cholecystectomy for chronic cholecystitis and cholelithiasis, a rather unremarkable postoperative course can generally be anticipated. In contrast, if the patient needs a cholecystectomy and drainage of the common duct because of acute suppurative cholangitis, the likelihood of significant bacterial contamination at the time of surgery with a potential for postoperative intraabdominal infection is much more pronounced. At even greater risk for postoperative intraabdominal infection is the patient who has sustained a gunshot wound to the left colon in which there has been significant fecal spillage or a patient whose duodenal ulcer has perforated and has not been brought to medical attention until 12 or more hours after the perforation, by which time considerable peritoneal soilage has occurred.

The clinical course of postoperative intraabdominal infection will depend on the size and the virulence of the bacterial inoculum. If contamination is quantitatively small, the patient's host defenses may be sufficient to bring about its resolution. A larger inoculum may severely stress the patient's defense mechanisms so that a diffuse peritonitis results, requiring immediate surgery and meticulous cleansing of the abdominal cavity with appropriate management of the underlying source of infection. In selective circumstances, intraabdominal drains may also require placement. More commonly, however, the inflammatory process tends to become localized through the development of protective adhesions that result in the formation of one or more abscesses. Since the clinical appearance of any of these forms of intra-abdominal infection is initially vague so that the ultimate outcome is uncertain, any suggestion that an intraabdominal etiology is responsible for postoperative infection should result in the prompt administration of parenteral antibiotics. Since the majority of pathogens isolated from peritonitis usually includes those harbored in the colon, intestine, or biliary tract, a broad-spectrum antibiotic regimen that adequately covers both aerobic and anaerobic gram-negative rods should be used. Often a cephamycin like cefoxitin will prove adequate, although it is not unusual that multiple antibiotics are required to provide a more complete spectrum of protection for the patient at risk.

If the suspected infection is caused by minor bacterial contamination during previous surgery, this therapeutic approach is usually satisfactory. Continuing evidence of infection indicates either the presence of peritonitis or the development of an intraabdominal abscess. The latter occurrence is more common but is much more difficult to diagnose. In contrast to peritonitis in which the physical examination characteristically demonstrates diffuse tenderness, involuntary muscle guarding, and often diffuse abdominal wall rigidity, the examination in the patient with an abscess is frequently unrevealing except for a localized area of tenderness, which is often difficult to distingush from normal incision discomfort. Rarely is the abscess mass itself palpable unless it has localized in the pelvis, in which case a gloved finger inserted into the rectum may demonstrate its presence. Because of the difficulty in identifying an intraabdominal abscess, a number of radiologic tests may be necessary to make the diagnosis more definite. If the abscess is localized below one of the diaphragms, a pleural effusion, an elevated hemidiaphragm, or evidence of extraluminal air are helpful radiologic hints. Not infrequently, abdominal ultrasound may facilitate diagnosis, particularly in the hands of an experienced ultrasonographer. In recent years, computerized tomography has evolved into another useful diagnostic aid and may ultimately prove to be the procedure of choice in delineating the presence or absence of intraabdominal infections.

If the clinical course strongly suggests the existence of an intra-abdominal abscess, whether or not radiologic confirmation exists, abdominal exploration is indicated since complete evacuation of the abscess cavity is the only effective treatment for this entity. For abscesses localizing in the pelvis, drainage through the anterior rectal wall is often adequate, particularly if a firm synthesis exists between the abscess and the rectum. Abscesses localized in a subdiaphragmatic space can usually be drained extraperitoneally using a posterior approach in which the twelfth rib is also usually removed. In other portions of the abdomen, however, a more formal intraabdominal approach is usually necessary to ensure the breakdown of abscess loculations and complete drainage. This approach also avoids the possibility of missing a second or third abscess that is not uncommonly present when intraabdominal infection develops.

Miscellaneous Infections

Although the foregoing discussion has considered the usual causes of postoperative infection, in reality many other causes can exist. For this reason, the surgeon must always maintain an open mind and frequently reexamine the patient to look for clues if the underlying source of infection has remained elusive. An unexplained heart murmur may be a tip-off for endocarditis, whereas unusual obtundation may be secondary to undiagnosed meningitis or brain abscess. Occasionally trauma patients who have sustained multiple injuries develop a pyarthrosis from open-joint injuries. Parotitis from an obstructed salivary gland duct may also be the incipient source, or the fever may not be caused by an infection at all but may be secondary to a drug reaction or may be an allergic reaction to a blood transfusion.

Finally, an additional type of infectious process is the intrinsic infections of the gastrointestinal tract that may occur occasionally following surgery, but they are by no means limited to the postoperative setting. The most common manifestations are fever and diarrhea. In many instances the diarrhea is related to enteral feedings and has nothing to do with the fever. Occasionally, however, a patient may acquire nosocomially a classic enteric pathogen. An example is the case of salmonellosis acquired from contaminated poultry or eggs, from enteral feedings, or from other patients during an outbreak of this disease.

Of more concern to the surgeon is the patient who has received antibiotic therapy and then has developed diarrhea. In many instances, this diarrhea is caused by an overgrowth of *Clostridium difficile,* which produces a cytotoxin. Antibiotics that are notably linked with antibiotic-associated enterocolitis (AAC) include ampicillin, cephalosporins, and lincomycins such as clindamycin, but most antibiotics have been shown to elicit this syndrome. AAC may be accompanied by fever and toxicity and is frequently overlooked as the potential source of postoperative fever. The cornerstone of diagnosis includes a stool culture for the presence of *Clostridium difficile* and, less important, an assessment of stool for the presence of *Clostridium difficile* cytotoxin. The fecal leukocyte examination may be positive, but, if negative, it does not exclude AAC. Finally, sigmoidoscopy may reveal the typical pseudomembranous lesions associated with this entity. After diagnosis, therapy is oral vancomycin—125 mg four times daily for 10 days.[18] Parenteral vancomycin is not recommended because the object of therapy is to obtain intraluminal levels of antibiotic, which I.V. vancomycin does not provide. An alternative therapeutic option is oral or I.V. metronidazole since both routes of administration are effective.[32] Because *Clostridium* spores may survive a course of vancomycin or metronidazole, relapses of AAC do occur, but they are treated simply by an additional course of the same antimicrobial agent.

THE ROLE OF THE LABORATORY IN INFECTION DIAGNOSIS

A variety of laboratory tests may be helpful in determining the timing of therapeutic interventions in the patient with proven or suspected infection. Many surgical infections are characterized by leukocytosis with a left shift in the differential count. A perfectly normal white count and differential, particularly if repeated and still found to be normal, should generate caution about diagnosing a bacterial infection. However, white blood cell counts by themselves can be misleading, especially in the elderly or compromised host. Elderly patients may only manifest vague symptoms and signs of infection, and the only clue to serious disease, such as an infarcted bowel, may be a normal number of white blood cells with a differential count that is markedly shifted to the left. Although many infected patients have some degree of coagulopathy, its absence does not exclude infection so that this laboratory parameter has not proven to be a discriminating finding. Likewise, overreliance on metabolic markers to define sepsis may be hazardous; in fact, it may lead to a delay in therapy. For instance, septic patients often demonstrate glucose intolerance, but they need not; some patients with sepsis may be initially seen with hypoglycemia.[28] Liver function studies may support a diagnosis of ascending cholangitis, cholecystitis, liver abscess, or hepatitis, but the range of overlap in liver function derangements in fundamentally different disease states is so high that the wise physician only places emphasis on extremes of liver function abnormalities. For example, exceedingly high aminotransferase levels (i.e., in the thousands) is virtually diagnostic of hepatitis (usually A, B, or non-A/non-B), but lower levels (i.e., in the hundreds) can be seen in hepatitis, cytomegalovirus infections, Epstein-Barr viral disease, syphilis, and toxoplasmosis. These lower levels can also be seen in alcoholic hepatitis, liver abscess, and occasionally gall bladder disease among other disease states.

The possibility of posttransfusion hepatitis should prompt the ordering of more specific serum tests, such as hepatitis B surface antigen and cytomegalovirus titers. Serum bilirubin and alkaline phosphatase elevations, on the other hand, have broad differentials that include many noninfectious conditions of the postoperative state and therefore can be difficult to interpret. The possibility of ascending cholangitis in an infected patient with hyperbilirubinemia should always be considered because of the emergent need to treat this condition with surgical intervention and adjunctive antibiotic therapy; however, this diagnosis is most often overlooked on medical, not surgical, services. The rapid appearance of jaundice secondary to a hemolytic process may indicate alpha toxin production by *Clostridium perfringens,* and recognition of this now uncommon condition might lead to life-saving surgery to evacuate infected tissue (e.g., hysterectomy).

Some tests are more specific and of pivotal importance in the decision to operate. Rising white blood cell counts may be the tip-off that a vague abdominal problem seen clinically may, in fact, be a surgically remedial condition. Chest radiograms, ultrasound of the abdomen and pelvis, and abdominal computerized axial tomography (CAT) scans are examples of technology that have permitted more specific preoperative diagnoses, but these tests are still associated with such a sufficiently high level of false positivity and negativity that collaborating evidence for underlying infection is usually sought before proceeding with surgery.

From the point of view of the infectious disease specialist, the laboratory helps in defining a locus of infection, isolating a specific organism or group of organisms, and providing data that support the worthiness of antimicrobial treatment in terms of ensuring both the killing of the organism and minimum toxicity from the drug chosen. Although the history, physical examination, and sometimes radiographic tests are valuable in defining the focus of infection, specifying the offending organism depends on relevant cultures and simple stains of relevant material. The operative word here is "relevant," and the deceiving word is "simple." Many surgical infections occur adjacent to mucous membranes or other areas where *colonizing* flora may be confused with *causal* flora. Classic examples of inappropriate and irrelevant cultures are as follows: culturing sputum for anaerobes in necrotizing pneumonia; culturing chest tube contents rather than percutaneously obtained pleural space material when empyema is suspected; culturing catheter tips instead of blood when catheter-site infection with bacteremia is suspected; swabbing wounds for culture rather than aspirating underlying abscesses through intact skin or cellulitic areas; and culturing sinus tracts rather than obtaining bone biopsies without contamination from the tract when osteomyelitis is suspected.

The Gram's stain is a deceivingly simple procedure. It is underused in surgical practice because its interpretation is not simple. With experience, however, many causative agents can be predicted, and the Gram's stain result can guide empiric therapy. For instance, clumps of staphylococci are clearly different from chains of streptococci. Clostridial species have a characteristic appearance of plump, gram-positive rods. Among surgical infections, mixed anaerobic-aerobic infections are common, and the Gram's stain result may be the only clue to the presence of an anaerobe that may fail to grow in culture. Busy surgeons frequently do not take the time to look at the stain results themselves so that they may interpret them in the light of the clinical situation. Instead they rely on the report of a microbiology technician who faithfully describes the individual organisms but who renders a description that is too often sterile of clinical judgment (as, legally, it must be). In this context, the infectious disease practitioner can be of invaluable service to the surgeon in guiding empiric therapy in difficult cases.

Blood should always be cultured as well as the local site of suspected infection when possible. The hope in these maneuvers is to have an organism available in the laboratory so that a number of tests can be performed on it to verify that correct antibiotics have been chosen and to point the way to an appropriate change in antibiotic coverage if the organism proves to be resistant. To predict antibiotic susceptibility of an organism, most microbiology laboratories use the disk diffusion test in which an antibiotic impregnated in a paper disk diffuses into an agar plate on which a lawn of organisms has been seeded. In 24 hours a sizeable clear zone (no growth) around the disk indicates that the organism is susceptible to that antibiotic. It must be noted, however, that the amount of antibiotic in a disk has been chosen so that the result of the test will predict that an organism *in the bloodstream* can be killed or its growth inhibited by concentrations of antibiotic achievable in the bloodstream. The minimum inhibitory concentration must be *exceeded* in the bloodstream to penetrate an abscess and kill susceptible organisms. Conversely, a urinary tract infection caused by an "antibiotic-resistant" organism may actually be cured by that antibiotic because the antibiotic is excreted, and thereby concentrated, in the urine. The apparent susceptibilities of certain organisms are subject to the exact number of organisms seeded onto the agar plate (i.e., inoculum effect). Susceptibilities of organisms such as *Pseudomonas aeruginosa* are very dependent on control of the cationic content of the media. Finally, a slow-growing organism may appear susceptible by disk diffusion testing when it is not.

In serious infections such as osteomyelitis and endocarditis more detailed information about antibiotic susceptibility is obtained by tube dilution susceptibility testing. Some hospitals perform this kind of test by automation. A highly controlled inoculum (often in serum to control the effects of protein binding) is exposed to specific antibiotics in twofold dilutions. The minimum inhibitory concentration (MIC) and minimum bactericidal concentration (MBC) of the antibiotic can then be defined and related to the measured or anticipated concentration of antibiotic achieved or achievable in target tissues. This kind of data is useful when the duration of antibiotic therapy is long and if another antibiotic must be substituted because of the development of adverse reactions. Making such a substitution can therefore be based on objective data.

In many clinical situations the blood concentration of an antibiotic cannot be determined because the techniques are not available. When an estimate of achieved antibiotic levels is desired to guarantee a positive therapeutic outcome, a so-called serum bactericidal titer can be determined. A sample of serum is drawn at the anticipated peak and trough of serum antibiotic levels. The serum is then diluted twofold, and a defined inoculum of the patient's infecting organism is added. The dilution that inhibits (and kills) the inoculum is called the serum inhibitory (and bactericidal) titer. In patients with osteomyelitis and bacterial endocarditis, it is generally advisable to maintain a trough serum bactericidal titer at 1:8 or higher. Serum bactericidal titers appear to be useful in infections caused by aerobic gram-positive cocci, but they are not reliable in predicting outcome of gram-negative bacterial infections. Most surgical infections can be managed well by using standard disk diffusion antibiotic susceptibility data and providing dosages of standard amounts of antibiotic as specified in references such as the *Physicians' Desk Reference* or hospital formularies. One very important exception to this rule is the apparent susceptibility of methicillin resistant *Staphylococcus aureus* (MRSA) to cephalosporins when tested by the disk diffusion method.[3] MRSA may appear to be susceptible, but when checked by tube dilution susceptibility testing, the minimum inhibitory concentrations are found to be high. Consequently, clinical failures can occur when MRSA is treated with even high doses of cephalosporins. For this reason, many laboratories will no longer report the cephalosporin susceptibility of MSRA.

Other potentially useful and rapidly performed tests are currently on the horizon that may ultimately prove beneficial in the diagnosis of infection. Some are already available, such as assessing blood, cerebrospinal fluid, and urine by counter-current immunoelectrophoresis or using latex agglutination testing for the presence of antigens of pathogens such as *Streptococcus pneumoniae, Haemophilus influenzae,* or *Neisseria meningitidis.* The surgeon is much more interested in organisms such as normal flora that may be causing infection; for them, the most useful rapid technology includes blood culturing systems that rely on radioactive glucose use, with turnaround times measured in hours. Other techniques such as gas-liquid chromatography promise to identify the footprints (e.g., short-chain fatty acids of anaerobes) of select pathogens, but such technology is not yet readily available.

PATHOGENS RESPONSIBLE FOR SURGICAL INFECTION

A common approach to characterizing surgical infection is to list the microbial agents that cause such infections. Considering the phenomenal number of organisms that can infect compromised hosts, a list of "surgical microbes" becomes merely a weak attempt at a review of the entire field of microbiology. Equally inappropriate are lists of microbes and the preferred antimicrobial agents to treat them. Memorizing such lists is a relatively fruitless exercise because many surgical infections are polymicrobic; thus the surgeon must more realistically design an empiric therapy with a broad-spectrum agent or a combination of agents. The rational approach to surgical microbiology is to learn those microbes that can singly cause important infections and that may have classic clinical presentations. Also the surgeon must learn the combinations of microbes that are frequently encountered in surgical situations so that empiric therapy can be instituted until the results of appropriate Gram's stains and cultures are available. Table 6-4 is a brief exposure to the most common and important bacterial pathogens that are of relevance to the surgeon.

Among the fungi, *Candida albicans* is the most impor-

Table 6-4 **SELECTED FEATURES OF BACTERIA IN SURGICAL INFECTION**

Organism	Frequency of Organism Seen in Surgical Infection	Likelihood of Single-Pathogen Surgical Infection	Types of Surgical Infection	Comments	Future Considerations
AEROBIC BACTERIA					
Gram-positive cocci					
Staphylococcus aureus	High	High	Skin and wound abscess, cellulitis, infected I.V. catheter site, bacteremia, endocarditis, infected prosthetic device, pneumonia, postneurosurgery meningitis, osteomyelitis, infected joint	Methicillin resistant (MRSA) strains common in large teaching hospitals	New antibiotics such as the carboxyquinolones may become an alternative to vancomycin to treat MRSA
Staphylococcus epidermis	Moderate	Low	Usually mixed infection but can cause bacteremia, ventriculoperitoneal shunt infection, endocarditis, skin infection	Frequently methicillin resistant (MRSE)	Endocarditis caused by MRSE may require combination therapy—vancomycin, rifampin, and an aminoglycoside

Table 6-4 **SELECTED FEATURES OF BACTERIA IN SURGICAL INFECTION—cont'd**

Organism	Frequency of Organism Seen in Surgical Infection	Likelihood of Single-Pathogen Surgical Infection	Types of Surgical Infection	Comments	Future Considerations
Streptococcus pneumoniae	Moderate	High	Pneumonia, bacteremia, infected joint	Penicillin resistance not common in U.S. but should be recognized as possibility; vaccination available. Special risk for first 2 yr after splenectomy for trauma	Vancomycin may become drug of choice if resistance increases
"Enterococci"	High	Low	Usually mixed infection—wound and intra-abdominal abscess, endocarditis, urinary tract infection (UTI)	Often do not need specific therapy for "enterococcus" in drained and debrided mixed infection in which other organisms are treated	Unlicensed, extremely broad-spectrum antibiotic (imipenem) retains antienterococcus activity
Other *Streptococcus* species	Moderate	Low	Usually mixed infection—skin and wound infection, intra-abdominal abscess	Group B *Streptococcus* occasionally the single pathogen in elderly patient after trauma	Speciation may help to associate isolation of certain *Streptococci* species with underlying medical conditions (e.g., *Streptococcus bovis* and bowel malignancy)
Gram-negative cocci					
Neisseria gonorrhoeae	Low	Moderate	Tubo-ovarian abscess; mixed infection with anaerobes, enteric bacilli, and *Chlamydia* is common	Penicillinase production (PPNG) among some isolates	If PPNG does become numerically important, empiric therapy needs to include cefoxitin, cefotaxime, or spectinomycin
Neisseria meningitidis	Low	High	Bacteremia, pneumonia (especially Group Y)	Uncommon role in surgical infection	Should remain an uncommon surgical problem
Branhamella catarrhalis	Low	Moderate	Pneumonia (usually community acquired)	Elaborates penicillinase; role in postoperative pneumonia is uncertain	Should remain an uncommon surgical problem
Gram-positive bacilli					
Bacillus species (especially *cereus*)	Low	High	Usually contaminant; may cause bacteremia, endophthalmitis	Occasional cause of sepsis in compromised host	Empiric use of clindamycin, which penetrates vitreous fluid, may lead to salvage of infected eye
"JK-Diphtheroids"	Low	High	Bacteremia	Occasional cause of sepsis in compromised host	Because of this organism and MRSA, vancomycin will enjoy more empiric usage in compromised hosts
Gram-negative bacilli					
Escherichia coli	High	Moderate	Bacteremia, UTI, pneumonia; often in mixed infection—wound, intra-abdominal and pelvic abscess	Often susceptible to many antibiotics, but ampicillin resistance is rising	Multiply resistant strains; may cause outbreaks in large hospitals

Continued.

Table 6-4 SELECTED FEATURES OF BACTERIA IN SURGICAL INFECTION—cont'd

Organism	Frequency of Organism Seen in Surgical Infection	Likelihood of Single-Pathogen Surgical Infection	Types of Surgical Infection	Comments	Future Considerations
AEROBIC BACTERIA—cont'd					
Gram-positive bacilli—cont'd					
Other *Enterobacteriaceae*					
Klebsiella- Enterobacter, Proteus, Morganella	High	Low	Mixed infection such as wound, intra-abdominal, and pelvic abscess; occasional bacteremia, UTI, pneumonia	Antibiotic susceptibilities vary among genera and species; multiply resistant strains can be a problem	Newer cephalosporins and other beta-lactam antibiotics may supplant use of aminoglycosides
Serratia and *Providencia*	Moderate	Moderate	Occasional bacteremia, pneumonia, UTI	Patient is usually compromised host; red pigmentation not present in all strains of *Serratia*	With advent of extraordinarily broad-spectrum antibiotics, watch for developing resistance
Non-*Enterobacteriaceae*					
Pseudomonas aeruginosa	Moderate	High	Bacteremia, pneumonia, wound infection (especially burn)	Patient often compromised host; exotoxin production and perivascular infiltration of organisms may contribute to mortality	Newer cephalosporins (e.g., ceftazidime) have anti-*Pseudomonas* activity, but in vivo development of resistance (such as with the anti-*Pseudomonas* penicillins) may limit use as single agents
Gram-negative coccobacilli					
Haemophilis influenzae	Low	High	Pneumonia, sinusitis	Beta-lactamase production dictates antibiotic coverage	Will become better recognized as disease cause in elderly patients and postoperative pneumonia
Acinetobacter	Low	Moderate	Often mixed infection; may cause UTI, pneumonia, intra-abdominal and wound infection, bacteremia	In respiratory specimens Gram's stain appearance may be confused with commensural *Neisseria;* tobramycin predictably least efficacious of the aminoglycosides	Highly resistant strains may plague large hospitals; only the newest beta-lactam antibiotics will prove useful (e.g., ceftazidime, imipenem)
ANAEROBIC BACTERIA					
Gram-positive cocci					
Peptococcus, Peptostreptococcus, anaerobic *Streptococci*	Moderate	Low	Mixed infection, genitourinary infections, fasciitis	Complicated taxonomy; bacteremia may lead to brain abscess	The clinical impact of lack of activity of metronidazole against these organisms may never be proven because genitourinary infections are usually drained, and most organisms in mixed infection are treated
Gram-positive bacilli					
Clostridium perfringens	High	Moderate to low	Usually mixed infection (wound, intra-abdominal), gas gangrene, occasional devastating sepsis in genitourinary infection	Alpha-toxin may cause severe hemolysis necessitating aggressive surgical intervention (e.g., hysterectomy)	Was more commonly seen as single agent in past; trend should continue

Table 6-4 **SELECTED FEATURES OF BACTERIA IN SURGICAL INFECTION—cont'd**

Organism	Frequency of Organism Seen in Surgical Infection	Likelihood of Single-Pathogen Surgical Infection	Types of Surgical Infection	Comments	Future Considerations
Clostridium tetani	Low	High	Causes tetanus	Occasional problem in elderly (especially female) unvaccinated population or in neonates when mother unvaccinated	Use of intrathecal tetanus immune globulin to prevent progression of localized to generalized tetanus is controversial but worth considering
Clostridium difficile	Low	High	Causes antibiotic-associated enterocolitis	Most antibiotics have a causal role—notably cephalosporins, ampicillin, clindamycin	Nosocomial outbreaks may occur; metronidazole is probably reasonable alternative to oral vancomycin
Clostridium botulinum	Low	High	Causes wound botulism	Recognition and use of antitoxins are key	Should remain an uncommon event
Gram-negative bacilli					
Bacteroides fragilis	High	Moderate	Usually mixed infection	Heparinase production may lead to local thrombosis; capsular virulence factor aids in establishing synergistic infection	May see complications of inadequate therapy when practitioners fail to recognize many newer cephalosporins do NOT have adequate activity against *B. fragilis*
Other *Bacteroides* species	High	Low	Mixed infection	Many make penicillinase	The clinical axion, "above-the-belt anaerobes are sensitive to penicillin G," may die slowly; may see penicillin G therapeutic failures in necrotizing pneumonia
Fusobacteria	Moderate	Low	Mixed infection	Easily recognized by needle shape on Gram's stain	Underscores the clinical usefulness of a Gram's stain even if culture for anaerobes is not performed

tant and is not infrequently involved in intravenous catheter-related fungemia. In general, there has been a movement to try oral ketoconazole instead of amphotericin B in situations that are not overtly life-threatening. In compromised hosts, however, amphotericin B is clearly superior to ketoconazole in treating *C. albicans* syndromes, and ketoconazole is not effective against nonalbicans species of *Candida*. The easiest way to control *Candida* infections in routine surgical practice is to prevent its occurrence by choosing the most narrow-spectrum antibiotic or combination of antibiotics and using them for the briefest duration consistent with guaranteed clinical success. Other fungal agents, including *Aspergillus* and *Mucor,* are still occasional problems for the surgeon and may cause systemic infections in debilitated patients. The source of these infections (e.g., the burn wound or diabetic abscess) will require aggressive surgical excision in conjunction with high-dose (as much as 1.0 mg/kg/day for the first week) amphotericin B if effective treatment is to be rendered. Aspergillus species may only be colonizers, but when they do infect, they tend to invade vessels and cause local thrombosis, necrosis, and cavitation. Mucor species do not often infect, but when they do, they tend to invade vessels and spread along adipoidal tissue planes; the extent of infection is often much greater than is clinically apparent.

The role of viruses in surgical infection is poorly studied

except for the blood-borne hepatitides such as hepatitis B, cytomegalovirus, and non-A/non-B hepatitis. Cytomegalovirus infection has proven to be poorly recognized and underdiagnosed as a cause of fever in postoperative trauma patients.[2] Also, cytomegalovirus is a common problem in transplant patients. Presently no effective therapy exists for cytomegalovirus, but new agents are being tested.

Herpes simplex and herpes zoster infections are marginally involved in surgical practice. Rectal infection with herpes simplex virus can cause urinary bladder retention and come to the attention of the urologist. Rarely, generalized *Herpesvirus* infections complicate the management of a burn patient or other compromised hosts. In these patients, use of the antiviral agent acyclovir has become an important treatment modality. In surgical practice, *Herpesvirus* is much more likely to be a problem for surgical or nursing personnel when it causes a herpetic whitlow.

Parasitic infections are occasionally very important to the surgeon. The classic example is the huge solitary liver abscess in the right lobe of the liver. In such cases amoebic disease must be suspected and confirmed rapidly by an amoeba serology test; then metronidazole must be instituted before surgery. Unless such abscesses threaten to burst, however, they are usually managed with antimicrobial agents alone, and surgery or percutaneous drainage is generally not necessary.[17] When hydatid disease is suspected, it should be confirmed serologically, and serious consideration should be given to treating the patient with albendazole before surgery.[35] Finally, a number of parasites that are not commonly seen, including *Pneumocystis carinii* and *Toxoplasma gondii,* are encountered routinely in AIDS patients and are obliging all physicians, including surgeons, to become reacquainted with their clinical appearances.

ROLE OF ANTIBIOTICS IN INFECTION MANAGEMENT

It is beyond the scope of this chapter to discuss in any comprehensive fashion the mechanisms by which antibiotics mediate their antibacterial effects. It should be emphasized, however, that differing modes of action are responsible for the differing effects of antibiotics against various microorganisms. Penicillins, for example, characteristically inhibit cell wall synthesis, probably by interfering with transpeptidase activity and thereby preventing normal cross-linkage. Thus a circumstance is created in which water from isotonic body fluids is able to move freely into bacteria because of the high osmotic pressure, ultimately creating a bursting effect. The aminoglycosides, on the other hand, inhibit protein synthesis through a primary action on ribosomes, which results in the misreading of messenger RNA and the subsequent interference with amino acid replication. Through still another mode of action, polymyxin affects cell membrane permeability by its cationic detergent action, as well as interfering with cellular oxidative phosphorylation. Finally, agents such as the sulfonamides inhibit nucleotide synthesis and therefore DNA synthesis. The extent to which these various antibiotic effects prevent bacterial growth will often influence the efficacy of an antibiotic under a given set of clinical conditions. A bacteriocidal antibiotic, which actually kills bacteria, is often preferable to a bacteriostatic antibiotic, which inhibits growth or multiplication of bacteria and allows normal host defenses to actually effect bacterial destruction. In an immunocompromised patient in whom host defenses may be severely depleted, a bacteriocidal drug is usually preferred.

In the same way that antibiotics differ in their modes of action, microorganisms develop bacterial resistance in a variety of ways. These ways may include mutation to a resistant strain or the production of an enzyme such as penicillinase or beta-lactamase that can destroy the antibiotic effects of penicillins and cephalosporins, respectively. In addition, a given pathogen may activate a latent biochemical process or acquire by transfer a chromosome-like factor, known as a resistance factor, that may block the mode of action of a particular antibiotic. It is for these reasons that an antibiotic, although once effective therapeutically against a specific pathogen, may lose its efficacy.

An antibiotic may be administered prophylactically to prevent the subsequent development of an infection or therapeutically to treat an infection when it has actually occurred. The following discussion outlines a rational approach to each of these types of antibiotic usage.

Prophylactic Use

The use of antibiotics to prevent wound infections is an exceedingly complicated topic. An approach to prophylaxis is outlined in Table 6-1. The underlying principle, however, is to use adjunctive mechanical means, whenever possible, to decrease the concentration of infective organisms that could ultimately give rise to a wound infection. For example, in operations involving the large bowel, a period of mechanical cleaning through the use of cathartics and/or enemas before surgery can go far to decrease the enteric bacterial count and thereby lessen the risk of infection. In such clean/contaminated cases, antibiotics are administered shortly before or at the time of contamination and are continued, in most instances, for only a few perioperative dosages. Such dosages are kept high to ensure adequate tissue penetration. Antibiotics are chosen for their efficacy against the contaminating flora, and this choice must take into account the likelihood of resistant hospital flora. If methicillin-resistant *Staphylococcus aureus* or *epidermidis* was a common colonizer in a given hospital setting, methicillin would obviously be contraindicated and another prophylactic antibiotic such as vancomycin[5,23,38] should be substituted.

Sometimes antibiotics that are intended to prevent infection can be administered after contamination has occurred. An example would be a gunshot wound to the abdomen in which a colon injury has occurred without the luxury of preoperative mechanical cleaning. The thesis underlying this concept is that antibiotics are begun within 2 to 3 hours of contamination during the so-called *effective period.* During this period mediators of inflammation have already been set into motion, but the use of a short course of antibiotics can still prevent clinical infection from developing. Use of antibiotics in this fashion is more appropriately called short-term therapy than prophylaxis and forms the basis of antibiotic treatment in contaminated wounds.

When indicated during cesarean section, antibiotics can be administered immediately after the cord is clamped—that is, after contamination has occurred. This ensures that the use of antibiotics does not interfere with the evaluation of the neonate and that the antibiotics are administered in time to be of benefit to the mother. When the patient with a gunshot wound penetrating the peritoneal cavity is managed with early aggressive surgery and the expeditious (within 2 to 3 hours after the gunshot) administration of appropriate antibiotics, usually one dose of the antibiotic chosen suffices for low-risk patients (no bowel penetration or significant injury to liver, spleen, or pancreas and no problem with homeostasis). Even high-risk patients can be managed with only 3 days of antibiotic therapy, possibly less.[31,34] When antibiotics can be started in the effective period and the concentration of potentially infecting contaminants can be diminished, the use of a full course (7 to 10 days) of antibiotics in contaminated cases can no longer be recommended since it contributes to excessive hospital costs and risks of superinfection.

Although antibiotic prophylaxis has clearly reduced the risk of infection in many clinical situations (e.g., in the case of penetrating abdominal trauma—placebo controlled trials in this setting are now considered unethical), the prevention of wound and other postoperative infections is by no means limited theoretically to the exercise of good infectious disease principles. Other risk factors in the development of infection have already been discussed and include the following: the age of the patient, the degree of injury as quantitated by blood loss (which also relates to the presence of a fertile ground for bacterial culture [e.g., hematoma]), the presence of intercurrent disease, the underlying nutritional status, and the presence or absence of trauma (e.g., colonic injury, which implies a high load of potential contaminants[11,30]). This multiplicity of risk factors demands excellent surgical technique—debridement of devitalized tissues, proper management of wounds that are suspected to be heavily colonized, and aggressive management of host factors postoperatively, most notably to include attention to the nutritional status of the patient. Even before the advent of antibiotics and sophisticated approaches such as total parenteral nutrition, adherence to classic surgical techniques had led to a substantial decrease in wound infection rates.

Therapeutic Use

Principles governing the therapeutic use of antibiotics are outlined in the boxed material below. Suggested therapy for common surgical infections, pending results of cultures, is indicated in Table 6-5, and recommendations for antibiotic therapy of selected pathogens are included in Table 6-6. A recent therapeutic trend has been the use of new broad-spectrum cephalosporins as substitutes for aminoglycosides in the treatment of aerobic gram-negative bacilli. These organisms are usually a part of a mixed aerobic-anaerobic flora causing surgical infection. Although the new cephalosporins generally are quite potent against aerobic gram-negative bacilli, a fair generalization is that they may sacrifice gram-positive as well as anaerobic coverage. For this reason, they may not serve well as a single therapy for serious conditions. New antibiotics such as imipenem may prove to be acceptable as a single therapeutic agent even for infections acquired in large

PRINCIPLES OF ANTIBIOTIC THERAPY

1. *The organism should be sensitive to the antibiotic chosen.* Obtain an appropriate culture with susceptibility testing to guide possible changes in antibiotic coverage. Recall in vitro/in vivo disparity in susceptibility of some organisms (e.g., cephalosporins are *not* effective in vivo against methicillin-resistant *Staphylococcus aureus*).
2. *Antibiotics should be in doses that ensure adequate peak concentrations and tissue penetration.* Blood levels should exceed minimum inhibitory concentration by 2 to 3 times to ensure penetration of infected tissues.
3. *The antibiotic must come in contact with the organism.* The blood-brain, prostatic, obstructed bile, and other barriers prevent penetration of some antibiotics.
4. *Frequency of administration is based on the half-life and the route of elimination of the antibiotic.* Inadequate antibiotic serum concentrations at the end of a dosing interval may lead to "break-through" bacteremia. With developing renal or hepatic dysfunction, the dosing interval is lengthened and, as function improves, is shortened again.
5. *Choose a bacteriocidal antibiotic when appropriate.* Endocarditis, osteomyelitis, and the infected compromised host with neutropenia require bacterio*cidal* antibiotics.
6. *Use synergistic therapy when appropriate. Pseudomonas* infections (especially compromised host), serious enterococcal infection, *Staphylococcus epidermidis* endocarditis, or ventriculoperitoneal shunt infections deserve synergistic therapy.
7. *Avoid antagonistic combinations of antibiotics.* Antagonism is most likely when two "bacteriostatic" antibiotics are used together.
8. *Choose the most narrow-spectrum antibiotic.* Superinfection is minimized. Often cost is less.
9. *Avoid side effects when possible.* Decreasing the side effects should dictate choice of antibiotic more than cost or convenience of administration. Many antibiotics may interact adversely with other drugs (e.g., metronidazole with ethanol).
10. *Control potential interfering conditions or substances.* Acidic pus may render an antibiotic useless; therefore drain pus. Organisms may survive an antibiotic when a foreign body is present; therefore remove the foreign body.
11. *Ensure the proper duration of therapy.* For many surgical infections, continuing antibiotics 3 or 4 days past the day of afebrility will suffice; however, undrained pus may require very long therapy, and an unremoved foreign body (e.g., infected vascular graft) may require therapy for life.

Table 6-5 **APPROACH TO EMPIRIC THERAPY (PENDING RESULTS OF CULTURES) FOR SERIOUS SURGICAL INFECTION**

			Antibiotic	
Type of Infection	**Usual Organism**	**Usual Gram's Stain Result**	**Large Teaching Hospital***	**Small Community Hospital**
Wound infection	*Staphylococcus aureus*	Gram-positive cocci in clusters	Vancomycin—500 mg I.V. q6hr	Nafcillin—1 g I.V. q4hr
	Mixed anaerobes and enteric aerobic gram-negative bacilli	Mixed flora	Clindamycin—900 mg I.V. q8hr plus tobramycin 1.5 mg/kg I.V. q8hr or ceftazidime—2 g I.V. q8hr	Cefoxitin—1 g I.V. q4hr
Intraabdominal abscess	Mixed anaerobes and enteric aerobic gram-negative bacilli	Mixed flora	Clindamycin—900 mg I.V. q8hr plus tobramycin—1.5 mg/kg I.V. q8hr or ceftazidime—2 g I.V. q8hr	Cefoxitin—1.0-2.0 g I.V. q4hr
Ascending cholangitis	Enteric aerobic gram-negative bacilli, anaerobes, *streptococci*	Usually not available	Ampicillin—1-1.5 g I.V. q4hr plus tobramycin 1.5 mg/kg I.V. q8hr or ceftazidime—2 g I.V. q8hr	Ampicillin—1-1.5 g I.V. q4hr plus cefuroxime—1.5 g I.V. q8hr (or third generation cephalosporin)†
Pneumonia	*Streptococcus pneumoniae*	Gram-positive lancet-shaped diplococci	Penicillin G—0.5-1 megaunits I.V. q4hr	Same
	Haemophilus influenzae	Pleomorphic gram-negative coccobacilli	Cefuroxime—1.5 g q8hr	Same
	Staphylococcus aureus	Gram-positive cocci in clusters	Vancomycin—500 mg I.V. q6hr	Nafcillin—1.5 g I.V. q4hr
	Aspiration pneumonia (hospital-acquired)	Mixed flora	Clindamycin—900 mg I.V. q8hr plus tobramycin—1.5 mg/kg I.V. q8hr or ceftazidime—2 g I.V. q8hr	Cefuroxime—1.5 g I.V. q8hr (or third generation cephalosporin)†
	Aerobic gram-negative bacilli (e.g., *Escherichia coli, Klebsiella, Enterobacter, Pseudomonas*)	Gram-negative bacilli	Mezlocillin—5 g I.V. q6hr plus tobramycin—1.5 mg/kg I.V. q8hr or ceftazidime—2 g I.V. q8hr	Same
Urinary tract infection	Enteric aerobic gram-negative bacilli	Gram-negative bacilli	Tobramycin—1-1.5 mg/kg I.V. q8hr or ceftazidime—1-2 g I.V. q8hr	Cefuroxime—750-1500 mg I.V. q8hr (or third generation cephalosporin)†
	Enterococcus	Gram-positive cocci	Ampicillin—0.5-1 g I.V. q4hr	Same

*Aztreonam (recently released for use) may prove to be a substitute for aminoglycosides.
†Includes cefotaxime or cefoperazone—2 g I.V. q8hr.

Table 6-5 **APPROACH TO EMPIRIC THERAPY (PENDING RESULTS OF CULTURES) FOR SERIOUS SURGICAL INFECTION—cont'd**

Type of Infection	Usual Organism	Usual Gram's Stain Result	Antibiotic: Large Teaching Hospital*	Antibiotic: Small Community Hospital
Sepsis	Enteric aerobic gram-negative bacilli, *Staphylococcus, Pseudomonas*	Usually not available	Mezlocillin—5 g I.V. q8hr plus vancomycin—500 mg I.V. q6hr plus tobramycin—1.5 mg/kg I.V. q8hr or ceftazidime—2 g I.V. q8hr	May substitute nafcillin—1.5 g I.V. q4hr for vancomycin
Infected intravenous catheter site	*Staphylococcus aureus*	Gram-positive cocci in clusters	Vancomycin—500 mg I.V. q6hr	Nafcillin—1.5 g I.V. q4hr
	Enteric aerobic gram-negative bacilli, *Pseudomonas*	Gram-negative bacilli	Tobramycin—1.5 mg/kg I.V. q8hr of ceftazidime—2 g I.V. q8hr	Same

Table 6-6 **SUGGESTED EMPIRIC ANTIBIOTICS FOR SELECTED BACTERIA COMMON IN SURGICAL INFECTIONS**

Organism	Antibiotics: Large Teaching Hospital	Antibiotics: Small Community Hospital
Aerobic Bacteria		
Gram-positive		
Streptococci (nonenterococcus)	Penicillin G	Same
"Enterococci"	Ampicillin, penicillin G plus an aminoglycoside, or vancomycin	Same
Staphylococci	Vancomycin	Nafcillin
Gram-negative		
Enteric bacilli *(Escherichia coli, Klebsiella-Enterobacter, Proteus)*	Aminoglycoside, ceftazidime, or imipenem	Cefuroxime, cefotaxime, or cefoperazone
*Pseudomonas aeruginosa**	Mezlocillin plus aminoglycoside, ceftazidime, or imipenem	Same
Anaerobic Bacteria		
Gram-positive		
Peptococcus, Peptostreptococcus, Clostridia	Penicillin G or clindamycin	Same
Gram-negative		
Bacteroides fragilis	Clindamycin, chloramphenicol, or metronidazole	Same

*Many authorities adding aminoglycoside to ceftazidime or imipenem.

teaching hospitals where the development of antimicrobial resistance is common. Presently such centers are ill-advised to use a single drug such as cefoxitin, which does have excellent anti-gram–positive, anti-gram–negative, and antianaerobic activity but fails to control multiply-resistant gram-negative bacilli for which even aminoglycosides may not suffice.

There are an ever increasing number of cephalosporin derivatives from which to choose. The recommendations in Tables 6-5 and 6-6 are merely one approach to the rational use of these broad-spectrum beta–lactam antibiotics. The bias presented in these tables is that second generation cephalosporins such as cefuroxime probably do have a role, particularly in smaller hospitals, and that third generation cephalosporins, particularly in teaching hospitals, may not be as useful when compared to new agents such as ceftazidime that maintain excellent gram-negative coverage as well as add anti-pseudomonal coverage. In smaller community hospitals where resistant organisms are not frequently seen, second or third generation cephalosporins will suffice even for serious infections.

Finally, it cannot be emphasized too strongly that the use of antibiotics in most surgical infections is really an adjunct to the proper management of the locus of infection. Thus abscesses need to be drained, devitalized tissue needs to be debrided, and grossly contaminated wounds need to be packed and left open to heal by secondary intention. Equally important, the infected patient must be supported nutritionally. It is not uncommon for a patient with surgical infection to be grossly malnourished. In providing optimum care, this component of therapy is just as important as the choice of antibiotic.

SUMMARY

Despite advances in surgical management and antibiotic therapy, infection continues to be the most important cause of morbidity and mortality in postoperative surgical patients, leading to prolonged length of hospitalization and a consequent increased cost of hospital care. The most common surgical infections are hospital-acquired, and the responsible microorganisms are usually endogenous. If the development of such infections is to be minimized, efforts at preventing derangements in host-defense mechanisms must be ensured, and meticulous surgical techniques must be employed. When infections do occur, rational treatment should stress the importance of accurate identification of the responsible microorganism, logical investigation of the underlying source of infection, and adherence to sound principles governing antibiotic prophylaxis and treatment. The application of these guidelines to the clinical management of the surgical patient should lead to substantial improvements in the outcome of surgical disorders that are complicated by infection in terms of both a reduction in complications and an enhancement of survival.

REFERENCES

1. Altemeier, W.A., et al., editors: American College of Surgeons, Committee on Control of Surgical Infections of the Committee on Pre- and Postoperative Care: manual on control of infection in surgical patients, ed. 2, Philadelphia, 1984, J.B. Lippincott Co.
2. Baumgartner, J.D., et al.: Severe cytomegalovirus infection in mutiply transfused, splenectomized, trauma patients, Lancet **2**:63, 1982.
3. Benner, E.J., and Morthland, V.: Methicillin-resistant *Staphylococcus aureus:* antimicrobial susceptibility, N. Engl. J. Med. **277**:678, 1967.
4. Beutler, S.M., et al.: Delayed complications of candidemia (abstract no. 496), Twenty-second Interscience Conference on Antimicrobial Agents and Chemotherapy, Miami, 1982.
5. Boyce, J.M., and Causey, W.A.: Increasing occurrence of methicillin-resistant *Staphylococcus aureus* in the United States, Infect. Control **3**:377, 1982.
6. Charnley, J., and Eftekhar, N.: Postoperative infection in total prosthetic replacement arthroplasty of the hip joint, Br. J. Surg. **56**:641, 1969.
7. Copeland, E.M., MacFadyen, B.V., and Dudrick, S.J.: Effect of intravenous hyperalimentation on established delayed hypersensitivity in the cancer patient, Ann. Surg. **184**:60, 1976.
8. Cruse, P.J.E.: Surgical wound sepsis, Can. Med. Assoc. J. **102**:251, 1970.
9. Cruse, P.J.E.: Incidence of wound infection on the surgical services, Surg. Clin. North Am. **55**:1269, 1975.
10. Cruse, P.J.E., and Foord, R.: A five-year prospective study of 23,649 surgical wounds, Arch. Surg. **107**:206, 1973.
11. Dellinger, E.P., et al.: Risk of infection following laparotomy for penetrating abdominal injury, Arch. Surg. **119**:20, 1984.
12. Dumoulin, G.C., et al.: Aspiration of gastric bacteria in antacid-treated patients: a frequent cause of postoperative colonization of the airway, Lancet **1**:242, 1982.
13. Haley, R.W., et al.: Nosocomial infections in U.S. hospitals, 1975-1976, Am. J. Med. **70**:947, 1981.
14. Harley, D.P., et al.: Pulmonary embolism secondary to venous thrombosis of the arm, Am. J. Surg. **147**:221, 1984.
15. Hill, G.L., et al.: Malnutrition in surgical patients: an unrecognized problem, Lancet **1**:689, 1977.
16. Howard, R.J.: Host defense against infection, Parts I and II, Curr. Probl. Surg. **17**:267, 1980.
17. Katzenstein, D., Rickerson, V., and Brande, A.: New concepts of amebic liver abscess derived from hepatic imaging serodiagnosis and hepatic enzymes in 67 consecutive cases in San Diego, Medicine **61**:237, 1982.
18. Keighley, M.R.B., et al.: Randomized controlled trial of vancomycin for pseudomembranous colitis and postoperative diarrhea, Br. Med. J. **2**:1667, 1978.
19. Krizek, T.J., and Robson, M.C.: Biology of surgical infection, Surg. Clin. North Am. **55**:1261, 1975.
20. Kune, G.A.: Life-threatening surgical infection: its development and prediction, Ann. R. Coll. Surg. Engl. **60**:92, 1978.
21. Law, D.K., Dudrick, S.J., and Abdou, N.I.: The effect of protein-calorie malnutrition on immune competence of the surgical patient, Surg. Gynecol. Obstet. **139**:257, 1974.
22. Levison, M.E., et al.: Clindamycin compared with penicillin for the treatment of anaerobic lung abscess, Ann. Intern. Med. **98**:466, 1983.
23. Lowy, F.D., and Hammer S.M.: *Staphylococcus epidermidis* infections, Ann. Intern. Med. **99**:834, 1983.
24. MacLean, L.D., et al.: Host resistance in sepsis and trauma, Ann. Surg. **182**:207, 1975.
25. Maki, D.G., Weise, C.E., and Sarafin, H.A.: A semi-quantitative method for identifying intravenous catheter-related infection, N. Engl. J. Med. **296**:1305, 1977.

26. Meakins, J.L., et al.: Delayed hypersensitivity: indicator of acquired failure of host defenses in sepsis and trauma, Ann. Surg. **186:**242, 1977.
27. Melly, M.A., Thomison, J.B., and Rogers, D.B.: Fate of staphylococci within human leukocytes, J. Exp. Med. **112:**1121, 1960.
28. Miller, S.I., et al.: Hypoglycemia as a manifestation of sepsis, Am. J. Med. **68:**649, 1980.
29. Munster, A.M.: Septic thrombophlebitis: a surgical disorder, JAMA **230:**1010, 1974.
30. Nichols, R.L., et al.: Risk of infection after penetrating abdominal trauma, N. Engl. J. Med. **311:**1065, 1984.
31. Oreskovich, M.R., et al.: Duration of preventive antibiotic administration for penetrating abdominal trauma, Arch. Surg. **117:**200, 1982.
32. Pashby, B.J., Bolton, R.P., and Sheriff, R.J.: Oral metronidazole in *Clostridium difficile* colitis, Br. Med. J. **1:**1605, 1979.
33. Pietsch, J.B., Meakins, J.L., and Maclean, L.D.: The delayed hypersensitivity response: application in clinical surgery, Surgery **82:**349, 1977.
34. Rowlands, B.J., and Ericsson, C.D.: Comparative studies of antibiotic therapy after penetrating abdominal trauma, Am. J. Surg. **148:**791, 1984.
35. Saimot, A.G., et al.: Albendazole as a potential treatment for human hydratidosis, Lancet **2:**652, 1983.
36. Tarck, M., and Stamm, W.: Nosocomial infection of the urinary tract, Am. J. Med. **70:**65, 1981.
37. Tuazon, C.U., et al.: *Staphylococcus aureus* bacteremia: a relationship between formation of antibodies to teichoic acid and development of metastatic abscesses, J. Infect. Dis. **137:**57, 1978.
38. Watanakunakorn, C.: Treatment of infection due to methicillin-resistant *Staphylococcus aureus,* Ann. Int. Med. **97:**376, 1982.
39. Watanakunakorn, C., and Baird, I.M.: *Staphylococcus aureus* bacteremia and endocarditis associated with a curable infected intravenous device, Am. J. Med. **63:**253, 1977.
40. Wolfe, J.E., Bone, R.C., and Ruth, W.E.: Effects of corticosteroids in the treatment of patients with gastric aspiration, Am. J. Med. **63:**719, 1977.
41. Wynne, J.W., and Modell, J.H.: Respiratory aspiration of stomach contents, Ann. Int. Med. **87:**466, 1977.

7 G. Patrick Clagett

Hemostasis in Surgical Patients

"Hemostasis is usually taken for granted because it is such a highly perfected physiologic mechanism that it seldom fails. Yet, when it does, the lack of basic understanding of how the body is protected against loss of blood becomes strikingly apparent."—A.J. Quick[33]

The safe conduct of surgery depends on normal hemostasis. Surgeons challenge the hemostatic mechanism every day, and it is important that they have fundamental knowledge of the physiologic principles of hemostasis as well as derangements that precipitate bleeding. Because increasing numbers of operations, both routine and complex, are being performed on patients who have diseases and medical treatments that alter hemostasis, the frequency of abnormal bleeding in surgical patients can be expected to increase.[8]

HEMOSTASIS: PHYSIOLOGIC PRINCIPLES

Fluidity of circulating blood is normally maintained without appreciable evidence of platelet activation, blood coagulation, or hemorrhage. As a reaction to vascular injury, the hemostatic response occurs to arrest hemorrhage. A unique feature of this response is its confinement to the site of injury. This occurs through efficient, finely tuned interactions among circulating proteins (coagulation factors and inhibitors), cellular elements (platelets and white blood cells), and vascular endothelium. Despite all elements of the hemostatic mechanism being disseminated throughout the circulation, local hemorrhage is controlled with local clotting because of multiple checks and balances in the system. Thus normal hemostasis is concerned with vascular patency as well as the staunching of blood flow from the site of vascular injury. Circulating hemostatic elements and their properties are listed in Table 7-1.

Following transection of a vessel, vasoconstriction occurs because of intrinsic contractile responses of vascular smooth muscle, elasticity of the vessel wall, and chemicals secreted by platelets that promote vasoconstriction. Platelets rapidly adhere and aggregate at the site of injury and form a platelet plug that temporarily stops blood flow from the constricted vessel. The initial platelet plug is fragile, however, and rebleeding is likely to occur with relaxation of vasoconstriction unless fibrin formation occurs by activation of coagulation pathways. A fibrin network fortifies the platelet plug, makes it a more lasting seal, and provides a frame for fibroblastic ingrowth and ultimate healing of the injury.

Platelets are anucleate cells produced in the bone marrow by fragmentation of megakaryocytes. They normally circulate as round, disk-shaped cells with a life-span of 8 to 10 days. In this state, they do not adhere to other platelets, circulating blood cells, or normal endothelium. When platelets are activated by physical and chemical stimuli, they undergo a change in shape (become spherical), develop pseudopodia, and become sticky. Platelet adherence to surfaces and to other platelets is a unique function of this cell; it is stimulated by loss of endothelium or exposure to artificial surfaces (Fig. 7-1). Among the subendothelial components to which platelets adhere are collagen and basement membrane. A necessary cofactor for platelet adhesion to subendothelium is plasma von Willebrand's factor (VIIIR:VWF), the high-molecular-weight glycoprotein that circulates in association with factor VIII and is lacking in von Willebrand's disease. Von Willebrand's factor acts as a bridge between the subendothelium—where it binds spontaneously—and the platelet membrane, where it binds to specific high-affinity receptor sites made available during platelet activation. Platelet adherence to other platelets (platelet aggregation) also depends on membrane receptors. For this function, fibrinogen acts as a bridge between platelets by binding to receptors that are made available by the action of adenosine diphosphate (ADP), epinephrine, and perhaps other stimuli.

If the stimulus is sufficiently intense, the platelet release reaction occurs, in which platelets extrude into the microenvironment biologically active substances that are stored in intracytoplasmic granules. Platelet-dense granules contain ADP, serotonin, calcium, and other substances. Release of ADP leads to aggregation of other platelets in the area, thereby amplifying the response (see Fig. 7-1). Platelet alpha granules, which also release their contents during the platelet release reaction, contain a variety of proteins whose physiologic significance is not fully understood. One of these is platelet factor 4 (PF4), which can neutralize some of the anticoagulant effects of heparin. Another is platelet-derived growth factor (PDGF), a mitogen for smooth muscle cells and fibroblasts that may be important in healing and repair of vascular injury.[12] PDGF has also been cited as a pathogenetic factor for the development of atherosclerosis because it may stimulate hyperplasia of smooth muscle cells in vessels.

Pathways for platelet activation leading to the platelet release reaction are shown in Fig. 7-2. In the first pathway, stimulation of platelets by chemical and mechanical means results in the activation of phospholipases that hydrolyze membrane phospholipids and liberate arachidonic acid.[40] The membrane-bound enzyme cyclo-oxygenase converts arachidonic acid to prostaglandin endoperoxides. Cyclo-oxygenase is inhibited by aspirin and other nonsteroidal anti-inflammatory agents. Prostaglandin endoperoxides are then converted to thromboxane A_2, a labile substance that is a potent stimulus for platelet aggregation and

Table 7-1 **CIRCULATING HEMOSTATIC ELEMENTS**

					Minimum Levels Required in Surgical Patients		
Name	**Common Synonyms**	**In Vivo Half-life**	**Stability in Bank Blood**	**Agents Available for Replacement**	**Maintenance**	**Routine Surgery**	**Major Trauma, Extensive Surgery**
I	Fibrinogen	4-5 days	Stable	Whole blood, fresh frozen plasma, concentrated fibrinogen, cryoprecipitate	>50 mg/100 ml	>150 mg/100 ml	>200 mg/100 ml
II	Prothrombin	3-4 days	Stable	Whole blood, fresh frozen plasma, concentrated preparation	>20%	>40%	>50%
V	Proaccelevin, labile factor, accelerator globulin	1-3 days	Labile (50% activity at 1 week)	Fresh frozen plasma, whole blood <1 week old	>10%	>25%	>50%
VII	Proconvertin	4-6 hr	Stable	Whole blood, fresh frozen plasma, concentrated preparation	>10%	>10%	>50%
VIII	Antihemophilic factor (AHF), antihemophilic globulin	8-12 hr	Labile (30% activity at 1 week)	AHF concentrate, cryoprecipitate, fresh frozen plasma	>10%	>20%	>50%
IX	Christmas factor, plasma thromboplastin component (PTC)	24 hr	Stable	Whole blood, fresh frozen plasma, concentrated preparation	>10%	>20%	>50%
X	Stuart factor	48-60 hr	Stable	Whole blood, fresh frozen plasma, concentrated preparation	>10%	>20%	>50%
XI	Plasma thromboplastin antecedent (PTA)	60 hr	Stable	Whole blood, fresh frozen plasma	>10%	>20%	>50%
XII	Hageman factor	50-70 hr	Stable	Replacement unnecessary	—	—	—
XIII	Fibrin stabilizing factor	3-5 days	Stable	Whole blood, fresh frozen plasma	2%-3% of normal (?)	?	?
Platelets	—	8-11 days (lifespan)	Labile (no effective platelets at 48 hr)	Platelet concentrate	>10,000/mm^3	60-100,000/mm^3	>100,000/mm^3

vasoconstriction. Thromboxane A_2 leads to mobilization of intracellular calcium stores and triggers the platelet release reaction. Arachidonic acid can be metabolized by another membrane-bound enzyme, lipoxygenase. The products of lipoxygenase action on arachidonic acid include substances that may modulate platelet aggregation and promote chemotaxis of leukocytes. There are other (prostaglandin-independent) pathways for platelet release and aggregation, the most important of which is activated by thrombin. Thrombin stimulates prostaglandin synthesis in platelets, but this is not necessary for thrombin's induction of platelet release and aggregation. This reaction is illustrated by a simple experiment in which platelets treated with aspirin aggregate and undergo complete release when stimulated with thrombin. In vivo, it is likely that thrombin-induced platelet aggregation is the most important pathway in hemostatic platelet plug formation.

Fibrin formation is the end product of coagulation reactions, which classically have been divided into the intrinsic and extrinsic systems[4] (Fig. 7-3). The coagulation factors circulate in the form of inactive precursors known as zymogens or proenzymes. Each zymogen is converted to an

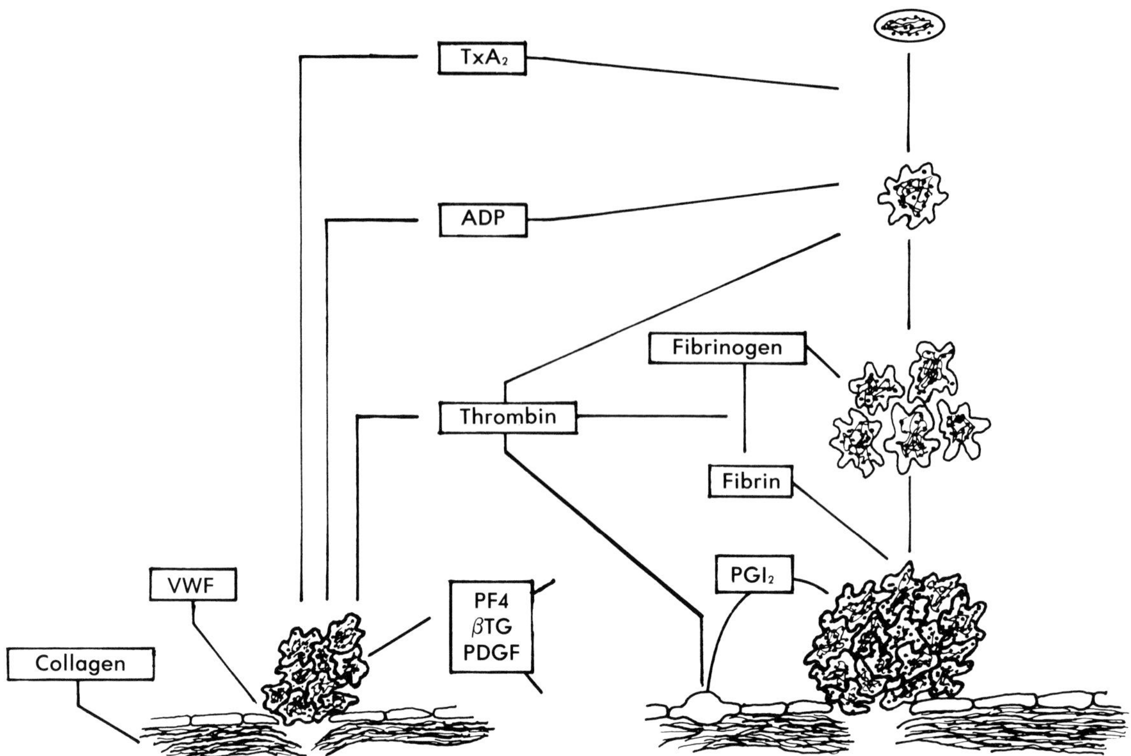

Fig. 7-1 Formation of platelet plug. The early reactions leading to formation of an unstable, reversible platelet plug are shown on the left of the figure. The later events, leading to the formation of a stable platelet plug, are shown on the right. Immediately following vascular injury with loss of endothelium, platelets adhere to exposed collagen and other subendothelial components. Platelet adherence is facilitated by plasma von Willebrand's factor *(VWF)*. Activation of platelets leads to generation of thromboxane A_2 *(TxA_2)* and platelet release of adenosine diphosphate *(ADP)*, which aggregates other platelets in the area and increases the bulk of the platelet plug. Other substances extruded into the microenvironment during the platelet release reaction include platelet factor 4 *(PF4)*, beta-thromboglobulin *(βTG)*, and platelet-derived growth factor *(PDGF)*. Activation of the intrinsic and extrinsic coagulation systems at the site of injury leads to thrombin generation, which also stimulates platelet aggregation and leads to fibrin formation, which in turn fortifies the platelet mass. Thrombin also stimulates prostacyclin *(PGI_2)* formation by endothelium, which limits the growth of the platelet plug.

active form and in turn activates the next clotting factor in the sequence. Five of the seven proteins in this cascade that leads to the generation of thrombin are activated during the coagulation process, and the other two proteins (V and VIII) are cofactors for their activation. There is good evidence that activation of factors XII, XI, IX, X, and prothrombin is accomplished by a common mechanism: each enzyme precursor is activated when it releases a protein-cutting enzyme that has the amino acid serine at its active center. These activated factors are known as serine proteases. The intrinsic pathway is designed for amplification in that the initiating proteins have a plasma concentration approximately 1/500 that of the final substrate fibrinogen. Initiation of the intrinsic pathway (termed "contract activation") involves a complex interaction in which factor XII undergoes a conformational change following exposure to nonendothelialized surfaces. The activation of factor XII occurs principally through the action of kallikrein, with high-molecular-weight kininogen acting as a necessary cofactor. This complicated surface-mediated series of reactions can lead not only to clotting, but also to kinin formation, complement activation, and fibrinolysis. In fact, the higher reactions in the intrinsic coagulation cascade are probably more important in triggering inflammatory responses and other defense reactions than they are in hemostasis. Patients with factor XII deficiency have no bleeding diathesis, and patients with factor XI deficiency generally have only mild bleeding.

The extrinsic coagulation system reactions leading to fibrin formation are much faster than those of the intrinsic system, and the extrinsic system is the dominant coagulation pathway in hemostasis. Almost all cells, including endothelial cells, contain a lipoprotein termed tissue thromboplastin, which is released with tissue trauma and cellular disruption. Circulating white cells are also rich in thromboplastic activity. The availability of tissue thromboplastin is a regulating factor in the expression of factor VII activity. Factor VII is the only coagulation factor that possesses

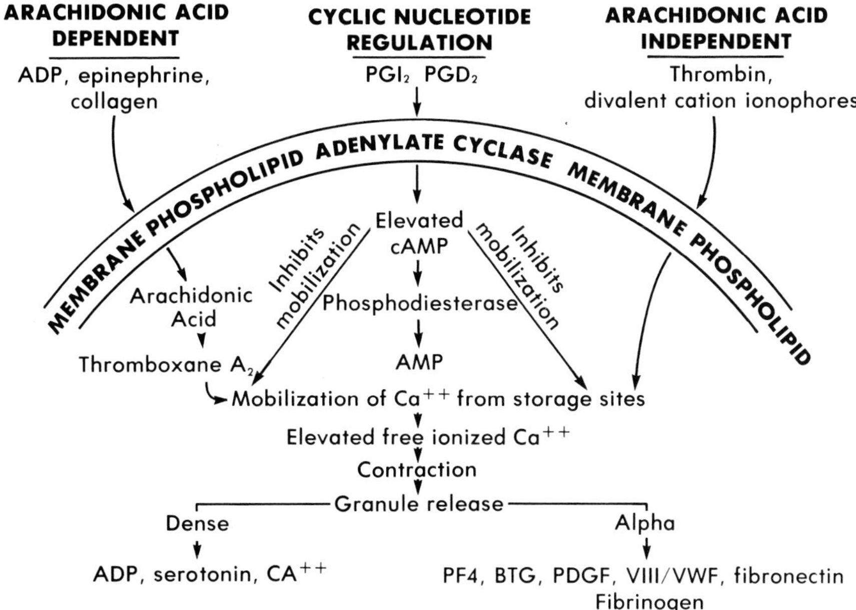

Fig. 7-2 Pathways for platelet activation. On the left is the arachidonic acid pathway, in which membrane phospholipids are converted to arachidonic acid, which in turn is converted by cyclo-oxygenase to prostaglandin endoperoxides and thromboxane A_2. Thromboxane A_2 leads to changes in intracellular Ca^{++}, which triggers contraction of platelet myofilaments and the extrusion of platelet dense–and alpha-granule contents into the surrounding microenvironment. There are other pathways (shown on the right) leading to platelet release that do not require arachidonic acid metabolism. The most important of these is thrombin activation of platelets, and this is probably the dominant physiologic pathway for platelet activation in normal hemostatsis. Elevation of platelet intracellular cAMP inhibits these activation pathways and abolishes the platelet release reaction. PGI_2 and other compounds inhibit platelet release and paralyze platelet function by stimulating membrane-bound adenylate cyclase.

enzyme activity without being subjected to limited proteolysis. However, factor VII is active only when tissue thromboplastin is present to act as a cofactor. The activation of factor X by factor VII, tissue thromboplastin, and calcium has represented the classical extrinsic pathway. This concept has been altered by the discovery of the activation of factor IX by factor VII[32] (Fig. 7-3). As with the activation of factor X, tissue thromboplastin is a necessary cofactor. This reaction sequence, in which the extrinsic pathway in effect activates the intrinsic pathway, lessens the distinction between the classical intrinsic and extrinsic systems and underscores the importance of the extrinsic system in normal hemostasis.

The activation of factor X by the intrinsic and extrinsic systems is the final common pathway to thrombin generation and fibrin formation. The conversion of prothrombin to thrombin by Xa is markedly accelerated by the presence of factor V, platelets, and calcium. Once generated, thrombin cleaves two pairs of arginine peptide bonds in fibrinogen, leading to the formation of fibrin monomer and fibrinopeptides. Fibrin monomer is then polymerized to a fibrin clot by factor XIII, a transamidase activated by thrombin. The cross-linked fibrin clot is comparatively stable and more resistant to lysis.

There was a tendency in the past to consider coagulation and platelet reactions as separate and distinct physiologic

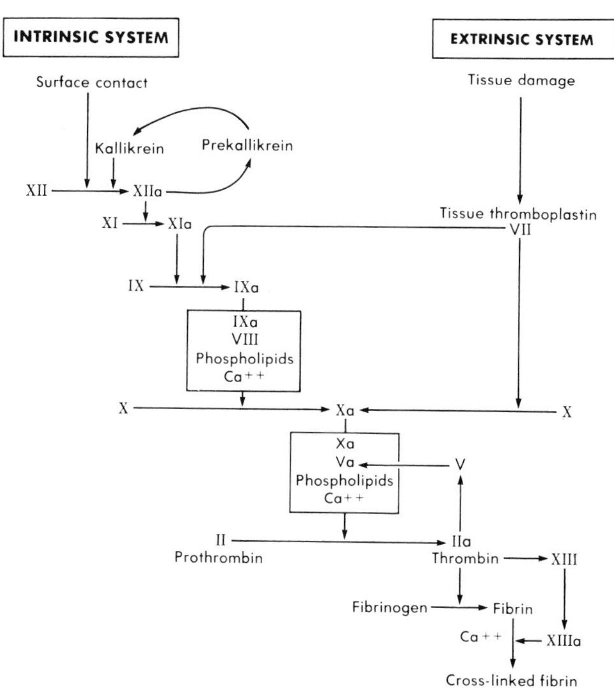

Fig. 7-3 The intrinsic and extrinsic coagulation protein reactions leading to thrombin generation and fibrin formation. Refer to text for details.

functions. This tendency was engendered in part by the necessities of in vitro laboratory investigation, in which the coagulation and platelet components of hemostasis were studied separately in purified systems. However, in vivo, platelet function and blood coagulation are intimately linked, and platelets are specifically and actively involved in providing essential catalytic and protective functions in coagulation reactions. Platelets provide a relatively stable surface on which coagulation proteins can interact. Since platelets adhere to the site of vascular injury, where hemostasis is needed, they in effect aid in locally concentrating activated coagulation factors, which might otherwise be swept away in the flowing blood. The areas in squares in the coagulation cascade shown in Fig. 7-3 are areas at which the phospholipid platelet membrane catalyzes the enzymatic coagulation reactions. In the first area, factor IXa forms a complex with factors VIII and X in the presence of calcium ions at the platelet surface. This complex is called the factor X activating complex. In the second area, activated factor X (Xa), whether produced by the intrinsic or the extrinsic pathway, attaches to the platelet membrane by activated factor V, which acts as a receptor for Xa (Fig. 7-4). This complex, termed the prothrombinase complex, then converts prothrombin to thrombin. The physiologic importance of the attachment of Xa to the platelet membrane is readily appreciated given that the prothrombin-activating potential of Xa is increased 300,000-fold. When bound to the platelet membrane, Xa is also protected against inactivation by the serine protease inhibitor antithrombin III. Platelets may also have a role in activating the upper levels of the intrinsic system. Evidence has accumulated that platelets stimulated by ADP can activate factor XII, and that platelets stimulated by collagen can activate factor XI. Thus platelets aggregating at the site of vascular injury may trigger intrinsic coagulation.

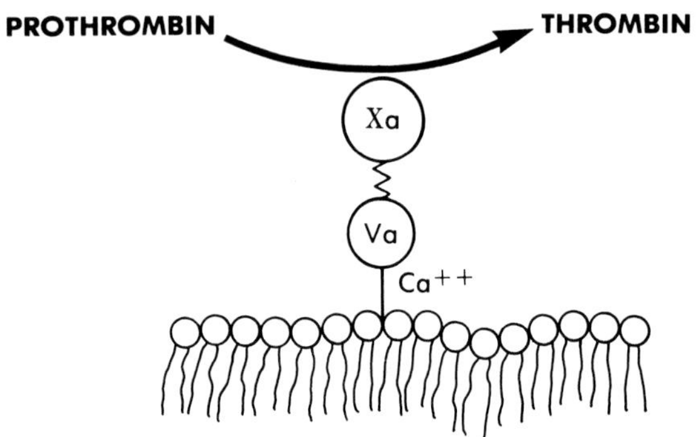

Fig. 7-4 Prothrombin activating complex. Activated factor V *(Va)* attached to the platelet phospholipid membrane acts as a receptor for activated factor X *(Xa),* which in turn converts prothrombin to thrombin. The activity of Xa is increased by 300,000-fold when complexed in this form with the platelet membrane.

The interdependence of the platelet and coagulation systems in the hemostatic response is illustrated schematically in Fig. 7-5. These physiologic concepts are particularly relevant to coagulopathies that develop in surgical patients whose disorders of hemostasis are usually acquired and complex. Only rarely are the hemostatic defects isolated, i.e., involving either platelet or coagulation mechanisms; most often the defects are multiple, have various intensities, and involve several aspects of both systems. An important concept in managing these coagulopathies is that mild defects, which have little impact on hemostasis when they are isolated, can lead to severe bleeding when they are multiple and involve both platelet and coagulation mechanisms. The effects are generally summative, and therapy must be based on correction of as many of the defects as possible.[8]

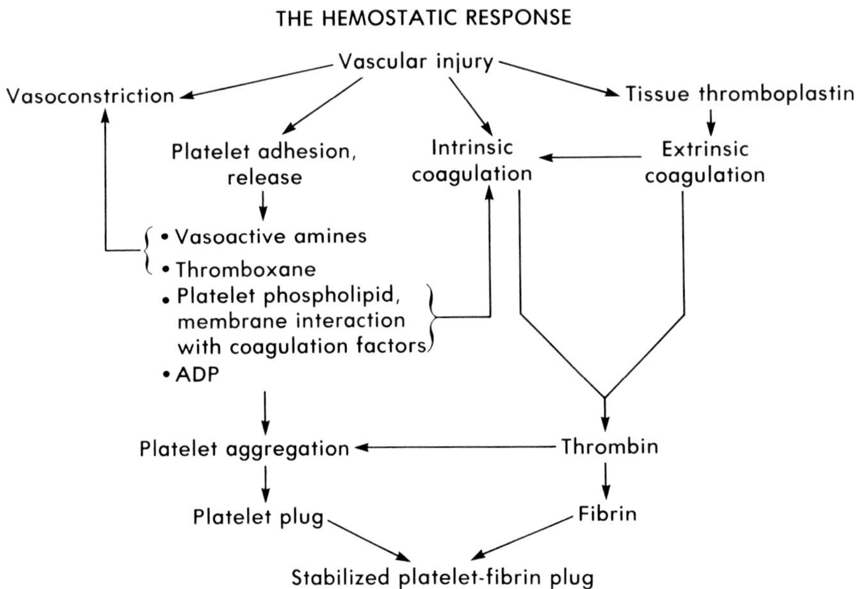

Fig. 7-5 The integrated hemostatic response depends on platelet and coagulation reactions, which proceed simultaneously. Both platelet and coagulation systems interact at multiple levels, and reactions in one accelerate reactions in the other.

Fibrinolysis and mechanisms that inhibit clotting limit the hemostatic response and maintain vascular patency. Fibrinolysis is stimulated by vascular injury and release of plasminogen activator from endothelial cells. A variety of tissue activators of plasminogen are present throughout the body and are released during tissue trauma (Fig. 7-6). Stimulation of fibrinolysis also occurs through activation of factor XII. Through these and other mechanisms, the inactive plasma precursor molecule plasminogen is converted to the proteolytic enzyme plasmin, which can digest fibrin, fibrinogen, and other coagulation proteins. Plasmin also acts on native plasminogen, liberates a portion of this molecule, and converts glu-plasminogen to lys-plasminogen. Lys-plasminogen selectively binds to fibrin during clotting and is more easily activated to plasmin than is native plasminogen. Selective incorporation of lys-plasminogen into the gel clot also protects the subsequent conversion product plasmin from the natural inhibitor alpha$_2$-antiplasmin, which efficiently neutralizes plasmin in the fluid phase only. Thus the action of plasmin is localized to the site of clotting or thrombus formation, where fibrin is digested. Free plasmin is thus prevented from escaping into the general circulation. Small amounts of plasmin that leak into the circulation or are generated in flowing blood are rapidly inactivated by the action of alpha$_2$-antiplasmin and other inhibitors. When plasminogen activator or plasmin is present in excess, the unchecked action of plasmin impairs hemostasis by digesting fibrinogen and other coagulation proteins. The products of plasmin action on fibrinogen and fibrin, particularly fragments X and Y, possess striking anticoagulant properties, principally interference with fibrin monomer polymerization (Fig. 7-7). These fragments also impair hemostasis by inhibiting platelet formation.

Endothelial cells possess a number of properties and functions that limit the hemostatic response (Fig. 7-8). A cyclo-oxygenase enzyme system that is present in the endothelial cell membrane can oxidize arachidonic acid to prostaglandin endoperoxides.[40] These intermediates, together with endoperoxides produced by stimulated platelets in the area, can be converted to prostacyclin, a potent platelet anti-aggregatory substance that also causes vasodilation. Thrombin stimulates endothelial production of prostacyclin, which inhibits platelet adherence and aggregation by elevating intraplatelet cAMP through stimulation of adenylate cyclase (Fig. 7-2). Endothelium also possesses a thrombin receptor, thrombomodulin, that serves as a cofactor together with thrombin for the activation of circulating protein C, an inhibitory blood-clotting protein.[16] Protein C is a vitamin K–dependent protein that is

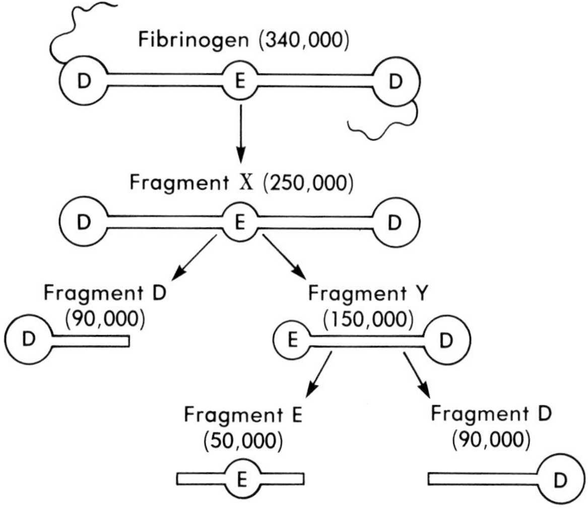

Fig. 7-7 Fibrinogen is cleaved into several fragments (molecular weights in parentheses) by the action of plasmin.

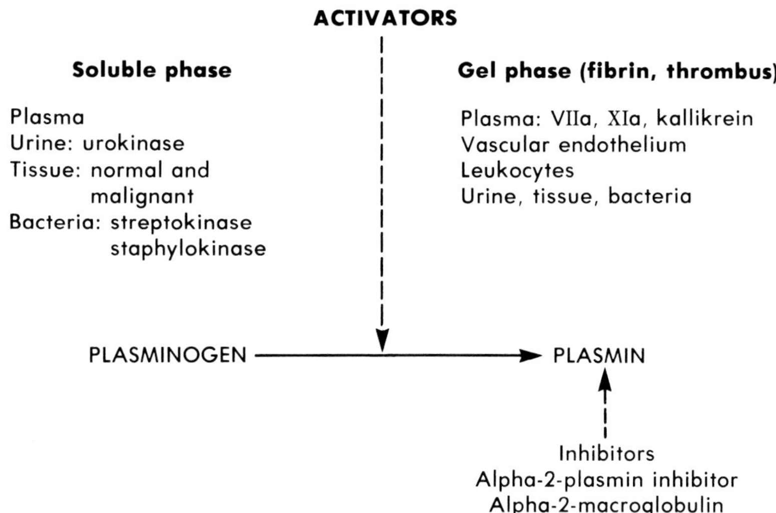

Fig. 7-6 Activators of plasminogen are categorized as soluble (found circulating or in body fluids) and gel (localized to fibrin clot or tissue). Plasmin is neutralized principally by alpha$_2$-antiplasmin and alpha$_2$-macroglobulin. Of the two inhibitors, alpha$_2$-antiplasmin reacts with plasmin much more rapidly and is the predominant circulating inhibitor preventing free generation of plasmin.

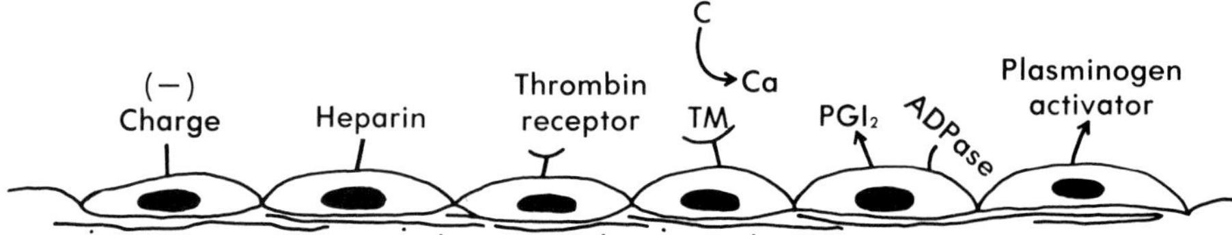

Fig. 7-8 Endothelial cells have several mechanisms that limit thrombus formation. There is a net negative charge that repels cellular elements. Proteoglycans (heparan sulfate) are synthesized by endothelial cells that have anticoagulant activity (accelerate antithrombin III reactions). There are thrombin receptors on the cell surface that bind and inactivate thrombin and activate protein C by the thrombomodulin *(TM)* complex. Platelet activation is limited by endothelial prostacyclin *(PGI_2)* production and by the action of endothelial ADPase, which degrades ADP that has been released by platelets and from other sources in the area of vascular injury. Finally, endothelium is the principal source of plasminogen activator, which is released by damage to endothelial cells.

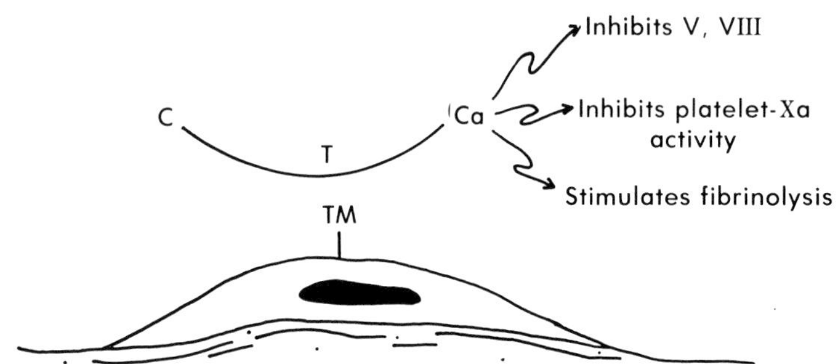

Fig. 7-9 When thrombin *(T)* binds to a specific receptor—termed thrombomodulin *(TM)*—on the endothelial cell surface, the resulting complex is able to activate protein C. Activated protein C *(Ca)* acts as a potent anticoagulant by inhibiting factors V and VIII, neutralizes Xa activity, and stimulates fibrinolysis.

made in the liver. When activated by the endothelium-thrombomodulin-thrombin complex, it acts as a potent anticoagulant and also stimulates fibrinolysis (Fig. 7-9). Endothelium is also a rich source of plasminogen activator, which is released with local endothelial trauma. Other properties of endothelial cells that may have physiologic importance include the presence of a net negative charge on the endothelial surface and the presence of an enzyme (endothelial ADPase) capable of degrading ADP; this may limit platelet aggregation. A recent discovery is the importance of heparin sulfate (a glycosaminoglycan with anticoagulant properties) on the endothelial cell surface.[36] This substance, synthesized by endothelial and smooth muscle cells, is capable of activating antithrombin III. This interaction may be physiologically important in maintaining blood fluidity and preventing clotting at the endothelial surface.

An important plasma mechanism for limiting clotting and modulating hemostasis is the presence of plasma serine protease inhibitors, the most important of which is antithrombin III. Antithrombin III inhibits not only thrombin but also the activated coagulation factors XIIa, XIa, IXa, and Xa. Plasma kallikrein and plasmin are also inhibited by antithrombin III. Antithrombin III is unique in that its inhibitory activity is dramatically increased by the presence of the anticoagulant heparin.[35] The reaction between antithrombin III and thrombin or factor Xa is enhanced at least 1000-fold by heparin.

PREOPERATIVE ASSESSMENT

Evaluation of hemostatic competence is mandatory in all preoperative patients, regardless of the magnitude of the proposed operation. Even a "minor" surgical procedure in a patient with impaired hemostasis is a major undertaking; a diligent search for occult bleeding disorders should be a routine part of the preoperative assessment. This does not require an expensive battery of laboratory tests in the vast majority of patients. Emphasis should be placed on a careful history and physical examination, with specific inquiries directed at a history of abnormal bleeding. The history should elicit whether the patient bleeds unusually in response to minor trauma or spontaneously in the absence of trauma. The responses to major and minor surgery and to dental extractions are particularly helpful. A patient who has recently undergone surgery without bleeding complications has had a far better test of hemostasis than any laboratory can provide. The manifestations of abnormal bleeding can provide clues to the nature of the underlying hemostatic defect. Easy bruisability, ecchymoses, petechial hemorrhages, nosebleeds, and oral mucosal and gingival bleeding generally indicate thrombocytopenia or a qualitative platelet disorder, whereas joint hemorrhages, deep muscular hematomas, and retroperitoneal bleeds are usually signs of a coagulation defect (congenital factor deficiency or anticoagulant use). The family history is relevant, and a pedigree chart of a familial bleeding tendency may provide important clues. Classic hemophilia (factor

Table 7-2 **LABORATORY TESTS AND HEMOSTATIC DISORDERS**

Bleeding Diathesis	APTT	PT	Bleeding Time	Platelet Count	Fibrinogen	Possible Defects
Absent	Abnormal	Normal	Normal	Normal	Normal	HMW kininogen, prekallikrein, factor XII, lupus anticoagulant
Present	Abnormal	Normal	Normal	Normal	Normal	XI, IX, VIII, heparin
Present	Abnormal	Abnormal	Normal	Normal	Normal	V, X, II, dysfibrinogenemia, heparin, malnutrition, warfarin
Present	Normal	Abnormal	Normal	Normal	Normal	VII
Present	Abnormal	Normal	Abnormal	Normal	Normal	von Willebrand's disease
Present	Abnormal	Abnormal	Abnormal	Normal	Low	Afibrinogenemia, hyperfibrinolysis
Present	Normal	Normal	Abnormal	Abnormal	Normal	Thrombocytopenia
Present	Normal	Normal	Abnormal	Normal	Normal	Qualitative platelet disorder (aspirin, other drugs, thrombopathy)
Present	Normal	Normal	Normal	Normal	Normal	Factor XIII
Present	Abnormal	Abnormal	Abnormal	Abnormal	Abnormal	DIC, severe liver disease

VIII deficiency) and Christmas disease (factor IX deficiency) are transmitted as X-linked traits, whereas all other inherited deficiencies of coagulation factors affect both sexes. A careful drug history is particularly important. All patients should be asked specifically about the ingestion of aspirin and other drugs that interfere with platelet function.

In healthy patients having elective surgery, the only preoperative laboratory test needed is a simple platelet estimate based on a stained blood smear (normally 6 to 10 platelets per high-powered field are seen). This is important because thrombocytopenia can be occult, can stem from multiple causes, and is the most common cause of abnormal bleeding seen in general medical practice. Screening tests of coagulation such as the prothrombin time (PT) and the activated partial thromboplastin time (APTT) are generally unnecessary and are no substitute for a thorough history and physical examination directed toward bleeding disorders.[15] However, in preoperative patients with systemic, debilitating illnesses, patients scheduled to undergo cardiopulmonary bypass, and patients with an abnormal bleeding history, a more extensive laboratory evaluation is necessary.[5] General screening tests including APTT, PT, bleeding time, platelet count, and fibrinogen level are helpful in these situations. Possible interpretations or abnormal screening test results are shown in Table 7-2.

CONGENITAL BLEEDING DISORDERS

The most common congenital bleeding disorders are covered in this section. They include hemophilias A and B and von Willebrand's disease.[19]

Hemophilia A (factor VIII deficiency, classic hemophilia) is an X-linked, recessive bleeding disorder in which there is a molecular defect in the factor VIII molecule. The protein is present in normal amounts in patients with hemophilia A when measured by immunologic methods (normal levels of factor VIII antigen, VIII:Ag) but has impaired function because its procoagulant portion is defective or absent (decreased levels of factor VIII coagulant activity, VIII:C). The disease occurs only in males, with a frequency of approximately 1 per 10,000 male births. The sons of affected males will be free of the disease; daughters will be asymptomatic carriers of the trait. The severity of bleeding in patients with hemophilia A roughly correlates with factor VIII levels measured by functional assays (normal level = 50% to 100%). Individuals with factor VIII levels <1% are severely affected and have major bleeding episodes requiring therapy two to four times monthly. Those with levels between 1% and 5% are classified as having moderately severe disease and also suffer multiple spontaneous bleeds. Hemophiliacs with factor VIII levels greater than 5% of normal are mildly affected and usually hemorrhage only during surgery or trauma. Whereas patients with severe forms of the disease are usually diagnosed shortly after birth, those with mild disease may escape detection until adulthood.

Hemophilia B (factor IX deficiency, Christmas disease) is also an X-linked, recessive bleeding disorder. The clinical manifestations are identical to those of hemophilia A. However, the disease is much less common than hemophilia A, which comprises approximately 80% of all hemophilias. Some patients with hemophilia B synthesize an abnormal factor IX molecule that lacks procoagulant activity; others have no detectable factor IX antigenic material level in their blood and have a true deficiency of factor IX.

Clinically, abnormal bleeding in patients with hemophilias A and B is most frequently characterized by painful joint and muscle hemorrhages that lead to disabling long-term sequelae. Because platelet plug formation is normal, excessive hemorrhage from minor cuts and abrasions is unusual. Easy bruisability and bleeding into soft tissues are frequent, however, and are hallmarks of the disease. Hemarthroses appear in childhood shortly after the child begins to walk. The joints most frequently involved are (in descending order of frequency) the knees, elbows, ankles, shoulders, hips, and wrists. Joint hemorrhages lead to chronic synovitis, which predisposes a patient to further episodes of hemarthrosis and ultimately to established hemophilic arthropathy characterized by chronic pain, limitation of motion, disuse atrophy of local muscle groups, bony cysts, and fibrous or bony ankylosis of large joints. To prevent these disabling sequelae, aggressive factor replacement therapy is necessary at the first signs of joint hemorrhage; in some severe cases prophylactic treatment may be appropriate. Intramuscular hematomas are common in hemophiliacs and may lead to compression of adjacent nerves or other important structures. Hematomas of the psoas muscle cause abdominal pain, fever, and leukocytosis and thus may mimic acute appendicitis or other intra-abdominal surgical emergencies. Bleeding into musculofascial compartments can lead to compartment syndromes; in the forearm this may be manifested by median or ulnar nerve paralysis or Volkmann's ischemic contracture of the hand. Intracranial bleeding leads to death in 25% of hemophiliacs and may be subdural, epidural, subarachnoid, and intracerebral. Intraspinal bleeding with acute spinal cord syndromes can also occur.

Elective and emergency operations are hazardous undertakings in hemophiliacs and should be performed only in centers where expert care is available. This requires a coordinated team effort involving surgeon, hematologist, and blood bank and coagulation laboratory personnel. Adequate replacement therapy with meticulous laboratory monitoring of factor levels until complete healing occurs is the hallmark of safe surgery in patients with hemophilia. Replacement sources for factor VIII include cryoprecipitate and factor VIII concentrates. Because the half-life of factor VIII in plasma is between 8 and 12 hours, infusions are usually given every 8 to 12 hours. For major surgery, the factor VIII level should be >80% just before surgery and then maintained above 30% for 10 to 14 days. For extensive orthopedic surgery, 4 to 6 weeks of replacement therapy may be necessary. In hemophilia B, fresh frozen plasma can be used for a replacement source, but its use is limited by the volume necessary to achieve adequate factor IX levels. When circulatory overload is a concern, prothrombin complex concentrates (containing factors II, VII, IX, and X) can be used. For major surgery, the factor IX level should be >60% at the time of surgery and then should be kept above 30% for 10 to 14 days.

Certain perioperative guidelines should be observed for operations on hemophiliacs. Aspirin produces a marked prolongation of the bleeding time in hemophiliacs and can produce disastrous bleeding. Medications containing aspirin are contraindicated. Intramuscular injections should also be avoided. Generally, surgery should be scheduled early in the week to take advantage of the best availability of laboratory resources. Because of the great expense of hospitalization and replacement therapy in these individuals, one should consider performing minor necessary procedures such as dental extractions at the same time as major operations. During the operation, meticulous attention to hemostasis is critical. Ligation of small bleeders is used in preference to electrocoagulation because rebleeding may occur after the cauterized ends of vessels slough.

A particularly hazardous situation arises when a patient with hemophilia A develops an inhibitor to factor VIII as a complication of transfusion therapy. This occurs in 6% to 8% of patients with severe hemophilia. Factor VIII inhibitors neutralize factor VIII, act as anticoagulants, and increase with infusions of factor VIII. Factor VIII preparations are therefore avoided in such individuals with minor bleeds. In life-threatening bleeding, when vigorous plasmapheresis is used to reduce the inhibitor titer, it may be followed by large doses of factor VIII concentrate. Prothrombin complex concentrates may also be used to control severe bleeding in patients with inhibitors. The beneficial action of these concentrates is probably the result of small amounts of activated coagulation factors, the procoagulant activity of which bypasses the factor VIII–dependent clotting reactions. Factor VIII inhibitors have also been described in the following: in nonhemophiliacs, most commonly in patients with immunologic disorders such as systemic lupus erythematosus, rheumatoid arthritis, regional enteritis, and ulcerative colitis; in postpartum females, and, on rare occasions, in elderly patients of either sex.

After hemophilia, von Willebrand's disease is the congenital bleeding disorder that appears most commonly in adult life. The disease is transmitted as an autosomal trait, with dominant and recessive modes of inheritance. Von Willebrand's disease is characterized by a dual hemostatic defect. First, there is a deficiency or absence of von Willebrand factor (VIIIR:VWF), which is important in platelet adhesion to subendothelial surfaces. This defect causes impaired platelet plug formation and results in prolongation of the bleeding time. Ristocetin cofactor activity (VIIIR:RCo), the activity necessary for ristocetin-induced platelet aggregation, may in part reflect the plasma levels of VIIIR:VWF. Second, there is usually a deficiency of factor VIII procoagulant activity (VIII:C) that contributes to the hemostatic defect. It is uncertain whether these activities reside in the same or different molecules (circulating in complexed form), but it is clear that the primary defect results from either decreased quantities of the entire factor VIII–von Willebrand factor protein complex or its presence in dysfunctional form.

In severe von Willebrand's disease, abnormal bleeding is present in early childhood; in less severe forms, the disease may not be apparent before adulthood. Mucosal and cutaneous hemorrhages are characteristic of the disorder. Epistaxis, gingival bleeding, and gastrointestinal bleeding are common, and menorrhagia is frequent. Excessive bleeding after tonsillectomy, other surgery, or dental extraction, and after otherwise normal pregnancy and delivery is frequently the first manifestation of the disease. In contrast to hemophilias A and B, joint and muscle hemorrhages are rare, except in severe forms of von Willebrand's disease. The mainstay of therapy for von Willebrand's disease is transfusion of cryoprecipitate containing all of the molecular forms of the factor VIII–von Willebrand factor complex. Therapy should be directed at normalizing the bleeding time and attaining normal levels of VIIIR:RCo. Factor VIII concentrates that contain large amounts of VIII:C do not contain sufficient VIIIR:VWF to efficiently restore the bleeding time to normal, so they should not be used. Cryoprecipitate both corrects the bleeding time and restores adequate levels of VIII:C. In preparing patients for surgery, replacement therapy should begin 1 day before operation. Aspirin should be avoided under all circumstances, and the same general guidelines for surgery on patients with hemophilia should be observed.

Table 7-3 **PATTERNS OF SCREENING TESTS IN COMMON ACUTE BLEEDING DISORDERS**

Disorder	Platelets	Prothrombin Time	Activated Partial Thromboplastin Time	Thrombin Time	Fibrinogen
Massive transfusion	↓	N or ↑	↑	N	N
Disseminated intravascular coagulation	↓	↑	↑	↑	↓
Liver disease	N or ↓	↑	↑	↑	N or ↓
Vitamin K deficiency and coumarin drugs	N	↑	↑	N	N
Circulating heparin	N	N or ↑	↑	↑	N
Hyperfibrinolysis	N	↑	↑	↑	↓

N, normal; ↑, increased; ↓, decreased.

ACQUIRED HEMOSTATIC DISORDERS

General Treatment Principles

In surgical patients, the vast majority of coagulopathies are acute and acquired and are frequently associated with specific clinical settings, such as massive trauma with large transfusion requirements, shock, sepsis, extensive malignancy, and deranged liver function. Abnormal bleeding may first be recognized intraoperatively. Early recognition is important; at the first hint of intraoperative coagulopathy, the surgeon and the anesthesiologist should work together to diagnose the bleeding disorder and to alert those who will be needed to manage the problem (laboratory, blood bank, clinical pathologist, and hematologist). Getting these people involved early can prevent confrontations, delays, and inconveniences should the need for blood component therapy arise later. The surgeon should remain flexible and keep in mind that he or she may have to alter the operative plan and may even have to abort the procedure. Until the situation is clarified, maneuvers that commit to extensive dissections and larger, complex procedures should be avoided. For example, a simple loop colostomy with exteriorization of the lesion would be preferable to colonic resection with primary anastomosis in this setting.

The first sign of intraoperative coagulopathy is persistent oozing of blood from raw surfaces that previously had been dry. During vascular surgical procedures, this may be manifested by generalized, slow oozing through interstices of a knitted Dacron prosthesis that previously had been adequately preclotted and was bloodtight. In more advanced and obvious cases, the surgeon may note that blood welling up in the field fails to clot. The anesthesiologist may first recognize coagulopathy by noting the onset of bleeding from intravenous sites, from the nose at the site of nasogastric tube insertion, from the oropharynx, and from the endotracheal tube. Blood should immediately be drawn for determination of platelet count, prothrombin time, activated partial thromboplastin time, thrombin time, and fibrinogen level. Most acute, acquired coagulopathies can be defined within an hour with these simple screening tests (Table 7-3). Depending on the severity of bleeding, therapy need not be withheld pending the results of these tests. Therapy is often empiric and based on the clinical setting. The value of blood tests lies as much in assessing progress in treating coagulopathy as in making a specific diagnosis. Additionally, it is wise to obtain extra blood samples at the onset of coagulopathy so that citrated plasma can be stored for more detailed laboratory analyses later, if needed.

Many acute coagulopathies are transient and require no specific treatment. Major attention should focus on maintaining blood volume and hemodynamic stability. Avoidance of hypotension and shock states that promote coagulopathy is a mainstay of therapy. If blood is being transfused at the onset of coagulopathy, it should be stopped immediately on the assumption that incompatible blood with major transfusion reaction might be etiologic. Heparinized solutions being infused through radial and pulmonary arterial catheters to maintain patency should also be changed. It is possible that a dosage error was made in mixing solutions, resulting in inadvertent systemic heparinization.

For more complex coagulopathies, management is frequently complicated by lack of precise diagnosis, coupled with logistic problems in obtaining blood component therapy. The vast majority of intraoperative coagulopathies are treated with platelet concentrate, which is not always readily available. Thrombocytopenia and platelet dysfunction are especially important to correct, and proper therapy depends on infusion of platelets in amounts adequate to restore hemostasis. The strain on blood bank resources is a legitimate concern of hematologists or clinical pathologists who, in most hospitals, control these resources. This concern is often interpreted by the surgical team as an unsympathetic and uncooperative attitude, and the confrontation that results is counterproductive in solving the problem at hand.

A frequent error on the part of clinical pathologists and hematologists is that they require the results of diagnostic coagulation tests deranged to a certain minimum degree before they will release blood components from the blood bank. This approach is wrong from several standpoints. First, valuable time is wasted in awaiting the results of blood tests to establish a precise diagnosis. The clinical setting (e.g., severe trauma, massive transfusion, sepsis, liver disease) determines the diagnosis and directs therapy as much as do specific blood tests. If the coagulopathy is life-threatening, component therapy should be initiated before the results of the coagulation screen are available. Bleeding that continues while the surgeon awaits blood test results will only exacerbate the coagulopathy. Second, as emphasized previously, unexpected intraoperative coagulopathies are usually acquired (as opposed to congenital) disorders of hemostasis and as such are complex, involving platelet and coagulation mechanisms. Individual coagulation tests may be only mildly deranged and may not reflect the hemostatic instability in a bleeding patient. For example, a bleeding patient with massive transfusion and a dilutional coagulopathy may have a platelet count of 90,000/mm^3 and only mild prolongations of the prothrombin time and the activated partial thromboplastin time. Withholding component therapy in such a patient because of unimpressive laboratory results may be dangerous.

With the onset of severe coagulopathy, further blood transfusions should generally be in the form of whole blood. Fresh warm blood is optimal but rarely available. Packed red cells coupled with crystalloid infusions do not replenish coagulation factors and should be used only if whole blood is unavailable. Whole blood contains normal amounts of all hemostatic elements with the exception of factors V and VIII and platelets (see Table 7-1). If volume overload is a concern, packed red cells can be infused together with limited amounts of fresh frozen plasma (FFP). The most common major underlying defects in unexpected intraoperative coagulopathy are thrombocytopenia and platelet dysfunction, and infusions of platelet concentrate are the cornerstone of therapy. However, every attempt should be made to correct coagulation abnormalities first, and this usually requires infusion of two to four units of FFP. Such an approach provides an optimal in vivo setting for the platelets to function hemostatically and minimizes the amount of platelets required. Because of the ready availability of FFP, legitimate concerns have been raised about the overuse of this component and the increased potential for disease transmission (hepatitis and acquired immunodeficiency syndrome [AIDS]). FFP should be used only when clinical or laboratory evidence of coagulopathy is present or the patient's life is at risk from further bleeding from nonmechanical, nonsurgically correctable sources; indiscriminate use of this component should be discouraged.

Most acute, acquired bleeding disorders of moderate severity that develop intraoperatively can be managed successfully with component therapy. However, in some cases of severe coagulopathy—particularly those associated with major trauma, massive transfusion, shock, and disseminated intravascular coagulation—bleeding may be refractory. In such cases, the hemostatic defect is uncorrectable because of continued surgical blood loss. A vicious cycle is established in which it is impossible to replenish circulating hemostatic elements because of the rapidity of hemorrhage. This situation often leads to death.

In cases of severe refractory coagulopathy, the wisest course may be to terminate the operation after ligating all major bleeding vessels and to pack the abdominal cavity tightly with gauze pads.[38] Before this is done, vessels necessary for survival should be repaired, open ends of bowel and other hollow organs should be ligated with purse-string sutures, and the spleen and kidney should be removed if they are bleeding. The peritoneal cavity is closed securely (watertight) with running fascial sutures, and the patient is returned to the intensive care unit for stabilization. A concerted effort is made to correct the coagulopathy, after which the patient is returned to the operating room (usually 12 to 24 hours later) for definitive surgery. Because of increased intra-abdominal pressure and elevated diaphragms, positive pressure ventilation is mandatory in these patients. The principle of temporary abdominal tamponade with correction of hemostatic defects can be life-saving because it effectively halts blood loss and stabilizes the blood volume so that hemostatic levels of platelets and coagulation factors can be achieved with infusions of blood components.

Massive Transfusion

The principle underlying the pathogenesis of coagulopathy associated with massive transfusion is dilution.[10] Stored blood that is more than 48 hours old is deficient in platelets and clotting factors V and VIII (Table 7-1); replacement of the patient's blood with this blood impairs hemostasis. Because of large body reserves, deficiencies of factors V and VIII in the patient's blood are rarely severe—this explains the minimally prolonged prothrombin and activated partial thromboplastin times seen in this disorder. On the other hand, thrombocytopenia may be marked.[9] In most studies of trauma patients, the platelet count falls to 100,000/mm^3 after a 10-U blood transfusion (Fig. 7-10). Thrombocytopenia of this degree is tolerated in most individuals. However, when thrombocytopenia combines with mild clotting factor deficiencies in patients with surgical and traumatic wounds in whom further transfusion is anticipated, hemostasis may rapidly decompensate. Correction of thrombocytopenia is the mainstay of treatment.

Coagulation defects other than simple dilution of hemostatic elements may complicate some cases of massive transfusion. Disseminated intravascular coagulation (DIC) can develop, particularly when shock, extensive trauma, multiple long-bone fractures, or penetrating brain injury is present with massive transfusion. Laboratory assessment is helpful (Table 7-3), and the presence of a low fibrinogen level, markedly prolonged activated partial thromboplastin time, prolonged thrombin time, and elevated fibrin split products is strong evidence of DIC. Another abnormality frequently encountered in massive transfusion is qualitative platelet dysfunction. Most studies document prolongation of the bleeding time disproportionate to the degree of thrombocytopenia present.[29] The prevalence of this finding and the nature of the platelet defect are controversial, but the clinical relevance is that platelet transfusions may be needed even though the systemic platelet count is at "hemostatically safe levels." One should aim for a platelet count of at least 100,000/mm^3 in patients with established transfusion coagulopathy.

In rare cases, it may be possible to prevent coagulopathy associated with massive transfusion by the judicious prophylactic use of blood components. All too often, attempts at restoring hemostasis are not begun until the onset of clinically overt coagulopathy. In patients in whom massive transfusion is inevitable, 6 to 10 U of platelet concentrate should be given after the first 10 U of blood have been

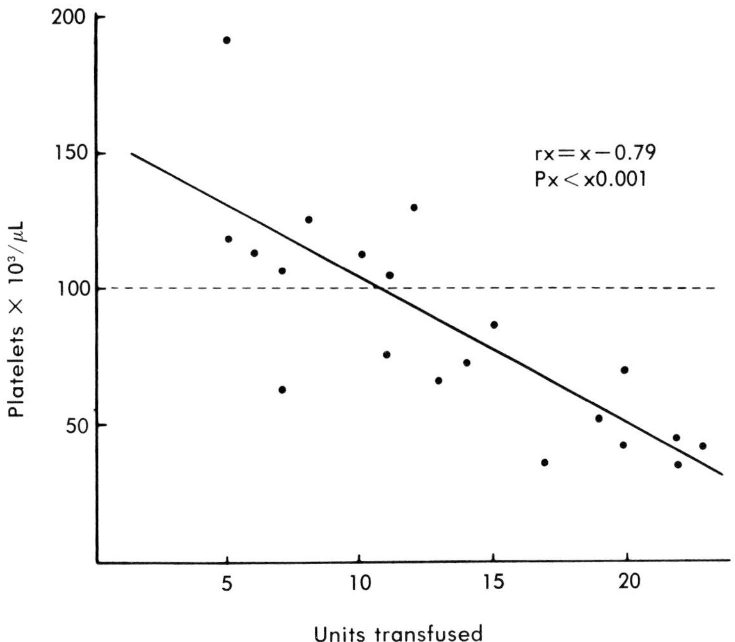

Fig. 7-10 Relationship between units of blood transfused and platelet count in patients with trauma. (From Clagett, G.P., and Olsen, W.R., Ann. Surg. **187:**369, 1978.)

administered and for every successive 10 U of blood. To replenish clotting factor deficiencies, 1 U of FFP should be given for every 3 to 4 U of infused blood. An alternative approach is to give fresh whole blood in a ratio to stored blood of 1:2 to 1:4. This is the ideal, but fresh blood is rarely available in emergencies. In established massive transfusion coagulopathy, 2 to 4 U of FFP should be infused, followed by 8 to 10 U of platelet concentrate. The following formula is useful in guiding platelet transfusion therapy:

$$\text{No. of bags of platelet concentrate} = \frac{\text{Desired increment} \times \text{Body surface area } (M^2)}{10{,}000}$$

In patients with low fibrinogen levels, infusion of cryoprecipitate may be appropriate. Each bag contains 150 to 250 mg of fibrinogen, but only 50% to 60% is functional. To raise the level of circulating effective fibrinogen by 100 mg/dl, four bags of cryoprecipitate are required for every 10 kg of body weight.

Disseminated Intravascular Coagulation

DIC is an acute manifestation of a disease process that may have many different underlying causes. Bleeding from DIC results from consumption of hemostatic elements (principally fibrinogen, factors V and VIII, and platelets), stimulation of excessive fibrinolysis, and formation of fibrin(ogen) degradation products that interfere with fibrin polymerization and impair platelet function. The clinical presentation is variable, depending on the intensity of the triggering stimulus (acute, fulminant vs. chronic, compensated DIC), the location of the site of stimulus (localized intravascular or extravascular vs. systemic consumption of hemostatic elements), and the nature of the stimulus and its predominant effect on the hemostatic balance (excessive coagulation vs. excessive fibrinolysis). There are few if any specific diagnostic laboratory tests in routine clinical practice, and the presence or absence of DIC depends largely on the clinical setting in which abnormal coagulation tests are found. In addition to the tests listed in Table 7-3, a stained blood smear demonstrating fragmented red cells, and tests documenting elevated fibrin(ogen) split products, are helpful.

In surgical patients, multiple clinical settings are associated with DIC and intraoperative coagulopathy.[11] Severe bacterial infections with septicemia and endotoxemia, often stemming from gram-negative gut organisms, frequently trigger DIC. Gram-positive bacterial infections also can be etiologic. Massive tissue trauma, especially when associated with shock, can flood the circulation with thromboplastic and procoagulant substances and lead to acute consumption of hemostatic elements sufficient to incite bleeding. Localized trauma in the form of brain injury (usually severe and penetrating)[20] and long-bone fractures can trigger DIC by similar mechanisms. Many tumors, particularly mucin-secreting adenocarcinomas, are rich in thromboplastic substances and specific procoagulants (for example, factor X–activating protein), and DIC is always a potential hazard when the tumor is large or widely metastatic. Pancreatic and prostatic adenocarcinomas are particularly vulnerable to this complication, but any disseminated malignancy can cause the problem. DIC associated with malignancy is frequently chronic and partially compensated, and it may lead to thromboembolic events that require surgical intervention, such as arterial thromboembolectomy. The surgeon should be alert to the possibility of underlying chronic DIC in such patients because surgery can trigger uncompensated DIC with hemorrhagic complications. Similarly, chronic partially compensated DIC can occur with aortic aneurysms,[30] and it has been estimated that 4% to 5% of patients with large aortic aneurysms have this complication.[18] Ecchymoses seen at the preoperative hospital examination are a cardinal feature of DIC and should prompt laboratory confirmation. Aortic surgery in such patients can be associated with severe bleeding; specific measures, such as the use of nonporous vascular prostheses (e.g., woven Dacron) and having blood components for use intraoperatively and postoperatively, are important in minimizing complications.

One of the more common causes of sudden, unexpected coagulopathy is DIC caused by hemolysis from a major transfusion reaction. This can occur with the infusion of as little as 25 ml of mismatched blood. The clinical manifestations—shaking chills, fever, and back pain—are obscured by general anesthesia, and sudden hypotension and diffuse bleeding may be the only clues of intraoperative transfusion reaction. The diagnosis is subtle in this setting and should be suspected in any operative patient who develops sudden bleeding and hypotension while receiving blood. Treatment is directed at (1) stopping transfusion, (2) restoring normal blood pressure and volume with crystalloid and appropriate pharmacologic support, (3) alkalinization with sodium bicarbonate, and (4) administering mannitol to protect against renal tubular necrosis. Fortunately, the DIC that attends a major transfusion reaction is transient and usually requires no treatment once the causative agent has been stopped.

The treatment of all forms of DIC occurring intraoperatively is aimed primarily at supporting normal blood volume and pressure and expeditious removal of the stimulus for DIC.[27] Specific therapies directed against DIC, such as heparinization, have no place in an acutely bleeding patient and are contraindicated in this setting.[17] Likewise, antifibrinolytic agents such as epsilon amino-caproic acid (EACA) are ill-advised because a degree of fibrinolysis protects against occlusive thrombosis of capillaries and prevents organ ischemia.[7] Most authorities believe that EACA should not be used for DIC unless the patient is heparinized. In a patient with DIC undergoing operation, control of bleeding must by necessity be effected by infusions of FFP (to replace fibrinogen and factors V and VIII), cryoprecipitate (to replace fibrinogen), and platelets. The fear of "fueling the fire" and making the process worse has been overemphasized in the past. Component therapy can be life-saving in this difficult clinical circumstance.

Cardiopulmonary Bypass

Of the many factors contributing to the transient bleeding diathesis induced by cardiopulmonary bypass, platelet dysfunction most consistently correlates with the clinical bleeding seen in 2% to 5% of patients. The bleeding time is markedly prolonged during and shortly after bypass, bears little relationship to the circulating platelet count, and remains abnormal in patients who bleed.[22,28] Although the qualitative platelet defect has not been precisely defined, the central underlying event is extensive contact between blood and foreign surfaces of the extracorporeal circuit.[2] This leads to platelet activation characterized by platelet adhesion, formation of platelet aggregates, platelet thromboxane synthesis, partial release of platelet alpha and dense granule products, decreased density of circulating platelets, membrane abnormalities, and diminished sensitivity of platelets to standard agonists. Platelet function may be further impaired by hypothermia, heparin and other drugs used during the procedure, and preexisting hemostatic abnormalities. Thrombocytopenia from dilution, consumption, and sequestration of platelets in the reticuloendothelial system also prolongs the bleeding time. Other abnormalities that contribute to impaired hemostasis during cardiopulmonary bypass and are less-frequent causes of bleeding include dilutional reductions in coagulation factors, activation of fibrinolysis, and incomplete reversal of heparin.[3] DIC has been observed rarely, usually in patients with severely depressed cardiac output or in patients in whom inadequate amounts of heparin were administered during cardiopulmonary bypass.[6]

Immediately following cardiac surgery, the patient should have a platelet count, prothrombin time, and partial thromboplastin time. The blood for these tests should be drawn by fresh venipuncture and not from injection ports of intravascular catheters. Moderate thrombocytopenia (100,000 to 150,000/mm^3) from consumption, and mild prolongations of the PT and APTT resulting from small quantities of circulating heparin or from increases in circulating fibrin(ogen) degradation products, are frequently seen immediately after cardiopulmonary bypass. In the absence of excessive bleeding, these mild abnormalities need not be treated. However, if bleeding is excessive (>100 ml/hr from mediastinal drainage tubes), or if the initial screening test results are markedly abnormal, further evaluation and treatment are necessary. With massive hemorrhage, a mechanical source for bleeding should be suspected; clotting studies should be drawn but should not delay the return of the patient to the operating room. Marked prolongations in the APTT and activated clotting time (ACT) are usually the result of excess heparin, which should be treated with protamine sulfate, 25 to 50 mg; the response should be noted with repeat determinations of the APTT and ACT. If there is thrombocytopenia (<75 to 100,000/mm^3) and bleeding, 8 to 12 U of platelet concentrate should be transfused. In some cases, generalized bleeding occurs in the absence of major abnormalities in clotting tests and in thrombocytopenia. In these cases, defects in platelet function are usually etiologic, and platelet transfusions should be administered. It is not necessary to document platelet dysfunction before giving platelet transfusions in this circumstance. The bleeding time is unreliable because of vasoconstriction. Platelet dysfunction is always present to some degree after cardiopulmonary bypass and is a contributory factor to coagulopathy even if it is not primarily etiologic. In the rare patient with DIC from cardiopulmonary bypass, laboratory abnormalities with prolongations of clotting times not correctable with protamine, low fibrinogen levels, and elevated fibrin(ogen) degradation products are seen. With DIC and generalized bleeding, treatment with platelet transfusion, FFP, and cryoprecipitate may be necessary. In all cases of abnormal bleeding following cardiopulmonary bypass, diagnosis and treatment of coagulopathy must proceed rapidly. If laboratory test results are relatively normal after treatment and if bleeding continues, a mechanical source for hemorrhage is probably present and prompt reexploration is necessary.

Liver Disease and Vitamin K Deficiency States

The liver is an important organ in blood coagulation and hemostasis: it is the major site of synthesis for 12 blood coagulation proteins (fibrinogen, prothrombin, prekallikrein, high-molecular-weight kininogen, protein C, and factors V, VII, IX, X, XI, XII, and XIII), prime components of the fibrinolytic system (plasmininogen and alpha$_2$-antiplasmin), and the important serine protease inhibitor antithrombin III.[25] It also serves an important filtering function in that it clears activated coagulation factors and plasminogen activators from the circulation. The derangement of hemostasis that can occur with advanced liver disease is complex, serious, and difficult to manage. Defective synthesis of fibrinogen and other coagulation factors accompanied by hyperfibrinolysis are further complicated by thrombocytopenia that may result from congestive splenomegaly. Platelet function may also be impaired because of the deleterious effects of fibrin(ogen) digestion products on platelet aggregation and other poorly understood mechanisms.[39] Finally, DIC is believed to complicate some cases of severe liver disease because of (1) activation of coagulation by release of thromboplastin into the circulation during hepatic necrosis, (2) defective clearance of activated coagulation factors, and (3) decreased levels of antithrombin III.

Coagulopathies in surgical patients with severe liver disease are very difficult to treat. Laboratory tests are important in determining whether DIC is present and/or hyperfibrinolysis is operative. With coagulopathy developing during surgery in a patient with liver disease, therapy with FFP should be instituted immediately. One to 1.5 L of FFP will usually correct the factor deficiencies. If large amounts of stored blood (more than 8 U) have been infused before the onset of coagulopathy, or if thrombocytopenia was present preoperatively, platelet transfusions will also be necessary. Cryoprecipitate may also be needed if the fibrinogen is low. While these measures are being instituted, blood should be drawn for laboratory determinations of the presence of DIC and/or hyperfibrinolysis. Most laboratories can perform a euglobulin lysis time. If no test of fibrinolysis is available in an emergency situation, one can simply allow 1 ml of whole blood to clot in a glass tube, incubate it at 37° C, and observe it for lysis. Spontaneous lysis within 1 to 2 hours is evidence of severe fibrinolysis (a normal clot takes 24 hours to lyse). Most often, intensive component therapy will control the coagulopathy. In desperate situations, EACA therapy may be required for hyperfibrinolysis. One must be extremely cautious with this agent, however, because if DIC is present, microcirculatory thrombosis can be potentiated. The use of prothrombin complex concentrates (concentrated factors II, VII, IX, and X) is generally contraindicated in this setting. These concentrates contain activated coagulation factors that are poorly tolerated in liver disease because of low levels of antithrombin III and decreased hepatic clearance of activated factors. DIC can be initiated or exacerbated by such agents, and fatal large-vessel thrombosis has been reported as well.

Vitamin K deficiency states should be recognized and treated preoperatively. Prolonged starvation, malnutrition, biliary obstruction and fistulas, malabsorption syndromes, liver disease, drug therapy with warfarin, and the use of gut-sterilizing and other broad-spectrum antibiotics can reduce the level of vitamin K–dependent coagulation factors (II, VII, IX, and X) to hemostatically unsafe levels. Parenteral vitamin K_1 (10 to 15 mg per day for 3 to 4 days) should be administered with daily monitoring of prothrombin times. In urgent situations, 10 to 25 mg of vitamin K_1 should be administered intravenously. Parenteral vitamin K_1 usually restores effective hemostasis in 6 hours; normal prothrombin times are achieved in 24 to 36 hours. In emergency situations, FFP (2 to 4 U) can be administered to achieve immediate restoration of hemostasis.

Quantitative and Qualitative Platelet Abnormalities

Thrombocytopenia is common in surgical patients and is often occult. Adequate preoperative evaluation, which includes a platelet count, will identify these patients. Thrombocytopenias are classified according to disorders of platelet production, destruction, and sequestration. Among surgical patients, defective platelet production is found with aplastic anemia, marrow infiltration (carcinoma, leukemia, myeloproliferative disorders, and tuberculosis), myelosuppressive drugs used in cancer chemotherapy, nutritional deficiencies (vitamin B_{12}, folic acid, and possibly iron), viral infections, and drugs that affect platelet production (thiazide diuretics, alcohol, and estrogens). Abnormal destruction of platelet sufficient to impair hemostasis is particularly common and develops from nonimmune sources (infection, DIC, extracorporeal circulation, and drugs) and immune sources (idiopathic thrombocytopenia purpura, drugs, posttransfusion purpura, and some allergies). Drug-related thrombocytopenias are particularly noteworthy because platelet transfusion is rarely necessary if the offending agent is removed. Common drugs associated with thrombocytopenia in surgical patients include:

Acetaminophen (Tylenol)
Alcohol
Alpha-methyldopa
Ampicillin
Aspirin
Cephalothin
Chlorpropramide (Diabinese)
Chlorthalidone (Hygroton)
Cimetidine
Digitoxin
Estrogens
Furosamide
Gold salts
Heparin
Isoniazid (INH)
Lincomycin
Meprobamate
Nitrofurantoin
Nitroglycerin
Oxytetracycline
Para-aminosalicylic acid (PAS)
Penicillin
Phenylbutazone
Phenytoin (Dilantin)
Propylthiouracil
Quinidine
Quinine
Spironolactone
Streptomycin
Sulfonamides
Thiazides
Tolbutamide (Orinase)

Platelet sequestration occurs with hypersplenism from multiple causes.

The treatment for surgical patients with thrombocytopenias is platelet transfusion. The need for platelet transfusion is determined by the platelet count, the functional capabilities of circulating platelets (best assessed with a bleeding time), and the magnitude of the operative procedure. Patients with disorders of platelet destruction who have accelerated platelet turnover rates (for example, idiopathic thrombocytopenic purpura) tend to have near-normal bleeding times because the circulating platelets are young, robust, and hemostatically effective.[21] These patients generally require platelet transfusions less often than do patients with disorders of platelet production (e.g., alcoholism or marrow infiltration). At equivalent low platelet counts, the latter patients have longer bleeding times and are more at risk of bleeding during surgical procedures. In all patients with thrombocytopenia, drugs that impair platelet function should be avoided. In performing splenectomy on patients with idiopathic thrombocytopenia purpura and splenic sequestration disorders, it is important to withhold platelet transfusion until after ligation of the splenic artery or removal of the spleen, because the majority of infused platelets will immediately be removed from the circulation by the spleen. In many of these patients, platelet transfusion following spleen removal is unnecessary. If transfusion is required before control of the splenic artery is achieved, it usually requires three times the amount of platelet concentrate used for other thrombocytopenias. Patients with bleeding and infection-induced thrombocytopenia and other consumptive processes also frequently require greater-than-expected amounts of platelet concentrate. In all other patients with thrombocytopenia, the previously described formula serves well as a rough guideline for increasing the platelet count to a hemostatically safe level.

During vascular surgical procedures, reversal of heparin with protamine sulfate can lead to a transient decrease in platelet counts of 20% to 50%. This often causes a paradoxical oozing immediately after protamine administration. The mild thrombocytopenia, presumably caused by the protamine-heparin complex, occurs because of transient sequestration of platelets in the reticuloendothelial system of the liver and spleen. The oozing lasts only minutes, is rarely troublesome, and requires no treatment.

Acquired platelet dysfunction is common and occurs with several medical illnesses as well as with ingestion of drugs that impair platelet function.[26] Clinically significant bleeding stemming from platelet defects has been described in uremia, myeloproliferative disorders (essential thrombocythemia, polycythemia vera, myeloid metaplasia, and acute nonlymphocytic leukemias),[37] dysproteinemias (multiple myeloma, macroglobulinemia), and liver disease. Surgical procedures on uremic patients are frequently complicated by abnormal bleeding. The pathogenesis appears to be related to the buildup of guanidinosuccinic acid and other compounds toxic to platelets.[34] Defective platelet function is corrected by peritoneal dialysis or hemodialysis, and adequate preoperative and postoperative dialysis is mandatory in all uremic patients undergoing surgical procedures. Platelet transfusion is ineffective in uremia unless thrombocytopenia is also present. Infusion of 10 bags of cryoprecipitate will immediately correct the prolonged bleeding time in uremia; the beneficial effects lasts for 24 hours.[24] The mechanism by which cryoprecipitate corrects platelet dysfunction in uremia is unknown. Cryoprecipitate can be very helpful in emergency operations on uremic patients who are incompletely dialyzed.

The following drugs affect platelet function and produce a mild defect in hemostasis that is measurable by prolongation of the bleeding time:

- Anti-inflammatory agents
  - Aspirin
  - Other nonsteroidal anti-inflammatory agents
- Antibiotics
  - Penicillin G (high dose)
  - Carbenicillin
  - Ticarcillin
  - Nitrofurantoin
- Tranquilizers, antipsychotic agents
  - Phenothiazines
  - Tricyclic antidepressants
- Phosphodiesterase inhibitors
  - Dipyridamole
  - Aminophyllin
  - Papaverine
- Miscellaneous agents
  - Dextran
  - Furosemide
  - Antihistamines
  - Sulfinpyrazone

In otherwise healthy patients, drug-induced platelet dysfunction rarely causes clinically significant intraoperative hemorrhage. However, when such dysfunction combines with other mild hemostatic abnormalities frequently encountered in surgical patients (such as uremia, mild thrombocytopenia, and coagulation defects produced by liver disease, malnutrition, or mini-dose heparin), the effects on hemostasis are summative, and serious bleeding can result.

Aspirin is the most commonly ingested drug that impairs platelet function. Nonprescription, over-the-counter drugs containing aspirin are listed in Table 7-4. The mode of action is through acetylation and inactivation of cyclo-oxygenase, an enzyme responsible for conversion of membrane arachidonic acid to prostaglandin endoperoxides and thromboxane A_2. Platelet release is inhibited, and platelet aggregation is impaired. Since the acetylation reaction is irreversible, and since platelets lack the nuclear machinery to replenish the enzyme, all platelets exposed to a single dose of aspirin are affected for their life-span. Clinically, this translates into a prolonged bleeding time and the potential for bleeding during surgical procedures for up to 3 to 4 days after the last dose of aspirin. In most individuals, the aspirin-induced bleeding tendency is mild and causes no problems during surgical procedures; however, in some, bleeding can be pronounced and troublesome.

Other nonsteroidal anti-inflammatory drugs produce a defect in platelet release similar to that caused by aspirin, but their effects are transient and are present only while the drug is circulating. Interestingly, alcohol in moderate

Table 7-4 **NONPRESCRIPTION, OVER-THE-COUNTER DRUGS CONTAINING ASPIRIN**

Drug	Aspirin Content (mg)	Manufacturer	Drug	Aspirin Content (mg)	Manufacturer	Drug	Aspirin Content (mg)	Manufacturer
Alka-Seltzer	324	Miles	Buffex	325	Mallard	4-Way Cold Tablets	324	Bristol-Myers
Anacin	400	Whitehall	Buffinol	325	Otis-Clapp	Gemnisyn	325	Rorer
Anacin, Max. Strength	500	Whitehall	Buf-Tabs	324	Halsey	Goody's Headache Powders	520	Goody's
Anodynos Tabs	357.3	Berlex	Cama	500	Dorsey	Hiprin	487.5	Blaine
Arthritis Pain Formula	487.5	Whitehall	Congespirin	81	Bristol-Myers	Measurin	650	Winthrop-Breon
Arthritis Pain Formula	500	Whitehall	Cope	420	Glenbrook	Midol	454	Glenbrook
ASA Enseals	325	Lilly	Cp-2 Tab	390	Century	Momentum Tab	162.5	Whitehall
Ascriptin	325	Rorer	Coricidin	325	Schering	Panalgesic	*	Poythress
Ascriptin A/D	325	Rorer	Cosprin	325	Glenbrook	Persistin	165	Fisons
Asperbuff	324	Bowman	Cosprin	650	Glenbrook	Presalin	260	Mallard
Aspergum	227.5	Plough, Inc.	Dasin Caps	130	Beecham Labs.	Sine-Off	325	Menley & James
BC Tabs	325	Block Drug Co., Inc.	Duradyne Tabs	230	Forest Pharmaceuticals	Stanback	324	Stanback
BC Powder	650	Block Drug Co., Inc.	Ecotrin	325	Menley & James	Stanback	648	Stanback
Buffaprin	325	Buffington	Ecotrin, Max. Strength	500	Menley & James	Supac	230	Mission
Buff-A	324	Mayrand	Emagrin Tabs	260	Clapp	Synalgos	356.4	Wyeth
Buffered aspirin	325	[Various]	Empirin	325	Burroughs Wellcome	Triaminicin Tablets	450	Dorsey
Bufferin	325	Bristol-Myers	Empirin Compound	233	Burroughs Wellcome	Vanquish	227	Glenbrook
Bufferin, Arthritis Strength	486	Bristol-Myers	Excedrin	250	Bristol-Myers	Wesprin Buffered	325	Wesley
			Extra Strength Bufferin	500	Bristol-Myers			

*8% by weight.

doses, which has no effect on platelet function,[14,23] potentiates the effect of aspirin on the bleeding time.[13] In the context of the alcoholic with upper gastrointestinal hemorrhage who ingests aspirin, the combined effect may be important. The deleterious effect of aspirin on hemostasis is corrected rapidly and easily with platelet transfusion. Six to 10 U of platelet concentrate will immediately reverse the prolonged bleeding time and restore normal hemostasis.

Of the drugs other than aspirin listed above, the antibiotics penicillin G, carbenicillin, and ticarcillin have been most often associated with bleeding. These drugs produce dose-dependent inhibition of platelets and appear to act by blocking platelet receptors for ADP and epinephrine. High doses of these antibiotics in sick patients who have other platelet disorders (especially thrombocytopenia or uremia) or mild coagulation impairment can lead to serious intraoperative bleeding. If possible, the drugs should be stopped a few days before surgery because the effects on platelet function linger beyond the time the antibiotics are in the circulation. Further treatment requires transfusion with platelet concentrate. Dextran, used frequently as an antithrombotic agent in surgical patients, impairs platelet function and produces defective fibrin polymerization. The effect on platelets is unclear but appears to be related to lowering the level of circulating von Willebrand's factor.[1] Preparations with an average molecular weight of 40,000 rarely cause bleeding, but as the molecular weight increases, the effects on platelets and the incidence of bleeding increase. It has been suggested that clinically significant bleeding associated with dextran might be treated with infusions of cryoprecipitate or factor VIII concentrate.

Hyperfibrinolysis

Systemic hyperfibrinolysis can occur with massive release of endothelial cell plasminogen activator, which converts plasminogen to plasmin. Plasmin lyses hemostatic fibrin plugs and degrades fibrinogen to degradation products that have potent anticoagulant and antiplatelet properties. The hemostatic balance is severely disturbed, and bleeding can be profuse. Systemic hyperfibrinolysis has been reported with heatstroke, cardiac arrest, and cardiopulmonary bypass and frequently is a manifestation of DIC, particularly in patients with severe hepatic decompensation. Whether isolated hyperfibrinolysis can occur (in the absence of administration of urokinase or streptokinase) is unclear, and most authorities believe that underlying DIC is responsible for most reported cases. This is important because antifibrinolytic therapy with EACA is contraindicated[31] unless the patient is systemically heparinized. EACA therapy alone should not be used unless laboratory studies have documented the absence of DIC.

Pharmacologic induction of systemic fibrinolysis with streptokinase and urokinase is being increasingly employed to dissolve thrombi in the arterial and venous circulations. Even with so-called "regional" use—perfusion of a single arterial bed with low doses of fibrinolytic agents—systemic fibrinolysis frequently occurs, with impairment of hemostasis. Emergency surgical procedures may be necessary in such patients because the ischemic process—for which fibrinolytic therapy has been initiated—worsens, and emergency coronary or vascular surgery becomes necessary. Because of the current enthusiasm for fibrinolytic therapy, general, vascular, and cardiac surgeons can expect to be confronted with this problem and the need to restore the hemostatic balance rapidly. The goals should be to stop the fibrinolytic process, allow clearance of the degradation products by the reticuloendothelial system (half-life = 2 to 6 hours), and restore normal fibrinogen levels. EACA can be used to halt the action of free plasmin; the standard regimen is 5 g given intravenously as a loading dose, followed by 1 g per hour for 2 to 4 hours. Fibrinogen levels are restored most efficiently by rapid infusions of cryoprecipitate, using the rough guideline that four bags per 10 kg of body weight will increase the effective fibrinogen level by 100 mg/dl. If blood transfusion is necessary, whole blood should be employed because of its fibrinogen content.

SUMMARY

Because increasing numbers of routine and complex operations are being performed on patients who have diseases that alter hemostasis, the frequency of abnormal bleeding in surgical patients can be expected to increase. Knowledge of the physiologic principles underlying hemostasis and of derangements that precipitate bleeding is important in modern surgical care. Hemostasis depends on interactions among circulating proteins (coagulation factors and inhibitors), cellular elements (platelets and white blood cells), and vascular endothelium and smooth muscle. In the early stages of hemostasis, platelets rapidly adhere and aggregate at the site of vascular injury and form a platelet plug that temporarily stops blood flow. At the same time, the intrinsic and extrinsic coagulation pathways are activated, resulting in a fibrin network that fortifies the platelet plug and provides a frame for fibroblastic ingrowth and ultimate healing of the injury. The hemostatic response is finely regulated to limit clotting to the site of injury and thereby to maintain vascular patency. Inhibitory mechanisms include the fibrinolytic system, plasma serine protease inhibitors (the most important of which is antithrombin 3), and the antithrombotic properties and functions of endothelial cells. Derangements in hemostatic mechanisms can be both congenital and acquired. In surgical patients, acquired bleeding disorders are far more common than congenital ones. To diagnose and treat such disorders adequately, preoperative assessment of hemostatic competence is mandatory in all surgical patients. The keystone to preoperative evaluation for all bleeding disorders is a thorough history and physical examination.

SUGGESTED READINGS

Coleman, R.W., et al., editors: Hemostasis and thrombosis, Philadelphia, 1982, J.B. Lippincott Co.

Williams, W.J., et al., editors: Hematology, New York, 1977, McGraw-Hill Book Co.

REFERENCES

1. Aberg, M., Hedner, U., and Bergentz, S.: Effect of dextran on factor VIII (anti-hemophilic factor) and platelet function, Ann. Surg. **189:**243, 1979.
2. Addonizio, V.P., and Colman, R.W.: Platelets and extracorporeal circulation, Biomaterials **3:**9, 1982.
3. Bachmann, F., et al.: The hemostatic mechanism after openheart surgery. I. Studies on plasma coagulation factors and fibrinolysis in 512 patients after extracorporeal circulation, J. Thorac. Cardiovasc. Surg. **70:**76, 1975.
4. Bennett, J.S.: Blood coagulation and coagulation tests, Med. Clin. North Am. **68:**557, 1984.
5. Bowie, E.J.W., and Owen, C.A.: The significance of abnormal preoperative hemostatic tests. In Spaet, T.H., editor: Progress in hemostasis and thrombosis, New York, 1980, Grune & Stratton Inc.
6. Boyd, A.D., et al.: Disseminated intravascular coagulation following extracorporeal circulation, J. Thorac. Cardiovasc. Surg. **64:**685, 1972.
7. Charytan, C., and Purtilo, D.: Glomerular capillary thrombosis and acute renal failure after epsilonamino caproic acid therapy, N. Engl. J. Med. **280:**1102, 1969.
8. Clagett, G.P.: Unexpected coagulopathies during surgery, Probl. Gen. Surg. **1:**200, 1984.
9. Clagett, G.P., and Olsen, W.R.: Non-mechanical hemorrhage in severe liver injury, Ann. Surg. **187:**369, 1978.
10. Counts, R.B., et al.: Hemostasis in massively transfused trauma patients, Ann. Surg. **190:**91, 1979.
11. Damus, P.S., and Salzman, E.W.: Disseminated intravascular coagulation, Arch. Surg. **104:**262, 1972.
12. Deuel, T.F., and Huang, J.S.: Platelet-derived growth factor: structure, function, and roles in normal and transformed cells, J. Clin. Invest. **74:**669, 1984.
13. Deykin, D., Janson, P., and McMahon, L.: Ethanol potentiation of aspirin-induced prolongation of the bleeding time, N. Engl. J. Med. **306:**852, 1982.
14. Dunn, E.L., et al.: Acute alcohol ingestion and platelet function, Arch. Surg. **116:**1082, 1981.
15. Eisenberg, J.M., Clarke, J.R., and Sussman, S.A.: Prothrombin and partial thromboplastin times as preoperative screening tests, Arch. Surg. **117:**48, 1982.
16. Esmon, C.T.: Protein-C: biochemistry, physiology, and clinical implications, Blood **62:**1155, 1983.
17. Feinstein, D.I.: Diagnosis and management of disseminated intravascular coagulation: the role of heparin therapy, Blood **60:**284, 1982.
18. Fisher, D.F., Jr., Yawn, D.H., and Crawford, E.S.: Preoperative DIC associated with aortic aneurysms: a prospective study of 76 cases, Arch. Surg. **118:**1252, 1983.
19. Gill, F.M.: Congenital bleeding disorders: hemophilia and von Willebrand's disease, Med. Clin. North Am. **68:**601, 1984.
20. Goodnight, S.H., et al.: Defibrination after brain-tissue destruction: a serious complication of head injury, N. Engl. J. Med. **290:**1043, 1974.
21. Harker, L.A., and Slichter, S.J.: The bleeding time as a screening test for evaluation of platelet function, N. Engl. J. Med. **287:**155, 1972.

22. Harker, L.A., et al.: Mechanism of abnormal bleeding in patients undergoing cardiopulmonary bypass: acquired transient platelet dysfunction associated with selective α-granule release, Blood **56:**824, 1980.
23. Haut, M.J., and Cowan, D.H.: The effect of ethanol on hemostatic properties of human blood platelets, Am. J. Med. **56:**22, 1974.
24. Janson, P.A., et al.: Treatment of bleeding tendency in uremia with cryoprecipitate, N. Engl. J. Med. **303:**1318, 1980.
25. Losowsky, M.S., Simmons, A.V., and Miloszewski, K.: Coagulation abnormalities in liver disease, Postgrad. Med. **53:**147, 1973.
26. Malpass, T.W., and Harker, L.A.: Acquired disorders of platelet function, Semin. Hematol. **17:**242, 1980.
27. Mant, M.J., and King, E.G.: Severe acute disseminated intravascular coagulation: a reappraisal of its pathophysiology, clinical significance and therapy based on 47 patients, Am. J. Med. **67:**557, 1979.
28. McKenna, R., et al.: The hemostatic mechanism after open-heart surgery. II. Frequency of abnormal platelet functions during and after extracorporeal circulation, J. Thorac. Cardiovasc. Surg. **70:**298, 1975.
29. Miller, R.D., et al.: Coagulation defects associated with massive blood transfusions, Ann. Surg. **174:**794, 1971.
30. Mulcare, R.J., Royster, T.S., and Phillips, L.L.: Intravascular coagulation in surgical procedures on the abdominal aorta, Surg. Gynecol. Obstet. **143:**730, 1976.
31. Naeye, R.L.: Thrombotic state after a hemorrhagic diathesis, a possible complication of therapy with epsilon-amino caproic acid, Blood **19:**694, 1962.
32. Osterud, B.: Activation pathways of the coagulation system in normal haemostasis, Scand. J. Haematol. **32:**337, 1984.
33. Quick, A.J.: Hemostasis in surgical procedures, Surg. Gynecol. Obstet. **128:**523, 1969.
34. Rabiner, S.F.: Uremic bleeding. In Spaet, T.H., editor: Progress in hemostasis and thrombosis, New York, 1972, Grune & Stratton Inc.
35. Rosenberg, R.D.: Actions and interactions of antithrombin and heparin, N. Engl. J. Med. **292:**146, 1975.
36. Rosenberg, R.D., and Rosenberg, J.S.: Natural anticoagulant mechanisms, J. Clin. Invest. **74:**1, 1984.
37. Schafer, A.I.: Bleeding and thrombosis in the myeloproliferative disorders, Blood **64:**1, 1984.
38. Stone, H.H., Strom, P.R., and Mullins, R.J.: Management of the major coagulopathy with onset during laparotomy, Ann. Surg. **197:**532, 1983.
39. Thomas, D.P., Ream, J., and Stuart, R.K.: Platelet aggregation in patients with Laennec's cirrhosis of the liver, N. Engl. J. Med. **276:**1344, 1967.
40. Weksler, B.B.: Prostaglandins and vascular function, Circulation **70**(suppl. III):III-63, 1984.

8

A. Gerson Greenburg

Pathophysiology of Shock

"Shock" is defined as a state of altered tissue perfusion severe enough to induce derangements in normal cellular metabolic function. It occurs when the blood flow to organs and tissues is insufficient to provide necessary nutrients and oxygen and to remove the waste products resulting from their metabolism. If left untreated, the cellular dysfunction that attends shock will ultimately lead to death. Since shock represents the end result of circulatory failure, an understanding of its clinical presentation is mandatory if aggressive and expeditious treatment is to be rendered. It is not unusual for a patient in shock to require rapid restoration of an effective circulating blood volume within a short period of time (often within minutes), if there is to be any hope of survival. This treatment involves both a thorough understanding of the pathophysiologic derangements associated with shock and the distinguishing characteristics of the various etiologies responsible for its development.

TYPES OF SHOCK

Although shock has been classified in a number of ways, from an etiologic standpoint, four types of shock have been recognized and described (Table 8-1). These are hypovolemic shock, septic shock, cardiogenic shock, and neurogenic shock. It is important to remember, however, that a given patient may not fit conveniently into one of these four categories, but rather may have components of more than one category contributing to his shock-like state. For example, a patient with compromised cardiac reserve from atherosclerotic heart disease is commonly a victim of an automobile accident in which there is blood loss from a ruptured spleen and/or a long bone fracture. Although the initial presentation to the emergency suite may be primarily one of hypovolemic shock, the compromised cardiac reserve may result in myocardial failure, in which case cardiogenic shock would also be a major factor contributing to the patient's shock state. Realizing the potential interplay of the various etiologies in a given patient is crucial if effective treatment is to be instituted. Further, it cannot be stressed too strongly that, independent of etiology, altered tissue perfusion with impaired oxygen delivery and/or oxygen use is common to all forms of shock.[13,37] A more physiologically oriented schema for classifying shock is detailed in Table 8-2. By considering the physiologic derangements that occur in shock, one can direct treatment at correcting these perturbations with appropriate interventions.

Hypovolemic Shock

Hypovolemic shock is the circulatory failure that results from a decrease in intravascular blood volume. This decrease in "effective circulation" results in a corresponding decrease in both the cardiac output and tissue perfusion. This form of shock may be caused by the loss of blood or plasma volume or both from the circulation. Hemorrhage (e.g., from the gastrointestinal tract, injuries), vomiting, diarrhea, and sequestration of fluid (as may occur intraluminally in bowel obstruction, intraperitoneally in pancreatitis or peritonitis, and interstitially in burns) may all lead to a decrease in intravascular volume.

Table 8-1 **ETIOLOGIC CLASSIFICATION OF SHOCK**

Type of Shock	Primary Etiology
Hypovolemic	Hemorrhage, vomiting, diarrhea, intraperitoneal fluid sequestration (e.g., pancreatitis), intraluminal fluid sequestration (e.g., bowel obstruction), interstitial fluid sequestration (e.g., burns and traumatized tissues)
Cardiogenic	Intrinsic to the heart: myocardial infarction, myocarditis, ventricular aneurysms, valve prolapse, arrhythmias
	Extrinsic to the heart: pericardial tamponade, pericarditis, tension pneumothorax, pulmonary embolus
Septic	Bacterial, viral, or fungal sepsis; endotoxin from bacterial wall breakdown
Neurogenic	Spinal cord trauma, gastric dilation, spinal anesthesia

Table 8-2 **PHYSIOLOGIC CLASSIFICATION OF SHOCK**

Type of Shock	Primary Etiology
Hypovolemic	
Exogenous losses	Diarrhea, vomiting, dehydration, burns and hemorrhage (i.e., blood, plasma, or water losses)
Endogenous losses	Inflammation, trauma, tourniquet
Cardiogenic	
Focal power failure	Myocardial infarction, ventricular aneurysm, cardiac valve prolapse
Generalized power failure	Viral, drug, or chemical myocarditis
Distributive	
Normal or high peripheral vascular resistance	Sepsis, endotoxin
Low peripheral vascular resistance	Sepsis, CNS/spinal cord injury, anaphylaxis, spinal anesthesia

In the early stages of hypovolemic shock, blood is diverted from the skin so that perfusion to such organs as the liver, kidneys, brain, and heart will be maintained. Generally the only clinical findings will include a postural increase in the patient's pulse and blood pressure in the sitting or standing position, compared with the supine posture. In addition, the skin may be pale and cool, and the neck veins may be flat. If the hypovolemia continues, further redistribution of blood flow will occur from such organs as the kidneys and gut to ensure adequate flow to the heart and brain. At this stage in shock development, the patient will usually be thirsty, the urine will become concentrated, and its volume will decrease. A tachycardia is usually present, and the blood pressure is more labile. If hypovolemia worsens further, blood flow to the brain and heart will become compromised. This circumstance is characterized clinically by restlessness, agitation, confusion, and occasionally even obtundation. The measurable blood pressure is lower, and the pulse becomes more rapid, weak, and often irregular. Respiration is also compromised and is characterized by deep, rapid breathing. Ultimately cardiac arrest and death will ensue if this sequence of events is not reversed. A summary of the clinical signs associated with a form of hypovolemic shock (e.g., hemorrhage), based on the magnitude of blood volume loss, is detailed in Table 8-3.

Since hypovolemic shock represents a deficit in circulating blood volume, the goals in treatment should include identification of the source of the plasma or blood loss, an attempt at controlling this loss, and efforts to restore the volume of effective circulation. As discussed later in this chapter, this volume restoration will include infusion of balanced salt solutions and blood, if hemorrhage is present.

Septic Shock

Septic shock usually occurs under conditions of severe infection and is characterized by a decrease in peripheral vascular resistance and a hyperdynamic circulatory state. Although the exact sequence of events responsible for these findings remains to be defined, the pathogenetic organisms associated with this form of shock appear to increase the circulation at the site of the infectious process. Organisms commonly involved include gram-negative pathogens such as *Escherichia coli, Klebsiella pneumoniae, Aerobacter aerogenes, Pseudomonas aeruginosa,* and at times *Proteus* organisms and *Bacteroides* species. On occasion, gram-positive organisms such as *Staphylococcus aureus* and fungal agents such as *Candida albicans* may also be implicated. In addition to the direct effects that bacteria may have on the cardiovascular system and cellular metabolism, endotoxin, a lipopolysaccharide component of cell walls of gram-negative bacteria, apparently activates the complement system, releasing biologically active amines that regulate release of vasoactive and cardiotonic factors. This outpouring of vasoactive and metabolically inhibiting factors leads to a hyperdynamic state, resulting in peripheral vasodilation and increased cardiac output. Oxygen use is blocked at the subcellular level with accumulation of lactic acid, despite the adequacy of oxygen delivery to cells and the high blood-flow state that usually exists. Clinically, such patients appear with fever; a rapid, bounding pulse; and, usually, a normal blood pressure. The respiration rate is often rapid, and the neck veins are normal. Because of the enhanced blood flow peripherally, the skin is warm and usually somewhat flushed. If this *hyperdynamic state* continues and is maintained, the urine output is usually adequate. As the septic process continues, however, fluid will be lost from the intravascular space into the interstitial and cellular spaces and will ultimately give rise to *hypodynamic septic shock.* When this form of septic shock occurs, it appears clinically much like hypovolemic shock. Thus the skin becomes cold and clammy, the neck veins are flat, the pulse continues to be rapid but now becomes weak, the blood pressure lowers, and the urinary output decreases. If this shock is not successfully treated, confusion followed by obtundation, coma, and death will eventually supervene.

The treatment of this form of shock will almost always require identification of the septic focus with appropriate antibiotic coverage and definitive surgical drainage. Until drainage of the septic focus has been accomplished, therapy is at best supportive and symptomatic. Besides broad-spectrum antimicrobial coverage, this will include fluid replacement and inotropic drugs to maintain ventricular function so that adequate tissue perfusion is ensured.

Table 8-3 **CLINICAL SIGNS RELATED TO MAGNITUDE OF BLOOD VOLUME LOST**

Decrease in Blood Volume (%)	Approximate Blood Loss (ml)	Signs
0-10	0-500	None; slight tachycardia
10-20	500-1200	Slight tachycardia, decreased blood pressure, peripheral vasoconstriction
20-30	1200-1800	Tachycardia (>120 beats/min), hypotension, vasoconstriction, diaphoresis, postural hypotension, anxiety, restlessness, oliguria
30+	1800-3000	Hypotension (BP <70 systolic), diaphoresis, obtundation, anuria

Cardiogenic Shock

Cardiogenic shock occurs when tissue perfusion is impaired because of underlying heart failure. Conditions leading to this form of shock include compromised ventricular function secondary to atherosclerotic coronary artery disease, myocardial infarction, mechanical obstruction of venous return (as occurs in pericardial tamponade or tension pneumothorax), ineffective cardiac contraction (as may occur in various arrhythmic states), and pulmonary embolism. Clinically, these patients appear much like those with hypovolemic shock. The pulse is usually rapid and weak, the blood pressure is low, the skin is cold and clammy, and the respiration rate is rapid. Urinary output is also low, but unlike the case in other forms of shock, the neck veins are distended. If the shock is secondary to pericardial tamponade, a paradoxical pulse may also be present. If a tension pneumothorax is responsible for this shock, the trachea may be shifted away from the involved side with hyperresonance on percussion of that side.

Treatment of this form of shock consists of supporting the failing circulation with an adequate circulating blood volume through the administration of intravenous fluids, and providing appropriate cardiotonic agents to support the failing heart. If cardiac tamponade is responsible for the shock, pericardiocentesis is indicated. Similarly, chest tube placement will be necessary in a tension pneumothorax. If pulmonary embolus is the underlying etiology, a surgical embolectomy may become necessary. For a more in-depth discussion of this form of shock, see Chapter 37.

Neurogenic Shock

Neurogenic shock is the result of a reduction in vasomotor tone from a loss of sympathetic innervation. This form of shock is most commonly encountered from some impairment of the central nervous system, usually spinal cord trauma. It also can occur following the administration of a high spinal anesthetic, and on occasion secondary to acute gastric dilation. Although severe forms of neurogenic shock may result in inadequate cardiac output and poor tissue perfusion, as noted in other forms of shock, the clinical picture with this entity is usually appreciably different. Although the pulse rate may be rapid and the blood pressure may be low, the common clinical picture is one of a slow pulse rate, a warm, dry skin, and only mild hypotension. In addition, the mental status is usually normal, respiratory function is undisturbed, and the neck veins are flat. Often, elevating the legs for a short period of time may be all that is needed to correct this problem, particularly if it has been induced from a spinal anesthetic. If neurogenic shock is secondary to spinal cord injury, increasing an effective circulating blood volume with a balanced salt solution will generally prove to be sufficient treatment. On rare occasions, vasoconstrictive agents may be needed to increase the vasomotor tone.

THE PATHOPHYSIOLOGIC RESPONSE TO SHOCK

Since shock indicates a state of tissue perfusion inadequate to maintain nutrition of cells and remove metabolic waste products, it is not surprising that a common pathophysiologic response occurs in all shock states to avert these derangements. The components of this response may differ somewhat depending on the form of shock encountered, but the compensatory mechanisms called into play are virtually identical. It is primarily the magnitude of these mechanisms that differs among the various forms of shock. In hypovolemic shock, for example, these mechanisms are quite pronounced because tissue perfusion is severely compromised in this state, whereas in neurogenic shock they may be minimal or absent because impairment of tissue perfusion is only mildly affected. Because the overall pathophysiologic response to shock is similar for all etiologies, an understanding of this response is paramount if appropriate treatment is to be rendered.

Neuroendocrine Response

A complex neuroendocrine response is triggered to various degrees in the different shock states to assuage the ineffective circulating blood volume (Fig. 8-1).[12,17,25,34,38] The decrease in circulating volume is sensed by low-pressure stretch receptors in the right atrium and by high-pressure baroreceptors in the aorta and the carotid arteries. As blood volume, venous return, and cardiac output decrease, baroreceptor activity is also attenuated, resulting in loss of the tonic inhibition of the central and sympathetic nervous

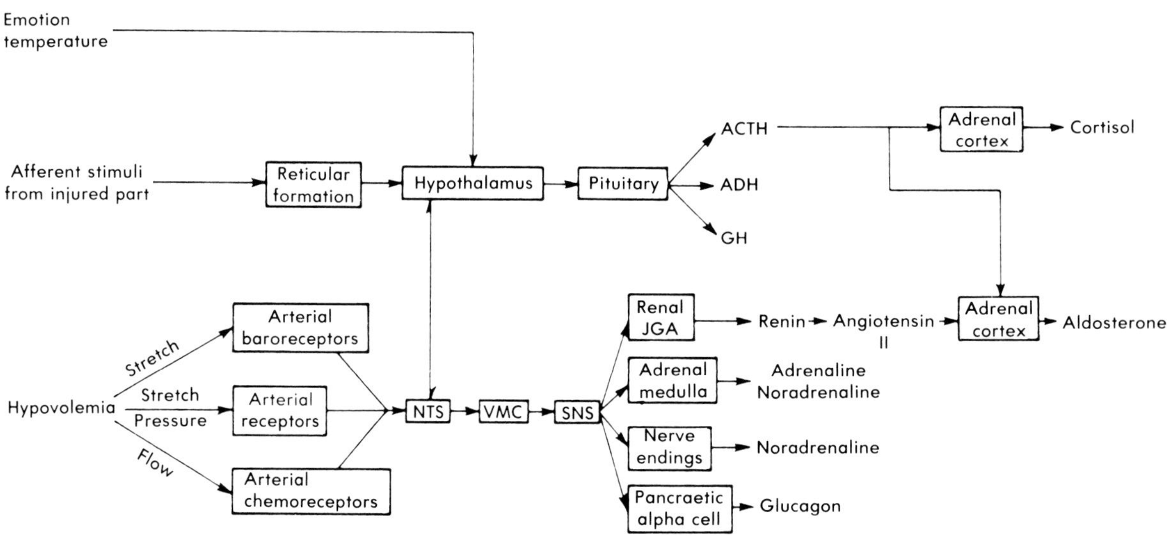

Fig. 8-1 Schematic representation of the neuroendocrine response to ineffective circulating blood volume, as seen in hypovolemic shock. *NTS,* nuclei of the solitary tract; *VMC,* vasomotor center; *SNS,* sympathetic nervous system; *JGA,* juxtaglomerular apparatus. (From Pardy, B.J.: Trauma and shock. In Burnett, W., editor: Clinical science for surgeons, Boston, 1981, Butterworth Publishers, Inc.)

systems. Such a loss triggers increased secretion of adrenocorticotropic hormone (ACTH), antidiuretic hormone (ADH), and growth hormone by the pituitary gland through central hypothalamic pathways, and of epinephrine and norepinephrine secretion by the adrenal medulla through peripheral sympathetic pathways. Additional hormonal interactions arising from the adrenal cortex include stimulation of cortisol release by ACTH, and aldosterone release by both ACTH and by way of the renin-angiotensin system secondary to decreased renal perfusion. Glucagon and insulin are also released by the pancreas in shock, but because of the antagonism of epinephrine, cortisol, and glucagon against the metabolic effects of insulin, a relative insulin deficiency is usually present. Fear or anxiety will augment this neuroendocrine response through stimulation of the limbic areas of the brain. Limbic system projections to the hypothalamus and lower brainstem nuclei lead to increased hypothalamic, adrenomedullary, and adrenocortical activity (see Fig. 8-1). Abnormalities in both body and ambient temperatures produce similar changes along identical pathways. An additional entry into this response pathway includes stimulation of chemoreceptors located in the aortic and carotid bodies. Changes in the concentration of oxygen, hydrogen ion, or carbon dioxide in the blood will result in further neuroendocrine perturbations. The net result of this interplay of hormonal interactions is arteriolar vasoconstriction (i.e., increased peripheral vascular resistance), renal conservation of both water and salt, and the provision of circulating glucose adequate to maintain the nutritional needs of such vital organs as the heart and brain.

Hemodynamic Perturbations

The primary function of the neuroendocrine response to shock is to correct inadequate tissue perfusion. This response is particularly pronounced in patients with hypovolemic shock and those with the hypodynamic form of septic shock. It is directed at all elements of the circulation, including the heart, peripheral vasculature, and blood volume. Mechanisms responsible for restoring cardiovascular homeostasis include: (1) augmentation of cardiac output, (2) redistribution of blood flow, and (3) restoration of intravascular volume.

Cardiac output, the principal determinant of tissue perfusion, is directly proportional to venous return.[12,17,25,34,38] The increase in the end-diastolic stretch of ventricular muscle fibers (preload) results in a stronger contraction during systole and therefore an increased ejection of blood. The compensatory mechanism by which venous return is increased in shock—with a corresponding preload increase—is through decreasing venous capacitance, which restores an effective circulating blood volume. Decreased venous capacitance occurs secondary to specific organ vasoconstriction. The vasoconstriction is mediated by sympathetic nerves, circulating catecholamines, angiotensin II (via the renin-angiotensin system), and vasopressin (also called ADH).[12,17,25,34,38] Blood flow to the heart, brain, and adrenal and pituitary glands is protected by vasodilation of their vessels. Blood flow to skin, skeletal muscles, and the splanchnic circulation is decreased, with the degree of vasoconstriction being proportional to the deficit in circulating blood volume. These alterations are particularly pronounced in hemorrhage, with changes in hepatic and renal blood flow varying in direct proportion with the degree of hemorrhage. For example, following mild hemorrhage, portal blood flow decreases secondary to vasoconstriction of the splanchnic circulation. The hepatic arteries initially dilate, but total hepatic blood flow is decreased following even minor blood loss. In cases of moderate to severe hemorrhage, this arterial autoregulation is lost and the hepatic arteries actually vasoconstrict. Renal blood flow is only compromised following loss of a large volume of blood.[12,17,25,34,38] With continued blood loss, the mechanisms responsible for maintaining blood flow to the heart and brain will also be compromised and will eventually fail.

Systemic arterial resistance increases secondary to arteriolar constriction and is also mediated by sympathetic nerves, circulating catecholamines, angiotensin II, and vasopressin.[12,17,25,34,38] This increase in afterload results in a net decrease in cardiac output. However, blood flow to the heart and lung is maintained at near normal levels through redistribution of available cardiac output to these critical, nonconstricted areas of the circulation. The increase in systemic arterial resistance is most pronounced in hypovolemic shock. It is also seen in cardiogenic shock and the hypodynamic phase of septic shock. In contrast, in the early, hyperdynamic phase of septic shock, a decrease in peripheral arterial resistance is seen. This is probably related to the direct effects of bacteria and endotoxin on the cardiovascular system and cellular metabolism.

The other determinants of cardiac output are contractility and heart rate. Increases in contractility will result in direct increases in cardiac output. Increased heart rate also increases cardiac output, but the response to this mechanism is limited. A heart rate beyond 180 beats/minute is associated with a decreased cardiac output secondary to a reduced diastolic filling time. Increases in both contractility and heart rate occur secondary to stimulation of cardiac sympathetic nerves and by the action of circulating catecholamines. Other vasoactive substances that are known to circulate in shock include enkephalins, endorphins, arachidonic acid metabolites, serotonin, kinins, and histamine, but the physiologic importance of these substances in mediating the hemodynamic response to shock remains to be determined. The overall hemodynamic perturbations are summarized in Fig. 8-2.

Restitution of an effective circulating blood volume, in addition to the compensatory changes already noted, is important in preventing the deleterious effects of shock (i.e., tissue ischemia and death). According to Gann and Amaral,[12] this blood volume restoration occurs in two phases: an initial transcapillary refill phase and a plasma protein restitution phase. These responses are particularly pronounced in patients with hypovolemic shock secondary to hemorrhage. Acute blood loss, for example, results in a decrease in capillary pressure initiated by hypotension and augmented by sympathetically mediated precapillary arteriolar constriction. The resultant decrease in capillary hydrostatic pressure promotes movement of fluid from the

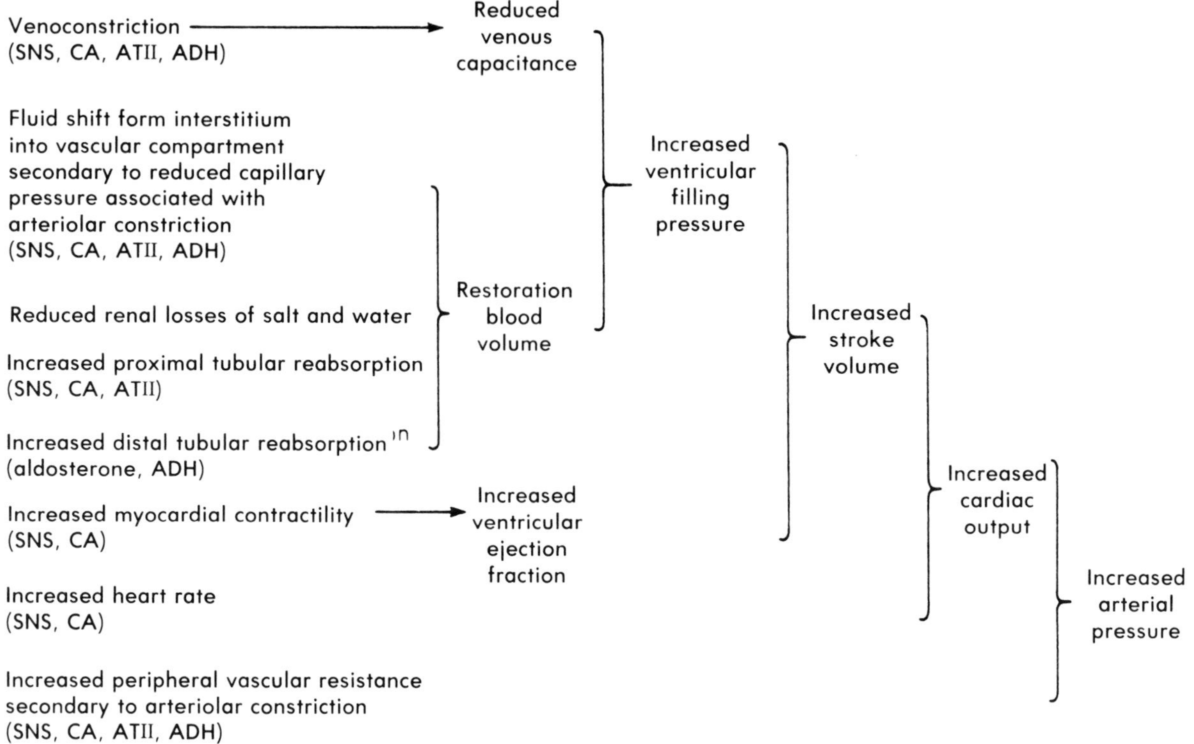

Fig. 8-2 Hemodynamic responses to ineffective circulating blood volume, as seen in hypovolemic shock. *SNS*, sympathetic nervous system; *CA*, catecholamines; *ATII*, angiotensin II. (From Pardy, B.J.: Trauma and shock. In Burnett, W., editor: Clinical science for surgeons, Boston, 1981, Butterworth Publishers, Inc.)

interstitial space into the capillary bed. This extracellular fluid shift to the vascular compartment may restore up to 50% of the lost blood volume.

The second phase of vascular restitution begins with increases in the serum osmolality. The liver is the primary source of the solutes contributing to this hyperosmolality, which include glucose, phosphate, lactate, pyruvate, amino acids, and urea. The elevation in serum osmolality is proportional to both the degree and the rate of hemorrhage. The rise in plasma osmolality results in an increase in osmolality in the interstitial space. Interstitial hyperosmolality leads to an osmotic gradient, with a resultant movement of water from the cells. The increased interstitial volume results in an increase in interstitial pressure, promoting a transcapillary movement of albumin from the interstitial space to the intravascular compartment. Complete restoration of blood volume depends on this restitution of plasma protein.

Metabolic Perturbations

The ineffective circulating blood volume that occurs in shock and the corresponding reduction in cardiac output result in an increased extraction of oxygen by the tissues from arterial blood (see boxed material at right). The cellular hypoperfusion and hypoxia result in a shift to anaerobic glycolysis. Instead of entering the citric acid cycle through coenzyme A, pyruvate is converted to lactic acid. This cellular acidosis is transmitted to the circulation, as reflected in the increased blood lactic acid levels that are commonly observed in patients in shock. Each mole of lactic acid releases one mole of hydrogen ion to body fluids, with a corresponding reduction of buffering capacity and a resultant systemic acidosis. If not treated, this acidosis will offset the normal hemodynamic responses and lead to irreversible shock and death.

Hyperglycemia also occurs in response to shock. Changes in carbohydrate metabolism arise secondary to the action of catecholamines, cortisol, glucagon, and growth hormone. Although insulin secretion is also increased in shock, its anabolic effects—at least acutely—are antagonized by these substances so that a state of catabolism ensues.[17] The hyperglycemic response is mediated by these various agents and is secondary to increased hepatic production of glucose through (1) glycogen breakdown; (2) stimulation of gluconeogenesis from breakdown of skeletal

METABOLIC PERTURBATIONS IN SHOCK

Hyperglycemia
Fat mobilization (i.e., increased free fatty acids in the blood)
Protein catabolism
- Increased synthesis of urea
- Increased aromatic amino acids

Decreased synthesis of acute phase reactants
Increased extracellular osmolality

muscle protein into amino acids and the conversion of these amino acids in the liver into glucose; and (3) impaired peripheral uptake of glucose by tissues.[17] Further, epinephrine selectively inhibits insulin secretion. This metabolic response is primarily invoked to provide glucose to the cerebral circulation since this substance is the only metabolic fuel that can be used effectively by brain tissue.

In addition to the alterations in glucose metabolism that occur in shock, cortisol and glucagon, in conjunction with catecholamines, stimulate lipolysis and thereby increase plasma concentrations of free fatty acids.[17] This lipolytic action, which is also antagonistic to the effects of insulin, is another mechanism by which additional fuel and energy substrate are provided at a time of increased metabolic demand.

Other metabolically and hemodynamically active agents are released in various shock states. The known elevation in blood levels of endorphins, opiate-like agents, may contribute to the hypotension and myocardial depression seen in those forms of shock in which hypovolemia is not a major underlying etiologic factor.[2] Elevations of arachidonic acid metabolites, particularly thromboxane A_2 and prostacyclin, have also been observed in both clinical and experimental shock.[19] Since these agents have opposite physiologic effects (thromboxane A_2 aggregates platelets and is a vasoconstrictor, whereas prostacyclin inhibits platelet aggregation and is a vasodilator), and since both are generally elevated in shock, the net effect will depend on which one dominates. In addition, since both agents have relatively short half-lives, their importance probably lies in regulating the microcirculatory alterations that occur in shock (see the next section).

Other hormones may also play a role in shock, but experimental information to date is too meager to allow any meaningful conclusions. In particular, the thyroid and parathyroid glands do not receive much basal blood flow, and in shock they could undergo further compromise, leading to tissue hypoxia and cell damage. Since thyroxin plays an important role in regulating oxygen consumption of tissues, a deficit of this hormone could contribute to the impaired oxygen utilization seen in some shock states. Similarly, alterations in calcium metabolism, caused by changes in the synthesis and/or release of parathormone or thyrocalcitonin, may impair important metabolic functions necessary for cellular viability.[41]

Effects of Shock at the Cellular Level

The Microcirculation

The microcirculation is that component of the vasculature that provides nutrient blood flow directly to tissues and is involved with the removal of metabolic waste products. Although much more needs to be learned about the physiology of the microcirculation and what derangements actually exist in the various shock states, considerable useful pathophysiologic information has been obtained in recent years from the study of various laboratory animals under normal and shock conditions. Just as the neurohumoral response to shock produces changes in various hemodynamic parameters (e.g., tachycardia, altered peripheral resistance) that are potentially detrimental to some organs (e.g., kidney and gut) and protective of others (e.g., heart and brain), corresponding changes also occur in the microcirculation that may be either protective or detrimental.

Various vascular mediators released during shock (i.e., angiotensin II, arachidonic acid metabolites, kinins) appear to act selectively at the level of afferent arterioles or efferent venules. These agents may induce arteriovenous shunting, occlusion of capillary beds, and altered pressure-flow relationships in oxygen delivery to cells. Such vascular aberrations, coupled with the low flow state induced by hypovolemia or cardiac failure, often lead to platelet aggregation and thrombus formation. A variety of vasoactive substances (e.g., prostanoids, serotonin) are then liberated as the clot forms. These agents, together with the resulting anoxia, produce endothelial damage and increased capillary permeability, which then result in the formation of edema and further restriction and redistribution of blood flow.

Although it is uncertain which of these precipitating events is most important, it is known that anoxia has a direct effect on vascular endothelium and may indeed be the mechanism responsible for the increased capillary permeability.[33] Like other cells, endothelium appears to require oxygen to function; when oxygen is deprived, a leaky capillary membrane ensues. The leak results from a widening of cell-to-cell junctions, with aggressive fluid movement into the interstitium. This effective increase in interstitial fluid is noticeable in a number of organs but can be especially pronounced in the lungs, particularly during septic shock. In fact, monitoring lung water has proved helpful in assessing the presence and magnitude of this capillary leak, independent of the underlying etiology of shock.[39] Other investigators have suggested that this capillary leak may not be caused by the anoxia per se, but rather may be related to the release of oxygen-derived free radicals associated with rapid volume expansion and oxygen delivery during shock resuscitation. It is known, for example, that the superoxide anion, a major component of this oxygen radical system, directly damages cells and cell membranes. If oxygen radicals are ultimately shown to play a major role in the microcirculatory events during shock and its resuscitation, future pharmacologic therapy may include measures directed at attenuating or eliminating the effects of these toxic anions.[10,18]

The Cell

The primary pathophysiology of shock at the cellular level is a change in metabolism affecting energy production and function. Crucial to cell function is the need for oxygen as basic fuel. Aerobic metabolism more efficiently replenishes the high-energy phosphates required for ongoing metabolism. Under low-flow, poor perfusion states, less oxygen is delivered, and the cells are forced into a state of anaerobic metabolism. In this situation, fewer high-energy bonds are created, and cellular efficiency is reduced as the acidosis generated anaerobically alters normal enzyme kinetics.[28,34,38] This observation serves as the basis for ATP–$MgCl_2$ therapy (discussed later in this chapter).

The major protective mechanism of a cell is its membrane.[6] This bi-lipid layer, which is composed of fatty acids, is responsible for the ionic differential that exists between the cell and its surrounding environment and maintains the high potassium and low sodium intracellular concentrations. Malfunction of this membrane ultimately sets the stage for cellular death. When this occurs, sodium moves into the cell, drawing with it a volume of water appropriate to maintain osmotic equilibrium with the surrounding interstitial space. The resulting cellular edema ultimately impairs normal intracellular metabolism, causing cell death. Cell membrane damage may be the result of a primary insult from endotoxin, complement, or some other unidentified agent that may accumulate during shock. Membrane injury may also occur secondarily from deranged intracellular metabolism that fails to regulate the sodium/potassium ratio within the cell or its corresponding concentration of calcium, a substance necessary for normal enzyme function. Failure of mitochondrial oxidative phosphorylation, and the accumulation of lactic acid and other anions within the cell, also produce intracellular and membrane damage. In general, the accumulation of hydrogen ion in the cell results in intracellular acidosis and is detrimental to all cellular organelle function. In addition to the ion and water changes that may occur within the cell when its membrane loses its integrity, such disruption may also alter normal responses to various circulating agents such as catecholamines, corticosteroids, insulin, and glucagon, substances that play important roles in normal cellular metabolism. Thus an ''expected response'' may be attenuated or exaggerated, depending on the state of cellular enzymes at the time of the shock injury.

Although the cell and microcirculation have been considered separately in this discussion, it must be remembered that any perturbations in their function secondary to shock are intimately related. Thus alterations in the microcirculation secondary to a low flow state generally result in derangements in normal cellular metabolism because of the absence of adequate oxygen and nutrients to maintain cell function. Similarly, aberrations in cellular physiology alter the surrounding microcirculation secondary to the accumulation of hydrogen ion and the release of such lysosomal enzymes as acid phosphatases and dehydrogenases.

Organ Failure in Shock

With the exception of neurogenic shock, which is usually mild and easily controlled, all forms of shock, if severe enough, can result in major organ dysfunction. The pattern of this dysfunction relates to (1) the various abilities of organs to withstand hypoxia and low flow, (2) the type of shock insult (hypovolemic vs. septic), and (3) the underlying basic metabolic rate. This dysfunction is further influenced by the degree of ''organ reserve'' and the innate ability of a particular organ to withstand a metabolic insult. If preexisting or intercurrent disease is present, the ability of a given organ to withstand the detrimental effects of low flow and hypoxia will be further compromised.

The *kidney* is a flow-sensitive organ which, as previously noted, is involved in the basic compensatory response to shock, acting to conserve sodium and water. The mechanisms responsible for this action include the renin-angiotensin system, release of ADH from the pituitary gland, and intrinsic regulatory alterations within the kidney tubules themselves. If shock is severe enough, a considerable redistribution of blood flow away from the kidney may occur to provide a more effective circulation to other organs, such as the heart and brain. In this circumstance, the kidney may sustain an ischemic insult as a result of the accompanying poor perfusion. Sepsis and other factors (e.g., nephrotoxic drugs) may further aggravate this insult. When renal function is impaired secondary to shock, one of two responses may occur: oliguric renal failure or high-output (i.e., non-oliguric) renal failure. These two clinical presentations probably represent different points on a continuum of acute renal failure. The exact mechanisms underlying these different presentations are not known, but it is generally accepted that in oliguric failure, poor perfusion and anoxia alter glomerular function, which is reflected in a lower glomerular filtration rate and a decrease in urine output. In non-oliguric renal failure, a diuretic form of renal dysfunction occurs, presumably from a lesser insult to the glomerulus and renal tubules.

The *liver* has a high metabolic rate and plays a prominent role in protein synthesis, among other functions. The liver depends on an adequate blood flow: under normal conditions approximately 30% of the cardiac output is directed to this organ by way of the hepatic artery (systemic circulation) and portal vein (splanchnic circulation). In hypovolemic states, the liver ''autotransfuses'' its vascular contents by mechanically shunting inflow to the hepatic sinusoids. In moderate to severe states of shock, the splanchnic blood flow may decrease significantly (by as much as 40% to 50%, resulting in a corresponding decrease in flow to the hepatic Kupffer cells, the name given to the hepatic reticuloendothelial system. As a consequence of this event, the filtration of debris and bacteria by the liver is impaired, allowing toxic material to pass through it to the lungs. Although significant morphologic damage can be detected in the liver soon after shock—particularly shock occurring after hemorrhage—clinical evidence of hepatic dysfunction is often absent. Generally, only a modest increase in serum bilirubin concentration is noted, whereas other indices of liver function remain normal or show only modest abnormalities. Thus, if a patient is successfully resuscitated from shock, liver dysfunction is only minor in terms of clinical significance. In shock patients in whom sepsis is a major underlying etiology, pronounced liver failure may occur, with serum bilirubin concentrations reaching levels as high as 15 to 20 mg/100 ml. Histologic examination of such livers has usually revealed fatty infiltration. Although impaired perfusion probably plays a role in the pathogenesis of this failure, the exact mechanisms responsible for it remain ill-defined. Interestingly, in septic and/or endotoxin-infused animal models simulating septic shock, hepatic lactate use is diminished. Thus the use of a lactated Ringer's solution in patients with septic shock is probably contraindicated; an acetate-based solution should be used in its place.[15]

The *pancreas* and *gastrointestinal tract,* other organs that are very active metabolically, may also be adversely affected in shock. The changes in insulin and glucagon release that occur during sepsis and hypovolemia indicate that the pancreas is influenced by the shock state. Whether these responses are primarily protective mechanisms to assist the body in meeting its metabolic demands, or whether they occur because of impaired perfusion to the pancreas, remains to be determined. There is some evidence that the pancreas releases a myocardial depressant factor during shock that is directly related to impaired blood flow to this organ.

In contrast to the uncertain effects of shock on the pancreas, both sepsis and hypovolemia have been shown to have adverse effects on the gastric mucosa through impaired blood flow. The resulting erosive gastritis may produce profound hemorrhage that by itself is life-threatening. It is now known that buffering gastric acid with topical antacids and antisecretory agents such as cimetidine can significantly lessen this risk. The potentially adverse effect of shock on blood flow to the intestinal mucosa is less certain. Since this epithelial surface forms a barrier to protect the host from its luminal environment, it seems likely that its breakdown in response to ischemia could allow a sudden influx of bacteria and toxins to cross the intestinal wall and translocate to other organs. There is some experimental evidence to suggest that such a breakdown can occur in severe states of shock (particularly hemorrhagic) and can be responsible for the delayed sepsis that can occur following initial resuscitation.[4]

The response of the *lungs* to shock has been studied extensively. Critical for survival following any shock insult is the lungs' basic function of oxygenation. It is now clearly recognized that the lung may suffer profoundly adverse effects from shock and its resuscitation, and that pulmonary failure is a major complication contributing to mortality and morbidity in shock. This relates to the lung's function as a natural filter for intravenous debris, cellular aggregates, lipids, and bone marrow particles. When these materials lodge deep in the pulmonary capillaries, they initiate an intensely inflammatory response, with increased local capillary permeability and edema formation that may reach substantial proportions. Implicated in this cascade is the role of complement activation and other vasoactive substances originating in white cells. The factors that can cause the pulmonary vascular bed to leak are all associated with, or made worse by, the presence of sepsis and infection. Anoxia, various vascular mediators released in shock, and direct alveolar wall damage all initiate changes in pulmonary capillary permeability and can be seen in various shock states. With relatively normal perfusion, the lungs can clear an excess of fluid accumulating in the interstitial space. Generally, increases in lung water sufficient to impair oxygenation are not observed in pure hypovolemia alone, but rather are seen only in patients with sepsis and cardiac failure. In these latter conditions, significant impairment in lung blood flow can result. The precise mechanisms responsible for lung damage in these various shock states remain to be defined. Lysosomal enzyme release from leukocytes, the generation of superoxide anions in ischemic tissue, and the release of calcium-mediated cyclic nucleotides and prostanoids are all under investigation as potentially key mediators in the production of lung damage in shock.

The *host-defense system* is exquisitely sensitive to both hypovolemic and septic insults. This extensive filter system removes unwanted antigens and potentially toxic particles from the circulation. There are many components to this system, including fixed and circulating macrophages, leukocytes, and opsonic proteins. In both sepsis and hypovolemic shock, a depression in the production of opsonic protein and fibronectin may occur, indicating impairment in normal clearance mechanisms. Because of the impaired clearance of bacteria and particles normally removed by the spleen and liver, the lung becomes a target, resulting in localized pulmonary inflammation with edema formation and the potential for pulmonary failure.[7,23,29]

Although dysfunction of any of these organ systems may occur alone or in various combinations in response to shock, the lungs and kidneys are particularly susceptible to insult, and in profound shock the liver is also commonly involved. If shock has been severe and resuscitation has been unusually difficult, a sequence of organs may fail in succession; the term "multiple organ failure" syndrome has been applied to this circumstance. The associated mortality is extremely high. For more detailed discussions of the effects of hypovolemia and sepsis on the organs discussed here the reader is referred to other sections of this book.

The Concept of Irreversible Shock

Occasionally a shock insult is so severe that it does not respond to standard therapeutic interventions. When this occurs, the shock is defined as "irreversible." Since irreversibility implies a fatal outcome, it is extremely important that every treatment option be exhausted before a patient is assigned to this category. Thus assessment of a patient with unresponsive shock (preferable to "irreversible shock") requires an appreciation of the potential occult causes of persistent physiologic alterations (see the boxed material below).

CORRECTABLE CAUSES OF "IRREVERSIBLE" SHOCK

- Failure to assess response to a fluid challenge
- Inadequate fluid resuscitation
  - Volume need underappreciated
  - Presumption of overload when cardiac disease is present
- Hypoxia caused by inadequate ventilation
  - Or barotrauma to the lung
  - Or iatrogenic pneumothorax or cardiac tamponade
- Inadequately treated sepsis
- Drug toxicity or drug-drug interactions with exaggerated effects
- Ongoing acid-base abnormalities, uncorrected
- Electrolyte abnormalities resulting from inadequate or inappropriate replacement of perceived derangements
- Endocrine failure, e.g., adrenal insufficiency, acute hypothyroidism

Table 8-4 **DESIRABLE PHYSIOLOGIC END POINTS RELATIVE TO NORMAL VALUES**

Variable	Normal Value or Range	Preferred Value in Shock Treatment
Hemodynamics		
Blood pressure (BP)	120/80 mm Hg	Systolic >100 mm Hg
Mean BP	96 mm Hg	Systolic >80 mm Hg
Heart rate	70-80 beats/min	75-100/min
Central venous pressure	3-6 cm water	>4 cm water
Cardiac index (CO/BSA*)	3-4 L/min	>4 L/min
Pulmonary capillary wedge pressure (PCWP)	7-10 mm Hg	11-18 mm Hg
System vascular resistance index	1900-2100 dyne-sec/ cm^5/M^2	>1500 dyne-sec/ cm^5/M^2
Pulmonary extravascular water	180-200 ml	<260 ml
Oxygenation and Gas Exchange		
Hemoglobin	12-15 g%	>12 g%
Po_2 room air	80-100 mm Hg	>70 mm Hg
O_2 content (100% O_2)	18-20 ml O_2/100 ml	>18 ml O_2/100 ml
O_2 delivery	500-600 ml/min/m^2	>550 ml/min/m^2
O_2 consumption	115-165 ml/min/m^2	>170 ml/min/m^2
P_{50}†	25-28 mm Hg	>25 mm Hg
Mixed venous Po_2	35-40 mm Hg	>25 mm Hg
Arterial-venous O_2 difference	4-5 ml O_2/100 ml	4-6 ml O_2/100 ml
Pco_2	37-45 mm Hg	33-46 mm Hg
Arterial pH	7.35-7.45	>7.35
Miscellaneous		
Urine flow	30-50 ml/hr	>25 ml/hr
Temperature	37-38° C	39.5° C
Blood volume		
Males	3.2 L/m	>3.8 L/m
Females	2.8 L/m	>3.2 L/m

*CO, Cardiac output; BSA, body surface area (m^2).
†P_{50}, Partial pressure of O_2 at which blood is 50% saturated.

MANAGEMENT OF THE PATIENT IN SHOCK

Because of the complexity of the pathophysiologic response to "shock," criteria-based, goal-oriented therapy with defined end points represents the most rational approach to managing a patient in shock. Thus treatment is directed toward the correction of defined abnormalities as determined by monitoring specific hemodynamic and clinical variables. Such therapy requires a thorough understanding of the pathophysiology underlying the various types of shock and their attendant sequelae.

In defining treatment end points, "normal" or "normal range" may not be the desired goal. Restoration of all variables to only "normal" may leave an organ or particular body system in an uncompensated state, incapable of sustaining adequate function. Consequently, the concept of an "optimal" end point becomes more relevant. This value may exceed the normal range, and it represents what is usually necessary to achieve a desired objective in terms of the restoration of organ function. Thus a seriously ill patient may require higher cardiac filling pressures, a greater cardiac output, or supplemental oxygen to achieve a desired physiologic objective and still maintain a degree of "reserve" to compensate for any further insult (Table 8-4).

Rapid restoration of deficits is the goal of shock therapy. Since shock is fundamentally an impairment of tissue perfusion secondary to inadequate cardiac output, the basic elements in shock management are (1) attention to ventilation and perfusion abnormalities to ensure adequate tissue oxygenation, and (2) the provision of nutrients. Once these fundamental considerations are addressed, pharmacologic interventions to correct and optimize specific physiologic aberrations can be entertained. In any case, management of the patient in shock must be deliberate and systematic. Although the cellular response to the different forms of shock is basically the same, etiology has to be considered to avoid treating only signs, symptoms, and laboratory data. Many elements of therapy are common in the various shock states, but failure to appreciate their differences and to adapt treatment to the underlying etiology may add significantly to morbidity and mortality. The basic hemodynamic and metabolic abnormalities seen in the major types of shock are summarized in Table 8-5.

Monitoring Parameters During Shock Resuscitation

The degree and extent of monitoring in shock patients, both during and following resuscitation, will depend on the magnitude of shock, the urgency of resuscitation, and the patient's course thereafter.[1,16] Assessment parameters during acute shock should generally be restricted to basic hemodynamic monitoring. This includes measurement of arterial blood pressure, pulse rate, respiratory rate, and the adequacy of urine output. If time permits, a central venous catheter should be placed to monitor central venous pressure at the same time that access routes are being positioned to infuse intravenous fluids. Blood samples to measure hemoglobin, blood urea nitrogen, plasma electrolytes, and arterial blood gases should also be obtained initially as baseline information from which further treatment measures can be guided. The objective for resuscitation must be to restore hemodynamic and respiratory variables to acceptable levels. If these symptoms can be normalized, oxygen delivery will be optimized and the ravages of hypoxia will be minimized.

Following initial resuscitation, when time constraints are less critical, more sophisticated monitoring to determine ongoing hemodynamic derangements or response to therapy will generally be indicated. If not already in place, a central venous pressure monitor should be positioned at this time. If the magnitude of shock has been substantial, a pulmonary arterial catheter (i.e., Swan-Ganz) for measuring pulmonary capillary wedge pressure and cardiac output directly may prove invaluable in following hemodynamic responses to treatment. In patients in severe shock who have already had substantial impairment of tissue perfusion for a prolonged period, and in whom signif-

Table 8-5 **BASIC HEMODYNAMIC AND METABOLIC ABNORMALITIES SEEN IN SHOCK**

Indicator	Status* in the following type of shock:			
			Septic	
	Hypovolemic	Cardiogenic	Hyperdynamic	Hypodynamic
Blood pressure	−	−/N/+	−	− −
Pulse rate	+ +	+	+ + +	+
Central venous pressure (CVP)	− −	N/+	N/+	−
Respiration rate	+	+ +	+ + + +	+ +
Urinary output	−	−	+/−	−
Cardiac index	−	− −	+ +	−
Pulmonary capillary wedge pressure	− −	+ +	−/N	−/N
Peripheral resistance	+ + +	+	− − −	− −
Arterial-venous oxygen difference	+ +	+	− −	−
Po_2	−	−	−	−
Pco_2	−	+/−	−/+	+ +
Arterial pH	−	−	−/N	−
Arterial lactate	+ +	+	−/N	+/−
Response to volume load†	+ + +	−	+	− −
Skin temperature	Cold	Cold	Warm	Cold
Skin sensation to touch	Clammy	Clammy	Dry	Clammy

*Symbols: −, decreased, +, increased, *N*, normal. The relative magnitude of change is shown by multiple plus or minus signs.
†Usually 250 to 500 ml of balanced salt solution; this will increase blood pressure, decrease heart rate, and increase cardiac output.

icant capillary leaking is likely to occur, wedge pressures must be kept near normal (6 to 10 mm Hg). In less pronounced forms of shock, higher pressures may be tolerated to ensure peripheral perfusion. This may require pressures approaching 20 mm Hg. An indwelling arterial line is advocated in most patients in shock to measure arterial pressure, so that inaccuracies introduced by the blood pressure cuff in hypovolemic, vasoconstrictive patients with narrow pulse pressures are eliminated. Moreover, this line provides access to arterial blood, facilitating blood gas analyses while avoiding frequent and risky arterial punctures.

Frequent determinations of heart rate and rhythm are of particular value in assessing a patient's volume status and the effectiveness of cardiac output. Changes in heart rate often reflect corresponding changes in sympathetic tone. Abrupt rate changes usually represent compensatory responses for alterations in vascular volume or resistance and may be the first sign that effective circulating blood volume has not been maintained. Similarly, the respiration rate—providing a patient does not need ventilator assistance—is often an important index of the adequacy of tissue oxygenation. Hyperventilation, for example, suggests a response to the metabolic acidosis that frequently arises when tissue hypoperfusion exists. Arterial blood gas measurements will determine the adequacy of gas exchange.

Since successful resuscitation in shock depends, in the final analysis, on the adequacy of tissue oxygenation, a sufficient red-cell mass to ensure adequate amounts of hemoglobin to carry oxygen is paramount in any treatment scheme.[35] Thus hemoglobin should be checked at least hourly during ongoing resuscitation, and at frequent intervals thereafter. For effective resuscitation to occur, a hemoglobin level in excess of 12 g/100 ml is generally necessary.

Although the various monitoring techniques discussed above are important in assessing a response to therapy, two clinical indices that cannot be overemphasized are urine output and sensorium. Generally, a urine output greater than 0.5 ml per kg of body weight per hour indicates a well-perfused kidney and thus indirectly indicates good peripheral blood flow. In addition, the level of consciousness reflects the adequacy of oxygen delivery to the brain. With very few exceptions, the sensorium is altered with hypoxia, poor cerebral perfusion, or the accumulation of toxic metabolites that commonly circulate in shock and septic states. A normal sensorium generally indicates adequate tissue perfusion.

Treatment Considerations

Ventilation

Failure of respiratory gas exchange is one of the most frequent causes of death in patients with shock. Thus the first priority in treating shock is to ensure effective ventilation. Maintenance of adequate oxygen and carbon dioxide exchange is essential to survival. In the traumatized, septic, or hypovolemic patient, there is a significantly higher oxygen demand that often reaches twice normal. Under most circumstances, hyperventilation provides an effective means of increasing oxygen delivery when needed. The shock patient, however, has difficulty exerting this additional effort and rapidly develops signs of respiratory failure together with respiratory acidosis. Depending on the magnitude of shock, supplemental oxygen may help to maintain efficient oxygen delivery. In more severe situations, endotracheal intubation and ventilatory assistance may be warranted, as discussed elsewhere in this book and summarized in the boxed material on p. 164. Critically ill patients must be intubated early to avoid respiratory failure—especially comatose and lethargic patients.

The goals of ventilator therapy, when it is needed, are relatively specific. Respiratory alkalosis must be avoided.

INDICATIONS FOR INTUBATION AND VENTILATORY SUPPORT

Respiration rate of 30 per minute or greater
P_{CO_2} greater than 45 mm Hg with metabolic acidosis
P_{CO_2} greater than 50 mm Hg with normal bicarbonate levels
P_{O_2} less than 60 mm Hg on 40% O_2
Tidal volume less than 5 ml/kg
Vital capacity less than 10 ml/kg
Minute ventilation less than 8 L/min
Excessive ventilatory effort

Adjusting the respiratory rate to ensure a P_{CO_2} of 35 to 40 mm Hg maintains cerebral perfusion and avoids a left shift of the oxyhemoglobin dissociation curve, which results in an increased affinity of oxygen for hemoglobin (see Chapter 33). Such a left shift represents a significant decrease in oxygen availability to tissues and requires a hemodynamic compensation by way of increased cardiac output to maintain adequate tissue oxygenation. Generally, the arterial P_{O_2} is maintained at 80 to 100 mm Hg through provision of an inspired oxygen concentration that is as low as possible. Failure to achieve this goal requires additional inspired oxygen or the use of end-expiratory pressure to improve oxygenation by increasing the functional residual capacity of the lungs. Peak inspiratory pressure is minimized to avoid barotrauma (i.e., pneumothorax), pressures less than 20 to 22 cm of water being desirable. A tidal volume of 9 to 13 ml per kg of body weight, which exceeds normal by 50% or more, is generally needed to respond to the increased metabolic and oxygenation demands in shock patients.

Perfusion

After adequate ventilation is assured, aggressive restoration of an "effective" circulating blood volume becomes the central focus of therapy. Volume resuscitation brings about a rapid improvement in circulatory status and oxygen delivery.[13] At the same time that fluid is being administered to restore blood volume, pharmacologic intervention may prove useful. There is mounting evidence that many of the hemodynamic aberrations induced by shock are amenable to pharmacologic manipulation.

The improved cardiac output that follows such maneuvers enhances oxygen delivery and tissue perfusion, as described by the relationship between cardiac output (CO), arterial oxygen content (CaO_2), and oxygen delivery:

$$\text{Oxygen delivery} = \text{CO (ml/min)} \times CaO_2 \text{ (ml of } O_2 \text{ per ml of blood)}$$

Oxygen content is described in terms of hemoglobin (Hb) concentration, oxygen saturation (SO_2), and arterial oxygen pressure (P_{O_2}) by the relation:

$$CaO_2 = Hb \times SO_2 \times 1.34 + Hb \times 0.00034\ P_{O_2}$$

Both saturation and P_{O_2} depend at least partially on the FI_{O_2} (inspired oxygen content) and the pulmonary status of a patient in terms of gas exchange. Increases in oxygen content (by way of blood transfusion or supplemental oxygen administration) and/or flow (cardiac output) enhance oxygen delivery. The rapid restoration of vascular volume in the hypovolemic patient increases cardiac output and thus oxygen delivery. Increasing the volume of a hypovolemic patient by 25% to 35% frequently increases cardiac output by more than 100%. In response to this enhanced output, normalization of oxygen consumption occurs, which indicates restoration of tissue perfusion.[37]

Table 8-6 **ENDOGENOUS RESPONSE TO LOSS OF CIRCULATING BLOOD VOLUME**

Mechanism	Time Frame (With No Therapeutic Intervention)
Restoration/maintenance of hemodynamic stability; redistribution of flow	Seconds to minutes
Restoration of vascular volume; transcapillary refill, primarily from interstitial fluid compartment	3-4 hr
Restoration of vascular volume with albumin stores	18-24 hr
Addition of new (i.e., synthesized) albumin	24-36 hr
Replacement of lost red-cell mass	3-5 weeks

The sequence of events assumes that the loss of blood volume was mild to moderate and that survival does not depend on therapeutic intervention.

RESUSCITATION FLUIDS. Balanced salt solutions are effective volume expanders for the initial resuscitation of patients from shock. If hypovolemia from the loss of fluid (e.g., diarrhea) or blood (e.g., gastrointestinal hemorrhage) is the underlying cause of the shock, a volume of solution in excess of measured losses is generally required to effect improved function and survival.[33,34] The additional fluid, 1 to 1.5 times the fluid lost, replaces the extracellular fluid deficit that results from the rapid equilibration of plasma volume with interstitial fluid (Table 8-6). For most patients, Ringer's lactate solution is the preferred resuscitation solution. The lactate ion acts as a buffer, eventually being metabolized to carbon dioxide and water. Septic patients, and those with significant hepatic dysfunction, do not metabolize lactate well.[15] For these individuals, balanced salt solutions with acetate as the major anion are preferred.

Initially, the hypovolemic patient is given 2 to 3 L of crystalloid, and the response of pulse rate, blood pressure, and urinary output is observed. If this therapy fails to correct hemodynamic abnormalities, as may occur in patients sustaining significant blood losses, additional crystalloid followed by type-specific blood is indicated, especially if an urgent operation is anticipated to control the blood loss. It must be remembered that crystalloids in large quantities will ultimately provoke a dilutional effect that can significantly decrease the blood's oxygen-carrying capacity. Even in this setting, delivery of oxygen to tissues may be improved because of the restored vascular volume and the accompanying increase in cardiac output through the mechanisms discussed in "Perfusion" section. Nevertheless, even though a young, nondiseased heart can mount a sustained increase in cardiac output in response to this excess fluid, an older patient with coronary arteriosclerotic disease is generally unable to do so and may develop myocardial failure or infarction from this added stress. In these older patients, red cell blood transfusions should be given early in the resuscitation to obviate this problem.

Although crystalloids are the preferred solution for resuscitation in shock, with the use of red cells as indicated for massive or ongoing blood losses, colloid solutions such as albumin have also been advocated in shock treatment. Colloid solutions, however, are expensive and have no apparent advantage over crystalloids, provided similar physiologic end points are measured. In addition, there is some evidence that colloids may be detrimental in treating shock.[27,44] When given to equivalent cardiac filling pressures during elective surgical procedures, for example, these solutions are effective for volume replacement, and no apparent differences in pulmonary function—presumably from increased lung water—can be detected. However, such resuscitation is actually controlled volume replacement, a model not really comparable to the hypovolemia and ischemia that occur in shock. Real differences are apparent, though, in septic patients in whom the leak of proteins across a damaged pulmonary membrane can be demonstrated with colloids. Albumin, for example, produces a significant oncotic effect, drawing and holding water in the alveoli and impairing cellular function. On the other hand, there are no firm data to support the idea of a decrease in oncotic pressure being detrimental in the shock state, provided the vascular pressures are not allowed to exceed acceptable levels. It may be that a difference in the hydrostatic and oncotic pressures is more important for fluid flux into the lungs or other tissues than is an absolute level of either. Based on these considerations, colloids are not recommended as being of any major importance in the treatment of shock. Only in patients with marked hypoproteinemia (i.e., serum albumin less than 2.5 g/100 ml) is it reasonable to provide colloid in the resuscitation regimen.

The role of hypertonic salt resuscitation in shock management remains undefined. This form of treatment has been tested in patients undergoing elective major vascular surgery, and it appears effective.[31] To date it has not been tested in shock resuscitation. The concept of hypertonic resuscitation is based on the aim of refilling the intravascular space with interstitial fluid by drawing on the body's reserves to augment intravascular volume.[43] In elective, well-hydrated patients, this aim may be valid. In hypotensive, hypovolemic patients, it may not achieve the desired results because the interstitial space is already contracted and cannot serve as a reserve.

Starches can also be used for volume expansion and have been employed successfully in the treatment of shock. These agents are nonprotein plant derivatives that have little antigenicity. On the basis of molecular size and weight, they effect an oncotic pressure by binding plasma water or by drawing interstitial fluid into the vascular space and thus rearranging water distribution in much the same way that hypertonic saline does. Two particular starches, dextran and hydroxyethyl starch (HES), have been shown to improve capillary perfusion by augmentation of cardiac output and flow and also by lowering viscosity. HES has fewer problems than dextran in the clinical setting and is an effective and safe volume expander and resuscitative agent.[32] Despite their ability to resuscitate shock patients, there is no evidence that starch solutions are more effective than crystalloids in this regard, and the starches are considerably more expensive.

Transfusion of Blood and Blood Products

General principles. Although intravenous infusion of balanced salt solutions is an appropriate therapeutic modality in the early treatment of shock, transfusion of blood and/or blood products is eventually required in hypovolemic shock secondary to hemorrhage. Because of the many physiologic functions of blood, its importance in the treatment of hemorrhagic shock cannot be overemphasized. Unlike salt solutions, whose primary role in shock is to reestablish an effective circulating blood volume, blood, in addition to this function, possesses the unique ability to transport oxygen and also provides coagulation factors that will ultimately become depleted if hemorrhage continues.

Since so much of the body's physiology depends on oxygen delivery, this function must be supported to avoid any significant hemodynamic or respiratory compromise in already stressed patients. Maintenance of near-normal levels of hemoglobin may have a benefit in providing reserve when an additional stress is encountered. The intimate relationship between hemoglobin concentration and the adequacy of oxygen consumption at the tissue level is well established[30] and underscores the importance of maintaining normal levels of hemoglobin in circulating blood. Since increases in oxygen availability can be provided only by increasing blood flow to tissues or by enhancing the blood's oxygen-carrying capacity, red-blood-cell transfusions are particularly useful in this subset of shock patients. In hemorrhagic shock, excessive loss of blood or massive ongoing losses (i.e., 100 ml/min) often occur. In such patients, it is desirable to maintain hemoglobin concentrations at 10 g/100 ml or better so as to provide some reserve in the oxygen delivery system while preparations are being made to control the etiologic factor(s) responsible for the blood loss.

In contrast to a decade ago, when whole-blood transfusions were fashionable in the treatment of hemorrhagic shock, only red-cell transfusions are recommended today to provide an adequate hemoglobin concentration, with concurrent supplementation of crystalloid solutions to maintain an adequate circulating blood volume. The other blood components can then be used to benefit patients who do not require red cells but who have a particular need for a specific component to treat an underlying physiologic deficit, such as a clotting deficiency. Only when multiple (i.e., 4 or 5) units of red cells are required to maintain an adequate hemoglobin concentration should a unit of whole blood be considered to replace lost coagulation factors. Table 8-7 gives the primary components of blood, their forms and storage modalities, and the defects corrected by their administration.

Table 8-7 **BLOOD COMPONENTS**

Component	Volume (ml) Administered	Expected Increase in (70-kg Patient)	Deficit Corrected
Oxygen carriers			
Whole blood	500	2%-3%, Hematocrit	Anemia, plasma volume
Red cells, packed	250-300	3%-4%, Hematocrit	Anemia
frozen	200	2%-3%, Hematocrit	Anemia
WBC poor	200	2%-3%, Hematocrit	Anemia
Coagulation factors			
Platelets	35-50	5-10,000/U of platelets	Thrombocytopenia (absolute, functional)
Fresh frozen plasma	210-250	3%-4%, Factor VIII	Coagulation factors; fibrinogen
Cryoprecipitate	10-25	2%-3%, Factor VIII; 10-30 mg fibronectin	Coagulation factors; fibrinogen; Factor VIII; fibronectin
Oncotic agents			
Albumin			
Standard	250	—	Plasma volume expansion
Salt-poor	25	—	Plasma volume expansion
Plasma protein factor	250	—	Plasma volume expansion
Other			
Granulocyte	50-75	2-500/unit	Leukopenia
Gamma globulin	100-300	3%-5%/unit	Compromised immune system

Because of the rapidity of blood loss in hemorrhagic shock, and the need to correct the diminished oxygen-carrying capacity quickly, *stored* red cells are generally transfused. Depending on the age of these cells, optimum oxygen delivery to tissues may not be as ideal as one wishes, since stored red cells develop a specific defect in energy metabolism (i.e., a loss of 2,3-diphosphoglyceric acid and ATP) that results in an increased affinity of oxygen for hemoglobin and an accompanying shift in the oxyhemoglobin dissociation curve to the left (see Chapter 33). If this shift is significant, a hemodynamic compensation (i.e., increased cardiac output) may be required to ensure adequate oxygen delivery to ischemic tissues. In such blood, there is sufficient oxygen present, but it is not "available" because of the tight binding of oxygen to hemoglobin. Large quantities of old, banked red cells can induce this effect, which usually corrects itself within 24 hours of infusion. The exact physiologic impact of high-oxygen-affinity blood remains controversial. By itself the effect may be minimal, but when coupled with existing hemodynamic, metabolic, and cardiac abnormalities it may be significant. Newer blood preservation techniques have addressed the issue of red-cell energy loss so that shelf storage can be enhanced and prolonged without compromising patient care.[8] Older blood is usually used during the period of ongoing blood loss, despite the potential metabolic defect. Fresher red cells are preferred once the blood loss has been controlled, as these cells will last longer and provide more efficient oxygen delivery.

In a number of trauma centers, autologous blood has been used to replace ongoing blood losses in shock patients, together with attempts at operative correction of the bleeding site. This autotransfusion of lost blood has proved to be an effective and useful therapeutic tool in selected cases of hemorrhagic shock. Although the risk of transfusion reactions is virtually eliminated with this approach, contamination is a potentially serious problem since the collected blood is often mixed with other body secretions and thus requires careful filtering before its infusion.

Although the ideal in transfusion therapy is the use of fresh frozen blood, its availability is often limited. Further, the time required to thaw and prepare it for infusion often limits its usefulness in a patient who requires blood quickly. Finally, once thawed, fresh frozen blood has a shelf life of only 24 hours. Thus in most situations this form of blood is not applicable for treatment in the majority of shock patients requiring urgent transfusion.

Unless life-threatening blood loss is encountered, blood should not be administered until definitive typing and cross-matching have been done. Only if resuscitation with salt solutions is not efficacious should emergency blood transfusions be given. In this circumstance, type-specific blood may prove to be life-saving until the cross-match has been completed.

Consequences of transfusion therapy. Although blood transfusions are necessary in the treatment of most patients sustaining hemorrhagic shock (unless the bleeding is mild and stops spontaneously), it must be remembered that transfusion therapy is not without risks. Thus in deciding to transfuse a patient, one must be fully aware of the potential complications and prepared to manage them should they occur. The morbidity and mortality associated with transfusion therapy are directly related to the volume of blood infused (i.e., the greater the volume infused, the greater the risk). Posttransfusion fatalities generally result from clerical errors and are usually associated with a single-unit transfusion that is not compatible with the patient's own blood type. Despite occasional human error during infusion of blood, transfusion reactions are relatively rare (less than 0.05%). The transmission of disease by infused blood, once thought to be 10% to 12%, is probably less but is clearly related to the donor population.

Citrate toxicity and hypothermia are rate related. The infusion of stored blood, unwarmed, at a rate in excess of

100 ml/min results in the binding of ionized serum calcium, which produces myocardial depression and dysrhythmias. High levels of citrate, seen with rapid infusion, sensitize the myocardium to the effects of potassium. Each unit of old, banked blood or red cells contains 10 to 20 mEq or more of potassium. In the presence of excess citrate, the myocardium is in peril. Calcium chloride, 2.5 mEq/U, is given when the rate of infusion exceeds 100 ml/min. Hypothermia likewise ensues when cold blood is infused too rapidly. Hypothermia also induces a sensitive myocardium which, in the face of altered calcium and potassium concentrations, may precipitate arrhythmias with untoward hemodynamic consequences.

A dilutional coagulopathy can be seen after massive blood transfusions.[9] This is primarily a thrombocytopenia and is corrected with infusion of platelets once the major bleeding site is controlled. One unit of platelets raises the peripheral platelet count by 5000 to 10,000 cells. Therapy for counts over 60,000 is usually not necessary.

Various diseases can also be transmitted by blood (e.g., hepatitis, AIDS, parasites). There is likewise the possibility of infusing bacteria or contaminated blood products, resulting in septicemia. Emboli to the lungs (i.e., air and microembolic debris) are similarly possible during blood transfusion, with a potentially dire outcome. This latter complication is considered a technical problem during administration and should be preventable if appropriate care is exercised.

Immunologically modulated transfusion reactions can be immediate or delayed and have been traced to virtually every component of blood. Immediate hemolytic reactions are almost always the result of a clerical error in which mismatched blood is infused. Bleeding, fever, hypotension, pain in the back (referred from kidneys), and a constricting feeling in the chest are all possible clinical signs of a transfusion reaction. The patient in the operating room and asleep may manifest only a slight coagulopathy; the hemolysis resulting from such a reaction may be fatal. If the reaction occurs, the transfusion should be stopped immediately, all clerical information should be rechecked, and the typing and cross-match should be repeated. Specific therapy includes maintaining adequate renal blood flow and treatment of any hypotension, both with intravenous crystalloid solutions. A diuretic can be added to aid in the renal clearance of toxins developing from the transfusion reactions. In terms of renal damage, the red-cell stroma (i.e., cell wall), not the hemoglobin, is the primary offending agent. If renal failure ensues, prompt dialysis is indicated.

White cells, platelets, and proteins can also induce immediate or delayed immunologic reactions, all modulated by the immune system. Graft vs. host disease, a rare complication of blood transfusion, is seen primarily in immunosuppressed patients.

Blockade of the host-defense system and immune mechanisms may also be a consequence of transfusion therapy. In the severely ill patient, it is unwise to compromise this important system. Debris from red-cell transfusions can lodge in the pulmonary circuit, producing local inflammation and infiltrates. The exact effects are not usually apparent in terms of altered clinical function; this probably reflects our lack of sensitivity in detecting such abnormalities.

Pharmacologic Interventions

In the historical development of recommended treatment modalities for shock, both vasoconstrictive and vasodilatory drugs have been in vogue at different times as potentially useful agents. It was thought that vasoconstrictor drugs could assist in increasing blood pressure until effective circulating blood volume was restored. It is now known that the already compromised tissue perfusion is further aggravated by such vasoconstriction, which therefore actually compounds the shock state rather than assisting in its control. Similarly, vasodilator drugs were thought advantageous in improving flow to tissues at the microcirculatory level. Despite the logic of this concept, the clinical use of these agents did not bring improvement and actually resulted in peripheral pooling of blood, with adverse effects on cardiac output. As the pathophysiology of shock has become more clearly understood, both of these treatment approaches have been abandoned.

The major role of vasoactive drugs in modern shock treatment relates to their potentially useful inotropic and chronotropic effects on the heart. Since an appropriate cardiac output is desirable in patients with shock, factors that govern heart rate and stroke volume can be manipulated to improve peripheral blood flow. Although such therapy cannot be justified as appropriate routine treatment, it may prove efficacious in patients with compromised cardiac reserve.

As discussed in more detail in Chapter 36, stroke volume is governed by ventricular preload, afterload, and contractility. Although preload is primarily influenced by the volume of circulating blood, both afterload and contractility can be manipulated by a number of pharmacologic agents. Afterload reduction may prove efficacious in the patient who has a relatively normal or slightly depressed arterial blood pressure, but in whom the cardiac output is low and the pulmonary arterial wedge pressure is high (>18 mm Hg). Nitroprusside is especially useful for this circumstance and has balanced vasodilating effects on both the arterial and venous circulations, so that adverse affects on arterial blood pressure are minimized. Nitroglycerin has also been used for this purpose, but its action is primarily to dilate the venous capacitance vessels—specifically the pulmonary vasculature—and it has only minimal effects on systemic vasodilation. Recent studies have also suggested that prostaglandin E_2 may be an effective reducer of cardiac afterload, but the precise effects of this agent, which appear to be directed primarily on the pulmonary circulation, require further investigation.[19] Ganglionic blocking agents have also been employed to reduce afterload, but since their effects are primarily on the arterioles, systemic hypotension has been a major side effect. If used appropriately, afterload reduction—particularly with an agent such as nitroprusside, which is easy to titrate—should result in an effective increase in cardiac output, with little or no change in arterial blood pressure.

A number of agents have been shown to effectively improve cardiac contractility by their inotropic effects.[37] The major agents used for this purpose today are dopamine, dobutamine, isoproterenol, and digoxin. Each of these agents has specific properties that can prove useful in altering hemodynamics to obtain the desired therapeutic effect. Dopamine, for example, effectively increases both blood pressure and cardiac output and thus improves oxygen delivery to tissues. Dopamine appears to have specific effects on renal blood flow (presumably through dopamine receptors) and thus can be especially beneficial when the clinical situation suggests that renal perfusion is a problem. Dopamine has been used effectively in the treatment of both cardiogenic and hypovolemic shock, with minimal side effects. Its use in septic shock has been less impressive. Failure to respond to dopamine is most likely the result of inadequate cyclic AMP (cAMP) in tissues, which is necessary for membrane function and receptor integrity, or to the presence of alkalosis. Both conditions are frequently seen in septic patients. Dobutamine is similar to dopamine in its inotropic effects and has proved useful in situations in which dopamine has not been effective.

Isoproterenol and epinephrine have also been shown to be effective inotropic agents. Isoproterenol not only improves ventricular contraction but increases the heart rate as well. Because it also decreases peripheral resistance, it is a very useful agent when this effect is desired in combination with the drug's cardiac effects. Epinephrine is likewise an effective inotropic and chronotropic agent, but it can cause increases in peripheral resistance as well as ventricular irritability. Thus it must be administered more cautiously than isoproterenol and is probably contraindicated in hypovolemic patients. Norepinephrine also has both inotropic and chronotropic effectis, but unfortunately its peripheral effects of increased vascular resistance and inoreased afterload augment and exaggerate its potentially beneficial effects on cardiac contraction. Some investigators have proposed that an alpha-adrenergic blocking agent be used in combination with norepinephrine to enhance its cardiac effects, but with the availability of other agents, this is generally considered inappropriate and potentially dangerous.

Although digitalis compounds, and particularly digoxin, are the mainstay of drugs used to enhance cardiac contractility, their use in acute situations such as shock is limited because it takes considerable time for even the more rapid-acting compounds to have an effect. Consequently, another inotropic drug is usually required if cardiac support needs to be assured more expeditiously. In less acute situations, digoxin is the most appropriate drug and is quite effective when there is a need for a prolonged increase in cardiac contractility.

Occasionally, the blood-ionized calcium levels may be low in shock patients, particularly those in whom a septic component is present. This calcium depletion may have adverse effects on cardiac hemodynamics. In patients in septic shock with low calcium levels, cautious infusion of ionized calcium is effective in enhancing cardiac output.

Glucagon also has inotropic effects, but compared with the agents discussed previously, its action is weak. Its effects are most likely mediated through mobilization of stored glycogen. In addition, glucagon also has slight direct vasoconstrictor activity. As a routine inotropic drug, glucagon has no advantage over other agents and thus is not recommended by most clinicians.

Over the years, steroids have been intermittently recommended as an effective adjunctive measure in the treatment of shock, particularly in patients with septic shock. The physiologic basis for using steroids stems from experimental observations in various animal models in which these agents have been shown to have a protective effective against gram-negative organisms and/or their endotoxins, presumably through membrane and lysosomal stabilization. Since experimental evidence suggests that the most opportune time to give steroids is early in the pathogenesis of septic shock, at a time when the glucocorticoid and mineralocorticoid response to shock is maximal, it is unlikely that exogenous administration of these agents would offer any additional benefit. In those studies that have addressed this issue in some systematic fashion, there has been virtually no evidence to support the claim that steroids should be used in the treatment of shock.

The use of antibiotics in the treatment of shock depends on the underlying etiology. For most forms of hypovolemic and cardiogenic shock, antibiotic coverage cannot be justified. If tissue injury produces the shock, as may occur from vascular disruption secondary to penetrating trauma, antibiotics may prove efficacious in preventing the subsequent development of wound infections and/or abscesses. In this circumstance, a broad-spectrum antibiotic should be administered as early as possible after wounding and should be continued for 2 or 3 days thereafter. In contrast to their relative significance in hypovolemic or cardiogenic shock, antibiotics form an important component of therapy in the management of patiens with septic shock. In fact, the antibiotic selected for the patient with sepsis is the most important determinant of subsequent morbidity and mortality. Thus every effort needs to be made to select an antibiotic against the organism that seems most likely to be responsible for the underlying infection. In general, the antibiotic should have broad-spectrum properties and should be administered intravenously to ensure adequate blood levels. Frequently a combination of antibiotics will be needed. For gram-negative infections, an aminoglycoside is an appropriate first-line defense agent. If the infection is thought to be gram-positive in origin, particularly if cocci are involved, intravenous penicillin should be administered. When the antibiotic sensitivities have been determined from the cultured sources thought to be responsible for the infection, appropriate alterations in antibiotic coverage can be instituted as needed. Since surgical drainage will ultimately be necessary in most patients to eradicate the source of infection, it is important that high blood levels of antibiotics be established before operative intervention and continued for a reasonable period of time thereafter (usually 7 to 10 days).

Mast Trousers

Mast trousers, or the mast suit, is a pneumatic antishock garment that is placed on a patient much as a pair of pants would be and then is filled with air to a predetermined pressure. First introduced during the Vietnam war, its purpose is to maintain effective circulating blood volume by reducing perfusion to the lower half of the body and increasing peripheral resistance so that blood flow is directed centrally to maintain flow to oxygen-sensitive organs such as the heart and brain. Although the logic underlying its use is quite simple, its effect on prolonging survival in seriously ill patients in hypovolemic shock remains to be determined. Its major use in most trauma centers has been in stabilizing pelvic and long bone fractures to reduce the severe blood loss accompanying these disorders until other resuscitative efforts can be effectively administered. Problems relating to its use include restriction of rib cage motion by the abdominal portion of the garment because of the compression of the abdominal contents and elevation of the diaphragm. Such restriction can markedly reduce the vital capacity of the lungs. In addition, the increased blood pressure that often occurs following application of this garment may lead to increased bleeding above the level of the trousers. Since most reports summarizing the efficacy of mast trousers in the treatment of hypovolemic shock are based on anecdotal accounts, its role in shock treatment must await further studies.

Future Therapeutic Modalities

Blood Substitutes

Red-cell substitutes. Since the major function of red blood cells in the treatment of shock relates to their oxygen-carrying capacity, considerable interest has been generated in recent years in developing red-cell substitutes. One approach has used enzymatic cleavage of specific-blood-type antigens from the surface of red cells, creating in effect a universal blood donor. The merit of this approach is that it eliminates the need to type and cross-match blood before infusion. Experimental work so far has demonstrated that cells modified in this fashion have altered function and a markedly decreased half-life.

Another approach has used the oxygen-carrying capacity of fluorocarbons. These substances are dense organic chemicals that carry oxygen in proportion to ambient oxygen pressure that varies from one fluorocarbon to another, depending on the underlying molecular structure. Unfortunately, fluorocarbons are toxic in their pure form, primarily because of an accompanying vapor pressure, and are also insoluble in water. Even though oxygen is more soluble in fluorocarbons than in water by a factor of 10 to 20 times, the oxygen-carrying capacity of a fluorocarbon emulsion equals that of blood only at 100% inspired oxygen, an udnesirable therapeutic modality. The emulsification that is necessary to reduce the toxicity of fluorocarbons before their infusion contributes to a limited circulating half-time that is generally on the order of hours to days. Since the clearance of fluorocarbons from the bloodstream is primarily by way of the reticuloendothelial system (RES), and since dwell time in this system may be months or longer, a long-term toxicity problem is potentially posed, the significance of which remains unknown. Further, RES clearance introduces another major problem because this system is also stressed and impaired in septic and hypovolemic shock. The fact that it does not seem wise to further impair this vital system, coupled with the observation that fluorocarbons are not biologically inert in either their native or emulsified form,[21] makes it questionable whether they will ever be clinically useful in the treatment of shock.

Interestingly, the efficacy of a 20% fluorocarbon emulsion in carrying oxygen has been reported in a small population of patients.[22] At best, the solution proved to be a moderate volume expander, but its ability to carry oxygen and to effect an improvement in tissue perfusion in ischemic or low flow states was far from convincingly documented. In another study, involving seven severely anemic patients, it was noted that at ambient oxygen tensions, fluorocarbon acted primarily as a volume expander, whereas only at higher tensions (>300 mm Hg) did it contribute substantially to effective oxygen delivery.[40]

In animal studies evaluating fluorocarbons, adequate hemodynamic resuscitation following shock has been demonstrated, but the complication of coagulation problems, particularly thrombocytopenia, has been noted.[14,15] Other abnormalities at the microcirculatory level have been encountered, including white-cell clumping and platelet aggregation. Further, in baboons with hematocrits as low as zero, fluorocarbons were shown to have no clear advantage over stroma-free hemoglobin in terms of oxygen delivery characteristics (see following paragraph). Thus despite the initial enthusiasm for the use of fluorocarbons as red-cell substitutes, these animal studies, as well as available human data, have failed to substantiate any significant clinical role for these agents.

Stroma-free hemoglobin. In contrast to other red-cell substitutes, which to date have not demonstrated features that would allow them to be used clinically, stroma-free hemoglobin (SFH) possesses many properties that are desirable in a blood substitute. It carries and releases oxygen in a cooperative fashion, has virtually no antigenic properties, is not nephrotoxic, and is oncotically active. When properly prepared it is neither an anticoagulant nor a procoagulant, and it can be stored for reasonable periods of time. Finally, at ambient Po_2 it has been shown to preserve life function as an efficient and effective resuscitation fluid in total blood exchange and hemorrhagic shock animal models. Further, SFH effects an excellent hemodynamic resuscitation and affords improved tissue oxygenation as measured by hepatic mitochondrial function during the post-resuscitation period.[14] Despite these desirable characteristics, two major problems have kept SFH in the laboratory and have detained clinical study. These are: (1) a profound affinity for oxygen by SFH, and (2) the perception on the part of potential users of this agent clinically that its intravascular persistence is too short to be of therapeutic usefulness.[11]

An appreciation of hemoglobin biophysics and the basic structure-function relationships that determine the metabolic fate of free hemoglobin led to attempts to modify SFH to solve these problems. Both intermolecular and intramolecular chemical modifications of SFH have been attempted. Polymerizing SFH (i.e., intermolecular modification) to increase its molecular weight has been reported to improve its intravascular persistence (for 2 to 3 days) and to maintain near normal oxyhemoglobin affinity.[24] Although most SFH is excreted by the kidneys, no one can predict the impact that these larger molecules may have on the RES. These polyhemoglobins may follow different metabolic pathways and excretory routes that could be detrimental and might result in RES blockade, a particularly undesirable side effect in the polytraumatized patient.

Intramolecular modifications of SFH have also been undertaken to improve intravascular persistence without increasing oxyhemoglobin affinity. These chemical modifications have used various phosphate analogs to bind to various sites on the beta chains of the hemoglobin molecule, normally occupied by 2,3-diphosphoglycerate, the key intracellular phosphate in hemoglobin that is involved intimately with oxyhemoglobin affinity. SFH chemically modified with a number of phosphorylated dialdehydes has been shown in dogs to persist intravascularly for as long as 12 hours (a sixfold increase over unmodified SFH), with maintenance of normal oxyhemoglobin affinity.[14] Moreover, resuscitation with these modified SFHs has demonstrated a beneficial effect. Further, this intramolecularly modified SFH is not a polyhemoglobin, and thus may be less of a problem to the RES. In one study of hemorrhagic shock resuscitation followed 5 days later by septic challenge, modified-SFH animals did not demonstrate any impairment in defense mechanisms.

The concept of a neohemocyte is also being evaluated. The idea underlying this approach is to encapsulate SFH with a modifier to improve its functional capacity. Although this appears technically feasible, how these artificial cells will react in the circulation remains unknown. What little information is available indicates that these artificial cells would function as a foreign body and probably would be cleared rapidly by the RES. Consequently, only with repeated infusions of neohemocytes would a sufficient concentration be obtained in the blood to afford effective oxygen delivery.

On the basis of current knowledge, chemically modified SFH continues to evolve as the most useful of the potential red-cell substitutes. Although considerable clinical testing needs to be undertaken to ensure the safety and efficacy of modified SFH, research to date has been most encouraging. As an oxygen-carrying colloid suspended in a balanced salt solution, it may very well prove to be the ultimate resuscitation fluid.

Metabolic Manipulations

As additional information is obtained concerning the altered mechanisms that underlie the various shock states, more specific metabolic manipulations to prevent these derangements can be anticipated. A more beneficial outcome is likely to result from either blocking the detrimental aspects of these processes or augmenting those responses that are clearly protective. In this regard, several investigative observations have been noted in recent years that may directly influence shock management in the near future. For example, the endogenous opiate, beta-endorphin appears to be involved in the hypotension and impaired tissue perfusion that commonly occur in both hypovolemic and septic shock states; elevations in this substance can be demonstrated at the time these physiologic aberrations occur.[2]

Naloxone, an inhibitor of endorphin activity, has been studied as a possible agent to prevent these alterations. Although it has no effect on the cardiovascular system under normal circumstances, naloxone has been shown in animal studies to elevate blood pressure and cardiac output, and to significantly improve survival in septic, endotoxin, and hemorrhagic shock models.[2] Early clinical studies with this agent in shock patients have also demonstrated its potential efficacy as a therapeutic tool.[26]

Another approach to shock management has involved the use of various metabolic substrates to improve cell function and thus to allow better toleration of shock and/or ischemia. It is well known that a clear relationship exists between ATP depletion and organ dysfunction in shock and ischemia and that intravenous infusion of ATP complexed with $MgCl_2$ can promote "survival" in both hemorrhagic and septic animal shock models.[5,6] Whether these highly charged molecules can cross cell membranes (either damaged or intact) is still unresolved, but the presumed energy that they provide in shock situations has definitely influenced outcome. Derangements in hepatic metabolism secondary to shock have been especially responsive to ATP–$MgCl_2$.[20] Beneficial effects have also been achieved in various shock models by providing solutions of tissue substrates such as pyruvate, inosine, adenosine, and creatine phosphate.[42] These moieties presumably provide the substrate necessary for the synthesis of high-energy phosphates. Solutions of glucose, insulin, and potassium have likewise been shown to be efficacious, apparently by providing substrate necessary for cells in need.[3] Whether these approaches will be useful in the treatment of human shock states remains to be determined.

Cyclic AMP (cAMP), the "second messenger" that instructs the cell to respond to a stimulus when its membrane is activated by a specific hormone, is depleted in septic and hemorrhagic shock.[36] Defects in cAMP metabolism produce dysfunctional cells and thereby impair normal beneficial homeostatic responses. Administration of cAMP to experimental animals has yielded varied beneficial results. Cellular membrane stabilization aimed at preserving adenyl cyclase will likely be as effective as cAMP alone in maintaining cellular integrity.

Many of the cellular deficits in various shock states result from increased cell membrane permeability.[6] In shock, control of the large and small channels within cell membranes directly relates to cell viability. If membrane integrity is preserved, intracellular homeostasis is maintained. Future therapy for shock may involve pharmacologic manipulation of calcium, sodium, and potassium flux as a means of preserving cellular function and structure in the face of the shock insult.

Alterations in the metabolism of prostaglandins in shock have been recently recognized. These ubiquitous, vasoactive lipids with short half-lives may play a role in the pathophysiology of shock by vasodilation or vasoconstriction of the microcirculation with shunting of blood. In addition, prostaglandins probably play a role in coagulation and regulation of white cells by preventing them from releasing toxic or vasoactive substances.[19] The therapeutic role of prostaglandins in shock management is not yet defined.

Finally, beneficial effects have been achieved by using antisera in the treatment of gram-negative sepsis.[45] This passive augmentation of the host defense system has a rational basis in the treatment of shock because of the variety of immune defects that have been documented in the various shock states.

SUMMARY

''Shock'' is a state of altered tissue perfusion that occurs when the cardiac output is inadequate to maintain effective blood flow to organs and tissues sufficient to provide necessary nutrients and oxygen, and the removal of waste products resulting from their metabolism. Etiologically, four types of shock have been recognized: hypovolemic, septic, cardiogenic, and neurogenic. Despite its underlying etiology, a basic neuroendocrine response is evoked when shock occurs that results in redistribution of the body's blood flow to ensure adequate perfusion to such vital organs as the heart and brain. In addition, a number of metabolic aberrations ensure adequate nutrients (e.g., glucose) to maintain normal cellular function. The magnitude of these responses depends on the severity of shock, but they can be particularly pronounced in those forms of shock secondary to hypovolemia and/or sepsis.

The successful treatment of shock involves a thorough understanding of these pathophysiologic derangements and the distinguishing characteristics of the various etiologies that can give rise to its development. By careful hemodynamic monitoring and the re-establishment of an effective circulating blood volume (through the infusion of intravenous fluids and/or blood, and by various pharmacologic manipulations), adequate tissue perfusion and oxygen-carrying capacity of blood can be assured under most shock conditions. Metabolic abnormalities usually are not treated directly, but rather tend to resolve when the underlying source of shock is corrected. With such physiologically directed therapy, many more patients survive their shock insult today than did as recently as 5 or 10 years ago. As knowledge in this area continues to improve, we can expect even greater advances.

REFERENCES

1. Bland, R., Shoemaker, W.C., and Shabot, M.M.: Physiologic monitoring goals for the critically ill patient, Surg. Gynecol. Obstet. **147:**833, 1978.
2. Bone, R.C., et al.: Endorphins in endotoxin shock, Microcirculation **1:**265, 1981.
3. Bronsveld, W., et al.: Effects of glucose-insulin-potassium (GIK) on myocardial blood flow metabolism in canine endotoxin shock, Circ. Shock **13:**325, 1984.
4. Carrico, C.J., et al.: Multiple-organ-failure syndrome, Arch. Surg. **121:**196, 1986.
5. Chaudry, I.H., Sayeed, M.M., and Baue, A.E.: Effect of adenosine triphosphate-magnesium chloride administration in shock, Surgery **75:**220, 1974.
6. Chaudry, I.H., Clemens, M.G., and Baue, A.E.: Alterations in cell function with ischemia and shock and their correction, Arch. Surg. **116:**1309, 1981.
7. Christou, N.V., Meakins, J.L., and Superina, R.: Host defenses, sepsis and the critically ill patient. In Bartlet, R.H., Whitehouse, W.M., and Turcotte, J.C., editors: Life support systems in intensive care, Chicago, 1984, Year Book Medical Publishers.
8. Collins, J.A.: Pertinent recent developments in blood banking, Surg. Clin. North Am. **63:**483, 1983.
9. Counts, R.B., et al.: Hemostasis in massively transfused trauma patients, Ann. Surg. **190:**91, 1979.
10. Del Maestro, R.F., Bjork, J., and Arfars, K.E.: Free radicals and microvascular permeability. In Autar, A.P., editor: Pathology of oxygen, New York, 1982, Academic Press, Inc.
11. DeVenuto, F., et al.: Appraisal of hemoglobin solution as a blood substitute, Surg. Gyn. Obstetr. **149:**417, 1979.
12. Gann, D.S., and Amaral, J.F.: Pathophysiology of trauma and shock. In Zuidema, G.D., Rutherford, R.D., and Ballinger, W.F., editors: The management of trauma, Philadelphia, 1985, W.B. Saunders & Co.
13. Gould, S.A., Rice, C.L., and Moss, G.S.: The physiologic basis of the use of blood and blood products, Surg. Ann. **16:**13, 1984.
14. Greenburg, A.G.: Blood substitutes: Where are we? Surg. Ann. **15:**13, 1983.
15. Greenburg, A.G., and Peskin, G.W.: Blood, salt and water: recent advances. In Bartlett, R.H., Whitehouse, W.M., and Turcotte, J.G., editors: Life support systems in intensive care, Chicago, 1984, Year Book Publishers, Inc.
16. Greenburg, A.G., and Peskin, G.W.: Monitoring in the recovery room and surgical intensive care unit. In Saidman, L.J. and Smith, N.T., editors: Monitoring in anesthesia, ed. 2, Boston, 1984, Butterworth Publishers, Inc.
17. Gump, F.E.: Whole body metabolism. In Altura, B.M., Lefer, A.M., and Schumer, W., editors: Handbook of shock and trauma, vol. I: Basic sciences, New York, 1983, Raven Press.
18. Halliwell, B.: Oxygen is poisonous: the nature and medical importance of oxygen radicals, Med. Lab. Sci. **4:**157, 1984.
19. Hechtman, H.B., et al.: Prostaglandin and thromboxane mediation of cardipulmonary failure, Surg. Clin. North Am. **63:**263, 1983.
20. Hirasawa, H., et al.: Improved survival and reticuloendothelial function with intravenous ATP-$MgCl_2$ following hemorrhagic shock, Circ. Shock **11:**141, 1983.
21. Hoyt, D.B., et al.: Intra-abdominal sepsis and perfluorocarbons: mechanisms of protection and pulmonary response, Surg. Forum **32:**51, 1981.
22. Mitsuno, T., Ohyanogi, H., and Naito, R.: Clinical studies of a perfluorocarbon whole blood substitute: Fluosol DA-20, Ann. Surg. **195:**60, 1982.
23. Mosher, D.F.: Physiology of fibronectin, Annu. Rev. Med. **35:**361, 1984.
24. Moss, G.S., Gould, S.A., and Sehgal, L.R.: Hemoglobin solutions—from tetramer to polymer, Surgery **95:**249, 1984.
25. Pardy, B.J.: Trauma and shock. In Burnett, W., editor: Science for surgeons, Boston, 1981, Butterworth Publishers, Inc.
26. Peters, W.P., et al.: Pressor effect of naloxane in septic shock, Lancet **ii:**529, 1981.
27. Poole, G.U., et al.: Comparison of colloids and crystalloids in resuscitation from hemorrhagic shock, Surg. Gyn. Obstet. **154:**577, 1982.
28. Rhodes, R.S., and DePalma, R.G.: Mitrochondrial dysfunction of the liver and hypoglycemia in hemorrhagic shock, Surg. Gyn. Obstet. **150:**347, 1980.
29. Saba, T.M.: Reversal of plasma fibronectin deficiency in septic-injured patients by cryoprecipitate infusion. In Collins, J.A., Mugawski, D., and Shafer, A.W., editors: Massive transfusion in surgery and trauma, New York, 1983, Alan R. Liss, Inc.
30. Schneider, A.J., Stockman, J.A., and Oski, F.A.: Transfusion nomogram: an application of physiology to clinical decisions regarding the use of blood, Crit. Care Med. **9:**469, 1981.
31. Shackford, S.R., et al.: Hypertonic sodium lactate versus lactated Ringer's solution for intravenous fluid therapy in operations on the abdominal aorta, Surgery **94:**41, 1983.
32. Shatney, C.H., et al.: Efficacy of hetastarch in the resuscitation of patients with multisystem trauma and shock, Arch. Surg. **118:**804, 1983.
33. Shires, G.T., Williams, J., and Brown, F.: Acute change in extracellular fluids associated with major surgical procedures, Ann. Surg. **154:**803, 1961.
34. Shires, G.T., Carrico, C.J., and Canizaro, P.C.: Shock, Philadelphia, 1973, W.B. Saunders Co.

35. Shoemaker, W.C., and Czer, L.S.C.: Evaluation of the biologic importance of various hemodynamic and oxygen transport variables, Crit. Care Med. **7**:424, 1979.
36. Sibbald, W.J., et al.: Variations in plasma levels of adenosine 3′-5′ monophosphate during clinical sepsis, Surg. Gyn. Obstet. **144:**199, 1977.
37. Sibbald, W.J., et al.: Concepts in the pharmacologic and nonpharmacologic support of cardiovascular function in critically ill patients. Surg. Clin. North Am. **63:**455, 1983.
38. Trachte, G.J.: Endocrinology of shock. In Altura, B.M., Lefer, A.M., and Schumer, W., editors: Handbook of shock and trauma, vol. I: Basic science, New York, 1983, Raven Press.
39. Tranbaugh, R.F., et al.: Lung water changes after thermal injury: the effects of crystalloid resuscitation and sepsis, Ann. Surg. **192:**479, 1980.
40. Tremper, K.K., et al.: The preoperative treatment of severely anemic patients with a perfluorochemical oxygen transport fluid, Fluosol-DA, N. Engl. J. Med. **307:**277, 1982.
41. Trunkey, D.D., Holcroft, J., and Carpenter, M.A.: Calcium flux during hemorrhagic shock in baboons. J. Trauma **16:**633, 1976.
42. Valeri, C.R., and Zarvoulis, C.G.: Rejuvenation and freezing of outdated stored human red cells, N. Engl. J. Med. **287:**1307, 1972.
43. Velasco, I.T., et al.: Hyperosmotic NaCl and severe hemorrhagic shock, Am. J. Physiol. **239**(Heart Circ. Physiol. 8):H664, 1980.
44. Virgilio, R.W., et al.: Crystalloid versus colloid resuscitation: is one better? Surgery **85:**129, 1979.
45. Ziegler, E.J., et al.: Treatment of gram-negative bacteremia and shock with human antiserum to a mutant E. coli, N. Engl. J. Med. **307:**1125, 1982.

9

John E. Niederhuber and David N. Shapiro

Neoplastic Disease: Pathophysiology and Rationale for Treatment

Our understanding of both the cellular and molecular aspects of neoplasia has been significantly enhanced by recent studies of clonogenic tumor cells in tissue culture and by the recent discovery of the activation of certain cellular genes (oncogenes) in human tumors.[80,98,109] From these studies it has been proposed that a cancer growth can be regarded as a mixture of cells that have the capacity to renew themselves ("stem cells") and maintain the tumor. Although the majority of cells in the tumor are derived from the stem cells, they are committed to clonal expansion and differentiation.[106,130,157]

Evidence is increasing that proliferative potential is directly dependent on the expression of specific genes and that oncogenes are involved in the regulation of the expression of the genes controlling proliferation in both normal and neoplastic stem cells. On the basis of several lines of evidence, it is reasonable to postulate that transformation of normal stem cells may represent a defect in the gene(s) regulating cell proliferation.

These advances in our understanding of tumor cell proliferation and transformation of normal cells have great importance in the design of rational therapy using multiple treatment modalities. Clearly, the best therapy available to a cancer patient will involve the application of surgery, radiation therapy, chemotherapy, and agents capable of modifying the host response (biologic response modifiers). These modalities must be used by specialists well trained in the basic concepts and current knowledge of tumor cell biology. The basis for such knowledge begins with a study of normal cell growth and comparison to growth of neoplastic transformed cells.

NORMAL GROWTH OF CELLS AND CELL CYCLE KINETICS

A fundamental principle of tumor cell biology is that cancer develops from the subset of cells in any tissue that can divide and replace themselves (stem cells).[107,130] Most cells are in a quiescent state; some for the lifetime of the organism. Such cells are in a terminal state of differentiation and are often referred to as "end-stage" cells. The "end-stage" cells are in the G_0 phase of the cell cycle and cannot, under normal conditions, continue to divide.[163] Replacement of these cells occurs when a stem cell in the tissue is activated to divide, resulting in two daughter cells, one of which replaces the original stem cell, whereas the other enters a phase of proliferation and differentiation to replace the lost "end-stage" cell. The result is a delicate balance of replacement that depends on sensitive regulatory mechanisms. During the growth of a cancer, the rate of cell division and replacement exceeds cell loss as a consequence of the loss of normal growth regulation. In some cases, the balance may be only slightly shifted toward increased cell division, and as a result a cancer may develop over many years.

Both normal cells and cancer cells proliferate by an identical process termed the cell division cycle.[90] The classic cycle of cell division can be divided into four stages: G_1, S (DNA synthesis), G_2, and M (mitosis) (Fig. 9-1).[112,156,173] G_1 is the "gap" between completion of cell division and the beginning of DNA synthesis that occurs in the S phase. Daughter cells generated by mitosis reside in either G_1 or G_0 and retain a diploid set of chromosomes. Cells in culture usually spend several hours in G_1. For example, NIH-3T3 cells typically have a G_1 of 6 hours, whereas another cell line, L cells, has a G_1 of 12 hours. The G_1 transit time, however, is highly variable even from one cell to another within the same culture, and it is during this phase of the cycle that the cell is most affected by external conditions. Studies of cell cycle kinetics suggest that a specific control event (restriction point) exists within G_1 that determines whether a cell can progress to DNA synthesis.[112]

If the cell is not triggered to DNA synthesis, it may be shunted into a resting state termed G_0, from which the cell can reenter G_1 when conditions are appropriate. Tumor cells or transformed cells in culture, however, rarely enter G_0. Nevertheless, the variable time in G_1 has the effect of protecting some tumor cells from being killed by phase-specific chemotherapy active during S phase.[74]

During the S phase, cells synthesize DNA, and chromosomal replication begins.[91] The average duration of the S phase of NIH-3T3 cells is 8 hours, and at the completion of DNA synthesis the cell has replicated its entire complement of genetic material and therefore has two diploid sets of chromosomes. The S phase is followed by a second gap termed G_2, averaging approximately 3 hours for NIH-3T3 cells in culture. The daughter chromosomes generated during the S phase remain intimately associated with their partner until mitosis. During G_1, S, and G_2, the interphase of the cell cycle, RNA and protein synthesis are steadily increasing with duplication of all organelles, including ribosomes and mitochrondria. Mitosis represents the culmination of cell growth that has occurred during G_1, S, and G_2 and is the process by which a cell distributes two sets of chromosomes to the two daughter cells. As noted, the most variable period of the cell cycle is the first gap—G_1.

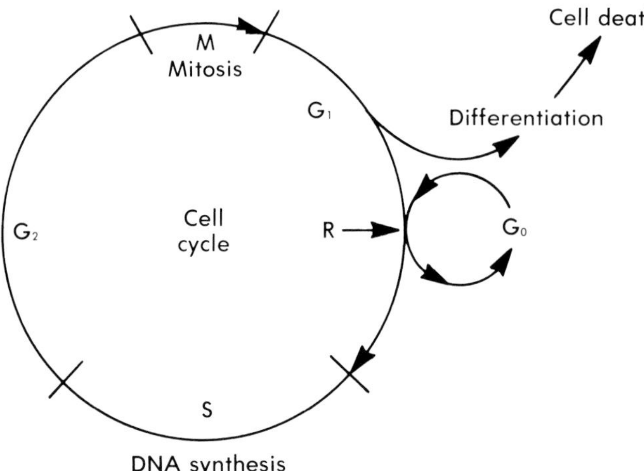

Fig. 9-1 The cycle of cell division is divided into two parts: interphase and mitosis *(M)*. Interphase can be divided into three parts: gap 1 *(G_1)*, phase of DNA synthesis *(S)*, and gap 2 *(G_2)*. A point, restriction point *(R)*, exists in G_1 and determines whether a cell can progress to *S*. If a cell is not triggered to DNA synthesis, it may be shunted to a resting place G_o. The amount of time that is spent in each phase of the cycle is unique to the particular cell type.

G_1 essentially determines the length of the cycle by responding or not responding to intrinsic or extrinsic signals that trigger entry into the S phase.[18,124]

In vitro studies of cultured normal and transformed cells have indicated that there are a number of significant differences between them. Normal cells placed in culture have a limited growth potential. Their most striking property is density-dependent inhibition of growth.[12] For example, normal cells do not grow across one another but line up in an even monolayer, with the resultant cessation of cell division and DNA synthesis once this monolayer covers the surface of the culture flask.[2] Normal cells also are much more dependent than tumor cells on exogenous growth factors, including serum concentration present in the medium.

The most striking characteristic of transformed cells is their loss of contact growth inhibition. Transformed cells in culture can grow across one another, form dense piled-up colonies, and usually manifest unlimited growth potential. Frequently, transformed cells lose their requirement for surface attachment (loss of anchorage) and grow in suspension or soft agar.[11] Generally, transformed cells require less serum in the culture media and demonstrate decreased adhesiveness.

Loss of adhesiveness by transformed cells is associated with decreased glycosylation of surface glycoproteins, loss of cell surface fibronectin, decreased intracellular cAMP, decreased microfilament bundles, increased microvilli on the cell surface, and increased agglutination with plant lectins such as concanavalin A and wheat germ agglutinin. Not all of these phenotypic changes, however, may be manifest in a given transformed cell, and no single property of a transformed cultured cell ensures that it will be capable of inducing a tumor when placed in vivo. Transformed cells with several of these phenotypic changes, especially loss of anchorage, are more likely to possess the ability to form an in vivo tumor.

The growth of both normal and transformed cells depends on the presence of specific growth factors and cell surface receptors for these proteins. Genes that code for these factors, their receptors, and the intracellular proteins involved in transmitting their signals to the nucleus are critical to an orderly proliferation of cells. Abnormalities that occur in the genes that code for growth factor receptors and transmitter proteins will obviously have much influence on the control of cell division and the state of abnormal cell transformation. The characterization of these genes and their products represents one of the most exciting new developments in cancer biology.

MOLECULAR BASIS OF NEOPLASIA

Viral and Cellular Oncogenes

Concepts concerning the cause of malignancy have been revolutionized by the identification in most, if not all, vertebrates of a series of genes that are closely related to the oncogenic genes of certain RNA tumor viruses (retroviruses) and by the finding that alterations in the structure and expression of these genes are associated with cellular transformation.[1,52,76,168] Retroviruses as a family have been shown to retain structural homology (Fig. 9-2), consisting of two sequences of RNA nucleotides (one at each end), which contain genetic signals for starting and stopping transcription and for enhancing gene expression (long terminal repeat [*LTR*]). Intact retroviruses have three internal genes in series: one for internal viral core proteins *(gag)*; one for the enzyme reverse transcriptase *(pol)* that transcribes DNA from RNA; and one for an envelope protein *(env)*.[16,43] These three genes code for proteins required for replication of an infectious virus within its host.

The life cycle of these retroviruses consists of several stages (Fig. 9-2). The mature, encapsulated RNA virus enters a host cell and is transcribed into DNA by a reverse transcriptase *(pol)* into a DNA copy, which integrates into the DNA of the host. The integrated viral DNA is then used to generate more RNA copies, which are encapsulated in a protein coat. These copies bud through the membrane of the cell to yield mature progeny.[15]

Some retroviruses rapidly induce malignant change when they enter an animal cell (acute transforming retroviruses). Tumor induction by retroviruses is a phenomenon unrelated to the virus' own propagation; however, the effect on the cell can be devastating. The structural component of the virus responsible for tumor induction is a fourth gene, unrelated to *gag, pol* or *env*. Because of its ability to induce malignant change, this fourth gene is designated the viral oncogene (v-*onc*).[43] In some retroviruses the oncogene is found in addition to intact *gag, pol,* and *env* genes; in other viruses, the oncogene replaces part or all of one or more of the *gag, pol,* and *env* structural genes. In the latter circumstance, the virus is defective and cannot replicate alone because it lacks critical genetic information for generating appropriate enzymes and structural proteins. These replication-defective viruses require co-infection with a related "helper" virus that supplies the missing genetic information for virus replication.

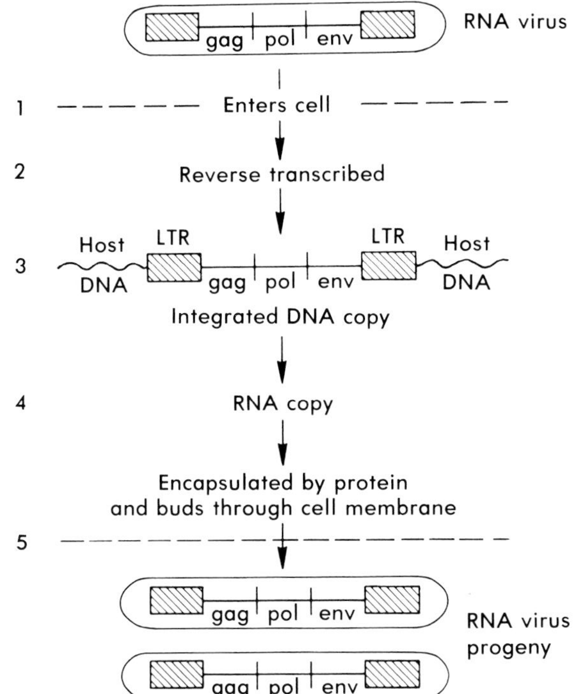

Fig. 9-2 RNA tumor viruses contain genes for internal proteins *(gag)*, reverse transcriptase *(pol)*, and envelope proteins *(env)*. When a tumor virus enters a cell, its RNA is reverse transcribed to DNA within the cytoplasm and enters the nucleus. Viral DNA containing two identical sequences at each end long terminal repeats *(LTR)* integrates into the DNA of the host cell. The viral DNA directs synthesis of viral messenger RNA, which in turn directs synthesis of viral proteins. Viral RNA is encapsulated by protein and mature progeny virus bud through the cell membrane.

The viral oncogenes in retroviruses are responsible for the induction of malignant transformation in the cells of various vertebrates.* Viral oncogenes were initially thought to be of viral origin and to be required for some purpose important to the life cycle of the virus. However, this model did not easily explain why some retroviruses lacked oncogenes and still propagated in a satisfactory manner. Only when tissues from normal, uninfected animals were examined did it become apparent that genes similar to viral oncogenes were a normal constituent of the cells of many vertebrate species.

The first studies reported the presence of genes similar to the oncogene of the Rous sarcoma virus in cells of normal chickens.[158] Similar genes related to the Rous sarcoma virus were later identified not only in the cells of birds, but also in those of mice, rats, and other mammals, including humans. There rapidly followed the identification of cellular genes more or less corresponding to the oncogenes of over 20 different retroviruses.[35,52] For each of the viral oncogenes there is a corresponding gene in the cells of many vertebrate species. Some of these genes have been found in all species examined. The cellular genes homologous to the viral oncogenes are designated cellular oncogenes (c-*onc*).[52] In some instances the cellular oncogenes are essentially identical in structure to the corresponding viral oncogenes; in other cases there has been some divergence in structure between viral and animal genes during the course of evolution.

After the discovery of cellular oncogenes in uninfected cells, the first logical interpretation was that they represented genetic sequences acquired sometime in the early evolution of animals during the course of infection by viruses. However, the converse proved to be true, and it is now known that the cellular oncogenes are normal genetic components of all vertebrate cells and that some of these cellular genes have been incorporated into retroviruses in the course of an infection during evolution. Therefore the direction of transmission of genetic information is thought to be from animals cells to viruses and not the reverse.[16]

Cellular oncogenes are phylogenetically ancient and have been found in all vertebrates thus far examined. Related genes are even found in invertebrates such as the fruit fly and in primitive nucleated cells of yeast.[149] Preservation of cellular oncogenes through phylogeny with relatively little structural change suggests that these genes code for essential cellular proteins.[72] Recently, a novel class of human retroviruses, the human T-cell leukemia viruses (HTLVs) have been shown to be responsible for a group of human T-cell diseases commonly termed adult T-cell leukemia (ATL).[121,127] However, they differ from other retroviruses because no substantial homology exists between HTLV and other animal viruses or with cellular oncogene sequences present in normal animals or humans. HTLV is expressed when neoplastic T cells from patients with ATL-related diseases are cultured in the presence of T-cell growth factor. Analysis of the HTLV genome demonstrated the usual genes of a retrovirus required for viral replication (i.e., *gag, pol,* and *env*) and an additional set of sequences termed *Px* located 3′ to *env*.[144,145,170] As yet, a *Px* protein has not been found, but evidence suggests that the *Px* product may be essential to initiation of transformation by HTLV. *Px,* however, does not fit the definition of a true viral oncogene since no homologous DNA sequences are present in normal animals or humans.

Functions of Cellular Oncogenes

The functions of the cellular oncogenes are not known, although some clues have been obtained from the study of proteins encoded by structurally similar viral oncogenes. DNA sequence analysis, functional activity, and DNA-mediated gene transfer (transfection) experiments have been used to classify the viral oncogenes into specific families. These include the *src*-related oncogenes with identified protein kinase activity, the *src*-related oncogenes that have not yet been shown to have protein kinase activity but have sequence homology to *src,* the *ras* oncogene family that binds guanine nucleotides, the *myc* oncogene family that has DNA-binding activity, the *sis* oncogene family that encodes for cellular growth factors, and unrelated oncogenes (Table 9-1).

Several viral oncogenes encode proteins that act as enzymes that add phosphate groups to amino acid residues in proteins—a process known as phosphorylation. Many

*References 17, 28, 31, 38, 40, 48, 66, 68, 96, 100, 123, 164.

Table 9-1 **CLASSIFICATION OF VIRAL ONCOGENES**

Retroviral Source	Viral Oncogene	Tumor Induced by Viral Oncogene	Oncogene Product	
			Activity*	Localization
Avian species	v-*src*	Sarcoma	PK(tyr)	Plasma membrane
Avian species	v-*fps*	Sarcoma	PK(tyr)	Plasma membrane
Avian species	v-*yes*	Sarcoma	PK(tyr)	Not known
Avian species	v-*ros*	Sarcoma	PK(tyr)	Not known
Avian species	v-*myc*	Sarcoma, carcinoma, leukemia	DNA binding	Nucleus
Avian species	v-*erb*^{B}	Sarcoma, leukemia	Related to receptor for epidermal growth factor	Not known
Avian species	v-*myb*	Myeloid leukemia	Not known	Nucleus
Avian species	v-*rel*	Lymphoid leukemia	Not known	Not known
Avian species	v-*ski*	Not known	Not known	Not known
Murine species	v-*raf*	Not known	Not known	Not known
Murine species	v-*mos*	Sarcoma	Not known	Cytoplasm
Murine species	v-*bas*	Sarcoma	Not known	Not known
Murine species	v-*abl*	Lymphoid leukemia	PK(tyr)	Plasma membrane
Murine species	v-*ras*^{Ha}	Sarcoma, erythroleukemia	PK(thr), GTP binding	Plasma membrane
Murine species	v-*ras*^{Ki}	Sarcoma, erythroleukemia	PK(thr), GTP binding	Plasma membrane
Murine species	v-*fos*	Sarcoma	Not known	Nucleus
Cats	v-*fes*	Sarcoma	PK(tyr)	Plasma membrane
Cats	v-*fms*	Sarcoma	Not known	Intracellular membrane
Woolly monkey	v-*sis*	Sarcoma	Related to platelet-derived growth factor	Cytoplasm

**PK(tyr),* protein kinase phosphorylating tyrosine; *PK(thr),* protein kinase phosphorylating threonine; *GPT,* guanosine triphosphate.

phosphokinases found in normal cells phosphorylate serine or threonine residues in protein, whereas some oncogene phosphokinases phosphorylate tyrosine residues in proteins.[33] These phosphokinases resemble certain normal cell membrane-bound hormone receptors that function as enzymes. When these receptors are activated by hormone or growth factor binding, they act as tyrosine phosphokinases transducing membrane signals into the cytoplasm.[32]

Only the eight *src* viral oncogene proteins have been shown to act as phosphokinases; the other oncoproteins have different and less well understood functions. For example, the *ras* genes encode for proteins that bind guanine nucleotides with high affinity and stimulate protein phosphorylation on threonine residues.[148] The product of the *sis* gene is a cellular growth factor that is equivalent to platelet-derived growth factor (PDGF) and stimulates proliferation of fibroblasts.[166] The *myc* gene encodes a protein that binds to DNA,[135] whereas the *erb-B* gene product has close similarity to the truncated receptor for epidermal growth factor.[50]

Although their functions are unknown, the association of viral oncogenes with malignant cellular proliferation suggests that cellular oncogenes may play a role in cell proliferation.[72] Furthermore, the association of certain viral oncogenes with specific cell lineages also suggests a possible role for some normal cellular oncogenes in cellular differentiation. In addition, studies of cellular oncogene expression during mammalian embryonic development has shown some oncogenes to be maximally expressed at specific stages of embryonic development.[114,115] For example, c-*myc* is maximally expressed at a time when the hematopoietic system is rapidly expanding in the fetal liver, spleen, and then bone marrow. Still other oncogenes seem to have a specific association with the rapidly proliferating cells of the placenta and fetal membranes. However, the precise role of these oncogenes in embryonic development is uncertain. It is tempting to speculate that some oncogenes code for proteins that instruct other lineages of cells to divide, proliferate, and differentiate.

Malignancy Induced by Cellular Oncogenes

Under some circumstances cellular oncogenes can induce normal cells to undergo malignant transformation. This phenomenon is not surprising in view of the structural similarity of cellular oncogenes with the oncogenes of retroviruses that cause tumors. The evidence for the induction of malignancy by cellular oncogenes can be summarized in four ways. First, a class of retroviruses, known as avian leukosis virus, induces lymphomas in chickens after latent periods of many months. These viruses have *gag, pol,* and *env* sequences but lack identifiable viral oncogene sequences that characterize other acutely transforming retroviruses that induce tumors rapidly. The mechanism of tumor induction by avian leukosis virus seems to involve many cycles of viral replication and spread to adjacent cells until, by chance, viral DNA is inserted near the cellular c-*myc* oncogene and activation of this gene occurs.[82] Activation of c-*myc,* and perhaps of other as yet unidentified oncogenes, results in transformation of the infected cells to the malignant state. Second, when certain cellular oncogenes such as c-*mos* and c-*ras* are isolated, cloned, linked to an active promoter of gene expression, and introduced into tissue culture cells, they induce malignant transformation.[17,38] The third piece of evidence has as its

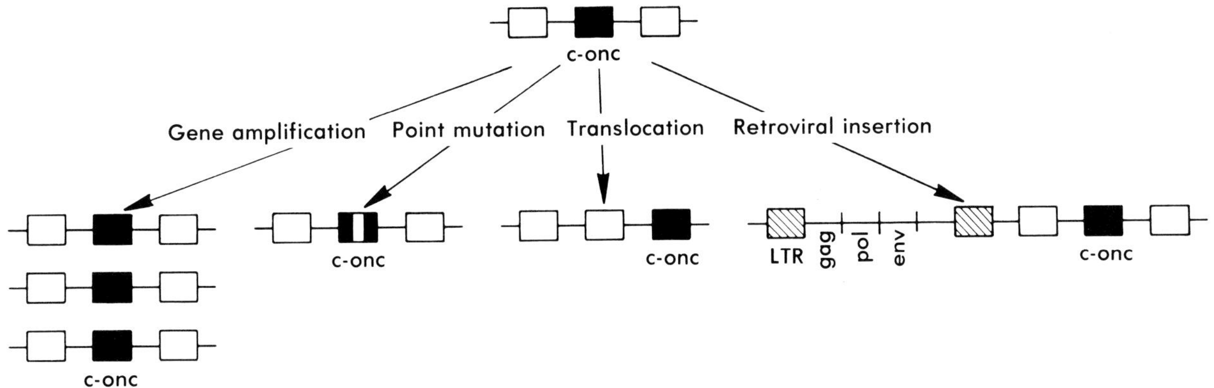

Fig. 9-3 Cellular oncogenes *(c-onc)* can be activated, and their expression increased by gene amplification, point mutation, chromosomal translocation, or retroviral insertion. Note that only point mutation actually involves structural alteration of cellular oncogenes. The other mechanisms of cellular oncogene activation may involve control by unrelated regulatory sequences of other genes such as an immunoglobulin promoter or retroviral long terminal repeats *(LTR)*.

basis the introduction of cellular oncogenes into a line of mouse fibroblasts designated NIH-3T3 cells. Normally these cells grow in sheets with the characteristic flattened appearance of fibroblasts. When they undergo malignant transformation, the cells show unrestrained growth, become rounder, and pile up on one another. The NIH-3T3 cells can therefore be used as a model of cancer induction.[35] Specific gene sequences capable of inducing malignant transformation have been identified in bladder, colon, and lung cancer cell lines, as well as in fresh tumors.[30,42,108,147,151] In these cases the tumor gene sequences were further characterized and identified as belonging to a cellular oncogene family. For example, the *ras* gene family has frequently been implicated as inducing malignant transformation in the in vitro NIH-3T3 model system. Malignant-transforming genes have also been isolated from B-cell lymphomas of humans and chickens.[46] Finally, transformation of NIH-3T3 cells has been accomplished by direct microinjection of cloned p21 protein, the product of the *ras* cellular oncogene.[154] Similar results have also been obtained by the coordinate action of a c-*sis* product (PDGF) and epidermal growth factor.[9] These studies clearly identify the products of cellular oncogenes as being directly responsible for morphologic and growth-related changes observed in cells transformed by these respective oncogenes.

Current thinking suggests that NIH-3T3 cells are already partially transformed toward the malignant state and that the insertion of a single oncogene induces true neoplasia. In contrast, if normal cells such as embryonic fibroblasts are used, the concerted and coordinate action of two or more oncogenes is required to induce malignant transformation.[97] It is clear that under some circumstances cellular oncogenes can induce cells to undergo neoplastic transformation. How cellular oncogenes induce this change is still uncertain.

Mechanisms of Activation of Cellular Oncogenes

The cellular oncogenes and the proteins that they specify form a structurally and functionally heterogeneous group. It is therefore not surprising that various molecular mechanisms are involved in activation of these genes (Fig. 9-3). In fact, five separate mechanisms of cellular oncogene activation have been found.[97]

The first mechanism to be documented involves overexpression of a cellular oncogene following acquisition of a unique transcriptional promoter. Both the *myc* and *erb-B* cellular oncogenes present in several avian hematopoietic neoplasias have become activated after adjacent integration of an avian leukosis proviral DNA segment. This viral segment provides a strong transcriptional promoter that replaces the indigenous promoters of these genes.[65,82] Many retroviruses may activate acquired cellular genes by forcing overexpression through the viral transcriptional promoter.

A second mechanism of activation involves overexpression caused by amplification of the cellular oncogene. The *myc* cellular oncogene is amplified 30 to 50 times in the human promyelocytic leukemia cell line HL-60 and in some lung cancer lines.[37,106,169] The C-ras^{Ki} gene is amplified three to five times in a human colon carcinoma cell line.[108] Recently 30 to 100 copies of a newly discovered relative of the *myc* gene, termed N-*myc,* were found in a number of human neuroblastomas.[143] In these cases the increased gene copy number is presumed to cause corresponding increases in transcript and gene product.

A third mechanism influences levels of transcription and, in turn, the amount of gene product. This mechanism depends on the poorly understood mechanism of action of "enhancer" sequences, which can increase use of transcriptional promoters to which they become linked. The linked promoter may be as far as several kilobases away, the enhancer element may be positioned upstream or downstream of the promoter. One example of this is the presence of retrovirus genome fragments downstream from the *myc* gene in avian lymphomas.[125] Here the retrovirus element appears to act by contributing not a promoter but an enhancer sequence.

Another mechanism by which cellular oncogene expression may be increased is by chromosomal translocation. In

Burkitt's lymphoma there is often a translocation of the c-*myc* gene from its normal position on chromosome 8 to the region on chromosome 14 containing the immunoglobulin heavy chain genes.[6,36,101] This appears to result in deregulation of the *myc* gene, which loses regulatory sequences of its own and instead acquires normally unlinked sequences involved in immunoglobulin production. The levels of c-*myc* transcripts in Burkitt cells are increased fivefold compared with normal lymphoblastoid cells, which have no such chromosomal rearrangement. A number of variant translocations of the c-*myc* gene in association with B-cell lymphomas have been recently reported. Other examples of cellular oncogene translocation have been characterized; e.g., in chronic myelocytic leukemia there is a reciprocal translocation of c-*sis* from chromosome 22 and c-*abl* from chromosome 9, resulting in high levels of c-*abl* expression.[39,77]

Of interest is the observation that many of the described nonrandom translocations involving oncogenes appear to be in characteristic chromosomal regions known as "fragile sites."[99,172] Fragile sites tend to be expressed as gaps or breaks during routine chromosome preparations and presumably represent chromosome segments that do not undergo compaction during mitosis. Whether this is a predisposing factor for chromosomal rearrangement involving cellular oncogenes is yet to be determined.

The fifth mechanism depends on alteration of the oncogene protein. This mechanism is best documented in the case of the oncogene proteins encoded by the *ras* genes. In the case of the human bladder carcinoma oncogene of the T24/EJ cell line, it is clear that a simple point mutation converted the normal, nontransforming c-*ras*^{Ha} oncogene into a potent oncogene. This point mutation results in a single amino acid substitution at position 12 of the transforming p21 protein.[23,136,160] This is a change in a single amino acid, but it can yield a significant difference in the structure of the protein.[142]

A slightly different result comes from the study of a human lung carcinoma c-*ras*^{Ha} oncogene that carries a mutation affecting amino acid 61 of the p21 protein.[171] It appears that these changes do not affect the levels of expression of these genes, only the structure of the encoded proteins. These results, along with recent evidence demonstrating somatic alteration of c-*ras*^{Ha} in actual human bladder tumors obtained from patients, suggest that the codons specifying residues 12 and 61 represent critical sites that, when mutated, will often create oncogenic alleles.[64] Point mutations in presumed oncogene suppressors may also be critical in the development of certain other malignancies such as retinoblastoma and Wilms' tumor.[116,120] It seems likely that point mutations elsewhere in the cellular oncogenes may also serve to inactivate these genes instead of converting them into potent oncogenes.

Malignancy as a Multistep Process

One of the most important points emerging from current investigations of oncogene activation in malignancy is that multiple sequential steps involving alterations in oncogene structure and expression are involved in oncogenesis. For example, chromosomal translocation and enhanced c-*myc* expression are observed in the majority of Burkitt's lymphomas[6]; however, the precipitating event triggering the cascade may be related to antecedent Epstein-Barr virus infection in certain cases.[85] Similarly, recent work has demonstrated that tumor cells could be created in a two-step process involving initial cellular immortalization by a chemical carcinogen followed by introduction of a cloned oncogene.[118] The progression of tumors from precancerous growths such as papillomas and adenomas into autonomously growing cancers may also have an underlying molecular basis involving oncogenes. Clearly, environmental factors such as exposure to radiation or mutagenic chemicals may be important in initiating the multistep process resulting in malignant transformation. Further, inherited chromosomal fragile sites[99,172] may be the locations where the earliest cellular derangement occurs.

This is not to say that all aspects of the cancer process will be readily understood in terms of the oncogenes with which we are now familiar. Cancer cells can modulate their antigenicity to evade immune defenses. They can also acquire an ability to break off from a primary tumor and seed secondary growths at distant sites. Such cancer phenotypes do not represent initial derangements in growth control, but rather secondary adaptations that favor survival and clonal expansion. The precedent of oncogenes leads us to the belief that even these secondary biologic phenomena responsible for the true malignancy of a tumor will also be traced back to the alteration of specific genes.

The eventual development of unique therapeutic strategies against cancer cells will require discovery of agents that recognize targets that are present only in the cancer cell and are at the same time essential for the continued growth of this cell. Oncogenes and their proteins represent good candidates for targets of this sort.[31,100] These deviant forms of cellular oncogenes may be specific to cancer cells and, unlike a variety of other cancer traits such as certain surface antigens, maybe indispensable for the ongoing growth of the tumor cell. By learning how oncogene-encoded proteins function, we may learn how to specifically antagonize their function and the mechanism by which oncogenes and their products interact to yield malignancy.

CHARACTERISTICS OF TUMOR GROWTH

Tumors appear to grow exponentially. However, with increasing size the doubling time also increases.[34,162] This relationship, in which the rate of growth decreases as the tumor grows, is described mathematically as a Gompertzian function.[105,141] The decreasing growth rate with increasing tumor size prohibits determining the date of tumor origin from a simple extrapolation of metastatic tumor doubling time. But, despite the Gompertzian growth curve, useful information is obtained from knowledge of the doubling time of measurable tumor. Although the same tumor type may grow at markedly different rates when studied in different patients, the various metastatic lesions in an individual patient show a very uniform rate of growth—a rate that appears to be more rapid than the primary tumor.[27] For most human tumors, such predicted growth rates are only an approximation because they cannot accurately account for tumor cell loss caused by cell death and exfoliation. The growth of human tumors results in increased size, leading to areas of inadequate tumor blood supply and partial necrosis. Thus the rate of cell proliferation may vary considerably even within the tumor.

A critical event in the history of a tumor and what may separate a slow-growing (almost dormant) in situ cancer from an invasive neoplasm is the process of neovascularization.[61] The vascularization of the cancer, perhaps stimulated by a specific factor(s), results in increased growth, leading to compression of surrounding tissues, invasion through the basement membrane, and distant seeding (metastases) of tumor cells in other body tissues.

The establishment of a secondary tumor appears to be a multistep process, and the likelihood that each step will proceed without interruption by host defenses is more uncommon than thought. Although the biology of tumor metastasis remains largely hypothetic, interesting experimental models have begun to clarify mechanisms of tumor-organ interaction that lead to the establishment of metastatic tumors.[53] Although the direct shedding of tumor cells into body cavities to form secondary tumor implants is easily understood, it is more difficult to envision the mechanisms by which tumor cells develop secondary spread by invasion of capillaries, venules, and lymphatic vessels. The invading tumor cells appear to form tumor emboli within the vessel by clumping with other tumor cells and with platelets. Fibrin deposition occurs, and, from this site of intravessel invasion, cells or clumps of cells shed and circulate through the body and its organ systems.[21,103]

It should be noted that tumor cells that enter the circulation through the lymphatic vessels and travel to regional nodes are not necessarily "trapped" in these nodes but may pass to higher nodes or enter the vascular circulation at the lymph node.[89] The vascular and lymphatic systems have extensive communication, especially within the lymph node, with the result that tumor cells entering either circulation are freely exchanged between the two systems.[41,58] Although there are many innate properties of the tumor cell that affect metastatic potential, there are also a variety of host defenses that can modify metastatic spread. It appears that the process of metastasis can be divided into two phases: escape of cells from the primary tumor and the establishment of growth at a secondary site.

A number of experimental models have attempted to define mechanisms involved in these two phases of the metastatic process.[103,104,138] Perhaps the most informative experiments have been those of Fidler involving the B-16 mouse melanoma.[53] He demonstrated an impressive clonal heterogeneity in metastatic tumor cells by injecting melanoma cells intravenously and subsequently isolating only the lung metastases. The isolated metastatic tumor cells from the lung were cultured in vitro and then reinjected. The process of isolation from the lung, culture, and reinjection was repeated multiple times until essentially only lung metastases would develop when the harvested tumor cells were injected. In addition, these lung-specific tumor cells could be shown to adhere better to lung cells in aggregation assays. Similar methods were used to select for metastatic tumor cells specific for the brain and the ovary.[19,20]

Perhaps even more important than the observation of metastatic heterogeneity of the secondary tumor when compared to the primary was the additional finding that other phenotypic properties also showed variability.[54] The important clinical implication of this heterogeneity is that different metastatic cell populations will vary widely in their response to chemotherapeutic agents. There is also evidence that, as susceptible subclones of a metastatic cell mass are selectively killed by a cytostatic drug, the remaining clones become more unstable and begin to drift, giving rise to an even greater heterogeneity.[128] Other experiments have addressed the question of whether cell surface determinants were directly involved in selecting the site of metastatic spread. For example, membrane vesicles prepared from lung-colonizing B-16 melanoma lines and cultured on the surface of nonspecific melanoma lines resulted in an enhanced rate of lung metastases.[129]

Another model of tumor spread has involved selecting metastatic cells with surface mutations induced by exposure to lethal concentrations of lectins such as wheat germ agglutinin. Metastasizing melanoma cells selected for resistance to wheat germ agglutinin were found to be poorly metastasizing cells.[155,161] These mutant cells demonstrated a loss of two of four terminal sialic acid residues from membrane oligosaccharides and a gain of two fucose residues.[57,94] In addition, these mutant cells had a seventy-fold increase in fucosyltransferase activity. Of interest was the observation that the treatment of these mutant cells with other lectins such as ricin or lotus tetragonolobus produced revertants that had regained their terminal sialic acid residues and their metastatic potential.[56] Such correlations of changes in molecular characteristics with function are needed to determine the relevance of specific phenotypic changes to the metastatic process.

It is important to note that the experiments with the B-16 melanoma, which demonstrated selection of organ-specific metastasizing cells, did not show any alteration in dissemination of the cells. As a result, explanations for organ specificity could include both preferential organ invasion and tissue-specific survival. In fact, experiments have shown that liver-specific melanoma cells grow much better on hepatocyte feeder layers than do melanoma cells lacking this metastatic potential.[111] Thus tissue-specific survival and growth promotion are additional mechanisms that must be considered as effecting the process of tumor metastasis.[55]

Admittedly, our present knowledge regarding the spread of cancer cells is derived from highly structured in vitro and in vivo models and does not take into account active and passive host defenses. Therefore, it is possible that these models have little relevance to the events of a spontaneous in vivo metastatic process. Considerably more information relating the metastatic events described by these models to the occurrence of spontaneous tumor spread is necessary.

TUMOR IMMUNITY IN HOST RESISTANCE

Since the 1900s it has been postulated that tumors express surface antigens that could distinguish them from normal cells. These original conclusions were derived from experiments that demonstrated the rejection of tumors transplanted between outbred mice. The realization that tumor rejection in outbred mice was caused by immune rec-

ANTIGENS DETECTED ON CANCER CELLS

- Class I transplantation antigens
- Tumor-specific transplantation antigens
- Tumor-associated antigens
  - Virus antigens
  - Embryonic antigens
  - Differentiation antigens
- Transformation-specific antigens

ognition of normal alloantigens resulted in much skepticism about the presence of tumor-specific antigens. In 1943, Gross[75] demonstrated immunity to a methylcholanthrene-induced sarcoma in inbred mice. In the intervening years, tumor-specific antigens or tumor-associated antigens have been demonstrated to be a feature of most, if not all, cancers.[10,78,79,132,150] More recently, the use of precise, highly specific monoclonal antibodies has made it possible to define a number of antigens that appear to be relatively specific for certain types of tumors.[84] For example, monoclonal antibodies have been found that are specific for antigens on melanoma cells,[159] colorectal adenocarcinoma,[88] neuroblastoma,[95] and lymphoid leukemia cells.[29]

The biochemical structure of tumor-specific antigens has not been well defined. However, it is clear that these tumor-specific transplantation antigens (TSTAs) are expressed as an integral part of the cell membrane. TSTAs are unique (i.e., antigenically distinct) for each carcinogen-induced tumor, suggesting that they arise from mutational events altering the normal cell membrane. In contrast, the TSTAs demonstrated on the cell membranes of virally induced tumors are not unique and are shared by all cells transformed by that virus.

Tumor cells may also express other types of tumor-specific antigens such as "oncofetal" antigens. These surface markers have been demonstrated to be embryonic or fetal cell antigens that are reexpressed on membranes of transformed cells. The most common examples include carcinoembryonic antigen and alpha-fetoprotein.[7,69] Even though carcinoembryonic antigen and α-fetoprotein lack some degree of specificity, they have proven to be extremely useful markers for the presence of their respective tumors. DNA tumor viruses produce yet another tumor-specific antigen (T antigen) in transformed cells.[152] The T antigen is an antigen unrelated to the structural proteins of the virus and is present on the nuclear membrane of DNA virus–transformed tumor cells. Its location in the nucleus makes it useful as a marker but not as an important antigen in tumor immunity.

The uniqueness of these tumor-specific antigens or the degree to which these neotumor structures are more "non-self" than "self" is the basis by which the body's immune system responds to tumors (see boxed material above). In experimental models, tumor-specific antigens can stimulate an immune response that results in resistance to tumor growth. This protection against tumor growth can be adoptively transferred to syngeneic animals to afford similar protection. Although tumor antigens associated with oncogenic viruses or ultraviolet-light exposure generate strong resistance, chemically induced tumors have weaker antigens, and tumors that arise spontaneously produce little or no detectable immune response.[71]

In addition to the acquired response of the immune system to antigens on transformed cells, the host also has innate mechanisms that can destroy tumor cells. The relationship between these two components of the host defense mechanism is unclear, but it is possible that the latter may be of greater significance. For example, there is considerable interest in the function and importance of the natural killer (NK) lymphoid cell, which is similar in many respects to the T cell involved in antibody-dependent cytolysis.[87] NK cells are spontaneously cytolytic for a number of (but not all) tumor lines in vitro, as well as for a significant number of virally infected cells. NK cells are present in athymic nude mice but recently have been found to be impaired or absent in Beige-J (C57/BL/6J/bg^J) mice.[137] The cytolytic activity of NK cells is not restricted by MHC Class I or II molecules, and NK cells do not demonstrate clonal expansion in response to specific antigenic challenge. The activity and number of NK cells, however, is increased by gamma interferon, and their activity inhibited by prostaglandin-E.[86,122] NK cells also possess Fc receptors and can kill antibody-coated target cells in vitro. It is not clear what the NK cell recognizes as the specific target on the tumor cell. However, in mice there is evidence that the differentiation antigen Ly-5 is part of the NK receptor.[67] The importance of NK cells to tumor resistance remains to be established. In humans there is a relationship between the level of NK cells found in peripheral blood and the extent of tumor growth. Different strains of mice appear to have differences in the numbers and activity of NK cells, and high NK strains have a lower incidence of spontaneous and induced tumors.[122]

Potentially NK cells offer passive protection; in addition, macrophages activated by T cell–derived lymphokines, bacterial lipopolysaccharide, double-stranded RNA, and *Bacille bilié de Calmette-Guérin* will also nonspecifically kill tumor cells.[4] Little is known about the capacity of in vivo activated macrophages to provide innate protection for the host, but many tumors appear to harbor increased numbers of monocytes or macrophage-like cells. Although it is difficult to extract these cells from viable tumor for use in experiments, there is some evidence that macrophages resident in tumors can be activated to kill the tumor cells in vitro.[4]

The T-lymphocyte population is involved in the immune response to tumor antigens through subsets of positive and negative regulatory cells and the generation of cytolytic T lymphocytes (CTLs).[25,117] The subset of T cells providing positive regulation, termed helper T cells (T_H), is involved in tumor antigen recognition and release of lymphokines such as gamma interferon. As in the immune response to soluble antigens, the response to tumor antigens results in negative regulation through suppressor T cells (T_s).[14] The third subset of T cells involved in tumor immunity is the CTLs. CTLs are clonally restricted, possess memory to previous antigenic stimulation, and recognize tumor-specific antigens in the context of self-class I molecules of the major histocompatibility complex (MHC). Although the CTL lysis of tumor target cells can be blocked by monoclonal antibody to the Class I determinant, the exact mechanism for T-cell recognition of the target cell is not known.

As noted, tumor-specific antigens can be recognized by the immune system as nonself, and such recognition can result in the production of tumor-specific antibody by B lymphocytes. Antibodies specific for tumor cells can destroy those cells by complement–dependent cytotoxicity and antibody-dependent cellular cytotoxicity.[113] Specific antibody can also bind to soluble tumor antigens to form antigen-antibody complexes, and these complexes have been shown to block immune function in an antigen-restricted fashion.[83]

The immune response to synchronous and metachronous tumor antigens involves the cells just described in a number of very complex cellular interactions. Cell-cell communication and resultant triggering of specific cellular functions have the potential for both positive antitumor effects and negative modulation, which may protect tumor cells from immune destruction. The immune response to soluble foreign proteins or membrane antigens requires that the antigen be presented to T_H cells by a macrophage that expresses MHC Class II molecules. The foreign antigen is in some way associated on the surface of the macrophage with the Class II MHC determinant, and the T_H cell "sees" both antigen and self-class II molecule in an extremely restricted interaction.[102,146,153] This interaction between macrophage and T_H cell sets the stage for the interaction of the T_H cell with B cells to induce specific antibody formation.

Negative regulation of this immune response involves the generation of both antigen-specific and nonspecific suppressor T lymphocytes.[13] These T_s cells have been found to be present in animals with actively growing tumors and, when adoptively transferred to syngeneic tumor-bearing recipients, enhance tumor growth.[62,63,73,119] The enhanced tumor growth appears to be linked to the ability of T_s cells to inhibit effector antitumor responses, including development of CTLs. The induction of T_s cells seems to be favored when the T cell encounters foreign antigen in a form that is not associated with Class II molecules on macrophages. T_s cells "down regulate" the response through the production of soluble mediators that act directly to suppress T_H and B cells.[49]

Antigen presentation by macrophages is not involved in the generation of tumor immunity by CTLs. Instead, the surface antigens are seen directly by a cytotoxic T-cell precursor that induces the generation of CTLs specific for the tumor antigen and for the self-Class I MHC molecule.[92,174] These cytotoxic T cells will only kill tumor cells that have the same tumor antigen and the same Class I MHC molecules used in immunizing the precursor cells. Thus T-cell interactions are MHC restricted whether they are cytotoxic T cells, helper T cells, or suppressor T cells. In each instance, the T cell has a receptor that recognizes a self MHC molecule and a foreign antigen. In the human, cytotoxic T cells and suppressor T cells express a differentiation antigen recognized by a monoclonal antibody, termed OKT8. Helper T cells express a different surface marker called OKT4.[110]

With the recent use of antigen-specific T-cell clones and monoclonal antibodies specific for the clone, it has been possible to precipitate a T-cell receptor molecule of 80,000 to 89,000 daltons. Under reducing conditions, this molecule is composed of two chains of 40,000 and 41,000 daltons.[3,81,140] Both of these chains have variable and constant regions. Much work remains to determine how these two glycoproteins function to recognize antigen and the MHC molecule and how such mechanisms may be used to enhance the effect of the immune response in controlling tumor growth.

As noted earlier, there is ample evidence to suggest that most, if not all, human tumors contain tumor-specific or at least tumor-associated antigens. Despite the presence of these unique "nonself" antigens on the tumor, manipulations of the host immune response and adoptive immunotherapy have been disappointingly ineffective in controlling tumor growth. The possible explanations for the inability to control tumor growth include:

1. Tumor antigens are poor stimulators of the immune system.
2. Tumor antigens may cause tolerance or favor stimulation of the suppressor T-cell circuit.
3. Cancer patients have or develop defects in immune responsiveness.
4. Tumors elaborate immunosuppressive "factors," including antigen-antibody complexes.
5. The rapid growth of large masses of metastatic tumor exceeds the capacity of the immune system.

Despite these disappointments, efforts by tumor immunologists continue to relate the elucidation of specific immune response functions to effective antitumor therapy. Although nonspecific stimulation of the response by such adjuvants as *Bacille bilié de Calmette-Guérin* and *Corynebacterium parvum* have largely been abandoned, there continues to be interest in the use of cell vaccines, lymphokines produced by activated macrophages and T cells, antigen-specific cloned cytolytic T cells, and monoclonal antibodies produced with the use of murine myeloma cells as fusion partners.[5,93,117,139] Monoclonal antibodies have potential applications in: (1) tumor imaging; (2) in vitro purification of bone marrow before autologous transplantation; (3) in vivo passive serotherapy; and (4) conjugation to anticancer agents for target-specific delivery. Recently there have been efforts to achieve human B-cell fusions with human myeloma cells to avoid some of the problems encountered with in vivo administration of murine protein. Human-human cell fusions, however, have tended to be more unstable than rodent hybridomas and to produce relatively low amounts of antibody.

Although the administration of monoclonal antibodies specific for hematopoietic cells has been associated with a transient decrease in circulating leukemic target cells and encouraging responses, the same has not been true for solid tumors. It would appear that, in the case of nonhematogenous tumors, monoclonal antibodies will need to function as the carrier of anticancer drug or radioisotopes to be effective.

BIOLOGIC RATIONALE FOR THERAPY

Chemotherapy

General Considerations

In spite of intensive efforts on the part of many investigators, our understanding of the malignant process and of fundamental structural or functional differences between normal and malignant cells is still rudimentary, and our ability to exploit aspects of these differences remains limited. Therefore many of the considerations related to the clinical use of chemotherapeutic agents tend to revolve around their toxicity, the object usually being to combine agents that do not have overlapping toxic effects so that each can be given in fully effective doses. Toxicity is also a determinant of the frequency with which chemotherapy courses can be given since the patient must be permitted to recover from the toxic effects of prior cycles of treatment.

Despite these limitations, our ability to identify antitumor agents has been enhanced by insight into the patterns of growth of normal and neoplastic cells. A picture is emerging that divides the cell population into proliferating stem cells and nonproliferating cells, which may be resting, differentiated, or nonviable. The most fully characterized portions of the normal cell cycle are the S phase and mitosis. Most of the active chemotherapeutic agents developed to date are designed to inhibit processes occurring during these two phases of the cell cycle, and these drugs are in general more effective against rapidly dividing cells (in which a larger fraction of each cycle is devoted to DNA synthesis and mitosis) than slowly dividing cells.

The synthesis of DNA is a multistep process, using various enzyme pathways. Agents have been developed that, when combined, can inhibit the process at several points simultaneously, thereby enhancing the cytocidal effect. As knowledge of the other phases of the cell cycle increases and as other factors effecting the growth of normal and malignant tissues become better understood, the ability to develop new antitumor agents with different mechanisms of action will undoubtedly improve, as will our ability to develop more effective multiple-agent chemotherapy regimens. A variety of general strategies can be used to this end, including sequential blockade of different steps in the same biosynthetic pathway, concurrent blockade of different pathways for the synthesis of necessary compounds, complimentary inhibition of biochemical processes (whereby repair processes that circumvent chemotherapeutic damage are inhibited), and metabolic sensitization of intracellular constituents to chemotherapeutic effects by prior exposure to drugs that render the cells more susceptible.[167] Examples of each of these approaches have been described.[45,70,131] Characterization of the mitotic phase of the cell cycle, although morphologically clear, is still missing the biochemical level of insight and understanding that has been achieved with respect to nucleic acid structure and biosynthesis. Therefore relatively fewer chemotherapeutic agents have been identified that are specifically active at this phase of the cycle, although current efforts to characterize the macromolecular structures involved will undoubtedly lead to a larger number of active agents and to improved synergistic combinations with agents active in other phases of the cell cycle. Other considerations in the use of chemotherapeutic agents and the design of chemotherapy regimens include the emergence of drug-resistant cells (either by selection of insensitive clones or by the induction of cellular changes that result in drug resistance). The presence of sites that are inaccessible to drug effect on a physiologic or anatomic basis and the relative distribution of biologically effective drug between tumor cells and normal tissues determines the balance between toxic and therapeutic drug effects.

There have been many studies related to the origins of chemotherapeutic resistance. Recent advances of particular promise include the direct demonstration of the genetic origin of some types of drug resistance and the development of in vitro methods of evaluating clones of human tumor stem cells.[8,165] The latter technique has also shown promise as a chemotherapeutic screening procedure for individual patients that may permit correlations between in vitro cytotoxicity (as measured by decreased numbers of colony-forming units or clonogenic stem cells from the patient's tumor) and the in vivo chemotherapeutic response of that patient. The concept of this in vitro screening is very attractive, although the early results suggest that the value of this assay may be as a negative predictor of in vivo drug response (i.e., drug resistance).

Studies of drug penetrance into anatomically or physiologically protected sites (those relatively inaccessible to drug such as the central nervous system or testis) have led to the design of chemotherapy regimens that aim to improve drug penetrance, to the study of derivatives of known antineoplastic agents that have improved access to such privileged sites, and to the development of new agents and vehicles that can either alter the characteristics of the pharmacologic barrier or the ability of active drug to achieve pharmacologic concentrations within the privileged site.

Combination Chemotherapy

One of the major advances in cancer chemotherapy has been the use of combinations of drugs. This assertion is supported by extensive experimental and clinical evidence.[45,70] Some of the most striking results of combination chemotherapy have been achieved in childhood lymphoblastic leukemia and Hodgkin's disease. There are three generally accepted guidelines to choosing drugs for combination chemotherapy:

1. Select drugs that are active against the tumor when used alone.
2. Select drugs that have different mechanisms of action.
3. Select drugs that have minimally overlapping toxicities.

If these guidelines are followed, dosages that are close to the maximally tolerable dosages for each drug can be used in an intermittent drug treatment schedule designed to optimize the cytotoxic effect of each drug. For example, the administration of a drug whose action is not as dependent on the proliferative state of a cell population can be used to effect a significant cell kill and subsequent recruitment of resting G_0 cells followed by a drug with a cell cycle phase–specific activity. The total cell kill in such a regimen would be potentially greater than the killing effect of either drug alone.

Mechanisms of action of the anticancer drugs are summarized in Table 9-2. In general, anticancer drugs can be divided into two principal classes: (1) those that interact directly with DNA to alter the template for DNA replication or RNA transcription, and (2) those that inhibit nucleic acid synthesis by blocking the pathways for purine and pyrimidine nucleotide formation or by interference with action of nucleic acid polymerases. A unique anticancer drug not included in these two categories is L-Asparaginase, an enzyme that blocks protein synthesis by hydrolyzing an amino acid essential for the growth of certain tumors. A number of subcategories, based on the type of biochemical disruption produced, exist within the group of drugs that interact with DNA. The alkylating agents, for example, primarily alkylate purine bases and may produce cross-links between the two DNA strands; whereas many of the antitumor antibiotics intercalate between the bases as they are stacked in the DNA double helix. The mechanism of action of these two types of "template-active" drugs is different enough to allow these two classes to be combined in a combination drug regimen. Similarly, drugs that block nucleotide formation at different steps or by different mechanisms have been combined into clinically advantageous therapeutic regimens.

Adjuvant Chemotherapy

The use of drugs as adjuvants to surgery or irradiation has led to significant advances in the chemotherapy of cancer.[44] Many times the primary localized tumor mass can be removed by surgery or destroyed by irradiation. But even if the diagnosis has been made relatively early, with certain tumors it is quite probable that small, clinically undetectable metastases have already occurred. With the available diagnostic techniques, the most common solid tumors (breast, lung, and colon carcinomas) are usually not detectable until the tumor attains a mass 1 cm in diameter. By this time about 10^9 cells are present, and the tumor has already doubled in mass about 30 times. Since the chance for cell shedding into the lymphatic system or the bloodstream increases with each doubling in tumor mass, there is a significant chance that a few cells have already metastasized by the time a tumor can be detected by palpation or available x-ray film techniques. Thus in many cases patients have metastatic disease at the time of diagnosis of the primary tumor. It is not usually practical to eliminate small metastatic foci by surgery or irradiation;

Table 9-2 **ANTICANCER DRUGS**

Site of Inhibition	Drug	Mechanism of Action
Purine synthesis	Methotrexate	Inhibits one-carbon transfer required for purine ring synthesis
	6-Mercaptopurine and 6-Thioguanine	Inhibit purine ring Synthesis and intro-conversion of purines
	Hydroxyurea	Inhibits conversion of ribonucleotides to deoxyribonucleotides
Primary synthesis	Methotrexate	Inhibits one-carbon transfer required for synthesis of dTMP from dUMP
	5-Fluorouracil	Inhibits dTMP formation by blocking thymidylate synthesis
DNA polymerase	Azacytidine Cytarabine	Competitively inhibits incorporation of dCTP into DNA
DNA (direct interaction)	Melphalan Cyclophosphamide Chlorambucil *cis*-Platinum Nitrogen mustards Nitrosoureas Busulfan Dacarbazine Thiotepa Mitomycin C	React convalently with DNA, often cross-linking strands
	Bleomycin	Cause DNA breakage
	Doxorubicin Daunorubicin Actinomycin D	Intercalate between DNA basis
Spindle inhibitors	Vincristine Vinblastine Epipodophyllotoxins (VP-16, VM-26)	Bind to tubulin in microtubules
	L-Asparaginase	Hydrolyzes L-Asparagine

thus chemotherapy is usually the treatment of choice in metastatic disease.

The principles for the use of drugs with surgery or radiotherapy are similar to those for the use of drugs in combination regimens. Drugs without a demonstrable activity against the tumor when used alone should not be used in adjuvant trials. A single drug with a demonstrated activity against advanced disease may have an enhanced antitumor effect after surgery or irradiation has produced a large decrease in total tumor bulk (debulking). If combinations of drugs have been shown to be effective in patients with advanced disease, they may also be used in adjuvant therapy. Another important consideration is that the drug or the drug combination must be relatively low in general toxicity. Since a significant number of patients may remain free of disease with surgery or radiotherapy alone, the added risk of drug toxicity (and in some cases the induction of secondary malignancies such as leukemia) must be carefully weighed against the potential benefit.

Clearly, cancer chemotherapy will continue to benefit from the development of new agents and improved schedules of administration and effective drug combinations. The rational design of new drugs may reduce dose-limiting toxicity such as the cardiotoxicity of anthracycline antibiotics. In addition, the targeting of chemotherapeutic agents coupled to monoclonal antibodies or enclosed in liposomes may offer the possibility of improved delivery while minimizing side effects by sparing normal tissues.

Radiation Therapy

General Considerations

The radiosensitivity of a large variety of tissues, both normal and malignant, has now been studied. A typical mammalian cell-survival curve is shown in Fig. 9-4.[126,134] These data are derived from the exposure of clonogenic cells to single radiation doses. The curve consists of two portions: an initial "shoulder", which is thought to represent a dosage range in which repair of sublethal injury takes place; and an experimental portion, in which a given dose of radiation kills a constant proportion of cells. The slope of the experimental portion of the curve is $-1/D_o$, where D_o is the dose of radiation that reduces the surviving fraction of irradiated cells to 37% of its former value and n, the "extrapolation number" or the value obtained when the experimental portion of the curve is extrapolated back to the ordinate.

Radiosensitivity of cells is usually defined in terms in D_o. Although such tumors as seminomas or lymphomas are uniquely sensitive, most adenocarcinomas and squamous cell carcinomas have D_os that are very similar and in the range of 120 to 160 rad. Moreover, normal cells have D_os in the same range. Differences in the radioresponsiveness of various tumors and in the number of tumor vs. normal cells killed must be explained in terms other than those of inherent radiosensitivity. The phenomena of repair, reoxygenation, repopulation, and redistribution are among the mechanisms invoked to account for these differences. If radiotherapy is given in one dose but in two or more fractions, repair of sublethal damage takes place between radiation treatments. The total dosage required for a given level of cell kill after fractionated radiotherapy is

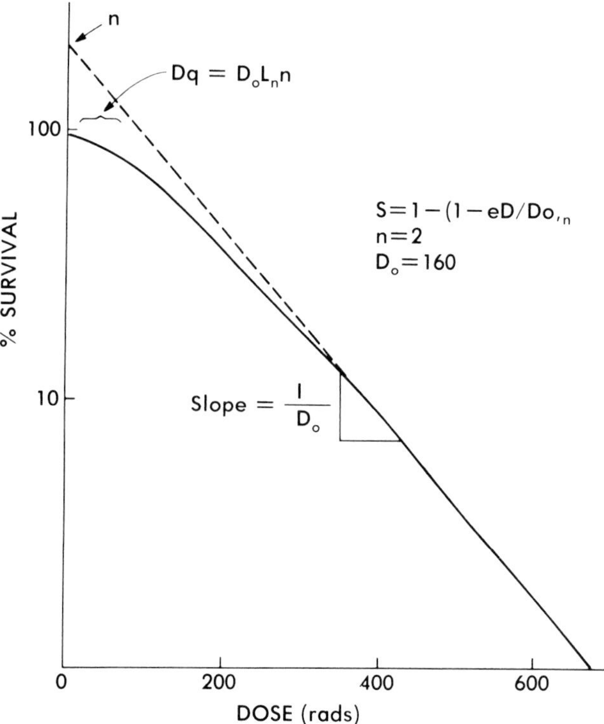

Fig. 9-4 Theoretic cell survival curve for mammalian cells exposed to a single dose of radiation. D_q denotes the quasi-threshold dose, D_o the dose of radiation that reduces the surviving fraction of irradiated cells to 37% of its former value, or the extrapolation number, $L_n n$ the natural logarithm of n, D the dose of radiation, and S the surviving fraction.

greater than that required when radiation is delivered in a single treatment. The strategy of treating tumors with multiple fractions of radiation is based on the supposition that sublethal radiation injury is repaired more effectively in normal tissue than in tumors.

Selection of an optimal time-dosage pattern for treating tumors is, however, a complex problem. It is unlikely that one time-dosage prescription is optimal for a wide variety of kinetically different tumors located in different anatomic areas. The determination of fraction size, overall treatment time, and total dosage that is best for the control of various tumors constitutes a major research problem confronting radiotherapists at the present time. It is based on several factors such as the inherent radiosensitivity of the tumor and surrounding normal tissues, tumor blood supply, and use of concomitant adjuvant therapy.

Although tumor type has limited effect on inherent radiosensitivity, lack of oxygen has a profound influence. Hypoxic cells are 2.5 to three times more resistant to radiation than are well-oxygenated cells. The presence of hypoxic cells within human tumors is thought to limit the effectiveness of radiation. There have been many attempts to overcome the hypoxic cell problem, including the use of hyperbaric oxygen, electron affinity compounds that selectively sensitize hypoxic cells, densely ionizing or high-energy transfer radiation such as neutrons or pi-mesons, optimization of the time-dosage schedule to increase reoxygenation between radiation doses, and hyperthermia.[24,26,51]

Mechanism of Radiation Cell Kill

Therapeutic radiation is ionizing—it ejects electrons from atoms or molecules with which it interacts. The energy transfer from radiation to tissue by this ionization process is immediate. The biologic manifestation of this physical transfer is, however, highly complex. The cellular target of ionizing radiation is believed to be DNA, and the meaningful biologic end point, at least in terms of cancer therapy, is loss of cellular reproductive capability. Although the molecular interactions of radiation are rapid, the time to cell death is variable, depending on normal tissue and tumor kinetics. Tumor regression will depend not only on the proportion of cells killed but also on the proliferation kinetics of the irradiated cells and on cell-loss factors.[47] Furthermore, the rate of tumor regression does not necessarily correlate with the likelihood of tumor control.

Since cell survival after irradiation is an exponential function of dosage, the amount of radiation required for a given level of cell kill is directly proportional to the logarithm of the number of clonogenic cells irradiated. In clinical terms, tumor size is a critical factor in determining the likelihood of cure with a given radiation dose. It has been demonstrated in a wide variety of clinical situations that 5000 rad administered over 5 weeks controls (kills) subclinical, or microscopic, disease in 90% to 95% of cases.[59] Tumors up to 3 cm in size are usually cured locally by radiation dosages in the range of 6000 to 7000 rad over 6 to 7 weeks. The probability of tumor control (elimination of all clonogenic cells) with these dosages, which are generally the maximum tolerable by contiguous normal tissues, declines with increasing tumor size.

Radiation Oncology

Radiotherapy has three major roles in cancer treatment. It may be used singly as the primary curative method. It may be used as "adjuvant" therapy with surgery (either before or after operation) or with chemotherapy or both. Finally, radiation serves to palliate the symptoms of locally advanced or metastatic disease.

As a single method of treatment undertaken with curative intent, radiotherapy is a local or regional form of therapy that is often competitive with surgery. If the probability of cure is equivalent for the two methods, a choice between them will often be made on the basis of which carries the lower risk of morbidity. In the case of large tumors, surgery usually has a higher likelihood of tumor cure. However, primary radiotherapy is often used in neoplasms that are technically unresectable or that require surgery that is excessively mutilating. There has been a recent trend toward combining radiotherapy with surgery in more advanced tumors.[60] The rationale is to enhance the chance for cure and to improve functional results by resecting clinically apparent disease and delivering moderate radiation dosages to potential foci of residual microscopic tumors in the primary site or regional nodal areas or both.

Many clinical demonstrations of this principle are now available. Adjuvant radiotherapy to clinically uninvolved lymph nodes in carcinoma of the breast, head and neck, testicle, prostate, and bladder is effective in controlling potential disease in these nodes, obviating the need for "prophylactic" nodal dissection in the great majority of instances.[60] Dissection may still be necessary for grossly involved nodes or to obtain prognostic information as a guide to systemic adjuvant treatment.

As chemotherapy becomes more effective, radiation may have more of a role to play as an adjuvant to this treatment. A notable example is Hodgkin's disease, in which supplemental radiotherapy administered to patients with advanced disease who have achieved a complete remission with chemotherapy and directed toward initial sites of involvement appears to increase the cure rate, because of the high probability that microscopic foci remain at initial sites of disease.[133] A similar situation may exist with respect to small-cell carcinoma of the lung, in cases in which patients appear to be failing locally in the chest, despite some very favorable initial responses to chemotherapy.[22] Adjuvant radiotherapy is also of value for the treatment of subclinical disease in "sanctuary" sites not usually accessible to systemic chemotherapy such as the brain or testis.

Local control of cancer is likely to remain an important clinical problem. Thus radiotherapy, chemotherapy, and surgery should be viewed as complementary and not competitive methods of cancer management. The number of new investigative approaches in radiotherapeutic trials aimed at improving disease control has increased dramatically. These include hypoxic cell sensitizers, radiation protectors, hyperthermia, intraoperative radiotherapy, particle irradiation, altered fractionation, and improved diagnostic imaging for tumor localization. It is to be hoped that intelligent integration of improved radiotherapy, along with chemotherapy and surgery, will prove beneficial in the treatment of cancer.

Surgical Oncology

Surgery is generally recognized as the original cancer therapy and until recent years offered the only opportunity for cure. During the past two decades, however, there has been a tremendous advancement in the development of effective nonsurgical methods of treating cancer, and this has greatly changed the role of surgery. Perhaps one of the most important advances in cancer surgery has been related to an understanding of the biology of cancer growth and metastases. The original concept of a local tumor spreading contiguously to surrounding tissues and to regional lymph nodes led to more and more radical operations. Now it is recognized that at the time of cancer diagnosis some 70% of all solid tumors are already systemic. This understanding of the cancer process has helped the surgeon rethink the role of primary surgery and better define realistic margins of resection integrated into a multimodality approach to treatment.

The surgeon is most often the primary physician conducting the evaluation of the patient suspected of having cancer and as such must assume responsibility for obtaining appropriate tissue for histologic review. This requires that the surgeon have a thorough knowledge of the natural history of the tumors treated and must know the amount of tissue required and its proper handling to ensure accurate diagnosis. Placement of biopsy incisions so as not to compromise primary surgical treatment and avoidance of techniques that might risk unwanted seeding of tumor cells in violated tissue planes are the surgeon's responsibility. The surgeon must work closely with the pathologist so that maximum advantage can be taken of special techniques for accurate histologic evaluation. The biopsy may be the only time when appropriate tumor markers can be evaluated or such procedures as electron microscopy performed. Whether the biopsy specimen is placed in formalin, liquid nitrogen, or tissue culture media is critical to gaining the maximum amount of useful information about a given malignancy.

As the primary physician, the surgeon must assume the responsibility for identifying which patients can be potentially cured by local resection alone and which should have added adjuvant treatment. The surgeon must also decide the extent of resectional therapy, balancing the potential for cure through local control with the morbidity of extensive tissue resection. Although one can list a number of examples of tumors in which primary resection with sufficient margins of normal tissue can provide cure without additional treatment, today the use of surgery as the sole treatment for a given cancer is primarily determined by the stage of the tumor and not by its histology. Thus the surgeon has a critical role in providing accurate clinical staging of the disease, often using operative intervention to accomplish this assignment in such malignancies as cancer of the ovary, esophagus, lung, bowel, and Hodgkin's disease.

The surgeon is also frequently involved in treating patients with large, extensive tumors and patients with metastatic disease. The decision to resect isolated metastases or to attempt debulking of large tumor masses is always difficult. Although the resection of certain metastatic tumors such as isolated liver tumors and metastatic sarcoma in the lung may in fact extend the life of an individual patient, there is little evidence that ultimate survival is changed. The decision to attempt such procedures depends largely on the availability of other effective treatment modalities for the tumor in question and has little, if any, value otherwise.

In recent years, the cancer surgeon has been called upon to provide chronic vascular access for administration of sclerotic chemotherapy, hematologic support, and occasionally nutritional support. The implementation of chronic vascular access has allowed the use of more aggressive treatment involving multiple drugs given over complicated schedules. To meet this need, a number of new implantable catheter systems and drug delivery pumps have been developed. Although the reliability and patient acceptance of these devices is proving to be quite good, their successful use depends largely on the dedicated and skilled surgeon responsible for this aspect of the interdisciplinary oncology program.

The surgeon is also called on to handle a variety of surgical emergencies related to the advancing cancer or the use of aggressive therapy. Hemorrhage, sepsis, perforation of viscera, and obstruction of the gastrointestinal tract are examples of problems requiring surgical intervention. These emergencies require a thoughtful and caring physician who understands not only the need to solve the problem at hand but also the delicate balance between helping and not helping.

Today's surgical specialist involved in cancer diagnosis and treatment has a far greater responsibility for understanding the biology of the cancer process, the natural history of specific tumors, the current status of integrated treatment options for each tumor, and the investigative options that may be important to the patient than has existed previously. The role of the surgeon assuming these responsibilities is best defined as that of a member of a multidisciplinary oncology team, skilled in various treatment modalities, and dedicated to experimental research that can lead to new diagnostic and treatment options.

SUMMARY

The past decade has witnessed exciting advances in cell biology and molecular genetics. These new developments in modern biomedical research have shed new light on the processes involved in transformation of normal cells into neoplastic cells, tumor cell proliferation, and the biology of tumor metastasis. Today's surgeon must have a thorough understanding of these processes and their relationship to therapy in order to participate as a key member of an integrated, multidisciplinary oncology research and treatment program. This chapter has reviewed and highlighted the genetic regulation of abnormal cell growth, the development of metastases, the host response, and the rationale for the integration of treatment options on the basis of our current understanding of those mechanisms responsible for oncogenesis.

REFERENCES

1. Aaronson, S.: Unique aspects of the interactions of retroviruses with vertebrate cells: C.P. Rhoads Memorial Lecture, Cancer Res. **43**:1, 1983.
2. Abercrombie, M.: Contact inhibition and malignancy, Nature **281**:259, 1979.
3. Acuto, O., et al.: The α and β subunits of the human T cell receptor: their appearance in ontogeny and biochemical relationship to one another on IL-2 dependent clones and T cell tumors, Cell **34**:717, 1983.
4. Adams, D.O., and Hamilton, T.A.: The cell biology of macrophage activation, Annu. Rev. Immunol. **2**:283, 1984.
5. Adams, D.O., Johnson, W.J., and Marino, P.A.: Mechanisms of target recognition and destruction in macrophage-mediated tumor cytotoxicity, Fed. Proc. **41**:2212, 1982.
6. Alpert, M.E.: Alphafetoglobulins in the diagnosis of human hepatoma, N. Engl. J. Med. **278**:984, 1968.
7. Al-Rushdi, A., et al.: Differential expression of the translocated and the untranslocated c-*myc* oncogene in Burkitt lymphoma, Science **222**:390, 1983.
8. Alt, F.W., Kellems, R.E., and Schimke, R.T.: Synthesis and degradation of folate reductase in sensitive and resistant lines of S-180 cells, J. Biol. Chem. **251**:3063, 1976.
9. Assoian, R.K., et al.: Cellular transformation by coordinated action of three peptide growth factors from human platelets, Nature **309**:804, 1984.
10. Baldwin, R.W.: Immunity to methylcholanthrene-induced tumors in inbred rats following implantation and regression of implanted tumors, Br. J. Cancer **9**:652, 1955.
11. Barrett, J.C., and Ts'o, P.O.: Evidence for the progressive nature of neoplastic transformation in vitro, Proc. Natl. Acad. Sci. (USA) **75**:3761, 1978.
12. Baserga, R.: The cell cycle, N. Engl. J. Med. **304**:453, 1981.
13. Benacerraf, B.: Genetic control of the specificity of T lymphocytes and their regulatory products, Prog. Immunol. **4**:420, 1980.

14. Berendt, M.J., and North, R.J.: T-cell mediated suppression of anti-tumor immunity, J. Exp. Med. **151:**69, 1980.
15. Bishop, J.M.: The molecular biology of RNA tumor viruses: a physician's guide, N. Engl. J. Med. **303:** 675, 1980.
16. Bishop, J.M.: Oncogenes, Sci. Am. **246:**80, 1982.
17. Blair, D.G., et al.: Activation of the transforming potential of a normal cell sequence: a molecular model for oncogenesis, Science **212:**941, 1981.
18. Brooks, R.F., Bennett, D.C., and Smith, J.A.: Mammalian cell cycles need two random transitions, Cell **19:**493, 1980.
19. Brunson, K.W., Beattie, G., and Nicolson, G.L.: Selection and altered properties of brain colonizing metastatic melanoma, Nature **272:**543, 1978.
20. Brunson, K.W., and Nicolson, G.L.: Selection of malignant melanoma variant cell lines for ovary colonization, J. Supramol. Struct. **11:**517, 1979.
21. Butler, T.P., and Gullino, P.M.: Quantitation of cell shedding into efferent blood of mammary adenocarcinoma, Cancer Res. **35:**513, 1975.
22. Byhardt, R.W., Libnock, J.A., and Cox, J.D.: Local control of intrathoracic disease with chemotherapy and the role of prophylactic cranial irradiation in small-cell carcinoma of the lung, Cancer **47:**2239, 1981.
23. Capon, D.J., et al.: Complete nucleotide sequence of the T24 human bladder carcinoma and its normal homologue, Nature **302:**33, 1983.
24. Castro, J.R.: Particle radiation therapy: the first forty years, Semin. Oncol. **8:**103, 1981.
25. Cerrottini, J.C., and Brunner, K.T.: Cell-mediated cytotoxicity, allograft rejection and tumor immunity, Adv. Immunol. **18:**67, 1974.
26. Chapman, J.D.: Hypoxic sensitizers—implications for radiation therapy, N. Engl. J. Med. **301:**1429, 1979.
27. Charbit, A., Malaise, E., and Tubiana, M.: Relation between the pathological nature and growth rate of human tumours, Eur. J. Cancer **7:**307, 1971.
28. Chen, I.S., et al.: Characterization of reticuloendotheliosis virus strain T DNA and isolation of a novel variant of reticuloendotheliosis virus strain T by molecular cloning, J. Virol. **40:**800, 1981.
29. Chessels, J.M., Hardesty, R.M., and Rapson, N.T.: Acute lymphoblastic leukemia in children, classification and progress, Lancet **2:**1307, 1977.
30. Chung, E.H., et al.: Tumorigenic transformation of mammalian cells induced by a normal human gene homologous to the oncogene of Harvey murine sarcoma virus, Nature **297:**474, 1982.
31. Cline, M.J., Slamon, D.J., and Lipsick, J.L.: Oncogenes, implication for diagnosis and treatment of cancer, Ann. Int. Med. **101:**223, 1984.
32. Cohen, S.: The epidermal growth factor (EGF), Cancer **51:**1787, 1983.
33. Collett, M.S., and Erikson, R.L.: Protein kinase activity associated with the avian sarcoma virus *src* gene product, Proc. Natl. Acad. Sci. (USA), **75:**2021, 1978.
34. Collins, V.P., Leoffler, R.K., and Twey, H.: Observation on growth rates of human tumours, Am. J. Roentgen. **76:**988, 1956.
35. Cooper, G.M.: Cellular transforming genes, Science **218:**801, 1982.
36. Dalla-Favera, R., et al.: Human c-*myc* onc gene is located in the region of chromosome 8 that is translocated in Burkitt lymphoma cells, Proc. Natl. Acad. Sci. (USA) **79:**824, 1982.
37. Dalla-Favera, R., Wong-Staal, F., and Gallo, R.G.: Oncogene amplification in promyelocytic leukemia cell line HL-60 and primary leukemic cells of the same patients, Nature **299:**61, 1982.
38. DeFeo, D., Gonda, M.A., and Young, H.A.: Analysis of two divergent rat genomic clones homologous to the transforming gene of harvey murine sarcoma virus, Proc. Natl. Acad. Sci. (USA) **78:**3328, 1981.
39. DeKlein, A., VanKessel, A.G., and Grosveld, G.: A cellular oncogene is translocated to the Philadelphia chromosome in chronic myelocytic leukemia, Nature **300:**765, 1982.
40. Delorbe, W.J., et al.: Molecular cloning and characterization of avian sarcoma virus circular DNA molecules, J. Virol. **36:**50, 1980.
41. dek Regato, J.A.: Pathways of metastatic spread of malignant tumors, Semin. Oncol. **4:**33, 1977.
42. Der, C.J., Krontiris, T.G., and Cooper, G.M.: Transforming genes of human bladder and lung carcinoma cell lines are homologous to the *ras* genes of Harvey and Kirsten sarcoma viruses, Proc. Natl. Acad. Sci. (USA) **79:**3637, 1981.
43. Dernhardt, F.: Biology of primate retrovirus. In Klein, G., editor: *Viral oncology,* New York, 1980, Raven Press.
44. DeVita, V.T.: Principles of chemotherapy. In DeVita, V.T., Hellman, S., and Rosenberg, S.A., editors: *Cancer: principles and practice of oncology,* Philadelphia, 1982, J.B. Lippincott Co.
45. DeVita, V.T., Young, R.L., and Canellos, G.P.: Combination versus single agent chemotherapy: a review of the basis for selection of drug treatment of cancer, Cancer **35:**96, 1975.
46. Diamond, A., Devine, J.M., and Cooper, G.M.: Nucleotide sequence of a human B-*lym* transforming gene activated in Burkitt's lymphoma, Science **225:**516, 1984.
47. Dische, S., et al.: Tumor regression as a guide to prognosis: a clinical study, Br. J. Radiol. **53:**454, 1980.
48. Donner, L., et al.: McDonough feline sarcoma virus: characterization of the molecularly cloned provirus and its feline oncogene (v-*fms*), J. Virol. **41:**489, 1982.
49. Dorf, M.E., and Benacerraf, B.: Suppressor cells and immunoregulation, Annu. Rev. Immunol. **2:**127, 1984.
50. Downward, J., et al.: Close similarity of epidermal growth factor receptor and v-*erb*-B oncogene protein sequences, Nature **37:**521, 1984.
51. Dritschilo, A., and Piro, A.J.: Therapeutic implications of heat as related to radiation therapy, Semin. Oncol. **8:**83, 1981.
52. Duesberg, P.H.: Retroviral transforming genes in normal cells? Nature **304:**219, 1983.
53. Fidler, I.J.: Selection of successive tumor lines for metastasis, Nature **242:**148, 1973.
54. Fidler, I.J.: Recent concepts of cancer metastasis and their implications for therapy, Cancer Treat. Rep. **68:**193, 1984.
55. Fidler, I.J., and Kripke, M.L.: Metastasis results from pre-existing variant cells within a malignant tumor, Science **197:**893, 1979.
56. Finne, J., Burger, M.M., and Prieels, J.P.: Enzymatic basis for a lectin-resistant phenotype: increase in a fluosyltransferase in mouse melanoma cells, J. Cell Biol. **92:**277, 1982.
57. Finne, J., Too, T.W., and Burger, M.M.: Carbohydrate changes in glycoproteins of a poorly metastasizing wheat germ agglutinin-resistant melanoma clone, Cancer Res. **40:**2580, 1980.
58. Fisher, B., and Fisher, E.R.: The interrelationship of hematogenous and lymphatic tumor cell dissemination, Surg. Gynecol. Obstet. **122:**791, 1966.
59. Fletcher, G.H.: Clinical dose-response curves of human malignant epithelial tumours, Br. J. Radiol. **46:**1, 1973.
60. Fletcher, G.H.: The evolution of the basic concepts underlying the practice of radiotherapy from 1949 to 1977, Radiology **127:**3, 1978.
61. Folkman, J.: The vascularization of tumors, Sci. Am. **234:**58, 1976.
62. Fujimoto, S., Green, M.I., and Sheon, A.H.: Regulation of the immune response to tumor antigens. I. Immunosuppressor cells in tumor-bearing hosts, J. Immunol. **116:**791, 1976.
63. Fujimoto, S., Green, M.I., and Sheon, A.H.: Regulation of the immune response to tumor antigens. II. The nature of immunosuppressor cells in tumor-bearing hosts, J. Immunol. **116:**800, 1976.
64. Fujita, J., et al.: Ha-*ras* oncogenes are activated by somatic alterations in human urinary tract tumors, Nature **309:**464, 1984.
65. Fung, Y-K, et al.: Activation of the cellular oncogene c-*erb-B* by LTR insertion: molecular basis for induction of erythroblastosis by human leukosis virus, Cell **33:**357, 1983.
66. Gelmann, E.P., et al.: Molecular cloning and comparative analyses of the genomes of simian sarcoma virus and its associated helper virus, Proc. Natl. Acad. Sci. (USA) **78:**3373, 1981.
67. Glimcher, L., Shen, F.W., and Cantor, H.: Identification of a cell surface antigen selectively expressed on the natural killer cell, J. Exp. Med. **145:**1, 1977.
68. Goff, S.P., et al.: Structure of the Abelson murine leukemia virus genome and the homologous cellular gene: studies with cloned viral DNA, Cell **22:**777, 1980.
69. Gold, P., and Freedman, S.O.: Specific carcinoembryonic antigens of the human digestive system, J. Exp. Med. **22:**467, 1965.

70. Goldin, A., Venditti, J.M., and Mantel, M.: Combination chemotherapy: basic considerations. In Sartorelli, A.C., and Johns, D.G., editors: Antineoplastic and immunosuppressive agents, part I, Berlin, 1974, Springer-Verlag, Inc.
71. Gorelik, E.: Concomitant tumor immunity and the resistance to a second tumor challenge, Adv. Cancer Res. **39**:71, 1983.
72. Goyette, M., et al.: Expression of a cellular oncogene during liver regeneration, Science **219**:510, 1983.
73. Greene, M.I., Fujimoto, S., and Sheon, A.H.: Regulation of the immune response to tumor antigens. III. Characterization of thymic suppressor factor(s) produced by tumor-bearing hosts, J. Immunol. **119**:764, 1977.
74. Griswold, D.P., Jr.: Altered sensitivity of a hamster plasmacytoma to cytosine arabinoside, Cancer Chemother. Rep. **54**:337, 1970.
75. Gross, L.: Intradermal immunization of C3H mice against a sarcoma that originated in an animal of the same line, Cancer Res. **3**:326, 1943.
76. Gross, L.: Oncogenic viruses, Oxford, 1983, Pergamon Press.
77. Grotten, J., et al.: C-*sis* is translocated from chromosome 22 to chromosome 9 in chronic myelocytic leukemia, J. Exp. Med. **158**:9, 1983.
78. Habel, K.: Resistance of polyoma virus immune animals to transplanted polyoma tumors, Proc. Soc. Exp. Biol. Med. **106**:772, 1961.
79. Hakomori, S.: Tumor-associated carbohydrate antigens, Annu. Rev. Immunol. **2**:103, 1984.
80. Hamburger, A.W., and Salmon, S.E.: Primary bioassay of human tumor stem cells, Science **197**:461, 1977.
81. Haskins, K., Kappler, J., and Marrack, P.: The major histocompatibility complex-restricted antigen receptor on T cells, Annu. Rev. Immunol. **2**:51, 1984.
82. Hayward, W.S., and Neel, B.G.: Insertion activation of a cellular oncogene by promoter insertion in ALV-induced lymphoid leukosis, Nature **240**:475, 1981.
83. Hellstrom, I., and Hellstrom, K.E.: Colony inhibition studies on blocking and nonblocking serum effects on cellular immunity to Moloney sarcomas, Int. J. Cancer **5**:195, 1970.
84. Hellstrom, K.E., Brown, J.P., and Hellstrom, I.: Monoclonal antibodies to tumor antigens, Contemp. Top. Immunobiol. **11**:117, 1980.
85. Henderson, A., et al.: Chromosome site for Epstein-Barr virus DNA in a Burkitt tumor cell line and in lymphocytes growth-transformed in vitro, Proc. Natl. Acad. Sci. (USA) **80**:1987, 1983.
86. Herberman, R.: Overview and perspectives: natural resistance mechanisms. In Normann, S.J., and Sorkin, E., editors: Macrophages and natural killer cells, New York, 1982, Plenum Publishing Corp.
87. Herberman, R.B., and Ortaldo, J.R.: Natural killer cells: their role in defenses against disease, Science **214**:24, 1981.
88. Herlyn, M., et al.: Colorectal carcinoma specific antigen: detection by means of monoclonal antibodies, Proc. Natl. Acad. Sci. (USA) **76**:1438, 1979.
89. Hewitt, H.B., and Blake, E.: Quantitative studies of translymphoidal passage of tumour cells naturally disseminated from a nonimmunogenic murine squamous carcinoma, Br. J. Cancer **31**:25, 1975.
90. Howard, A., and Pelc, S.: Nuclear incorporation of ^{32}P as demonstrated by autoradiographs, Exp. Cell. Res. **2**:178, 1951.
91. Howard, A., and Pelc, S.: Synthesis of DNA in normal and irradiated cells and its relation to chromosome breakage, Heredity **6**(suppl.):261, 1953.
92. Hunt, P., and Sears, D.: CTL crossreactivities reveal shared immunodominant determinants created by structural homologous regions of MHC class I antigens, J. Immunol. **130**:1439, 1983.
93. Johnson, W.J., Somers, S.D., and Adams, D.O.: Activation of macrophage from tumor cytotoxicity, Contemp. Top. Immunobiol. **14**:127, 1983.
94. Jumblatt, J.E., et al.: Altered surface glycoproteins in melanoma cell variants with reduced metastasizing capacity selected for resistance to wheat germ agglutinin, Biochem. Biophys. Res. Commun. **95**:111, 1980.
95. Kennett, R.H., and Gilbert, F.: Hybrid myelomas producing antibodies against a human neuroblastoma antigen present on fetal brain, Science **203**:1120, 1979.
96. Kitamura, M., et al.: Avian sarcoma virus Y73 genome sequence and structural similarity of its transforming gene product to that of rouse sarcoma virus, Nature **297**:303, 1982.
97. Land, H., Parada, L.F., and Weinberg, R.A.: Cellular oncogenes and multistep carcinogenesis, Science **222**:771, 1983.
98. Land, H., Parada, L.F., and Weinberg, R.A.: Tumorigenic conversion of primary embryo fibroblasts requires at least two cooperating oncogenes, Nature **304**:596, 1983.
99. LeBeau, M.M., and Rowley, J.D.: Heritable fragile sites in cancer, Nature **308**:607, 1984.
100. Lebowitz, P.: Oncogenes: their potential role in human malignancy, J. Clin. Oncol. **1**:657, 1983.
101. Leder, R., et al.: Translocation among antibody genes in human cancer, Science **222**:765, 1983.
102. Lin, C.-C., et al.: Selective loss of antigen-specific *Ir* gene function in I-A mutant B6.C-H-2^{bm12} is an antigen-presenting cell defect, Proc. Natl. Acad. Sci. (USA) **78**:6406, 1981.
103. Liotta, L.A., et al.: Degradation of basement membrane by murine tumor cells, J. Natl. Cancer Inst. **58**:1427, 1977.
104. Liotta, L.A., Kleinerman, J., and Saidel, G.M.: Quantitative relationships of intravascular tumor cells, tumor vesicles, and pulmonary metastases following tumor implantation, Cancer Res. **34**:997, 1974.
105. Lird, A.K.: The dynamics of tumour growth, Br. J. Cancer **28**:490, 1966.
106. Little, C.D., et al.: Amplification and expression of the c-*myc* oncogene in human lung cancer cell lines, Nature **306**:194, 1983.
107. Mackillop, W.J., et al.: A stem cell model of human tumor growth; implications for tumor cell clonogenic assays, J. Natl. Cancer Inst. **70**:9, 1983.
108. McCoy, M., et al.: Characterization of a human colon/lung carcinoma gene, Nature **302**:79, 1983.
109. McCulloch, E.A.: Abnormal myelopoietic clones in man, J. Natl. Cancer Inst. **63**:884, 1979.
110. Meuer, S.C., et al.: The human T-cell receptor, Annu. Rev. Immunol. **2**:23, 1984.
111. Misevic, G.N., et al.: Model macromolecules for cell-cell recognition: can specificity arise from two independent molecular interactions? Prog. Clin. Biol. Res. **102**:475, 1982.
112. Mitchison, J.M.: The biology of the cell cycle, London, 1971, Cambridge University Press.
113. Moller, E.: Contact-induced cytotoxicity by lymphoid cells containing foreign isoantigens, Science **147**:873, 1965.
114. Muller, R., et al.: Differentiated expression of cellular oncogenes during pre- and postnatal development of the mouse, Nature **299**:640, 1982.
115. Muller, R., Slamon, D.J., and Adamson, E.D.: Transcription of c-ras^k and c-*fms* during mouse development, Mol. Cell. Biol. **3**:1062, 1983.
116. Murphee, A.L., and Benedict, W.F.: Retinoblastoma: clues to human oncogenesis, Science **223**:1028, 1984.
117. Nabholz, M., and MacDonald, H.R.: Cytolytic T lymphocytes, Annu. Rev. Immunol. **1**:273, 1983.
118. Newbold, R.F., and Overell, P.W.: Fibroblast immortality is a prerequisit- for transformation by EJ C-Ha-ras oncogene, Nature **304**:648, 1983.
119. North, R.J.: Cyclophosphamide-facilitated adoptive immunotherapy of an established tumor depends on elimination of tumor-induced suppressor T cells, J. Exp. Med. **155**:1063, 1982.
120. Orkin, S.H., Goldman, D.S., and Sallan, S.E.: Development of homozygosity for chromosome 11p markers in Wilms' tumor, Nature **309**:172, 1984.
121. Oroszlan, S., Sarngudharan, M.G., and Copeland, J.D.: Primary structure analysis of the major internal protein p24 of human Type C T-cell leukemia virus, Proc. Natl. Acad. Sci. (USA) **79**:1291, 1982.
122. Ortaldo, J.R., and Herberman, R.B.: Herterogeneity of natural killer cells, Annu. Rev. Immunol. **2**:359, 1984.
123. Oskarsson, M., et al.: Properties of normal mouse cell DNA sequence (sarc) homologous to the *src* sequence of moloney sarcoma virus, Science **207**:1222, 1980.
124. Pardee, A.B.: A restriction point for control of normal animal cell proliferation, Proc. Natl. Acad. Sci. (USA) **71**:1286, 1974.

125. Payne, G.S., Bishop, J.M., and Varmus, H.E.: Multiple arrangements of viral DNA and an activated host oncogene in bursal lymphomas, Nature **295**:209, 1982.
126. Peschel, R.E., and Fischer, J.J.: Optimization of the time-dose relationship, Semin. Oncol. **8**:38, 1981.
127. Poiesz, B.M.J., et al.: Detection and isolation of type C retrovirus particles from fresh and cultured lymphocytes of a patient with cutaneous T cell lymphoma, Proc. Natl. Acad. Sci. (USA) **77**:7415, 1980.
128. Poste, G., Doll, J., and Fidler, I.J.: Interactions among clonal subpopulations affect stability of the metastatic phenotype in polyclonal populations of B16 melanoma cells, Proc. Natl. Acad. Sci. (USA) **78**:6226, 1981.
129. Poste, G., and Nicolson, G.L.: Arrest and metastasis of blood-borne tumor cells are modified by fusion of plasma membrane vesicles from highly metastatic cells, Proc. Natl. Acad. Sci. (USA) **77**:399, 1980.
130. Potten, C.S., Schofield, R., and Lajtha, L.G.: A comparison of cell replacement in bone marrow, testis and three regions of surface epithelium, Biochim. Biophys. Acta **560**:281, 1979.
131. Pratt, W.B., and Ruddon, R.W.: The anticancer drugs, New York, 1979, Oxford University Press.
132. Prehn, R.T., and Main, J.M.: Immunity to methycholanthrene-induced sarcomas, J. Natl. Cancer Inst. **18**:769, 1957.
133. Prosnitz, L.B., et al.: Long-term remissions with combined modality therapy for advanced Hodgkin's disease, Cancer **37**:2826, 1976.
134. Prosnitz, L.R., Kapp, D.S., and Weissberg, J.B.: Radiotherapy, N. Engl. J. Med. **309**:771, 1983.
135. Ramsay, G., Evan, G.I., and Bishop, J.M.: The protein encoded by the human proto-oncogene c-*myc*, Proc. Natl. Acad. Sci. (USA) **81**:7242, 1984.
136. Reddy, E.P., et al.: A point mutation is responsible for acquisition of transforming properties by the T24 human bladder carcinoma oncogene, Nature **300**:149, 1982.
137. Roder, J., and Duwe, J.: The *beige* mutation in the mouse selectively impairs natural killer cell function, Nature **278**:451, 1979.
138. Roos, E., et al.: Invasion of lymphosarcoma cells into the perfused mouse liver, J. Natl. Cancer Inst. **58**:1427, 1977.
139. Rosenberg, S.A.: Potential use of expanded T lymphoid cells and T-cell clones for the immunotherapy of cancer. In Fathman, C.G., and Fitch, F.W., editors: Isolation, characterization, and utilization of T lymphocyte clones, New York, 1982, Academic Press, Inc.
140. Saito, H., et al.: Complete primary structure of a heterodimeric T-cell receptor deduced from cDNA sequences, Nature **309**:757, 1984.
141. Salmon, S.E., and Smith, B.A.: Immunoglobulin synthesis and total body tumour cell number in IgG multiple myeloma, J. Clin. Invest. **49**:1114, 1970.
142. Santos, E., et al.: Spontaneous activation of a human proto-oncogene, Proc. Natl. Acad. Sci. (USA) **80**:4679, 1983.
143. Schwab, M., et al.: Amplified DNA with limited homology to *myc* cellular oncogene is shared by human neuroblastoma cell lines and a neuroblastoma tumor, Nature **304**:245, 1983.
144. Seiki, M., et al.: Adult T-cell leukemia virus: complete nucleotide sequence of the provirus genome integrated in leukemia cell DNA, Proc. Natl. Acad. Sci. (USA) **80**:3618, 1983.
145. Seiki, M., Hattori, S., and Yoshida, M.: Human adult T-cell leukemia virus: molecular cloning of the provirus DNA and the unique terminal structure, Proc. Natl. Acad. Sci. (USA) **79**:6899, 1982.
146. Shevach, E.M., Paul, W.E., and Green, I.: Histocompatibility-linked immune response gene function in guinea pigs: specific inhibition of antigen induced lymphocyte proliferation by allo-antisera, J. Exp. Med. **136**:1207, 1972.
147. Shih, C., et al.: Transforming genes of carcinomas and neuroblastomas introduced into mouse fibroblasts, Nature **390**:261, 1981.
148. Shih, C., et al.: Guanine nucleotide binding and autophosphorylating activities associated with the p21 *src* protein of harvey murine sarcoma virus, Nature **287**:686, 1980.
149. Shilo, B.Z., and Weinberg, R.A.: DNA sequences homologous to vertebrate oncogenes are conserved in Drosophila melanogaster, Proc. Natl. Acad. Sci. (USA) **78**:6789, 1982.
150. Sjogren, H.O., et al.: Resistance of polyoma virus immunized mice to transplantation of established polyoma tumor, Exp. Cell Res. **23**:204, 1961.
151. Slamon, D.J., et al.: Expression of cellular oncogenes in human malignancy, Science **224**:256, 1984.
152. Springer, G.F., et al.: Proposed molecular basis of murine tumor cell-hepatocyte interaction, J. Biol. Chem. **258**:5702, 1983.
153. Sredni, B., et al.: Antigen-specific T cell clones restricted to unique F_1 major histocompatibility complex determinants: inhibition of proliferation with a monoclonal anti-Ia-antibody, J. Exp. Med. **153**:677, 1981.
154. Stacey, D.W., and Kung, H-F.: Transformation of NIH-3T3 cells by microinjection of Ha-*ras* p21 protein, Nature **310**:508, 1984.
155. Stanley, P.: Surface carbohydrate alterations of mutant mammalian cells selected for resistance to plant lectins. In Lennarz, W.J., editor: The biochemistry of glycoproteins and proteoglycans, New York, 1980, Plenum Press.
156. Stanners, C.P., and Till, J.E.: DNA synthesis in individual L strain mouse cell, Biochim. Biophys. Acta **37**:406, 1960.
157. Steel, G.G.: Growth kinetics of tumors, Oxford, 1977, Clarendon Press.
158. Stehelin, D., et al.: DNA related to the transforming gene(s) of avian sarcoma virus is present in normal avian DNA, Nature **260**:170, 1976.
159. Steplewski, Z., et al.: Reactivity of monoclonal anti-melanoma antibodies with melanoma cells freshly isolated from primary and metastatic melanoma, Eur. J. Immunol. **9**:94, 1979.
160. Tabin, C.J., et al.: Mechanism of activation of a human oncogene, Nature **300**:143, 1982.
161. Too, T.W., and Burger, M.M.: Non-metastasizing variants selected from metastasizing melanoma cells, Nature **270**:437, 1977.
162. Tubiana, M., and Malaise, E.P.: Growth rate and cell kinetics in human tumours: some prognostic and therapeutic implications. In Symington, T., and Carter, R.L., editors: Scientific foundations of oncology, Chicago, 1976, Year Book Medical Publishers, Inc.
163. Tudaro, G.J., Lazar, G.U., and Green, H.: The initiation of cell division in a contact inhibited mammalian cell line, J. Cell. Physiol. **66**:325, 1965.
164. Vennstrom, V., et al.: Molecular cloning of the avian myelocytomatosis virus genome and recovery of infectious virus by transfection of chicken cells, J. Virol. **39**:625, 1981.
165. VonHoff, D.O., Johnson, G.E., and Glaubiger, D.L.: Initial experience with the human tumor stem cell assay. In Salmon, S.E., editor: Human tumor cloning in vitro, New York, 1980, Grune and Stratton, Inc.
166. Waterfield, M.D., et al.: Platelet-derived growth factor is structurally related to the putative transforming protein p28 *sis* of simian sarcoma virus, Nature **304**:35, 1983.
167. Weber, G.: Biochemical Strategy of cancer cells and the design of chemotherapy: G.H.A. Clones Memorial Lectures, Cancer Res. **43**:3466, 1983.
168. Weiss, R.A.: The search for human RNA tumor viruses. In Weiss, R., et al., editors: RNA tumor viruses, Cold Spring Harbor, 1982, Cold Spring Harbor Laboratory.
169. Westin, E.H., et al.: Expression of cellular homologous of retroviral onc genes in human hematopoietic cells, Proc. Natl. Acad. Sci. (USA) **79**:2490, 1982.
170. Yoshida, M., Miyoshi, I., and Hinuma, Y.: Isolation and characterization of retrovirus from cell lines of human adult T-cell leukemia and its implication in the disease, Proc. Natl. Acad. Sci. (USA) **79**:2031, 1982.
171. Yuasa, Y., et al.: Acquisition of transforming properties by alternative point mutations within c-bas/has human proto-oncogene, Nature **303**:775, 1983.
172. Yunis, J.J., and Soreng, A.L.: Constitutive fragile sites and cancer, Science **226**:1199, 1984.
173. Zetterberg, A.: Nuclear and cytoplasmic growth during interphase in mammalian cells, Adv. Cell. Biol. **1**:211, 1970.
174. Zinkernagel, R.M., and Doherty, P.C.: Restriction of an in vitro T cell–mediated cytoxicity in lymphocyte choriomeningitis within a syngeneic or semiallogeneic system, Nature **248**:701, 1974.

10

Jeffrey Katz

Physiology of Anesthesia

Since Horace Wells demonstrated in 1844 that teeth could be pulled painlessly if the patient inhaled nitrous oxide, anesthesiologists have been dedicated to improving surgical care from the perspective of both patient and surgeon. A direct translation of *anesthesia,* which is Greek in origin, is "without feeling"; this is one of the four basic requirements for a general anesthetic. The other three are amnesia, relaxation, and loss of consciousness.

Numerous agents provide varying degrees of anesthesia when inhaled. Nitrous oxide was the first to be administered clinically. William T.G. Morton demonstrated the amazing effects of inhaled ether to a meeting of the Massachusetts General Hospital on Oct. 16, 1846, when a tumor was removed painlessly from a patient's jaw. The next inhalation agent introduced was chloroform, and many others followed. Not until 1934 did J.S. Lundy of the Mayo Clinic introduce thiopentone, the first anesthetic agent that could be injected intravenously.

Currently, anesthetic techniques are broadly classified in two areas. These include conduction and general anesthesia.

1. *Conduction anesthesia* includes both local and regional anesthesia. With this approach, chemicals that temporarily block normal nerve function are injected into the area immediately surrounding the nerve and induce anesthesia for a limited time.
2. *General anesthesia,* on the other hand, involves anesthesia administered by inhalation and intravenous routes. Inhalation anesthetics induce anesthesia with varying degrees of amnesia, relaxation, and loss of consciousness when a vapor is inhaled along with oxygen. Intravenous anesthesia, also called balanced anesthesia, provides the four basic anesthetic requirements with a combination of drugs especially used for those purposes (e.g., D-tubocurarine for relaxation [paralysis], thiopentone for loss of consciousness, a narcotic for analgesia, and nitrous oxide, which enhances the analgesia and provides unconsciousness/amnesia).

This chapter will review in detail these various approaches to anesthesia, the physiologic principles underlying the use of anesthetics, and the various clinical settings in which each is used.

ANESTHETIC TECHNIQUES

Local Anesthesia

Local anesthesia is administered by injecting an anesthetic solution into the tissues immediately surrounding a peripheral nerve or group of peripheral nerves so that the area supplied by those nerves is rendered totally insensible. Any interruption in function along a nerve from where an impulse is initiated to where it is perceived (i.e., the brain) is a form of local anesthesia.

Physiology of Nerve Conduction

The single most important structure in the propagation of neural impulses is the cell membrane of the neuron. The bimolecular membrane layer, the myelin sheath, and the nodes of Ranvier all play a role in setting up an electrical gradient between the axoplasm within the cell and the extracellular environment. The arrival of an action potential along a nerve fiber changes the permeability of the cell membrane to sodium ions. These ions then move down a concentration gradient into the cell, which in turn changes the voltage difference across the cell membrane from a negative to a positive charge. It is now widely believed that the sodium ions pass through the cell membrane by transversing small pores called sodium channels. It is also accepted that some kind of structural gate to this passage exists and that this gate is opened by the arrival of an action potential.

Pharmacology of Blocking Agents

A local anesthetic action must be totally reversible within a predictable period of time. Local anesthetics tem-

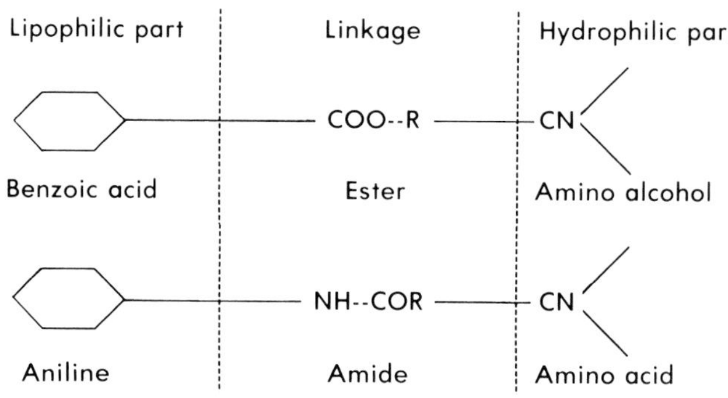

Fig. 10-1 Basic structures of two types of local anesthetics in clinical use. Ester structure is shown above, and amide below.

COMMONLY USED LOCAL ANESTHETICS

Esters	Amides
Cocaine	Lidocaine
Procaine	Bupivacaine
2-Chloroprocaine	Prilocaine
Tetracaine	Mepivacaine
	Etidocaine

porarily block neuronal function by interfering with the movement of sodium ions through the fast sodium channels.

Local anesthetics are all tertiary amines; i.e., they are ammonia molecules with each of the three hydrogen atoms replaced by organic groups. The general configuration of the molecule comprises two structural components. The lipophilic component, which imparts lipid solubility, comprises the largest part of the molecule. Its aromatic structure is commonly derived from benzoic acid or aniline. The hydrophilic component, which imparts water solubility, is an amino derivative of either ethyl alcohol or acetic acid. These two components are joined by an intermediate hydrocarbon chain that is either an amide or an ester (Fig. 10-1). The drugs are thus characterized as either amides or esters. Commonly used drugs within each group are listed in the boxed material on p. 190.

Toxic and Allergic Reactions

One significant difference between the amide and ester anesthetic agents is their potential to cause allergic responses. All esters are broken down into para-amino benzoic acid (PABA), which is highly allergenic in humans, but the amides are rarely implicated in allergic reactions. Toxic reactions to local anesthetics occur when the blood concentration rises above the toxic threshold for a given patient. Local anesthetics enter the intravascular compartment by being absorbed from infiltration sites or by being erroneously injected directly into vessels. Although tolerable doses for various agents have been calculated,[39] responses vary widely from patient to patient, and extreme conservatism appears to be the wisest path.

Initial signs of local anesthetic toxicity are auditory hallucinations and vague paresthesias around the mouth. At higher doses convulsions are typical; left untreated and with blood levels of the drug remaining high, stupor, coma, and respiratory arrest follow. Central nervous system signs occur at lower doses; cardiovascular symptoms occur at higher doses. Hypotension secondary to peripheral circulatory collapse is followed by direct myocardial depression and arrhythmias resulting from conduction aberrations. Fatalities from local anesthesia[1] toxicity are rare (Table 10-1).

The clinical manifestations of local anesthetic toxicity are caused by the ability of these drugs to depress the central nervous system. Although the earlier signs of toxicity (hallucinations and seizures) appear excitatory in nature, they are related to early depression of inhibitory pathways in the brain. As the blood level rises, more pathways are depressed until coma and respiratory arrest result. In the heart, the local anesthetics are very highly protein bound, and the contractile proteins appear to be no exception. Consequently, these contractile proteins do not perform normally, and myocardial depression and hypotension result.

The successful treatment of toxicity requires most importantly that the patient be adequately ventilated. This may entail controlling the seizure with thiopentone, diazepam, or a muscle relaxant such as succinylcholine. Once the seizure has been controlled, the airway is cleared, and ventilation supported; a paralyzed patient almost always needs intubation (see boxed material below). Cardiovascular collapse is treated with appropriate inotropic and chronotropic agents to maintain optimal cardiac funtion.

Local anesthetic toxicity is more likely to occur when drugs are injected into highly vascular areas such as the head and neck or the epidural space. The addition of dilute epinephrine to the local anesthetic solution slows the onset of action and the absorption of the anesthetic from the tissues; however, it also increases the duration of action. Care should be exercised when using epinephrine in patients with hypertensive or ischemic heart disease.

Regional Anesthesia

A local anesthetic affects a peripheral nerve or group of nerves; in contrast, regional anesthesia requires that a local anesthetic solution be injected into the vicinity of a nerve trunk that supplies an entire anatomic region, e.g., a brachial plexus block for anesthesia of the upper limb. The two most commonly used regional techniques are: (1) the use of a spinal anesthetic, which blocks the lower part of the trunk and the legs; and (2) the use of epidural anesthetic, which blocks a similar region but is more flexible in that a catheter can be left at the site of action so that additional doses of anesthetic can be given.

Spinal Anesthesia

Spinal anesthesia refers to the block obtained when local anesthetics are injected through a lumbar puncture needle into the cerebrospinal fluid. The drug acts on the nerve roots as they leave the spinal cord before they enter the foramina. There is evidence that, when local anesthetics

Table 10-1 **SYMPTOMS OF LOCAL ANESTHETIC TOXICITY**

Level	Symptoms
High	Cardiovascular collapse
↑	Hypotension
	Respiratory arrest
Local	Coma
anesthetic	Stupor
blood	Grand mal convulsion
level	Localized seizure activity
		Auditory hallucinations (tinnitus)
		Confusion, anxiety
Low	Circumoral tongue parasthesias

TREATMENT OF LOCAL ANESTHETIC TOXICITY

Oxygenate	Thiopentone	50-75 mg
	Diazepam	5-10 mg
	Succinylcholine	50-100 mg
	Ventilate	
Cardiovascular collapse	Cardiopulmonary resuscitation (CPR)	
	Inotropes	
	Chronotropes	
	Antiarrhythmics	

Table 10-2 **ORDER OF DIFFERENTIAL BLOCKADE IN LOCAL ANESTHESIA**

Conduction Speed	Nerve Function	Dose
Fast ↑	Motor	High ↑
	Touch/pressure	
	Proprioception	
	Pain (fast)/ temperature	
	Pain (slow)/ temperature	
	Autonomic/preganglionic (sympathetic)	
Slow	Autonomic postganglionic	Low

are injected directly into nerve tissues, significant irreversible damage can occur. Therefore, before drugs are injected, it must be possible to easily aspirate cerebrospinal fluid through the spinal needle. The extent of the spinal block (i.e., the level of the blockade) and its duration are related to the type of anesthetic used and the dose administered.

Although spinal anesthetics are safe and relatively easy to administer, careful patient selection is necessary. Patients with obvious infection in the area, documented clotting problems, and previous back problems are not appropriate candidates for spinal anesthesia.

Different nerve fibers blocked during spinal anesthesia have different sensitivities to local anesthetics. It appears that the order of differential blockade is consistent as shown in Table 10-2. Unmyelinated autonomic fibers are blocked at the lowest concentration of local anesthetic. Therefore, even though a local anesthetic is injected at a specific level and lack of sensation can be detected up to that level, sympathetic block can occur up to four vertebral levels higher. If a spinal anesthetic provides loss of sensation as high as thoracic level 4 (T4), the sympathetic fibers of levels T1 through T3 might also be blocked. This would constitute a total sympathectomy (sympathetic fibers come off spinal cord levels T1 through L5), which would remove the patient's ability to control blood pressure by changing the tone of the peripheral vasculature. Thus one of the most severe problems associated with spinal anesthesia is profound hypotension. Patients should, therefore, receive at least 1 L of crystalloid solution intravenously before receiving a spinal anesthetic.

Epidural Anesthesia

Two types of epidural anesthesia exist: (1) lumbar epidural anesthesia, in which the anesthetic solution is injected into the epidural space in the lumbar area, and (2) caudal anesthesia, in which the drug is injected into the epidural space in the caudal region at the sacral hiatus. Thin plastic catheters can be placed in either location and left there for additional injections. The site of action for these techniques is at the nerve roots as they cross the epidural space.

Although the physiology of epidural and spinal anesthesia is similar, certain basic differences are relevant to this discussion. The epidural space is potentially large and contains many blood vessels that can absorb anesthetic solution. Further, the dosage of anesthetics and the volume of drug injected are much larger than those for spinal anesthesia. Finally, because the dosage of anesthetic is so much larger, the potential for high blood levels and thus for local anesthetic toxicity is much greater.

The popularity of epidural anesthesia is related to its ability to provide continuous anesthesia for as long as the situation demands. Hence, continuous lumbar epidural anesthesia is frequently used in obstetric practice; anesthesia can be provided during labor and the dosage increased to cover the pelvic area during the delivery.

General Anesthesia

Although many interesting facts concerning the mode and site of action of general anesthetics are known,[26] the ultimate mechanism whereby patients lose consciousness and become analgesic remains unclear. Two helpful facts have emerged in studies of this question. The first is that very high barometric pressures (50 to 100 atm)[27] can reverse the effects of general anesthesia in certain animal models, probably because of the effects of pressure on molecular configuration. Second, in 1969 Eger and Saidman showed that the oil/gas partition coefficient multiplied by the minimum alveolar concentration of any inhalation agent consistently gave a product of 2.1.[16] The oil/gas partition coefficient is a measure of the distribution of the inhalation agent between two phases, in this case the inhalation gases in the lung and the fatty component of the brain. Minimum alveolar concentration, a measure of potency, is the anesthetic concentration at which 50% of patients do not move in response to a noxious stimulus. Basically, Eger and Saidman's description relates anesthetic potency to the agent's solubility in fat.

Preoperative Considerations

An understanding of the patient's complaints and symptoms, the surgical diagnosis, and the intended procedure are essential components of a thorough anesthetic plan. Preparing the patient for what is to come can be achieved only when an intelligent plan has been made. Most important is the patient's history of previous anesthesia and current and past drug intake. Potential problems such as difficulty with airway management, sensitivity to drugs, and anatomic problems in placing needles and endotracheal tubes can be detected during a preoperative visit.

Airway Management

Most anesthetic complications are associated with airway mishaps. Proper placement of an artificial airway such as an endotracheal tube or tracheostomy tube depends on knowledge of the anatomy of the mouth, nasopharynx, esophagus, and larynx. Essential to competent airway control is the ability to ventilate the patient with a reservoir bag and mask since many patients do not require endotracheal intubation.

Airway management is closely related to the anesthetic technique chosen. Administration of general anesthesia includes three phases: induction, maintenance, and emergence/recovery. Induction includes the establishment of a secure airway. Anesthesia is commonly induced with a rapid-acting potent intravenous barbiturate such as thiopentone. After the patient loses consciousness, the airway is the first priority. Maintenance of anesthesia can either be provided by allowing the patient to inhale anesthetic agents mixed with oxygen or by injecting selected intravenous agents that are tailored to the patient's requirements. Most patients are ventilated with oxygen/nitrous oxide mixtures that are combined with either intravenous or inhalation agents as required.

Mechanisms and Stages of General Anesthesia

Although theories on the mechanism of action of general anesthetics abound, this burning question remains unanswered. It is not even clear whether various anesthetic agents whose structures vary considerably are, in fact, bringing about the same state, although they are recognized under one term, i.e., general anesthesia. It is understood that narcotics render patients analgesic by occupying specific receptors in the brain and spinal cord and that benzodiazepines induce their effects by reacting with central nervous system receptors. But these are individual effects and only components of general anesthesia. Further, receptor antagonists that reverse the effects of these drugs do not reverse general anesthetics.

However, anesthesiologists do not differ on what constitutes general anesthesia and when patients are suitably anesthetized for surgery to take place. General anesthetics exert their main action, which is depressant, producing unconsciousness and abolishing reflexes, on the central nervous system; and through this action they modify every system. By their action on the various centers (e.g., respiratory center) and reflexes, phenomena are produced, the study of which enables a competent anesthesiologist to judge accurately at any moment the depth of anesthesia present. From commencement of induction to the point of death, anesthesia is divided into four stages:

Stage 1: This is the stage of analgesia, and is characterized by a progressive decrease in response to painful stimuli and progressive loss of consciousness.

Stage 2: During this phase delirium becomes manifest, with incoherent talking and struggling. Patients are unconscious and amnestic. Respiration is irregular and reflexes are inclined to be exaggerated.

Stage 3: This is heralded by muscular depression sufficient to prevent the patient from moving his limbs in response to stimuli. Surgical anesthesia is indicated by the onset of: (1) automatic respiration, and (2) loss of eyelid reflex. Stage 3 is subdivided into four planes:

- Plane 1: There is progressive decrease in the range and rapidity of eyeball movement.
- Plane 2: Eye is in a central position, and the intercostal muscles and diaphragm retain function.
- Plane 3: Thoracic movement is depressed until only diaphragmatic function remains.
- Plane 4: Respiratory effort is absent.

Stage 4: The heart beats, and the patient remains alive if oxygenated. As depth increases, pupils become dilated and irregular. This is an overdose.

Stage 3, plane 3, is commonly thought to represent the ideal anesthetic state for most surgery.

CHOICE OF AN ANESTHETIC

Two important decisions face the anesthesiologist when confronted with a new patient. One is what type of anesthetic technique to use (i.e., general, regional, or local), and the second concerns what pharmacologic agents to use.

Several factors play a part in the first decision. Frequently, if the surgery is to be performed on a small localized part of the body that is amenable to neural blockade, local anesthesia would seem appropriate. Other indications for local anesthesia include patient preference and the type of illness that a given patient may have that could make a more invasive technique potentially dangerous. In those situations in which more than one technique would be equally suitable, the anesthesiologist considers patient preference, his own familiarity with the regional technique, the surgeon's preference, the need to discuss the pathology during surgery, and whether teaching will take place intraoperatively. But even though all factors might indicate that a regional technique is best, the degree of familiarity of the anesthesiologist with that technique should play an important role in the decision.

There are persuasive arguments for general anesthesia in some situations: (1) when a skin or bone graft from a location removed from the primary surgical site is planned, requiring two injections; and (2) when the sound of some procedures such as heavy orthopedic manipulations of sawing or chiseling might be very disturbing to the awake patient.

In patients who have potentially difficult airways to manage, regional anesthesia is often recommended. However, it is wise to remember that the difficult airway is best managed electively; and if a spinal should ascend too high or a cervical block paralyze the vocal cords, the difficult airway might have to be managed in an emergency situation. In patients who will need blood transfusions, perhaps under pressure, general anesthesia is preferred because pushing blood intravenously under pressure can be painful and very uncomfortable to the patient.

In conclusion, many factors play a role in the anesthesiologist's decision as to what technique to use. Sometimes the need to teach a particular technique dictates that it be used, especially if there are no reasons to avoid that technique. What is important is that these decisions are made in full harmony with the surgeon and the patient, so that all are happy with the way things are progressing.

The second decision regarding the anesthetic agent to be used depends more heavily on the preexisting medical and surgical conditions found in the patient and is more fully discussed in a subsequent section of this chapter. Briefly, an important consideration in the selection of anesthetic agents is the route by which they are metabolized and excreted. Although most drugs are metabolized in the liver and excreted in the urine, some are degraded to active or toxic products. It is now believed that halothane hepatitis is related to the toxic metabolites of nonoxidative degradation of halothane in the liver. Care should also be taken to avoid agents that produce distortion or mask valuable signs. For example, it is well known that nitrous oxide expands gas-containing cavities, thereby distorting anatomy by massive dilation. Similarly, sedatives interfere with neurologic assessments, narcotics cause spasm of the sphincter of Oddi, and general anesthesia can mask intra-abdominal pain following viscus perforation. With few exceptions, general anesthetics are regarded as myocardial depressants. Careful selection of anesthetic technique is therefore necessary with patients who have a history of heart disease.

Most anesthetic complications occur during induction and emergence; thus airway management is as important during emergence and recovery as it is at the beginning of a procedure. Other potential postoperative problems related to anesthetics include arrhythmias, bleeding problems, renal failure, clotting of vascular grafts, malignant hyperthermia, and changes in the level of consciousness.

PATIENT MONITORING

As computers have become smaller and more widely available, many automated systems have been developed for patient monitoring during anesthesia. Nevertheless, there is no substitute for careful hands-on monitoring of surgical patients. Certain techniques have become standard and are considered minimum requirements for good patient care. These include the monitoring of blood pressure, heart rate, cardiac electrical activity, temperature, breath sounds, heart sounds, and inspired oxygen concentration.

Direct monitoring of blood pressure from an arterial catheter allows continuous evaluation of mean arterial, systolic, or diastolic pressure and makes arterial blood easily available for measuring arterial blood gases. If large changes in central blood volume are expected, central venous pressure monitoring might be indicated. Although urine output, heart rate, and blood pressure give relevant information, central venous pressure allows the anesthesiologist to closely follow changes in volume and observe the effect of volume infusions. However, central venous pressure reflects the volume and compliance of the right side of the heart most accurately. If systemic blood volume and left ventricular function measurements are required, a pulmonary artery catheter is the only currently available device that provides measurement of central venous pressure, pulmonary artery pressure, and pulmonary capillary wedge pressure. This catheter also allows sampling of mixed venous blood, thermodilution measurement of cardiac output, and monitoring of cardiac electric activity or pacing of the heart. Pulmonary capillary wedge pressure reflects left atrial pressure, which in turn reflects left ventricular filling pressure and volume. Further, with the use of the Starling principle, a ventricular function curve can be constructed that allows optimal volume loading, of special value in patients with a compromised left ventricle.

A pulmonary artery catheter is recommended for patients undergoing cardiac surgery or any patient with severe heart disease undergoing other types of surgery. Additional indications for pulmonary artery catheterization are: (1) major surgery involving massive blood and fluid replacement, and (2) any procedure associated with circulatory instability (e.g., massive trauma, extensive burns, hypotensive shock, severe sepsis, aortic surgery requiring clamping, pulmonary embolus, major portal surgery).

The end-expired carbon dioxide tension is a measurement that is used extensively in neurosurgical procedures. Apart from the very early detection of significant occlusion of pulmonary artery outflow caused by air embolism, as evidenced by a drop in end-expired P_{CO_2}, the end-expired P_{CO_2} is also an indication of cardiac output. Computer technology has made it possible to measure the somatosensory-evoked potential that accurately measures spinal cord function during surgery when spinal cord integrity might be threatened.

Electroencephalography, a measure of adequacy of cerebral perfusion and oxygenation, is now commonly used in the operating room during procedures in which cerebral blood flow might be compromised.

DISEASE-RELATED CONSIDERATIONS IN ANESTHETIC PRACTICE

Trauma

Anesthetic management of trauma patients is primarily directed toward airway control and maintenance of cardiovascular stability until bleeding is controlled and blood loss has been replaced. Trauma patients are often young and therefore more likely to have normal cardiovascular systems than the usual surgical population. Therapeutic priorities in these patients are delineated in Fig. 10-2.

Special Problems

There are a number of unique constraints that affect the treatment of victims of severe trauma:

- Frequently they are unable to give any history regarding their medical status or their drug intake.
- Because of the high incidence of occult cervical vertebral fractures associated with traumatic head injury,

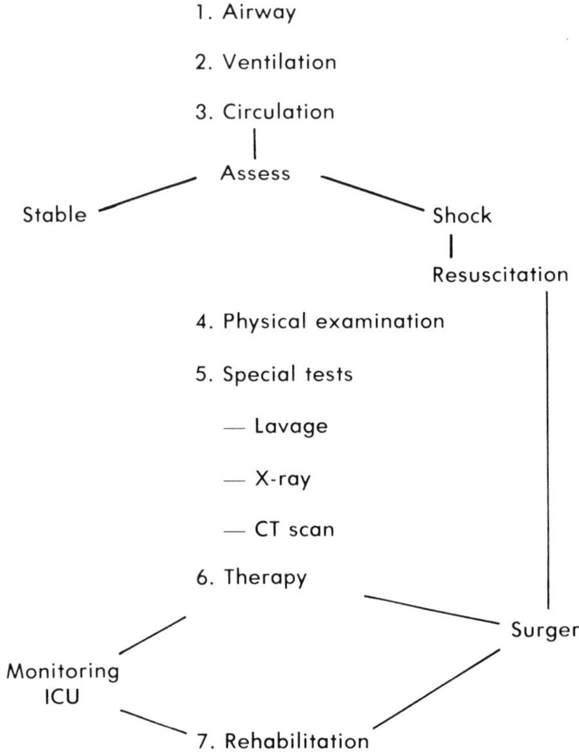

Fig. 10-2 Order of management of traumatized patient.

the neck must be treated as fractured until radiologic evidence to the contrary is available.

- All trauma patients are considered to have full stomachs which affects airway management; and many are under the influence of alcohol or drugs.
- Trauma patients are often bleeding actively and must be assumed to be in hemorrhagic, hypovolemic shock.
- Trauma patients are inclined to be maximally sympathetically stimulated and thus peripherally vasoconstricted, making intravenous access difficult, especially when the patient is also hypothermic.

Anesthetic Management

Hypothermia is common in trauma patients, especially in areas of the country that have severe winters. Efforts must be made to warm these patients as rapidly as is physiologically safe. Although hypothermia may impart some cerebral protection from hypoxia, depending on the rate of cooling, it is associated with a number of physiologic aberrations.

During periods of decreased cardiovascular function, hypothermia might be beneficial because metabolic activity is decreased, which in turn lessens oxygen requirements at the same time that oxygen delivery is reduced. This is especially true of the brain, which can survive a much longer period of ischemia if cooled first. However, at 30° C (86° F) premature ventricular contractions become manifest and further degenerate to ventricular fibrillation at 28° C (82° F) or below. Further, with oxygen delivery threatened, blood viscosity increases with decreasing temperature, and shivering increases oxygen demand by as much as 300%. Despite the fact that induced hypothermia has been used with some success clinically, uncontrolled hypothermia is detrimental since most body functions become depressed as temperature drops (see the boxed material below).

Gastric emptying stops as soon as sympathetic activity is stimulated by the occurrence of an accident. Therefore, no matter when the trauma occurred, the stomach is judged to be full, and the airway receives maximal protection from the possibility of aspiration of gastric contents. If general anesthesia is undertaken, induction should follow a definite sequence designed to minimize the chances of aspiration as shown in Table 10-3.

Trunkey has stated that 99% of trauma victims may be intubated orally.[50] In an emergency, cricothyrotomy[43] can be temporarily life-saving until a more permanent artificial airway can be established. If the anesthesiologist believes that intubation might be difficult, the patient should not be anesthetized until the airway has been secured[7] since induction of general anesthesia and the resulting paralysis can simultaneously impair the reflexes that protect the airway and eliminate all respiratory effort.

Maintenance of anesthesia should be directed toward providing good operating conditions while maintaining cardiovascular stability so that vital organ perfusion is assured. Following induction, anesthesia is maintained with agents that minimize cardiovascular depression. Frequently, paralysis is provided with intravenous pancuronium while the patient is ventilated with 100% oxygen. Analgesia is provided with intravenous narcotics that are titrated against the patient's blood pressure. Because as many as 40% of trauma patients are awake during trauma surgery,[4] the use of an amnestic sedative without cardiac depressive effects (e.g., lorazepam)[32] should be considered.

Monitoring should include use of a central venous pressure catheter, an electrocardiogram, an arterial line, and a urinary catheter and blood pressure checks. Blood should be replaced as quickly as possible through blood warmers to minimize hypothermia, and microfilters used to lessen the particulate matter trapped in the lung that appears to be a major factor in the development of the adult respiratory distress syndrome following multiple transfusions.

Cardiothoracic Disease

Over the last 20 years the number of open-heart procedures has increased markedly. The pulmonary artery catheter has revolutionized the management of patients with cardiovascular disease by allowing the anesthesiologist to optimally manipulate preload and afterload so that the myocardium is allowed to work at maximum efficiency within the constraints of its oxygen supply.

Preoperative Evaluation

Simple questions can establish the patient's exercise tolerance, the presence of orthopnea, and the frequency of chest pain. A history of hypertension, rheumatic fever, di-

EFFECTS OF HYPOTHERMIA

1. Reduced oxygen consumption and basal metabolic rate
2. Central nervous system depression leading to coma
3. Arrhythmias: PVCs (premature ventricular contractions) (30° C) (86° F)
   Ventricular fibrillation (28° C) (82° F)
4. Oxygen dissociation curve shift to left
5. Coagulopathy (28° C) (82° F)
6. Shivering (32°-24° C) (89.6°-75.2° F) and increased oxygen consumption
7. Increased blood viscosity (28° C) (82° F)
8. Respiratory depression—apnea at 23° C (73.4° F)
9. Hyperglycemia
10. Metabolic acidosis
11. Slow drug biotransformation
12. Depressed renal function—ceases at 20° C (68° F)
13. Arteriolar paralysis 32° C (89.6° F)

Table 10-3 **RAPID SEQUENCE INDUCTION (AIRWAY PROTECTION)**

Preparation	Suction	
	Laryngoscopes (two blades)	
	Tubes (three sizes)	
	Preoxygenation (3 min)	
	Precurarization (curare 3 mg)	
Induction	Thiopentone (3-5 mg/kg)	Cricoid pressure
	Succinylcholine (1-1.5 mg/kg)	Cricoid pressure
Airway	Intubate	Cricoid pressure
	Ventilate (check right and left)	Cricoid pressure
	Secure tube well	

abetes mellitus, smoking, obesity, inactivity, and family cardiac disease all tend to increase the patient's chances of myocardial infarction during surgery. It is important to determine what drugs the patient takes (e.g., digitalis), their effect, and serum drug levels. Cardiac patients should come to the operating room relaxed, pain free, and if necessary with supplemental oxygen. They should be sedated enough to comfortably tolerate the placement of intra-arterial, pulmonary artery, and peripheral intravenous catheters while awake.

Anesthetic Management

As the drive for the ideal cardiac anesthetic technique has progressed, two approaches have emerged. The first is related to the fact that inhalation agents are generally profound vasodilators that therefore routinely decrease afterload. Because they are also significant myocardial depressants,[3] they act maximally to decrease cardiac work and thus oxygen consumption. The problem with these agents is that they can cause hypotension so severe that coronary artery perfusion is inadequate for myocardial requirements. The second approach depends on the synthetic narcotic fentanyl, which has minimal cardiac depressant activity.[46] In very high doses[5] (50 to 100 μg/kg vs. 3 to 5 μg/kg in balanced anesthesia) fentanyl is currently the anesthetic of choice for cardiac surgery; patients are ventilated with 100% oxygen and given a relaxant such as metacurine that has no cardiac side effects and a benzodiazepine that acts as a hypnotic and amnestic agent.

Hypotension or hypertension are frequently seen on weaning from cardiopulmonary bypass. The anesthesiologist should be prepared to vasodilate, vasoconstrict, stimulate heart rate, slow it, or manipulate all cardiac performance indices to promote an adequate oxygen supply/demand ratio with satisfactory cardiac output.

In summary, invasive monitoring and the pulmonary artery catheter have enabled anesthesiologists to accurately determine all indices of cardiac performance and to tailor anesthetic management to protect the ailing myocardium from ischemic assault.

Chronic Pulmonary Disease

Much controversy surrounds the anesthetic management of patients with advanced lung diseases. Should they have regional anesthetics when possible? Should intubation be avoided? Should they be paralyzed? In general, these patients remain stable as long as no change occurs. Typical changes are simple upper respiratory tract infection, the onset of an unrelated disease process, or a significant change in climate.

Preoperative Evaluation

Determining exercise tolerance in these patients is of great importance since incapacitated patients are more likely to have problems postoperatively. The cessation of smoking before surgery[42,51] is of benefit both in terms of oxygen delivery and postoperative morbidity. However, because the chronic smoker's airway is more reactive, attempts should be made to avoid airway irritation. Dependence on bronchodilators is also associated with postoperative difficulties. Patients taking theophylline derivatives should have serum levels of these drugs within therapeutic range at all times. Dependence on steroids to control bronchospasm dictates the additional use of steroids during the stressful perioperative period.

If surgery is imminent, pulmonary function tests are more valuable as a predictor of postoperative problems than as aids in planning anesthetic technique. If there is time to act on what pulmonary function tests show, bronchodilators or chest physiotherapy can be prescribed as the situation demands. The most commonly used indicator of pulmonary function is the measurement of forced expiratory volume in 1 second (FEV_1). This test places patients with obstructive disease in one of three groups: (1) because of their considerable pulmonary reserve, patients with an FEV_1 greater than 50% of that predicted and normal arterial blood gases do not have an increased risk of perioperative problems; (2) patients with FEV_1 within 25% to 50% of that predicted are at significant risk for postoperative morbidity and should be evaluated with a view to achieving the best possible preoperative condition; and (3) patients with FEV_1 below 25% of predicted are hypoxemic, at high risk, and should have surgery only for life-threatening conditions.[30]

Anesthetic Management

General anesthesia for patients with chronic pulmonary disease is associated with decreased clearing of pulmonary secretions, increased alveolar atelectasis, increased intrapulmonary shunting, and significant changes in the ventilation/perfusion ratio.[29] Furthermore, paralysis is associated with increased ventilation perfusion mismatching.[19]

Studies on patients with normal pulmonary function[15] have failed to demonstrate any positive correlation between anesthetic technique and incidence of postoperative pulmonary complications. Similar studies on patients with chronic obstructive pulmonary disease have shown a much higher incidence of postoperative respiratory failure in patients receiving general anesthesia[49] than those receiving regional anesthesia. Ventilatory impairment is related to the anatomic site of surgery in patients with and without pulmonary disease. Upper abdominal and thoracic procedures are associated with significant degrees of impairment in vital capacity.[12]

When general anesthesia is used in patients with pulmonary disease, it should be tailored to compensate as much as possible for the abnormal airway architecture, the disturbed ventilation/perfusion ratios, the increased sensitivity to ventilatory depressants, the limited ability to mobilize secretions over a poorly functioning mucociliary escalator, and the restricted potential for humidifying inspired gases. Arterial blood gases should be monitored frequently to ensure adequate gas exchange. Finally, gases should be humidified to prevent the extreme drying of airways that follows prolonged ventilation with dry gases. Assuming that a general anesthetic technique has been chosen, the specific pharmacologic agents administered do not appear to affect the outcome.

Efforts should be directed to extubating patients as soon as possible after surgery. There is a tendency to leave these patients in surgical intensive care units for prolonged periods while they are being weaned off ventilators. The longer they depend on assisted ventilation, the greater their morbidity.

Liver Disease

There are four important considerations in managing surgical patients with liver disease. These are: (1) worsening of the liver disease, (2) extrahepatic complications, (3) impairment of liver synthetic activity, and (4) alteration of drug disposition.

Anesthetic Risk Factors

Although hard evidence does not exist, it can be assumed intuitively that surgery and anesthesia worsen preexisting liver disease. Spinal anesthesia is known to decrease hepatic blood flow if hypotension develops. Moreover, studies have shown that spinal anesthesia, cyclopropane, and ether anesthesia are all associated with the same degree of postoperative hepatic dysfunction in patients with liver disease.[18] Similar studies have not been made with the modern inhalation anesthetics such as halothane, enflurane, and isoflurane.

Extrahepatic complications include encephalopathy, which lowers anesthetic requirements; esophageal varices; and ascites. Bleeding esophageal varices represent the most serious anesthetic risk factor in patients with liver disease because of the dual threat of aspiration of blood and hypovolemia. Many of the principles of trauma management apply equally well to this type of surgical emergency.

Hypoxemia is common in patients with portal hypertension and ascites. Ascites reduces diaphragmatic excursion, compresses the lungs, and decreases the ventilation perfusion ratio in basilar sections of the lungs. Because of vena caval compression, ascites also can impair venous return to the heart, causing hypotension, which further complicates the hypovolemia of bleeding varices. Finally, ascites increases the volume of distribution of anesthetic drugs. Ascitic fluid is isolated from the circulation and can serve as a sink for drugs, delaying the onset and prolonging the duration of their action.

Anesthetic Management

Destruction of liver cells can impair the ability of the liver to synthesize compounds such as plasma proteins, plasma pseudocholinesterase, and clotting factors, which are vital to anesthetic management. Since a number of drugs used for anesthesia are significantly bound to plasma proteins, decreased levels of these proteins can cause altered pharmacokinetics and dynamics. Pseudocholinesterase is the enzyme responsible for metabolizing succinylcholine and all ester local anesthetics. Although significant hepatic destruction must be present before the metabolism of these drugs is affected, the duration of action of succinylcholine, an ultrashort-acting relaxant, can be significantly prolonged in patients with substantial liver disease. In such a setting of reduced plasma pseudocholinesterase activity, neuromuscular function could take hours to return to normal instead of the expected 5 minutes. Finally, the decreased production of clotting factors that occurs in liver disease could also pose significant problems in anesthetic management, particularly in the patient who is hypovolemic from bleeding varices.

Many factors interact to alter the half-life of drugs used in anesthetic practice. These include altered synthesis of plasma proteins with changes in albumin/globulin ratio, decreased hepatic biotransformation, decreased hepatic blood flow, and changes in the volume of distribution. Furthermore, anesthesia itself may decrease hepatic blood flow and can inhibit the action of hepatic microsomal oxidative enzymes.[6]

Local anesthetics of the amide type, which depend on liver metabolism for their breakdown, are inclined to clear the blood less rapidly than in normal patients. Thus the tendency toward local anesthetic toxicity with these agents is increased, and caution should be exercised when using them.

Diabetes Mellitus

Infection is the leading cause of death in diabetic surgical patients. In the past it was thought that patients would remain stable if they were hyperglycemic but not ketotic during surgery. Although short durations of hyperglycemia to levels of 400 to 600 mg/100 ml will not be harmful to diabetics, hypoglycemia of similar duration can cause severe and irreversible brain damage. It is obvious that hypoglycemia would be very difficult to detect clinically during administration of general anesthesia. Therefore the tendency toward hyperglycemia grew in popularity. Recent evidence, however, indicates that diabetics with normal blood glucose levels have a lower incidence of morbidity.[11]

Preoperative Evaluation

Evaluation of the diabetic patient before surgery must include consideration of the duration and severity of the illness and present medications. Juvenile diabetics have lower circulating insulin levels and are more difficult to control perioperatively. The maturity-onset diabetic is more likely to have a decreased fasting blood sugar without ketosis when starved preoperatively. The hypoglycemic agent prescribed, its dosage, and the frequency of administration will predict both peak effect and potential for hypoglycemia in the patient. Long-acting insulins or oral agents such as chlorpropamide can still have an effect on the morning of surgery, even when the last dose was given 24 hours before the operation. A morning fasting glucose should always be drawn before induction of anesthesia.

Anesthetic Management

In the interest of maintaining near normal glucose levels intraoperatively, many protocols have been developed. The tendency to avoid hypoglycemia led to an approach based on minimal interference during the operation. No glucose or insulin was given on the day of surgery, and insulin was used only to treat severe hyperglycemia and/or ketosis.[9] More recently, a partial dose of the normal insulin requirement was given on the morning of surgery.

Blood sugars were followed intraoperatively and treated appropriately, the glucose was added as necessary until the patient tolerated tube or oral feeding postoperatively. Currently, intravenous insulin, either by injection or continuous intravenous infusion, is given with intravenous dextrose during surgery. The insulin dose is either adjusted to the glucose infusion rate or titrated by frequent blood glucose measurements.[47] No single protocol can be expected to manage all diabetic patients adequately. Frequent blood analysis with appropriate insulin therapy is probably the most reliable method available.

Inhalation anesthetics tend to increase blood sugar.[23] An anesthetic for diabetic patients is tailored more toward the manifestations of the disease (e.g., renal failure) than toward the disease itself. If neuropathy and/or infections are present, spinal or epidural anesthesia is relatively contraindicated. Because of the need for repeated venous blood samples, monitoring intraoperative blood sugars is easier in unconscious patients than in awake patients. Adherence to the concepts described here should allow any general anesthetic technique to be used safely.

Renal Failure

Acute renal failure is the abrupt impairment of renal function, whereas chronic renal failure implies a more permanent functional impairment that has profound systemic effects such that, if there were no method of clearing the blood of toxic metabolites, death would surely follow.

Medical Complications

Infection and sepsis are the leading causes of mortality in anephric patients.[47] These problems are aggravated in transplant recipients who are receiving immunosuppressive drugs such as steroids. A meticulous sterile technique should be used whenever catheters are placed. Invasive monitoring techniques should be used sparingly since the incidence of thrombophlebitis is high. In patients who depend on flow through arteriovenous shunts for dialysis, strict criteria for inserting arterial catheters should be developed.

Patients in renal failure have a high incidence of cardiovascular disease. Hypertension is common, and signs of left ventricular hypertrophy are frequent. The murmurs of aortic and mitral insufficiency occur as a result of hypertension, anemia, and fluid overload. However, these murmurs often resolve with dialysis. Uremia is also associated with cardiomyopathy and pericardial effusions. Hypertension is either related to fluid overload or increased plasma renin levels. Although functionally overloaded, anephric patients behave as though they are volume-depleted during anesthesia. Hypotension can occur with minimal blood loss or vasodilation. The temptation to fill up the dilated vascular bed can cause severe hypertension following surgery and tends to push the patient into volume overload. The management of fluids in these patients is extremely precarious. Although the tendency is to err on the side of hypovolemia, hypotension should be treated early.

Dialysis is associated with several problems that can affect anesthesia. Patients may be placed on the dialysis machine in fluid overload and hypertensive yet come off hypovolemic and hypotensive. The date of the most recent dialysis, postdialysis laboratory values, and weight loss must be determined before surgery. Dialysis is associated with anemia in renal failure patients, with typical hematocrits ranging between 20% and 25%. Although the anemia is well tolerated, there are acceptable limits to its severity before anesthesia. These limits have not been definitively established, but hematocrits of 20% to 25% represent an oxygen-carrying capacity of 50% or less of normal. Cardiac output is usually increased to compensate for this decreased oxygen-carrying capacity.

Anesthetic Management

It is best to avoid anesthetic agents that depend on renal function for elimination. Thiopentone tends to have a longer duration of action in patients with uremia. Narcotics also appear to have prolonged effects. D-Tubocurarine is the only relaxant that has a route of elimination through an organ other than the kidney (i.e., the liver) and therefore is the relaxant of choice in these patients. Atracurium besylate is a new shorter acting nondepolarizing relaxant that is eliminated from the body by processes not requiring intact renal function. This drug is becoming more popular for patients in chronic renal failure. Inhalation anesthesia is the safest technique, because inhalant drugs are only minimally metabolized and do not depend on renal excretion for cessation of their action.

Pediatric Diseases

Two primary differences between a child and adult influence the treatment of pediatric patients. First, although the child's surface area is one twentieth that of adults, his surface-to-volume ratio is 70 times greater.[24] The most obvious effect of this circumstance is the increase in heat loss that children undergo and thus the increased caloric requirements needed to maintain body temperature. The other important difference is that children usually have no insight into their problem, do not cooperate, and feel threatened and alienated, especially when coming to the operating room.

Physiologic Considerations

Basic differences in cardiovascular function do exist but are not so significant that the principles of safe management change. Infants up to 6 months of age tend to have right ventricular hypertrophy as a leftover from the fetal circulation. To compensate for the lower oxygen-carrying capacity of fetal hemoglobin, the infants have a cardiac output that is 30% to 50% greater than in adults. Arterial pressure also varies with age. Neonates tend to have pressures around 60 to 70 mm Hg systolic, which increase to systolic pressures of approximately 100 by the age of 12. Finally, children also have an increased blood volume. During the first month of life blood volume is approximately 85 ml/kg.[36] By age 14 it has decreased to 68 to 75 ml/kg.

For anatomic reasons, atelectasis is more likely to occur in infants. Their alveoli are smaller, and their chest wall is very compliant. A term infant has a wasted ventilation of 40% that decreases to adult levels of 30% by 1 month of age. Oxygen requirements in children are up to twice that of adults (6 ml/kg).[37] When combined with the very small vital capacity of infants, this high oxygen requirement can rapidly lead to hypoxia and cyanosis during oxygen deprivation.

Renal function is poorly developed in newborns but is adequate to meet their metabolic needs. Infants have difficulty reabsorbing bicarbonate from their urine and, in effect, have renal tubular acidosis.[14] Only when their protein intake increases are they able to secrete hydrogen ions and ammonia. Neonates are unable to concentrate their urine as well as adults, although they can increase this ability when stressed.

One significant difference between neonates and adults is how they maintain body temperature. Infants metabolize brown fat, which is located between the scapulae, around the heart, and around vital structures in the neck as a source of calories.[45] Neonates are unable to shiver. Because of their enormous surface area–to–body weight ratio they have a tendency to lose temperature to the environment, especially when uncovered or wet.[44] Cold operating rooms, hypoglycemia, exposure of abdominal and thoracic contents, and ventilation with cold dry gases compound this problem. Thus temperature must be carefully monitored in children.

Anesthetic Management

Most children come to the operating room without intravenous access. The current technique used in pediatric anesthesia is an inhalation induction followed by placement of an intravenous line as soon as the patient has lost consciousness. Once this access is secured, the anesthetic management is similar to that used in the adult.

The pediatric larynx is somewhat different from that of adults. The narrowest part of the larynx in the adult is the glottis, whereas in the child the cricoid ring is the limiting factor. The larynx is somewhat higher in the neck (i.e., at C2 as opposed to C3 to C6 in the adult). Children are generally easier to intubate with a straight laryngoscope blade than with a curved one. No cuffs are needed on pediatric tubes since the cricoid ring seals the tube in the larynx.

Finally, children tend to emerge rapidly from anesthesia and need early support and encouragement until they are reunited with their parents.

ANESTHETIC EMERGENCIES

Cardiac Arrest

Three main groups of etiologic factors are associated with cardiac arrest[13]: (1) impairment of cardiac electrical activity, which is usually manifested by some arrhythmia; the most common of these is ventricular fibrillation, but ventricular tachycardia, asystole, and complete heart block are also seen; (2) disorders of myocardial contractility following hypoxia, myocardial infarction, cardiac failure, acidosis, electrolyte abnormalities, or drug effects; and (3) entities associated with decreased venous return, including hypovolemia, tamponade, pulmonary embolus, myocardial rupture, dissecting aneurysm, or vena caval compression. During anesthesia, all cardiac arrests are viewed as hypoxia until proved otherwise. By far the most prevalant of anesthetic accidents is the disconnection of the patient from the ventilatory source, resulting in hypoxic cardiac arrest.

Although the treatment of cardiac arrest is aimed at correcting the cause, the initial phases of cardiopulmonary resuscitation are similar for all arrests. All patients should be ventilated with 100% oxygen. A 5- to 10-ml amount of epinephrine at a ratio of 1:10,000 intravenously can elevate perfusion pressure; change fine to coarse fibrillation, which is more responsive to defibrillation; and stimulate spontaneous or more forceful cardiac contraction. Sodium bicarbonate is given intravenously to combat metabolic acidosis in initial doses of 1 mEq/kg. A dosage of 5 to 7 mg/kg of 10% calcium chloride infused intravenously is also a reliable inotropic agent. Lidocaine can be given to suppress ventricular ectopy in doses of 1 mg/kg intravenously. Atropine in 0.5 mg doses repeated to a desired effect is used in third-degree heart block and asystole to accelerate heart rate. Isoproterenol can be infused to treat third-degree block or electromechanical dissociation.

Cardiac arrest that occurs in the operating room usually responds to this sequence of therapy. If arrest occurs during induction and the patient is successfully resuscitated, surgery should be postponed. If it occurs intraoperatively and is reversed, every effort should be made to end the procedure as soon as possible.

Pneumothorax

One of the complications of positive pressure ventilation is the development of pulmonary interstitial emphysema. Pulmonary interstitial emphysema may or may not be accompanied by pneumothorax.[35] Several surgical factors increase the chances of pneumothorax: (1) surgery deep in the flank in the kidney position, (2) any trauma surgery in which projectiles have passed through the diaphragm, and (3) any type of surgery performed near the diaphragm.

Although pneumothorax itself may not necessarily lead to an anesthetic emergency, the onset of tension pneumothorax is a potentially fatal emergency if not swiftly relieved. Tension pneumothorax occurs when a one-way valve effect is set up, allowing air to enter the pleural space but not to leave. If this air and gas are being driven into the chest under pressure, as occurs with mechanical ventilation, the potential for disaster is large. Signs of pneumothorax include high inflation pressures, sudden shift of the mediastinum to the opposite side, circulatory collapse, subcutaneous emphysema, and coughing of serosanguinous material. In these situations immediate decompression of the pleural space is required and can be accomplished by inserting a large bore needle or chest tube into the pleural space.

The use of nitrous oxide further complicates the entrapment of air in any cavity such as the chest. Nitrous oxide expands these cavities relatively quickly and increases the circulatory and respiratory compromise caused by pneumothorax.[16]

Tension pneumothorax can occur spontaneously. When hypotension occurs and no obvious cause is seen, suspicion of tension pneumothorax may save a life that would otherwise have been lost.

Malignant Hyperthermia

Malignant hyperthermia is a disease of muscle tissue, which, when triggered by various anesthetic agents, sets off a chain of events leading to uncontrollable muscle hypermetabolism, rampant metabolic acidosis, and severe hypoxia. It is a genetically determined disease, more common in children and young adults. The incidence of malignant hyperthermia in children is estimated to be about 1:14,000 anesthetics. It is more common in individuals having muscular abnormalities such as joint hypermobility, kyphoscoliosis, ptosis, squint, clubbed feet, and history of muscle cramps. The mortality rate associated with malignant hyperthermia approaches 50%.

The disease is usually reported to be initiated by the administration of either halothane or succinylcholine.[22] Failure of the jaw to relax after succinylcholine administration is associated with the disease.[17] Other early clinical signs include tachycardia and metabolic acidosis. Fever is a later finding, and the disorder is severe when it occurs. Arrhythmias, tachypnea, and an increase in tidal volume indicate the tremendously high carbon dioxide tensions manifested by these patients. The skin becomes mottled, and the tissues of the wound and viscera may feel hot. Profound sweating may occur. P_{CO_2} is usually very high, often over 100 mm Hg. Hypoxia may or may not be present. Disseminated intravascular coagulopathy may follow. An elevated creatine phosphokinase level in the serum is present in 70% of patients with this condition.[31] To make the diagnosis in susceptible patients, a muscle biopsy that includes evaluation of caffeine-induced contractures with and without halothane is the most useful test.[28]

A protocol for the management of this condition should be summarized and taped to every anesthetic machine. A separate box and cart labeled "hyperthermia emergency kit" should be available in all operating room suites. Dantrolene, the current specific treatment for this disease, probably works by decreasing the amount of transmitter released by the excitation-contraction coupling process within muscle, thus indirectly reducing the amount of calcium released. The following list shows the sequence of treatment in this disease (see boxed material below left).

Late complications of the disease include renal failure, myoglobinuria, and hypotension (prerenal failure); consumption coagulopathies are treated with fresh frozen plasma and platelets; and central nervous system damage, which may become apparent only later.

TREATMENT OF MALIGNANT HYPERTHERMIA

1. Stop administration of all anesthetics and end surgery as soon as possible.
2. Send for help.
3. Replace the anesthesia machine with a nonrebreathing circuit, free of anesthetic vapors.
4. Begin mixing dantrolene sodium (20 mg/60 ml water) and give 1-2 mg/kg i.v.
5. Treat acidosis with sodium bicarbonate according to formula:

   Base deficit =
   0.3 × weight (kg) × base excess in (mEq/L)
6. Treat hypotension by correcting pH and giving cold crystalloid loading.
7. External cooling should be vigorous. Cool room and bathe patient in ice packs and wet towels soaked in alcohol.
8. Monitor all laboratory values. Treat hyperkalemia with glucose and insulin if necessary.
9. Admit to an intensive care unit and continue dantrolene and other therapy.

Venous Air Embolism

Although the pathophysiology of the various types of pulmonary venous emboli are similar, air embolism can occur rapidly and without warning in the operating room. The entry of air into the venous system occurs regularly when bubbles enter the veins through intravenous infusions. However, these small volumes are usually filtered out[8] or absorbed without causing any sequelae. In any procedure in which the wound is higher than the right atrium, a gravity gradient exists between the wound site and the right atrium, permitting entrainment of air. This complication is most commonly seen in neurosurgical procedures performed with the patient in the sitting position, but it has been reported after head and neck surgery,[2] dilation and curettage (D & C), hysterectomy,[34] and the placement of subclavian central venous catheters.[41]

Once air has entered the venous system, it is carried to the right atrium. As the volume of gas increases, the bubbles move to the right ventricle and then to the pulmonary artery where they block the pulmonary artery outflow tract, inducing acute right ventricular failure.

When surgical patients must be in positions in which air embolism is a possible complication, certain preparations can aid the diagnosis and treatment of this condition. Initially, a right atrial central catheter can be placed to monitor central venous pressure; it must be located so that air bubbles can be aspirated conveniently. Bubbles in the blood cause turbulence as they pass through the heart. As little as 0.5 ml of air can be detected with an ultrasound chest doppler placed over the right atrium. When any type of pulmonary embolism occurs, some degree of occlusion of the pulmonary outflow tract is usually present. Thus perfusion of the lung by venous blood is decreased, and the blood retains carbon dioxide that would have been eliminated in the alveoli. Hence the arterial P_{CO_2} increases, whereas the end expiratory carbon dioxide decreases. These changes can be monitored on a capnograph, which is a reliable form of monitoring for pulmonary ve-

TREATMENT OF VENOUS AIR EMBOLISM

1. Inform surgeon, who can cover wound with saline-soaked sponges and prevent further air entrainment.
2. Send for help.
3. Discontinue nitrous oxide.
4. Aspirate right atrial catheter.
5. Change height of wound in relation to the right atrium, if possible.
6. Treat cardiovascular depression supportively.

nous embolism. Treatment is described in the boxed material on p. 200.

Electrolyte Disturbances

Calcium and potassium ions are intimately involved with the generation of action potentials in the excitable tissue of the heart. The presence of these electrolytes in abnormal concentrations thus is reflected in abnormal electrocardiograms and arrhythmias, some of which may herald the onset of critical conduction defects.

Hypocalcemia

Normal serum calcium levels are between 8 and 10.5 mEq/L. Membrane function, neuromuscular function, and myocardial contractility depend on the amount of ionized calcium in extracellular fluid. The ionized portion of the serum calcium in turn depends on the pH (decreasing pH increases ionized calcium) and plasma proteins (decreased protein decreases ionized calcium). The causes of acute severe hypocalcemia are massive transfusion (citrate intoxication), severe alkalosis, and parathyroidectomy. Severe respiratory alkalosis may be the cause of true tetanic muscle spasms similar to those seen in hypocalcemic tetany following parathyroidectomy. In the operating room hypocalcemia is associated with hypotension, electrocardiographic abnormalities (Fig. 10-3, *A*), and cardiac arrest in diastole if calcium levels drop too low. Severe hypocalcemia is best treated with calcium chloride in dosages of 1 g as a slow intravenous infusion over several minutes.

Hypercalcemia

Hypercalcemia is a much rarer phenomenon and results in calcium levels of 17 to 20 mg/100 ml or even higher, a severe and sometimes fatal problem. These levels are usually seen only in patients with severe hyperparathyroidism or metastatic bone cancer. Extracellular fluid expansion, chelating agents, steroids, and dialysis sometimes fail to control hypercalcemia. Electrocardiographic aberrations are seen, with cardiac arrest occurring in systole. See Fig. 10-3, *B*.

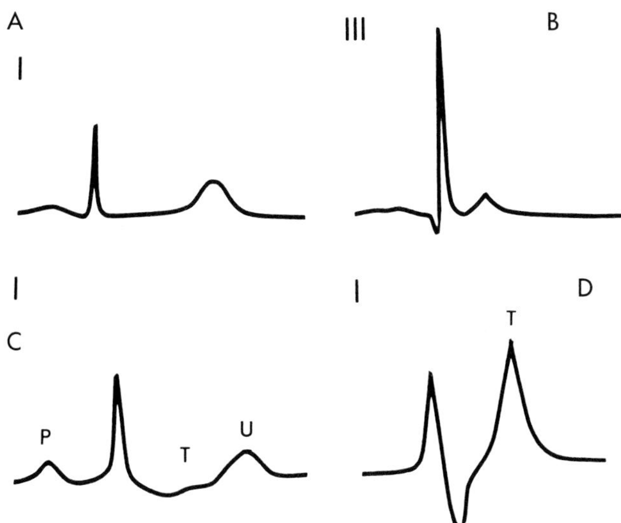

Fig. 10-3 Electrocardiographic changes in various electrolyte abnormalities. **A,** Hypocalcemia: Most obvious feature is prolonged Q-T interval and late T-wave. Lead I. **B,** Hypercalcemia: Note shortened Q-T interval and shortened S-T segment. Lead III. **C,** Hypokalemia: Exaggeration of U-wave, depression of S-T segment, and fusion of T-wave with U-wave. Lead I. **D,** Hyperkalemia: Peaked and tall T-waves, widening of QRS, and decreased Q-T interval. Lead I.

Hypokalemia

Normal extracellular fluid potassium levels vary between 4 and 5 mEq/L. This accounts for 2% of total body potassium, the rest of which is intracellular (150 mEq/L). Potassium is shifted intracellularly by alkalosis, hyperventilation, and glucose-insulin therapy. The three most common causes of hypokalemia in surgical patients include excessive renal losses, unreplaced losses from gastrointestinal secretions, and movement of potassium ions into the cells. Most of the commonly used diuretics, especially the thiazides, are associated with increased potassium loss through the urine.

Hypokalemia results in poor contractile strength in skeletal, smooth, and cardiac muscle. It is recommended that anesthesia not be administered when potassium levels are below 3 mEq/L.[21] In surgical emergencies potassium can be replaced at a rate not to exceed 0.5 mEq/kg/hour. Cardiac electrical activity and urine output should be monitored during replacement, and levels should be checked frequently. During anesthesia, hyperventilation, which reduces potassium levels even further, should be avoided. Electrocardiographic changes are shown in Fig. 10-3, *C*.

Hyperkalemia

Arrhythmias, resistance to digitalis, and high-peaked T waves on electrocardiograms are the typical cardiac effects of hyperkalemia (Fig. 10-3, *D*). Usual causes include impaired excretion of potassium in renal failure and massive blood transfusions. Anesthesia should be postponed if potassium levels are over 6 mEq/L. The combination of hyperkalemia and arrhythmogenic anesthetics such as halothane is unwise. Potentially fatal hyperkalemia can occur after the administration of succinylcholine in certain conditions including major burns, massive trauma, and neurologic injury.[25] Peak potassium levels of 10 to 15 mEq/L are associated with dangerous arrhythmias, including ventricular tachycardia and ventricular fibrillation.

RECENT ADVANCES AND FUTURE CONSIDERATIONS

Monitoring

The future thrust in monitoring technology will be in the area of noninvasive techniques. Computer miniaturization has permitted the development of sophisticated equipment for operating room use. Mass spectrometry allows monitoring concentrations of multiple anesthetic and physiologic gases. Equipment now available enables one observer at a central console in the operating room to monitor the expired gas concentrations of six to 12 rooms concurrently. Problems such as hypercarbia, hypoxia, and anesthetic overdose can be detected rapidly with the use of this system. The equipment is extremely sensitive in detecting air embolism. Further, anesthetic gas concentrations can be monitored, and dangerous errors corrected.

Transesophageal echocardiography is another new technique used for intraoperative monitoring. This technique has emerged as a reliable method of detecting a patent foramen ovale[33] and the presence of foreign substances in the chambers of the heart. In the past the equipment for echocardiography was too large and awkward; however, this equipment is now rapidly approaching a size that will make it practical for operating room use. Several reports describe the use of an echocardiogram with a transesophageal transmitter to successfully locate air bubbles in the right and left sides of the heart.[10] Although expense presently prohibits the routine use of this equipment, it is one way in which paradoxic air embolism through a probe patent foramen ovale[20] might be detected early.

Agents

The most profound development has occurred in the production and synthesis of newer ultrapotent narcotic agents. Derivatives of fentanyl (i.e., alfentanil and sufentanil) are more potent than fentanyl, which is in turn ten times more potent than morphine. Further, these new narcotics have a more rapid onset and shorter duration of action than fentanyl, yet apparently they have minimal cardiac depressant activity.[40] Many researchers are confident that new ultrapotent narcotics under investigation will change the way anesthesia is practiced in the future.

SUMMARY

An important component of surgical care relates to the ability to adequately anesthetize that portion of the body being subjected to operation. Currently two broad categories of anesthetic technique are recognized: conduction anesthesia in which chemicals are injected to areas immediately surrounding nerves to temporarily block their normal function; and general anesthesia in which inhalant substances elicit an anesthetic state by inducing varying degrees of amnesia, relaxation, and loss of consciousness. In choosing an anesthetic for a given patient, the anesthesiologist is confronted with two important decisions: (1) what type of technique to use, and (2) what pharmacologic agent to use to induce anesthesia once the technique has been decided on. Factors affecting these decisions include the part of the body being subjected to operation, the type of illness that a given patient may have, the patient's particular preference, and the expertise and familiarity of the anesthesiologist when considering the appropriateness of a given technique in a particular situation. In all cases, flexibility should be the rule, and a knowledge of the advantages and disadvantages of a given anesthetic in a specific clinical setting thoroughly understood so as to choose the optimal approach for each patient and thereby minimize the incidence of both intraoperative and postoperative problems.

REFERENCES

1. Albright, G.A.: Cardiac arrest following regional anesthesia with etidocaine or bupivacaine, Anesthesiology **51:**285, 1979.
2. Amussat, J.Z.: Recherches sur l'introduction accidentelle de l'air dans les veins, Paris, 1839, Germer Bailliere.
3. Bahlman, S.H., et al.: The cardiovascular effects of halothane in man during spontaneous ventilation, Anesthesiology **36:**494, 1972.
4. Bogetz, M.S., and Katz, J.A.: Recall of surgery in victims of major trauma: effect of anesthetic dose, Anesthesiology **57:**A331, 1982.
5. Bovill, J.G., and Sebel, P.S.: Pharmacokinetics of high-dose fentanyl: a study in patients undergoing cardiac surgery, Br. J. Anaesth. **52:**795, 1980.
6. Brown, B.R., Jr.: The diphasic action of halothane on the oxidative metabolism of drugs by the liver: an in vitro study in the rat, Anesthesiology **35:**241, 1971.
7. Burtner, D.D., and Goodman, M.: Anesthetic and operative management of potential upper airway obstruction, Arch. Otolaryngol. **104:**657, 1978.
8. Butler, B.D., and Hills, B.A.: The lung as a filter for microbubbles, J. Appl. Physiol. **47:**537, 1978.
9. Crawley, B.E., and Seager, R.: Monitoring of blood sugar during surgery, Anaesthesia **25:**73, 1970.
10. Cucchiara, R.F., et al.: Air embolism in upright neurosurgical patients: detection and localization by two-dimensional transesophageal echocardiography, Anesthesiology **60:**353, 1984.
11. Davidson, M.B.: The case for control in diabetes mellitus, West. J. Med. **129:**193, 1978.
12. Diament, M.L., and Palmer, K.N.V.: Postoperative changes in gas tensions of arterial blood and in ventilatory function, Lancet **2:**180, 1966.
13. Donegan, J.H.: Cardiopulmonary resuscitation. In Miller, R.D., editor: Anesthesia, New York, 1981, Churchill Livingstone.
14. Edelman, C.M., Jr., et al.: Renal bicarbonate reabsorption and hydrogen ion excretion in normal infants, J. Clin. Invest. **46:**1309, 1967.
15. Egbert, L.D., Laver, M.B., and Bendixen, H.H.: The effect of site of operation and type of anesthesia upon the ability to cough in the postoperative period, Surg. Gynecol. Obstet. **115:**295, 1962.
16. Eger, E.I., II, and Saidman, L.J.: Hazards of nitrous oxide anesthesia in bowel obstruction and pneumothorax, Anesthesiology **26:**61, 1965.
17. Ellis, F.R., and Halball, P.J.: Suxemethonium spasm: a differential diagnosis conundrum, Br. J. Anaesth. **567:**381, 1984.
18. French, A.B., et al.: Metabolic effects of anesthesia in man. V. A comparison of the effects of ether and cyclopropane anesthesia on the abnormal liver, Ann. Surg. **135:**145, 1952.
19. Froese, A.B., and Bryan, A.C.: Effects of anesthesia and paralysis on diaphragmatic mechanics in man, Anesthesiology **41:**242, 1974.
20. Furuya, H., and Okumura, F.: Detection of paradoxical air embolism by transesophageal echocardiography, Anesthesiology **60:**374, 1984.
21. Goldstein, G.: Serum potassium levels and anesthesia, Curr. Rev. Clin. Anesth. **1**(21):169, 1981.
22. Goron, R.A., Britt, B.A., and Kalow, W.: International symposium on malignant hyperthermia, Springfield, Ill., 1973, Charles C Thomas, Publisher.
23. Green, N.M.: Insulin and anesthesia, Anesthesiology **41:**75, 1974.
24. Gregory, G.A.: Pediatric anesthesia. In Miller, R.D., editor: Anesthesia, New York, 1981, Churchill Livingstone.
25. Gronert, G., and Theye, R.A.: Pathophysiology of hyperkalemia induced by succinylcholine, Anesthesiology **43:**89, 1975.
26. Halsey, M.J.: Mechanisms of general anesthesia. In Eger, E.I., II, editor: Anesthetic uptake and action, Baltimore, Md., 1974, The Williams and Wilkins Co.
27. Halsey, M.J., Wardley-Smith, B., and Green, C.J.: Pressure reversal of general anesthesia: a multi-site expansion hypothesis, Br. J. Anaesth. **50:**1091, 1978.
28. Harrison, G.G.: A pharmacological in vitro model of hyperpyrexia, S. Afr. Med. J. **47:**774, 1973.

29. Heironimus, T.W., III: The anesthetic management of the pulmonary cripple. In Hershey, S.G., editor: ASA refresher courses in anesthesiology, vol. 3, Park Ridge, Ill., 1975, American Society of Anesthesiologists.
30. Hensley, M.J., and Fencl, V.: Lungs and respiration. In Vandam, L.D.: To make the patient ready for anesthesia: medical care of the surgical patient, Menlo Park, Calif., 1980, Medical/Nursing Division, Addison-Wesley Publishing Co., Inc.
31. Isaacs, H., and Barlow, M.B.: Malignant hyperpyrexia: further muscle studies in asymptomatic carriers identified by creatinine phosphokinase screening, J. Neurol. Neurosurg. Psychiatry **36:**228, 1973.
32. Katz, J., et al.: Safety of lorazepam in hypovolemic shock, Anesthesiology **59:**A96, 1983.
33. Kronik, G., and Mosslacher, H.: Positive contrast echocardiography in patients with patent foramen ovale and normal right heart hemodynamics, Am. J. Cardiol. **49:**1806, 1982.
34. Lembke, W.: Ueber erfolgreiche Behandlung einer schweren Luftembolie durch Herzkammerpunktion, Chirung **17-18:**31-35, 1946.
35. Lenaghan, R., Silva, Y.J., and Walt, A.J.: Hemodynamic alterations associated with expansion rupture of the lung, Arch. Surg. **99:**339, 1969.
36. Linderkamp, O., et al.: Estimation and prediction of blood volume in infants and children, Eur. J. Pediatr. **125:**227, 1977.
37. Lister, G., Hoffman, J.I.E., and Rudolph, A.M.: Oxygen uptake in infants and children: A simple method for measurement, Pediatrics **53:**656, 1974.
38. Reference deleted in proofs.
39. Munson, E.S., et al.: Etidocaine, bupivacaine, and lidocaine seizure thresholds in monkeys, Anesthesiology **42:**471, 1975.
40. Naute, J., et al.: Anesthetic induction with alfentanil: a new short-acting narcotic analgesic, Anesth. Analg. **61:**267, 1982.
41. Ordivay, C.G.: Air embolus via CVP catheter without positive pressure: presentation of a case and review, Ann. Surg. **179:**479, 1974.
42. Pearce, A.C., and Jones, R.M.: Smoking and anesthesia: preoperative abstinence and perioperative morbidity, Anesthesiology **61:**576, 1984.
43. Sauderi, P.E., McLeskey, C.H., and Comer, P.B.: Emergency percutaneous transtracheal ventilation during anesthesia using readily available equipment, Anesth. Analg. **61:**867, 1982.
44. Silverman, W.A., and Sinclair, J.C.: Temperature regulation in the newborn, N. Engl. J. Med. **274:**92, 1966.
45. Sinclair, J.C.: Heat production and thermoregulation in small infants, Pediatr. Clin. North Am. **17:**1:147, 1970.
46. Stanley, T.H., and Webster, C.R.: Anesthetic requirements and cardiovascular effects of fentanyl-oxygen and fentanyl-diazepam-oxygen anesthesia in man, Anesth. Analg. **57:**411, 1978.
47. Taitelman, U., Reece, E.A., and Bessman, A.N.: Insulin in the management of the diabetic surgical patient: continuous intravenous infusion versus subcutaneous administration, JAMA **237:**658, 1977.
48. Tapia, H.R., et al.: Causes of death after renal transplantation, Arch. Intern. Med. **131:**204, 1973.
49. Tarhan, S., et al.: Risk of anesthesia and surgery in patients with chronic bronchitis and chronic obstructive pulmonary disease, Surgery **74:**720, 1973.
50. Trunkey, D.D.: Resuscitation of the trauma victim, Surg. Profiles, Feb. 1982.
51. Warner, M.A., Tinker, J.H., and Divertie, M.B.: Preoperative cessation of smoking and pulmonary complications in pulmonary dysfunction, Anesthesiology **59:**A60, 1983.

11

Frank G. Zavisca and Charles W. Lloyd

Pharmacokinetics and Drug Metabolism

Clinical pharmacology involves the study of structure-activity relationships of drugs, their mechanism of action, clinical uses, adverse actions, and when the use of a given drug may be contraindicated. *Pharmacokinetics* is the study of changing drug and metabolite concentrations in various body fluids (often plasma) and tissues over time. The major areas of interest are absorption, distribution, metabolism, and elimination (ADME) of drugs. *Pharmacodynamics* is the study of the mechanism of drug action and the relationship between drug concentration and effect. Ideally, a constant therapeutic drug level is desirable but seldom possible. However, pharmacokinetic data can aid in predicting peak and trough concentrations of a drug, thus helping to avoid toxic or subtherapeutic drug levels. An understanding of clinical pharmacokinetics and pharmacodynamics will enable the surgeon to better evaluate information on drug action, to foster a skeptical attitude toward claims about drugs, and to optimize therapy.

Historically, the development of surgery is intimately involved with that of pharmacology. Although the discovery of anesthisia was of fundamental importance in this development, the introduction of antibiotics and many other drugs, blood transfusion therapy, and new medical devices, has played a crucial role in making modern surgery possible. Today, complex surgery on very ill patients is commonplace. The cliche "he's too sick to operate on" has become "he's too sick not to operate on." The modern surgeon, in addition to having technical expertise, must possess a working knowledge of the basics of pharmacology and understand the principles underlying drug action. Only in this way will the surgeon be able to effectively communicate with colleagues in other medical disciplines and coordinate the expertise of anesthesiologists, internists, other medical specialists, and other members of the health care team to provide the optimum care for patients.

PRINCIPLES OF DRUG ADMINISTRATION

Pharmacokinetics describes, quantitatively, what the investigator thinks will happen to a drug in the body and thus is a guide to therapy. It uses a model* that is a simplified description (often mathematic or graphic or both) of what might happen to a drug in the body; the model is constructed and based on previous experimental observations and refined as necessary after further observations. If agreement between the model and observation is satisfactory, the model may be used to predict optimum drug dosage under a variety of conditions. The model highlights the four major processes of drug disposition (ADME) and allows for a better understanding of how each process can affect drug action.

The chemical and mathematical procedures used to describe what happens to a drug are often complex. In this discussion, with the use of several simple models, attention will be focused on the basic principles used to describe the time-course of drug concentration in the body. This material will then be used to describe how variations in the condition of the patient can alter these parameters. Knowledge of these factors may then be used to optimize therapy.

Time-Course of Drug Effects

One-Compartment Model

The simplest model of the time-course of drug concentration is the one-compartment open model (Fig. 11-1, *A*). This model[7,9,15] assumes that an intravenous bolus of drug results in complete, instantaneous mixing and uniform distribution. Vd is the apparent volume of distribution (see later discussion). The rate of change of drug concentration is proportional to the concentration of drug at a given time; i.e., a constant *proportion* of drug is eliminated irreversibly per unit time (Fig. 11-1, *A*). This type of elimination is known as first order, and Fig. 11-1, *B* illustrates the

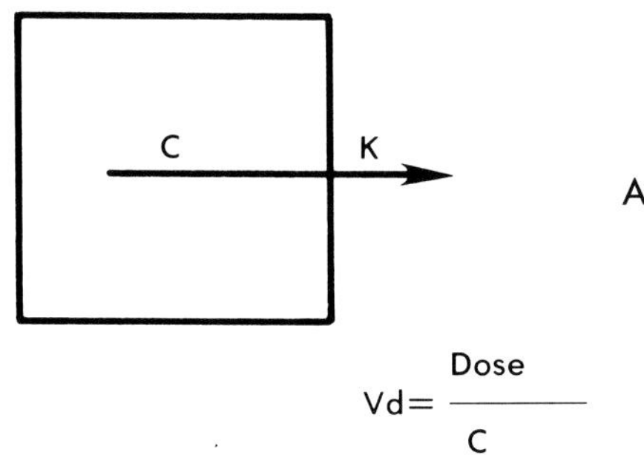

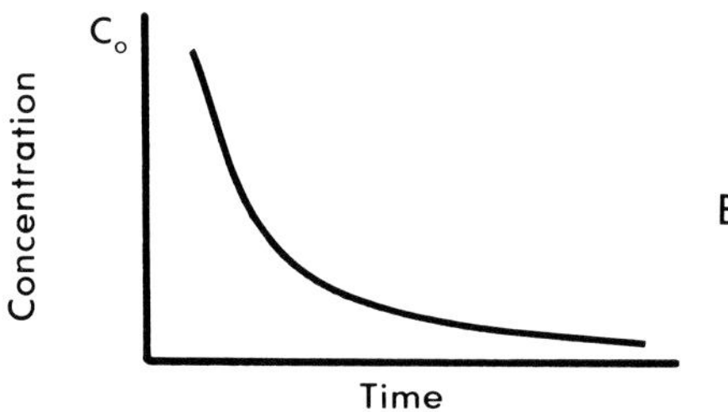

Fig. 11-1 Model and linear plot of a one-compartment open model. *C*, Concentration of drug at any given time; *Co*, concentration of drug at time zero; *k*, first order elimination rate constant; *Vd*, volume of distribution; *dose*, amount of drug given. (See text for discussion.)

*References 2,6,7,9,10, and 15.

concentration-time relationship for this model. This relationship can be expressed by the equation:

$$\Delta c/\Delta f = -kc$$

where c is the concentration of drug at a given time; k is the first-order elimination rate constant; t refers to time; and $\Delta c/\Delta f$ is the rate of change in concentration of drug over a given time (i.e., dc is the delta or change in concentration and dt is the delta time over which the change takes place.)

This equation illustrates that a constant proportion (rather than a constant amount) of drug is eliminated per unit time (i.e., 50% of the drug is eliminated per hour if the half-time for elimination is 1 hour). Elimination is proportional to concentration. Mathematically, this equation describes an exponential line. Thus this equation can be converted logarithmically into a form that describes a straight line (Fig. 11-2) as shown by the expression:

$$\log Ct = \log Co - \frac{k \times t}{2.303}$$

where Ct is the concentration at time t after starting at time zero; Co is the concentration at time zero; 2.303 is the constant required for conversion to common logarithms; and k is the first-order elimination rate constant.

This second equation allows the exponential relationship (see Fig. 11-1, *B*) to be expressed as a straight line (see Fig. 11-2) with log *C* plotted against time. The y-intercept is Co and represents the concentration immediately after the completion of the intravenous bolus, assuming instantaneous, complete mixing. The slope of the line is given by k/2.303 and is constant over time. This negative slope represents the rate of drug elimination. The actual amount eliminated per unit time would depend on the initial Co. A larger dose would produce an elimination curve that has the same slope but would be graphically above and parallel to curve *B*. Thus a constant *proportion* of drug is eliminated per unit time, regardless of the initial Co.

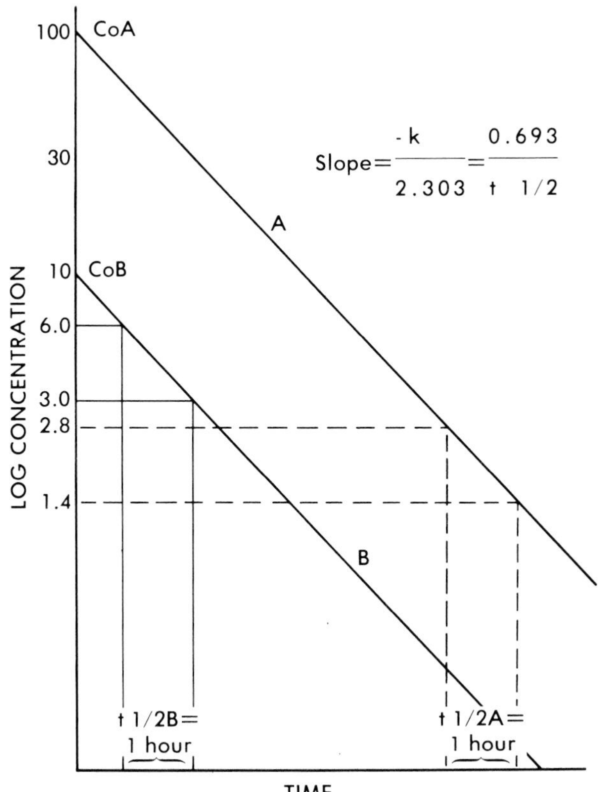

Fig. 11-2 Semilogarithmic drug concentration graph for one-compartment open model. For different initial concentrations, the same terminal half-life can be determined because a constant proportion of drug is eliminated per unit time. (See text for discussion.)

Elimination Rate Constant—Additivity of First-Order Processes. The overall measured elimination rate constant (k) may represent a number of first-order processes (k_1, k_2, k_3) occurring simultaneously. The effect of multiple first-order processes acting concurrently on the same quantity of drug can be represented by the algebraic sum of their individual rate constants. Thus one measured k may represent the sum of renal excretion and hepatic metabolism, both occurring by first-order processes, and this k gives a reasonably accurate pharmacokinetic parameter with which to work.

Volume of Distribution. The true physiologic volume of distribution (Vd) is defined as the sum of the concentration of free drug times the volume associated with it plus the concentration of drug bound to the various proteins and tissues times each of those volumes (see Fig. 11-1, *A*). A more commonly used volume of distribution, known as the extrapolated volume of distribution (Vd Ext), is determined by the equation:

$$\text{Vd Ext} = \frac{\text{Dose}}{\text{Cpo}}$$

where Dose is the amount of drug given; and Co is the initial peak concentration after intravenous bolus infusion. This relationship between volume, amount, and concentration is useful in the clinical setting when Vd is known for a particular drug. By rearranging the equation, the concentration or dose can be predicted as follows:

$$\text{Cpo} = \text{Dose/Vd}$$
$$\text{Dose} = \text{Cpo} \times \text{Vd}$$

The degree to which a drug is bound to tissue or plasma protein helps determine the Vd. A drug that is strongly bound would have a very large Vd, whereas one poorly bound to tissue or plasma proteins does not. Thus a drug such as digoxin, which is strongly bound to tissues, has a Vd that even exceeds the actual total body weight; because of this binding, the drug is stored or pooled in the peripheral compartments, and its elimination is prolonged. On the other hand, a poorly bound drug such as gentamicin or tobramycin would have a Vd approximating only total body water and a corresponding rapid elimination. A drug strongly bound only to plasma proteins (i.e., warfarin) would have a Vd of 10 to 15 L, greater than the plasma volume but less than that of digitalis.

Concept of Half-Life. Half-life is the time in which 50% of the remaining drug is eliminated. For example, once the first 50% of the drug is eliminated, then 50% of the remaining 50% (i.e., 25% of the original amount) is eliminated during the second half, and so on for subsequent

Table 11-1 **RELATIONSHIP OF HALF-LIVES TO AMOUNT OF DRUG ELIMINATED BY A FIRST-ORDER REACTION**

Number of Half-Lives	Fraction Remaining (%)	Fraction Lost (%)
0	100.0	0.0
1	50.0	50.0
2	25.0	75.0
3	12.5	87.5
4	6.2	93.8
5	3.1	96.9
6	1.6	98.4

half-lives. The half-life of a first-order process may be approximated by selecting any concentration on a semilogarithmic plot of drug elimination (see Fig. 11-2) and then determining the time interval required to reach one-half that value. The half-life can also be calculated from the equation:

$$t\ ½ = 0.693/k$$

where k is the first-order elimination rate constant; and 0.693 is the natural logarithm of 2. The relationship of t ½ to the percentage of drug elimination is illustrated in Table 11-1. Approximately six half-lives are required to eliminate 98% of a drug. When instituting drug therapy it should be noted that if a loading dose is not given, approximately six half-lives will be needed to achieve a maximum concentration or steady state.

NONLINEAR KINETICS. For drugs like ethyl alcohol, aspirin, phenytoin, and phenylbutazone, elimination from the plasma is not a first-order process; rather, a constant amount, not a constant proportion, of remaining drug is eliminated per unit time. This process, called zero-order or Michaelis-Menten Kinetics, usually occurs when the major mechanism of drug elimination becomes saturated with drug (i.e., alcohol saturates the liver enzyme alcohol dehydrogenase, and only about 10 ml/hr is metabolized, regardless of the concentration in the blood) and elimination proceeds at its maximum possible rate. In such cases, a true half-life for these drugs cannot be determined because the velocity of the elimination changes over time, until maximum velocity (Vmax) is achieved.[2,9,15]

Two-Compartment Model

The two-compartment model (Fig. 11-3) more accurately describes the disposition of many drugs and also illustrates principles that may be applied to more complex models. Again, an intravenous bolus with complete, instantaneous mixing is assumed. Absorption from oral or other routes would require addition of another compartment, but the same basic principles apply. After rapid infusion, the drug is first distributed from a central (V_1) to a peripheral (V_2) compartment (k_{12}) and back again (k_{21}) by first-order processes. The drug is also assumed to be eliminated (k_3) by another first-order process, only by way of the central compartment.

Plasma concentrations may be representative of drugs in the central compartment. The highest concentration of drug (Cpo) occurs at time zero and is determined by the

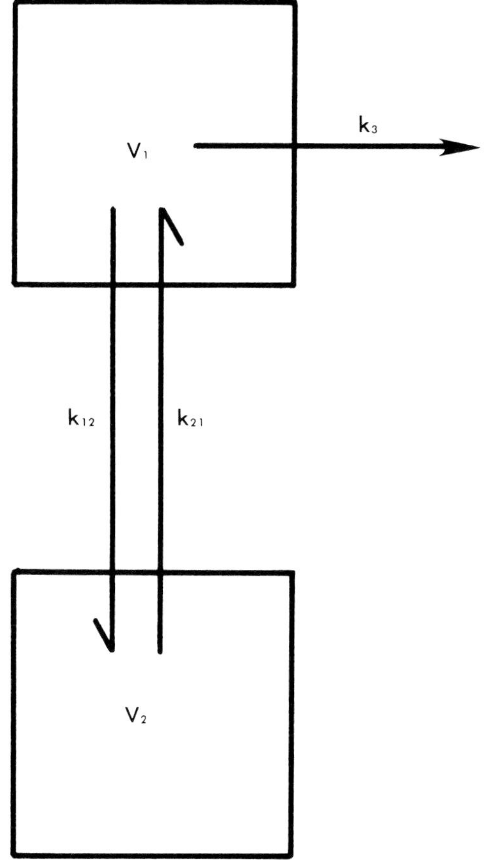

Fig. 11-3 Two-compartment open model of drug distribution and elimination. (See text for discussion.)

dose and the volume of distribution of the central compartment (V_1) in which it is diluted. This may be represented by:

$$Cpo = \frac{Dose}{V_1}$$

where Cpo is the concentration of drug after mixing; dose is the dose of drug administered intravenously; and V_1 is the volume of distribution of the central compartment. The central compartment is defined in terms of an *apparent* volume (V_1) and consists of plasma and those tissues in rapid equilibrium with plasma (such as brain, heart, lung, liver, and kidneys). V_1 differs for each drug and depends largely on physicochemical factors.

The plasma concentration of a drug is affected by its rate of entry into the peripheral compartment (redistribution) and its rate of elimination from the body. Both processes begin immediately as a drug enters the circulation, but the elimination process plays the more significant role in the later decline of the plasma concentration. For most drugs the contribution of redistribution to declining plasma levels is short-lived because of the exchange of drugs between central and peripheral compartments. Initially, the concentration gradient is from the central to the peripheral compartment at the maximum possible rate (k_{12}), as determined by the drug's tissue-blood permeability coefficient (i.e., the ratio of solubility in tissues to that in blood), and blood flow to the tissues. After a period of time, equilibrium is approached and the concentrations of the central and peripheral compartments are nearly equal. Eventually, elimination of the drug from the central compartment (k_3) causes a shift in the concentration gradient between the central and peripheral compartments; the shift favors transfer toward the central compartment.

The practical significance of the peripheral compartment can be illustrated for the ultra-short–acting barbiturate, sodium thiopental.[12] Even though redistribution is short-lived, it may exert a major influence on drug levels. The peripheral component is defined only in terms of its apparent volume of distribution (V_2), which is very large for thiopental. Because of its lipid solubility, it is taken up rapidly (large k_{12}) into muscle, fat, and other tissues, where it is temporarily stored. Thus, after an intravenous bolus, thiopental is immediately redistributed to other tissues (large k_{12} and large V_2), rapidly reducing the plasma concentration and thereby accounting for its ultra-short action. However, after repeated or continuous thiopental administration, the equilibrium point may be reached, where enough drug is "stored" so that re-entry of the drug into the central compartment can actually maintain plasma concentrations. The residual drug present in the peripheral compartment will inhibit the distributive process and lead to more intense and prolonged effects after multiple doses and possibly even produce a "hangover."

Drug disposition in a two-compartment model can be represented graphically by plotting the log concentration vs. time (Fig. 11-4). This produces a biexponential curve representing the two distinct phases of redistribution and elimination. The terminal elimination portion of the curve is linear and can be described by a beta (β) line and its intercept B when the curve is extrapolated back to the Y-axis. Since elimination begins immediately, it is justifiable to extrapolate the line back to zero time. The slope of the β line allows calculation of the terminal elimination half-life and the y-intercept B, which represents the concentraion of drug that would be present in the first phase of elimination, allowing calculation of the apparent volume of distribution of the elimination phase. The initial (redistribution) portion of the curve represents the combined effects of distribution and elimination. To determine the slope of this part of the curve, the contribution of the elimination phase must be subtracted by the back-projection technique; this yields another straight line characterized by an alpha (α) line and its y-intercept A, at time zero. This extrapolated line represents the first-order kinetics of redistribution. The y-intercept A represents the concentration of drug that would be present in the first phase of redistribution.

Analysis of this biexponential curve allows determination of factors important for optimization of therapy.[4,5] These include: (1) volume of distribution for the distribution phase, Vdα; (2) volume of distribution for the elimination phase, Vdβ; (3) half-life for distribution, t ½α; and (4) half-life for elimination, t ½β. These four parameters can then be used to calculate clearance (CLT), defined as the volume of blood that is completely filtered out of the drug per unit time, as shown below:

$$\text{CLT} = \frac{\text{Vd}\beta}{1.44 \times \text{t } 1/2} = \frac{\text{Vd}\beta(0.693)}{\text{t } 1/2} = k_3 \times \text{Vd}$$

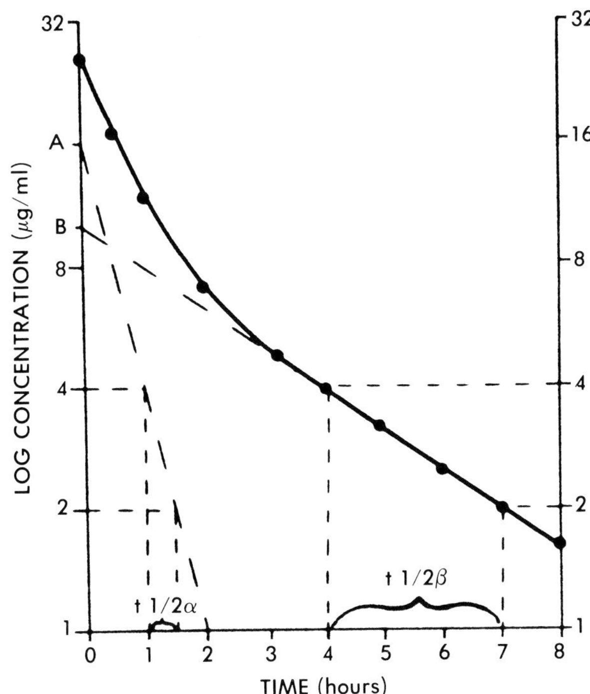

Fig. 11-4 Semilogarithmic drug concentration–elimination graph for two-compartment open model. At time zero a drug is administered intravenously. The dots represent the experimentally measured concentrations, and the curvilinear solid line connecting them can be described as the sum of two straight lines. Note that the terminal portion of the curve is linear and can be described by its slope (β) and its intercept *(B)* when the line is extrapolated back to the ordinate. The t 1/2 β is 3 hours and represents the half-time of drug elimination. If the values represented by the extrapolated portion of the line are subtracted from the actual measured values on the initial curved portion of the solid line, another straight line can be plotted with a slope (α) and an ordinal intercept *(A)*. The t 1/2 α is 0.5 hours and represents the half-time of distribution. (See text for further discussion.) (Reprinted with permission from the International Anesthesia and Research Society from Hug, C.C.: Pharmacokinetics of drugs administered intravenously, Anesth. Analg. **57**:715, 1978.)

where k_3 is the elimination rate constant; and 1.44 refers to a constant equal to 1 divided by 0.693.

The clinical significance of this analysis depends on the assumption that plasma levels are related to drug concentrations at the site of drug action.[2,6,15] This relationship may be modified by several factors, including: (1) an active metabolite, having different kinetics than the parent drug, may be formed; (2) the drug may reach the site of action slowly because of limited transport across membranes or low blood flow to the site; (3) after large doses of the drug, maximum effects may occur; (4) alterations in protein binding may alter the amount of active drug, whereas chemical assays may measure total amounts of the drug.

Relationships For Variations in Dosage

Single Doses

Effects of a single dose of drug[2] may be characterized by latency, time to peak effect, magnitude of peak effect, and duration (Fig. 11-5). Latency is defined as the time

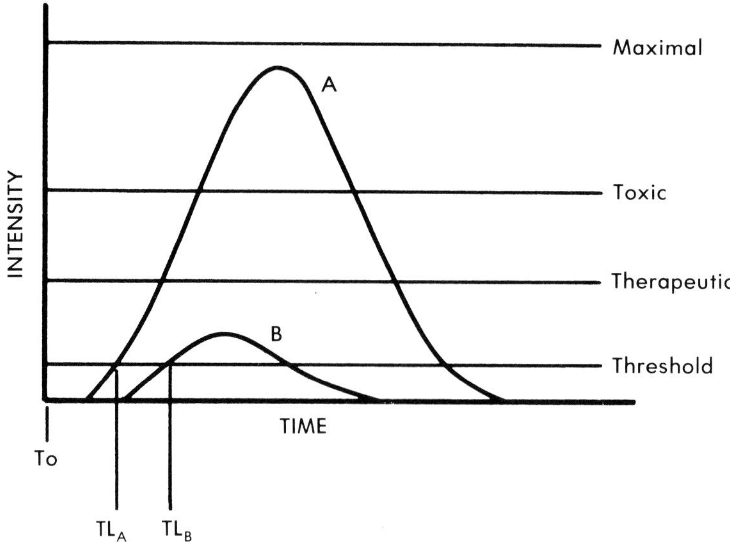

Fig. 11-5 Time relationships of intensity of drug effect after different doses. TL_A and TL_B are latencies for larger *(A)* and *(B)* doses of a drug. (See text for discussion.) (From DiPalma, J.R., editor: Drill's pharmacology in medicine, ed. 4, New York, 1971, McGraw-Hill Book Co.)

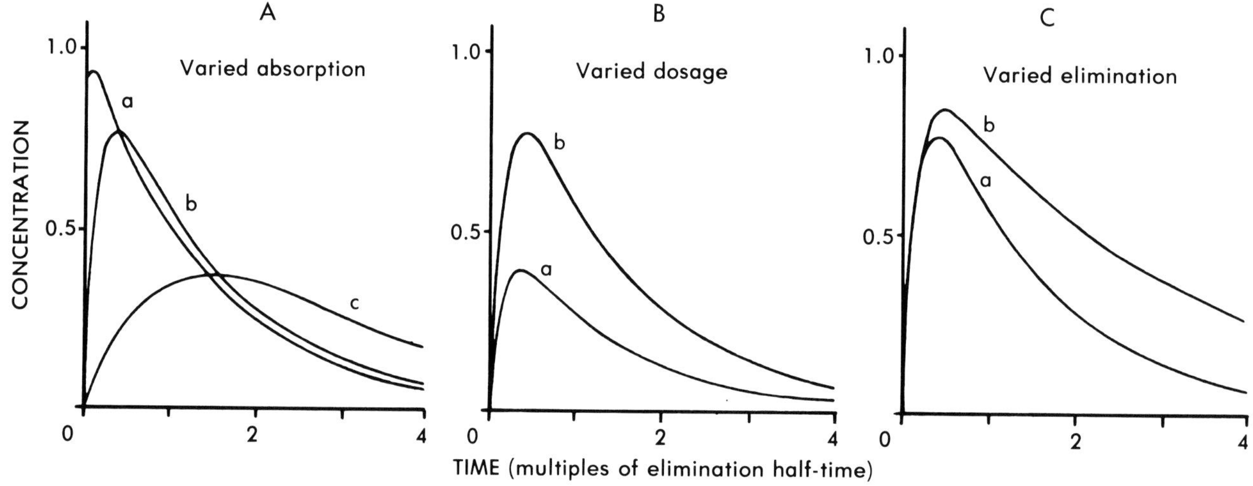

Fig. 11-6 Influence of absorption, dosage, and rate of elimination of drug levels. **A,** Influence of absorption—*a,* 100 times as rapid; *b,* 10 times as rapid; *c,* equal to elimination. **B,** Influence of dosage—*a,* basal dose; *b,* twice basal dose. **C,** Influence of rate of elimination—*a,* basal rate; *b,* twice basal rate. (From Gilman, A.G., Goodman, L.S., and Gilman, A., editors: The pharmacological basis of therapeutics, ed. 6, New York, Copyright © by 1980 Macmillan Publishing Co.)

from administration to a demonstrable threshold therapeutic effect. For a larger dose (see Fig. 11-5), the latency and time to peak effect are shorter, the duration of all effects is larger, and the chances for toxicity are greater.

Differences in absorption (Fig. 11-6, *A*) may result from different routes of administration or different dosage forms.[9] When absorption is rapid relative to elimination, differences in rate of absorption are of less consequence; the peak effects approach that achieved after intravenous administration, and latency and time of peak effect are determined primarily by the rate of absorption. With increased dosage (Fig. 11-6, *B*), latency decreases, and the peak effect increases without changing the time of peak effect. Duration of effect is increased proportionally less than the peak effect. Reduced elimination results in the expected prolongation of drug effect (Fig. 11-6, *C*). If the drug is rapidly absorbed, differences in rate of elimination have a relatively minor influence on the peak effect.

Repeated Doses

During repeated administration of a drug, its concentration is characterized by the time course of accumulation, the maximum amount of accumulation, fluctuations resulting from the dosage interval, and the elimination of half-life (Fig. 11-7). Because five or six half-lives are required for nearly complete elimination of a drug (see Table 11-1), any shorter interval leads to accumulation.[9] During repeat administration, drug accumulation continues until the rate of elimination and administration are equal. This follows from the principle that, in first-order elimination, the

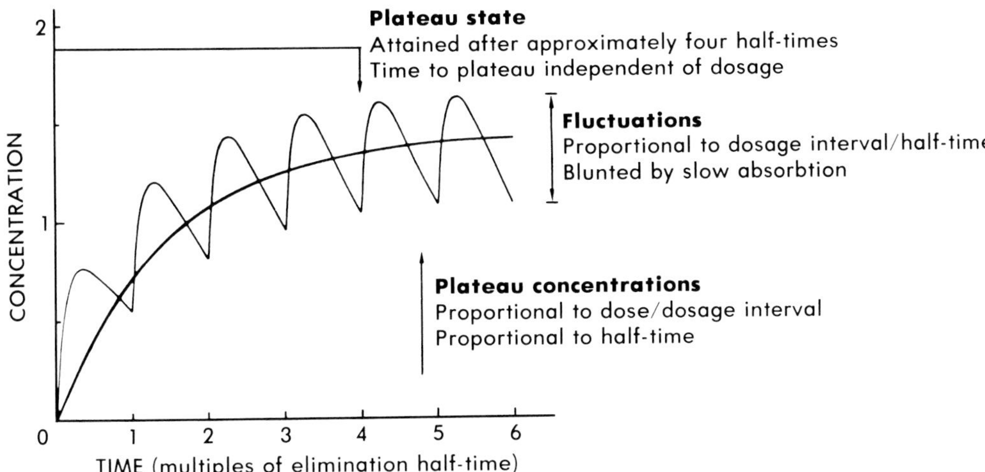

Fig. 11-7 Fundamental pharmacokinetic relationships for repeated administration of drugs. The light line is the pattern of drug accumulation during repeated administration of a drug at intervals equal to its elimination half-time, when drug absorption is 10 times as rapid as elimination. As the relative rate of absorption increases, the concentration maxima approach *2*, and the concentration minima approach *1* during the plateau state. The heavy line depicts the pattern during administration of equivalent dosage by continuous intravenous infusion. Curves are based on a one-compartment model. (See text for discussion.) (From Gilman, A.G., Goodman, L.S., and Gilman, A., editors: The pharmacological basis of therapeutics, ed. 6, New York, Copyright © by 1980 Macmillan Publishing Co.)

rate of elimination is proportional to the dose. Thus, after repeated or continuous administration, the total body stores increase exponentially to a plateau, with a half-life of increase equal to the elimination of half-life. Accordingly, maximum accumulation occurs after five or six half-lives, when elimination equals administration.

The total body store of drug at equilibrium (plateau phase) is a function of the maintenance dose and the elimination half-life and is about 1.5 times the amount administered per elimination half-life. During the plateau phase, fluctuations in levels are proportional to the ratio of dosage interval and the elimination half-life (Fig. 11-7). Less fluctuation in drug concentration would occur by slow absorption or redistribution from body stores or both. When a rapidly absorbed drug is administered at intervals equal to its elimination half-time, the ratio of peak to minimal concentration between doses is nearly twice as great. Half-doses at half-intervals will maintain the same average concentration with smaller fluctuations, which becomes more important if the margin of safety is small. The margin of safety is the ratio of unacceptably toxic levels to therapeutic levels.

Choice of Dosage Interval. The dosage interval should be selected with the intent of avoiding fluctuations in drug levels leading to toxicity or loss of efficacy.[4,5,9] Thus an interval less than the elimination half-life is usually recommended. However, larger intervals are acceptable if larger fluctuations are tolerable or if absorption is slow. Also, dosage interval may be chosen for convenience or to ensure patient compliance. For example, penicillin, with a safety-toxicity ratio of 100:1, may be given at intervals much greater than its half-life (t ½ = 1 hr), whereas digoxin has a ratio of approximately 2:1, so dosage is more critical. Gentamicin has a half-life of t ½ = 2 hours and is given every 8 hours to ensure sufficient time for excretion of the accumulated drug.

Loading Dose. Therapeutic doses may be given initially if a delay in effect of four to six half-lives is tolerable. With a larger loading dose, a more rapid effect occurs, but caution must be exercised so this larger dose is not continued. After the first four to six half-lives, the plateau concentration becomes independent of the loading dose.

ABSORPTION, DISTRIBUTION AND ELIMINATION OF DRUGS: ROLE OF CELL MEMBRANES

Absorption, distribution, and elimination of drugs and their metabolites occur across cell membranes,[9] which include: (1) a lipoid barrier structure, more permeable to lipid soluble, unionized molecules than to other substances; (2) pores of varying sizes, permitting passage of small water-soluble molecules; and (3) channels, formed by proteins permeating the lipoid structure, where molecules are transported (actively or passively) by specific carriers (Fig. 11-8). Drugs are usually metabolized to a less lipid-soluble form, which then is less readily reabsorbed across renal tubular membranes and is therefore excreted.

Drugs and other molecules are transported across membranes throughout the body by both passive and active mechanisms. Passive transport can include filtration, passive diffusion, or carrier-facilitated transport. In *filtration* a drug crosses a cell membrane by way of bulk flow of water through aqueous pores, driven by hydrostatic and osmotic gradients (e.g., across capillary walls). With *passive diffusion* a drug moves across a membrane by driving forces of concentration and charge gradients. This can occur through aqueous pores (small, water-soluble molecules such as alcohol) or through the lipoid interior (lipid-soluble

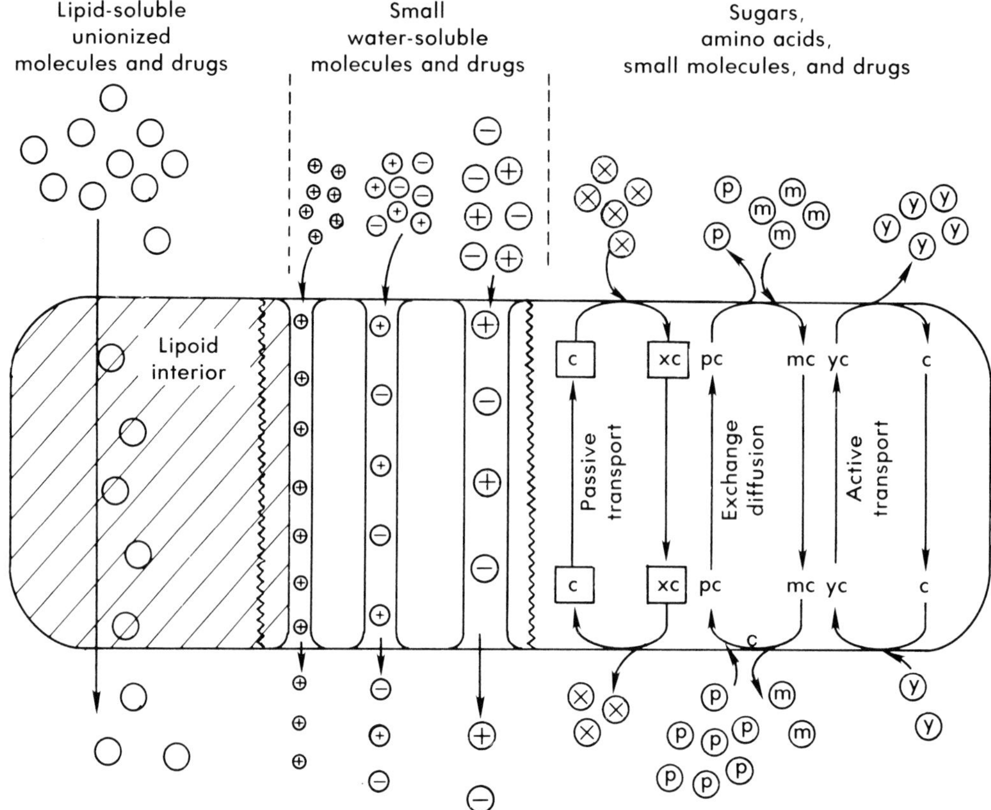

Fig. 11-8 Role of cell membranes in drug transport. (See text for discussion.)

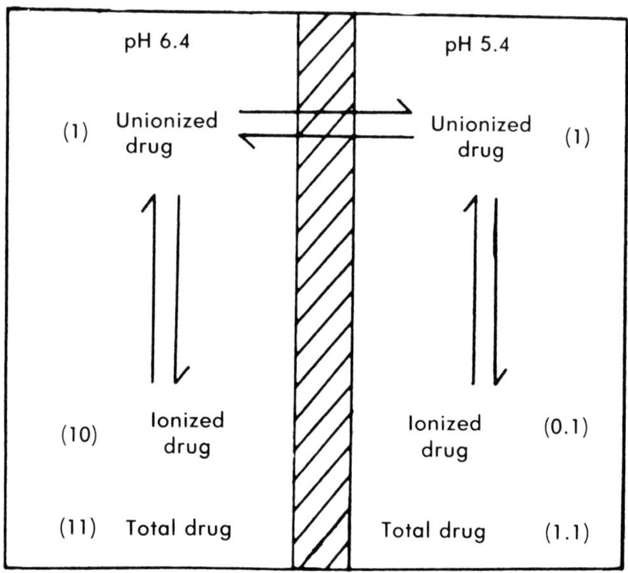

Fig. 11-9 Drug transport of pH-induced changes in concentration of ionized forms. A drug with a pKa of 6.4 is partially ionized as a weak acid ($RH \longleftrightarrow R^- + H^+$). The membrane is permeable only to the unionized drug. Therefore at steady state the amount of ionized drug in the compartment with the higher pH is 10 times higher than in the other compartment, whereas the concentration of unionized drug is equal in both compartments. (Reprinted with permission from the International Anesthesia and Research Society from Hug, C.C.: Pharmacokinetics of drugs administered intravenously, Anesth. Analg. **57:**706, 1978.)

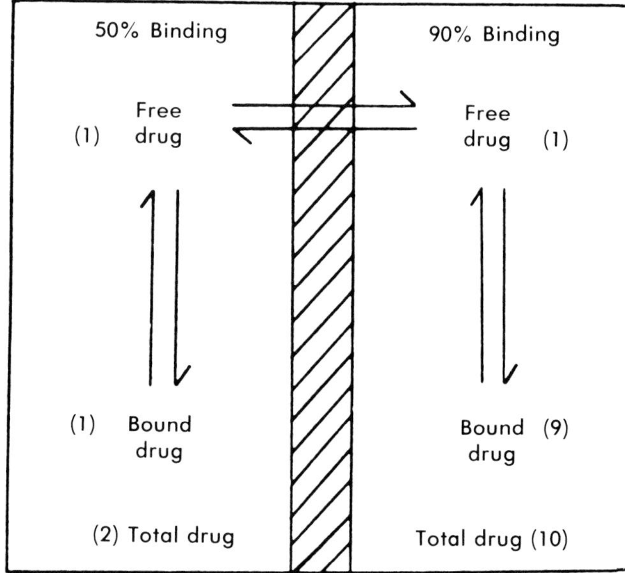

Fig. 11-10 Effect of protein binding on drug transport. A membrane permeable only to free drugs separates the compartments. The degree of binding of the drug to macromolecules differs in the two compartments. Therefore at steady state the total amount of drug in one compartment is five times greater than in the other, whereas the concentration of free drug is equal in both compartments. (Reprinted with permission from the International Anesthesia and Research Society from Hug, C.C.: Pharmacokinetics of drugs administered intravenously, Anesth. Analg. **57:**707, 1978.)

molecules such as halothane and digoxin). For weak acids and bases, the unionized form is transported across a cell membrane because the concentration of this form may differ on each side of the membrane. Similarly, some drugs may be transported by this mechanism (Fig. 11-9).[7] Because cell membranes are impermeable to proteins, the amount of drug bound to proteins differs on both sides in the steady state. In similar fashion, drug binding may affect the *rate* of equilibrium of the unbound form (Fig. 11-10)[7] and thereby affect drug concentration. Thus transport by diffusion may be affected by ionization because of pH gradients, protein binding, lipid-water partition, and concentration gradients.

Carrier-facilitated transport may be either passive or active. *Passive* carrier–facilitated diffusion occurs by way of a specific carrier but only along a concentration gradient. It is specific, saturated at high concentrations of a drug, and may be reversibly inhibited by a similar compound. Exchange diffusion occurs when the same carrier picks up a second, similar molecule after release of the first one and transports it back to the original side of the cell membrane. This type of transport always occurs down concentration gradients. *Active* carrier–facilitated transport also is mediated by specific carriers and occurs by mechanisms similar to carrier-mediated passive transport, but it can also occur against a concentration gradient and therefore requires energy.

ROUTE OF DRUG ADMINISTRATION

Following administration, the uptake of a drug in a given tissue is affected by its molecular size, shape, and charge, its solubility in lipids or aqueous solutions, the degree to which it ionizes, the surface area available for its absorption, the adequacy of the circulation to the absorption site, and various local conditions including its concentration in the perfusing vessels with respect to its target tissue.[9] *Bioavailability* (or physiologic availability) is defined as a measure of the extent of absorption and the rate at which the drug reaches the general circulation. Bioavailability has become a critical term since the 1960s when there was a trend toward writing prescriptions generically, changes in government policy on purchasing drugs based on price, and the repeal of antisubstitution laws. All generic drugs are not equal. Thus the clinician must use his or her own judgment regarding which preparation is best for the patient, based on a knowledge of basic pharmacokinetic principles and the available information on the preparation in question.

Equally important as these considerations is the route chosen to administer a drug because this will influence the efficiency of drug uptake. No one route is perfect or ideal for all situations. Consequently, a knowledge of the advantages and disadvantages of the various routes employed is mandatory if a drug is to provide optimum effects in a given clinical situation.

Oral Route

The overwhelming advantages of this route are convenience, economy, the absence of pain, and the lack of a need for special equipment. Because absorption is slow, toxicity occurs slowly, allowing time for therapy; residual drug can often be inactivated or removed by inducing vomiting. On the other hand, variations in gastrointestinal (GI) motility, complicated by food, insolubility at acid pH, and degradation, may lead to erratic absorption of a drug when this route is employed. In addition, some drugs have an unacceptable taste, and may cause nausea and vomiting resulting from gastric irritation. After oral administration, absorption may be too slow for use in emergency situations, and this route generally cannot be used in unconscious patients. In the perioperative period, GI function is often disturbed, also making absorption unpredictable. In patients with liver disease, the amount of blood flow from the GI tract that bypasses the liver may increase, decreasing hepatic metabolism and thus increasing bioavailability.

For drugs absorbed in the stomach, absorption occurs mainly by simple diffusion. The stomach has tight intercellular junctions and small membrane pores. Thus small neutral water-soluble molecules (such as alcohol) are rapidly absorbed and limited only by gastric emptying. The absorption of weak acids depends on the pH gradient between gastric juice and plasma (see Fig. 11-9). Weak acids and neutral molecules, unionized at usual gastric pH levels ($pH<4$), are well absorbed. For example, aspirin, a weak acid, is well absorbed from the stomach when the intragastric pH is 3 or less, but with buffering it becomes more ionized and hence poorly absorbed. In contrast, weak bases, such as some narcotics, may actually be excreted into the stomach because of the pH gradient between gastric juice and plasma, with the gastric lumen acting as a reservoir for such drugs. The narcotic may then be later reabsorbed into the plasma in the postoperative period, leading to potentially untoward complications. Further, the alkaline pH of the small intestine may also favor absorption of weak bases.

Other External Routes

Sublingual-Buccal. This route is convenient for potent, nonionic, lipid-soluble drugs such as nitroglycerine, even though absorption may be irregular. Because nitroglycerine is metabolized in the liver after absorption into the portal circulation, it is ineffective when administered orally. However, because veins from the oral cavity drain directly into the superior vena cava, the liver is bypassed.

Rectal. This route is convenient in the unconscious patient when nausea and vomiting prevent oral administration and in the uncooperative child. However, rectal absorption may be irregular, and local irritation may precipitate expulsion of the drug.

Nasal. This route is convenient for certain types of drugs because of the large vascular surface area in the nose and the fact that venous drainage bypasses the liver. Thus antidiuretic hormone, pitocin, codeine, and snuff may be given nasally. As with the sublingual-buccal and rectal routes, however, absorption may be irregular and irritation is frequent.

Lungs. The alveoli provide such a large absorptive surface that even some ionized compounds such as sympathomimetics may be absorbed by this route. Nicotine, other products of tobacco smoke, and many environmental toxins can be absorbed from the lungs. However, the frequent, intense reaction to local irritation prevents the lungs from being a useful route for systemic drug administration.

OTHER SURFACES. Drug absorption occurs from other membranes including the skin, eyes, placenta, vagina, urethra, bladder, and colon. Absorption by these routes is important since drug toxicity may result from systemic absorption of drugs administered to these surfaces to treat local conditions.

Parenteral Routes

INTRAVENOUS. The intravenous (IV) route allows quick, accurate administration of a drug, and with the more rapidly acting agents (such as IV anesthetics and some vasodilators), moment-to-moment control of the individual patient's response is possible. Some drugs too irritating to administer by other routes may be given intravenously. Further, the IV route may be used in patients with nausea and vomiting, in patients during the postoperative period when GI function is disturbed, and in the unconscious or uncooperative patient. However, IV administration may rapidly lead to toxicity, and obviously the drug cannot be withdrawn after being given by this route. Most oil-based drugs and those that cause hemolysis cannot be given intravenously. Also, after rapid IV administration, allergic reactions to drugs may be severe. Finally, IV drug administration may be painful, expensive, inconvenient, require special equipment and sterility, and may be technically complex. These considerations also apply, in part, to other parenteral routes.

INTRAMUSCULAR AND SUBCUTANEOUS. Absorption from intramuscular (IM) and subcutaneous (Subcu) injections occurs by diffusion of the drug across the interstitial fluid (ISF) to the microcirculation and is limited by its solubility in the interstitial fluid and local blood flow. Large aqueous channels in the endothelial membrane account for rapid diffusion of molecules, despite low lipid solubility. Oily suspensions and pellets (designed to produce slow absorption) can be given by these routes. Absorption may be increased by local massage, heat, and hyaluronidase and decreased by local cooling or vasoconstriction. Thus absorption is often irregular.

INTRAPERITONEAL. Intraperitoneal (IP) administration may be used when a large absorptive surface is needed or when a large volume of fluid is given (as for peritoneal dialysis). However, drugs administered in this fashion enter the portal circulation and thus are metabolized by the liver. Technical problems such as adhesions and infection are common after peritoneal dialysis.

INTRATHECAL. Antibiotics, antitumor agents, and other drugs can be given intrathecally to treat local diseases. Because ionized compounds do not readily cross the blood-brain barrier, very little of the administered drug enters the systemic circulation.

OTHER. Drugs given locally (such as local anesthetics to nerves) can produce toxicity when systemic absorption occurs.

DISTRIBUTION OF DRUGS WITHIN TISSUES

After absorption a drug is simultaneously distributed to its site of action and other sites.[9,15] Initially, distribution is limited primarily by blood flow to tissues. In the surgical patient, many factors (e.g., anesthetics, fluid shifts, endogenous catecholamines, tissue inflammation, sepsis, and coexisting diseases) may affect tissue blood flow and help explain some of the unexpected drug reactions not uncommonly encountered.[1] In addition to tissue blood flow, final distribution of a drug to tissues is determined by the storage capacity for the drug, which represents a composite of its transport across cell membranes, pH gradients, protein binding (Fig. 11-10), and the lipid-water partition.

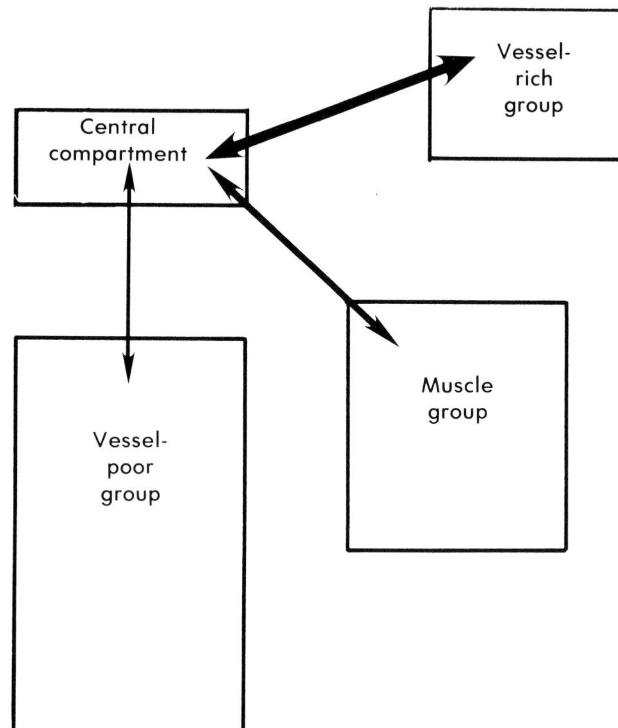

Fig. 11-11 Distribution of drugs. (See text for discussion.)

Distribution of drugs to tissues by way of the central circulation may be divided into several tissue groups, based on blood flow and drug storage capacity (Fig. 11-11). These include a vessel-rich group, a muscle group, and a vessel-poor group. The *vessel-rich group* represents a tissue with high blood flow and low storage capacity. A given drug initially reaches this group of tissues, which includes the heart, lungs, liver, kidney, and brain. After distribution to the vessel-rich group, a drug reaches the *muscle group,* which is characterized by a lower blood flow and large capacity because of great tissue mass. Muscle, skin, and gut comprise this group. Finally, a drug reaches the *vessel-poor group* (bone, cartilage, and fat) after distribution to other tissues. This group is characterized by a very low blood flow and varying storage capacity.

A more detailed description of the distribution of sodium thiopental, an example discussed earlier, may now be formulated.[12] After an IV bolus, the drug rapidly reaches the brain. Simultaneously it reaches other organs in the vessel-rich group, such as the heart, and may produce some myocardial depression. This depression of the heart, as well as the thiopental-induced anesthesia, is short-lived because the concentration gradient favors transfer from the vessel-rich group to the muscle group. This transfer is delayed because the circulation to the muscle group is less dominant initially. Because of the large drug storage capacity of the muscle group, the plasma concentration (and hence, the concentrations of drug in the brain and heart, which are in rapid equilibrium with plasma) decreases rapidly. After multiple doses, thiopental may accumulate also in the vessel-poor group, providing a reservoir, which accounts for the slow-release and "hangover" effect seen after additional doses. Although metabolism and renal excretion are needed to totally eliminate thiopental from the body, these actions occur much more slowly than redistribution, which primarily accounts for the initial effects of the drug. These concepts, although requiring more complex pharmacokinetic models to explain in detail, follow readily as an extension of the one- and two-compartment models discussed earlier. Other lipid-soluble drugs (such as fentanyl) may act in a similar manner.[7]

ELIMINATION OF DRUGS FROM THE BODY

The elimination of a drug from the body is often a complex process. The following discussion, which details those processes that interplay in drug removal, will help the reader understand this complexity.

Biotransformation

Many drugs are lipid-soluble, weak organic acids and bases, readily absorbed by the kidney. After conversion to more polar compounds, they are less well absorbed, and hence more readily excreted. This increased polarity also reduces their volume of distribution, further facilitating excretion.[9] Some metabolites may be pharmacologically active and their elimination kinetics may be different from the parent drugs; this characteristic increases the complexity of interpreting data. Biotransformation occurs largely by microsomal enzymes in the liver and other tissues. Nonsynthetic reactions include *oxidation, reduction,* and *hydrolysis*. Synthetic (also called *conjugation*) reactions involve coupling the drug (or metabolite) with an endogenous substrate, such as a carbohydrate (e.g., glucuronic acid), an amino acid or its derivative, an acetic acid, or an inorganic sulfate. Drugs absorbed from the intestine (e.g., propranolol) may be subject to the *first-pass effect*. This represents the combined action of a gastrointestinal epithelial enzyme or hepatic drug-metabolizing enzyme or both which may prevent the appearance of significant amounts of the drug in the circulation.

Enterohepatic Circulation

After biliary excretion, a lipid-soluble drug may be partially reabsorbed into the gut, as well as back into the renal tubule. This slows the excretion rate from the body. If the drug were polar, renal or fecal excretion or both would occur. After formation of a water-soluble glucuronide in the liver and its subsequent biliary excretion, the glucuronide may be split by glucuronidase in the intestinal lumen. The less polar parent drug then reforms and is readily reabsorbed into the intestine. The drug may then be reconjugated, split, and reabsorbed several more times before final excretion by the kidney.

Renal Excretion

The kidney accounts for most drug excretion, although the lung can excrete some volatile compounds (e.g., paraldehyde, alcohol, anesthetic agents, and industrial solvents). The kidney eliminates drugs by three major mechanisms. The first is *glomerular filtration,* which is affected by the rate of filtration and the degree to which a drug is bound to protein. The second mechanism is *active tubular secretion* (e.g., organic anions and cations), and the third is *passive tubular absorption,* which would occur with unionized, lipid-soluble drugs. This example shows the importance of the kidney: after administration of toxic doses of weak acids (e.g., salicylates and barbiturates), renal excretion may be increased by giving bicarbonate, which makes the urine more alkaline. This alkalinity increases the ionization of the drug, which in turn decreases renal tubular reabsorption.

Other Mechanisms of Terminating Drug Action

Termination of drug action may occur without actual drug metabolism or excretion. A drug may *redistribute* itself if its elimination phase is much slower than the redistribution phase. Examples include norepinephrine and exogenous catecholamines whose action is terminated by reuptake into nerve terminals. Changes induced by a drug may require a *repair process,* which may lag considerably behind the actual elimination of the drug from the body. Thus coumadin's anticoagulant action persists until protein synthesis replaces depleted clotting factors; phenoxybenzamine irreversibly alkylates alpha receptors, and new receptors must be synthesized to restore normal physiology; following chronic beta blockade, receptor supersensitivity persists long after drug elimination. *Pharmacologic antagonism* may obviate the effects of a drug; this occurs when naloxone is used as an antidote for morphine. Finally, *physiologic compensation* may terminate a drug's action. For example, baroreceptor reflexes occur after vasodilator administration, plasma volume may increase after antihypertensive therapy, and chronic narcotic therapy may lead to tolerance. In the latter circumstance, the resulting tachyphylaxis produces physiologic responses that counteract the effects of the narcotic, increasing the complexity of therapy.

BALANCING THERAPEUTIC DRUG EFFECTS AGAINST SIDE EFFECTS

Some drugs having a narrow margin of safety (e.g., cardiac glycosides and aminoglycoside antibiotics) may inadvertently produce toxic effects without eliciting clear-cut clinical signs of impending toxicity. Because many unknown factors may affect serum drug levels (especially in very ill patients), the only reliable way to determine these levels in individual patients is to measure them.[1,4,5,10] Determination of such levels may be of practical use for therapy if guidelines have been established for therapeutic versus toxic levels. By measuring drug levels serially, the desired plasma levels may be maintained in individual patients. Drugs currently monitored clinically include aminoglycoside antibiotics, which are associated with eighth cranial nerve and kidney damage; antiepileptic medications, which produce adverse effects in the liver, kidney, and heart; and digoxin and theophylline, which can elicit potentially lethal cardiac rhythm abnormalities.

For clinical interpretation of drug levels, certain pharmacokinetic information must be considered. This includes: (1) the reliability of the assay measuring the drug; (2) the interindividual variation of therapeutic and toxic serum levels; (3) the interval since last dose (i.e., t ½, clearance ranges, which help determine what plateau levels should be [see Fig. 11-7]); (4) the presence and kinetics of active metabolites; (5) concurrent medications the patient may be receiving; (6) the protein-binding characteristics of the drug; (7) the diseases states affecting pharmacokinetics (e.g., kidney, heart, and liver diseases); and (8) factors modifying the concentration-effect relationship (e.g., tolerance, supersensitivity, physiologic compensation, other drugs). When doses of a given drug are adjusted to give similar serum levels, pharmacologic variation in a population may decrease, suggesting that pharmacokinetic effects may account for much interindividual variation in drug effects.[1,4,5,10]

The practical clinical application of these pharmacokintic principles can best be illustrated by discussing the use of plasma levels in managing patients receiving two common types of drugs, cardiac glycosides and aminoglycoside antibiotics.

Cardiac Glycosides

For digoxin, the elimination half-life, which mainly results from renal excretion, is approximately 1 to 2 days. This prolonged effect occurs since digoxin is extensively bound to body tissues because of its lipid solubility, leading to a volume of distribution much larger than the total body water.[3,4,5] This large volume must be cleared by the kidney, resulting in prolonged excretion. When digoxin is administered by the oral route without a loading dose, approximately 1 week is required to produce a therapeutic effect. Initially, the gradient of drug concentration favors transfer from the central compartment (plasma) into the large peripheral compartment. After the peripheral compartment is partially filled, the plasma levels rise to the therapeutic range. Since digoxin has a narrow margin of safety and may produce serious toxicity, the patient must be observed carefully, and frequent electrocardiograms must be performed to watch for dysrhythmic effects. Even then, impending toxicity may not be evident. Additional information, such as plasma digoxin levels, may be useful to optimize therapy. The maintenance dosage must be equal to the daily loss. After the maintenance dosage has been given a sufficient amount to time (4 to 6 times the half-life), the concentration in plasma and the total body stores will be determined solely by the maintenance dosage; however, this amount varies in individuals given the same amount because of a variety of factors that are difficult to control. Thus measurement of digoxin levels may be useful in the following clinical situations:

- In the presence of cardiac arrhythmias in patients taking digoxin, serum levels greater than 20 mg/ml indicate that digoxin is a likely cause of the observed arrhythmia. This can be a very difficult diagnostic problem because digoxin toxicity can lead to almost every common arrhythmia.
- In patients with renal failure, published formulas suggest loading and maintenance dosage schedules; however, many factors affect the pharmacokinetics of digoxin in individual patients. Therefore the only reliable method of determining if therapeutic levels of the drug are present is to measure them. As always in medicine, these laboratory measurements must be considered as a part of the total clinical situation.

Aminoglycoside Antibiotics

Aminoglycosides are a group of bactericidal antibiotics used to treat many serious bacterial infections. These antibiotics include streptomycin, kanamycin, gentamicin, tobramycin, amikacin, and netilmicin, which are the more common ones; neomycin and paromomycin, the most toxic of the group, are no longer used systemically.

Nephrotoxicity and ototoxicity have been noted with all the aminoglycosides. These drugs are removed by glomerular filtration and are highly concentrated in the renal cortex. Nephrotoxicity may occur at any time in therapy[4,5,11,14] and is not always dose-dependent. Renal failure is usually nonoliguric, and is characterized by a high urine-to-plasma ratio of urea nitrogen, progressive azotemia in the face of normal daily urine volumes, impaired glomerular filtration rates, and reduced tubular concentrating capacity. Renal failure may also occur with hyperkalemia, hypocalcemia, mild metabolic acidosis with a concurrent widening of the anion gap, and possible hematuria or proteinuria or both. In most situations, the most commonly used indirect parameter for estimating renal function and therefore for defining aminoglycoside-associated nephrotoxicity, is serum creatinine.

Nephrotoxicity may be assumed to be caused by aminoglycosides when other common causes are precluded. The most useful monitoring parameter for therapy to avoid this complication, which may be insidious in nature, remains the serum aminoglycoside concentration (SAC). It is thought that peak concentrations of 4 to 8 μg/ml should produce an optimum therapeutic response and that peak concentrations greater than 12 μg/ml should be avoided to decrease the risk of nephrotoxicity. Serum levels may be needed several times per week during initiation of therapy, especially in seriously ill patients; thereafter less frequent measurements are necessary.

EFFECTS OF DISEASE ON PHARMACOKINETICS

Disease may affect the pharmacokinetics of many drugs.[1] Because the liver and kidneys are the most important organs for drug elimination, the effect of disease of these organs on pharmacokinetics will be discussed.

Liver Disease

The liver converts lipid-soluble drugs to a more water-soluble form that is more readily excreted into the bile or removed by the kidney. Because the liver has so much reserve, considerable damage must occur before drug disposition is significantly changed.[4,5,13] In cirrhosis, portal hypertension causes development of collateral channels around the liver; this decreases blood flow to the metabolizing cells. Therefore certain drugs extensively metabolized by the liver after oral ingestion (first-pass effect), such as propranolol, meperidine, and verapamil, are more effective when given orally in cirrhosis, and toxicity may result. Also in cirrhosis, excess lymph flows and may overwhelm lymphatic drainage channels, leading to its weeping into the peritoneal cavity and causing ascites. This ascitic fluid contains proteins, leading to a decrease in serum proteins and decreased binding of many drugs. Thus altered drug disposition resulting from liver disease depends on the relative importance of protein binding, liver blood flow, and hepatic enzymatic activity in the disposition of that drug. In addition, patients with severe liver disease may have altered renal function, causing further alterations in drug disposition.[8]

The hepatic clearance (Cl_H) of a drug is the amount of drug per unit time that is irreversibly removed by the liver. It is determined by both the fraction of drug removed or extracted from the blood during passage through the liver (E) and hepatic blood flow (Q_H). Thus:

$$Cl_H = Q_H \times E$$

where Cl_H represents hepatic clearance: Q_H is hepatic blood flow; and E, is the fraction of drug extracted by the liver.

Extraction of a drug by the liver is dependent on three factors. These are: (1) the activity of hepatic enzymes and transport mechanisms (Cl_{int}, intrinsic clearance); (2) the fraction of total drug free to interact with the elimination mechanism; and (3) hepatic blood flow. Drugs may be classified according to how liver disease might alter their disposition. Identification of and discussion about three groups of drugs follows.

Flow-Limited Drugs

When total intrinsic clearance (Cl_{int}) is large relative to hepatic blood flow (Q_H), the clearance depends on hepatic blood flow. Thus metabolism of these drugs (e.g., propranolol, morphine, verapamil) will be altered in cirrhosis (see earlier discussion) and following other diseases affecting hepatic blood flow.

Enzyme-Limited Drugs

When total intrinsic clearance (CL_{int}) of a drug is small relative to hepatic blood flow (Q_H), the flow is no longer the limiting factor in drug metabolism. The clearance then becomes dependent on liver enzyme and transport mechanisms. This class is further subdivided according to the extent of protein binding of the drugs. For enzyme-limited drugs in which less than 50% of the drug is bound to plasma proteins, changes in binding have little influence on hepatic drug elimination. Consequently, these drugs (e.g., amobarbital, caffeine, theophylline) are affected primarily by factors that change the activity of the liver enzymes responsible for their elimination (Cl_{int}). In contrast, for enzyme-limited drugs in which greater than 85% of the drug is bound to plasma proteins, the hepatic clearance is sensitive to both changes in protein binding in the blood and liver enzyme activity (e.g., benzodiazepines, indomethacin, tolbutamide, and warfarin).

Flow-Enzyme Sensitive Drugs

A drug's disposition may be affected by *both* hepatic blood flow and enzymes. The clearance of these drugs, therefore, may be sensitive to changes in liver blood flow, the intrinsic clearance of the liver, and protein binding (e.g., acetominophen, cloramphenicol, chlorpromazine, meperidine, and quinidine).

Because the percentage of each mechanism of drug elimination impaired by liver disease varies among patients, it would seem advisable to avoid drugs that are extensively metabolized by the liver in patients with hepatic dysfunction. Fortunately, glucuronide conjugation seems to be spared, even in severe liver disease. If drugs eliminated by the liver must be used in patients with hepatic disease, lowered doses may be advisable. Because drug levels in individual patients are affected by so many factors, measurement of such levels is often advisable to avoid the ''hills'' and ''valleys'' of toxicity and inadequate therapy.

Renal Disease

In patients with renal failure, the major pharmacokinetic problem is readjustment of maintenance doses and intervals. Reducing doses according to established guidelines, careful clinical and physiologic monitoring for signs of toxicity, and measuring blood levels of drugs when available can aid therapy in these patients.[4,5,8] The effectiveness and safety of drugs in renal failure depend on bioavailability, route of elimination, activity of metabolites, adaptive changes of the kidney to nephron loss, the margin of safety of the drug, the consequences of high drug levels, and the possibility of removing excesses by dialysis. In acute renal failure, ammonia buffering can lead to increased gastric pH and consequently affect absorption of certain drugs. During various shock states, hepatic, as well as renal, damage may occur, compounding the problem of drug therapy. Fortunately, since hepatic and renal diseases do not greatly affect initial disposition of a drug, loading doses are not adversely influenced.

Since peak drug concentration relates directly to dose and bioavailability and inversely to the distribution space, distribution may be rapid in uremia, partly because of increased permeability of cell membranes throughout the body. Following this rapid redistribution (alpha phase), the slower beta phase correlates with the elimination rate. In uremia, total body water is increased, which increases the volume of distribution of drugs, leading to decreased peak concentration after a given dose. Extracellular fluid is also increased in uremia, leading to a further increase in the distribution space of some drugs bound to plasma proteins (e.g., phenytoin). Protein binding is likewise reduced in uremia, leading to a lower total plasma concentration of these drugs (less bound drug is present) and a higher apparent volume of distribution, but a higher plasma water concentration. Therefore potentially more pharmacologic activity (and therefore more toxicity) may occur in uremic patients, and more rapid hepatic elimination may occur (for drugs also metabolized by this route). Consequently, the dosage interval may need adjustment.

For drugs eliminated by the kidney, the decreased elimination rate overrides the fractional increases in availability for elimination. Some drugs (such as digoxin) have larger apparent volumes of distribution, often exceeding body mass, and have a low plasma concentration.[3] Despite high clearances, these drugs are eliminated slowly because the reservoir is so large. Uremia decreases intracellular binding of digoxin, increasing plasma concentration but decreasing the fraction in myocardium.

In renal failure achieving high renal or urinary concentration of drugs (such as antibiotics) may not be possible except at the expense of high (often toxic) plasma levels. Further, metabolites (e.g., normeperidine) of drugs normally eliminated by the liver (e.g., meperidine) may accumulate in toxic amounts in patients with renal dysfunction.

Clinically, drug clearance by the kidney is not normally measured. Frequently, plasma creatinine, which bears an inverse relationship to the elimination rate of many drugs, may be used in formulas to adjust drug doses. However, in acute renal failure, plasma creatinine concentration is not a good estimate of renal function because the equilibrium concentration has not been reached. With stable, chronic renal failure, however, the plasma creatinine concentration correlates directly with the prolongation of half-life of drugs. In any case, measurement of sequential plasma levels of creatinine allows more accurate therapy.

SUMMARY

The study of pharmacokinetics, pharmacodynamics, and other aspects of pharmacology is essential for the physician caring for patients whose physiology has been altered by anesthesia, surgery, and the perioperative period. During this time, disposition of drugs by the usual mechanisms may be greatly altered; therefore knowledge of the differences in disposition of drugs administered by different routes is essential. In addition, knowledge of how the patient's underlying illness affects drug disposition is crucial to the effective use of drugs in the perioperative period.

No one physician can be expected to know all the relevant information concerning drug therapy of complex surgical patients. Because the surgeon frequently must coordinate the care of sick surgical patients, he or she must frequently obtain advice from other specialists concerning drug therapy. It is hoped that the surgeon will be able to communicate more effectively with these other specialists by learning some of the fundamentals of drug therapy presented in this chapter.

REFERENCES

1. Chernow, B., and Lake, C.R., editors: The pharmacologic approach to the critically ill patient, Baltimore, 1983, Williams & Wilkins.
2. Condouris, G.A.: The natural laws concerning the use of drugs in man and animals. In DiPalma, J.R., editor: Drill's pharmacology in medicine, ed. 4, New York, 1971, McGraw-Hill Book Co.
3. Doherty, J.E.: Digitalis glycosides: pharmacokinetics and their clinical implications, Ann. Int. Med. **79:**229, 1973.
4. Evans, W.E., Schentag, J.J., and Jusko, W.J., editors: Applied pharmacokinetics: principles of therapeutic drug monitoring, San Francisco, 1985, Applied Therapeutics, Inc.
5. Gibaldi, M., editor: Biopharmaceutics and clinical pharmacokinetics, ed. 3, Philadelphia, 1984, Lea & Febiger.
6. Gilman, A.G., Mayer, S.E., and Melmon, K.C.: Pharmacodynamics: mechanisms of drug action and the relationship between drug concentration and effect. In Gilman, A.G., Goodman, L.S., and Gilman, A., editors: The pharmacological basis of therapeutics, ed. 6, New York, 1980, Macmillan Publishing Co.
7. Hug, C.C.: Pharmacokinetics of drugs administered intravenously, Anesth. Analg. **57:**704, 1978.
8. Maher, J.F.: Adjustment of medications in renal failure. In Chernow, B., and Lake, C.R., editors: The pharmacologic approach to the critically ill patient. Baltimore, 1983, Williams & Wilkins.
9. Mayer, S.E., Melmon, K.C., and Gilman, A.G.: Introduction: the dynamics of drug absorption, distribution, and elimination. In Gilman, A.G., Goodman, L.S., and Gilman, A., editors: The pharmacological basis of therapeutics, ed. 6, New York, 1980, Macmillan Publishing Co.
10. Melmon, K.C., Gilman, A.G., and Mayer, S.E.: Principles of therapeutics. In Gilman, A.G., Goodman, L.S., and Gilman, A., editors: The pharmacological basis of therapeutics, ed. 6, New York, 1980, Macmillan Publishing Co.
11. Noone, P., et al.: Experience in monitoring gentamycin therapy during treatment of serious gram-negative sepsis, Br. Med. J. **1:**477, 1974.
12. Price, H.C.: A dynamic concept of the distribution of thiopental in the human body, Anesthesiology **21:**40, 1960.
13. Wedlund, P.J., and Branch, R.A.: Adjustment of medications in liver failure. In Chernow, B., and Lake, C.R., editors: The pharmacologic approach to the critically ill patient, Baltimore, 1983, Williams & Wilkins.
14. Whelton, A., and Neu, H., editors: The aminoglycosides: microbiology, clinical use and toxicology, New York, 1981, Marcel Dekker, Inc.
15. Winter, M.E., Katcher, B.S., and Koda-Kimble, M.A., editors: Basic clinical pharmacokinetics, San Francisco, 1980, Applied Therapeutics, Inc.

12 Physiology and Management of Pain

Philip Gildenberg

Pain is important in that it makes survival possible by identifying injury or disease. Yet when felt inappropriately, pain can be one of the most challenging and frustrating problems to confront both the physician and the patient. Pain is not a simple sensation such as sight, hearing, touch, temperature, taste, or proprioception. Rather, it is a perception. Although usually precipitated by a noxious or potentially injury-producing stimulus, it is modified by many other factors, both physical and emotional.

Clinically, pain should be divided into three categories: acute pain, cancer pain, and chronic pain of benign origin. These designations represent three totally different entities, and the management of one is entirely different from the management of the other two.[9] The usual classification, however, consists of acute pain and chronic pain. The latter class is further divided into pain of benign origin and cancer pain. Not only is this classification confusing, but it tends to group patients together whose management is dissimilar.

Using my classification, *acute pain* is an appropriate physiologic perception in response to tissue damage or potential tissue damage, such as pin prick, heat, pinch, cutting, inflammation, or tissue anoxia. The management of acute pain is directed to the management of the underlying cause such as immobilizing a fracture, treating the cause of inflammation, lancing an abscess to relieve the mechanical pressure and inflammation, or allowing time for healing to occur. Analgesics have been designed for use over a brief period as part of the management of acute pain and are inappropriate when used indiscriminately in other types of pain.

Cancer pain can be considered a continually recurring acute pain and probably involves repeated stimulation of the nociceptive pathways. Cancer pain also takes on some of the characteristics of chronic pain in that the pain is markedly increased by depression and anxiety. The ideal in management is to treat the underlying cause, but if that is not possible, the pain itself requires treatment, first with analgesics in increasing doses as tolerance develops, without regard to addiction. If this approach is not effective, it may be necessary to perform a surgical procedure to modify pain perception, usually by interrupting a pain pathway.

Chronic pain of benign origin is neither cancer pain nor acute pain and must be recognized as a separate entity. The treatment is the opposite of that of cancer or acute pain in that medications are withdrawn and ablative procedures are not used. Indeed, since all analgesics have been designed for the acute pain model, their use in chronic pain adds significantly to the patient's depression and pain perception and causes physiologic addiction and withdrawal problems. In patients with chronic pain, anxiety and depression increase pain perception and must be treated. Regression and immobility interfere with rehabilitation. Consequently, an important goal in treatment is to increase gradually the patient's physical activity and self care.

PHYSIOLOGIC BASIS OF PAIN

Peripheral Receptors

A noxious stimulus is one that has the potential for producing tissue damage. Specific receptors exist in the skin that respond to noxious stimulation and are called *nociceptors*. There are two main classes of cutaneous nociceptors: A-delta mechanical nociceptors and C polymodal nociceptors, named after the diameter of nerve fibers that innervate them. The A-delta nociceptors are innervated by nerves in the A-delta range that have a mean conduction velocity of 15 to 25 m/sec. These receptors possess a specific sensitivity to mechanical but not thermal or chemical noxious stimuli.[23] They consist of bare nerve endings, and their unmyelinated fine terminals are associated with Schwann cells at the junction of the dermis and epidermis.[24] They are present in both hairy and glabrous skin, and the threshold to mechanical stimulation may be anywhere from 5 to 1000 times the threshold for nonpainful mechanical sensation.[23]

C polymodal nociceptors are innervated by unmyelinated C fibers (conduction velocity less than 2.5 m/sec.) and respond to noxious mechanical, thermal, or chemical stimuli.[3] These receptors respond to approximately the same threshold of mechanical stimulation as the A-delta receptors. For example, they respond in a graded fashion to noxious heat stimuli[2] until frank tissue damage has occurred. A number of chemical substances have been identified that excite these receptors. Although most of these substances are nonspecific, such as acetylcholine, histamine, serotonin, bradykinin, prostaglandins, and potassium ions, substance P appears to be specific for pain perception. Bradykinin and prostaglandin cause a sensitization of the C polymodal nociceptors. Substance P causes an increased vascular permeability that may allow increased transmission of blood-borne chemicals to areas of pain.[30] The information about noxious stimulation is transmitted to the spinal cord by the A-delta and C nerve fibers, which constitute the small nerves that enter the dorsal root laterally to become part of the Melzack-Wall "gate" (see p. 220).[21]

Nociceptors have been identified in other tissues besides skin. Both A-delta and C fibers are present in the heart. A release of bradykinin or prostaglandin during ischemia of cardiac muscle may sensitize these fibers to produce angina pectoris.[30] Two types of nociceptors also exist in the respiratory passages. A-delta fibers innervate the epithelial lining and are excited by noxious mechanical stimulation in aerosols and inhalants. Type J receptors are found next to capillaries and are excited by pulmonary congestion, pulmonary edema, embolization, or blood-borne irritants.[30]

Specific nociceptor endings have not been found in the gastrointestinal tract, which may explain why noxious stimuli that cause pain when applied to the skin do not cause pain when applied to the intestine. Instead, pain results from distention, contraction, traction, or inflammation.

Peripheral Nerves

The three major types of peripheral nerve fibers are designated A, B, and C, according to diameter, which regulates conduction velocity[27] (Table 12-1). Type A fibers are myelinated somatic fibers, both afferent and efferent, and constitute the bulk of peripheral nerves. These fibers have a wide variety of diameters (and consequently a wide variety of conduction velocities). They are subdivided into alpha, beta, and delta groups, delta being the smallest. For somatic afferent fibers, A-alpha have a diameter of 6 to 17 μm while A-delta fibers have axons 1 to 6 μm in diameter. Noxious stimulation activates the A-delta fibers, which conduct at a speed of 2.5 to 3.6 m/sec. They can also be

Table 12-1 **PROPERTIES OF MAMMALIAN NERVE FIBERS**

Property	A	B	sC*	drC*
Fiber diameter (μm)	1-22	≤3	0.3-1.3	0.4-1.2
Conduction speed (msec)	5-120	3-15	0.7-2.3	0.6-2
Spike duration (msec)	0.4-0.5	1.2	2	2
Absolute refractory period (msec)	0.4-1	1.2	2	2
Negative afterpotential amplitude (% of spike)	3-5	None	3-5	None
Duration (msec)	12-20	—	50-80	—
Positive afterpotential amplitude, (% of spike)	0.2	1.5-4	1.5	—
Duration (msec)	40-60	100-300	300-1000	—
Order of susceptibility to asphyxia	2	1	3	3
Velocity-diameter ratio	6	?	?	1.73 average

From Ruch, T.C., Patton, H.D., and Towe, A.L.: Neurophysiology, Philadelphia, 1965, W.B. Saunders Co.
*sC, Sympathetic C fiber, drC, dorsal root fiber.

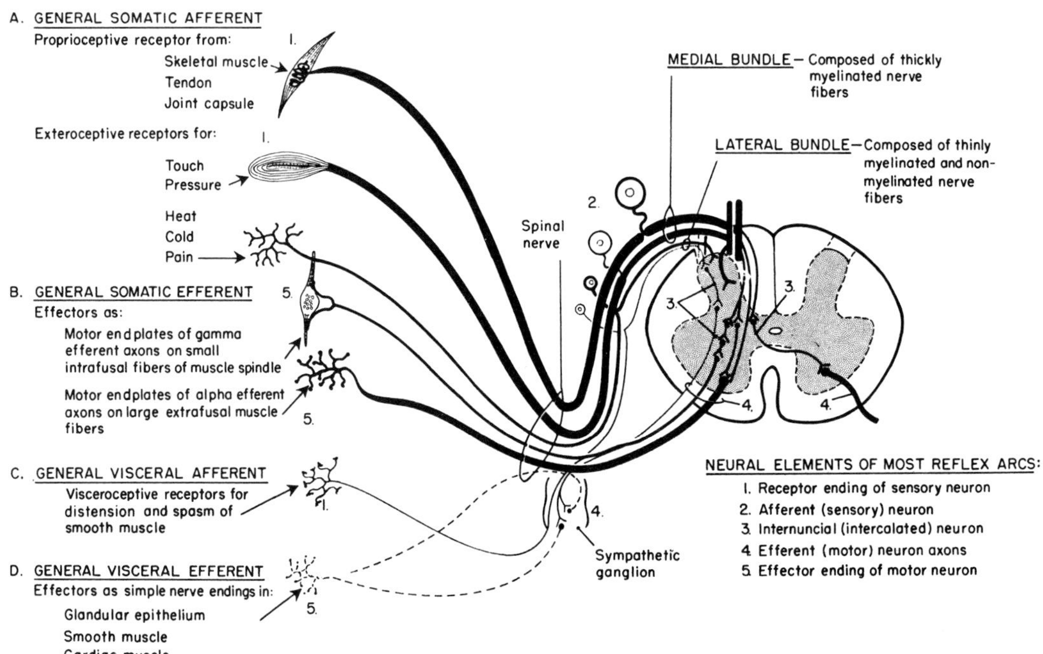

Fig. 12-1 Types and distribution of afferent fibers in the human spinal cord. (From Carpenter, M.B.: Human neuroanatomy, ed. 7, Baltimore, 1976, The Williams & Wilkins Co.)

fired by low-threshold mechanical receptor afferents or by cooling. Type B fibers are myelinated efferent preganglionic autonomic nerve fibers and are not concerned with somatic sensation. Type C fibers are unmyelinated with a diameter of 0.4 to 1.2 μm and a conduction velocity of 0.6 to 2 m/sec. Some are small afferent axons from peripheral nerves, and others are efferent postganglionic sympathetic axons. Only the former are concerned with somatic sensation, and they fire almost exclusively in response to noxious or thermal stimuli. Furthermore, they are also thought to be involved in the mediation of vascular and visceral pain.

Ascending Pathways

When the afferent fibers enter the spinal cord through the dorsal root, they distribute themselves with the larger fibers dorsomedial and the smaller fibers ventrolateral (Fig. 12-1). The somatosensory fibers ascend in the dorsal columns of the spinal cord but send collaterals to the area of the dorsal horn near the substantia gelatinosa where they participate in the formation of a pain gate (see p. 220) that begins to discriminate the sensation of pain even at segmental spinal levels. The smaller A-delta and C fibers enter the spinal cord from the lateral edge of the dorsal root. They synapse in the dorsal root entry zone and also participate in the gate. From those areas of the spinal cord, neurons originate that ascend as the various nociceptive pathways, primarily the spinothalamic tract, the spinoreticular tract, and the spinomesencephalic tract. All of these pathways ascend in the anterolateral quadrant.

The *neospinothalamic,* or *lateral spinothalamic, tract* is the best known of the ascending pathways. Fibers decussate in midline in the anterior white commissure within a few segments and ascend to various levels of the brainstem (Fig. 12-2). Those fibers projecting to the ventroposterolateral nucleus originate in Rexed's laminae I and V, while

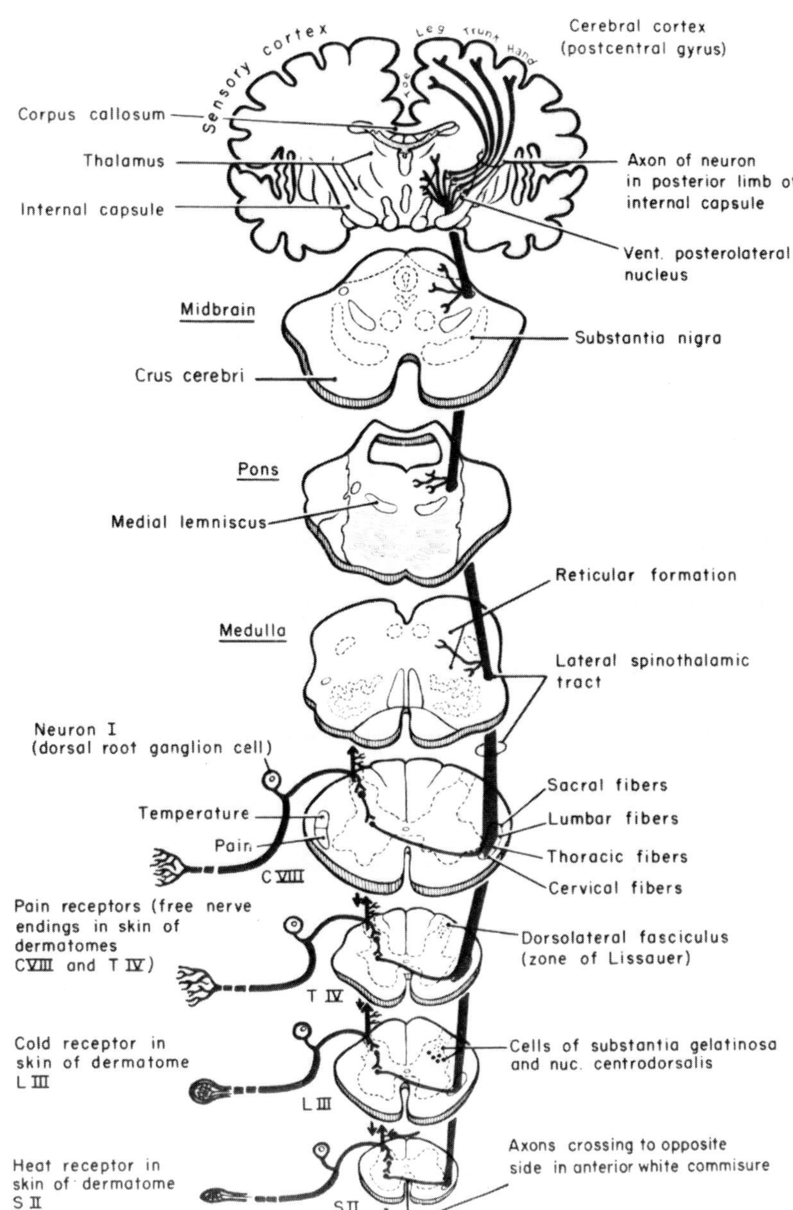

Fig. 12-2 Pathways of the lateral spinothalamic tract in the human spinal cord. (From Carpenter, M.B.: Human neuroanatomy, ed. 7, Baltimore, 1976, The Williams & Wilkins Co.)

those projecting to the centrum medianum and intralaminar nuclei originate further toward the ventral horn and project bilaterally.[31]

The neospinothalamic tract can be interrupted surgically in the anterolateral quadrant of the spinal cord to produce analgesia and loss of pain sensation in the contralateral lower body without affecting other sensory modalities. The same pathway can be interrupted selectively at medullary or midbrain levels to afford analgesia to the entire contralateral body and face and head.[8] In the brainstem, the neospinothalamic tracts are gathered lateral to the central gray matter and are organized somatotopically with the most caudal fibers more lateral and those from the head and neck more medial.[22] Their termination in the ventrolateral nucleus of the thalamus is intermingled with the termination of fibers subserving other sensory modalities. It appears that pain is brought to consciousness at thalamic levels or below, but fine discrimination of the location and character of the pain may require participation of the cortex to which the thalamic fibers project.

The *paleospinothalamic tract* begins as fibers ascending in the anterolateral quadrant of the spinal cord along with the neospinothalamic fibers but projects to the reticular formation in the brainstem, sometimes as spinoreticular fibers and sometimes as collaterals from spinothalamic neurons (Fig. 12-3). This multisynaptic pathway then ascends to areas concerned with emotions, such as the hypothalamus, the intraluminar nuclei of the thalamus, the centrum medianum, the parafascicularis, and the limbic lobe, which includes the cingulate gyrus, hippocampus, and amygdala.[7] Because the projection is bilateral, a unilateral lesion may affect perception of pain on both sides of the body, and it may be necessary to make bilateral lesions for successful pain treatment. The effects of a lesion in the paleospinothalamic tract are somewhat different from those in the neospinothalamic tract. Interruption of the neospinothalamic pathway causes loss of pain perception so that a patient tested with a pin no longer feels sharpness. Interruption of the paleospinothalamic tract may afford relief from cancer pain, but perception of a pin stick sensation is maintained.[6]

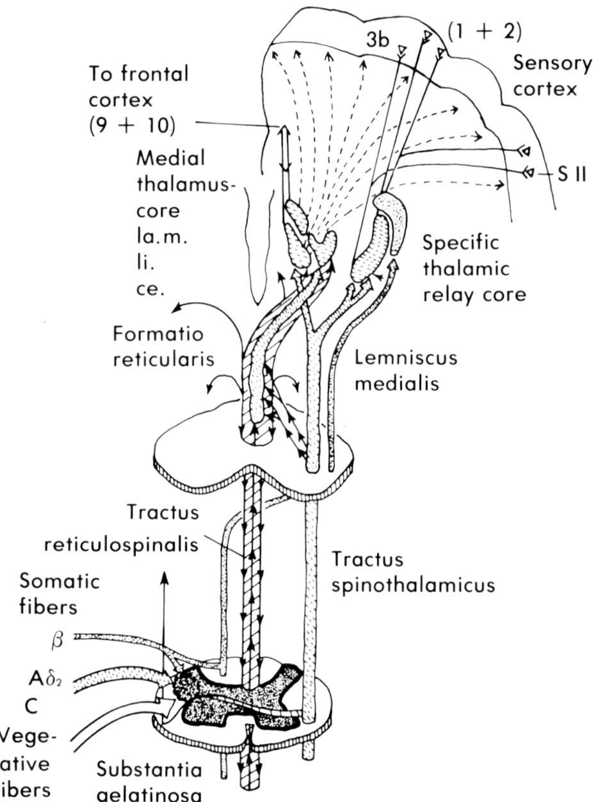

Fig. 12-3 Schematic diagram of the reception, conduction, and assimilation of pain stimuli according to functional aspects. Arrows on the left side symbolize the afferent impulse from skin, deep tissues, and the intestines, assimilation of it in spinal or bulbar control centers, and conduction of it to the neocortex. Arrows at right represent the ascending and descending reticular pain controls and the somatic, vegetative, and psychic reactions to pain stimuli. (From Struppler, A.: Processing in the central nervous system mediators and efferent modulation: central nervous assimilation and afferent influence. In Payne, J.P., and Burt, R.A., editors: Pain: basic principles—pharmacology—therapy. London, 1972, Churchill Livingstone.)

The *archispinothalamic pathway* is phylogenetically the oldest and least well defined. It is presumably a multisynaptic pathway that ascends through the entire length of the spinal cord and reticular formation and perhaps to the same areas of the thalamus and cerebrum as the paleospinothalamic tract, especially the limbic and hypothalamic areas. Because of the multisynaptic, diffuse nature of this pathway, it defies strict delineation by the usual anatomic or neurophysiologic techniques, but there is indirect evidence that it may ascend as a relatively compact bundle around the central canal of the spinal cord. Interruption of this pathway at spinal or lower-brainstem levels may provide the same type of relief as paleospinothalamic lesions, which may be particularly helpful for bilateral or midline pelvic pain.[10,12,28]

The Gate Theory

The gate theory was originally proposed by Melzack and Wall in 1965.[21] Although it has proved inaccurate in many respects, it serves several important functions. First, it helps to explain that pain is more complex than the other sensory modalities and consequently needs a more elaborate network to express itself. Second, it reinforces the observation that pain is not necessarily perceived in proportion to the noxious stimulation applied. There are many things that may modify pain perception, such as the application of a nonpainful stimulus or a difference in one's emotional tone. Such gating mechanisms undoubtedly occur not only at spinal cord levels, as proposed in the original theory, but at higher levels as well.

The gate theory is based on the observation that large nerve fibers (which carry nonpainful sensations) enter the spinal cord through segmental roots dorsomedial to the smaller pain fibers (Fig. 12-4). At the dorsal root entry zone there is a neurophysiologic arrangement that forms the gate. If firing of the small fibers predominates, the gate is open and pain is perceived. However, if firing of the large fibers increases, interneurons may presynaptically inhibit the transmission of pain. The gate theory suggests that both the larger and smaller fibers synapse on substantia gelatinosa (SG) cells. The SG cells are stimulated by collaterals from the large fibers but are inhibited by collaterals from the small fibers. If the balance is such that the large neuron firing predominates, SG cells fire and in turn inhibit the nociceptor cells from which the ascending pain pathways originate. If the small neurons predominate, the SG cells are inhibited and fail to suppress the firing of the pain pathways.

The gate theory provides an opportunity for management of pain that may be inhibited when large fibers are stimulated by nonpainful stimulation such as rubbing or massage ("if you rub it, it feels better"). This approach can be taken one step further with the use of an electronic unit controlled by the patient for transcutaneous electronic nerve stimulation (TENS) (see p. 233), which preferentially stimulates the lower threshold large fibers to close the gate.

Pain is transmitted from the spinal cord to various areas of the brain that Melzack and Wall[21] term the sensory-discriminative system and the motivational-affective system. The sensory-discriminative system is concerned with those parts of the brain that participate in the conscious perception of pain. The motivational-affective system, which is linked with those areas of the brain that are involved with emotions or the sympathetic responses to stress, monitors the intensity of pain perception and is concerned with the suffering component of pain. The perception of pain is further influenced by central control processes that allow distraction or motivation to affect the perceived intensity.

Descending Pathways

It has been shown in rats that stimulation of the brain in the area around the aqueduct at midbrain levels or around the posterior part of the ventricular system produces analgesia, so-called stimulation-produced analgesia (SPA).[19] During stimulation of this region, the rats no longer respond to noxious stimulants, particularly those applied to lower parts of the body. This exciting observation has led to the concept that there are systems within the brain that inhibit the perception of pain. It has been further demonstrated that stimulation of these areas in humans can inhibit cancer pain or chronic pain of benign origin and consequently can be employed therapeutically now that fully implantable electronic stimulators have been developed.[25]

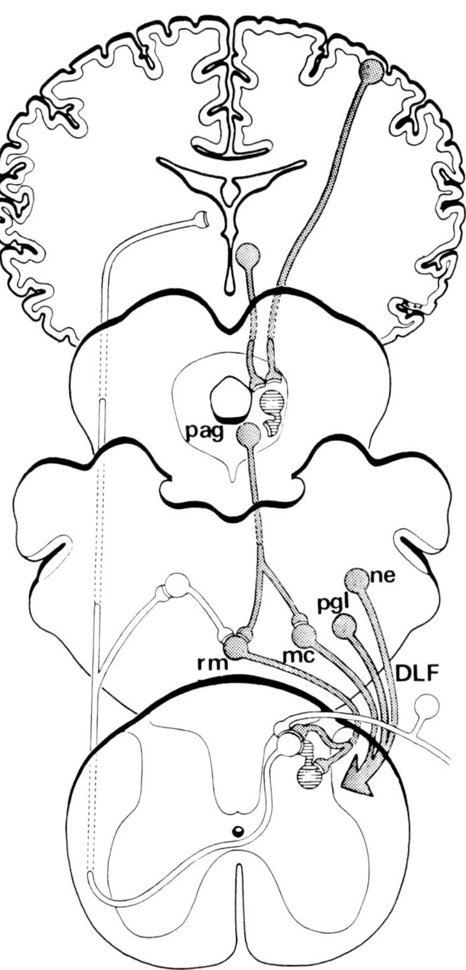

Fig. 12-5 Pain modulating network. Diagram of critical structures that contribute to control of pain-transmission neurons. The network includes connections from midbrain periaqueductal grey *(pag)* to medullary nucleus raphe magnus *(rm)* recticularis magnocellularis *(mc)* and, through the dorsolateral funiculus *(DLF)*, to the spinal cord dorsal horn. Additional bulbospinal pathways potentially relevant to analgesia arise from the nucleus paragigantocellularis *(pgl)*, which also receives input from *pag* and the noradrenergic medullary cell groups *(ne)* lateral to *pgl*.

In addition to this brain stem to spinal cord network, connections from neocortex and hypothalamus to the *pag* have recently been documented. Hypothalamic stimulation produces analgesia, but the role of the cortex in pain modulation has not been elucidated.

At the spinal level descending pathways inhibit nociceptive projection neurons through direct connections, as well as through interneurons in the superficial layers of the dorsal horn.

There is evidence that endorphin-containing interneurons (cross hatched) in *pag* and dorsal horn play an active role in pain modulation. (See text.) (From Fields, H.L., and Basbaum, A.I.: Endogenous pain control mechanisms. In Wall, P.D., and Melzack, R., editors: Textbook of pain, Edinburgh, 1984, Churchill Livingstone.)

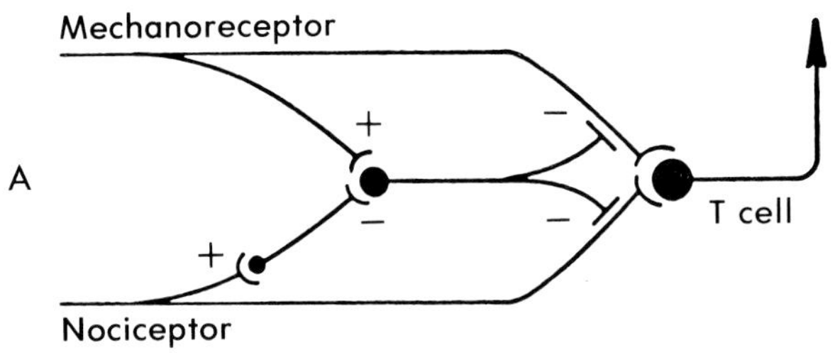

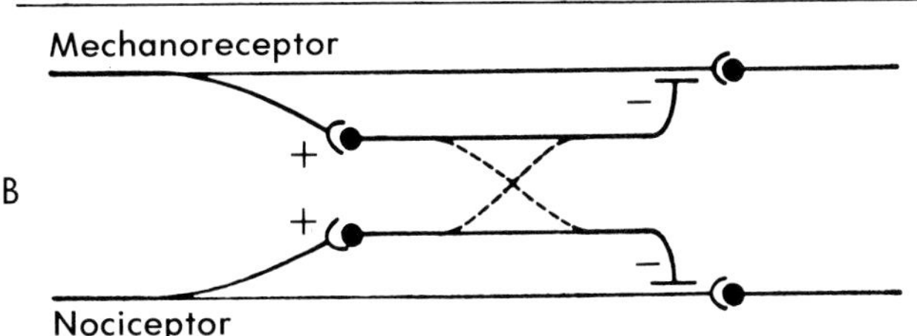

Fig. 12-4 Classic **(A)** and current **(B)** concepts of gating mechanisms in the spinal cord. (From Eyzaguirre, C., and Fidone, S.J.: Physiology of the nervous system; Chicago, 1975, Yearbook Medical Publishers, Inc. Reproduced with permission.)

The descending pain modulating system has only recently been elaborated. It primarily involves the periventricular and periaqueductal gray area where endogenous morphine-like substances, endorphins, are found in large concentrations. Neurons from those areas run to the nucleus raphe magnus and from there into the spinal cord through the dorsolateral funiculus. A lesion in the nucleus raphe magnus blocks SPA. This nucleus contains neurons that use serotonin as a neurotransmitter, and it can be demonstrated that SPA is diminished when serotonin is blocked or depleted. Conversely, drugs that stimulate the serotonin system, such as 5-hydroxytryptophane, enhance stimulation-produced analgesia[1] (Fig. 12-5). Of further interest, one of the areas in the reticular formation to which pain transmission neurons project is the nucleus reticulogigantocellularis, which in turn projects to the periaqueductal gray matter and nucleus raphe magnus to establish a negative feedback loop.[1]

Opiate analgesia and SPA have so many similar characteristics that they may operate through a common mechanism. Those sites that have been found to be most effective for SPA are also where opiate receptors have been found and where microinjection of morphine can produce pain relief in experimental animals. Presumably these same areas around the ventricles are those that are involved in pain relief on infusion of minute doses of morphine into the ventricles and possibly around the spinal cord as well. It has been demonstrated that enkephalins are released into the fluid of the third ventricle on the production of SPA, and the release of such substances may be related to the ensuing pain relief. Narcotic antagonists, such as naloxone, may block the action of such enkephalins, and it has also been demonstrated that they may block SPA as well. There is considerable cross-tolerance between SPA and opiate analgesia.[18] Animals that become tolerant to repeated administration of morphine may also lose the pain-relieving effects of stimulation of the brain. If deep-brain stimulation is used continually, it gradually loses its effect, similar to morphine tolerance, but regains its effect when it has been discontinued for a period of several days or weeks.

CLINICAL CONSIDERATIONS RELATING TO PAIN

Threshold vs. Tolerance

There is considerable confusion about the difference between *pain threshold* and *pain tolerance,* but both can be illustrated by a relatively simple experimental protocol. A stimulus of gradually increasing intensity such as a heat stimulus is applied to the center of the forehead. The subject is asked to report when the stimulus becomes painful. He is also provided with a button that will interrupt the stimulus and told to push the button only when he can no longer tolerate the pain. Pain threshold is indicated when the subject reports that the stimulus is painful. Pain tolerance is indicated by the amount of time it takes for the subject to push the button to interrupt the stimulus.

There is an amazing consistency in pain threshold among subjects tested, generally between 44.0° and 44.5° C, which is, not coincidentally, the temperature at which tissue damage begins to occur. However, there is a tremendous variability in the temperature at which subjects press the button to interrupt the stimulus, illustrating that tolerance to pain is extremely variable among subjects and even in the same subject under different conditions. Some subjects require interruption of the stimulus as soon as pain is perceived. Others may hold out until frank tissue damage occurs, particularly if they are well motivated to do so. An individual will have less tolerance during a period of stress or depression than when he is relaxed or optimistic. Translated into clinical terms, the variability in patients' pain response is the difference in pain tolerance based on emotion, motivation, cultural background, depression, or anxiety. By controlling some of these factors, the pain perception is minimized,[9] and thus the physician may help the patient tolerate pain much better.

The Three P's of Pain

Acute or cancer pain generally involves stimulation of nociceptive nerve endings and its transmission through the gate to those areas of the brain that concern conscious perception of sensation. Pain may also be perceived when injury or malfunction of sensory pathways causes aberrant neuronal firing to make the pain pathways fire abnormally. Finally, under the appropriate psychiatric circumstances (e.g., anxiety, depression) or after the peripheral nociceptive stimulus has resolved, pain can be perceived where no noxious stimulation exists. Thus in properly approaching an individual patient with chronic pain and determining appropriate treatment the physician can gain much insight by elucidating what portion of the pain is *physiologic, pathologic,* or *psychologic.*[9]

Physiologic pain is the appropriate perception of pain on application of a noxious stimulus, whether it be from injury, inflammation, or surgery. The nervous system is working appropriately to allow the patient to perceive a sensation that is primarily protective in its function.

Pathologic pain, in this context, refers to an aberrant perception of pain caused by an underlying pathologic process in the nervous system. If the nervous system is not functioning properly, pain may be perceived even in the absence of a noxious stimulus. A classic example is pain of peripheral neuropathy, wherein the large nerves may not be firing adequately so that a predominance of small-nerve firing occurs, opening the gate to pain perception. Peripheral nerve injury or a peripheral neuroma may cause the nerve to fire, even when no noxious cutaneous stimulation exists. Spinal cord injury or multiple sclerosis may cause a distortion of incoming sensation so that the resultant "static" causes the pain-perceiving part of the nervous system to fire and the patient to feel pain. In the thalamic syndrome a stroke may destroy part of the brain that presumably is concerned with inhibiting the perception of pain so that persistent and spontaneous pain exists.

In contrast to physiologic or pathologic pain, *psychologic pain* is pain that occurs or is magnified by psychologic factors. Firing of the pain perception system may or may not occur. Frequently psychologic pain occurs because of a magnification of pain perception, as in the patient who is totally disabled from a minor injury or the individual whose pain is magnified by depression. In the hysterical patient the perception of pain may exist even though there is no evidence of a pathologic condition.

Analgesics

Most analgesics used in the treatment of pain belong to the narcotic family of drugs. Those that are not true narcotics chemically behave analgesically as if they were and appear to mediate their effects through similar biochemical pathways. Although aspirin-like drugs have a mild analgesic action, they are primarily anti-inflammatory and antipyretic agents and thus will not be considered true analgesic drugs in this discussion.

In order to prescribe analgesics properly, the physician must remember that *all analgesics were designed around an acute pain model*. It is appropriate to use analgesics on a short-term basis for acute pain while the underlying disease process is brought under control. If the use of analgesics is limited to a maximum of 1 to 2 weeks, tolerance and addiction are minimized. However, patients who become addicted or enjoy the soporific effects of the narcotics request them even after the acute problem has resolved. Thus the desire for analgesics may be strong enough to perpetuate the perception of pain.

Analgesics are also the primary mode of treatment of cancer pain. Because tolerance develops, the dose must be adjusted upward regularly. Although addiction develops, the patient will probably remain on the narcotics for the rest of his limited life so that withdrawal is not an issue of concern.

In contrast to acute pain and cancer pain, *analgesics make chronic pain worse*. Pain that lasts more than a few weeks no longer derives benefit from analgesics. Virtually all analgesics are designed on molecules related to narcotics, and many of the narcotics are converted in the body to morphine-like molecules. Consequently they all share not only the analgesic properties of morphine but also the side effects of tolerance and addiction and its attendant withdrawal, all of which become serious problems if such drugs are used in the management of chronic pain.[9]

The exact physiologic mechanism responsible for withdrawal is not clearly understood. The theory that seems most tenable is that the administration of exogenous morphine or related drugs causes suppression of production of endogenous morphine-like substances within the brain. These endorphins appear to be involved with the naturally occurring pain modulating system designed to suppress the perception of pain. Thus if a patient is receiving a narcotic-like drug on a protracted basis, the chronic suppression of endorphin production disrupts its pain-modulating effects between periods of drug administration resulting in withdrawal and the need for either more frequent or higher doses of drugs to adequately provide analgesia. Evidence that endogenous endorphins may be involved in pain control stems from the observation that stimulation of certain areas in the deep brain suppresses pain. Interestingly, these areas are rich in endorphins and such stimulation promotes their release.[13]

Clinically, one of the first manifestations of withdrawal from narcotics is a decrease in pain tolerance and an increase in pain perception. If this is managed by increasing drug dosage, recurrent withdrawal will ultimately become a problem-causing potentiation of the chronic pain. As an example, picture the scenario of the patient who has been taking narcotics every 4 hours for several weeks and who has become physiologically addicted. About 3 hours after the last dose of the analgesic the patient begins to go into withdrawal. As the pain becomes worse, the patient becomes dysphoric and agitated and may try to hold off taking the next dose. Finally the distress becomes severe enough that he requests and is given more medication, which promptly aborts the withdrawal symptoms. Both patient and physician interpret this response as pain relief, even though it was the withdrawal that caused the pain in the first place. The patient may recognize that the relief is not total but say that it "takes the edge off." The repetition of the withdrawal state makes the pain increasingly worse over a period of time. The only way to stop recurrent withdrawal is to stop the medication completely, warning the patient that he will feel worse before he feels better. Indeed, for the first few days the patient may have intensified pain, be unable to sleep, feel depressed, agitated, and dysphoric. By 7 to 10 days the patient may find that the pain is markedly diminished and that no further analgesics are needed.

It is more than coincidence that patients with addiction-prone personalities are those most likely to develop chronic pain, conceivably in order to have a sanctioned reason for taking narcotics. It is not difficult for such patients to convince themselves and their physicians that they have pain. They may also feel the need for their drug when they are anxious, depressed, or under stress. It is not uncommon to see a chronic pain patient respond to a stressful confrontation by popping a pain pill. It is also unfortunately not uncommon to see a physician prescribing a narcotic for agitation, a significant misuse of such drugs. Because many physicians do not understand the relationship between drug withdrawal and potentiation of pain, iatrogenic addiction is one of the most common causes of chronic pain.

Placebo

A placebo (from the Latin "I shall please") is usually an inert substance given to a patient who believes he is receiving an active drug. A physician may give the patient a placebo in an attempt to see if the patient has "real" or "imaginary" pain. This naive concept ignores the fact that one third of patients with "real" or well-documented organic pain obtain relief from an inert medication they believe to be an analgesic. It is the placebo effect that makes drug trials difficult to interpret, but this very real effect demonstrates how strong the descending pain modulation system can be when set into play by conscious thinking.[5]

An interesting related observation is that side effects can be placebo effects as well. It is common in drug trials that patients who receive placebos have significant side effects. These may be subjective, such as unsteadiness, headache, or nausea, or objective physiologic changes such as flushing and changes in blood pressure.

The physician is strongly advised not to employ placebos to attempt to fool the patient into receiving less analgesics. If the patient discovers this ruse, he will lose confidence in the physician and may thereafter doubt even accurate, important clinical information. Rather than administering placebos, the physician should take the time to discuss with the patient the need for less medication and make it clearly understood that manipulation on the patient's part will not be rewarded by inappropriate analgesics.

Types of Pain

A number of terms are used in the description of physiologic pain that may have considerable clinical implications. These include the designations somatic pain, visceral pain, referred pain, projected pain, neuropathic pain, and vascular pain.

Somatic pain is the general term for acute pain from musculoskeletal or cutaneous structures that is the result of a noxious stimulus. It denotes tissue injury or potential injury and is an important protective sensation. It consists of an early and a late component. The *early pain* occurs almost immediately on application of the stimulus and is very sharply localized and well defined. The nature of the pain is a function of the type of stimulus, e.g., hot, sharp, cutting, burning. A few seconds after the actual injury *secondary pain* may occur. It is more diffuse and extends beyond the area of actual injury. It is more often burning in nature and seems to have more of the quality of suffering involved. Because of the wide distribution of the pain, its slow onset, gradual resolution, and diffusely burning character, it may result from the local or regional release of tissue substances such as histamine or bradykinin rather than the direct stimulation of nerve endings.

Visceral pain, which is pain sensation from the abdominal viscera, especially the gastrointestinal tract from the stomach to the midportion of the descending colon, is transmitted to a large extent through afferent fibers that travel with fine sympathetic nerves through the abdominal ganglia and from there through the splanchnic sympathetic pathways to their cell bodies located in the dorsal roots in the spinal cord. Once sensation has reached the cord it appears to travel along the same pathways as somatic sensation in the spinothalamic tracts. Vascular pain from the extremities may likewise be carried along sympathetic fibers that innervate the blood vessels and be transmitted to the spinal cord through the sympathetic nervous system. Consequently, interruption of the sympathetic chain or dissection of the abdominal sympathetic ganglia may alleviate the pain arising from both abdominal viscera and blood vessels.

Referred pain is pain felt in a different body part than where the underlying pathology arises. The most common example is the pain of a myocardial infarction that is felt in the left arm. Another example is myofascial pain that originates in the lumbar muscles and may be referred down the ipsilateral leg; it does not follow a radicular pattern nor does it ordinarily extend below the knee. There are several theories about why referred pain occurs. The most commonly accepted theory is that pain is perceived in the entire segment from which a structure originates. A striking example is stomach pain referred to the top of the shoulder. Both the stomach and shoulder represent C4 innervation, the segment at which the stomach originates embryologically before it descends into its abdominal position. Referred pain is not to be confused with *projected pain,* which is neuropathic in origin. An example of projected pain would be a herniated intravertebral disk compressing the L5 nerve root that causes pain that is projected along the entire L5 dermatomal distribution.

Neuropathic pain is caused by injury, particularly compression, to nervous tissue. It has distinctive qualities and may be described as "the feeling you get when you hit your funny bone." The most common example is the leg pain accompanying nerve root compression from a herniated lumbar disk. A frequent manifestation of neuropathic pain is *dysesthesia* wherein, with some injuries to peripheral nerves, even a nonpainful stimulus may be interpreted as being painful and the slightest touch may cause severe pain. This is different from *paresthesia* in which peripheral nerve injury is accompanied by tingling or numbness, particularly on application of a nonnoxious stimulus.

Vascular or *ischemic pain* results from anoxia. Most tissues respond to oxygen deprivation by producing pain, the major exception being the brain. A standard means of producing pain experimentally is to apply a blood pressure cuff inflated to a pressure greater than systolic and then to exercise the arm. The anoxic muscles soon produce extreme pain, presumably from the accumulation of metabolites since it disappears almost immediately on reestablishment of blood flow. Intermittent claudication has a similar mechanism wherein pain occurs when oxygen demand exceeds supply but is then alleviated when the extremity is put at rest to decrease the metabolic demand below oxygen availability. Another related example of vascular pain is that of angina pectoris from localized myocardial ischemia. Pain at rest signifies the decrease of oxygen availability to the point where it no longer is adequate for the tissue, even when no increased demand of activity is placed on it.

MANAGEMENT OF PAIN

General Considerations

There is considerable disagreement, confusion, and uncertainty about the treatment of pain. Since pain is such a common problem, it would seem to be a simple matter to establish a protocol to evaluate a given treatment for a particular type of pain. There are a number of reasons why this is not the case. These include:

1. *There are no measurements for pain.* Despite numerous attempts to devise a "dolorimeter," pain is not quantitatible. It must be continually stressed that pain is not a sensation, but a perception. Although it is possible to quantitate an experimental stimulus that can produce pain, different patients perceive a given pain quite differently because so many factors influence the perception of pain. In evaluating pain the physician must rely totally on the patient's subjective report, which is colored by many factors not directly related to the pathologic condition.

2. *Psychologic factors can influence pain and its management.* A patient who happens to be depressed from some unrelated factor may not respond to an appropriate treatment regimen for pain.

3. *Pain medications may help or hinder treatment of pain.* Since most pain medications produce a psychologic

response or a soporific effect, the desire for more medication may convince an individual patient that he still has the pain to justify continuing the treatment. This is particularly a problem in patients with an addictive personality or those who have become addicted to pain medications.

4. *Stressful situations modify the intensity of pain and the response to treatment.* Many painful conditions involve pain of muscular origin that is influenced by emotional tension. Thus the pain is aggravated by the stress of pain that increases muscle tension, which in turn increases the muscle pain, which causes more stress, and so forth. Response to treatment is much different in a patient under stress than in one who is relaxed and handles stress well.

5. *Any study involving the management of chronic pain must, by its very nature, include a heterogenous group of patients.* Although there are many things that patients with chronic pain have in common, there are also many differences, particularly emotional factors that cannot be quantitated. In such a study it is not possible to define or control the components of the patient population. For example, if patients with a large psychologic component to their pain were included, the results of an analgesic study would be much different from a study in which the patient population included primarily patients with a physiologic component.

6. *The physician's attitude toward pain will also influence its evaluation and treatment.* The surgeon often has an emotional makeup or personal prejudices that influence the evaluation of the pain patient. Surgeons in general are neither trained nor inclined to consider the psychologic problems of their patients except sometimes in a derisive manner. The idea that there must be an identifiable cause or the surgical mind-set that "I must do something" often leads to unnecessary operations that not only fail to solve the problem but add to the patient's difficulties. Most of the patients I see in our Chronic Pain Unit with psychogenic abdominal pain have had numerous laparotomies for "adhesions," a finding that should be considered unrelated to the problem of chronic pain unless it causes frank intestinal obstruction.

Specific Treatment Approaches

Acute Pain

The management of acute pain is primarily rest and the administration of analgesics on a short-term basis while the underlying cause is brought under control. Since all analgesics have been designed for acute pain and ordinarily will be required for only a brief period, there is insufficient time for tolerance and addiction to become a problem. Even so, the least amount of analgesia necessary to control pain should be employed. Nonnarcotic analgesics are usually the choice if the pain is not excessive. Narcotics should be employed in adequate doses to obtain reasonable pain relief after surgery or severe injury, but a strict limit should be placed on how long those doses are maintained. It is inappropriate and counterproductive to continue narcotics past the acute phase of convalescence (generally 5 to 10 days) even though some patients have difficulty giving up their drugs by that time.

Cancer Pain

Medical Treatment. Cancer pain can be considered continually recurring acute pain, although it shares some characteristics with chronic pain as well. The first line of management of cancer pain is pharmacologic. Because the patient's life expectancy is limited and it is anticipated that this individual will be taking analgesics for the rest of his life, addiction is not ordinarily a concern, and the regulation of analgesia should be determined by the magnitude of the pain. Because the cancer is most likely to cause progressive pain with increasing severity and because of the development of analgesic tolerance, it will be necessary to increase the dosage of analgesia as the requirement arises. However, the dose of a given drug should not be increased beyond the level required because tolerance to the drug may progress more rapidly, prematurely using up the patient's pharmacologic possibilities for continued drug management of pain.

Most orally administered narcotics are poorly absorbed or are detoxified by the liver so that it is necessary to adjust the dose accordingly. One of the difficulties encountered with the administration of narcotics for cancer pain on an as needed basis is the peaks and valleys in the blood levels of the drug. During the peak effect after administration of the drug, the patient may be oversedated and somnolent. As the effect of the drug wears off, the patient passes through a period of satisfactory analgesia and then enters another period of inadequate analgesia and withdrawal, with its attendant dysphoria, increase in pain perception, and depression. A large dose is then usually administered when the distress is intolerable, and the cycle is repeated. Unless the cancer patient can be instructed and relied on to take the pain medication before withdrawal occurs, scheduled doses are often more effective than intermittent ones in controlling pain, to prevent not only the peaks and valleys but the recurrent withdrawal as well.

If the patient reaches the point where he can no longer be comfortable with frequent small doses of the usual medications, one of the longer acting narcotics might be considered. Methadone has been extremely useful in this circumstance. Its long duration of action prevents the usual peaks and valleys of narcotic effect. Methadone is also absorbed almost completely by mouth and is not detoxified by the liver on first passage through it. Further, it seems to have the greatest analgesic effect for the amount of hypnosis or dysphoria of any available agent. Since the duration of action exceeds 8 hours it may be effective throughout the night and can be administered on a schedule of every 8 hours, or if necessary, every 6 hours. If a patient had been taking injectable narcotics at the time the methadone is prescribed, the methadone dose, scheduled in three divided doses at 8-hour intervals, should be equivalent to the dose of morphine necessary for pain relief over a 24-hour period.

A new form of slow-release morphine, MS Contin, in a wax medium may also prove very helpful in these patients. With this drug it is often possible to obtain good analgesia at a lower total dose mainly because it avoids the peaks and valleys. Like methadone, it can be administered every 6 hours or even every 8 hours. Finally, it may prove more convenient than methadone, which is often difficult to obtain because of the government regulations restricting its availability.

As a rule, the long-acting narcotics should not be given on an as-needed basis. They are slow to take effect and were not designed for that purpose. It is generally best to prescribe them on a scheduled basis with a "rescue" as-needed dose of another analgesic if pain management is not effective, at least until the dosage schedule for the longer acting narcotic is well established.

Narcotics should not be used as tranquilizers; analgesics are for analgesia. Accordingly, they are not appropriate drugs for agitation or depression and may make such problems worse. The psychiatric problems must be recognized and dealt with by counseling and the administration of antidepressants or tranquilizers as appropriate. Narcotic requirements usually decrease significantly when agitation, depression, and anxiety are managed by other means.

Because depression is so often a concomitant of pain in cancer patients and is an unfortunate side effect of almost all analgesics, it is frequently useful to give antidepressant agents along with analgesics. The total daily dose of an antidepressant may be given at bedtime, which may also help reestablish a normal sleep pattern in a frequently insomniac patient. Patients with cancer pain often respond to relatively low doses of tricyclic antidepressants (e.g., amitriptyline, 50 to 75 mg by mouth daily); if a higher dose is needed, it can be increased gradually until a therapeutic response is observed.

Surgical Ablation Techniques. If the patient still has intolerable pain despite the medical treatment program, a *neurosurgical procedure* might be considered. Usually for the cancer patient this involves an ablation technique, a procedure to interrupt one or several of the pain pathways described earlier in this chapter. The choice of procedure is determined by the distribution of the pain more than its specific characteristics and by whether the patient has so much emotional turmoil that a target should be selected that includes psychiatric relief as well.

The following general rules are formulated to select the most appropriate operation for those cancer patients who require an ablative procedure.[6]

1. It is preferable that the procedure affect only the most caudal or peripheral area that includes the region of pain.
2. If the patient has minor pain in an area other than the region of major pain, particularly on the contralateral side, the minor pain will probably increase when the major pain is alleviated.
3. The least change in sensory function is desirable. Thus procedures that leave an area totally insensitive should be avoided since patients may then develop a painful dysesthesia in this region. A cordotomy (see p. 227) that provides analgesia but preserves sensation is preferable to a procedure that causes numbness. The operative goal is to produce analgesia in the smallest area compatible with good pain relief.
4. Patients should not be talked into having a pain procedure. No pain procedure is ideal and all represent a trade-off for some other potential problem. If the pain is not so severe that the patient insists that something be done or if the patient is so depressed and anxious that he would not tolerate any procedure, it is best that none be performed.
5. Patients should be told of potential side effects of a proposed ablative procedure in detail. Once the pain is gone, side effects that seemed minor when described may become extremely distressing.
6. Disappointment following an ablative procedure should be anticipated. Patients often blame all of their disability on the pain and expect that once the pain is alleviated surgically, they will feel as they did before they had cancer. If the pain is alleviated and they still feel seriously ill and weak, all the consequences of a major illness must be faced. It is important therefore that both the physician and the patient have realistic goals when considering an ablative procedure for pain.

Most of the procedures for cancer pain involve interruption of the neospinothalamic tract. For bilateral, midline, or diffuse pain, interruption of the paleospinothalamic pathways may be more beneficial. If the pain involves the head or neck, the procedure must be done in the brain. If the pain involves the viscera, interruption of the archispinothalamic pathway in the spinal cord or the sympathetic pathway may be the procedure of choice.

Dorsal or sensory *rhizotomy* involves interruption of the dorsal nerve root as it enters the spinal cord (Fig. 12-6). Since the dorsal root involves fibers conducting all sensory modalities, total sensory loss occurs in those dermatomes affected, although there is some overlap between dermatomes. This procedure should be reserved for those patients with well localized pain involvement, usually with entrapment of the nerve itself. Dorsal rhizotomy is amazingly unsuccessful in many patients with pain following a thoracotomy, even though logic would dictate otherwise. To cut the dorsal roots as they enter the spinal cord, a laminectomy is required. Because the interruption lies

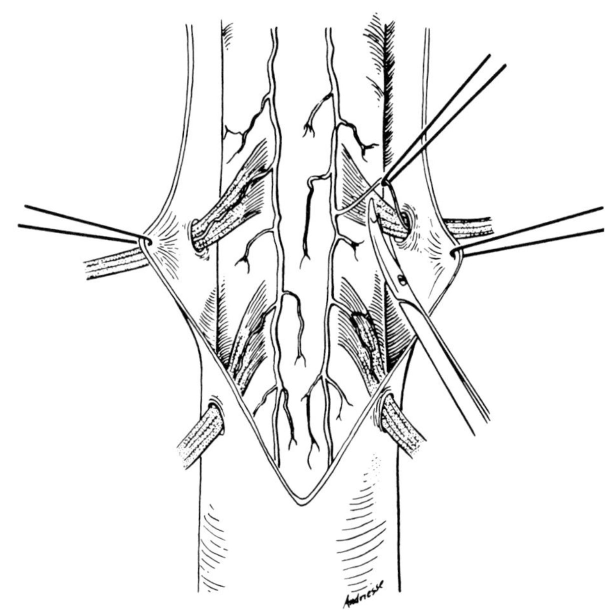

Fig. 12-6 Technique of dorsal rhizotomy. This approach spares important feeding arteries that accompany some of the posterior roots of the spinal cord. (From Loeser, J.D.: Dorsal rhizotomy. In Youmans, J., Neurological surgery, Philadelphia, 1982, W.B. Saunders Co.)

proximal to the cell bodies of the cut nerves, regeneration does not occur.

Another type of rhizotomy can be considered for rectal pain. When asked to describe the pain, some patients say that "it feels like I am sitting on a rock" or that "it feels like I always have to move my bowels." This sensation does not appear to be true pain conducted by well recognized pain pathways, even though it may be just as distressing to the patient; rather, it appears to be a distorted visceral sensation. Bilateral cordotomy, even with good analgesia, may not result in relief of this type of pain. If bowel and bladder function have already been lost because of the cancer or its therapy, a fairly simple procedure may be considered: *phenol sacral rhizotomy*. The patient is asked to sit at the side of the bed and a lumbar puncture is performed. Phenol crystals (500 mg) are dissolved in 2 ml of Pantopaque, which is very hyperbaric. When instilled through the lumbar puncture needle, it falls to the bottom of the thecal sac where it fixes the lower sacral nerve roots, frequently with excellent relief of pain. An occasional patient will also have some weakness of the hamstring muscles. It may be necessary to repeat the procedure if the pain returns in a few days, but usually the second dose of phenol provides permanent relief.[6]

After entering the spinal cord the neospinothalamic pain fibers cross to the other side before ascending to the brain. *Commissural myelotomy* involves interrupting those crossing fibers by bisecting the spinal cord over those segments involved with pain (Fig. 12-7). It is reserved for bilateral or midline body pain where pelvic metastases have occurred. A multilevel laminectomy is performed, and using the operating microscope, the surgeon divides the spinal cord over the appropriate number of segments corresponding to the patient's pain. The use of the operating microscope and the recognition that even bilateral cordotomies often do not help midline pelvic pain has led to renewed interest in this procedure.

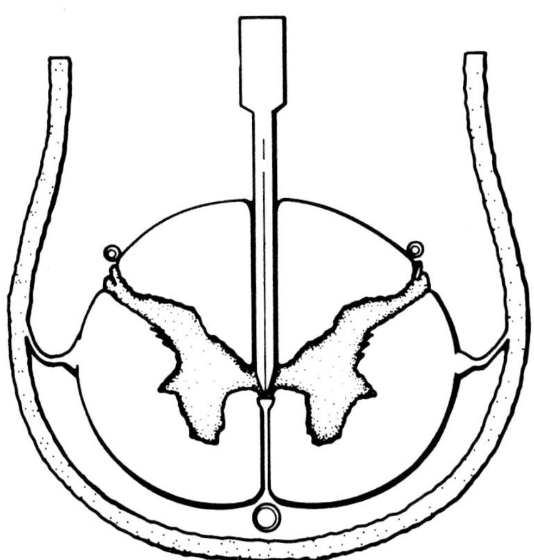

Fig. 12-7 Technique of myelotomy. The dissector is inserted through the midline of the spinal cord so that a mechanical lesion is made around the area of the central canal. (From Gildenberg, P.L., and Hirshberg, R.M.: Limited myelotomy for the treatment of intractable cancer pain, J. Neurol. Neurosurg. Psychiatry **47**:94, 1984.)

Many patients have excellent relief of pain after commissural myelotomy surgery, even though the area where nerve supply has been interrupted is not rendered completely analgetic. It has been theorized that perhaps the pain relief after myelotomy is not always the result of interruption of the decussating pain fibers but instead may be caused by trauma to the archispinothalamic pathways, which lie in the middle of the spinal cord. With this in mind, *limited myelotomy* involves making a lesion at the center of the cord at the C1 or midthoracic level. In many cases excellent relief of visceral or rectal pain can be obtained. For this procedure a one-level laminectomy is performed and a lesion created in the center of the cord either mechanically or with a radiofrequency electrode (see Fig. 12-7). The procedure at the C1 level is done stereotactically, wherein an electrode is inserted into the center of the spinal cord near the medulla under x-ray guidance, and the extralemniscal pathway is interrupted by a radiofrequency current.[10]

Cordotomy involves interruption of the lateral spinothalamic tract opposite the site of the pain within the spinal cord where it lies in the anterolateral quadrant away from fibers subserving other sensations (see Fig. 12-2). This is the most commonly used ablative procedure for cancer pain and is the procedure of choice for unilateral pain involving the lower part of the body. When used for this purpose, it is done at the T1 to T2 spinal level. Although primarily used for relief of unilateral pain, cordotomy can be performed bilaterally; but the patient must be advised, of course, that this could interfere with normal bladder, bowel, and sexual function. If the arm or shoulder is involved in the pain process, the cordotomy may be performed at the C2 level, but high cervical cordotomy should not be undertaken bilaterally because of the risk to the respiratory fibers that are intermingled with the pain fibers above the C4 level. Classically, cordotomy involves a laminectomy to expose the spinal cord several segments above the area of pain. The anterolateral quandrant is cut with a blade or a hook. Satisfactory relief can be anticipated in 85% of patients with cancer pain following cordotomy.

Recently, percutaneous cervical cordotomy has become the procedure of choice when cordotomy needs to be performed, since it can be done with the patient awake under local anesthesia obviating the need for general anesthesia, which is of particular concern in cancer patients who are often too debilitated for major surgery. Under x-ray guidance an electrode is inserted into the anterolateral quadrant of the spinal cord at the C1 to C2 level. The position of the electrode is tested with stimulation, and a radiofrequency lesion is made to interrupt the lateral spinothalamic tract. Because the patient is awake, a gradually progressive lesion can be made depending on the extent of the patient's pain.[26] Since bilateral cordotomy should not be done at the C2 level, an alternate percutaneous cervical cordotomy has been described to relieve bilateral pain involving the arms or shoulders wherein the needle is passed diagonally through the intervertebral disk in a lower cervical level. The angle of insertion can be calculated from anteroposterior and lateral x-rays of the neck.[17] With this approach bilateral pain relief can be achieved without concomitantly compromising respiratory function.

If pain involves the head, neck, or shoulder or if the patient has respiratory impairment and would not tolerate a cordotomy, satisfactory relief of cancer pain may be obtained by *mesencephalotomy,* interruption of the lateral spinothalamic tract at the level of the midbrain. The effect is essentially that of a cordotomy since the same pathway, the lateral spinothalamic tract, is interrupted but at a higher level. Thus the patient may have loss of pain sensation, not only over the contralateral half of the body, but the face and head as well. This procedure is generally performed stereotactically, using a stereotactic apparatus to guide an electrode accurately to any anatomical target (Fig. 12-8). With the patient under local anesthesia, the electrode is inserted into the lateral part of the midbrain at the level of the aqueduct. Electrical stimulation is applied to verify that the electrode lies within the lateral spinothalamic tract, in which case the patient has sensation projected to the opposite side of the body. The nerves in that area are somatotopically oriented with the face medial and the feet lateral. Pain relief can be obtained more consistently if the lesion also encroaches on the periaqueductal gray matter, paleospinothalamic and archispinothalamic fibers that lie just medial to the fibers concerned with sensation from the face. Because oculomotor fibers are in

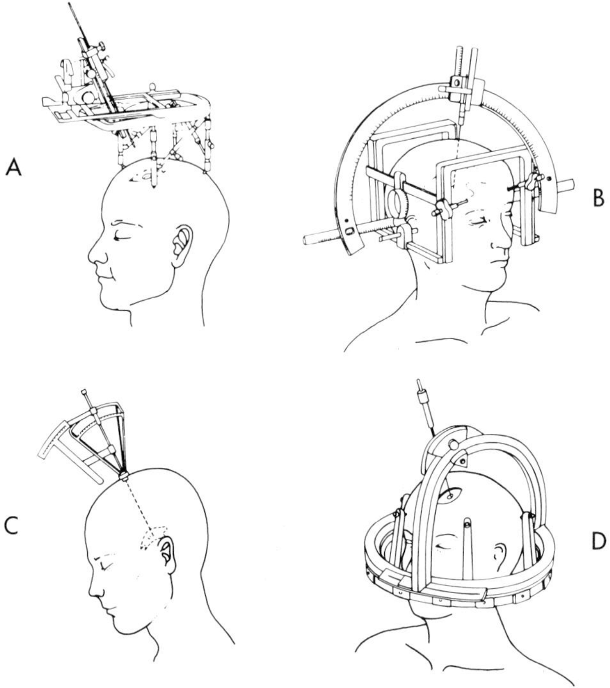

Fig. 12-8 Different types of stereotactic apparatus used in stereotactic neurosurgery. **A,** The rectilinear type, provides for the longitudinal and vertical movements of the electrode by simple linear mechanical adjustments. **C** is the swing type and consists of a ball joint screw into a burr hole, allowing the electrode to be pointed at a target and advanced into it. **B** and **D** represent two kinds of one type in which the target point lies at the center of an arc along which the electrode holder moves. (From Gildenberg, P.L.: Functional neurosurgery. In Schmidek, H.H., and Sweet, W.H., editors: Operative neurosurgical techniques, vol. 2, New York, 1982, Grune and Stratton, Inc.)

close opposition to that area, stimulation is also necessary to ensure that eye movements will not be adversely affected by the lesion.[8]

There are also several types of *thalamotomy* that can be surgically employed for pain relief, particularly cancer pain.[6] The convergence of the various neural pathways that relate to the different aspects of pathologic pain makes it possible to tailor the lesion within the thalamus to the needs of a given patient. The nonspecific fibers concerned with the paleospinothalamic and archispinothalamic systems ascend to the medial portion of the thalamus where they may be interrupted without sacrificing the lemniscal or neospinothalamic pathways. Such lesions may afford pain relief without significantly altering somatic sensation. Pain that lasts a long time, such as cancer pain, has several components to it. One is the pain sensation itself, which is a direct reflection of tissue injury. The other is "suffering," which indicates how intolerable the pain may be at any given time and need not be directly related to pain intensity. Thus under certain circumstances even relatively low-intensity pain can be intolerable and cause much suffering, whereas under other conditions a great deal of pain may be borne with very little suffering. The lemniscal or neospinothalamic pathways carry pain perception per se, whereas the nonspecific fibers of the paleospinothalamic and archispinothalamic systems are concerned with "suffering" and protect those parts of the brain that are concerned with the expression of emotion or with autonomic or sympathetic responses. It is now recognized that a great deal of relief may be obtained by alleviating the suffering component, even though it may not be possible to lessen pain sensation itself.

Basal thalamotomy (Fig. 12-9) involves the production of a small, discrete lesion to interrupt the archispinothalamic and paleospinothalamic fibers as they ascend toward the intralaminar nuclei, the centrum medianum, and the parafascicular nucleus. It can be used for cancer patients who have a large component of suffering. A prime example is the patient with Pancoast syndrome who may in addition to somatic pain have an intensely disagreeable distorted sensation, and who may not be significantly improved if only the somatic pain is alleviated. If it is desirable to alleviate both the suffering and the somatic pain sensation, basal thalamotomy may be combined with mesencephalotomy since the lesions are very close to each other. The basal thalamotomy lesion may also encroach on the neospinothalamic tract to provide the same result.

Medial thalamotomy (see Fig. 12-9) involves the production of a somewhat larger lesion to interrupt these same fibers at their termination in the intralaminar nuclei and centrum medianum. Although physicians originally hoped that basal thalamotomy would more efficiently produce longer-lasting and more complete pain relief than medial thalamotomy, the indications and results following these two procedures are comparable. Indeed, since it is usually desirable to make asymmetrical lesions if bilateral thalamotomy is indicated, perhaps the best chance for pain relief is to produce a unilateral intralaminar lesion with extension to the same level as the basal thalamotomy on the side opposite the greatest pain, and perform a dorsomedian thalamotomy on the alternate side. If necessary, the second side can be done in 3 to 6 weeks. Results for cancer pain have been good with this approach, early pain relief being achieved in 80% to 90% of patients.

Dorsomedian thalamotomy (Fig. 12-9) involves the production of a lesion in the dorsomedian nucleus to interrupt the origin of those fibers that project to the frontal lobe. It is generally employed for those patients with cancer pain who have a great deal of emotional distress (anxiety or depression as a result of having a terminal illness) in addition to the pain and its resultant suffering. This is the same thalamic lesion that has been employed for the treatment of various affective disorders (such as intractable depression or obsessive-compulsive behavior). Successful alleviation of pain has also been reported after bilateral lesions in the centrum medianum. In addition, lesions of the intralaminar nuclei have been successfully combined with lesions of the parafascicular complex for successful pain relief. This combination provides pain relief without analgesia, and the effects are similar to frontal leukotomy or cingulotomy, which have also been recognized as helpful surgical procedures to relieve cancer pain.

If pain involves only the face or head, it is quite difficult to obtain satisfactory relief from interruption of the trigeminal nerve because the area near the pharynx and middle ear are also supplied by the glossopharyngeal and vagus nerves and a portion of the area at the base of the skull is supplied by the second through fourth cervical nerve roots. In addition, interruption of the trigeminal nerve is frequently followed by dysesthesia or disagreeable anesthesia. Nonetheless, pain relief can often be obtained by a *medullary trigeminal tractotomy*, which interrupts the pain fibers in the descending tract of the nucleus caudalis of the trigeminal nerve at the level of the medulla or the upper cervical spinal cord (Fig. 12-10).[8] The procedure can be done by exposing the lateral medulla through a suboccipital craniectomy and C1 laminectomy. The fibers lie just below the surface anterior to the plane of emergence of the spinal accessory nerve. Alternately, an electrode can be inserted stereotactically and the lesion made under local anesthesia with radiofrequency current.[8]

Several conditions may benefit from *sympathectomy*, which not only interrupts the transmission of pain but also improves blood supply. One of the primary indications for sympathectomy is pain of vascular origin, particularly if pain persists after everything possible has been done to correct the vascular insufficiency. Sympathectomy may be especially useful for the pain of reflex sympathetic dystrophy, a condition whose mechanism is poorly understood and which may result from injury to a peripheral nerve (especially the median or sciatic nerve) to cause excruciating causalgia-type pain of an extremity (see p. 235). It is sometimes helpful to determine whether a patient may be a candidate for a surgical sympathectomy by performing a sympathetic block. However, failure to obtain pain relief from a block is not a definite indication that the patient would not benefit from a surgical sympathectomy. On the other hand, a patient sometimes has permanent relief of pain following repeated sympathetic blocks under local anesthesia obviating the need for sympathectomy.

For pain in the lower extremity, the lumbar sympathetic chain can be approached through a retroperitoneal dissection. It lies on the lateral surface of the upper lumbar vertebral bodies. To assure adequate sympathetic denervation, it is necessary to remove at least two ganglia and the intervening chain. Adequate denervation for relief of upper extremity pain can be accomplished with cervical sympathectomy without causing Horner's syndrome if the superior cervical ganglion is left untouched. There are various

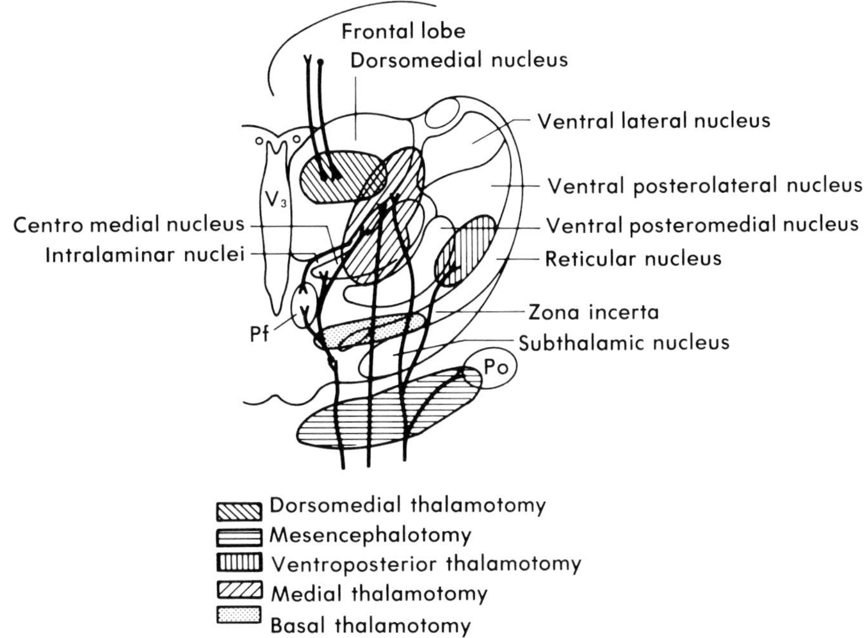

Fig. 12-9 Anatomic regions that are ablated during different types of thalamotomy. (From Gildenberg, P.L.: Functional neurosurgery. In Schmidek, H.H., and Sweet, W.H., editors: Operative neurosurgical techniques, vol. 2, New York, 1982, Grune & Stratton, Inc.)

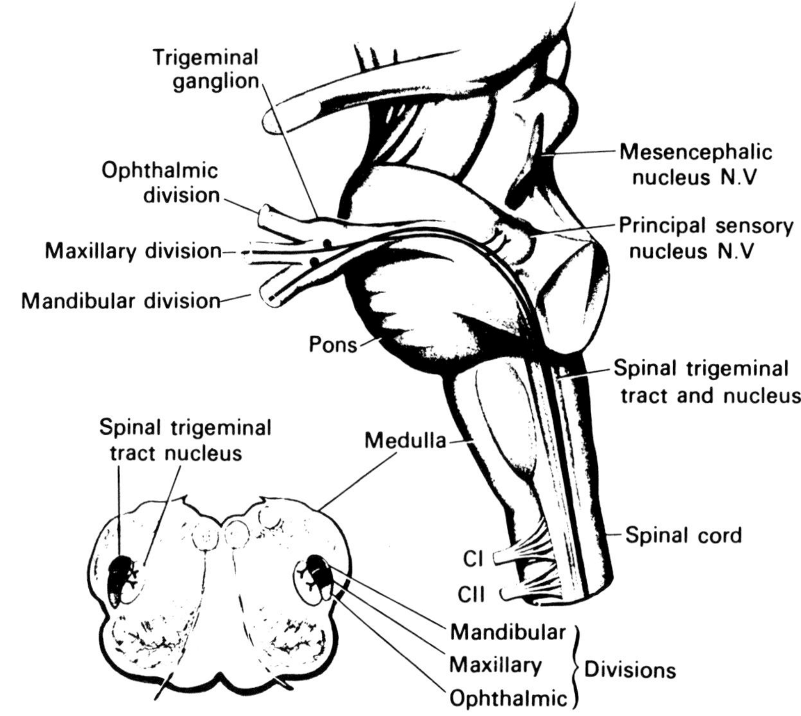

Fig. 12-10 Anatomic basis of medullary trigeminal tractotomy. (Reproduced with permission from Carpenter, M.B.: Human neuroanatomy, ed. 7, Baltimore, 1976, The Williams & Wilkins Co.)

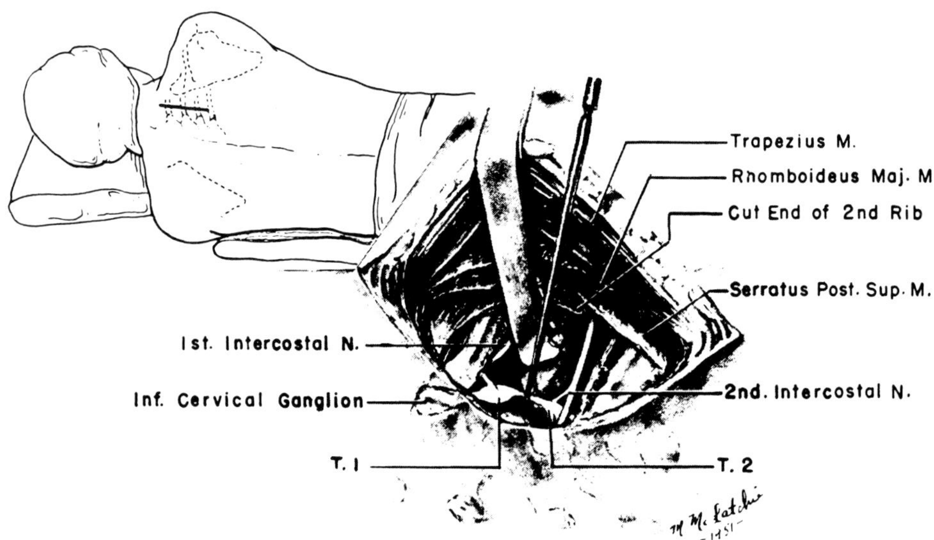

Fig. 12-11 Surgical approach to cervical sympathectomy. (From White, J.C., and Sweet, W.H.: Pain and the neurosurgeon, Springfield, Ill., 1969, Charles C Thomas.)

routes to the sympathetic chain in this area. Perhaps the most common route is the transaxillary approach where the brachial plexus is followed to the level of the sympathetic chain. However, I prefer the dorsal approach wherein a short piece of the proximal portion of the second rib is removed, and the ganglia just above and just below that exposed area are removed with the intervening chain (Fig. 12-11). With the good visualization and exposure obtained by this approach, it is almost always possible to perform an adequate sympathectomy without creating Horner's syndrome.

The pain resulting from carcinoma of the pancreas or retroperitoneal metastases can be severe, unremitting, and resistant to analgesics. In addition, it can be precipitated by eating, which may deprive the patient of adequate nutrition and hasten an already deteriorating state. Pain per-

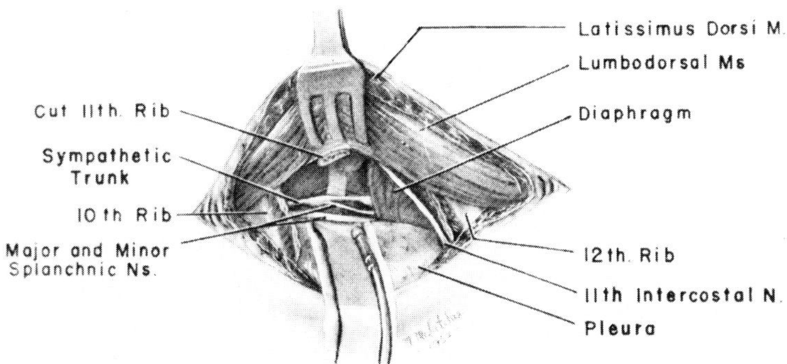

Fig. 12-12 Surgical approach to splanchnicectomy. (From White, J.C., and Sweet, W.H.: Pain and the neurosurgeon, Springfield, Ill, 1969, Charles C Thomas.)

ception of the pancreas is mediated through the abdominal sympathetic nerves, especially the small nerves from the celiac ganglion. The nerves responsible for this pain travel from that ganglion and join the three splanchnic nerves that supply sympathetic innervation to large parts of the abdominal viscera. Those three sympathetic nerves then join the sympathetic chain at or near the level of the diaphragm.

Pancreatic pain responds well to denervation in a majority of cases. When laparotomy is undertaken to make the diagnosis of pancreatic cancer, the opportunity is sometimes availed to perform a retroperitoneal dissection of the celiac plexus in an attempt to denervate the pancreas, a procedure called *celiac ganglionectomy*. Although this procedure often is successful in alleviating pain, not all surgeons routinely include it as part of their operative protocol in the management of pancreatic cancer. Further, even when ganglionectomy is performed, complete denervation is sometimes difficult because the plexus is a multitude of hardly visible, diffuse fibers. More complete denervation can be anticipated if section is performed above the diaphragm by sectioning the splanchnic nerves, a *splanchnicectomy* (Fig. 12-12). These nerves are readily accessible by removing the proximal portion of the eleventh rib. Usually two of the three splanchnic nerves are seen at that level, the greater and middle. The least splanchnic nerve often joins the sympathetic chain as it passes through the diaphragm. In order to assure denervation of that nerve as well, the sympathetic chain is divided and total denervation is accomplished by removing the two adjacent ganglia. It is generally advisable to perform splanchnicectomy as soon as it is certain that the patient has severe enough pain to warrant such a procedure rather than waiting until profound clinical deterioration from the underlying disease makes the risk of surgery prohibitive.

Chronic Pain of Benign Origin

The management of chronic pain of benign origin poses challenges that uniquely set it apart from the approaches that have been used to treat acute pain or cancer pain. Although any recognized derangements in normal physiology that may be contributing to chronic pain need to be addressed in any treatment protocol, the significant role that anxiety and depression play fostering this pain and influencing its effective management must be clearly understood. Thus for any chronic pain program to be successful and for a chronic pain patient to believe that his treatment has been successful, *realistic goals should be set* at the beginning of therapy. Many chronic pain patients have formulated no goals at all and merely drift from day to day; others may have as their goal an unrealistic return to a physical condition that may have existed years before and is no longer achievable; still others may have as their goal continued pain and disability.

Administration of narcotics to chronic pain patients produces dependency, tolerance and recurrent withdrawal, and adds significantly to depression, all of which interfere with any effective rehabilitation effort. Consequently, *narcotics should be withdrawn* at the start of a chronic pain management program. Most patients can be withdrawn abruptly, even though they may go through a period of increased pain during the withdrawal state. In time the pain tolerance increases and the pain perception diminishes so the patient usually ends up with much less pain when not taking the medication than he had while taking it. Other drugs that cause withdrawal problems and/or depression should also be discontinued, although barbiturates or diazepams must be withdrawn more gradually to avoid seizures.

The key to any successful treatment program for chronic pain is *the management of depression*. The hallmark of chronic pain and the one manifestation that is the most amenable to therapy is depression. It is normal for a patient to feel depressed when he is disabled, uncertain about the future, and in pain. However, the depression heightens pain perception and makes the pain much worse, which in turn causes increased depression. In addition, virtually all narcotics and tranquilizers used to manage acute pain have depression as a side effect and consequently make the pain worse. Patients who are depressed have little optimism or motivation for a rehabilitation program, which is the cornerstone of chronic pain management.[9,16,29]

One factor that adds significantly to depression in a surprising portion of chronic pain patients is unresolved grief. The death of a family member may have occurred several years before, but unless the patient has successfully navigated through the various stages of grief, the grieving process may remain unresolved and express itself as depression and chronic pain. This can be compounded when the person who was lost died of a painful condition with which the patient identifies.[4]

Depression can usually be managed with a combination of counseling and antidepressant medications. Following treatment of depression, patients frequently have a significant alleviation of their chronic pain. Interestingly, antidepressant medications appear to have a beneficial effect on chronic pain in general, even if the patient is not depressed, although the mechanism for this action is very poorly understood. It is only after alleviating chronic pain that the patient's downhill course can be reversed and rehabilitation efforts begun.

Chronic pain patients frequently have a dramatic decrease in physical activity. Thus they require a scheduled *remobilization program*. Many of the patients that I see in our Chronic Pain Unit have spent months sitting in front of a television set or lying in bed so that even normal physical activity provokes pain. Since these individuals already have a poor pain tolerance, any pain on even modest remobilization drives the patient back to the couch of immobility. Unfortunately, this process is often reinforced by the physician. It is appropriate to advise the patient with an acute pain problem to rest, but when a patient has chronic pain, the goal is for gradual and progressive mobilization.

Regression is the withdrawal of the patient from the responsibilities of adult behavior. A patient is sanctioned by society to "be taken care of" by a physician and family. Many patients who settle into a chronic pain state find this regressed posture more comfortable than that of responsible adulthood, particularly if the responsibilities they are escaping had been overwhelming to them before. The patient should be encouraged (or coerced) to become more physically active and consequently more independent. Behavioral modification is the key wherein the patient is rewarded with attention and approval for being up and independently active. If the patient regresses and becomes less active, the punishment is ordinarily lack of attention or approval.

One of the problems treating chronic pain patients in the acute care hospital setting is that the orientation of the program must be totally different. In the acute care setting nurses and hospital personnel are attuned to taking care of patients rather than promoting independence. Consequently it is virtually impossible to treat regression in the usual hospital environment.

Most patients with chronic pain have become withdrawn from friends and society and spend an inordinate amount of time sitting alone thinking about their pain. Patients can begin their *resocialization* process by interacting with other patients and eventually extending those social activities to relatives and friends.

Both *occupational* and *physical therapy* may be useful adjuncts in the management of chronic pain patients. Occupational therapy is helpful in breaking the pattern of regression. Most chronic pain patients need to relearn (or sometimes learn for the first time) recreational skills and activities of daily living. The specific requirements for *physical therapy* depend on the patient's individual pain problems. Since more than half of patients in Chronic Pain Units have low back problems, physical therapy uses the usual modalities directed at treating that area. In addition, remobilization involves an exercise program that begins extremely slowly but proceeds with relentless progression.

Biofeedback and *relaxation training* are necessary components of any chronic pain program. A vicious cycle occurs in chronic pain patients wherein stress causes the patient's subconscious to reflexly increase muscle tone. This is part of the "fight or flight" reaction, but it is an inappropriate response to stress. In the usual scenario the patient has stress either from the pain itself or from some external factor. This causes a stress reaction that involves a reflex increase in muscle tone, including muscles involved with myofascial pain. The increased muscle tone causes more pain, which in turn causes more stress, which heightens the muscle tone to cause more pain, and so forth.

To break this pattern it is necessary to attack the cycle in as many places as possible. The physical aspects are managed with physical therapy, especially massage or ultrasound, although trigger point blocks may sometimes be necessary. The stress-related feedback may be dealt with by a program of biofeedback. The patient receives a signal from an apparatus (usually an electromyographic electrode applied to the forehead) that indicates muscle tension. A tone or visual cue tells the patient how much muscle tension there is. The patient is then asked to decrease the signal and hence the muscle tone by conscious effort. The initial phase of biofeedback is presentation of the biofeedback signal. The second phase allows the patient to reduce muscle tone by using the same techniques when not connected to the biofeedback apparatus. In the third phase the patient unconsciously decreases muscle tone during stressful situations.

Closely akin to biofeedback is relaxation training. The patient does not receive a biofeedback signal but rather uses a preplanned procedure. An example would be a series of recordings in which the patient is instructed to relax one part of his body and then another in a conscious fashion or to imagine scenes or situations of relaxation. Physical techniques can also be incorporated into such relaxation sessions. Since it is possible to relax a muscle group more efficiently if it is first contracted isometrically and then relaxed, the patient is instructed to go through a series of physical maneuvers in which muscle groups in various parts of the body are first contracted and then relaxed.[15] Patients can also readily learn techniques to induce a state of self-hypnosis while still retaining consciousness for both relaxation and reduction of the perception of pain. All of these techniques are particularly helpful for pain of myofascial origin such as chronic low back strain with or without a preexisting injury, muscle tension headaches, atypical fascial pain (which often involves teeth clenching and a resultant temporomandibular joint dysfunction), or pain following a "whiplash" injury that frequently persists for a considerable period of time.

Specific Procedures in Chronic Pain of Benign Origin. It is inappropriate to treat chronic pain of benign origin by interrupting pain pathways since the pain almost invariably returns in patients who have been subjected to these procedures within 3 months to 2 years. Although it is suspected that other pain pathways assume the role of transmitting the painful impulses, it must also be speculated that much of the recurrence involves the motivational-affective system. Many patients with chronic pain have psychologic reasons why they need their pain and can adjust to the pain-free state only temporarily. Even if the physical cause for the pain is successfully alleviated, these patients are very often unable to return to a nondisabled state because they need their pain to cope with the world around them. Since the nervous system learns very well, those areas of the brain concerned with the perception of pain may continue to be active even after the peripheral stimulation is removed.

Approximately 20% of chronic pain patients are resistant to pain management. We call this group the "need to suffer" group. These patients have a lifelong history of recurrent disasters such as failed marriages, marriages to abusive spouses, multiple accidents, inability to retain satisfactory employment, working in an abusive situation. The pain fulfills a psychologic need for them. The pain of surgery is inviting to them, and many of these patients have had multiple operations of many types such as repeated laminectomies and negative exploratory laparotomies for "adhesions" or multiple injuries. Each surgical procedure is followed by a period of pain relief usually lasting 3 to 6 weeks, which only serves to entice the surgeon into performing more operations. Many patients classified as having Munchausen's syndrome fall into this category. This condition is characterized by habitual presentation for hospital treatment of an apparent, acute illness, given with a plausible and dramatic history, all of which is knowingly false.

Does this mean that there are no surgical procedures that can help patients with chronic pain of benign origin? Certainly not. However, the following rules must be followed in considering a surgical approach for pain control in chronic pain patients:

1. Before any surgical procedure is considered, the patient should undergo a program of conservative management. The patient's pain may be relieved so well with a nonsurgical approach that surgery becomes unnecessary, or it may become so apparent that the patient has so much need for his pain that any procedure will be unsuccessful.
2. Evaluation should be made only after the patient is no longer depressed, addicted, or regressed.
3. If the pain is of a specific nature and has a specific therapy, such therapy should be incorporated into an overall comprehensive pain program.
4. Goals must be appropriate. Not all pain patients can be freed from their pain, but the goal must be to allow the patient to live the least disabled and most drug-free life possible.
5. Only if a specific cause exists and psychiatric factors are controlled should a pain procedure be considered.

A stimulation rather than ablative procedure is the only surgical approach generally indicated for the management of chronic pain of benign origin. Stimulation procedures take advantage of the gating mechanisms to modify pain perception. Advantages of chronic stimulation are as follows:

1. Since pain pathways are not interrupted, there is no permanent alteration of sensation.
2. Side effects such as dysesthesia that occur following ablation procedures are quite rare.
3. Tolerance ordinarily does not develop unless the patient uses the stimulator constantly. If tolerance should develop, a period of time away from the stimulator will generally return effectiveness.
4. The patient himself controls the stimulation. Having some control over the situation may in and of itself afford the patient considerable pain relief.
5. It must be recognized that stimulation procedures for the control of pain are not magical nor do they cure the underlying problem. They are a helpful adjunct to a comprehensive treatment program but do not take the place of any other part of the program.
6. Perhaps the major reason why stimulation procedures may fail is improper patient selection. Patients who are depressed are not inclined to respond to any treatment and patients who are addicted rarely have pain relief.

Based on these considerations, certain types of stimulation have become important in the management of chronic pain of benign origin.

Transcutaneous stimulation. The gate theory indicates that stimulation of large sensory fibers, those subserving sensations other than pain, close the gate and inhibit pain perception. This theory led to the development of transcutaneous electronic neurologic stimulators (TENS) that could be taped to the skin over the painful area. The patient adjusts the voltage until a sensation is felt but does not feel painful. By definition this is the voltage at which large fibers, but not small fibers, are stimulated. TENS units have been found helpful in many conditions, both acute and chronic. They can also be applied adjacent to a surgical incision to minimize postoperative pain, which may decrease the narcotic requirements and thereby enable more effective breathing and diminish the incidence of postoperative atelectasis.

Spinal cord stimulation. If the pain involves a larger area than can be treated with a transcutaneous stimulator, a more efficient mode of stimulation must be sought. Large nerve fibers concerned with touch and proprioception ascend in the posterior columns of the spinal cord. Each fiber sends off a collateral to the substantia gelatinosa to close the gate. Thus an accident of nature provides that the dorsal spinal cord consists almost entirely of large nerve fibers concerned with nonpainful sensation. If the dorsal columns are stimulated, the impulse goes in both directions, up the spinal cord to the brain to be perceived as sensation and down the spinal cord to each of the collaterals at lower spinal cord segments to participate in gate control of pain in an inhibitory fashion. Consequently it was theorized that stimulation of the dorsal columns would inhibit transmission of pain in all of the segments below that region stimulated.

Spinal cord stimulation can be used to treat pain particularly in the lower part of the body. It has been found especially helpful for neuropathic pain such as multiple radiculopathy secondary to adhesive arachnoiditis or peripheral neuropathy. Pain of intermittent claudication can be dramatically relieved allowing the patient far more mobility. There is some evidence, particularly from studies performed in Europe, that spinal cord stimulation may also improve blood flow in patients with peripheral vascular disease to allow healing of vascular ulcers, but this has not yet been well documented in the United States.[20] In patients treated with spinal cord stimulation epidural electrodes are connected to a radio receiver implanted subcutaneously. The patient controls the stimulation with a hand-held radio transmitter.

Deep brain stimulation. Another technique that is being used in some centers for the management of chronic pain of benign origin is deep brain stimulation. An electrode, usually with multiple contacts, is inserted stereotactically into those areas of the brain that have been identified as producing the perception of analgesia on stimulation. These include the somatosensory area of the thalamus and the posterior limb of the internal capsule. Although frank analgesia is not produced, alleviation of chronic pain of various types has been documented.

Generally for chronic pain of benign origin and in some cases the pain of malignancy, an electrode is inserted into the periaqueductal gray matter or the posterior part of the periventricular gray matter near the posterior part of the third ventricle. It is from this area that fibers descend to the nucleus raphe magnus. The electrode is connected through subcutaneous leads to a radio receiver similar to the one used for spinal cord stimulation and is usually implanted in the subcutaneous fascia just below the clavicle. Response to such stimulation varies greatly, which has led to considerable disagreement about the effectiveness of deep brain stimulation as a treatment modality.[25]

Pain of neurogenic or central origin may be relieved by stimulation of the somatosensory areas of the thalamus, the ventral posterior nuclear area, or possibly the internal capsule. Presumably much neuropathic pain or denervation pain exists because parts of the nervous system fire inappropriately when deprived of their normal input. Stimulation above those areas may provide an artificial but nonpainful input where none existed before.[13,14]

OTHER SPECIFIC PAIN-RELATED PROBLEMS

A number of specific problems that are related to pain are encountered commonly enough in surgical practice to warrant further discussion. Perhaps the most common of these problems encountered by the general surgeon is *adhesions*. This diagnosis is frequently attached to patients who fit the classical psychiatric criteria for chronic pain on an emotional basis and happen to localize their pain to the abdomen. The mechanism for abdominal pain secondary to adhesions is physiologically obscure unless it specifically involves obstruction, inflammation, or perforation of a viscus. By far, most patients with chronic pain presumably caused by adhesions are individiuals who may or may not have a history of an identified intra-abdominal lesion that was diagnosed on objective criteria. Previously they have either had surgery for a specific intra-abdominal lesion or may have been subjected to exploratory laparotomy because of continued complaints of abdominal pain, in light of negative studies. Indeed, most of the patients that I have seen in the Chronic Pain Clinic have had anywhere from three to twelve abdominal procedures to look for an elusive cause for their chronic abdominal pain. After the first procedure adhesions are frequently found since they are often part of the natural healing process; they then become a handy diagnosis to explain future pain even though they may not be responsible for it. It is especially important therefore to avoid administering narcotics to this group of patients since one of the manifestations of recurrent withdrawal is intestinal hyperactivity alternating with suppression of peristalsis. This drug-induced intestinal disturbance can intensify the problem of abdominal pain, making management even more difficult.

Phantom limb pain is also not infrequently encountered in surgical practice. There are several theories to explain its physiology. The most popular is that, in the absence of naturally occurring somatosensory input from an extremity the central nervous system has a tendency to provide the missing information. However, this information may be distorted. The patient may perceive the extremity being held in a disagreeably painful position. An extremity lost early in life is ordinarily not associated with chronic pain. An extremity lost under a very painful circumstance, especially with a crushing or physically disruptive injury where pain has persisted for some time before the amputation was performed, is more likely to involve phantom pain than an extremity that is suddenly and cleanly lost. This evidence suggests that the learning process is very much involved with phantom limb pain. If a particular pathway is repeatedly stimulated, subsequent stimulation of the pathway can occur at a lower threshold, which appears to be the basis for much short-term learning. If the pathways involving pain from an extremity have been stimulated repeatedly over a protracted period, the threshold to such painful stimulation may be so low that the pain pathway fires spontaneously.

Because of these considerations, most procedures that have been designed to manage phantom limb pain involve stimulating the somatosensory system that ordinarily would supply the missing extremity. Stimulation of individual peripheral nerves in a chronic manner with an implanted stimulator has been employed, but ordinarily phantom limb pain involves more than just a single nerve distribution. Stimulation of the spinal cord has been used successfully to combat phantom limb pain, particularly when the perceived sensation goes into the missing extremity. Deep brain stimulation, either in the somatosensory or the periventricular areas, may also be successful.

It is important to differentiate between stump pain and phantom limb pain. Stump pain can more often be managed with a comprehensive pain program and local treatment. Although it is popular to perceive a neuroma in the stump as the cause of stump pain in many patients, this finding is actually a rare occurrence. Such a diagnosis should only be entertained if the pain is very sharp and localized to a single area and can be precipitated very specifically by local palpation with repeated alleviation of the tenderness by local anesthetic. Even so, patients with a neuroma may not have alleviation of pain because the local anesthetic does not distribute evenly in the scarred tissue. After many futile experiences at trying to find neuromas in incisions or stumps, I have come to the conclusion that such a search should generally not be undertaken. The individual nerve going to the area causing stump pain should be identified proximal to the scar tissue and sectioned at that point.

Although *myofascial pain* has been discussed earlier in this chapter, some additional comments are in order. Myofascial pain is the most common type of problem that involves chronic pain. In the Pain Clinic, approximately 55% of patients bear that diagnosis. The typical history of myofascial pain involves an accident that causes sudden pulling of muscles, e.g., a sudden deceleration injury that causes sudden stretch of posterior cervical muscles or excessively heavy lifting that causes a sudden stretch of the lumbar muscles. The patient is immediately aware that something happened, but it may not be until several hours later or even the next day that the pain becomes severe. This is unfortunately used by unknowledgeable or unscrupulous lawyers and/or insurance companies to "prove" that the patient's pain is not the direct result of a particular injury. The pain does not generally follow a radicular distribution, although it may be referred to the proximal part of the adjacent extremity. Thus a lumbar myofascial pain usually involves the muscle where it attaches to the crest of the sacrum or ilium, and when severe may radiate to the proximal leg, but ordinarily not below the knee. In contrast, pain of a herniated disk usually follows a radicular distribution when it extends into the leg, as it usually does.

The injury presumably involves tearing of muscle fibers. This may set up an area where the muscle spindles, which regulate muscle tone, become injured or hyperactive; the myotatic reflex causes a local increase in muscle tone, usually to the point where the sustained muscle contraction causes pain and sometimes to the point where frank muscle spasm ensues. This local area of injury is a trigger point since it triggers muscle spasm that may then spread over a large area of adjacent muscles. During physical examination the trigger point can often be identified by local tenderness on deep palpation and can be further identified by alleviation of the pain (and often muscle spasm) when the trigger point is injected with very small amounts of local anesthetic.

The treatment of chronic myofascial pain involves a chronic pain program. Biofeedback and relaxation training are particularly helpful, and trigger point blocks may also be necessary. There are a number of contrasting protocols for the administration of such a block. In my experience, after identification of the trigger point on deep palpation, it should be possible to block it with no more than 1 ml of local anesthetic. An individual patient, however, may have a number of trigger points but usually no more than four or six. Once the trigger points are identified, they may be dealt with by applying local deep massage or vibration; on occasion, ultrasound may help to break up the local muscle spasm. Trigger point blocks can be performed every 1 to 2 weeks, starting with local anesthetic and then adding equal amounts of a steroid preparation such as triamcinolone. If progress is being made but the trigger points are still resistant, an injection with 1 ml of local anesthetic followed by 1 ml of 10% phenol may allow long-term anesthesia of the involved muscle spindles and enable the patient to recover from the chronic pain syndrome.[9]

Pain following thoracotomy is the most common pain following incision, which is not surprising when the mechanics of a rib spreader are considered. It may result from compression of the intercostal nerve or injury at the costotransverse process joint. The pain is usually described as radiating along the incision, although it may incorporate only one part of the incision. Searching for a neuroma along the incision is most often a futile pastime. The pain can sometimes be controlled by interrupting the intercostal nerve as far proximal as possible. Unfortunately, by the time this procedure is considered, most patients are already depressed and addicted, and incorporation into a comprehensive chronic pain program is frequently necessary in addition to the intercostal neurectomy.

One of the most severe and devastating clinical pain syndromes is *reflex sympathetic dystrophy*. It occurs most frequently following injury to the median nerve in the arm or the sciatic nerve in the leg but can occur with injury to other nerves as well. The exact physiologic mechanism is not understood, but a reflex appears to be set up that results in spasm of the small blood vessels in the distal part of the extremity. The pain is severe and dysesthetic in nature. It can be precipitated by even the lightest touch or by a breeze blowing across the hand or foot. Trophic changes occur with the skin appearing shiny and atrophic and on occasion becoming cold and somewhat cyanotic. Typically the patient has a drawn and haggard expression as, for example, he cradles one hand over the other in order to protect the dystrophic extremity.

Relief can be dramatic on interruption of sympathetic innervation. One or several sympathetic blocks may help disrupt the reflex pattern and lead to permanent pain relief. If surgical sympathectomy is necessary, good relief may be obtained by removal of the first and second thoracic ganglia for the upper extremity or the lowest three lumbar ganglia for lower extremity pain. Because of the consistency of pain relief on sympathetic denervation, it appears that the sympathetic fibers act not only to produce the vascular spasm but also may be the pathway through which pain is transmitted to the brain.[11]

SUMMARY

Pain cannot be considered a simple sensation such as touch or temperature, and it becomes especially complex when the number of factors that may influence its perception in various clinical situations are considered. There are several different pathways by which pain sensation is transmitted through the nervous system, and these project to many different brain areas. Consequently the concept that it is possible to treat chronic pain by merely interrupting the "pain pathway" is incorrect and should be abandoned.

To determine the optimum program for managing pain, it is necessary to consider whether pain is acute pain, chronic pain of benign origin, or cancer pain. Acute pain is managed by administering analgesics on a short-term basis and treating the underlying cause. Cancer pain is managed by giving analgesics, possibly in increasing doses, and by interrupting pain pathways when pharmacologic response has been exceeded. Chronic pain of benign origin is treated by strict avoidance of analgesics and surgical procedures to interrupt pain pathways, by management of depression, regression, and addiction, and occasionally by chronic stimulation of the nervous system. Some particular types of pain may require specific procedures directed at the cause of the pain, but these patients must be selected with care.

REFERENCES

1. Basubaum, A.I., and Fields, H.L.: Endogenous pain control mechanisms: review and hypothesis, Ann. Neurol. **4:**451, 1978.
2. Beitel, R.E., and Dubner, R.: The response of unmyelinated (C) polymodal nociceptors to thermal stimuli applied to the monkey's face, J. Neurophysiol **39:**1160, 1976.
3. Bessou, P., and Perl, E.R.: Response of cutaneous sensory unit with unmyelinated fibers to noxious stimuli, J. Neurophysiol. **32:**1025, 1969.
4. DeVaul, R.A., and Zisook, S.: Unresolved grief, clinical considerations, Postgrad. Med. **5:**267, 1976.
5. Evan, F.J.: The placebo response in pain reduction. In Bonica, J.J., editor: Pain, Adv. Neurol. **4:**289, 1974.
6. Gildenberg, P.L.: Functional neurosurgery. In Schmidek, H.H., and Sweet, W.H., editors: Operative neurosurgical techniques, vol. 2, New York, 1982, Grune & Stratton, Inc.
7. Gildenberg, P.L.: Neuromuscular physiology and pain control. In Peters, R.M., Peacock, E.E., Jr., and Benfield, J.R., editors: Science applied to surgery, New York, 1983, Little, Brown & Co., Inc.
8. Gildenberg, P.L.: Mesencephalic and medullary tractotomy. In Bonica, J.J., et al., editors: The management of pain in clinical practice, ed. 2, Philadelphia, 1987, Lea & Febiger.
9. Gildenberg, P.L., and DeVaul, R.A.: The chronic pain patient: evaluation and management, Basel, 1985, S. Karger.
10. Gildenberg, P.L., and Hirshberg, R.M.: Limited myelotomy for the treatment of intractable pain, J. Neurol. Neurosurg. Psychiatry **47:**94, 1984.
11. Hardy, R.W., Jr.: Surgery of the sympathetic nervous system. In Schmidek, H.H., and Sweet, W.H., editors: Operative neurosurgical techniques, New York, 1982, Grune & Stratton, Inc.
12. Hitchcock, E.R.: Stereotactic cervical myelotomy, J. Neurol. Neurosurg. Psychiatry **33:**224, 1970.
13. Hosobuchi, Y., Adams, J.E., and Linchitz, R.: Pain relief by electrical stimulation of the central gray matter in humans and its reversal by naloxone, Science **197:**183, 1977.
14. Hosobuchi, Y., Adams, J.E., and Rutkins, B.: Chronic thalamic stimulation for the control of facial anesthesia dolorosa, Arch. Neurol. **29:**158, 1973.
15. Jacobson, E.: Modern treatment of tense patients, Springfield, Ill., 1970, Charles C Thomas, Publisher.
16. Liebeskind, J.C., and Paul, L.A.: Psychological and physiological mechanisms of pain, Annu. Rev. Physiol. **28:**41, 1977.
17. Lin, P., Gildenberg, P.L., and Polakoff, P.P.: An anterior approach to percutaneous lower cervical cordotomy, J. Neurosurg. **25:**553, 1966.
18. Mayer, D.J., and Hayes, R.L.: Stimulation-produced analgesia: development of tolerance and cross-tolerance to morphine, Science **188:**941, 1975.
19. Mayer, D.J., and Liebeskind, J.C.: Pain reduction by focal electrical stimulation of the brain: an anatomical and behavioral analysis, Brain Res. **68:**73, 1974.
20. Meglio, M., Cioni, B., and Dal Lago, A.: Pain control and improvement in peripheral blood flow following epidural spinal cord stimulation, J. Neurosurg. **54:**821, 1981.
21. Melzack, R., and Wall, P.D.: Pain mechanisms: a new theory, Science **150:**971, 1965.
22. Nashold, B.S., Jr.: Extensive cephalic and oral pain relieved by midbrain tractotomy, Confin. Neurol. **34:**382, 1972.
23. Perl, E.R.: Myelinated afferent fibers innervating the primate skin and their response to noxious stimuli, J. Physiol. **197:**593, 1968.
24. Perl, E.R.: Characterization of nociceptors and their activation of neurons in the superifical dorsal horn: first steps for the sensation of pain, Adv. Pain Res. Ther. **6:**23, 1984.
25. Richardson, D.E., and Akil, H.: Pain reduction by electrical brain stimulation in man. II. Chronic self-administration in the periventricular gray matter, J. Neurosurg. **47:**184, 1977.
26. Rosomoff, H.L., Brown, C.J., and Sheptak, P.: Percutaneous radiofrequency cervical cordotomy, J. Neurosurg. **23:**639, 1965.
27. Ruch, T.C., and Patton, H.D.: Physiology and biophysics, Philadelphia, 1965, W.B. Saunders Co.
28. Schvarz, J.R.: Spinal cord stereotactic techniques. Re: Trigeminal nucleotomy and extralemniscal myelotomy, Appl. Neurophysiol. **41:**99, 1978.
29. Sternbach, R.A.: Pain and depression. In Kiev, R., editor: Somatic manifestations of depressive disorders, Amsterdam, 1974, Excerpta Medica Foundation.
30. Willis, W.D.: The pain system: the neural basis of nociceptive transmission in the mammalian nervous system, Basel, 1985, S. Karger.
31. Willis, W.D., Kenshalo, D.R., Jr., and Leonard, R.B.: The cells of origin of the primate spinothalamic tract, J. Comp. Neurol. **188:**543, 1979.

13 Richard P. Saik

Physiologic Principles in Preparing a Patient for Surgery

Making the decision to perform a surgical procedure is one of the most complicated and controversial aspects of surgical practice. When no other alternative offers an optimum outcome for the patient with a given disease process, the decision to perform surgery is clear-cut. In other cases the timing, type, and efficacy of a surgical procedure in controlling or alleviating disease will involve weighing the risks and benefits of a given procedure for an individual patient. In many instances alternative surgical or medical therapies are available to treat a disease, and the physician must consider these factors in determining the patient's best interest. For example, many advocate nonsurgical methods (radiation, chemotherapy) in the treatment of breast cancer instead of surgery. At the same time many surgical options are currently available to treat breast cancer, each with its exponents and many with similar survival statistics, including simple removal of the breast lump with or without axillary node biopsy, total mastectomy, partial mastectomy, radical mastectomy, modified radical mastectomy, or extended radical mastectomy.

Better understanding of the natural history of disease and advances in surgical and medical techniques make some management decisions clearer but others more complex. The surgical procedure ultimately chosen for a given patient will depend not only on the particular disease being treated, but also on the patient's general health at surgery and the presence or absence of associated disease unrelated to the primary disorder. Thus appropriate preoperative preparation is absolutely mandatory to determine the best therapeutic approach and also to minimize risks and lessen complications that can adversely influence even the best technically performed operative procedure.

GENERAL ASPECTS OF PREOPERATIVE PREPARATION

History and Physical Examination

The basic history and physical examination (H and P) is important because it points to the diagnosis of a given disease and often identifies associated factors that could complicate a surgical procedure. The omission of some detail may adversely influence the course of a surgical procedure or the patient's postoperative convalescence. To patients, an H and P is usually the springboard for either inspiring confidence or doubt in the physician and for assessing the physician's sympathy for their problems.

Usually it is inadvisable to discontinue previous medications and start new ones immediately before surgery without adequate justification. New drugs may complicate the anesthetic management, and patients usually have some degree of confidence in the rationale and effectiveness of medications they have been using.

Extremes of age, i.e., less than 1 year or more than 70 years, are associated with an increased surgical risk. Operative mortality for an infant in the first year of life is four times that for young adults. Operative mortality rates generally increase with age, and the person over 70 has a 10 times greater risk than the young adult.[49] (See Chapter 66.)

Physical status should be assessed preoperatively; such variables as the type of procedure and age of the patient are critical factors in modifying the risk of anesthesia. These factors can be accurately estimated according to the American Society of Anesthesiologists' physical status system (Table 13-1).[43]

Surgical Consent

The details of a given procedure should be discussed with the patient and the family before the surgery. Discussion should cover the diagnosis, prognosis, business details, risks, benefits, family role, fears, potential problems, and the various roles of physicians and nurses perioperatively and postoperatively.

The standard "consent form" should be explained so that the patient understands the limitations, risks, and potential needs for further therapy. Repetition is necessary. Some preparation is expected by the patient, i.e., instructions regarding showers, dietary changes. Most patients are new to the hospital environment, are afraid, and may wish to deny their illness and its implications. The physician must be available to explain as many details and answer as many questions as necessary to dispel any anxiety that the patient or the family may have, although it is probably impossible to be too detailed or to answer too many questions about "what it will be like."[53]

Second Opinion

The request for another opinion should be viewed postively by both surgeon and patient and may help to relieve anxiety. Many medical insurance policies now require second opinions as a condition for full coverage for a given surgical procedure. It is in the patient's and the surgeon's interest to maximize insurance coverage. If the second opinion differs from the original recommendation, it is always better to obtain such disagreement preoperatively rather than when the patient has experienced a postopera-

Table 13-1 **CLASSIFICATION OF ANESTHETIC RISK BASED ON PHYSICAL STATUS ACCORDING TO THE AMERICAN SOCIETY OF ANESTHESIOLOGISTS**

Class*	Description	Examples
1	Normally healthy patient	No significant systemic disease
2	Patient with mild systemic disease	Mild anemia Controlled systemic arterial hypertension Mild chronic obstructive pulmonary disease (COPD) Minimally decreased renal function
3	Patient with severe systemic disease that is not incapacitating	Severe hypertension Coronary disease with stable angina or previous myocardial infarction Compensated congestive heart failure Moderate COPD "Brittle" insulin-dependent diabetes Moderate renal failure Cirrhosis without encephalopathy
4	Patients with incapacitating systemic disease that is a constant threat to life	Hypertensive encephalopathy Coronary disease with unstable angina or recent myocardial infarction Uncompensated heart failure with pulmonary edema and/or decreased cardiac output Severe COPD with respiratory failure Severe renal failure with metabolic and electrolyte abnormalities Acute hepatic necrosis or cirrhosis with encephalopathy
5	Moribund patient who is not expected to survive for 24 hr with or without surgery	Ruptured aortic aneurysm Ruptured intracranial aneurysm Massive trauma with severe shock Cardiac arrest

Reprinted from Chambers, D.: Anesthesia: methods, effects, and risks in the medical patient. In Lubin, M.F., Walker, H.K., and Smith, R.B., editors: Medical management of the surgical patient, Stoneham, Mass., 1982, Butterworth Publishers. With permission from the publisher.

*Emergency cases are designated by adding the letter E to the appropriate classification number.

tive complication or unsatisfactory outcome from unnecessary or inappropriate surgery.

Skin Preparation

Skin preparation should be performed to minimize infectious complications caused by endogenous microflora of the skin. Removal of excessive hair and scrubbing with detergent eradicates foreign material and loose epithelial cells, but shaving the skin causes nicks and cuts, which are colonized by pathogenic organisms in the hospital environment over time. Thus it is preferable to shave the operative site just before the procedure rather than the previous day or evening. The use of electric clippers and depilatories may have advantages with respect to skin trauma but are cumbersome and require more personnel time, thus limiting their practicality.

A 10-minute surgical scrub with hexachlorophene, chlorhexidine, or povidone-iodine is effective in reducing the bacterial count of the skin, and all these drugs possess a prolonged action. Antibiotic agents are more effective, but excessive cost makes their routine use prohibitive and impractical.[61] Rarely will a patient develop a hypersensitivity reaction to these cleaning agents. Iodine can be irritating if left on the skin for a prolonged time or if it puddles underneath the patient. An infected site near the planned incision, such as a furuncle or open wound, should be treated before undertaking the operative procedure.

Colon Preparation

Colon preparation for surgery of the large bowel is performed both to cleanse the bowel mechanically and to reduce the intraluminal bacterial count. Many different regimens have been advocated to achieve these goals and employ a combination of dietary restriction, purgation, enemas, and nonabsorbable antibiotics active against enteric organisms. A standard 3-day bowel preparation follows:

Day 1	Low-residue diet Castor oil or magnesium sulfate (30 ml of 50%) in morning
Day 2	Low-residue diet Magnesium sulfate (30 ml) in morning and afternoon Saline enemas in afternoon
Day 3	Clear liquids until evening before surgery Magnesium sulfate in morning Neomycin, 1 g orally at 1, 6, and 10 PM Erythromycin, 1 g at 1, 6, and 10 PM Saline enema in afternoon Intravenous fluid replacement (optional) Nothing orally after midnight
Day 4	Surgery

Elemental diets (clear liquid regimen) may be used instead of this low-residue diet but have no definite advantage. Recently it has become popular to substitute large quantities of electrolyte solutions orally (Golytely) for saline enemas and cathartics to induce purgation, but this technique should be used cautiously in the elderly or when subacute intestinal obstruction is suspected. Although controversial, most surgeons use some antibiotic preparation 1 day before surgery and stress the importance of the mechanical preparation already outlined.[57] Although many antibiotic preparations have been advocated, the oral combination of neomycin and erythromycin given in three doses the day before surgery has proved efficacious and has gained acceptance among most intestinal surgeons.

Prophylactic Antibiotics

Prophylactic antibiotics account for up to 25% of all hospital antimicrobial usage in the United States.[66] In many cases the use of antibiotics is based on presumptive data and theoretic considerations rather than solid evidence that a patient is at risk for the development of infection. In one large study assessing the risk of infection in surgical patients, infection of the wound was used as the measure of the rate of infection.[13] In 62,939 surgical cases the overall wound infection rate was 4.7%, with 1.5% in clean cases and 7.7% after clean-contaminated cases (a hollow viscus opened).[13] Infection rates in contaminated cases (perforated viscus) rose to 15.2%, and in contaminated cases where pus was encountered, this rate rose to 40%. If prophylactic antibiotics can diminish these rates, they should be employed because wound and other nosocomial infections have serious economic consequences in that they increase the length and cost of hospitalization, not to mention the risks to the patient and the possibility of a fatal outcome.[28]

A review of the literature indicates that the use of prophylactic antibiotics to minimize the risk of infectious complications following surgery is far from standardized. Britt and associates[6] reviewed 2782 patients and found that only 9% received antibiotics beginning within 6 hours of surgery and ending within 48 hours, a period when antibiotics should be most effective. In 34% of patients the antibiotics were begun after the procedure and were continued for longer than 48 hours in more than half of these patients. Gardner, Jones, and Polk[22] noted similar uses and abuses in 300 consecutive surgical patients in their hospital. Problems identified included beginning the drug after surgery (23 cases), continuing therapy for too long or too short a period (14 cases), or insufficient indications for its use (39 cases).

In determining the usefulness of antibiotics prophylactically, one should consider the type of procedure to be performed, the potential risk of the patient to develop infection, and the cost-benefit ratio of the antibiotic to be employed. Clean surgical cases constitute approximately 75% of all procedures, and the risk of infection is sufficiently small that the benefit of prophylactic antibiotics is difficult to demonstrate.[63] Antibiotics are useful in the other categories of surgery where the risk of bacterial contamination is high or the patient is immunologically compromised. Patients with malignancies or those receiving steroid therapy or immunosuppressive drugs fall into the latter category, where antimicrobial prophylaxis becomes warranted.[10] In addition, increased rates of infection occur in obese patients, presumably because adipose tissue has a poor blood supply, which warrants consideration for prophylactic antibiosis.[59]

Cephalosporins have been the most frequently studied systemic antibiotics for prophylaxis and are used widely in gastrointestinal and biliary surgery.[31] The effectiveness of antibiotics in preventing infection is greatest when they are in the wound at the time of bacterial inoculation. Most investigators agree than adequate tissue levels should be present when the incision is made and that "prophylaxis" after the procedure is valueless.[36,59] Peak tissue levels for most antibiotics are reached 1 to 2 hours after intravenous administration. Despite these considerations, it must be emphasized that a danger of the emergence of resistant bacteria or drug sensitivity exists if therapy is begun too early or is unduly prolonged after surgery.

Obesity

Obesity is a common condition, with less than 5% of all patients having a definable organic cause.[7] Results of dietary, behavioral, and pharmacologic treatment have been discouraging, and a high relapse rate following initial success with each of these modalities has been consistently noted. The surgical treatment of obesity is still evolving but has almost exclusively been reserved for those who are morbidly overweight (see Chapter 67). Surgical treatment is not available for widespread use outside of study centers.

Obese people undergo surgical procedures relatively frequently. They are especially at risk for the development of gallbladder disease and obstetric complications when pregnant. The incidence of cholelithiasis is three times greater in obese people than in those of normal weight, although the basic mechanism for this is not clear.[47] Tracy and Miller[74] studied obstetric patients weighing more than 250 pounds and noted such complications as toxemia, pyelonephritis, and diabetes in 62%; surgical intervention before term delivery was required in 35%, a higher frequency than would be normally expected.

Most studies reveal a high chance for complications following surgical procedures in patients.[9,65] A method for assessing risk is based on the *ponderal index (PI),* where the PI is equal to height (inches) divided by the cube root of weight in pounds (Fig. 13-1).[65] Mild obesity is associated with only slightly increased mortality, but as the magnitude of obesity increases, the risk rises exponentially. The problems noted most often in these patients are related to pulmonary and wound complications.

The physical examination of an obese patient is always a difficult challenge. Masses are difficult to palpate, and diagnostic signs are blunted. Although often inadequate, a thorough examination, especially of the pulmonary and cardiovascular system, should be carefully undertaken. Electrocardiogram, chest x-ray, and pulmonary function testing should be done for all obese patients. Preoperative pulmonary status may be improved by the use of bronchodilators, breathing exercises, and the cessation of smoking. Although controversial, low-dose heparin may be useful in reducing phlebitis and the increased incidence

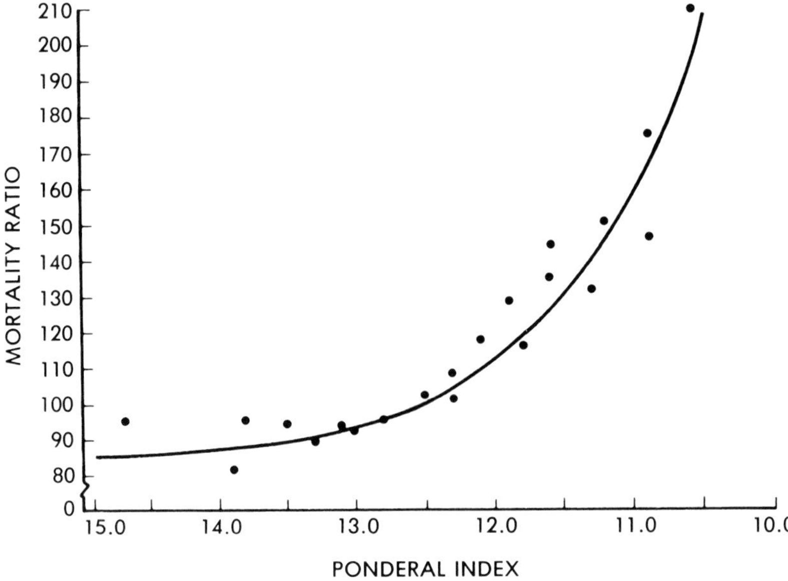

Fig. 13-1 Association of mortality with ponderal index (PI) for males, ages 40 to 49 years. (From Seltzer, C.C.: Reprinted by permission of N. Engl. J. Med. **274:**254, 1966.)

Table 13-2 **RECOMMENDED DAILY ALLOWANCES (RDA) FOR "REFERENCE" MAN AND WOMAN***

	Enteral			Parenteral	
Nutrient	**RDA (men)**	**Range†**	**RDA (women)**	**RDA (men)**	**RDA (women)**
Water (L)				2.1	1.7
Energy (kcal)	2700		2000	2100	1740
Protein (g)	56		44	39	33
Retinol equivalents (vitamin A)‡	1000		800	47	39
Vitamin D (μg)	5		5	3	2
Vitamin E (mg)	10		8	142	118
Vitamin K (μg)		70-140			
Ascorbic acid (mg)	60		60	35	29
Biotin (μg)		100-200			
Folacin (μg)	400		400	210	174
Niacin (mg)	18		13	14	12
Riboflavin (mg)	1.6		1.2	2.1	1.7
Thiamine (mg)	1.4		1	1.4	1.2
Vitamin B_6 (mg)	2.2		2	2.1	1.7
Vitamin B_{12} (μg)	3		3	2.1	1.7
Pantothenic acid (mg)		4-7		14	12
Calcium (mg)	800		800	310	310
Phosphorus (mg)	800		800	325	270
Iodine (μg)	150		150	133	110
Iron (mg)	10		18	4	3
Magnesium (mg)	350		300	68	56
Zinc (mg)	15		15	1	1
Copper (mg)		2-3		3	3
Potassium (mg)		1875-5625		2185	1810
Sodium (mg)		1100-3300		1930	1600
Chloride (mg)		1700-5100		3975	3295
Chromium (μg)		0.05-0.2			
Manganese (mg)		2.5-5		2.3	1.9
Molybdenum (μg)		0.15-0.5			
Selenium (μg)		0.05-0.2			
Fluoride (mg)		1.5-4			

Modified from Horowitz, J., et al.: In Lubin, M., Walker, H.K., Smith, R.B., editors: Medical management of the surgical patient, Boston, 1982, Butterworth Publishers.
*Reference man, 35 years old, 70 kg, 172 cm, moderately active, temperate climate; reference woman, 35 years old, 58 kg, 162 cm, moderately active, temperate climate.
†Recommended ranges for both sexes since more specific information not available.
‡1 Retinol equivalent equals 1 μg retinol or 6 μg beta-carotene.

of thrombopulmonary embolism postoperatively, which is sometimes observed in these patients.[39]

SPECIFIC ASPECTS OF PREOPERATIVE PREPARATION

Risks of Malnutrition

Patients with surgical disorders can be divided into three groups with respect to nutritional needs. Those in the first group are normally nourished and perioperatively will only require maintenance levels of calories and proteins. Since most elective surgery will necessitate only a short period of diminished nutrient intake orally, it will have little impact on nutritional stores in these patients, with resumption of normal alimentation 5 to 7 days following surgery. The second group of patients has preexisting moderate or severe malnutrition, usually secondary to their disease process, and may require a period of nutritional support to restore lean body mass. The third group comprises those who may be normally nourished but who have sustained some type of severe trauma (e.g., gunshot wound to abdomen or burns) or who develop complications that prolong their postoperative recovery. These patients can be expected to benefit from nutritional support that prevents further erosion of their lean body mass. The risks and benefits of nutritional support and the principles governing the use of enteral and parenteral nutrition in a broad spectrum of surgical disease is discussed in more detail in Chapter 3.

The expected daily nutritional requirements for an adult are listed in Table 13-2.[37] Major surgery, trauma, and burns raise the resting metabolic rate and result in a greater breakdown in muscle mass, which is reflected in increased excretion of urinary urea.[22] The goal of the physician should be to ensure an adequate nutritional state before elective surgery. Patients undergoing surgery may lose 4% to 15% of their body weight postoperatively depending on their preoperative nutritional status. Nutritional assessment may be performed using objective measurements such as triceps skinfold, serum albumin, serum transferrin, midarm muscle area, and skin test reactions to various recall antigens (see Chapter 3). Full objective nutritional assessment should be performed on those patients who are less than 80% of ideal body weight, have had an unintentional weight loss greater than 10 pounds, have a serum albumin concentration that is 3.4 or less, and have a total lymphocyte count of less than 1500.[37] Patients with sepsis, trauma, burns, and disease processes that preclude adequate nutrition or in whom excessive losses of nutrients may occur (e.g., from enteric fistulas, malabsorption, or diarrhea from ulcerative colitis) should also have careful assessment and management of their nutritional deficits.

Mullen and associates[55] have developed a formula for assessing a *prognostic nutritional index (PNI)* that identifies patients at risk for developing complications caused by their surgical disease (see boxed material at right). This index uses measurement of the triceps skinfold, which is the simplest index of endogenous fat stores, and serum levels of albumin and transferrin, which estimate visceral protein stores. In a prospective study of 148 patients these investigators demonstrated that preoperative nutritional support was beneficial only in the high-risk group (i.e., PNI > 50%). Despite a 9% operative mortality and a 23% complication rate in the nutritionally supported group, there was a 2.5-fold reduction in complications, a sixfold reduction in sepsis, and a fivefold reduction in mortality when compared to the control group who did not receive preoperative nutritional therapy.

CALCULATION OF PROGNOSTIC NUTRITIONAL INDEX (PNI) IN HYPOTHETIC, WELL-NOURISHED PATIENT

PNI = 158% − 16.6 (albumin) − 0.78 (triceps skinfold) − 0.2 (transferrin) − 5.8 (delayed cutaneous hypersensitivity reactivity)

Example:

Albumin → 4.8 gt/100 ml × 16.6	=	79.9
Triceps skinfold → 14 mm × 0.78	=	10.9
Transferring → 250 gt/100 ml × 0.20	=	50.0
Skin test reactivity → 2 × 5.8	=	11.6
TOTAL		152.2

PNI = 158% − 152.2% = 5.8%

The predicted risk of complications in this patient is 5.8%.

Modified from Mullen, J., et al.: Ann. Surg. **192:**604, 1980.

Nutritional support may be given orally, intravenously, or through the gastrointestinal tract. The latter route should be used if the patient's gastrointestinal tract is functional. Enteral products may be administered through intestinal tubes, gastrostomy, or feeding jejunostomy. Enteral alimentation is usually well tolerated, economic, and simple to administer. Many products are available, each of which is suitable for certain specific needs (see Chapter 3). Complications of enteral nutrition are rare but include such problems as aspiration, clogged tubing, esophageal erosion, gastrointestinal problems (vomiting, diarrhea), and metabolic derangements (hyperglycemia, edema, electrolyte abnormalities). The complications of prolonged intravenous hyperalimentation are usually more serious (see Chapter 3).[37] Many result from technical problems caused by the placement of the central venous catheter or from biochemical abnormalities caused by administration of hyperosmotic solutions. If appropriate protocols for central line insertion and fluid administration are followed, however, the benefits outweigh the risks.

Risks of Cardiovascular Disease

Cardiac Status

An evaluation of the cardiac status of all patients is mandatory before surgery that involves general or spinal anesthesia. In taking a history, the physician must phrase questions so as to search for evidence of chest pain, dyspnea, syncope, wheezing, peripheral edema, transient ischemic attacks, palpitations, previous rheumatic fever, myocardial infarction, arrhythmias, heart failure, or congenital heart disease. All antihypertensive, cardiotonic, diuretic, and antiarrhythmic medications should be noted.

A complete cardiac physical examination, chest x-ray films, and electrocardiogram are of use both for diagnosis and as a baseline. Additional studies in patients suspected of having cardiac disease (i.e., treadmill exercise tests to identify ischemia; echocardiography to provide information of chamber size, wall motion, and valve function) may also be useful. Myocardial scintographic studies and coronary angiography are indicated if these other procedures raise a high index of suspicion for ischemic heart disease.

Functional impairment is best assessed by the patient's activity capabilities. The ability to walk up two flights of stairs without stopping or developing angina, dyspnea, or excessive tachycardia is of great important and indicates considerable cardiac reserve. The patient with heart disease not only lacks this reserve but is susceptible to additional stress during surgery (i.e., the risks of pulmonary or peripheral emboli caused by mural thrombi and cardiac ischemia caused by anemia associated with blood loss). Cardiac reserve may be further compromised by overhydration or excessive transfusion during surgery or postoperatively and thus may set the stage for cardiac failure.

Hemodynamic Monitoring

Preoperatively, monitoring of hemodynamic stability can be assessed noninvasively by recording heart rate, systemic blood pressure, electrocardiograms, and urine output. In emergency cases when shock, fluid and electrolyte abnormalities, and hemodynamic instability exist, more sophisticated measurements are required, such as arterial pressure, central venous pressure (CVP), pulmonary capillary wedge pressure (PCWP), and cardiac output.

Arterial Pressure. Arterial catheters are indicated in an unstable patient when frequent pressure measurements and multiple blood gas analysis are required. Arterial catheters may be placed in the radial, brachial, or femoral vessels. Although major complications are rare (less than 1%),[17] minor problems such as hematoma and a decrease in peripheral pulsation may occur. When the radial artery is used, an Allen test should be performed to assess ulnar-palmar circulation. Teflon catheters are preferred because they are inert and cause less tissue reaction and arterial occlusion.[2] Aseptic technique is mandatory for both percutaneous or cutdown methods.

Central Venous and Pulmonary Capillary Wedge Pressures. A dynamic interrelationship exists between cardiac contractility, vascular tone, and blood volume. In the absence of impaired cardiac function, CVP measurement is a good reflection of right ventricular end-diastolic pressure, whereas the PCWP is a good estimate of the left ventricular end-diastolic filling pressure. Generally the values for these two measurements (i.e., CVP = 5 to 50 mm Hg and PCWP = 6 to 12 mm Hg) are comparable. Major differences between the CVP and PCWP indicate variations in the function of the right and left ventricles, which might occur secondary to myocardial infarction. For example, Rappaport and Scheinman[60] found normal or low CVP values in 30% of postinfarction patients in whom acute left ventricular failure and pulmonary edema were clearly present.

Both CVP and PCWP monitoring are useful in determining the timing of elective surgery in a patient with heart disease or in following an unstable patient who requires emergency surgery. Because PCWP monitoring is more invasive than CVP and requires the placement of a pulmonary artery (PA) catheter for its measurement, indications for its use have been more restrictive. Accepted indications for PCWP measurement include patients with chronic obstructive lung disease (increased pulmonary resistance); coronary artery disease requiring fluid replacement; decreased left ventricular function secondary to anoxia, acidosis, and electrolyte imbalance; decompensated cirrhosis; severe pancreatitis; generalized peritonitis; or multisystem trauma. PCWP measurements are also indicated in patients receiving massive transfusions, those with a high CVP and poor peripheral perfusion, those with suspected ventricular dysfunction, and those requiring cardiac surgery or sustaining cardiac trauma.[8]

Cardiac Output. Cardiac output measurements may be made using dye dilution (indocyanine green) or thermodilution techniques. The most frequently used techniques, thermodilution, measures a change in temperature of a bolus of cold saline injected into the superior vena cava and sampled in the pulmonary artery by thermistors incorporated into a PA catheter. The cardiac output is inversely proportional to the fall in temperature. This method uses a physiologic indicator, no blood is withdrawn, and no recirculation is required.[75]

Drug Therapy

Antihypertensives and/or antiarrhythmic drugs can be maintained throughout the perioperative period, thus lowering the anesthetic and operative mortality. The preoperative use of digitalis is controversial; in high-risk patients its use has been justified to offset the anticipated myocardial depressant effect of general anesthesia. However, no evidence exists to support prophylactic digitalization in a functionally normal individual to prevent postoperative congestive cardiac failure.[35] Administration without proper indication may complicate postoperative clinical assessment and management. Appropriate monitoring after surgery should give sufficient warning of deteriorating cardiac function and the appearance of arrhythmias.

Patients taking propranolol (propanolol) preoperatively can continue the drug to within 12 to 24 hours of surgery without risk of hypotension or bradycardia.[41] If withdrawn, the dose should be tapered over 2 or 3 days to avoid myocardial infarction, which may result from abrupt discrimination.[51]

Cardiovascular Problems

Coronary Artery Disease. Less than 1% of adults will experience a postoperative myocardiac infarction if there is no antecedent episode.[68,73] The smaller the interval between a previous myocardial infarction and surgery, the greater is the risk. Within 3 months of a myocardial infarction, the reinfarction rate is 27% to 37%; after 3 to 6 months, 11% to 16%; and after 6 months, 4% to 6%, where the rate remains thereafter.[53] Thus, in a patient with a previous myocardial infarction, elective surgery should be delayed until at least 6 months have elapsed. Interestingly the risk of reinfarction is not affected by the duration or type of anesthesia (spinal vs. general).[50,68,73] For a given patient the cardiac risk can be expressed as an index derived from the initial physical examination and laboratory examination (Tables 13-3 and 13-4).[26] The greater the number of "points," the greater is the risk.

Mitral Stenosis. Most patient with significant mitral stenosis can be expected to have a reduction in left ventricular end-diastolic filling pressure. The resultant increase in left atrial pressure can be transmitted to the pulmonary vascular bed, leading to pulmonary hypertension and right ventricular failure. Interstitial lung edema may occur initially with exercise, but later the patient may become symptomatic at rest. Patients with mitral stenosis have a high incidence of atrial arrhythmias, and the fast ventricular response that typically results may lead to acute pulmonary edema during or following surgery. Excessive tachycardia should be avoided because this may result in a decreased diastolic filling period. Preoperative digitalis is recommended to slow the ventricular response in atrial fibrillation and to allow better diastolic filling.

Mitral Insufficiency. In mitral insufficiency a decrease in left ventricular output is caused by regurgitation of much of the stroke volume into the left atrium. Despite a high left ventricular end-diastolic volume, the left ventricular end-diastolic pressure may be normal because of compliance and dilation of the left atrium. Because of this dilation, left atrial pressures may be only moderately increased. For the same reason, pulmonary vascular complications develop more slowly than with mitral stenosis. Afterload reduction with vasodilators (e.g., sodium nitroprusside) improves hemodynamics by decreasing left ventricular end-diastolic pressure and increasing stroke volume with an increase in cardiac output.[52] Inotropic drugs will also reduce heart size and mitral regurgitation.

Aortic Stenosis. Aortic stenosis may be valvular, subvalvular, or supravalvular. In patients over 65 years of age, the usual cause is degeneration of a normal tricuspid aortic valve with fibrosis and calcification. Chronic pressure overload of the left ventricle occurs, resulting in hypertrophy, increased oxygen consumption, and poststenotic dilation of the aortic root. Significant pulmonary hypertension is unusual. The timing of left atrial contraction is crucial in these patients because atrial systole contributes about 30% of the total left ventricular end-diastolic

Table 13-3 **POINT ASSESSMENT FOR COMPILATION OF CARDIAC RISK INDEX BASED ON PHYSICAL STATUS**

Criteria*	Multivariant-Discriminant Function Coefficient	"Points"
1. History		
a. Age > 70 yr	0.191	5
b. MI in previous 6 mo	0.384	10
2. Physical examination		
a. S_3 gallop or JVD	0.451	11
b. Important VAS	0.119	3
3. Electrocardiogram		
a. Rhythm other than sinus or PACs on last preoperative ECG	0.283	7
b. >5 PVCs/min documented at any time before surgery	0.278	7
4. General status:		
$Po_2 < 60$ or $Pco_2 > 50$ mm Hg, $K < 3.0$ or $HCO_3 < 20$ mEq/L, BUN > 50 or Cr > 3.0 mg/100 ml, abnormal SGOT, signs of chronic liver disease, or patient bedridden from noncardiac causes	0.132	3
5. Surgery		
a. Intraperitoneal, intrathoracic, or aortic procedure	0.123	3
b. Emergency surgery	0.167	4
TOTAL POSSIBLE		53

From Goldman, L., et al.: Reprinted by permission of N. Engl. J. Med. **297**:845, 1977.
*MI, Myocardial infarction; JVD, jugular vein distention; VAS, valvular aortic stenosis; PACs, premature atrial contractions; ECG, electrocardiogram; PVCs, premature ventricular contractions; Po_2, partial pressure of oxygen; Pco_2 partial pressure of carbon dioxide; K, potassium; HCO_3, bicarbonate; BUN, blood urea nitrogen; Cr, creatinine; SGOT, serum glutamic-oxaloacetic transaminase.

Table 13-4 **RISKS OF COMPLICATIONS AND DEATH BASED ON CARDIAC ASSESSMENT***

Class	Point Total	No or Only Minor Complications (n = 943)	Life-threatening Complication† (n = 39)	Cardiac Deaths (n = 19)
I (n = 573)	0-5	532 (99)‡	4 (0.7)‡	1 (0.2)‡
II (n = 316)	6-12	295 (93)	16 (5)	5 (2)
III (n = 130)	13-25	112 (86)	15 (11)	3 (2)
IV (n = 18)	>26	4 (22)	4 (22)	10 (56)

From Goldman, L., et al.: Reprinted by permission of N. Engl. J. Med. **297**:845, 1977.
*Refer to Table 13-3 for calculation of points.
†Documented intraoperative or postoperative myocardial infarction, pulmonary edema, or ventricular tachycardia without progression to cardiac death.
‡Figures in parentheses denote percentage.

volume. Atrial fibrillation may be fatal,[64] and angina is common in these patients.

Moderate or mild aortic stenosis is tolerated well, but severe aortic stenosis incurs the risk of sudden ventricular fibrillation and death under anesthesia. Preservation of sinus rhythm is essential. Correction of hypokalemia that may predispose to arrhythmias is important, especially in patients receiving digitalis. Adequate monitoring and preoperative digitalization are essential. Tachycardia or increased myocardial oxygen consumption should be treated with small doses of intravenous propranolol.

Aortic Insufficiency. Patients with aortic valvular disease experience an increase in left ventricular volume that leads to hypertrophy—or an increase in cardiac work and oxygen requirements—and a reduction in coronary artery blood flow. Cardiac output eventually decreases. Use of PCWP monitoring is important since patients may need higher left ventricular filling pressures because of the reduced left ventricular contractility. Improvement in myocardial function is likely following afterload reduction. Additional treatment should include coronary artery dilators to improve myocardial perfusion.

Prosthetic Valves. Most patients with prosthetic valves are well compensated and are candidates for elective surgical procedures. Complications that may occur include systemic embolization of valvular thrombi, infective endocarditis, hemolysis of red blood cells, and dysfuncton of the valve. Patients taking coumadin should be converted to heparin anticoagulation before surgery which can be reversed easily with protamine. All patients with valvular heart disease or prosthetic valves should receive antibiotic prophylaxis to reduce the risk of endocarditis.

Congestive Heart Failure. Patients with left ventricular dysfunction are vulnerable to complications of anesthesia, trauma, shock, hemorrhage, temperature elevation, and the stress of major surgery. A depression in the contractility of the myocardium reduces the response to a demand for increased cardiac function. Patients with congestive heart failure especially should be assessed carefully preoperatively. Exercise tolerance, the degree of cardiac enlargement, and respiratory function with exercise must be evaluated and therapy (e.g., diuretics and digitalis) instituted to improve preexisting cardiac failure. One study of 144 patients with overt heart failure on admission reported an operative mortality of 5.5% after satisfactory preoperative control,[30] an acceptable mortality in these severely compromised patients.

Hypertension. Hypertension is common among patients undergoing elective or emergency surgery, but its contribution to the mortality and morbidity of anesthesia and surgery varies, depending on the population evaluated, the surgical procedure performed, and the anesthesia given.[54] Skinner and Pearce[67] documented a 13% mortality rate for 293 noncardiac surgical patients with hypertensive heart disease. However, Nachlas, Abrams, and Goldberg[56] noted no increased mortality in 6000 patients, and Dana and Ohler[14] noted no mortality in 20 elderly males with hypertension undergoing major noncardiac surgery. These differences in mortality and morbidity are clearly related to hypertensive damage to target organs such as hypertensive heart disease and renal compromise. Uncomplicated and untreated mild hypertension, where preoperative diastolic pressures are 110 mm Hg or less, result in no adverse effects.[25]

The patient with detectable hypertension should be carefully screened for evidence of organ dysfunction. Hypertension is the leading cause of congestive heart failure, and 5-year survival rates in untreated patients may approach 50%.[40] The findings of left ventricular hypertrophy (physical examination, chest x-ray films, ECG, echocardiography), and congestive heart failure (distended neck veins, S_3 gallop, or pleural effusions) should be searched for and documented. Premature ventricular contractions (PVCs) and premature atrial contractions (PACs) should also be noted since these findings carry an increased risk of cardiac death following surgery.[26] Renal failure in hypertensive patients is usually caused by nephrosclerosis and may give rise to proteinuria, hematuria, or pyuria on urinalysis. A serum creatinine concentration of 1.7 mg/100 ml or higher usually indicates renal insufficiency. Hemorrhages or exudates seen on retinal examination indicate the presence of moderate to severe hypertension. The existence of hypertension secondary to pheochromocytoma should be eliminated in hypertensive patients with headaches, palpitations, and excessive sweating by measuring urinary catecholamines, vanillylmandelic acid (VMA), and metanephrines. Patients undergoing surgical procedures with unsuspected pheochromocytoma may have a mortality rate in excess of 50%.[72]

A patient with essential hypertension may have a lower than normal blood volume, an elevated total peripheral resistance, a reduced or low cardiac output, and baroreceptor reflexes accommodated to untreated hypertension.[19,20,21] Preoperative therapy should reduce diastolic pressures to below 110 mm Hg, as measured over 24 hours. Thiazide diuretics may have antihypertensive effects for up to 4 weeks following cessation of therapy. Plasma volume expansion may be required to avoid hypotension at induction of anesthesia. Hypokalemia, as a result of diuretic therapy, should be corrected preoperatively to avoid arrhythmias, ileus, the potentiation of muscle relaxants, and respiratory depression. Proportional losses of intracellular and extracellular potassium may make it difficult to predict the respiratory responses to the use of nondepolarizing muscle relaxants.[71] Hypokalemia most often leads to PVCs and PACs and sensitizes the myocardium to the irritable effects of digitalis and succinylcholine, sometimes resulting in asystole.[1]

Reserpine and other *Rauwolfia* compounds are often discontinued before surgery because their action is to deplete tissue stores of norepinephrine. Nonetheless, most circulating reflexes remain intact with reserpine activity,[42] and controlled trials show that the risk of hypotension is no greater in patients taking reserpine than in untreated hypertensive patients or those who had the drug discontinued preoperatively.[29]

Methyldopa (Aldomet) is a centrally acting sympatholytic agent and can be administered until the time of surgery. Guanethidine, which is used in severe hypertension, has a long half-life; its effect persists for 7 days following discontinuation. Propranolol (Inderal), a nonselective beta-blocker, may cause intraoperative hypotension, decreases in cardiac output, and atropine-resistant bradycardia[23]; thus therapy should be stopped the evening before surgery. Clonidine (Catapres), another centrally acting sympatholytic agent, may precipitate an acute hypertensive crisis when discontinued abruptly,[76] and therefore oral or intramuscular therapy is continued until just before surgery. Untreated hypertensive patients should be given antihypertensive therapy and have their hypertension controlled preoperatively to reduce the risk of major blood pressure changes and dysrhythmias during surgery. Uncontrolled hypertension may be as dangerous as profound hypotension during surgical procedures.

Risks of Pulmonary Disease

Respiratory Evaluation

Pulmonary complications typically occur in the postoperative period, especially in cigarette smokers and patients with chronic obstructive lung disease.[15] Incisions close to the diaphragm interfere most with pulmonary function. Cuffed endotracheal tubes and dry anesthetic gases depress the mucociliary action of the tracheobronchial tree. This, together with lack of deep breathing and coughing postoperatively, leads to bronchial mucous plugs, segmental atelectasis, and pneumonia. The incidence of atelectasis increases with duration of anesthesia, patient age,[12] and obesity. Daily consumption of more than 20 cigarettes is associated with a fourfold increase in atelectasis.[34]

A routine history is essential but may not be reliable in predicting the patient at risk. Specific questions should be asked about cigarette consumption, cough and sputum production, previous bronchitis or asthma, recurrent pulmonary infections, exposure to toxic inhalants, previous chest injuries or surgery, and current level of exercise tolerance. These queries may reveal mild, moderate, or severe respiratory debility.

Any dyspnea or cyanosis should be noted. Walking up one flight of stairs with patients is an excellent indication of their respiratory reserve capacity. The examiner should look for absence of breath sounds, wheezes, clubbing of fingers, and coarse or fine rhonchi and rales. The chest x-ray film is a static routine picture that is helpful in determining anatomic abnormalities and parenchymal disease. Arterial blood gases measure efficiency of ventilation and gas exchange, as well as acid/base status. Pulmonary function tests and arterial blood gas analysis can be used to quantitate respiratory dysfunction and assess the risk of surgery (Table 13-5).[15]

Table 13-5 **RISK OF POSTOPERATIVE PULMONARY COMPLICATIONS IN PATIENTS UNDERGOING MAJOR SURGERY**

Measurement*	Low	Moderate	High
FVC (liters)	1-1.5	0.6-1	0.6
FEV_1 (L/sec)	0.5-1	0.3-0.5	0.3
MMF (L/sec)	100-200	50-100	50
$Paco_2$ (mmHg)	40-45	45-55	55
Pao_2 (mmHg)	60-70	50-60	50

Modified from Wellmann, J.: In Lubin, M., Walker, H.K., and Smith, R.B., editors: Medical management of the surgical patient, Boston, 1982, Butterworth Publishers.

*FVC, Forced vital capacity; FEV_1, forced expiratory volume in 1 second; MMF, maximum midexpiratory flow; $Paco_2$, arterial carbon dioxide tension; Pao_2, arterial oxygen tension.

Pulmonary Function Analysis

Because of variations in pulmonary function resulting from age, sex, and height, values obtained during measurement of pulmonary function are expressed as the percentage of a predicted value. Values less than 70% of normal are considered abnormal. Analysis of forced expiration (Fig. 13-2) requires the patient to inspire to total lung capacity and then breath out to residual volume as rapidly as possible. Expiratory effort should last at least 6 seconds. Reduction in this forced vital capacity (FVC) occurs in both obstructive and restrictive pulmonary disease. The forced expiratory volume in 1 second (FEV_1) is reduced considerably with restrictive disease. Thus a decrease in the ratio of FEV_1/FVC serves as measure of airway obstruction. Maximum expiratory flow (MEF) is measured in liters per second by the slope of a line joining points at 200 ml and 1200 ml after the start of expiration (Fig. 13-2).[34] Maximum midexpiratory flow (MMF) is obtained by measuring in liters per second the slope of a line joining points at 25% and at 75% of FVC and depends less on the effort made by the patient (Fig. 13-2).[34] These measurements give an indication of the amount of both obstructive and restrictive disease present.

Functional residual capacity (FRC) and lung compliance decreases during general anesthesia. The cephalad shift of the diaphragm caused by displacement of the abdominal contents, atelectasis with air trapping, and accumulation of lung water all contribute to a decrease in compliance. Redistribution of pulmonary blood flow during anesthesia is

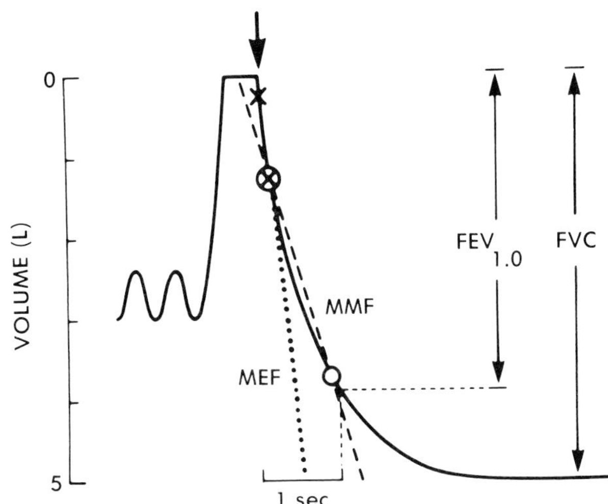

Fig. 13-2 Analysis of forced expiratory spirogram for maximum expiratory flow (*MEF*, slope of line joining points at 200 ml and 1200 ml after start of expiration) and of maximum midexpiratory flow (*MMF*, slope of a line joining points of 25% and 75% of forced vital capacity, *FVC*). Arrow indicates start of forced expiration. (From Hensley, M.J., and Fencl, V.: Lungs and respiration. In Vandam, L.D., editor: To make the patient ready for anesthesia: medical care of the surgical patient, Menlo Park, Calif., 1984, Addison-Wesley Publishing Co., Inc.)

mainly determined by gravity, with a higher perfusion of the dependent parts of the lung. The ventilation/perfusion ratio (V/Q) is inefficient, and effective gas exchange is decreased. The use of ventilation with positive end-expiratory pressure (PEEP) may decrease the degree of V/Q shunting and improve oxygenation of arterial blood.[27] The simplest measure of adequate gas exchange is obtained from analysis of arterial blood gases, and in normal patients the alveolar oxygen pressure (PA_{O_2}) is 10 to 15 mm Hg greater than the arterial oxygen pressure (Pa_{O_2}). Physiologic shunts represent the fraction of mixed venous blood that is blended with blood that has been equilibrated with PA_{O_2} to produce the measured Pa_{O_2}.

Respiratory Therapy

A systematic preoperative respiratory program can significantly reduce postoperative complications.[33,61,70] A standard program should include the cessation of smoking; respiratory physical therapy, including breathing exercises and bronchodilators to rid the tracheobronchial tree of retained secretions; oxygen therapy; and antibiotics if infection is present. Bronchodilators include theophylline derivatives and beta-adrenergic stimulators. Some patients may be receiving maintenance corticosteroid therapy, and this should be continued during surgery. Steroids given in high doses may help with unmanageable bronchospasm over brief periods (1 week). Fiberoptic bronchoscopy and tracheostomy may be necessary to improve bronchial toilet in selected patients. Broad-spectrum antibiotics can be used in those patients with chronic bronchitis or sputum production and when clinical deterioration suggests an underlying infection.[46]

Risks of Liver Disease

Evaluation of Hepatic Function

Liver function and reserve may be evaluated preoperatively by measuring both excretory and secretory capabilities and assessing for the presence or absence of hepatocellular injury (see boxed material below). Serum bilirubin is elevated in both extrahepatic obstruction and intrahepatic cholestasis resulting from intrinsic liver disease. With intrinsic liver disease both conjugated and unconjugated bilirubin concentrations rise. In contrast, with hemolysis elevations mainly occur in the unconjugated fraction, and with extrahepatic obstruction as the primary disorder rises occur in the conjugated fraction. Whereas bilirubin alterations can reflect both acute and chronic liver disease, changes in synthetic function are not as sensitive an indicator of acute liver impairment but are useful in helping to diagnose chronic hepatic disease (e.g., cirrhosis). The transaminase tests assess hepatocellular injury. Based on these considerations, liver function abnormalities can be grouped into four major clinical patterns: (1) hepatocellular injury, (2) cholestasis, (3) infiltrative disease, and (4) mixed, which can be helpful in the prediction of response to the stress of anesthesia and surgery (Table 13-6).[32,34]

Liver function tests do not provide a specific diagnosis

LABORATORY EVALUATION OF HEPATIC FUNCTION

TESTS OF HEPATIC EXCRETORY ABILITY
Bilirubin
Bromosulfophthalein (BSP)

TESTS OF HEPATIC SYNTHETIC ABILITY
Prothrombin time
Serum albumin

TESTS INDICATING HEPATOCELLULAR DAMAGE
Serum glutamic-oxaloacetic and serum glutamic-pyruvic transaminases (SGOT, SGPT)
Lactic dehydrogenase (LDH)
Alkaline phosphatase
Gamma-glutamyl transpeptidase (GGT)

Modified from Lamont, J.T.: In Vandam, L., editor: To make the patient ready for anesthesia: medical care of the surgical patient, Menlo Park, Calif., 1980, Addison-Wesley Publishing Co., Inc.

Table 13-6 **CATEGORIZATION OF LIVER DISEASE BASED ON LIVER FUNCTION TESTING**

Abnormality	Total Bilirubin (Normal = Less than 1.5 mg/100 ml)	Alkaline Phosphatase (Normal = 2 to 12 King-Armstrong Units)	Transaminases (Normal = Less than 45 units)	Albumin (Normal = 3.5 to 5 g/100 ml)	Prothrombin Time (Normal = 90% to 100%)	Example
Hepatocellular injury	2-10	1-2 times normal	>200	Decreased in severe cases	Increased in severe cases	Viral hepatitis
Cholestasis	10-30	2-4 times normal	<200	Normal	Increased in chronic cholestasis but correctable by vitamin K injection	Common duct stones
Infiltrative disease	<2	1-3 times normal	<100	Normal	Normal	Metastatic carcinoma
Mixed	2-20	1-3 times normal	100-500	Generally decreased	Increased but not correctable by vitamin K injection	Cirrhosis

Modified from Lamont, J.T.: In Vandam, L., editor: To make the patient ready for anesthesia: medical care of the surgical patient, Menlo Park, Calif., 1980, Addison-Wesley Publishing Co., Inc.

but allow definition of the pattern of disease and its etiology. These tests also are useful in predicting outcome of surgery and anesthesia, as in Child's Classification of liver function in cirrhotic patients (see Chapter 24). Decreased synthetic function reflects a reduced functional hepatocyte mass and indicates that stress (e.g. infection, blood loss, anesthesia, or surgery) will be poorly tolerated. In contrast, patients with a high-grade extrahepatic cholestasis usually tolerate surgical procedures well, especially if the obstruction is relieved. Unrelieved obstructive jaundice may eventually result in biliary cirrhosis, as manifested by hepatosplenomegaly, deep jaundice, and impaired synthetic function. (For more detailed discussions on the operative risks associated with portal hypertension and obstructive jaundice, see Chapters 25 and 29.)

Hepatitis

A careful history should document previous episodes of jaundice or exposure to toxins, drug abuse, and sexual promiscuity, all of which are associated with hepatitis. Serologic tests for hepatitis B and A are now available. Responses in both immunoglobulins G and M (IgG and IgM) occur with hepatitis A. IgM levels peak 30 days after exposure to hepatitis A and persist about 6 days after jaundice appears. Later the antibody response of IgG peaks, so that the initial high IgM/IgG ratio diminishes 30 to 90 days after exposure. Hepatitis B surface antigen is the best marker for identification of acute B infection and can be detected in the blood by radioimmunoassay. Hepatitis B core antibody appears soon after the surface antigen and is an important marker for exposure to virus B of long persistence. Many cases of hepatitis have neither antigen nor antibody and are referred to as non-A and non-B. In patients with acute hepatitis requiring emergency surgery, complications and deaths appear to be higher than expected, suggesting that the diseased liver cannot adequately handle the stress of surgery.[48] Thus elective procedures should be deferred in patients with hepatitis until clinical and laboratory evidence document the resumption of normal liver function.

Risks of Kidney Disease

The morbidity and mortality of surgical procedures are closely related to the degree of renal impairment. The kidney eliminates nitrogenous waste; regulates body water, electrolytes, and acid-base balance; helps control blood pressure, red blood cell count, and calcium; and serves as the route of excretion and degradation of many hormones and drugs. Some changes in renal physiology can be expected during the trauma and stress of surgery. These changes are mediated by the release of various hormones. Adrenocorticotropic hormone (ACTH) release stimulates the adrenal release of hydrocortisone and to some extent aldosterone. The usual regulation of antidiuretic hormone (ADH) by osmoreceptors is superseded by the direct influence of traumatic stimuli on the hypothalamus, resulting in fluid retention despite extracellular hypotonicity. Sodium and chloride retention results in urinary sodium declining to less than 5 mEq/day following surgery.[4] Dilutional hyponatremia is generally noted and results from water retention exceeding sodium retention. Increased potassium excretion parallels increased catabolism, cellular breakdown, and excretion of nitrogen, and the negative potassium balance is accentuated by the effect of aldosterone on the distal tubule.

A prolongation and exaggeration of the usual hormonal effects in response to surgery may be seen in kidney disease.[3] Although the hydrocortisone response to ACTH in renal failure appears to be normal, a diseased kidney may not respond to the release of ADH, and diabetes insipidus with sodium and water loss may evolve. Changes in fluid balance can lead to convulsions or coma. Urinary potassium loss caused by the catabolic response to surgery may not be great enough to maintain normal serum potassium concentrations, and the resultant hyperkalemia may lead to life-threatening arrhythmias.

Routine investigation of renal function preoperatively should include determinations of serum creatinine, blood urea nitrogen (BUN), electrolytes, and SMA-12 (particularly calcium and phosphate), as well as a urinalysis. Approximately 50% of renal function must be lost before any elevation in BUN or creatinine occurs. Because of these abnormalities, a urine osmolality and creatinine clearance should also be assessed. In patients with compromised renal function efforts should be directed to preventing further renal damage and avoiding precipitation of acute renal failure during surgery or postoperatively following hypovolemia, impaired cardiac function, peripheral vasodilation, or increased vascular resistance. Recent studies indicate that maintenance of renal perfusion with salt and water loading may prevent acute tubular necrosis (ATN) or reduce its severity if it develops.[5,69] The efficacy of diuretics in this regard is uncertain but appears to be beneficial. Furosemide (Lasix) is the diuretic of choice because of its effects on intrarenal prostaglandin production and the resulting improvement in renal blood flow and glomerular filtration rate.[4]

Patients with renal dysfunction may have several extrarenal complications. The associated anemia may be caused by decreased production of erythropoietin or uremic toxins, which suppress the bone marrow production of erythrocytes. Renal acidosis may help compensate for the anemia, however, by causing a shift of the oxygen dissociation curve to the right, resulting in enhanced tissue oxygenation. Because the plasma volume is often elevated in these patients, preoperative blood transfusion is rarely needed.[16] The hyperphosphatemia of renal failure leads to increased red blood cell production because of increases in 2,3-diphosphoglycerate (2,3-DPG) and adenosine triphosphate, thereby increasing the oxygen-carrying capacity of hemoglobin.[3]

Systemic hypertension is the most common cardiovascular complication of renal failure and is usually a manifestation of intravascular volume overload. Diuresis or dialysis usually restores normotension, but antihypertensive medication may be required preoperatively. Coronary artery disease is also frequently encountered in patients with renal dysfunction; routine electrocardiograms may help identify individuals at risk. The lower resistance to infection seen in patients with renal disease may result from a reduction in the chemotactic ability of white blood cells. Of the infections found in these patients, those involving the lung are most common.[16]

Drug therapy must be adjusted in patients with renal disease since decreased renal clearance will prolong the half-life of many medications, such as the aminoglycoside antibiotics. Nomograms have been developed to adjust the dosage according to the degree of renal impairment and properties of the drug. Sedation and hypnotics excreted primarily by the kidney should be avoided. Mortality rates approaching 2% to 4% and complications involving as many as 60% of patients may be expected with major surgery for renal disease.[16] Hyperkalemia, infection, and thrombosis of vascular access sites for hemodialysis are the most frequent problems. Dialysis before surgery helps correct any electrolyte abnormalities. Appropriate antibiosis of ongoing infections, as well as prophylactic treatment when substantial risk of infection exists, should be considered.

Risks of Endocrine Disease

Diabetes Mellitus

Insulin regulates a number of complex metabolic processes, including glucose hemostasis, lipoprotein balance, amino acid flux, and growth. Insulin-dependent diabetes mellitus occurs when the beta-cell mass is reduced and is insufficient to meet normal needs. This may occur as a result of genetic susceptibility, cellular destruction (mumps, rubella), or autoimmunity. In contrast, non-insulin-dependent diabetes represents a deficit of insulin action at the end organ. The normal daily insulin requirements of an adult of ideal body weight is about 33 units (U), or approximately 1 U/hour over 24 hours with an additional 3 to 5 U during each meal.[58] One's weight, diet and endogenous hormones (cortisol, glucagon) can adversely influence the insulin receptor, increasing the need for insulin. At times of stress, increases in ACTH, cortisol, epinephrine, norepinephrine, growth hormone, and glucagon secretion occur, all of which have an antagonistic effect on insulin. These hormones have a protective effect against the induction of hypoglycemia following excessive insulin release but can aggravate glucose homeostasis in patients with diabetes. The stress of surgery is also a factor in impaired glucose tolerance in diabetic patients.

In diabetic patients requiring emergency surgery, both hypoglycemia and diabetic ketoacidosis may be encountered. Hypoglycemia can be corrected quickly by administration of intravenous glucose and should not delay emergency surgery for long. Ketoacidosis involves a fluid and electrolyte imbalance and should be sufficiently corrected before surgery by insulin and fluid administration to achieve a plasma pH greater than 7.3 and a bicarbonate concentration greater than 20 mEq/L. Potassium supplements should also be given as needed to ensure balance of this electrolyte.

Several complications of diabetes may adversely affect the outcome of surgery and must be identified preoperatively. Nephropathy results in a high renal threshold to glucose, and a negative urine glucose can occur, with serum levels in excess of 300 mg/100 ml, which can greatly alter glucose homeostasis in the diabetic patient. Thus the adequacy of renal function needs to be known before these individuals undergo surgery. The risk of urinary tract infection is high in diabetes and must be detected and treated before the procedure; infectious complications often occur in these patients and are associated with significant mortality rates. Before the antibiotic era, the operative mortality for diabetes was about 7.3%. This has now dropped to 2%, as reviewed in a study of 16,352 surgical procedures at the New England Deaconess Hospital.[38] Despite the improvement, this mortality rate is still twice that of nondiabetic patients and primarily is caused by increased risk of infection.[11] Finally, vascular disease is frequently encountered in diabetes, and the risk of sudden death from a myocardial infarction or a stroke (cerebrovascular accident) is substantial,[77] indicating the importance of maintaining fluid balance, minimizing blood loss, and preventing unnecessary stress both during surgery and postoperatively in this highly vulnerable group of patients.

Cortisol Metabolic Dysfunction

Physiologic stress is perhaps the most important stimulus to ACTH and cortisol secretion. The cortisol response during surgery may be blocked by epidural anesthesia. Similarly, preanesthetic medications such as pentobarbital and diazepam effectively decrease cortisol levels. Patients with adrenal insufficiency, either from primary adrenal disease or secondary to suppression of adrenal function because of previous steroid therapy, lack this response and require steroid replacement during surgical stress.

The symptoms of adrenal insufficiency include weakness, weight loss, nausea, vomiting, and diarrhea. Orthostatic hypotension and dizziness are common. Acute insufficiency results in shock, sepsis, delirium, coma, and hyperthermia. Hyponatremia, hyperkalemia, and eosinophilia may also be seen. Serum cortisol and urinary 17-hydroxycorticosteroids or cortisol can be measured preoperatively in patients thought to be at risk. In addition, an ACTH stimulation test may prove helpful to evaluate adrenal reserve in patients receiving previous steroid replacement. Elderly patients may also be at risk for the development of adrenal dysfunction, as noted by Clark.[11] In a series of elderly patients without an antecedent history of adrenal disease, he observed the spontaneous development of adrenal hemorrhage in a substantial number within 33 days following various abdominal procedures. The explanation for this is uncertain.

Pheochromocytoma

A history of severe headaches, sweating, palpitations, anxiety, and unexplained increases in blood pressure, particularly induced by exercise, should raise the suspicion of a pheochromocytoma. The diagnosis can be confirmed by measuring plasma catecholamines, urinary vanillylmandelic acid (VMA), and metanephrines. Appropriate therapy, including surgery, should be instituted before performing other elective procedures.[62] (See Chapters 57 and 60 for a more detailed discussion of this disease.)

Thyroid Dysfunction

Surgical stress will produce a variety of changes in circulating thyroid hormone concentrations. Triiodothyronine (T_3) levels were noted to decrease by 50% postoperatively in eight euthyroid patients undergoing uncomplicated abdominal surgery.[18] Thyroxine (T_4) levels rose or were stable and a fall in thyroid-stimulating hormone (TSH) was observed in the first 24 hours following surgery. Similar changes have been noted in hyperthyroid patients undergoing cholecystectomy.[78] The stress of preoperative fasting and stress-induced cortisol release tend to potentiate these changes. Cortisol has been known to have inhibitory effects on the conversion of T_4 and T_3 and on the TSH response to thyrotropin-releasing factor (TRF).

Patients who have untreated hyperthyroidism may have significant morbidity during induction of anesthesia. These problems range from simple anxiety and tachycardia to thyroid storm. No correlation exists between severity of these reactions and the magnitude of the procedure performed. Control of hyperthyroidism preoperatively is achieved with oral antithyroid drugs such as prophylthiouracil or methimazole. Tachycardia, palpitations, anxiety, and restlessness are treated with beta-blockers (such as propranolol). When emergency surgery becomes necessary, rapid control is best achieved with intravenous propranolol and sodium iodide. If hyperthyroidism is untreated before surgery, thyroid storm, as manifested by hyperthermia (106° F), tachycardia, and hypotension, may occur unpredictably and result in death.

The increased morbidity associated with surgical hypothyroidism results primarily from anesthesia and the drugs involved in maintaining the anesthetized state. The heart rate may slow, and cardiac contractility may be less forceful. Cardiac output may decrease sufficiently to cause hypotension. Cardiomegaly and a pericardial effusion may exist with cardiomyopathy and conduction defects in hypothyroidism. Hypercholesterolemia and atherosclerosis are stigmata of hypothyroid patients, who tend to be obese and have reduced maximum breathing capacity with upper airway problems and reduced alveolar ventilation. Most respiratory problems can usually be reversed by thyroid replacement.[24] More than 50% of hypothyroid patients have hyponatremia resulting from impairment of free water excretion because of inappropriate ADH secretion,[78] but this is reversible with thyroid supplementation.

Hypothyroid patients are intolerant of cold and exhibit dry puffy skin, constipation, lethargy, slow speech, and a hoarse voice. They often have periorbital edema, dry thin hair, bradycardia, and muscle weakness. Diagnosis of hypothyroidism is confirmed by the finding of low levels of circulating thyroid hormones. With primary disease, TSH is elevated. Thyroxine is initiated in slowly increasing doses to avoid the sudden onset of cardiac problems[45]; 4 weeks may be required before adequate daily replacement is achieved. If surgery is mandated before optimum replacement therapy can be achieved, the use of sedatives and narcotics should be guarded and minimized and adequate ventilatory support provided. Some patients with myxedema may have a depressed adrenal reserve and require hydrocortisone supplementation.

Risks of Hematologic Disease

Anemia

Although the erythrocyte occupies an important position in oxygen transport, anemia poses no absolute contraindication to urgent or semiurgent surgery because it can be remedied by transfusion of whole blood or red cells.[45] Other mechanisms that interfere with delivery of oxygen to tissue, such as a reduction in blood flow, interference with the exchange of oxygen in the lungs, or inability of tissue to take up available oxygen, may be more important problems than the presence of anemia alone.

Anemia is usually defined as a hemoglobin concentration less than 12.5 g/100 ml of blood in a female and less than 14.0 g/100 ml in a male. Occasionally a patient may be hypoxic but not anemic. The shifting of the oxygen dissociation curve of hemoglobin can decrease the ability of hemoglobin to release oxygen to the tissues. This may occur with various hemoglobinopathies and in states of acid-balance imbalance where alkalosis is a problem. Physiologic compensation for anemia occurs naturally by means of increased tissue perfusion through an increased cardiac output, a decrease in blood viscosity, and decreased peripheral resistance. Elevation of 2,3-DPG, which increases the erythrocyte oxygen-binding capacity and shifts the dissociation curve to the right, may also improve oxygenation.

A depression of ventricular function occurs when the hematocrit is reduced to 24% to 31%.[45] This consideration, along with surgical threats to the oxygen delivery system, possible increased oxygen demands, and the expectation of some blood loss, have resulted in the recommendation that a minimum of 10 g/100 ml of hemoglobin exists before elective surgery. Preoperatively, if surgery is elective, a cause for anemia should be investigated before transfusion or therapy that may obscure the testing (Table 13-7).[70] The most common cause of anemia is blood loss, but if iron deficiency is diagnosed, it may take 7 to 10 days to achieve a peak in reticulocyte production with therapy and a rise in hemoglobin thereafter of 0.1 to 0.2 g/100 ml/day.

Polycythemia

An excess in red cells with a hemoglobin concentration greater than 18 in males or 16 in females can be documented by measuring red cell mass with chromium 51. Decreases in plasma volume can result in an increase in serum hemoglobin and should be considered in the differential diagnosis. Erythrogenin released by the hypoxic kidney acts on a plasma protein to produce erythropoietin, which stimulates production of red cell precursors. The increased blood viscosity in polycythemia can lead to poor tissue oxygenation and/or thrombosis. This is of particular concern in patients with hematocrits greater than 60%. Causes of polycythemia are summarized in the boxed material on p. 250.

The preoperative approach to the surgical patient with

Table 13-7 **DIAGNOSIS OF ANEMIA**

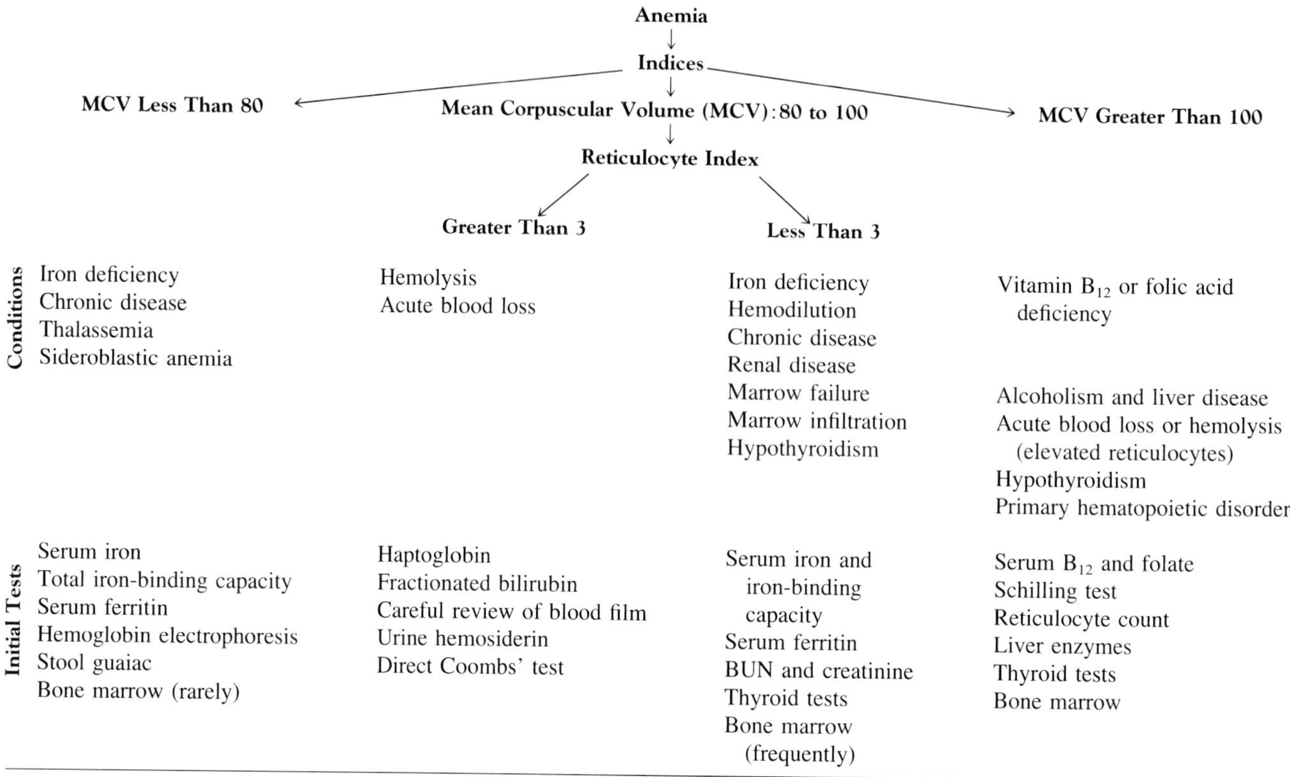

	MCV Less Than 80	MCV 80 to 100, Reticulocyte Index Greater Than 3	MCV 80 to 100, Reticulocyte Index Less Than 3	MCV Greater Than 100
Conditions	Iron deficiency Chronic disease Thalassemia Sideroblastic anemia	Hemolysis Acute blood loss	Iron deficiency Hemodilution Chronic disease Renal disease Marrow failure Marrow infiltration Hypothyroidism	Vitamin B_{12} or folic acid deficiency Alcoholism and liver disease Acute blood loss or hemolysis (elevated reticulocytes) Hypothyroidism Primary hematopoietic disorders
Initial Tests	Serum iron Total iron-binding capacity Serum ferritin Hemoglobin electrophoresis Stool guaiac Bone marrow (rarely)	Haptoglobin Fractionated bilirubin Careful review of blood film Urine hemosiderin Direct Coombs' test	Serum iron and iron-binding capacity Serum ferritin BUN and creatinine Thyroid tests Bone marrow (frequently)	Serum B_{12} and folate Schilling test Reticulocyte count Liver enzymes Thyroid tests Bone marrow

Reprinted from Keller, J.W.: Surgery in the patient with hematopoietic disease. In Lubin, M.F., Walker, H.K., and Smith, R.B., editors: Medical management of the surgical patient, Stoneham, Mass., 1982, Butterworth Publishers. With permission from the publisher.

CAUSES OF POLYCYTHEMIA

MISIDENTIFICATION
Dehydration
Spurious laboratory samples

APPROPRIATE ERYTHROPOIETIN RELEASE: HYPOXIA
Right-to-left shunts with cardiac disease
Chronic pulmonary disease
High altitude
Pickwickian syndrome
Abnormal hemoglobin with high oxygen affinity
Elevated carboxyhemoglobin
Postural hypoventilation

INAPPROPRIATE ERYTHROPOIETIN RELEASE
Renal cyst or hydronephrosis
Uterine fibroids
Malignancies: hypernephroma, hepatoma, adrenal carcinoma, ovarian carcinoma, pheochromocytoma

AUTONOMOUS: POLYCYTHEMIA VERA

Modified from Keller, J.W.: Surgery in the patient with hematopoietic disease. In Lubin, M., Walker, H.K., and Smith, R.B., editors: Medical management of the surgical patient, Boston, 1982, Butterworth Publishers.

polycythemia should deal with the underlying disease. In most cases this involves a pulmonary problem or dehydration. Phlebotomy will not help chronic lung problems. In patients with malignancies or polycythemia vera, phlebotomy should be undertaken to remove only 200 to 300 ml twice weekly[45] and generally less in the elderly patient.

White Blood Cell Disorders

Specific problems in patients undergoing surgery with myelodeficient and immunodeficient states may be encountered. Problems of infection related to granulocytopenia or immunodeficiency occur more frequently in such patients. Those patients with white counts as low as 500 to 1000/mm^3 are particularly at increased risk for the development of infection. Frequently encountered diseases that may require specific therapy before elective surgery are detailed in the boxed material on p. 251. No absolute contraindication exists to surgery in the patient with a granulocytopenia, but prognosis of the underlying disease must be balanced against the surgical benefits.

Platelet Disorders

Disorders of platelets typically take one of two forms: quantitative reduction or qualitative dysfunction. Patients with these disorders usually have petechiae or purpura with bleeding from mucous membranes, in contrast to patients with coagulation defects, who have soft tissue or joint

DISEASES ASSOCIATED WITH MYELODEFICIENT AND IMMUNODEFICIENT STATES

Lymphoproliferative Diseases

Solid tumors
- Hodgkin's disease
- Non-Hodgkin's disease

Leukemias
- Acute lymphocytic
- Chronic lymphocytic
- Hairy cell

Immunosecretors
- Plasma cell myeloma
- Waldenström's macroglobulinemia
- Heavy chain diseases

Myeloproliferative Diseases

Leukemias
- Acute nonlymphocytic
- Chronic myelocytic
- Erythroleukemia

Myelofibrosis

Idiopathic thrombocytosis

Granulocytopenias

Secondary to reduced production
- Hypoplasia: drugs, radiation, idiopathic
- Infiltrative processes: leukemia, myeloma, lymphoma, metastatic carcinoma, myelofibrosis
- Maturation defects: vitamin B_{12} and folic acid deficiency

Secondary to increased destruction or sequestration
- Hypersplenism
- Sepsis
- Antibodies
  - Drugs
  - Diseases, especially collagen vascular

Modified from Keller, J.W.: Surgery in the patient with hematopoietic disease. In Lubin, M., Walker, H.K., and Smith, R.B., editors: Medical management of the surgical patient, Boston, 1982, Butterworth Publishers.

CAUSES OF THROMBOCYTOPENIA

Increased Destruction of Platelets

Immune
- Idiopathic thrombocytopenic purpura (ITP)
- Collagen vascular diseases
- Lymphoma
- Transfusion-related conditions
- Drugs: quinidine, quinine, sulfonamide, digoxin, and so on

Disseminated intravascular coagulation (DIC)

Thrombotic thrombocytopenic purpura (TTP)

Infection

Hemorrhage

Extracorporeal perfusion

Sequestration (hypersplenism)

Decreased Formation of Platelets

Vitamin B_{12} and folate deficiency

Marrow hypoplasia
- Aplastic anemia
- Drug induced, especially chemotherapy
- Radiation induced

Marrow replacement
- Leukemias
- Lymphomas
- Myelofibrosis
- Myeloma
- Infections, tuberculosis
- Carcinoma

Congenital

Modified from Keller, J.W.: Surgery in the patient with hematopoietic disease. In Lubin, M., Walker, H.K., and Smith, R.B., editors: Medical management of the surgical patient, Boston, 1982, Butterworth Publishers.

bleeding. Platelet aggregation is stimulated by exposure to raw surfaces and collagen. Adenosine diphosphate (ADP) is released by platelet granules, resulting in more platelet aggregation and the formation of a plug. Platelets also stimulate the formation of fibrinogen and factor V, which promote clotting by way of thrombin. Platelet levels below 20,000 are associated with spontaneous bleeding, and counts greater than 50,000 are generally sufficient to avoid any noticeable excess bleeding during a surgical procedure. Causes of thrombocytopenia are listed in the boxed material at above right.

Qualitative abnormalities in platelet function have also been well recognized for many years. Platelet aggregation tests must be examined if total counts are normal to identify such patients. Causes of platelet function abnormalities are listed in the boxed material at right.

Other abnormalities may result in purpura but actually are vascular disorders rather than platelet abnormalities. These include vitamin C deficiency, vasculitis, Marfan's syndrome, and Rendu-Osler-Weber disease (hereditary hemorrhagic telangiectasia). Tests that assess platelet func-

CAUSES OF PLATELET FUNCTION ABNORMALITIES

Drugs

Salicylates (e.g., aspirin)

Pyrazolon derivatives (e.g., phenylbutazone)

Antidepressants (e.g., amitriptyline)

Indomethacin

Disease States

Renal disease

Myeloproliferative syndromes

Macroglobulinemia

Liver disease

Congenital

Storage pool disease

Defective ADP release

Wiskott-Aldrich syndrome

Bernard-Soulier syndrome

Thrombasthenia

von Willebrand's disease

Modified from Keller, J.W.: Surgery in the patient with hematopoietic disease. In Lubin, M., Walker, H.K., and Smith, R.B., editors: Medical management of the surgical patient, Boston, 1982, Butterworth Publishers.

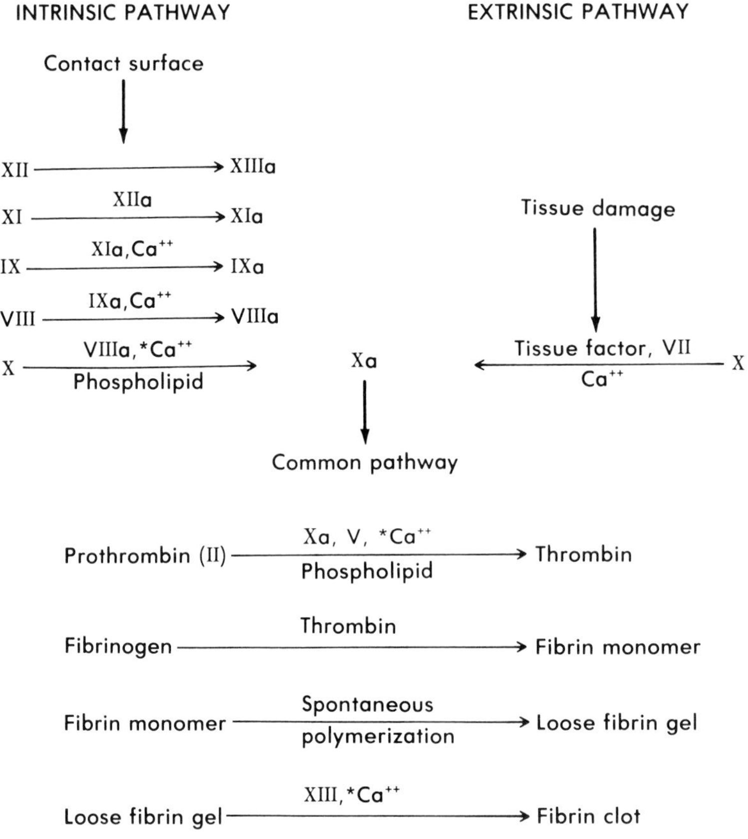

Fig. 13-3 Coagulation cascade. (From Keller, J.W.: Surgery in the patient with hematopoietic disease. In Lubin, M.F., Walker, H.K., and Smith, R.B., editors: Medical management of the surgical patient, Boston, 1982, Butterworth Publishers.)

tion include clot retraction, prothrombin consumption, the tourniquet test, platelet aggregation with various agents, and template bleeding times.

Preoperative transfusions are often helpful in correcting thrombocytopenia. For every platelet pack infused, a rise of 10,000 to 12,000/mm^3 would be expected in 1 hour. The underlying cause of thrombocytopenia should be first addressed (e.g., infection, vitamin deficiency, uremia, or local hemorrhage) since platelet transfusions are not useful in immune-mediated states or those in which rapid consumption of platelets occur, such as disseminated intravascular coagulation (DIC) and thrombotic thrombocytopenic purpura (TTP). The use of corticosteroids in treating thrombocytopenia is not clear. Most drug-related problems causing platelet abnormalities are reversible when the agent is discontinued. Aspirin effects have been noted for as long as 5 to 7 days; thus discontinuation of this drug must be initiated at least 1 week before surgery to ensure that no continuing adverse effects on platelet function occur.

Coagulation Defects

All clotting factors are largely synthesized in the liver, except factor VIII, which is derived from endothelial cells. The source of factors XI, XII, and XIII is not clear. Several of the factors can be ''consumed'' during coagulation, resulting in a disease state such as DIC. Vitamin K is one of the few natural substances that can influence the coagulation scheme; it is found in the diet and is also manufactured in the gut by gastrointestinal bacteria. Few drugs adversely affect coagulation, with the exceptions of warfarin (Coumadin) and heparin.

An understanding of the *coagulation cascade* (Fig. 13-3) will provide a solid conceptual basis for the various problems and defects that the surgical patient may have preoperatively or encounter postoperatively.[45] In general the cause of bleeding intraoperatively or postoperatively is from local or technical causes rather than a systemic bleeding diathesis, but several mechanisms can lead to deficiency in clotting that should be noted before surgery to prevent troublesome bleeding during the procedure and postoperatively. Examples include a genetic reduction in clotting factors and activity, such as von Willebrand's disease, or a genetic defect in activity but no actual decrease in concentration of the clotting factor, such as hemophilia. Decreased synthesis of clotting factors related to liver disease or lack of vitamin K may occur. Of course, patients taking warfarin or heparin should be readily identifiable.

Increased destruction or consumption of platelets (e.g., DIC) or circulating antagonists of clotting may be more difficult to uncover.

The laboratory tests most often used to evaluate the intactness of the clotting cascade are the *prothrombin time (PT)* and the *partial thromboplastin time (PTT)*. These tests will generally appear normal if the clotting factors are equal to or greater than 25% of normal. The PT is standardized and reproducible and detects problems with factors VII, X, II, and I. The PTT should be within 8 to 10 seconds of the control; if not, a problem may exist in either the intrinsic or common pathway, especially involving factors XII, X, IX, and VIII.

In detecting clotting problems, emphasis should be placed on the history of the patient. Bleeding disorders may have been noted recently (acquired), or a long personal or family history may be present. In general, surgical intervention can proceed after appropriate replacement therapy has been given.

SUMMARY

Preparation of a patient for surgery demands a thorough preoperative assessment to minimize operative risk and to ensure a smooth postoperative convalescence. A careful history as well as a thorough physical examination will usually identify the presence of associated disease and the need for further laboratory or radiologic evaluation. Although the risk of surgery will vary depending on the health status of a patient and the presence or absence of other complicating diseases, appropriate preoperative preparation will greatly minimize this risk and assist in the timing, type, and determination of efficacy for a particular surgical procedure in controlling or alleviating disease in an individual patient. Occasionally an alternate surgical or medical approach may be appropriate for a given disease process because of the undue risk of an associated health problem and the minimum benefits to be gained by the operative procedure being considered. Approaching the patient as an integrated organism in whom multiple systems interplay, rather than focusing on a specific disease that may or may not be best approached surgically, will minimize derangements in normal physiology and ensure that the ultimate therapeutic approach chosen will be in the patient's best interests in terms of the risk/benefit ratio.

REFERENCES

1. Alper, M.H., Flache, W., and Kraye, O.: Pharmacology of reserpine and its implications for anesthesia, Anesthesiology **24**:524, 1963.
2. Bar, P.O.: Percutaneous puncture of the radial artery with a multipurpose Teflon catheter for indwelling use, Acta Physiol. Scand. **51**:343, 1973.
3. Brenner, B.M., and Humes, H.D.: Mechanics of glomerular ultrafiltration, N. Engl. J. Med. **297**:148, 1977.
4. Brenner, B.M., and Rector, F.C.: The kidney, Philadelphia, 1981, W.B. Saunders Co.
5. Brenowitz, J., Williams, C., and Edwards, W.: Major surgery in patients with chronic renal failure, Am. J. Surg. **134**:765, 1977.
6. Britt, M.R., et al.: A 1979 statewide study to the "non-usage" of perioperative antibiotics in surgical prophylaxis—a continuing problem, Clin. Res. **28**:43, 1980.
7. Brook, C.G., Huntley, R.M., and Slade, J.: Influence of heredity and environment in determination of skinfold thickness in children, Br. Med. J. **2**:719, 1975.
8. Carrico, C.J., and Horowitz, J.: Monitoring the critically ill surgical patient. In Advances in surgery, vol. II, Chicago, 1977, Year Book Medical Publishers, Inc.
9. Chase, H.F.: To operate or not to operate—what is the risk? Resident Staff Physician **24**:65, 1975.
10. Chodak, G.N., and Plant, M.E.: Use of systemic antibiotic for prophylaxis in surgery—a critical review, Arch. Surg. **112**:326, 1977.
11. Clark, O.H.: Postoperative adrenal hemorrhage, Ann. Surg. **182**:124, 1975.
12. Collins, C.D., Drake, C.S., and Knowelden, J.: Chest complications after upper abdominal surgery: their anticipation and prevention, Br. Med. J. **1**:401, 1968.
13. Cruse, P.J., and Foord, R.: The epidemiology of wound infection—a 10 year prospective study of 62,939 wounds, Surg. Clin. North Am. **60**:27, 1980.
14. Dana, J.B., and Ohler, R.L.: Influence of heart disease on surgical risk, JAMA **162**:878, 1956.
15. Davis, P.G., and Spence, A.A.: Postoperative hypoxemia and age, Anesthesiology **37**:663, 1972.
16. Delcher, H., and Siddig, K.: Surgery in the patient with endocrine disorders. In Lubin, M., Walker, H.K., and Smith, R.B., editors: Medical management of the surgical patient, Boston, 1982, Butterworth Publishers.
17. Donno, J.B., Rodistein, P.D., and Klein, E.F.: Hazards of radial artery catheterization, Anesthesiology **38**:283, 1973.
18. Engler, D., Donaldson, E.B., and Stockigt, J.R.: Effect of surgical stress on serum thyroid hormones in hyperthyroidism, Aust. N. Z. J. Med. **8**:131, 1975.
19. Feldman, S.A.: Effects of changes in electrolytes, hydration and pH upon the reactions to muscle relaxants, Br. J. Anaesth. **35**:546, 1963.
20. Felner, J.: Noncardiac surgery for the cardiac patient. In Lubin, M., Walker, H.K., and Smith, R.B., editors: Medical management of the surgical patient, Boston, 1982, Butterworth Publishers.
21. Frohlick, E.D., Tarazi, R.C., and Dustan, H.P.: Reexamination of the hemodynamics of hypertension, Am. J. Med. Sci. **257**:9, 1969.
22. Gardner, F.T., Jones, C.E., and Polk, H.C., Jr.: Further definition of antibiotic use and abuse in the surgical setting, Arch. Surg. **114**:883, 1979.
23. Goldberg, A.D., Wilkinson, P.R., and Raftery, E.B.: The over-root phenomenon on withdrawal of cloridine therapy, Postgrad. Med. J. **52**(7):128, 1976.
24. Goldberg, M., and Rewich, M.: Studies on the mechanism of hyponatremia and impaired water excretion in myxedema, Ann. Intern. Med. **56**:120, 1962.
25. Goldman, L., and Caldera, D.L.: Risks of general anesthesia and elective operation in the hypertensive patient, Anesthesiology **50**:285, 1979.
26. Goldman, L., et al: Multifactorial index of cardiac risk in noncardiac surgical procedures, N. Engl. J. Med. **297**:845, 1977.
27. Gracey, D.R., Divetie, M.B., and Didrer, E.P.: Preoperative pulmonary preparation of patients with chronic obstructive pulmonary disease: a prospective study, Chest **76**:123, 1979.
28. Green, J.W., and Wenzel, R.P.: Postoperative wound infection: a controlled study of the increased duration of hospital stay and direct cost of hospitalization, Ann. Surg. **85**:264, 1977.
29. Hall, W.D.: Hypertension in the surgical patient: preoperative, intraoperative, and postoperative evaluation and management. In Lubin, M., Walker, H.K., and Smith, R.B., editors: Medical management of the surgical patient, Boston, 1982, Butterworth Publishers.
30. Hamilton, B.E.: Chronic cardiac or surgical risk, Surg. Clin. North Am. **6**:621, 1926.
31. Harley, D.L., Howard, P. Jr., and Hahn, H.N.: Perioperative prophylactic antibiotics in abdominal surgery—preview and recent progress, Surg. Clin. North Am. **59**:919, 1979.
32. Harville, D.D., and Summerskill, W.H.: Surgery in acute hepatitis: cause and effects, JAMA **184**:257, 1963.
33. Hechtman, H., et al.: Preoperative assessment and the high risk surgical patient, Surg. Clin. North Am. **60**:1349, 1980.
34. Hensley, M., and Fencl, V.: In Lungs and respiration. Vandam, L., editor: To make the patient ready for anesthesia: medical care of the surgical patient, Menlo Park, Calif., 1980, Addison-Wesley Publishing Co., Inc.

35. Hillis, D., and Cohn, P.: Noncardiac surgery in patients with coronary artery disease, Arch. Intern. Med. **138**:972, 1978.
36. Hirschmann, J.V., and Imir, T.S.: Antimicrobial prophylaxis: a critique of recent trial, Rev. Infect. Dis. **2**:1, 1980.
37. Horowitz, J., et al.: In Lubin, M., Walker, H.K., and Smith, R.B., editors: Medical management of the surgical patient, Boston, 1982, Butterworth Publishers.
38. Kahn, O., Wagner, W., and Bessman, A.N.: Mortality of diabetic patients treated surgically for lower back infection and/or gangrene, Diabetes **23**:287, 1974.
39. Kakkar, V.V., Corrigan, T.P., and Fossard, D.P.: Prevention of fatal post-operative pulmonary embolism by low doses of heparin: an international symposium, Lancet **2**:45, 1975.
40. Kannel, W.B., et al.: Role of blood pressure in the development of congestive heart failure: The Framingham study, N. Engl. J. Med. **287**:781, 1972.
41. Kaplan, J., and Dunbar, R.: Propranolol and surgical anesthesia, Anesth. Analg. **55**:1, 1976.
42. Katz, R.L.: Hazardous effects of drugs in hypertensive patients scheduled for elective surgery, Cardiovasc. Med. **3**:1185, 1978.
43. Keats, A.S.: The ASA classification of physical status—a recapitulation, Anesthesiology **49**:233, 1978.
44. Kehlet, H., Klauber, P.V., and Weeke, J.: Thyrotropin, free and total triiodolthyrone and thyroxine in serum during surgery, Clin. Endocrinol. **10**:131, 979.
45. Keller, J.W.: Surgery in the patient with hematopoietic disease. In Lubin, M., Walker, H.K., and Smith, R.B., editors: Medical management of the surgical patient, Boston, 1982, Butterworth Publishers.
46. Lamont, J.T.: The liver. In Vandam, L., editor: To make the patient ready for anesthesia: medical care of the surgical patient, Menlo Park, Calif. 1980, Addison-Wesley Publishing Co., Inc.
47. Mabee, T.M., et al.: The mechanism of increased gallstone formation in obese human subjects, Surgery **79**:460, 1976.
48. Mars, R.: Surgery in the patient with renal disease. In Lubin, M., Walker, H.K., and Smith, R.B., editors: Medical management of the surgical patient, Boston, 1982, Butterworth Publishers.
49. Marx, G.F., Mateo, C.F., and Orkin, L.R.: Computer analysis of post-anesthetic deaths, Anesthesiology **39**:54, 1973.
50. Miller, R., Silvag, G., and Lumb, P.D.: Anesthesia, surgery, and myocardial infarction: a review, Anesth. Rev. **6**:14, 1979.
51. Miller, R., et al.: Propranolol—withdrawal rebound phenomenon: exacerbation of coronary events after abrupt cessation of anti-angina therapy, N. Engl. J. Med. **293**:416, 1975.
52. Miller, R., et al.: Sustained reduction of cardiac impedance and preload in congestive heart failure with the antihypertensive vasodilator prazosim, N. Engl. J. Med. **297**:303, 1977.
53. Moore, F.: In American College of Surgeons: Manual of preoperative and postoperative care, Philadelphia, 1983, W.B. Saunders Co.
54. Moyer, C.A., and Key, J.A.: Estimated operative risk in 1955, JAMA **160**:853, 1956.
55. Mullen, J., et al.: Reduction of operative morbidity and mortality by combined preoperative and postoperative nutritional support, Ann. Surg. **192**:604, 1980.
56. Nachlas, M.M., Abrams, S.J., and Goldberg, M.M.: The influence of arteriosclerotic heart disease on surgical risk, Am. J. Surg. **101**:447, 1961.
57. Nichols, R.L., et al.: Effect of preoperative neomycin-erythromycin intestinal preparation on the incidence of infectious complications following colon surgery, Ann. Surg. **178**:453, 1973.
58. Palumbo, P.J., et al.: Diabetic mellitus: incidence, prevalence, survivorship, and causes of death in Rochester, Minnesota 1945-1970, Diabetes **25**:566, 1976.
59. Pollock, A.W.: Surgical wound sepsis, Lancet **1**:1283, 1979.
60. Rappaport, E., and Scheinman, M.: Rationale and limitations of hemodynamic measurements in patients with aorto myocardial infarction, Med. Concepts Cardiovasc. Dis. **38**:55, 1969.
61. Saik, R.P., Waltz, C., and Rhoads, J.E.: Evaluation of a bacitracin-neomycin surgical skin preparation, Am. J. Surg. **121**:557, 1971.
62. Samaan, H.A.: Risk of operation in a patient with unsuspected pheochromocytoma, Br. J. Surg. **57**:462, 1970.
63. Sandusky, W.R.: Use of prophylactic antibiotics in surgical patients, Surg. Clin. North Am. **60**:83, 1980.
64. Schlant, R.C., and Nutter, D.O.: Heart failure in valvular heart disease, Medicine **50**:421, 1971.
65. Seltzer, C.C.: Some re-evaluation of the build and blood pressure study, 1959, as related to ponderal index, somatotype and mortality, N. Engl. J. Med. **274**:254, 1966.
66. Shapiro, M., et al.: Use of antimicrobial drugs in general hospitals: pattern of prophylaxis, N. Engl. J. Med. **301**:351, 1979.
67. Skinner, J.F., and Pearce, M.L.: Surgical risk in the cardiac patient, J. Chronic Dis. **17**:57, 1964.
68. Steen, P.A., Tinker, J.A., and Tarhan, S.: Myocardial reinfarction after anesthesia and surgery, JAMA **239**:2566, 1978.
69. Stein, J.H., Lifschitz, M.D., and Barnes, L.D.: Current concepts on the pathophysiology of acute renal failure, Am. J. Physiol. **234**:171, 1978.
70. Stein, M., and Cassan, E.L.: Preoperative pulmonary evaluation and therapy for surgery patients, JAMA **211**:787, 1970.
71. Sumikawa, K., and Mitsya, K.: Succinylcholine-induced cardiac asystole in a patient with acute hypokalemia, Med. J. Osaka Univ. **28**:359, 1978.
72. Tarazi, R.C., Frohlick, E.D., and Dustan, H.P.: Plasma volume in men with essential hypertension, N. Engl. J. Med. **278**:762, 1968.
73. Topkins, M.J., and Artesio, J.F., Jr.: Myocardial infarction and surgery: a five-year study, Cleve. Anesth. Arch. **43**:716, 1964
74. Tracy, T.A., and Miller, G.L.: Obstetric problems of the massively obese, Obstet. Gynecol. **33**:204, 1969.
75. Weisel, R.D.: Measurements of cardiac output by thermodilution, N. Engl. J. Med. **292**:682, 1975.
76. Wellman, J.: In Lubin, M., Walker, H.K., and Smith, R.B., editors: Medical management of the surgical patient, Boston, 1982, Butterworth Publishers.
77. Younger, D., and Hadley, W.: Infection and diabetes. In Marble, A., et al., editors: Joslin's diabetes mellitus, Philadelphia, 1971, Lea & Febiger.
78. Zwillich, C.W., et al.: Ventilating control in myxedema and hypothyroidism, N. Engl. J. Med. **292**:662, 1975.

14 *Mark B. Orringer*

Physiologic Dysfunction of the Esophagus

In recent years major improvements in the surgical treatment of esophageal disease have paralleled refinements in the methods of assessing normal and abnormal physiology. Until relatively recently, most benign esophageal disease was approached somewhat empirically with attempts to correct abnormal anatomy rather than deranged physiology. Thus the merits of one-stage vs. two-stage operations to treat pharyngoesophageal (Zenker's) diverticula were discussed rather than the abnormal cricopharyngeal motor function responsible for their formation. "Reflux esophagitis" as a clinical entity was described in 1951,[1] but emphasis was placed on the anatomic correction of the often-associated hiatal hernia rather than on the abnormal distal esophageal sphincter mechanism in these patients. Surgery for benign esophageal disease has become more of a science with the improvements in manometric techniques and the ability to document gastroesophageal reflux objectively with the intraesophageal pH electrode. Thus esophageal manometry and intraesophageal pH reflux testing have become basic tools in the preoperative assessment of most patients with benign esophageal disease, and such studies are being performed postoperatively to document objectively the results of operations designed to improve patients with deranged esophageal physiology. These tests of esophageal function, however, are not infallible and must be viewed as only one facet of the evaluation of these patients—along with obtaining a careful history, a barium esophagram, and esophagoscopy. This chapter will describe the investigation of physiologic dysfunction of the esophagus as well as the physiologic basis for the surgical treatment of common esophageal disorders.

ASSESSMENT OF ESOPHAGEAL FUNCTION

History

As is true in so many disease processes, obtaining a careful history is the most valuable method for diagnosing an abnormality in esophageal function. The most common symptom of esophageal dysfunction is *dysphagia* (difficulty in swallowing). This complaint requires precise assessment in each individual patient concerning its duration, frequency, location, and associated symptoms. Intermittent dysphagia of several years' duration is more typical of benign functional disease than of esophageal carcinoma, which tends to cause progressive, constant difficulty in swallowing. Esophageal lesions producing mechanical obstruction (benign strictures or tumors) elicit constant dysphagia that the patient can localize with one finger to a specific retrosternal area, whereas motor dysfunction (e.g., esophageal spasm) produces vague intermittent retrosternal "slow emptying" that the patient is unable to pinpoint. Documentation of the patient's weight and any recent loss or gain is often helpful in differentiating benign from malignant esophageal disease. Food lodging in the lower esophagus may produce *hiccoughs* or retrosternal pain that radiates "straight through" to the interscapular region of the back. Patients with esophagitis often experience *odynophagia*—painful swallowing as food or hot or cold drinks pass the inflamed mucosa. *Regurgitation* is often indicative of esophageal disease but also has distinguishing characteristics in different conditions. In achalasia, for example, undigested food that is retained in the esophagus is regurgitated, whereas in esophageal spasm food is seldom regurgitated during the episodes of pain; instead, saliva, often described by the patient as "foam" or "phlegm" is regurgitated. All effortless regurgitation aggravated by the supine position is not caused by gastroesophageal reflux. The megaesophagus of a patient with achalasia may have a capacity of 1 to 2 L, and esophageal reflux of stagnating food in this patient is quite different from acid regurgitation that occurs in the patient with gastroesophageal reflux.

Heartburn is a common complaint of patients with upper-gastrointestinal disease. However, heartburn from peptic ulcer disease is characteristically exacerbated when the stomach is empty and is relieved by eating. When it is caused by gastroesophageal reflux, however, heartburn occurs shortly after the patient has eaten when the stomach is full and regurgitation has begun, and it is aggravated by the supine position or bending forward. It is a common misconception that heartburn in a patient with symptoms of gastroesophageal reflux is indicative of esophagitis. Heartburn merely reflects an acid-sensitive esophagus; esophagitis is an endoscopic diagnosis.

Chest pain may be the predominant symptom in patients with diffuse esophageal spasm and is often indistinguishable clinically from angina pectoris caused by coronary artery disease. The pain may radiate to the jaw or down the left arm and may be relieved by sublingual nitroglycerin, further obscuring the exact etiology of the pain. Radiation of the pain to the interscapular region, however, or a history of associated dysphagia, no matter how mild, should raise the possibility of an esophageal motor abnormality. In some patients, esophageal pain may be felt in the epigastrium or either upper quadrant of the abdomen. A host of *respiratory symptoms* may be associated with esophageal disease: (1) hoarseness caused by recurrent laryngitis that follows inhalation of refluxed gastric or esophageal contents into the airway; (2) nocturnal choking with a feeling of ''hot acid'' in the throat and lungs during an episode of gastroesophageal reflux and secondary aspiration; and (3) a vague feeling of cervical or retrosternal ''tightness'' often described as ''shortness of breath'' that occurs during episodes of esophageal spasm.

Barium Esophagram

After a patient's history is obtained that suggests the presence of esophageal disease, the next step in the evaluation is a barium esophagram. Unfortunately, an ''upper-gastrointestinal series'' focuses on just that—the stomach and intestines—and does *not* routinely include a thorough evaluation of the esophagus. A barium-swallow examination should be requested when evaluating the patient with esophageal symptoms. Although a relatively crude indicator of esophageal function, the barium esophagram with fluoroscopic assessment provides extremely vital information: (1) general anatomy (the presence of dilation, obstruction, or diverticulum); (2) the length and roentgenographic characteristics of an obstructing lesion; (3) the presence of impaired peristalsis (e.g., tertiary contractions of diffuse esophageal spasm or the abnormal motor activity of scleroderma or achalasia); and (4) the existence of a hiatal hernia and its type. The usual adult esophagus has a maximum diameter of 2.5 cm, and an esophagus that measures 3 cm or more on a barium study is clearly dilated. Benign esophageal strictures have typical radiographic characteristics; they are smooth, often tapered, and not associated with mucosal irregularity. Carcinomas, on the other hand, produce an irregular ''shelf'' of tumor that protrudes into the lumen and gives rise to a typical ''applecore'' or polypoid appearance. Esophageal dilation is more apt to be seen roentgenographically in an obstruction caused by benign disease because carcinomas are not present long enough for dilation to occur. These ''rules,'' however, are only guidelines, and it should always be remembered that x-rays are shadows, not histologic documentation of a diagnosis. Although surgeons may infer that a stricture is benign or malignant on the basis of its radiograph appearance, esophagoscopy and biopsy are mandatory procedures in the evaluation of *every* obstructing esophageal lesion to exclude the presence of carcinoma, which can occur even in association with a dilated esophagus or a smooth, tapered-appearing stenosis.

A skilled fluoroscopist can correctly diagnose esophageal motor abnormalities, but esophageal manometry provides the most objective assessment of such disorders. Similarly, the radiographic detection of abnormal gastroesophageal reflux is directly related to the experience and aggressiveness of the radiologist performing the study. Reflux of thick viscous barium is not the same as regurgitation of watery gastric acid from the stomach into the esophagus. Thus in a patient with significant symptoms of gastroesophageal reflux but a barium esophagram showing ''no hiatal hernia or reflux,'' the assumption should *not* be made that there is no organic disease. Rather, the physician should next turn to esophageal function tests using the intraesophageal pH probe to document reflux more objectively.

Esophagoscopy

Esophagoscopy is among the most vital diagnostic tools in the assessment of patients with esophageal symptoms from any cause and should be performed to exclude carcinoma in any patient with progressive dysphagia, irrespective of the findings of the barium esophagram. Although the development of the flexible fiberoptic esophagoscope has resulted in a greater number of these studies being performed on a more casual outpatient basis, it should always be borne in mind that esophagoscopy is among the most dangerous operations performed and that the disastrous physiologic results of a perforation are among the most horrendous problems encountered in surgery.

Although esophagoscopy provides little information about esophageal motor function, direct assessment of the interior of the esophagus provides data that is essential for the esophageal surgeon and is thus mandatory in every patient undergoing an esophageal operation. The combination of esophagoscopy and biopsy with brushings for cytologic evaluation establishes a diagnosis of carcinoma in 95% of patients with malignant strictures.[4,17] In the evaluation of patients with symptoms of gastroesophageal reflux, esophagoscopy provides the only accurate means of establishing the presence and extent of esophagitis. There is an extremely poor correlation between symptoms of reflux and the severity of endoscopic esophagitis. Many young patients with incapacitating pyrosis have only minimum erythema of the distal esophageal mucosa when seen during esophagoscopy; on the other hand, elderly patients may initially be seen with dysphagia from an established peptic stricture, which is the end result of reflux esophagitis, having never had significant reflux symptoms to warrant their seeking earlier medical care. Thus esophagoscopy is vitally important in the assessment of patients with abnormal gastroesophageal reflux if esophagitis is to be detected in its earlier stages when the results of surgical correction are more apt to be successful.

There is a wide variation in interpretation of endoscopic findings between different individuals using the traditional descriptions of ''mild,'' ''moderate,'' and ''severe'' esophagitis. The endoscopic grading system for reflux esophagitis proposed by Belsey provides a more objective description of the pathologic changes seen and allows more consistent evaluation of patients at different times and by different endoscopists.[37] The various grades of esophagitis that can be distinguished endoscopically using this system are as follows.

Grade I — Distal esophageal mucosal erythema—may obscure the esophagogastric squamocolumnar junction

Grade II — Mucosal erythema with superficial ulceration—typically linear and vertical with an overlying fibrinous membranous exudate that is easily wiped away leaving a bleeding surface (often misinterpreted as "scope trauma" by the inexperienced endoscopist)

Grade III Mucosal erythema with superficial ulceration and associated submucosal fibrosis—a dilatable "early" stricture

Grade IV Extensive ulceration and fibrous luminal stenosis—may represent irreversible panmural fibrosis

On the basis of this grading system, it should be apparent that an "early" stricture represents an *advanced* pathophysiologic stage of reflux esophagitis. A physician should not be lulled into a feeling of security that the disease process has been detected in a timely fashion when the radiologist reports finding a "mild" or "early" stricture associated with a hiatal hernia or with gastroesophageal reflux during a barium-swallow examination.

Two important questions regarding every radiographic esophageal stricture are answered by esophagoscopy—is the stricture benign or malignant, and can the stricture be dilated? Although the flexible fiberoptic esophagoscope provides superior optical magnification and assessment of mucosal detail, the pliability and the extent of esophageal stenoses are best determined by direct gentle probing of the stenosis with flexible gum-tipped dilators passed through a rigid esophagoscope. Such an examination is simply not possible with the flexible instruments. Passage of dilators through the rigid esophagoscope while viewed directly rather than "blindly" through the mouth is a far safer method of dilation of severe high-grade stenoses. In addition, use of the rigid esophagoscope is much more efficient in evacuating retained intraesophageal food and debris in the patient with the megaesophagus of achalasia and for removal of esophageal foreign bodies. Thus although the flexible instrument has the advantage of greater patient comfort and ease of instrumentation, it has its definite limitations in the assessment and management of esophageal disease. The flexible and rigid esophagoscopes, therefore, should be viewed as complementary but not mutually exclusive instruments, and ideally, the endoscopist should be trained in the use of both and have each at his disposal.

Esophageal Function Tests

Esophageal manometry is the direct recording of intraesophageal pressure phenomena such as the amplitude and length of the upper and lower sphincters, the extent and duration of relaxation of these sphincters during swallowing, and the characteristics of peristaltic activity in the body of the esophagus. Such intraluminal esophageal pressure measurements are obtained clinically in a variety of ways through small tubes swallowed by the patient. The recently available micropressure transducers are quite costly and are difficult to maintain in comparison to the more commonly used triple lumen, constantly perfused polyethylene or polyvinyl tubing through which pressure changes are transmitted to externally located transducers and then to a recording system.

The development of the intraesophageal pH electrode[39] has permitted the most direct and objective assessment of gastroesophageal reflux yet available. When combined, the esophageal pH electrode and the motility catheter form the basis for a series of tests of esophageal function that have become basic in the evaluation of patients with disordered esophageal motor activity and reflux (Fig. 14-1).[38] These esophageal function tests are: (1) manometry; (2) the acid reflux test; (3) the acid clearing test; and (4) the acid perfusion (Bernstein) test. *Manometry* documents the speed and amplitude of esophageal peristalsis, the location of the upper- and lower-esophageal sphincters in centimeters from the nostrils, and the extent and duration of relaxation of these sphincters during swallowing. In the *acid reflux test,* 200 to 300 ml of 0.1N HC1 are placed in the stomach; the pH electrode is then positioned 5 cm above the lower-esophageal sphincter as determined by previous manometric evaluation, and the presence of abnormal gastroesophageal reflux is documented by the fall of intraesophageal pH below a reading of four during a series of standardized respiratory and postural maneuvers. This study is far more accurate than the barium esophagram in detecting gastroesophageal reflux and is very useful in identifying patients with atypical chest pain caused by gastroesophageal reflux. In the *acid clearing test,* 15 ml of

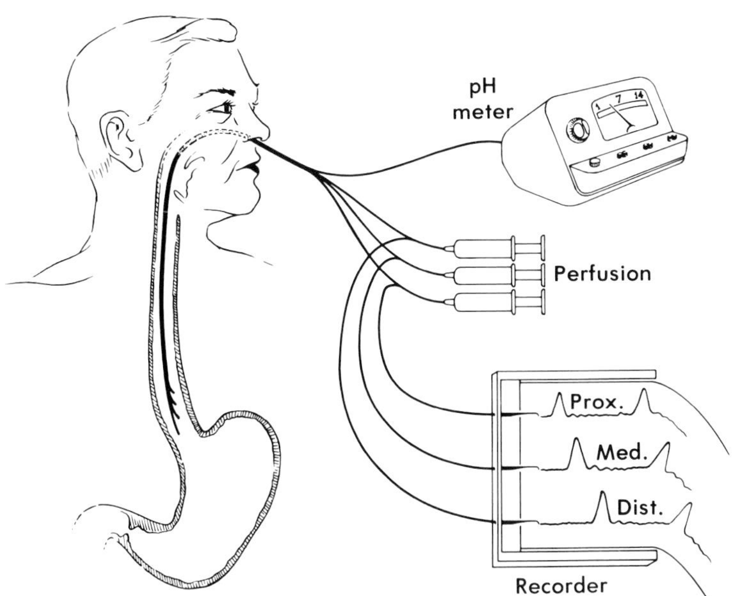

Fig. 14-1 Combined manometric pH recording system used for performing esophageal function tests. Intraluminal esophageal pressures are measured simultaneously from three levels with each separated from the next by 5 cm. Measurements are made from the nostril to the proximal opening of the recording catheter *(Prox.)*. The medial catheter *(Med.)* records pressures 5 cm distal to the proximal opening, and the distal catheter *(Dist.)*, 5 cm below this. The intraesophageal pH electrode is used to document gastroesophageal reflux. (From Orringer, M.B.: The esophagus. In Sabiston, D., editor: Textbook of surgery, ed. 13, Philadelphia, 1986, W.B. Saunders Co.)

0.1N HCl are instilled into the distal esophagus, and the patient is asked to swallow at 30-second intervals. The number of swallows required to "clear" the acid from the esophagus and raise the intraesophageal pH to five is recorded. Patients with normal esophageal motor function can generally clear the acid from the esophagus in 10 swallows or less. The *acid perfusion or Bernstein test* is a recording of subjective symptoms experienced by the patient as acid is dripped into the distal esophagus. This test is regarded as "positive" when the patient's complaints of heartburn or chest pain are induced by the acid infusion. A positive acid perfusion test, however, indicates *only* that the patient has an acid-sensitive esophagus, *not* that the patient has a hiatal hernia, gastroesophageal reflux, or esophagitis.

More recent additions to the armamentarium of objective tests of esophageal function include the bethanechol (Urecholine) "challenge" for esophageal spasm and 24-hour monitoring of distal esophageal pH.[5,16] In the former, the patient receives a subcutaneous injection, usually 5 mg, of a vagomimetic drug (bethanechol), followed 10 minutes later by a second 5-mg dose, and esophageal motor function is recorded from the body of the esophagus while the patient's subjective complaints are noted. In some patients with intermittent esophageal spasm that is not apparent on standard manometric recordings performed when the patient is having no pain, the vagomimetic drug will trigger an episode of both manometric and subjective spasm, both of which are eliminated with an intravenous injection of 0.4 mg of atropine. This correlation of chest pain with the objective manometric criteria of spasm is diagnostic of diffuse esophageal spasm. Finally, 24-hour monitoring of distal esophageal pH, now possible using a completely portable recording system in the ambulatory patient, is the most sensitive currently available means of documenting abnormal gastroesophageal reflux.

THE PHYSIOLOGY OF NORMAL SWALLOWING

The act of swallowing involves both voluntary and involuntary muscles and begins with a voluntary movement of the tongue. This motion initiates an involuntary peristaltic wave that quickly transverses the pharynx and reaches the upper-esophageal sphincter. A brisk upper-esophageal sphincter relaxation then occurs, followed by a sustained postdeglutitive contraction (Fig. 14-2). The upper-esophageal sphincter has an average length of 3 cm and a mean resting pressure of 20 to 60 mm Hg. Its duration of relaxation during swallowing is 0.5 to 1 second. The postdeglutitive contraction has a duration of 2 to 4 seconds and an amplitude of 70 to 100 mm Hg.

A *primary* peristaltic wave is initiated in the body of the esophagus as the swallowed bolus enters from above, and the swallowed material is normally propelled from the

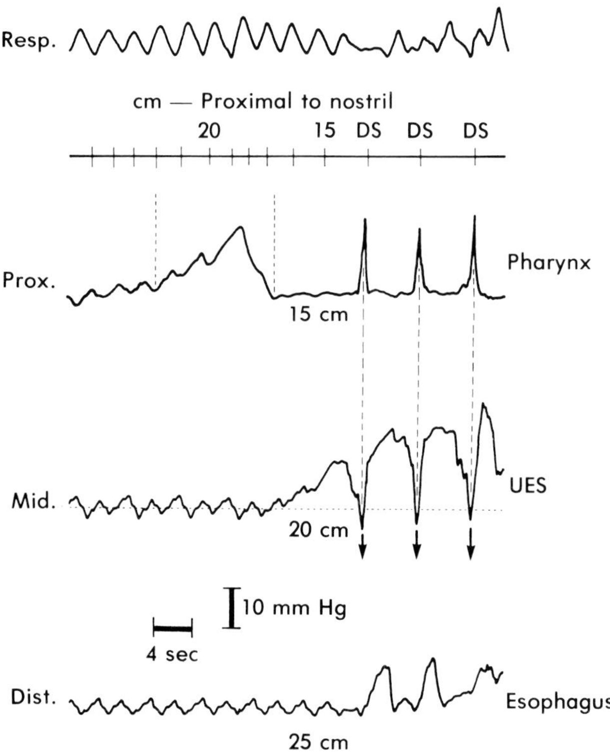

Fig. 14-2 Motility tracing of normal upper-esophageal sphincter *(UES)*. As the catheter is withdrawn, the proximal recording port passes through the upper-esophageal sphincter. Withdrawal is continued until the middle port is within the upper-esophageal sphincter. Each dry swallow *(DS)* results in pharyngeal contraction (proximal catheter), cricopharyngeal relaxation (middle catheter, *arrows*), and a peristaltic wave propagated by the swallow (distal catheter). (*Prox.*, proximal; *Mid.*, middle; *Dist.*, distal; *Resp.*, respiration.) (From Orringer, M.B.: The esophagus. In Sabiston, D., editor: Textbook of surgery, ed. 13, Philadelphia, 1986, W.B. Saunders Co.)

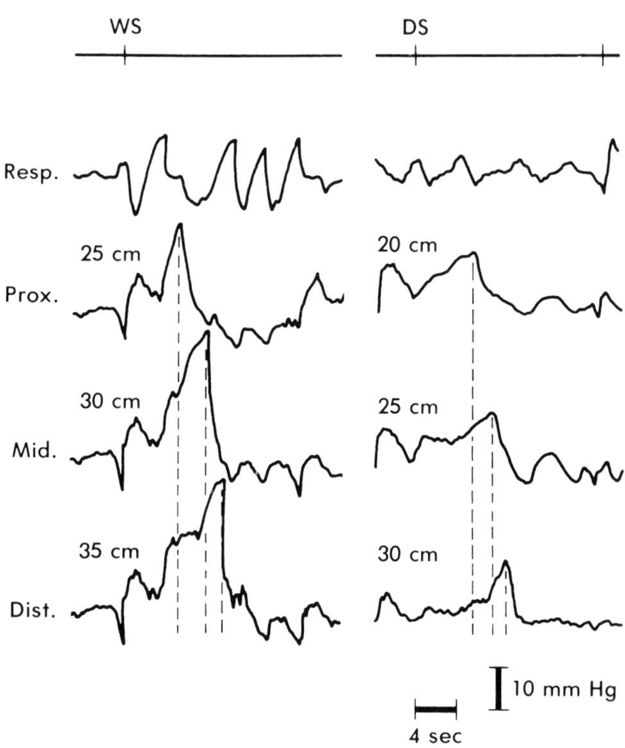

Fig. 14-3 Motility tracing of normal progressive peristaltic contractions that pass first by the proximal *(Prox.)*, then the middle *(Mid.)*, and finally the distal *(Dist.)* recording ports. (*WS*, wet swallow; *DS*, dry swallow; *Resp.*, respiration.) (From Orringer, M.B.: The esophagus. In Sabiston, D., editor: Textbook of surgery, ed. 13, Philadelphia, 1986, W.B. Saunders Co.)

pharynx into the stomach in 4 to 8 seconds in an orderly, progressive fashion (Fig. 14-3). In the chest, esophageal pressures reflect intrathoracic pressure dynamics and are maximally negative (−5 to −10 mm Hg) during inspiration and highest (0 to +5 mm Hg) during expiration. Peristaltic waves in the body of the esophagus have an amplitude of 25 to 80 mm Hg and a duration of 2 to 4 seconds. A *secondary* peristaltic wave is initiated by local distention of the esophagus rather than by a voluntary swallow and occurs if the swallowed bolus of food does not empty from the esophagus into the stomach. Secondary contractions, like the primary waves, are progressive and sequential but begin in the smooth muscle portion of the esophagus (near the level of the aortic arch) and persist until the retained intraesophageal contents are emptied into the stomach. *Tertiary* contractions are simultaneous, nonprogressive, nonperistaltic, and monophasic or multiphasic waves that represent incoordinated contractions of the smooth muscle and result in the radiographic appearance of the "corkscrew" esophagus seen during barium swallow examination.

The lower-esophageal sphincter is a *functional* rather than an *anatomic* sphincter and is thus more correctly referred to as the distal esophageal high-pressure zone (HPZ). A variety of factors, not all of which are known, contribute to the competence of the lower-esophageal sphincter mechanism, but one of the most important factors is the presence of an intra-abdominal segment of distal esophagus under the influence of positive intra-abdominal pressure. Although "normal" resting HPZ pressures range from 10 to 20 mm Hg, incompetence of the lower-esophageal sphincter mechanism cannot be diagnosed on the basis of an absolute HPZ value. Although patients with HPZ pressures of 0 to 5 mm Hg are more likely to have incompetence of the lower-esophageal sphincter and gastroesophageal reflux, many patients with pressures in this range do not have reflux. This is because of the anatomic variation between individuals and the radial asymmetry of the lower sphincter, which result in varied readings during "pull-through" determinations depending on the orientation of the catheter recording port. The intraesophageal pH electrode, not a manometrically determined HPZ value, is the most reliable indicator of lower-esophageal sphincter competence. HPZ length normally varies from 3 to 5 cm (Figs. 14-4 and 14-5). Relaxation occurs within 1.5 to 2.5 seconds after a swallow is initiated and lasts 4 to 6 seconds. Postdeglutitive contractions last 7 to 10 seconds during which HPZ pressures of 25 to 35 mm Hg are generated. Factors influencing distal HPZ pressures are shown in Table 14-1.

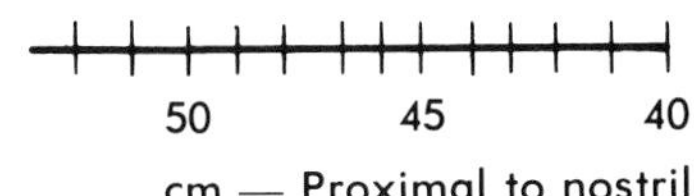

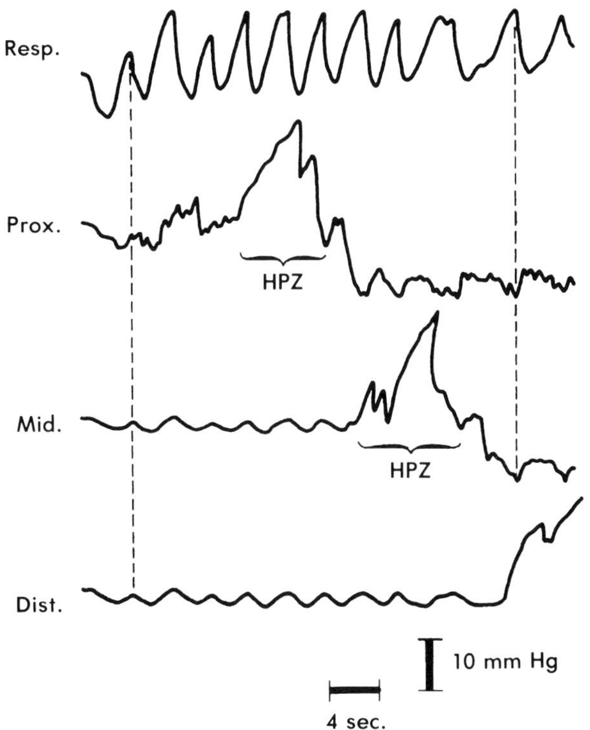

Fig. 14-4 Motility tracing of normal distal sphincter or high-pressure zone *(HPZ)*. Each of the three recording ports passes through the high-pressure zone as the catheter is withdrawn from the stomach into the esophagus. (*Resp.*, respiration; *Prox.*, proximal; *Mid.*, middle; *Dist.*, distal.) (From Orringer, M.B.: The esophagus. In Sabiston, D., editor: Textbook of surgery, ed. 13, Philadelphia, 1986, W.B. Saunders Co.)

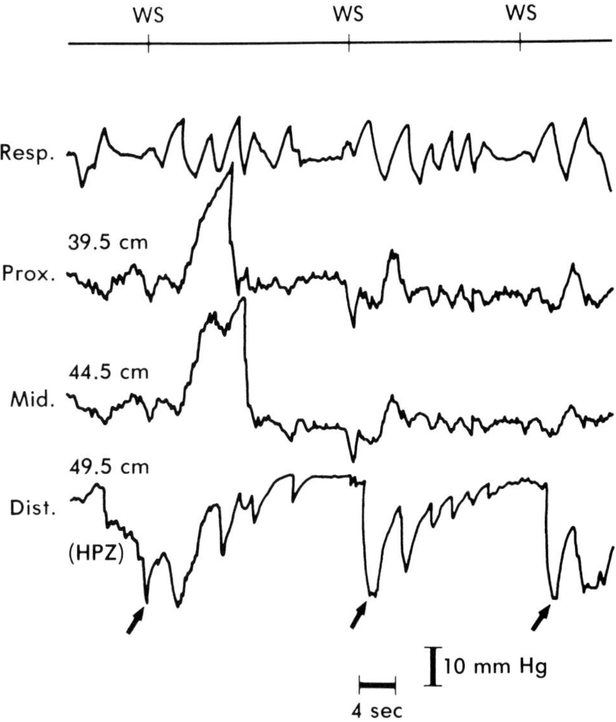

Fig. 14-5 Motility tracing showing normal high-pressure zone *(HPZ)* relaxation with swallowing. The distal recording port is within the high-pressure zone (49.5 cm from the nostrils). Each wet swallow *(WS)* generates a peristaltic wave and relaxation of the high-pressure zone *(arrows)* followed by a sustained postdeglutitive contaction. (*Resp.*, respiration; *Prox.*, proximal; *Mid.*, middle; *Dist.*, distal.) (From Orringer, M.B.: The esophagus. In Sabiston, D., editor: Textbook of surgery, ed. 13, Philadelphia, 1986, W.B. Saunders Co.)

Table 14-1 **FACTORS AFFECTING DISTAL HIGH-PRESSURE ZONE (HPZ) TONE**

Factors	Increased HPZ Tone	Decreased HPZ Tone
Hormonal	Gastrin Motilin Prostaglandin $F_2\alpha$ Bombesin	Secretin Cholecystokinin Glucagon Progesterone Estrogen Prostaglandin E_1, E_2, A_2 Vasoactive intestinal polypeptide
Drugs	Alpha-adrenergic agents Norepinephrine Phenylephrine Anticholinesterase Edrophonium Cholinergic agents Bethanechol (Urecholine) Methacholine (Mecholyl) Betazole Metaclopramide	Alpha-adrenergic blockers Phentolamine Anticholinergics Atropine Theophylline Beta-adrenergic blockers Isoproterenol Ethanol Nicotine Nitroglycerin
Foods	Protein meal	Fatty meal Chocolate
Myogenic	Normal resting muscle tone	? Aging ? Diabetes mellitus
Mechanical	Antireflux surgery	Hiatal hernia Abnormal phrenoesophageal ligament insertion Short or absent intra-abdominal distal segment Nasogastric tube
Miscellaneous	Gastric alkalinization Gastric distention	Gastric acidification Gastrectomy Hypoglycemia Hypothyroidism Amyloidosis Pernicious anemia

Modified from Hurwitz, A.L., Duranceau, A., and Haddad, J.K. In Smith, L.H., Jr.: Major problems in internal medicine, Philadelphia, 1979, W.B. Saunders Co.

CAUSES OF CRICOPHARYNGEAL MOTOR DYSFUNCTION

NEUROGENIC
Central
- Parkinson's disease
- Bulbar poliomyelitis
- Brain tumor
- Midbrain stroke—basilar artery thrombosis
- Amyotrophic lateral sclerosis
- Huntington's chorea
- Multiple sclerosis

PERIPHERAL
- Recurrent laryngeal nerve injury—either operative or secondary to inflammatory neuritis or to neuropathy
- Superior laryngeal nerve injury

Mixed—myasthenia gravis
Reflex
- Associated with gastroesophageal reflux
- Other distal esophageal disease (e.g., tumor and achalasia)

MYOGENIC
Polymyositis
Congenital oculopharyngeal myotonic dystrophy
Thyrotoxicosis

Modified from Hurwitz, A.L., Duranceau, A., and Haddad, J.K. In Smith, L.H., Jr.: Major problems in internal medicine, Philadelphia, 1979, W.B. Saunders Co.

SWALLOWING DISORDERS

Functional disorders of the esophagus are those conditions that interfere with the normal act of swallowing or produce dysphagia without any associated intraluminal organic obstruction or extrinsic compression of the esophagus.[2] These conditions have been more precisely defined as a result of the wider use of esophageal function tests, underscoring the importance of understanding both normal and abnormal esophageal physiology in these patients.

Upper-Esophageal Sphincter or Cricopharyngeal Dysfunction

The upper-esophageal sphincter is unique to the gastrointestinal tract, representing a sling rather than a ring of muscle (cricopharyngeus) arising from the cricoid cartilage and inserting into the median raphe of the posterior pharynx. Its anatomic configuration, the normal laryngeal excursions during the act of swallowing, and the rapidity of neuromotor events in the pharynx during deglutition are responsible for the failure to define precisely and consistently the manometric abnormalities in patients with cricopharyngeal motor function. Therefore such terms as cricopharyngeal achalasia, chalasia, or spasm generally lack objective basis since standard manometric techniques usually fail to show specific abnormalities of upper-esophageal sphincter function in patients with these conditions. Nevertheless, the diagnosis of globus hystericus in the patient with cervical dysphagia is a diagnosis of exclusion since most of these patients have a consistent history that is indicative or organic rather than psychologic disease. A variety of neural and myogenic processes affects the upper-esophageal sphincter (see boxed material above).[15] This sphincter, however, is limited in its response to these multiple conditions; the resulting syndrome of *cricopharyngeal dysfunction* has a remarkably constant clinical appearance that includes cervical dysphagia, expectoration of saliva, hoarseness, and weight loss.[22] Since gastroesophageal reflux or any condition that affects the lower esophagus may induce reflex upper-esophageal sphincter dysfunction, the physician should not limit his evaluation of the patient with cervical dysphagia to the throat; instead, he should examine the *entire* esophagus radiographically, endoscopically, and with esophageal function tests.

The barium esophagram of a patient with cricopharyngeal dysfunction may be normal if the patient has intermittent symptoms and is asymptomatic at the time of his radiograph evaluation. Alternatively, there may be hypertonicity of the upper sphincter, a typical posterior cricopharyngeal bar, or a pharyngoesophageal (Zenker's) diverticulum (Figs. 14-6 to 14-8). As indicated previously, manometry

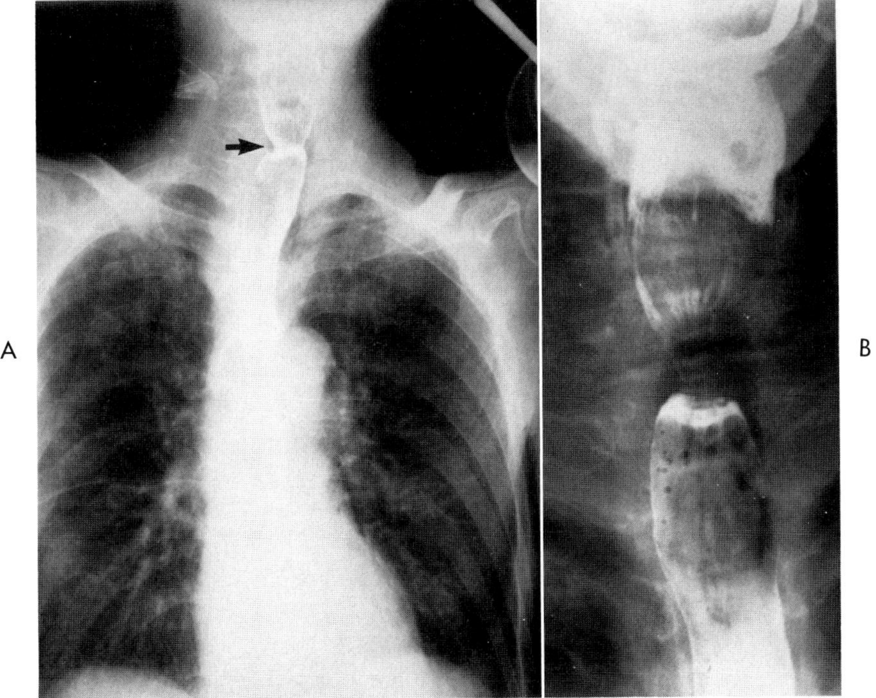

Fig. 14-6 **A,** Prominence of the cricopharyngeal sphincter *(arrow)* in a patient with cervical dysphagia and gastroesophageal reflux. **B,** Detail of cervical esophagus. (From Orringer, M.B.: J. Thorac. Cardiovasc. Surg. **80:**669, 1980.)

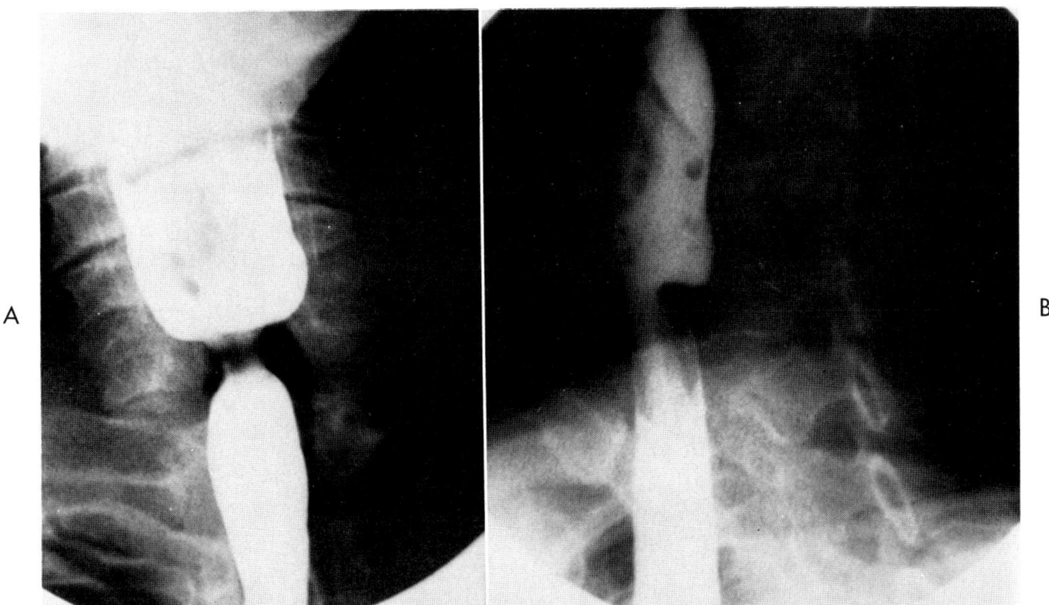

Fig. 14-7 **A,** Hypertrophic cricopharyngeal sphincter (anteroposterior view). **B,** Typical posterior cricopharyngeal bar (lateral view). (From Orringer, M.B.: J. Thorac. Cardiovasc. Surg. **80:**669, 1980.)

may fail to demonstrate spasm, hypotonicity, or lack of upper-esophageal sphincter relaxation, but incoordination of the temporal relaxation between pharyngeal contraction and cricopharyngeal relaxation has been shown in these patients.[10] Gastroesophageal reflux is detected with the intraesophageal pH electrode in at least one third of the patients. The patient with a pharyngoesophageal diverticulum categorically has abnormality of cricopharyngeal motor function. This pouch invariably occurs proximal to the upper-esophageal sphincter muscle within the inferior pharyngeal constrictor at the transition between the oblique fibers of the thyropharyngeus muscle and the more horizontal fibers of the cricopharyngeus muscle (Fig. 14-9). The transition in the direction of these muscle fibers (Killian's triangle) is a point of potential weakness in the posterior pharynx. As the swallowed bolus exerts pressure within the pharynx, the mucosa herniates through the anatomically weak area above the cricopharyngeus muscle. The diverticulum enlarges, drapes over the cricopharyngeus, and dissects inferiorly in the prevertebral space behind the esophagus and eventually into the superior mediastinum.

The treatment of cricopharyngeal motor dysfunction must be individualized and is as varied as the numerous conditions with which it is associated. Patients with reflux symptoms and associated cervical dysphagia may have their swallowing problem disappear with the institution of a strict medical antireflux regimen. Outpatient esophageal dilation to the range of 54 to 56 French dilator may provide relief from cervical dysphagia in patients with Parkinson's disease or the residual symptoms of a midbrain stroke. In the presence of incapacitating cervical dysphagia and aspiration, a radiographically or manometrically documented abnormal upper-esophageal sphincter, or particularly a pharyngoesophageal diverticulum, a cervical eso-

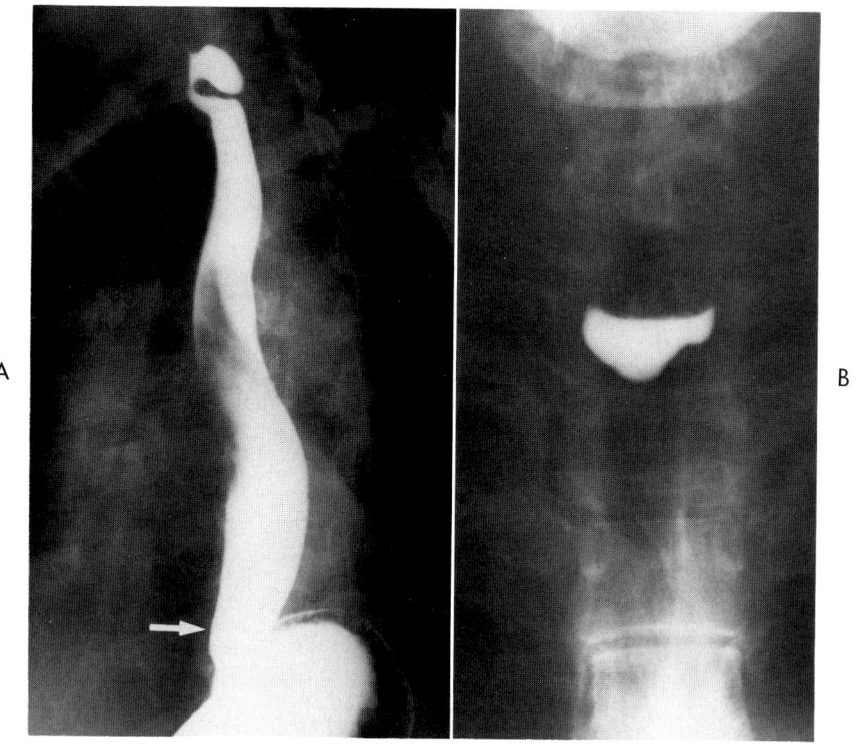

Fig. 14-8 **A,** Zenker's (pharyngoesophageal) diverticulum in a patient with a "patulous cardia" *(arrow)* and gastroesophageal reflux. **B,** Residual barium in the 2.5-cm pouch. (From Orringer, M.B.: J. Thorac. Cardiovasc. Surg. **80:**669, 1980.)

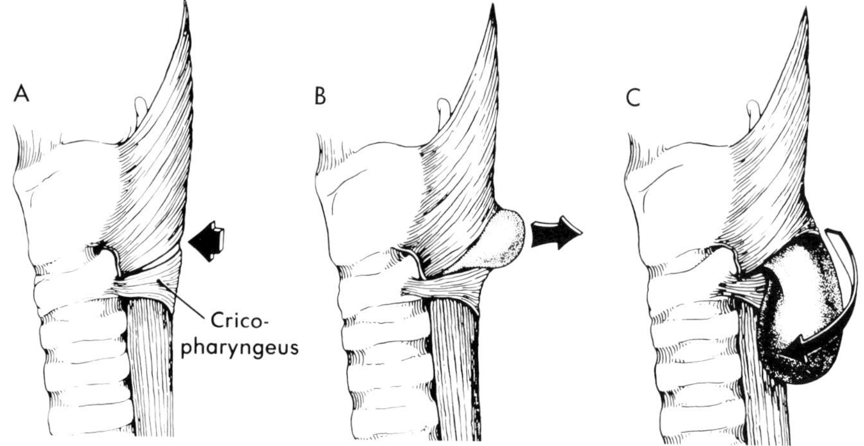

Fig. 14-9 Formation of Zenker's diverticulum. **A,** Herniation of the mucosa and submucosa occurs at the transition *(arrow)* between the oblique fibers of the thyropharyngeus muscle and the horizontal cricopharyngeus muscle fibers. **B** and **C,** The diverticulum enlarges and dissects toward the left side and downward into the superior mediastinum in the prevertebral space. (From Orringer, M.B.: The esophagus. In Sabiston, D., editor: Textbook of surgery, ed. 13, Philadelphia, 1986, W.B. Saunders Co.)

phagomyotomy relieves the relative obstruction from the incoordinated sphincter (Fig. 14-10). Diverticula 1 to 2 cm in diameter need not be excised since they simply disappear into the adjacent bulging mucosa after the cervical esophagomyotomy. Larger pouches are excised using an automatic stapler, but an esophagomyotomy *must* be performed (Fig. 14-11). This concept bears emphasis—the surgical treatment of the pharyngoesophageal diverticulum, like that of *every* pulsion diverticulum, must be directed at the underlying motor abnormality responsible for formation of the pouch and not at the pouch per se. In the neck, this means division of the cricopharyngeal sphincter. Simply resecting the diverticulum without dividing the underlying incoordinated sphincter leaves the potential for recurrence of the diverticulum and suture-line disruption. Cervical esophagomyotomy for cricopharyngeal dysfunction is successful in 65% to 85% of patients, especially those with pharyngoesophageal diverticula.[14,22]

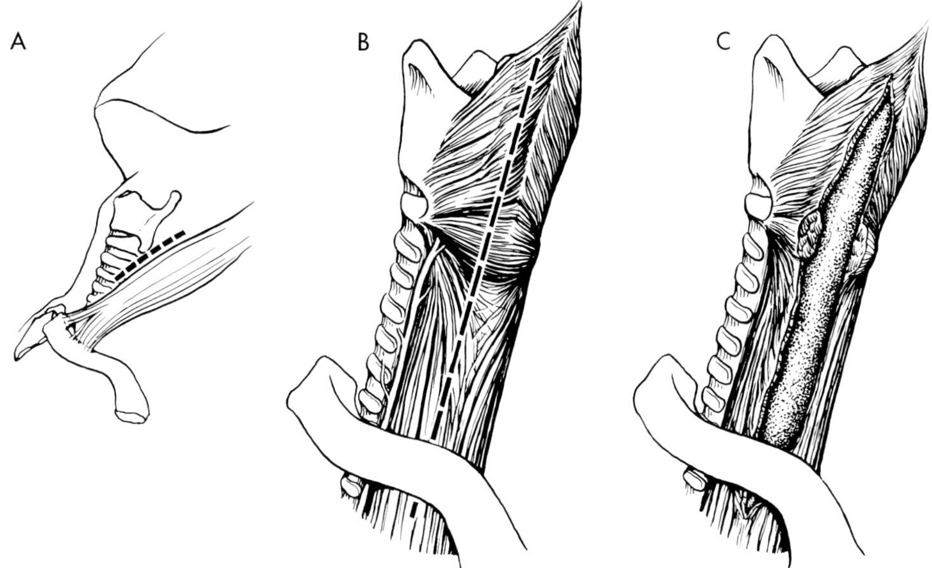

Fig. 14-10 Cervical esophagomyotomy for cricopharyngeal dysfunction is performed through a 5-cm oblique skin incision, **A,** anterior to the left sternocleidomastoid muscle and centered over the cricoid cartilage. **B,** Esophagomyotomy is performed on the left posterolateral aspect of the esophagus, avoiding injury to the recurrent laryngeal nerve in the tracheoesophageal groove. **C,** Completed myotomy extends from the level of the superior cornu of the thyroid cartilage to a point 1 to 2 cm behind the clavicle. (From Orringer, M.B.: J. Thorac. Cardiovasc. Surg. **80:**669, 1980.)

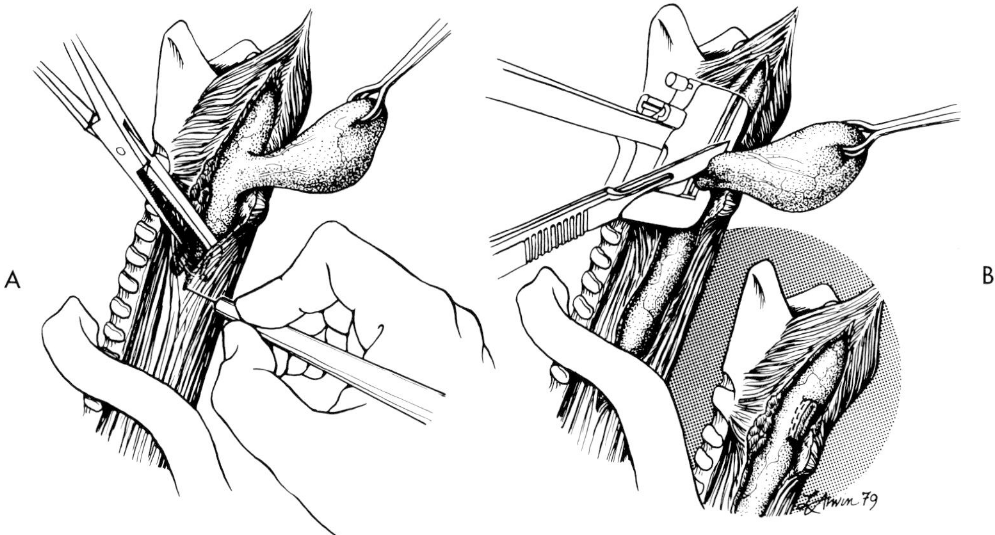

Fig. 14-11 Cervical esophagomyotomy and concomitant resection of a Zenker's diverticulum. **A,** Pouch is mobilized, and esophagomyotomy is performed from its base for the same distance shown in Fig. 14-10. **B,** Base of the pouch is crossed with a surgical stapler and is amputated. (From Orringer, M.B.: J. Thorac. Cardiovasc. Surg. **80:**669, 1980.)

Motor Disorders of the Body of the Esophagus

Motor disorders of the body of the esophagus are best viewed as a continuum with hypomotility (achalasia) at one extreme and hypermotility (diffuse esophageal spasm) at the other. Between these extremes are a variety of less well-characterized esophageal neuromotor disorders (vigorous achalasia and "curling") and nonspecific abnormal peristalsis associated with collagen vascular disease (scleroderma and dermatomyositis), peripheral neuropathy (diabetes and alcoholism), multiple sclerosis, myasthenia gravis, and other disorders.

Achalasia

Achalasia is a Greek term that literally means "failure or lack of relaxation" and refers to the failure of the lower-esophageal sphincter to relax normally when the patient swallows. This term, however, focuses solely on the distal sphincter when, in fact, this is a condition that involves the entire body of the esophagus. In South America, achalasia is associated with Chagas' disease, which is caused by parasitic infestation by the leishmanial forms of *Trypanosoma cruzi*. This parasite destroys the ganglion cells of Auerbach's plexus resulting in motor dysfunction and progressive dilation, not only of the esophagus, but also of the colon, ureters, and other viscera as well. In patients with achalasia unrelated to Chagas' disease, the esophageal ganglionic cells are similarly reduced in number. Because achalasia may follow a variety of conditions (e.g., infection and physical and emotional stress), it would appear that, just as with the upper-esophageal sphincter, there is only a limited number of ways in which the esophagus can respond to factors affecting either its central or peripheral vagal innervation or the ganglion cells of Auerbach's plexus.

The patient with achalasia is initially seen with a classic triad of symptoms—dysphagia, regurgitation, and weight loss. The difficulty swallowing is typically aggravated by stress or by ingestion of cold liquids. Large amounts of water are swallowed with meals to wash food into the stomach. Retrosternal fullness increases as the meal progresses, and the patient will often twist the upper torso or walk around the room in an effort to force down solids. Either the column of fluid within the esophagus becomes heavy enough to force open the lower-esophageal sphincter and allow emptying into the stomach or the patient must regurgitate for relief. Retrosternal pain is uncommon in achalasia and is more typical of diffuse spasm. When the esophagus becomes dilated, foul-smelling stagnating intraesophageal contents may be regurgitated, and the patient may experience nocturnal aspiration that results in recurrent respiratory infections. Weight loss in these patients is

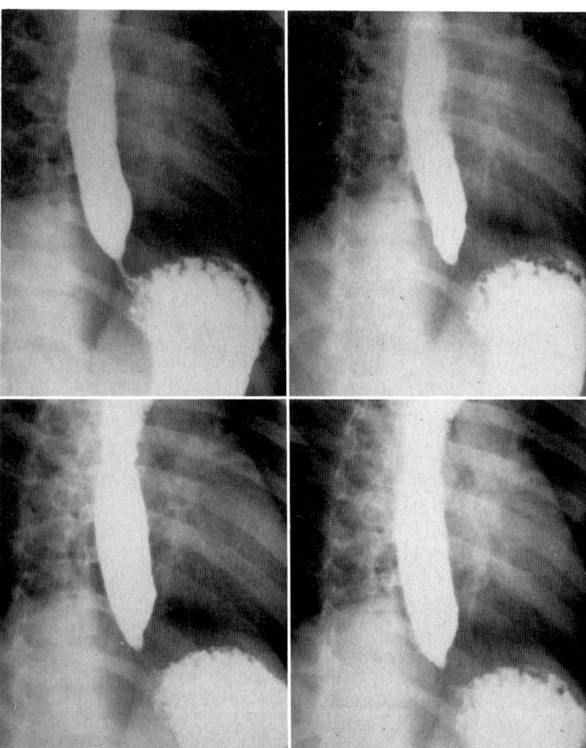

Fig. 14-12 Multiple views from cine esophagram showing typical bird-beak taper at the esophagogastric junction, delayed emptying, and mild esophageal dilation of early achalasia. (From Orringer, M.B.: The esophagus. In Sabiston, D., editor: Textbook of surgery, ed. 13, Philadelphia, 1986, W.B. Saunders Co.)

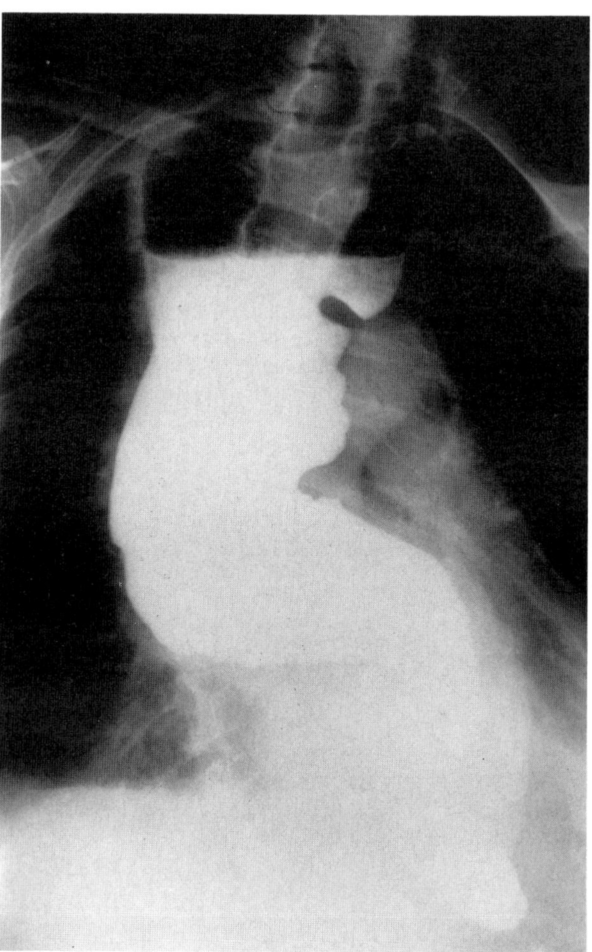

Fig. 14-13 Massively dilated megaesophagus of advanced achalasia showing retained secretions and air-fluid level high in thorax. This patient was experiencing nocturnal aspiration and recurrent pneumonia. (From Orringer, M.B.: The esophagus. In Sabiston, D., editor: Textbook of surgery, ed. 13, Philadelphia, 1986, W.B. Saunders Co.)

common. Achalasia is a premalignant lesion of the esophagus with carcinoma developing in 1% to 10% of patients who have this condition. The carcinoma is believed to be the result of severe mucosal irritation and the subsequent metaplasia induced by retention esophagitis from the putrifying intraesophageal contents.

Radiographically, the esophagus in patients with achalasia varies with the extent of the disease, showing mild dilation in the early stages (Fig. 14-12) and massive dilation, tortuosity, and a distal sigmoid configuration later (Fig. 14-13). Retained secretions are commonly seen, and peristalsis becomes progressively disordered and eventually disappears in patients with a megaesophagus. The "bird-beak" taper of the esophagogastric junction is the roentgenographic hallmark of achalasia. Manometrically, the lower-esophageal sphincter fails to relax during swallowing, and there is no progressive peristalsis throughout the length of the esophagus (Fig. 14-14). In early achalasia, contractions after swallowing may be of normal amplitude, but they are synchronous and simultaneous (Fig. 14-15). Later, contractions are either weak, simultaneous, or totally absent (Fig. 14-16). HPZ pressure is usually normal or slightly elevated but is not markedly hypertensive as seen in spasm. Esophagoscopy is necessary but extremely dangerous in the patient with achalasia with the risk of aspiration of retained esophageal contents being of utmost concern. It is my belief that patients with a megaesophagus should undergo esophagoscopy while under general anesthesia after their airway has been protected by the use of an endotracheal tube cuff. The rigid esophagoscope can then be used to evacuate intraesophageal debris. Esophagoscopy is necessary in achalasia: (1) to assess the presence of retention esophagitis, which might complicate surgery; (2) to exclude an associated esophageal malignancy; and (3) to determine if there is a distal stricture

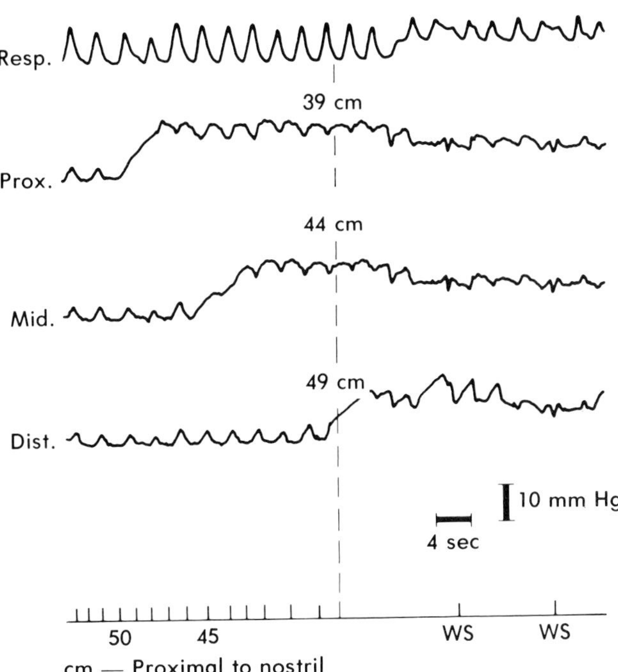

Fig. 14-14 Motility tracing of the distal high-pressure zone in achalasia showing elevated basal intraesophageal pressure relative to the stomach and lack of high-pressure zone relaxation with swallowing. The distal recording port is in the high-pressure zone. There is no evidence of peristalsis with swallowing. (*WS*, wet swallow; *Resp.*, respiration; *Prox.*, proximal; *Mid.*, middle; *Dist.*, distal.) (From Orringer, M.B.: The esophagus. In Sabiston, D., editor: Textbook of surgery, ed. 13, Philadelphia, 1986, W.B. Saunders Co.)

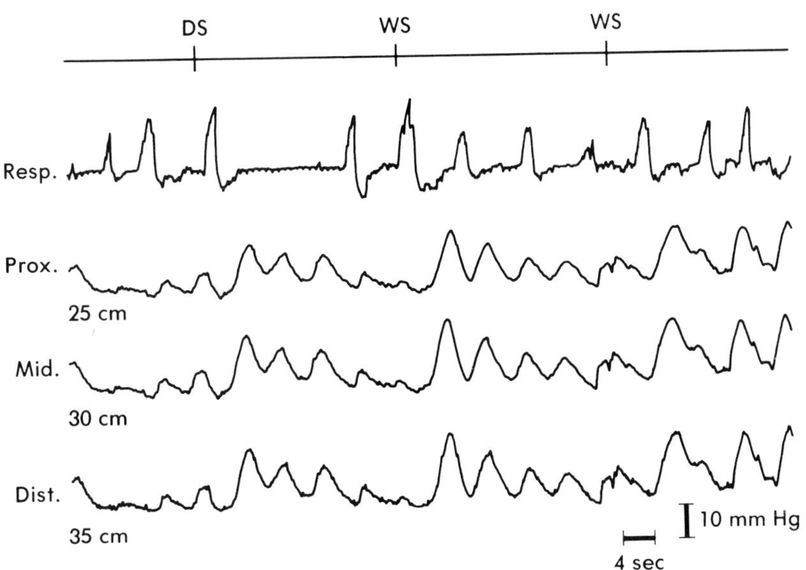

Fig. 14-15 Motility tracing in early achalasia showing normal amplitude esophageal contractions after swallowing, which are nonprogressive, simultaneous, and multiphasic. (*WS*, wet swallow; *DS*, dry swallow; *Resp.*, respiration; *Prox.*, proximal; *Mid.*, middle; *Dist.*, distal.) (From Orringer, M.B.: The esophagus. In Sabiston, D., editor: Textbook of surgery, ed. 13, Philadelphia, 1986, W.B. Saunders Co.)

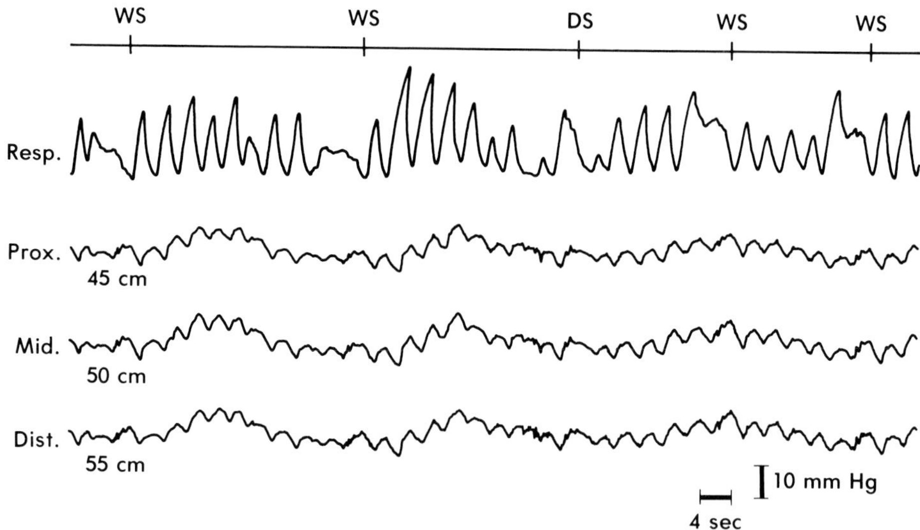

Fig. 14-16 Motility tracing in advanced achalasia with megaesophagus showing that virtually no esophageal contractions are generated by swallowing. (*DS,* dry swallow; *WS,* wet swallow; *Resp.,* respiration; *Prox.,* proximal; *Mid.,* middle; *Dist.,* distal.) (From Orringer, M.B.: The esophagus. In Sabiston, D., editor: Textbook of surgery, ed. 13, Philadelphia, 1986, W.B. Saunders Co.)

resulting from reflux esophagitis that may have followed previous forceful dilations or from an esophagomyotomy that destroyed the lower-esophageal sphincter mechanism.

The therapeutic options in achalasia are generally either forceful dilation (pneumatic or hydrostatic) or distal thoracic esophagomyotomy. An occasional patient with early achalasia may respond to sublingual nitroglycerin before meals or to passage of Maloney esophageal dilators. Regardless of the therapy, achalasia is currently an incurable disease; the derangement in motor function in these patients never returns to normal. Treatment is therefore palliative and directed at relieving the distal obstruction. The Mayo Clinic has the most extensive experience in the world with both forceful dilation and extramucosal distal esophagomyotomy for achalasia.[21] Its recently reported results are summarized in Table 14-2. Thoracic esophagomyotomy may be performed either through a thoracotomy or an abdominal incision and involves a 7- to 10-cm incision through the longitudinal and circular muscle fibers of the esophagus from the level of the inferior pulmonary vein above through the distal sphincter below.[8] Despite the demonstrated superiority of esophagomyotomy in terms of mortality, incidence of perforation, and long-term relief of dysphagia, there still is ample justification for using forceful dilation, which is successful in 65% of the cases when used as the primary treatment in these patients, reserving surgery for those patients in whom dilation is unsuccessful or not applicable. Few physicians, however, gain the required experience to become skillful in forceful dilation for achalasia; thus disruption of the incoordinated lower-esophageal members while under direct vision has greater appeal and safety in most cases.

One of the unresolved aspects of the surgical management of these patients is whether there is a need for an antireflux operation to be performed in association with the esophagomyotomy. In the Mayo Clinic experience in which an antireflux procedure was not routinely used after the esophagomyotomy, there was only a three-percent incidence of late serious complications of gastroesophageal reflux.[21] Other surgeons, however, believe that complete relief of the obstruction caused by the incoordinated lower-esophageal sphincter can only be achieved by rendering it incompetent (i.e., extending the esophagomyotomy through the entire sphincter and onto the stomach for 1 to 2 cm). A 20% to 25% incidence of significant gastroesophageal reflux after esophagomyotomy has been used as justification for the addition of either a modified Belsey or Nissen fundoplication.[3,18,19] Although it is commonly taught in the United States that a fundoplication will obstruct an atonic esophagus that lacks progressive peristal-

Table 14-2 **COMPARISON OF RESULTS OF HYDROSTATIC DILATION AND ESOPHAGOMYOTOMY (1949-1975)**

Factors	Dilation (431 patients)	Esophagomyotomy (468 patients)
Mortality	2 patients (0.5%)	1 patient (0.2%)
Esophageal perforation	19 patients (4%)	5 patients (1%)
Requiring surgery	10 patients	3 patients
Follow-up		
Duration	1-18 years	1-17 years
Number patients	311 patients (72%)	456 patients (97%)
Result		
Excellent	28% } 65%*	50% } 85%*
Good	37% }	35% }
Fair	16%	9%
Poor	19%	6%

From Okike, N., et al.: Ann. Thorac. Surg. **28:**119, 1979.
*Significantly different ($p < 0.001$).

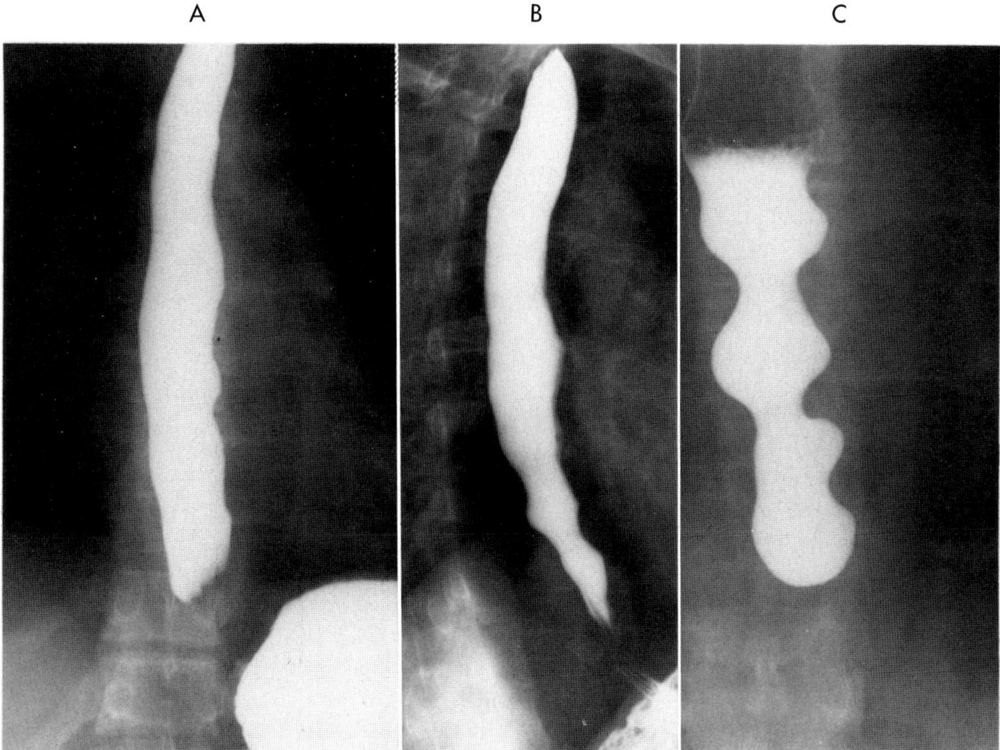

Fig. 14-17 Three views from barium esophagrams in the same patient with intermittent diffuse esophageal spasm showing the variability of roentgenographic findings in this condition. **A,** Virtually normal appearance; **B,** distal taper suggesting achalasia; and **C,** typical "cork-screw" esophagus. Esophageal manometry is essential for establishing a diagnosis in such a patient. (From Orringer, M.B.: The esophagus. In Sabiston, D., editor: Textbook of surgery, ed. 13, Philadelphia, 1986, W.B. Saunders Co.)

sis, in Europe a 360-degree fundoplication has been used in association with a transabdominal esophagomyotomy for achalasia for years with excellent results.[36] In my experience, as long as the esophagus is not greatly dilated (beyond 6 to 7 cm), a short 2-cm 360-degree Nissen fundoplication performed over a 46 French bougie provides a very satisfactory antireflux mechanism after esophagomyotomy for achalasia without producing esophageal obstruction.

In patients with recurrent esophageal obstruction after a previous esophagomyotomy or with a peptic stricture from reflux that has followed either esophagomyotomy or a forceful dilation, a further esophagomyotomy is unlikely to provide long-term relief from dysphagia. In such patients, esophageal resection and visceral esophageal substitution, usually with stomach, definitively eliminates the esophageal problem and premalignant potential and can be performed transhiatally without the need to open the thorax.[25]

Diffuse Esophageal Spasm

Diffuse esophageal spasm (DES) is a poorly understood hypermotility disorder in which the patient experiences chest pain and/or dysphagia as a result of repetitive, simultaneous, high-amplitude esophageal contractions. The etiology of DES is unknown. The patient with DES is typically, but not always, a young anxious woman with chest pain that is not consistently related to eating, activity, or position. The differential diagnosis is that of angina pectoris of cardiac origin, with the chest pain often described as squeezing, oppressive retrosternal pressure radiating toward the jaw, down the arms, or "straight through" to the interscapular region of the back. As with achalasia, symptoms are often worse under emotional stress; but in contrast to achalasia, although "slow emptying" of the esophagus may be felt, regurgitation is uncommon, and pain is the predominant complaint. These patients have often undergone an extensive cardiac evaluation before the possibility of an esophageal etiology for their pain has been considered. Gastroesophageal reflux as well as other associated intra-abdominal pathology (e.g., cholelithiasis and gastric or duodenal ulcer disease) may trigger DES and should therefore be excluded.

The barium swallow findings in patients with DES may be quite variable depending on the degree of symptoms being experienced at the time of the study (Fig. 14-17). Little if any abnormality may be apparent if the patient is having no pain during the barium swallow; at other times, "curling" or a "cork-screw" esophagus caused by segmental contractions of the circular muscle is seen. A hiatal hernia or gastroesophageal reflux may be seen. If an esophageal pulsion diverticulum of the mid- or lower-esophagus is seen on the barium esophagram, particularly if the patient has angina-like symptoms, the diagnosis of

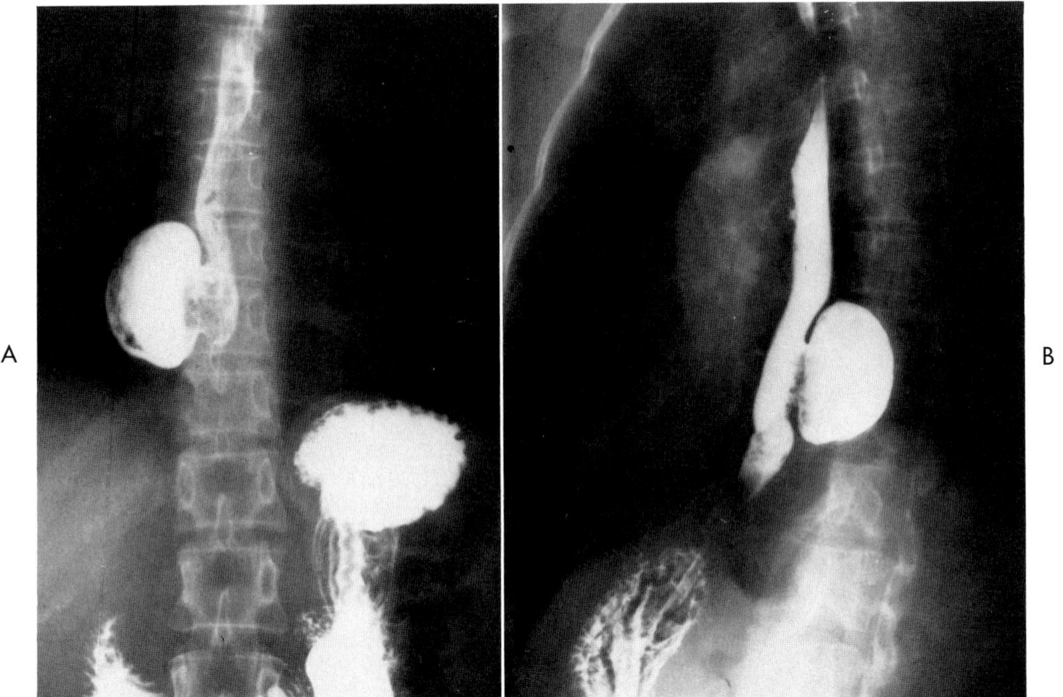

Fig. 14-18 **A,** Posteroanterior and, **B,** lateral views of barium esophagrams showing a midesophageal pulsion diverticulum in a patient with periodic chest pain and manometric esophageal spasm. (From Orringer, M.B.: The esophagus. In Sabiston, D., editor: Textbook of surgery, ed. 13, Philadelphia, 1986, W.B. Saunders Co.)

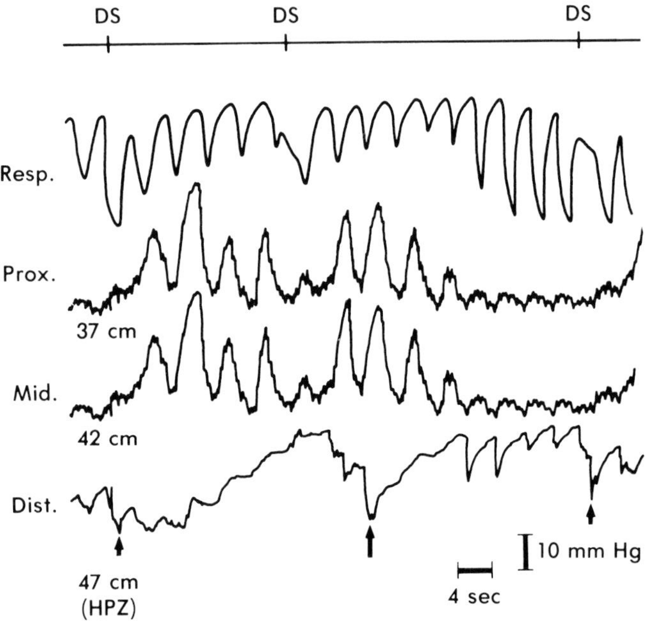

Fig. 14-19 Motility tracing in diffuse esophageal spasm showing simultaneous, multiphasic nonprogressive esophageal contractions after swallowing. Unlike with achalasia, high-pressure zone relaxation with swallowing *(arrows)* still occurs (*DS*, dry swallow; *Resp.*, respiration; Prox., proximal; *Mid.*, middle; *Dist.*, distal.) (From Orringer, M.B.: The esophagus. In Sabiston, D., editor: Textbook of surgery, ed. 13, Philadelphia, 1986, W.B. Saunders Co.)

diffuse esophageal spasm is virtually assured (Fig. 14-18). Just as with pharyngoesophageal diverticula, midesophageal and epiphrenic diverticula form only if there is distal obstruction caused either by an organic stenosis or, more commonly, by an abnormality of motor function.

Use of esophagoscopy is indicated in patients with diffuse esophageal spasm since a distal esophageal stenosis may produce proximal tertiary contractions that may be confused with diffuse esophageal spasm during a barium study; an infiltrating tumor, benign fibrous stricture, or reflux esophagitis should therefore be excluded. Although esophageal manometry is the classic means of diagnosing diffuse esophageal spasm, unless the patient is experiencing pain at the time of the evaluation, just as with the barium esophagram, the results may be entirely normal. During the manometric procedure, diffuse esophageal spasm is characterized by simultaneous, multiphasic, and repetitive high-amplitude contractions that occur after a swallow spontaneously in the smooth muscle portion of the esophagus (Fig. 14-19). Progressive peristalsis is seen in the upper one third and occasionally in the lower two thirds of the esophagus as well. Upper- and lower-sphincter resting pressures and relaxation during swallowing are usually normal, although a hypertensive lower-esophageal sphincter may be seen. The acid reflux test demonstrates abnormal gastroesophageal reflux in nearly one third of these patients. If standard manometry fails to demonstrate diffuse esophageal spasm, evocative maneuvers, including ice-water or hydrochloric-acid intraesophageal infusions, may induce the motility disorder. Administration of a vagomimetic drug (e.g., 10 mg of bethanechol administered

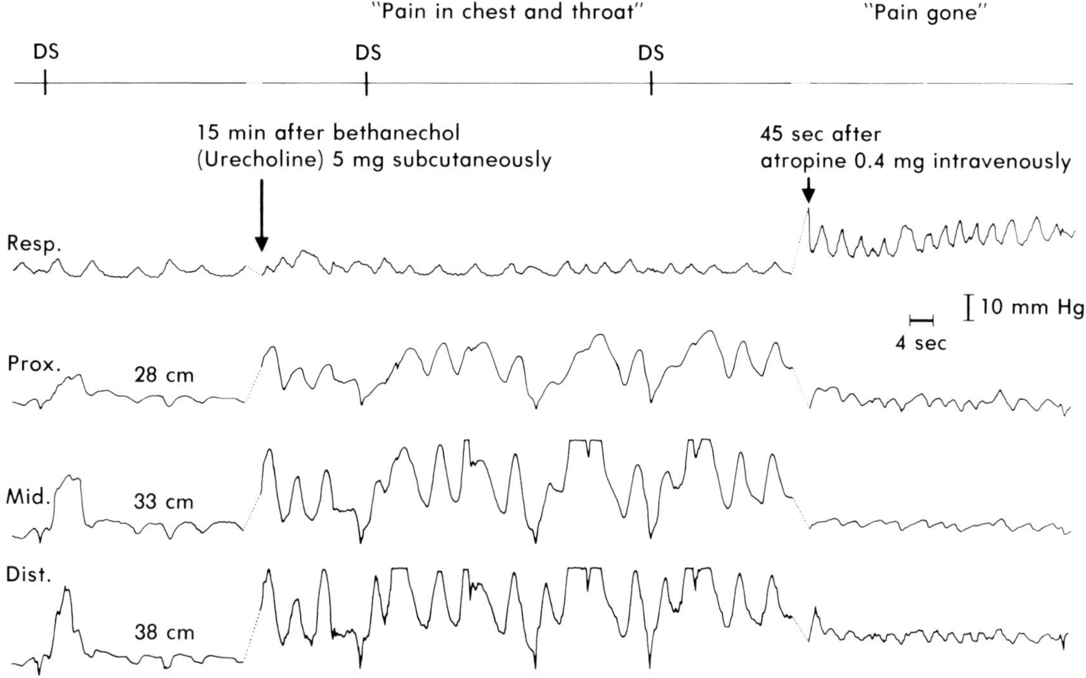

Fig. 14-20 Bethanechol (Urecholine) evocative test for esophageal spasm. Manometric and symptomatic esophageal spasm occur in response to this vagomimetic drug and are eliminated with atropine. (*DS,* dry swallow; *Resp.,* respiration; *Prox.,* proximal; *Mid.,* middle; *Dist.,* distal.) (From Orringer, M.B.: The esophagus. In Sabiston, D., editor: Textbook of surgery, ed. 13, Philadelphia, 1986, W.B. Saunders Co.)

subcutaneously) may result in both symptomatic and objective diffuse esophageal spasm in more than one third of these patients, and a positive "bethanechol (Urecholine) challenge" is thus the diagnostic hallmark of diffuse esophageal spasm (Fig. 14-20).

Because knowledge of the etiology of diffuse esophageal spasm is lacking, therapy is unsatisfactory in most cases. Many of these patients, extremely anxious individuals, have an underlying psychiatric abnormality and often have a history of functional bowel disease (irritable or spastic colon). These individuals are but another example of the sensitivity, in general, of the gut to emotional stress. Simply establishing an esophageal etiology for the pain in these patients and providing reassurance may have great therapeutic benefit. Stress at mealtime and "trigger" foods or drinks should be avoided. Gastroesophageal reflux, if documented with the acid reflux test, should be treated medically, but it should not be assumed that reflux is present or is the cause of the spasm in these patients. Cimetidine may be helpful in those patients with reflux. Anticholinergic antispasmodics may help at times. Sublingual nitroglycerin and long-acting nitrates may provide dramatic relief of esophageal spasm. The calcium blockers (e.g., nifedipine) have had variable efficiency in patients with diffuse esophageal spasm. Esophageal dilation with tapered Maloney bougies (in the range of size 50 to 60 French) may relieve both the dysphagia and the chest pain from diffuse esophageal spasm for weeks to months; if this is the case, consideration should be given to self dilations at home.

The advocated surgical treatment of diffuse esophageal spasm consists of a long esophagomyotomy extending from the level of the aortic arch to the lower-esophageal sphincter.[9] Unfortunately, this approach is successful in only 50% to 60% of these patients, who may continue to complain of chest pain and slow esophageal emptying despite objective evidence of improvement in the manometric and radiographic indicators of diffuse esophageal spasm. For this reason, in these often emotionally labile patients only in the most *extenuating circumstances*—incapacitating chest pain, dysphagia, or with a pulsion diverticulum of the intrathoracic esophagus—should an esophagomyotomy be performed for diffuse esophageal spasm. The technique is similar to that used for achalasia except that the extramucosal esophagomyotomy is longer. Again controversy surrounds the need to divide the lower-esophageal sphincter completely in these patients when performing the esophagomyotomy. Again I endorse Belsey's view that only complete division of all distal esophageal circular muscle fibers ensures relief from the obstruction caused by motor disease[2]; therefore either a modified Belsey Mark IV operation or a short 2-cm Nissen fundoplication performed over a 46-French bougie should be performed after the esophagomyotomy for diffuse esophageal spasm.

Scleroderma

Scleroderma, or systemic sclerosis, is a collagen vascular disease of unknown etiology that is characterized by induration of the skin, fibrosis of the smooth muscle of internal organs, and progressive loss of visceral and cutaneous function. Disruption of normal esophageal peristalsis is so common that it is regarded as a major diagnostic sign of scleroderma, particularly in the type of the disease associated with Raynaud's phenomenon (Fig. 14-21). Initially these patients with slow emptying of the esophagus are required to wash down their food with large quantities of water. As distal esophageal fibrosis progresses, however, the distal high-pressure zone loses its tone, and normal response to swallowing and gastroesophageal reflux occurs (Figs. 14-22 and 14-23). Thus reflux symptoms become the recurrent esophageal complaints in these patients.

The derangements in normal physiology in the patient with esophageal scleroderma are responsible for one of the most dramatic natural history studies of fulminant reflux esophagitis encountered in medicine.[31] The combination of gastroesophageal reflux and the impaired ability of the atonic esophagus to clear the refluxed acid back into the stomach results in prolonged contact between the refluxed gastric contents and the esophageal mucosa. This contact can result in the progression within a few years from a virtually normal-appearing barium esophagram to one showing a distal stricture (Fig. 14-24, *A* and *B*). The barium swallow shows varying degrees of diminished esophageal peristalsis but often fails to demonstrate gastroesophageal reflux. Esophageal function studies define both the motility disorder and the abnormal gastroesophageal reflux

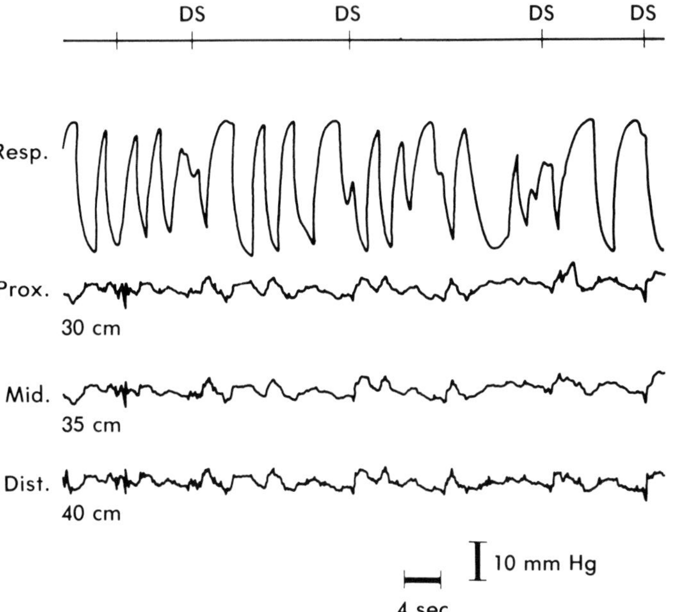

Fig. 14-21 Motility tracing showing lack of peristalsis in esophageal scleroderma. (*DS*, dry swallow; *Resp.*, respiration; *Prox.*, proximal; *Mid.*, middle; *Dist.*, distal.) (From Orringer, M.B., et al.: Ann. Thorac. Surg. **22:**120, 1976.)

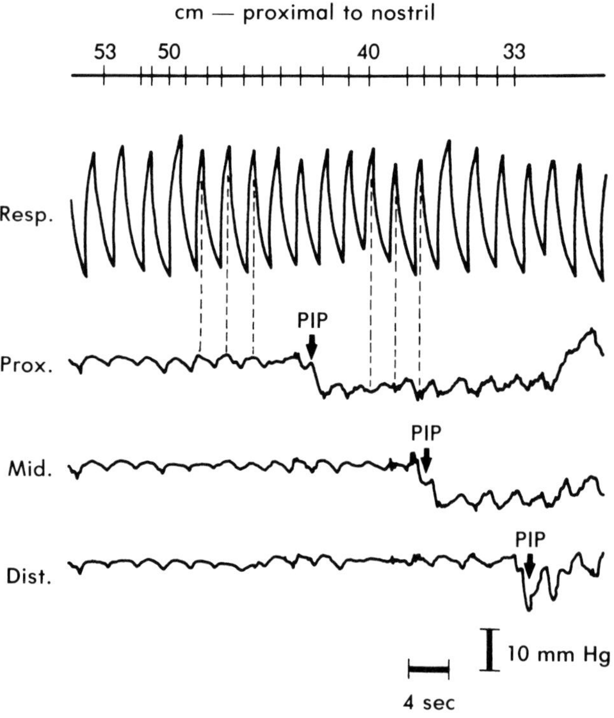

Fig. 14-22 Motility tracing showing lack of a distal esophageal high-pressure zone *(HPZ)* on pull-back determinations in a patient with esophageal scleroderma. The thoracic esophagus is entered at the pressure inversion point *(PIP)*, and the pH electrode is positioned 5 cm above the PIP for the acid reflux test (see Fig. 14-23). (*Prox.*, proximal; *Resp.*, respiration; *Mid.*, middle; *Dist.*, distal.) (From Orringer, M.B., et al.: Ann. Thorac. Surg. **22:**120, 1976.)

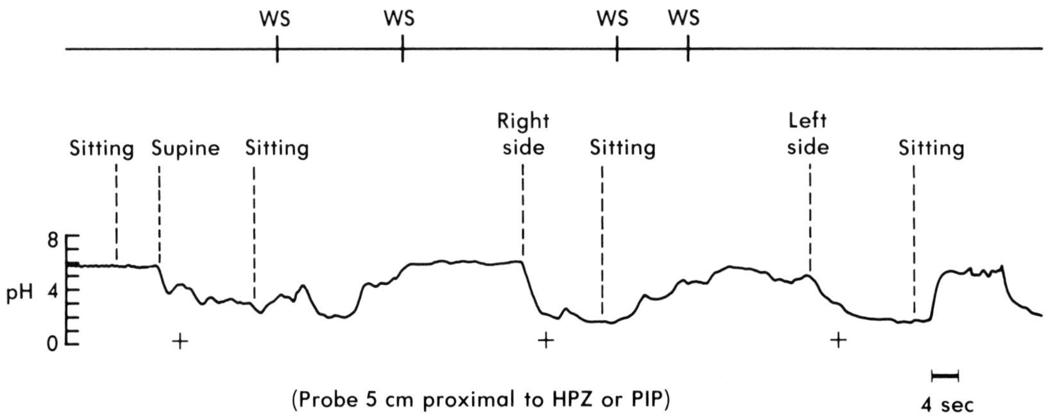

Fig. 14-23 Strongly positive acid reflux test in esophageal scleroderma. Gastroesophageal reflux (+) is indicated by drops in intraesophageal pH below four and occurs with the patient supine and on both sides. (*WS*, wet swallow; *HPZ*, high-pressure zone; *PIP*, pressure inversion point.) (From Orringer, M.B., et al.: Ann. Thorac. Surg. **22:**120, 1976.)

in these patients. Esophagoscopy typically demonstrates ulcerative distal esophagitis with or without stricture.

Intensive medical therapy for reflux should be instituted in patients with esophageal scleroderma. If severe symptoms of ulcerative esophagitis persist, however, surgical control of gastroesophageal reflux should be undertaken if the patient's general condition permits. Despite problems with poor wound healing in the ulcerated finger tips of patients with scleroderma, the healing of thoracic and abdominal incisions in these patients is usually quite adequate, and many can successfully undergo antireflux surgery without an increased rate of complications. In patients with ulcerative esophagitis and only mild-to-moderate esophageal dilation, dilation of an associated stricture performed with a combined Collis gastroplasty-fundoplication procedure is very successful.[13,32] In advanced esophageal scleroderma with marked dilation or a dense stricture that is unlikely to improve appreciably after antireflux surgery, transhiatal esophagectomy without thoracotomy and construction of a cervical esophagogastric anastomosis restores comfortable swallowing and eliminates clinically significant gastroesophageal reflux.[25]

Gastroesophageal Reflux and Hiatal Hernia

In 1951 Allison first used the term *reflux esophagitis* to define the etiology of the symptoms in patients with gastroesophageal reflux associated with a hiatal hernia.[1] He and his contemporaries subsequently developed a variety of operations designed to correct the anatomic defect (i.e., the hiatal hernia) in these patients—the so-called *hiatal hernia* operations. The concept of the fundoplication—wrapping stomach around an intra-abdominal segment of distal esophagus to create a valve mechanism (high-pressure zone)—was developed independently by Nissen[20] and Belsey[37] in 1955 and ushered in the era of anitreflux operations. Since that time, emphasis has been placed on the abnormal physiology responsible for gastroesophageal reflux and on methods for restoring a functional valve mechanism in these patients. Far greater sophistication in thinking about the subject of hiatal hernias and gastroesophageal reflux has developed since Harrington's treatise on diaphragmatic hernias (1928), which discussed sliding, paraesophageal, and traumatic diaphragmatic hernias with little distinction.[11]

Several basic principles regarding hiatal hernias and gastroesophageal reflux bear emphasis.

1. All hiatal hernias are not the same. Ninety-five percent of hiatal hernias are of the sliding (Type I) variety in which the gastroesophageal junction has herniated into the chest and is the leading point of the hernia. In the Type II or pure paraesophageal hernia, the gastroesophageal junction is fixed at its usual location within the diaphragmatic hiatus, but the gas-

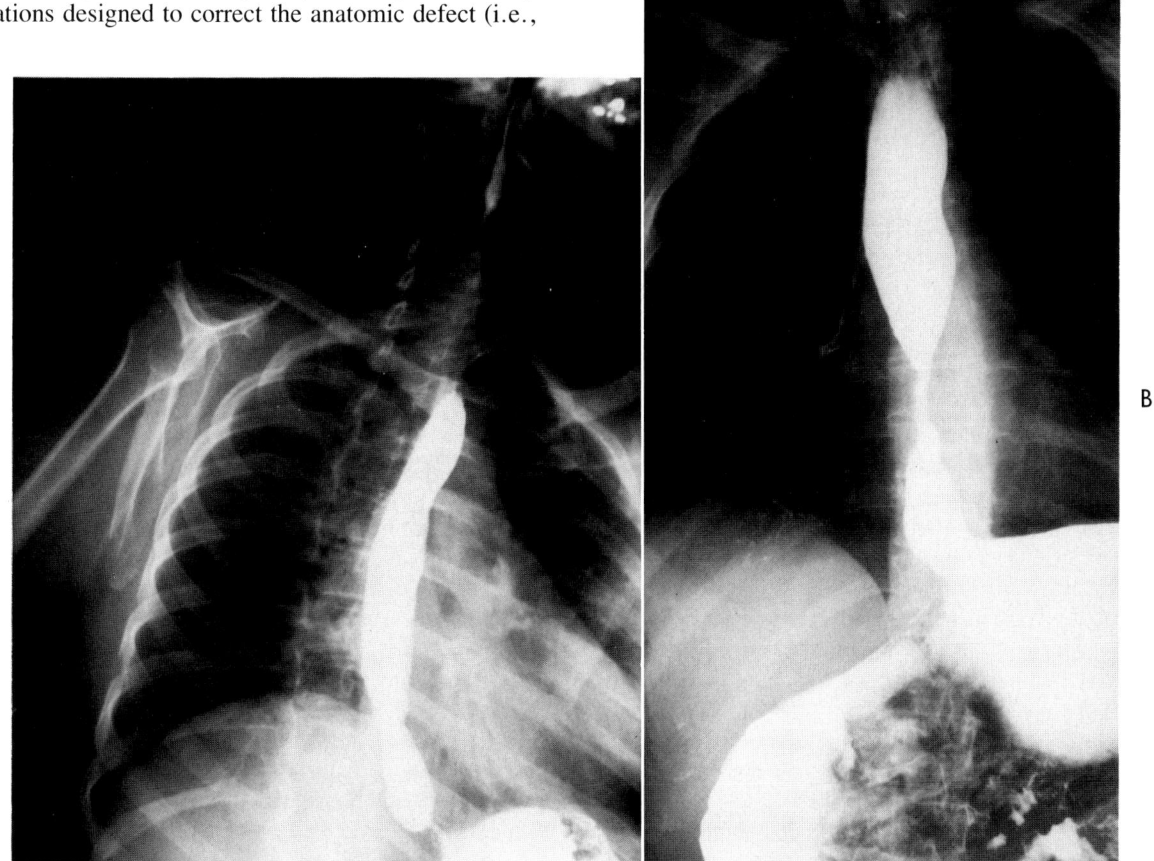

Fig. 14-24 Progression of reflux esophagitis in scleroderma. **A,** Normal esophagram when scleroderma was diagnosed. **B,** Same patient 5 years later with an esophageal stricture, proximal dilation secondary to the obstruction, and aspiration of barium into the right middle lobe bronchus. (From Orringer, M.B., et al.: Ann. Thorac. Surg. **22:**120, 1976.)

tric fundus herniates through the left anterolateral aspect of hiatus into the chest alongside the distal esophagus. This type of hernia is exceedingly rare. The majority of so-called "paraesophageal" hiatal hernia actually are the Type III or combined variety in which the esophagogastric junction is in the chest; but the herniated intrathoracic stomach is also in a paraesophageal location. In the Type IV hernia, other organs such as the spleen, colon, or small intestine are present along with the stomach in the hernia sac. Whereas gastroesophageal reflux is most common with the Type I hernia, the mechanical complications of hernia (incarceration, strangulation, bleeding, and perforation) occur with the other types. Thus the precise definition of the *type* of hernia the patient has is more than academic—an asymptomatic giant Type III hernia is completely unpredictable and may constitute a threat to the patient's life if strangulation occurs.

2. Hiatal hernia and gastroesophageal reflux are not synonymous terms, and each condition may occur in the absence of the other. Thus not every patient who has a hiatal hernia has gastroesophageal reflux, and conversely, not every patient with incompetence of the lower-esophageal sphincter mechanism and gastroesophageal reflux has a hiatal hernia.
3. In patients with reflux associated with a sliding hiatal hernia, it is the reflux not the hernia per se that causes symptoms. That is, the patient with severe pyrosis and acid regurgitation has symptomatic gastroesophageal reflux, not a "bad hiatal hernia."
4. The extent of existing reflux esophagitis correlates poorly with the degree of symptoms the patient manifests. Patients with severe heartburn and acid regurgitation may have little visible endoscopic esophagitis; others with dysphagia from an established peptic stricture may have a history of little, if any, heartburn or regurgitation of gastric contents. Thus it should not be inferred that the patient with severe heartburn and acid regurgitation has severe "esophagitis"; more correctly, such a patient has very symptomatic gastroesophageal reflux.

Gastroesophageal reflux is readily diagnosed in at least 75% of patients with this problem on the basis of a history of retrosternal burning pain ("heartburn") and effortless regurgitation of gastric acid and food aggravated by assuming the recumbent position or bending forward. Approximately one fourth of patients with gastroesophageal reflux are initially seen with atypical symptoms—chest or abdominal pain or cervical dysphagia—that require more sophisticated evaluation to establish a diagnosis. Although generally considered an extremely common and relatively benign condition, gastroesophageal reflux may be responsible for a number of complications—dysphagia, pulmonary symptoms, and bleeding. Dysphagia may occur with gastroesophageal reflux as a result of reflux-induced motor dysfunction involving the cricopharyngeal sphincter or any portion of the thoracic esophagus or because of the development of a stricture. Pulmonary symptoms occur in approximately 20% of patients with gastroesophageal reflux and include complaints of shortness of breath, recurrent pneumonia, bronchitis, bronchiectasis, asthma, lung abscess, and hemoptysis associated with chronic aspiration. Bleeding from reflux esophagitis is seldom massive and is most often seen as chronic blood loss anemia that may be exceedingly difficult to localize.

Although the diagnosis of gastroesophageal reflux is inferred on the basis of the history obtained from the patient, the barium swallow fails to demonstrate reflux in as many as 50% of patients subsequently proven to have this abnormality. If, however, spontaneous gastroesophageal reflux is seen during the barium study, the physician can be fairly certain that abnormal reflux is in fact present. As indicated previously, esophagoscopy is the only reliable means of diagnosing ulcerative esophagitis before the process progresses to stricture formation. Thus this procedure is an important part of the evaluation of every patient with symptomatic reflux that fails to respond to medical therapy. Esophageal function tests have become a basic part of my evaluation of patients with symptoms of gastroesophageal reflux, not only to document objectively the amplitude of the distal high-pressure zone and the degree of abnormal reflux as determined by the intraesophageal pH electrode but also to allow detection of any unsuspected motor abnormality and to provide a baseline against which subsequent postoperative studies can be compared.[24,27] Twenty-four–hour monitoring of the distal esophageal pH allows the demonstration of abnormal gastroesophageal reflux in patients with atypical symptoms as well as a determination of the positions in which reflux occurs.[5,16]

Medical therapy for gastroesophageal reflux is successful in alleviating symptoms in approximately 75% to 80% of patients and includes elevation of the head of the bed on 4- to 6-inch blocks, taking antacids before meals and at bedtime, avoiding eating for several hours before retiring at night, avoiding tight-fitting garments, and weight reduction when applicable. Patients with dysphagia caused by peptic strictures and with few if any symptoms of reflux may be treated with outpatient dilations and medical therapy with excellent symptomatic results. Patients with ulcerative reflux esophagitis during endoscopic evaluation or with very symptomatic gastroesophageal reflux that fails to respond to medical therapy are candidates for surgical control of reflux.

The leading antireflux operations—the Hill median arcuate ligament repair, the Belsey Mark IV repair, and the Nissen fundoplication—rely for their success on the restoration to the abdomen of a 3- to 5-cm segment of distal esophagus that is then enwrapped to varying degrees by the gastric fundus. This distal esophageal segment, under the influence of positive intra-abdominal pressure, serves as the high-pressure zone, which helps prevent reflux. Each of these operations requires sutures into either the distal esophagus or periesophageal tissues; the long-term success of these operations must therefore be jeopardized by the presence of any factors that either increase tension on the repair or interfere with the healing of sutures placed during the performance of the repair. It has been shown, for example, that the presence of a stricture or of periesophagitis from reflux at the time of performance of the Belsey Mark IV operation results in a recurrence rate of 45% to 75%.[6,30]

In an effort to minimize the incidence of recurrent gastroesophageal reflux after surgical reconstruction of the esophagogastric junction, the combination of an esophageal-lengthening Collis gastroplasty with either a Belsey- or Nissen-type fundoplication has been advocated.[12,24,34] With the Collis-Nissen procedure, the functional distal esophageal tube is lengthened by using a small portion of adjacent stomach (Fig. 14-25). A fundoplication is then performed around this new distal esophagus, which is then reduced beneath the diaphragm (Figs. 14-26 and 14-27). This procedure avoids the need for any sutures into the inflamed distal esophagus and eliminates tension on the repair, which results when an attempt is made to affix the esophagogastric junction of a shortened, inflamed esophagus below the diaphragm. The Collis-Nissen procedure is advocated for use in patients with severe reflux esophagitis, esophageal shortening, or marked obesity, all predisposing factors for recurrence after standard antireflux operations. Objective follow-up of patients undergoing either the Collis-Nissen procedure[24] or the combined Collis-Belsey operation[33] indicates generally excellent results. These operations represent technical modifications that have been developed in response to the recognized impact of reflux esophagitis on the healing of standard antireflux repairs.

Esophageal Carcinoma

Esophageal carcinoma remains among the most dismal visceral malignancies and occurs in epidemic proportion in parts of Iran, South Africa, and Russia, and the Linksien province of China. In the United States, the incidence of esophageal carcinoma is nine cases per 100,000 population per year.[35] This tumor is two to five times more common in men than in women and occurs predominantly in the sixth and seventh decades of life. Although the etiology of esophageal carcinoma is unknown, certain predisposing factors have been incriminated—alcohol, tobacco, nitrosamines, malnutrition, poor oral hygiene, previous gastric surgery, chronic ingestion of hot foods or beverages, and familial keratosis (tylosis). A number of esophageal lesions are believed to be premalignant—achalasia, reflux esophagitis, Barrett's (columnar-lined) lower esophagus, radiation esophagitis, caustic burns, Plummer-Vinson syndrome, leukoplakia, esophageal diverticula, and ectopic gastric mucosa. Histologically, 95% of esophageal carcinomas are squamous cell, and the remainder are adenocar-

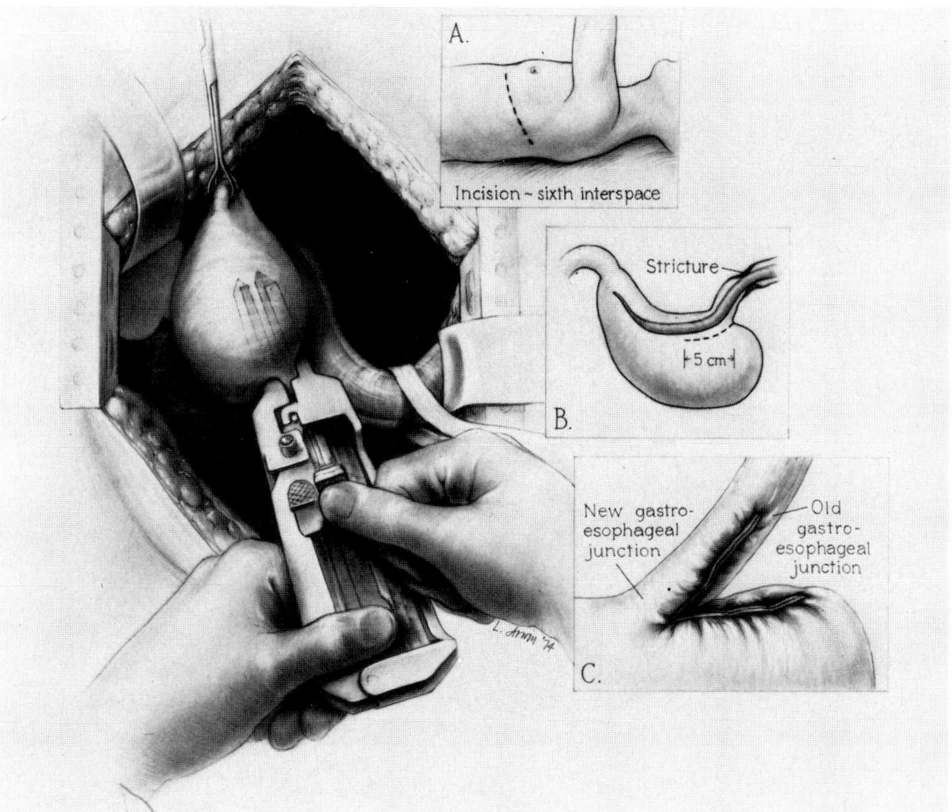

Fig. 14-25 Construction of the Collis-gastroplasty tube with GIA surgical stapler. **A,** The distal esophagus, cardia, and gastric fundus are mobilized through a sixth- or seventh-interspace left thoracotomy. **B,** A 54 or 56 French Maloney dilator is displaced against the lesser curvature of the stomach as the stapler is applied. The knife assembly is advanced, and the stapler is removed. **C,** A 5-cm long gastric tube extension of the functional esophagus is created. The staple suture line is oversewn with a running 4-0 Prolene Lembert stitch. (From Orringer, M.B., and Sloan, H.: J. Thorac. Cardiovasc. Surg. **71:**295, 1976.)

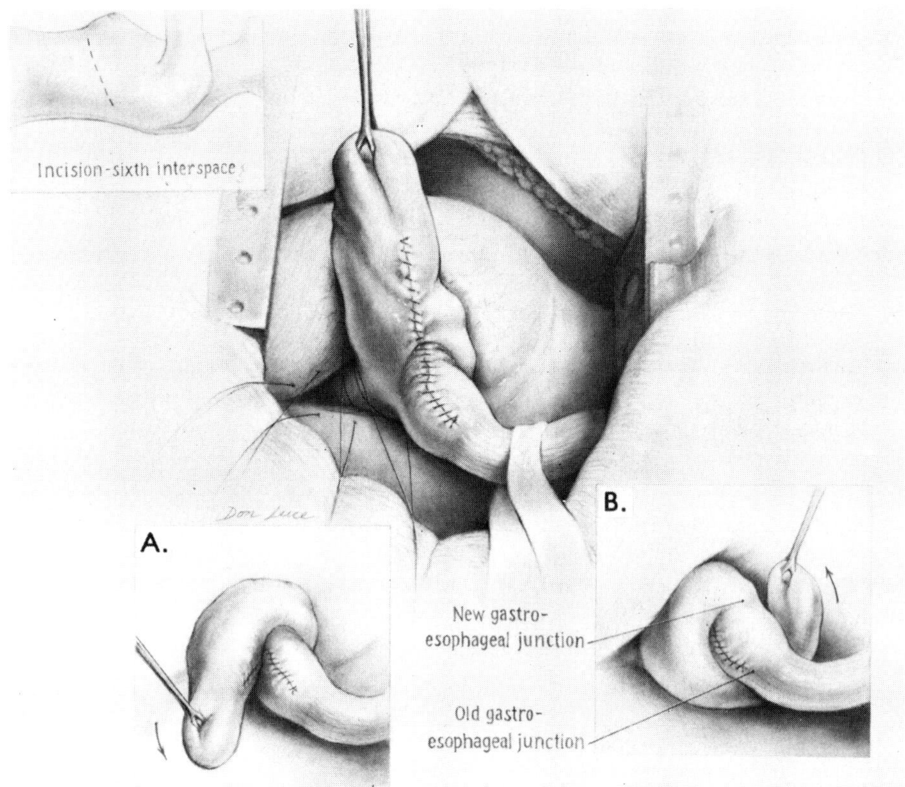

Fig. 14-26 Combined Collis-Nissen reconstruction of the esophagogastric junction. The elongated gastric fundus remaining after construction of the gastroplasty tube is passed around the tube and the adjacent stomach, **A** and **B.** (From Orringer, M.B., and Sloan, H.: Ann. Thorac. Surg. **25:**16, 1978.)

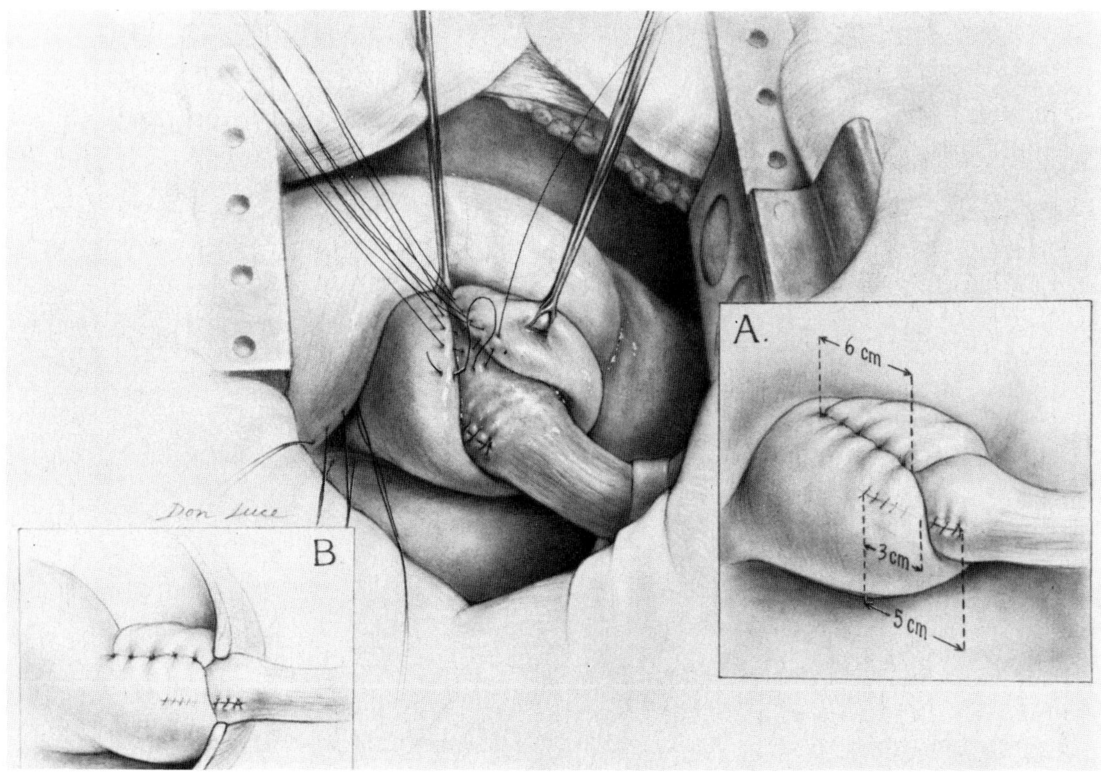

Fig. 14-27 Completion of the Collis-Nissen operation. Seromuscular sutures are placed from gastric fundus to adjacent gastroplasty tube to fundus again. **A,** A 3-cm long fundoplication is performed without the need to suture to the inflamed distal esophagus. **B,** The fundoplication is reduced beneath the diagram, and the previously placed crural sutures are tied. Tension on the repair is avoided because of the additional length provided by the gastroplasty tube. (From Orringer, M.B., and Sloan, H.: Ann. Thorac. Surg. **25:**16, 1978.)

cinomas arising at the cardia, in Barrett's mucosa associated with reflux esophagitis, or in the ectopic gastric mucosa. Squamous cell carcinoma is most frequent in the upper two thirds of the esophagus, next in the lower third, and least common in the cervical esophagus. Hematogenous and lymphatic spread are the rule with esophageal carcinoma, and mediastinal, supraclavicular, or celiac lymph node metastases occur in at least 75% of these patients. Esophageal carcinoma typically produces progressive dysphagia, weight loss, odynophagia, and chest pain. Any patient who complains of progressive dysphagia warrants *both* a barium esophagram and esophagoscopy to exclude carcinoma. The combination of esophageal biopsy and brushings for cytologic evaluation establishes a diagnosis of carcinoma in 95% of the patients with malignant strictures.[4,17]

Few diseases have the profound physiologic impact of esophageal obstruction caused by carcinoma, which results in malnutrition, negative nitrogen balance, and pulmonary complications resulting from chronic aspiration. Despite the fact that most patients with esophageal carcinoma are incurable when the disease is first diagnosed, of the possible modalities of therapy, surgery offers the most efficient and expeditious palliation. Neither a feeding tube nor a cervical esophagostomy relieves dysphagia or allows comfortable swallowing. Removal of the obstructed esophagus and restoration of continuity of the alimentary tract, generally by using the stomach, is the time-honored surgical approach. Nevertheless, despite improvements in preoperative assessment, operative and anesthetic techniques, and postoperative care, esophageal resection and reconstruction remain a formidable undertaking with an average mortality rate of 29% in a recent comprehensive review of modern surgical series.[7] By far, the two leading causes of death following standard transthoracic esophagectomy and an intrathoracic esophagogastric anastomosis are: (1) respiratory insufficiency associated with splinting from thoracic and abdominal incisions, and (2) sepsis from mediastinitis associated with an intrathoracic anastomotic disruption.

To minimize the factors responsible for the majority of poor results from esophageal resection and reconstruction, transhiatal "blunt" esophagectomy without thoracotomy has been advocated.[26,28] Regardless of the level of the tumor, the entire thoracic esophagus is resected and is replaced whenever possible with the stomach, which is anastomosed to the remaining cervical esophagus. The procedure is performed through an upper-midline abdominal incision and a cervical incision and involves resection of the thoracic esophagus through the diaphragmatic hiatus and the neck. The mobilized stomach is based on the right gastric and right gastroepiploic vascular arcades after dividing the left gastric and gastroepiploic vessels (Fig. 14-28). Performance of a pyloromyotomy and a feeding jeju-

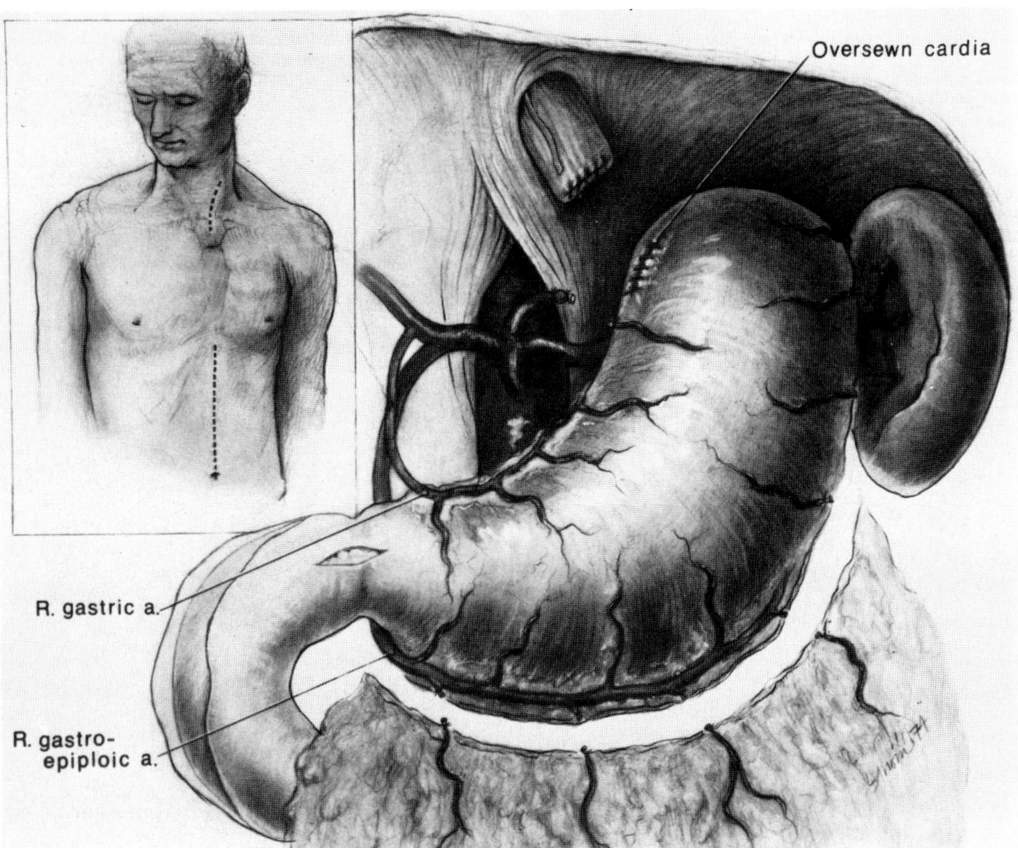

Fig. 14-28 Mobilization of the stomach for esophageal replacement after transhiatal esophagectomy without thoracotomy. The right gastric and right gastroepiploic vessels are preserved, a Kocher maneuver and a pyloromyotomy are performed, and the divided cardia is stapled and oversewn. (From Orringer, M.B., and Sloan, H.: J. Thorac. Cardiovasc. Surg. **70:**836, 1975.)

nostomy is routine. The entire thoracic esophagus from the level of the clavicles to the cardia is resected, and the intra-arterial blood pressure is continually monitored to avoid prolonged hypotension from cardiac displacement during the transhiatal esophageal dissection (Figs. 14-29 and 14-30). The stomach is then transposed to the posterior mediastinum, positioned in the original esophageal bed, and anastomosed to the cervical esophagus (Fig. 14-31). This procedure is also applicable for tumors involving the cardia and esophagogastric junction (Fig 14-32).

The advantages of this approach are: (1) a thoracotomy is avoided, thereby minimizing the physiologic insult to the patient; (2) an intrathoracic anastomosis with its potential for mediastinitis if a leak should occur is avoided (if a cervical anastomotic leak does occur, it is far more easily managed and is not fatal); (3) intra-abdominal and intrathoracic gastrointestinal suture lines are avoided in contrast to the situation with jejunal or colonic interposition; and (4) clinically significant gastroesophageal reflux that occurs in at least 40% of patients with an intrathoracic esophagogastric anastomosis seldom occurs with a cervical anastomosis. In my experience, this technique of esophagectomy has been possible in 100 of 104 consecutive operations for esophageal carcinoma.[23] The normal stomach has reached to the neck for a cervical anastomosis in every case. There have been no intraoperative deaths, intraoperative blood loss has averaged less than 1000 ml, and 85% of the patients have been discharged and have been able to swallow within 2 to 3 weeks of surgery. The hospital mortality rate has been 6%, and survival has been as good as that reported in many series of standard transthoracic esophagectomy for carcinoma. I believe that survival after resection of esophageal carcinoma is more a function of individual tumor biology and host resistance than of the extent of the resection performed, and if a thoracotomy is avoided in these debilitated patients, no less of a "cancer operation" has been performed.

Miscellaneous Disorders of Swallowing

Esophageal Webs and Rings

Sideropenic dysphagia (Plummer-Vinson syndrome or Paterson-Kelly syndrome) refers to the development of cervical dysphagia in patients with iron deficiency anemia. The patients are typically edentulous women over 40 years of age who have atrophic oral mucosa and brittle spoon-shaped fingernails. The dysphagia is usually, but not al-

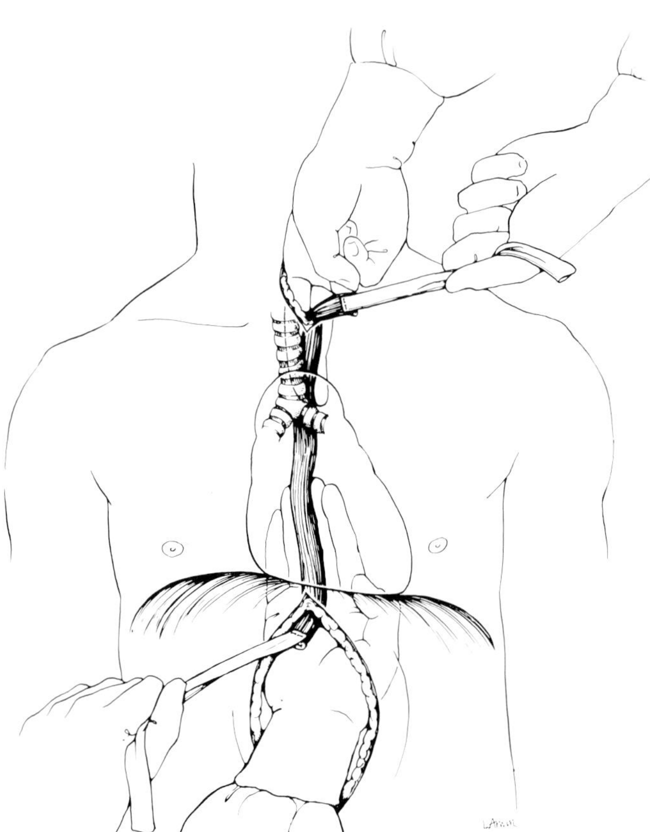

Fig. 14-29 Transhiatal dissection of the esophagus is performed through an upper-midline abdominal incision using Penrose drains sutured to either end of the divided esophagus for traction. The upper-thoracic esophagus is mobilized through a cervical incision. (From Orringer, M.B., and Sloan, H.: J. Thorac. Cardiovasc. Surg. **76:**643, 1978.)

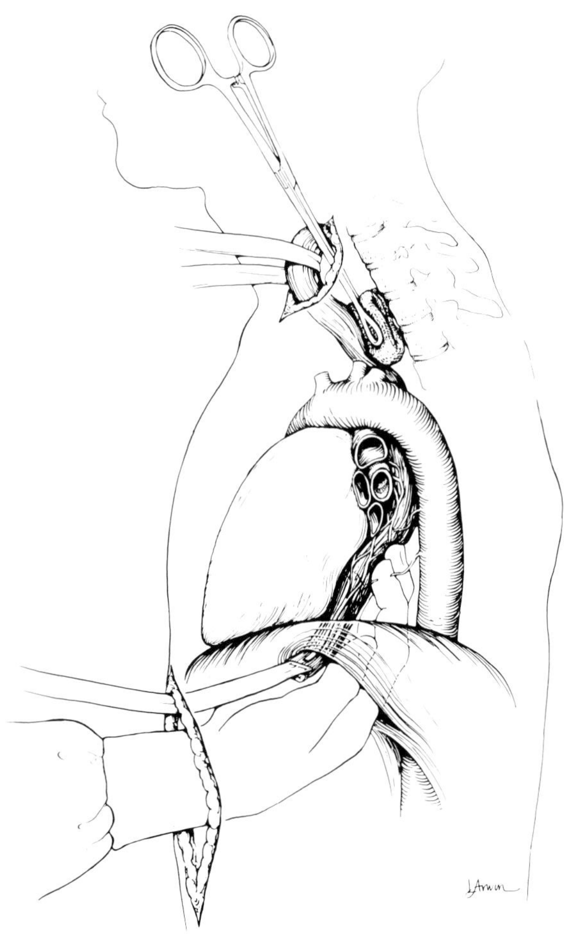

Fig. 14-30 Intra-arterial blood pressure is continually monitored through a radial artery catheter to avoid prolonged hypotension that may result from cardiac displacement during the transhiatal esophageal dissection. (From Orringer, M.B., and Sloan, H.: J. Thorac. Cardiovasc. Surg. **76:**643, 1978.)

ways, caused by a cervical esophageal web (Fig. 14-33). This condition, which is prevalent in Great Britain and Scandinavia, is a premalignant lesion with 10% of the patients so affected developing malignancies of the hypopharynx, oral cavity, or esophagus.[40] Plummer-Vinson syndrome is treated by esophageal dilation and correction of the anemia.

Distal esophageal webs (Schatzki ring) occur at the esophagogastric junction in patients with a sliding hiatal hernia (Fig. 14-34), and they cause dysphagia when their diameter is 13 mm or less. Histologically, the rings correspond to the squamocolumnar epithelial junction, and there is a slight amount of underlying submucosal fibrosis.[35] A Schatzki ring indicates only that a hiatal hernia is present, not that there is either reflux or esophagitis. Differentiation from a localized peptic stricture may be difficult. Patients who have a symptomatic Schatzki ring without associated reflux symptoms respond well to esophageal dilations. In those patients with severe reflux symptoms, intraoperative dilation of the ring in association with an antireflux procedure relieves symptoms as long as reflux control is achieved. Resection of the ring alone without repair of the associated hiatal hernia should not be performed.

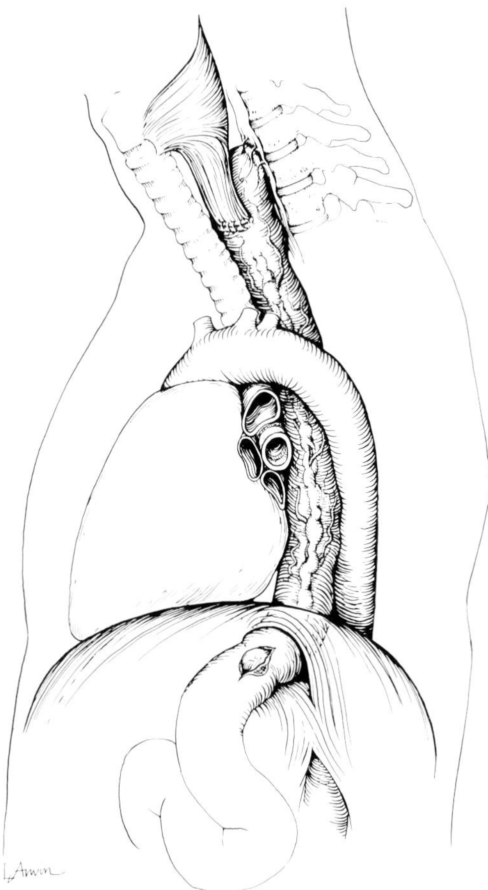

Fig. 14-31 After transhiatal esophagectomy and pyloromyotomy, the stomach is mobilized through the posterior mediastinum, the fundus is sutured to the cervical prevertebral fascia, and an end-to-side esophagogastrostomy is performed. (From Orringer, M.B., and Sloan, H.: J. Thorac. Cardiovasc. Surg. **76:**643, 1978.)

Monilial Esophagitis

Candida ablicans is a fungus, which is normally found in the human mouth, oropharynx, and gastrointestinal tract. In debilitated and immunosuppressed patients, the fungus may become pathogenic, and as a result of the use of more potent broad-spectrum antibiotics, chemotherapy in oncology patients, and immunosuppressants following organ transplantation, the incidence of monilial esophagitis is increasing.[29] In the acute form, as mucosal ulceration occurs, the patient complains of painful swallowing. Treatment is oral nystatin (Mycostatin), 400,000 to 600,000 U of the suspension every six hours. If the infection advances and intramural invasion of the thoracic esophagus by the fungus occurs and if the patients survives the underlying disease, a chronic stricture may follow healing of the inflamed esophagus. Strictures caused by monilial esophagitis tend to occur in the upper half of the thoracic esophagus where the esophageal submucosal

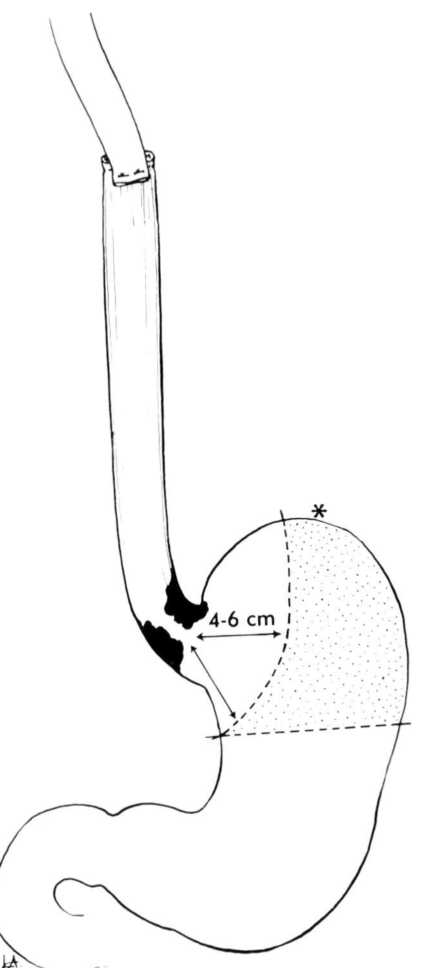

Fig. 14-32 For distal third carcinomas limited to the cardia and high-proximal stomach, a total thoracic esophagectomy and a proximal partial gastrectomy are performed, preserving the entire greater curvature of the gastric fundus and that point (*) that reaches most cephalad to the neck. A proximal hemigastrectomy for such tumors wastes valuable stomach *(stipled area)* that can be used for esophageal replacement. (From Orringer, M.B., and Sloan, H.: J. Thorac. Cardiovasc. Surg. **76:**643, 1978.)

glands predominate. If these glands become inflamed from infection, stasis, or distal obstruction, they become dilated and give the radiographic appearance of "intramural esophageal pseudodiverticulosis" (Fig. 14-35). Because postinflammatory strictures can occur, patients recovering from acute monilial esophagitis warrant serial barium swallow examinations during the first year to permit early detection of a developing stricture and prompt institution of bougienage therapy.

SUMMARY

Knowledge of the physiology of normal swallowing is basic to the understanding of the pathophysiology of disordered swallowing and to the ability to render optimum care to patients with these problems. Despite refinements in medical technology, obtaining a careful history remains the most valuable diagnostic tool in the assessment of abnormal swallowing. The history, a barium esophagram, an esophagoscopy, and esophageal function tests constitute

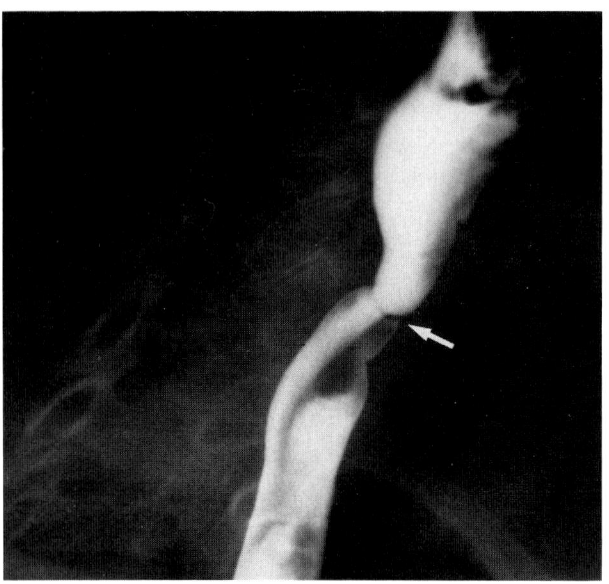

Fig. 14-33 Cervical esophageal web *(arrow)* in a woman with Plummer-Vinson syndrome. (From Orringer, M.B.: The esophagus. In Sabiston, D., editor: Textbook of surgery, ed. 13, Philadelphia, 1986, W.B. Saunders Co.)

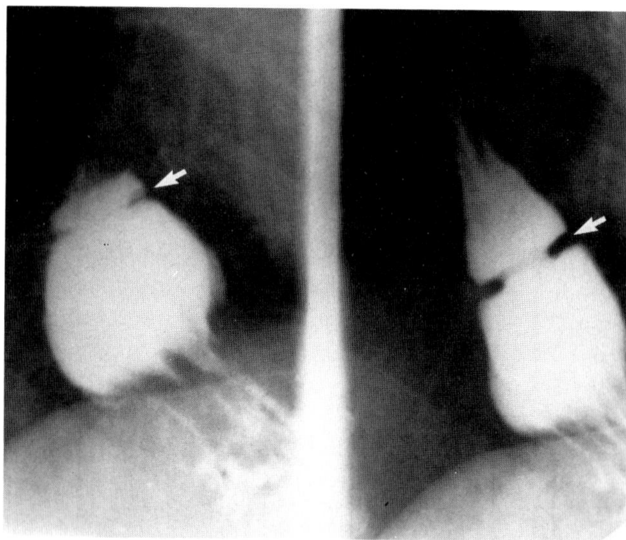

Fig. 14-34 Distal esophageal (Schatzki) ring *(arrows)* always occurs at the esophagogastric junction above a sliding hiatal hernia. (From Orringer, M.B.: The esophagus. In Sabiston, D., editor: Textbook of surgery, ed. 13, Philadelphia, 1986, W.B. Saunders Co.)

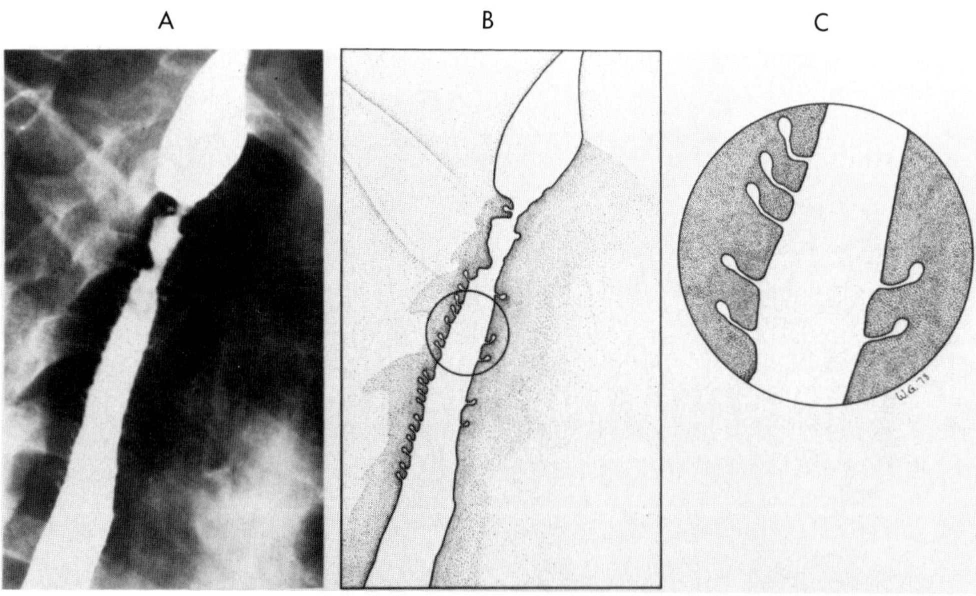

Fig. 14-35 **A,** Esophagram and, **B** and **C,** line interpretations of irregular upper-thoracic esophageal stricture from monilial esophagitis. The pattern of intramural pseudodiverticulosis results from dilation of the submucosal esophageal glands. (From Orringer, M.B., and Sloan, H.: Ann. Thorac. Surg. **26:**364, 1978.)

the minimum elements of a complete evaluation of esophageal motor dysfunction, but the results of these tests must be considered *together* since *none* is infallible and absolutely diagnostic of a specific abnormality. Even with the modern emphasis on the need to perform esophageal manometry in the patient with disordered swallowing, the limitations of this study must be stressed: (1) lower-esophageal sphincter pressure per se does not establish competence or incompetence of the valve mechanism; (2) patients with intermittent diffuse esophageal spasm may have perfectly normal esophageal peristalsis if manometry is performed when they are having no pain; (3) any esophageal obstruction (e.g., caused by a tumor or a benign stricture) may result in a manometric tracing that suggests esophageal spasm. Esophagoscopy *must* be performed in the patient with constant dysphagia, and the esophagoscope should never be passed without obtaining a barium esophagram first to define the level and anatomy of any abnormality present.

Esophageal carcinoma remains for the most part an incurable disease with "early detection" an ideal that is seldom realized in the United States. Current surgical advances in the treatment of this condition have focused on methods of achieving palliation of dysphagia in the safest and most efficient manner and avoiding a thoracotomy and an intrathoracic esophageal anastomosis whenever possible. The achievement of long-term survival in these patients will almost certainly depend on future discoveries in oncology and tumor biology.

REFERENCES

1. Allison, P.R.: Reflux esophagitis, sliding hiatal hernia, and the anatomy of repair, Surg. Gynecol. Obstet. **92:**149, 1951.
2. Belsey, R.: Functional disease of the esophagus, J. Thorac. Cardiovasc. Surg. **52:**164, 1966.
3. Black, J., Vorbach, A.N., and Collis, J.L.: Results of Heller's operation for achalasia of the esophagus: the importance of hiatal hernia repair, Br. J. Surg. **63:**949, 1976.
4. Bruni, H.C., and Nelson, R.S.: Carcinoma of the esophagus and cardia, J. Thorac. Cardiovasc. Surg. **70:**367, 1975.
5. DeMeester, T.R., et al.: Technique, indications, and clinical use of 24-hour esophageal pH monitoring, J. Thorac. Cardiovasc. Surg. **79:**656, 1980.
6. Donnelly, R.J., Deverall, P.B., and Watson, D.A.: Hiatus hernia with and without esophageal strictures; experience with the Belsey Mark IV repair, Ann. Thorac. Surg. **16:**301, 1973.
7. Earlam, R., and Cunha-Melo, J.R.: Oesophageal squamous cell carcinoma. I. A critical review of surgery, Br. J. Surg. **67:**381, 1980.
8. Ellis, F.H., Jr., and Olsen, A.M.: Achalasia of the esophagus, Philadelphia, 1969, W.B. Saunders Co.
9. Ellis, F.H., Jr., et al.: Surgical treatment of esophageal hypermotility disturbances, JAMA **188:**862, 1964.
10. Ellis, F.H., Jr., et al.: Cricopharyngeal myotomy for pharyngoesophageal diverticulum, Ann. Surg. **170:**3450, 1969.
11. Harrington, S.W.: Diaphragmatic hernia, Arch. Surg. **16:**386, 1928.
12. Henderson, R.D.: Reflux control following gastroplasty, Ann. Thorac. Surg. **24:**206, 1977.
13. Henderson, R.D., and Pearson, F.G.: Surgical management of esophageal scleroderma, J. Thorac. Cardiovasc. Surg. **66:**686, 1973.
14. Henderson, R.D., and Marryatt, G.: Cricopharyngeal myotomy as a method of treating cricopharyngeal dysphagia secondary to gastroesophageal reflux, J. Thorac. Cardiovasc. Surg. **74:**271, 1977.
15. Hurwitz, A.L., Duranceau, A., and Haddad, J.K.: Disorders of esophageal motility. In Smith, L.H., Jr.: Major problems in internal medicine, Philadelphia, 1979, W.B. Saunders Co.
16. Johnson, L.F., and DeMeester, T.R.: Twenty-four hour pH monitoring of the distal esophagus: a quantitative measurement of gastroesophageal reflux, Am. J. Gastroenterol. **62:**325, 1974.
17. Kobayashi, S., et al.: Improved endoscopic diagnosis of gastroesophageal malignancy: combined use of direct vision brushing cytology and biopsy, JAMA **212:**2086, 1976.
18. Lobello, R., Edwards, D.A.W., and Gummer, J.W.P.: The antireflux mechanism after cardiomyotomy, Thorax **33:**569, 1978.
19. Nemir, P., Jr., et al.: A study of the cause of failure of esophagocardiomyotomy for achalasia, Am. J. Surg. **121:**143, 1971.
20. Nissen, R.: Gastropexy and "fundoplication" in surgical treatment of hiatal hernia, Am. J. Dig. Dis. **6:**954, 1961.
21. Okikie, N., et al.: Esophagomyotomy versus forceful dilation for achalasia of the esophagus: results in 899 patients, Ann. Thorac. Surg. **28:**119, 1979.
22. Orringer, M.B.: Extended cervical esophagomyotomy for cricopharyngeal dysfunction, J. Thorac. Cardiovasc. Surg. **80:**669, 1980.
23. Orringer, M.B.: Transhiatal esophagectomy without thoracotomy for carcinoma of the thoracic esophagus, Ann. Surg. **200:** 282, 1984.
24. Orringer, M.B., and Orringer, J.S.: The combined Collis-Nissen operation: early assessment of reflux control, Ann. Thorac. Surg. **33:**534, 1982.
25. Orringer, M.B., and Orringer, J.S.: Esophagectomy: definitive treatment for esophageal neuromotor dysfunction, Ann. Thorac. Surg. **34:**237, 1982.
26. Orringer, M.B., and Orringer, J.S.: Transhiatal esophagectomy without thoracotomy: a dangerous operation? J. Thorac. Cardiovasc. Surg. **85:**72, 1983.
27. Orringer, M.B., and Sloan, H.: Complications and failings of the combined Collis-Belsey operation, J. Thorac. Cardiovasc. Surg. **74:**726, 1977.
28. Orringer, M.B., and Sloan, H.: Esophagectomy without thoracotomy, J. Thorac. Cardiovasc. Surg. **76:**643, 1978.
29. Orringer, M.B., and Sloan, H.: Monilial esophagitis: an increasingly frequent cause of esophageal stenosis? Ann. Thorac. Surg. **26:**364, 1978.
30. Orringer, M.B., Skinner, D.B., and Belsey, R.H.R.: Long-term results of the Mark IV operation for hiatal hernia and analysis of recurrences and their treatment, J. Thorac. Cardiovasc. Surg. **63:**25, 1972.
31. Orringer, M.B., et al.: Gastroesophageal reflux in esophageal scleroderma: diagnosis and implications, Ann. Thorac. Surg. **12:**120, 1976.
32. Orringer, M.B., et al.: Combined Collis-gastroplasty fundoplication operations for scleroderma reflux esophagitis, Surgery **90:**624, 1981.
33. Pearson, F.G., Henderson, R.D.: Long-term follow-up of peptic strictures managed by dilation, modified Collis gastroplasty, and Belsey hiatus hernia, Surgery **80:**391, 1976.
34. Pearson, F.G., Tanger, B., and Henderson, R.D.: Gastroplasty and Belsey hiatal hernia repair, J. Thorac. Cardiovasc. Surg. **61:**50, 1971.
35. Postlethwait, R.W.: Surgery of the esophagus, New York, 1979, Appleton-Century-Crofts.
36. Rossetti, M.: Esophagocardiomyotomy and fundoplication: a physiologic operation for cardiospasm and megaesophagus, Schweiz. Med. Wochenschr. **93:**925, 1963.
37. Skinner, D.B., and Belsey, R.H.: Surgical management of esophageal reflux and hiatus hernia, J. Thorac. Cardiovasc. Surg. **53:**33, 1967.
38. Skinner, D.B., et al., editors: Gastroesophageal reflux and hiatal hernia, Boston, 1972, Little, Brown, & Co. Inc.
39. Tuttle, S.G., and Grossman, M.I.: Detection of gastroesophageal reflux by simultaneous measurement of intraluminal pressures and pH, Proc. Soc. Exp. Biol. Med. **98:**225, 1958.
40. Wynder, E.L., et al.: Environmental factors in cancer of the upper alimentary tract: a Swedish study with special reference to Plummer-Vinson (Paterson-Kelly) syndrome, Cancer **10:**470, 1957.

15 *Haile T. Debas*

Physiology of Gastric Secretion and Emptying

Control of gastric secretion and emptying is brought about by complex interactions of nerves and humoral agents. The action of nerves at the effector cell (e.g., smooth muscle, oxyntic cell, gastric cell) requires the release of neurotransmitters, which, in addition to the classic cholinergic and adrenergic substances, include neuropeptides, amines (e.g., serotonin) and adenosine diphosphate (ADP). Some of the neuropeptides from nerve endings may be secreted into the interstitial fluid through which they may be spread to adjacent cells: neurocrine transmission. The humoral agents arrive at their target cells not only by the classic endocrine (blood-borne) pathway, but also by diffusion through the interstitial fluid after their local secretion by endocrine cells within the wall of the stomach: paracrine transmission. Thus any response to a given stimulant or inhibitor is modulated by the ambient concentrations of paracrine and neurocrine agents in the local milieu of the target cells. The concept of local modulation, therefore, must be taken into consideration when interpreting gastric secretory or motor responses to exogenous stimulants. In general much more is known about processes that stimulate secretion than those that inhibit it. Also, mechanisms that control gastric secretion have been defined better than those that regulate motility. Thus any review of this subject must indicate not only the degree of knowledge achieved but also the state of ignorance that remains.

The aim of this chapter is to summarize the current knowledge of the physiology of gastric secretion and emptying in a manner relevant to the surgery of this organ. Before discussion of gastric function, a brief review of the physiologic anatomy of the stomach is appropriate.

PHYSIOLOGIC ANATOMY

The traditional division of the stomach into three regions (the cardia, the body [corpus], and the antrum) is useful, but only for describing gross pathology. In the past, the body has been regarded as the exocrine organ concerned with the secretion of acid and pepsin; the antrum as the endocrine organ for the release of gastrin; and the cardia as that buffer zone between the esophagus and the gastric corpus with no particular function. In truth, the entire stomach functions as both an endocrine and exocrine organ.

The esophagus enters the abdomen at the diaphragmatic hiatus, which is at the level of the T12 vertebra. The pyloroduodenal junction is at the level of the L1 vertebra. The stomach is fixed at these two points from which it hangs in a J-shaped manner. The close proximity of the gastroesophageal junction and the pylorus should be appreciated.

Muscle Coat

The main muscle coat of the stomach consists of an outer longitudinal, middle circular, and inner oblique layer. The longitudinal muscle coat is concentrated along the lesser and greater curvatures of the stomach. The fibers of the middle circular layer are disposed at right angles to those of the longitudinal layer and completely encircle the stomach and become progressively thicker toward the pylorus. The inner oblique layer is concentrated largely over the anterior and posterior surfaces of the stomach and is deficient at the greater and lesser curvatures. At the pylorus there is an impressive thickening of the circular muscle layer, defining a distinct anatomic sphincter.

Mucosal Lining

The mucosal lining of the cardia of the stomach contains glands made up of simple columnar cells. No parietal or chief cells are present. The mucosa of the body of the stomach is characterized by the acid-secreting oxyntic cells and the pepsin-secreting chief cells. On the surface, the mucosa of the corpus contains gastric pits, each draining several gastric glands. The pits themselves are lined with mucus-neck cells that maintain a thin layer of mucous gel over the surface of the entire mucosa. The oxyntic (parietal) cells are the most striking cells of the gastric glands of the proximal stomach. They contain large amounts of mitochondria in their cytoplasm, indicative of the high energy requirements of acid secretion. In terms of their mitochondrial content, the oxyntic cells are only second to the cells of the myocardium, another organ with high energy requirements. A most impressive morphologic transformation occurs in the oxyntic cell when it is stimulated. At rest the cell is filled with smooth membrane structures (tubulovesicles). On stimulation, these structures decrease and become replaced by an expansion of the secretory canaliculus in the form of microvilli containing H^+K^+-ATPase, the proton pump.[38]

The antrum is lined by pyloric gland mucosa containing principally mucus-secreting cells. A few scattered parietal cells are also found. In the human, unlike the dog, no pepsin is secreted in the antrum. In the midzone of the pyloric glands are scattered gastrin-secreting cells (G cells) (Fig. 15-1). The G cells are of the open type; i.e., they open into the lumen of the glands, and their apical surface is thrown into microvilli that come in contact with the contents of the gastric lumen. These microvilli are thought to represent chemical and pH sensors for the G cell.

Several other endocrine cells are scattered throughout the gastric mucosa from the cardia to the pylorus. In the proximal stomach of humans at least five endocrine cells have been identified: D cells, which secrete somatostatin and some other unknown peptide; EC cells, which secrete serotonin and various other peptides; the ECL cells, whose secretory product is unknown; and P and X cells, whose function is also unknown.[39] The human antral mucosa also contains D, EC, and P cells but no ECL or X cells. The somatostatin (D) cells in the antrum have long processes that end in fusiform swellings abutting on G cells. Somatostatin is considered an important paracrine inhibitor of gastrin release. A list of both the exocrine and endocrine cells of the stomach is provided in Table 15-1.

Neural Supply

The extrinsic innervation of the stomach derives from the vagi and the sympathetic nervous system. It is no longer accurate to describe these nerves as cholinergic and adrenergic, respectively, because in truth both systems contain peptidergic and purinergic nerves. In addition, a certain number of adrenergic nerves are present in the vagi, and parasympathetic (cholinergic) nerves in the sympathetic fibers. Over 80% of the fibers in the vagi are afferent neurons carrying information back to the brain.

The anterior (left) and posterior (right) vagus nerves enter the abdomen at the esophageal hiatus (Fig. 15-2). On the anterior surface of the abdominal esophagus, the anterior vagus is present as a single trunk 60% of the time and

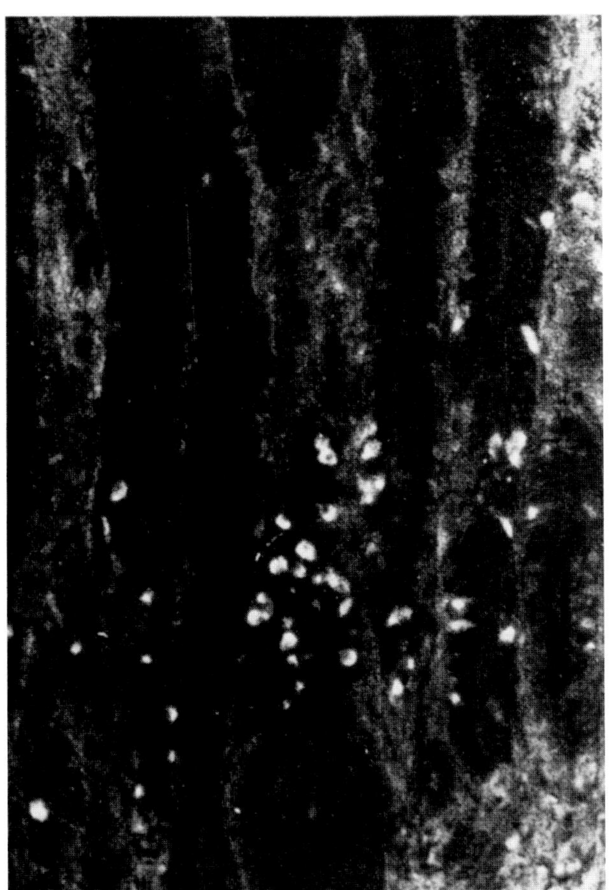

Fig. 15-1 Immunofluorescence study showing gastrin-secreting cells in the midzone of the antrum. (From Walsh, J.H., and Grossman, M.I. Reprinted by permission of N. Engl. J. Med. **292**(25):1324, 1975.)

Table 15-1 **THE EXOCRINE AND ENDOCRINE CELLS OF THE STOMACH AND THEIR SECRETORY PRODUCTS**

	Cells	Secretory Products
Exocrine	Mucous	Mucus
	Oxyntic	Acid
	Chief	Pepsin
Endocrine	G	Gastrin
	D	Somatostatin
	A*	Glucagon
	EC	Serotonin plus various peptides
	ECL	Unknown
	P	Unknown
	X	Unknown

*In fetus or newborn; only exceptionally found in adults.

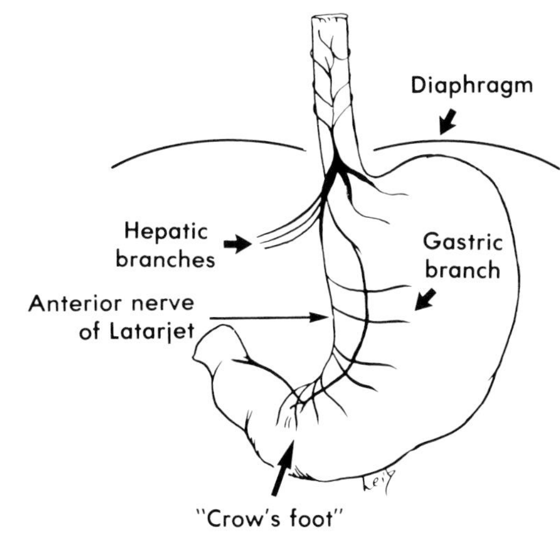

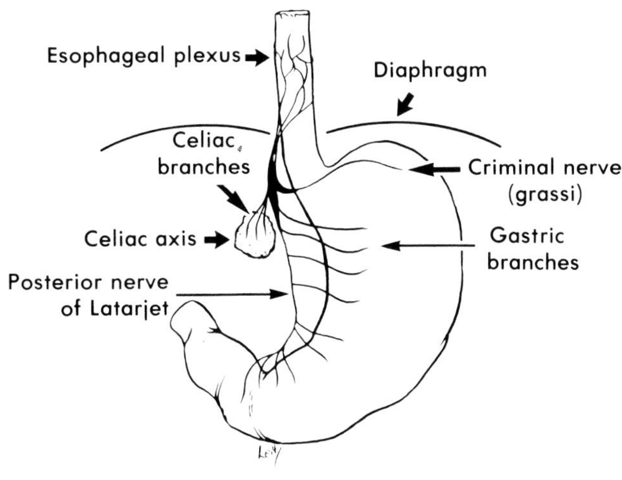

Fig. 15-2 Distribution of subdiaphragmatic vagi with their major branches.

as two or more trunks 40% of the time. By contrast, the posterior vagus, often found in the interval between the esophagus and the right diaphragmatic crus, is a single trunk in over 95% of cases. The extragastric vagal nerves come off the vagi proximal to or at the esophagogastric junction: the hepatic division from the anterior vagus coursing toward the liver high in the lesser omentum, and the celiac division from the posterior vagus running to the celial axis in proximity to the left gastric artery. These two branches are nearly always constant in their location and serve as useful guides to the identification of the main vagal trunks. Both vagi then give off gastric branches to the proximal stomach and continue on to the antrum as the nerves of Latarjet.

The sympathetic nerve distribution of the stomach, on the other hand, does not proceed along easily defined pathways as does the vagal distribution. Sympathetic preganglionic neurons from the fifth to the tenth thoracic segments reach the celiac axis through the greater splanchnic nerve. Neurons with cell bodies in the celiac ganglion innervate the stomach. Sympathetic fibers are distributed to the stomach in the adventitia of the arterial supply and form a meshwork within the gastric wall.* Adrenergic fibers innervate the three muscle layers (longitudinal, circular, and muscularis mucosa), but this innervation is sparse. Sympathetic innervation is more dense to the pyloric sphincter, and in a number of species a rich network of substance P–staining fibers are found, raising the possibility that substance P neurons (see discussion of substance P that follows) may mediate the relaxation of the pylorus. The major distribution of sympathetic fibers in the stomach is to the vasculature.

Much attention has been given recently to the "enteric nervous system (ENS)," which exhibits anatomic and physiologic independence from the central nervous system. In humans, the ENS of the entire gastrointestinal tract contains over 10^8 neurons compared to the number of efferent vagal fibers at the diaphragm of less than 2×10^3.[14] Therefore most enteric ganglion cells probably receive no vagal input. The ENS consists primarily of two main ganglionated plexuses (myenteric [Auerbach's] and Meissner's). The myenteric plexus lies between the circular and longitudinal muscle layers and forms more than one network of fibers connected to the ganglia. Several types of neurons have been identified in the ENS and are listed below:

A. Cholinergic (choline acetate transferase-staining)
B. Serotinergic (containing or activated by serotonin)
C. Peptidergic
   1. Vasoactive intestinal polypeptide (VIP)
   2. Substance P
   3. Somatostatin
   4. Enkephalins
   5. Neurotensin
   6. Other peptides: cholecystokinin (CCK), gastrin, pancreatic polypeptide

*Therefore it must be remembered that, with proximal gastric vagotomy in which thorough vagal denervation is accomplished by devascularizing the lesser curvature of the proximal stomach, not only vagotomy but also partial sympathectomy is performed.

These peptidergic neurons are considered important in modulating the control of the microcirculation and of secretory and motor functions.

Blood Supply

The rich blood supply to the stomach is known to every surgeon and is derived from the celiac axis. The left gastric artery courses to the lesser curve near the gastroesophageal junction and curves downward to anastomose with the right gastric artery, the first branch of the hepatic artery. The greater curvature is supplied through the right and left gastroepiploic arteries. The right gastroepiploic is a branch of the gastroduodenal artery, and the left a branch of the splenic artery. In addition, the splenic artery gives off the short gastric arteries that supply the fundus. Venous drainage is along the right and left gastric veins that join directly the portal vein and along the short gastric veins and the left gastroepiploic veins that join the splenic vein. The right gastroepiploic vein drains into the superior mesenteric vein.

The rich blood supply to the stomach is what makes bleeding from gastric ulcers such a serious problem, requiring surgical intervention much more commonly than bleeding from duodenal ulcers. Less than 10% of patients bleeding from a duodenal ulcer will require surgical control; invariably the ulcer in these patients has eroded into the gastroduodenal artery. When bleeding from duodenal ulcer is initially controlled medically and the patient then rebleeds while receiving medical treatment, the bleeding is nearly always from the gastroduodenal artery and requires immediate surgery.

NORMAL PHYSIOLOGY OF THE STOMACH

Motor Function

Electrical Activity

The stomach, like the heart, has a natural pacemaker.[45] The gastric pacemaker is located high on the greater curvature of the body of the stomach and is composed of a group of specialized smooth muscle cells that generate cyclic changes in potential, called pacesetter potentials. These electrical cycles appear regularly at a frequency of 3 cycles per minute in humans and propagate distally from the pacemaker to the antrum. The pacesetter potential depolarizes smooth muscle cells as it spreads caudad and causes the cells to come close to their threshold for action potentials. Thus the pacesetter potential controls the frequency, rhythm, direction of propagation, and velocity of contraction. The action potential is associated with mechanical contractions and determines the strength of the contraction. The gastric electrical activity is summarized in Fig. 15-3. If the proximal pacemaker is destroyed surgically, secondary pacemakers develop distally.

During fasting, gastric motility demonstrates interdigestive motor cycles that occur every 1 to 2 hours.[5] Each interdigestive motor cycle consists of three phases. The quiescent period when there is no motor activity is Phase I, followed by Phase II in which irregular contractile activity is seen, followed by Phase III when sweeping bursts of contractions occur (Fig. 15-4). The interdigestive motor complex has been called "the housekeeper potential" be-

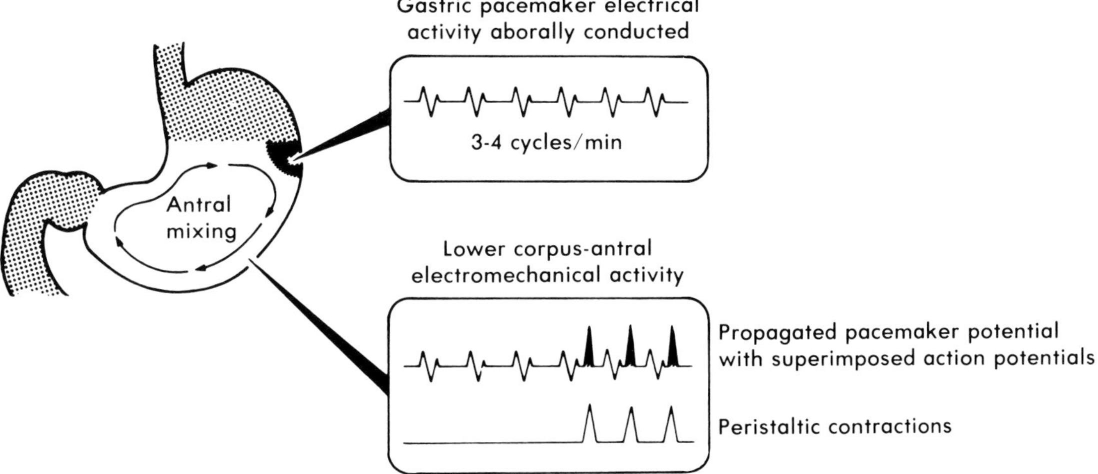

Fig. 15-3 Electrical activity of the stomach and the motor activity of the distal stomach responsible for gastric emptying of solids. Peristaltic contractions triturate digestible solids to near liquefied form before they are emptied. (Reprinted by permission of Elsevier Science Publishing Co., Inc. from Minami, H., and McCallum, R.W.: Gastroenterology **86:**1592, 1984. Copyright 1984 by The American Gastroenterological Association.)

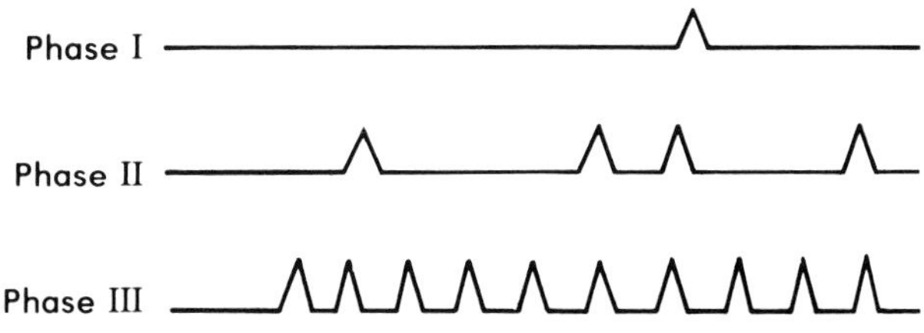

Fig. 15-4 The Migrating Myoelectric Complex (MMC) is initiated in the proximal stomach, and contractions during Phase III sweep down to the pylorus, clearing the stomach of residue; hence the term "housekeeper potential" applied to it. Phase I is the quiescent phase, and contractions start to appear in Phase II before they become numerous and repetitive in Phase III.

cause the Phase III contractions have the effect of clearing the stomach of its contents every 1 to 2 hours regularly.

Feeding disrupts the fasting cyclic motor activity; and the stomach responds to the neural, humoral, and mechanical stimulation imposed by the meal. The motor activities in the stomach are then directed toward delivering the gastric contents into the duodenum in appropriate volumes and particle sizes.

Mechanical Activity

The stomach is normally collapsed when empty. Feeding initiates "receptive relaxation" primarily of the fundus and upper body so that the meal is accepted without precipitous rise in intragastric pressure. Vagotomy interferes with this receptive relaxation so that the arrival of food to the stomach is associated with relatively higher increases in intragastric pressure. Gastric emptying of liquids is thought to be primarily controlled by the proximal stomach. Low-amplitude tonic fundic contractions increase the intragastric pressure sufficiently to create a pressure gradient between the stomach and the duodenum. Liquids are thus squeezed out of the stomach much like wine is squeezed out of a Spanish bota bag. By contrast, the emptying of solid meals is under the control of the distal stomach and is associated with strong antral and antropyloric contractions. When solids are present in the stomach, ring contractions are stimulated to develop in the midbody, generating intraluminal pressures as high as 100 mm Hg.[4] These advance toward the pylorus, propelling the gastric contents caudad and pushing the food against a closed pylorus. The effect is propulsion and retropulsion of the food, ensuring good mixing with the liquid phase. The strong muscular contractions of the antropylorus region grind down solids into small particles. Only particles less than 1 mm in diameter are emptied into the duodenum. The ability of the stomach to discriminate between particle sizes is remarkable and a phenomenon not fully explained.

In summary, the ingestion of food is associated with disruption of the interdigestive motor complex and receptive relaxation of the proximal stomach. Emptying of liquids is controlled primarily by the proximal stomach and involves low-pressure tonic contractions. The emptying of solids, on the other hand, is a function of the distal stomach and is associated with contraction rings, high pressures, propulsion and retropulsion, and grinding down of food particles by the "antral pump." This classic view of assigning control for emptying liquids to the proximal stomach and solids to the distal stomach may not be entirely accurate; some evidence is already emerging that the distal stomach may also play a role in the emptying of liquids.

Regulation of Gastric Emptying

The mechanisms that control and regulate gastric emptying involve both neural and humoral components. The receptive relaxation of the proximal stomach to feeding is mediated through vagal inhibitory reflexes, with the sensory receptors being located in the distal esophagus. The transmitter(s) involved in receptive relaxation are unknown, but they are neither adrenergic nor cholinergic. Evidence has been produced that both dopamine and enkephalin may play a role. The main determinants of gastric emptying are: (1) whether a meal is solid or liquid; and (2) its nutrient content, acidity, and osmolality. Both osmoreceptors and pH-sensitive receptors are present in the upper small intestine. These factors are important in activating feedback inhibition of gastric emptying through neurohumoral pathways. Although a number of peptides, including gastric inhibitory polypeptide, glucagon, vasoactive intestinal polypeptide, and neurotensin, have been proposed as mediators, only cholecystokinin (CCK) has been shown to inhibit gastric emptying in physiologic doses.[8] CCK is released from the duodenum and upper jejunum by protein digests, fat, acid, and perhaps also by high osmolality. Brain centers are probably also involved in the regulation of gastric emptying. Mechanoreceptors in the stomach that respond to distention and glucoreceptors in the first portion of the duodenum have been shown to influence the activity of neurons in the medulla (the nucleus tractus solitarius and the dorsal vagal nucleus).[12] The centers probably relay signals for both satiety and gastric emptying. In the duodenum, pH and osmoreceptors are present, and activation of these receptors delays gastric emptying. It is possible that CCK release may mediate in part the effect of low pH and high osmolality in slowing gastric emptying. A suggestion has also been made that the caloric content of the food passing into the duodenum may be important. It is possible that the receptors for all these mechanisms activate afferent vagal discharge. Therefore the effects of vagotomy on gastric emptying that must be considered are both the gastric effects of the operation and the interruption of afferent vagal input from duodenal pH and osmoreceptors. We know a fair amount about the former but little of the latter. Two important effects of truncal vagotomy on the stomach are the loss of receptive relaxation and accommodation of the proximal stomach and loss of the relaxing effect on the pyloric sphincter. The result is that there is marked inhibition of emptying of both liquids and solids unless the pyloric sphincter is either destroyed or bypassed, in which case gastric emptying of liquids is accelerated as a result of an increased luminal pressure gradient between the stomach and the duodenum or jejunum and relatively normal emptying of solids. Proximal gastric vagotomy that preserves the innervation of the antropyloric mechanism has little permanent effect on gastric emptying of either liquids or solids.

Measurement of Gastric Emptying[26]

Current methods for measuring gastric emptying all have inherent problems, but progressive refinement has made available a number of useful techniques. These techniques are of three types: intubative, radiologic, and radioisotopic. Intubative techniques are more useful for measuring emptying of liquids. In the most common one, "Hunt's Test," a nasogastric tube is used, and 700 ml of saline containing either phenol red or polyethylene glycol as nonabsorbable markers is instilled. The residual volume is aspirated 30 minutes later. If gastric emptying is normal, the residual volume in the stomach should be less than 350 ml. This test is useful in following patients with emptying problems on the ward and, though less accurate, can be used without the nonabsorbable markers as a bedside test. With more sophisticated intubation techniques, both gastric and duodenal intubation are used. Perfusion of different markers into the stomach and duodenum allows for the evaluation of both gastric emptying and duodenogastric reflux.

Radiologic techniques, with both liquid barium and barium-impregnated solids, can be used to measure emptying of liquids or solids. These techniques have never been adequately validated but could provide rough estimates of gastric emptying. Radioisotope tests have now replaced radiologic tests. With the use of two different isotopes, one for liquid and the other for solid, emptying of liquids and solids can be studied simultaneously after the ingestion of a mixed meal. The commonly used markers are technetium-99m (^{99m}Tc) and indium-111. The problem of nuclide marker dissociation from the meal has been overcome by administering ^{99m}Tc-sulfur colloid to chickens in vivo and killing them 30 minutes later to obtain their livers to use as a solid meal. The marker is taken up by Kupfer cells in the liver. The upper abdomen is scanned by a gamma camera immediately after ingestion and at 5-minute intervals for 2 hours. Minute-by-minute evaluation of emptying is made possible by interfacing a computer with the gamma camera. See Minami and McCallum[26] for a discussion of the limitations of these various tests.

Secretory Functions

Endocrine Stomach

As previously indicated, it is no longer valid to consider the distal stomach as an endocrine organ and the proximal stomach as an exocrine organ. Endocrine cells are found throughout the stomach. In addition, peptides and amines are found in neural elements within the wall of the stomach.[17] Peptides arrive at their target site, whether this be the parietal cell or a smooth muscle cell, in one of three ways.

ENDOCRINE. Peptides are secreted through the basolateral membrane into the circulation. They circulate and arrive at the target cell through the bloodstream. This appears to be the mechanism by which gastrin is delivered to the parietal cell. Clearly, peptides secreted by the endocrine cells of the intestine (e.g., CCK, secretin, gastric inhibitory polypeptide ([GIP]), and neurotensin) arrive at the parietal cell through the blood.

PARACRINE. Some humoral agents are evanescent in the circulation, and they may reach their target cells by diffusion after being secreted into the interstitial fluid. Prime examples of paracrine agents are histamine and prostaglandins. In addition, a number of peptides may use this mode of delivery. The most important of these are somatostatin and vasoactive intestinal polypeptide (VIP).

NEUROCRINE. Peptides are secreted from nerve endings and cross a small synaptic gap to the end plate or receptor to cause their actions. A prime example is bombesin or its mammalian counterpart, gastrin-releasing polypeptide (GRP). Another peptide that probably also acts as a neurotransmitter is substance P. Some peptides, e.g., somatostatin and VIP, may use more than one method of delivery. A number of peptides (CCK, somatostatin, VIP, and substance P) are present in and secreted down the axons of the vagus nerves. What function these vagally-transported peptides play is as yet undetermined.

In physiologic studies, peptides are usually administered into the bloodstream to determine their action. Our inability to deliver them at the neural terminal or interstitial fluid of the target organ represents a serious limitation in our ability to study any neurocrine or paracrine function they might have. From this discussion, it should be obvious that the target cells, e.g., the oxyntic cells, operate within a milieu in which a number of neural and humoral stimuli operate. Therefore in vivo responses represent reactions more to a perturbation of this chemical milieu than to that of a pure stimulus.

Gastric Peptides

The peptides found in measurable quantities in the stomach include gastrin, somatostatin, GRP, VIP, glucagon, and substance P. In addition, a number of other peptides (e.g., neurotensin) are found in detectable quantities.

Gastrin. Gastrin is the most important hormone in the control of acid secretion. A second significant function relates to its trophic action on the parietal cell mucosa. In the Zollinger-Ellison syndrome (ZES) the marked hypertrophy of the rugi of the proximal stomach is caused by the trophic effect of high levels of circulating gastrin.

Biosynthesis and molecular heterogeneity of gastrin. Gastrin is synthesized as a prepropeptide that has the gastrin molecule sandwiched between extensions at both amino and carboxy terminals. Processing of this preprogastrin liberates glycine-extended progastrin, which then undergoes alpha-amidation to form the gastrin molecule with an amino terminal. Not one but a number of gastrin molecules are formed.[10] The important molecular forms of gastrin include; (1) *big gastrin,* a 34–amino acid residue (i.e., G-34) with a molecular weight of 3839 daltons; (2) *little gastrin,* with 17 amino acid residues (i.e., G-17) and a molecular weight of 2098; and (3) *minigastrin,* with 14 amino acids (i.e., G-14) and a molecular weight of 1833. All molecular forms of gastrin are found in both antral tissue and the circulation in both the sulfated and unsulfated forms. In the circulation, however, G-34 predominates primarily because of its longer metabolic half-life, 9 to 15 minutes for G-34 vs. 3 minutes for G-17.

Release of gastrin. The release of gastrin is regulated in a complex manner that is not completely understood.[9] Gastrin is released from the antrum by luminal protein digests and amino acids.[23] Gastric distention and vagal stimulation are additional important stimulants of release. The mechanism by which protein digests release gastrin is thought to be by direct chemical action on the microvilli of the G-cell, which reach the lumen of the antral glands, although neural reflex mechanisms with chemical sensors on the mucosal surface may also be involved. Release of gastrin by distention is largely mediated by acetylcholine and is blocked by atropine. By contrast, vagal release of gastrin is not mediated by acetylcholine. Although the neurotransmitter for vagal release of gastrin has not been definitively identified, GRP is the prime candidate. Calcium and prolonged alkalization (>8 hr) also release gastrin. Inhibition of gastrin is accomplished in several ways. The most important is by an acid negative feedback mechanism. When the pH in the antral lumen falls below 2.5, gastrin release is inhibited. Somatostatin, present in the antrum, is now thought to be an important modulator of gastrin release. The release of somatostatin from antral tissue in vitro and antral veins in vivo has been shown to be reciprocal to that of gastrin. Somatostatin inhibits gastrin release, and in situ inactivation of somatostatin by somatostatin antiserum results in augmented release of gastrin.[34] Vagal stimulation by sham feeding, insulin hypoglycemia, or direct electrical stimulation of the vagus results in the release of gastrin, but all forms of vagotomy also result in increased release of gastrin. Postvagotomy hypergastrinemia probably results not only as a consequence of reduced acid secretion, but also because of withdrawal of other vagal inhibitory influences.[18]

Actions of gastrin. Gastrin has a wide range of actions, but many of these effects are seen at pharmacologic doses. In pharmacologic doses gastrin has the following effects: increase of the lower esophageal sphincter pressure, stimulation of pepsinogen and intrinsic factor secretion, stimulation of motility of the intestine and the gallbladder, and stimulation of pancreatic enzyme secretion. The action of gastrin that is known to occur at physiologic levels of the peptide is acid secretion, but indirect evidence also suggests that the trophic action of gastrin on the parietal cell is also physiologic.

Somatostatin. Somatostatin[21] is found both in the antrum and fundus of the stomach, where it is present both in endocrine cells and in nerve endings. It exists in two forms: somatostatin-14, with 14 amino acid residues; and somatostatin-28, with an extra 14 amino acid extension of the amino terminus of the tetradecapeptide. Somatostatin is released by food, antral acidification, vagal stimulation, and intravenous infusion of gastrin. The gastrin effects of somatostatin include: (1) inhibition of gastric acid; and (2) pepsin responses to gastrin, cholinergic stimulation, and, to a lesser degree, histamine stimulation. It inhibits basal, postprandial-, and vagal-stimulated gastrin release. It also blocks the trophic effect of gastrin in the stomach. Contradictory effects on gastric emptying have been described. It is likely that the most important action of somatostatin is regulation of gastrin release. Somatostatin cells also contain receptors for gastrin, and gastrin can release somatostatin. It is possible that such release in the oxyntic mucosa may exert a paracrine inhibitory modulation of acid secretion.

Gastrin-Releasing Peptide. Erspamer and co-workers[11] first isolated a tetradecapeptide with potent acid and gastrin-stimulating action from the frog, *Bombina bombina.* Subsequently, bombesin-like immunoreactivity was shown in the mammalian brain and gut. More recently, MacDonald and associates[25] have isolated from intestinal extracts a 27–amino acid peptide with nine of the 10 C-terminal residues identical to bombesin. They called it gastrin-releasing peptide (GRP), the mammalian counterpart of bombesin; it is also a potent releasor of gastrin and stimulant of acid secretion. Stimulation of acid secretion by bombesin and GRP is secondary to the release of gastrin. In the mammalian stomach GRP is probably exclusively localized in nerves and not in endocrine cells and therefore is likely to act as a neurotransmitter. As indicated previously, the prime action of GRP is probably to act as the neurotransmitter by which vagal stimulation releases gastrin. GRP and bombesin are potent inhibitors of gastric motor activity in the dog. When administered into the cisterna magna or the lateral ventricle of a number of animal species, bombesin causes inhibition of acid secretion, lowering of body temperature, and hyperglycemia.[41]

VASOACTIVE INTESTINAL POLYPEPTIDE. Vasoactive intestinal polypeptide (VIP) was initially isolated from hog intestinal extracts by Mutt and Said[28] and subsequently chemically characterized as a 27–amino acid peptide with strong homology to secretin, glucagon, and gastric inhibitory polypeptide (GIP). In the stomach, VIP is present mainly in nerves, and the VIP-containing fibers are concentrated particularly at the gastroesophageal and pyloric sphincters and around the blood vessels of the lamina propria. It is highly likely that the actions of VIP in the stomach are neurocrine and paracrine. Its effects in the stomach include inhibition of gastric acid secretion and gastrin release, stimulation of pepsin, decrease in mucosal blood flow, relaxation of the lower esophageal sphincter, inhibition of antral smooth muscle contraction, and relaxation of the proximal stomach.

SUBSTANCE P. Substance P is widely distributed throughout the gut and central nervous system. It is found in the vagus nerves and in the stomach. It is present in neurons in the muscle layers. Its precise role in the physiology of the stomach is unknown, but it probably functions as a neurotransmitter in control of blood flow, muscle contraction, and mediation of pain.

GLUCAGON. This 29–amino acid peptide[19] has been shown to be present in A cells in the oxyntic mucosa of a number of species. Although present in significant quantities in the human fetus, it is present only in small quantities in the human adult. Its physiologic significance, if any, in the stomach is unknown, although glucagon administered intravenously is known to inhibit gastric acid secretion and gastric motor activity.

Other Local Agents

Other local agents important in the control of gastric physiology include prostaglandins and histamine. In addition, dopamine and other vasoactive amines are present in the wall of the stomach, although their physiologic role has not been fully determined. The role of prostaglandins in the control of gastric function will be discussed elsewhere in this book. The physiologic significance of histamine will be discussed in the section that follows.

Exocrine Stomach

CONTROL MECHANISMS OF ACID SECRETION

Basal acid secretion. The human stomach secretes small amounts of acid under conditions of no apparent stimulation. The normal subject secretes 1 to 5 mmol of HCl per hour under basal conditions (mean = 2.5 mmol/hour).[27] Both atropine and vagotomy reduce basal acid secretion by 75% to 90%, indicating the importance of vagal-cholinergic control of basal secretion. The H_2 receptor antagonists, cimetidine and ranitidine, reduce basal acid secretion by greater than 90%, demonstrating an important role for histamine. Potentially important roles for the other neurocrine and paracrine substances discussed in the regulation of basal acid secretion have not yet been clearly defined. By contrast, there is no evidence that gastrin plays an important role in this control.

Table 15-2 **SUMMARY OF MECHANISMS REGULATING ACID SECRETION**

Phase	Pathway	Mediator
STIMULATION OF ACID		
Cephalic	Vagus	Acetylcholine Gastrin
Gastric	Neural reflexes Hormonal	Acetylcholine Gastrin
Intestinal	Hormonal ?Neural	*Enteroxyntin** ?
Postabsorptive	Blood	Amino acids
INHIBITION OF ACID		
Cephalic	Vagus Central	*Vagogastrone* *Neuropeptides*
Gastric	Luminal acid Distention reflexes Paracrine	? Somatostatin ? Somatostatin, ? prostaglandins
Intestinal	Hormonal Neural	*Enterogastrone, bulbogastrone,* secretin, GIP, neurotensin ?
Colonic	Hormonal	"Cologastrone," peptide YY (PYY)

*Substances in italics have yet to be chemically characterized.

Stimulated acid secretion. The most important physiologic stimulus of acid secretion is food. Eating brings into play cephalic, gastric, and intestinal factors that stimulate acid secretion[32] (Table 15-2). The thought, sight, smell, and taste of food stimulates several brain centers. The message is then transferred through the hypothalamus, mesencephalon, and brainstem to the vagal dorsal motor nucleus, whence efferent stimulation is sent to the oxyntic cell mucosa through the vagi. Vagal stimulation results in the direct activation of the oxyntic cell through the release of acetylcholine. In addition, vagal stimulation releases from the antrum small amounts of gastrin, which has a potentiating interaction with acetylcholine to cause the oxyntic cell to secrete acid. The cephalic phase of acid secretion in humans can be estimated from studies that stimulate vagal centers either by modified sham feeding (chew-and-spit technique) or by insulin-hypoglycemia or 2-deoxyglucose. Modified sham feeding is by far the most physiologic test of the cephalic phase. The average response of healthy human individuals is about 50% of their maximum acid response to exogenous gastrin or histamine.

Once food enters the stomach, both distention and the action of the chemical constituents of the food result in the stimulation of acid secretion. Distention activates both long vagovagal reflexes and short reflexes completed within the wall of the stomach.[15] In dogs provided with pouches of their proximal and distal stomachs, it is possible to show that distention of fundic antral pouches causes reflex stimulation of acid, suggesting the presence of both oxynto-oxyntic and pyloro-oxyntic reflexes.[10] Attempts to reproduce these studies in humans by balloon distention of various portions of the intact stomach have been unsuccessful. From studies in humans using glucose meals with intragastric titration, the distention factor has been estimated to account for 20% to 50% of the maximal acid response to a peptone meal. Food in the stomach also stimulates by virtue of its chemical composition. Protein digests and amino acids (but not carbohydrates or fats) stimulate the G cell to secrete gastrin. A significant part of the acid response to a meal (60%) is caused by circulating gastrin.[22] An additional mechanism by which amino acids and protein can stimulate acid secretion is by direct action of the oxyntic cell. However, direct chemical stimulation of the parietal cells is artifactual; i.e., it is explained by carbonic acid production as a result of trapping of mucosal carbon dioxide by the highly buffered food in the lumen. If food chemicals stimulate the parietal cell directly, the contribution of this stimulation to the overall secretion of acid must be small.

Once chyme enters the intestine, two additional phases of acid secretion are initiated: the intestinal phase and the postabsorption phase. The intestinal phase is presumed to be caused by release of "enteroxyntin," a stimulant of acid secretion originating from the intestine. Enteroxyntin has not been fully isolated or chemically characterized.[29,44] When liver extract is infused into the intestine of dogs with vagally denervated (Heidenhain) pouches of the proximal stomach, acid secretion from the pouches is stimulated only weakly. However, if intestinal perfusion of liver extract is combined with background stimulation with intravenous pentagastrin or histamine, there is marked potentiation with maximum acid production greater than the total of that obtained with liver extract alone and pentagastrin or histamine alone.[7] The postabsorptive phase of acid secretion is caused by absorbed amino acids. Intravenous infusion of amino acids in humans is capable of stimulating acid secretory rates of 30% to 35% of maximum without increasing plasma gastrin concentrations.[20]

Inhibition of acid secretion. Much more is known about the mechanisms that stimulate acid secretion than those that inhibit it. The stimulus for inhibition of acid may arise in the head (cephalic), the stomach, the small intestine, and the colon (see Table 15-2). The cephalic phase of inhibition is adduced from experiments in animals that show that sham feeding inhibits pentagastrin-stimulated acid secretion and that vagotomy increases Heidenhain pouch acid secretion.[31,37] Grossman[16] has named the presumed mediator of inhibition "vagogastrone." Neither the nature of vagogastrone nor whether it plays a role in regulation of acid secretion under physiologic conditions is known. When some neuropeptides (bombesin, corticotropin-releasing factor) are injected into the cisterna magna or the lateral cerebral ventricle, strong inhibition of gastric acid secretion is observed. Whether these observations have physiologic relevance has yet to be established. The best characterized inhibitory mechanism is the negative feedback inhibition of gastrin by acid in the lumen of the stomach.[33] When intragastric pH reaches 2, gastrin release by food is shut off. The mechanism by which luminal acid inhibits the release of gastrin is unknown but may involve somatostatin. Antral distention both stimulates and inhibits acid secretion. The inhibitory mechanism(s) of distention are unknown but may involve the release of a fundic inhibitor from the oxyntic mucosa that is a powerful inhibitor of both acid secretion and gastrin release.[6] Somatostatin is also present in the proximal stomach, and to what extent it might play a paracrine inhibitory role during normal gastric function is unknown.

When chyme enters the small intestine, a number of inhibitory mechanisms, both neural and humoral, are activated. The presence of acid and hyperosmolar solutions in the duodenum inhibit acid secretion. However, the most potent inhibitor of gastric acid secretion is fat in the upper intestine.[22] The mediator of fat-induced inhibition has been called "enterogastrone," but to date its chemical nature has not been defined. GIP is an excellent candidate enterogastrone because it is released by fat, but studies both in humans and animals have shown that GIP is not an important enterogastrone.[24,46] Another candidate enterogastrone is neurotensin. A number of other intestinal peptides, including secretin, VIP, glucagon, and CCK, are capable of inhibiting acid secretion. CCK stimulates acid when given alone but inhibits competitively the response to gastrin. To what extent these inhibitory peptides play a role in the physiologic regulation of gastric acid secretion is not known. Recently the colon has been identified as an endocrine organ. Both in dogs and humans, colonic perfusion with liver extract, peptone, or fats inhibits acid secretion.[36,40] Seal and Debas[36] have suggested the name "cologastrone" to designate this colon-derived inhibitor of the stomach. More recently, peptide YY (PYY), a peptide with strong structural homology to pancreatic polypeptide, has been found in abundance in the colon and terminal ileum.[30] Intravenous injection of PYY inhibits both acid and pancreatic secretion.[30] It is not known if PYY is the only cologastrone.

Cellular and Subcellular Mechanisms of Acid Secretion.[33] The oxyntic cell has three distinct receptors for stimulants of acid secretion on its surface. These receptors are for acetylcholine, gastrin, and histamine. Receptors are specific proteins that bind to specific stimulants. They are synthesized by the cell and in many instances can be recycled. When the stimulants (ligands) bind to their specific receptors and form hormone-receptor complexes, intracellular mechanisms are activated that eventually result in the secretion of hydrogen ions into secretory canaliculi. Fig. 15-5 summarizes the intracellular events in acid secretion. That histamine works through generation of cAMP is well established. Similarly, it is generally accepted that, when acetylcholine binds to its receptor, mobilization of intracellular calcium and increased plasma membrane permeability result in the increase in intracellular calcium that, through the calmodulin pathway, triggers the process that culminates in acid secretion. Gastrin is thought to act in a manner similar to acetylcholine, but this has not been proven. Whatever cell surface receptor is activated and whichever intracellular pathway is used, the final event is the generation and activation of H^+K^+-ATPase, which finds its way to the microvilli of the secretory vesicles. The H^+K^+-ATPase is the proton pump that regulates the

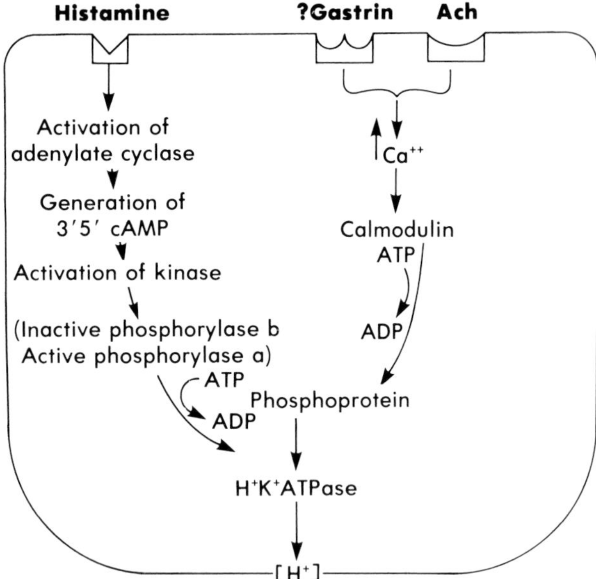

Fig. 15-5 Model for cellular basis of acid secretion showing cell surface receptors for histamine, acetylcholine *(Ach)*, and gastrin. Activation of cAMP generation when histamine binds its receptors and the increase in intracellular Ca^{++} by acetycholine are well established. Gastrin probably also acts by the Ca^{++} pathway. Subsequent intracellular events that eventually lead to generation of H^+K^+-ATPase, the proton pump, are, however, not fully established. Steps indicated in this diagram distal to cAMP and Ca^{++} conform to most of the present findings and thought but are likely to change as intracellular events are better elucidated.

final step of secretion of H^+. Hence, an inhibitor of the proton pump will inhibit acid secretion caused by whatever stimulus is applied to the oxyntic cell.

Function of Gastric Acid. The interposition of a highly acid medium between the environment and the intestinal tract serves to protect against colonization of the stomach and upper small intestine by bacteria. Bacterial colonization of the stomach and duodenum is known to occur in achlorhydric states, and achlorhydria is probably a factor in the cause of gastric malignancy, allowing the generation of nitrosamines. In addition, H^+ is necessary to convert pepsinogen into pepsin, which is required for the initial hydrolysis of protein into polypeptides. Acid is also required as a stimulus of secretin release from the duodenum so that a bicarbonate-rich watery pancreatic flow can occur.

Pepsin Secretion. Pepsin is secreted by chief cells in the proenzyme form, pepsinogen, a protein with a molecular weight of 42,500. Two immunologically distinct groups of pepsinogens have been described by Samloff.[35] Group I pepsinogens (composed of five types of pepsinogen) are found only in the oxyntic mucosa in the peptic and mucus-neck cells. Group II pepsinogens (two types) are found in the oxyntic, antral, and duodenal mucosa. Group II pepsinogen have a higher pH optimum of action. Both groups of pepsinogens are released into the circulation where they may be measured by specific radioimmunoassay techniques. More recently, Samloff[35] has identified another peptic protein he has called ''slow-moving protease,'' (SMP), on agar gel electrophoresis. The significance of SMP is yet to be described. Pepsinogen is converted to pepsin by acid, and thereafter pepsin autocatalyzes its generation.

Much less is known about the mechanisms that control pepsin secretion than those that control acid secretion. Vagal stimulation and cholinomimetic drugs are the most potent stimuli of pepsin secretion in humans. Gastrin and, to a lesser extent, histamine also stimulate pepsin secretion. Secretion is a potent stimulant of pepsin secretion and an inhibitor of acid production. Atropine and vagotomy are the most potent inhibitors of pepsin secretion.

Intrinsic Factor Secretion. Intrinsic factor[3] is secreted by the oxyntic cell in humans, and its secretion generally parallels that of acid. It is a 60,000 dalton mucoprotein that forms a complex with vitamin B_{12}, facilitating the absorption of the vitamin in the distal ileum. Intrinsic factor deficiency develops after total gastrectomy and in pernicious anemia. In the latter condition most patient have antibodies to intrinsic factor.

Secretion of Gastric Mucus and Bicarbonate. Two additional exocrine secretory products of the stomach are mucus and bicarbonate. The stomach is lined by a mucous gel composed of protein, glycoproteins, and mucopolysaccharides.[1] The mucous gel is thought to protect the gastric mucosa from mechanical damage by food. Because of its ability to retain water, the mucous gel maintains a perpetual aqueous environment for the mucosal surface. It may also retain an alkaline atmosphere on the mucosal surface by trapping bicarbonate secreted by mucosal cells. Thus the mucous gel might slow H^+ permeability, and this may be of importance in the so-called protection by the ''mucobicarbonate barrier.'' Mucus is also thought to be important in maintaining the normal gastrointestinal flora while at the same time providing antibacterial and antiviral protection. The mucous gel is in a dynamic equilibrium, being continually solubilized by luminal pepsin on the one hand and secreted by mucosal cells on the other. The mechanisms that control mucous production are poorly understood.

Bicarbonate secretion by the gastric mucosa is a topic of recent great interest.[13] In vitro studies have shown that active bicarbonate secretion takes place in the oxyntic mucosa, whereas both active and passive secretion occurs in the antrum. In vitro, calcium, carbachol, prostaglandins, glucagon, and dibutyryl-cGMP stimulate bicarbonate production. Secretin has been shown to stimulate gastric bicarbonate production in humans. In vitro inhibitors of bicarbonate secretion include acetylsalicylate, indomethacin, ethanol, alpha adrenergic agents, glucagon, and parathormone. The magnitude of bicarbonate secretion relative to acid is small. Hence, any potential protective role of bicarbonate against gastric injury probably derives from provision of an alkaline medium within or deep to the mucous gel at the mucosal cell surface.

ABNORMAL PHYSIOLOGY

Abnormal motor and secretory function of the stomach develops as a result of either disease or surgical interventions of the stomach or of its innervation.

Motor Abnormalities

Transient Delay in Gastric Emptying

A transient delay in gastric emptying is seen most frequently in postoperative patients and in patients who have pancreatitis or peritonitis. The mechanism for this delay is unknown but is generally thought to involve neural reflexes or norepinephrine release. Usually gastric motor function returns with the resolution of the underlying disease, although protracted gastric atony lasting weeks to months is sometimes seen in acute pancreatitis. Transient delay in gastric emptying may also have metabolic causes, including hypokalemia, hypercalcemia and hypocalcemia, hypomagnesemia, hypothyroidism, uremia, hepatic coma, and hyperglycemia. Correction of the metabolic abnormality usually restores normal gastric emptying.

Chronic Impairment in Gastric Emptying

Diabetic Gastroparesis. Diabetic gastroparesis, usually in individuals with insulin-dependent diabetes, may be present in symptomatic or asymptomatic form. Asymptomatic patients may become symptomatic following major abdominal surgery. The basic defect in diabetic gastroparesis appears to be one of impaired neural control with loss of Phase III activity in the stomach (see Fig. 15-3). Although many of these patients have an element of vagal neuropathy, it is probably not appropriate to ascribe diabetic gastroparesis to autovagotomy. Metoclopramide (a drug that enhances gastric contraction) is often effective in improving gastric emptying in these patients.

Postoperative Delay in Gastric Emptying. Distressing problems in gastric emptying are occasionally seen after vagotomy and/or gastrectomy in the absence of gastric outlet obstruction.

Truncal vagotomy without drainage in dogs causes impairment of gastric emptying of both liquids and solids. When pyloroplasty is added, the emptying of liquids is accelerated, whereas the emptying of solids becomes normal. Similar changes are observed in humans when vagotomy was initially performed without a drainage procedure. About 30% to 40% of patients with vagotomy but without drainage develop significant impairment of gastric emptying. After vagotomy and drainage, about 5% of patients develop prolonged postoperative gastric stasis. Proximal gastric vagotomy in duodenal ulcer patients without drainage causes remarkably little impairment of gastric emptying. This is caused in part by the fact that the antropyloric mechanism is intact and in part perhaps by concomitant sympathectomy of the proximal stomach. Antrectomy causes rapid emptying of solids with minimal increase in liquid emptying. The addition of vagotomy to antrectomy tends to delay emptying of solids. About 5% to 10% of patients have significant emptying problems following this operation.

Accelerated Gastric Emptying

A Billroth II gastrectomy (anastamosis of the gastric remnant to the proximal jejunum) and vagotomy with drainage or with antrectomy occasionally result in accelerated gastric emptying leading to the dumping syndrome. The rapid entry of a hyperosmolar load into the jejunum or duodenum results in a rapid fluid shift from the intravascular space into the intestinal lumen and initiation of vasomotor symptoms that are in part caused by the release of bradykinin and serotonin. Fortunately, although the incidence of dumping early following surgery is high, only 5% of patients develop the complication after gastric surgery for ulcer. Avoiding rich carbohydrates in the diet, lying down for 20 minutes after eating, and avoiding drinking fluids with eating are elements in the conservative treatment of dumping. In experimental animals, Becker and associates[2] have shown that electrical pacing of the proximal small intestine through electrodes implanted on the serosa slows gastric emptying and ameliorates the dumping syndrome after vagotomy. This ingenious approach is yet to be tested in the clinical situation.

Tachygastria

An unusual cause of gastric atony develops when ectopic pacemakers appear in the stomach, leading to an irregular rhythm. In this situation the stomach behaves much like the heart with ventricular fibrillation and is incapable of effective contractions that would lead to gastric emptying. The condition can occur de novo or may appear with postoperative ileus, with gastric carcinoma, and after vagotomy. Again in animals, Telander and co-workers[43] have shown that electrical pacing can overdrive the pacemakers, abolish the tachygastria, and return the gastric electrical pattern to its regular, rhythmic pattern.

Gastric Emptying Patterns in Peptic Ulcer Disease

Several investigators have reported delayed gastric emptying in gastric ulcer. The abnormality is more common in Type II (prepyloric) ulcers and for the emptying of solids. Impaired gastric emptying, however, is by no means a universal finding in gastric ulcer. By contrast, accelerated gastric emptying is a common feature in duodenal ulcer and one that may be genetically transmitted.

Secretory Abnormalities

Secretory abnormalities can involve both the endocrine and exocrine stomach. Both hypersecretory and hyposecretory states may result.

Ulcerogenic Hypergastrinemic States

Conditions of hypergastrinemia associated with peptic ulceration include the Zollinger-Ellison syndrome (ZES), G-cell hyperplasia or hyperfunction, the retained antrum, and the short-gut syndromes. In ZES a gastrin-producing tumor is present usually in the pancreas and occasionally in the duodenum or elsewhere. In G-cell hyperplasia the number of gastrin-secreting cells in the antrum is increased. In G-cell hyperfunction the number of antral G cells is normal, but the cells hyperfunction. The latter two conditions are inherited as autosomal-dominant diseases and are associated with hyperpepsinogenemia I.[42] In the retained antrum, G cells are excluded from the acid stream of the stomach and exposed to alkaline pancreatic and biliary secretion in the "duodenal stump." This condition occurs in patients undergoing Billroth II gastrectomy and results in hypersecretion of gastrin and recurrent peptic ulcer. These conditions can be distinguished from each other by performing the secretin and meal tests. In response to a bolus intravenous injection of secretin (2 U/kg), patients with ZES have a paradoxic rise in their serum gastrin (>125 pg/ml), whereas those in G-cell hyperplasia or hyperfunction and those with retained antrum have either no change or a decrease in their serum gastrin. By contrast, after the ingestion of a meal, patients with ZES have an increase in their serum gastrin less than 10% of the basal, whereas those with G-cell hyperplasia or hyperfunction have exaggerated rises. Patients with retained antrum respond little or not at all to this meal.

Nonulcerogenic Hypergastrinemic States

Achlorhydric or hypochlorhydric conditions are associated with hypergastrinemia. The most important causes are pernicious anemia, previous proximal gastrectomy, and previous vagotomy (all types). Postvagotomy hypergastrinemia rarely results in elevation of serum gastrin beyond two or three times normal; but, if a patient has a recurrent ulcer after vagotomy, ZES must be ruled out by the secretin test. Another cause of hypergastrinemia is renal failure when serum gastrin elevation is caused by failure of renal elimination of gastrin.

SUMMARY

The aims of this chapter have been to: (1) outline the normal anatomy of the stomach to indicate the complex neuroendocrine design of the gut; (2) describe the physiologic mechanisms that control the secretory and motor functions of the stomach; and (3) discuss abnormalities of secretion and motility. The transport of a number of peptides down the vagus and the presence of peptides in vagal nerve terminals within the stomach wall have been described. The point has been made that peptides that control gastric function arrive at their target cell not only through the blood, as do classic endocrine substances, but also as neurocrine agents secreted in proximity to receptors on target cells and as paracrine agents diffusing to the target cells through the interstitial fluid after their secretion from neurons or endocrine cells.

In the control of the motor function of the stomach, the presence of the gastric pacemaker; the control of frequency, rhythm, and direction of propagation of electrical activity and the ensuing velocity of contraction; and the role of the interdigestive motor complex that appears to sweep down the stomach regularly every 1 to 2 hours have been discussed. The mechanisms that regulate gastric emptying of liquids and solids and the methods for measuring gastric emptying have been outlined.

The complexity of the control of acid secretion has been addressed. It has been suggested that vagal stimulation causes acid secretion by direct cholinergic action on the oxyntic cell and by release of antral gastrin, which potentiates the direct cholinergic action. Gastrin is the most important hormone in the control of acid secretion; its molecular heterogeneity and the regulation of its release have been discussed. The mechanisms of inhibition of acid secretion have been discussed, and the cephalic (vagal), gastric, and intestinal components have been outlined. The cellular and subcellular mechanisms of acid secretion have been outlined, and the imperfection of our understanding of intracellular events has been emphasized. A number of motor and secretory abnormalities of the stomach have also been discussed to show the importance of understanding normal physiology in order to understand the abnormal. The advances that have been made in gastric physiology are impressive. But many serious gaps in our knowledge remain, and the reader must appraise the literature critically to see where major potential contributions can be made.

REFERENCES

1. Allen, A., and Snarz, D.: The structure and function of gastric mucus, Gut **13:**666, 1972.
2. Becker, J.M., et al.: Intestinal pacing for canine postgastrectomy dumping, Gastroenterology **84:**383, 1983.
3. Binder, J.J., and Donaldson, R.M.: Effect of cimetidine on intrinsic factor and pepsin secretion in man, Gastroenterology **74:**535, 1978.
4. Carlson, H.C., Code, C.F., and Nelson, R.A.: Motor action of the canine gastroduodenal function: a cineradiographic, pressure and electric study, Am. J. Dig. Dis. **11:**155, 1966.
5. Code, C.F., and Marlett, J.A.: The interdigestive myoelectric complex of the stomach and small bowel of dogs, J. Physiol. (Lond.) **246:**289, 1975.
6. Debas, H.T.: Proximal gastric vagotomy interferes with a fundic inhibitory mechanism, Am. J. Surg. **146:**51, 1983.
7. Debas, H.T., Slaff, G.F., and Grossman, M.I.: Intestinal phase of gastric acid secretion: augmentation of maximal response of Heidenhain pouch to gastrin and histamine, Gastroenterology **68:**691, 1975.
8. Debas, H.T., Farooq, O., and Grossman, M.I.: Inhibition of gastric emptying as a physiological action of cholecystokinin, Gastroenterology **68:**1211, 1975.
9. Debas, H.T., et al.: Release of antral gastrin. In Chey, W.Y., and Brooks, F.P., editors: Endocrinology of the gut, Thorofare, New Jersey, 1974, Charles B. Slack, Inc.
10. Debas, H.T., et al.: Proof of a pyloro-oxyntic reflex for stimulation of acid secretion, Gastroenterology **66:**526, 1974.
11. Erspamer, V., et al.: Occurrence of bombesin and alytesin in extracts of the skin of three European discoglossid frogs and pharmacological actions of bombesin on extravascular smooth muscle, Br. J. Pharmacol. **45:**333, 1972.
12. Ewart, W.R., and Wingate, D.: Cholecystokinin octapeptide and gastric mechanoreceptor activity in rat brain, Am. J. Physiol. **244G:**613, 1983.
13. Felmstrom, G.: Active alkalinization of amphibian gastric fundic mucosa in vitro, Am. J. Physiol. **233**(suppl. E):1, 1977.
14. Furness, J.B., and Costa, M.: Types of nerves in the enteric nervous system, Neuroscience **5:**1, 1980.
15. Grossman, M.I.: Secretion of acid and pepsin in response to distension of vagally-innervated fundic gland area in dogs, Gastroenterology **41:**718, 1962.
16. Grossman, M.I.: Candidate hormones of the gut, Gastroenterology **67:**1016, 1974.
17. Hokfelt, T., et al.: Peptidergic neurons, Nature **284:**515, 1978.
18. Hollinshead, J.W., et al.: Hypergastrinemia develops within 24 hours of truncal vagotomy in dogs, Gastroenterology **88:**35, 1985.
19. Holst, J.J.: Extrapancreatic glucagons, Digestion **17:**168, 1978.
20. Isenberg, J.I., and Maxwell, V.: Intravenous infusion of amino acids stimulates gastric acid secretion in man, N. Engl. J. Med. **298:**27, 1978.
21. Konturek, S.J.: Somatostatin and the digestive system, Gastroenterol. Clin. Biol. **1:**849, 1977.
22. Kosaka, T., and Lim, R.K.S.: Demonstration of the humoral agent in fat inhibition of gastric secretion, Proc. Soc. Exp. Biol. Med. **27:**890, 1930.
23. Lam, S.K., et al.: Gastric acid secretion is abnormally sensitive to endogenous gastrin released after peptone test meals in duodenal ulcer patients, J. Clin. Invest. **65:**555, 1980.
24. Maxwell, V., et al.: Effect of gastric inhibitory polypeptide on pentagastrin-stimulated acid secretion in man, Dig. Dis. Sci. **25:**113, 1980.

25. McDonald, T.J., et al.: A gastrin releasing peptide from the porcine nonantral gastric tissue, Gut **19:**767, 1978.
26. Minami, H., and McCallum, R.W.: The physiology and pathophysiology of gastric emptying in humans, Gastroenterology **86:**1592, 1984.
27. Moore, J.G., and Englert, E.: Circadian rhythm of gastric acid secretion in man, Nature **226:**1261, 1970.
28. Mutt, V., and Said, S.I.: Structure of procine vasoactive intestinal octacosapeptide: the amino acid sequence: use of kallikrein in its determination, Eur. J. Biochem. **42:**581, 1974.
29. Orloff, M.J., Guillemin, R.C.L., and Nakaji, N.T.: Isolation of the hormone responsible for the intestinal phase of gastric secretion, Gastroenterology **72:**820, 1977.
30. Pappas, T.N., et al.: Peptide YY inhibits meal-stimulated pancreatic and gastric secretion, Am. J. Physiol. (in press).
31. Preshaw, R.M.: Inhibition of pentagastrin-stimulated acid output by sham feeding, Fed. Proc. **32:**410, 1973.
32. Richardson, C.T., et al.: Studies in the mechanisms of food-stimulated gastric acid secretion in normal human subjects, J. Clin. Invest. **58:**623, 1976.
33. Sachs, G., and Berglindh, T.: Physiology of the parietal cell. In Johnson, L.R., et al., editors: Physiology of the gastrointestinal tract, New York, 1981, Raven Press.
34. Saffouri, B., et al.: Gastrin and somatostatin secretion by perfused rat stomach: functional linkage of antral peptides, Am. J. Physiol. **238G:**495, 1980.
35. Samloff, I.M.: Pepsinogen, pepsins and pepsin inhibitors, Gastroenterology **60:**586, 1971.
36. Seal, A.M., and Debas, H.T.: Colonic inhibition of gastric acid secretion in the dog, Gastroenterology **79:**823, 1980.
37. Sjodin, L.: Inhibition of gastrin-stimulated canine acid secretion by sham feeding. Scand. J. Gastroenterol. **10:**73, 1975.
38. Smolka, A., Helander, H.F., and Sachs, G.: Monoclonal antibodies against gastric H^+K^+-ATPase, Am. J. Physiol. **245G:**589, 1983.
39. Solcia, E., et al.: Human GEP endocrine-paracrine cells: Lausanne 1977 classification revisited. Cellular basis of chemical messengers in the digestive system, New York, 1980, Academic Press, Inc.
40. Soon-Shiong, P., Debas, H.T., and Seal, A.M.: Colonic inhibition of gastric acid secretion in man, Surg. Forum **31:**152, 1980.
41. Tache, Y.: Nature and biological actions of gastrointestinal peptides: current status, Clin. Biochem. **17:**77, 1984.
42. Taylor, I.L., et al.: Hypergastrinemic and hyperpepsinogenemic I duodenal ulcer disease, Ann. Intern. Med. **95:**421, 1981.
43. Telander, R.L., et al.: Human gastric atony with tachygastria and gastric retention, Gastroenterology **75:**497, 1978.
44. Vagne, M., and Mutt, V.: Entero-oxyntin: a stimulant of gastric acid secretion extracted from porcine intestine, Scand. J. Gastroenterol. **15:**17, 1980.
45. Weber, J., Jr., and Kohatsu, S.: Pacemaker localization and electrical conduction patterns in the canine stomach, Gastroenterology **59:**717, 1970.
46. Yamagishi, T., and Debas, H.T.: Gastric Inhibitory Peptide (GIP) is not the primary mediator of the enterogastrone action of fat in the dog, Gastroenterology **78:**931, 1980.

16

Stanley W. Ashley and Laurence Y. Cheung

Gastritis and Peptic Ulceration

Although there have been many recent major advances in the study of the pathophysiology of the upper gastrointestinal tract, our understanding of this subject is still far from complete. Despite the apparent complexity of normal gastric physiology, disorders in this system of integrated functions appear primarily as some form of injury to the gastroduodenal mucosa. The two derangements of major importance to the surgeon are gastritis and peptic ulceration. Each of these processes can be conceptualized as a disturbance in the normal interplay between acid-pepsin secretion and gastroduodenal mucosal defense. This central theme of a balance between these two factors provides a useful framework in which to organize the sometimes diverse clinical and laboratory data regarding pathogenesis and treatment. However, beyond this very basic similarity, gastritis and peptic ulcer differ greatly. In fact, each of the two general categories actually represents a heterogenous group of disorders with widely varying characteristics.

The pathologic entities discussed in the following pages will be characterized first in terms of the direction in which they disturb this normal balance between the mucosal defense and acid-pepsin secretion. The spectrum extends from acute lesions, which predominantly stem from a defect in defense mechanisms, through gastric and duodenal ulcer, to the Zollinger-Ellison syndrome, which is the most flagrant example of acid hypersecretion. Since the fairly similar medical and surgical therapies for these disorders primarily represent attempts to artificially restore this balance, they will be approached first of all in terms of this concept and secondarily as they relate to the specific disease processes. Finally, recurrent ulceration after surgery will be presented as an illustrative failure in these attempts to reestablish the normal interplay of secretion and defense.

PATHOPHYSIOLOGY OF GASTRITIS AND PEPTIC ULCERATION

The distinction between gastritis and ulceration is an important one. In general terms, gastritis represents inflammation confined to the mucosa of the stomach and can occur in both acute and chronic forms. Chronic gastritis is only rarely of direct significance for the surgeon and in this chapter is discussed only in the context of its role in the pathogenesis of chronic gastric ulcer. Acute gastritis, on the other hand, is a commonly encountered problem for anyone involved in the care of the seriously ill. It occurs frequently after major physical or thermal trauma, shock, sepsis, head injury, and ingestion of a variety of chemical agents such as aspirin and alcohol. This lesion is generally classified under the generic term stress erosion. Stress ulcer has been used synonymously, although this designation actually represents a misnomer. True ulcers extend through the muscularis mucosa into the submucosa and muscularis (Fig. 16-1). Although this extension may occur occasionally in acute erosive gastritis, thereby initiating massive hemorrhage from a large submucosal vessel, ulceration is usually chronic in nature. In fact, chronic gastric and duodenal ulcers are distinguished by the presence of an established inflammatory reaction.

Both gastric and peptic ulcers have presented major obstacles to experimental study. Stress erosions usually occur in the setting of severe illness; the management of the illness often supersedes any efforts to examine the pathogenesis of the erosions. However, a number of fairly good animal models exist for acute lesions and have made possible an investigation of the factors responsible for this type of disorder. On the other hand, peptic ulceration is by nature a chronic and recurrent disease, and this has permitted a variety of clinical studies. Investigators have made a very thorough examination of disturbances in acid secretion and its control in these patients. A major difficulty in these studies arises in the distinction between abnormalities of etiologic significance and those that merely represent a consequence of the ulcer diathesis itself. Further understanding of the pathogenesis of chronic ulceration has been hampered by the lack of a really satisfactory animal model. Although secretory abnormalities have been accessible through clinical studies, little is known about the role of mucosal defense mechanisms in chronic lesions, and investigators have been forced to rely on inferences from the findings of acute animal preparations.

Acute Gastritis

Although the precise mechanisms involved in the pathogenesis of acute gastric erosions are not known, current evidence suggests a multifactorial cause.[6] Stress erosions are usually multiple, small, punctate lesions situated in the proximal acid-secreting portion of the stomach, although they may occasionally extend into the antrum and even the duodenum. They occur in three main clinical settings, two of which are associated with a reduction in the ability of the gastric mucosa to protect itself against injury. First, patients with severe illness, trauma, burns, or sepsis, may all develop these lesions, although they achieve clinical significance only in a small percentage. When they extend into larger submucosal vessels, life-threatening hemorrhage can result. In the setting of thermal injury, acute erosions have been distinguished as Curling's ulcers, although no real pathologic difference exists. Patients in this seriously ill group have multiple reasons for a depression of normal defense mechanisms, although, as will be discussed, mucosal ischemia seems to be the predominant

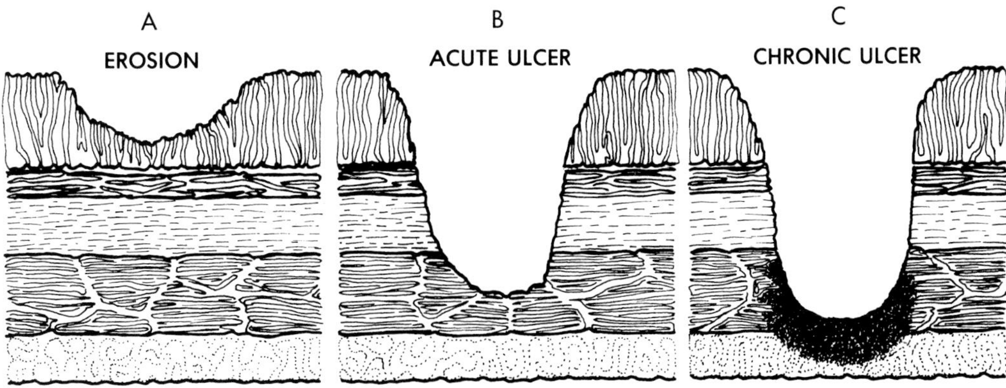

Fig. 16-1 Schematic representation of the distinction between acute erosion **(A)**, acute ulcer **(B)**, and chronic ulcer **(C)**. Erosions are confined to the mucosa, whereas ulcerations extend through the muscularis mucosa to the submucosa and muscularis. Chronic ulceration is distinguished by the presence of established inflammatory reaction.

factor. The second setting for acute erosions occurs in the context of drug and chemical ingestion. Aspirin, a variety of nonsteroidal anti-inflammatory agents, and alcohol may all produce an acute erosive gastritis. These agents presumably directly alter gastric mucosal resistance, allowing back diffusion of acid and further damage. It has been suggested that at least a portion of the caustic effects of these anti-inflammatory drugs stems from inhibition of the synthesis of prostaglandins that appear to have multiple roles in the preservation of normal mucosal integrity. The third underlying condition associated with acute lesions, i.e., central nervous system trauma, is not so clearly related to a defect in mucosal defense. In fact, these patients have elevated levels of serum gastrin and, most likely, a secondary increase in acid secretion. This lesion, Cushing's ulcer, is characteristically deeper than other acute erosions and more frequently perforates.

Pathogenesis

Recent experimental observations have identified a number of factors that appear to contribute to acute erosive gastritis. Most reduce the ability of the stomach to protect itself against acute injury rather than increasing the amount of acid secretion. In fact, experimental evidence suggests that hemorrhagic shock and sepsis may actually result in a reduction in acid secretion. In general, however, Schwarz's "no acid, no ulcer" dictum remains valid, and almost all experimentally induced erosions under conditions resembling clinical settings require low gastric luminal pH.[48]

Given that the presence of luminal acid is a necessary but not sufficient prerequisite for the development of stress lesions, it seems reasonable to postulate that some mechanisms may result in an increased back diffusion of hydrogen ion into the tissue. Davenport and Barr[10] noted that substances such as aspirin, bile salts, and alcohol reduced the normal barrier function of the gastric mucosa, increasing the efflux of sodium ions and the backflux of hydrogen ions. He postulated that this back diffusion might produce histamine release, vasodilation, and eventual bleeding (Fig. 16-2). This concept of a gastric mucosal barrier has

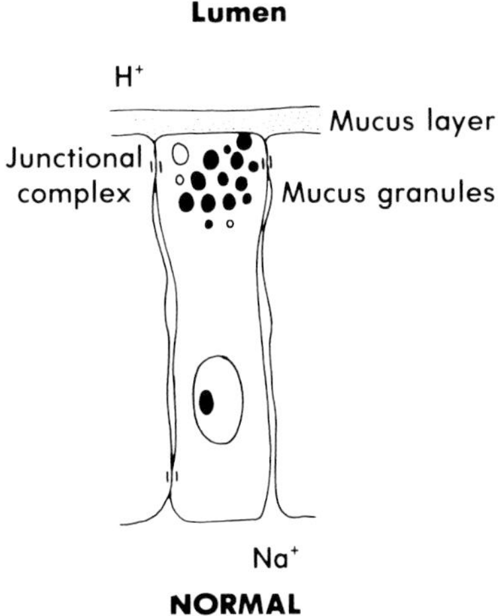

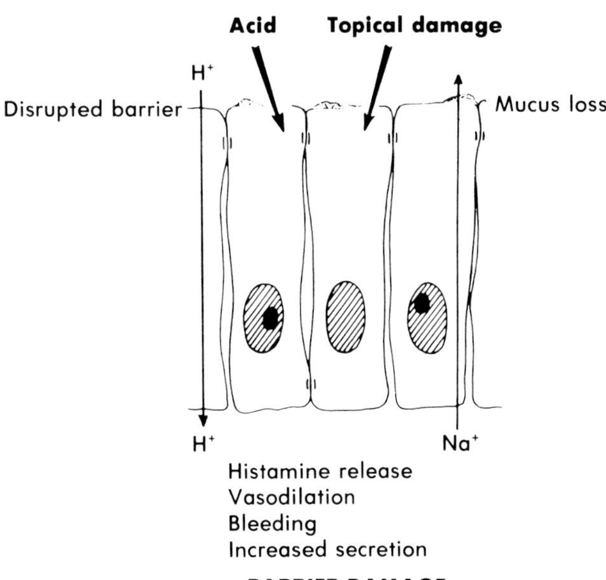

Fig. 16-2 Intact and disrupted gastric mucosal barrier. (From Sircus, W., and Smith, A.N., editors: Scientific foundations of gastroenterology, Philadelphia, 1980, W.B. Saunders Co.)

been supported by a number of subsequent experimental studies with chemical-induced erosion. However, other models for stress lesions suggest that barrier disruption may not be an essential component of the pathologic process in all types of lesions. For example, hemorrhagic shock and endotoxemia can produce lesions without overt evidence of a defect in the barrier.[7] Even in these instances, however, back diffusion of a smaller magnitude probably occurs. In severely traumatized or septic patients, endogenous bile salts may chemically disrupt the barrier. Clinical observations suggest that reflux of bile from duodenum to stomach is more common in critically ill patients, probably as a result of the adynamic ileus. Ritchie[45] has shown that the combination of acid, bile salts, and mucosal ischemia is remarkably ulcerogenic and that it is the concentration of both bile salts and acid that causes great damage.

There is a general consensus among most investigators that mucosal ischemia is a critical pathogenic factor. Most patients have experienced an episode of shock from hemorrhage, sepsis, or cardiac dysfunction, and decreased mucosal blood flow is a common denominator in many experimental models for stress erosion. It remains uncertain what the exact role of blood flow is in maintaining mucosal defense. The leading hypothesis is that it somehow functions to dispose of or buffer acid entering the tissue. Ischemia reduces this capacity, lowering intramucosal pH. Menguy[34] has also suggested that it may reduce mucosal resistance by secondarily producing a deficit of mucosal adenosine triphosphate and other high-energy phosphate intermediates. His animal experiments have demonstrated that this deficit is greater in the fundus than the antrum, possibly explaining the predisposition of this region to stress erosion. It is also greater in the fasted state when energy sources are presumably depleted.

Recent studies also indicate important roles for both systemic and gastric acid/base balance. Acidosis has been shown to reduce the ability of the gastric mucosa to protect itself against injury in animal studies. The secretory status of the mucosa itself may be a critical factor. In concert with acid secretion, bicarbonate is released into the tissue, the so-called "alkaline tide." O'Brien ad Silen[37] have recently demonstrated the importance of this release in mucosal protection. The actively secreting stomach in animal studies appears to be much more resistant to luminal acid than it is under conditions of secretory inhibition.

Mucus normally covers the gastric mucosa, and the possibility that this somehow has a protective role has stimulated considerable interest. It has been postulated that the mucus layer over surface epithelial cells may serve as an unstirred layer in which actively secreted bicarbonate neutralizes luminal acid before it can reach and damage the cells. However, the exact role of mucus and bicarbonate secretion in protecting the mucosa against acute lesions is as yet incompletely defined. The rate of epithelial renewal may also be a factor, presumably preventing the appearance of injury by replacing damaged mucosal cells. Gastrin and epidermal growth factor, a peptide found in salivary secretions, have both been shown to have trophic effects on the gastric epithelium. These agents inhibit the formation of erosions. Prostaglandins exert a protective effect in the gastric mucosa, and the inhibition of their production by aspirin and other nonsteroidal anti-inflammatory agents may be a primary mechanism for gastric injury. Prostaglandins in high doses inhibit acid secretion, but even at lower concentrations they seem to exert what has been termed a "cytoprotective" effect. Experimental evidence suggests several possible mechanisms.[35] These agents increase mucosal blood flow and, in addition, they have been shown to stimulate bicarbonate secretion, presumably providing a luminal buffer.

The recognition of these pathogenic mechanisms has provided a rationale for the prevention of stress erosions by bolstering mucosal defenses in critically ill patients. As a result, in recent years the incidence of these lesions has notably decreased. The prerequisite for acid secretion provides a rationale for the regular use of antacid prophylaxis, the efficacy of which has been demonstrated in a number of clinical trials. Cimetidine has not proved quite so effective, possibly because the secretory inhibition is accompanied by both a decrease in mucosal blood flow and a reduction of bicarbonate release into the tissue. The correction of abnormalities in cardiac output and intravascular volume may be critical in the prevention of mucosal ischemia. Adequate nutritional therapy is suggested by the concept of a mucosal energy deficit. Finally, the correction of systemic acid/base balance may also have a role. Hopefully, as we continue to improve our management of at-risk patients, the incidence of this lesion will further decrease.

Clinical Manifestations and Diagnosis

The predominant clinical manifestation of erosive gastritis is gastrointestinal bleeding. Prodromal signs such as abdominal pain are infrequent. Massive bleeding usually occurs 7 to 10 days after the initial insult when the superficial erosion extends into larger submucosal vessels. Only rarely do erosions perforate. If a high index of suspicion is maintained in conditions that predispose to this illness, diagnosis is usually fairly straightforward. Routine upper gastrointestinal series are of little value—the critical condition of these patients often precludes a good quality study, the erosions are usually too superficial to visualize, and, should angiography become necessary, the contrast material may interfere. Upper endoscopy is the procedure of choice and is diagnostic in nearly 90% of patients.[5] Additionally, radionuclide scanning and visceral angiography may prove useful.

These patients are usually critically ill, and it is essential to stabilize and correct any predisposing conditions at the same time diagnostic maneuvers are being performed. Hypovolemia and coagulopathies should be identified and treated as early as possible. Large-bore nasogastric intubation with an Ewald tube decompresses the stomach, eliminating the stimulating effects of distention and blood on acid secretion. In addition, it provides information about the rate of bleeding, clears the stomach for endoscopy, and allows saline lavage that alone will control the bleeding in greater than 80% of patients.[29] Although suggested by some, the efficacy of lavage with iced solutions and levarterenol for their vasoconstrictor effects has not yet been demonstrated. Once the diagnosis is established, further steps in medical and, possibly, surgical management should be instituted.

Chronic Peptic Ulcer

The physiologic mechanisms involved in chronic gastric and duodenal ulcer are very different and will be treated separately in the following discussion. However, despite attempts to make distinctions on the basis of such parameters as the type of pain, their clinical presentation and diagnosis are remarkably similar and will be presented together.

Pathogenesis of Gastric Ulcer

Gastric ulcer is the next entity in this spectrum of gastroduodenal mucosal injury. Three forms are commonly recognized. Type I is the primary gastric ulcer, usually located in the proximal antrum and constituting the majority of gastric ulcers. Its pathogenesis has also been generally associated with a disturbance in mucosal defense and a characteristic hyposecretion of gastric acid. Type II gastric ulcer, which arises secondary to duodenal ulcer with pyloric stenosis, and Type III, the prepyloric and channel ulcer, are often associated with acid hypersecretion and are assumed to share a common cause with duodenal ulcer. Only Type I ulcerations will be considered here.

As mentioned earlier, no really good experimental model exists for chronic peptic ulceration, and much of our current knowledge of its pathogenesis stems from epidemologic and genetic studies.[57] In many instances the links between this body of information and the pathophysiology of chronic ulceration are speculative. For example, no explanation has been provided for the relative shift in disease prevalence over the last century. In the late 1800s the incidence of gastric ulcer greatly exceeded that of duodenal ulcer, whereas today the reverse is true. Likewise, the suggested role of dietary factors in the greater prevalence of gastric ulcer in Japan is unsubstantiated. In Australia, an increased incidence among lower class women has been explained by their heavy aspirin consumption.[19] The greater frequency of this lesion with advancing age may be related causally to an increased incidence of gastritis in the elderly. In addition, genetic factors seem to have a role. There is a definite familial aggregation of both gastric and duodenal ulcer.[46] However, unlike duodenal ulcer, as yet no genetic markers have been identified for this disease.

A number of risk factors have been recognized, although their direct relationship to the pathogenesis of this disorder is for the most part unconfirmed. There appears to be a correlation with cigarette smoking.[58] Nicotine reduces pyloric sphincter pressure and increases duodenogastric reflux. As will be discussed, this reflux may be an important factor in the development of gastric ulceration. There are as yet no data to support the popular belief that irritants such as spices and curries may damage the gastric mucosa. One epidemiologic study has implicated coffee and soft drinks in ulcerogenesis but did not distinguish between gastric and duodenal disease.[40] In addition to its role in acute gastritis, aspirin has been clearly associated with chronic gastric ulceration. Little is known about the difference between the action of aspirin in chronic ulcer and that effect seen in acute lesions in which it appears to cause both direct mucosal injury and an inhibition of prostaglandin synthesis. Although most gastric ulcer patients have an element of chronic gastritis in association with their ulcer, studies of gastrectomy specimens have revealed that habitual aspirin users may develop ulcers in otherwise normal mucosa. Though a relationship between psychologic factors and chronic ulceration has been suggested, patient studies have not been particularly revealing. No one personality pattern has been identified, and there are rather conflicting findings regarding the role of stressful life events.

Current theories suggest that there are two major but closely related physiologic abnormalities in gastric ulcer—duodenogastric reflux and damage to mucosal defenses.[44] In contrast to the hypersecretion noted in duodenal ulcer, gastric ulcer patients secrete in a range from normal to barely detectable. Although a few subjects have been reported with no detectable acid secretion or achlorhydria, in general it is believed that at least some acid-pepsin is required for ulceration. However, it is clear that the defect in these patients must include a significant disorder of defense.

It has been speculated that the most basic abnormality in gastric ulcer is a reflux of duodenal contents (i.e., biliary and pancreatic secretions) into the stomach, resulting in gastritis and eventual ulceration. Barium fluoroscopy and marker studies have in general demonstrated increased reflux in these patients, probably because of pyloric sphincter dysfunction.[16] Normally the pylorus has a low resting pressure that increases in response to acid, fat, amino acids, and cholecystokinin from the duodenum. In some gastric ulcer patients, low basal pressures have been documented, and in others pressure increases in response to duodenal infusion of acid or fat are significantly less than those of control (Fig. 16-3). Pressure also rises less in response to exogenous cholecystokinin and secretin. It has been suggested that when these two hormones are released endogenously by acids or fat in the duodenum, the lack of response to them may be the primary mechanism for all these abnormalities. The pyloric malfunction presumably explains the increase in duodenogastric reflux.

The physiologic link between reflux and gastric ulceration has not been clearly established. Drainage of duodenal contents into the stomach in experimental animals will produce a superficial gastritis that is worst in the antrum.[11] However, it has not been shown to result in chronic ulceration. Some gastric ulcer patients do have an increase in bile acid conjugates in the stomach, both in the fasting state and after meals; and the severity of their gastritis seems to correlate with the concentration.[12] Bile acids (particularly deoxycholate and taurocholate), lysolecithin, and pancreatic secretions are the agents in duodenal contents speculated to have the most damaging consequences. It is believed that they damage the mucosa topically, disturbing the surface mucus layer and somehow producing a low-grade disruption of the gastric mucosal barrier. Aspirin seems to have similar effects. Ion transport and metabolic processes such as adenosine triphosphate production may be altered. It has been suggested that gastric ulcer patients are predisposed to this alteration by some inherent

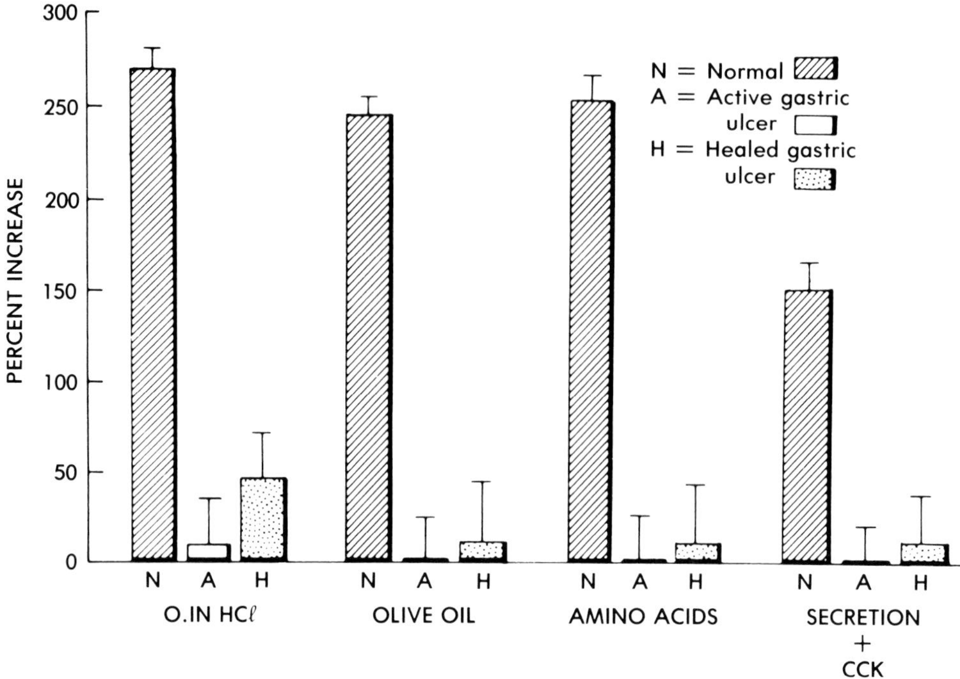

Fig. 16-3 Pyloric pressure responses to intraduodenal stimuli and exogenous hormonal administration in normal persons and patients with gastric ulcer before and after healing. Pyloric pressure is expressed as the percentage increase above basal pressure. In normal individuals, hydrochloric acid, olive oil, amino acids, and intravenous secretin all increase pyloric pressure. In gastric ulcer these agents fail to produce a significant rise both before and after ulcer healing. (From Fisher, R.S., and Cohen, S.: Reprinted by permission of the New England Journal of Medicine [N. Engl. J. Med.] **288:** 273, 1983.)

abnormality in mucus or bicarbonate secretion. Some data support a decrease in mucus secretion with atrophic gastritis, but it is very difficult to distinguish which disorder is the primary one.[3] No definite defect in the composition of gastric mucus has yet been demonstrated.

Chronic gastritis is the widely assumed intermediary step between the repeated injury to the gastric mucosal barrier by refluxing duodenal contents and the development of gastric ulceration. This concept of gastritis producing ulceration is unproven, and chronic atrophic gastritis is very common in the elderly, found in approximately 40% of persons over the age of 50.[4] Although gastritis is usually associated with chronic ulcers, the primary event has not been clearly established. Gastritis may be limited to only the area around the ulcer, but it usually persists after ulcer healing. The extension of the usual antral pattern of gastritis into the fundus helps to explain the generally low rates of acid secretion in gastric ulcer patients. In addition, some increase in basal hydrogen ion back diffusion may also play a role. Gastrin cells are apparently spared the gastritis because, in response to the reduced acidity, fasting serum gastrin levels are usually slightly elevated and may double the normal increase after a meal.[54]

The pathologic anatomy of gastric ulceration has provided some insight into its pathogenesis. These ulcers usually occur along the lesser curvature at the angularis, on the antral side of the junction between the corpus and antrum. Several possible explanations for this have been proposed.[38] Near the angularis there are prominent muscle bundles underlying the mucosa that might somehow predispose to ulceration. With advancing age, the corpus-antral junction migrates cephalad; this occurs most rapidly along the lesser curvature. It has been suggested that ulcers develop when this junction overlies the muscle bundles. The bundles may somehow constrict the mucosal blood supply, increasing the susceptibility of the mucosa to acid-peptic injury. The concept that changes in mucosal blood flow may have a role in chronic ulceration is only conjecture. However, the blood supply is different on the lesser curvature. There mucosal capillaries and submucosal arteries are end vessels arising directly from the left gastric artery, whereas in the rest of the stomach they arise from an extensive submucosal plexus. Muscular contractions may constrict these end arteries and, without the usual system of anastomosing vessels, produce areas of focal mucosal ischemia.

In summary, gastric ulcer seems to result from a defect in gastric mucosal defense against digestion by acid-pepsin. Physiologic defects that may contribute to gastric ulcer are:

A. Normosecretion or hyposecretion of acid
B. Duodenogastric reflux
   1. Pyloric sphincter dysfunction
C. Damaged gastric mucosal defenses
   1. Chronic gastritis
   2. Gastric mucosal barrier disruption
   3. Focal mucosal ischemia
   4. Defects in mucus or bicarbonate secretion

Hypersecretion cannot be incriminated in its pathogenesis. There is evolving evidence that pyloric dysfunction, acting through duodenogastric reflux, allows endogenous agents to exert injurious effects on the mucosa. These agents, in combination with acid-pepsin, produce ulceration in areas of reduced mucosal resistance.

Pathogenesis of Duodenal Ulcer

Duodenal ulcer primarily represents a disorder in acid-pepsin secretion, and more than 95% of duodenal ulcers occur in the first part of the duodenum, most within 3 cm of the junction between pyloric and duodenal mucosa.[20] This distribution suggests that the role of gastric acid is crucial in their pathogenesis. However, recent refinements in our knowledge have been made to complicate this theory.

As with gastric ulcer, much of our knowledge of the pathogenesis of duodenal ulcer stems from the indirect evidence of epidemiologic and genetic studies. For example, in India, duodenal ulcer, often in conjunction with pyloric obstruction, is more common in the rice-eating south than in the northern regions where wheat is the primary staple. This difference has been linked by suggestion to an increase in salivary secretion with the wheat diet. Saliva does have a high concentration of epidermal growth factor, which inhibits acid secretion and stimulates epithelial renewal. Another study from York, England suggested a higher incidence among urban than country dwellers, supporting the common belief that urbanization may play a role.[28] There is considerable controversy regarding recent trends in the incidence of duodenal ulcer.[26] Several studies have reported major declines in the number of hospitalizations, complications, operations, and mortality figures for duodenal ulcer, perhaps implying some basic difference in the pathophysiology of the disease. However, others have disputed these suggested trends, implying that these changes may be more a reflection of other factors such as differences in hospital disease classifications, an increase in patient self-medication with antacids, a greater willingness to treat ulcer on an outpatient basis, and an improved diagnostic approach with the advent of more widespread endoscopy.[50]

A number of risk factors have also been identified. Smoking is associated with an increased incidence and also appears to impair the healing of duodenal ulcers. Nicotine decreases pancreatic secretion, and it has been proposed but not proved that the loss of this neutralizing factor may be partially responsible for the effect of tobacco. In another study in college students, milk consumption was correlated with a decrease and coffee and soft drinks with an increase in the later development of ulcers.[40] Despite popular belief, there is no good evidence that a change in diet has a major effect on the disease.

There have been attempts to associate duodenal ulcer with a number of other chronic diseases, but as yet no common pathophysiologic mechanism has been identified. The increased incidence of duodenal ulcer in patients with chronic lung disease appears unrelated to the degree or treatment of the pulmonary disease, and, in fact, the ulcer often precedes the development of respiratory problems.[46] Cirrhosis seems to be associated with duodenal ulcer, and the finding that acid secretion is normal in these patients has led to the suggestion that a portal hypertension-induced alteration in mucosal blood flow may be involved.[25] Duodenal ulcers probably occur with increased frequency after renal transplantation, and this has generated some speculation regarding a relationship between steroids and ulcerogenesis.[39]

There is now very strong evidence that genetic factors play an important role in the pathogenesis of duodenal ulcer.[21] Until quite recently it was thought that peptic ulcer was a single polygenic disease, the result of complex interactions between many different genes and environmental factors. However, the recent recognition of several distinct, genetically determined subcategories of peptic ulcer has suggested instead that it is a heterogenous group of distinctly different diseases, in some instances the result of simple Mendelian genetics, all of which present as an ulcer of the gastroduodenum.[32] Initial evidence for a genetic basis came from familial aggregation and twin concordance studies, but this has been strengthened by the recognition of a number of rare genetic syndromes that all produce duodenal ulcer as a component of the phenotype. These include, among others, multiple endocrine adenoma Type I, which frequently presents as the Zollinger-Ellison syndrome; systemic mastocytosis; and an autosomal dominant disorder of tremor, nystagmus, narcolepsy, and ulcer.[2] In addition to this evidence, a number of discrete genetic subtypes of common duodenal ulcer have been identified by means of both biochemical and physiologic markers.[47] There is a group of duodenal ulcer patients who all have an elevated serum pepsinogen I, the inactive precursor for pepsin, a characteristic that seems to be transmitted by an autosomal dominant pattern of inheritance. The risk of ulcer is increased only in hyperpepsinogenemic siblings. Other genetic subgroups have been identified by normopepsinogenemia, a pattern of rapid gastric emptying, and antral gastrin cell hyperplasia.

Empiric observations have repeatedly suggested that stressful life events and anxiety-producing situations affect the course of individual patient's illnesses and may even be important in the initial pathogenesis.[56] A number of studies, particularly in chronic gastric fistula patients, have demonstrated that emotions have an important effect on both gastric acid secretion and blood flow. But, although animal studies with restraint and avoidance models implicate a role for stress in acute lesions, such a role has been nearly impossible to evaluate or clearly document in human studies. Attempts to identify an ulcer personality have not proven particularly fruitful.

In addition to this rather indirect knowledge of the pathophysiology of duodenal ulcer, a wide variety of functional disturbances has been identified in patient groups. This variation provides further evidence for the concept of heterogeneity in duodenal ulcer disease. At the opposite end of the spectrum from the defects in mucosal defense identified in acute lesions, the most important factor in duodenal ulceration seems to be a disorder in acid secretion, although in some subsets disturbances in motility or acid disposal may be primary.

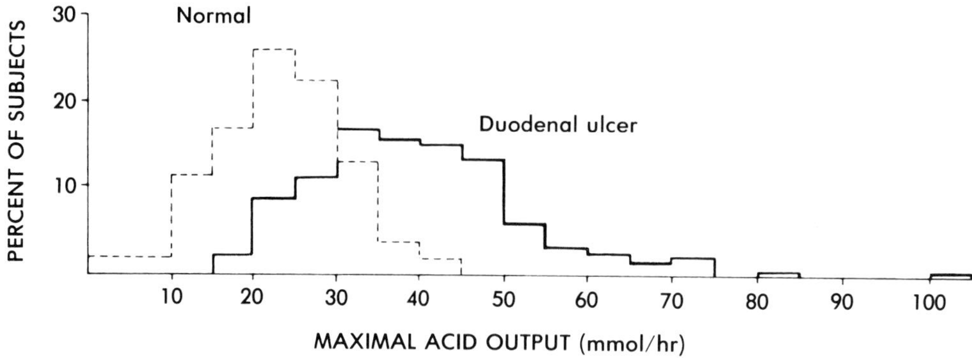

Fig. 16-4 Maximal acid response to intravenous infusion of histamine in normal men and men with duodenal ulcer. The median value is significantly greater in the patients with duodenal ulcer, although overlap is considerable, and approximately 70% of duodenal ulcer patients fall within the normal range. (Data from Kirkpatrick, et al. Reproduced with permission from Grossman, M.I., editor: Peptic ulcer: a guide for the practicing physician, Chicago, 1981, Year Book Medical Publishers, Inc. Copyright © 1981 by the CURE foundation.)

In general duodenal ulcer is associated with hypersecretion of acid. Patients with duodenal ulcer tend to secrete more both at rest and in response to stimulation than do normal controls (Fig. 16-4).[20] However, there is considerable overlap, and in fact there appears to be no direct relationship between the degree of acid hypersecretion and the severity of the ulcer diathesis. Multiple sources for this increase in acid secretion have been identified. Duodenal ulcer patients have an average of 1.8 billion parietal cells as compared with 1 billion in controls.[8] Chief cell numbers increase in parallel, although the role of their secretory product, pepsin, in ulcerogenesis has not yet been clearly proved. Several explanations have been provided for this increase in secretory mass. In at least one subset of patients, i.e., those distinguished by hyperpepsinogenemia I, it probably occurs on a genetic basis. In others, it may be the acquired result of an increase in the release of trophic factors such as gastrin and histamine.[22] Partial pyloric obstruction in rats has been shown to elevate gastrin levels as a result of antral distention and probably as a consequence produces an increase in secretory mass. Likewise, the elevated histamine levels of systemic mastocytosis seem to exert a trophic effect. It may be that in some patients there is an increase not only in cell numbers but also in the capacity of the individual cell to secrete; this is a very difficult hypothesis to test. Secretory capacity tends to increase with longer duration of the disease, although it returns to control levels after ulcer healing.[50] The cause-and-effect relationship between this increase in secretory capacity and duodenal ulcer is by no means established.

There is also evidence that acid hypersecretion in some patients results from an increase in stimulation. There is an increase both in basal secretion that might reflect only the increase in secretory capacity and in the ratio of basal secretion to total secretory capacity, suggesting that there is some increase in the background stimulus to acid secretion. Basal secretion probably results primarily from a combination of steady-state vagal and histamine stimulation. Dragstedt[11] originally suggested that vagal hyperactivity might be the physiologic basis for duodenal ulcer. Studies demonstrating an increase in the acid secretory response to sham feeding and to insulin-induced hypoglycemia in duodenal ulcer patients, both of which are believed to be mediated through the vagus, provide some support for this hypothesis.[15] Because there is no satisfactory method for measuring gastric histamine release, it is very difficult to evaluate the suggestion that an increase in basal histamine stimulation is involved. One study did report a decrease in the histamine content and in the activity of histamine methyltransferase in the fundus of duodenal ulcer patients, although this finding is very difficult to interpret.[41]

Duodenal ulcer patients also secrete more acid in response to exogenous stimuli. With meals, some studies have demonstrated an increase in peak secretion, whereas others demonstrate a more prolonged response.[30] Although basal serum gastrin levels are usually not elevated and the actual gastrin content of the duodenal mucosa is normal, the increase of acid in response to meals seems to be greater. A decrease in gastrin degradation or a defect in inhibition rather than an increase in release could be occurring. Hyperacidity should inhibit antral gastrin secretion; thus gastrin levels in these patients may be inappropriately high in relation to their secretory capacity. Studies have variously shown defects in inhibition of both acid secretion and gastrin release in response to instilled acid or amino acids,[30] possibly reflecting defects in the intestinal phase of acid secretion. A host of disorders in secretory stimulation or inhibition by regulatory peptides, gut hormones, or absorbed food products may potentially be identified. There is also evidence of an increase in parietal cell sensitivity to secretogogues. For example, the dose of pentagastrin required to produce a half-maximal response is much reduced.[27] Explanations for this such as an increase in parietal cell receptors or more efficient stimulation-secretory coupling are merely speculative.

In addition to these disorders in acid secretion, some duodenal ulcer patients have a motility abnormality. There is more rapid gastric emptying of meals, particularly liquids, and acid and food in the duodenum slow emptying to a lesser extent than in controls.[30] The etiologic basis for this rapid emptying is unclear. In some patients, as mentioned, there is evidence for a genetic pattern, whereas in others bulbar inflammation and ulceration may reduce the effectiveness of acid or food-sensitive mechanisms.

Thus both the tendency to secrete more acid and to empty it more rapidly contribute to an increase in the amount of acid delivered to the duodenum, lowering bulbar pH. As yet no definite defect in duodenal acid disposal has been identified. Despite the concept that duodenal ulcer, at least to a greater extent than gastric ulcer, represents a disorder in acid secretion, most patients secrete within the normal range. This has led some investigators to propose an additional defect in duodenal defense. Studies to document this have had various results. Impaired motility of the proximal duodenum, decreased production of prostaglandins, reduced bulbar mucosal blood flow, and defects in mucus or bicarbonate secretion have all been hypothesized. Chronic duodenitis has been noted in much the same way that gastritis has been associated with gastric ulcer, prompting the theory that this inflammation somehow weakens the mucosa.

In summary, consistent with current concepts of duodenal ulcer as a heterogenous group of disorders, a wide variety of abnormal physiologic patterns has been described as outlined here:

A. Hypersecretion or normosecretion of acid
   1. Increase in parietal cell mass
   2. Increase in basal and stimulated secretion
   3. Decrease in secretory inhibition
B. Rapid gastric emptying
C. Defect in duodenal acid disposal or mucosal defense

The most striking defects involve some disorder in basic acid secretory mechanisms and their control. In addition, at least in some patients, rapid gastric emptying may play a role. Defects in duodenal disposal of acid and mucosal defense have not yet been completely ruled out.

Clinical Presentation and Diagnosis of Peptic Ulcer

The physiologic manifestations and diagnostic possibilities in peptic ulcer disease are extensive and are discussed only briefly here. Gastric and duodenal ulcer often present in a very similar fashion. Classically, gastric ulcer has been associated with a gnawing or burning epigastric pain brought on by or closely following the secretory stimulus of eating. On the other hand, duodenal ulcer pain is supposedly relieved by food or alkali and usually develops several hours after a meal when food has passed the duodenum and the crater is exposed to unbuffered gastric secretion. In fact, symptoms in these two processes are very nonspecific, and even the correlation of pain with the actual presence of peptic ulceration is a poor one.[50] Although intractable pain is generally considered an indication for surgery in peptic ulcer, because of its nonspecific nature intractable pain is very difficult to define. The actual physiology of ulcer pain is not known, although two explanations have been suggested. Acidic luminal contents may irritate afferent nerves within the ulcer crater itself or, alternatively, peristaltic waves passing through the ulcer might produce discomfort. The relative importance of these two possibilities has not been determined. Pain symptomatology in both gastric and duodenal ulcer tends to be chronic and recurrent. Usually these ulcers cannot be differentiated on the basis of clinical findings, although the mean age of gastric ulcer patients is approximately 10 years greater than that of patients with duodenal lesions.[44] Gastric ulcers have a peak incidence from ages 50 to 65 years, whereas most duodenal ulcers develop in the fourth decade of life. Other common symptoms include nausea and weight loss, even in the absence of pyloric obstruction, and mild epigastric tenderness.

Diagnosis is usually fairly straightforward. Routine laboratory studies add little to the diagnostic workup. In the future, measurement of serum pepsinogen I by radioimmunoassay may prove useful in distinguishing familial ulcer disease.[47] Because of the overlap in rates between ulcer patients and controls, secretory studies are not usually indicated. The two mainstays of diagnosis are upper gastrointestinal radiography and endoscopy. The decision of when to study a patient with dyspepsia is a complex issue requiring consideration of the character, severity, and duration of symptoms. The choice between radiography and endoscopy is not a simple one. However, at present radiography is the more cost-effective procedure and, with optimal double-contrast studies, greater than 90% of gastric and duodenal ulcer craters will be detected, a sensitivity rate comparable to that achieved with endoscopy.[50] Endoscopy is indicated in the case of a poor-quality x-ray film study. The question of malignancy in gastric ulcer complicates the decision, and, because 3% to 7% of gastric malignancies appear benign on x-ray film studies, endoscopy in all cases has been recommended.[44] Other clinicians have suggested that endoscopy and biopsy are only necessary when gastric ulcers do not appear typically benign on standard x-ray films, are large, or fail to heal with standard therapy.

Peptic ulcer may produce one of three main complications—hemorrhage, perforation, or obstruction. These can develop without any premonitory symptoms but typically appear as an abrupt change from preexisting dyspepsia. The pathophysiology of these complications is relatively simple; all basically result from the extension of ulceration and the accompanying inflammation deeper into the wall of the gastroduodenum.

When the crater extends into a major vessel, significant hemorrhage may result. About 15% to 20% of patients with peptic ulcer at some point develop gross bleeding, and occult blood loss is even more common.[44] Emergent bleeding requiring operation is most often the result of posterior erosion of a duodenal ulcer into the gastroduodenal artery. Bleeding gastric ulcers appear with hematemesis or melena in about equal frequency, whereas duodenal ulcers tend to produce melena alone.[50] Other symptoms stem from the resultant hypovolemia—patients have presented with transient ischemic attacks (TIAs) and other neurologic complaints, myocardial infarction, and intestinal ischemia. As with acute gastritis, it is important to stabilize the patient at the same time diagnostic maneuvers are performed. The diagnosis of upper gastrointestinal hemorrhage is confirmed by passage of a nasogastric tube. However, bleeding peptic ulcer accounts for only about a third of massive upper gastrointestinal bleeds; endoscopy is therefore indicated to identify the nature and site of the lesion.[52]

When the ulcer erodes through the full thickness of the gastroduodenum, it may produce a perforation or a penetration into surrounding structures. This occurs in 5% to 10% of patients with peptic ulcer.[52] With perforation, the spilled gastric juice incites both peritonitis and consequent catastrophic abdominal pain, marked tenderness, and ileus. This peritoneal irritation also is responsible for the accompanying leukocytosis and hypovolemia from fluid sequestration. Pneumoperitoneum is present in 75% of patients.[55] Diagnosis is usually obvious. However, it may be more difficult if the perforation seals quickly—these patients occasionally seek medical attention only after a localized intra-abdominal abscess develops. If the perforation is diverted by the falciform ligament into the right colic gutter, it may infrequently be confused with appendicitis. Penetration into the biliary tract or colon can produce a gastric or duodenal fistula.

Gastric outlet obstruction develops, usually in the context of chronic ulcer disease, when secondary edema or scarring occludes the lumen. If edema is the result of a major lesion, the episode may be reversible either spontaneously or with a short course of intensive medical therapy, including nasogastric suction. However, if inflammatory scarring is the basis, improvement is unlikely. Obstruction develops in less than 5% of patients, usually with duodenal but occasionally gastric ulcer.[55] Onset is insidious, but patients usually present with nausea, vomiting, and abdominal distention. Vomiting of hydrochloric acid may produce a severe dehydration and a metabolic alkalosis. This is perpetuated by a paradoxic aciduria as the kidney retains bicarbonate with sodium to maintain electroneutrality in the absence of the chloride lost in the vomitus. The diagnosis can be documented with barium x-ray films, the saline load test consisting of a 400 ml residual one-half hour after gastric instillation of 750 ml of saline, or sequential Scintiscanning with technetium-labeled liquids or solids. Endoscopy can differentiate atony from true obstruction when the diagnosis is in question.

Zollinger-Ellison Syndrome

Although uncommon, (i.e., it occurs in 0.1% to 1.0% of all patients with peptic ulcer), Zollinger-Ellison syndrome is the best understood form of gastroduodenal mucosal injury.[33] Physiologic abnormalities have been directly related to clinical manifestations and have provided the basis for very refined diagnostic maneuvers.

Pathogenesis

This syndrome represents the extremes in the pathophysiologic spectrum, extending from disturbances in mucosal defense to those in acid secretion. Ulceration results from massive hypersecretion of acid, which is stimulated by ectopic gastrin production from a nonbeta islet cell tumor, the gastrinoma. These tumors produce several forms of gastrin: the predominant form in the tumor is gastrin-17, whereas gastrin-34 with its longer half-life is the major circulating form. Gastrinomas are most often located in the pancreas but have also been identified in the duodenum. Generally, they are assumed to represent ectopic lesions. The cells are histologically distinct from those in the antrum that normally produce gastrin, and gastrin cells have not been identified in the normal pancreas. Accompanying islet cell hyperplasia has been recognized, although its significance is not yet clear. In about 25% of patients, there is an association with the multiple endocrine neoplasia syndrome Type I.[43] In this group the disease has a genetic basis. At least 50% of gastrinomas are multiple, and more than two thirds are malignant.[36] However, in general, they are very slow-growing, indolent tumors.

The parietal cell mass is expanded enormously, probably as a result of the trophic effects of gastrin. It has been estimated to be at least three to six times as large as that in normal individuals.[33] The physiologic effects of the resulting massive gastric secretion are most easily discussed in terms of the clinical features.

Clinical Manifestations and Diagnosis

More than 90% of patients with gastrinoma develop peptic ulcer during the course of their disease.[55] Symptoms tend to be more severe, unrelenting, and less responsive to therapy than those of usual ulcers. Most ulcers are located in the proximal duodenum. However, probably because of the greater acid secretion, gastric and more distal ulcerations also occur. Lesions are usually single and small, but multiple and giant ulcers have been described with greater frequency than in common duodenal ulcer.

Diarrhea is also a frequent symptom and may occur in the absence of gross ulceration. This is probably a result of the large quantities of hydrochloric acid. In addition, it has been suggested that gastrin may contribute by inhibiting intestinal transport of water and electrolytes.[33] There are frequently morphologic abnormalities throughout the small bowel with stunted villi and mucosal inflammatory infiltrates. Brunner's glands, usually limited to the proximal duodenum, have been found as far distally as the ligament of Treitz. Steatorrhea is also a finding and probably results from two mechanisms. The low pH inactivates pancreatic lipase, impairing hydrolysis of dietary fats. In addition, bile salts are precipitated at low pH, reducing the formation of the micelles required for lipid absorption. Acidic conditions also appear to interfere with B_{12} absorption, although intrinsic factor secretion by the stomach is normal.

The diagnosis of gastrinoma has become increasingly refined. A search for this syndrome is warranted in patients with multiple, giant, or distal ulcers; ulcer disease refractory to the usual medical therapy; and recurrences after adequate surgery for peptic ulcer. Diagnostic techniques of some use include acid secretory studies and contrast radiography. These patients usually have elevated acid secretion, and basal acid output is usually greater than 60% of maximal.[36] However, there is considerable overlap with normal patients and common duodenal ulcer patients. Upper gastrointestinal x-ray films can reveal ulceration, prominent rugal folds indicating stimulated hypertrophy, dilated small intestine, and even the occasional tumor in the duodenum. Determination of basal serum gastrin levels by radioimmunoassay can be diagnostic; however, elevations may also be detected in several other pathologic conditions. In pernicious anemia, which is an atrophic and inflammatory gastric process that reduces the number of parietal cells but typically spares the antrum, hypergastrinemia results from both an increase in the number of gastrin cells and a loss of the normal acid feedback inhibition of secretion. Patients with renal insufficiency also develop elevated serum gastrins, although the mechanism has not yet been defined and gastrin clearance is normal even in anephric patients.[33] Antral gastrin-cell hyperplasia or hyperfunction occurs in a small proportion of patients with duodenal ulcer. These patients have hypergastrinemia and hypersecretion, although an actual increase in the number of gastrin cells has not been proved.

Three provocative tests have improved the specificity of biochemical diagnosis. In the secretin test, 2 U/kg of secretin is given intravenously over 30 seconds, and serum gastrin is measured 5 minutes before, immediately before, and at 5-minute-intervals for one-half hour after injection. In normal patients and patients with duodenal ulcer, secretin has no significant effect, but in patients with Zollinger-Ellison syndrome there is a dramatic increase in serum gastrin levels. The mechanism for this is unknown, although it has been suggested that secretin may release gastrin by a direct local effect on blood flow in the tumor. In the calcium infusion test, calcium gluconate is given intravenously at a rate of 5 mg/kg for a 3-hour period, and serum gastrin levels are determined 30 minutes before and at half-hour intervals for 4 hours. In Zollinger-Ellison patients there is usually more than a 400 pg/ml increase, possibly through release of peptide hormone through the calmodulin system, whereas much smaller increases occur in duodenal ulcer and other conditions. A third provocative test, the use of a standard meal, produces little change from basal levels in gastrinoma patients when compared with the marked increase produced in control subjects or in patients with gastrin-cell hyperplasia. The secretion of the gastrinoma is independent of normal control mechanisms. Neither angiography per se nor computerized tomographic scanning has provided much assistance in the diagnosis of gastrinoma. However, the recently described technique of percutaneous transhepatic portopancreatic venous sampling has provided additional information for localization of the tumor.

PHYSIOLOGIC BASIS FOR TREATMENT IN GASTRITIS AND PEPTIC ULCER

Consistent with the general concept of a disturbance in the interplay between acid secretion and mucosal defense as the basis for these syndromes of gastroduodenal mucosal injury, the medical and surgical therapies of gastritis and peptic ulceration represent attempts to artificially restore this balance. Most treatments have approached this by methods designed to reduce acid secretion, although a few have been devised to improve mucosal resistance. These therapies will be discussed first generally in terms of their physiologic mechanism of action and then briefly related to the specific disease entities.

Medical Therapy

In the past a variety of measures, generally unrelated to the pathophysiology of these lesions, was adapted empirically as part of the treatment regimen. Dietary therapy with frequent feeding of bland foods has not been shown to be particularly effective and has little if any effect on gastric acid secretion. Milk, another home remedy, is actually a strong secretory stimulus. Similarly, hospitalization for peptic ulcer was believed to improve healing, although recent evidence suggests that there is little, if any, added benefit.[44] On the other hand, several general measures probably are useful. Cigarette smoking has clearly been shown to retard ulcer healing and should be avoided.[50] Likewise, aspirin has a detrimental effect on mucosal resistance and should not be prescribed. Coffee strongly stimulates acid secretion, and alcohol may damage the mucosa; at least moderation in their consumption should be suggested.

Pharmacologic therapy has been developed to restore the balance of secretion by three general mechanisms: neutralization of gastric secretion, inhibition of secretion, or protection of the gastric mucosa from further injury. Table 16-1 summarizes the classes of drugs available. A combination of drugs acting by different mechanisms may have more than an additive effect in improving ulcer healing.

Antacids are the oldest therapy. They reduce gastric acidity by reacting with hydrochloric acid to form a salt and water; inhibit peptic activity by the increase in pH; and bind bile acids, which may have a special role in the treatment of gastritis and gastric ulcer. Various antacids differ

Table 16-1 **DRUGS FOR THE TREATMENT OF GASTRITIS AND PEPTIC ULCER**

Class	Example	Mode of Action
Antacids	Aluminum hydroxide	Acid neutralization
H_2-receptor antagonists	Cimetidine	Secretory inhibition
Anticholinergics	Propantheline bromide (Probanthine)	Secretory inhibition
Tricyclics	Pirenzepine	Secretory inhibition
Substituted benzimidazoles	Omeprazole	H^+/K^+-ATPase inhibition
Prostaglandins	E_2 Prostaglandins	Secretory inhibition, "cytoprotection," increase of blood flow
Sulfated disaccharides	Sucralfate	Protective coating, antipeptic activity
Colloidal bismuth	Bismuthate	Protective coating, antipeptic activity
Licorice extracts	Carbenoxolone	Increase of mucus, antipeptic activity

Modified from Stabile, B.E., and Passaro, E., Jr.: Curr. Probl. Surg. **21**:1, 1984.

greatly in their buffering strength, absorption, taste, and side effects. Magnesium antacids tend to be the best buffers but cause significant diarrhea by a cathartic action. Aluminum antacids precipitate with phosphorus, resulting in occasional hypophosphatemia and, in addition, may produce significant constipation. Calcium compounds can cause a delayed acid secretory rebound, felt largely to result from the effect of absorbed calcium ion itself. For each equivalent of hydrochloric acid neutralized, bicarbonate is released in the tissue, and all these drugs may produce a systemic alkalosis. Normal renal function usually prevents this from becoming significant. Antacids are best taken an hour after meals because the food tends to prolong emptying.

The H_2-receptor antagonists are a relatively new class of agents that have revolutionized the treatment of peptic ulcer by directly reducing acid secretion. There are actually two types of gastric histamine receptors: (1) H_1, located on smooth muscle cells, and (2) H_2, located on the parietal cells. This class of agents was devised to specifically block the histamine-H_2 receptor. Recent isolated cell studies indicate that there are three independent but mutually augmenting parietal cell receptors for histamine, acetylcholine, and gastrin.[49] Thus inhibition of the histamine receptor alone also reduces the effects of acetylcholine and gastrin. These drugs all consist of a five-member organic ring and a side chain similar to histamine itself. Lengthening and alteration of the side chain has produced agents of increasing antagonistic potency. The physiologic effects include a decrease in both basal and stimulated acid secretion by what is believed to be competitive inhibition at the parietal cell level.[42] Pepsin output is also reduced. The decrease in antral acidity elevates serum gastrin levels, although there is no evidence as yet that this elevation results in a trophic increase in parietal cell numbers. These agents also reduce gastric blood flow, a finding that may explain the observation that they are less effective than antacids in preventing stress erosions when the protective effect of mucosal blood flow has been clearly demonstrated. Cimetidine is the most widely used H_2-receptor antagonist. It is a potent inhibitor of acid secretion with a half-life of approximately 2 hours, requiring a dosage schedule of four tablets per day. Patient compliance is generally much improved over antacids. However, a number of significant side effects, including a reduction in sperm counts, gynecomastia, and a reversible central nervous system toxicity have been recently described. This has led to the development of ranitidine, a new longer-acting agent that appears to be free of some of the side effects of cimetidine; however, studies are preliminary, and it is likely to have some toxicity of its own.

The anticholinergic agents act to inhibit the action of acetylcholine at muscarinic receptors. In the stomach they are believed to act directly at the parietal cell level. Atropine and probanthine are typical anticholinergic agents that, at equal doses, are even more potent than H_2-receptor antagonists.[42] However, side effects, including urinary retention, blurred vision, dry mouth, delayed gastric emptying, and mental disturbances, permit their use only at lower, less effective doses. The tricyclic agents, including those with an antidepressant activity, are also thought to reduce acid secretion by an anticholinergic mechanism. Pirenzepine, which lacks antidepressant activity, appears to be as effective as cimetidine in the treatment of duodenal ulcer.[9]

Very recently an exciting new class of secretory inhibitors, i.e., the substituted benzimidazoles, has been developed. These agents selectively inhibit parietal cell H^+/K^+-ATPase, the enzyme responsible for acid secretion. Omeprazole, the member that has been introduced first clinically, seems to be a highly potent agent that may be effective even in refractory gastrinoma. Long-term side effects may become evident, but at present the potential for this group of agents is enormous.

Four different agents seem to be effective by improving gastric mucosal resistance. The prostaglandins are naturally occurring fatty acids that prevent or heal mucosal injury by several mechanisms.[35] The methylated E_2 analogs are absorbed orally and significantly inhibit gastric acid secretion. However, at doses required for this effect, they also produce dramatic diarrhea. At lesser doses they still exert a "cytoprotective" action, probably by increasing bicarbonate and mucus secretion and mucosal blood flow. Use of these agents is still experimental.

Sucralfate is a new, sulfated disaccharide related structurally to heparin, although it has no anticoagulant effects. Its unique mechanism of action is proving very effective in the treatment of established ulcer disease, and this drug is the only one of these agents presently in widespread clinical use that acts by enhancing resistance. It is an aluminum salt of sulfated sucrose that dissociates under the acidic condition in the stomach. It has been proposed that the sucrose polymerizes and binds to proteins in the ulcer crater, producing a kind of protective coating that lasts up to 6 hours.[42] The liberated aluminum hydroxide may have some slight additional antacid effect. Little of this is absorbed, so side effects are minimal. Colloidal bismuth likewise coats exposed protein. It is the salt that chelates under acidic conditions and has been shown to protect against acute mucosal lesions in a variety of experimental models. An additional antipeptic activity has also been postulated to explain its effectiveness.

Licorice extracts, the most frequently used of which is carbenoxolone, a synthetic derivative, also act to enhance mucosal defense.[50] Glycyrrhetic acid appears to be the active moiety in these agents. They have no effect on acid secretion but actually enhance gastric mucus production and its thickness. This seems to reduce hydrogen ion back diffusion. They also appear to decrease pepsin secretion and inhibit peptic activity. Finally, they may increase epithelial cell half-lives. However, this drug is absorbed systemically and has significant aldosterone-like effects, including sodium retention, hypertension, and hypokalemia, which have limited its use clinically.

Surgical Therapy

The primary goal in the surgical treatment of gastritis or peptic ulcer is to eliminate the pathologic lesion while minimizing the consequent disruption of normal gastroduodenal physiology. Obviously, treatment must be individualized, depending on the specific type of lesion and its mode of presentation. However, the common theme be-

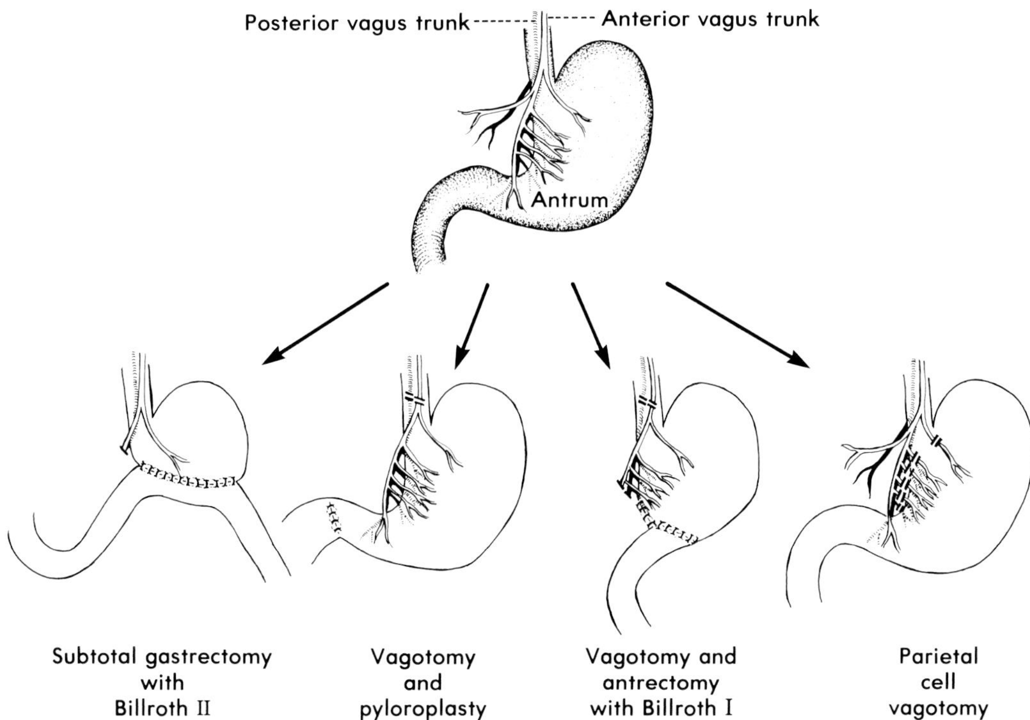

Fig. 16-5 Four most commonly used operative procedures for reduction of gastric acid secretion.

hind all these procedures is to restore the normal balance between secretion and mucosal resistance. Until quite recently, it has been impossible to alter the poorly understood mechanisms of mucosal defense from a surgical standpoint, and therefore all previous procedures have approached these diseases by attempting to reduce acid secretion as follows: (1) by decreasing the number of parietal cells, (2) by eliminating the hormonal stimulation from the antrum, or (3) by sectioning the vagus nerve. Basically four general operations have been devised to produce these results (Fig. 16-5). These are subtotal gastrectomy, vagotomy and drainage, vagotomy and antrectomy, and parietal cell vagotomy. A discussion of the physiologic rationale and consequences of these procedures would be impossible without at least briefly mentioning some of their undesirable side effects, i.e., the so-called postgastrectomy syndromes.

Subtotal gastrectomy, in the past probably the most commonly performed procedure, is based on the reduction of acid and pepsin secretion by several mechanisms. It removes not only a major portion of the parietal and chief cells in the corpus but also the antral gastrin cells, eliminating the gastrin stimulus to secretion and also its trophic effects, resulting in atrophy of the remaining mucosa. This operation reduces basal and stimulated secretion by about 75% and 50%, respectively.[24] It also eliminates the antral-pyloric mixing mechanism or trituration by which food is reduced to chyme before entering the duodenum. In addition, emptying of both liquids and solids is more rapid. With removal of the pylorus, increased reflux of intestinal contents into the stomach may have major consequences in terms of the development of reflux gastritis. The choice between Billroth I reconstruction to the duodenal stump vs. Billroth II anastomosis to a more distal loop of jejunum has important physiologic consequences that should be considered in addition to their respective complications. Billroth II eliminates the added stimulus to acid secretion from duodenal release of gastrin in response to passing chyme. However, it also prevents the meal from reaching pH and osmoreceptors in the proximal duodenum, which normally slow gastric emptying.

The rationale for truncal vagotomy is based on the elimination of direct cholinergic stimuli to acid-pepsin secretion. This withdrawal also makes parietal cells less responsive to histamine and gastrin and abolishes the vagal stimulus to release of antral gastrin. Basal and stimulated acid secretion are reduced by 80% and 50%, respectively.[21] Gastrin levels actually increase, probably as a result of a reduction in the normal acid inhibition of antral gastrin cells. Vagotomy also markedly alters gastric motility patterns. Both receptive relaxation and trituration are impaired. Gastric emptying of liquids is speeded, whereas solid evacuation slows significantly, leading to overt gastric stasis. As a result, some form of emptying procedure (i.e., pyloroplasty or gastrojejunostomy) must be performed. These drainage operations also have important physiologic consequences. Pyloroplasty further speeds gastric emptying and, by reducing the period of contact between gastric contents and the antral mucosa, decreases acid secretion mediated through the direct gastric phase of stimulation. Gastroenterostomy may actually enhance secretion by producing antral gastrin release and eliminating the secretion of inhibitory factors normally generated by the passage of chyme through the duodenum. An increase in gastrin levels may result because of stasis in the partially excluded antrum and because the gastroenterostomy allows acid to empty and be neutralized before it can bathe the antrum. Both procedures eliminate the pyloric sphincter and produce duodenogastric reflux.

Vagotomy with antrectomy seems to combine some of the advantages of both these procedures. The simultaneous effects of vagotomy and antrectomy remove both the cholinergic and the gastrin stimulus to acid secretion. Basal acid secretion is virtually abolished, whereas stimulated acid secretion is decreased by nearly 80%.[24] The rationale for this procedure was to preserve some of the reservoir function eliminated by a more subtotal gastrectomy. Dumping complications, the subject of the next chapter, seem to be slightly less frequent than after more complete resection. Unlike reconstruction after a subtotal resection in which a Billroth II seems to be preferable both in terms of suture line tension and recurrence rates, experience has suggested that restoration of normal continuity with a Billroth I is more desirable after vagotomy and antrectomy.

The fairly recent development of parietal cell vagotomy is a prime example of the application of modern physiologic principles to the design of a practical surgical procedure. The rationale for this procedure is to eliminate vagal stimulation to the acid-secreting portion of the stomach without interrupting supply to the antrum or more distal gastrointestinal tract. Basically, the operation involves severing all the branches of the vagus along the lesser curvature that innervate the corpus and fundus. Basal and stimulated acid are reduced by greater than 75% and 50%, respectively.[21] In addition it reduces the secretion of acid in response to gastric distention. Basal serum gastrin is increased, although the response to a meal is reduced. Receptive relaxation is again impaired, and emptying of liquids is more rapid than normal. However, antral peristalsis, trituration, and sphincter function are preserved. The emptying of solids is normal. The normal small bowel innervation preserves intestinal motility patterns and reduces the incidence of diarrhea and dumping. However, the lower complication rates are balanced by a somewhat higher incidence of recurrence.

The choice among surgical procedures is a very complex one. The most important single factor is the nature of the disease process itself, and this will be considered in the following section. Although an elective procedure can be aimed directly at eliminating the pathophysiologic process in an emergent situation, attention must of necessity be directed to the morphologic lesion. Other considerations in the choice among procedures include the respective operative mortalities and postoperative morbidities, the incidence of recurrent ulceration, the postgastrectomy side effects of the procedure, the long-term metabolic consequences of the operation (in terms of weight loss, bone disease, and anemia), and even the possible risk of gastric carcinoma. In addition, the familiarity of the operative surgeon himself with the techniques of various operative procedures is a crucial consideration.

Reliable data on the results of various operations have really only been generated over the last decade and a half. Published series in general have used different criteria for patient selection and have varied in how vigorously the incidence of side effects were pursued. Subtotal gastrectomy alone offers no advantage over the other procedures and is probably not as widely used as the other procedures. Table 16-2 summarizes the data on the other three procedures. Briefly, mortality is lowest for highly selective vagotomy and greatest for vagotomy and antrectomy. The relative incidence of side effects is about the same for vagotomy with antrectomy or drainage and lower for the parietal cell operations. On the other hand, the incidence of recurrence is significantly lower with vagotomy and antrectomy. Thus truncal vagotomy has both the high recurrence rate of parietal cell vagotomy and the unfavorable incidence of side effects of vagotomy and antrectomy. In general, vagotomy and drainage should have little place in the elective therapy of peptic ulcer. But even though this procedure is controversial, there is probably still a role for it in the emergent treatment of a patient for whom time is a critical factor; it can be performed considerably more quickly than a resection or the somewhat tedious parietal cell procedure.

Table 16-2 **MORTALITY, SIDE EFFECTS, AND RECURRENCE RATES FOR THE THREE MOST COMMON ACID-REDUCING OPERATIONS**

Operation	Mortality (%)	Side Effects (%)	Recurrence (%)
Vagotomy and antrectomy	2	5	1
Vagotomy and drainage	1	5	10
Highly selective vagotomy	0.2	1	10

Modified from Grossman, M.I., editor: Peptic ulcer: a guide for the practicing physician, Chicago, 1981, Yearbook Medical Publishers, Inc.

Treatment for Specific Entities

An exhaustive discussion of the specific treatment for each of these pathologic entities is beyond the scope of this chapter and has been provided elsewhere. What follows is a brief discussion of the basic principles of therapy in relation to the specific physiologic abnormalities of each disease. The various procedures are summarized in Table 16-3.

Acute Gastritis

As mentioned previously, gastric evacuation and lavage will halt bleeding in most patients with stress erosions. In addition, antacid administration is useful in preventing the development of further hemorrhage. The pH of gastric contents should be checked regularly, probably every hour; and magnesium or aluminum antacids that are insoluble and remain in the stomach for prolonged periods should be instilled to keep the pH above 5. One prospective randomized study comparing efficacies demonstrated antacid to be superior to cimetidine in the prevention of bleeding in critically ill patients.[42] Anticholinergics have not been believed to be effective in controlling erosive bleeding except in head trauma patients who hypersecrete; they are probably contraindicated in the seriously ill because of the major

Table 16-3 **CHOICE OF OPERATIVE PROCEDURE BASED ON INDICATION**

Indication	Procedure
Acute gastritis	Vagotomy and pyloroplasty with oversewing of erosions or near-total gastrectomy
Gastric ulcer	Subtotal gastrectomy with ulcer excision
Duodenal ulcer	
Intractable pain	Parietal cell vagotomy
Perforation	Simple closure or closure and parietal cell vagotomy
Bleeding	Vagotomy and antrectomy with suture ligation of bleeding vessel or Vagotomy and pyloroplasty with suture ligation
Obstruction	Vagotomy and antrectomy
Zollinger-Ellison syndrome	Tumor resection or parietal cell vagotomy or total gastrectomy

side effects. Intra-arterial infusion of vasopressin controls hemorrhage in approximately 80% of patients.[1] A variety of other medical therapies, including prostaglandins, trans-arterial embolization, and endoscopic coagulation, have been suggested but as yet have not been adequately proven.

Surgery should be considered when the bleeding exceeds 6 to 8 U over 48 hours, but the underlying condition of the patient should enter this decision. Mortality for surgery in this group of patients is in the range of 40%, and there is much controversy over the type of operation that offers the best chance of success.[5] No really good prospective trial has been performed, but some surgeons have advocated near-total gastrectomy in preference to the lesser procedures of vagotomy and pyloroplasty with oversewing of the bleeding erosions or partial gastrectomy with vagotomy. Generally, if the lesser procedures are successful, they are associated with a reduced morbidity and mortality but a greater incidence of rebleeding. Vagotomy is effective by reducing acid secretion and perhaps also by acutely decreasing mucosal blood flow. The oversewing of a few bleeding erosions is effective because, although there is most often a diffuse gastritis, only a few of these erosions have progressed into the deeper submucosal vessels, and it is these lesions that are responsible for the significant hemorrhage. Fairly satisfactory results have been obtained with the use of vagotomy and pyloroplasty with oversewing of bleeding erosions as the initial procedure, reserving total resection for those who rebleed.

Gastric Ulcer

Trials of medical therapy for chronic gastric ulcer have not been as distinctly successful as those for duodenal ulcer. Several conclusive clinical studies have shown cimetidine to be significantly more effective than placebo in healing gastric ulcers, although prior investigators were unable to demonstrate this statistically.[44] Two considerations are important in evaluating the therapy for chronic ulcer—healing and pain relief. There is a trend to better pain relief with cimetidine in most studies of gastric ulcer. On the other hand, antacids have not been shown to be effective; the physiologic reasons for this difference still are unclear. Likewise, the anticholinergics have not proved particularly useful in chronic gastric ulcer. Sucralfate appears to speed healing but at least in one study was less effective than cimetidine.[31] Current recommendations suggest that these patients should be started on cimetidine initially.[44] After 2 weeks, if pain relief has not been achieved, a second medication should be added. At 8 weeks, follow-up x-ray films or endoscopy should be performed. If the ulcer is not completely healed, these studies should be repeated again at 12 and 15 weeks. Patients whose ulcers have not healed by this time should be offered surgery.

In the past, gastric ulcer has generally been treated with surgery somewhat earlier than duodenal ulcer. There are several, somewhat unjustified reasons for this approach. One is the fear of malignancy in benign-appearing ulcers. Improvements in the endoscopic diagnosis of cancer have reduced this risk, however. In addition, most data indicate that gastric ulcer patients are more often hospitalized for their illness than duodenal ulcer patients, suggesting that gastric ulcer may be a somewhat more virulent disease. Finally, the older gastric ulcer patient has a distinctly higher mortality for a complication of his ulcer than the corresponding younger patient with a duodenal lesion.[21] Generally, surgery is recommended for the recurrent ulcer refractory to medical therapy, the ulcer that recurs during treatment with cimetidine, the ulcer that fails to heal within 12 to 15 weeks, or one of the complications of ulcer disease.

The elective surgical decisions in gastric ulcer are somewhat simpler than those in duodenal ulcer. As mentioned, prepyloric ulcers or those in association with duodenal ulcers share a common cause with duodenal lesions and should be treated as such. For usual gastric ulcers, gastric resection with or without vagotomy has proved effective. Usually it is unnecessary to remove a large amount of stomach for elective treatment of gastric lesions. The ulcer itself should be excised completely and submitted for pathology. Because gastric ulcer does not primarily result from a secretory disturbance, the use of vagotomy has been questioned. The specific operations for complications of gastric ulcer are similar in rationale to those performed for duodenal ulcer and will be discussed in the following section.

Duodenal Ulcer

In many instances duodenal ulceration is an easily manageable disease entity, and some patients are able to self-medicate their disease with over-the-counter drugs, never seeking formal medical therapy. Of those who come to professional treatment, greater than 80% will be controlled by pharmacologic therapy designed to reduce acid secretion.[50] Antacids are extremely effective, but their inconvenience has made cimetidine the drug of choice. Combination therapy is usually necessary only in refractory patients; antacids or cimetidine alone will heal all but about 25% of duodenal ulcers within 4 weeks.[21] Neither of these regimens affects the natural history of the disease process itself. With cessation of therapy, ulcers will recur within 6 months in about 80% of patients.[50] Continuation of cimetidine at lower, perhaps only once daily, doses after healing has been shown to significantly reduce the risk of recurrence.[17] Sucralfate appears similar in efficacy to cimetidine, and there has been some conflicting evidence that it may reduce recurrence rates.[31] Colloidal bismuth, in a few small clinical trials, also appears to equal the H_2-receptor antagonist. There is some question as to whether an actual ulcer crater need be documented by x-ray film or endoscopy before starting therapy; in fact, it has been suggested that the symptoms and potential complications should be the most important factors in determining treatment. Many ulcers heal, and most symptoms disappear with placebo.[13] However, even though pharmacologic treatment is more expensive, the more rapid response and greater probability of healing probably justify it. After healing, the relative merits of maintenance therapy vs. intermittent treatment for recurrences are still controversial and probably depend on the individual patient. The ultimate effect of routine medical therapy and maintenance treatment on the complication rate has not yet been determined.

Classically the four indications for surgery include intractability and the complications of hemorrhage, perforation, and obstruction. Elective operation for intractability has become an increasingly rare occurrence because current medical therapy is so effective. The decision entails weighing the relative risks and benefits of both medical and surgical therapy. However, really good long-term data on these characteristics of treatment with the very recently developed H_2-receptor antagonists or parietal cell vagotomy—the best alternatives for elective therapy—do not yet exist.

The choice of an operative procedure and its ultimate results depends critically on the indication for surgery and its specific pathophysiology. In the treatment of intractable pain, surgery is elective, the patient is adequately prepared for the procedure, time is not a crucial factor, and there is little justification for exposing the patient to the potential for severe early or late postoperative complications. Under these circumstances, parietal cell vagotomy is probably the procedure of choice. The lumen of the gastrointestinal tract is not entered, reducing the risk of septic complications. In addition, because the normal functional anatomy of the stomach and pylorus are preserved and because distal vagal innervation is not interrupted, the potential for the serious long-term side effects of dumping and diarrhea is greatly reduced.

Hemorrhage is the principle cause of death from duodenal ulcer[23]; the current choice of operations remains difficult. These patients are critically ill and often have significant associated medical problems delaying the decision for surgery, although most studies indicate that early operation is the only way to reduce mortality and complications.[52] After preoperative stabilization, choice of procedure in these patients is usually limited to two possibilities. Initially the bleeding lesion itself should be addressed directly by control through suture ligation after pyloroduodenotomy. The choice between vagotomy and drainage vs. vagotomy and antrectomy is a controversial one. Vagotomy and pyloroplasty can be performed quickly and simply in the patient unable to tolerate any additional procedure. However, the addition of antrectomy, particularly with modern stapling techniques, does not add much in terms of time or morbidity and significantly reduces the risk of what may be a fatal recurrence.

In the past perforation was treated by simple closure, occasionally reinforced with omentum. This is a rapid, often effective treatment and is still recommended for patients with preoperative shock, perforation exceeding 48 hours, and significant coexistent medical problems.[23] However, recent studies suggest that, of those treated with simple closure, 80% will develop a recurrence and one third will require another operation.[53] Several recent studies have shown that, with proper patient selection, definitive treatment can be performed.[23] Both vagotomy and pyloroplasty and parietal cell vagotomy have been suggested. The latter seems to be receiving greater support.

Treatment for obstruction should both relieve this lesion and deal with the ulcer diathesis. Although there has been some hesitation in using vagotomy in the presence of already disturbed motility patterns, it should probably be included in the definitive operation. Vagotomy with antrectomy, resecting the scarred pylorus, is the procedure of choice, although vagotomy with drainage has been applied by some surgeons.

Zollinger-Ellison Syndrome

Treatment of gastrinoma has taken some interesting turns in relation to our understanding of methods of control for this secondary disturbance in gastric physiology. In the past, the recognition that these tumors were frequently multicentric and metastatic though slow growing led to the use of the only operation believed to reliably and consistently reduce acid secretion: the total gastrectomy. Subsequently, with the advent of cimetidine most clinicians adopted this pharmacologic therapy in preference to such a major procedure with its considerable accompanying morbidity and mortality. More recently there has been a trend back to surgery for several reasons. First, a number of trials have suggested that up to 25% of gastrinoma patients on maintenance cimetidine therapy will develop a complication of acid hypersecretion.[36] In addition, compliance problems and the recognition of long-term side effects with cimetidine have raised valid doubts about the desirability of continuing medical therapy. It has been suggested that, because there are a percentage of patients in whom the lesion is solitary and resectable, particularly if they develop in the duodenum, most patients deserve an exploration. Preliminary studies indicate that the use of transhepatic portovenous sampling may assist in improving the removal of pancreatic tumors. Recently it has been proposed that, at least in those deemed unresectable, a parietal cell vagotomy may shift the dose-response curve of cimetidine, preventing breakthrough secretion.[36] Preliminary reports indicate that both ranitidine and omeprazole may be effective in treating those refractory to cimetidine without the adverse side effects. Because of the generally low grade of this malignancy, if acid secretion is negated, long-term survival is possible. Little other effective treatment, (e.g., radiotherapy or chemotherapy) is yet available.

RECURRENT ULCER AFTER SURGERY

Recurrent ulceration after surgery represents a failure of these attempts to restore the normal balance between acid secretion and mucosal defense and provides an interesting concluding perspective on the physiology of acid-peptic disease. Ulceration recurs in approximately 5% of patients who undergo surgery for peptic ulcer disease, although this incidence may be increasing as parietal cell vagotomy is applied with greater frequency in an attempt to reduce the general mortality and morbidity of ulcer surgery.[15] Ninety-five percent occur after surgery for duodenal ulcer; only a few ulcerations recur after gastric ulcer operations. In the past the vast majority were stomal ulcers, although with increasing use of parietal cell vagotomy duodenal ulcers are becoming more common.[51]

Pathogenesis

Multiple factors have been implicated in the pathophysiology of recurrent ulceration. However, an incomplete primary surgical procedure, which possibly results in an inadequate reduction in acid-pepsin secretion despite a technically sufficient operation, is by far the most frequent cause.[14] In these instances the wrong primary operation was chosen. On the other hand, the basis may be some failure in the original technique. Recurrences are more frequent when a new operation is used; specifically the experience of the surgeon seems to play an important role. The high incidence of incomplete vagotomy in some series has led to suggestions of intraoperative testing for completeness. After truncal vagotomy it is usually the right trunk that has been missed, whereas after a parietal cell operation fibers on the distal esophagus (i.e., the nerves of Grassi) are usually responsible. The high incidence of recurrence in some preliminary series with parietal cell vagotomy has been reduced as more experience with the operation is gained. In subtotal gastrectomy without vagotomy, insufficient resection of the acid-secreting region has been implicated. Retained antrum was a frequent cause for recurrence that has been eliminated by recognition and careful avoidance. This entity may still occur after antrectomy and Billroth II reconstruction when a portion of antrum is retained in the duodenal stump, sequestered from the inhibiting effects of gastric acid and thus still capable of stimulating acid secretion in the remaining stomach through release of the hormone gastrin.

Inadequate gastric drainage with stasis and distention-induced secretion has also been implicated as a cause of recurrent ulcer. Long afferent loops after Billroth II anastomoses that increase the distance between the stoma and the neutralizing effects of pancreatic and duodenal bicarbonate have been incriminated. Nonabsorbable sutures at the site of gastroenterostomy may also play a role in recurrent ulcer.

Several etiologic sources for recurrent ulcer formation have been identified, unrelated to the original procedure. Two entities, gastrinoma and antral gastrin cell hyperplasia, can result in enough acid hypersecretion that ulceration results despite the adequacy of the initial operation. In addition, ingestion of aspirin, other anti-inflammatory agents, and even alcohol may damage the mucosa enough to allow ulcer recurrence. Malignancy may also appear as recurrent ulceration.

Clinical Manifestations and Diagnosis

Abdominal pain is the most common presentation.[14] In some instances it may be suggestive of ulcer; however, because of the disturbance in normal anatomy, it can be very atypical and difficult to distinguish from other postoperative symptoms. Approximately one half of patients may develop chronic or acute bleeding.[14] Others have presented with weight loss, nausea and vomiting, gastric outlet obstruction, free perforation, and gastrojejunocolic fistula. Some degree of localized perforation is common.

Diagnosis is often difficult both in terms of the ulcer itself and its cause. Barium studies only detect 50% to 65% of recurrences—postoperative inflammatory changes can be very hard to distinguish from ulceration.[14] Endoscopy has been the procedure of choice for identification of the ulcer and can be diagnostic in the case of malignancy. Serum gastrin levels suggest the presence of gastrinoma or gastrin cell hyperplasia, which can be differentiated by secretin or calcium infusion tests. Acid secretory studies are not very helpful for two reasons. First, seldom have they been performed before surgery to know whether operation has altered the secretory capacity of the stomach, and, second, it has not been determined to what extent acid production must be decreased to indicate completeness of vagotomy. The Hollander insulin test has been shown to cause dangerous hypoglycemia, hypokalemia, and catecholamine release; in addition, it is frequently unreliable. Sham feeding–induced secretion, mediated through vagal pathways, appears to be a fairly good alternative test for completeness of vagotomy in the few published studies in which it has been used.

Treatment

Treatment for recurrence remains somewhat controversial. Before the availability of cimetidine, less than a third of ulcers healed with medical therapy, and about 40% of those recurred.[51] Cimetidine heals the majority of recurrences, however, and maintenance therapy may prevent redevelopment.[14] Surgery is indicated if the recurrent ulcer fails to heal or again recurs on medical therapy, if a complication develops, or if a compliance problem exists.

Two main approaches have been taken in the surgical therapy for recurrence. Sometimes the operative choice is made on the basis of the preliminary procedure. For example, if subtotal resection was performed, vagotomy may be added. Others specifically tailor the operation to the suspected cause. For suspected incomplete vagotomy, revagotomy is performed. Basically three options exist: vagotomy or revagotomy, resection or reresection, or the combination of vagotomy and antrectomy or gastrectomy. When no attempt is made to reduce acid secretion (e.g., after simple closure of a perforation) the recurrence rate is almost 50%.[14] Revagotomy alone has an approximate 15% recurrence rate whereas the combination of revagotomy and resection has rates ranging from 1% to 12%.[18] The patient's general medical condition should play a role in decisions regarding therapy. For the poor-risk patient, transthoracic vagotomy may be the safest alternative. However, if the ulcer is large or some other lesion is suspected, laparotomy is mandatory. Gastric recurrence usually indicates that alkaline reflux gastritis plays a role and surgery should include a Roux loop diversion. In a few instances, examination of the duodenal stump and resection of retained antrum may be all that is necessary.

SUMMARY

In the past three decades significant advances have been made in the understanding of basic gastric physiology and its disturbance in various disease states. A variety of experimental and clinical studies has helped to elucidate the factors responsible for acid secretion and for the capacity of the mucosa to withstand acid-pepsin digestion. Many of these principles have been successfully applied to our clinical management of the various syndromes of gastroduodenal mucosal injury. For example, the findings from a variety of experimental models for acute gastric injury have been used successfully in the preventive management of critically ill patients at risk for development of stress erosions. Likewise, in peptic ulcer the development of a host of therapeutic agents, especially H_2-receptor antagonists, was only possible after elucidation of the physiologic mechanisms of acid secretion and mucosal defense. Progress in the surgical management of acid-peptic disease is a prime example of the successful application of new physiologic principles to the development of more specific therapies. Thus the experimental definition of the importance of vagal pathways and antral gastrin in the control of gastric secretion has prompted the abandonment of the somewhat crudely oblative gastrectomy in favor of the more directed vagotomy and antrectomy. Quite recently these principles in the control of acid secretion were combined with an understanding of the pathogenic importance of disruptions in vagal innervation and gastrointestinal continuity to the development of postoperative side effects known as the postgastrectomy syndromes. This led to the parietal cell vagotomy, probably the best example of the implications of scientific principles for the development of new surgical procedures.

Very recent advances offer exciting possibilities for the future treatment of these disorders. For example, the study of duodenal mucosal defense mechanisms and bicarbonate and mucus secretion are still really in infancy. The recent recognition of the heterogeneity of duodenal ulcer raises the possibility of individualizing therapy on the basis of the specific pathophysiologic mechanisms of each subset of chronic disease. Recent studies of the intestinal endocrine control of gastric secretion have revealed a host of new mechanisms that may be exploited to improve the treatment of these disorders. New cellular and subcellular studies have permitted the characterization of the specific machinery of acid secretion, the H^+/K^+-ATPase, and the application of this knowledge to the development of specific inhibitors, i.e., the substituted benzimidazoles. There is every indication that this physiologic approach to gastritis and peptic ulceration will continue to enhance our clinical management.

REFERENCES

1. Athanasoulis, et al.: Control of acute gastric mucosal hemorrhage. Intraarterial infusion of posterior pituitary extract, N. Engl. J. Med. **290:**597, 1974.
2. Balard, H.S., Frame, B., and Hansock, R.J.: Familial multiple endocrine adenoma-peptic ulcer complex, Medicine **43:**481, 1964.
3. Baron, J.H.: Current views on pathogenesis of peptic ulcer, Scand. J. Gastroenterol. **170**(suppl 80):1, 1982.
4. Carter, D.C.: Aetiology of peptic ulcer. In Sircus, W., and Smith, A.N., editors: Scientific foundations of gastroenterology, Philadelphia, 1980, W.B. Saunders Co.
5. Cheung, L.Y.: Treatment of established stress ulcer disease, World J. Surg. **5:**235, 1981.
6. Cheung, L.Y.: Pathophysiology of stress-induced gastric mucosal erosions: an update, Surg. Gastroenterol. **1:**235, 1982.
7. Cheung, L.Y., Reese, R.S., and Moody, F.G.: Direct effect of endotoxin on the gastric mucosal microcirculation and electrical gradient, Surgery **79:**564, 1976.
8. Cox, A.J.: Stomach size and its relation to chronic peptic ulcer, Arch. Pathol. **54:**403, 1952.
9. Dal Monte, P.R., et al.: Pirenzipine versus cimetidine in duodenal ulcer: a double-blind placebo-controlled short-term clinical trial, Hepatogastroenterology **27**(suppl):48, 1980.
10. Davenport, H.W., and Barr, L.L.: Failure of ischemia to break the dog's gastric mucosal barrier, Gastroenterology **65:**619, 1973.
11. Dragstedt, L.R.: The pathogenesis of duodenal and gastric ulcers, Am.J. Surg. **136:**286, 1978.
12. Du Plessis, D.J.: Pathogenesis of gastric ulceration, Lancet **1:**974, 1965.
13. Eshelman, F., Sanzari, N., and DeFelice, S.: "Placebo" responsiveness of peptic ulcers (Letter), Gastroenterology **74:**159, 1978.
14. Feldman, M.: Postoperative recurrent ulcer, N. Engl. J. Med. **302:**749, 1980.
15. Feldman, M., Richardson, C.T., and Fordtran, S.: Effect of sham feeding on gastric acid secretion in healthy subjects and duodenal ulcer patients: evidence for increased vagal tone in some ulcer patients, Gastroenterology **79:**796, 1980.
16. Fisher, R.S., and Cohen, S.: Pyloric sphincter dysfunction in patients with gastric ulcer, N. Engl. J. Med. **288:**273, 1976.
17. Fitzpatrick, W.J.F., Blackwood, W.S., and Northfield, T.C.: Bedtime cimetidine maintenance treatment: optimum dose and effect on subsequent natural history of duodenal ulcer, Gut **23:**239, 1982.
18. Fromm, D.: Complications of gastric surgery, New York, 1977, John Wiley & Sons, Inc.
19. Gillies, M.A., and Skyring, A.: Gastric and duodenal ulcer, the association between aspirin ingestion, smoking, and family history of ulcer, Med. J. Aust. **2:**280, 1969.
20. Grossman, M.I. (moderator): UCLA Conference: Peptic ulcer: new therapies, new diseases, Ann. Intern. Med. **95:**609, 1981.
21. Grossman, M.I., editor: Peptic ulcer: a guide for the practicing physician, Chicago, 1981, Year Book Medical Publishers, Inc.
22. Johnson, L.R.: The trophic action of gastrointestinal hormones, Gastroenterology **70:**278, 1976.
23. Jordan, P.H., Jr.: Peptic ulcer disease and early postoperative complications. In Sleisenger, M.H., and Fordtran, J.S., editors: Gastrointestinal disease: pathophysiology diagnosis management, Philadelphia, 1983, W.B. Saunders Co.
24. Kelly, K.A., and Hinder, R.A.: Evaluation of surgical procedures. In Sircus, W., and Smith, A.N., editors: Scientific foundations of gastroenterology, Philadelphia, 1980, W.B. Saunders Co.
25. Kirk, A.P., Dooley, J.S., and Hunt, R.H.: Peptic ulceration in patients with chronic liver disease, Dig. Dis. Sci. **25:**756, 1980.
26. Kurato, J.H., Honda, G.D., and Frankl, H.: Hospitalization and mortality rates for peptic ulcers: a comparison of a large health maintenance organization and United States data, Gastroenterology **83:**1008, 1982.
27. Lam, S.K., et al.: Gastric acid secretion is abnormally sensitive to exogenous gastrin released after peptone test meals in duodenal ulcer patients, J. Clin. Invest. **65:**555, 1980.

28. Langman, M.J.S.: The epidemiology of chronic digestive disease, Chicago, 1979, Year Book Medical Publisher, Inc.
29. Lucas, C.E., Sugawa, C., and Riddle, J.: Natural history and surgical dilemma of "stress" gastric bleeding, Arch. Surg. **102:**266, 1971.
30. Malagelada, J.R., et al.: Gastric secretion and emptying after normal meals in duodenal ulcer, Gastroenterology **73:**981, 1977.
31. Marks, I.N., et al.: Ulcer healing and relapse rates after initial treatment with cimetidine or sucralfate, J. Clin. Gastroenterol. **3**(suppl. 2):163, 1981.
32. McCarthy, D.M.: Peptic ulcer heterogeneity and clinical implications (editorial), Ann. Intern. Med. **95:**507, 1981.
33. McGuigan, J.E.: The Zollinger-Ellison syndrome. In Sleisenger, M.H., and Fordtran, J.S., editors: Gastrointestinal disease: pathophysiology diagnosis management, Philadelphia, 1983, W.B. Saunders Co.
34. Menguy, R.: Role of gastric mucosal energy metabolism in the etiology of stress ulceration, World J. Surg. **5:**175, 1981.
35. Miller, T.A., and Jacobson, E.D.: Gastrointestinal cytoprotection by prostaglandins, Gut **20:**75, 1979.
36. Modlin, I.M., and Brennan, M.F.: The diagnosis and management of gastrinoma, Surg. Gynecol. Obstet. **158:**97, 1984.
37. O'Brien, P., and Silen, W.: Influence of acid secretory state on the gastric mucosal tolerance to back diffusion of H^+, Gastroenterology **71:**760, 1976.
38. Oi, M., Oshida, K., and Sugimura, S.: The location of gastric ulcer, Gastroenterology **36:**45, 1959.
39. Owens, M.L., et al.: Treatment of peptic ulcer disease in the renal transplant patient, Ann. Surg. **186:**17, 1977.
40. Paffenbarger, R.S., Jr., Wing, A.L., and Hyde, R.T.: Chronic disease in former college students. XIII. Early precursors of peptic ulcer, Am. J. Epidemiol. **100:**307, 1974.
41. Peden, N.R., et al.: Gastric mucosal histamine and histamine methyltransferase in patients with duodenal ulcers, Gut **23:**56, 1982.
42. Peterson, W.L., and Richardson, C.T.: Pharmacology and side effects of drugs used to treat peptic ulcer. In Sleisenger, M.H., and Fordtran, J.S., editors: Gastrointestinal disease: pathophysiology diagnosis management, Philadelphia, 1983, W.B. Saunders Co.
43. Priebe, H.J., et al.: Antacid versus cimetidine in preventing acute gastrointestinal bleeding: a randomized trial in 75 critically ill patients, N. Engl. J. Med. **302:**426, 1980.
44. Richardson, C.T.: Gastric ulcer. In Sleisenger, M.H., and Fordtran, J.S., editors: Gastrointestinal disease: pathophysiology diagnosis management, Philadelphia, 1983, W.B. Saunders Co.
45. Ritchie, W.P., Jr.: Acute gastric mucosal damage produced by bile salts, acid and ischemia, Gastroenterology **68:**699, 1975.
46. Rotter, J.I.: The genetics of peptic ulcer: more than one gene, more than one disease, Prog. Med. Genet. **4:**1, 1980.
47. Samloff, I.M.: Pepsinogens and their relationship to peptic ulcer. In Rotter, J.L., Samloff, I.M., and Rimoin, D.L., editors: The genetics and heterogeneity of common gastrointestinal disorders, New York, 1980, Academic Press, Inc.
48. Schwarz, K.: Ueber penetrierende Magen-und Jejunalgeschwure, Beitr. Klin. Chir. **67:**96, 1910.
49. Soll, A.H., and Grossman, M.I.: The interaction of stimulants on the function of isolated canine parietal cells, Philos. Trans. R. Soc. Lond. (Biol.) **296:**5, 1981.
50. Soll, A.H., and Isenberg, J.I.: Duodenal ulcer diseases. In Sleisenger, M.H., and Fordtran, J.S., editors: Gastrointestinal disease: pathophysiology diagnosis management, Philadelphia, 1983, W.B. Saunders Co.
51. Stabile, B.E., and Passaro, E., Jr.: Recurrent peptic ulcer, Gastroenterology **70:**124, 1976.
52. Stabile, B.E., and Passaro, E., Jr.: Duodenal ulcer: a disease in evolution, Current Probl. Surg. **21:**1, 1984.
53. Steiger, E., and Cooperman, A.M.: Considerations in the management of perforated peptic ulcers, Surg. Clin. North Am. **56:**1395, 1976.
54. Trudeau, W.L., and McGuigan, J.E.: Relations between serum gastrin levels and rates of gastric hydrochloric acid secretion, N. Engl. J. Med. **284:**408, 1971.
55. Walker, C.: Complications of peptic ulcer disease and indications for surgery. In Sleisenger, M.H., and Fordtran, J.S., editors: Gastrointestinal disease: pathophysiology diagnosis managment, Philadelphia, 1983, W.B. Saunders Co.
56. Wolf, S.: Peptic ulcer: Psychosomatic illness review: no. 3 in a series, Psychosomatics **23:**1101, 1982.
57. Wormsley, K.G.: The pathophysiology of duodenal ulceration, Gut **15:**59, 1974.
58. Wormsley, K.G.: Smoking and duodenal ulcer (editorial), Gastroenterology **75:**139, 1978.

17 *Thomas A. Miller*

Gastric Neoplasia

In addition to acid-peptic disease, the other major disorder of surgical significance involving the stomach is that of neoplasia. Both benign and malignant lesions may arise in the stomach, but malignancies are clearly more commonly encountered and comprise approximately 90% of all gastric tumors. For inapparent reasons, the incidence of gastric malignancy in the United States has decreased dramatically over the last 50 years. In 1930, for example, gastric cancer was diagnosed in approximately 29 per 100,000 population, compared to 1980 in which only seven per 100,000 population had this disease.[51] Efforts to explain this phenomenon have been unrevealing; most authorities believe that a true decrease in the incidence of this disease has occurred rather than improvements in its prevention and treatment. A similar decline has been noted in Great Britain and much of western Europe. By contrast, gastric cancer is increasing in Japan, Chile, and Iceland and continues to be a major health problem in many of the Scandinavian countries and eastern Europe. The explanation for this observation has been equally elusive. Despite the decline of gastric cancer in the United States, surgical therapy is presently the only means of potentially effecting cure. Thus an understanding of its clinical presentation and the physiologic principles underlying treatment are essential to good surgical practice.

TYPES OF GASTRIC TUMORS AND THEIR PATHOLOGIC FEATURES

Benign Tumors

Benign tumors of the stomach comprise between 5% and 10% of all gastric neoplasms and arise primarily in the epithelium or underlying submucosa.[3,19] Those tumors of epithelial origin present clinically as polypoid lesions and may either be sessile or pedunculated. Unless they are located in the distal stomach where they may alter normal gastric emptying, they are usually asymptomatic and often discovered as incidental findings on upper gastrointestinal endoscopy or barium study. Their major importance surgically is that they may harbor an underlying malignancy.

Polyps arising from the epithelium may be hyperplastic or adenomatous.[41,57] The hyperplastic variety constitutes approximately 80% of cases and actually is not a true neoplasm at all since it represents on overgrowth of normal epithelium. Lesions of this type usually occur in the body and fundus of the stomach, rarely exceed 2 cm in diameter, and are often multiple. Adenomatous polyps, on the other hand, are true neoplasms, are usually single, and most commonly occur in the antrum. Histologically, the adenomatous polyp is similar to a colonic adenoma, particularly the villous variety, and has been observed to harbor an underlying malignancy in as many as 25% to 50% of cases, depending on its size. Whether the malignancy was always present or developed from an underlying benign polyp remains unsettled. Adenomatous polyps are common in areas of the stomach where there is intestinal metaplasia or chronic gastritis. Lesions in excess of 2 cm in diameter are at particular risk for an underlying malignancy. Gastric polyps are often seen in patients with the Peutz-Jeghers or Gardner's syndromes and may be of the hyperplastic or adenomatous variety.

Benign tumors arising from the submucosa are commonly found within the gastric wall and almost invariably represent smooth muscle tumors known as leiomyomas. These lesions are generally of little clinical significance unless they compromise the blood supply to the overlying epithelium secondary to excessive growth. When this occurs, a central ulceration of the epithelium and underlying leiomyoma develops that has been known to culminate in a massive upper gastrointestinal hemorrhage. Distinguishing lesions of this nature from their malignant counterparts may be very difficult.

Other benign tumors of the stomach may also occur. Generally they are asymptomatic and discovered as incidental findings at autopsy, on endoscopy, or during radiologic studies of the stomach. Examples include neurofibromas, lipomas, carcinoid tumors, and occasionally a remnant of a pancreatic rest (i.e., ectopic pancreas).

Malignant Tumors

Adenocarcinoma is by far the most common gastric malignancy, accounting for 95% of all cancers of the stomach.[12] Lymphomas and leiomyosarcomas constitute the rest. On rare occasions the stomach may be the source of a tumor such as a squamous cell carcinoma, rhabdomyosarcoma, teratoma, angiosarcoma, or a metastasis from an adjacent or distant organ.

Adenocarcinoma

Adenocarcinoma of the stomach usually originates from the progenitor cells at the base of the gastric pits. This neoplasm may arise anywhere within the stomach, but most tumors develop in the pyloric and antral regions, generally along the lesser curvature. Although various classifications have been proposed to distinguish the different histologic presentations of this tumor,[9,32,40] from the standpoint of biologic behavior four types have been recognized:

1. Superficial spreading
2. Polypoid or fungating
3. Ulcerative
4. Infiltrating (scirrhosis—linitis plastica)

The most favorable form of carcinoma is the superficial spreading type in which the neoplastic process is confined to the mucosa and is not associated with any breakdown

TNM CLASSIFICATION

Primary Tumor (T)

T_1 Limitation of the tumor to mucosa and submucosa, regardless of its extent or location

T_2 Tumor involvement of the mucosa and submucosa (including the muscularis propria), with extension to or into the serosa but not penetration through the serosa

T_3 Tumor penetration through the serosa without invasion of contiguous structures

T_4 Tumor penetration through the serosa and invasion of contiguous structures

Nodal Involvement (N)

N_0 Absence of regional lymph node metastases

N_1 Perigastric lymph node involvement within 3 cm of the primary tumor along the lesser or greater curvature

N_2 Regional lymph node involvement more than 3 cm from the primary tumor, which can be removed at surgery, including those nodes located along the left gastric, splenic, celiac, and common hepatic arteries

N_3 Other intraabdominal lymph node involvement that cannot be adequately removed at surgery such as the paraaortic, hepatoduodenal, retropancreatic, and mesenteric nodes

Distant Metastasis (M)

M_0 No known evidence of distant metastases

M_1 Distant metastases are present

of the epithelium or chronic ulceration. Unfortunately at the time of diagnosis most gastric cancers in this country are noted to be infiltrating lesions that penetrate deep into the gastric wall. The luminal portion of the tumor may be polypoid in appearance, at times even bulky, or flat and more ulcerating. This latter presentation may be confused with a benign gastric ulcer. Although less frequent than these other manifestations, gastric carcinoma may actually infiltrate the gastric wall diffusely, producing a rigid, nondistensible stomach in the region of involvement. This type of cancer is known as linitis plastica and produces a peculiar "leather-bottle" appearance on barium contrast study of the stomach.

Gastric cancer may spread by lymphatics, bloodstream, peritoneal seeding, or direct extension. Gastric adenocarcinoma has a tendency toward intramural extension by lymphatic channels. Tumors of the gastric antrum spread along subserosal lymphatics to the duodenum, whereas tumors of the fundus and cardia spread into the esophagus along submucosal lymphatics. Thus it is not unusual for invasion of the regional lymphatics to occur, and as many as 50% to 70% of patients will have evidence of lymphatic spread at the time they seek medical therapy and a curative operation is attempted. Hematogenous spread is primarily by means of the portal vein to the liver or through the systemic circulation to the lungs, bones, and other distant sites. If the serosa of the stomach is invaded by tumor, neoplastic cells may become seeded directly into the peritoneal cavity and form serosal implants. The firm metastatic mass that results from implants in the rectovesical or rectouterine cul-de-sac is referred to as a Blumer's shelf and is an indication of advanced carcinomatosis. Ovarian implants are known as Krukenberg's tumor.

Although the size, location, and degree of tumor differentiation (the less differentiated, the less favorable) directly influence the prognosis in gastric cancer, the two major factors influencing survival in potentially resectable tumors are the *extent of spread* through the gastric wall and the presence or absence of regional *lymph node involvement*. The TNM system of classifying gastric carcinoma emphasizes these two prognostic factors and is currently the major system of staging this disease in the United States (see boxed material above).[14,28] With this staging scheme, the extent of disease is defined in terms of the degree of penetration of the primary tumor through the gastric wall, designated by the letter T; the extent of regional lymph node involvement, designated by the letter N; and the presence or absence of distant metastases, designated by the letter M.

Lymphomas and Leiomyosarcomas

Comprising approximately 4% of gastric malignancies, lymphomas may occur as an isolated neoplasm confined to the stomach or represent a component of a more widespread disease.[4,22] Such lesions may assume the gross characteristics of a carcinoma, in which case they usually present as a tumor mass, or, as more commonly occurs, they present as a thickening of the epithelial folds secondary to their lymphocytic infiltration within the submucosa. Histologically, they are similar to lymphomas in other organs and regions of the body. Leiomyosarcomas are submucosal malignancies representing approximately 1% of all gastric malignancies.[4,35] Like carcinomas, these lesions may extend into the lumen of the stomach or be confined primarily to the gastric wall. Like leiomyomas, they may compromise the blood supply of the overlying epithelium and result in hemorrhage. Occasionally these tumors may extend primarily into the abdominal cavity and become adherent to adjacent organs such as the liver or pancreas.

ETIOLOGIC CONSIDERATIONS

The cause of both benign and malignant tumors of the stomach has remained elusive. Despite this uncertainty, a number of interesting correlations have identified several possible causal agents that may be of importance in the development of gastric neoplasia, particularly adenocarcinoma. These include environmental, dietary, and hereditary influences.

As already noted, the incidence of gastric cancer has steadily decreased in the United States and several other countries over the last 50 years, whereas it continues to be an important malignancy in Japan and the Scandinavian countries, suggesting that environment itself may be a risk factor. That environmental factors may indeed play a role in the development of gastric cancer is underscored by the observation that first-generation Japanese who migrated to Hawaii had a similar incidence of gastric cancer to those of the same generation remaining in Japan, whereas second-generation Japanese, born and reared in Hawaii, actually had a lower incidence of this neoplasm.[20] In a recent epidemiologic study in which the incidence of gastric cancer was compared between Hawaiians of Japanese extraction and native Hawaiians, no differences were observed.[51] Studies of this nature suggest that exposure to environmental factors early in life may play a role in the subsequent development of gastric malignancy. What these factors are remains to be determined, but the possibility of inhaled or ingested carcinogens must be considered.[54]

Various dietary factors have likewise been implicated in the development of gastric cancer. Increased salt consumption and the ingestion of starch, pickled vegetables, and salted fish and meat have all been positively correlated with the development of gastric cancer.[24,25] Dietary nitrates may also be causative agents. When ingested, these substances can be reduced to nitrites by various enteric bacteria, which then may combine with dietary amines and amides to form various nitrosourea compounds such as nitrosamines and nitrosamides.[23] These latter substances have been demonstrated experimentally to have potent carcinogenic properties. In one population at high risk for gastric malignancy, a higher than average intake of nitrates has been demonstrated.[8]

Various genetic factors may be of importance. There is at least a twofold risk of developing gastric cancer among first-degree relatives of patients with this neoplasm.[27] In addition, individuals with blood group A appear to have a 20% greater risk of developing gastric cancer when compared with other blood groupings.[1,33] Of equal note is the higher frequency of gastric cancer among men than women and among blacks than whites, suggesting genetic factors relating to sex and race.[12,38] Finally, kindreds having adenocarcinoma exclusively of the stomach are known,[59] again implicating the potential importance of genetics in the pathogenesis of gastric cancer.

A number of other factors appear to be potential precursors for the development of gastric malignancy. As already noted, carcinoma is quite commonly found in an adenomatous polyp and may be a precursor of cancer. Chronic atrophic gastritis and pernicious anemia also appear to be predisposing risk factors.[13,55] In atrophic gastritis gastric glands are decreased or absent and often coexist with areas of intestinal metaplasia in which the gastric epithelium is replaced by mucosa that resembles that of the small intestine.[7,55] Because of these epithelial changes, patients with this condition are frequently hypochlorhydric or achlorhydric. Evidence linking this condition with the development of gastric cancer includes: (1) the increased incidence of chronic atrophic gastritis in countries like Japan where an increased incidence of gastric cancer also occurs[7]; (2) the observation that this entity precedes the development of malignancy in various experimental models[7]; and (3) the finding that, correcting for other factors, 10% of patients with this condition, when followed for 20 or more years, subsequently develop gastric cancer.[52,55] The potential risk of developing gastric carcinoma in patients with pernicious anemia likewise appears to be real.[13] Although the extent of this risk remains debatable, the incidence of gastric cancer in patients with pernicious anemia appears to be clearly increased over control patients when this disease has been present for 5 years or longer.

Over the past decade a number of reports have suggested an association between previous gastric surgery for benign conditions such as ulcer disease and the subsequent development of gastric cancer.* Most cases have occurred in the gastric remnant following a Billroth II gastrectomy, as long as 20 years or more after the original surgical procedure. Unfortunately the majority of these reports have been retrospective in nature and suffer from a lack of appropriately matched control populations. Three prospective studies have addressed this issue both in the United States and abroad.[15,48,58] Critical statistical assessment of patients undergoing a previous gastric procedure and developing a carcinoma in the gastric remnant have failed to demonstrate an increased risk of gastric cancer following gastric resection when compared to the normal incidence of carcinoma in a control population. Thus it would appear that the initial concern for this problem is unwarranted.

Ménétrier's disease, also called hypertrophic gastropathy, is a clinical condition characterized by giant hypertrophy of the gastric rugae, excessive loss of protein from the thickened mucosa, and usually an accompanying hypochlorhydria. Although in most patients this disease follows a benign course, careful follow-up has revealed that some cases gradually evolve into atrophic gastritis or undergo a malignant change as a late complication.[49] The malignant potential of this disease continues to be debated but may complicate its course in as many as 10% of cases.

Finally the issue of whether a benign gastric ulcer may ultimately undergo carcinomatous change continues to be hotly debated. Careful studies by Morson and Dawson[43] have indicated that, if such changes do in fact occur, the incidence is probably 1% or less. Thus, if biopsy of a gastric ulcer reveals evidence of malignancy, it was most likely malignant from the time of onset.

CLINICAL PRESENTATION AND DIAGNOSIS OF GASTRIC NEOPLASIA

Unfortunately a gastric tumor may initially be asymptomatic, even though at subsequent diagnosis its size indicates that it has been present for a considerable period of time. Often the earliest clinical symptoms are vague and are no different than the indigestion and/or mild abdominal pain that most individuals experience at various times throughout life. It is for this reason that gastric tumors are often diagnosed late in their development and, if malignant, have already advanced to a state at which surgical cure is unlikely.

For gastric polyps the initial presentation may be one of unexplained anemia or mild upper gastrointestinal bleeding. Occasionally a polyp in the distal stomach may intermittently create a gastric outlet obstruction resulting from prolapse of the polyp through the pylorus. Leiomyomas

*References 10, 11, 17, 21, 42, 45, 46.

are almost always asymptomatic until they reach a diameter of 3 to 4 cm or greater, in which case they compromise blood supply to the overlying epithelium and present as unexplained bleeding.

The clinical presentation in the initial stages of development of gastric cancer is often vague and nondescript. It is for this reason that early diagnosis is infrequent. As the disease becomes more advanced, it may interfere with the motor activity of a portion of the stomach wall. When such derangements occur, postprandial fullness, loss of appetite, and heartburn may ensue. In those tumors arising in the distal stomach, particularly near the pylorus, obstructive symptoms such as vomiting and pain may actually appear secondary to gastric distention and attempts of the stomach to empty its contents. In fact, pain is usually the symptom that brings the patient with gastric cancer to a physician. In the earlier stages of cancer, this pain may be similar to what is commonly noted with a peptic ulcer (i.e., postprandial, nocturnal, relieved by eating); as the malignant process becomes more extensive, the pain is often more continuous, may actually be aggravated by eating, and may extend into the substernal and precordial regions. If the pain is associated with eating, the patient may actually eat less frequently in an effort to lessen its magnitude and persistence. This results in weight loss and evidence of obvious protein-calorie malnutrition. Occasionally, an ulcerating tumor will set into motion a state of chronic blood loss. The resulting anemia will add to the weakness that already exists from the malnutrition. In rare instances the tumor may actually bleed quite briskly and require emergency surgical intervention for control.

On occasion, symptoms referable to distant spread will be the first evidence that a gastric malignancy is present. Thus a palpable supraclavicular node (especially on the left, known as Virchow's node) or a Blummer's shelf may herald the diagnosis. Other patients may complain of abdominal swelling secondary to malignant ascites from peritoneal metastases. Still other patients may first appear with an enlarged liver, demonstrating firm nodularity suggestive of metastatic disease. Finally, a dermatologic disorder known as acanthosis nigricans is strongly associated with gastric carcinoma and often precedes its clinical appearance by many years.[34] It is characterized by the presence of hyperpigmented, roughened skin in the groins, below the breasts, and in the axillae.

Diagnosis of gastric cancer, especially if it is to be identified in its early stages, will depend on a high index of suspicion in patients with gastrointestinal complaints. Unfortunately, the cost-benefit ratio of performing intensive diagnostic evaluations on all patients with gastrointestinal complaints is not practical when the low incidence of gastric cancer in the general population is considered. This problem obviously contributes to its late diagnosis. Nonetheless, if one is familiar with those patient groups at risk, as discussed earlier, more extensive study of such populations can be undertaken when nondescript and ill-defined symptoms develop.

The first diagnostic test obtained in individuals with upper gastrointestinal symptoms should be radiologic examination of the stomach after ingestion of a barium meal. When this is performed in combination with the introduction of air, enhanced detail of the gastric mucosal surface supervenes. Suggestive evidence that a gastric tumor, and possibly a malignancy, may be present includes the demonstration of a polypoid mass protruding into the gastric lumen, nondistensibility of a portion of the gastric wall, effacement of normal gastric folds, and an ulcer crater. The presence of any of these findings warrants further evaluation by gastroscopy. The ready availability of fiberoptic endoscopes makes it now possible to visualize and carefully examine virtually any region in the stomach. With this technique, biopsy and histologic evaluation of any suspicious area should be undertaken. To ensure a high probability of accurate diagnosis, as many as eight to ten biopsies should be obtained in an area of suspicion.[47] Combining endoscopic biopsy with the collection of cytologic specimens obtained by brushing the area in question results in a diagnostic accuracy of identifying gastric cancer that approaches 97% to 100%.[2,5,31]

Routine laboratory studies are generally of little help in the diagnosis of gastric neoplasia. If chronic blood loss from the tumor has occurred, the hematocrit may be depressed, and stool examinations for occult blood may be positive. Similarly, liver function tests are usually abnormal if hepatic metastases are present, but this is distinctly uncommon in the early stages of gastric malignancy. Chest x-ray films are also usually normal unless the malignant process is advanced, in which case evidence of pulmonary spread may be demonstrable.

Other diagnostic maneuvers that may prove useful under selective circumstances when the diagnosis of gastric malignancy is uncertain include gastric secretory studies and the measurement of various tumor markers. Achlorhydria in a patient with ulcer disease indicates the presence of a gastric malignancy until proven otherwise. Elevated serum pepsinogen I levels are a marker for intestinal metaplasia of the gastric epithelium, a histologic alteration that appears to be a precursor of gastric malignancy.[53] Finally, measurement of carcinoembryonic antigen in gastric juice may prove useful.[16,56] From a practical standpoint, however, these additional diagnostic maneuvers are usually unnecessary, and the findings obtained on gastroscopic biopsy and brushings will provide the information needed to establish a diagnosis of gastric cancer.

Once the diagnosis has been confirmed, the role of preoperative staging in gastric cancer remains an unsettled issue. Moss and associates[44] have shown that findings on preoperative abdominal computerized axial tomography (CAT) scanning correlate quite closely with the extent of disease detected at operation. They have suggested that CAT scan results should be used to determine the suitability of undertaking an operation and have stressed that knowing this information will avoid unnecessary surgery in some patients. The logic of this argument is untenable if, as McFee and Aust[39] have emphasized, the belief is held that most patients should be explored, not only with the intention of effecting care if this is possible, but also with the notion that surgery can provide the best palliation against the development of complications such as obstruction, hemorrhage, and perforation. Most surgeons, including the author, would agree with this latter position and believe that, even if distant disease exists, this circumstance in no way obviates the potential benefits that can be derived from surgery.

RATIONAL APPROACH TO TREATMENT

Surgical Options

For both benign and malignant tumors of the stomach, some form of surgical excision is the treatment of choice. Because therapeutic decisions differ somewhat between benign and malignant lesions, each type will be discussed separately.

Benign Tumors

As previously noted, benign tumors are usually demonstrated during barium studies of the stomach or at the time of gastroscopy. If the lesion is a polyp, every attempt should be made to remove it or at the very least adequately perform a biopsy on it because of the potential of underlying malignancy, particularly in the adenomatous variety. If the polyp is predunculated, biopsy can usually be accomplished endoscopically with a snare and electrocautery. Pedunculated polyps as large as 3 to 4 cm in diameter not uncommonly lend themselves to this approach. For sessile lesions or larger pedunculated lesions, debate exists as to whether biopsy is adequate or actual surgical excision should be carried out. As a general rule, polyps 2 cm or greater in diameter should be removed because of the increased incidence of malignancy in these larger lesions. Such removal will usually require an exploratory laparotomy to effect a generous excision of the lesion (Fig. 17-1). For smaller lesions multiple biopsies to rule out an underlying malignancy are generally an appropriate approach to management, as long as the patient can be followed periodically with repeat endoscopic examin ation. However, even smaller lesions should be removed if they have been the cause of gastric bleeding or obstruction.

When a leiomyoma is discovered, formal excision during laparotomy is almost always indicated, not only to relieve associated symptoms if present but also to rule out the possibility of an occult leiomyosarcoma. A similar approach is recommended for other benign tumors, including fibromas, lipomas, and other benign lesions.

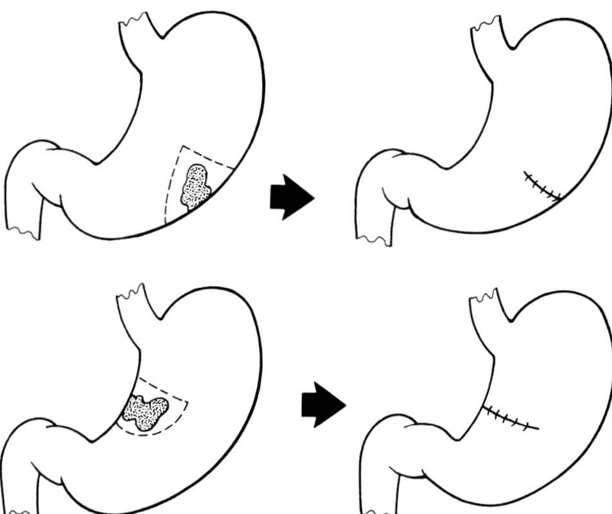

Fig. 17-1 Surgical approach to excision of benign lesions of stomach that cannot be removed endoscopically to rule out an underlying malignancy.

Malignant Tumors

ADENOCARCINOMA. At the present time, surgical excision provides the only chance for cure in a patient with gastric adenocarcinoma. Although historically total gastrectomy was used to accomplish this goal, there is general agreement among most authorities that subtotal gastric resection is the procedure of choice for most cancers of the stomach. This consensus has been reached on the basis of the observation that survival rates following subtotal resection have been as good, if not better, than those following total gastrectomy and that both operative mortality and associated morbidity are considerably less with subtotal resection.* In a given patient, however, the operative approach will depend on whether the procedure can be performed under elective circumstances or needs to be carried out on an emergency basis, what is observed at the time of operation in terms of the potential for curability, and if adequate margins can be ensured on either side of the tumor with a subtotal resection or if the more extensive total gastrectomy will be necessary.

Assuming that preoperative workup of the patient has failed to reveal any evidence of distant metastases, the most important initial concern of the operating surgeon should be the determination of whether the tumor can be resected for cure. If evidence of distant disease within the abdomen such as metastases to the liver, peritoneal implants, and widespread nodal involvement is present, a curative procedure is not possible. In addition, direct extension of the tumor into contiguous organs such as the pancreas, transverse colon, and liver also mitigates against curative resection. However, care must be taken to ensure that extension of the tumor through the serosa has indeed occurred or that what appears to be extension may in fact only be adherence to a contiguous structure resulting in an inflammatory response to the tumor. If this latter circumstance exists, the tumor may still be amenable to curative resection. Similarly, lymph node involvement per se does not exclude curability. Although long-term survival is clearly related to the extent of node involvement (see boxed material on p. 311) curative resections (i.e., excision of tumor plus lymph node drainage routes) for positive nodes within 3 cm of the neoplasm (i.e., N_1 nodes) or even those further away in the region of common hepatic artery, celiac axis, and splenic hilum (i.e., N_2 nodes) have been associated with significant survival advantages when compared with palliative resection of the tumor alone (i.e., in some series 5-year survival rates approaching 20% to 25%).[5,14,26] Thus curative resection should not be restricted under these conditions. In contrast, evidence of nodal spread to more distant regions such as the porta hepatis and along the para-aortic and retropancreatic nodes (i.e., N_3 nodes) has a much more dismal prognosis and indicates that only a palliative procedure is of value.

If exploration indicates that a potential for cure exists, a generous subtotal gastrectomy for midstomach and distal

---

*References 12, 18, 29, 30, 36, 37.

gastric lesions should be performed. This should include en bloc removal of the greater and lesser omenta to ensure excision of lymph node drainage routes[6] (Figs. 17-2 and 17-3). For lesions in the more proximal stomach, a more proximal subtotal gastrectomy is recommended, leaving a remnant of the antrum for anastomosis to the distal esophagus. If the more proximal tumor is along the greater curvature, splenectomy is also recommended in combination with the gastrectomy because of the propensity for tumors in this area to spread along the pancreaticolienal group of nodes. Some authorities also believe that the body and tail of the pancreas should be included in the resected specimen for tumors in this area, particularly if the cancer adheres to the pancreas posteriorly or if enlarged lymph nodes exist along the superior border of the pancreas. This latter approach is open to debate. Some authorities also believe that a total gastrectomy should be performed for proximal gastric lesions, particularly those near the cardia. As already indicated, the problems associated with this more extended resection mitigate against its routine use. A total gastrectomy should clearly be reserved for patients in whom a cure is in fact strongly anticipated.

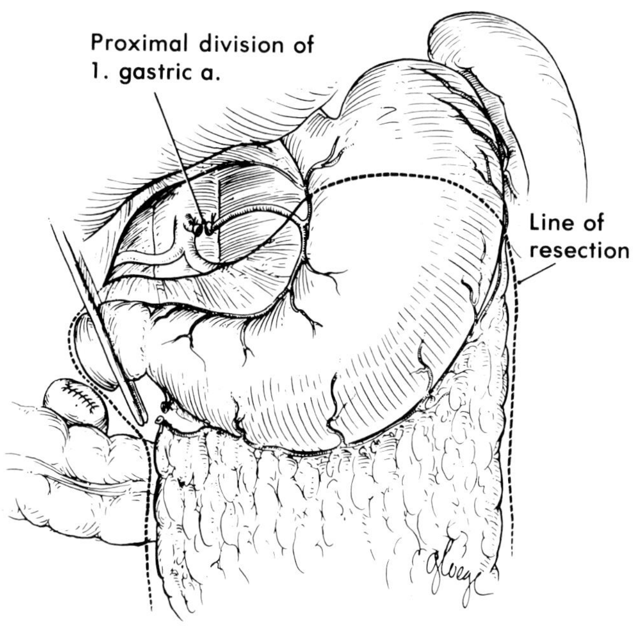

Fig. 17-2 "Standard" type of subtotal gastric resection for cancer of the distal portion of the stomach. For a midstomach lesion, the proximal line of resection would be more proximal. (From Fink, A.S., and Longmire, W.P., Jr.: Carcinoma of the stomach. In Sabiston, D.C., editor: Textbook of surgery, ed. 13, Philadelphia, 1986, W.B. Saunders Co.)

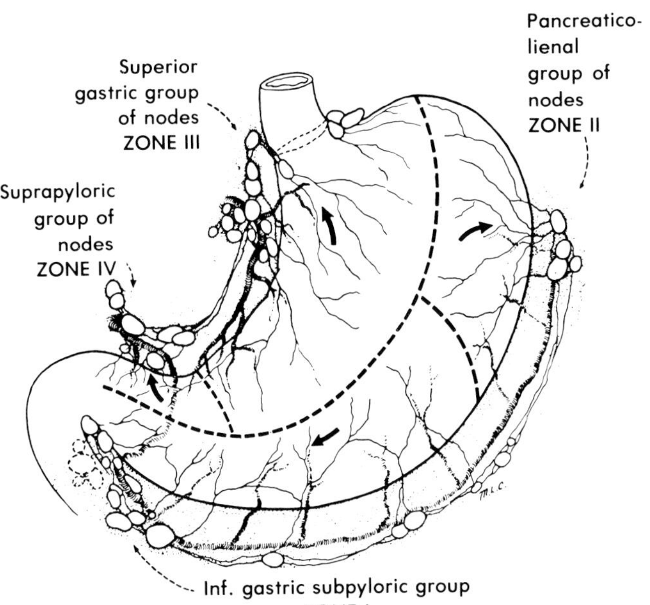

Fig. 17-3 Routes of lymphatic spread for carcinoma of stomach. (From Coller, F.A., Kay, E.B., and McIntyre, R.S.: Arch. Surg. **43:**748, Copyright 1941, American Medical Association.)

The extent of gastric resection for gastric cancer remains an unsettled issue. Proximal extension of the tumor, mainly through the submucosal lymphatics, has been shown to extend as far as 6 cm from the tumor itself.[60] Similar extensions distally have also been noted.[61] For this reason it is usually recommended that at least a 6-cm margin of resection on either side of the tumor be ensured. If the primary tumor happens to be in the distal stomach, this resection should include the proximal duodenum and be extended as far distally as possible, particularly if the tumor reaches the pylorus. For more proximal tumors in which esophageal invasion is likely, a generous portion of the distal esophagus should be removed. Under most circumstances, it is advisable to obtain frozen section examination of the margins to ensure the absence of residual tumor. If tumor cells are seen, additional resection is indicated.

For tumors of the midbody and distal stomach in which a subtotal gastrectomy is performed, a Billroth II recon-

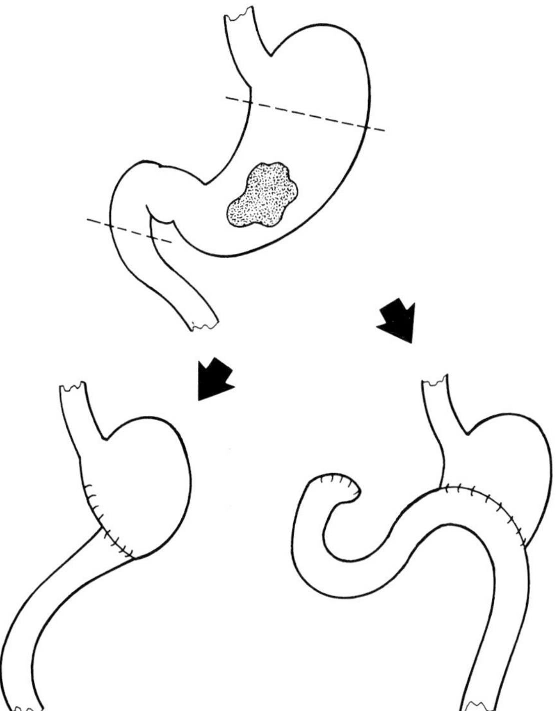

Fig. 17-4 Types of gastrointestinal reconstruction following subtotal gastrectomy for cancer of the distal and midstomachs. Darkened area in the top part of the figure represents a malignancy.

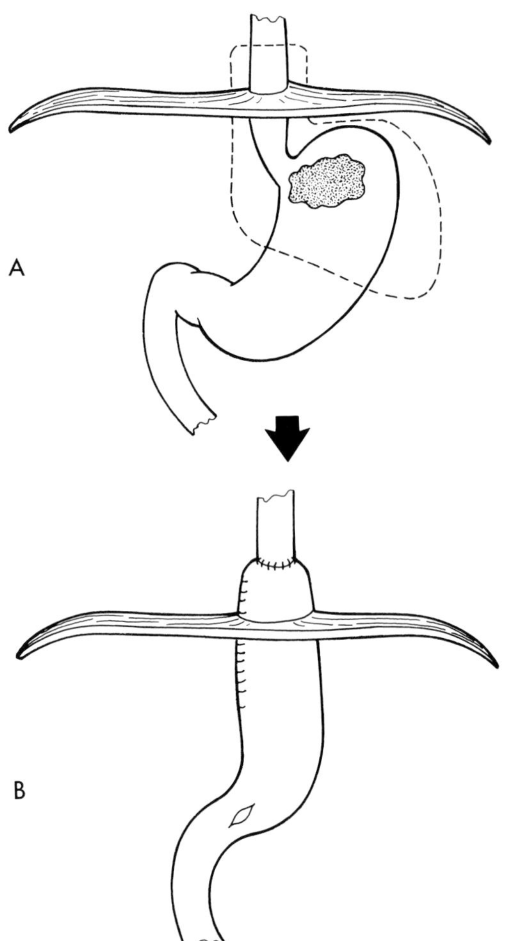

Fig. 17-5 Type of alimentary tract reconstruction when subtotal gastrectomy is used for cancer of the proximal stomach. **A,** Darkened area represents the tumor, and broken line represents the part of stomach and distal esophagus removed. **B,** Distal stomach remnant is anastomosed to the esophagus, and a pyloromyotomy is performed to prevent gastric outlet obstruction.

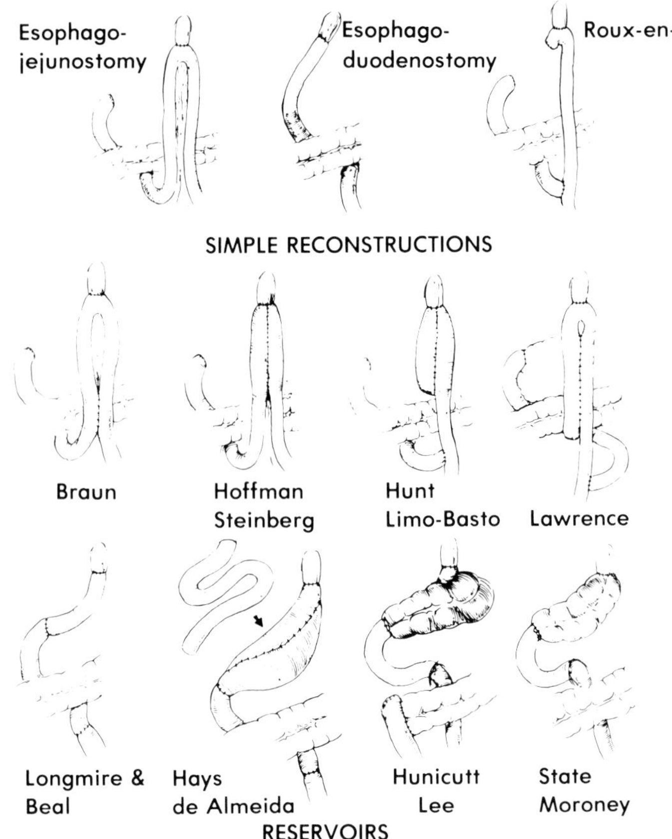

Fig. 17-6 Types of reconstruction procedures following total gastrectomy. (From Nora, P.F., editor: Operative surgery, ed. 2, Philadelphia, 1972, Lea & Febiger.)

struction is generally used to reestablish gastrointestinal continuity (Fig. 17-4). This does not mean that the Billroth I reconstruction is inappropriate but that a Billroth II reconstruction can usually be carried out with less technical difficulty. If a subtotal gastrectomy is used for a more proximal lesion in which a distal gastric remnant is left, the remaining distal esophagus is reimplanted into the distal stomach, and a pyloromyotomy is performed to prevent gastric outlet obstruction (Fig. 17-5). In those special circumstances when a total gastrectomy has been used, a Roux-en-Y esophagojejunostomy or some other modification is recommended for the establishment of alimentary tract continuity (Fig. 17-6).

For those patients in whom curative resection is not possible because of distant disease discovered at operation or known before surgery, some type of palliation is usually indicated. The reason for this relates to the fact that many of these tumors will either bleed or cause obstructive problems and occasionally even perforate if not resected. Thus, in the remaining months or years that the patient may have to live, a palliative procedure can do much to enhance the quality of life. The type of procedure performed will depend on the extent of tumor found at operation and the facility with which an operative procedure can be performed. Ideally, limited gastric resection is the procedure of choice. When this is not possible, a variety of bypass procedures can be fashioned. The various options available are demonstrated in Fig. 17-7.

In the rare circumstance in which emergency surgery is indicated to manage a complication of a gastric malignancy (i.e., bleeding, obstruction, or perforation), the major consideration should be the alleviation of the complication, followed by a determination as to whether cure can be effected. None of these complications necessarily indicates incurability. However, because of other risk factors associated with an emergent procedure, the technical aspects and length of time necessary to perform a curative procedure may not be possible. Obviously, situations of this nature will need to be individualized.

Other Malignancies. As with adenocarcinomas, the treatment of choice for other malignancies is also surgical resection. This should generally be a subtotal gastric resection to include en bloc removal of regional lymph nodes. In the case of lymphomas, it should be remembered that they are often large and bulky, giving the initial impression of unresectability. This finding, as well as the pres-

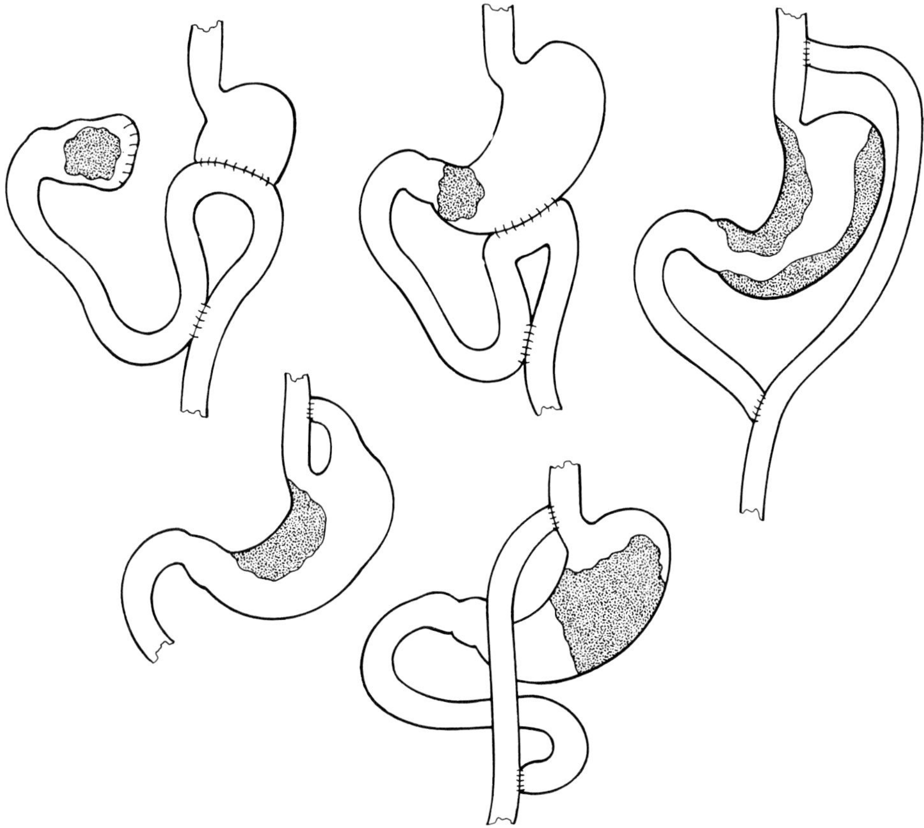

Fig. 17-7 Various types of surgical procedures used for palliation when curative resection cannot be successfully accomplished. Darkened areas represent the unresectable tumor.

ence of large lymph nodes (which are often hyperplastic), should not discourage the performance of a curative resection since the prognosis with this disease is considerably better than that of carcinoma.[4,22] Similarly, leiomyosarcomas may grow to a large size and extend beyond the gastric wall.[4,35] Even if a radical resection is required for this neoplasm, such efforts should be used since survival rates have generally been quite good. Because of their rarity, the surgical management of other malignancies will need to be individualized, but generally an aggressive approach should be used, and every effort undertaken to accomplish surgical resection.

Other Therapeutic Modalities

The role of adjunctive therapeutic modalities such as chemotherapy and radiation treatment will depend on the type of underlying malignancy. Generally the response of adenocarcinomas to radiation treatment has been disappointing. Other than the occasional case of a tumor of this histologic type demonstrating radiosensitivity, there is no convincing evidence at the present time that radiation therapy is of any value in enhancing survival with this neoplasm. On the other hand, a number of recent studies suggest that adjuvant chemotherapy may be of value in prolonging survival not only when used in combination with curative surgery but also for more advanced disease.[5,14,50] Generally these studies have shown that various chemotherapeutic agents, when used in combination with one another, are more efficacious than single-agent therapy. Despite these encouraging findings, the exact role of chemotherapy in the management of gastric carcinoma remains to be determined.

Neither palliative nor adjuvant chemotherapy or x-ray film therapy has been shown to be of any benefit in the treatment of leiomyosarcoma. In contrast, radiation treatment may be of considerable benefit in the management of gastric lymphoma. With the use of a combination of surgical resection and postoperative radiotherapy, 5-year survival rates have ranged from 45% to 90%, depending on the extent of disease at diagnosis and the histologic type.[5] For more advanced disease, adjuvant chemotherapy also appears to be of value.[5,50]

Outcome

At the present time, the overall 5-year survival rate for gastric carcinoma in the United States is about 12%.[5,12,14,36,37] This is directly related to the extent of spread of disease at the time of diagnosis. Even though most patients with carcinoma are surgical candidates, at least half of them will be found to have unresectable tumors for "cure" at the time of exploration. Of those subjected to potentially curable procedures, the resected specimen will often demonstrate microscopic evidence of extensive disease. Thus the importance of early diagnosis becomes obvious. This is exemplified by the observation that if this neoplasm is limited to the mucosa, 5-year survivals approach 85% to 90%, whereas widespread involvement of nodes or distant disease diminishes the likelihood of survival to virtually zero.

Lymphomas and leiomyosarcomas fare more favorably. Generally, 50% or more of patients with lymphomas will be alive at 5 years without evidence of disease.[4,5,22] Factors influencing survival include stage of disease, histologic type, and extent of penetration of gastric wall. Similar results can be expected with leiomyosarcomas where 5-year survivals range from 35% to 55%.[4,5,35] This relates to the fact that these tumors are usually well localized, with invasion of adjacent organs or metastatic spread occurring late.

SUMMARY

Compared with acid-peptic diseases of the stomach, gastric tumors are relatively uncommon. Nonetheless, because the majority of these neoplastic lesions are malignant and diagnosis is usually late, an understanding of their clinical presentation, populations at risk for their development, and the treatment options available is mandatory if any hope of cure is to be realized. Currently the treatment of choice for gastric cancer is surgical resection of the neoplasm to include en bloc removal of lymph node drainage routes. Under most circumstances a subtotal gastrectomy should be performed, not only because the morbidity and mortality associated with this procedure is less than with total gastrectomy but also because survival rates have been at least as good, if not better, than those with the more extensive procedure. Since most gastric malignancies occur in the midbody or distal portions of the stomach, a subtotal resection can generally be performed without undue technical difficulty. Even for more proximal lesions, a subtotal gastrectomy is recommended; alimentary tract continuity is reestablished by anastomosing the distal esophagus to the gastric antral remnant. Some authorities recommend that a total gastrectomy be performed for more proximal lesions, although the potential advantages of this procedure are debatable. Even with an aggressive surgical approach, the 5-year survival rate for adenocarcinoma, which comprises 95% of gastric malignancies, is only 12%. For rarer lesions such as lymphoma and leiomyosarcoma, 5-year survival rates are more encouraging and approach 50%. Until other treatment modalities such as radiation therapy and chemotherapy prove efficacious in the treatment of gastric cancer, the overall outcome will probably remain dismal since there are no specific symptoms or signs distinguishing this gastric malady from other problems of the stomach and thereby ensuring earlier diagnosis. Perhaps the most optimistic thing that can be said about gastric cancer is its steady decrease in incidence over the last 50 years in this country as well as throughout many other parts of the world. Hopefully this trend will continue.

REFERENCES

1. Aird, I., and Bentall, H.H.: A relationship between cancer of the stomach and the ABO blood groups, Br. Med. J. **1**:799, 1953.
2. Au, F.C., et al.: The role of cytology in the diagnosis of carcinoma of the stomach, Surg. Gynecol. Obstet. **151**:601, 1980.
3. Beard, R.J., et al.: Noncarcinomatous tumors of the stomach, Br. J. Surg. **55**:535, 1968.
4. Bedikian, A.U., et al.: Primary lymphomas and sarcomas of the stomach, South. Med. J. **73**:21, 1980.
5. Coit, D.G., and Brennan, M.F.: Gastric cancer. In Moody, F.G., et al., editors: Surgical treatment of digestive disease, Chicago, 1986, Year Book Medical Publishers, Inc.
6. Coller, F.A., Kay, E.B., and McIntyre, R.S.: Regional lymphatic metastases of carcinoma of the stomach, Arch. Surg. **43**:748, 1941.
7. Crespi, M., and Munoz, N.: Gastric precancer states. In Fielding, J.W.L., et al., editors: Gastric cancer, Oxford, 1981, Pergamon Press.
8. Cuello, C., et al.: Gastric cancer in Columbia. I. Cancer risk and suspect environmental agents, J. Natl. Cancer Inst. **57**:1015, 1976.
9. Day, D.W.: Histopathology of gastric cancer. In Fielding, J.W.L., et al., editors: Gastric cancer, Oxford, 1981, Pergamon Press.
10. Domellof, L., Eriksson, S., and Jaunger, K.G.: Late precancerous changes and carcinoma of the gastric stump after Billroth II resection, Am. J. Surg. **132**:26, 1976.
11. Domellof, L., Eriksson, S., and Jaunger, K.G.: Carcinoma and possible precancerous changes of the gastric stump after Billroth II resection, Gastroenterology **73**:462, 1977.
12. Dupont, J.B., Jr., et al.: Adenocarcinoma of the stomach: review of 1,497 cases, Cancer **41**:941, 1978.
13. Elsborg, L., and Mosbech, J.: Pernicious anemia as a risk factor in gastric cancer, Acta Med. Scand. **206**:315, 1979.
14. Fink, A.S., and Longmire, W.P., Jr.: Carcinoma of the stomach. In Sabiston, D.C., editor: Textbook of surgery, ed. 13, Philadelphia, 1986, W.B. Saunders Co.
15. Fisher, A.S., Graham, N., and Jensen, O.N.: Risk of gastric cancer after Billroth II resection for duodenal ulcer, Br. J. Surg. **70**:552, 1983.
16. Fujimoto, S., Kitsukawa, Y., and Itoh, K.: Carcinoembryonic antigen (CEA) in gastric juice as an aid in the diagnosis of gastrointestinal cancer, Ann. Surg. **189**:34, 1979.
17. Geboes, K., et al.: Histologic appearance of endoscopic gastric mucosal biopsies 10 to 20 years after partial gastrectomy, Ann. Surg. **192**:179, 1980.
18. Gilbertson, V.A.: Results of treatment of stomach cancer. An appraisal of efforts for more extensive surgery and a report of 1,983 cases, Cancer **23**:1305, 1969.
19. Grafe, W., Thorbjarnason, B., and Pearce, J.M.: Benign neoplasms of the stomach, Am. J. Surg. **100**:561, 1960.
20. Haenszel, W., et al.: Stomach cancer among Japanese in Hawaii, J. Natl. Cancer Inst. **49**:969, 1972.
21. Hankland, H., and Johnson, J.A.: Gastric cancer after vagotomy and excision for gastric cancer, Eur. Surg. Res. **13**:371, 1981.
22. Hertzer, N.R., and Hoerr, S.O.: An interpretive review of lymphoma of the stomach, Surg. Gynecol. Obstet. **143**:113, 1976.
23. Hill, M.: Nitrates and bacteriology. Are these important etiologic factors in gastric carcinogenesis? In Fielding, J.W.L., et al., editors: Gastric cancer, Oxford, 1981, Pergamon Press.
24. Hirayama, T.: Changing patterns in the incidence of gastric cancer. In Fielding, J.W.L., et al., editors: Gastric cancer, Oxford, 1981, Pergamon Press.
25. Joosens, J.V., and Geboers, J.: Nutrition and gastric cancer, Proc. Nutr. Soc. **40**:37, 1981.
26. Kajitani, T., and Miwa, K., editors: Treatment results of stomach cancer in Japan, 1963-1966, WHO Monograph No. 2, 1979, WHO Collaborating Center for Evaluation of Methods of Diagnosis and Treatment of Stomach Cancer.
27. Kawai, K., Kizu, M., and Miyaoka, T.: Epidemiology and pathogenesis of gastric cancer, Front. Gastrointest. Res. **6**:71, 1980.
28. Kennedy, B.J.: TNM classification for stomach cancer, Cancer **26**:971, 1970.
29. Kock, N.G., Lewin, E., and Petterson, S.: Partial or total gastrectomy for adenocarcinoma of the cardia, Acta Chir. Scand. **135**:340, 1969.
30. Koga, S., et al.: Prognostic significance of combined splenectomy or pancreatosplenectomy in total and proximal gastrectomy for gastric cancer, Am. J. Surg. **142**:546, 1981.
31. Landres, R.T., and Strum, W.D.: Endoscopic techniques in the diagnosis of gastric adenocarcinoma, Gastrointest. Endosc. **23**:203, 1977.
32. Lauren, P.: The two histological main types of gastric carcinoma: diffuse and so-called intestinal-type carcinoma: an attempt at a his-

tological classification, Acta. Pathol. Microbiol. Scand. **64:**31, 1965.
33. Lee, Y.T.N.: The ABO blood groups and cancer, Surg. Gynecol. Obstet. **132:**1093, 1971.
34. Leviatan, A., et al.: Malignant acanthosis nigricans, Arch. Dermatol. **114:**281, 1978.
35. Lindsay, P., Ordonez, N., and Raaf, J.: Gastric leiomyosarcoma: clinical and pathological review of fifty patients, J. Surg. Oncol. **18:**399, 1981.
36. Longmire, W.P., Jr.: The place of radical surgery in gastric cancer. In Fielding, J.W.L., et al., editors: Gastric cancer, Oxford, 1981, Pergamon Press.
37. Longmire, W.P., Jr., Kuzma, J.W., and Dixon, W.J.: The use of triethylenethiophosphoramide as an adjuvant to the surgical treatment of gastric carcinoma, Ann. Surg. **167:**293, 1968.
38. Lumpkin, W.M., et al.: Carcinoma of the stomach: review of 1035 cases, Ann. Surg. **159:**919, 1964.
39. McFee, A.S., and Aust, J.B.: Gastric carcinoma and the CAT scan, Gastroenterology **80:**196, 1981.
40. Ming, S.C.: Gastric carcinoma: a pathobiological classification, Cancer **39:**2475, 1977.
41. Ming, S.C., and Goldman, H.: Gastric polyps: a histogenetic classification and its relation to carcinoma, Cancer **18:**721, 1965.
42. Morgenstern, L., Yamkawa, T., and Setzer, D.: Carcinoma of the gastric stump, Am. J. Surg. **125:**29, 1973.
43. Morson, B.C., and Dawson, I.M.P.: Gastrointestinal pathology, London, 1979, Blackwell Scientific Publications.
44. Moss, A.A., et al.: Gastric adenocarcinoma: a comparison of the accuracy and economics of staging by computed tomography and surgery, Gastroenterology **80:**45, 1981.
45. Nicholls, J.C.: Stump cancer following gastric surgery, World J. Surg. **3:**731, 1979.
46. Papachristo, D.N., Agnanti, N., and Fortner, J.G.: Gastric carcinoma after treatment of ulcer, Am. J. Surg. **139:**193, 1980.
47. Sancho-Poch, F.J., et al.: An evaluation of gastric biopsy in the diagnosis of gastric cancer, Gastrointest. Endosc. **24:**281, 1978.
48. Schafer, L., et al.: The risk of gastric carcinoma after surgical treatment for benign ulcer disease, N. Engl. J. Med. **309:**1210, 1983.
49. Scharschmidt, B.F.: The natural history of hypertrophic gastropathy (Ménétrier's disease). Report of a case with 16 years follow-up and review of 120 cases from the literature, Am. J. Med. **63:**644, 1977.
50. Schein, P.S., Coffey, R., Jr., and Smith, F.P.: Chemotherapy and combined modality treatment for gastric cancer. In Fielding, J.W.L., et al., editors: Gastric cancer, Oxford, 1981, Pergamon Press.
51. Silverberg, E.: Cancer statistics, 1984, Cancer **34:**7, 1984.
52. Siurala, M.: Gastritis, its fate and sequelae, Ann. Clin. Res. **13:**111, 1981.
53. Stemmermann, G.N., et al.: Serum pepsinogen I and gastrin in relation to extent and location of intestinal metaplasia in the surgically resected stomach, Dig. Dis. **25:**680, 1980.
54. Stocks, P., and Davies, R.I.: Zinc and copper content of soils associated with the incidence of cancer of the stomach and other organs, Br. J. Cancer **18:**14, 1964.
55. Strickland, R.G., and MacKay, I.R.: A reappraisal of the nature and significance of chronic atrophic gastritis, Am. J. Dig. Dis. **18:**426, 1973.
56. Tatsuta, M., et al.: Carcinoembryonic antigen in gastric juice as an aid in diagnosis of early gastric cancer, Cancer **46:**2686, 1980.
57. Tomasulo, J.: Gastric polyps: histologic types and their relationship to gastric carcinoma, Cancer **27:**1354, 1971.
58. Welvart, K., and Warnsinck, H.: The incidence of carcinoma of the gastric remnant, J. Surg. Oncol. **21:**104, 1982.
59. Woolf, C.M., and Isaacson, E.A.: An analysis of 5 "stomach cancer families" in the state of Utah, Cancer **14:**1005, 1961.
60. Zinninger, M.M.: Extension of gastric cancer in the intramural lymphatics and its relation to gastrectomy, Am. J. Surg. **20:**920, 1954.
61. Zinninger, M.M., and Collis, W.T.: Extension of carcinoma of the stomach into the duodenum and esophagus, Ann. Surg. **130:**557, 1949.

18

Thomas A. Miller

Derangements in Gastric Function Secondary to Previous Surgery

Although operative procedures on the stomach are less commonly performed today than they were a decade or two ago because of the decreasing incidence of gastric cancer and the ability to manage most forms of acid-peptic disease with various pharmacologic manipulations, gastric procedures are still performed with sufficient frequency that an understanding of those derangements that may be surgically induced is paramount to good surgical practice. Virtually any type of gastric operation will be attended by some type of postoperative symptomatology; fortunately, the majority of these physiologic alterations can be managed with little patient inconvenience. Despite a surgeon's best efforts, however, a small percentage of patients subjected to gastric surgery will develop untoward sequelae that can be devastating not only to a patient's sense of well-being, but also to his ability to function in society and continue gainful employment. These physiologic aberrations can result from the loss of normal gastric reservoir function, transection of the vagus nerves, interruption of normal pyloric sphincter function, or be directly related to the procedure performed to restore normal gastrointestinal continuity following treatment of the underlying disease. An understanding of the pathophysiology responsible for these various derangements is mandatory if successful management is to be effectively rendered.

DERANGEMENTS RELATED TO GASTRIC RESECTION OR INTERRUPTION OF NORMAL PYLORIC SPHINCTER FUNCTION

Dumping Syndrome

The dumping syndrome refers to the symptom complex that occurs following the ingestion of a meal when a portion of the stomach has previously been removed or the normal pyloric sphincter mechanism has been disrupted. Both an early and late form of this syndrome have been described, with the early form occurring considerably more frequently.

Early Dumping

The early form of the dumping syndrome usually occurs within 10 to 30 minutes following the ingestion of a meal and is associated with both gastrointestinal and cardiovascular symptomatology. The gastrointestinal symptoms include nausea and vomiting, a sense of epigastric fullness, eructations, crampy abdominal pain, and often explosive diarrhea. The cardiovascular symptoms include palpitations, tachycardia, diaphoresis, fainting, dizziness, flushing, and occasionally blurred vision. Characteristically these symptoms occur while the patient is seated at the table eating or shortly after arising. This symptom complex can develop after any operation on the stomach, but it is especially common after partial gastrectomy with a Billroth II reconstruction in which as many as 50% to 60% of patients may be victims, especially if more than two thirds of the stomach has been removed. Less commonly it is observed after a Billroth I gastrectomy and in patients following vagotomy and drainage procedures, particularly if the type of drainage was a generous gastroenterostomy or a Finney-type pyloroplasty. Only rarely does this full-blown symptom complex supervene, and usually the gastrointestinal symptomatology is more frequently encountered than the vasomotor aberrations.

Although the exact sequence of events responsible for this syndrome remains to be defined, there is general agreement that it occurs because of the rapid passage of food of high osmolarity from the stomach into the small intestine.[20,43] This occurs because the previous gastric resection or interrupted pyloric sphincteric mechanism no longer allows the stomach to prepare its contents and deliver them to the proximal bowel in the form of small particles in isosmotic solution. Thus the resulting discharge of this hyperosmotic chyme into the small intestine induces a rapid shift of extracellular fluid into the intestinal lumen to achieve isotonicity. The luminal distention that follows and the autonomic responses induced by the resultant decrease in circulating plasma volume are thought to be responsible for many of the symptoms of this syndrome.

To what extent the contracted blood volume per se gives rise to the autonomic symptoms following dumping remains to be clarified since a number of studies have failed to demonstrate a clear correlation between the severity of symptoms and the magnitude of blood volume derangements.[20] On the other hand, several other studies have implicated a role for various vasoactive substances released in response to the intestinal distention. Serotonin, for example, is released from the intestine in response to distention, and serotonin antagonists have been shown to benefit some patients with dumping symptoms.[29,39] Evidence also exists that plasma levels of a bradykinin-like substance are elevated during dumping attacks and that bradykinin can reproduce many of the vasomotor components of the syndrome when administered exogenously.[54] Finally, plasma enteroglucagon concentrations are increased in symptomatic postgastrectomy patients following a glucose challenge, in contrast to nondumping controls.[5] In addition, this agent inhibits sodium and water absorption from the small intestine and through such a mechanism could account for the diarrhea that occurs in early dumping.

Generally the symptoms associated with dumping are sufficiently obvious that the diagnosis can be made on this basis alone. It must be emphasized, however, that in any group of patients complaining of dumpinglike symptoms, a high proportion of individuals with social problems, various neuroses, and occasionally alcoholism may be present.[16] Thus, if any doubt exists concerning the exact cause of the symptomatology, objective support for the diagnosis should be obtained, especially if a surgical procedure to correct the problem is potentially anticipated. This would include the demonstration of rapid gastric emptying on upper gastrointestinal barium study or by assessment with one of the currently available radionuclide techniques.[13] Another diagnostic approach is use of a provocation test in which a patient is given a meal of 200 ml of a 50% glucose solution in water.[33] In patients with the dumping syndrome, instillation of this liquid meal into the residual stomach has been shown to provoke the symptom complex concomitant with a fall in plasma volume.

It is of interest that the majority of patients subjected to gastric surgery will complain of some dumpinglike symptoms in the early months following surgery. Most of these individuals, however, will experience spontaneous relief and require no specific treatment.[9,48] Of those patients plagued with prolonged symptomatology, dietary measures alone can effect adequate management in most instances. Such measures should include avoiding foods containing large amounts of sugars, frequent feeding of small meals rich in protein and fat, and separating liquids from solids during a meal. If hot drinks elicit symptoms, as occurs in some patients, they should also be avoided. Lying down when symptoms do occur may likewise be beneficial since gravity can aggravate dumping symptomatology. In some patients, carbohydrate gelling agents such as pectin have been ingested with the meal and shown to be of some success[28]; unfortunately, these agents are rather unpalatable and not readily tolerated for long periods of time. Serotonin antagonists are the only pharmacologic agents that have proved to be of possible benefit in the relief of dumping symptoms. Both methysergide maleate (Sansert) and cyproheptadine (Periactin) have been helpful in some individuals when given before meals.[29] Usually large dosages of such agents are required, producing their own disagreeable side effects. Thus their use in any long-term fashion is limited.

In the few patients (1% or less) who fail to respond to these treatment measures, operative intervention may become necessary. The physiologic rationale behind surgery should be to improve gastric reservoir function, decrease the rapid gastric emptying, or hopefully accomplish both of these goals. Although a wide variety of surgical procedures have been used to manage dumping, the use of isoperistaltic or antiperistaltic jejunal segments has met with the greatest success in dealing with this problem in most centers (Fig. 18-1). With the former approach, a 10- to 20-cm loop of jejunum is interposed between the stomach and small intestine in an isoperistaltic fashion.[34,40] Over time this loop dilates and thereby promotes reservoir function. It also appears to delay gastric emptying, at least that of liquids. In the antiperistaltic approach a jejunal segment 10 cm in length is used, in which the jejunum is twisted on its mesentery so that its distal end is anastomosed to the stomach and its proximal end to the small intestine.[40,47] The resulting reversal in peristalsis permits the loop to act as a substitute pylorus, enabling it to slow the rate of gastric emptying and thereby allow more time for mixing and grinding of food before delivery into the small bowel. Published experience with this latter technique is now in excess of 10 years, demonstrating significant alleviation of symptoms in more than 90% of patients.[47] Another technique of recent interest is the creation of a long-limb Roux-en-Y anastomosis to delay gastric emptying (see Fig. 18-1).[27] It remains to be determined what long-term benefit this approach will offer, but early results have been encouraging.

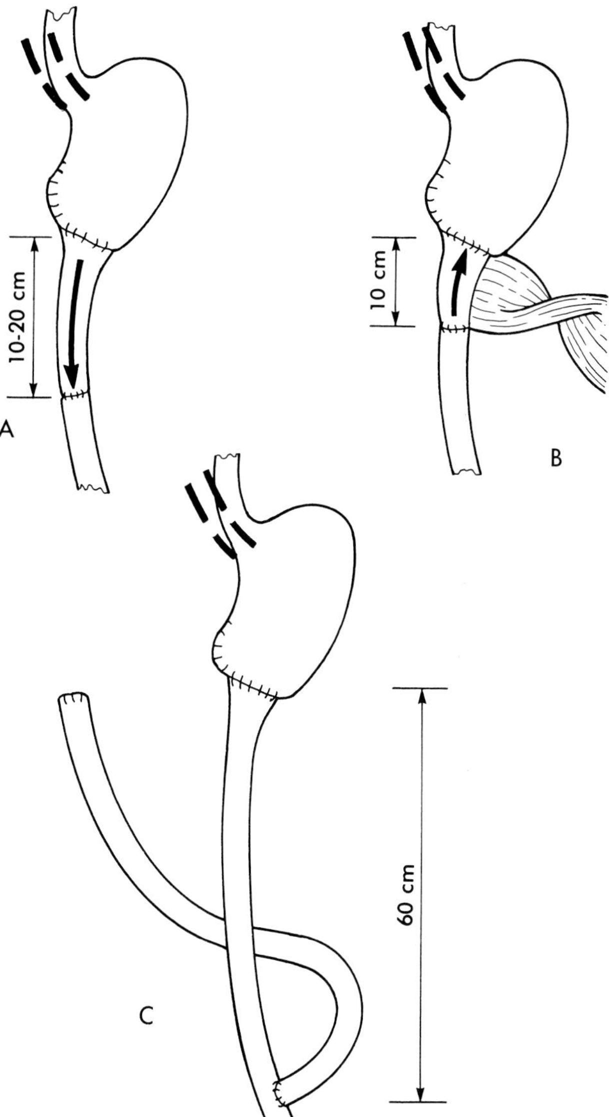

Fig. 18-1 Surgical approaches to treat the dumping syndrome. **A,** A 10- to 20-cm loop of jejunum is interposed between the stomach and the small intestine in an isoperistaltic fashion. **B,** A 10-cm loop of jejunum is twisted on its mesentery so that its distal end is anastomosed to the stomach, and its proximal end to the small intestine in an antiperistaltic fashion. **C,** A long-limb Roux-en-Y anastomosis where the jejunojejunostomy is fashioned approximately 60 cm from the gastrojejunostomy.

Late Dumping

Late dumping occurs 2 to 3 hours after a meal and is considerably less common than its early counterpart. Like early dumping, the basic defect in this disorder is also rapid gastric emptying. In this situation, however, it is related specifically to carbohydrates and can be induced by meals containing large amounts of monosaccharides or disaccharides. When these sugars are delivered rapidly to the small intestine, they are quickly absorbed. The resulting hyperglycemia triggers the release of large amounts of insulin to control the rising blood sugar. In the attempt to normalize blood sugar, an actual ''over-shooting'' occurs so that a profound hypoglycemia ensues.[20] Catecholamine released by the adrenal gland is then activated, with the resulting symptoms of diaphoresis, tremulousness, lightheadedness, tachycardia, and confusion. This symptom complex is indistinguishable from insulin shock.

As with early dumping, patients should be advised to ingest frequent small meals and markedly reduce their carbohydrate intake. Pectin has also been used in the treatment of this disorder, either alone or in combination with acarbose, an alpha-glucoside hydrolase inhibitor, a compound that delays carbohydrate absorption through impairment of intraluminal starch and sucrose digestion.[28,49] If these nonoperative approaches fail, the use of an antiperistaltic loop of jejunum between the residual gastric pouch and intestine has also been shown to effectively manage this problem (see Fig. 18-1). Not only does this loop delay gastric emptying, but it also results in a flattening of the glucose tolerance curve and an alleviation of the hypoglycemic symptomatology.[18]

Small Stomach Syndrome

If an excessive amount of the stomach has been removed, leaving only a small gastric pouch, some patients may develop the small stomach syndrome. This syndrome is characterized by extreme discomfort following the ingestion of even small amounts of food. Because of this unpleasant sensation and the fact that vomiting often occurs if any attempt is made to increase oral intake, patients with this disorder are frequently malnourished. The exact cause of this disorder is uncertain, but it probably develops because of the inability of the proximal stomach to dilate and receive a bolus of food without increasing intragastric pressure.[43] Normally the vagus nerve, which has been transsected in most of these patients, initiates distention of the stomach to allow accommodation of ingested food, a process known as receptive relaxation. If this vagally mediated action has been interrupted, such relaxation does not occur, and the intragastric pressure increases with distention on reception of food.

Unfortunately, treatment of this problem has remained extremely difficult. Although frequent small feedings and various liquid and enteral diets have been tried to alleviate symptoms, such nonoperative approaches have usually been unsuccessful. A number of operative approaches have

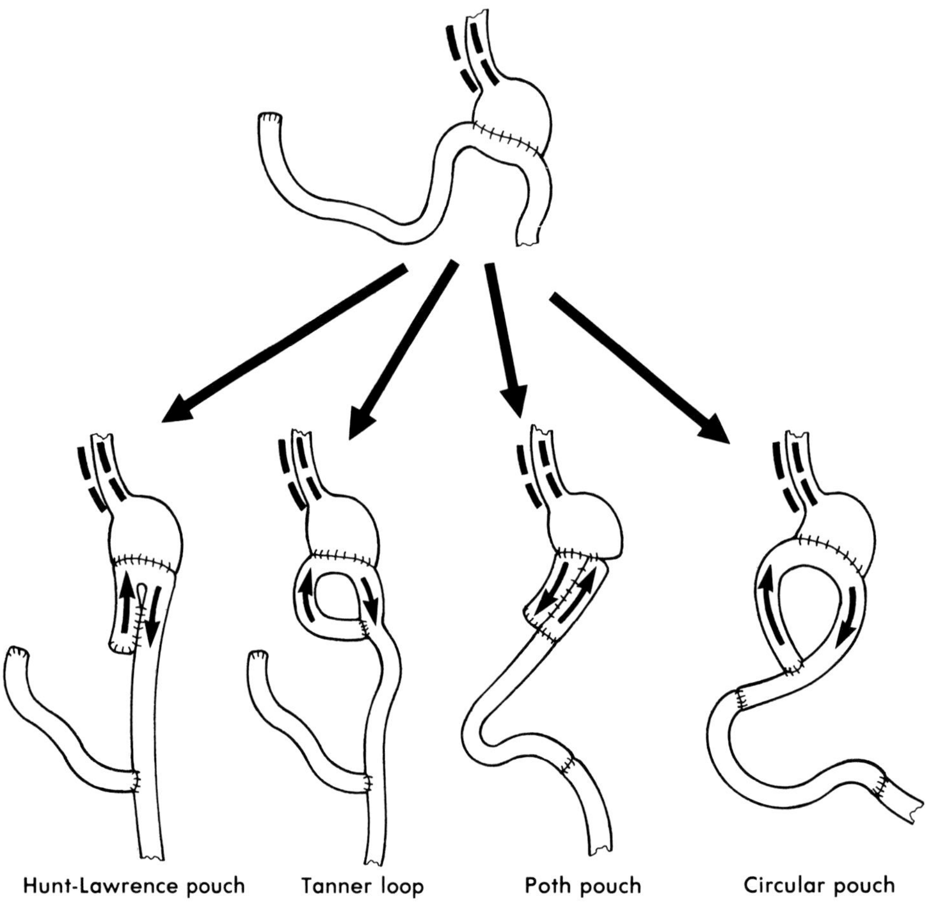

Fig. 18-2 Surgical management of the short stomach syndrome.

also been used with varying degrees of success. These have included procedures to enlarge the gastric reservoir through the creation of various pouches interposed between the stomach and intestine (Fig. 18-2).[46] Jejunal interposition with the use of an isoperistaltic limb has also been used to treat this disorder with reasonable success in alleviating symptoms and improving the underlying malnutrition problems.[11] In view of the difficulty in managing this disorder, the best approach is to prevent its development rather than to attempt to treat it when it occurs.

Gastric Stump Carcinoma

As discussed in Chapter 17, a number of reports over the past several decades have suggested that patients undergoing previous gastric operations (particularly gastric resections) are at increased risk for the development of carcinoma in the gastric stump. Unfortunately, most of these reports have been anecdotal in nature and lacking in appropriate control populations. However, several recent studies have prospectively followed such patients and have failed to demonstrate an increased incidence of carcinoma when compared with the population at large. Thus the original concern for this potential problem appears to be unwarranted.

Metabolic Disturbances

Metabolic problems may develop following any type of gastric procedure, but they are more common and serious after partial gastrectomy than after vagotomy, and the incidence following gastrectomy is much greater if a Billroth II rather than a Billroth I approach has been used in reconstruction.[1] As with dumping, the severity of these disturbances is directly related to the extent of the gastric resection.

Anemia is clearly the most common metabolic derangement. Two major types have been identified: (1) that related to a deficiency of iron, and (2) that related to an impairment in vitamin B_{12} metabolism. Of the two, iron deficiency is the more common, and over 30% to 50% of patients carefully evaluated will demonstrate this type of anemia following gastrectomy. The exact cause has remained elusive, but it appears to be related to a combination of: (1) decreased iron intake; (2) impaired iron absorption; and (3) chronic subliminal blood loss secondary to the hyperemic, friable gastric mucosa primarily involving the margins of the stoma where the stomach connects with the small intestine.[1,43] Generally the addition of iron supplements to the patient's diet will correct this problem.

A megaloblastic anemia can also occur following subtotal gastrectomy (50% or greater) but only rarely develops after partial gastric resection (e.g., antrectomy). This problem is caused by a deficiency of vitamin B_{12} secondary to poor absorption of this substance because of the lack of intrinsic factor secretion in the gastric juice.[1,43] The more extensive the gastric resection, the more likely is this deficiency; it always occurs following total gastrectomy. If a patient develops a macrocytic anemia, a serum B_{12} level should be obtained. If this is abnormal, the patient should be treated by intramuscular injection of cyanocobalamin every 3 to 4 months indefinitely since its administration orally is not a reliable route. The other cause of macrocytosis is a folate deficiency. This is a rare anemia following gastric resection, but it may coexist with an iron or B_{12} deficiency anemia. It is usually a consequence of inadequate oral intake and can generally be corrected by dietary supplementation.

Impaired absorption of fat is relatively common following any type of gastric operation, but the magnitude of fecal fat loss is usually small and of little importance clinically. Occasionally, steatorrhea is seen after a Billroth II gastrectomy and probably occurs as a result of inadequate mixing of bile salts and pancreatic lipase with ingested fat because of bypass of the duodenum. When this results, deficiencies in the uptake of fat-soluble vitamins may also be observed. For mild degrees of fat malabsorption, no treatment is indicated. If steatorrhea develops, pancreatic replacement enzymes are often effective in decreasing fat loss. Feeding with medium-chain triglycerides is also of value since these substances do not require bile and pancreatic lipase for absorption.

Occasionally, gastric resection is associated with the development of bone disease. Both osteoporosis and osteomalasia have been observed and appear to be caused by deficiencies in calcium absorption. If fat malabsorption is also present, the calcium problem is further aggravated since free fatty acids bind calcium; further, fat malabsorption also inhibits the absorption of vitamin D, an important component in normal calcium balance.[43] The incidence of this problem clearly increases with the extent of gastric resection and is mainly an aberration associated with a Billroth II gastrectomy.[1,37] Usually the bone disease develops insidiously, and symptoms are generally not seen until 4 or 5 years after surgery. Occasionally spontaneous fractures or unexplained aches and pains in the back or bones may be the only indication that a calcium deficiency exists. Treatment of this disorder is usually straightforward and includes the administration of calcium supplements (1 to 2 g/day) and vitamin D (500 to 5000 U daily). In patients developing postgastrectomy bone disease, serial serum calcium determinations are indicated, and adjustments in calcium supplementation and vitamin D administration are altered accordingly.

Weight loss is relatively common following surgical procedures on the stomach but is generally not a significant problem, except in those individuals who have had either all or substantial portions of their stomach removed, in which case considerable malnutrition may develop. The degree of weight loss correlates closely with such factors as the presence or absence of dumping, steatorrhea, diarrhea, abdominal discomfort during eating, and bilious vomiting.[38,55] Treatment of malnutrition is directed at improving nutritional balance by multiple small feedings, avoidance of factors that may precipitate the dumping syndrome, and dietary or pharmacologic management of diarrhea and/or steatorrhea. If such manipulations are not successful in treating this problem, some type of surgical procedure to delay gastric emptying and/or enhance the gastric reservoir effect, as outlined previously, may become necessary.

DERANGEMENTS RELATED TO GASTRIC RECONSTRUCTION

A number of disorders may develop following gastric resection that are directly related to the approach used to establish gastrointestinal continuity. All of these problems are more commonly encountered in patients who have had a Billroth II gastrectomy, and the afferent loop and retained antrum syndromes occur exclusively in patients with this type of gastrectomy.

Afferent Loop Syndrome

The afferent loop syndrome is a mechanical problem produced by partial obstruction of the afferent loop resulting in its inability to empty its contents. Consequently, it can only occur following gastrectomy with a Billroth II type of reconstruction. A variety of causes can give rise to this obstruction, including angulation of the anastomosis with kinking, herniation of the afferent loop posterior to the efferent loop, stenosis of the gastrojejunostomy, valvulus, and adhesions (Fig. 18-3). This disorder is nearly always associated with the presence of a long (greater than 30 to 40 cm) afferent limb that has been anastomosed to the gastric remnant in an anticolic fashion. Both acute and chronic forms of this disorder have been recognized, but chronic afferent loop obstruction is clearly more common.[30,36]

From a pathophysiologic standpoint, the syndrome occurs because of an accumulation of pancreatic and hepatobiliary secretions within the obstructed loop, resulting in its distention. The stimulus for such secretion is the presence of food in the gastric remnant and efferent loop, which elicits the various neurohumoral mechanisms involved in normal digestion. Such distention results in epigastric discomfort and cramping. If the loop is only partially obstructed, the increasing intraluminal pressure is usually capable of overcoming it, following which the afferent loop empties its contents into the stomach, resulting in forceful (and sometimes projectile) vomiting of bilious material with immediate relief of symptoms. The vomitus lacks food since any ingested meal has already passed into the efferent limb. If the obstruction is complete, necrosis and perforation of the loop can occur. This is a consequence of the surgical closure of the proximal duodenum that is performed during a Billroth II gastrectomy, resulting in a closed-loop type of obstruction. In this circumstance, constant abdominal pain is noted that can involve the entire upper abdomen, often more pronounced in the right upper quadrant, with radiation into the interscapular area. Unless this distention is surgically relieved, a lethal outcome may ensue from perforation and subsequent peritonitis.

In most patients suffering from the afferent loop syndrome, only partial obstruction of the afferent limb is present.[30,36] Symptoms may exist for months or sometimes even years. These symptoms are directly related to eating, at which time the hepatobiliary and pancreatic secretions distend the loop. Bile-stained material devoid of food is vomited after the meal has passed into the efferent limb, relieving symptoms; and the patient is relatively comfortable until the next meal. Obviously the degree of afferent loop obstruction will influence the extent to which the patient is incapacitated by his symptoms and the need to seek medical treatment. If partial afferent loop obstruction has been present for a long period, it may be aggravated by the development of the blind loop syndrome. In this condition, bacterial overgrowth of enteric organisms proliferates in the static loop and binds with vitamin B_{12} and deconjugated bile acids.[43] This results in a systemic deficiency of vitamin B_{12} with the development of a megaloblastic anemia and an inefficient micellization of fat that, if severe enough, can create steatorrhea.

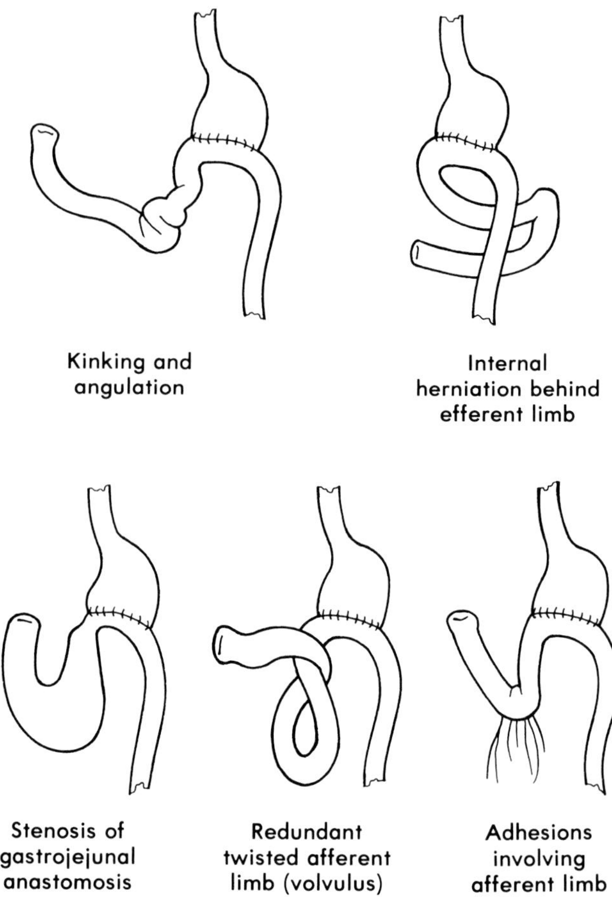

Fig. 18-3 Causes of the afferent loop syndrome.

The acute form of afferent loop obstruction may occur early after operation (within a few days) or may develop quite unexpectedly months to years following the Billroth II gastrectomy. In both circumstances it is caused by acute blockage of the afferent limb as may occur with volvulus or herniation of the afferent loop posterior to the efferent loop. Because of the resulting closed-loop type of obstruction, acute afferent loop obstruction needs to be corrected by immediate operation. Although physical findings are usually nonspecific with the exception of the occurrence of a palpable abdominal mass in about one third of patients,[43] the associated pain and tenderness are usually severe enough to indicate the necessity of urgent operative intervention. Even if the diagnosis may not have been made before surgery, findings at surgery will confirm the underlying cause.

In contrast to the diagnosis of the acute form, that of

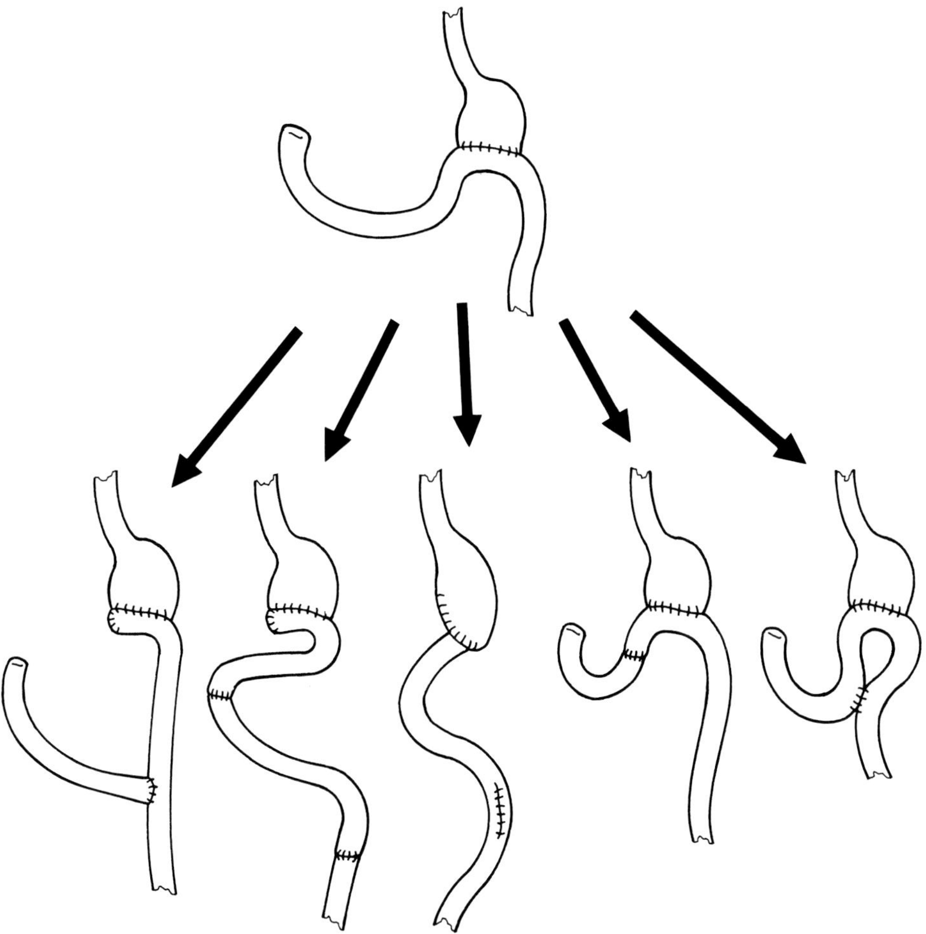

Fig. 18-4 Surgical management of the afferent loop syndrome.

chronic afferent loop obstruction may be more difficult. Although symptoms are often suggestive of this abnormality, confirmation of the diagnosis may be difficult. Usually the dilated afferent limb is not demonstrable on plain films of the abdomen, and only occasionally will contrast barium studies of the stomach delineate the presence of an obstructed loop. Failure to visualize the afferent limb on upper endoscopy is suggestive evidence for the diagnosis. Recently hepatobiliary radionuclide imaging techniques have been used with some success in diagnosing the afferent loop syndrome.[43] With this technique the hepatic excretion of a previously administered radionuclide is followed after giving a patient a fatty meal or the hormone cholecystokinin. If the nuclide fails to pass into the stomach or distal bowel after being excreted into the afferent limb, the possibility of an afferent loop obstruction needs to be considered. Although this technique shows diagnostic promise, its clinical usefulness remains to be determined.

Because the afferent loop syndrome, whether acute or chronic, is a mechanical problem, operation is the only effective treatment. With few exceptions, a long afferent limb is usually the underlying problem. Thus treatment will involve the elimination of this loop. A variety of procedures have been advocated to accomplish this feat, including the conversion of a Billroth II construction into a Billroth I anastomosis, enteroenterostomy below the stoma, and the use of a Roux-en-Y anastomosis (Fig. 18-4).[20] If the latter procedure is used, a concomitant vagotomy should also be performed to prevent marginal ulceration from the diversion of duodenal contents from the gastroenteric stoma.

Efferent Loop Obstruction

Compared to other derangements in gastric function following previous surgery, obstruction of the efferent limb of a gastrojejunostomy is relatively rare. Clearly the most common cause of such obstruction is herniation of the limb behind the anastomosis in a right-to-left direction.[45] This problem occurs because of the space that exists posterior to the anastomosis after construction of a gastrojejunostomy and has been described with both antecolic and retrocolic gastrojejunostomies. The preference for herniation in the right-to-left direction most likely results from the fact that the gastrojejunostomy lies to the left of the main mass of small intestine, thus making it mechanically easier for herniation to occur from right to left.[20] Although obstruction of the efferent loop is the usual circumstance with this type of herniation, it may also compress the mesentery of the afferent limb and thereby compromise its blood supply and/or obstruct the afferent limb as well.

Efferent limb obstruction following gastrojejunostomy from a retroanastomotic hernia may occur at any time following surgery, but more than half of the patients who develop this disorder do so within the first postoperative month. Diagnosis is frequently difficult. Initial complaints include colicky left upper quadrant pain; copious, bilious vomiting; and abdominal distention. Usually the most helpful diagnostic maneuver is a contrast barium study of the stomach in which barium fails to enter the efferent limb. Operative therapy is virtually always required and consists of reducing the retroanastomotic hernia and ensuring that the retroanastomic space is securely closed to prevent recurrence of this condition.

Alkaline Reflux Gastritis

Reflux of bile into the stomach is relatively common following surgical procedures on this organ. In a small percentage of patients this reflux is associated with severe, continuous, unrelenting epigastric pain and bilious vomiting and weight loss.[6,8,12,41-43] Occasionally this pain is substernal in nature, but, despite its location, it is characteristically not relieved by food or antacids. The bilious vomiting may occur at any time during the day or night and not uncommonly awakens a patient from sleep. On endoscopic examination of the stomach, the mucosa is noted to be beefy red, friable, and frequently demonstrating superficial erosions that may extend into the distal esophagus. Microscopically both parietal and chief cells are greatly diminished, and superficial mucosal ulcerations are common with evidence of hemorrhage, atrophy, and intestinalization of the epithelial surface. It is not uncommon for achlorhydria to be present in many of these patients; and little, if any, response is elicited following stimulation with a secretagogue such as pentagastrin. Associated with these findings is the frequent demonstration of an iron deficiency anemia and weight loss. Since patients with this constellation of signs and symptoms are lacking in other explainable causes, the association of an alkaline gastric content, endoscopic gastritis in combination with bile reflux, and histologic confirmation of mucosal injury has been termed alkaline reflux gastritis.[41-43]

In most patients who develop alkaline reflux gastritis, gastric resection with restoration of gastrointestinal continuity with a Billroth II approach has been used.[43] The syndrome has also been reported after gastroduodenostomy or gastroenterostomy and in a few patients who have undergone vagotomy and drainage procedures.[8] Symptoms may develop any time following operation and have been observed as late as 20 years following surgery. Although bile reflux appears to be the inciting event, a number of problems remain unanswered with respect to the role of bile in its pathogenesis.[41-43] For example, both clinical and experimental reports indicate that enterogastric reflux is quite common following gastric surgery, although gastric mucosal injury is not an invariable consequence of this circumstance. In addition, asymptomatic patients frequently demonstrate histologic and endoscopic changes in the gastric epithelium not unlike those with symptoms of alkaline reflux gastritis. Finally, a clear correlation between the volume of bile and its composition (i.e., primary and secondary bile acid components) and the subsequent development of alkaline gastritis has never been proved. Thus, although it appears that the syndrome does in fact exist, caution must be exercised to be sure that it is not overdiagnosed.

Although a variety of approaches have been used to manage the symptoms of alkaline reflux gastritis, medical treatment has usually failed in this condition. Antacids, cimetidine, anticholinergics, and cholestyramine have all been tried to relieve symptoms without consistently demonstrating efficacious results. Consequently, patients who have intractable problems with this disorder should undergo surgery. The principle underlying surgery is to divert the bile and pancreatic secretions away from the stomach. Although a large number of approaches have been used to accomplish this feat, the most effective operative procedure in terms of relieving symptoms, promoting weight gain, and reversing the findings seen in alkaline gastritis has been achieved with the use of a Roux-en-Y gastrojejunostomy in which the Roux limb has been 41 to 46 cm in length.[21,42,43]

Retained Antrum Syndrome

Occasionally inadequate resection of the gastric antrum may occur during partial gastrectomy, even though the resection was carried beyond the pyloric sphincter. This happens because the antral mucosa may extend past the pyloric muscle for a distance of 0.5 cm.[44] The significance in remembering this is that a Billroth II anastomosis can result in the development of a retained antrum syndrome if residual antrum is included in the duodenal stump. This circumstance allows the retained antrum to be continually exposed to an alkaline pH from the duodenal, pancreatic, and biliary juices that may in turn stimulate the release of large amounts of gastrin with a corresponding continuous hypersecretion of hydrochloric acid in the gastric remnant. This highly ulcerogenic preparation is responsible for about 9% of recurrent ulcers following previous surgery for peptic ulcer disease and is associated with an incidence of recurrent ulceration as high as 80%.[3,50] This potential problem can virtually be eliminated if biopsy confirmation of duodenal mucosa is obtained during resection of the proximal duodenum at the time of a Billroth II gastrectomy.

If a patient develops a recurrent ulcer following previous gastrectomy for ulcer disease in which a Billroth II anastomosis was fashioned, the possibility of a retained antrum must be entertained. To exclude this possibility, a technetium scan may prove helpful.[10] In patients having a retained antrum, this scan demonstrates a hot spot that is adjacent to the area where normal uptake of technetium by the gastric mucosa of the remaining stomach occurs. Antral cuffs as small as 1 cm have been detected experimentally with this technique.[10] If a retained antrum is diagnosed, pharmacologic management with an H_2 receptor blocker may prove helpful in controlling the acid hypersecretion. If this is not effective, either conversion of the Billroth II anastomosis to a Billroth I reconstruction or excision of the retained antral tissue in the duodenal stump with reclosure should obviate the problem.

Jejunogastric Intussusception

Jejunogastric intussusception is a rare entity that results when the afferent or efferent limb intussuscepts into the stomach or residual gastric pouch. It may occur in any patient whose stomach has been anastomosed to the jejunum but has been most commonly seen following simple gastroenterostomy. Both acute and chronic variants have been described.[53] Although surgical intervention is the treatment of choice for both types of the disease, it is a surgical emergency in the acute variety to prevent strangulation of the intussuscepted bowel. Foster[19] has summarized the important features of diagnosis and has emphasized that any patient who has had gastric surgery (i.e., gastric resection or gastroenterostomy) and who subsequently develops the following should be suspected of having jejunogastric intussusception until proven otherwise:

1. Severe epigastric pain
2. Persistent vomiting (either bile-stained or bloody)
3. A palpable epigastric mass
4. Tenderness over the epigastrium
5. Any combination of these signs or symptoms

The more chronic form of the disease is less dramatic clinically and usually presents as recurrent episodes of vague upper abdominal pain that is exacerbated by meals. The pain ceases after eating because the intussuscepted limb reduces itself. Although jejunogastric intussusception may involve either the afferent or efferent limbs, the efferent limb is the more common intussuscipiens and is responsible for more than 80% of the reported cases.[53] Depending on findings at surgery, surgical approaches may include reduction of the intussuscepted intestine and/or its resection, takedown of the anastomosis, or its revision. Generally the afferent and efferent limbs of jejunum are also fixed to adjacent tissue such as the mesocolon, colon, or stomach to prevent recurrence.

DERANGEMENTS RELATED TO VAGAL TRANSECTION

Postvagotomy Diarrhea

Diarrhea of varying degrees is relatively common following gastric surgery, and, if carefully questioned, 30% or more of patients will indicate some difficulty with this problem.[25] Fortunately, it is not severe in the majority of individuals and often disappears within the first 3 or 4 months following surgery. In many patients with diarrhea, it is part of the dumping syndrome. As the patient develops more discriminating eating habits, the dumping improves along with the diarrhea. Distinct from the diarrhea associated with an inadequate gastric reservoir, vagotomy itself is associated with alterations in stool frequency. As many as 30% to 70% of patients report an increased frequency in daily bowel movements following truncal vagotomy.[14,22-24,32] For a previously constipated patient, this is often viewed as beneficial. In some patients, actual diarrhea develops that may occur two to three times weekly or manifest itself once or twice a month at which times it lasts 3 or 4 days. In others, it may be more explosive, resulting in the soiling of clothing. Between attacks, bowel movements may be entirely normal. Fortunately, most patients developing diarrhea following vagotomy find a diminution in this problem with time.

The mechanisms responsible for postvagotomy diarrhea have remained elusive. That it indeed occurs is borne out by the Leeds/York trial, in which 7% of patients developed diarrhea following subtotal gastrectomy, compared to an impressive 23% who underwent resection of the same magnitude in combination with a truncal vagotomy.[22-24] Bacterial overgrowth in the upper gastrointestinal tract has been proposed as one possible mechanism on the basis of the observation that colonization of the jejunum with aerobic and anaerobic bacteria is relatively common following vagotomy. The problem with this hypothesis is that the degree of overgrowth does not appear to be different in patients developing postvagotomy diarrhea and those who are asymptomatic.[7] Denervation of the intestine in dogs following truncal vagotomy was shown to enhance the movement of small intestinal contents into the colon through a loss of the sphinteric mechanism of the ileal cecal valve.[2] Although a similar circumstance may occur in humans, data relative to that issue are unknown. However, other experimental observations have failed to uncover differences in small intestinal morphology, small intestinal fluxes of fluid and electrolytes, or the fecal output of fat in patients with and without vagotomy.[20] Some studies have suggested a more rapid gastric emptying in patients developing postvagotomy diarrhea compared with those without this problem, but consensus on this issue is far from uniform.[20] Although the incidence of postvagotomy diarrhea in patients who are subjected to selective vagotomy was initially reported as being less than a comparable group receiving truncal vagotomy, further follow-up with larger groups of patients has not borne out this contention.[20,31]

From a therapeutic standpoint, it is known that cholestyramine, an anionic exchange resin that absorbs bile salts and thereby renders them unabsorbable and inactive, can significantly decrease the severity of diarrhea in patients developing this problem following vagotomy.[4] The possible explanation for this relates to the finding of Allan, Gerskovitch, and Russell[2] who noted that, although the total bile acid content in the stools of patients was not significantly greater in the presence or absence of diarrhea, those with postvagotomy diarrhea excreted more than twice the amount of chenodeoxycholic acid than vagotomy patients without diarrhea.

Because postvagotomy diarrhea is usually a self-limited disease, treatment should be symptomatic. In the 5% of patients in whom symptoms are severe and interfere drastically with life-style, cholestyramine is the treatment of choice. Ayulo[4] noted improvement within 1 to 4 weeks of treatment with this agent in almost all patients receiving the drug. Significant decreases in urgency, frequency, and severity of diarrhea were all noted. Treatment consists of 4 g of cholestyramine with meals three times daily and adjusted to a maintenance dosage, allowing one to two well-formed bowel movements per day.[4]

Only in extremely rare instances is operative treatment justified for postvagotomy diarrhea. When diarrhea has remained incapacitating for at least 1 year following initial operation and fails to respond to cholestyramine therapy, remedial surgery is indicated. If patients are selected properly, this will involve no more than 1% of all patients undergoing vagotomy. The operative procedure of choice is to interpose a 10-cm segment of reversed jejunum 70 to

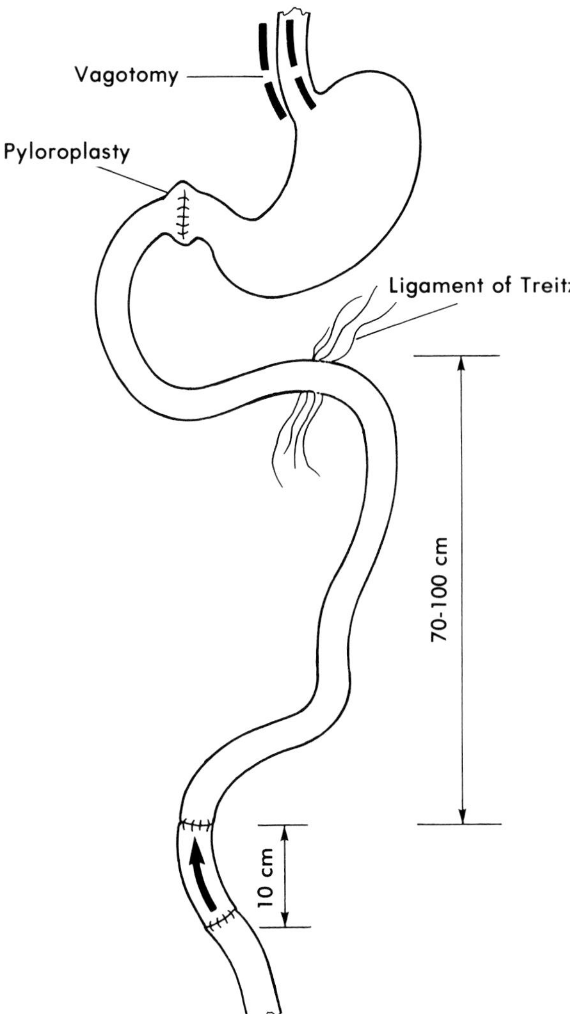

Fig. 18-5 Surgical management of postvagotomy diarrhea.

100 cm from the ligament of Treitz (Fig. 18-5).[26] In patients subjected to this operation, sustained relief from diarrhea has resulted.

Postvagotomy Dysphagia

Although it is rare, occasionally after vagotomy a patient will complain of dysphagia that is usually noted within the first 2 weeks following operation. It is probably related to edema or an intramural hematoma of the esophagus resulting from injury to the esophageal wall at the time of vagal section and is more commonly noted after the transthoracic approach of performing a vagotomy than following a transabdominal procedure.[15,51] Radiologically the disorder resembles achalasia; but, unlike this disease, liquids pass easily, whereas solids usually evoke symptoms. Esophagoscopic and manometric findings are usually normal, indicating that both esophageal sphincter function and peristalsis are intact. Treatment is usually symptomatic since the condition generally disappears spontaneously within 2 to 12 weeks of vagotomy. If dysphagia is particularly troublesome, esophageal dilation may be indicated with the use of a mercury-weighted bougie such as a Maloney dilator.

Postvagotomy Gastric Atony

Delayed gastric emptying is also a consequence of vagotomy, and it is for this reason that a drainage procedure needs to be performed when a truncal or selective vagotomy is performed. This relates to the normal function of the vagus in adjusting gastric tone to the volume of the stomach so that peristalsis is initiated and coordinated properly. Since parietal cell vagotomy does not disrupt this function because of the maintenance of antral innervation, postvagotomy atony is not a problem with this procedure.

Sometimes after vagotomy (i.e., truncal or selective) and an apparently adequately performed drainage procedure, a patient may have persistent and bothersome gastric stasis that causes food to be retained in the stomach for several hours. Usually this is accompanied by no more than a feeling of fullness in the midepigastrium. At times this will be associated with marked abdominal pain and rarer still with a functional gastric outlet obstruction. If endoscopic examination of the stomach reveals no evidence of a true anatomic obstruction, watchful waiting is usually the treatment of choice. Occasionally short-term treatment with metoclopramide is indicated to improve gastric tone.[35]

Incomplete Vagal Transection

Since vagotomy is an important component of the surgical treatment of peptic ulcer disease, it is important that vagal transection of the acid-secreting portion of the stomach be complete. If this is not ensured, the patient is predisposed to the possibility of recurrent ulcer formation. The type of vagotomy influences the likelihood of this circumstance. In highly selective vagotomy (i.e., parietal cell) in which meticulous vagal denervation of the stomach is accomplished, an incomplete vagotomy is rarely a problem. In contrast, truncal vagotomy may be associated with a high incidence of incomplete transection because of the variability in size of the two vagal trunks and their anatomic position. Although inadequate transection of either vagus may occur during truncal vagotomy, the right vagus is inadequately transected three times more frequently than the left vagus.[17,52] This relates to the fact that the right vagus is frequently buried in the right periesophageal fibroareolar tissue in contrast to the left vagus, which usually hugs the anterior esophageal surface. The likelihood of incomplete vagotomy can be greatly lessened by confirming vagal transection histologically at the time of operation by frozen section examination of excised nerve tissue.

SUMMARY

Derangements in gastric function are common following operations on the stomach. These aberrations in normal physiology can result from a loss of gastric reservoir function when a portion of the stomach has been removed, from motility disturbances secondary to transection of the vagus nerves, or from interruption of the normal pyloric sphincter mechanism secondary to pyloroplasty; or they can be directly related to the type of reconstructive procedure that has been undertaken to restore normal gastrointestinal continuity. Although most patients will experience some type of postoperative symptomatology following a gastric operation, many of these problems are short-lived and will abate with time. In a small percentage of patients, however, significant untoward sequelae will result that may require substantial dietary manipulation and occasionally pharmacologic management to alleviate distressing signs and symptoms and enable a patient to function adequately in society. Occasionally reoperation will become necessary to correct the underlying physiologic dysfunction. Fortunately, patients in this latter category are less commonly seen today than they were a decade or so ago because of the decreasing incidence of gastric cancer and the development of new strategies to manage acid-peptic diseases of the stomach, both of which have resulted in fewer operative procedures involving the stomach.

REFERENCES

1. Alexander-Williams, J., and Donovan, I.A.: Postgastrectomy and postvagotomy syndromes and their management. In Glass, G.B.J., and Sherlock, P., editors: Progress in gastroenterology, vol. IV, New York, 1983, Grune & Stratton, Inc.
2. Allan, J.C., Gerskovitch, V.P., and Russell, R.I.: The role of bile acids in the pathogenesis of postvagotomy diarrhea, Br. J. Surg. **61**:516, 1974.
3. Allen, W.A., and Welch, C.E.: Gastric resection for duodenal ulcer, Ann. Surg. **115**:530, 1942.
4. Ayulo, J.A.: Cholestyramine in postvagotomy syndrome, Am. J. Gastroenterol. **57**:207, 1972.
5. Bloom, S.R., Rorpton, C.M.S., Thomson, J.P.S.: Enteroglucagon release in the dumping syndrome, Lancet **2**:789, 1972.
6. Boren, C.H., and Way, L.H.: Alkaline reflux gastritis: a reevaluation, Am. J. Surg. **140**:40, 1980.
7. Browning, G.C., Buchanan, K.A., and MacKay, C.: Clinical and laboratory study of postvagotomy diarrhea, Gut **15**:644, 1974.
8. Bushkin, F.L., et al.: Postoperative alkaline reflux gastritis, Surg. Gynecol. Obstet. **138**:933, 1974.
9. Chaimoff, C.H., and Dintsman, M.: The long-term fate of patients with dumping syndrome, Arch. Surg. **105**:554, 1972.
10. Chaudhuri, T.K., et al.: Radioisotopic scan—a possible aid in differentiating retained antrum from Zollinger-Ellison syndrome in patients with recurrent peptic ulcer, Gastroenterology **65**:697, 1973.
11. Cuschieri, A.: Long-term evaluation of a reservoir jejunal interposition with an isoperistaltic conduit in the management of patients with small stomach syndrome, Br. J. Surg. **69**:386, 1982.
12. Davidson, E.D., and Hersh, T.: The surgical treatment of bile reflux gastritis: a study of 59 patients, Ann. Surg. **192**:175, 1980.
13. Donovan, I.A.: The different components of gastric emptying after gastric surgery, Ann. R. Coll. Surg. Engl. **58**:368, 1976.
14. Duthie, H.L., and Kwong, N.K.: Vagotomy or gastrectomy for gastric ulcer, Br. Med. J. **4**:79, 1973.
15. Edwards, D.A.: Postvagotomy dysphagia, Lancet **2**:90, 1970.
16. Eldkh, J., et al.: Long-term results of surgical treatment for dumping after partial gastrectomy, Br. J. Surg. **61**:90, 1974.
17. Fawcett, A.N., Johnston, D., and Duthie, H.L.: Revagotomy for recurrent ulcer after vagotomy and drainage for duodenal ulcer, Br. J. Surg. **56**:111, 1969.
18. Fink, W.J., et al.: Treatment of postoperative reactive hypoglycemia by a reversed intestinal segment, Am. J. Surg. **131**:19, 1976.
19. Foster, D.G.: Retrograde jejunogastric intussusception—rare cause of hematemesis, Arch. Surg. **73**:1009, 1956.
20. Fromm, D.: Complications of gastric surgery, New York, 1977, John Wiley & Sons, Inc.
21. Fromm, D.: Ulceration of the stomach and duodenum. In Fromm, D., editor: Gastrointestinal surgery, New York, 1985, Churchill Livingstone.
22. Goligher, J.C., et al.: Five to eight year results of Leeds/York controlled trial of elective surgery for duodenal ulcer, Br. Med. J. **2**:781, 1968.
23. Goligher, J.C., et al.: Clinical comparison of vagotomy and pyloroplasty with other forms of elective surgery for duodenal ulcer, Br. Med. J. **2**:787, 1968.
24. Goligher, J.C., et al.: Five to eight year results of truncal vagotomy and pyloroplasty for duodenal ulcer, Br. Med. J. **1**:7, 1972.
25. Goligher, J.C., et al.: Several standard elective operations for duodenal ulcer: ten to 16 year clinical results, Ann. Surg. **189**:18, 1978.
26. Herrington, J.L., et al.: Treatment of severe postgastrectomy diarrhea by reversed jejunal segment, Ann. Surg. **168**:522, 1968.
27. Hocking, M.P., et al.: Delayed gastric emptying of liquids and solids following Roux-en-Y biliary diversion, Ann. Surg. **194**:494, 1981.
28. Jenkins, D.J.A., et al.: Effect of dietary fiber on complications of gastric surgery: prevention of post-prandial hypoglycemia by pectin, Gastroenterology **72**:215, 1977.
29. Johnson, L.P., et al.: Serotonin antagonists in experimental and clinical "dumping," Ann. Surg. **156**:537, 1962.
30. Jordon, G.L., Jr.: The afferent loop syndrome, Surgery **38**:1027, 1955.
31. Kennedy, T.: The vagus and the consequences of vagotomy, Med. Clin. North Am. **58**:1231, 1974.
32. Kronborg, O.: Clinical results 6 to 8 years after truncal vagotomy and drainage for duodenal ulcer in 500 patients, Acta Chir. Scand. **141**:657, 1975.
33. Lawson-Smith, C., and Thomson, J.P.S.: A dumping provocation test, Br. J. Surg. **62**:153, 1975.
34. Mackie, C.R., et al.: The effect of isoperistaltic jejunal interposition upon gastric emptying, Surg. Gynecol. Obstet. **153**:813, 1981.
35. McClelland, R.N., and Horton, J.W.: Relief of acute, persistent postvagotomy atony by metoclopramide, Ann. Surg. **188**:439, 1978.
36. Mitty, W.E., Jr., Grossi, C., and Nealon, T.F., Jr.: Chronic afferent loop syndrome, Ann. Surg. **172**:996, 1970.
37. Morgan, D.B., et al.: Search for osteomalasia in 1228 patients after gastrectomy and other operations on the stomach, Lancet **2**:1085, 1965.
38. Pryor, J.P., et al.: The long-term metabolic consequences of partial gastrectomy, Am. J. Med. **51**:5, 1971.
39. Reichle, F.A., et al.: The effect of gastrectomy on serotonin metabolism in the human portal vein, Ann. Surg. **172**:585, 1970.
40. Remus, N.I., Williamson, R.C.N., and Johnston, D.: The use of jejunal interposition for intractable symptoms complicating peptic ulcer surgery, Br. J. Surg. **69**:265, 1982.
41. Ritchie, W.P., Jr.: Alkaline reflux gastritis: an objective assessment of its diagnosis and treatment, Ann. Surg. **192**:288, 1980.
42. Ritchie, W.P., Jr.: Alkaline reflux gastritis: a diagnosis in search of a disease, J. Clin. Surg. **1**:414, 1982.
43. Ritchie, W.P., Jr., and Perez, A.R.: Postgastrectomy syndromes. In Moody, F.G., et al., editors: Surgical treatment of digestive disease, Chicago, 1986, Year Book Medical Publishers, Inc.
44. Ruding, R., and Hirdes, W.H.: Extent of the gastric antrum and its significance, Surgery **53**:743, 1963.
45. Rutledge, R.H.: Retroanastomotic hernias after gastrojejunal anastomoses, Ann. Surg. **177**:547, 1973.
46. Sawyers, J.L.: Surgical management of post-gastrectomy syndrome, J. Miss. State Med. Assoc. **14**:28, 1974.
47. Sawyers, J.L., and Herrington, J.L.: Superiority of anti-peristaltic jejunal segments in management of severe dumping syndrome, Ann. Surg. **178**:311, 1973.
48. Silver, D., et al.: The mechanism of the dumping syndrome, Surg. Clin. North Am. **46**:425, 1966.
49. Speth, P.A.J., Jansen, J.B.M.J., and Lammers, C.B.H.W.: Effect of acarbose, pectin, a combination of acarbose with pectin, and placebo on postprandial reactive hypoglycemia after gastric surgery, Gut **24**:798, 1983.
50. Stabile, B.E., and Passaro, E.: Recurrent peptic ulcer, Gastroenterology **70**:124, 1976.
51. Suleiman, S.I., Maglad, S.A., and Hobsley, M.: Dysphagia following selective vagotomy, Br. J. Surg. **66**:607, 1979.
52. Venables, C.W.: The value of a combined pentagastrin/insulin test in studies of stomal ulceration, Br. J. Surg. **57**:757, 1970.
53. Wait, J.O., Beart, R.W., Jr., and Charboneau, W.: Jejunogastric intussusception, Arch. Surg. **115**:1449, 1980.
54. Wang, P.Y., et al.: Kallikrein-kinin system in postgastrectomy dumping syndrome, Ann. Intern. Med. **80**:577, 1974.
55. Wheldon, E.J., Venables, C.W., and Johnston, I.D.A.: Late metabolic sequelae of vagotomy and gastroenterostomy, Lancet **1**:437, 1970.

19

Joseph H. Sellin

Physiology of Digestion and Absorption

The physiology of digestion and absorption involves the transformation of the vast array of foodstuffs eaten by man into assimilable forms and then the transferal of these nutrients across an epithelial barrier. Considering the complexity of the task, it is somewhat surprising, and comforting, that the gut usually accomplishes these functions without difficulties. However, derangements of this normally well-regulated system do occur and present significant clinical problems. Therapeutic intervention is based on an understanding of normal gut function.

This chapter will describe the processes involved in the digestion and absorption of carbohydrate, protein, and fat; the mechanisms of intestinal fluid and electrolyte regulation; and the gastrointestinal tract's role in vitamin and mineral metabolism. Emphasis will be placed on the clinical relevance of a knowledge of normal physiology. Rational approaches to the evaluation and management of malabsorption and diarrhea are also outlined.

PROTEIN ABSORPTION

Dietary proteins normally comprise 15% of total caloric intake. These complex substances are broken down in a step-wise manner into oligopeptides and amino acids, which are absorbed primarily in the upper small bowel (duodenum and jejunum). Specific transport pathways in small bowel enterocytes mediate active transport of these nutrients, which cross the enterocytes and then enter the portal circulation.

Protein digestion begins in the stomach. Pepsinogen, secreted by gastric chief cells, is converted to pepsin in the acidic environment of the gastric lumen and begins the process of protein digestion by breaking down dietary protein into polypeptide subunits. However, pepsin is not essential for normal protein digestion and its ultimate absorption; individuals whose systems do not make pepsin (e.g., individuals with pernicious anemia and those who have had a gastrectomy) still absorb protein efficiently.

The bulk of protein digestion occurs in the upper small bowel. Polypeptides formed from digested protein within the intestinal lumen stimulate intestinal endocrine cells to release the hormone cholecystokinin-pancreozymin.* The pancreas responds to this hormonal stimulation by secreting peptidases, which serve to break the protein down to oligopeptides and amino acids. The endopeptidases, trypsin, chymotrypsin, and elastase, cleave the protein at specific interior sites. The exopeptidases, primarily carboxypeptidase, sequentially cleave off amino acids from a specific end of a polypeptide chain. The end result of this process of intraluminal digestion is a mixture of roughly equal amounts of amino acids and oligopeptides (Fig. 19-1).[37] Because these compounds are polar and water-soluble, they do not require bile salts and micelle formation in the absorptive process. However, because of their polar nature they cannot diffuse through cell membranes like lipids and require specific carriers to be transported across the mucosal membrane of the enterocyte.

Several distinct carrier proteins accomplish this task. Specific carrier systems appear to exist for neutral amino acids (e.g., leucine, phenylalanine, threonine) and others for basic amino acids (e.g., arginine, lysine, cystine). These systems involve the coupling of amino acids with sodium to mediate movement across the apical membrane. Sodium (Na) movement into the cell is generated by a favorable electrochemical gradient, i.e., it is "downhill"; the coupling of amino acids with Na allows them to accumulate in the cell against a concentration gradient (see Fig. 19-1). Once concentrated in the cell, diffusion across the basolateral membrane takes place.

Several factors may affect this absorptive system. In a mixture of amino acids within the intestinal lumen, competition for binding to the carrier proteins will be present. For example, amino acids with long side chains appear to have a high affinity for the carrier and may inhibit the absorption of other amino acids with shorter side chains. Although sodium is an absolute requirement for this carrier system, endogenous secretion of Na into the intestinal lumen is always sufficient for the system to be operative. Intraluminal pH affects this system only when extremely low (<2.5). Results regarding the effects of dietary deprivation on protein absorption have been conflicting. It appears that diabetes is associated with increased transport activity of both the neutral and basic amino acids.[35] Intestinal and renal epithelial cells share similar transport systems, and in inherited metabolic disorders such as cystinuria and Hartnup disease defects can be demonstrated in both organs.

Oligopeptides apparently can be absorbed intact by the intestine without first being broken down into individual

*Historically, cholecystokinin and pancreozymin were thought to be two separate hormones. Current evidence indicates that they are the same hormone. Many authors refer to cholecystokinin-pancreozymin as simply cholecystokinin (CCK).

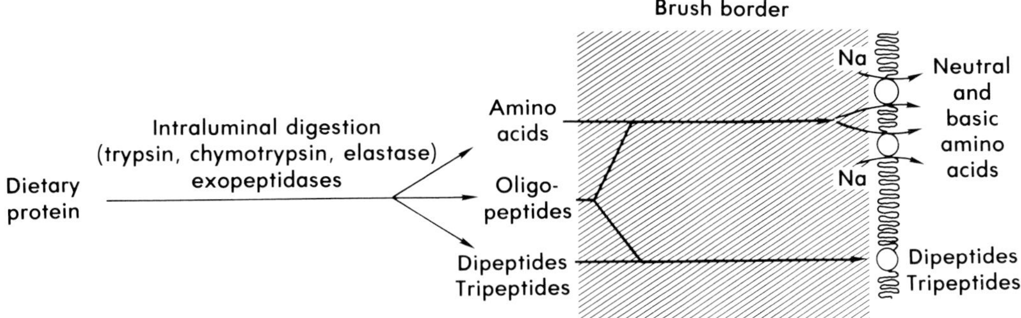

Fig. 19-1 Protein digestion and absorption. Intraluminal digestion of protein occurs primarily through the action of pancreatic enzymes *(left side of figure)*. Brush border enzymes play a relatively minor role and probably aid in the breakdown of residual oligopeptides *(cross-hatched area)*. Amino acids, dipeptides and tripeptides are then actively transported into the cell *(right side of figure)*.

amino acids. Dipeptides and tripeptides are absorbed by a carrier system(s) separate from that for amino acids. Tetrapeptides and larger protein digestive products are not absorbed intact. Although specific brush border dipeptidases and tripeptidases are on the small bowel mucosal membrane, the bulk of this enzyme activity is intracellular. Therefore it is likely that the majority of oligopeptides are absorbed and then subjected to intracellular hydrolysis[1,24] (see Fig. 19-1).

The presence of a specific transport system for oligopeptides has important physiologic and clinical implications because this may be a major mechanism for absorption of dietary proteins. This system exhibits a higher rate of maximal uptake than the amino acid carriers and probably is not influenced as much by diabetes or diet. Recognition of oligopeptide absorption is necessary for the rational design of formulas for enteral nutrition.

CARBOHYDRATE ABSORPTION

Absorption of carbohydrates depends on a sequence of orderly steps involving intraluminal digestion, uptake across the luminal membrane of small bowel enterocytes by specific carriers, and subsequent entry into the mesenteric tributaries to portal blood in a manner analogous to protein absorption. However, unlike proteins, intraluminal digestion of carbohydrates is incomplete and brush border enzymes are essential for the conversion of oligosaccharides into simple sugars that can be transported across the luminal membrane.

Carbohydrates are generally the chief source of calories. Starch, the major form of dietary carbohydrate, is a polymer of glucose with a molecular weight of 100,000 or greater; i.e., 1 molecule of starch will usually have more than 500 glucose subunits. The linkage between the glucose moieties determines the type of starch and its enzymatic degradation. Such types are classified by the spatial configuration of the glucosidic bond (α, β) and the carbon atoms involved in the linkage (1,4 or 1,6). Amylose is a straight chain of α-1,4 linked glucoses. The most common form of dietary starch is the branched starch amylopectin, which consists of α-1,4 chains and branch points created by α-1,6 linkages at every 20 to 25 residues (Fig. 19-2). Glycogen is a branched starch like amylopectin, but it has

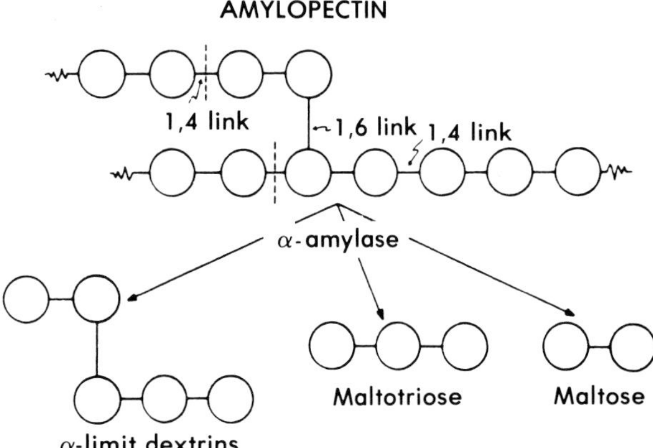

Fig. 19-2 Alpha-amylopectin and its final hydrolytic products are shown with glucose molecules *(circles)* joined by α-1,4 *(horizontal)* links or α-1,6 *(vertical)* links. (From Gray, G.M. Reprinted by permission of N. Engl. J. Med. **292:**1225, 1975.)

a greater frequency of α-1,6 linkages. Although only a minor dietary form of starch, it is the major storage form of carbohydrate within the body.

Disaccharides comprise approximately one third of dietary carbohydrate. The two principal disaccharides are sucrose (glucose-fructose) and lactose (glucose-galactose). Several types of nondigestible carbohydrates are in the diet, chiefly the various forms of fiber (cellulose, hemicellulose, and pectin) and oligosaccharides found in legumes such as beans and lentils (raffinose, stachyose).

Digestion of starch begins in the mouth with salivary amylase but comes to a rapid halt in the acid environment of the stomach. Carbohydrate digestion is completed in the upper small bowel (primarily jejunum) and consists of two phases: intraluminal breakdown of starch and brush border hydrolysis of oligosaccharides (Fig. 19-3). Pancreatic alpha-amylase is primarily responsible for intraluminal digestion of starch. Because it is secreted in great excess, clinically significant amylase deficiency is extremely rare, even in cases of severe steatorrhea* associated with pan-

*Steatorrhea refers to excessive amounts of fats in the feces in excess of 7 g/day when a patient is maintained on a 100 g fat diet.

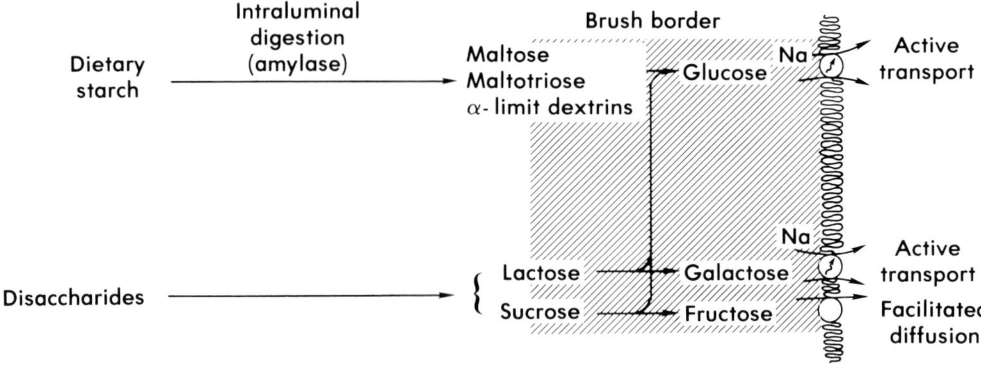

Fig. 19-3 Carbohydrate digestion and absorption. The principal intraluminal event is starch digestion by amylase *(left side of figure)*. The resulting maltose, maltotriose, and α-limit dextrins are broken down further by brush border enzymes, as are the disaccharides *(cross-hatched area)*. Specific active transport systems, coupled to Na, exist for glucose and galactose. Fructose is absorbed by facilitated diffusion.

creatic insufficiency. Alpha-amylase is active only at the interior α-1,4 bonds of starch. It cannot hydrolyze 1,6 links, 1,4 links next to branch points, or the terminal glucose-glucose links. Therefore the final products of amylase digestion are the disaccharide maltose, the trisaccharide maltotriose, and alpha-limit dextrins, i.e., larger oligosaccharides of 5 to 10 glucose units containing the branch points (Figs. 19-2 and 19-3). Human amylase is inactive against beta links; therefore cellulose, which is made up entirely of β-1,4 links, is not digested.

Maltose, maltotriose, and alpha-limit dextrins, along with dietary disaccharides, next are broken down into simple sugars by specific brush border enzymes.[11] The end products of this process are glucose, galactose, and fructose (Fig. 19-3). Glucose and galactose are transported across the luminal membrane of the cell by a carrier protein that couples the movement of two sugars to one Na ion.[18] This transport mechanism is similar to Na–amino acid absorption. In the later stages of absorption, intraluminal concentrations of sugars may decrease; however, because of the Na coupling, active transport of sugars against a concentration gradient can occur. Fructose absorption occurs by facilitated diffusion, i.e., carrier-mediated, but not active, transport.

Generally, transport into the cell is the rate-limiting step in this absorptive process. The hydrolytic capacity of the brush border enzymes provides an excess of monosaccharides for the transport carrier. The exception to this is lactose absorption, where the hydrolytic capacity of lactase is rate limiting. A complex regulatory mechanism appears to coordinate the activity of the brush border enzymes and the corresponding transport proteins.[33]

The overall design of carbohydrate absorption is to deliver maximum amounts of calories while introducing the least possible osmotic force into the duodenum and jejunum, where carbohydrates are primarily absorbed. A molecule of starch and glucose have the same osmotic effect but vastly different caloric value. Intraluminal digestion of starch stops at the oligosaccharide stage, limiting the osmotic effect. The rapid absorption of monosaccharides into the intestine after action by brush border enzymes minimizes the potential for drawing fluid into the jejunum and duodenum. Under normal conditions this system is extremely effective; when disrupted, malabsorption may be compounded by osmotic diarrhea.

FAT ABSORPTION

The absorption of fat is complex and depends on the integrated function of the pancreas, biliary system, and intestinal mucosa. Much of this complexity is created by the problem of delivering a water-insoluble nutrient into an aqueous environment. Fat composes approximately one third of the typical American diet, although the percentage of fat seems to be decreasing somewhat in recent years. The bulk of this fat is in the form of triglycerides (90%), phospholipids, cholesterol, fat-soluble vitamins, and other trace lipids.*

The intraluminal phase of digestion is crucial for fat absorption. Dietary fat is mechanically broken down, emulsified, and finally solubilized within the upper small bowel lumen before being presented to the intestinal mucosa for transport through the enterocyte and into the lymph. Microscopic observations have elucidated some of the complex physiochemical phases of the state of lipids within the intestinal lumen. The oil phase represents emulsified fat droplets of 2000 to 50,000 Å in size. Then enzymatic digestion by lipases forms calcium soaps (free fatty acids complexed with calcium) and a viscous isotropic phase of protonated fatty acids and monoglycerides. A fat droplet remnant of undetermined composition generally remains after formation of the viscous isotropic phase. The constituents of the viscous isotropic phase, fatty acids and monoglycerides, then interact with bile salts to form micelles.[27,28]

The primary enzymes responsible for fat digestion are lipase, phospholipase A_2, and nonspecific lipase (cholesterol esterase). Lipase has two sources: lingual and pancreatic. Lingual lipase is resistant to acid degradation in

*These poorly characterized nonpolar lipids may represent industrial pollutants, residues from fossil fuels, degradation products from high temperature cooking, natural products, and essential oils of plants; they account for the remainder of the fat in the diet.

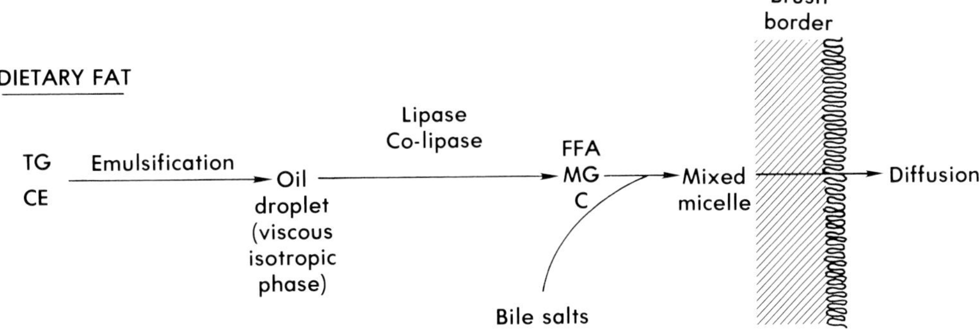

Fig. 19-4 Fat digestion and absorption. Dietary fats, triglycerides *(TG),* and cholesterol esters *(CE)* are emulsified to form fat droplets within the intestinal lumen. These droplets undergo a physiochemical transformation into a viscous isotrophic phase. At this stage, the triglyceride is digested by pancreatic lipase. The resultant free fatty acids *(FFA)* and monoglyceride *(MG),* along with cholesterol *(C),* form mixed micelles with bile salts. The micelle then diffuses to the apical membrane. There are no brush border enzymes on specific membrane transport systems for fat absorption.

the stomach and prepares dietary fat for more efficient intestinal degradation. Pancreatic lipase is the major digestive enzyme for triglycerides. Extrapolations from in vitro activity suggest that a 1000-fold excess of lipase is secreted to handle the average daily fat intake. Lipase acts by hydrolyzing the two outside arms of triglyceride, yielding two fatty acids and a monoglyceride (Fig. 19-4).

It has long been recognized that in the setting of severe lipase deficiency there may still be a wide range in the magnitude of fat malabsorption. Recent studies on colipase underscore the intricate nature of fat absorption and aid in our understanding of the variability of steatorrhea in these clinical states. Physiologic concentrations of bile salts in the upper gut inactivate pancreatic lipase by displacing it from its natural substrate, the triglyceride-containing fat droplet. Therefore, without some additional factor, lipase could not digest triglycerides in its natural environment. That added factor is colipase, which is secreted by the pancreas as a peptide chain of slightly over 100 amino acids (procolipase), which is then broken down to its active form (96 amino acids) by trypsin.[9]

Unlike lipase, colipase is not displaced from the surface of fat emulsions by bile salts. It appears that colipase binds to the triglyceride substrate, then binds lipase, and serves as the necessary bridge to link the enzymes to its target. Thus colipase plays a crucial role in intraluminal fat digestion (see Fig. 19-4). Recent evidence suggests that variations of colipase secretion in pancreatic insufficiency with severe lipase deficiency may account for some of the range of fat malabsorption.[10]

Dietary phospholipids are primarily derived from biologic membranes of food stuffs. They are structurally similar to triglycerides, possessing a glycerol backbone and two ester links to fatty acids. In the third position, however, there is an ester link to phosphoric acid, which is then linked to a nitrogen-containing base (choline, serine, ethonalamine). Phospholipids are relatively resistant to lipase and appear to be primarily degraded by phospholipase A_2, which requires calcium and bile salts as cofactors. An additional enzyme, nonspecific lipase, exhibits activity on cholesterol esters, monoglycerides, and trace fats.

One dietary source of fat comes replete with its own digestive enzyme. Human, but not cow, milk contains a nonspecific lipase that is acid resistant and therefore serves as an intestinal lipase for breast-fed infants. Considering the relatively low levels of lipase in the newborn, nature has provided an ingenious package to ensure that maximal nutritional benefit of human milk for the infant is achieved.

The products of enzymatic digestion of dietary fat remain relatively water-insoluble, primarily in the viscous isotropic phase (see Fig. 19-4). At this point bile salts and the formation of micelles provide the mechanism for bringing cholesterol, monoglycerides, fatty acids, and phospholipids into solution. Bile salts are detergents; like all detergents they are amphiphiles, possessing both hydrophilic and hydrophobic regions. Placed in an aqueous solution, bile salts spontaneously form into a particular three-dimensional arrangement called a micelle, in which the hydrophilic regions of the molecules are directed outward and the hydrophobic regions inward, thereby shielded from the aqueous environment. This formation occurs above a specific concentration of bile salts termed the critical micellar concentration (CMC). Depending on the types of bile salts involved, the CMC is generally in the range of 1 to 5 mM. Mixed micelles are formed with the products of lipase action shielded from the aqueous, polar environment of the intestinal lumen by the bile salts. Micelles are smaller (30 to 100 Å) than the fat emulsion and are in solution. Diglycerides and triglycerides are too bulky to be packaged in these micelles and must await lipase hydrolysis. Fat-soluble vitamins are solubilized by inclusion in mixed micelles.

Before absorption the mixed micelle and its constituent lipids must then diffuse through two functional barriers: the apical membrane of the intestinal cell and the unstirred water layer, that portion of intestinal fluid immediately adjacent to the epithelium not subject to the bulk mixing that occurs normally within the lumen. The rate of diffusion is dependent on the thickness of the unstirred water layer, the concentration gradient across it, and the permeability coefficient of the micelle.[40,41] The micelle probably dissociates at the apical membrane. Fatty acids, cholesterol, and monoglycerides can then permeate through the lipid regions of the apical membrane into the cell interior. Unlike amino acids and sugars, they do not require a specific carrier protein. Whereas most dietary fat is absorbed in the duodenum and upper jejunum, bile salts generally remain in the intestinal lumen until they are reabsorbed in the terminal ileum. Diffusion through the unstirred water layer is probably the rate-limiting step in fat absorption.

Once inside the enterocyte, the digestive process is essentially reversed; monoglycerides and fatty acids are resynthesized into triglyceride. Through a series of enzymatic steps in the endoplasmic reticulum, triglycerides are reformed and then accumulate within the Golgi apparatus. However, before exiting across the basolateral membrane of the cell, the triglycerides must be suitably packaged for transport in lymph. This process is chylomicron formation.

Chylomicrons are large spheres (1000 to 5000 Å) with a core of hydrophobic lipids, primarily triglycerides, but that also include cholesterol, cholesterol esters, fat-soluble vitamins, and trace fats. The surface is covered by phospholipids and specialized apolipoproteins. Although these apolipoproteins cover less than a quarter of the surface and account for about 1% of the mass, they are essential for chylomicron formation and transport. These proteins are made in the intestine; their rate of synthesis appears to be stimulated by fat absorption. Congenital absence of a certain apolipoprotein (abetalipoproteinemia) prevents the exit step of chylomicrons across the basolateral membrane of the cell.[31] Once in the subepithelial space, chylomicrons enter the central lacteal of the villus and the intestinal lymphatic system. Because of their size they cannot pass through the relatively tight junctions of the capillaries and are therefore excluded from the portal system.

However, one source of dietary fat is able to enter the portal system. Medium chain triglycerides (MCTs), with fatty acid moieties of 6 to 10 carbon atoms, are metabolized somewhat differently than their long chain counterparts. About one third of an oral dose of MCT can be absorbed intact. Pancreatic lipase acting at both the alpha and beta positions can yield 3 medium chain fatty acids. These fatty acids may be absorbed directly into the portal blood independent of chylomicrons. The therapeutic implications of this distinct metabolism of MCTs is self-evident.

ENTEROHEPATIC CIRCULATION

The process by which substances are recycled through biliary secretion, intestinal absorption, and hepatic uptake is termed enterohepatic circulation. Although some organic anions, drugs, and hormone metabolites undergo enterohepatic circulation, its principal constituents are bile acids. Bile acids are a family of steroids synthesized by the liver from cholesterol. They are the physiologically most significant component of bile and serve several important functions: stimulation of hepatic bile flow; solubilization and excretion of cholesterol; micellarization of dietary lipid; and stimulation of intestinal fluid secretion.

Bile acids may be classified in several different ways: by the number of hydroxyl groups, by where they are synthesized, and by their conjugation. The number of hydroxyl groups determines, to a large extent, how water-soluble the bile acid is; this, in turn, determines many of its functional characteristics. Cholic acid has three hydroxyl groups on its steroid nucleus, chenodeoxycholic and deoxycholic possess two, and lithocholic a single hydroxyl group. Primary bile acids (cholic, chenodeoxycholic) are synthesized in the liver. The secondary bile acids (deoxycholic, lithocholic) have had a hydroxyl group removed by anaerobic bacteria in the intestine. All bile acids secreted into bile by the liver are conjugated; the two major conjugates are glycine and taurine.

The underlying biochemical mechanisms of conjugation are poorly understood. It appears that the system prefers taurine conjugation; however, because the relative supply of glycine is much greater, approximately two thirds of bile acids are glycine conjugates. No major functional difference is apparent between the two conjugates. Lithocholate may also be sulfated in addition to being conjugated with glycine and taurine. A small fraction of bile acids is glucuronidated. Conjugation has several important effects. It makes the bile acids more polar and therefore more water soluble. Additionally, conjugated bile acids are less likely to precipitate in an acid environment or to complex with calcium. Intestinal bacteria are capable of deconjugating bile acids. Because the small bowel is relatively sterile, deconjugation normally occurs in the colon. Therefore bacteria have two major effects on intestinal bile acid metabolism: (1) dehydroxylation, i.e., conversion of primary to secondary bile acids, and (2) deconjugation.

There are two different mechanisms of intestinal absorption of bile acids: passive permeation, which occurs throughout the length of the gut, and active absorption, which is restricted to the terminal ileum. The difference in intestinal transport among the classes of bile acids is considerable, depending to a large extent on the acids' physical characteristics. The more polar (conjugated) bile salts are well absorbed by the active transport mechanism in the ileum. This absorption is dependent on Na and is similar to other Na-coupled transport systems in the small bowel that link the intracellular accumulation of a solute to the downhill movement of Na across the apical membrane. As the polarity of the bile salt decreases (i.e., fewer hydroxyl groups), its active transport decreases. Therefore lithocholate is minimally absorbed by this transport mechanism. In contrast, passive absorption is greater for the less polar bile salts. The rate of passive absorption depends on two factors: (1) the concentration of the bile salt monomer within the intestinal lumen and (2) the passive permeability coefficient, which is inversely related to the polarity. Therefore bile acids that are unconjugated, or have fewer hydroxyl groups, are more easily absorbed passively.

Within this framework the passage of the different bile acids through the enterohepatic circulation can be traced (Fig. 19-5). The primary bile acids, conjugated cholic and chenodeoxycholic acid, are poorly absorbed in the upper small bowel. Teleologically, there is a certain sense to this. Since a high concentration of bile salts is necessary for intraluminal fat digestion, it would be counter-productive to have bile acids absorbed in the jejunum. In the

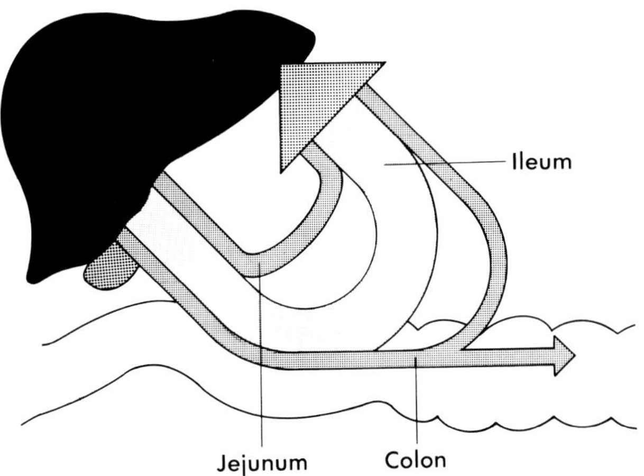

Fig. 19-5 Enterohepatic circulation. Bile acids secreted by the liver enter the intestine at the level of Vater's ampulla. In the jejunum, absorption occurs primarily by passive diffusion of conjugated bile acids. In the ileum, active transport of all bile acids occurs through an Na-dependent carrier. In the colon, passive diffusion of free bile acids occurs.

ileum, the active absorption of bile salts is efficient. The bile salts are transported across the ileal epithelium to the portal circulation and returned to the liver (see Fig. 19-5). At this level of the gut, the bacterial metabolism of bile salts becomes significant. Somewhat more than a quarter of ileal bile acid is either deconjugated or dehydroxylated (i.e., converted to secondary bile acids). These may then be absorbed passively and enter the enterohepatic circulation.

The fate of the two secondary bile acids is quite different. Deoxycholate, the dihydroxy bile acid formed from cholic acid, is well absorbed and, once conjugated in the liver, is handled by the enterohepatic circulation in a manner quite similar to the primary dihydroxy bile acid, chenodeoxycholate. Lithocholate, a monohydroxy bile acid, has limited passive reabsorption. On returning to the liver, it is reconjugated with glycine and taurine. Additionally, about two thirds of the lithocholate is also conjugated with sulfate. These conjugates are secreted through the bile into the intestinal lumen. The nonsulfated lithocholate is probably absorbed by the ileum, whereas the sulfated moieties pass into the colon. Here they may be deconjugated by bacteria; a fraction of this lithocholate will then be passively reabsorbed and will re-enter the enterohepatic circulation (see Fig. 19-5).

Normally, the enterohepatic circulation is well regulated. A bile salt pool of approximately 2 g cycles itself through the enterohepatic circulation approximately 6 times daily, resulting in an intestinal bile acid secretion rate of 12 g/day. Approximately 0.5 g is lost in the stool daily; this is matched by an equivalent rate of bile acid synthesis by the liver. The turnover rate for the various bile acids varies. As one might expect, given its inefficient intestinal absorption, the pool of lithocholate (60 mg) is entirely turned over every 24 hours. Between 20% and 30% of the other major bile salts are excreted in the stool each day.

Disruption of the enterohepatic circulation may result in malabsorption or diarrhea. Ileal resection or dysfunction (e.g., Crohn's disease) will block the reabsorption of bile acids. With small bowel resection of the ileum (<100 cm), the passage of bile acids into the colon is increased. The dihydroxy bile acids are potent cathartics; they alter intestinal permeability and stimulate active electrolyte secretion. Because there is considerable hepatic synthetic reserve, the increased fecal loss is compensated for by increased production. Therefore steatorrhea is mild, and the diarrhea that occurs is caused primarily by the colonic bile salts. With larger ileal resections (>10 cm), the liver can no longer produce enough bile acid to compensate for the fecal loss. Bile salt secretion drops significantly, and the steatorrhea becomes more severe (>20 g fat/day) because of inadequate micelle formation in the small bowel. Diarrhea results in this setting from the increase in colonic fatty acids, which, like bile salts, stimulate secretion.

The enterohepatic circulation may be significantly altered in additional clinical settings. Drugs such as the binding resin cholestyramine may sequester bile acids. In bacterial overgrowth, bile acid deconjugation in the small bowel is significant; therefore, because unconjugated bile salts are less soluble, there may be a drop below the critical micellar concentration required for fat absorption. In cholestasis the block in enterohepatic circulation occurs either in the liver or in the biliary tree. In this setting the pattern of hepatic conjugation of primary bile acids is changed; more sulfates are formed, and, subsequently, renal excretion is greater.

FLUID AND ELECTROLYTE TRANSPORT

The average adult individual produces approximately 100 to 200 ml of stool water daily. Considering that the gut normally handles almost 10 L of fluid daily, this organ exhibits a highly efficient mechanism for conserving salt and water. Oral intake comprises only a small portion, approximately 1 L, of the total amount of gut fluid. The remainder consists of endogenous secretion from the salivary glands, stomach, pancreas, biliary tree, and the intestine itself. Even minor aberrations in this finely tuned system will result in an increase in stool water and hence diarrhea.

The major factors involved in the gut's absorption of fluid are intestinal motility and epithelial transport. Traditionally, it was assumed that diarrhea was a consequence of hypermotility. The term diarrhea, derived from the Greek, means "to run through." Laxatives were presumed to be irritants that worked by increasing intestinal contractions, whereas antidiarrheals slowed motility. Over the last 15 years the pendulum has swung in the opposite direction. With the recognition that cholera toxin causes the intestinal epithelium to actively secrete fluid and that sugar-containing solutions can counter this effect,[6,17] the major research emphasis has been on the mechanisms involved in epithelial transport, delineating the carriers, channels, and pumps involved in movement of sodium (Na) and chloride (Cl). Although motility clearly is important, its role in diarrhea is, as yet, undefined (i.e., is hypermotility [hyperthyroidism] or hypomotility [diabetic diarrhea] more important as a cause of diarrhea?). The answer is unclear. The major emphasis of the remainder of this section will center on the role of epithelial transport.

Each section of the smoothly functioning intestine serves a special role in fluid absorption. The jejunum absorbs fluid isosmotically secondary to Na-coupled nutrient absorption. The ileum absorbs Na-Cl and secretes bicarbonate (HCO_3), again isosmotically. Generally, the small bowel absorbs large volumes of fluid but does not concentrate the intestinal luminal contents. The colon, primarily the distal colon, is capable of absorbing Na against a concentration gradient and therefore is well adapted for its role of conserving salt and water.

In crossing the intestinal epithelium, ions, solutes, and water face a series of barriers. One route is around the cells through the tight junctions. Water, low molecular weight solutes, and ions move through this paracellular route passively in response to electrochemical and osmotic gradients. These gradients are established by active transport of ions and solutes through the cell (transcelleular transport). Two-way traffic of ions occurs across the intestine. Fluxes occur in a serosal-to-mucosal direction, as well as from mucosa to serosa. Net transport depends on the magnitude of the opposing fluxes. Alterations in one or both of the unidirectional fluxes may result in absorptive or secretory changes. Water movement occurs in response to osmotic gradients. Na is the principal ion driving absorptive flows, whereas active Cl secretion promotes movement of water into the intestinal lumen. Nutrients may have a crucial role in determining the rate of water transport. Carbohydrate malabsorption causes luminal retention of considerable osmotic force, resulting in either inhibition of water absorption or actual secretion. On the other hand, well-absorbed sugars and amino acids enhance water absorption.

All transport epithelia possess similar characteristics: a polarity of membranes with distinct apical (luminal) and basolateral (serosal) membranes; an Na pump (ouabain-inhibitable Na-K-ATPase) located on the basolateral membrane, exchanging intracellular Na for extracellular potassium (K); a characteristic electrochemical potential profile, in which the intracellular potential difference is negative and the intracellular Na concentration is low. Na entry into the cell is therefore "downhill" because of the favorable electrical and chemical gradients, and the Na pump consumes energy (ATP) to extrude Na across the basolateral membrane (Fig. 19-6). Intracellular Cl is generally above its electrochemical equilibrium; this means that Cl exit from the cell does not require energy. Given these common characteristics, what distinguishes one section of the intestine from another are the specific entry mechanisms for Na across the apical membrane and the response to a variety of hormonal, bacterial, and pharmacologic mediators of transport.

There are three basic mechanisms of Na entry across the apical membrane: (1) solute-coupled Na transport, (2) chloride-coupled Na transport, and (3) electrogenic Na absorption independent of other ions or solutes. In all cases Na absorbed across the apical membrane is extruded across the basolateral membrane by the Na pump[36] (see Fig. 19-6). Solute-coupled Na absorption allows for accumulation of nutrients in the enterocyte against a concentration gra-

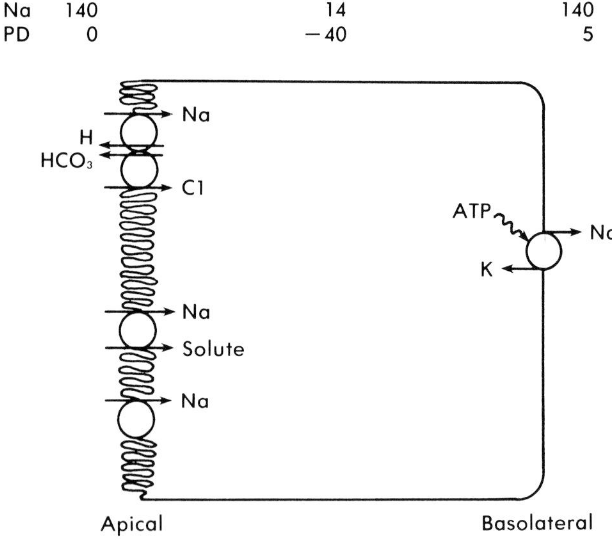

Fig. 19-6 Na absorptive pathways in the small bowel. A favorable electrochemical gradient exists for Na entry into the cell. The Na-K-ATPase on the basolateral border pumps Na out of the cell in exchange for K. Na enters the cell across the apical membrane through three different pathways: (1) coupled to Cl, in a system of Na-H, Cl-HCO_3 exchange, (2) coupled to solutes, such as glucose or amino acids, or (3) independently, in an electrogenic entry step. *Na,* sodium; H, hydrogen; *HCO_3*, bicarbonate; *Cl,* chloride; *K,* potassium; *PD,* potential difference. Numbers following Na and PD at top of figure refer to concentration of Na and PD in millivolts, respectively.

dient through linkage to downhill Na movement. Coupled transport mechanisms depend on the presence of both substances for the system (a carrier protein) to be operative. If only a single species is present, no transport will occur through that specific pathway. The addition of the cotransported substance will stimulate the transport of the first. The absorption of the solute does not directly use energy but depends on movement of Na into the enterocyte, which is favored by the low Na concentration and negative intracellular potential difference. This coupling has been termed *secondary active transport.* The transport may be electrogenic or electroneutral, depending on the charge of the cotransport solute. Glucose- and amino acid–coupled Na absorptions are found throughout the length of the small bowel but not in the colon. Specialized Na-coupled transport mechanisms such as those for bile acids may be restricted to a limited region of the intestine.

Na-Cl–coupled transport is found in a variety of epithelia. The nature of coupling is complex, and the existence of at least two different cotransport systems is probable. In the intestine Na-Cl absorption does not occur through a single transporter; instead, there are two coordinated, electrically neutral systems, one exchanging Na for H, the other Cl for HCO_3[7,22] (see Fig. 19-6). Since H + HCO_3 can combine to form water and CO_2, the net result is Na and Cl absorption. The two transporters are most likely synchronized by intracellular pH. Na-Cl–coupled transport is found in the jejunum and ileum and may also be present in the human colon.

Na absorption that is not coupled to a solute or chloride

Table 19-1 **INTESTINAL SECRETORY STIMULI**

Luminal	Serosal	Intracellular Mediator
Bacterial enterotoxins (cholera, *Escherichia coli* heat-labile toxins, *Shigella* organisms, *Staphlococcus aureus*) Laxatives (castor oil, diocytl sodium sulfosuccinate)	Vasoactive intestinal peptide Prostaglandins	Cyclic AMP
Bile acids Dihydroxy fatty acids		?
Bacterial enterotoxins (*E. coli* heat-stable toxin)		Cyclic GMP
Detergents (bile acids?)	Acetylcholine Serotonin Substance P Neurotensin Bombesin	Calcium

is electrogenic because it involves net transfer of positive charge. Unlike the coupled transport systems that involve specialized protein carriers, this type of Na transport occurs through selective channels in the membrane that allow the passage of Na but exclude other cations and anions. This absorptive pathway is most readily apparent in the distal colon and can be blocked by the diuretic amiloride.

Chloride, the principal ion governing secretion, accumulates within intestinal cells above its electrochemical equilibrium. The permeability (conductance) of the apical membrane for chloride determines the rate of the anion's movement across this membrane. The chloride conductance is controlled by three intracellular mediators—cyclic AMP (cAMP), cyclic GMP (cGMP), and calcium. Therefore stimuli that increase any of these three factors will cause active Cl secretion and, secondarily, movement of water into the intestinal lumen.[8] Enterocytes possess specific membrane receptors for a host of hormones, drugs, and toxins that activate the cellular machinery for secretion through these three mediators (Table 19-1).

cAMP, cGMP, and calcium have similar effects on specific transport pathways. In addition to increasing the chloride conductance of the apical membrane, they block the Na-Cl cotransport system. This antiabsorptive effect favors fluid accumulation within the intestinal lumen and an increase in diarrhea. However, these agents have no effect on Na absorption coupled to solutes such as sugars or amino acids. The therapeutic implications of this observation have been applied to the development of a specific oral rehydration therapy for cholera and other severe diarrheal diseases. In addition to having the requisite electrolytes, this solution has a high concentration of glucose. It does not reverse or inhibit cholera toxin–induced secretion; rather, it stimulates an independent, alternate (Na-glucose) absorptive pathway. The absorptive movement of Na and glucose tends to counter the osmotic effect of chloride secretion. This standoff between absorptive and secretory forces diminishes or eliminates water flow into the intestinal lumen.

The enterocyte has the capacity to either absorb or secrete. It is normally exposed to a vast array of absorbagogues and secretagogues, both from the luminal and serosal sides. The transport function of the epithelium depends on the net sum of these stimuli. Knowledge of the pathways and their regulation aid in understanding the pathophysiology of diarrheal states and designing successful therapeutic strategies.

Acute diarrheas are frequent and generally self-limited. The diagnostic workup is straightforward: a stool search for blood, pus, and pathogens. Chronic diarrheas are uncommon and demand a logical clinical approach based on defining whether the diarrhea is secretory or osmotic in nature. This "paint can workup" requires serial 24-hour stool collections for volume, electrolytes, osmolality, and fat. Frequently stool volumes will turn out to be normal, suggesting a functional cause and thereby shifting the emphasis of the workup. If stool volumes are increased (> 500 ml/day), examination of the electrolytes and osmolality will determine the type of diarrhea. In secretory diarrheas the osmolality can be accounted for by the ions in the stool water (calculated as the sum of Na and K, multiplied by 2). In osmotic diarrheas the osmolality is much greater than the concentration of measured ions.

Osmotic diarrheas may be caused by malabsorption of specific carbohydrates (lactose intolerance), ingestion of poorly absorbed solutes (laxatives containing magnesium), or unregulated entry of an osmotic load into the small bowel (postgastrectomy syndromes). Characteristically, in these conditions the diarrhea stops when nothing is taken by mouth. Secretory diarrheas may be caused by hormone-producing tumors. Vasoactive intestinal peptide, serotonin, calcitonin, gastrin, and prostaglandins have been implicated in the pathogenesis of tumor-related diarrheas. Bile salts, fatty acids, laxatives, and other drugs may produce a secretory diarrhea. Additionally, increased hydrostatic pressure or obstructed lymphatic drainage (Crohn's disease, lymphoma) may cause a similar clinical picture.

The clinical hallmark of a secretory diarrhea is continuation of the diarrhea while the patient is fasting. Hormone-induced diarrheas tend to be more voluminous than osmotic diarrheas, whereas those associated with lymphatic obstruction may have protein-losing enteropathy or lymphocytopenia. Once the presence of diarrhea and the broad category into which it falls have been established, attention can be focused on a more specific cause.

VITAMIN D AND MINERAL METABOLISM

The increasing recognition of the association between gastrointestinal dysfunction and metabolic bone disease serves to emphasize the importance of the gut and liver in the regulation of mineral metabolism.[15] Vitamin D and calcium are the two critical factors in mineral homeostasis; their metabolism and actions are intertwined, and both are dependent on normal intestinal absorptive function. The role of the multiple metabolites of vitamin D, which may more properly be considered a prohormone, has been extensively studied over the last decade. Significant questions remain over the physiologic role of some of the metabolites, the mechanisms of action of vitamin D, and the intestinal transport of calcium. Vitamin D has two major sources: (1) endogenous production, in which sterol precursors are converted to vitamin D by ultraviolet radiation; and (2) food that is either naturally rich in vitamin D (such as fatty fishes, eggs, and chicken liver) or has been fortified with vitamin D (such as milk).

Vitamin D itself is biologically inactive. It is sequentially metabolized by the liver (25-hydroxylation) and kidney (1-hydroxylation) to produce 1,25 $(OH)_2$ vitamin D, the most potent of the vitamin D metabolites. The major regulatory step in this pathway is the renal hydroxylation. Both parathormone and low serum phosphate concentrations stimulate 1-hydroxylation. There is a feedback inhibition loop in which 1,25 $(OH)_2$ vitamin D leads to preferential hydroxylation at the 24- rather than the 1-position. The biologic role of 24,25 $(OH)_2$ vitamin D is unknown; it may simply represent a degradation pathway.[3] The major circulating vitamin D metabolite is the 25-OH form; serum concentration generally reflects body stores. Both vitamin D and 25-OH vitamin D have relatively long half-lives (weeks to months) and are stored primarily in fat and muscle. Serum levels of 1,25 $(OH)_2$ vitamin D do not correspond well with the individual's vitamin status and may remain normal during deficiency.

Because it is fat soluble, dietary vitamin D depends on intestinal bile salts and micelle formation for absorption. Although 25-hydroxylation is a necessary step in vitamin D metabolism, little correlation exists between the severity of liver disease and 25-hydroxylation. Although vitamin D deficiency and metabolic bone disease are commonly seen in primary biliary cirrhosis, this may be caused more by the degree of steatorrhea. Drug-induced changes in hepatic enzyme activity may affect the liver's metabolism of vitamin D and be associated with a deficiency. The most notable clinical example of this is anticonvulsant therapy (e.g., dilantin).

An enterohepatic circulation of vitamin D occurs. Along with its more polar metabolites, vitamin D is excreted into bile and reabsorbed by the intestine. The importance of this enterohepatic circulation for overall vitamin D economy is unknown.

Calcium absorption depends on dietary intake, intraluminal factors, mucosal integrity, and hormonal status. The recommended minimal daily intake of calcium is 1000 mg; however, it is likely that a substantial portion of the population (the lactase deficient, the elderly) do not ingest even this amount. The principal food source for calcium is milk and milk products. Approximately one quarter of milk calcium is in the form of calcium citrate; the remainder appears to be in a colloidal calcium phosphate suspension. In other animal sources protein-bound calcium is present. In vegetables the predominant form is calcium salts (oxalates, phytates, or other organic anions).

Intraluminal factors, in addition to the source of the calcium, may determine the availability for absorption. To be absorbed, calcium must be ionized in the form of a soluble salt. Therefore, when complexed with a fatty acid, oxalate, phytate, or cholestyramine, calcium will not be absorbed. Intraluminal pH and gastric acid have been presumed to facilitate calcium absorption, promoting both the dissociation of food-calcium complexes and the solution of relatively insoluble calcium salts. For example, hydrochloric acid from gastric secretion can convert dietary calcium carbonate to calcium chloride, a salt from which ionized calcium may be absorbed. It is interesting to note, therefore, that recent studies have demonstrated that gastric acid secretion has a striking lack of effect on absorption of calcium salts,[4] thereby bringing into question the role of the stomach in calcium absorption. Intraluminal factors can also increase calcium absorption. Most notably sugars, especially lactose,[16,26,43] have been shown to increase intestinal calcium absorption, presumably secondary to changes in fluid transport. Bile acids, amino acids, and certain antibiotics such as penicillin and chloramphenicol facilitate calcium absorption by forming more soluble complexes.

Calcium transport across the intestinal epithelium occurs by both active and passive mechanisms. At low intraluminal calcium concentrations, vitamin D–responsive active transport is dominant. If intraluminal calcium concentration is increased sufficiently, passive transport can be demonstrated. Although vitamin D clearly stimulates production of several specific transport proteins (calcium-binding protein, calcium-dependent alkaline phosphatases, calcium-ATPase), its stimulatory effect on calcium absorption may be related to changes in membrane structure and phospholipid metabolism.[30,39]

Intestinal transport, bone resorption, and renal excretion form a triad of regulatory sites for maintenance of serum calcium. Changes at one site generally stimulate a compensatory response at another. Parathormone and 1,25 $(OH)_2$ vitamin D act in concert to increase serum calcium. Parathormone has no direct action on the intestine but may alter calcium absorption indirectly by affecting vitamin D metabolism. Other factors may also play an important role: growth hormone, prolactin, estrogens, and sarcoidosis may increase calcium absorption; glucocorticoids, thyroxine, thiazides, uremia, chronic acidosis, and aging decrease calcium absorption. These factors may act either directly on the intestine or alter vitamin D metabolism. Decreased calcium absorption is a common problem in gastrointestinal disease. Frequently dietary intake is inadequate; lactose intolerance may compound this difficulty. Steatorrhea may result in intraluminal saponification with calcium binding to fatty acids. Additionally, steatorrhea will be associated with vitamin D malabsorption. Loss of epithelial absorptive surface, either from resection or loss of mucosal integrity (e.g., in patients with sprue, inflammatory bowel disease, jejunoileal bypass) will impair calcium absorption. The principal liver disease associated with impaired calcium absorption is primary biliary cirrhosis, in which severe metabolic bone disease may be a crippling complication of the disease.

Magnesium deficiency is relatively uncommon because obligatory fecal loss is minimal and the renal conservation mechanisms are extremely effective. However, magnesium deficiency can develop in a setting of renal disease, ketoacidosis, and malabsorption. Alcoholics appear particularly prone to develop magnesium deficiency. Because magnesium is necessary for parathormone's release from the parathyroid gland and its action on bone, magnesium deficiency may be the underlying cause of hypocalcemia. Magnesium replacement should always be considered in cases of refractory hypocalcemia.

FOLIC ACID AND VITAMIN B_{12} METABOLISM

Folate and vitamin B_{12} are the two water-soluble vitamins that are potent hematinics; their intestinal absorption is complex but necessary for maintaining normal red cell production. Because isolated deficiencies of both these vitamins occur frequently, an understanding of their unique metabolic pathways is important.

Folic Acid

Folate functions as a methyl donor in several vital reactions including purine synthesis, amino acid metabolism, and initiation of protein synthesis. Folate deficiency leads to megaloblastic changes in both the hematopoeitic system and the intestinal epithelium.

Free folate consists of a pteroic acid moiety linked to L-glutamate. Most dietary folate is in a conjugated form, with a chain of several glutamates (polyglutamate folates). Absorption of folate depends on hydrolysis of the glutamic acid chain and subsequent transfer of the monoglutamyl product across the intestinal epithelium. The glutamic acid chain appears to be resistant to pancreatic digestive enzymes and is most likely broken down by brush border enzymes, which liberate free folic acid and amino acids. Polyglutamate folate, as such, is not absorbed.[32]

The rate-limiting step in folate absorption is entry across the apical membrane. At low luminal concentrations of folate, a saturable, carrier-mediated mechanism of facilitated diffusion exists. At high luminal concentrations, a component of passive diffusion becomes evident. Alterations in pH affect the rate of intestinal uptake of folate; the optimum is pH 6.5. Folate uptake across the apical membrane is mediated by an anion exchange mechanism. The role of Na in folate transport has not been delineated. The epithelial cells reduce methylate folate, releasing methyltetrahydrofolate into the portal blood.

The body stores of folate are limited, in the range of 5 to 20 mg. The liver, which is the major storage site, contains primarily polyglutamate folate. Folate is excreted into the bile as the monoglutamate and undergoes an enterohepatic circulation with intestinal reabsorption. Folate deficiency may result from either inadequate intake or intestinal disease. Because the body stores of folate are small, individuals on a diet low in leafy green vegetables are particularly prone to folate deficiency; these include alcoholics, elderly people on tea and toast diet, and younger individuals eating primarily "junk food." Intestinal diseases such as gluten enteropathy and nontropical sprue are important causes of folate deficiency. Because megaloblastic changes of the intestinal epithelium can by themselves induce malabsorption, folate replacement is an essential first step in evaluating these patients.

States of increased folate demand can result in folate deficiency; the most notable example of this is pregnancy. Drugs may also contribute to folate deficiency. Anticonvulsants, most frequently dilantin, have been implicated in folate deficiency. Sulfasalazine interferes with the intestinal absorption of folate; therefore individuals with inflammatory bowel disease who are taking this drug and may already have malabsorption or inadequate dietary intake are particularly prone to folate deficiency. Methotrexate blocks formation of the active form of folic acid (tetrahydrofolate) and therefore interferes with its biologic effects. Although diet is undoubtedly the major reason for folate deficiency in alcoholics, some evidence suggests that ethanol's toxic effect on the small bowel may impair folate absorption.[12] Because intestinal folate transport is inhibited by luminal alkalinization, patients with pancreatic insufficiency may exhibit supranormal folate absorption.

Vitamin B_{12}

Vitamin B_{12} (cobalamin) is an essential cofactor in the conversion of homocysteine to methionine. Cobalamin deficiency leads to a derangement in folic acid metabolism and subsequently DNA synthesis. This deficiency underlies the megaloblastic maturation pattern seen in hematopoietic and epithelial cells. Additionally, vitamin B_{12} is necessary for the conversion of methylmalonyl-CoA to succinyl-CoA. Disruption of this pathway causes accumulation of nonphysiologic fatty acids in neuronal lipids, the likely cause of the neurologic problems seen with vitamin B_{12} deficiency.

Because humans cannot synthesize vitamin B_{12}, dietary sources are required to meet the body's requirements. Since the vitamin is found only in animal products (meat and dairy foods), strict vegetarians are at risk for developing a deficiency. The body stores sufficient vitamin B_{12} to meet requirements for several years; therefore, unlike folic acid deficiency, vitamin B_{12} deficiency does not develop acutely. As a corollary, individuals may malabsorb vitamin B_{12} for an extended period of time while their serum levels remain normal.

The absorption of cobalamin is complex and dependent on gastric, pancreatic, and ileal function. Because vitamin B_{12} is relatively large (MW 1355) and bulky and possesses many polar groups, it cannot readily diffuse through membranes; therefore it depends on specific transport processes. A series of binding proteins is essential for vitamin B_{12} absorption: R proteins, intrinsic factor, and transcobalamin II. Considering the minute quantity of cobalamin in the diet ($\approx$ 10 μg/day), this system is highly efficient. The three binding proteins have a high affinity for cobalamin. Intrinsic factor is a glycoprotein produced by gastric parietal cells. It has two distinct binding sites, one for cobalamin and the other for an ileal brush border receptor. R proteins are a family of glycoproteins found in plasma, saliva, tears, bile, and gastric juice. The only distinct receptors for R proteins are found in the liver. Circulating R proteins are termed transcobalamin I and transcobalamin III. Transcobalamin II is a circulating polypeptide that facilitates uptake of vitamin B_{12} into rapidly dividing cells. For the purpose of this discussion, the focus will be only on the role of the gut in cobalamin absorption.

Cobalamin in food protein complexes is rapidly liberated in the acid environment of the stomach. Knowledge of the subsequent steps in cobalamin absorption has undergone some revision in recent years. In the classic view it was assumed that free cobalamin rapidly complexed with intrinsic factor. However, recent studies suggest that within the acid environment of the stomach, cobalamin binds to salivary and gastric R proteins, in preference to intrinsic factor. In the duodenum the increased intraluminal pH decreases the affinity of R protein for intrinsic factor. More significantly, pancreatic proteases degrade R proteins, liberating the cobalamin to bind with intrinsic factor.[2] The intrinsic factor-cobalamin complex, which is resistant to proteolytic digestion, proceeds to the distal ileum. Specific receptors on the brush border of distal ileum recognize and bind the complex. This process is dependent on a neutral pH and calcium but does not clearly require energy. Cobalamin then enters the ileal cell; the fate of intrinsic factor during this internalization has not been determined. Cobalamin exits the ileal cell across the basolateral border into the portal circulation bound to transcobalamin II.

Although the role of R proteins in cobalamin absorption has been delineated, their significance is unknown. R proteins do not recognize the ileal cobalamin–intrinsic factor receptor, and therefore cannot mediate absorption. Individuals with R protein deficiency have been identified; no hematologic derangements are apparent in this condition. In pancreatic insufficiency, transfer of cobalamin from R proteins to intrinsic factor may be defective. This may cause an abnormal Schilling test (see later discussion), but it generally does not result in either a vitamin deficiency or megaloblastic changes. The most attractive hypothesis concerning their function centers on the possible protective role of R proteins.[19] In addition to vitamin B_{12}, bacteria produce many inactive cobalamin analogs. R proteins bind to these inactive analogs with a high affinity, whereas intrinsic factor is fairly specific for the bioactive cobalamins. Therefore R proteins may serve to bind and divert these unwanted cobalamin analogs.

Evaluation of cobalamin absorption is easily accomplished with a Schilling test. By using dual-labeled Co^{57} and Co^{58}, vitamin B_{12}, with and without intrinsic factor, can be administered orally at the same time and the relative rates of absorption can be calculated by measuring the 24-hour urinary excretion of the two isotopes. Given the complexity of cobalamin absorption, several different pathologic entities may cause an abnormal Schilling test. Atrophic gastritis with achlorhydria may be associated with a failure of intrinsic factor production. Additionally, in atrophic gastritis, antibodies directed at either of the two intrinsic factor binding sites (for B_{12} or the ileal receptor) may be found. Gastric resection may remove the source of intrinsic factor production, while ileal resection may eliminate the site for intestinal absorption. Either pancreatic insufficiency or Zollinger-Ellison syndrome may impair transfer of cobalamin to intrinsic factor. Bacterial overgrowth may provide a competitive site for cobalamin uptake. Rare congenital deficiencies of either intrinsic factor of transcobalamin II will inhibit absorption. Megaloblastic changes associated with folic acid deficiency may also affect the results. After appropriate clinical assessment, a modified Schilling test with either a course of antibiotics to treat overgrowth or pancreatic enzyme replacement may elucidate the cause of the cobalamin malabsorption.

WATER-SOLUBLE VITAMINS

Contrary to common thought, most water-soluble vitamins are not absorbed from the intestine by simple diffusion. These substances are relatively large, not freely diffusible in lipid because of their polar side chains, and found in the intestinal lumen in low concentrations; therefore they are ideal candidates for carrier-mediated transport. Recent studies suggest that ascorbic acid, biotin, nicotinic acid, and thiamine all possess Na-dependent active transport processes. Studies with riboflavin suggest a carrier-mediated absorption, whereas pyridoxine exhibits a nonspecific transport process. Intestinal metabolism of pyridoxine, riboflavin, and thiamine appears to involve a phosphorylation step. Isolated malabsorption of these water-soluble vitamins is rare but in global malabsorption or dietary deprivation deficiencies may become clinically significant.

Thiamine acts as a coenzyme involved in the metabolism of pyruvate and alpha ketoglutarate and in other reactions involving the cleavage of carbon-carbon bonds. In addition to its role in intermediate metabolism, thiamine may have a specific role in nerve conduction. Clinical thiamine deficiency (beriberi) may appear as congestive heart failure or may have neurologic derangements such as peripheral neuropathy, Wernicke's encephalopathy, and the Korsakoff's syndrome. Wernicke's encephalopathy may appear with horizontal nystagmus, lateral rectus muscle palsies, confusion, or coma. Korsakoff's syndrome involves recent memory loss with a compensatory, often colorful, confabulation. Clinically significant thiamine deficiency is found most frequently in alcoholics or globally malnourished individuals, including patients with gastric partitioning.

Daily thiamine requirement may vary with the diet composition, increasing with more carbohydrates, decreasing with more fat. Therefore it is possible to precipitate overt signs of thiamine deficiency in a marginally compensated individual by administration of a large carbohydrate load. Routine administration of thiamine to alcoholics who go to a medical facility for care is aimed at preventing such an occurrence.

Deficiencies of other water-soluble vitamins, such as ascorbic acid, biotin, nicotinic acid, pyridoxine, and riboflavin, are sufficiently rare not to warrant any detailed discussion. For a review of the clinical manifestations associated with deficiencies of these vitamins, the reader is referred to standard textbooks of nutrition.

IRON

Because the mechanisms of iron (Fe) excretion, through either bile or kidney, are extremely limited, intestinal iron absorption is central to iron homeostasis. In adult males approximately 1 mg of Fe is absorbed daily, matching intestinal losses. In women absorption is somewhat higher, 1.5 mg/day. Rates of intestinal absorption clearly adapt to the body's overall needs; in states of Fe deficiency, the intestine increases its rates of absorption. The mechanisms for this autoregulation have yet to be definitively elucidated despite intensive investigation.

The type of iron ingested and a variety of intraluminal events play major roles in Fe absorption. Dietary iron may be plant iron, heme, or inorganic salts (pharmacologic replacement). Heme iron is more efficiently absorbed by mechanisms different from nonheme iron and is not affected by intraluminal events.[29] In contrast, nonheme iron absorption is influenced by intraluminal factors that either increase or decrease its solubility.[34]

The chemical form of dietary iron is important. A ferrous (Fe^{2+}) compound is absorbed better than a ferric (Fe^{3+}) one. This may be related to the fact that $FeCl_2$ is much more soluble than $FeCl_3$ at neutral pH. Therefore factors that tend to reduce Fe, such as gastric acid, tend to increase its absorption. In pancreatic insufficiency, increased iron absorption may be found; this is probably related to the high phosphate and bicarbonate concentrations found in normal pancreatic secretions, which alter the chemical form of Fe. Ascorbic acid also increases Fe absorption. In part, this results from its action as a reducing agent. Additionally, it may form a soluble complex with Fe, maintaining it in a more absorbable form. Other factors, such as bile, amino acids, and succinic acid, further assist Fe absorption.

A variety of intraluminal binding agents may decrease Fe absorption. Phytate, phosphates, oxalate, and carbonate inhibit Fe absorption by forming insoluble complexes. Dietary fiber may also function as an intraluminal binder. There is evidence that other metallic cations such as cobalt and manganese (but not calcium or magnesium) may inhibit Fe absorption.

The chief site of Fe absorption is in the duodenum. Hemoglobin is split into its two constituent moieties within the intestinal lumen; heme is then taken up in an intact form by the epithelium. Once within the cell, the iron is enzymatically released and enters the cellular Fe pool. The mechanisms of nonheme iron transfer across the intestinal epithelium are less clearly defined. Entry across the apical membrane is carrier-mediated, saturable, and energy-dependent.[23] Within the cell, Fe may either enter the portal circulation bound to transferrin or complex with ferritin and remain within the epithelial cell. Fe retained within epithelial cells will eventually be excreted after the cells exfoliate.

Although the epithelium clearly adapts to the body's need for Fe and the degree of erythropoesis, the specific factors responsible for this adaptation have not been identified. Ferritin, plasma transferrin saturation, and iron content of mucosal cells have all been proposed as possible regulatory mechanisms, but evidence in the literature supporting these various possibilities is conflicting.

Fe deficiency may occasionally result from an inadequate diet (almost exclusively observed in infants), achlorhydria, malabsorption syndromes, duodenal bypass and/or resection, or increased metabolic demands (e.g., in pregnancy). As a practical matter, however, Fe deficiency must be assumed to be caused by blood loss until proven otherwise. Approximately half of the body's Fe stores is found in red blood cells (2500 mg). One ml of packed red cells contains 1 mg of Fe. Since the rate of mobilization of Fe from nonheme stores is relatively slow, the only compensation for acute blood loss is limited.

Iron overload syndromes may result from excessive Fe absorption. In hemochromatosis, Fe absorption may be as high as 4 mg/day. Because of the limited excretory mechanisms for this substance, total body Fe stores gradually and inexorably increase. Excessive Fe absorption is found in states of ineffective erythropoesis or hemolysis. Increased dietary Fe can rarely cause overload; the classic example is the Bantu tribe in South Africa, who brew their beer in iron pots.

CLINICAL APPROACH TO MALABSORPTION

By combining a modicum of clinical acumen with the rational use of diagnostic tests, physicians can establish a diagnosis of malabsorption, pinpoint a cause, and establish a rational therapeutic plan. Crucial to accomplishing this is an understanding of the pathophysiology of malabsorption and the principles underlying the diagnostic tests.[42]

Individual patients may exhibit either global malabsorption or malabsorption of a specific nutrient; their initial clinical appearance will vary accordingly. The cardinal symptom of global malabsorption is weight loss. Diarrhea is a common finding, but it is important to remember that not all diarrhea implies malabsorption and, conversely, global malabsorption is not always accompanied by diarrhea. The development of bulky, floating stools suggests malabsorption. The presence of oily or foul smelling stools or both is a less reliable indicator. Fatigue and lethargy are frequently present. The clinical appearance of malabsorption of a specific nutrient (e.g., vitamin B_{12}, lactose) may be more subtle and depends on the particular substance involved.

Generally, the first step is to confirm the presence of malabsorption by documenting the presence of steatorrhea. Fecal fat, rather than carbohydrate or protein, is used as the sensitive indicator of malabsorption for two fundamental reasons: successful fat absorption requires the pancreas, biliary system, and intestinal mucosa and therefore reflects the normal functioning of all three components. Additionally, and on a more pragmatic level, a reasonable correlation exists between unabsorbed dietary fat and fecal fat, whereas unabsorbed carbohydrate and protein are rapidly degraded by bacteria into ammonia, hydrogen, carbon dioxide, and short-chain fatty acids, disrupting the relationship between the actual unabsorbed and fecal components. Although it has generally been assumed that fatty acids are not attacked by bacteria,[14] recent studies of fecal fat suggest that there may be bacterial metabolism of fat.[27]

Several methods are used to detect fecal fat. The gold standard is a quantitative fecal fat collected over 72 hours while the patient is ingesting a 80 to 100 g fat diet. A

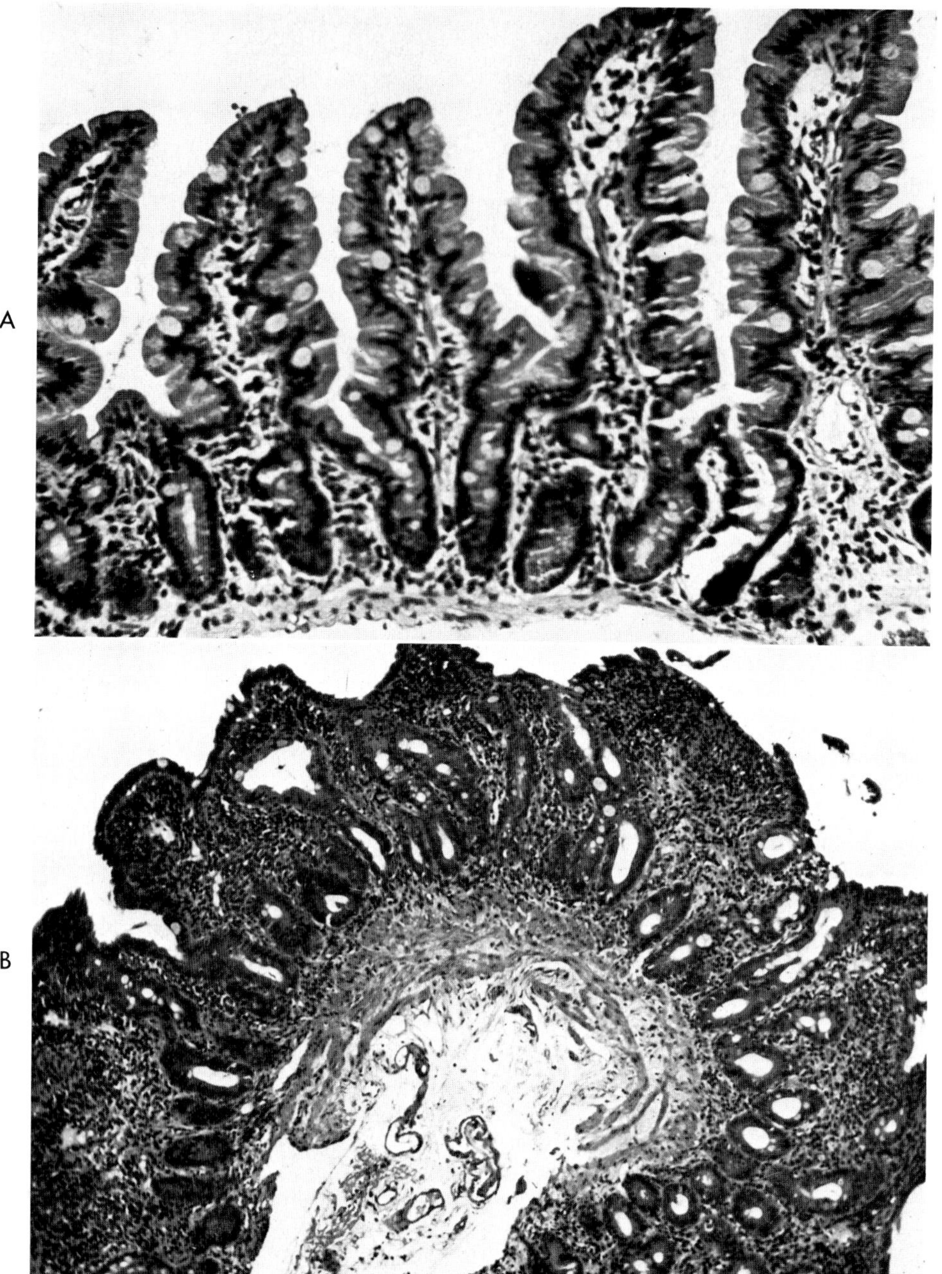

Fig. 19-7 Small bowel histology obtained by biopsy. **A,** Normal small bowel, with long slender villi, modest crypts, and a minimal number of inflammatory cells in the interstitium. **B,** Partial villous atrophy. The villi are clubbed and the crypts elongated.

qualitative estimate of steatorrhea can be obtained with a Sudan stain of a stool sample. The C^{14}-triolein breath test represents a promising advance at quantifying steatorrhea without the cumbersome approach of 3-day stool collections.[25]

Once the presence of steatorrhea is established, the next series of tests are designed to differentiate between mucosal and intraluminal defects. Intraluminal defects are associated with loss of pancreatic or biliary secretions or both or the failure of digestive enzymes to mix with food within the intestinal lumen. Mucosal defects imply a disruption of the normal epithelial function, either by loss of surface area or by disruption of the absorptive machinery of the epithelial cells. The classic tests for mucosal function include D-xylose absorption, small bowel x-rays, and small bowel biopsy. D-xylose is a poorly absorbed five-carbon sugar. Because xylose does not require intraluminal digestion by pancreatic enzymes, it is generally regarded as an indicator of intestinal mucosal disease. Since the test is inexpensive, essentially risk-free, and accurate, it is one of the primary tests in assessing malabsorption. After drinking a solution containing 25 g of D-xylose, urine is collected over a 5-hour period. Urinary excretion of 5 g or greater of D-xylose is normal. Severe bacterial overgrowth can sometimes lead to a falsely positive test because intraluminal bacteria successfully compete with the mucosa for

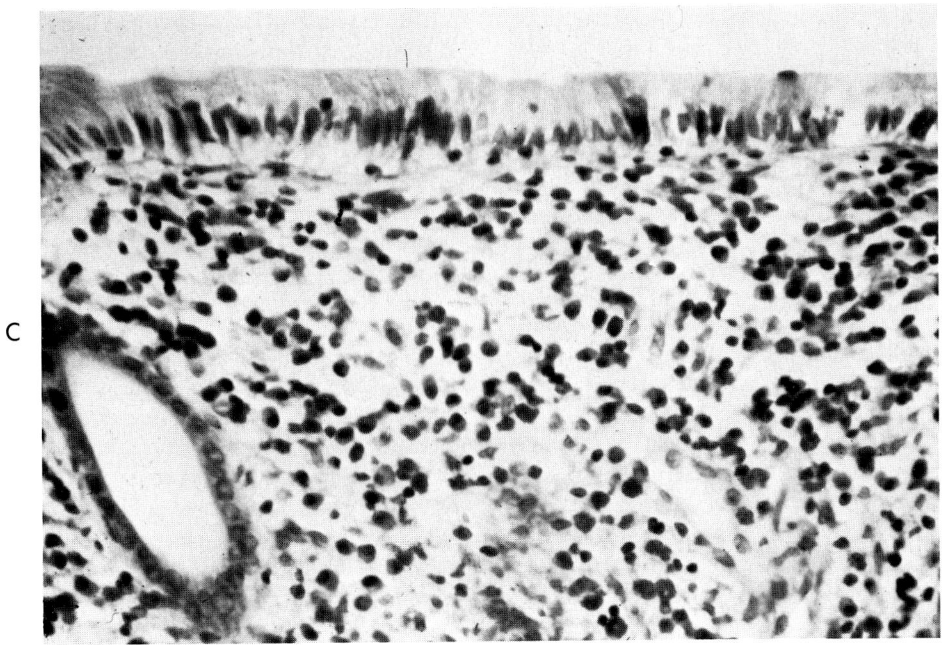

Fig. 19-7, cont'd **C,** Subtotal villous atrophy. Villi are absent suggesting a "flat mucosa."

the sugar. After treatment for overgrowth, D-xylose absorption should return to normal.

Barium contrast studies of the small bowel are essential for diagnosing specific anatomic defects (e.g., strictures, jejunal diverticulum) and for assessing the mucosal pattern of the small bowel. The cardinal findings in intestinal disease include dilation of the intestinal lumen, thickening of mucosal folds, dilution of barium, and segmentation of the head of the barium column.[20] Thickening of folds generally indicates an infiltrative process (amyloidosis) or a response to hypoproteinemia. The new improved barium sulfate now used in contrast studies is "nondispersible"; therefore flocculation is no longer a reliable or common sign in malabsorption. Dilution of the barium is secondary to increased water within the intestinal lumen, a common finding in diarrhea associated with malabsorption. X-ray studies may indicate fairly specific abnormalities such as lymphonodular hyperplasia or inflammatory bowel disease that may elucidate the etiology of a particular case of malabsorption. The small bowel series is an important diagnostic tool in a malabsorption workup; one proviso, however, is necessary: barium studies should be held in abeyance until all stool collections are complete.

The small bowel biopsy provides histologic confirmation of mucosal disease and frequently enables a specific diagnosis to be made.[38] Uncommon diseases such as abetalipoproteinemia, Whipple's disease, and immunodeficiency syndromes have diffuse lesions that are pathognomonic on small intestinal biopsy. Diagnostic small intestinal biopsies may also be obtained in diseases with patchy lesions (e.g., lymphoma, eosinophilic enteritis, amyloidosis, and Crohn's disease). The small bowel biopsy is probably most useful in the diagnosis of gluten enteropathy (nontropical sprue) (Fig. 19-7). In this disease the normal villous pattern is replaced by a "flat" mucosa in which the villi are absent, the crypts hypertrophied, and the lamina propria contain increased numbers of inflammatory cells. Since sprue involves primarily the proximal small bowel, it is amenable to diagnosis by biopsy. However, subtotal villous atrophy occasionally can occur in tropical sprue and therefore, by itself, is not pathognomonic. Clinical and histologic improvement after withdrawal of dietary gluten can confirm the diagnosis. Partial villous atrophy is characterized by shortened, clubbed villi and increased numbers of inflammatory cells in the lamina propria and interepithelial spaces (see Fig. 19-7). It is found in a number of intestinal diseases including tropical sprue, severe bacterial overgrowth, and radiation enteritis.

When considering a diagnosis that produces a patchy mucosal lesion, multiple biopsies are necessary. Normal results from a small bowel biopsy provide useful clinical information because they direct the malabsorption workup toward intraluminal defects caused by pancreatic insufficiency, bacterial overgrowth, and short bowel syndrome. Examples of the kinds of information that small bowel biopsy can provide are demonstrated in Fig. 19-7.

Accurate clinical assessment of pancreatic function is difficult and notoriously insensitive. The standard pancreatic secretion test assesses the increase in duodenal fluid and bicarbonate and pancreatic enzymes in response to secretion stimulated by secretin or CCK or both. In severe chronic pancreatitis, both bicarbonate and volume are reduced. In carcinoma of the head of the pancreas, similar reductions may be found. In partial duct obstruction, bicarbonate secretion may be maintained while volume is decreased. Mild to moderate pancreatic insufficiency and carcinomas of the body and tail generally do not cause abnormalities in the pancreatic secretion tests.

Because of this insensitivity attempts at developing tubeless pancreatic function tests have been numerous. Probably the two most promising are the dual-label pancreatic Schilling test and the bentiromide absorption test.

The pancreatic Schilling test compares the rates of absorption of vitamin B_{12} bound to intrinsic factor and to R protein. Because dissociation of the B_{12}–R protein complex depends on pancreatic proteases, in contradistinction to the B_{12}–intrinsic factor complex, the relative rates of absorption of these two complexes provides an assessment of pancreatic secretory function.[5] In a similar manner, bentiromide absorption depends on peptide cleavage by chymotrypsin, which liberates *p*-aminobenzoic acid (PABA). PABA is subsequently absorbed and excreted into the urine, where it can be easily measured.[21] Since both tests are relatively new, their clinical utility will have to be proven as their use becomes more widespread.

The introduction of breath tests into clinical medicine has enhanced the physician's acumen in diagnosing malabsorption.[13] Although there is a wide array of breath tests, they are based on common principles: nutrients are absorbed in the small bowel, which is relatively sterile; therefore they normally escape bacterial degradation. However, if unabsorbed nutrients pass into the colon or if there is significant bacterial contamination of the small bowel, intraluminal bacterial metabolism of the nutrients will produce a gas (either carbon dioxide [CO_2] or hydrogen [H_2]) that is freely diffusible across the gut wall into the systemic circulation. The gas will then be excreted by the lungs.

Because hydrogen is not normally expired, an increase in breath hydrogen can be used as a sensitive signal for malabsorption. The situation is somewhat more complicated for CO_2. Because CO_2 is a normal constituent of expired air, a labeled form of carbon is necessary to detect CO_2 of gut origin. This can be accomplished by using either a radioactive isotope of carbon (^{14}C) that can be detected by standard scintillation counting techniques or a nonradioactive stable isotope (^{13}C). However, because the stable isotope is not as readily available and requires specialized mass spectroscopy for detection, this technology will most likely be restricted to research centers.

The hydrogen breath test has been used primarily to detect carbohydrate malabsorption. It has proven extremely useful in detecting lactase deficiency. In this situation, an oral load of lactose is not absorbed because of a lack of the brush border disaccharidase enzyme. The sugar passes into the colon where bacterial metabolism yields 2- and 3- carbon fragments, CO_2 and H_2. An increase in the amount of H_2 in expired air indicates malabsorption. Because the test is noninvasive, does not use radioisotopes, does not require blood-drawing, and uses relatively simple equipment, it is ideal for assessing carbohydrate intolerance in children and pregnant women. This methodology can be easily applied to the study of other carbohydrates, including xylose, fructose, and glucose.

By radiolabeling one of the carbon atoms in the glycine conjugate of a bile acid, the enterohepatic circulation of bile salts can be assessed. Normally the terminal ileum efficiently absorbs the bile salts presented to it. However, if there is significant ileal dysfunction or small bowel bacterial overgrowth, the bile salt will be deconjugated, the glycine metabolized, and the $^{14}CO_2$ thus produced will be excreted by the lungs. Therefore an abnormal ^{14}C–bile salt breath test can indicate ileal dysfunction or bacterial overgrowth. It cannot reliably distinguish between the two conditions.

The triolein breath test has been proposed as a substitute for a quantitative fecal fat collection. ^{14}C-triolein is given with a standard oral fat load. Normal fat absorption results in a significant increase in expired $^{14}CO_2$, whereas steatorrhea is suggested by the lack of a $^{14}CO_2$ peak. This test differs from other breath tests in that the signal is found in normal results and does not depend on bacterial metabolism of the nutrient.

Compared to recent technologic advances, the standard Schilling test may appear rather staid. Nevertheless, it can prove extremely useful in a general malabsorption workup in addition to its obvious application in detecting vitamin B_{12} malabsorption. It should be kept in mind that a Schilling test may be abnormal in bacterial overgrowth (caused by bacterial metabolism of cobalamin), pancreatic insufficiency (secondary to lack of protease action on R protein), and ileal disease (with lack of the specific transporter). Because it is a sensitive indicator of malabsorption and readily available to every clinician, it remains a useful diagnostic tool.

A malabsorption workup can proceed in a rational fashion, applying diagnostic tests to answer a series of progressive questions:

Is global malabsorption (steatorrhea) present?
Is there any evidence of mucosal disease?
Is pancreatic function intact?
Is there malabsorption of a specific nutrient?

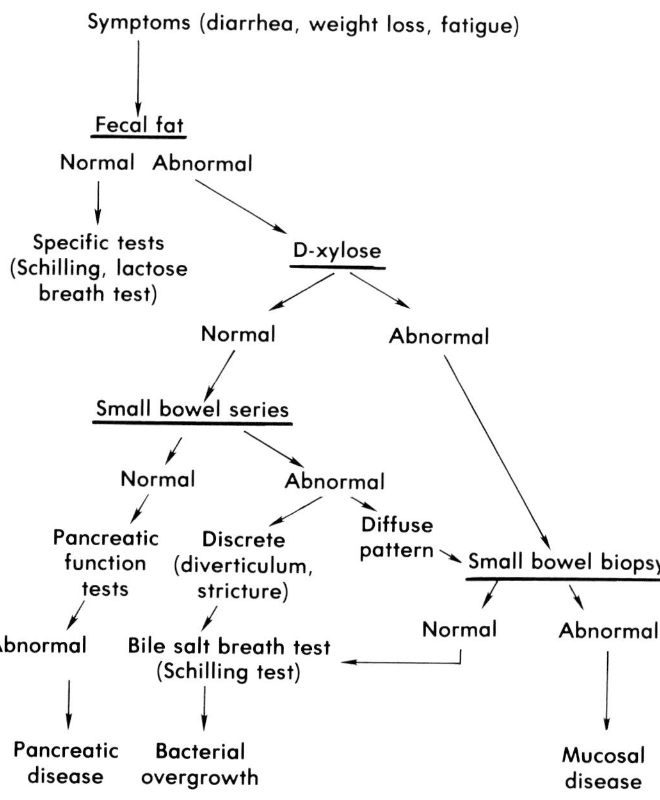

Fig. 19-8 Algorithm for a clinical approach to malabsorption.

By following a standard algorithm, such as the one summarized in Fig. 19-8, the physician can proceed through a malabsorption workup quite efficiently.

DISORDERS OF MALDIGESTION AND MALABSORPTION ENCOUNTERED IN SURGICAL PATIENTS

The majority of diseases giving rise to malabsorption or maldigestion in surgical patients occur in situations in which a previous operation on the intestinal tract has been performed. For example, excessive overgrowth of bacteria in the small intestine occasionally occurs in a patient undergoing a Billroth-II gastrectomy in which the afferent loop becomes obstructed. The accompanying diarrhea may adversely affect the digestion and absorption of all kinds of foodstuffs including fats, protein, and carbohydrates. In addition, bacteria compete for vitamin B_{12} and thereby can potentially alter the absorption of this substance, giving rise to a megaloblastic anemia. Another example of a surgically induced maldigestive syndrome results when extensive intestinal resection becomes necessary as occasionally occurs in patients with inflammatory bowel disorders or following intestinal infarction secondary to embolization of the superior mesenteric artery. Depending on the extent of intestinal resection, severe disturbances in the normal physiology of digestion and absorption may ensue. For a more detailed discussion of surgically induced disorders of malabsorption and maldigestion, the reader is referred to the chapter on derangements in intestinal function secondary to previous surgery.

In addition to surgically induced disease, other conditions may also give rise to derangements in intestinal function in surgical patients. Inflammatory bowel disease of the ileum (Crohn's disease) may severely alter the normal transport and absorptive mechanisms of the distal ileum affecting vitamin B_{12} absorption and the enterohepatic circulation. More extensive involvement of the small intestine may result in an abnormality in calcium absorption with attendant hypocalcemia and bone pain from osteomalacia or osteoporosis or both. On occasion, deficiencies in vitamin K and iron may also be encountered with the accompanying sequelae resulting therefrom. Because Crohn's disease is associated with involvement of the entire thickness of the bowel wall, resulting in transmural inflammation, a wide variety of effects on nutrient transport can be observed; these are directly related to the length of intestine involved with this disease.

In patients with various neoplastic disorders in which radiation comprised a major component of treatment, malabsorption is occasionally observed because of the resulting fibrosis and endarteritis, which affects the full thickness of the intestinal wall and alters nutrient transport. Lymphomatous involvement of the intestinal tract may also cause malabsorption. Again, the length of intestine involved in these disorders will influence the magnitude of the maldigestive problem. Other diseases, more commonly encountered by internists than surgeons, that can greatly alter digestion and absorption include celiac sprue, tropical sprue, and Whipple's disease. Because these disorders are only rarely seen by surgeons, the reader is referred to standard gastroenterology textbooks for a detailed discussion of their clinical appearance.

SUMMARY

Efficient absorption and digestion depend on integration of a series of complex events both within the intestinal lumen and at the epithelial border. Of the three major categories of food, only fat requires emulsification and solubilization by micelles within the intestinal lumen before passive absorption across the epithelium. The products of carbohydrate and protein digestion use specific transport carriers at the apical border of the intestinal epithelium.

The movement of water is secondary to the active transport of ions. Specifically, sodium is the major ion determining osmotic gradients favorable for water absorption, whereas chloride is the usual driving force for secretion. A host of hormones, peptides, drugs, and bacterial toxins regulate the traffic of ions and water across the intestinal epithelium.

Diarrhea and malabsorption are the major clinical manifestations of dysfunction of the intestinal epithelium. An orderly clinical approach coupled with judicious use of basic diagnostic tests will usually clarify the etiology of diarrhea (osmotic vs. secretory) or malabsorption (maldigestion vs. epithelial disease).

REFERENCES

1. Adibi, S.A., and Kim, Y.S.: Peptide absorption and hydrolysis. In Johnson, L.R., editor: Physiology of the gastrointestinal tract, New York, 1981, Raven Press.
2. Allen, R.H., et al.: Effect of proteolytic enzymes on the binding of cobalamin to R protein and intrinsic factor, J. Clin. Invest. **61**:47, 1978.
3. Avioli, L.V., and Haddad, J.G.: The vitamin D family revisited, N. Engl. J. Med. **311**:47, 1984.
4. Bo-Linn, G.W., et al.: Evaluation of importance of gastric acid secretion in the absorption of dietary calcium, J. Clin. Invest. 640, 1984.
5. Brugge, W., et al.: Development of a dual label Schilling test for pancreatic exocrine function based on the differential absorption of cobalamin bound to intrinsic factor and R protein, Gastroenterology **78**:937, 1980.
6. Carpenter, C.C., et al.: Site and characteristics of electrolyte loss and effect of intraluminal glucose in experimental canine cholera, J. Clin. Invest. **47**:1210, 1968.
7. Fordtran, J.S., Rector, F.C., and Carter, N.W.: Mechanisms of sodium absorption in the human small intestine, J. Clin. Invest. **47**:884, 1968.
8. Frizzell, R.A., Heintze, K., and Stewart, C.P.: Mechanisms of intestinal chloride secretion. In Field, M., Fordtran, J.S., and Schultz, S.G., editors: Secretory diarrhea, Bethesda, Md., 1980, American Physiological Society.
9. Gaskin, K.J., et al.: Colipase and maximally activated pancreatic lipase in normal subjects and patients with steatorrhea, J. Clin. Invest. **69**:427, 1982.
10. Gaskin, K.J., et al.: Colipase and lipase secretion in childhood-onset pancreatic insufficiency, Gastroenterology **86**:1, 1984.
11. Gray, G.M.: Carbohydrate digestion and absorption, N. Engl. J. Med. **292**:1225, 1975.
12. Green, P.H.R., and Tall, A.R.: Drugs, alcohol, and malabsorption, Am. J. Med. **67**:1066, 1979.
13. Hepner, G.W.: Breath tests in gastroenterology, Adv. Intern. Med. **18**:25, 1978.
14. Hoffman, A.F.: Fat absorption and malabsorption, Viewpoints Dig. Dis. **9**:13, 1977.
15. Kaplan, M.M.: Metabolic bone disease associated with gastrointestinal diseases, Viewpoints Dig. Dis. **15**:9, 1983.

16. Kelly, S.E., et al.: Effect of meal composition on calcium absorption: enhancing effect of carbohydrate polymers, Gastroenterology **87**:596, 1984.
17. Kimberg, D.V., et al.: Stimulation of intestinal mucosal adenylate cyclase by cholera enterotoxin and prostaglandins, J. Clin. Invest. **50**:1218, 1971.
18. Kimmich, G.A., and Randles, J.: Evidence for an intestinal Na^+: sugar transport coupling stoichiometry of 2.0, Biochim. Biophys. Acta **596**:439, 1980.
19. Kolhouse, J.F., and Allen, R.H.: Absorption, plasma transport and cellular transport of cobalamin analogues in the rabbit, J. Clin. Invest. **60**:1381, 1977.
20. Kumar, P., and Bertram, C.I.: Relevance of the barium follow through examination in the diagnosis of adult celiac disease, Gastrointest. Radiol. **4**:285, 1979.
21. Lankisch, P.G.: Tubeless pancreatic function tests, Hepatogastroenterology **28**:333, 1981.
22. Liedtke, C.M., and Hopfer, U.: Mechanism of Cl translocation across small intestinal brush border membrane, Am. J. Physiol. **243**:G263, 1982.
23. Manis, J., and Schacter, D.: Active transport of iron by intestine, Am. J. Physiol. **203**:73, 1962.
24. Matthews, D.M., and Adibi, S.A.: Peptic absorption, Gastroenterology **71**:151, 1976.
25. Newcomer, A.D., et al.: Triolein breath test, Gastroenterology **76**:6, 1979.
26. Norman, D.A., Morawski, S.G., and Fordtran, J.S.: Influence of glucose, fructose, and water movement on calcium absorption in jejunum, Gastroenterology **78**:22, 1980.
27. Patton, J.S.: Gastrointestinal lipid digestion. In Johnston, L.R., editor: Physiology of the gastrointestinal tract, New York, 1981, Raven Press.
28. Patton, J.S., and Carey, M.C.: Watching fat digestion, Science **204**:145, 1979.
29. Prasad, A.S., editor: Trace elements and Fe metabolism, New York, 1978, Plenum Publishing Corp.
30. Rasmussen, H., et al.: Role of changes in membrane lipid structure in the action of 1.25 dihydroxy-vitamin D_3, Fed. Proc. **41**:72, 1982.
31. Riley, J.W., and Glickman, R.M.: Fat malabsorption—advances in our understanding, Am. J. Med. **67**:980, 1979.
32. Rosenberg, I.H.: Intestinal absorption of folate. In Johnson, L.R., editor: Physiology of the gastrointestinal tract, New York, 1981, Raven Press.
33. Rosensweig, N.S., and Herman, R.H.: Control of jejunal sucrase and maltase activity by dietary sucrose or fructose in man, J. Clin. Invest. **46**:186, 1967.
34. Schade, S.G., Cohen, R.J., and Conrad, H.E.: Effect of hydrochloric acid on iron absorption, N. Engl. J. Med. **279**:672, 1968.
35. Schedl, H.P., Wenger, J., and Adibi, S.A.: Diglycine absorption in streptozoticin diabetic rats, Am. J. Physiol. **235**:E457, 1978.
36. Schultz, S.G.: Cellular models of sodium and chloride absorption by mammalian small and large intestine. In Field, M., Fordtran, J.S., and Schultz, S.G., editors: Secretory diarrhea, Bethesda, Md., 1980, American Physiological Society.
37. Sleisenger, M.H., and Kim, Y.S.: Protein digestion and absorption, N. Engl. J. Med. **300**:659, 1979.
38. Trier, J.S.: Diagnostic value of peroral biopsy at the small intestine, N. Engl. J. Med. **85**:1470, 1971.
39. Wasserman, R.H., et al.: Evidence for multiple effects of vitamin D_3 on calcium absorption, Proc. Natl. Acad. Sci. USA **79**:7939, 1982.
40. Westergaard, H., and Dietschy, J.M.: Delineation of the dimensions and permeability characteristics of the two major diffusion barriers to passive mucosal uptake in the rabbit intestine, J. Clin. Invest. **54**:718, 1974.
41. Wilson, F.A., and Dietschy, J.M.: Characterization of bile acid absorption across the unstirred water layer and brush border of the rat jejunum, J. Clin. Invest. **51**:3015, 1972.
42. Wilson, F.A., and Dietschy, J.M.: Differential diagnostic approach to clinical problems of malabsorption, Gastroenterology **61**:911, 1971.
43. Ziegler, E.E., and Fomon, S.T.: Lactose enhances mineral absorption in infancy, J. Pediatr. Gastroenterol. Nutr. **2**:288, 1983.

20 *James M. Becker*

Normal Peristalsis and Abnormalities in Intestinal Motility

In 1899 Bayliss and Starling wrote, "In no subject in physiology do we meet with so many discrepancies of fact and opinion as in that of the physiology of the intestinal movements." Although medical professionals have greater knowledge about intestinal motility today, much uncertainty and lack of understanding still exist. The movement of ingested food and secretions through the gastrointestinal (GI) tract and its appendages depends on a highly integrated and coordinated response of the smooth muscle contained within the wall of the gut. This chapter wil consider in detail the various myogenic, neurogenic, endocrine, and paracrine factors that contribute to the usual aborad propulsion of GI contents. Clinical problems associated with disorders of motility of the GI tract, which are extremely common and, in general, refractory to medical or surgical management, will also be discussed. Although physicians now better understand the physiology of gut motility, the relationship of normal and abnormal physiology to symptom complexes remains unclear. Therefore treatment is empiric and often not specific.

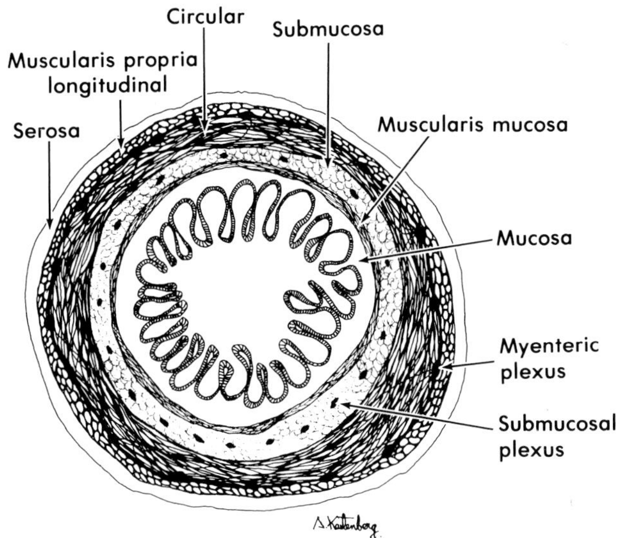

Fig. 20-1 Neuromuscular anatomy of the alimentary tract. Muscularis propria consists of both longitudinal and circular muscle groups.

GENERAL CONSIDERATIONS IN GASTROINTESTINAL MOTILITY

The primary role of the GI tract is to absorb water, electrolytes, minerals, vitamins, and nutrients. In human beings and other higher forms muscular activity of the wall of the GI tract is vitally important in directing the ingested material to the appropriate anatomic site for absorption. The motor action, or *motility,* of the GI tract therefore serves several major functions, including propulsion, mixing, and storage. Ingested foods and fluid, as well as secretions and desquamated cells, are *propulsed* through the alimentary canal in a well-controlled fashion to deliver the intraluminal content to the absorptive cells and propel the undigested material into and through the colon. During this process the chyme undergoes a thorough *mixing,* resulting in mechanical dispersion that increases surface area and facilitates contact with the digestive secretions and absorptive mucosal cells. Secretions from the stomach, pancreas, and biliary system are mixed with the chyme as it passes through the GI tract. The alimentary tract also serves a very important *reservoir* or *storage* function. The reservoir capacity of the stomach and gallbladder are discussed in Chapters 15 and 26. The colon stores unabsorbed small intestinal contents while it acts to reabsorb electrolytes, and it then eliminates the residual by the process of defecation.

The integration and regulation of intestinal motility depend on the interaction of extrinsic and intrinsic neural, humoral, and myogenic factors. Coordinated by electric patterns of intestinal smooth muscle, the myogenic factors appear to be the most fundamental. Neural control is exerted by intrinsic and extrinsic nerves of the GI tract. Humoral control is exerted by various endogenous chemicals that act either directly on the smooth muscle cells or on the nerves. As discussed in the next section, myogenic control mechanisms determine the temporal and spatial patterns of contractions, whereas neural and humoral control mechanisms determine whether contractions will occur at a given site.

Relatively consistent neuromuscular anatomy exists throughout the alimentary tract (Fig. 20-1). With the exception of the oropharynx, proximal esophagus, and external anal sphincter, the musculature of the GI tract is smooth muscle. In general, the smooth muscle of the alimentary canal is arranged in three layers. These include an inner muscularis mucosa surrounded by the circular layer of smooth muscle and finally an outer longitudinal layer with fibers running parallel to the axis of the bowel. Between these muscle layers are the interconnecting plexuses of the enteric nervous system composed of ganglia and nerve fibers. The myenteric (Auerbach's) plexus is located between the longitudinal and circular muscle layers. The submucosal (Meissner's) plexus is located between the muscularis mucosa and the circular muscle layer. The en-

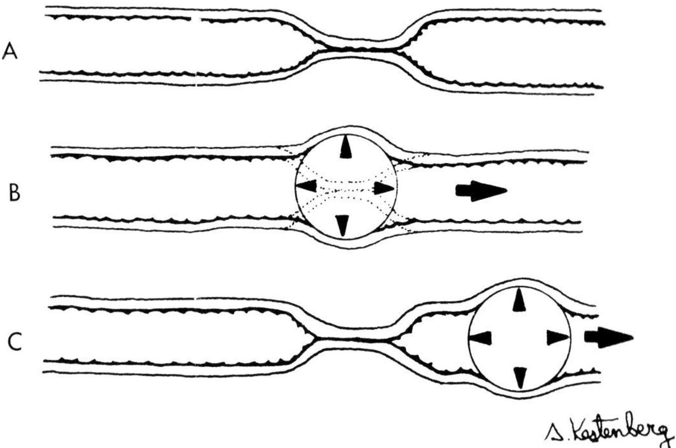

Fig. 20-2 Responses of gastrointestinal sphincters to intraluminal content. **A,** Tonic contraction of the sphincter at rest. **B,** Relaxation of the sphincter associated with passage of intraluminal content. **C,** Reestablishment of tonic contraction of the sphincter with aborad passage of the intraluminal bolus.

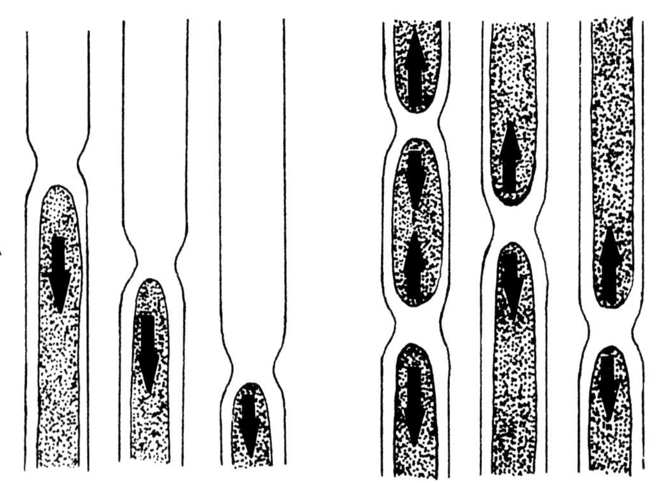

Fig. 20-3 **A,** Aborad movement of an intestinal peristaltic contraction. **B,** Segmental contraction of the bowel.

teric nervous system receives input from local receptors in the mucosa and smooth muscle, as well as from the central nervous system through the autonomic nervous system. These elements of the nervous system interact with neuropeptides and classic GI hormones and together help integrate sensory information for control of motor activity.

Motility of the GI tract can be simplified into major patterns of muscle contraction. In general, three types of motor activity of the gut occur: (1) tonic contractions, (2) peristaltic waves, and (3) segmenting contractions. *Tonic contractions* are sustained and generally produce low pressure (Fig. 20-2). They are most often observed in sphincter segments but are also necessary for emptying the fundus of the stomach and the gallbladder. The basic propulsive motor activity of the GI tract is *peristalsis,* which consists of rings of contraction moving in an aborad direction (Fig. 20-3, *A*). The major stimulus for the initiation of peristalsis is distention of the bowel. As first described by Cannon, the law of the intestine dictates that contraction occurs above and relaxation below the point of distention (Fig. 20-4). *Segmental contractions* are primarily responsible for intraluminal mixing (Fig. 20-3, *B*). Whereas peristaltic activity occurs throughout the GI tract, segmentation is confined to the small intestine and colon.

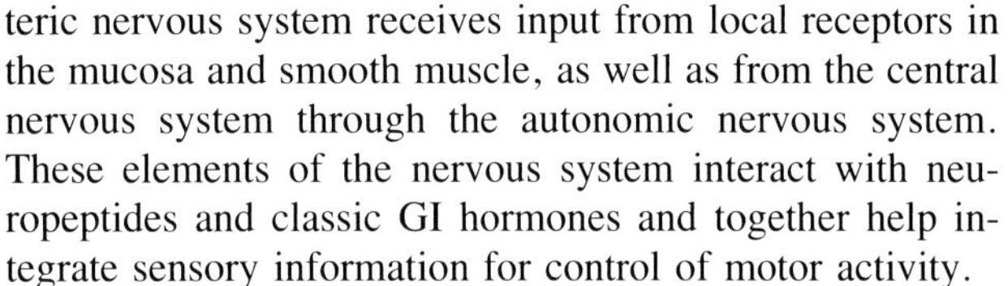

MYOELECTRIC CONTROL OF INTESTINAL MOTILITY

As first described by Alvarez,[2] one of the intrinsic properties of GI smooth muscle is the spontaneous generation of electropotential charges. These electric oscillations in membrane potential are seen as either bursts of fast spike activity; slower, rhythmic variations in potential; or both. The slow pattern is an omnipresent, cyclically recurring, rhythmic depolarization in smooth muscle potential usually designated as the *slow wave, basic electric rhythm (BER),* or *electric control activity (ECA).* It is present when the muscle is at rest or when it is contracting. The second

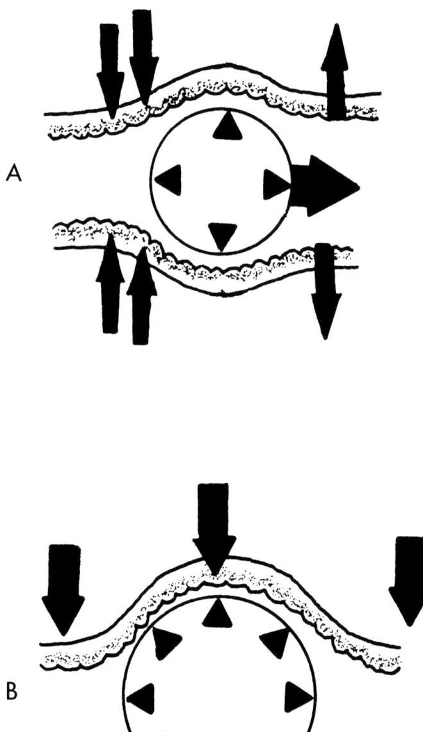

Fig. 20-4 **A,** According to Cannon's Law of the Intestine, physiologic distention of the bowel results in contraction orad to that point and relaxation aborad from that point with net aborad flow of intraluminal contents. **B,** Pathologic intraluminal distention of the bowel results in spasm and defective peristalsis with little or no aborad flow.

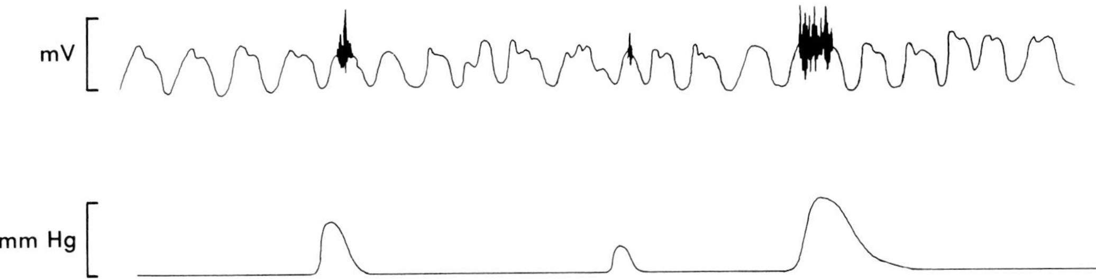

Fig. 20-5 Myoelectric slow waves with superimposed spike potentials *(upper tracing)*. In general, slow waves determine the timing of spike potentials, which then initiate smooth muscle contractions *(lower tracing)*. Recent evidence suggests that slow waves alone may induce contractions in certain regions of the gut.

component consists of bursts of rapid fluctuation in potential superimposed on the slow wave and is referred to as *spikes, spike potentials, action potentials,* or *electric response activity (ERA)*. Spike potentials represent rapid, complete depolarizations of smooth muscle cells and are usually followed by visible or measurable mechanical contractions.[6,8]

Slow Waves

Although controversy still exists about the significance and function of intestinal slow waves, the current prevailing concept is that they are myogenic in origin and that, by coordinating spike activity, they establish both the rhythmicity and the polarity of intestinal contractions. Slow waves consist of periodic depolarizations of intestinal muscle cells (Fig. 20-5). In the upper GI tract the slow-wave potential most likely originates in the longitudinal muscle of the bowel wall. It then spreads electrotonically into the circular muscle layer in an aborad direction. For this to occur, the muscle cells of the two layers must be electrically coupled by means of low-resistance pathways. The anatomic basis for such coupling is thought to be provided by nexus or gap junctions.[34]

The frequency of the slow wave determines the maximum frequency of contraction of the bowel in the following manner: contractile activity is triggered by spike potentials that occur in bursts occupying a specific segment of the slow wave. Since only one burst occurs with each slow wave and thus only one contraction, the slow-wave frequency of a segment of bowel is also its maximum contractile frequency. Thus the slow wave serves as the pacesetter for a particular segment of bowel (see Fig. 20-5). Each oscillation lasts 2 to 3 seconds and, as shown by intracellular recordings, results in a rhythmic change of membrane potential from about −70 to −25 or −30 mV. The intestine may be characterized on the basis of its particular frequency of slow-wave oscillations.[12,13] In human beings the slow-wave frequency of the stomach in vivo is 3/minute, the duodenum 12/minute, the jejunum 10/minute, and the ileum 8/minute. A gradient of frequency of rhythmic segmentation in an aborad direction is thus seen.

The regular intrinsic frequency of slow-wave electric activity can be compared to a *relaxation oscillator*.[55] This conceptual model can be the solution to a mathematic equation or an electronic circuit. An illustrative example is a device that consists of a container fastened to one arm of a balance and maintained in position by a weight on the other arm. The container is slowly filled with water until the weight of the water exceeds the weight on the opposite arm. The container then empties, returns to its balanced position, and begins to refill. The sequence occurs again and again. The relaxation oscillator model was first used to describe the inherent rhythmic activity in the smooth muscle of the heart. This pattern of relaxation-oscillation gives a recurrent waveform at a steady frequency similar to the slow-wave electric activity of smooth muscle of the intestine. When two such oscillators are coupled, they influence one another. The one with the lower intrinsic frequency shows an increase in frequency so that a pacemaker effect can be produced. By choosing appropriate intrinsic frequencies and coupling factors, a chain of oscillators can be set up that gives slow waves of the pattern found in the small intestine.[39] When the chain is broken, the waves above and below the break mirror the results seen when the gut is cut across. In the stomach a network or matrix instead of a chain of oscillators is used to model the experimental findings. Still another arrangement of oscillators is needed to produce wave patterns similar to those found in the human colon.

Spike Potentials

Superimposed on the relatively slow membrane potentials are rapid depolarization-repolarization cycles, usually referred to as action or spike potentials (see Fig. 20-5). Spike potentials occur only during slow-wave depolarization after a critical or threshold potential is attained.[16] Since not all slow waves are associated with spike activity, it appears that those that are associated usually have greater amplitude than those without spikes. Action potentials initiate phasic contractions of the smooth muscle fibers, apparently by effecting this process of excitation-contraction coupling by stimulating actinmyosin–adenosine triphosphatase (ATPase) activity through release of troponin inhibition. Thus, whereas the slow wave may be present in mechanically inactive bowel, spike potentials are responsible for smooth muscle contraction. One slow wave may be associated with many spikes, a *burst,* resulting in a band or wave front of smooth muscle cell contraction passing along the intestine. Because action potentials are conducted for only short distances in smooth muscle, three to four cell lengths, the basic slow wave organizes the wave front of smooth muscle contraction over long distances. This is not the peristaltic reflex per se, but rather the stratum for part of its organization. Conceptually the slow change in membrane potential is in a depolarizing direction, and the maintenance of this low voltage for several seconds may be regarded as a platform on which action potentials are superimposed.

Thus the slow wave serves as pacemaker or phasing unit for spike potentials and thus mechanical activity. The presence or absence of spike activity in phase with the slow-potential oscillations of smooth muscle cells is the modulation exerted by superimposed excitatory or inhibitory systems. The maximum slow-wave frequency is also the maximum peristaltic frequency of the intestine. Thus the gradients in peristaltic frequency noted in the intestine have as their basis and reflect the corresponding gradient in slow-wave frequencies. The modulation of spike activity with each slow wave is a fundamental control feature.

Although applicable to most of the alimentary canal, this concept has recently been challenged in some anatomic segments. It appears that, in the stomach and colon, motor activity may be associated with slow waves without spikes. This conflict may be resolved by reports suggesting that both slow waves and spikes result primarily from smooth muscle cellular influx of calcium, which, if it results in sufficient membrane depolarization, will result in contraction.

The modulation of spike activity with slow-wave activity is organized to effect propulsion of intestinal contents. This organization is produced by an intrinsic reflex arc of the intestine with an afferent and efferent limb. Thus a second order of control is established. This is responsible for the law of the intestine alluded to previously (see Fig. 20-4). A third order of control of intestinal motility is centrally mediated and is responsible for extrinsic intestinal reflexes. The afferent and efferent limbs of these central neural reflexes lie in both vagal and splanchnic nerve tracts. The intestinal receptors appear to lie within the mucosa and muscular layers. Among other things, the extrinsic neural pathways are responsible for the intestinal-intestinal inhibitory reflex. Electric correlates of this reflex have not been clearly elucidated.

Myoelectric Patterns in the Duodenum and Small Bowel

Slow waves show a clear and consistent pattern along the duodenum. As in other intestinal smooth muscle, duodenal slow waves arise in the longitudinal muscle coat and are transmitted to the circular layer. When multiple electrodes are placed at close intervals along the duodenum, a frequency plateau of 12 cycles/minute in human beings and 18 cycles/minute in dogs is found, with slow-wave frequency identical at multiple sites along the duodenum. This frequency is driven by a pacemaker located in the wall of the first 5 to 6 mm of the duodenum. The localization of the pacemaker was demonstrated in elegant studies by Herman-Taylor and Code,[23] who recorded duodenal electric activity sequentially along the duodenum after annular myotomy at varying levels. The pacemaker is the site of greatest intrinsic frequency of the slow wave. Beyond this duodenal plateau, over a segment of proximal jejunum approximately 5 to 6 cm long, a stepped gradient in the intrinsic frequency of the slow wave is found.

The more rapid frequency of the duodenal pacemaker ensures that under normal conditions the slow wave is propagated in a distal direction from the pacemaker site over the rest of the duodenum. Such distal propagation can organize action potentials and therefore motor activity into a peristaltic sweep along the duodenum. Physical or physiologic separation of the distal duodenum from the proximal pacemaker area exposes the slower intrinsic slow-wave frequency of the distal segment. The site of origin and direction of conduction of the slow wave then becomes more inconstant. Retrograde propagation of the slow wave and associated action potential (i.e., antiperistalsis) is not observed in the normal duodenum.[23] Clinical electromyographic techniques are now identifying conditions in which duoedenal propagation is clearly abnormal. For example, duodenal trauma or inflammatory disease can lead to functional loss of the duodenal pacemaker with resultant retrograde or disjointed peristalsis. Vagotomy may lead to gastric and duodenal antiperistalsis with resultant aberrations of gastric emptying.

The frequency of the slow waves gradually decreases beyond the duodenum to reach 6 to 9 cycles/minute in the ileum in human beings. Two alternate patterns of frequency decline have been hypothesized: (1) a succession of plateaus of variable lengths and decreasing frequency to reach 12 cycles/minute in the ileum or (2) a gradually decreasing frequency along the small bowel to the ileum.[18] Experimental differences may be the result of the different preparations employed in data collection. Most investigators now support the concept of linked frequency plateaus. The gradient of slow-wave frequency in the small intestine agrees quantitatively with the gradient of maximum frequency of rhythmic contractions along the bowel. In addition, the progression of slow waves along the gut with superimposed spike activity causes the movement of rings of contraction caudad and thus establishes the velocity of peristaltic sequences.

Migrating Motor Complex

Characteristic patterns of motility occur in the small intestine of human beings and many other species during fasting and after feeding. During fasting, activity follows a cyclic pattern called the *interdigestive myoelectric complex (IDMEC)* or the migrating motor complex (MMC) (Fig. 20-6). As originally described by Szurszewski in 1969,[52] each cycle has four phases. Phase I has little or no contractile activity or electric spike activity. Phase II has intermittent spike activity and thus intermittent contractile activity. Phase III has maximum spike activity superimposed on every slow wave; this is associated with regular, strong contractile activity. Phase III is usually followed by a brief period of intermittent spike activity known as Phase IV. This serves as a transition phase between the phase of regular contractile activity and the quiescent phase. The duration of an entire cycle is approximately 2 hours in the dog and 90 to 120 minutes in the human being. Each phase appears first in the distal esophagus, stomach, and duodenum and migrates down the small intestine. The migration takes about 2 hours. Eating abolishes the interdiges-

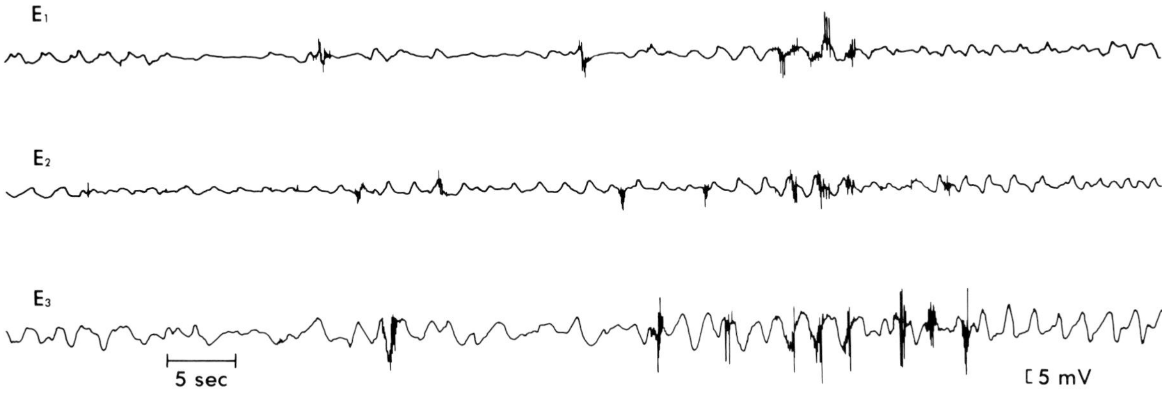

Fig. 20-6 Interdigestive myoelectric complex (IDMEC) recorded from sequential bipolar electrodes (i.e., E_1, E_2, and E_3) from the feline small intestine. Each cycle has four phases: Phase I has little or no electric spike activity; Phase II has intermittent spike activity; Phase III has maximum spike activity, with spikes superimposed on every slow wave; and Phase IV is again a period of only intermittent or absent spike activity.

tive cycles and in their place induces a pattern of intermittent contractile activity. The physiologic significance of the MMC is not completely understood because the complexes are present only in the fasted state and in most species they have no apparent role in the mixing or propulsion of ingested meals. Code and Marlett[14] proposed that these complexes may act as ''housekeepers of the small intestine,'' in the sense that they may purge the small bowel of residual foods, secretions, and desquamated cells during the interdigestive state. It is reported that the MMC may also serve to limit the overgrowth of bacteria in the distal small bowel.[58] This was supported by further work in rats by Scott and Cahall.[46]

Vantrappen, Peeters, and Janssens[57] demonstrated that the development of Phase III of the MMC in human beings is also associated with increased secretion of pepsin and hydrochloric acid by the stomach and of amylase and bicarbonate by the pancreas. The association of bile secretion with the MMC has been suggested by experiments in human subjects and laboratory animals that have demonstrated increasing duodenal output of bile acid and bilirubin during Phase II of the MMC, which peaked just before Phase III activity and decreased again during Phase I.[25,31] Increased myoelectric and spike activity has also been demonstrated from the sphincter of Oddi of the opossum and other species in coordination with the MMC of the stomach and small bowel.[5]

The factors controlling the initiation and migration of the patterns of intestinal motor and secretory activity are incompletely understood. Several investigators have found that concentrations of plasma motilin, a GI peptide found in high concentrations in the duodenal and jejunal epithelium, vary cyclically in association with the duodenal MMC in dog and in human beings, with plasma concentration peaks found during duodenal Phase III activity and troughs during Phase I. Moreover, exogenous infusions of motilin have induced premature Phase III activity in the stomach and duodenum. Although still controversial, motilin has been suggested to be the ''interdigestive hormone'' that regulates the initiation of cyclic motor activity in the small intestine.[44] Further studies on the relationship between the occurrence of Phase III activity and motilin cycling have demonstrated that a 1:1 relationship does not always exist between motilin cycles and MMC cycles.[27,32,36] Motilin cycling therefore may not be essential for the cycling of the MMC. In addition, recent studies have suggested that motilin is not the only substance capable of initiating premature Phase III–like activity. Morphine, somatostatin, substance P, substance K, and isoproterenol have been shown to initiate premature MMCs.[10,40,50,53,54] Recent studies by Sarna and associates[43] using morphine injections to initiate MMC cycling have suggested tht motilin cycling may not be the cause but rather the effect of MMC cycling.

Most investigators now share the view that extrinsic neural control of MMC activity is comparatively slight and that the major roles are played by myogenic or intrinsic nerve mechanisms mediated by the myenteric nerve plexuses. Early studies suggested that extrinsic nerves and especially the vagus nerve played a key role in controlling initiation and propagation of MMC activity.[11,59] These studies were based on preparations using Thiry-Vella loops with intact intrinsic innervation. Subsequent studies, however, have clearly demonstrated that neither vagotomy nor sympathectomy abolish the initiation or propagation of the MMC.[9,24,30] Although not playing a key role in initiation or propagation, the extrinsic nerves may modulate other mechanisms that could control the MMC.

Evidence exists that the site, smell, and ingestion of food into the stomach inhibit the migrating complexes. The exact mechanism whereby feeding abolishes the complexes and induces the so-called fed pattern is not known. Work by Heppell and associates[22] has suggested that perfusion of a jejunal loop with postprandial duodenal chyme inhibits interdigestive myoelectric complexes in the canine duodenum.

Colon Motility

The patterns of colon motor activity and specifically the control mechanisms of colonic motility are complex and poorly understood. The major motor functions of the colon are mixing, temporary storage, and very slow distal pro-

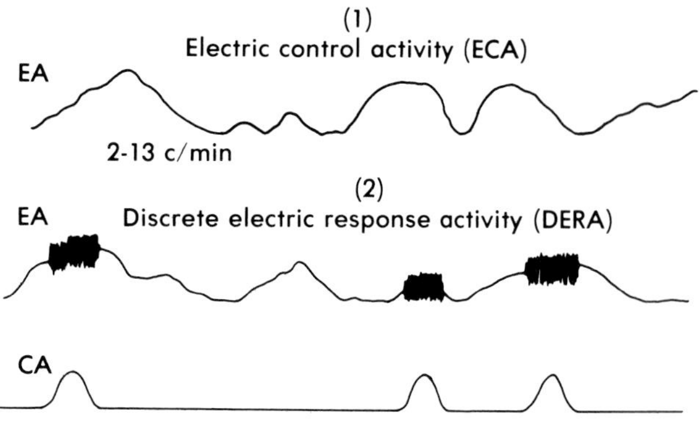

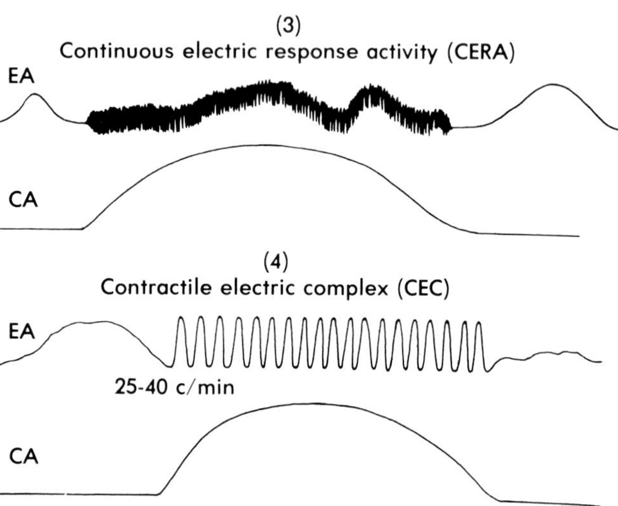

Fig. 20-7 Types of electric and contractile activity in the colon. *EA,* Electric activity; *CA,* contractile activity. (Modified from Sarna, S.: The control of colonic motility. In Chey, W.Y., editor: Functional disorders of the digestive tract, New York, 1983, Raven Press.)

pulsion. Sarna[37,38] has recently summarized current knowledge about the electric control activity of the colon and its relationship to colonic propulsion. As described by Sarna, the smooth muscle of the colon has four types of myoelectric activity: (1) electric control activity, (2) discrete electric response activity, (3) continuous electric response activity, and (4) the contractile electric complex (Fig. 20-7).

Electric control activity (ECA) is similar to the slow waves already described and identified in the stomach and small bowel. In the colon both the amplitude and the frequency of ECA are variable. In the human colon ECA is present in both a low-frequency range of 2 to 9 cycles/minute and a higher-frequency range of 9 to 13 cycles/minute.[42] The lower-frequency ECA is generally found in the ascending and sigmoid colon, whereas the higher-frequency ECA is more often observed in the transverse and descending colon. ECA by itself is not associated with colonic contractile activity unless there is superimposed spiking activity.

Discrete electric response activity (DERA) is analogous to the spike potentials and spike bursts observed in the upper GI tract. DERA occurs as discrete spike bursts on the individual ECA potentials. The occurrence of DERA in the colon thus is organized and controlled by ECA. Because the ECA pattern is disorganized, both the DERA and the associated contractile activity of the colon are also disorganized.

The third type of colonic myoelectric activity, *continuous electric response activity (CERA),* is very different from the myoelectric activity of the small intestine or stomach. In this pattern a continuous burst of spike potentials is seen to span one or more control wave cycles. This activity is independent of the ECA. It is associated with tonic contractions of the colon that are in general nonpropagating.

The final type of colonic myoelectric activity is the *contractile electric complex (CEC).* This consists of oscillations of potential with a frequency range of 25 to 40 cycles/minute. This activity is directly associated with tonic contractions of the colon. These tonic contractions are propagating and quite powerful and appear to result in the propulsion of intraluminal content within the colon. Thus the rhythmic to-and-fro contractions of the colon that result in mixing of stool are a result of the ECA with its superimposed discrete electric response, spike-burst activity. On the other hand, stool propagation within the colon is primarily a result of the propagating CECs.

NEUROHUMORAL CONTROL OF INTESTINAL MOTILITY

Neural control of motor activity of the GI tract is exerted at two levels. The first consists of stimuli from the central nervous system through the autonomic nervous system; peripheral neural reflex arcs with synaptic connections in the prevertebral ganglia are also present. The second level of neural control of gut motility is the enteric nervous system. As mentioned earlier, this has been divided on an anatomic basis into myenteric and submucosal ganglia and plexuses. Of the two levels, it appears that the enteric nervous system is much more important in control of gut motility.

The extrinsic neural pathways to the GI tract include parasympathetic, sympathetic, and purinergic inputs. The branches of the vagus nerve supply the parasympathetic input to the esophagus, stomach, small intestine, and proximal colon. The pelvic nerves supply the parasympathetic input to the distal colon. The splanchnic nerves, by way of the celiac ganglion, supply the sympathetic input to the esophagus, stomach, small bowel, and proximal colon, whereas the hypogastric nerves from the superior and inferior mesenteric ganglia supply the sympathetic input to the remainder of the colon. The organization of the enteric nervous system is complex and largely unknown. The enteric nervous system sends not only excitatory and inhibitory messages to the muscles of the bowel but also contains in the interneurons of the ganglia the control mechanisms for the well-recognized patterns of intestinal motor activity.

Even less is known about the effect of endocrine and paracrine agents on intestinal motility. In the last several decades many new peptide hormones have been isolated from the GI tract. Many of these gut peptides have been shown in either physiologic or pharmacologic doses to af-

Table 20-1 **REPRESENTATIVE GUT PEPTIDES**

Peptide	Site of Production	Endocrine or Paracrine Cell of Origin	Motor Action: Physiologic or Pharmacologic?
Gastrin	Antrum Duodenum	G	↑ Antral contractions
Cholecystokinin (CCK)	Intestine, central nervous system (CNS)	I	↑ Gallbladder contraction Intestinal motility
Secretin	Intestine	S	↓ Gastroduodenal motility
Vasoactive intestinal peptide (VIP)	Intestine, CNS	Nerve	Intestinal motility ↓ Smooth muscle tone
Motilin	Intestine, CNS	Mo	↑ Gastric fundic pressure
Somatostatin	Gut, CNS	D	↓ GI hormone release
Enkephalins	Gut, CNS	Nerve	↓ Peristalsis ↑ Mixing

fect gut motility either directly or through neural pathways. These gut peptides are released by neural, paracrine, and endocrine cells to act on both nerves and smooth muscle cells to facilitate or inhibit smooth muscle excitability and result in contraction. This effect is modulated by myogenic and neural input. The physiologic role of most of these peptides, however, is still unknown (Table 20-1).

DISORDERS OF INTESTINAL MOTOR FUNCTION

Disorders of gut motility spare no anatomic segment of the GI tract. The esophagus and stomach are responsible for a substantial proportion of GI motility problems (see Chapters 14 and 15). Small bowel motility disorders probably cause many GI symptoms and may be associated with systemic diseases such as scleroderma and diabetes mellitus (see the boxed material at right). Some of these disorders are known to affect primarily the intestine, but in others the effect on small bowel motility is only one part of a more generalized condition.

Abdominal surgery can have two effects on GI motor activity and the orderly propulsion of intestinal contents. The first effect, *postoperative ileus,* is generally of short duration and is related to surgically entering the abdomen, handling the intra-abdominal contents, and dissecting the bowel. The second effect is related to the *type of procedure* performed such as vagotomy, resection, or enterotomy and is often of long duration. Another group of patients will have intestinal pseudo-obstruction, thought to be caused by poorly defined abnormalities of intestinal smooth muscle or the enteric autonomic nervous system.

Perhaps the most ubiquitous, yet poorly defined, disorders of GI motility involve the colon. With modern diagnostic techniques, including GI manometry and electrophysiology, radioscintigraphy, and tissue histology, physicians are now able to more specifically identify these disorders.

DISEASES ASSOCIATED WITH SMALL INTESTINAL MOTOR DISORDERS

- Chronic idiopathic intestinal pseudo-obstruction syndromes
  - Myopathies
  - Visceral neuropathies
- Paralytic ileus (acute intestinal pseudo-obstruction)
  - Acute abdomen
  - Abdominal surgery
  - Electrolyte disturbances
  - Drug toxicity
- Mechanical obstruction
- Autonomic neuropathies
  - Diabetes mellitus
  - Chagas' disease
  - Shy-Drager syndrome
- Collagen vascular diseases
  - Progressive systemic sclerosis
- Myotonic dystrophy
- Thyroid disorders
- Miscellaneous
  - Prophyrias
  - Amyloidosis

Systemic Diseases Producing Intestinal Motor Dysfunction

Vantrappen and Janssens[56] have recently proposed a classification of motor abnormalities of the small intestine based on the well-established motility patterns previously described in this chapter. They suggested that the motility pattern disorders be classified by abnormalities of slow-wave rhythm and abnormalities of interdigestive patterns.

Abnormalities of slow-wave rhythm include tachyarrhythmias and bradyarrhythmias that are related to hyperthyroidism with diarrhea and hypothyroidism with constipation. The underlying mechanism might be associated with the effect of thyroid hormone on intestinal slow waves. Patients with hyperthyroidism have been shown to have increased duodenal slow-wave frequency and a prolonged duodenal frequency plateau. Patients with hypothyroidism have shown the opposite pattern.

Foster and co-workers[19] also recently described a pattern of small bowel dysmotility that they have labeled *paroxysmal tachyarrhythmia (Q complex)* and identified in several patients with GI disease. This disorder was characterized by discrete bursts of regular contractile waves of high amplitude and high frequency. It was associated with abdominal pain at irregular intervals in some patients. This was believed to result from paroxysmal slow-wave tachyarrhythmia. Inversion of the slow-wave frequency gradient in the small intestine has also been identified and is thought to be associated with retrograde peristalsis.

Finally, patients have been identified in whom small bowel slow activity is absent during the interdigestive period, apparently as a result of hypopolarization of the intestinal smooth muscle.

Vantrappen and Janssens[56] also described *abnormalities in interdigestive patterns*. They have found a number of patients with absent MMC activity. In all these patients an associated jejunal bacterial overgrowth was found. The authors believed that the overgrowth resulted from this disordered motility pattern, although they did not establish a clear cause-and-effect relationship. Other studies in experimental animals have supported this concept. Pharmacologic studies in animals have demonstrated nonmigrating, Phase III–like activity. Presumably this could also occur in clinical situations. Other reports have demonstrated that morphine and other pharmacologic agents and peptides can induce premature MMC-like activity. These premature activity fronts have occurred spontaneously in some situations. The opposite effect, i.e., disruption of the MMC, has been shown to occur with use of castor oil and ricinoleic acid and has been associated with diarrhea. Other experimental studies have suggested that various enterotoxins, such as those produced by cholera and other noninvasive organisms, may disrupt the MMC patterns of the small intestine. Clear abnormalities of motility in the postprandial or fed state have not been well described.

Intestinal Pseudo-obstruction

Chronic idiopathic intestinal pseudo-obstruction is a syndrome characterized by chronic or recurrent symptoms and signs of intestinal obstruction, occurring in the absence of both organic luminal obstruction and a recognized underlying disease. It is important for the surgeon to make a diagnosis of pseudo-obstruction in these patients since surgery is contraindicated. The surgeon also must not overlook an organic cause of the obstruction. The syndrome can either occur sporadically or be familial. The clinical manifestations of the syndrome result from delayed GI transit caused by disordered motility. Although all portions of the alimentary tract can be affected, these symptoms most often result from bowel dysmotility. The condition is often associated with smooth muscle dysfunction of the urinary tract and other smooth muscle regions.

In some cases of pseudo-obstruction no pathologic abnormality can be found. In other cases histologic examination has shown two distinct pathologic abnormalities. One pathologic subtype includes degeneration of intramural neurons, frequently associated with specific derangements in the myenteric plexus, the celiac ganglia, the spinal cord, and in some cases the brain. Chronic pseudo-obstruction has been labeled *visceral neuropathy* in this situation. A second pattern has been that of degeneration of intestinal smooth muscle cells, or *hollow visceral myopathy*. Histologic studies in these patients have demonstrated vacuolization of the smooth muscle and atrophy of muscle fibers in both the longitudinal and the circular muscle layers. Electron microscopic evaluation has confirmed destruction of the smooth muscle cells. Hollow visceral myopathy appears to be transmitted in a genetic manner as a dominant trait.[47] Summers, Anuras, and Green[49] have recently reported jejunal manometry patterns in patients with idiopathic intestinal pseudo-obstruction. These patients were found to have absent MMCs. Some patients had rare low-amplitude contractions before and after eating, whereas other patients had multiple aborally migrating clustered contractions. Sullivan and associates[48] studied GI myoelectric activity in idiopathic intestinal pseudo-obstruction and found that duodenal spike and motor activity was normal in the basal state. Spike activity was significantly inhibited, however, after water distention of the duodenum or after secretin administration.

Patients with idiopathic intestinal pseudo-obstruction appear clinically with abdominal pain and distention and other nonspecific alterations in bowel habit. In general the patients have a long history of GI symptomatology. They may complain of both constipation and diarrhea, the latter occurring if secondary bacterial overgrowth is present. When these patients are in the acute state, they will have prominent abdominal distention. Abdominal plain x-ray films or barium studies will confirm dilation of the small bowel and often the colon. It may be difficult, however, to differentiate between idiopathic pseudo-obstruction and organic or mechanical bowel obstruction. Tests must be done in this situation to rule out systemic or mechanical causes for obstruction. It is important to separate the reversible causes of obstruction from pseudo-obstruction since they can be treated directly, although in many cases unsuccessfully. If true pseudo-obstruction is identified, attempts should be made to classify this as a neural or smooth muscle dysfunction. When an underlying disorder of the autonomic nervous system is suspected, direct attempts can be made to manipulate the cholinergic tone of the bowel. Stimulation of GI smooth muscle by acetylcholinesterase inhibitors, acetylcholine analogs, metoclopramide, or the newer benzimides may be useful, although in general the results with these drugs have been discouraging. Nutritional support has been helpful in the form of parenteral hyperalimentation and, more recently, long-term home hyperalimentation. Surgery is to be avoided if possible and is rarely of benefit. Surgery may be required, however, if acute decompensation in the patient's condition such as volvulus or intussusception develops.[45]

Functional Disorders of Colonic Motility

Abnormalities of colonic motility are generally believed to exist in many disorders, frequently labeled as "functional," of which the most common is the irritable bowel syndrome. Some believe that colonic diverticular disease is a motility disorder. Simple constipation and diarrhea are frequent manifestations of colonic dysmotility. Despite the many clinical conditions in which disordered colonic motor activity is important, definition and description of abnormalities have not yet been achieved. As already described, this is probably because so little is known about normal colonic motility.

Irritable Bowel Syndrome

The irritable bowel syndrome is a functional disorder involving primarily the colon and sometimes more proximal parts of the GI tract. Clinically it is characterized by abdominal pain and distention, constipation, and/or diarrhea. Although psychologic factors are generally thought to be important in the cause of irritable bowel syndrome, not all patients manifest neurotic behavior.

Colonic motility studies have recently identified clear abnormalities in patients with irritable bowel syndrome. Manometric studies of the colon have demonstrated that patients with irritable bowel syndrome react aberrantly to distending stimuli, reporting pain at lower distending volumes and pressures than control subjects. Some evidence suggests, however, that hyposegmentation rather than hypersegmentation of the sigmoid colon may occur in patients with irritable bowel syndrome. In studying myoelectric patterns in patients with this syndrome, several investigators have demonstrated a greater prevalence of the slow-frequency electric control activity (3 cycles/minute). Although various studies have corroborated this finding, it has not been possible to correlate the dominant 3 cycles/minute frequency with specific symptom complexes.[29]

Severe Idiopathic Constipation

It is generally accepted that chronic constipation is associated with hypersegmentation of the colon and that chronic functional diarrhea is associated with hyposegmentation. Investigators have reasoned that excessive local contractions impede the distal transit of colonic contents, resulting in constipation. Hyposegmentation of the bowel would result in mass movement of stool and diarrhea. Very little experimental data exist to support this concept. Recently, however, distinctive abnormalities of the colonic myenteric plexus have been identified in selected patients with severe idiopathic constipation.

Krishnamurthy and associates[26] have recently described a small proportion of patients with constipation in whom the condition is much more severe, persistent, and unresponsive to fiber and laxatives and for which no cause can be found. These patients will often have stool frequencies of less than one per week despite the use of fiber and laxatives but are otherwise in good health without major psychiatric problems. Manometric evaluations of the esophagus and anal sphincter mechanism have demonstrated no abnormalities. Colonic transit studies have shown a clear delay in transit of markers through the colon. At the time of subtotal colectomy, histologic evaluation of the neural elements with silver stains has revealed abnormalities within the myenteric plexus. Further studies of this subgroup of patients may identify those who will benefit from colon resection.

Colonic Diverticulosis

Researchers have hypothesized in the last several decades that colonic diverticulosis is a direct result of high intraluminal pressures that cause herniation of the mucosa through the colonic wall. Studies of postmortem material and surgical resection specimens have demonstrated that the colonic muscle in patients with diverticulosis is thickened and that the luminal diameter of the colon is narrowed. The diverticuli occur between the mesenteric and antimesenteric teniae coli in association with the transit of blood vessels through the colon wall. The diverticuli consist of colonic mucosa and a layer of muscularis mucosa. Manometric studies have confirmed that intraluminal pressures in the sigmoid colon in patients with colonic diverticulosis are higher than in control subjects both physiologically and with pharmacologic stimulation. Studies of myoelectric activity in patients with diverticulosis, however, have shown no difference in myoelectric patterns from control subjects. It is currently accepted from epidemiologic studies and therapeutic trials that low fecal volume resulting from our refined Western diet is a major contributing factor to diverticulosis. Therapy has therefore been directed toward altering this diet.[29]

Postoperative Motor Dysfunction

Vagotomy

As described in Chapter 15, vagotomy has a profound effect on gastric motility. It might be expected that small intestinal motility would be similarly impaired after vagotomy. Diarrhea and hyperirritability of the small bowel do follow vagotomy in animals and human beings. Nevertheless, the precise effects of vagotomy on intestinal motility have been difficult to elucidate. Although vagotomy has been demonstrated to affect intestinal slow waves and spike potentials, the effects of vagotomy on fasting or fed myoelectric motor patterns have been variable. In dogs vagotomy has resulted in no change in the interdigestive pattern and no decrease in cycle length with an increase in cycle variability.[60] In human beings no change in MMC has been demonstrated after vagotomy. In all species, however, alterations in conversion to the fed pattern or in the fed pattern itself have been observed. These alterations may explain the changes in jejunal and ileal transit time observed after vagotomy.

The effects of vagotomy on colon motility are even less certain. Some have suggested that truncal vagotomy reduces the length of periods of active colon contractile activity and the amplitude of contractile waves and intraluminal pressures; such changes do *not* occur after selective or proximal gastric vagotomy. A marked increase in colonic contractile activity after a liquid meal is observed after both truncal and selective vagotomy, suggesting that postvagotomy changes may more accurately reflect changes in gastric emptying than direct effects on colonic motility.

The incidence of postoperative diarrhea following vagotomy ranges from 2% to 13% after proximal gastric vagotomy to 8% to 60% after selective vagotomy and drainage and 20% to 67% after truncal vagotomy and drainage. The pathophysiology of postvagotomy diarrhea has not been clearly elucidated, but little support exists for the view that diarrhea after vagotomy is a consequence of parasympathetic denervation of the small intestine. Proposed mechanisms have included[4]:

1. Bacterial colonization of the small bowel, with resulting direct irritation of the mucosa or deconjugation of bile salts
2. Unmasking of nontropical sprue or lactose malabsorption
3. Pancreatic insufficiency
4. Early gastric emptying of fluids
5. Increased presence of bile acids in the intestine caused by changes in biliary kinetics
6. Rapid small bowel transit of bile acids, with incomplete absorption, subsequent colonic irritation, and diarrhea[4]

Ileus

Ileus has been defined as a period of functional intestinal aperistalsis that is expected to follow nearly all major abdominal operations. It is also associated with such pathologic conditions as peritonitis and mechanical intestinal obstruction. Clinically, ileus is characterized by diminished bowel sounds and accumulation of gas and fluid within the lumen of the bowel, resulting in a lack of propulsion of intestinal content.

The pathophysiology of ileus is poorly understood. Several conditions associated with surgical procedures have been implicated in the pathogenesis of postoperative ileus. These have included preoperative medication, anesthetic agents, analgesics, manipulation of the bowel, mechanical or chemical irritation of the peritoneum, and postoperative electrolyte or metabolic disturbances. Since preoperative medication regimens include anticholinergics, these drugs probably have a profound effect on postoperative intestinal motility. Studies have demonstrated that anesthetic agents most likely contribute little to postoperative ileus. Laparotomy seems to be fundamentally important in the pathogenesis of postoperative ileus. In contrast, the duration of surgery or the extent of small bowel handling appear to have little effect on the duration of postoperative ileus.[21,61]

Regardless of the extent of handling and exposure of the bowel, small intestinal contractile activity returns to normal within 5 to 10 hours after abdominal surgery. Gastric motility returns to normal within 24 hours, and colonic motility within 24 to 60 hours. Other studies have demonstrated that laparotomy does not affect small bowel slow-wave frequency or its gradient along the small intestine. However, laparotomy does appear to affect cycling of the small intestinal MMC, with an omission of the complexes for 1 to 2 days after laparotomy.

Analgesics administered to patients postoperatively have been long associated with postoperative ileus. As described, opioid agents have a profound effect on motor activity of the bowel. Morphine stimulates MMC-like activity in the small bowel. Codeine appears to depress small bowel function. Meperidine and codeine depress contractile frequency in the colon, although morphine appears to have little effect on colonic contraction. Opioid agents have been used for some time as antidiarrheal agents.[15]

Small Bowel Transection

As one would predict, small bowel transection has a profound effect on small intestinal myoelectric and motor activity. Transection would be expected to affect both myogenic and intrinsic neural control mechanisms. As explained by the theory of coupled-relaxation oscillators, if the bowel is divided, the slow-wave frequency distal to the site of transection will decrease, and that proximal to the site of transection will remain the same. It would then be expected that the contractile frequency of the distal bowel would decrease. Although this change of myoelectric pattern has been observed in human beings after surgical transection and reanastomosis of the bowel, no apparent clinical effect on intestinal motility has been observed. Sarna, Condon, and Cowles[41] have recently demonstrated that small bowel transection also apparently interrupts the intrinsic neural network. They found that, after small bowel transection, MMC cycles occurred proximal and distal to the site of transection independent of one another. This effect lasted approximately 30 to 40 days after intestinal transection, after which regeneration of intrinsic nerves began to couple the MMC cycles across the reanastomosis. At approximately 100 days after surgery, the MMC migrated over the entire length of the small bowel. The clinical relevance of this observation remains uncertain.[38]

Acute Intestinal Obstruction

Acute intestinal obstruction remains a frequently encountered and difficult-to-manage condition for the clinical surgeon. Intestinal obstruction is manifested by paroxysmal, crampy, abdominal pain and distention that is aggravated by eating and partially relieved by vomiting. It has been generally thought, based on clinical observations, intraluminal balloons, and direct observation of the gut, that motor activity is greatly increased proximal to the obstruction. Only recently has this been carefully assessed using manometric and electromyographic techniques.

Summers and co-workers[51] demonstrated experimentally that proximal to the site of obstruction spike-burst frequency increased markedly, whereas distal to that obstruction spiking was depressed. When the obstruction was continued for more than 5 hours, the inhibition persisted distally, but proximal myoelectric spike activity and contractile activity gradually fell to control levels. After prolonged obstruction, the investigators observed clusters of regular intense spike bursts, preceded and followed by lengthening periods of absent motor activity. Further work from this group suggested that changes in luminal contents and nervous activity both contribute to the intestinal motility changes that accompany obstruction. Increased motor activity proximal to obstruction appeared to be mediated by cholinergic nerves. Some of the distal inhibition of spike bursts may be mediated by noncholinergic, nonadrenergic pathways, and some may result from diminished intraluminal contents.[33]

TREATMENT OF INTESTINAL MOTOR DYSFUNCTION

With the uncertainty surrounding the pathophysiology of gut motility disorders, the development of effective drugs to treat these problems has been slow. Potentially, drugs can alter gut motility by several mechanisms (see boxed material on p. 357):

1. Interacting with receptors in the central nervous system with neural stimulation in the gut
2. Enhancing or inhibiting neural transmission
3. Affecting submucosal pressure-sensitive receptors in the gut
4. Interacting with specific peptide receptors, intramural nerves, or smooth muscle cells
5. Influencing the intracellular contents of smooth muscle cells

Although cholinergic stimulants and inhibitors have been used for some time, major new entries into the pharmacology of gut motility disorders include the benzimide agents metoclopramide, domperidone, and cisapride; prostaglandin inhibitors; and the intracellularly acting calcium channel blockers.

Metoclopramide

Of the promotility agents, metoclopramide is the only one currently available for use in the treatment of GI motility disorders in the United States. As shown in Fig. 20-8, metoclopramide's chemical structure is methoxy-2-chloro-5-procainamide. Justin-Besançon and associates[24a] first described it in the early 1960s. Although originally introduced for the treatment of the nausea and vomiting of pregnancy, metoclopramide now has wide application to the GI tract and other organ systems. Its effect on GI smooth muscle is not entirely understood. However, metoclopramide lowers the pressure threshold for the occurrence of the peristaltic reflex, reduces appearance of muscle fatigue, and enhances the frequency and amplitude of longitudinal muscle contraction. Its uniqueness lies in its ability to coordinate gastric, pyloric, and duodenal motor activity to result in net aborad movement of GI chyme.

Metoclopramide is not a cholinomimetic agent in the usual sense, but its mechanism of action appears to depend on intramural cholinergic neurons. Its GI smooth muscle action was thought until recently to result from antagonism of the inhibitory neurotransmitter dopamine. It now appears that metoclopramide acts to enhance GI motility primarily by augmenting release of acetylcholine and perhaps by inhibition of serotonin release. Its antiemetic effect, however, is probably central. Metoclopramide has been shown to increase resting lower esophageal sphincter pressure in control subjects and in patients with gastroesophageal reflux and also to decrease symptoms in this latter group. It clearly increases gastric emptying and has been useful in patients with diabetic gastroparesis and those with postoperative gastric dysmotility. Metoclopramide may be useful in patients with intestinal pseudo-obstruction and colonic hypomotility.[1]

In addition, metoclopramide has been used to treat postoperative ileus. Davidson and associates,[17] in a randomized double-blind study using metoclopramide and placebo in many patients after laparotomy, found less nausea and vomiting and a better tolerance to solid food in the metoclopramide-treated group. However, no statistically significant difference was found in other parameters, such as abdominal pain, return of bowel sounds, and passage of flatus and stool. Other studies have shown similar or even better results, although further prospective and controlled observations are clearly needed.

POTENTIAL MECHANISMS OF DRUG EFFECTS ON INTESTINAL MOTILITY

INTERACTION WITH RECEPTORS IN CENTRAL NERVOUS SYSTEM WITH NEURAL STIMULATION OF GUT

EFFECTS ON NEUROTRANSMISSION

Enhancement by:
1. Increased neurotransmitter synthesis
2. Increased neurotransmitter release
3. Decreased inhibition or destruction of neurotransmitter

Inhibition by:
1. Decreased synthesis of neurotransmitter
2. Decreased storage of neurotransmitter
3. Decreased release of neurotransmitter

EFFECTS ON SUBMUCOSAL PRESSURE-SENSITIVE RECEPTORS IN THE GUT

INTERACTION WITH THE FOLLOWING SPECIFIC RECEPTORS ON INTRAMURAL NERVES

Cholinergic (nicotinic) receptors
5-Hydroxytryptamine receptors
Prostaglandin receptors
Vasoactive intestinal peptide receptors
Substance P receptors
Somatostatin receptors
Opiate receptors

INTERACTION WITH THE FOLLOWING SPECIFIC RECEPTORS ON THE SMOOTH MUSCLE CELL

Beta-adrenergic receptors
Cholinergic (muscarinic) receptors
5-Hydroxytryptamine receptors
Prostaglandin receptors
Vasoactive intestinal peptide receptors
Substance P receptors
Opiate receptors

EFFECTS ON INTRACELLULAR CONTENTS OF SMOOTH MUSCLE CELL, INCLUDING CA^{++} FLUX

From Farrar, J.T.: Clin. Gastroenterol. **11**(3):674, 1982.

Domperidone

Domperidone, a benzimidazole derivative, shares with metoclopramide an antidopaminergic action. It appears to increase gastric antral contractile activity and to accelerate gastric emptying. It may also be useful as an antiemetic agent. Its role in small bowel or colonic dysmotility is unclear.[28]

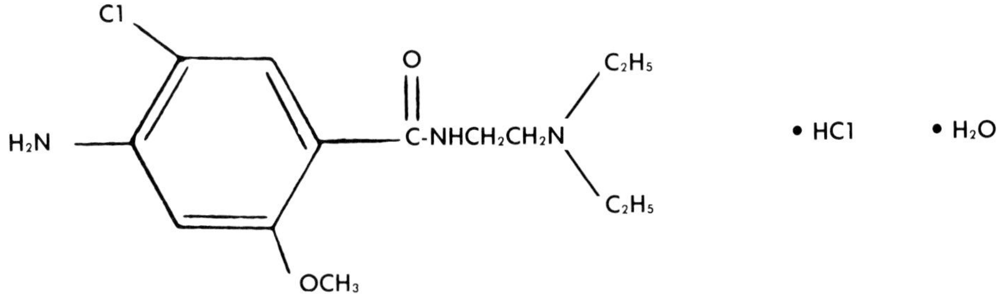

Cl
H_2N
$C\text{-}NHCH_2CH_2N$
O
C_2H_5
C_2H_5
OCH_3
• HCl • H_2O

Fig. 20-8 Chemical structure of the promotility agent, metoclopramide (methoxy-2-chloro-5-procainamide).

Cisapride

Cisapride is a newly developed benzimide that stimulates GI motility, most likely through facilitation of acetylcholine release from myenteric nerves. Unlike metoclopramide and domperidone, cisapride possesses no antidopaminergic properties. Unlike other cholinergic agents, cisapride appears to have no effect on GI secretion. Potentially the substance could be useful in a variety of pathologic conditions. It has been shown experimentally to increase lower esophageal sphincter pressure, to accelerate gastric emptying, and to increase colonic transit. Further clinical studies of this exciting new promotility agent are needed.

Anticholinergics and Opiates

Both anticholinergics and opiates have been used therapeutically to inhibit GI motility. Anticholinergics, as would be expected, delay gastric emptying and generally inhibit gut contractile activity. These drugs may be of use in patients with intestinal hypermotility states associated with myenteric plexus disease or autonomic myopathy.

It is well known that opiates cause constipation, but the level in the gut at which their action predominates is unclear. Their constipating action may be partly attributable to a direct antimotility effect on the stomach and small intestine. Opiates such as loperamide decrease pancreatobiliary secretion and exhibit intestinal antisecretory effects that may contribute largely to their antidiarrheal properties. Opiates also have an effect on colonic motility, as previously described. Loperamide may also increase the resting tone of the internal anal sphincter. Systemically acting opioides are probably contraindicated in most intestinal motor disorders because of their central side effects and propensity toward addiction. However, peripherally acting drugs such as loperamide can be used in patients with gastroparesis and pseudo-obstruction, particularly those in whom diarrhea and uncontrolled motor activity predominate. Loperamide has also been useful in patients with high ileostomy output, with short bowel syndrome, and after ileoanal anastomosis.[35]

Intestinal Pacing

An exciting new approach to gut motility disorders is intestinal pacing. Experimental work has demonstrated that electric pacing can alter the frequency and direction of propagation of the enteric myoelectric pacesetter potential or slow wave, thereby affecting intestinal motility, transit, and absorption.[3] In experimental animals retrograde intestinal pacing has effectively ameliorated the postgastrectomy dumping syndrome[7] and the short bowel syndrome.[20] Antegrade pacing might be expected to enhance gastric emptying and further inhibit bile reflux in patients after Roux-en-Y conversion. In addition, antegrade pacing might be expected to play some role in other disorders of intestinal atony or stasis.

Rapid improvement in technology and materials has made it possible to consider human implantation of an intestinal pacing unit in the near future in patients with gastrointestinal motility disorders. Further, if the units could be placed on the bowel nonsurgically, several conditions now refractory to currently available therapy might be readily treated by an intestinal pacing device.

SUMMARY

Motility of the gastrointestinal tract depends on a highly integrated and coordinated response of the smooth muscle contained within the wall of the bowel. Small and large intestinal motility is controlled by three basic control mechanisms: myogenic, neural, and humoral. The organization of these control mechanisms is different in different anatomic sections of the GI tract. Understanding of these control mechanisms in both the physiologic and the pathologic state is incomplete, although this is improving rapidly with modern electrophysiologic, manometric, and histologic techniques. Motor disorders affect the entire GI tract. The disorders can be intrinsic to the alimentary canal, may reflect a generalized neural or myogenic dysfunction, or can result from surgical manipulation of the bowel or nervous system. These disorders are difficult to diagnose and treat.

Surgical therapy is seldom indicated for these disorders of motility; however, groups of patients are being identified with specific motor dysfunctions of the esophagus, stomach, and colon who may be amenable to surgical therapy. Several new promotility agents, including metoclopramide, domperidone, and cisapride, may be useful in the treatment of many hypomotility disorders. Opiates effectively delay GI transit and control diarrhea. Intestinal pacing is effective in experimental motility disorders and may ultimately be applicable to clinical disorders of intestinal motor function.

REFERENCES

1. Albibi, R., and McCallum, R.W.: Metoclopramide: pharmacology and clinical application, Ann. Intern. Med. **98:**86, 1983.
2. Alvarez, W.C.: The mechanics of the digestive tract, ed. 2, New York, 1928, Hoeber, Inc.
3. Becker, J.M.: Electrical pacing for post-surgical disorders of gastric motility. In Akkermans, L.M.A., Johnson, A.G., and Read, N.W., editors: Gastric and gastroduodenal motility. Surgical science series, vol. 4, East Sussex, U.K., 1984, Praeger Publishers.
4. Becker, J.M., and Kelly, K.A.: Implications of vagotomy. In Carter, D.C., editor: Clinical surgery international: peptic ulcer, vol. 7, Edinburgh, 1983, Churchill Livingstone, Inc.
5. Becker, J.M., and Moody, F.G.: Sphincter of Oddi and biliary motility. In Condon, R.E., and DeCosse, J.J., editors: Surgical care II, Philadelphia, 1985, Lea & Febiger.
6. Becker, J.M., Duff, W.M., and Moody, F.G.: Myoelectric control of gastrointestinal and biliary motility: a review, Surgery **89:**466, 1981.
7. Becker, J.M., et al.: Intestinal pacing for canine post-gastrectomy dumping, Gastroenterology **84:**383, 1983.
8. Bortoff, A.: Myogenic control of intestinal motility, Physiol. Rev. **56:**418, 1976.
9. Bueno, L., Pradduade, F., and Ruckebusch, Y.: Propagation of electrical spiking activity along the small intestine: intrinsic versus extrinsic neural influences, J. Physiol. (Lond.) **292:**15, 1979.
10. Bueno, L., et al.: Effects of motilin, somatostatin, and pancreatic polypeptide on the migrating myoelectric complex in pig and dog, Gastroenterology **82:**1395, 1982.
11. Carlson, G.M., Bedi, B.S., and Code, C.F.: Mechanism of propagation of intestinal interdigestive myoelectric complex, Am. J. Physiol. **222:**1027, 1972.
12. Christensen, J.: The controls of gastrointestinal movements: some old and new views, N. Engl. J. Med. **285:**85, 1971.

13. Christensen, J., Schedl, H.P., and Clifton, J.A.: The small intestinal basic electrical rhythm (slow wave) frequency gradient in normal men and in patients with a variety of diseases, Gastroenterology **50:**309, 1966.
14. Code, C.F., and Marlett, J.A.: The interdigestive myoelectric complex of the stomach and small bowel of dogs, J. Physiol. (Lond.) **246:**298, 1975.
15. Condon, R.E., and Sarna, S.K.: Motility after abdominal surgery, Clin. Gastroenterol. **11:**609, 1982.
16. Daniel, E.E.: Electrical activity of the longitudinal muscle of the dog small intestine studied in vivo using microelectrodes, Am. J. Physiol. **198:**113, 1960.
17. Davidson, E.D., et al.: The effects of metoclopramide on postoperative ileus: a randomized double-blind study, Ann. Surg. **190:**27, 1979.
18. Diamant, N.E., and Bortoff, A.: Effects of transection on intestinal slow wave gradient, Am. J. Physiol. **216:**734, 1969.
19. Foster, G.E., et al.: Abnormal jejunal motility in gastrointestinal disease: the Q complex. In Wienbeck, M., editor: Motility of the digestive tract, New York, 1982, Raven Press.
20. Gladden, H.E., and Kelly, K.A.: Electrical pacing for short bowel syndrome, Surg. Gynecol. Obstet. **153:**697, 1981.
21. Graber, J.N., et al.: Relationship of duration of postoperative ileus to extent and site of operative dissection, Surgery **92:**87, 1982.
22. Heppell, J., et al.: Postprandial inhibition of canine enteric interdigestive myoelectric complex, Am. J. Physiol. **244:**G160, 1983.
23. Herman-Taylor, J., and Code, C.F.: Localization of the duodenal pacemaker and its role in the organization of duodenal myoelectrical activity, Gut **12:**40, 1971.
24. Itoh, Z., Aizawa, I., and Takeuchi, S.: Neural regulation of interdigestive motor activity in canine jejunum, Am. J. Physiol. **240:**G324, 1981.
24a. Justin-Besançon, L., and Laville, C.: Action du métoclopramide sur le système nerveux autonome. C.R. Soc. Biol (Paris) **158:**1016, 1964.
25. Keane, F.B., et al.: Relationships among canine interdigestive exocrine pancreatic and biliary flow, duodenal motor activity, plasma pancreatic polypeptide, and motilin, Gastroenterology **78:**310, 1978.
26. Krishnamurthy, S., et al.: Severe idiopathic constipation associated with a distinctive abnormality of the colonic myenteric plexus, Gastroenterology **88:**26, 1985.
27. Lee, K.Y., Kim, M.S., and Chey, W.Y.: Effects of a meal and gut hormones on plasma motilin and duodenal motility in dog, Am. J. Physiol. **238:**G280, 1980.
28. Malajalada, J.R.: Potential and pharmacologic approaches to management of gut motility disorders, Scand. J. Gastroenterol. (Suppl.) **19:**111, 1984.
29. Misiewicz, J.J.: Human colonic motility, Scand. J. Gastroenterol. (Suppl.) **93:**43, 1984.
30. Ormsbee, H.S., et al.: Mechanism of propagation of canine migrating motor complex: a reappraisal, Am. J. Physiol. **240:**G141, 1981.
31. Peeters, T.L., Vantrappen, G., and Janssens, J.: Bile acid output and the interdigestive migrating motor complex in normals and in cholecystectomy patients, Gastroenterology **79:**678, 1980.
32. Poitras, P., et al.: Motilin-independent ectopic fronts of the interdigestive myoelectric complex in dogs, Am. J. Physiol. **239:**G215, 1980.
33. Prihoda, M., Flatt, A., and Summers, R.W.: Mechanisms of motility changes during acute intestinal obstruction in the dog, Am. J. Physiol. **247:**G37, 1984.
34. Prosser, C.L., Burnstock, G., and Kahn, J.: Conduction in smooth muscle: comparative structural properties, Am. J. Physiol. **199:**545, 1960.
35. Raymond, J., et al.: Stool output following colectomy, mucosal proctectomy, and endorectal ileoanal pull-through (abstract), Gastroenterology **88:**1550, 1985.
36. Rees, W.D.W., et al.: Human interdigestive and postprandial gastrointestinal motor and gastrointestinal hormone patterns, Dig. Dis. Sci. **27:**321, 1982.
37. Sarna, S.: The control of colonic motility. In Chey, W.Y., editor: Functional disorders of the digestive tract, New York, 1983, Raven Press.
38. Sarna, S.K.: Small and large bowel motility and postoperative disorders. In Condon, R.E., and DeCosse, J.J., editors: Surgical care II, Philadelphia, 1985, Lea & Febiger.
39. Sarna, S.K., Daniel, E.E., and Kingma, G.J.: Stimulation of slow-wave electrical activity of small intestine, Am. J. Physiol. **221:**166, 1971.
40. Sarna, S., Northcott, P., and Belbeck, L.: Mechanism of cycling of migrating myoelectric complexes: effect of morphine, Am. J. Physiol. **242:**G588, 1982.
41. Sarna, S., Condon, R.E., and Cowles, V.E.: Enteric mechanisms of initiation of migrating myoelectric complexes in dogs, Gastroenterology **84:**814, 1983.
42. Sarna, S.K., et al.: Human colonic electrical control activity (ECA), Gastroenterology **78:**1526, 1980.
43. Sarna, S.K., et al.: The cause-and-effect relationship between motilin and migrating myoelectric complexes, Am. J. Physiol. **245:**G277, 1983.
44. Sarr, M.G., Kelly, K.A., and Go, V.L.W.: Motilin regulation of canine interdigestive intestinal motility, Dig. Dis. Sci. **28:**249, 1983.
45. Schuffler, M.D., and Deitch, E.A.: Chronic idiopathic intestinal pseudo-obstruction: a surgical approach, Ann. Surg. **192:**752, 1980.
46. Scott, L.D., and Cahall, D.L.: Influence of the interdigestive myoelectric complex on enteric flora in the rat, Gastroenterology **82:**37, 1982.
47. Smout, A.J.P.M., et al.: Chronic idiopathic intestinal pseudo-obstruction: coexistence of smooth muscle and neuronal abnormalities, Dig. Dis. Sci. **30:**282, 1985.
48. Sullivan, M.A., et al.: Gastrointestinal myoelectrical activity in idiopathic intestinal pseudo-obstruction, N. Engl. J. Med. **297:**233, 1977.
49. Summers, R.W., Anuras, S., and Green, J.: Jejunal manometry patterns in health, partial intestinal obstruction, and pseudo-obstruction, Gastroenterology **85:**1290, 1983.
50. Summers, R.W., et al.: Evidence that somatostatin mediates isoproterenol-induced activity fronts in fed dogs, Gastroenterology **82:**1190, 1982.
51. Summers, R.W., et al.: Acute intestinal obstruction: an electromyographic study in dogs, Gastroenterology **85:**1301, 1983.
52. Szurszewski, J.H.: A migrating electric complex of the canine small intestine, Am. J. Physiol. **217:**1757, 1969.
53. Thor, P., et al.: Effect of somatostatin on myoelectrical activity of small bowel, Am. J. Physiol. **4:**E249, 1978.
54. Thor, P.J., Sendur, R., and Konturek, S.J.: Influence of substance P on myoelectric activity of the small bowel, Am. J. Physiol. **6:**G493, 1982.
55. Van der Pol, B.: Biological rhythms considered as relaxation oscillators, Phil. Mag. **2:**978, 1926.
56. Vantrappen, G.R., and Janssens, J.: Intestinal motility disorders, Dig. Dis. Sci. **29:**458, 1984.
57. Vantrappen, G.R., Peeters, T.L., and Janssens, J.: The secretory component of the interdigestive migrating motor complex in man, Scand. J. Gastroenterol. **14:**663, 1979.
58. Vantrappen, G., et al.: The interdigestive motor complex of normal subjects and patients with bacterial overgrowth of the small intestine, J. Clin. Invest. **59:**1158, 1977.
59. Weisbrodt, N.W., et al.: Nervous and humoral factors which influence the fasted and fed patterns of intestinal myoelectric activity. In Vantrappen, G., editor: Proceedings of the Fifth International Symposium on Gastrointestinal Motility, Herentals, Belgium, 1975, Typoff.
60. Weisbrodt, N.W., et al.: Effect of vagotomy on electrical activity of the small intestine of the dog, Am. J. Physiol. **288:**650, 1975.
61. Woods, J.H., et al.: Postoperative ileus: a colonic problem? Surgery **84:**527, 1978.

21

David W. McFadden and Michael J. Zinner

Intestinal Circulation and Vascular Disorders

Intestinal homeostasis is entirely dependent on an adequate blood supply. Abnormalities in the intestinal blood supply at the macrocirculatory level may lead to a wide spectrum of disorders ranging from mild postprandial abdominal pain (intestinal angina) to profound abnormalities such as intestinal gangrene.[55] Microcirculatory derangements can lead to impaired absorption, motility, and poor anastomotic healing. This chapter will discuss the normal anatomic and physiologic controls of intestinal blood flow and the various clinical methods of evaluating the integrity of the gastrointestinal circulation. A summary of the clinical manifestations of impaired gut circulation will also be considered, along with current concepts in its management.

ANATOMY AND PHYSIOLOGY OF THE INTESTINAL CIRCULATION

The intestine is perfused by three main arterial systems (Fig. 21-1). The celiac axis supplies the foregut structures primarily below the diaphragm. The superior mesenteric artery is the main supplier of intestinal blood flow from the duodenojejunal junction to the mid-transverse colon. The inferior mesenteric artery supplies the hindgut from mid-transverse colon to the rectum. An extensive but variable collateral system exists among these three vascular trunks. The gastroduodenal artery and its ramifications provide the major connection between the celiac and the superior mesenteric arteries. Several arterial channels, including the sigmoidal artery of Drummond and the arch of Riolan, provide a generous collateralization between the superior and inferior mesenteric systems. A total of over 50 collateral pathways have been described for intestinal arterial blood flow such that asymptomatic occlusion of any one of the three main trunks is often possible. Microscopically, extensive submucosal vascular plexi exist that serve a protective function at the cellular level.[24]

At rest, approximately 10% to 15% of total cardiac output is distributed to the intestines or between 30 to 70 ml/min per 100 g of tissue.[24] Of this, 70% to 90% perfuses the mucosal-submucosal layers, with the remainder supplying the muscularis-serosal coats. Wide variances in reported blood flows are caused by the various measurement techniques (radioactive microspheres, inert gas washouts) and animal preparations (innervated, fasted, awake, or anesthetized). The physiology of intestinal circulation is still an evolving and often controversial science, but most published data[24,35] implicate three large groups of circulatory determinants: intrinsic (local metabolic vs. myogenic), extrinsic (sympathetic and parasympathetic nervous systems), and circulating or local vasoactive or neurohumoral agents.

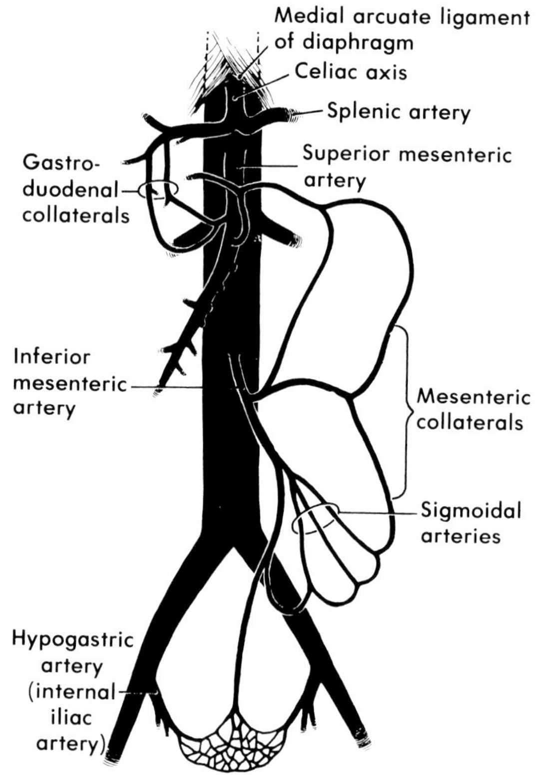

Fig. 21-1 Main arterial systems perfusing the gastrointestinal tract. (From Stoney, R.J., and Lusby, R.J.: Vascular surgery principles and techniques, ed. 2, East Norwalk, Conn., 1984, Appleton-Century-Crofts.)

The study of the intrinsic regulation of intestinal blood flow has long centered on the debate between metabolic and myogenic mechanisms. These interdependent mechanisms presumably control the immediate fluctuations in intestinal blood flow. Well-documented physiologic phenomena such as pressure-flow autoregulation, hypoxic vasodilation, and reactive hyperemia lend credence to the integral nature of intrinsic controls. The metabolic hypothesis of intrinsic regulation attributes the accumulation of various tissue metabolites, such as H^+, K^+, adenosine, and the adenosine nucleotides, as the modifiers of local blood flow. Any situation creating an imbalance between tissue oxygen supply and demand would raise the local concentrations of these local metabolites with resultant vasodilation. The metabolic theory therefore states that it is oxygen delivery, rather than blood flow per se, that regulates the intestinal circulation.[24] The myogenic theory assumes vascular resistance to be proportional to arteriolar transmural pressure,[28] requiring the existence of arteriolar tension receptors. The myogenic mechanism would therefore regulate and maintain a constant intestinal capillary pressure and transcapillary fluid exchange.[23] Although more solid evidence exists in favor of the myogenic regulation of intestinal blood flow, the consensus is that both intrinsic mechanisms serve important functions.

Blood flow autoregulation is a frequently used physiologic concept describing the inherent ability of an organ to maintain a constant blood flow despite wide variations in arterial (perfusion) pressures. Intestinal autoregulation is neither as intense as in other organs (heart, kidney) nor is it as experimentally reproducible. However, in "fed" animal preparations it does appear to exist as demonstrated by the constant blood flow that is maintained through a range of perfusion pressures between 40 and 125 mm Hg.[41] The precapillary resistance vessels (arteriole) appear to be the site of this pressure-flow autoregulation and also appear to be neurally independent.[24] An inherent sensitivity to oxygen concentration apparently is in effect in fasted animal preparations supporting a metabolic component as well.[23] Simple venous pressure increases appear to change blood flow by a myogenic mechanism as increased vascular transmural pressure leads to raised arteriolar tone and vasoconstriction. In contrast, the metabolic theory would predict blood stagnation, increased interstitial metabolic products, and vasodilation.

The intrinsic autoregulatory system is also demonstrated in both the hypoxic and hypercapnic vasodilatory response. An intestinal reactive hyperemia is well described that is proportional to the length of time of arterial occlusion. This reactive hyperemia appears to affect the muscularis more prominently in experimental occlusions of greater than 1 minute,[23,24] leading to increased motility after occlusion. Postprandial, or functional, hyperemia remains an unsettled phenomenon. In addition to metabolic and myogenic effects, the concomitant influence of locally produced hormones, neural reflexes, and changes in visceral smooth muscle tone have all been empirically implicated in this complex response.[23,24]

The extrinsic component of intestinal blood flow regulation comprises the generous sympathetic postganglionic vasoconstrictor fibers of the splanchnic intestinal nerves. Stimulation of these fibers leads to vasoconstriction and decreased blood flow. A well-documented autoregulatory "escape" in experimental cases of prolonged electrical splanchnic stimulation occurs within 1 to 2 minutes and may play a protective role in physiologic states of high sympathetic activity.[24] A reactive hyperemic response generally follows the cessation of sympathetic stimulation, concluding this triphasic response to splanchnic sympathetic activity.[24] At the present time there is scant evidence to support other neurologic effects (vagal, cholinergic, sympathetic, histaminergic) on intestinal blood flow, although motility is certainly affected.[24]

Numerous pharmacologic compounds affect intestinal blood flow when supplied intravascularly. The inherent difficulties in studying their effects and extrapolating them to possible physiologic roles is extremely complex and beyond the scope of this chapter. The boxed material above right lists the more thoroughly investigated compounds according to their proposed vascular effects.

The naturally occurring catecholamines, epinephrine and norepinephrine, stimulate intense splanchnic vasoconstriction. Low circulating levels of epinephrine dilate the splanchnic vascular tree by selectively activating vascular beta receptors, whereas higher doses cause vasoconstriction. Similarly, dopamine in low doses (10^{-6} to 10^{-4} M) causes mesenteric vasodilation because of its effect on specific splanchnic dopamine receptors. At higher doses its crossover interaction with alpha-adrenergic receptors leads to vasoconstriction. Endogenously released dopamine is generally thought to be overwhelmed by concomitant epinephrine and norepinephrine release, so its circulating physiologic role is perhaps limited.[24] Dopamine's role in mesenteric circulation during exogenous infusion for myocardial disease is more important. The exogenous administration of catecholamines as vasopressors is the most common clinical condition seen, and their debilitating effects on intestinal perfusion are clinically well documented. Acetylcholine is generally believed to be a splanchnic vasodilator, but at higher doses this effect is counteracted by intestinal smooth muscle compression of the vascular bed.[3] Atropine in doses up to 1.0 mg/kg is able to block the systemic effects of exogenously applied acetylcholine without demonstrable effects on intestinal vascular resistance.[3]

Histamine is an intestinal vasodilator that primarily mediates its effects by H_1 receptors, although the less numerous H_2 receptors in the small bowel may mediate a more sustained vasodilation. Vasopressin, as its name implies, is a potent constrictor of the mesenteric vasculature and may be physiologically important in the response to shock and hemorrhage.[24] Its action is nonspecific, and therefore

PHARMACOLOGIC COMPOUNDS AFFECTING INTESTINAL BLOOD FLOW

Decrease	Increase
Norepinephrine	Epinephrine (β-effect, low dose)
Epinephrine (α-effect, high dose)	Dopamine
Methoxamine	Isoproterenol
Metaraminol	Dobutamine
Phenylephrine	Acetylcholine
Dopamine (α-effect, high dose)	Histamine
Vasopressin	Bradykinin
Angiotensin	Sodium nitrate
Hexamethonium	Nitroprusside
Halothane	Aminophylline
Ouabain	Papaverine
Digoxin	Adenosine
Indomethacin	Caffeine
PGE_1 (rat)	Diazepam
PGE_2 (dogs)	Gastrin, pentagastrin
PGF_2 α or β	Secretin
	Glucagon
	Cholecystokinin
	VIP
	Substance P
	PGE_1 (rabbit)
	PGE_2 (pig)
	PGI_2 (dog)
	GIP

its value is primarily as a general vasoconstrictor and not as a specific mesenteric vasoconstrictor. Another proposed physiologic vasoconstrictor is angiotension. It appears to act by both its direct vascular effects and its potentiation of the catecholamine response to shock or blood loss.

The effect of circulating gastrointestinal hormones on the gastrointestinal circulation, as well as possible local effects by either localized agents (paracrine) or endoluminal secretion, remains an exciting new field of study. Difficulties in interpreting experimental data are generated by species' differences in response to individual gut hormones and the shortcomings of the various animal preparations in approximating a true physiologic condition. Gastrin, or pentagastrin, in addition to increasing gastric acid secretion, increases gastric mucosal blood flow and has a questionable effect on proximal small intestinal blood flow. Secretin and cholecystokinin vasodilate the small intestine in experimental animals, with selective mucosal hyperemia noted in cholecystokinin-infused animals. Glucagon is also a potent intestinal vasodilator in the cat, with vasodilating concentrations correlating well with those normally seen in the postprandial state. Serotonin, a potent stimulant of intestinal motility, does not appear to increase intestinal blood flow at normal circulating concentrations.[64] Substance P, VIP, and GIP all tend to be vasodilators at pharmacologic doses but not physiologic levels. Somatostatin, however, appears to be a relatively selective vasoconstrictor of the upper gastrointestinal circulation at pharmacologic doses. This recent finding may have clinical significance in the treatment of upper gastrointestinal bleeding. Numerous substances are found in the intestinal lumen either basally or after vagal stimulation (serotonin, substance P, motilin, gastrin, somatostatin, VIP, CCK), and the new findings of a neurally independent mucosal hyperemia caused by endoluminal substance P[62] has opened an entirely new field of study of intraluminal, paracrine (or local) controls of mucosal blood flow.

Prostaglandins are also released intraluminally into the small intestine and elicit a wide range of responses in the gastrointestinal circulation. Variable intestinal responses, clear species differences, and rigorous assay techniques make this a difficult field of investigation, but one reviewer states that the splanchnic microcirculation quite likely will be shown to be normally controlled by locally released prostaglandins.[19]

CLINICAL EVALUATION OF INTESTINAL BLOOD FLOW

The search for effective preoperative and intraoperative indicators of intestinal blood flow and viability has been an avid one for the general surgeon. Previously the presence of certain physical symptoms and signs (fever, constant rather than colicky pain, bloody stool, peritoneal signs) were used in a generally unsuccessful way to differentiate viability from nonviability. Later certain common laboratory parameters were used to make this same differentiation (leukocytosis, hyperamylasemia, acidosis) but with similarly inadequate results. Other esoteric biochemical measurements (venous and peritoneal phosphate, creatine phosphokinase) have been currently linked to intestinal ischemia, but a large prospective study in patients with bowel obstructions could find no differences between patients with viable and nonviable bowel in all the aforementioned categories.[52] In addition, this same study did not demonstrate any predictive value of a senior attending surgical staff member's preoperative impressions. In sum, although numerous physical and laboratory findings suggest bowel ischemia, their significance has not been documented clearly in the literature.

Abdominal x-ray films are generally nonspecific, but a "gasless" abdomen has been described in association with mesenteric ischemia caused by small bowel spasm with subsequent distention and ileus. Portal venous gas is rare and considered a terminal finding. Barium examinations may help by revealing a thumb-printing pattern caused by submucosal hemorrhage and superficial mucosal ulcerations (Fig. 21-2). If the diagnosis of mesenteric ischemia is suspected, rapid arteriography is considered the next step.[4,55] Arteriography is extremely helpful in differentiating the causes of intestinal ischemia. Acute thromboses usually involve the origin of any or all of the three main vessels, whereas embolic phenomena typically affect the superior mesenteric artery, usually several centimeters distal to its origin and often at the orifice of the middle colic artery. Nonocclusive ischemic disease characteristically shows segmental mesenteric arterial constriction, often

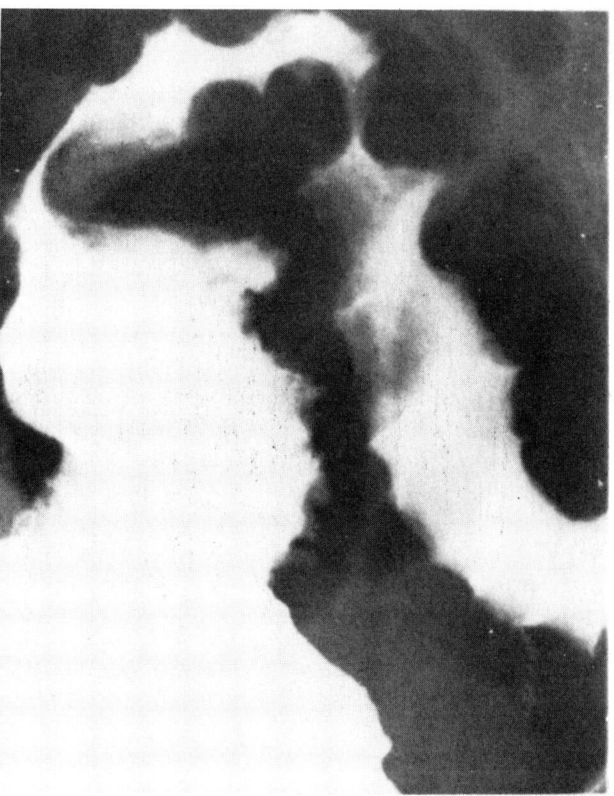

Fig. 21-2 Characteristic thumb-printing pattern seen in association with ischemic colitis. Spot-film taken during the filling phase of a barium enema. The smooth indentations ("thumbprints") are the result of hemorrhage and/or edema in the submucosa. (From Wittenberg, J.: Radiology of the colon, Baltimore, 1980, The Williams and Wilkins Co.)

with an associated proximal stenosis of the superior mesenteric artery. Both anteroposterior and anterolateral arteriographic views are necessary to adequately evaluate the arterial tree, and the selective infusion of vasodilating agents (papaverine 0.5 to 1.0 mg/min) has been advocated to maintain intestinal perfusion while other resuscitative measures are undertaken and the surgical team is assembled. In summary, current arteriographic techniques do not allow for quantitation of blood flow, but in the face of possible acute mesenteric ischemia, differentiation between occlusive and nonocclusive disease is necessary.[61]

Numerous techniques involving radiolabeled particles have been investigated as preoperative indicators of intestinal ischemia. Intravascular injections of technetium (^{99m}Te) labeled pyrophosphate, which binds to the extravasated extracellular calcium from ischemic cells, and ^{99m}Te–sulphur colloid labeled leukocytes, which migrate to areas of inflammation, have been used with moderate laboratory success, although clinical data remain unreported. The major shortcoming for both of these techniques is their need for advanced bowel ischemia, i.e., necrosis, to obtain isotope uptake and the characteristic "hotspots" on isotope imaging.[21] A new intraperitoneal injection technique using Xenon-133 (^{133}Xe), an inert gas usually dissolved in normal saline, has been reported to be successful in differentiating strangulated small bowel obstructions from nonstrangulated small bowel obstructions in laboratory animals.[9] Its elucidation of acute mesenteric ischemia in laboratory animals is also documented.[21] Intraperitoneally injected ^{133}Xe is quickly and equally absorbed by passive transperitoneal diffusion into ischemic and normal bowel.[21] It is promptly cleared by normally perfused bowel to the lungs. Poorly perfused intestine retains ^{133}Xe, which is easily detectable externally by gamma camera techniques. Diagnostic advantages include its safety, rapidity of results (30 to 90 minutes), ability to detect early ischemia, and lack of interference by adhesions and moderate ascites.[20] More quantitative washout curve analysis may be needed, especially in critically ill, hypotensive patients who may have associated asymptomatic reduced splanchnic blood flow. Nonetheless, this technique is an exciting new diagnostic tool, and appropriate clinical trials to test its efficacy are indicated.

The efficacy of any intraoperative method of assessing bowel circulation and viability must quite naturally be compared to experienced clinical judgment and be a technique that involves no sophisticated equipment or risk to the patient. Most surgeons use normal bowel color, peritoneal sheen, mesenteric arterial pulsations, and the presence of spontaneous peristalsis as criteria in this assessment based on experience and the obvious absence of these entities in infarcted bowel. The technique of applying warmed moist packs to bowel of questionable viability for varying lengths of time is almost universally accepted. The technique of second-look procedures, usually at 24 to 48 hours after the first laparotomy, is a time-honored one but subjects the patient, who frequently is critically ill, to additional anesthetic and metabolic stress. Simple transillumination of mesenteric vessels with a sterile light source has been suggested as an adjuvant naked-eye technique.[17] Reported attempts at clinical assessment of intestinal blood flow after ischemic insult have included various sophisticated but technically unwieldy methods, including electromyography, bowel wall pH determinations, and radioactive microsphere injections. At present, most clinical debate focuses on two relatively simple and safe methods of mesenteric circulatory assessment, Doppler ultrasound and intravenous sodium fluorescein administration.

The hand-held, pencil-like, sterile Doppler ultrasound flow probe is used by applying it to the antimesenteric border of the bowel walls and to discrete mesenteric vessels. The presence of a typical pulsatile arterial signal is claimed by its proponents as an indication of adequate blood flow to that particular bowel segment.[45] Although enthusiastically supported by animal studies[53] and small clinical experiences,[42] its drawbacks include a lack of sensitivity, especially for small patchy areas of inadequate circulation along the bowel wall. In addition, it clinically has been shown in a prospective study to be of little or no value in cases of mesenteric venous occlusion.[37] Nevertheless, its quickness and facility of application have made it a popular and generally useful tool for some surgeons.

Fluorescein dye is an organic compound that emits a gold-green fluorescence when exposed to ultraviolet light between 3600 and 4000 Å wavelengths. It readily enters extracellular fluid after intravenous injections, whereupon its entrance into viable tissue occurs within minutes. A maximal intensity is reached within a few minutes of administration with a gradual disappearance over 48 hours. It is nontoxic in normal dosage (10 to 15 mg/kg). Its success in experimental mesenteric arterial and venous occlusions is well documented.[38] In humans 2 ampules (1000 mg) of sodium fluorescein are intravenously injected over 30 to 60 seconds. After dimming the operating room lights, a Woods lamp (3600 Å) is used to illuminate the operative field. Viable bowel shows a confluent fluorescence, although a fine granular pattern may be noted. Nonviable intestine demonstrates an absence of fluorescence, with only a perivascular fluorescent pattern, or patches of nonfluorescence greater than 5 mm in diameter.[45] Because of sodium fluorescein's rapid transudation into the peritoneal cavity and its prolonged presence after injection, this test can really be performed only once, at least within 48 hours, making it a one-shot examination.[45] To date only two prospective trials have been published comparing the Doppler ultrasound flow probe analysis to sodium fluorescein injection in human mesenteric vascular disease[10,37]; both markedly support the fluorescein technique. The overall sensitivity and specificity of the sodium fluorescein technique was 100% and 100%, respectively, in the larger series[10]; the figures were 50% and 58% for the Doppler ultrasound. In fact, the clinical judgment of the senior operating surgeon in this study had a sensitivity and specificity of 82% and 91%, respectively, in identifying nonviable small intestine. At present, the use of intravenous sodium fluorescein appears to be the investigation of choice in assessing mesenteric blood flow or adequacy of bowel perfusion in the intraoperative setting. Table 21-1 compares the various techniques that are available to assess bowel viability.

Table 21-1 **TECHNIQUES OF ASSESSING BOWEL VIABILITY**

Method	Advantages	Disadvantages
Physical signs and symptoms	Rapid, inexpensive	Low sensitivity, low specificity
Common laboratory tests (WBC, amylase, pH)	Inexpensive	Low specificity
Plain radiographs	Inexpensive	Nonspecific
Arteriography	Diagnostic in majority of cases	Significant morbidity, time consuming
Radiolabeled techniques	Highly specific for late? ischemia or infarction	Clinically unproven, requires isotope scanning, only sensitive in late ischemia
^{133}Xe	Highly specific, rapid, safe	Clinically unproven at present
Intraoperative Doppler	Rapid, safe, easily interpretable	Low sensitivity for small ischemic areas, poor for venous disease
Intraoperative fluorescein	Safe, rapid, specific	Present for 48 hours, ''one-shot'' test
Intraoperative clinical judgment	Safe, inexpensive, 90% specific, 80% sensitive	Based on clinical experience

MESENTERIC VASCULAR DISEASE

Mesenteric occlusive vascular disease is classically divided into acute and chronic variants with the provision that many patients with acute manifestations are demonstrating sudden deteriorations of chronic, often asymptomatic, visceral vascular disease. For the purpose of clarity, this classification will be employed in the subsequent discussion.

Acute ischemic syndromes are the result of embolic occlusions of visceral branches of the abdominal aorta, thrombotic occlusions of a previously diseased branch of the mesenteric arterial system, mesenteric venous thrombosis, or nonocclusive mesenteric ischemia (''low-flow'' syndrome).[45,55] The usual result of any of these conditions is intestinal infarction with overall mortalities ranging from 40% to 70%. Acute mesenteric ischemia is responsible for 0.1% of all hospital admissions in the United States, and with the increase in the elderly proportion of the population an aggressive approach to early diagnosis and intervention is warranted. The mortality of these conditions is directly related to the presence of frank bowel infarctions and the frequent concomitant presence of significant cardiovascular disease. Attempts should be made to differentiate among the causes of acute mesenteric ischemia because both treatment and prognoses differ.

Nearly 70% of affected patients are over the age of 60, and over 90% in most series report the acute onset of abdominal pain, often crampy and epigastric or periumbilical in location, as the most prominent symptom. Most patients describe the pain as severe or violent and generally disproportionate to the lack of physical findings. Abdominal pain followed by spontaneous bowel evacuation without significant physical findings is frequently seen in early occlusive mesenteric ischemia. Typically, patients with nonocclusive mesenteric ischemia initially have pain in the absence of defecatory urge of evacuation.[55] Other clinical signs include vomiting, diarrhea, abdominal distention or tenderness, and melena. Bowel sounds range from hyperactivity in the early stages to absolute quiet as transmural necrosis proceeds. Occult blood is a frequent finding in stool examination. A history of preexisting postprandial abdominal pain, ''intestinal angina,'' is seen in about 10% of patients[26] and is an important diagnostic key. Shock, secondary to volume depletion or perforative sepsis, is seen in one fourth of patients at time of initial examination. Hemoconcentration and leukocytosis greater than 20,000/mm^3 are frequently seen, but no single test or combination of blood tests is diagnostic. Serum amylase is elevated in one third of patients with mesenteric ischemia. It should be stressed that acute, severe abdominal pain, especially in the elderly, in the absence of associated abdominal findings, is usually the clearest sign of early mesenteric ischemia, and at this stage most patients will not have progressed to intestinal infarction.[55] Furthermore, the development of abdominal or peritoneal signs implies infarction and significantly increases mortality. The use of plain and angiographic roentgenograms has already been mentioned as essential for diagnosis and is only noted here as a reminder for their rapid institution. Medical stabilization, metabolic correction, and invasive cardiovascular monitoring are integral efforts in these critically ill patients in the interim before surgery. Coexisting atherosclerotic heart disease, chronic airway disease, and diabetes mellitis are frequently encountered in these patients and require rapid investigation and physiologic normalization.

Acute Mesenteric Arterial Embolism

Sixty percent of acute mesenteric arterial embolic events are amenable to surgery, making them the most important surgical cause of intestinal ischemia, comprising 12% to 67% of all acute mesenteric vascular catastrophes.[26,49] Bergan's triad of acute abdominal crisis, significant cardiac disease, and spontaneous gastrointestinal emptying is used descriptively for this disorder.[2] Affected patients are often younger with no prior intestinal angina symptoms. Important historical or concomitant findings include arrhythmias in 70% of the patients; the majority of these are atrial tachyarrhythmias, recent myocardial infarctions, previous arterial emboli, rheumatic heart disease, and atherosclerotic heart disease.[5,45] The oblique takeoff of the superior mesenteric artery (SMA) favors embolization with a total of 5% of all peripheral arterial emboli involving this vessel or a distal branch. Usually emboli lodge several centimeters distal to the SMA origin, occluding the middle colic artery (55%), right colic artery (16%), ileocolic artery (7%), the SMA (15%), or smaller peripheral branches (4%).[14] The usual source of emboli is the heart but unusual emboli forms include those from bronchogenic carcinoma, atrial myxoma, aortic or mitral valvular prostheses, and the proximal aortic wall.[61]

Surgical management consists of four parts: (1) the identification and resuscitation of the high-risk patient; (2) arteriographic localization and confirmation of the vascular abnormality; (3) operative management; and (4) postoperative management that includes a possible second-look procedure. The identification of these patients is done by observation of the aforementioned signs, symptoms, and history. Resuscitation involves metabolic correction and monitored restoration of intravascular volume. Because of their constrictor effects on splanchnic blood flow, vasopressors and digitalis compounds should be avoided whenever possible. Antibiotic coverage for those for whom surgery is anticipated is recommended, and broad spectrum coverage is the rule.

After a brief but thorough resuscitative phase, early angiography is mandated. Lengthy delays before angiography not only allow for further bowel ischemia, but also obscure the radiologic diagnosis by allowing distal clot propagation. Femoral arterial access for angiographic evaluation is generally preferred with biplane selective injection of all three major splanchnic trunks. Some authorities recommend halving the usual dose of contrast because of these patients' tenuous fluid balance and to avoid renal failure.[5,30] Occlusion of the SMA or one of its branches with arterial spasm and a lack of collaterals (as seen with acute thrombosis) is the usual angiographic picture. The splanchnic vasoconstriction seen with SMA embolization is well documented,[49] and its persistence after embolectomy may be a reason for the frequent inability to restore adequate blood flow and for the frequent late reocclusions of distal vessels. Persistent precapillary arterial vasospasm is seen experimentally after just 2 hours of partial SMA occlusion[6]; this possibly reflects myogenic control mechanisms. Because of this distal vasospasm, selective arterial vasodilator administration is performed by most radiologists.[5,45] Tolazoline is used in an initial 25-mg bolus because of its rapid effect; further angiographic exposures are taken to ascertain its effect. If a vasodilation is noted, a continuous intra-arterial infusion of papaverine is begun at 30 to 60 mg/hour. Tolazoline is neither as safe nor as efficacious as papaverine for continuous infusion. The infusion is continued while surgical teams are assembled.

Operative management of this disorder is probably the least controversial aspect (Fig. 21-3). The SMA is dissected free through the base of the small bowel mesentery, and linear arteriotomies are made, followed by embolectomy and vein patch graft closure of the arteriotomy. Since vein is preferred for patching, both legs should be prepped and draped into the operative field. The presence of palpable pulses distal to the arteriotomy must be documented before proceeding to bowel evaluation and resection. Most patients require the resection of some intestine followed by standard end-to-end anastomoses. Observational criteria or the previously discussed fluorescein injection or Doppler ultrasound or all of these are used to select viable bowel for anastomosis and nonviable bowel for resection. Mortality is related to the amount of bowel resected, with greater than 50% resections approaching a 90% mortality.[5] The need for a second-look operation is decided on before

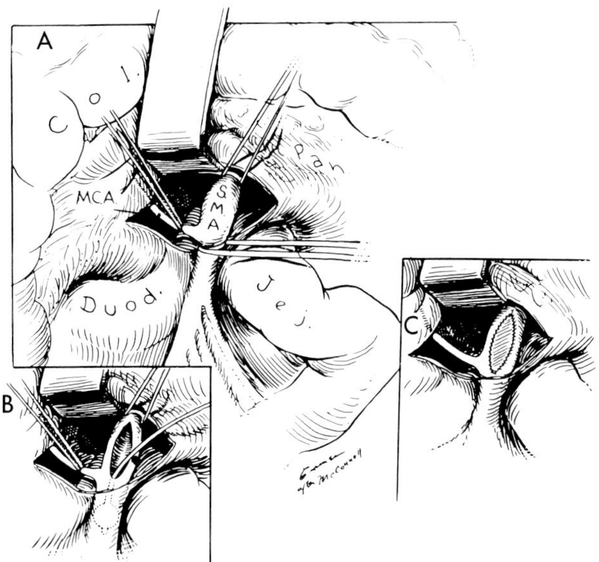

Fig. 21-3 Surgical management of embolism to the superior mesenteric artery. **A,** The artery has been isolated at the base of the transverse mesocolon and controlled with tapes. **B,** Longitudinal arteriotomy placed proximal to the origin of the middle colic artery. Fogarty catheter has been passed distally. **C,** Arteriotomy closure using a vein patch that may or may not be necessary. (From Boley, S.J., et al.: Surgery annual, New York, 1973, Appleton-Century-Crofts.)

closure; this decision is adhered to regardless of subsequent clinical improvement. Repeat angiography and postoperative continuation of intra-arterial papaverine is advocated by Boley,[5] whose 55% survival figures are the best reported.

The use of anticoagulants in SMA embolus is controversial.[2,5,43] The relative risks of significant intestinal bleeding versus the incidence of late postoperative thromboses leads most authorities to recommend some late (48 hours postoperatively) form of anticoagulation. In patients awaiting a second-look procedure, low molecular weight dextran has been cited for both its plasma volume expansion qualities and its antithrombotic properties.

A variety of postoperative problems, both early and late, may arise. Sepsis, gastrointestinal bleeding, acute renal failure, pulmonary insufficiency, and myocardial dysfunction are all common and mandate admission of these patients to an intensive care unit for several days. The findings of unexplained acidosis, sepsis of unexplained origin, or refractory cardiovascular instability suggest continuing bowel necrosis and may necessitate a second-look procedure.

Acute Mesenteric Thrombosis

Acute thrombosis of a previously atherosclerotic SMA, celiac trunk, or inferior mesenteric artery (in that order of frequency) is the most common cause of acute mesenteric ischemia. Various series report this entity as comprising 44% to 82% of all mesenteric ischemic disorders.[14,26,55] The preoperative and postoperative management of these patients is basically identical to that described in the earlier section, but several unique features of this condition merit further discussion.

Anatomically significant or complete atherosclerotic obstructions of any or all of the splanchnic major vessels are a frequent finding in a high proportion of patients undergoing arteriography for other vascular disorders.[14,26,55,61] The presence of significant, but usually hemodynamically incomplete, collateral systems is also noted. These collateral systems may allow for a longer "grace period" before infarction occurs, although survival statistics do not support this. They may also be responsible for the less dramatic clinical appearance of this disorder as compared to embolic phenomenona. Both the clinical and radiographic picture early on often simulate a bowel obstruction. Abdominal pain, again out of proportion to clinical findings, associated with a history of cardiovascular disase is often the only early finding, although fever, shock, and melena eventually develop in many. Both abdominal symptoms and angiographic evidence of ischemic disease are necessary before laparotomy for this condition should be performed.

Most of these patients will have had a significant gastrointestinal history. Between 50% and 70% will have had in the previous year a significant history of weight loss, diarrhea, abdominal pain, or the diagnosis of an abdominal bruit.[34] Many patients have had unsuccessful investigations in the preceding months for peptic ulcer or gallbladder disease, and many have the label of having psychiatric or functional abdominal pain. The exact percentage of patients with intestinal angina who progress to frank bowel infarction is unknown. Overall mortality of acute thromboses averages 80%, with almost two thirds of these patients in some series undergoing either an "open and close" laparotomy because of the extensive intestinal necrosis or heroic massive bowel resections.

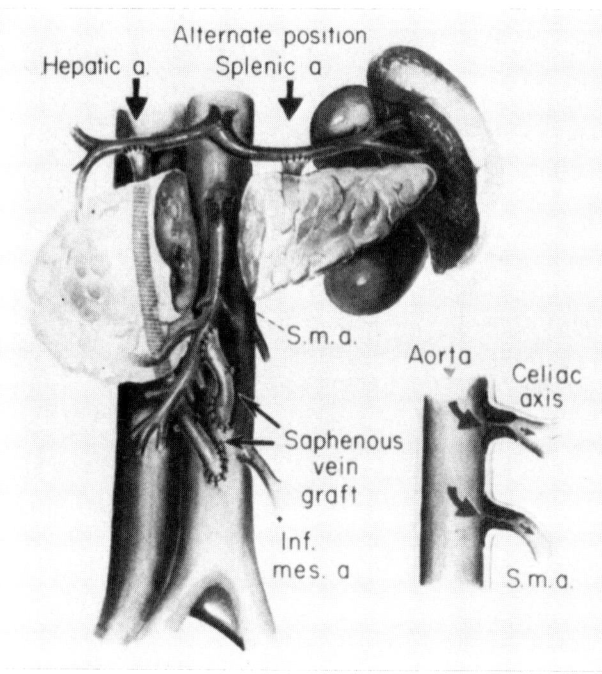

Fig. 21-4 Bypass of the atherosclerotic or thrombosed celiac or superior mesenteric artery. Artist's drawing showing saphenous bypass grafts to the celiac axis territory and superior mesenteric artery. The celiac axis graft passes behind the pancreas to connect with either the hepatic artery or the splenic artery. Atherosclerotic occlusions of the celiac axis and superior mesenteric artery are depicted in the lateral view of the aorta. (From Bergan, J.J., and Yao, J.S.T. In Rutherford, R.B., editor: Vascular surgery, ed. 2, Philadelphia, 1984, W.B. Saunders Co.)

Again, early arteriographic evaluation is necessary in these high-risk patients. The frequent concomitant obstruction of both celiac and superior mesenteric vessels is usually ameliorated by restoring blood flow through just one of the involved vessels. Operatively the SMA is more accessible and easier to manipulate than the celiac artery and is the preferred vessel for bypass. All mesenteric vessels have a reputation for friability[45] and handling them requires great care. The prompt relief of an obstructed SMA or celiac artery is the surgical goal. Although successful thromboendarterectomy has been reported,[48] most current authors favor venous graft or prosthetic bypass of the affected segment using the aorta or right iliac artery as the inflow vessel (Fig. 21-4). Postoperative management is similarly difficult because of the systemic nature of atherosclerosis and because most survivors succumb to some form of the disease.

Acute Mesenteric Ischemia After Aortic Surgery

Because of the significant association between aortic atherosclerotic disease and disease of the splanchnic arterial vessels, it is not uncommon for aortic revascularization procedures to create ischemic insults for the gut. Acute small intestinal or large intestinal ischemia, most commonly involving the left colon, may result from aortic surgery.[49] The reported incidence of significant colon ischemia varies between 1% and 10% with mortality averaging from 40% to 65%.[29,49] Small intestinal ischemia, usually associated with right colon ischemia as well, is much rarer, with an incidence of less than 0.1% but mortalities approaching 90%.[29] Intestinal ischemia (primarily left colon) is seen 10 times more frequently after aneurysm repair of the abdominal aorta than after occlusive aortic disease surgery. In the latter situation, the inferior mesenteric artery (IMA) is already occluded and the left colon receives its blood supply from collateral routes; in aneurysmal disease, inferior mesenteric flow is often intact and the colon receives its major blood supply through this vascular route.

Ischemia of the left colon may follow intraoperative ligation of the IMA if collateral circulation from above is compromised by coexistent SMA disease, by previous bowel resection, or by congenital interruption or absence of collateral routes. These congenital findings include aberrant take off of the middle colic artery (usually from the right colic artery) in 20% of cases and absence of the marginal artery of Drummond at the splenic flexure in 7%.[54] Other statistically implicated factors include prolonged cross-clamp time; ruptured aneurysm; the presence of hypoxemia, hypotension, or arrhythmias; operative colonic trauma; and digitalis toxicity.[32,54] Furthermore, internal iliac artery flow compromised by occlusive or aneurysmal disease additionally limits bowel collateral flow. Embolization of thrombotic and atheromatous debris also occurs.[49] An aortoiliac steel syndrome has been described after simultaneous aortic reconstructions and lumbar sympathectomies, resulting in a 40% to 70% decrease in IMA flow.[33] In sum, patients at high risk for ischemic colitis following aortic surgery are those with an absence or occlusion of the marginal artery at the splenic flexure, absent middle colic artery, internal iliac arterial inflow disease, or middle colic artery enlargement suggesting SMA occlusive disease.[54]

Infarction of the small intestine is usually related to inopportune ligation of the IMA when it supplies the majority of the gastrointestinal tract through the meandering mesenteric artery. Careful examination of the preoperative arteriogram, especially lateral views, should alert the surgeon to this risk. In this circumstance, revascularization, generally by aortosuperior mesenteric artery bypass grafting, should be planned.[49]

Left colon ischemia is prevented by ligation of the IMA immediately adjacent to the aorta to obviate interruption of its collateral channels. Careful vascular technique to avoid embolization is a must. Avoiding hypotension and ensuring patency of the hypogastric arteries are emphasized. If the left colon appears ischemic on IMA clamping or division, if the IMA is patent but has very little backflow, or if the IMA shows large ascending collateral vessels on preoperative angiographic examination,[16,49] an IMA reimplantation (Fig. 21-5) using Carrel button techniques or an aorto-IMA bypass should be performed.

If colonic ischemia occurs following surgery, symptoms are often late in appearing (48 to 72 hours). Left lower abdominal pain, bloody diarrhea, and systemic toxicity are the usual findings. Subclinical mucosal ischemia has been reported in 4% to 7% of patients,[16,49] but clinical ischemia reveals hemorrhagic ulcerations and mucosal edema with friability on sigmoidoscopy. If such findings occur, relaparotomy is necessary on an urgent basis.

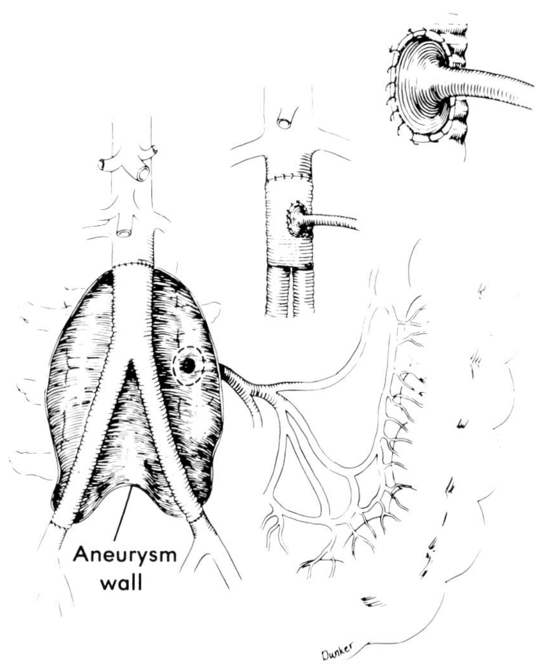

Fig. 21-5 Reimplantation of the inferior mesenteric artery (IMA) during abdominal aortic aneurysm surgery. Carrel path technique of IMA reconstruction. Excision of button of aneurysm wall surrounding IMA orifice facilitates repair. (From Ernst, C.B.: Complications in vascular surgery, ed. 2, Orlando, Fla., 1985, Grune & Stratton, Inc.)

Small bowel ischemia is treated similarly in an aggressive fashion although sigmoidoscopic findings may only reveal melena. Again, if clinical doubt exists, early relaparotomy is performed.

Mesenteric Venous Thrombosis

The syndrome of acute or subacute thrombosis of the mesenteric veins was first described in 1935 by Warren and Eberhard and now comprises approximately 10% of all cases of mesenteric ischemia.[59] The majority of patients lack predisposing conditions. Associated conditions include peritonitis or abdominal inflammation, abdominal trauma, portal hypertension, intra-abdominal tumors, adhesions, volvulus, sickle cell disease, polycythemia vera, coagulopathies (especially anti–thrombin III deficiencies), pregnancy, recent splenectomy, and the use of oral contraceptives.[45,55,61] Over 40% of patients will have had a previous deep vein thrombophlebitis of the lower extremity. The reported age range is from 11 months to 89 years, but most series report an average age of only 47 years.[31,51]

Patients may be divided into two categories: those with subacute and acute presentations.[40] The subacute category is far more common, often having a vague prodrome of crampy abdominal pain, distention, nausea, and lassitude lasting from a few days to several weeks. This group is considered to have thrombi that originated in small mesenteric veins or venules and then propagated proximally. The more acute presentations are thought to represent primary thrombosis of large, often named mesenteric veins.[40] Rarely are veins in the inferior mesenteric system involved. By the time of presentation, most patients have significant abdominal pain, tenderness, and distention. Laboratory investigations reveal a leukocytosis, hemoconcentration, and a copious bloody peritoneal transudate. As venous pressure increases, myogenic mechanisms stimulate arteriolar vasoconstriction, which leads to capillary distention and leakage with an abundant serosal transudation of bloody fluid. Additional anatomic findings include massive edema of the bowel wall as a result of interstitial edema, mesenteric arterial pulsations, compensatory mesenteric lymphatic engorgement, and mesenteric veins full of clot. Classic, but frequently overlooked, radiographic findings include rigid, thick-walled segments of edematous bowel in which a small gas collection remains fixed in a straight or curved lumen on different radiographs.[31] Early angiography can be diagnostic, showing a delay in filling the arterial phase, small artery spasm, poor emptying of arteries, failure of venous systems (including the portal vein) to opacify, and often opacification of thickened bowel wall as a result of transudation of contrast.[45,55,61]

Treatment is again similar to that discussed for other ischemic disorders of the splanchnic vasculature. Aggressive restoration of intravascular volume and antibiotics are administered before urgent laparotomy. A small bowel resection, averaging over 100 cm,[31] is virtually always necessary. If palpable clot is present, a venous thrombectomy is performed through the superior mesenteric vein controlled inferior to the pancreas. A transverse venotomy is performed and manual milking of the clot, as well as the use of Fogarty catheters, is employed to remove the thrombus. Most surgeons begin heparinization immediately, and warfarin compounds are continued for 3 to 6 months following surgery. If a predisposing coagulopathy exists, anticoagulation is continued indefinitely. Often only a bowel resection is necessary, but a wide mesenteric resection is performed to avoid leaving residual thrombotic veins behind that may later propagate clot.[12,31,40,51] Untreated, the mortality rate approaches 100%, but newer series report operative mortalities averaging 20%.[12,31,40,51] Rethrombosis is common, usually occurs early, is seen in about one third of cases, and has a higher mortality of 60% to 80%.[31] Some surgeons routinely advocate second-look procedures because of this high rethrombosis rate.[31] Certainly a high index of suspicion and intensive care monitoring of the patient are warranted.

Nonocclusive Mesenteric Ischemia

The entity of nonocclusive mesenteric ischemia is a diverse series of interrelated events that accounts for 20% to 50% of all mesenteric infarctions in which autopsy data are included.[12,31,40,51] It involves the distribution of the SMA almost exclusively and is usually the consequence of both an anatomic defect (SMA stenosis in greater than one third of patients) and some acute process that requires either an increase or a redistribution of cardiac output.[61] This results in a decrease in mesenteric perfusion pressure with an accompanying splanchnic vasoconstriction initiated by myogenic mechanisms. As splanchnic vasoconstriction occurs, the critical closing pressures of small arteries are surpassed, leading to segmental microvascular collapse. This circumstance favors microthrombus formation with a concomitant further reduction in blood flow.[55] If systemic hypotension also exists, increased endogenously or exogenously administered catecholamines or both may further constrict the splanchnic microcirculation with eventual ischemia and necrosis. Local acidosis and thrombus formation lead to capillary sludging and hemoconcentration. Bowel distention, often present, further decreases blood flow by mural pressure increases. This vicious physiologic circle continues until frank segmental bowel infarction occurs; untreated, this results in a mortality rate approaching 100%. A myriad of conditions has been associated with nonocclusive mesenteric ischemia. The majority of patients with this disease have some underlying cardiac abnormality.

Digitalis compounds are potent in vitro contractors of arterial and venous smooth muscle in the gut and simultaneously decrease splanchnic blood flow and oxygen consumption. Up to 83% of patients with nonocclusive mesenteric ischemia are taking digitalis compounds at the time of diagnosis. Other conditions associated with this disorder include congestive heart failure, arrhythmias, cardiopulmonary bypass, cardiogenic or septic shock, administration of vasopressors or intravenous calcium or both, major thermal injuries, and pancreatitis.

Patients are often hospitalized for these associated conditions when the disorder arises. Abdominal pain and evidence of a low output state are the major diagnostic aids. Frequently patients are examined for other acute abdominal processes including cholecystitis, appendicits, and bowel obstruction. The absence of abdominal pain in this condition is far more frequent than in occlusive mesenteric ischemia because of concomitant symptomatic conditions. Evidence of peripheral circulatory shutdown, acidosis, and hemoconcentration are often present. Plain abdominal roentgenograms often show only fluid-filled bowel loops. Arteriography is useful in distinguishing this condition from occlusive mesenteric ischemia. In addition, careful angiography may reveal segmental spastic arterial constriction (chain of sausages)[45] and there may be a failure to visualize mesenteric vascular arcades or intramural vessels. The intra-arterial infusion of vasodilators (papaverine, glucagon, prostaglandins) has been clinically reported with some success[12,50,55] while aggressive attempts to increase cardiac output and normalize intravascular volume are performed. Repeat angiography is performed after vasodilator therapy is begun to document improvement.

Unlike other types of acute mesenteric ischemia, immediate surgery is not indicated in nonocclusive ischemia. Further, anesthesia and intraoperative manipulation decrease intestinal blood flow. Generally, a scrutinous 8- to 12-hour observation of the patient while vasodilator therapy is administered and cardiac improvement is attempted is the initial treatment of choice. Following this, or sooner if evidence of infarcted bowel is suspected, laparotomy is performed in the majority of patients.

Chronic Intestinal Ischemia

Chronic intestinal ischemia and its manifestation as intestinal angina were first described by Mikkelson in 1958.[39] The importance of this entity lies not only in its production of physical disability for the individual patient, but also in its propensity to progress to life-threatening mesenteric infarction. Over 50% of patients dying of SMA thrombosis previously have had intestinal angina. These patients are classically in the sixth decade of life and are heavy smokers. Unlike other types of peripheral vascular disease, females outnumber males by a ratio of three to one. Over a third of these patients will have atherosclerotic disease of the aorta or renal arteries.

The classic triad of abdominal pain, weight loss, and diarrhea is seen in this condition.[22,49] Recurrent abdominal pain occurs 15 minutes to 1 hour postprandially; it is periumbilical, crampy, and lasts from 1 to 3 hours. Because this pain commences soon after eating, it often causes a fear of eating, which can lead to a significant weight loss that averages 20 to 25 pounds in most patients.[57,63] Diarrhea that is often occult blood positive is seen in about one third of patients. Malabsorption is frequently seen, but specific diagnostic tests are not usually helpful. An abdominal bruit is heard in 50% of patients but abdominal examination, even during attacks of pain, is frequently unremarkable. Atherosclerosis is the leading cause of the visceral artery stenoses that cause this syndrome, although extrinsic compression, neoplasms, and local inflammation have been implicated.[57] Because of the nature of the symptoms patients are often investigated for the presence of an occult gastrointestinal neoplasm.[13,22,55,57,63] Arteriography should be performed if the malignancy investigation results are negative. Lateral views are important in evaluating the celiac and SMA, whereas oblique views help demonstrate the IMA. Significant stenoses of both the celiac and the

SMA are seen in 85% of patients[57] and large collateral vessels are usually seen.

Treatment is reserved for patients with intestinal angina pain, weight loss that is documented, and angiographic evidence of advanced atherosclerosis. Treatment has evolved from simple thromboendarterectomy or reimplantation of the SMA to the current choices of transaortic endarterectomy or bypass grafting. Proponents of transaortic endarterectomy cite the high incidence of concomitant aortic atherosclerosis found at operation and the ease of doing simultaneous one or two vessel endarterectomy. Many surgeons favor aortovisceral artery bypass grafting because SMA atherosclerosis usually originates 5 to 15 mm from the main arterial ostium. Dacron grafts are preferred over saphenous vein grafts because of their resistance to kinking and better clinical results.[13,55,57] If gastrointestinal spillage or contamination occurs at the time of surgery, vein grafting would be preferred. Intraoperative pressure gradients greater than 35 mm Hg across the stenosed vessel are usually found, and although single vessel bypass (usually the SMA) generally leads to a good result, many surgeons recommend bifurcated grafts to both the celiac artery and the SMA because of substantial recurrence rates with a single bypass graft.[45] Pain relief is obtained in 90% of patients, and over 75% will regain lost weight and improve their malabsorption.

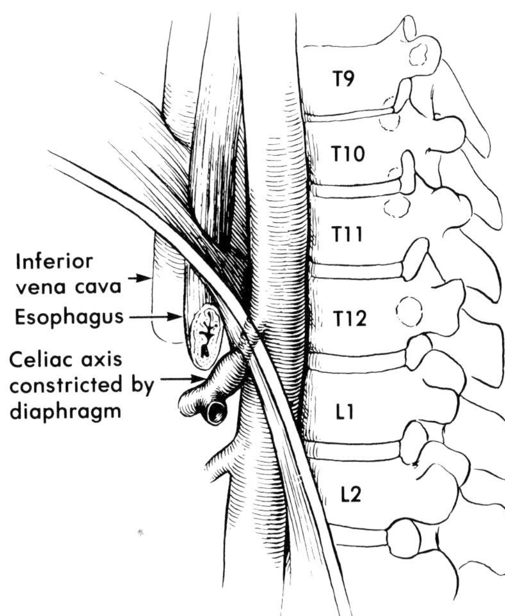

Fig. 21-6 Compression of celiac axis by median arcuate ligament of diaphragm. (From Stoney, R.J., and Lusby, R.J. In Haimovici, H., editor: Vascular surgery principles and techniques, ed. 2, East Norwalk, Conn., 1984, Appleton-Century-Crofts.)

MISCELLANEOUS DISORDERS OF THE INTESTINAL VASCULATURE

Several rare, interesting, and controversial disorders of the mesenteric circulation exist and will be discussed briefly.

Celiac Artery Compression Syndrome

The celiac artery compression syndrome, or median arcuate ligament syndrome, has been a controversial subject since its initial description in 1963 by Harjola.[25] It is briefly defined as compression of the celiac axis by either the median arcuate ligament of the diaphragm or fibrosed celiac ganglion tissue, leading to postprandial and often positional pain in the epigastrium, nausea, weight loss, and epigastric bruits. Women in the younger age groups are more often affected than men.[49] The variable anatomic positions of the celiac axis and median arcuate ligament may indeed lead to an anterior compression of the celiac axis, especially during expiration and various postural changes (Fig. 21-6). In addition, 50% of patients with this problem have a celiac ganglion that interconnects around the axis with retroperitoneal fibrous and fatty tissue that forms a thick and potentially compressing shield.[7] Both SMA and IMA systems normally provide excellent compensation for celiac arterial inflow decreases. In a series of 50 symptomatic patients undergoing arteriography, 24% were found to have at least a 50% stenosis of the celiac axis.[36] In addition, between 6% and 16% of normal people have epigastric bruits indicating compromised flow through the celiac artery.[7] One large literature review composed of 330 patients with the celiac artery compression syndrome could document postprandial abdominal pain in only 30% and weight loss in only 50%.[7] In addition, alarming postoperative recurrence rates of 50% to 86%[18,46,49] have been reported after careful follow-up. The possibility of splanchnic nerve pain secondary to pulsative compression of the celiac plexus by the celiac artery has been entertained as an explanation for this syndrome, with anecdotal reports of symptomatic relief after splanchnic ganglionectomy.[55,61]

Nevertheless, despite debate concerning the origin of this entity and the significance of compromised flow through the celiac axis, median arcuate ligament or celiac plexus compression of the celiac artery or both do exist and may well be the cause of the syndrome in a few patients with otherwise negative evaluations.[26,56] Lateral aortography should reveal a smooth asymmetrical narrowing of the superior aspect of the artery, often with inferior displacement. Patients with postural, exercise, or respiratory components of the pain may do better following surgery. Surgical correction usually entails simple division of the constricting median arcuate ligament of the celiac ganglion. Bypass or vein patch angioplasty of the compressed segment is occasionally performed.[49,56] It is clear that the debate over this entity's actual existence is far from over, and newer clinical blood flow studies during attacks of pain may help resolve the problem and its clinical significance.

Vascular Compression of the Duodenum

Vascular compression of the duodenum is known by several names: Wilkie's syndrome, superior mesenteric artery syndrome, and arteriomesenteric duodenal compression. First described by Rokitansky in 1861, it was later well delineated by Wilkie in a series of 75 patients in 1927.[60] The symptoms of postprandial distention and vomiting with associated weight loss are caused by duodenal compression between the SMA or one of its branches and

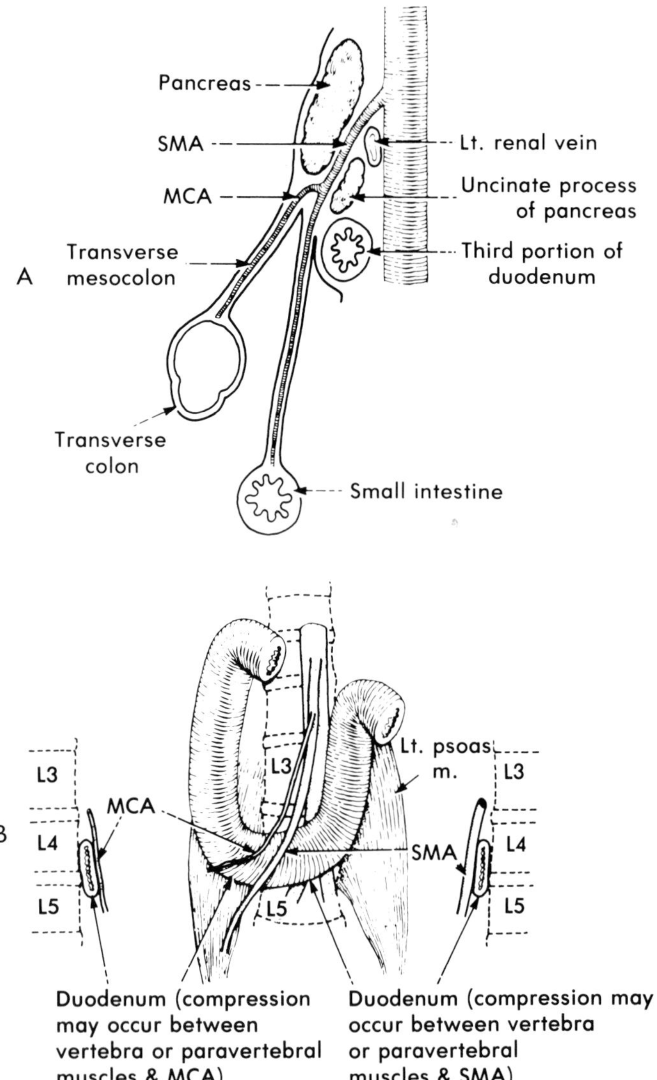

Fig. 21-7 Vascular compression of the duodenum by the superior mesenteric vessels. **A,** Diagrammatic sagittal section through the neck of the pancreas showing the relation of the third portion of the duodenum to the superior mesenteric artery (SMA), the middle colic artery (MCA), the aorta, and the mesentery. **B,** Anterior view of the duodenum, SMA, MCA, and the vertebral column. (From Akin, J.T., Gray, S.W., and Skandalakis, J.E.: Surgery **79:**515, 1976.)

the aorta and vertebral bodies. Probably owing to the attainment of an erect posture in humans, the SMA leaves the aorta at an acute angle through which pass the third and fourth portions of the duodenum[1] (Fig. 21-7).

The majority of patients are young (less than 40 years old), and 60% are female. Many claim that lying on the left side or in the knee-chest position alleviates the pain. Associated conditions are common: prolonged bed rest, body cast, scoliosis, acute weight losses, and anorexia nervosa.[1,44,47] No patient has been described as obese. Diagnosis is based on classic symptomatology and cineradiography. Cineradiography reveals the classic to-and-fro churning of the duodenal contents proximal to the crossing of the SMA with barium cascade over the incomplete obstruction.[1] Associated peptic ulcers are seen in 15% of patients.

Treatment is usually simple division of Treitz's ligament. Occasionally duodenojejunostomy will be required in chronic cases. Weight gains have been reported to cure the condition in anorexic patients. Removal of body casts and mobilization, if feasible, should be attempted initially in appropriate patients before initiating surgical intervention.

Visceral Artery Aneurysms

Of the visceral artery aneurysms, splenic arterial involvement is the most common, accounting for 41%.[58] The overall autopsy incidence is 0.78%, but these aneurysms are seen in 10% of geriatric patients and 7.1% of patients with portal hypertension. Splenic artery aneurysm is the third most common intra-abdominal aneurysm, exceeded in incidence only by aneurysms of the infrarenal aorta and iliac vessels. Normally diagnosed in the sixth decade of life, these aneurysms are four times more common in women. Since pregnancy accentuates splenic blood flow, it is thought to be an etiologic factor. Interestingly, 88% of female patients with this disease have had one or more pregnancies; 45% have had more than six.[11,49,58] The majority of patients are asymptomatic and are diagnosed incidentally by ultrasonography or the presence of "eggshell" calcifications in the left upper quadrant on plain abdominal radiographs. The development of referable symptoms implies impending rupture with an associated mortality of 25%. Rupture in pregnancy, usually occurring in the third trimester, carries a mortality of 68%.[49] The ability of the lesser sac to contain splenic arterial rupture accounts for the better survival in the nonpregnant patient.

Most splenic artery aneurysms are atherosclerotic in origin, and associated vascular disease in these patients is common. Two thirds of splenic artery aneurysms are located in the main splenic artery before its arborization, and 40% are multiple.[58] Their size ranges from 0.6 to 30 cm.[58] Elective surgery, usually entailing excision with accompanying splenectomy, is recommended for all symptomatic patients and asymptomatic women of childbearing age. Pregnant women should undergo elective excision, which has an operative mortality of less than 1%.[49,58] Asymptomatic aneurysms less than 2 to 3 cm in the elderly or high-risk patient should be watched.

Hepatic artery aneurysms account for 16% to 20% of visceral artery aneurysms. Approximately three fourths are extrahepatic and 10% are mycotic.[58] The most common symptom is rupture, which occurs in 44% of patients;[11,49] right upper quadrant pain simulating cholelithiasis is also common. Complete visceral angiography is necessary to elucidate the intrahepatic aneurysm, which may require hepatic resection for cure. Rupture is usually equally divided between free intraperitoneal bleeding or intrabiliary hemorrhage with resultant hemobilia and hematemesis. Surgery is recommended for all hepatic artery aneurysms, with excision and bypass grafting, usually with Dacron, being the favored procedure.

Celiac axis aneurysms account for only 3% of visceral artery aneurysms. Most are asymptomatic, but surgery is recommended if they are discovered because of their 80% rupture mortality rate.[11,49] Pancreaticoduodenal artery aneurysms are rare. Difficult exposure and identification at the time of surgery are the main problems in elective repair. Since 50% of these will ultimately rupture (generally into the peritoneal cavity), with an accompanying high mortality rate, surgical excision is the treatment of choice when they are diagnosed.

Intestinal Buerger's Disease

Less than a dozen verified cases of intestinal Buerger's disease, or thromboangiitis obliterans, have been reported to date since Buerger first described this disorder of the peripheral vascular tree in 1908.[8] The majority involve the small intestine[15]; a 40% mortality is reported. Peripheral ischemic complaints are generally absent or minimal in these patients, implying a selective involvement of the mesenteric vessels. Chronic or intermittent gastrointestinal complaints are common in these patients, often with associated weight loss. At the time of initial laparotomy, 40% had an intestinal perforation without any typical clinical picture to indicate its likelihood. The careful observation of these patients, especially those with abdominal complaints, and the realization that mesenteric disease acts independently of peripheral disease should be noted by the surgeon. Although it is suspected that cessation of smoking will alleviate the symptoms in these patients, clinical data supporting this assumption are lacking at present.

SUMMARY

The sophisticated array of intestinal functions relies on an intact vascular supply. In addition to the patency of a normal vascular tree, interdependent intrinsic and extrinsic regulatory mechanisms exist to effectively distribute the 10% to 15% of total cardiac output to the gut. Intrinsic mechanisms include both myogenic and metabolic regulatory systems. Extrinsic controls include the generous but poorly understood parasympathetic and sympathetic nerve supply and numerous hormonal and neurohumoral influences.

Vascular disorders of the intestine are significant for the diagnostic challenge that they present and for the substantial morbidity and mortality that they cause. For the operative clinician, a review of the clinical and experimental methods of determining intestinal viability supports intravenous fluorescein and experienced clinical judgment as the best intraoperative discriminators. Many vascular disorders are present with similar symptoms, but careful attention to appropriate diagnosis will lead to the best directed therapy.

REFERENCES

1. Akin, J.T., Gray, S.W., and Skandalakis, J.E.: Vascular compression of the duodenum: presentations of ten cases and review of the literature, Surgery **79:**515, 1976.
2. Bergan, J.J., et al.: Revascularization in treatment of mesenteric infarction, Ann. Surg. **187:**430, 1975.
3. Boatman, D.L., and Brody, M.J.: Affects of acetylcholine on the intestinal vasculature of the dog, J. Pharmacol. Exper. Therap. **7:**185, 1963.
4. Boley, S.J., Brandt, L.J., and Vieth, F.J.: Ischemic disorders of the intestines, Curr. Prob. Surg. **15:**1, 1978.
5. Boley, S.J., Feinstein, F.R., and Sammartano, R.: New concepts in the management of emboli of the superior mesenteric artery, Surg. Gynecol. Obstet. **153:**561, 1981.
6. Boley, S.J., et al.: Persistent vasoconstriction: a major factor in nonocclusive mesenteric ischemia, Curr. Top. Surg. Res. **3:**425, 1971.
7. Brandt, L.J., and Boley, S.J.: Celiac axis compression syndrome: a critical review, Dig. Dis. **23:**633, 1978.
8. Buerger, L.: Thromboangiitis obliterans: a story of the vascular lesions leading to presenile spontaneous gangrene, Am. J. Med. Sci. **136:**567, 1908.
9. Bulkley, G.B., et al.: The use of intraperitoneal Xenon 133 for imaging of intestinal strangulation in small bowel obstruction, Am. J. Surg. **141:**128, 1981.
10. Bulkley, G.B., et al.: Intraoperative determination of small intestinal Klacsman viability following ischemic injury, Ann. Surg. **193:**628, 1981.
11. Busuttil, R.W., and Brin, B.T.: The diagnosis and management of visceral artery aneurysms, Surgery **88:**619, 1980.
12. Bynum, T.E., and Jacobson, E.D.: Non-occlusive intestinal ischemia, Arch. Int. Med. **139:**281, 1979.
13. Connolly, J.E., and Dwaan, J.H.: Management of chronic visceral ischemia, Surg. Clin. North Am. **62:**345, 1982.
14. Crawford, E.S., et al.: Celiac axis, superior mesenteric artery, and inferior mesenteric arterial occlusion: surgical considerations, Surgery **82:**856, 1977.
15. Deitch, E.A., and Sikkema, W.W.: Intestinal manifestations of Buerger's disease, Am. Surg. **47:**326, 1981.
16. Ernst, C.B., et al.: Inferior mesenteric artery stump pressure, Ann. Surg. **187:**1, 1978.
17. Ersek, R.A.: Mesenteric transillumination for vascular 641-visualization, Surg. Gynecol. Obstet. **152:**339, 1981.
18. Evans, W.E.: Long-term evaluation of the celiac band syndrome, Surgery **76:**867, 1974.
19. Gallavan, R.H., and Jacobson, E.D.: Minireview: prostaglandins and the splanchnic circulation, Proc. Soc. Exper. Bio. Med. **20**(170):391, 1982.
20. Gharagozloo, F., et al.: Intraperitoneal Xenon for the detection of early intestinal ischemia: effects of ascites, adhesions, and misdirected injections, J. Surg. Res. **34:**581, 1983.
21. Gharagozloo, F., et al.: The use of intraperitoneal Xenon for early diagnosis of acute mesenteric ischemia, Surgery **95:**404, 1984.
22. Gluecklich, B., et al.: Chronic mesenteric ischemia masquerading as cancer, Surg. Gynecol. Obstet. **148:**49, 1979.
23. Granger, D.N., and Kvietys, P.R.: The splanchnic circulation: intrinsic regulation, Ann. Review Physiol. **43:**409, 1981.
24. Granger, D.N., et al.: Intestinal blood flow, Gastroenterology **78:**837, 1980.
25. Harjola, P.T.: A rate obstruction of the celiac axis, Acta Chir. Gynecol. Fenn. **52:**547, 1963.
26. Hildebrand, H.D., and Zierler, R.E.: Mesenteric vascular disease, Am. J. Surg. **139:**188, 1980.
27. Jacboson, E.D., Gallavan, R.H., and Fondacarro, J.D.: A model of the mesenteric circulation, Am. J. Physiol. **242:**G541, 1982.
28. Johnson, P.C.: Myogenic nature of increase in intestinal vascular resistance with venous pressure elevation, Circ. Res. **6:**992, 1959.
29. Johnson, W.C., and Nasbeth, D.C.: Visceral infarction following aortic surgery, Ann. Surg. **180:**312, 1974.
30. Kaufman, S.L., Harrington, D.P., and Siegelman, S.S.: Superior mesenteric artery embolization: an angiographic emergency, Radiology **124:**625, 1979.
31. Khodadadi, J., et al.: Mesenteric venous thrombosis: the importance of a second look operation, Arch. Surg. **115:**315, 1980.
32. Kim, M.W., et al.: Ischemic colitis after aortic aneurysmectomy, Am. J. Surg. **145:**392, 1983.
33. Kountz, S.L., Taub, D.R., and Connolly, J.E.: Aortoiliac steal syndrome, Arch. Surg. **92:**490, 1966.
34. Kwann, J.H.M., and Connolly, J.E.: Prevention of intestinal infarction resulting from mesenteric arterial occlusive disease, Surg. Gynecol. Obstet. **157:**321, 1983.
35. Lanciault, G., and Jacobson, E.D.: The gastrointestinal circulation, Gastroenterology **71:**851, 1976.
36. Levin, D.C., and Baltaxe, H.A.: High incidence of celiac axis narrowing in asymptomatic individuals, Am. J. Roentgenol. **46:**426, 1972.
37. Mann, A., Fazio, V.W., and Lucas, F.V.: A comparative study of the use of fluorescein and the Doppler device in the determination of intestinal viability, Surg. Gynecol. Obstet. **154:**53, 1982.

38. Marguggi, R.A., and Greenspan, M.: Reliable intraoperative prediction of intestinal viability using a fluorescent indicator, Surg. Gynecol. Obstet. **152:**33, 1981.
39. Mikkelson, W.P.: Intestinal angina: its surgical significance, Am. J. Surg. **94:**262, 1957.
40. Naitove, A., and Weissmann, R.: Primary mesenteric venous thrombosis, Ann. Surg. **161:**516, 1965.
41. Norris, C.P., et al.: Autoregulation of superior mesenteric flow in fasted and fed dogs, Am. J. Physiol. **237:**H174, 1979.
42. O'Donnell, J.A., and Hobson, R.W., II: Operative confirmation of Doppler ultrasound in evaluation of mesenteric ischemia, Surgery **87:**109, 1980.
43. Ottinger, L.W.: The surgical management of acute occlusion of the superior mesenteric artery, Ann. Surg. **188:**721, 1978.
44. Pentlow, B.D., and Dent, R.G.: Acute vascular compression of the duodenum in anorexia nervosa, Br. J. Surg. **68:**665, 1981.
45. Perler, B.A., and Zuidema, G.D.: Mesenteric vascular occlusive disease. In Cameron, J.L., editor: Current surgical therapy 1984-1985, St. Louis, 1984, The C.V. Mosby Co.
46. Plate, G., Eklof, B., and Vang, J.: The celiac compression syndrome: myth or reality? Acta Chir. Scand. **147:**201, 1981.
47. Price, P., and Clark, C.G.: Wilkie's syndrome, J. Royal Coll. Surg. Edinb. **24:**280, 1979.
48. Rob, C.: Surgical diseases of the celiac and mesenteric arteries, Arch. Surg. **93:**21, 1966.
49. Rogers, D.M., et al.: Mesenteric vascular problems: a 26 year experience, Ann. Surg. **195:**554, 1982.
50. Russ, J.E., et al.: Surgical therapy of non-occlusive mesenteric infarction, Am. J. Surg. **134:**638, 1977.
51. Sack, J., and Aldret, J.S.: Primary mesenteric venous thrombosis, Surg. Gynecol. Obstet. **154:**205, 1982.
52. Sarr, M.G., Bulkley, G.B., and Zuidema, G.D.: Pre-operative recognition of intestinal strangulation obstruction, Am. J. Surg. **145:**176, 1983.
53. Shah, S.D., and Andersen, C.A.: Prediction of small bowel viability using Doppler ultrasound, Ann. Surg. **194:**97, 1981.
54. Siddharth, P., and Smith, N.L.: An anatomic basis to prevent ischemia of the colon during operations upon the aorta, Surg. Gynecol. Obstet. **153:**71, 1981.
55. Siva, W.E.: Intestinal vascular disease. In Cutler, B.S., et al., editors: Manual of clinical problems in surgery, Boston, 1984, Little, Brown & Co.
56. Stanley, J.C., and Fry, W.J.: Median arcuate ugament syndrome, Arch. Surg. **103:**252, 1971.
57. Stoney, R.J., and Meacham, P.W.: Chronic intestinal ischemia caused by visceral atherosclerosis. In Cameron, J.L., editor: Current surgical therapy, 1984-1985, St. Louis, 1984, The C.V. Mosby Co.
58. Trastek, V.F., et al.: Splenic artery aneurysms, Surgery **91:**694, 1982.
59. Warren, S., and Eberhard, T.P.: Mesenteric venous thrombosis, Surg. Gynecol. Obstet. **61:**102, 1935.
60. Wilkie, D.P.D.: Chronic duodenal ileus, Am. J. Med. Sci. **173:**643, 1927.
61. Williams, L.F.: Vascular insufficiency of the intestines, Gastroenterology **61:**757, 1971.
62. Yeo, C.J., Jaffe, B.M., and Zinner, M.J.: Local regulation of blood flow in the feline jejunum. A possible role for edoluminally released substance P, J. Clin. Invest. **70:**1329, 1982.
63. Zelenock, G.B., et al.: Splanchnic arterio-sclerotic disease and intestinal angina, Arch. Surg. **115:**497, 1980.
64. Zinner, M.J., Kasher, F., and Jaffe, B.M.: The hemodynamic effects of intravenous infusions of serotonin in conscious dogs, J. Surg. Res. **34:**171, 1983.

22 *Thomas A. Miller*

Inflammatory, Neoplastic, and Mechanical Disorders of the Intestine, Rectum, and Anus

In addition to the ischemic disorders and motility disturbances discussed in Chapters 20 and 21, respectively, that may affect the intestinal tract, the small bowel, colon, rectum, and anus are also sites of a wide variety of other disease processes. These can be categorized under the broad headings of inflammatory, neoplastic, and mechanical disorders. This chapter summarizes the more important surgical disorders under each of these categories, again emphasizing the underlying physiologic dysfunction associated with each of them and the means by which normal physiology is restored when surgery becomes necessary.

INFLAMMATORY DISORDERS

Appendicitis

The most common inflammatory disorder of the intestinal tract is appendicitis. This disease may occur in any age group, but is especially common in patients younger than 15 years of age. The basic underlying cause is obstruction of the appendix, usually secondary to a fecalith that becomes impacted within the appendiceal lumen; other causes include mucous plugs, tumors, or foreign bodies.

The clinical presentation of appendicitis is one of anorexia, nausea (and occasionally vomiting), and periumbilical pain that ultimately migrates to the right lower quadrant over a period 8 to 12 hours following onset of the disease. Constipation is also frequently present because of a reflex ileus; and, due to the inflammatory process within the appendiceal wall, fever and leukocytosis are common features. Physical findings suggestive of appendicitis include right lower quadrant tenderness, guarding, and rebound. The point of maximum tenderness is usually at McBurney's point, an anatomic location one third of the distance from the anterior superior iliac spine on a line connecting this site to the umbilicus. It should be emphasized, however, that many of the aforementioned clinical findings may be absent, indicating the need for a high index of suspicion in a patient with unexplained abdominal pain and tenderness, particularly in the region of the right lower quadrant. Further, in the elderly patient the response to appendicitis may be quite mild, with little evidence of any infectious process, even though disease within the appendix may be quite suppurative.

The major problem associated with appendicitis is the risk of appendiceal perforation secondary to the increased intraluminal pressure that develops from the obstructive process. Thus abdominal exploration should be performed in any patient with signs and symptoms suggestive of appendicitis. This procedure can be carried out through a right lower quadrant incision. The appendix is amputated at its base, and the appendiceal stump inverted into the cecum by the placement of a number of seromuscular sutures (Fig. 22-1). If perforation has already occurred and an actual abscess has not formed, the purulent debris secondary to perforation is aggressively evacuated from the right lower quadrant, and an appendectomy still performed.[27] Broad-spectrum antibiotics are indicated. For patients with an appendiceal abscess, the abscess should generally be drained first, and an interval appendectomy

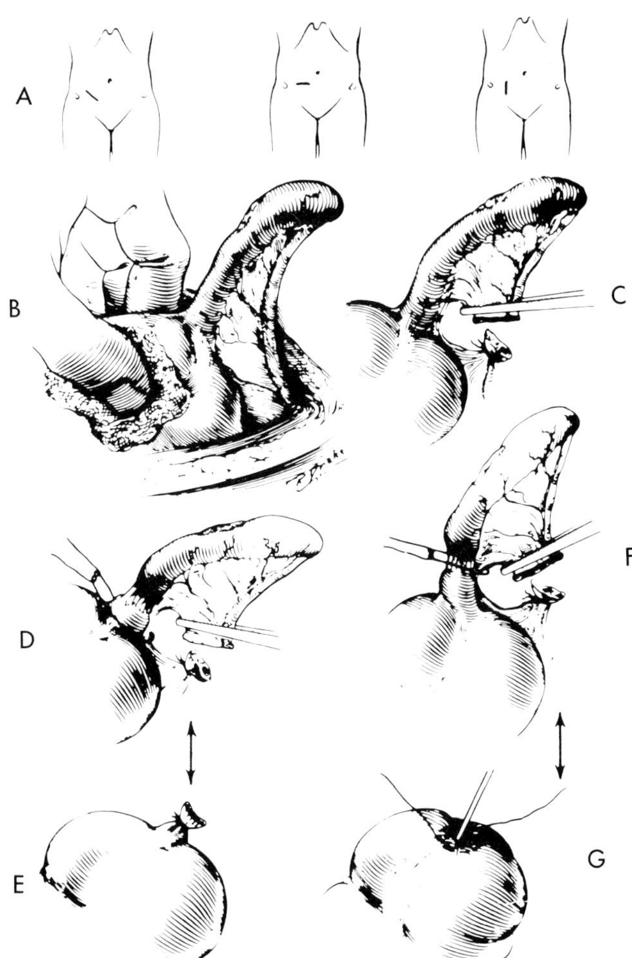

Fig. 22-1 Technique of appendectomy. **A,** Common incisions, oblique or transverse. **B,** Delivery of appendix. **C,** Ligation and division of mesoappendix. **D,** Ligation of base. **E,** Residual stump without inversion. **F,** Removal of appendix with ligation. **G,** Inversion of unligated stump. (From Sabiston, D.C., Jr., editor: Essentials of surgery, Philadelphia, 1987, W.B. Saunders Co.)

performed some weeks or months thereafter.[27] For a further discussion of the clinical presentation of appendicitis, see Chapter 32.

Meckel's Diverticulum

A Meckel's diverticulum represents a congenital remnant of the omphalomesenteric duct or yolk sac.[52] Anatomically, it appears as a blind diverticulum situated in the antimesenteric border of the ileum and includes all layers of the intestinal wall. In most patients it is located about 2 feet proximal to the ileocecal valve. Other interesting features of this congenital defect are its occurrence in 2% of the population, the presence of gastric mucosa in approximately 50% of patients, the fact that it becomes symptomatically apparent in the first two years of life in more than half the patients, and the observation that it is twice as frequent in males as females.

The inflammatory process associated with a Meckel's diverticulum is that of acute diverticulitis. Although uncommon because of the broad-based nature of most diverticula, if a narrow neck exists, obstruction may occur by the entrapment of food, scarring secondary to a healing ulcer within the gastric mucosa lining the diverticulum, torsion, external bands, or a nearby tumor. When diverticulitis occurs, its clinical presentation is not unlike that arising from acute appendicitis and includes such findings as right lower quadrant pain, anorexia, nausea and vomiting, abdominal tenderness, and fever and leukocytosis. If abdominal exploration to identify the cause of these symptoms fails to reveal an acute appendicitis, but demonstrates a Meckel's diverticulum, excision should generally be performed, particularly if the diverticulum possesses a narrow neck.[34]

Other complications of a Meckel's diverticulum include intestinal obstruction and hemorrhage. The obstruction may result from a volvulus around a persistent omphalomesenteric cord, entrapment of a loop of intestine behind the mesentery of the diverticulum, and intussusception of the diverticulum into the distal ileum. The clinical presentation secondary to all of these mechanisms is not unlike that arising from other causes of small bowel obstruction (see discussion later in chapter). Hemorrhage may occur secondary to the ectopic gastric mucosa and subsequent peptic ulceration. Usually this presents before the age of 2. Treatment is generally an emergency diverticulectomy, although bleeding can occasionally be controlled with an H_2-receptor blocking agent, permitting surgery to be performed under more elective circumstances.

Diverticular Disease of the Colon

In contrast to a Meckel's diverticulum, which is a congenital abnormality and involves all layers of the intestinal wall, diverticula of the colon are almost always acquired and represent protrusions of mucosa through the muscular wall, where in combination with the serosa of the bowel they form small sacs (Fig. 22-2). Because they do not involve all layers of the bowel wall, they are termed false diverticula. These diverticula are rarely seen in patients under 30 years of age. In contrast, as many as 50% of individuals over age 65 and 60% to 75% of those over 80 are affected.[1] Despite their commonality, colon diverticula

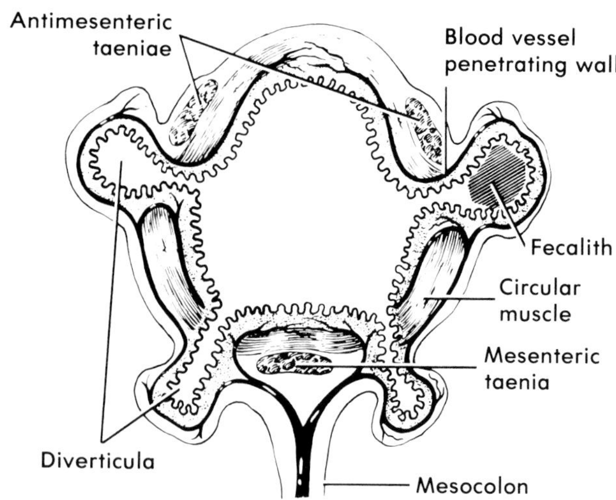

Fig. 22-2 Cross section of the colon depicting the sites where diverticula form. Note that the antimesenteric portion is spared. The longitudinal layer of muscle completely encircles the bowel and is not limited to the taeniae as depicted here. (From Way, L.W., editor: Current surgical diagnosis and treatment, ed. 7, Los Altos, Calif., 1985, Lange Medical Books.)

are frequently asymptomatic and discovered as incidental findings on barium contrast study of the large intestine. Whether symptomatic or not, diverticula may occur in any portion of the large bowel, but are most commonly seen in the sigmoid and descending colons.

Why colon diverticula develop has not been entirely agreed on by investigators studying their pathogenesis. Considerable evidence suggests that their development is related to localized areas of high intraluminal pressure that thereby allow herniation of colonic mucosa through weak spots in the colonic wall.[1,32] This theory is certainly consistent with the anatomic distribution of diverticula as outpouchings between the tenia at the point of entry of blood vessels within the circular musculature (see Fig. 22-2). It is also consistent with the sigmoid and descending colon distribution of diverticula where segmentation of the colonic musculature is most pronounced and development of localized areas of high intraluminal pressure commonly occur.[1,32] Of further interest is the observation that the irritable colon syndrome is frequently a precursor for the development of diverticulosis.[4] Patients with this abnormality have intermittent abdominal discomfort and altered bowel habits, presumably through excessive contraction of the colonic musculature. In a patient with unusually strong contractions, diverticula could easily develop over time.

Despite the convincing nature of these findings, many patients appear to have normal pressures within the sigmoid and no obvious abnormalities in motility patterns.[1,32] In fact, only 60% to 70% of resected colons containing diverticula have evidence of hypertrophied circular muscle (i.e., myochosis). These findings are consistent with the two types of diverticulosis that have been described. In the first type the diverticulosis is associated with a spastic colon characterized clinically by marked abdominal pain and altered bowel habits in which myochosis coli can be demonstrated and hypermotility patterns are present. The diverticula in this type are limited to the sigmoid or the

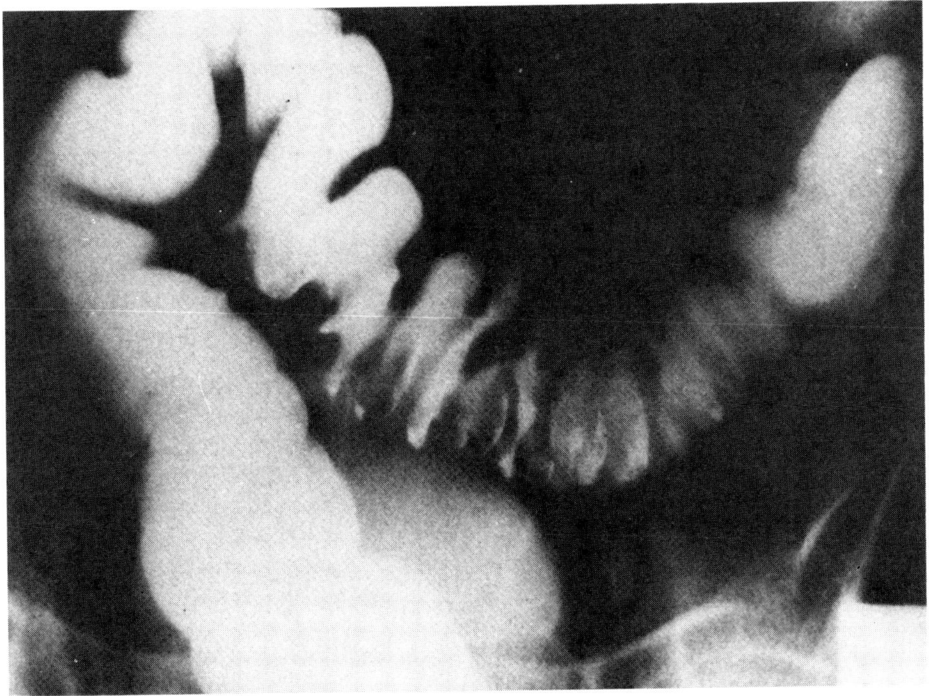

Fig. 22-3 X-ray film appearance typical of sawtoothed deformity. This was formerly considered pathognomonic of diverticulitis, but it may be the result of smooth muscle abnormality of diverticulosis. (From Hardy, J.D., editor: Rhoads textbook of surgery: principles and practice, ed. 5, Philadelphia, 1977, J.B. Lippincott Co.)

lower descending colon with the circular muscle heaped into thick spastic rolls, giving rise to the saw-toothed appearance seen on barium enema (Fig. 22-3). The second simple massed form of diverticulosis is present in individuals with relatively normal colonic muscle, no hypermotility patterns, the absence of any significant symptoms, and the distribution of diverticula throughout the colon. In contrast to the first form of diverticulosis in which a high intraluminal pressure appears to play a primary role, the diverticula in the second type probably develop in response to diffuse weaknesses throughout the colonic wall. This would explain the increased incidence of this disease in elderly patients and the lack of any associated symptoms.

From a surgical standpoint diverticular disease of the colon is important primarily because of the associated potential complications (Fig. 22-4). These include diverticulitis and lower gastrointestinal tract hemorrhage. With diverticulitis, an inflammation develops in the lining of the diverticula from entrapped fecaliths, which then may erode through the mucosa and allow infection to spread into the adjacent bowel wall. Depending on the magnitude of infection arising from this peridiverticulitis, the resultant abscess formation may be confined by adjacent structures or may enlarge and spread. Often antibiotic therapy will result in its resolution and the promotion of its drainage spontaneously into the lumen of the bowel. If the infection becomes more extensive, it may involve an adjacent viscus (such as the bladder) and form a fistula, rupture into the peritoneal cavity and produce generalized peritonitis, or result in a walled off abscess. Since most diverticula are limited to the sigmoid and left colon, the clinical presentation will be one of "left-sided appendicitis." Thus the

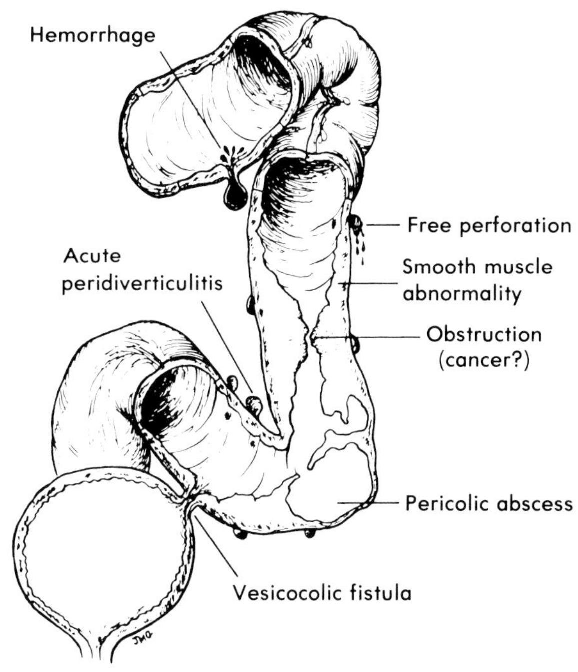

Fig. 22-4 Commonly occurring complications of diverticular disease. (From Hardy, J.D., editor: Rhoads textbook of surgery: principles and practice, ed. 5, Philadelphia, 1977, J.B. Lippincott Co.)

patient will experience left lower quadrant pain, tenderness and muscle guarding on palpation, and an associated fever and leukocytosis. Occasionally a tender mass may be palpable, representing the pericolonic inflammation and abscess formation. More commonly, a vague, tender fullness is encountered in the left lower quadrant.

The diagnosis of diverticulitis is usually convincing enough on clinical grounds alone that no specific maneuvers are indicated to confirm its presence. Certainly, contrast radiologic studies should be deferred until the acute inflammatory process abates. In situations in which the diagnosis is in doubt, a computed tomography (CT) scan may be helpful in showing a colonic mass.

In most patients treatment will consist of bowel rest and systemic antibiotic coverage. In the absence of a more pronounced complication such as abscess or perforation, clinical improvement with this approach will generally occur with subsidence of the inflammation and associated induration. If a palpable tender mass persists and/or the patient becomes septic, the likelihood of an abscess and the need for surgical intervention becomes a more crucial consideration. Under this circumstance, it is usually necessary to perform a temporary diverting colostomy in combination with abscess drainage. In a subsequent operation the affected portion of the intestine is resected, and an end-to-end anastomosis is accomplished. The colestomy is usually also taken down at this time. Additional situations where surgery may be indicated include recurrent attacks of diverticulitis or specific complications such as fistula formation and intestinal obstruction.

The other major complication of colonic diverticular disease is hemorrhage. Although bleeding seldom presents a problem in diverticulitis, massive blood loss may occur from simple, uncomplicated diverticulosis. Often this bleeding comes from the right colon, even though diverticula may exist diffusely throughout the large bowel. The close relationship of intramural vessels to the diverticula probably creates a shearing effect that is responsible for the bleeding (see Fig. 22-2). In most instances conservative measures can successfully manage hemorrhage. Specifically, embolization of the bleeding site angiographically is often helpful. If recurrent bleeding becomes a problem, localized colonic resection of the affected area is usually indicated. These considerations are discussed further in the chapter on gastrointestinal bleeding.

Inflammatory Bowel Disease

Although the disorders just described represent true inflammatory processes involving various anatomic regions of the intestinal tract, the term "inflammatory bowel disease" has generally been reserved for two specific diseases involving the small bowel and/or colon, i.e., granulomatous enterocolitis and ulcerative colitis.

Granulomatous Enterocolitis (Crohn's Disease)

Crohn's disease (also called regional enteritis, regional ileitis, regional ileocolitis, and transmucosal colitis, depending on the region of bowel involved) is a chronic progressive inflammatory disorder of the alimentary tract. Although it may affect any part of the gastrointestinal tract, the distal ileum is most frequently involved. Collected published experience with this disease indicates that the small bowel alone is involved in approximately 20% to 30% of patients, the distal ileum and colon in about 40% to 50%, and the large bowel alone in 20% to 30%.[12,35] The cause of Crohn's disease has remained elusive. Infectious, allergic, environmental, psychologic, and autoimmune causes have all been considered, but no one cause has held up under careful scientific scrutiny. A genetic influence is also suggested because of a family history of this disease in as many as 20% of patients.[13] Overall, the incidence of new cases annually is approximately three to five cases per 100,000 population, with a prevalence of approximately 25 to 50 cases per 100,000 population. The disease generally first appears between the second and fourth decades of life; no sex distribution has been noted.

Pathologically the earliest lesion appears to be hyperplasia of lymphoid follicles and Peyer's patches with subsequent alteration of the overlying intestinal mucosa.[42] The mucosal lesions are characterized by hemorrhagic, shallow ulcers and the formation of knifelike clefts known as fissures. Frequently surrounding these fissures and serpiginous ulcers are areas of normal intact mucosa, resulting in a cobblestone appearance to the mucosal surface. As the disease progresses, a transmural involvement of the intestinal wall occurs, characterized first by edema and later by thickening that can often progress to stricture formation.[42] It is this transmural feature that histologically distinguishes Crohn's disease of the colon from the primarily mucosal involvement typical of ulcerative colitis (see discussion that follows). In addition to these transmural changes, the associated mesentery becomes edematous, and the surrounding lymph nodes are hypertrophied. Granulomas are seen in the bowel wall in as many as 70% of patients and in the mesenteric nodes in as many as 25% to 30%. It is not infrequent for there to be discontinuous areas of disease within an intestinal segment such that normal bowel *(skip lesions)* exists between abnormal segments.

Depending on the amount of intestine involved, its regional distribution, the progression of the disease, and its duration, a patient with Crohn's disease may be relatively asymptomatic or present with a whole host of potential clinical derangements. These include diarrhea, malabsorption, various nutritional abnormalities (e.g., iron deficiency anemia, vitamin B_{12} or folate deficiency, steatorrhea), mechanical bowel obstruction, and fistulas either between the intestine and the skin, or between various loops of intestine or other viscera such as the bladder. Clinically, these aberrations may be manifest as abdominal pain, anemia, unexplained weight loss, fever, lassitude, and diarrhea. Of these presentations, abdominal pain, diarrhea, and weight loss are the most common.[12,35]

Since Crohn's disease can mimic other intestinal disorders such as appendicitis, diverticulitis, and ulcerative colitis, diagnosis will generally require a barium contrast study of both the upper and lower intestinal tracts to look for characteristic radiologic findings.[12,35] These include a thickened bowel wall with the classic "string sign" of the terminal ileum, indicating fibrosis and stricture formation; and flattening and raggedness of the mucosa with puddling of barium secondary to the longitudinal ulcerations, which as they deepen give rise to the cobblestone appearance. Evidence of fistula formation, abscess, and skip lesions are other diagnostic features of potential importance. In patients in whom the colon is involved, colonoscopic evaluation reveals the cobblestone appearance, with the demonstration of irregular ulcerations separated by normal-appearing mucosa. In contrast to ulcerative colitis, the rectum may be normal in as many as 50% to 60% of patients with this disease.[57] Not uncommonly the perianal skin may have a violaceous hue and demonstrate one or more fistulae.

The clinical course of Crohn's disease is one of remissions and relapses. Although there is no drug that has been demonstrated to cure Crohn's disease, a number of agents have been used to lessen acute flare-ups of the disorder and induce or prolong remission. Both prednisone and sulfasalazine have proven to be effective in controlling acute exacerbations of the disease.[23,24] Various immunosuppressive drugs such as azathioprine and mercaptopurine have been used alone and in combination with steroids to induce or prolong remission with reasonable success.[11,23,51] In addition to these drug approaches to treatment, a low-residue, milk-free, high-protein diet is generally recommended to provide adequate nutrition and minimize excessive stimulation of the bowel. In more nutritionally depleted patients, supplementation with either enteral or parenteral nutrition strategies may be necessary. Certainly if an operation is anticipated, nutrition should be optimized to the best state possible; in this regard, parenteral nutrition for 5 to 10 days before surgery may significantly reduce potential complications. If obvious vitamin deficiencies are present, these should be corrected with appropriate supplements. Finally, physical rest and alleviation of stress and/or family conflicts are also important components of therapy.

The role of surgery in the management of Crohn's disease is primarily limited to the development of complications. These include the drainage of abscesses (generally rare), alleviation of intestinal obstruction, resection of strictured areas of intestine, hemorrhage, and resection of fistulas that do not close with medical therapy. Occasionally a blind loop syndrome may develop in which intestinal resection is necessary for effective treatment. If radiologic findings are suspicious for neoplasia or dysplastic changes are noted on colonoscopic biopsy, resection of the involved segment of intestine may be indicated to prevent the subsequent development of cancer or assure its absence, an increased incidence of which has been demonstrated in this disease.[50] Finally, toxic megacolon may develop in patients with colonic Crohn's disease. This entity is characterized by acute, severe attacks of colitis, massive dilation of the colon, fever, leukocytosis, tachycardia, and hypoalbuminemia.[14] Not infrequently, severe electrolyte imbalance, anemia, shock, and a toxic psychosis may also be present, as well as signs of peritonitis. If peritonitis is absent, aggressive supportive therapy to include bowel rest, blood transfusions, fluid and electrolyte therapy to correct deficiencies in acid/base balance, adrenocorticotropic hormone (ACTH) treatment, and broad-spectrum antibiotics may prove helpful in treating this disorder. If response is not immediate and/or evidence of peritonitis is present, a total colectomy is usually considered the treatment of choice.[14]

Ulcerative Colitis

Ulcerative colitis is characterized pathologically by multiple ulcerations diffusely involving the colonic mucosa. Varying degrees of inflammation accompany these ulcers. As the disease becomes more pronounced, abscesses form in the intestinal crypts and glands and penetrate into the submucosa and muscularis.[42] These submucosal abscesses frequently spread in a horizontal direction, causing the overlying mucosa to slough. In regions where ulcers are present in the colonic mucosa, their margins are raised as mucosal tags. Such projections into the lumen give the impression of polyps, hence the term pseudopolyposis for the mucosal abnormalities seen in ulcerative colitis.[42] As the disease becomes more progressive and chronic, the resultant inflammatory changes give rise to fibrosis with eventual shortening and rigidity of the colon, even though its mesentery remains thin.

Although the cause of ulcerative colitis remains unknown, both psychic and environmental factors have been thought to play a role.[2,11] In many patients some form of acute psychic trauma has often preceded the onset of the disease, suggesting that tension and stress are somehow involved with its cause, although proof for this notion remains to be established. The other major hypothesis is that a patient becomes sensitized to various external agents such as microbes, viruses, or dietary factors that set into motion an immunologic response that precipitates an inflammatory reaction in the bowel wall. That a genetic predisposition may be involved is supported by the observation that as many as 20% to 40% of patients have a family history of ulcerative colitis and/or Crohn's disease, suggesting that the two diseases may be variants of a single disorder.[13] It is of interest that the disease manifests itself in two different age groups. The more prominent period of onset is between the ages of 15 and 30, with the second peak occurring in the sixth to eighth decades of life.[2,11] In most published series females are affected somewhat more commonly than males, with an incidence of 1.5:1.

Clinically ulcerative colitis commonly presents with crampy abdominal pain associated with diarrhea, rectal bleeding, and occasionally weight loss and tenesmus. Early in the onset of the disease diarrhea and bleeding may be minimal; but, as the disorder becomes more pronounced, patients may defecate as many as 20 times a day, losing considerable amounts of fluid and, not infrequently, blood. Therefore it is not unusual for these patients to be emaciated, anemic, and dehydrated.

In almost all patients with ulcerative colitis, the rectum is involved. The disorder then spreads proximally to affect the left colon, and, in as many as 30% to 40% of patients, the entire colon may be involved, in which case it is called pancolitis.[2,11] In approximately 40% to 50% of patients only the rectum is involved, where it is termed ulcerative proctitis. Because of the frequency of the disease in the rectum, diagnosis can usually be established by sigmoidoscopy. This examination will reveal the characteristic ulcers and will demonstrate the hyperemic, edematous, and friable mucosa so typical of this disease. In addition, oozing of blood, pus, and mucus are frequently seen on the mucosal surface. In questionable cases biopsy will generally confirm the diagnosis. Once the existence of ulcerative colitis is confirmed on sigmoidoscopy, the extent of colonic involvement is usually ascertained with a barium enema.

As with Crohn's disease, the initial treatment of ulcerative colitis is nonoperative.[23,24,51] In addition to measures

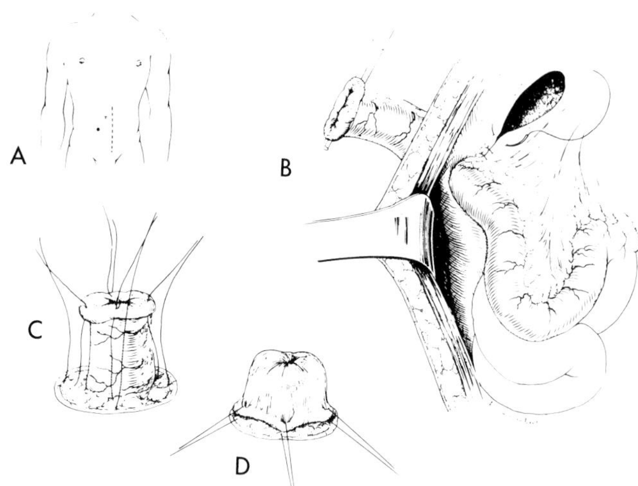

Fig. 22-5 Ileostomy after colectomy. **A,** Abdominal incision for colectomy is indicated by dotted line, and site of ileostomy by black dot. (A midline incision is favored by many surgeons instead of the left paramedian incision shown.) **B,** The ileum has been brought through the abdominal wall. **C** and **D,** The ileostomy stoma has been everted, and its margins sutured to the edges of the wound. (From Way, L.W., editor: Current surgical diagnosis and treatment, ed. 7, Los Altos, Calif., 1985, Lange Medical Books.)

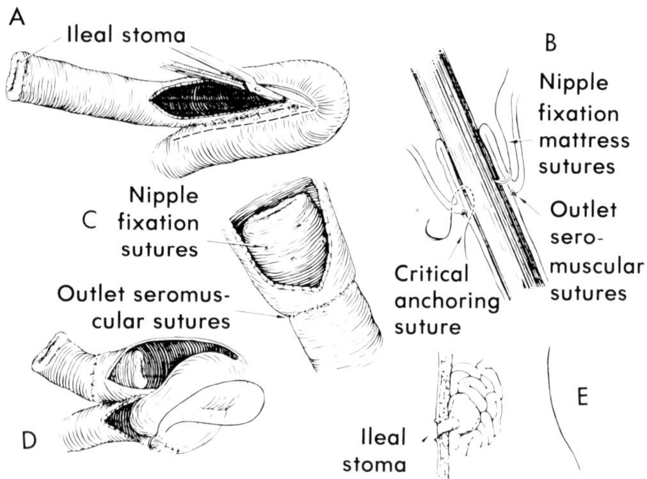

Fig. 22-6 Continent ileostomy. **A,** Formation of U limb. **B,** Placement of fixation sutures with temporary tube in place; **C,** Open view of nipple formation. **D,** Closure of reservoir. **E,** Sagittal view with ileostomy in place. (From Nora, P.F.: Operative surgery: principals and techniques, Philadelphia, 1980, Lea & Febiger.)

to support nutritional balance and correct dehydration, rest, sedation, and various antidiarrheal agents such as paregoric or diphenoxylate hydrochloride and atropine (Lomotil) are used to manage the diarrhea. Corticosteroids, ACTH, and sulfasalazine (Azulfidine) in various combinations have been used in the medical management of most patients, providing good-to-excellent palliation.

Surgical management is reserved for those patients with intractable disease or complications such as bleeding, perforation, and the development of toxic megacolon. This latter condition (which was discussed under the section on Crohn's disease) is a particularly ominous problem and results from the acute colonic dilation and necrosis of the bowel.[14] The treatment of choice for all of these complications is usually total proctocolectomy.[15] Depending on the medical status of a given patient, this operation may be performed in one or two stages. At the time of surgery, a permanent ileostomy is fashioned that is fully compatible with a normal life. This may be performed in the standard Brooke fashion (Fig. 22-5) or by constructing the continent ileostomy popularized by Kock (Fig. 22-6). This latter operation is especially attractive because it does not require the need for an ileostomy bag and can be drained two or three times a day. However, the performance of this procedure will require the skills of an experienced surgeon knowledgeable in the surgical technique. If such expertise is not available, the complication rate following this procedure is quite high.[33]

An alternative surgical approach in the treatment of ulcerative colitis is the ileoanal pull-through procedure. In this operation the entire abdominal colon is resected, the rectal mucosa is removed, and the terminal ileum is anastomosed to the anus. This procedure allows maintenance of good rectal function and therefore the absence of any need for an ileostomy and the assurance that the cancer-prone mucosa has been adequately removed. Experience with this approach to date has been most gratifying and has also proven useful in managing patients with Crohn's disease requiring proctocolectomy.[16]

A particular problem in patients with ulcerative colitis is the high incidence of colon cancer with long-standing disease.[25,45] Because of the aggressive nature of this neoplasm and its poor prognosis in this setting, early diagnosis is absolutely crucial. This can generally be assured only with colonoscopy and biopsy, since the accuracy of diagnosis with barium enema approaches only 50% as a result of the loss of radiologic mucosal signs suggestive of colon cancer because of the underlying colitic process. Patients at risk for carcinoma are those who have had ulcerative colitis in excess of 10 years. At this time in the disease process, there is a fourfold increase in the chance of developing cancer, with this incidence rising 2% per year thereafter. It is for this reason that patients with long-standing disease need to be carefully followed and at least undergo an annual colonoscopy with multiple biopsies in search of precancerous changes. It is now known that epithelial dysplasia is associated with the chance of finding cancer in the colon in as many as 50% of cases.[45] If such findings are demonstrated microscopically, further surveillance is unwarranted, and a proctocolectomy or ileoanal pull-through procedure should be performed.

NEOPLASTIC DISORDERS

Small Intestine

Compared to tumors arising in other portions of the gastrointestinal tract such as the stomach, colon, and rectum, neoplastic disease involving the small intestine is distinctly uncommon. Overall, small bowel tumors comprise about 1.5% of all gastrointestinal neoplasms, with roughly half of them being malignant.[37] Why the small intestine is generally spared from tumorogenicity when compared to other portions of the gastrointestinal tract remains unknown. A proposed mechanism is the abundant lymphoid tissue within the small bowel that could play an intrinsic protective role in preventing neoplastic formation.[37] For equally unexplained reasons, tumors arising in the small bowel are generally found in the duodenum, upper jejunum, and terminal ileum, with relative sparing of the distal jejunum and proximal ileum.

Types of Tumors

Benign Tumors. Virtually any type of tumor can develop in the small intestine, but epithelial tumors such as adenomas and papillomas and connective tissue tumors such as fibromas and leiomyomas are clearly the most commonly encountered. Although they may occur in any age group, the peak incidence for benign tumors is generally in the fourth decade of life. Of these tumors, 50% occur in the ileum, 30% in the jejunum, and approximately 20% in the duodenum.[37] An interesting subset of benign tumors that arise in the small intestine are those represented by hamartomatous polyps of the gastrointestinal tract. These hamartomas may be solitary or multiple. In the latter circumstance, they may be associated with the hereditary familial disease known as Peutz-Jeghers syndrome which is characterized by diffuse gastrointestinal polyposis and mucocutaneous pigmentation.[37] The hyperpigmentation is a result of melanin deposition and is most commonly observed on the lips, buccal mucosa, and nasomucosal membranes. The hamartomas associated with this syndrome are almost always benign and only rarely develop malignant alterations.

Malignant Tumors. Malignant tumors of the small bowel comprise four major groups and include carcinomas, carcinoid tumors, malignant lymphomas, and sarcomas. Of these, the adenocarcinoma is clearly the most common, the incidence ranging from 30% to almost 50% in most collected series.[37] The peak incidence of small bowel malignancies occurs between the fifth and sixth decades, with the exception of primary lymphomas, which tend to develop about 10 years earlier. As with benign tumors, the ileum is the favorite site for malignant growth in 50% or more cases. In addition to primary small bowel malignancies, a number of malignant tumors may directly metastasize to this organ. These include primary tumors arising in the uterine cervix, cutaneous melanomas, and primary neoplasia involving other portions of the gastrointestinal tract and kidney.

An especially unique malignancy that may develop in the small intestine is the carcinoid tumor. Although originally thought to be primarily benign, it is now fully recognized that carcinoid tumors do indeed have a true potential for biologic malignancy.[60] The appendix is the most common site of origin of carcinoid tumors, with a small intestinal location ranking second. When they occur in the small bowel, they are usually found within 2 or 3 feet of the ileocecal valve as hard, white nodules arising in the deep aspect of the mucosa. In contrast to appendiceal carcinoids, in which metastases are uncommon, as many as 35% to 40% of ileal carcinoids will have spread to regional nodes when first identified at surgery. The likelihood of metastases is related to their size, with tumors larger than 2 cm in diameter having metastasized in 80% to 90% of cases.[60]

Two other features of carcinoid tumors that merit consideration include their association with other malignancies and the carcinoid syndrome. Since carcinoid tumors arise from enterochromaffin cells throughout the gut, they are members of the amine precursor uptake and decarboxylase (APUD) family, as discussed in other portions of this book. Thus it is not surprising that they are associated with neoplasms involving other enterochromaffin tissues, including medullary carcinoma of the thyroid and pheochromocytoma. This coexistence of a second neoplasm has been noted in as many as 30% to 53% of patients with carcinoid tumors.[9,41]

Not uncommonly, the first indication that a carcinoid tumor is present may be the development of the carcinoid syndrome. This syndrome is characterized by episodic manifestations of cutaneous flushing, asthma, intestinal hyperperistalsis and diarrhea, and a variety of hemodynamic alterations that may result in vasomotor collapse. This constellation of symptoms occurs virtually only in the presence of metastases, especially those involving massive liver implants. The exact biochemical events responsible for this syndrome remain to be fully clarified, but an abnormality in serotonin metabolism has been clearly implicated.[60] Under normal conditions, approximately 1% of dietary tryptophan, the immediate precursor of serotonin, is metabolized to produce this substance. In contrast, as much as 50% to 60% of tryptophan may be diverted into the serotonin pathway with the presence of a functioning carcinoid tumor. Usually, any excess in serotonin production is broken down in the liver to 5-hydroxy-indoleacetic acid, which is then excreted in the urine. However, in patients with metastatic carcinoid tumor implants, this breakdown is impaired, with the subsequent release of serotonin into the systemic circulation. It is this enhanced release of serotonin and perhaps other unidentified substances that gives rise to the carcinoid syndrome. Since available liver parenchyma, even in the presence of metastatic implants, attempts to catalyze as much serotonin as possible, even though this event is not completely successful, levels of 5-hydroxy-indoleacetic acid in the urine are greatly increased. This urinary measurement provides the chemical basis for the diagnosis of a functioning carcinoid tumor.

Clinical Presentation

Because there are no specific symptoms or signs suggestive of a small bowel neoplasm, diagnosis will depend on a high index of suspicion when other more common causes have been excluded. Abdominal pain is usually the presenting symptom and is the initial complaint in as many as 50% of patients.[37] Because it is vague and nonspecific initially, the diagnosis of a possible underlying small bowel neoplasm is usually not considered. As the tumor enlarges, the pain is frequently aggravated by eating. Other common complaints include nausea and vomiting, a feeling of weakness, anorexia, and weight loss. Depending on the location of the tumor and its size, intestinal obstruction may result, often secondary to intussusception. An unexplained anemia may also be noted secondary to chronic blood loss from the tumor. Less frequently, a major gastrointestinal hemorrhage may supervene. Jaundice is rare with small bowel tumors except for those arising in the periampullary region of the duodenum. If a tumor has been present for a considerable period of time, particularly if it is a malignancy, the first evidence of its existence may be a palpable abdominal mass. This may be related to the tumor itself or represent dilated small bowel loops or intussusception secondary to obstruction. On rare occasions, a perforation may occur, giving rise to peritonitis. With tumors involving lymphoid tissue (an example being a malignant lymphoma), the primary symptoms may be intermittent fever and chills.

In a patient suspected of having a small bowel tumor, radiologic evaluation can be quite helpful.[31] A plain x-ray film of the abdomen, for example, may reveal the classic features of small bowel obstruction (see later discussion). If other factors have been excluded as potential causes for this obstruction, the possibility of a small bowel tumor should be entertained. Often, radiologic contrast studies will assist in confirming the diagnosis not only by establishing the point of obstruction, but not infrequently by identifying mucosal abnormalities in the region in question, which may make the diagnosis of a small bowel tumor more likely. In addition, the demonstration of intussusception would make this diagnosis more likely.

If obstructive symptoms are absent, but the presenting complaints are suggestive of a small bowel neoplasm, barium contrast studies may also be of value in this circumstance. Abnormalities in the mucosal pattern, evidence of space-occupying defects that appear to be pushing the bowel aside, and fixation of loops of small bowel and protruding masses in the intestinal lumen are all important clues that a small bowel neoplasm may indeed be present. For suspected lesions in the region of the duodenum, a variation of the standard small bowel study, called *hypotonic duodenography*, may be helpful.[31] This procedure uses the relaxing effects of glucagon on small bowel musculature to render the duodenum flaccid and relatively immobile so that a more accurate delineation of possible mucosal abnormalities can be obtained. Fiberoptic endoscopy may also prove helpful in the diagnosis of proximal small bowel lesions through direct visualization of the mucosa.

The role of angiography in the diagnosis of small bowel tumors remains to be established. Certainly if a tumor is bleeding at the time of investigation, angiography may be quite helpful. With certain connective tissue tumors such as angiomas, the blood supply may be increased relative to adjacent areas of intestine. This increase in vascularity may be observed as an increase in the opacification of the tumor during the venous phase, referred to as the *tumor blush* or *stain*. If the tumor is especially large, distortions in the normal arterial architecture of the bowel and adjacent blood vessels may create angulations and vascular contortions suggestive of an underlying neoplasm. The current availability of computed axial tomography may also be of value in the diagnosis of small bowel tumors, but its exact role remains to be defined.

For the most part, routine laboratory testing is of little value in the diagnosis of small bowel neoplasia. The detection of a hypochromic, microcytic anemia indicates the need for a systematic evaluation of possible sources of blood loss. Assuming that common causes have been excluded, the possibility of a small bowel tumor needs to be entertained. Similarly, stools with occult blood require a thorough evaluation for the underlying source. If clinical signs and symptoms suggest the possibility of the carcinoid syndrome, urinary 5-hydroxy-indoleacetic acid levels should be checked.

Management

Whether benign or malignant, the treatment of a small bowel neoplasm should be surgical excision, unless the lesion can be successfully removed through a fiberoptic duodenoscope as may occur with more proximal lesions. Generally, a segmental resection of the involved bowel with adjacent mesentery to include as many lymph nodes as are grossly identifiable should be performed. For obviously malignant or potentially malignant lesions, the margin on either side of the tumor should be generous (usually 20 cm of intestine on either side of the neoplasm).[37] Intestinal continuity is then reestablished by an end-to-end anastomosis. Even if the tumor is almost certainly benign, a limited intestinal resection should be carried out to prevent the risk of subsequent complications such as bowel obstruction and hemorrhage and to ensure the diagnosis of benignancy, which can be made with certainty only by microscopic examination of the resected tumor. In those situations in which there is evidence of widespread metastases, palliative bypass procedures are generally used to manage the obstruction or potential obstruction that may ultimately supervene. In lesions involving the periampullary region, a radical pancreaticoduodenectomy (Whipple operation) may be indicated if a cure seems possible.

Although various chemotherapeutic approaches have been used in combination with surgery to treat small bowel neoplasia, the role of chemotherapy remains to be defined for most types of small bowel malignancies.[37] The major exception is the carcinoid tumor of the small intestine in which streptozocin, either alone or in combination with other chemotherapeutic agents, appears to be of value in controlling patients with metastatic carcinoid tumors and the carcinoid syndrome.[38-40] In addition, serotonin antagonists have been of value in attempting to control many of the symptoms referable to this syndrome. Radiation therapy may have some beneficial effects in treating sarcomas, but has not been shown to be efficacious in the management of adenocarcinomas or carcinoid tumors.[37] In contrast, lymphomas of the small bowel have generally been quite responsive to radiation therapy.[37]

Large Bowel and Rectum

Of neoplastic disorders involving the large bowel and rectum, polyps and adenocarcinoma are clearly the most common and potentially life-threatening tumors arising in this region of the intestinal tract. Carcinoma of the colorectum is second only to lung cancer in men and breast cancer in women in terms of its incidence in the United States. During the next year, as many as 140,000 to 150,000 new people will develop carcinoma of the colorectum. Another 50,000 to 60,000 people will die of sequelae resulting from this disease. The importance of polyps surgically resides in the fact that they may harbor an underlying malignancy.

Polyps

The term "polyp" is a morphologic designation and refers to a wide variety of masses of tissue that project into the lumen of the colon and/or rectum with differing histologic characteristics. Polyps may be sessile or pedunculated, and as many as 70% of them develop in the region of the rectosigmoid. A detailed discussion of the various types of polyps is beyond the scope of this chapter. The more important types clinically include the adenomatous polyp, the villous polyp, and the juvenile polyp.

Adenomatous polyps are clearly the most commonly encountered neoplasms of the colon and rectum.[22] They are usually pedunculated, are more likely to be found in patients over 40, usually arise in the rectosigmoid region, and are often asymptomatic. The first clinical manifestation of their presence is often rectal bleeding. Polyps less than 1 cm in size are almost always benign, whereas those in excess of 2 cm are associated with a malignant potential approaching 20%.[22,43] Except for the smallest of lesions, most polyps should be removed. This can usually be accomplished through a sigmoidoscope (or a colonoscope for more proximal lesions), especially if the polyp is pedunculated. For more sessile polyps, complete surgical excision is usually indicated. This can be accomplished through a transanal approach if the lesion is in the rectum. For more proximal lesions a formal laparotomy is usually indicated, and the polyp is removed through an incision in the intestinal wall.

Villous polyps (also called adenomas) are velvety, broad-based tumors that are easily identified by their frond-like projections.[49] More than 80% of these polyps reside in the rectum and are rarely seen below the age of 40. Because of the large size of these tumors (often over 2.5 cm) and the reported incidence of associated malignancy approaching 30%,[49,58] the possibility of cancer must always be suspect with these lesions. Like adenomatous polyps, they are frequently asymptomatic and are first diagnosed when a patient is being evaluated for rectal bleeding. Occasionally these tumors are associated with excessive mucous production and diarrhea that give rise to severe fluid and electrolyte (particularly potassium) losses. Because of this problem and the high malignant potential of these lesions, complete excision is the treatment of choice. This can generally be accomplished through a transanal approach, unless the adenoma is more proximally located, in which case a formal laparotomy and resection is indicated. Because of the broad base of these tumors, endoscopic removal is rarely possible. If invasive cancer is noted histologically, a more radical operation will be required (e.g., an abdominoperineal resection for a rectal lesion).[49,58]

Juvenile polyps are really hamartomas rather than true neoplasms and occur predominantly in children under 12 years of age. Because of their hamartomatous nature, malignancy is not a problem. Clinically, they are usually first recognized because of an unexplained rectal bleeding. These polyps are nearly always pedunculated and thus lend themselves to easy removal through an endoscope. Interestingly, many of these polyps autoamputate or spontaneously disappear.

A number of interesting syndromes involve colorectal polyps. Among these is the entity known as *familial polyposis coli*.[8] This disease is a rare, inheritable trait that can be transmitted by either parent and is characterized by literally hundreds, sometimes thousands, of polyps that are distributed throughout the entire colon and rectum. These polyps are adenomatous histologically and can vary greatly in size and configuration. The disease becomes clinically apparent between the ages of 20 and 40 and is usually manifest by rectal bleeding and/or diarrhea. These polyps have a high propensity for malignant degeneration, and, if the disease is left untreated, colonic cancer will develop in 100% of cases. It is for this reason that total proctocolectomy with a permanent ileostomy is recommended as the treatment of choice to eliminate the risk of cancer.[8] Some authorities argue that this approach is too radical and that an abdominal colectomy, with anastomosis of the ileum to the proximal rectum to preserve normal rectal function, is an acceptable alternative. This approach, however, requires careful cancer surveillance with regular sigmoidoscopic examinations every 3 months to ensure the detection and destruction of any polyps that may develop. It has met with varying long-term success, with cancer developing in the rectum in as many as one third of patients followed over a period of 20 years.[56] A more recent alternative approach is the ileoanal pull-through procedure[3] discussed in the section on ulcerative colitis.

Another syndrome that is probably a variant of familial polyposis is *Gardner's syndrome*.[18] This entity is characterized by diffuse colorectal polyposis, but patients afflicted with it also have osteomas involving the mandibular skull, desmoid tumors, and multiple sebaceous cysts. Other features of this syndrome include an increased incidence of periampullary cancer and polyps throughout the small intestine. Because the colorectal polyps in Gardner's syndrome carry the same risk for the development of cancer as occurs in familial polyposis, the principles underlying treatment are basically the same.

In contrast to familial polyposis and Gardner's syndrome, the colonic polyps seen in the Peutz-Jeghers syndrome (see section on small bowel neoplasia for further discussion) are at minimal risk for the development of a malignancy, since these polyps are basically hamartomas. For this reason, removal is generally reserved for those that are symptomatic.

Colorectal Cancer

Cancer of the colon can involve any region of the colorectum.[47] Of these lesions, 70% arise distal to the splenic flexure, with 50% occurring in the rectosigmoid region. In most series rectal cancer is more commonly found in males, whereas colonic cancer is more common in females. Regardless of sex, the incidence clearly increases with age and rises sharply after the age of 45. For inapparent reasons, a progressive shift from the rectosigmoid region to the right colon has been noted over the last several decades. At the time of diagnosis, as many as 5% of patients may have two or more cancers occurring simultaneously, designated as *synchronous* lesions. In 2% to 3% of patients, a second primary lesion may develop in a patient who has undergone a previous resection procedure for colon cancer, in which case the new lesion is referred to as *metachronous* cancer. Histologically, 95% to 97% of colorectal cancers are adenocarcinomas.

The cause of colorectal cancer remains unknown. Since it is relatively common in highly industrialized regions of the world such as North America, Western Europe, and Australia, in contrast to more poorly developed countries, various environmental factors, particularly diet, have been thought to be important causative factors.[59] Research to date is inconclusive in this regard, but the observation by Burkitt[7] that countries subsisting on high-fiber, low-sugar diets have a relatively low incidence of colon and rectal cancers suggests that dietary fiber may play a protective role by increasing fecal bulk and thereby diluting the opportunity for carcinogens in excretory material to come in contact with the bowel mucosa. As already discussed, a genetic predisposition is clearly involved in the development of colorectal cancer in some patients as attested by the high incidence of this problem in familial polyposis and Gardner's syndrome.[8,18] In addition, a cancer family syndrome has also been noted in which there appears to be an increased tendency to develop cancer of the large intestine and other sites that seems to be transmitted as an autosomal dominant trait.[29,48] Further, ulcerative colitis and granulomatous colitis, both diseases presumably transmitted through genetic influences, are also associated with an increased incidence of colorectal cancer.

Pathologic Features. Regardless of the site of origin, adenocarcinomas of the colorectum tend to grow circumferentially. Because of the larger luminal caliber in the right colon, these tumors may become quite bulky and fungating, with extensive projection into the bowel lumen. This is in contrast to the left colon where more complete circumferential involvement occurs. As the neoplasm continues to grow, it penetrates the deeper layers of the bowel wall and may actually extend by contiguity into neighboring structures. In addition to direct extension, colorectal cancer spreads hematogenously through colonic veins and through regional lymphatics. Additional routes of spread include transperitoneal seeding, in which the tumor has extended through the serosa of the bowel wall, allowing tumor cells to separate from the bowel itself and to be carried to distant sites throughout the peritoneal cavity. Such seeding is responsible for the generalized abdominal carcinomatosis that is occasionally observed, as well as spread to the rectovesicle and rectouterine pouches. This means of spread is also responsible for the "frozen pelvis" that occurs when extensive tumor implants are present in the pelvis. Finally, tumor cells may be shed from the surface of the cancer into the intestinal lumen and carried distally through the fecal current. How important this route of spread is remains to be determined.

DUKES' CLASSIFICATION OF COLORECTAL CANCER

Stage A	Limited to bowel wall
Stage B	Extension of cancer through the bowel wall into pericolic tissues, but without lymph node involvement
Stage C	Cancer involving not only the bowel wall, but also extending into regional nodes

The prognosis in colorectal cancer is directly related to the extent of spread at the time of diagnosis. Although a number of staging procedures have been proposed over the last several decades, the original Dukes' classification continues to have considerable merit.[10] This classification is summarized in the boxed material at left and is based on the extent of disease and its confinement to the bowel wall or pericolic tissues, and the absence or presence of involved nodes. Involvement of regional nodes decreases the likelihood of survival by approximately 50% when patients are evaluated 5 years after diagnosis. Distant spread beyond regional nodes generally represents incurability, and very few patients are alive beyond 1 year following diagnosis. Other modifications of the Dukes' classification are shown in Table 22-1.

Clinical Presentation. Colorectal cancer may present in virtually any fashion; but changes in one's bowel habits, anemia, blood in the stools, and colonic obstruction represent the usual clinical findings that bring a patient to medical attention. Anemia is much more common in right

Table 22-1 **OTHER MODIFICATIONS OF THE DUKES' CLASSIFICATION OF COLORECTAL CANCER***

Stage	Astler, Coller—1954	Gunderson, Sosin—1974
A	Tumor limited to mucosa	Tumor limited to mucosa
B_1	Tumor extension into muscularis propria, but not through it	Tumor extension through mucosa, but still within bowel wall
B_2	Tumor extension through muscularis propria, but without nodal involvement	Tumor extension through entire bowel wall, but without nodal unvolvement
B_3	—	Tumor adherent to or invading adjacent organs, but without nodal involvement
C_1	Tumor limited to bowel wall, but nodes nevertheless positive	Tumor limited to bowel wall, but nodes nevertheless positive
C_2	Tumor extension through entire bowel wall, nodes also positive	Tumor extension through entire bowel wall, nodes also positive
C_3	—	Tumor adherent to or invading adjacent organs, nodes also positive

Modified from Astler, V.B., and Coller, F.A.: Ann. Surg. **139:**846,1954; and Gunderson, L.L., and Sosin, H.: Cancer **34:**1278,1974.
*None of these classifications include Stage D. Convention, however, assigns patients to Stage D if they have distant metastases or locally unresectable tumor.

colon lesions than in those involving the rectum, sigmoid, and descending colons, principally because these tumors are large and bulky and are constantly exposed to the caustic contents within the fecal stream. In contrast, tumors involving the left colon tend to obstruct because of their angular, circumferential growth characteristics and the generally narrower lumen in this region of the intestine. Unless the tumor has been present for a considerable period of time, allowing it to reach a size in which a palpable mass is present, physical findings are often absent. If the tumor is present in the rectum, it is often palpable on rectal examination. In addition, many tumors, if not grossly bleeding, are associated with occult blood in the stool.

In any patient suspected of having a colorectal cancer, a proctosigmoidoscopy should be performed. This allows adequate visualization of the anorectal and distal sigmoid regions and the opportunity for biopsy of any suspicious lesion. If a more proximal tumor is suspected, a barium contrast study of the colon is indicated. Lesions involving the left colon are usually noted as fixed filling defects and frequently demonstrate an angular configuration, known as the apple core effect (Fig. 22-7). Lesions involving more proximal portions of the colon, particularly the right colon, often demonstrate intraluminal masses. Once a barium contrast study has been performed, fiberoptic colonoscopy should be undertaken in any patient suspected or known to have cancer of the colon. This will allow opportunity for a biopsy of the lesion in question and histologic confirmation. In addition, the presence or absence of synchronous polyps or cancers can also be determined. Depending on the colonoscopic expertise available at an institution, some authorities feel that a barium enema is unnecessary and that, in any patient being evaluated for colorectal cancer, colonoscopy alone is a sufficient diagnostic maneuver.

Most routine laboratory tests are of little value in the workup of a patient with suspected colorectal cancer. Studies of particular value, however, include hemoglobin determination and tests to assess liver function. The hemoglobin indicates the presence or absence of anemia, a condition commonly seen with right colon cancers, and indicates the need for blood transfusion before definitive treatment. Liver function tests, if abnormal, are an index of possible hepatic metastases. When such abnormalities occur, radionuclide scans of the liver should be obtained to further delineate this possibility. Chest x-ray films are also a routine part in the workup of any patient with proven or suspected colon cancer and are not only of value in preparing the patient for surgery but also in excluding the possibility of pulmonary metastases.

A serum determination of carcinoembryonic antigen (CEA) is a useful tumor marker to follow patients with colorectal cancer.[62] This cell membrane glycoprotein is found in many tissues, including tissue involving malignancies of the colon and rectum. Although not specific for colorectal cancer, its elevation in serum correlates quite closely with the status of the disease. For example, an elevated CEA level (which occurs in 60% to 70% of patients with colorectal cancer) before surgery that fails to fall to normal levels after presumed curative resection implies a poor prognosis and the existence of residual disease. Conversely, a normal level before surgery that becomes elevated at some period following surgery or an elevated level before surgery that reverts to normal following surgery and then subsequently becomes elevated again suggests a high likelihood of recurrent cancer.

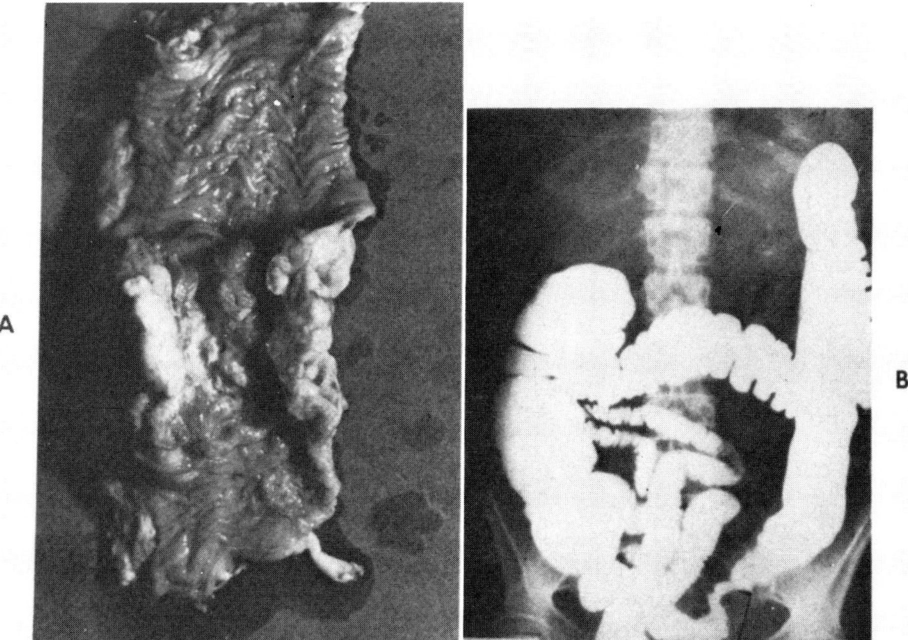

Fig. 22-7 **A,** Annular, constricting carcinoma of sigmoid colon. **B,** Barium enema outlining "apple core" defect of sigmoid carcinoma shown in **A.** (From Liechty, R.D., and Soper, R.T., editors: Synopsis of surgery, ed. 3, St. Louis, 1976, The C.V. Mosby Co.)

TREATMENT CONSIDERATIONS. Like other gastrointestinal cancers, the principal treatment of colorectal malignancies is surgical removal. Such treatment includes not only excision of the cancer itself with adequate margins on either side, but concomitant removal of areas of lymphatic spread and local extension. In the conduct of such a procedure, the venous drainage routes of the tumorous area are ligated early in the procedure, and ligatures encircling the bowel above and below the tumor are placed. These maneuvers help to minimize the dissemination of cancer cells during surgical manipulation of the malignancy.

Before surgery measures should be used to cleanse the bowel of its fecal contents and to decrease its bacterial content. In so doing, the incidence of postoperative infection is greatly diminished (e.g., wound infections, intraabdominal abscess). Maneuvers to accomplish these goals include the use of laxatives and enemas to mechanically cleanse the bowel, the institution of a clear liquid diet a day or two before surgery to decrease stool bulk, and the administration of preoperative antibiotics. Of these maneuvers, mechanical cleaning is clearly the most important.

The particular surgical procedure to be performed depends on the location of the neoplasm. For those malignancies involving the abdominal colon, resection of the tumor-bearing intestine in continuity with its lymphatic drainage routes is accomplished, following which intestinal continuity is reestablished either by a primary suture technique or by the use of one of the currently available staple guns. For lesions involving the rectum, the choice of surgical procedure depends on the height of the lesion above the anal verge. As long as a 2.5 cm margin of normal bowel can be resected below the tumor and not jeopardize the reestablishment of intestinal continuity, a low anterior resection of the rectum can be performed. This involves a primary resection of the proximal rectum and lymph node–bearing tissue through an abdominal incision. If such a margin cannot be obtained, an abdominoperineal resection of the rectum is undertaken. This is accomplished through a combined abdominal and perineal approach and includes resection of the distal sigmoid colon, the rectosigmoid, the rectum, and the anus. A permanent end sigmoid colostomy is then performed. These treatment considerations are summarized in Fig. 22-8.

Other approaches to rectal tumors have included various sphincter-preserving operations and fulguration. The two sphincter-saving procedures have included a posterior transacral approach and the pull-through operation. In the former, surgery is performed through a posterior approach, allowing resection of the tumor-bearing area and anastomosis of the proximal colon to the anus.[19,28] This procedure has been particularly useful in obese patients or in an individual with a narrow pelvis. In the pull-through procedure, an anorectal stump is everted, allowing anastomosis to be technically accomplished outside of the rectum itself. Unfortunately, bowel function following this procedure has not proven to be as good as originally thought.[19] In selected cases some rectal tumors have been treated by local fulguration with electrocautery. This procedure involves aggressive cauterization of the tumor, frequently in several sessions, under general anesthesia. It is primarily suited for lesions below the pelvic peritoneal reflection and is limited solely to removal of the rectal cancer rather than to removal of associated lymph node areas.[30] Its primary application has been in elderly, poor-risk patients who are believed not to be suitable candidates for more radical resective procedures.

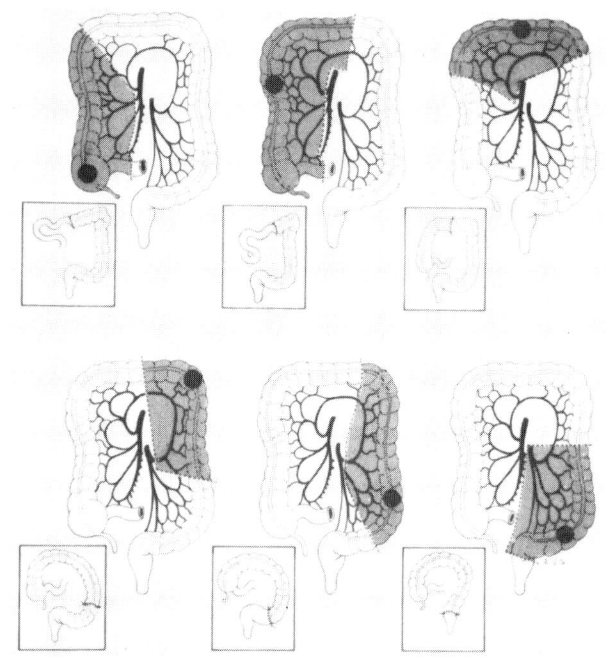

Fig. 22-8 Extent of surgical resection for cancer of the colon at various sites. The cancer is represented by a black disk. Anastomosis of the bowel remaining after resection is shown in the small insets. The extent of resection is determined by the distribution of the regional lymph nodes along the blood supply. The lymph nodes may contain metastatic cancer. (From Way, L.W., editor: Current surgical diagnosis and treatment, ed. 7, Los Altos, Calif., 1985, Lange Medical Books.)

If distal spread of colorectal cancer is encountered at the time of surgery, only a palliative procedure should be undertaken. This involves removal of the primary tumor to prevent subsequent complications such as bleeding and obstruction. Occasionally an isolated metastasis will be found in an organ such as the liver that may lend itself to resection. In the likelihood of that event, a more aggressive approach may be undertaken in which a standard curative resection of the primary colonic lesion is performed at the same time that hepatic resection of the metastasis is undertaken. This approach has demonstrated reasonably good results in selected patients.[61] However, more diffuse metastases in the liver obviate this approach, and only a palliative procedure should be undertaken in this circumstance.

It remains to be determined what role chemotherapy and immunotherapy will play in the treatment of colorectal cancer. Most studies to date evaluating these modalities have failed to demonstrate any significant benefit. In contrast, radiation therapy appears to be of potentially significant value in the management of rectal cancer. A number of approaches have been used, including intracavitary, external, and implantation radiation techniques that demonstrate an ability to shrink the tumor and kill cells in the regional lymphatics.[20,53] Such responses to radiotherapy have enabled subsequent surgical removal of lesions previously thought to be unresectable.

Prognosis. As with neoplastic disease in other organs, the prognosis of colorectal cancer will depend on a variety of factors, including the age of the patient at the time of diagnosis, the extent of the tumor, its location, the presence or absence of involved lymph nodes, and whether the disease arose in association with another disorder. Generally, the younger a patient is at the time of diagnosis, the more virulent the neoplasm. Cancers arising in association with diseases such as ulcerative colitis and familial polyposis are also generally more aggressive than those arising de novo. Rectal cancers do not fare as favorably as those arising in other parts of the colon, and cancers associated with intestinal obstruction usually have a more dismal prognosis than nonobstructive tumors. All other circumstances aside, the absence or presence of node involvement is clearly the most important determinant of outcome. For Dukes' A and B lesions, the 5-year survival rate approaches 80% and 60%, respectively. If lymph nodes are involved, this survival rate drops precipitously to approximately 30% to 35%. For more distant disease (e.g., lung, liver metastases), survival rates decrease to 5% or less.

Other Neoplastic Lesions of the Colon and Rectum

In addition to polyps and adenocarcinoma, a wide variety of other tumors have also been demonstrated to occur in the colon and rectum.[42,47] Most common among these other lesions are lymphomas, lipomas, and leiomyomas. Lymphomas are the most common noncarcinomatous malignant tumors, whereas lipomas and leiomyomas are the most frequently encountered benign lesions. Carcinoid tumors may also occur in the large bowel and rectum but are much less common than in other regions of the gastrointestinal tract.[60] Further, the carcinoid syndrome is extremely rare when carcinoids arise in this portion of the gastrointestinal tract.

MECHANICAL DISORDERS: OBSTRUCTIONS OF THE INTESTINE

Under normal circumstances food is propelled through the gastrointestinal tract without difficulty. Nutrients are absorbed at various places along the small intestinal mucosa, and those components of dietary intake of no metabolic or nutritional value are ultimately transported to the rectum, where they are excreted as waste materials. If the peristaltic activity of the intestine becomes ineffective or the caliber of the intestinal lumen becomes compromised by either an intrinsic or extrinsic process, intestinal obstruction is said to exist. Ineffective peristalsis has been referred to as adynamic ileus and is discussed in detail in Chapter 20. Obstruction caused by compromise of the size of the intestinal lumen is referred to as mechanical obstruction and forms the basis of this discussion.

Causes of Mechanical Obstruction

Obstruction of the intestinal lumen can occur anywhere throughout the small and large intestine but is clearly more common in the small bowel, with approximately 80% of all bowel obstructions involving this region of the intestinal tract. This obstruction can be secondary to intrinsic lesions within the intestinal lumen that compromise luminal size or secondary to extrinsic compression of the bowel wall. Depending on the degree of the lumen compromised, mechanical obstruction can be either partial or complete.

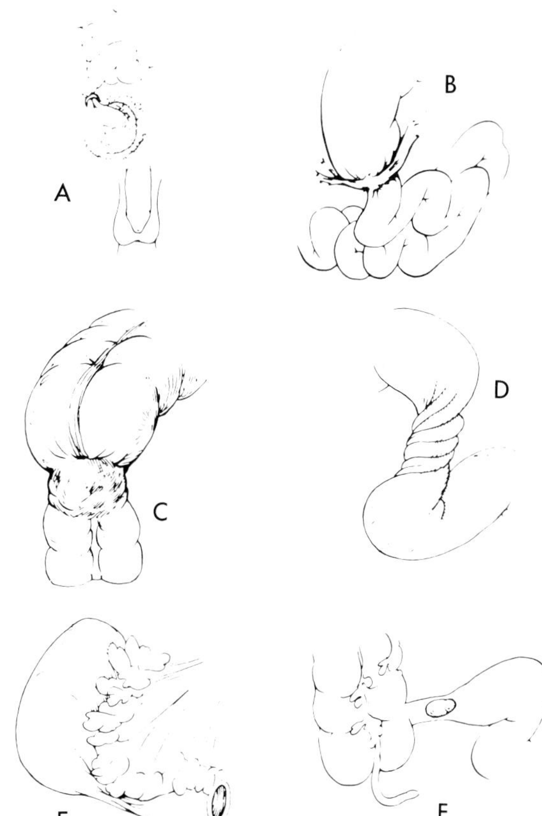

Fig. 22-9 Diagram of some representative causes of intestinal obstruction. **A,** Hernia. **B,** Adhesions. **C,** Tumor. **D,** Volvulus. **E,** Stricture. **F,** Foreign body. (From Polk, H.C., Jr., Stone, H.H., and Gardner, B., editors: Basic surgery, ed. 3, Norwalk, Conn., 1987, Appleton-Century-Crofts.

A wide variety of etiologic factors may be responsible for mechanical intestinal obstruction, but adhesions, hernias, and tumors are clearly the most common[26,55] (Fig. 22-9). In fact, hernias and adhesions together are responsible for about 65% to 70% of all bowel obstructions; the site of obstruction almost always involves the small bowel. Tumors account for an additional 15% to 20% and are more likely to be the cause when the obstruction occurs in the large bowel. Other less common causes of intestinal obstruction include volvulus; intussusception; various inflammatory lesions; and, less commonly still, obturation from materials within the gut lumen, including fecal impaction and gallstone ileus. In the pediatric population a number of congenital defects, discussed in further detail in Chapter 65, may be responsible for obstruction.

Adhesions

In a patient who has undergone a previous surgical procedure of the abdomen, adhesions are the most likely cause of the obstruction. Why adhesions develop continues to be the subject of considerable debate, but lower abdominal incisions appear to be more commonly associated with adhesive obstructions than those involving the upper abdomen. This circumstance probably relates to the shielding properties of the omentum in the upper abdomen that prevent adhesive bands from forming around the intestine. If these bands are pronounced enough, blood supply to the involved bowel may also be compromised, in which case the obstruction is said to be strangulating. On occasion, adhesions may form around a loop of intestine so that it is closed at both ends. When this occurs, the increasing pressure within this loop from intestinal secretions and gas may result in intestinal perforation if the obstructing band is not surgically released.

Hernias

Virtually any type of hernia can give rise to intestinal obstruction. The more common sites where this is likely to occur are the inguinal and umbilical regions. As with adhesions, a segment of intestine may become strangulated by its protrusion through the hernial defect. When this occurs, the hernial contents become tense, tender, and nonreducible. Treatment becomes a surgical emergency, often necessitating the resection of the involved bowel because of vascular compromise. A less common cause of intestinal obstruction arising from a hernia is that arising from a mesenteric defect. In this circumstance the hernia is actually internal and results because of protrusion of a portion of bowel through a mesenteric defect that then becomes incarcerated (nonreducible but blood supply not compromised) or strangulated. Generally, this type of obstruction is not diagnosed correctly before surgery and only becomes apparent at the time of surgery.

Neoplastic Disorders

Although various neoplastic disorders may obstruct the small or large bowel, neoplastic obstruction is more commonly encountered in the large bowel. A lesion arising in the left colon may result in considerable dilation of the proximal colon, particularly if the ileocecal valve is competent. Because of the tremendous pressure generated in the proximal colon, particularly the cecum, due to Laplace's law (which states that the tension in the wall of a tubular structure at a particular pressure is directly related to the diameter of that structure), perforation is imminent if surgical decompression is not forthcoming. It is for this reason that large bowel obstructions are generally considered surgical emergencies.

Inflammatory Lesions

Of the inflammatory lesions responsible for bowel obstruction, Crohn's disease of the small and/or large bowel and diverticulitis of the large bowel are clearly the more common causes. As indicated elsewhere in this chapter, Crohn's disease is often associated with strictured areas of the intestinal tract, which can result in severe compromise of the luminal size. Since the resulting strictured area is not reversible, surgical excision is frequently necessary. Diverticulitis may also result in mechanical obstruction, but because much of this obstruction is secondary to tissue edema within the bowel wall, it may become less of a problem once the inflammatory process is brought under control. Only when an irreversible strictured area results will surgical intervention become an important priority in management. Much less frequent inflammatory causes of intestinal obstruction include tuberculosis, ulcerative colitis, and amebiasis.

Other Causes of Mechanical Obstruction

Other potential causes of intestinal obstruction include intussusception and volvulus. Intussusception is primarily a childhood disorder and only rarely occurs in adults. This disorder is characterized by an invagination or telescoping of one segment of bowel into another. Intussusception usually occurs in the distal ileum in which this region of the small bowel telescopes into the cecum. The major threat with this problem is strangulation of the involved bowel caused by compromise of the blood supply of the portion of intestine that has intussuscepted. This disease is usually seen in children between the ages of 6 and 18 months. It is characterized by acute abdominal pain that occurs every 5 or 10 minutes during which the child doubles up, followed by a period of quietness. The intussuscepted bowel can often be palpated on abdominal examination as a tubular mass across the upper abdomen. Not uncommonly, the passage of a bloody stool resembling "currant jelly" is noted. Barium enema usually confirms the diagnosis and can often be successfully used to reduce the intussuscepted bowel. If this is not possible, surgical reduction and, on occasion, bowel resection, are required. In contrast to children in whom the cause of intussusception is rarely identified, it is usually secondary to some neoplastic process when it occurs in adults. For that reason, hydrostatic reduction with barium enema is not used in the adult population, and treatment involves abdominal exploration and resection of the affected bowel.

In contrast to intussusception, volvulus is commonly seen in adults. This disorder represents a condition in which the intestine twists on its mesentery with a resultant compromise in blood supply. Two types have been described. Sigmoid volvulus is clearly the more common of the two and results because of the long and redundant sigmoid mesentery. This disorder is particularly common in older, debilitated patients. Often, sigmoidoscopy can decompress this type of volvulus, allowing removal of the trapped gas and liquid feces. Because of the high recurrence rate in patients with this condition, surgical treatment is generally indicated, at which time the sigmoid colon is resected. The other type of volvulus involves the cecum. This occurs when the cecal mesentery is long, allowing its free movement within the peritoneal cavity. Schematic representations of these two types of volvulus and radiologic presentations are shown in Figs. 22-10 and 22-11. Small bowel volvulus may also occur and is almost always related to an adhesive band around a loop of small intestine. In this circumstance, the base of the loop is formed by an adhesion that joins two portions of the small bowel.

Clinical Presentation

The principal signs and symptoms of intestinal obstruction are abdominal pain, distention, vomiting, and the lack of flatus or defecation. The severity of these complaints and the likelihood that all may be present in a given patient

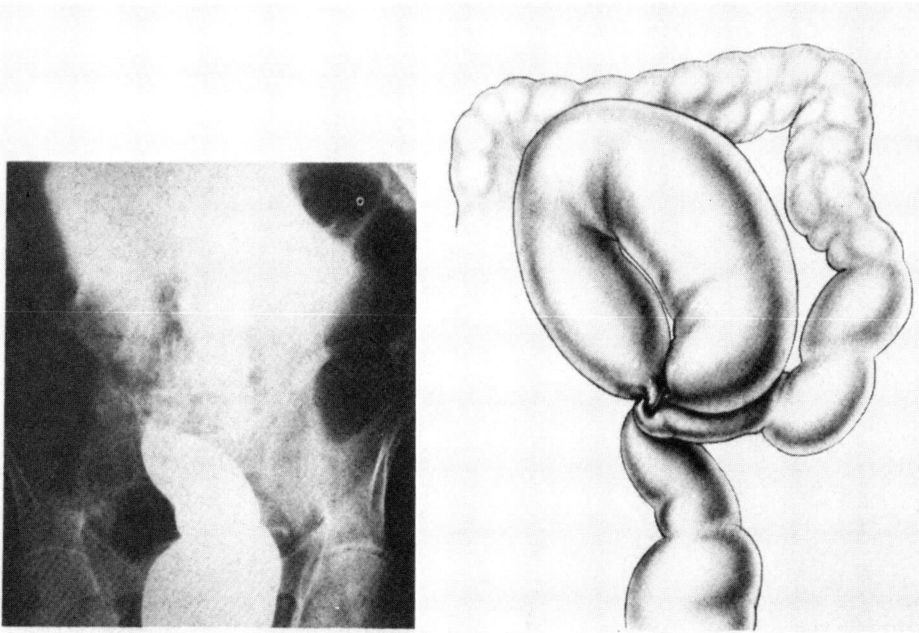

Fig. 22-10 Sigmoid volvulus. X-ray film shows large fluid-filled mass and typical bird-beak deformity outlined by barium in distal sigmoid colon. Diagram shows the twist. (From Liechty, R.D., and Soper, R.T., editors: Synopsis of surgery, ed. 3, St. Louis, 1976, The C.V. Mosby Co.)

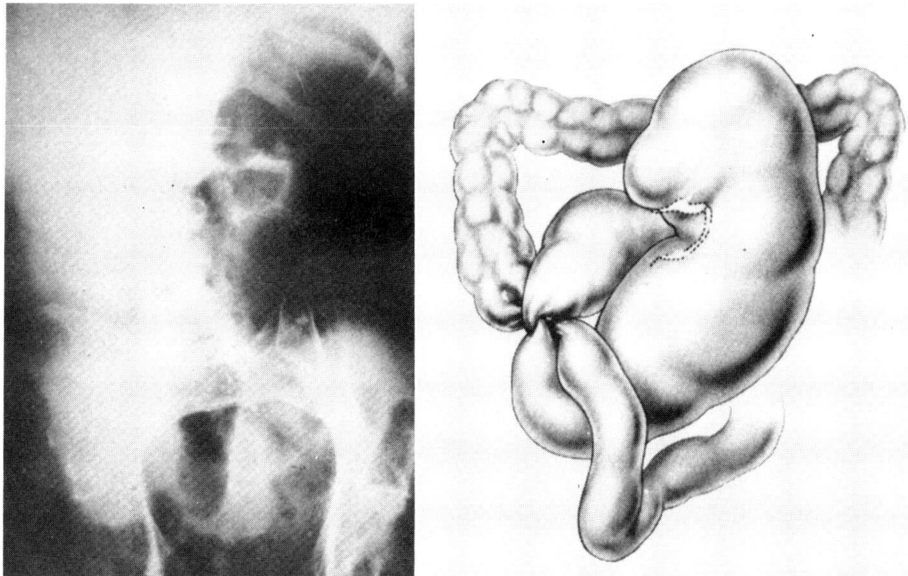

Fig. 22-11 Cecal volvulus. Note dilated, gas-filled cecum in left upper quadrant on x-ray film. Diagram shows the twist. (From Liechty, R.D., and Soper, R.T., editors: Synopsis of surgery, ed. 3, St. Louis, 1976, The C.V. Mosby Co.)

depends on the completeness of obstruction and the region of the intestinal tract involved. The pain of intestinal obstruction is typically crampy and intermittent. This results from the vigorous contraction of the bowel wall musculature in its attempts to push fluid and gas pass the point of obstruction. On auscultation of the abdomen, bowel sounds are usually hyperactive and high-pitched and often occur in rushes associated with the onset of the pain. Between these periods of hyperperistalsis, the abdomen is quiet, and the pain is usually less pronounced or absent entirely. Although pain occurs with both small and large bowel obstructions, the pain is usually of a longer interval when the colon is involved.

As with pain, distention virtually always accompanies obstruction. The more complete the obstruction, the more likely it is distention will be present. In addition, the level of obstruction will dictate the extent to which distention can be demonstrated clinically. In obstruction involving the proximal small bowel, distention is usually minimal. With lower intestinal obstruction, it is much more pronounced and can be massive because of the greater amount of bowel that is filled with gas and liquid. Actually, the more distended the abdomen, the more distal the obstruction will be.

The extent to which vomiting is a clinical feature of obstruction again relates to the completeness of obstruction and the level of intestine involved. Vomiting is frequently an early symptom of obstruction when the proximal bowel is involved because of the accumulation of bile and pancreatic and gastric juices in the obstructed segment, in addition to its own secretions. In more distal types of obstruction, vomiting is less pronounced or may be absent initially, particularly if the obstruction is not complete. With obstructions involving the distal ileum or colon, feculent vomiting often results. This occurs because the resident bacteria within the distal small bowel or colon undergo enhanced growth secondary to stagnation and the decomposition of intraluminal contents. This gives the vomitus a feculent odor and character.

Most patients with bowel obstruction will indicate some change in bowel habits preceding the onset of other symptoms. This may be noted as a change in the frequency of defecation or in the passage of flatus. The more complete the obstruction, the more likely it is that these findings will be observed. In patients with complete bowel obstruction, neither gas nor feces are passed.

From a laboratory standpoint, the most important aids in diagnosing intestinal obstruction are plain x-ray films of the abdomen to include views both in the upright and supine positions. The presence of air and fluid levels virtually assures the diagnosis of mechanical intestinal obstruction (Fig. 22-12). The pattern of these air/fluid levels will suggest the level of obstruction. If a high duodenal obstruction is present, the double bubble sign caused by an air/fluid level in the stomach and a second air/fluid level in the duodenum is often present. Beyond the point of obstruction there is no air. For more distal obstructions, multiple air/fluid levels will be demonstrated throughout the abdomen. The more air/fluid levels that are seen, however, the more difficult it becomes to differentiate between an obstruction in the small bowel or colon. In this circumstance a barium enema is often helpful to either exclude or confirm the colon as the site of obstruction.

In addition to demonstrating air/fluid levels and giving information concerning the site of obstruction, plain x-ray films of the abdomen may also be helpful in other respects. Free air in the peritoneal cavity, for example, indicates the presence of a perforation. In addition, calculi may be demonstrated in the renal fossa or biliary tree and help sort out underlying pathology in less clear cases in which a differentiation between paralytic ileus and mechanical obstruction is being considered. Other ways in which plain x-ray films of the abdomen may prove helpful is in the demonstration of fecaliths in the region of the appendix, various tumors, and the demonstration of radiopaque foreign bodies.

In any patient with suspected intestinal obstruction, a complete blood count, urinalysis, electrolyte profile, and blood urea nitrogen analysis should be obtained. Often the hemoglobin and hematocrit are elevated, indicating the underlying dehydration and hemoconcentration secondary to the intestinal obstruction. The white count may also be elevated and provide supporting evidence of a suspected underlying strangulation obstruction. If considerable fluid has been sequestered into the small bowel from the obstruction, a number of electrolyte abnormalities may supervene that can be demonstrated on the electrolyte profile. The urinalysis is also helpful in gaining information concerning the degree of fluid and electrolyte imbalance, since the specific gravity will usually be elevated in patients in whom the dehydration has been long-standing. In addition, if ketones are present in the urine, this finding generally indicates an accompanying metabolic acidosis.

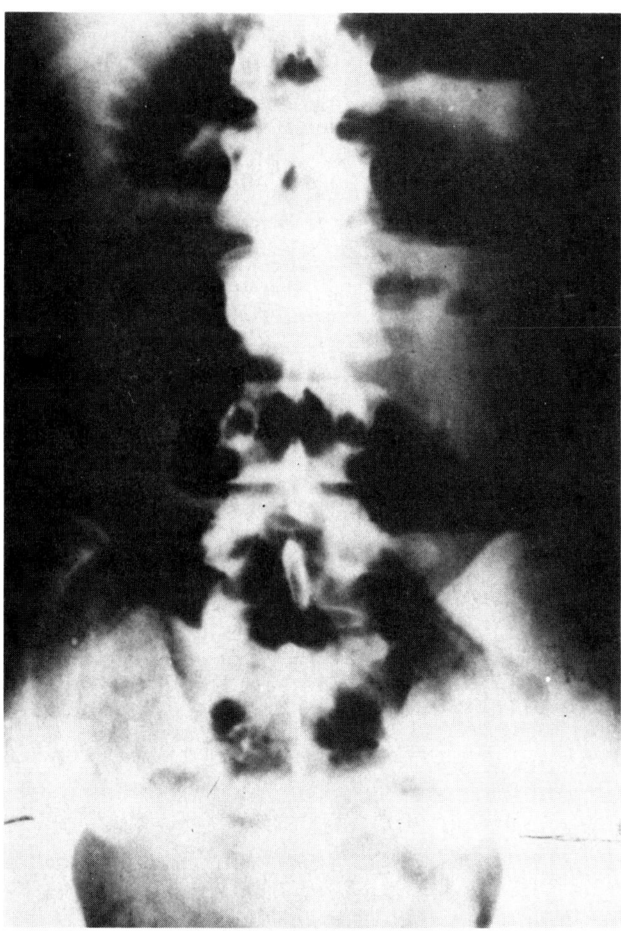

Fig. 22-12 Upright abdominal x-ray film in small bowel obstruction demonstrating multiple, centrally located air fluid levels and dilated bowel loops. (From Davis, J.H., editor: Clinical surgery, vol. 2, St. Louis, 1987, The C.V. Mosby Co.)

Management Strategies

Before specific treatment for presumed intestinal obstruction is instituted, it is important to ensure that this disorder does indeed exist and, providing it does, to determine the urgency of surgical intervention and its site of origin as precisely as possible. Although mechanical obstruction and paralytic ileus are generally easily distinguished from one another, it is important to exclude a paralytic ileus as the source of signs and symptoms to prevent an unnecessary operation. Where there may be confusion between these two entities, a number of features specific for each one should make their differentiation more evident. Of particular importance is the difference in clinical findings. In contrast to mechanical obstruction in which high-pitched, hyperactive bowel sounds are almost always present and accompanied by rather intense abdominal pain, the abdomen of the patient with paralytic ileus is silent and usually painless and nontender, unless the cause of the ileus is secondary to some source of peritoneal irritation such as pancreatitis, cholecystitis, pneumonitis, or trauma. Further, the radiologic picture of the two conditions is quite different. With mechanical obstruction, air/fluid levels are routinely noted proximal to the site of obstruction with the absence of gas distal to this site. In contrast, gas is generally evenly distributed throughout the large and small bowel in paralytic ileus. If the radiologic and clinical picture is sufficiently confusing to mandate the need for other information before surgery is undertaken, the administration of some contrast medium (such as thin barium) and evaluation of its serial movement through the intestinal tract can often give valuable information in terms of the presence or absence of obstruction. If no anatomic obstructive focus is present, the contrast medium should freely flow through the intestinal tract, albeit often slowly. If a true obstruction is present, the anatomic site will ultimately become identifiable.

Another feature of importance in managing bowel obstruction is the urgency with which surgery should be performed if a true mechanical obstruction is present. In most patients some period of preoperative preparation is appropriate to correct the underlying dehydration and any fluid and electrolyte abnormalities. However, if the possibility of strangulation is under serious consideration, surgical management becomes more urgent. A number of diagnostic indices are suggestive of strangulation obstruction. These include a change in the characteristics of pain from the usual intermittent, colicky type to a more unrelenting, steady type. Further, the development of abdominal tenderness, particularly in association with rebound tenderness, makes the possibility of strangulation obstruction a serious consideration, since tenderness is usually not a pronounced feature of intestinal obstruction. Other corroborating findings include the presence of an abdominal mass, laboratory findings such as an elevated white count, with a left shift (suggestive of inflammation), and an elevation in the temperature and pulse.

Finally, it is helpful to differentiate a small bowel obstruction from a colonic obstruction before surgery, since the treatment approaches are frequently different. If a large bowel obstruction is clearly present, a standard laparotomy is usually not indicated, since the immediate goal is to decrease the colonic distention with a colostomy. On the other hand, if a small bowel obstruction is present, a formal laparotomy is usually performed. Under most circumstances, these two types of obstruction can be differentiated from one another by the information provided on the plain abdominal x-ray films. In confusing cases a barium enema usually provides the additional information that is necessary to aid in distinguishing these two conditions.

Preoperative Preparation

With bowel obstruction, particularly if it has been present in excess of 24 hours, most patients will have a considerable amount of dehydration. This results from the absence of oral intake, the loss of fluid through vomiting, the sequestration of fluid within the intestinal tract lumen both because of impaired absorption and increased net secretion, the edema of the bowel wall proximal to the obstructing site, and any transudation of fluid into the peritoneal cavity.[36] These various sources of fluid loss are important to remember because they may be quite substantial. In its attempt to force bowel contents pass the obstructive site, the bowel immediately proximal to the site of obstruction becomes edematous quite quickly. Not only does this edematous wall lose its absorptive capabilities, but also its secretions and edema fluid increase.[36] These aberrations propagate more proximally the longer the obstruction exists.

Another problem secondary to these pathophysiologic alterations is the increased intraluminal pressure that builds proximal to the point of obstruction. In time, this pressure compromises blood flow to the bowel wall and eventually is able to exceed the capillary perfusion pressure.[36] If this sequence of events is not reversed, the consequent ischemia ultimately results in bowel wall necrosis, perforation, and peritonitis. When this state of affairs occurs, the contractile properties of the bowel musculature are lost, and the previous crampy abdominal pain with hyeractive bowel sound gives rise to an amazingly silent abdomen. When this develops, any intraluminal bacteria and toxins can escape across the bowel wall into the peritoneal cavity, giving rise to sepsis and endotoxic shock.

On the basis of the foregoing considerations, both correction of dehydration and alleviation of the intestinal distention are important priorities before surgical intervention. To relieve the distention, the passage of some type of large-bore nasogastric tube should be positioned immediately upon making the diagnosis of bowel obstruction. Through intermittent suction, such a tube provides a quite efficient means of removing air and intestinal fluid. Whether the passage of a long intestinal tube adds anything to the management of a patient being readied for surgery remains a debatable issue. Most clinicians, including myself, have not found such tubes to be of particular value.

Correction of the underlying dehydration can usually be accomplished with a balanced salt solution such as Ringer's lactate, with the addition of 20 to 30 mEq/L of potassium chloride. Depending on the magnitude of dehydration, several liters may be required before surgery to help reestablish fluid and electrolyte balance. Obviously the time interval over which the fluid that has been lost is replaced depends on the urgency of surgery. If the operation needs to be performed as quickly as possible because of a suspicion of strangulation, fluids should be infused equally rapidly by monitoring such parameters as urinary output, blood pressure, pulse, and central venous pressure. In a particularly fragile patient, a Swan-Ganz catheter may also be indicated for monitoring. In less urgent situations the fluid can be administered more slowly, and the adequacy of replacement determined by the urinary output. Generally, urine output should be in excess of 30 ml/hour, and the systolic blood pressure above 100 mm Hg before surgery is undertaken.

The role of antibiotics in bowel obstruction remains a

controversial issue.[6,26] Generally, the longer the obstruction has been present allowing distention of the bowel wall and the possibility of diapedesis of intestinal flora across it and into the bloodstream, the more likely antibiotics will be of value. Thus if bowel obstruction has been present in excess of 24 hours, broad-spectrum antibiotics should be administered before surgery and continued for 2 or 3 days thereafter.

Types of Bowel Obstruction

Small Bowel Obstruction. The usual cause of small bowel obstruction is some extrinsic problem such as adhesions or the entrapment of a portion of small bowel in a hernial defect. In either circumstance, the surgical approach is usually straightforward. Thus adhesions are lysed, or the bowel entrapped in a hernia is reduced. If there is any question at the time of surgery of the viability of a particular portion of intestine, resection should be undertaken with primary anastomosis. If small bowel volvulus is present, resection is usually indicated, since the volvulated intestine has usually had considerable vascular compromise. In the uncommon circumstance of intussusception, resection of the affected bowel is also indicated in most circumstances.

Large Bowel Obstruction. In contrast to obstructions involving the small intestine, most large bowel obstructions are caused by intrinsic lesions such as neoplasia. Most of these obstructions are in the left colon, particularly in the sigmoid area. The type of surgery will depend on the duration of the obstruction and the competency of the ileocecal valve. If an incompetent ileocecal valve exists, allowing regurgitation of the obstructed contents into the small bowel, management of the underlying problem becomes less formidable. If the obstruction is secondary to neoplastic disease, the causative lesion can generally be resected, and a colostomy performed. At a later second-stage operation, gastrointestinal continuity can be reestablished with a primary colon-to-colon anastomosis. In the event that the ileocecal valve is competent, which exists in about 50% of patients, the underlying obstruction is referred to as a closed loop obstruction. On radiologic evaluation, the abdomen shows gross dilation of the colon between the obstructing lesion and the ileocecal valve. Because this circumstance is associated with a high mortality rate due to the possibility of cecal perforation,[36,55] immediate surgical decompression is the treatment of choice. A proximal transverse colostomy is performed, through which decompression of the bowel is easily accomplished, and any intraluminal gas and feces are diverted through this new opening in the abdominal wall. Although cecostomy has also been recommended as an appropriate diverting procedure, it generally is ineffectual in providing a satisfactory evacuation of the intestinal contents. After the patient convalesces from the emergency colonic decompression, he can be returned to the operating room under elective circumstances for resection and management of the underlying cause of obstruction. If this is secondary to a colon carcinoma, the appropriate resective procedure can be accomplished at the second procedure with the reestablishment of gastrointestinal continuity.

ANUS AND RECTUM

In addition to inflammatory bowel disease and the various neoplastic disorders already described that may involve the rectum, a number of other diseases of surgical significance may arise in the anorectal region. For this reason every physical examination should include a careful evaluation of the anus and rectum by both inspection and digital exploration. If a specific disease process is suspected, further evaluation with an anoscope can be carried out to define more clearly the underlying pathology. Disorders of surgical significance include hemorrhoids, fissures, parianal and perirectal abscesses, anal fistula, rectal prolapse, and perianal malignancies. The anatomy of the anorectum is shown in Fig. 22-13.

Hemorrhoids

Of complaints involving the anorectum, hemorrhoidal disease is clearly the most common. This entity represents enlargement or dilation of the terminal veins of the external and internal hemorrhoidal plexus involving the anus and lower rectum. External hemorrhoids originate below the dentate line and are covered by a squamous epithelium that is well innervated. In contrast, internal hemorrhoids arise above the dentate line and are covered by a nonsen-

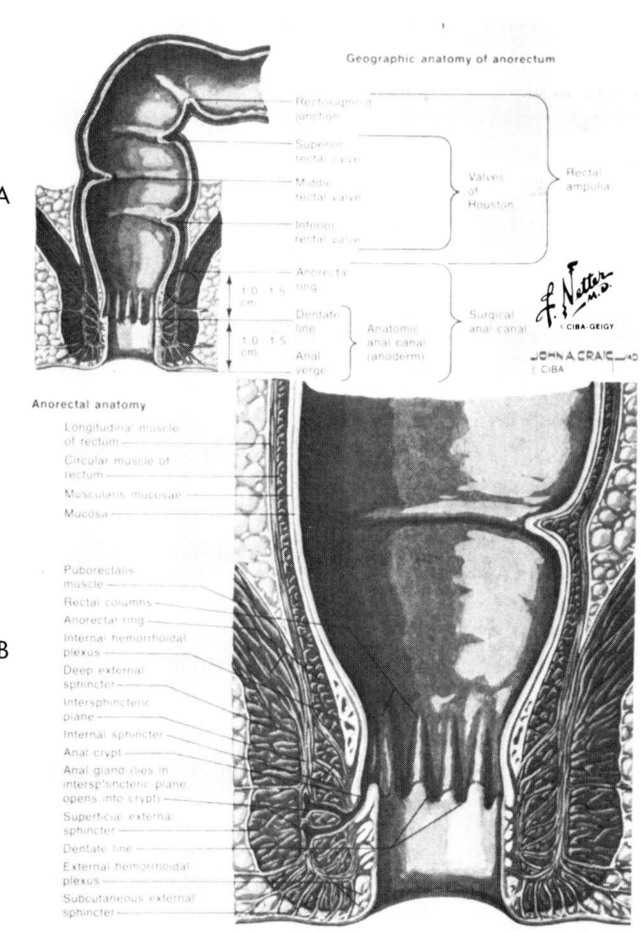

Fig. 22-13 Anatomy of anus and rectum. **A,** Geographic anatomy. **B,** Anorectal anatomy. (From Fry, R.D., and Kodner, I.J.: Clinical symposia: anorectal disease, vol. 37, West Caldwell, N.J., 1985, CIBA Pharmaceutical Co.)

sitive rectal mucosa. The symptoms related to hemorrhoids may vary considerably. Internal hemorrhoids frequently bleed and may first come to the attention of a patient when blood is noted on stooling or on the toilet paper during wiping. If the hemorrhoid is large enough, prolapse may occur. External hemorrhoids are usually of little significance clinically unless one of the external hemorrhoidal veins becomes thrombosed, in which case severe pain may develop.

It remains to be established why hemorrhoids develop, but excessive straining during stooling appears to be an important etiologic factor. The straining may be related to poor dietary habits (i.e., low-bulk diet), poor toilet habits, laxative abuse, and pregnancy. The lack of valves in the hemorrhoidal plexus probably plays a contributory role, but the extent to which this is an etiologic factor is uncertain, since many patients never develop a problem with hemorrhoidal disease. Similarly, the erect posture of the human being suggests possible gravity effects, but why this would be of importance in one person and not another remains unexplained.

From a surgical standpoint, hemorrhoidal disease is of significance when symptoms persist or become severe. For external hemorrhoids, the major indication for surgical intervention relates to the development of a thrombosed external hemorrhoidal vein. The thrombosis becomes demonstrable as a bluish, subcutaneous nodule underlying the perianal skin that is usually painful and tender to touch. Excision of the overlying skin with evacuation of the thrombus usually results in cure with no further problems. With regard to internal hemorrhoids, the need for surgical intervention will depend on the size of the hemorrhoids. To determine their clinical significance, a staging system has been developed.[17] First-degree internal hemorrhoids are generally small or only of moderate size and do not protrude below the dentate line when the patient is instructed to strain. Second-degree internal hemorrhoids are generally larger than first-degree hemorrhoids, but, because the submucosal supporting tissue is not able to hold the hemorrhoid in its normal position, it generally prolapses into the anal canal during defecation or on straining. After either of these maneuvers is completed, the hemorrhoid retracts to its normal position above the dentate line. Third-degree internal hemorrhoids represent further stretching of the submucosal supporting tissue and further prolapse on straining or defecation, requiring manual manipulation for reduction. With fourth-degree internal hemorrhoids, the rectal mucosa is redundant, and the overstretched submucosal attachments are no longer able to retain the internal hemorrhoids in their normal position. Thus prolapsing occurs almost continuously.

For first-degree hemorrhoids, most patients can be managed by local measures such as sitz baths and the use of bland suppositories. Education in bowel habits and the implementation of appropriate dietary changes are additional measures. Rarely will surgery be indicated. Similar measures can be used frequently in the management of second-degree hemorrhoids unless the prolapse becomes unusually bothersome. When that occurs, hemorrhoid banding is a highly successful technique to eliminate this problem. This technique uses a special ligating instrument that grasps the redundant hemorrhoidal tissue and ligates it with a rubber band. This instrument is passed through an anoscope. This procedure can easily be performed on an outpatient basis. The ligated tissue will usually slough by the third to fifth day, resulting in scarring and fixation of any residual hemorrhoidal disease. Third-degree internal hemorrhoids may also be managed successfully in most circumstances with hemorrhoidal banding, although on occasion a formal surgical hemorrhoidectomy may prove necessary. This latter procedure involves the actual excision of the hemorrhoid, with ligation of the accompanying hemorrhoidal veins. Fourth-degree hemorrhoids nearly always require formal hemorrhoidectomy. If the prolapsed hemorrhoidal tissue becomes strangulated, this procedure may need to be carried out under urgent circumstances.

Anal Fissures

An anal fissure represents a linear tear in the lining of the anal canal. This disruption usually occurs below the dentate line and commonly extends to the level of the anal verge. Patients with this condition complain of pain during defecation that may produce a sphincter spasm leading to constipation. If this occurs, defecation becomes even more difficult and painful, and the problem is further aggravated. In addition to the pain, the passage of bright red blood, either noted on toilet paper or covering the stool, is a frequent accompanying complaint.

The most frequent cause of an anal fissure is the passage of a dry, hard, large-caliber stool. Other causes include persistent diarrhea, Crohn's disease, and carcinoma of the anal canal. Most fissues occur in the anterior or posterior commisure. Those arising in other anatomic positions should raise the suspicion of a possible neoplastic process.

Most fissures will respond to conservative treatment, including steroid creams, bland suppositories, and local-anesthetics. Occasionally, stretching the anal sphincter under local anesthesia will become necessary, but usually effects cure. Anal fissures that persist and become more chronic will often require local excision because of the chronic ulceration that develops in the fissured tissue.

Perianal, Perirectal, and Anorectal Abscesses

Abscesses developing in the perianal and perirectal regions usually result from infections of the anal glands with erosion into adjacent tissues (Fig. 22-14). Those abscesses that spread directly downward to the anal margin are referred to as perianal and generally exhibit themselves with pain and localized tender swelling. In more severe situations the abscesses may erode into tissue spaces adjacent to the rectum such as the supralevator or ischiorectal spaces (Fig. 22-14). When this occurs, exquisite pain and tenderness may develop, with evidence of fever and leukocytosis. If the abscess has been present for any length of time, the patient may actually be quite toxic when first observed. Treatment of anal/rectal abscesses, whatever their anatomic location, involves formal surgical drainage in conjunction with antibiotic therapy. After surgery, sitz baths are also included, and dietary education given to ensure good bowel habits in the future.

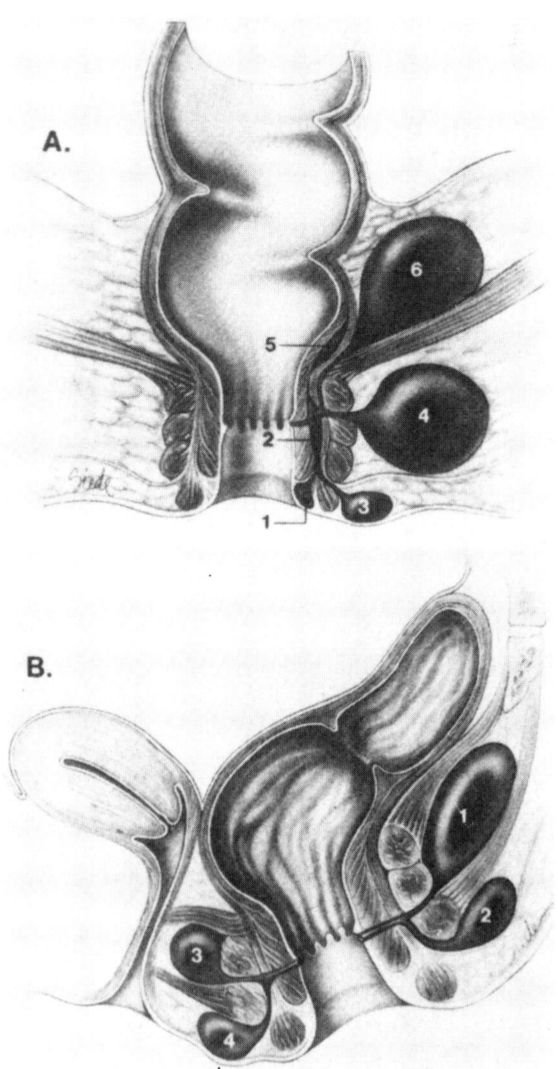

Fig. 22-14 Anorectal abscesses. **A,** Frontal. *1,* Subcutaneous; *2,* low intermuscular; *3,* perianal; *4,* ischioanal; *5,* high intermuscular; *6,* supralevator. **B,** Saggital. *1,* Deep postanal space; *2,* superficial postanal space; *3,* deep anterior space; *4,* superficial anterior space. (From Polk, H.C., Jr., Stone, H.H., and Gardner, B., editors: Basic surgery, ed. 3, Norwalk, Conn., 1987, Appleton-Century-Crofts.)

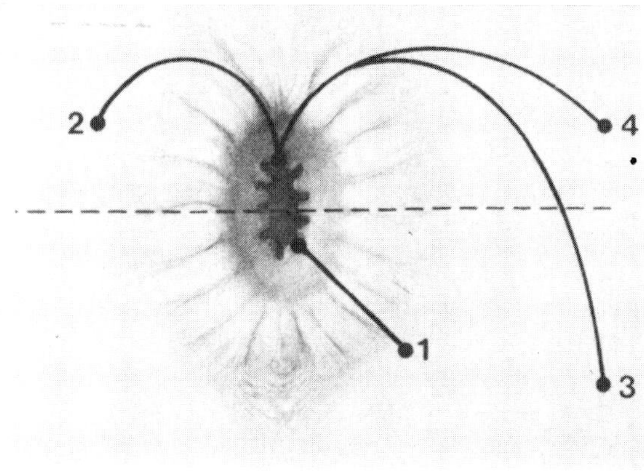

Fig. 22-15 Goodsall's rule (dotted line is the coronal plane). *1,* Anterior external opening; *2,* posterior external opening; *3,* anterior opening 5 cm from anal margin; *4,* posterior external opening. (From Polk, H.C., Jr., Stone, H.H., and Gardner, B., editors. Basic surgery, ed. 3, Norwalk, Conn., 1987, Appleton-Century-Crofts.)

Anal Fistula

A fistula-in-ano usually represents a connection of the anal glands and the skin that has resulted from a previous anorectal abscess. Clinically it presents as a sinus connecting the perianal skin with the anus. Depending on the origin of the anorectal abscess, the path of the sinus tract may vary considerably. Transsphincteric fistulas cross the external sphincter into the ischiorectal fossa, whereas suprasphincteric fistulas arise above the muscles responsible for anal continence. Fortunately, these two types of fistula are relatively rare compared to the intersphincteric fistula that passes downward along the bowel wall within the external sphincter. Usually, inspection of the perianal region can provide valuable information to the primary origin of the external opening. Using Goodsall's rule, a transverse line is drawn across the anal opening in the coronal plane. If the opening is anterior to this line, the primary opening in the anal crypt will be in a direct radial line to the nearest crypt. If the opening is posterior to the coronal line, the primary opening is almost always in a posterior midline crypt. If external openings are greater than 3 cm from the anal margin, the primary origin of the fistula will most likely arise in one of the posterior crypts (Fig. 22-15).

Rectal Prolapse

Rectal prolapse (also called procidentia) is a condition in which the full thickness of the rectum descends through the anus. Basically this condition represents a failure in one or more of the mechanisms responsible for normal rectal support. It occurs primarily in the two extremes of life (i.e., in children under 3 or in the elderly). In children anatomic abnormalities involving rectal attachments and formational derangements of the sacral curvature appear to be the major causes. Usually, conservative, nonsurgical measures prove successful in treating the prolapse in this patient population until such time as anatomic maturity occurs.

In adults the disorder is acquired and may be secondary to damage to the levator musculature, weakness, and attenuation of the rectal supporting tissues, muscular degeneration, and on occasion a neurologic disease such as paralysis of the canda equina. In this patient group treatment will be dictated by the extent of the prolapse and its effects on anal continence. A number of surgical procedures have been recommended to correct this abnormality, including resection of the redundant and prolapsing bowel, reconstruction of the peritoneal floor, suspension or fixation of the prolapsed bowel, and reduction in the size of the anus.[21,54] For individuals who are poor surgical risks, the subcutaneous passage of a silastic or synthetic loop or a steel suture wire will often achieve sufficient tightening of the anus, which thereby prevents further prolapse. Although this is a simple surgical approach, the loop or wire may break, resulting in a high failure rate. More definitive surgical approaches include transabdominal suspension of the rectum and excision of the redundant bowel through a peritoneal or low anterior approach. If a transabdominal procedure is planned, the Ripstein operation has generally been the procedure of choice. This operation fixes the rectum to the presacral fascia with the use of a synthetic mesh sling and has resulted in a recurrence rate of only 2% to 3%.[21,54] This operation can also be performed transanally, but the recurrence rate has generally been much higher.

Malignant Lesions of the Anus and Perianal Region

In contrast to malignancies of the colon and rectum, cancer of the anus and perianal region is distinctly uncommon and represents only about 2% to 3% of all tumors involving the colorectal region. These tumors arise from the epithelial surface distal to the mucocutaneous juncture separating the anus from the rectum. A variety of symptoms, most of which are nonspecific, may signal their presence, including pain, pruritis, bleeding, and occasionally a palpable mass. Since these symptoms are also characteristic of the multiple benign lesions afflicting the perianal region, early diagnosis usually depends on a high index of suspicion. Establishment of the presence of an anal or perianal neoplasm will ultimately require biopsy for histologic confirmation. Of those lesions involving this region, squamous cell carcinoma (epidermoid carcinoma) is clearly the most common tumor in this region and constitutes approximately 75% of reported tumors.[5,46] A variant of squamous cell carcinoma includes transitional cell, cloacogenic, mucoepidermoid, and basosquamous tumors.

The treatment of squamous cell carcinoma of the perianal region depends on the histologic stage of the tumor, its location, and the depth of invasion. Small (less than 2 cm), superficial, mobile lesions arising below the mucocutaneous junction can generally be adequately treated by wide local excision. Larger tumors, particularly if invasion of the anal sphincter or rectum exists, have been traditionally treated with an abdominoperineal resection (excision of the anus, rectum, and sigmoid colon). Recent results with combination therapy involving chemotherapy and external radiation have suggested that such radical surgery may not be appropriate for all patients. By administering 5-fluorouracil and mitomycin-C followed by 3000 rad of external radiation to the pelvis over a period of 3 weeks, Nigro and colleagues[44] reported that approximately 50% of lesions showed the absence of any residual tumor after treatment and many of the remaining tumors were sufficiently reduced in size that local excision could be performed in place of the more radical operation.

Like most neoplasia, the prognosis in patients with squamous cell carcinoma of the perianal region depends on the presence or absence of lymphatic spread. Since the major lymphatic drainage route for tumors arising in this region is primarily to the inguinal nodes, metastases in this region are important in determining prognosis. For patients with inguinal metastases at the time of diagnosis, the 5-year survival rate is quite dismal and approaches 5% or less. The absence of such metastases results in a 5-year survival rate of 75% or better.[5,46]

Several other tumors may also arise in the perianal region.[5,46] Of these, malignant melanoma is particularly virulent and is associated with a poor 5-year survival rate, despite the aggressiveness of treatment. In contrast, basal cell carcinoma with its "rodent ulcer" appearance can almost always be managed by local excision, since this tumor virtually never metastasizes. Extramammary Paget's disease of the anus is a gray, plaque-like lesion that may not have an underlying carcinoma like its counterpart in the breast. If an underlying tumor is absent, local excision is the treatment of choice; the presence of a tumor dictates more radical therapy, usually an abdominoperineal resection. Bowen's disease (intraepidermal carcinoma) is a dull, red, spreading, plaquelike eczematoid lesion that on biopsy reveals carcinoma in situ. Treatment generally consists of wide local excision, with the topical use of 5-fluorouracil cream or dinitrochlorobenzene. Interestingly, a variety of internal malignancies may be associated with this lesion, particularly tumors of the urogenital tract, and should be carefully searched for in the workup of patients with this lesion.

SUMMARY

A large number of inflammatory, neoplastic, and mechanical disorders may adversely influence the normal physiology of the small bowel, colon, rectum, and anus. The inflammatory disorders of surgical significance include appendicitis, Meckel's diverticulitis, diverticular disease of the colon, Crohn's disease, and ulcerative colitis. The impact that each of these disease processes has on intestinal function varies considerably in terms of disability and long-term sequelae. Appendectomy for appendicitis, for example, is usually associated with no long-term sequelae, in contrast to Crohn's disease in which a variety of maldigestive disorders may plague the patient for most of his life, depending upon the status of the disease, the frequency of relapses, the duration of remissions, and the type(s) of surgical management rendered. With neoplastic disorders of the intestine, rectum, and anus, altered physiology can usually be restored to normal or near normal following surgical resection of the underlying tumor, unless widespread metastases have taken place. In this circumstance life span is shortened; and, in addition to the primary disease, other organ systems are also adversely affected, allowing only supportive care rather than permanent reversal of the underlying pathophysiologic processes. Mechanical disorders of the intestinal tract represent those diseases in which normal digestion and absorption is impeded because of some obstructive process. In the small intestine such obstruction is usually related to adhesions or hernias; in contrast, obstructions involving the large intestine are usually secondary to neoplastic processes. The underlying pathophysiology with both types of obstruction is virtually the same. Understanding this physiologic derangement forms the basis for its correction and for those surgical procedures that must be used to restore intestinal function to normal.

REFERENCES

1. Almy, T.P., and Howell, D.A.: Diverticular disease of the colon (medical progress), N. Engl. J. Med. **302**:324, 1980.
2. Banks, P.A., Present, D.H., and Steiner, P., editors: The Crohn's disease and ulcerative colitis fact book. New York, 1983, Charles Scribner's Sons.
3. Becker, J.M., and Raymond, J.L.: Ileal pouch—anal anastomosis: a single surgeon's experience with 100 consecutive cases, Ann. Surg. **204**:375, 1986.

4. Berk, R.N.: Radiographic evaluation of spastic colon disease, diverticulosis, and diverticulitis, Gastroenterol. Endosc. **26:**265, 1980.
5. Boman, B.M., et al.: Carcinoma of the anal canal: a clinical and pathologic study of 188 cases, Cancer **54:**114, 1984.
6. Brolin, R.E.: Partial small bowel obstruction, Surgery **95:**145, 1984.
7. Burkitt, D.P.: Etiology and prevention of colorectal cancer, Hosp. Pract. **19:**67, Feb 1984.
8. Bussey, H.J.R.: Familial polyposis coli, Baltimore, 1975, Johns Hopkins University Press.
9. Crowder, B.L., Judd, E.S., and Dockerty, M.B.: Gastrointestinal carcinoids and the carcinoid syndrome: clinical characteristics and therapy, Surg. Clin. North Am. **47:**915, 1967.
10. Dukes, C.E.: Cancer of the rectum, J. Pathol. Bacteriol. **35:**323, 1932.
11. Farmer, R.G.: Medical aspects of inflammatory bowel disease. In Farmer, R.G., Achkar, E., and Fleshler, B., editors: Clinical gastroenterology, New York, 1983, Raven Press.
12. Farmer, R.G., Hawk, W.A., and Turnbull, R.B.: Clinical patterns in Crohn's disease: a statistical study of 615 cases, Gastroenterology **68:**627, 1975.
13. Farmer, R.G., Michener, W.M., and Mortimer, E.A.: Studies of family history among patients with inflammatory bowel disease, Clin. Gastroenterol. **92:**271, 1980.
14. Fazio, V.M.: Toxic megacolon in ulcerative colitis and Crohn's colitis, Clin. Gastroenterol. **9:**389, 1980.
15. Fazio, V.W.: Inflammatory bowel disease: Surgical aspects. In R.G., Farmer, E. Achkar, and B. Flashler, editors: Clinical gastroenterology, New York, 1983, Raven Press.
16. Fonkalsrud, E.W.: Endorectal ileoanal anastomosis with isoperistaltic ileal reservoir after colectomy and mucosal proctectomy, Ann. Surg. **199:**151, 1984.
17. Fry, R.D., and Kodner, I.J.: Clinical symposia: anorectal diseases, vol 37, West Caldwell, N.J., 1985, CIBA Pharmaceutical Co.
18. Gardner, E.J.: Familial polyposis coli and Gardner's syndrome—Is there a difference? In Prevention of hereditary large bowel cancer, New York, 1983, Alan R. Liss, Inc.
19. Goligher, J.C.: Modern trends in sphincter-saving operations for carcinoma of the rectum. In Najarian, J.S., and Delaney, J.P., editors: Gastrointestinal surgery, Chicago, 1979, Year Book Medical Publishers, Inc.
20. Higgins, G.A.: Current status of adjuvant therapy in the treatment of large bowel cancer, Surg. Clin. North Am. **63:**137, 1983.
21. Keighley, M.R.B., and Matheson, D.: Results of treatment for rectal prolapse and fecal incontinence, Dis. Colon Rectum **24:**449, 1981.
22. Konishi, F., et al.: Histopathologic comparison of colorectal adenomas in English and Japanese patients, Dis. Colon Rectum **27:**515, 1984.
23. Korelitz, B.I.: Therapy of inflammatory bowel disease including use of immunosuppressive agents, Clin. Gastroenterol. **9:**331, 1980.
24. Lennard-Jones, J.E.: Toward optimal use of corticosteroids in ulcerative colitis and Crohn's disease, Gut **24:**177, 1983.
25. Lennard-Jones, J.E., et al.: Cancer surveillance in ulcerative colitis: experience over 15 years, Lancet **2:**149, 1983.
26. Levine, B.A., and Aust, J.B.: Surgical disorders of the small intestine. In Sabiston, D.C., Jr., editor: Essentials of surgery, Philadelphia, 1987, W.B. Saunders Co.
27. Lewis, F.R., et al.: Appendicitis: a critical review of diagnosis and treatment in 1000 cases, Arch. Surg. **110:**677, 1975.
28. Localio, S.A.: Abdominal-transsacral resection and anastomosis from midrectal carcinoma, Surg. Gynecol. Obstet. **132:**123, 1971.
29. Lynch, H.T., et al.: Surveillance/management of an obligate gene carrier: the cancer family syndrome, Gastroenterology **84:**404, 1983.
30. Madden, J.L., and Kandalaft, S.I.: Electrocoagulation as a primary curative method in the treatment of carcinoma of the rectum, Surg. Gynecol. Obstet. **157:**164, 1983.
31. Marshak, R.H., and Lindner, A.E.: Radiology of the small intestine, Philadelphia, 1960, W.B. Saunders Co.
32. Marshak, R.H., Linder, A.E., and Maklansky, D.: Diverticulosis and diverticulitis of the colon, Mt. Sinai J. Med. **46:**261, 1979.
33. McLeod, R.S., and Fazio, V.W.: Quality of life with the continent ileostomy, World J. Surg. **8:**90, 1984.
34. Meckel's diverticulum: surgical guidelines at last? (Editorial) Lancet **2:**438, 1983.
35. Mekhjian, H.S., et al.: Clinical features and natural history of Crohn's disease, Gastroenterology **77:**898, 1979.
36. Miller, L.D., Mackie, J.A., and Rhoads, J.E.: The pathophysiology and management of intestinal obstruction. Surg. Clin. North Am. **42:**1285, 1962.
37. Miller, T.A.: Tumors of the duodenum, ampulla of Vater, and small bowel. In Copeland, E.M., III., editor: Surgical oncology, New York, 1983, John Wiley & Sons.
38. Moertel, C.G.: Clinical management of advanced gastrointestinal cancer, Cancer **36:**675, 1975.
39. Moertel, C.G.: Chemotherapy of gastrointestinal cancer, N. Engl. J. Med. **299:**1049, 1978.
40. Moertel, C.G., and Hanley, J.A.: Combination chemotherapy trials for metastatic carcinoid tumor, Proc. Am. Assoc. Cancer Res. Am. Soc. Clin. Oncol. **19:**322, 1978.
41. Moertel, C.G., et al.: Life history of the carcinoid tumor of the small intestine, Cancer **14:**901, 1961.
42. Morson, B.C., and Dawson, I.M.P.: Gastrointestinal pathology, Oxford, 1979, Blackwell Scientific Publications.
43. Morson, B.C., et al.: Histopathology and prognosis of malignant colorectal polyps treated by endoscopic polypectomy, Gut **25:**437, 1984.
44. Nigro, N.D., et al.: Combined preoperative radiation and chemotherapy for squamous cell carcinoma of the anal canal, Cancer **51:**1826, 1983.
45. Nugent, F.W., and Haggett, R.C.: Longterm followup, including cancer surveillance, for patients with ulcerative colitis, Clin. Gastroenterol. **9:**459, 1980.
46. Quan, S.: Anal and perianal tumors, Surg. Clin. North Am. **58:**591, 1978.
47. Ramming, K.P., and Haskell, C.M.: Colorectal malignancies. In Haskell, C.M., editor: Cancer treatment, ed. 2, Philadelphia, 1985, W.B. Saunders Co.
48. Sheehan, M.P., Metzmaker, C.O.: Cancer family syndrome manifested in an extended kindred, Surg. Gynecol. Obstet. **158:**450, 1984.
49. Shinya, H., and Wolff, W.I.: Morphology, anatomic distribution, and cancer potential of colonic polyps: an analysis of 7000 polyps endoscopically removed, Ann. Surg. **190:**679, 1979.
50. Shorter, R.G.: Risks of intestinal cancer in Crohn's disease, Dis. Colon Rectum **26:**686, 1983.
51. Singleton, J.W.: Medical treatment of inflammatory bowel disease, Med. Clin. North Am. **64:**1117, 1980.
52. Soltero, M.J., and Bill, A.H.: The natural history of Meckel's diverticulum and its relation to incidental removal: a study of 202 cases of diseased Meckel's diverticulum found in King County, Washington over a fifteen-year period, Am. J. Surg. **132:**168, 1976.
53. Tepper, J.E.: Radiation therapy of colorectal cancer, Cancer **51:**2528, 1983.
54. Veidenheimer, M.C.: Rectal prolapse, Surg. Clin. North Am. **60:**451, 1980.
55. Wangensteen, O.H.: Historical aspects of the management of acute intestinal obstruction, Surgery **65:**363, 1969.
56. Watne, A.L., et al.: The occurrence of carcinoma of the rectum following ileoproctostomy for familial polyposis, Ann. Surg. **197:**550, 1983.
57. Waye, J.D.: Endoscopy of inflammatory bowel disease, Clin. Gastroenterol. **9:**279, 1980.
58. Wheat, M.W., Jr., and Ackerman, L.V.: Villous adenomas of the large intestine: clinicopathologic evaluation of 50 cases of villous adenomas with emphasis on treatment, Ann. Surg. **147:**476, 1958.
59. Willett, W.C., and MacMahon, B.: Diet and cancer: an overview. N. Engl. J. Med. **310:**697, 1984.
60. Wilson, H., et al.: Carcinoid tumors. In Ravitch, M.M., editor: Current problems of surgery, Chicago, 1970, Year Book Medical Publishers, Inc.
61. Wilson, S.M., and Adson, M.A.: Surgical treatment of hepatic metastases from colorectal cancer, Arch. Surg. **111:**330, 1976.
62. Wolmark, N., et al.: The prognostic significance of preoperative carcinoembryonic antigen levels in colorectal cancer: results from NSABP clinical trials, Ann. Surg. **199:**375, 1984.
63. Zinkin, L.D.: A critical review of the classifications and staging of colorectal cancer, Dis. Colon Rectum **26:**37, 1983.

23 Andrew M. Seal

Derangements in Intestinal Function Secondary to Previous Surgery

The principal physiologic roles of the intestinal tract are digestion and absorption of fluid, electrolytes, nutrients, and vitamins. Digestion is a complex process requiring the integration of many neural and humoral mechanisms in which gastric, pancreatic, and biliary secretions are produced to render intraluminal contents suitable for absorption. Efficient absorption requires both adequate intestinal surface area and cellular absorptive function. Although much absorption occurs uniformly throughout the bowel, preferential absorption in specific regions of the gut for certain substances is well known. The duodenum and proximal jejunum absorb calcium, folate, and iron, whereas the distal ileum absorbs vitamin B_{12} and bile salts. Of the 10 L of fluid that enter the bowel each 24 hours from oral fluid intake and secretions of the stomach, pancreas, and biliary tree, approximately 9 L are absorbed in the ileum. Numerous intestinal diseases interfere with these processes, producing maldigestion and inevitable malabsorption states.[22,29]

This chapter will discuss those mechanisms involving previous surgical procedures on the intestinal tract that contribute to these derangements of normal intestinal physiology. (For a more thorough discussion of basic intestinal physiology, see Chapter 19.)

SHORT BOWEL SYNDROME

Extensive resection of the small bowel, with or without the colon, may result in a malabsorption state known as the short bowel syndrome (SBS).[38,40,46] The three most common clinical conditions in which this syndrome occurs are: (1) bowel infarction following vascular thrombosis or embolus, (2) unrelenting progressive inflammatory bowel (Crohn's) disease requiring multiple intestinal resections over many years, and (3) trauma in which compromised blood supply necessitates removal of intestine. Less frequent causes include volvulus, neoplasia, and infarcted bowel trapped in a strangulated hernia. Survival and the subsequent degree of morbidity secondary to pathophysiologic changes induced by removal of the intestine depend on many factors, including the site and extent of resection and the nature of the underlying disease. Up to 50% of the bowel can be resected with little disturbance in normal physiology provided that the duodenum, proximal jejunum, distal ileum, and colon have been spared. If resection includes the distal ileum and right colon, however, severe diarrhea and malabsorption will develop. Loss of the ileocecal valve undoubtedly increases morbidity because of the more rapid transit time of the residual small bowel contents and the ileal reflux of colonic flora into the small bowel, resulting in a superimposed blind loop syndrome (see later discussion in this chapter).

Pathophysiology

Fluid and Electrolytes

After small bowel resection in which the colon is intact, fluid and electrolyte losses may not be excessive because the colon has an absorptive reserve capacity of up to 5 L/day. However, if the resection includes a significant loss of ileum that results in the malabsorption of bile salts, these increased luminal bile salts will not only reduce the absorption of sodium and water in the colon, but also stimulate the colon to secrete, producing a secretory or cholerheic form of diarrhea.[40] Jejunal resection is well tolerated because the increased fluid and electrolyte load presented to the ileum is reabsorbed, with any excess taken up by the colon. When both ileum and colon have been resected and only a small jejunal remnant remains, this remaining bowel is unable to concentrate luminal contents. Such patients are subject to excessive losses of isotonic water and electrolytes, leading to dehydration and the potential for severe electolyte imbalance.

Fat

Dietary fats are mainly in the form of triglycerides that are water insoluble. Pancreatic lipase is responsible for their hydrolysis to fatty acids and monoglycerides, which are rendered soluble by the presence of bile salts. Bile salts are both hydrophobic and hydrophilic and exist as small, water-soluble aggregates known as *micelles*. Once the lipolytic products have been absorbed by the enterocytes, the bile salt micelles are returned to the intestinal lumen, where they are finally absorbed by an active transport mechanism in the distal ileum. They then return to the liver to be resecreted into the biliary canaliculi, the bile ducts, and the duodenum. This sequence of events is the so-called enterohepatic circulation of bile acids.[13]

Disorders of fat digestion and absorption are well recognized in the SBS and develop for two main reasons:

1. When more than 100 cm of ileum have been resected, bile salts are lost in the stool, and the liver is unable to synthesize sufficient bile acids to maintain the bile salt pool at a concentration high enough for intraluminal micellar solubilization of fat. The unabsorbed fatty acids pass into the colon where, acting as bile acids, they impair water and ion absorption and stimulate water secretion. The fatty acid–related diarrhea produced has been termed *steatorrhea,* an important clinical feature of the short gut syndrome.

2. Optimum absorption of fat and all nutrients requires sufficient numbers of intact enterocytes. After an extensive intestinal resection, mucosal uptake may be decreased secondary to loss of absorptive surface area.

Vitamins

Vitamins A, D, E, and K depend on micellar solubilization for their absorption since they are insoluble in aqueous solution. Their absorption is therefore impaired whenever the bile salt pool is diminished, as already described. Cobalamin (vitamin B_{12}) is absorbed in the distal ileum, where specific receptors exist for the intrinsic factor–vitamin B_{12} complex. Predictably, therefore, ileal resection results in vitamin B_{12} deficiency, and such patients require long-term vitamin B_{12} replacement.[22]

Oxalate Stones

Oxalate is a metabolic end product of glycine metabolism. In healthy individuals dietary oxalate is rapidly precipitated from solution as its insoluble calcium salt. In patients with ileal resections (or ileal bypass, as discussed later), because of the bile acid and fat malabsorption, hyperabsorption of dietary oxalate occurs. The oxalate is secreted in the urine, causing hyperoxaluria. If the solubility product of calcium oxalate is exceeded and crystal nucleation occurs, oxalate nephrolithiasis may develop.

The pathogenesis of enteric hyperoxaluria involves both intraluminal and mucosal abnormalities. Intraluminal bile salt concentration is reduced, resulting in the formation of insoluble calcium salts from excess fatty acids. The concentration of calcium ions in the aqueous phase falls. The oxalate thus remains in solution and passes into the colon, where it is easily absorbed because of increased colonic mucosal permeability for small molecules produced by excess bile acids.[13]

Gastric Acid Secretion

In animals with denervated gastric pouches, hypersecretion of gastric acid after massive small bowel resection is an invariable phenomenon. In dogs with fistulas of the totally innervated stomach, however, hypersecretion does not occur.[36] In human beings hypersecretion is not invariable following intestinal resection; achlorhydria, reduced or normal acid secretion, and hypersecretion have all been reported in this condition. Furthermore, hypersecretion, when it does occur, develops acutely and subsides within the first few days following resection.[44] The validity of a hypersecretory syndrome in the patient with a short gut now seems questionable.

Gastrointestinal Hormones

The number of hormones and peptide substances thought to possess humoral actions (i.e., candidate hormones) in the gastrointestinal (GI) tract is extensive. The gut has been described as the principal and most complex endocrine organ in the body. Since the various physiologic roles of many of these hormones are unknown, a clear understanding of how their absence after extensive intestinal resection might affect normal intestinal physiology is difficult to determine.

Serum gastrin has been reportedly both elevated and normal in separate animal and human studies following extensive intestinal resection.[36] In those studies in which hypersecretion of gastric acid has been demonstrated, the cause has been ascribed to a state of hypergastrinemia. Investigators have proposed that the small bowel is a major site for gastrin metabolism and that when hypergastrinemia develops after small bowel resection, it results from a decrease in gastrin catabolism occurring after removal of the small bowel. Gastrin metabolism, however, has recently been shown *not* to be influenced by extensive small bowel resection in the dog.[35] Furthermore, arterioportal differences in serum gastrin across the splanchnic bed are unaffected by small bowel resection.[26] The role of the small bowel in the metabolism of gastrin thus appears to be insignificant.

Several other GI hormones, including secretin, insulin, and pancreatic glucagon, have also been studied after extensive intestinal resection.[4] No good evidence exists, however, to show that changes in the tissue or serum concentrations of any of these hormones can be related to the pathophysiology observed in SBS.

Perhaps the most interesting GI peptide is enteroglucagon, which becomes elevated both peripherally and in colonic and ileal tissue after small bowel resection. Although no physiologic function has been ascribed to this peptide, it is currently the principal candidate for the unknown enterotropic factor believed to be partly responsible for postresectional intestinal hyperplasia (see following section on adaptation).[42]

Motility

Motility changes in SBS are well recognized, with distal small bowel resection producing a greater decrease in transit time than proximal resection. The ileocecal valve is known to have a regulating effect on small bowel emptying. Its removal decreases transit time, but in combination with a distal small bowel resection, intestinal transit is decreased even further.[46] In studies of intestinal motility adaptation after bowel resection in rats, Nygaard[24] has shown that adaptation occurs more rapidly after proximal than after distal resection, with intestinal transit time returning to near normal after a 75% proximal resection 2 weeks after surgery. This adaptive motility response is a factor to be considered in the known greater tolerance for proximal rather than distal bowel resection.

The association between steatorrhea and small bowel hypomotility has been known for more than 50 years. Spiller and associates[37] have recently shown that ileal perfusion with fat at concentrations seen in malabsorption inhibited jejunal motility and delayed caudal transit of jejunal contents in 24 normal human subjects. They termed this phenomenon the *ileal break*. Although they exercise caution in extrapolating these results to the pathophysiology of patients who have malabsorption states, they propose that this ileal breaking mechanism could account for the adaptive prolongation of small bowel transit time that follows proximal small bowel resection, as described by Nygaard.[24] Loss of this ileal break after an ileal resection could also explain reduced adaptive lengthening of intestinal transit time seen after distal bowel resection. The mechanism is at present unknown; however, as with other enteroenteric reflexes, neural and humoral factors are thought to be responsible.

Adaptation

After small bowel resection, adaptive changes occur in the remaining bowel that lead to improved nutritional absorption and ultimately prolonged survival. These changes are both structural and functional.[28,42] Mucosal epithelial cell hyperplasia develops and is associated with an increase in villus height and crypt depth most prominent distal to the site of resection. These changes are more pronounced in the ileum after a jejunal resection than in the jejunum after an ileal resection. Functional adaptation is demonstrated by increased nutrient absorption per centimeter of gut for monosaccharides, dissacharides, water, electrolytes, calcium, amino acids, bile acids, and vitamin B_{12}. This increased uptake is thought to result from an increase in absorptive cell number rather than improved absorptive activity.

Three main mechanisms for the regulation of intestinal adaptation have been proposed: humoral, pancreaticobiliary, and luminal. Existence of a *humoral mechanism* has been tested directly in studies of parabiotic rats. In rats linked by cutaneous and vascular parabiosis, intestinal hyperplasia can be demonstrated in the nonresected group following intestinal resection in the other. Gastrin, known to be trophic for gastric and duodenal mucosa, was thought to be the humoral agent responsible.[42] Compensatory ileal hyperplasia after jejunostomy, however, can be dissociated from both exogenously infused and endogenously released gastrin, providing evidence against gastrin having a major role in intestinal adaptation. One patient has been described with an enteroglucagon-producing tumor in which intestinal hyperplasia was present.[42] Since enteroglucagon is elevated after small bowel resection, it is considered a major candidate for the unknown enterotropic humoral factor.

The importance of *pancreaticobiliary secretions* in intestinal hyperplasia remains unproved.[42] Transplantation of the duodenal papilla to the distal ileum produces local mucosal hyperplasia. A villus-enlarging factor present in papillary secretions has been proposed but remains to be identified.

Exogenous nutrients within the bowel lumen appear to be essential for the development of cellular hyperplasia. In dogs and rats receiving only parenteral nutrition after extensive intestinal resection, no structural or functional changes are seen in the remaining bowel.[42] The mechanism whereby luminal nutrients stimulate postresectional intestinal hyperplasia is unknown. They may cause release of local and/or systemic enterotropic factors in addition to bile and pancreatic secretions, with adaptive hyperplasia the result of all factors acting together.[42]

After extensive small bowel resection, the colon plays an essential role in the absorption of water and electrolytes. It may also have an endocrine role, which is yet to be fully characterized.[7] Immunocytochemistry has shown that the colon possesses many endocrine cells containing enteroglucagon, somatostatin, and 5-hydroxytryptamine. The neural peptides vasoactive intestinal peptide (VIP) and substance P are also present in high concentrations in the distal bowel. Colonic perfusion with nutrients has been shown to inhibit both gastric and pancreatic secretion.[34,36] After massive bowel resection in which proximal jejunum is anastomosed to colon, the colon's endocrine potential could become functional, replacing lost humoral activity of the small bowel and promoting adaptation. Every effort should be made to spare the colon when small bowel resection is necessary, with the enterocolonic anastomosis performed as far proximal in the colon as technically possible.

Management

Nonsurgical Treatment

An understanding of the pathophysiology of the SBS allows appropriate therapy to be undertaken. Fluid and electrolyte changes require careful monitoring in the immediate postoperative period. These patients benefit from total parenteral nutrition (TPN), which should be started as soon as possible. Depending on the extent of resection, complete oral nutrition may not be possible for several months; during this time TPN is continued. In some cases this may continue indefinitely, with patients treating themselves at home as part of an outpatient TPN program. With more than 60 to 80 cm of small bowel remaining, a refeeding program should be progressively instituted in an effort to resume alimentation with a normal or modified oral diet. Initially, solutions of isotonic carbohydrate-electrolyte feedings should be used. If patients cannot tolerate natural foods, artificial formula-defined diets are used. Since these diets are hyperosmolar, they are diluted to one-third or one-quarter strength and given through a small feeding tube by continuous drip over a 24-hour period, gradually increasing to full strength. The type of natural diet to be reinstituted is controversial. Although some believe that a low-fat diet with medium-chain triglycerides is important, high-fat diets may be beneficial.[11,15,43,45]

The use of elemental diets in GI disease has been well reviewed by Koretz and Meyer.[19] As they indicate, no good evidence shows that in SBS elemental diets are superior to polymeric diets or whole food in providing the necessary luminal stimulation for the development of compensatory hyperplasia. When an elemental diet containing free amino acid as a nitrogen source was compared with a polymeric diet containing whole protein and fat, no differences could be identified in a prospective, controlled clinical trial in 70 patients with normal gastrointestinal function.[18] Such a study remains to be performed in the setting of SBS to determine the relative efficacies of elemental and polymeric diets in these patients.

Diarrhea is the most frequent problem in the SBS, and its treatment requires an understanding of its etiology. If less than 100 cm of ileum has been removed, diarrhea is caused by excess colonic bile salts, so-called cholerheic diarrhea. This can be managed by cholestyramine, 8 to 12 g daily, which binds the unabsorbed bile acids, preventing their secretory action on the colon.[40] If more extensive bowel resection has occurred, much of the diarrhea is caused by the colonic secretory effects of hydroxy fatty acids, so-called steatorrhea, in addition to the presence of bile salts, and the osmotic effects of other unabsorbed nutrients. Cholestyramine is of no benefit to these patients, who are best treated by fat restriction.

Specific deficiencies of minerals and vitamins may develop in SBS but can be prevented by appropriate replacement therapy. Calcium, magnesium, zinc, and vitamin D supplements are beneficial. Vitamins A and K should be monitored and replaced as necessary. When the ileum has been resected, vitamin B_{12} requires parenteral replacement. The water-soluble vitamins, including folic acid and vitamin C, are absorbed throughout the bowel and are rarely deficient unless only a small jejunal remnant remains. Twenty-four-hour urinary oxalate excretion should be measured by intervals. If hyperoxaluria is present, food high in oxalate (e.g., spinach, beans, coffee, cocoa, parsley, rhubarb) should be restricted. Fat restriction may also be beneficial. Cholestyramine may diminish oxalate absorption by reducing colonic bile acid concentration, thus preventing altered mucosal permeability.

If hypersecretion of gastric acid develops in the early postoperative phase, it is best controlled with an H_2-receptor antagonist such as cimetidine. Since this abnormality is almost always transient, gastric secretory function should be monitored, and the antagonist discontinued once gastric function has returned to normal. Because of the transient nature of gastric acid hypersecretion, vagotomy should not be considered.

Surgical Treatment

In patients with SBS who have not responded to dietary and medical management, various surgical procedures have been devised (1) to delay intestinal transit time by means of reversed interpositions and (2) to enhance absorptive capacity by means of recirculating loops (Fig. 23-1). These techniques have been well reviewed and studied by Barros D'Sa[3] and Barros D'Sa, Parks, and Roy,[5] who conclude that reversed segments produce the most favorable results. With the development of parenteral nutrition and home feeding programs, however, the role of surgery in the management of patients most resistant to medical therapy has become limited.

In the future, when the survival of patients on home feeding programs becomes jeopardized by catheter-related or venous access problems, they may become candidates for intestinal transplantation. Although no successful surviving human small bowel allografts have occurred to date, success in laboratory animals is now being reported. Using a combination of cyclosporine and prednisone to combat rejection, Diliz-Perez and associates[9] have reported successful small bowel allotransplantation in dogs, with two animals surviving 550 and 555 days, respectively. A high mortality has been reported in all studies, however, with the important causes of death related to technical aspects of the transplantation, rejection, and graft vs. host disease.[9,23] As pharmacologic and surgical techniques to overcome these problems are refined, successful human intestinal transplantation will undoubtedly become a reality.

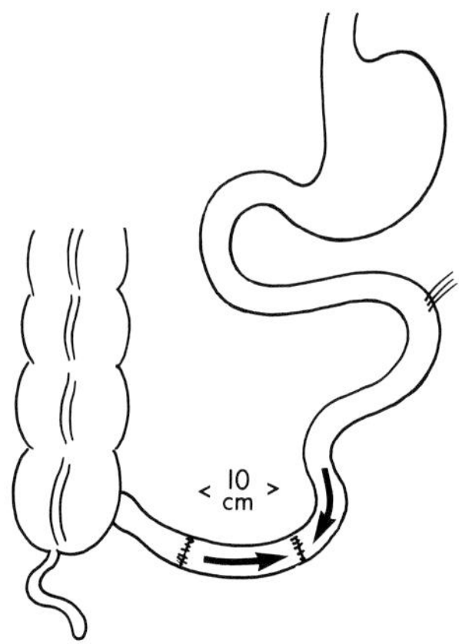

Fig. 23-1 Reversed intestinal interposition segments that may be used in the surgical management of short bowel syndrome (SBS).

INTESTINAL BYPASS

In SBS the pathophysiologic changes that occur depend on resection of a bowel that is primarily diseased. The purpose of jejunoileal bypass (JIB) surgery (Fig. 23-2) has been to produce pathophysiologic changes that will benefit the patient whose GI tract is otherwise normal. The patients who undergo this metabolic surgery have morbid obesity; the basis for their treatment is a surgically induced malabsorption state.[21] Since the subject of morbid obesity is presented in great detail in Chapter 67, this section will discuss only briefly the rationale for intestinal bypass surgery and consider its pathophysiology.

Morbid obesity has been defined as a two to three times increase in ideal body weight persistent for 5 years despite intensive nonsurgical efforts at weight reduction.[16] Such individuals are at increased risk for many disease processes and have serious social, psychologic, and economic problems. Historically the prototype procedure involved bypassing the small bowel by jejunocolic anastomosis. Mortality and morbidity were unacceptable with this procedure, however, and led to the development of JIB, as described by DeWind and Payne and associates.[8,25] The jejunum was transected 14 inches distal to Treitz's ligament, and the proximal end anastomosed end-to-side to the ileum 4 inches proximal to the ileocecal valve. Scott and co-workers[33] modified this by performing an end-to-end jejunoileal anastomosis. Several other variations have been described. The proximal end of the bypassed segment is oversewn, and its distal end anatomosed to various sites in the colon: cecum, ascending, transverse, or sigmoid (see Fig. 23-2).[27] Weight loss from these various procedures has been variable but averages 35% of the preoperative weight in the first year.

Pathophysiology and Complications

A wide array of complications associated with JIB have been described. In the obese patient the complications of any surgical procedure are more prevalent; however, those specific to intestinal bypass surgery relate to nutritional deficiencies and the excluded blind loop (see later discussion in this chapter).

Diarrhea

Diarrhea is universal in patients with JIB and commences shortly after surgery, with an initial stool frequency of up to 20 times per day. If no diarrhea is present, it can be assumed that the bypass has been inadequate. By the end of the first year, the frequency of diarrhea has usually decreased to two or three soft stools per day. In some patients the diarrhea persists, leading to severe fluid and electrolyte imbalance and necessitating reestablishment of normal anatomic intestinal continuity. The mechanisms thought to be responsible for this problem include loss of absorptive intestinal surface; excessive colonic bile and fatty acids, inducing a secretory diarrhea; and steatorrhea caused by fat malabsorption. Disaccharidase deficiency can also occur in these patients, with development of milk intolerance (suggesting a lactase deficiency) and leading to an osmotic diarrhea.

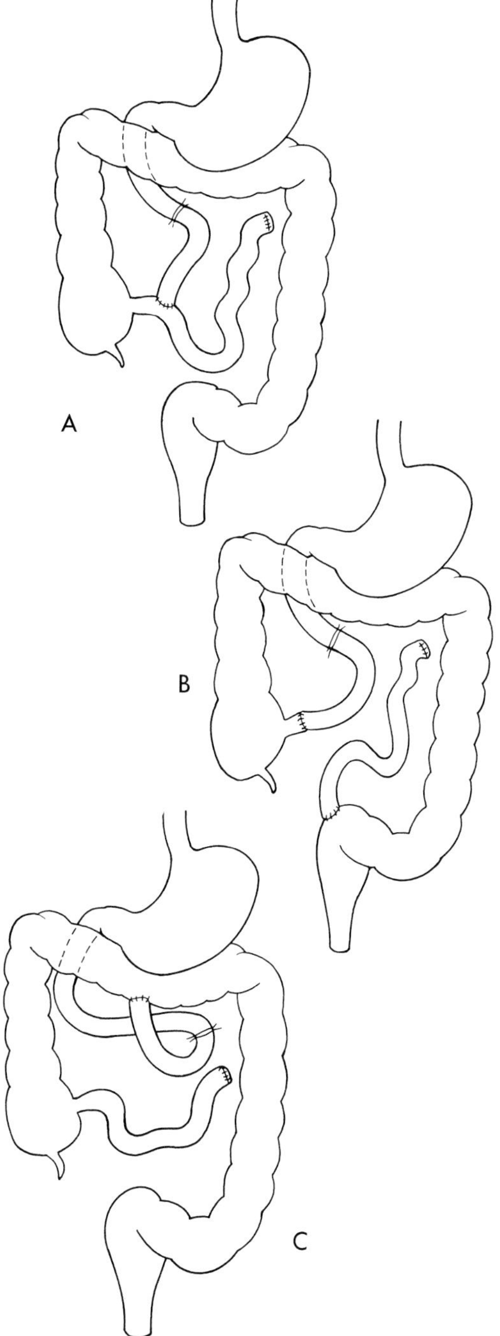

Fig. 23-2 Diagrammatic representation of various jejunoileal bypass (JIB) procedures used in the surgical treatment of morbid obesity. **A,** End-to-side jejunoileostomy. **B,** End-to-end jejunoileostomy and drainage of remaining small intestine into sigmoid colon. **C,** Jejuno-transverse colostomy.

Interestingly, although decreased stool frequency occurs with time, no evidence suggests that this can be related to changes in intestinal transit time. In a radiologic study of small bowel transit time in 10 patients before and after jejunoileostomy, preoperative times of 80 to 270 minutes were reduced postoperatively to 1 to 30 minutes. During the following 6 months, an immediate postoperative stool frequency of 6 to 12 movements per day was dramatically decreased, but transit time showed no significant tendency toward slowing. In two patients with no diarrhea at 4 years, transit times were still 2½ and 7½ minutes, compared to preoperative values of 240 and 90 minutes, respectively.[10]

Fluid, Electrolytes, Minerals, and Vitamins

Abnormalities in fluid and electrolytes are usually secondary to unrelenting diarrhea. Potassium deficiency is manifested by muscle pain, cramps, and lassitude. Potassium replacement is required until the bypass remnant is hypertrophied enough to absorb sufficient potassium from the diet. Calcium deficiency develops secondary to both malabsorption and increased saponification of excess bile acids. Patients may have acute tetany, requiring urgent intravenous calcium gluconate therapy. Long-term calcium replacement may become necessary. A magnesium deficiency that accompanies the calcium deficiency will also require appropriate replacement.

Serum vitamin B_{12} levels can be reduced by two-thirds normal after bypass surgery. Studies have demonstrated, however, that since vitamin B_{12} levels are a function of retained ileum, vitamin B_{12} deficiency may not develop if a significant length of ileum is conserved. Vitamin B_{12} deficiency was not a complication in the series by Payne and associates,[25] who suggested that reflux into the bypassed ileum may have been protective in these patients by maintaining absorption of this vitamin.

Vitamin D deficiency may also develop because of malabsorption and requires replacement.

Oxalate Stones

Hyperoxaluria typically occurs after JIB. As previously described, this is caused by hyperabsorption of dietary oxalate from the colon.[13] Urinary calculi and nephrocalcinosis occur in approximately 1% to 7% of patients after an average interval of 18 months following the bypass.

Gastric Acid Secretion

The variability of reports of altered gastric function in SBS also pertain to JIB; increased, normal, and decreased rates of acid secretion have all been described. MacLean[20] has reported the reduction of both basal and meal-stimulated acid secretion in a group of obese patients after bypass surgery. Hesselfeldt and associates,[12] using the technique of intragastric titration of a peptone meal, showed significant reduction in gastric acid secretion in five female patients after JIB. The mechanism for this reduction in meal-stimulated gastric acid secretion after JIB is not known. The concept of distal inhibition is an attractive hypothesis because, as described previously, colonic perfusion with various substances has been shown to inhibit pentagastrin-stimulated gastric acid secretion in both animals and human beings.[34,36] A reduction in gastric acid secretion after intestinal bypass thus may be partly explained by a distal intestinal inhibitory mechanism.

Gastrointestinal Hormones

In both gastric studies just mentioned,[12,20] serum gastrin levels were unchanged after bypass. Atkinson and colleagues,[1] however, have shown gastrin levels to be increased after bypass. In a large study by Sarson, Scopinaro, and Bloom[30] comparing gut hormone changes after jejunoileal and biliopancreatic bypass (see following section), serum gastrin levels were also elevated. Other GI peptides such as motilin and GIP were reduced, whereas both fasting and postprandial enteroglucagon and neurotensin levels were grossly elevated after bypass. As discussed earlier, how these changes in GI hormones relate to altered physiology has yet to be discovered.

Liver

Hepatic dysfunction is a well-recognized complication of intestinal bypass.[16] Approximately 5% of patients will develop some degree of liver failure, with 1% progressing to frank cirrhosis. Thus evidence of cirrhosis preoperatively has been a contraindication to surgery. Etiologic factors proposed to explain this hepatic dysfunction have included protein malnutrition, conversion of chenodeoxycholic acid to lithocholic acid (a known hepatotoxin), adverse intestinal bacterial metabolism of protein and bile acids, and impairment of branch-chain amino acid absorption, all of which have been shown to occur in JIB patients to varying degrees.[16]

Intestinal Complications

Other problems that may develop after JIB are related to the bypassed segment and involve mechanical or bacterial complications. The three mechanical problems described in the literature include intussusception, internal herniation through a mesenteric defect, and volvulus. Severe abdominal pain in a patient after intestinal bypass should alert the surgeon to one of these possibilities. Bypass enteritis, or the excluded loop syndrome, is caused by bacterial overgrowth in the bypassed limb. It may develop acutely in the postoperative period and be accompanied by pneumatosis cystoides intestinalis (intestinal emphysema), gangrene, and sepsis. Colonic pseudo-obstruction may be seen as a late complication and has been noted from 18 months to 3 years after bypass. The obstruction is always distal to the point in which the ileum is drained into the colon; the mechanism is unknown.[16,27]

Biliopancreatic Bypass

Scopinaro and colleagues[32] have described a method of intestinal bypass in which the jejunum is transected 20 cm distal to Treitz's ligament and the proximal jejunal loop anastomosed to the distal ileum. In addition, partial gastrectomy is performed, the duodenal stump closed, and a gastrojejunostomy created with the distal part of the transected jejunum (Fig. 23-3). Although experience with this procedure is limited, the physiologic principles underlying it are interesting. The rationale is to separate the biliopancreatic secretion from ingested food and thus produce selective maldigestion of starch and fat, leaving the enterohepatic circulation of bile acids undisturbed. Early results have been encouraging. None of the complications associated with JIB has been seen. Weight loss has reached 34% of preoperative weight at 12 months. The absence of both indiscriminant malabsorption and a long excluded loop are believed responsible for the lack of complications. The role of biliopancreatic bypass in obesity surgery awaits further evaluation.

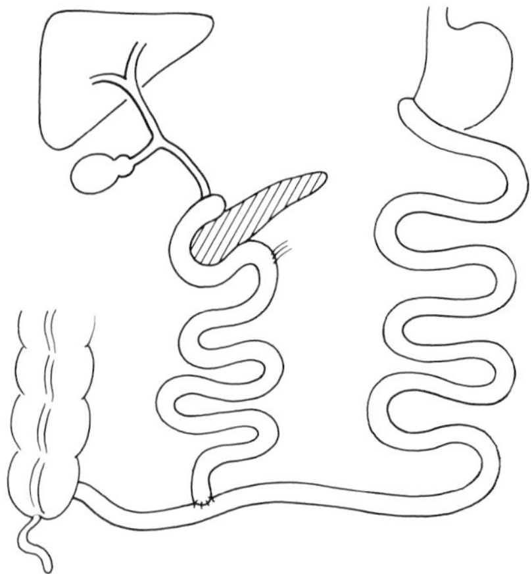

Fig. 23-3 Biliopancreatic bypass.

Adaptation

The functional, nonbypassed intestinal remnant undergoes hypertrophy, dilation, and elongation. Jejunal villi lengthen, and ileal crypts deepen. Although total intestinal absorptive surface area is reduced almost 90% after bypass, within 2 years the surface area available for absorption will have trebled. Mucosal disaccharidase, alkaline phosphatase, thymidine kinase, and fat transportation are all increased.[16] The mechanism for adaptation in this remnant remains unknown, but luminal secretory and humoral factors have been proposed.

Management

Correction of fluid, electrolyte, and mineral deficiency should be managed by replacement therapy. Diarrhea is treated by diphenoxylate and atropine (Lomotil), codeine phosphate, loperamide, and fat restriction. Liver failure requires treatment by enteral or parenteral nutrition. Since liver failure is reversible if normal intestinal anatomy is reestablished, it should be recognized early. Anatomic reconstruction for this complication accounts for 36% of second surgeries.

Future of Bypass Surgery

JIB has fallen into disfavor as an acceptable procedure in the surgical treatment of morbid obesity at most medical centers. Its prohibitive complications have discredited its usefulness and have led to the development of alternative procedures, particularly gastric bypass or partitioning (see Chapter 67). But these gastric procedures are not without significant complications, including anastomotic leaks, perforations, obstruction, hemorrhage, and the dumping syndrome. Biliopancreatic bypass appears to have fewer problems than JIB but has yet to gain wide acceptance. The role of surgery in the management of morbid obesity is thus unresolved and will require constant reevaluation in the future before its ultimate place is defined.

BLIND LOOP SYNDROME

Malabsorption of vitamin B_{12} (cobalamin) leading to a megaloblastic anemia, in association with steatorrhea secondary to fat malabsorption, are the two characteristic features of the blind loop syndrome (BLS).[39] This syndrome has also been called the *stagnant loop syndrome, contaminated small bowel syndrome,* and *bacterial overgrowth syndrome;* each title indicates an abnormality of intestinal function that leads to an increase in small bowel bacterial microflora. The syndrome can develop when the mechanisms controlling the size of the intestinal bacterial population are disturbed. The bacterial microflora of the small bowel under normal conditions consists of less than 10^4 organisms/ml of intestinal fluid. In the BLS this figure may reach as much as 10^{10} organisms/ml, with the organisms resembling those of colonic microflora and consisting predominantly of enteric coliforms and strict anaerobes. The mechanisms that control the small bowel bacterial population include gastric acid secretion and intestinal motility. The ileocecal valve is also an important functional barrier that keeps the anaerobic colonic contents from entering the small bowel.[14]

Surgical procedures associated with this bacterially induced malabsorption state include (Fig. 23-4):

1. Afferent loop stasis after Billroth II gastrectomy or gastroenterostomy
2. Blind loop secondary to obstructed or bypassed bowel
3. Enteroenterostomy
4. Jejunoileal bypass
5. Continent ileostomy (Koch pouch) after colectomy
6. Loss of ileocecal valve

Other predisposing conditions that may or may not be surgically induced include strictures (Crohn's disease, radiation, adhesions), fistulas (gastrojejunocolic), motility disturbances (scleroderma, pseudo-obstruction), achlorhydria, and diverticula (Meckel's, intestinal).

Bacterial overgrowth in the small bowel may lead to an extreme state of malnutrition with severe weight loss and protein deficiency that can resemble kwashiorkor. Patients usually have less advanced disease, however, and their signs and symptoms are primarily moderate weight loss, megaloblastic anemia, and diarrhea.

Pathophysiology

Fat

The excess bacteria in the small bowel, particularly anaerobes, deconjugate bile salts to liberate free unconjugated bile acids. The bile salt concentration then falls below the level critical for micellar formation, with resulting fat malabsorption and steatorrhea, as previously described.

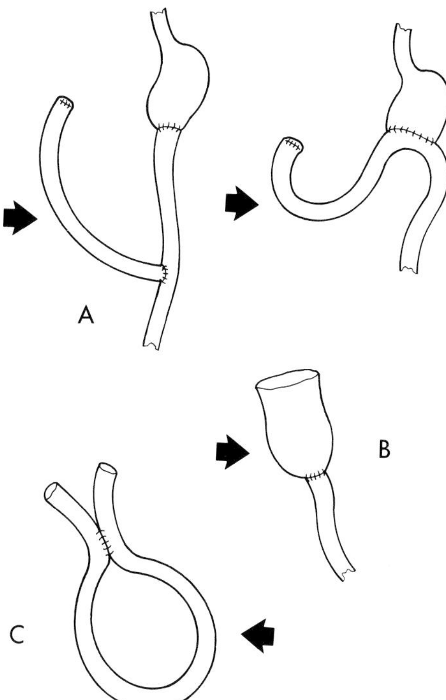

Fig. 23-4 Surgical procedures that may result in the development of a blind loop. Arrows indicate those areas possibly functioning as blind loops. **A,** Intestinal cul de sac. Blind loop syndrome from a cul-de-sac may develop if an obstruction of a Roux-en-Y limb or afferent loop occurs. **B,** Intestinal stricture. The bowel proximal to a strictured anastomosis may give rise to the blind loop syndrome. **C,** Blind loop intestine. An intentionally created blind loop to bypass a portion of intestine may give rise to blind loop syndrome.

Vitamin B_{12}

Vitamin B_{12} malabsorption in BLS is caused by the excessive anaerobic bacteria, particularly bacteroides, competing with intrinsic factor (IF) for available luminal vitamin B_{12}. The bacteria are also able to detach vitamin B_{12} bound to IF and internalize and metabolize it to inactive substances called cobamides. These latter substances are excreted in the gut and can combine with IF to block the ileal vitamin B_{12} receptor sites.[2]

Protein

Alterations in protein digestion and absorption can occur in BLS, although the mechanisms are not well understood.[6] Several factors that may contribute include (1) intraluminal bacterial catabolism, (2) decreased uptake and transport secondary to reduced brush border peptidase activity, (3) a decrease in enterokinase, and (4) loss of endogenous protein from mucosal defects. Impairment of albumin synthesis may be a nonspecific effect secondary to hepatic damage, as seen after JIB.

Carbohydrates

Malabsorption of carbohydrates occurs infrequently in BLS. When present, it may result from impaired disaccharidase activity and monosaccharide absorption secondary to mucosal damage. The resulting increased osmotic load can contribute to the diarrhea.

Motility

The human small intestine has a cyclic pattern of motor activity that has been divided into three phases: Phase I, the resting phase; Phase II, regular activity; and Phase III, regular rapid spikes of myoelectric activity that sustain an increase in intraluminal pressure over 1 to 3 minutes. Phase III is characterized by a wave of contraction moving down the small bowel on average once every 2 hours in fasting persons. This is known as the migrating myoelectric complex (MMC) and is under both neural and humoral control. Abnormalities in Phase III activity have been reported in patients[14,41] with the bacterial overgrowth syndrome in whom the MMCs were absent. Antibiotic therapy successfully corrected the syndrome, and Phase III activity was restored to normal.[14] (For a more extensive discussion of the MMC, see Chapter 20.)

Mucosal Damage

Morphologic changes in BLS include blunting and broadening of villi with brush border damage and an increase in mononuclear cells in the lamina propria.[14] The lesion may resemble glutin-sensitive enteropathy. Biochemical and functional abnormalities following these changes include decreased brush border activity, decreased intracellular enzymes, and defects in mucosal uptake of amino acids and sugars. The pathogenesis of mucosal injury is uncertain. Excess free bile acids and elastase-like enzymes produced by the intestinal bacteria are considered possible etiologic factors.[17]

Management

The therapeutic approaches to BLS are directed at reducing the altered abnormal intestinal flora, treating the malabsorption state, and correcting any surgically amenable abnormality where possible. Since BLS consists of several features, notably vitamin B_{12} deficiency and steatorrhea, their presence in a patient whose history includes previous intestinal surgery should alert the physician to the possibility of BLS.

Tests to demonstrate bacterial overgrowth include intestinal intubation for fluid analysis and specific breath analysis tests.[14,29,39] Aspiration of intestinal fluid allows direct examination of small bowel contents for qualification of the bacterial population. Breath tests are noninvasive and provide indirect evidence of intestinal bacterial overgrowth. The tests consist of the timed analysis of volatile metabolites produced by intestinal bacteria and excreted in the breath.

The bile acid test measures expired $^{14}CO_2$ released by bacterial cleavage of the amide bond linking ^{14}C-1 glycine in cholic acid. It has a 30% false-negative rate and has been partly replaced by the more sensitive xylose breath test. Xylose is normally entirely absorbed and excreted unmetabolized in the urine. In patients with BLS, after administration of 1 g of ^{14}C-xylose, 85% have elevated $^{14}CO_2$ levels in their breath within 60 minutes. Hydrogen breath analysis is also used and detects excess bacterial hydrogen production after administration of 50 g of glucose or 10 g of lactulose. This test also has a high false-negative rate. When the results of all breath tests are combined, however, accuracy approaches 90%. (These tests are discussed in greater detail in Chapter 19.)

Other tests of importance in patients with BLS include quantitative measurements of 72-hour fecal fat excretion to determine the presence of steatorrhea and the Schilling test for vitamin B_{12} and intrinsic factor absorption (see Chapter 19). Contrast radiologic studies of the small bowel will often demonstrate anatomic abnormalities of the mucosa and may be particularly helpful as a diagnostic modality in these patients.

Treatment of BLS may be divided into two main groups: surgical and medical.

Surgical

Surgical correction of the underlying cause is the ideal form of treatment because it is curative. The lesions amenable to surgical cure include short intestinal segments involved by diverticula, strictures, fistulas, and tumors; Billroth II anatomoses; and reversal of JIB.[2,31] Unfortunately most patients with BLS do not have surgically correctable lesions or are too debilitated to withstand surgery. Patients with generalized intestinal disorders such as systemic sclerosis, pseudo-obstruction, multiple intestinal diverticulosis, diabetic enteropathy, and scleroderma clearly are not surgical candidates.

Medical

Medical management employs antimicrobial therapy and nutritional replacement and support.[2,31,39] A broad-spectrum antibiotic is given, with tetracycline the usual drug of choice in a dose of 250 to 500 mg four times a day. Other agents used include metronidazole, chloramphenicol, erythromycin, and clindamycin. A single 10-day course with one of the antibiotics may often render a patient symptom free for many months. Other patients may require intermittent courses of therapy, alternating between two or three different antibiotics. The aim of therapy is to induce a remission of signs and symptoms, as judged by normalization of fat absorption studies and the Schilling test. Nutritional support includes fat restriction, lactose restriction, parenteral vitamin B_{12}, and supplements of fat-soluble vitamins A, D, and K as indicated. Calcium, magnesium, and zinc may also be necessary. If patients have unusually severe diarrhea, they may have excessive fluid and electrolyte losses that require intravenous replacement. Intravenous hyperalimentation may also be life saving for the patient with advanced malnutrition.

SUMMARY

Previous surgery on the intestinal tract may induce several derangements in intestinal physiology that may adversely affect the digestion and absorption of a variety of nutrients, including minerals and vitamins and that may result in malnutrition, vitamin deficiencies, and electrolyte imbalance. Such derangements can generally be grouped under the broad headings of short bowel syndrome, intestinal bypass, and the blind loop syndromes. Although management of these conditions can tax the ingenuity and clinical skills of the best physician, an understanding of their pathophysiology and the consequent alteration in normal physiology will provide a sound basis for appropriate treatment. Often a second surgical procedure will be required to restore normal physiology and eliminate symptoms. When this is not possible, various nonsurgical treatments will prove efficacious in most patients.

REFERENCES

1. Atkinson, R.L., et al.: Gastrin secretion after weight loss by dieting and intestinal bypass surgery, Gastroenterology **77**:696, 1979.
2. Banwell, J.G., et al.: Clinical conference: small intestinal bacterial overgrowth syndrome, Gastroenterology **80**:834, 1981.
3. Barros D'Sa, A.A.B.: An experimental evaluation of segmental reversal after massive small bowel resection, Br. J. Surg. **66**:493, 1979.
4. Barros D'Sa, A.A.B., and Buchanan, K.D.: Role of gastrointestinal hormones in the response to massive resection of the small bowel, Gut **18**:877, 1977.
5. Barros D'Sa, A.A.B., Parks, T.G., and Roy, A.D.: The problems of massive small bowel resection and difficulties encountered in management, Postgrad. Med. J. **54**:323, 1978.
6. Curtis, K.J., Prizont, R., and Kin, Y.S.: Protein digestion and absorption in the blind loop syndrome, Dig. Dis. Sci. **24**:929, 1979.
7. Debas, H.T.: The colon as an endocrine organ, (editorial), Dig. Dis. Sci. **26**:193, 1981.
8. DeWind, L.T., and Payne, J.H.: Intestinal bypass surgery for morbid obesity: long-term results, JAMA **236**:2298, 1976.
9. Diliz-Perez, H.S., et al.: Successful small bowel allotransplantation in dogs with cyclosporine and prednisone, Transplantation **37**(2):126, 1984.
10. Gothlin, J., Andersson, K.E., and Dencker, J.: Small bowel transit time and roentgenological changes in the intestinal mucosa after jejunoileostomy in obese patients, Acta Chir. Scand. **144**:45, 1978.
11. Greenberger, N.J.: State of the art: the management of the patient with short bowel syndrome, Am. J. Gastroenterol. **70**:528, 1978.
12. Hesselfeldt, P., et al.: Meal-stimulated gastric acid and gastrin secretion before and after jejuno-ileal shunt operation in obese patients, a preliminary report, Scand. J. Gastroenterol. **14**:13, 1979.
13. Hoffman, A.F.: The enterohepatic circulation of bile acids in health and disease. In Sleisenger, M.H., and Fordtran, J.S., editors: Gastrointestinal disease: pathophysiology, diagnosis, management, Philadelphia, 1983, W.B. Saunders Co.
14. Isaacs, P.E.T., and Kim, Y.S.: Blind loop syndrome and small bowel bacterial contamination, Clin. Gastroenterol. **12**:395, 1983.
15. Jeejeebhoy, K.N.: Therapy of the short-gut syndrome, Lancet **1**:1427, 1983.
16. Joffe, S.N.: Progress report: surgical management of morbid obesity, Gut **22**:242, 1981.
17. Jonas, A., and Forstner, C.G.: Pathogenesis of mucosal injury in the blind loop syndrome, Gastroenterology **75**:791, 1978.
18. Jones, B.J.M., et al.: Comparison of an elemental and polymeric enteral diet in patients with normal gastrointestinal function, Gut **24**:78, 1983.
19. Koretz, R.L., and Meyer, J.H.: Elemental diets—facts and fantasies, Gastroenterology **78**:393, 1980.
20. MacLean, L.D.: Intestinal bypass operations for obesity: a review, Can. J. Surg. **19**:387, 1976.
21. Mason, E.E.: Surgical treatment of obesity: major problems in clinical surgery, vol. 26, Philadelphia, 1981, W.B. Saunders Co.
22. May R.J., Nath, B.J., and Shapiro, R.H.: Altered gut absorption in disease. In Fisher, J.E., editor: Surgical nutrition, Boston, 1983, Little, Brown & Co.
23. Nordgren, S., et al.: Functional monitors of rejection in small intestinal transplants, Am. J. Surg. **147**:152, 1984.
24. Nygaard, K.: Resection of the small intestine in rats, Acta Chir. Scand. **133**:407, 1967.
25. Payne, J.H., et al.: Surgical treatment of morbid obesity: sixteen years of experience, Arch. Surg. **106**:432, 1973.
26. Pensler, J.M., et al.: The small intestine: not a significant source of gastrin metabolism, Surg. Forum **31**:177, 1980.
27. Phillips, R.B.: Small intestinal bypass for the treatment of morbid obesity, Surg. Gynecol. Obstet. **146**:455, 1978.
28. Robinson, J.W.L., Dowling, R.H., and Riecken, E.O., editors: Mechanisms of intestinal adaptation, Thirtieth Falk Symposium, Titisee, West Germany, 1981, Higham, 1982, MTP Press Ltd.
29. Ryan, M.E., and Olsen, W.A.: A diagnostic approach to malabsorption syndromes: a pathophysiological approach, Clin. Gastroenterol. **12**:533, 1983.
30. Sarson, D.L., Scopinaro, N., and Bloom, S.R.: Gut hormone changes after jejunoileal (JIB) and biliopancreatic (BPB) bypass surgery for morbid obesity, Int. J. Obes. **5**:471, 1981.
31. Savino, J.A.: Malabsorption secondary to Meckel's diverticulum, Am. J. Surg. **144**:588, 1982.
32. Scopinaro, N., et al.: Bilio-pancreatic bypass for obesity. II. Initial experience in man, Br. J. Surg. **66**:618, 1979.
33. Scott, H.W., et al.: New considerations in use of jejunoileal bypass in patients with morbid obesity, Ann. Surg. **177**:723, 1973.
34. Seal, A.M., and Debas, H.T.: Colonic inhibition of gastric acid secretion in the dog, Gastroenterology **79**:823, 1980.
35. Seal, A.M., Debas, H.T., and Taylor, I.L.: Small bowel resection does not affect gastrin metabolism in the dog, Ann. R. Coll. Phys. Surg. (Can.) **15**:292, 1982.
36. Seal, A.M., et al.: Gastric and pancreatic hyposecretion following massive small bowel resection, Dig. Dis. Sci. **27**:117, 1982.
37. Spiller, R.C., et al.: The ileal brake—inhibition of jejunal motility after ileal fat perfusion in man, Gut **25**:365, 1984.
38. Tilson, M.D.: Pathophysiology and treatment of the short bowel syndrome, Surg. Clin. North Am. **60**:1273, 1980.
39. Toskes, P.P., and Donaldson, R.M.: The blind loop syndrome. In Sleisenger, M.H., and Fordtran, J.S., editors: Gastrointestinal disease: pathophysiology, diagnosis, management, Philadelphia, 1983, W.B. Saunders Co.
40. Trier, J.S.: The short bowel syndrome. In Sleisenger, M.H., and Fordtran, J.S., editors: Gastrointestinal disease: pathophysiology, diagnosis, management, Philadelphia, 1983, W.B. Saunders Co.
41. Vantrappen G., et al.: The interdigestive motor complex of normal subjects and patients with bacterial overgrowth of the small intestine, J. Clin. Invest. **59**:1158, 1977.
42. Weser, E.: Nutritional aspects of malabsorption: short gut adaptation, Clin. Gastroenterol. **12**:443, 1983.
43. Weser, E., Fletcher, J.T., and Urban, E.: Clinical conference: short bowel syndrome, Gastroenterology **77**:572, 1979.
44. Windsor, C.W.O., Fejfar, J., and Woodward, D.A.K.: Gastric secretion after massive small bowel resection, Gut **10**:779, 1969.
45. Woolf, G.M., et al.: Diet for patients with a short bowel: high fat or high carbohydrate? Gastroenterology **84**:823, 1983.
46. Wright, H.K., and Tilson, M.D.: The short gut syndrome: pathophysiology and treatment. In Current problems in surgery, Chicago, 1971, Yearbook Medical Publishers.

24 Hepatic Physiology

Ronald C. Merrell

The liver has been regarded as a critical structure from the earliest time of written records. It was a vital feature of mummification in Egypt, studied by seers in the Roman rites of entrail reading, and regarded by the Galenic school as the seat of life. It is not an accident of etymology that the teutonic word "liver" reflects the importance to life attributed to the liver by teutonic and Gallic tribes. This chapter will present the metabolic importance of the liver on the basis of current biochemical knowledge. The liver is the gatekeeper separating the splanchnic or digestive intake circulation from the systemic circulation that reflects the consumption of this digestive intake. In its gatekeeper role the liver plays the most important role in homeostasis by ensuring flow of amino acid, lipid, and carbohydrate substrate to the systemic circulation over a wide range of fasting, fed, and starved circumstances. However, the liver is also the victim of most of the pathologic processes of the remainder of the body, and it must either heal itself or fail. That failure, if total, results in death.

HEPATIC ANATOMY

The liver is the largest organ in the body and weighs between 1200 to 1500 g. The liver primordium is an endodermal derivate that appears in the middle of the third week of embryonic life at the distal end of the foregut. This hepatic diverticulum invades the transverse septum between the pericardial cavity and the yolk sac as a rapidly growing cell mass. The anlage is invaded from the yolk sac by vitelline venous radicals that will ultimately form the portal venous system and by umbilical venous radicals from the placenta to form a capillary network of sinusoids along which the hepatocytes proliferate.[17]

After birth the umbilical vein obliterates, leaving the liver with two sources of blood: (1) the former vitelline network of splanchnic circulation through the portal vein and (2) the hepatic artery. The dual blood supply is entirely appropriate for the function of the liver as a digestive organ, enabling it to adequately respond to the metabolic demands of the whole organism. Substrate coming from the gastrointestinal tract through the portal vein is modulated by the liver in response to the requirements of systemic homeostasis communicated by hepatic artery plasma.

The dual blood supply merges in the hepatic sinusoids and is collected from this site into the hepatic veins. The blood supply divides the liver into left and right lobes, which cleave in a plane that passes through the bed of the gallbladder and inferior vena cava. The blood supply to the liver enters at the porta hepatis, and the three hepatic veins join the vena cava behind the liver. The arborization of the blood supply to the liver further divides the structure into anterior and posterior segments of the right lobe, the medial and lateral segments of the left lobe, the quadrate lobe anterior to the porta hepatis, and the caudate lobe posterior to the porta. The segments of the liver are divided by fissure planes not apparent on the surface of the liver, which are important surgically in planning partial hepatic resections. The falciform ligament attaches the liver to the anterior abdominal wall and diaphragm and contains the obliterated umbilical vein in the ligamentum teres hepatis. The liver is further attached to the diaphragm by the right and left triangular ligaments.[22]

From the porta hepatis radicals of the hepatic artery and portal vein and tributaries of the bile duct follow one another in a branching pattern to end in fibrous tracts called portal triads, which have a perpendicular orientation to the hepatic venous radicals (Fig. 24-1). Between the portal triads and the hepatic venules are the hepatic sinusoids lined by endothelium and highly specialized reticuloendothelial elements known as the Kupffer cells. The sinusoids traverse a column of 12 to 20 hepatocytes. Blood does not directly bathe hepatocytes because they are separated from it by the endothelium of the sinusoid and its basal lamina. This basal lamina, however, is quite porous, unlike other capillary basement membranes. Therefore the hepatocyte does not interact with an ultrafiltrate of blood but instead receives an abundant flow of plasma with a protein concentration of some 6 g/100 ml. The hepatocyte does not actually share the basal lamina of the sinusoid but is separated from it by the space of Disse, which receives the plasma filtrate from the sinusoid, allowing the sinusoidal aspect of the hepatocyte to interact with this fluid and ultimately deliver it to the lymphatics. Even though the degree of filtration is brisk, the sinusoid still obeys Starling's law of capillaries, resulting in a return of most fluid to the sinusoid at the low pressure end toward the hepatic venules. This large volume of filtration is only evident when hepatic venous pressure rises and high protein fluid accumulates in the form of ascites.[12]

Although hepatocytes are not subtended by the basal

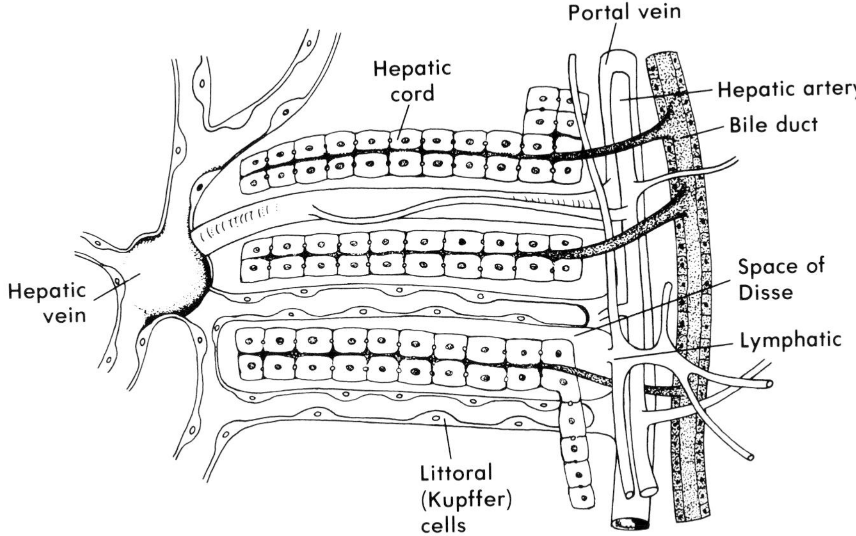

Fig. 24-1 Portal triad structures are at a right angle to hepatic vein tributaries. Between portal elements and the central vein are the hepatic sinusoids, the units of hepatic function.

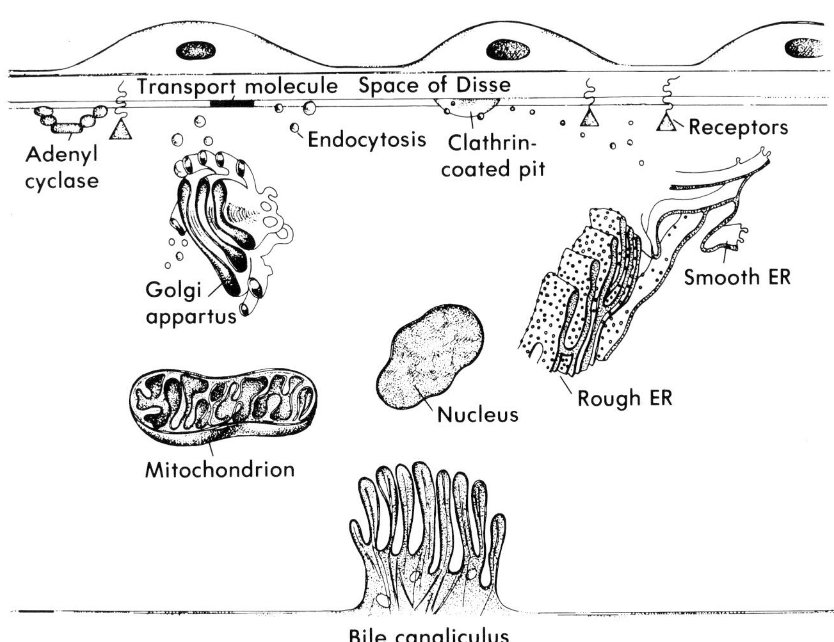

Fig. 24-2 The hepatocyte is a highly polar cell that relates (1) to the space of Disse, source of the plasma filtrate that reflects systemic metabolic requirements and incoming substrate, or (2) to the bile canaliculus, exit point for export of bile. Plasma relationship is quantitatively much more important, occupying much more surface area. The hepatocyte also communicates with adjacent adherent hepatocytes through gap junctions. *ER,* Endoplasmic reticulum.

lamina of the sinusoid, the cords of cells that they form are tightly bound to one another. These cords are drained by the bile canaliculi that gather that portion of hepatocyte secretions destined for bile. The hepatocyte is the major cell of the liver, and it uses the unique architecture of the liver to accomplish its function. Hepatocytes comprise 60% of all hepatic cells, representing approximately 1.7 $\times 10^5$ cells per milligram tissue. The hepatocyte is a large polyhedral cell with a diameter of 25 to 30 μm. These cells divide frequently and renew themselves continually; studies in rats have revealed their life span to be about 300 days.[22] The nucleus of the hepatocyte is usually single but is occasionally multiple. On the plasma side of the hepatocyte, a rich array of receptors gathers information and transports critical substrate, hormones, and carrier proteins into the cell. The hepatocyte then processes this information and dispenses appropriate metabolic products back into the plasma or into the bile canaliculi at the other side of the cell (Fig. 24-2). The number of Kupffer cells is about one fifth the number of hepatocytes. These cells are functionally macrophages and represent 30% of the total body fixed macrophages.

HEPATIC FUNCTIONS

Filtration (i.e., reticuloendothelial system)
- Process incoming substrate & vitamins

Metabolic Homeostasis
- ***Fundamental mechanisms***
  - Capture
  - Maintenance of intracellular metabolism
  - Storage
  - Release
- ***Metabolic substrates***
  - Carbohydrates—modulate glucose
  - Lipids—modulate free fatty acids
  - Amino acids—modulate amino acid pools

Specific Protein Synthesis
- Coagulation: Fibrinogen; Prothrombin; VII, IX, X
- Carrier proteins: Albumin; Transferrin; Lipoprotein

Lipid Phase Metabolism
- Drug metabolism
- Bile formation
- Lysosomal and nonlysosomal transport

NORMAL HEPATIC FUNCTIONS

The liver filters the incoming splanchnic blood to remove bacteria and to process transported substrate and vitamins (see boxed material above). It also processes systemic blood to monitor and maintain plasma levels of glucose, lipids, and amino acids by recognizing concentrations by means of mass action in intracellular enzyme pathways and by responding to humoral messengers or hormones by means of specific receptors. The most important of the hormones are insulin and glucagon, evoked by delivery of secretagogues to the pancreas. Maintenance of plasma levels of metabolic substrate relies on the phenomenal synthetic and degradative pathways of the hepatocytes. The liver also monitors plasma for an incredible array of chemicals (e.g., drugs) and frequently modifies them enzymatically to facilitate excretion. Hepatocytes secrete bile into the canalicular system and newly synthesized plasma proteins into the space of Disse. These proteins include albumin, carrier proteins for various substances, and clotting factors. The hepatocyte without question expresses phenotypically more of the human genome than any other cell of the body by using virtually every enzyme, receptor, and transport mechanism in the genetic library. The liver cannot be replaced by mechanical, physical, or biochemical supports that do not use viable hepatocytes themselves. The anhepatic state is not compatible with life for more than a few hours, and liver failure is a highly relative term in discussing compromise of any of its functions. If the liver truly fails, death follows shortly. But the human liver can replace itself even after massive subtotal resection with the vigor and precision of the salamander tail. Hepatic functions are outlined in the boxed material above and discussed more fully below.

Filtration

The reticuloendothelial activity of the Kupffer cells removes as much as 99% of bacteria from portal venous blood, which is fairly heavily contaminated with gastrointestinal flora. It also is able to clear endotoxin and fragments of fibrinolysis. However, the capacity of Kupffer cells to remove bacteria, especially bacilli, does not extend to viruses.[15]

By modulating the splanchnic presentation of ingested substrate and gastrointestinal hormones, the hepatocyte mass in large measure determines the systemic presentation of ingested foods and, more importantly, the systemic concentration of regulatory hormones such as insulin or glucagon. The effect of the liver on splanchnic substrate and peptides is precisely that of a filter.

Metabolic Homeostasis

Hepatic capacity to regulate general metabolism may be divided into four categories: capture, intracellular metabolism, storage, and release. Capture represents removal of substrate in the transit of blood across the liver, and this extraction is accomplished largely because active intracellular metabolism of the substrate generates a sharp gradient for the substrate across the hepatocyte plasma membrane. This gradient facilitates passive and active transport. The modified substrate can be stored as glycogen in the case of carbohydrate or accommodated in the metabolic pools in the case of amino acids. When plasma levels fall, the transhepatic gradient is reversed, and metabolites are released from the liver so that portal concentrations of, for example, glucose are lower than the concentration in the hepatic vein. All categories are modulated by (1) receptor-mediated variations in second messengers such as cAMP or calcium, (2) variations in gene expression with respect to enzymes or other receptors, or (3) mass action as the available substrate and metabolites regulate the direction and rate of the chemical reactions that are catalyzed by the enzymes pertinent to carbohydrate, lipid, and amino acid metabolism and their interrelationships.

Carbohydrates

The role of the liver in providing a steady flow of glucose is arguably the most important of its tasks. Certainly after subtotal hepatectomy the greatest early metabolic hazard is hypoglycemia. Between meals the liver exports 10 g of glucose per hour. After the ingestion of complex carbohydrates, splanchnic blood brings vast quantities of glucose, galactose, and fructose to the hepatocyte. Galactose freely enters the cell, but the rate of entry of glucose and fructose is greatly facilitated by phosphorylation at the plasma membrane. This phosphorylation in turn is activated by insulin in the portal plasma, which has a concentration 1 logarithm greater than that in systemic blood. Galactose can be converted to glucose enzymatically, and all of the hexose sugars can enter the glycolytic pathway or proceed to polymerization to glycogen. Two enzymes are critical to the liver for hexose capture and release: hexokinase and glucose-6-phosphatase. Both are present in the liver in enormous quantities. Hexokinase will phosphorylate all the common dietary monosaccharides and introduce them to glycolytic pathways. This phosphorylation is irre-

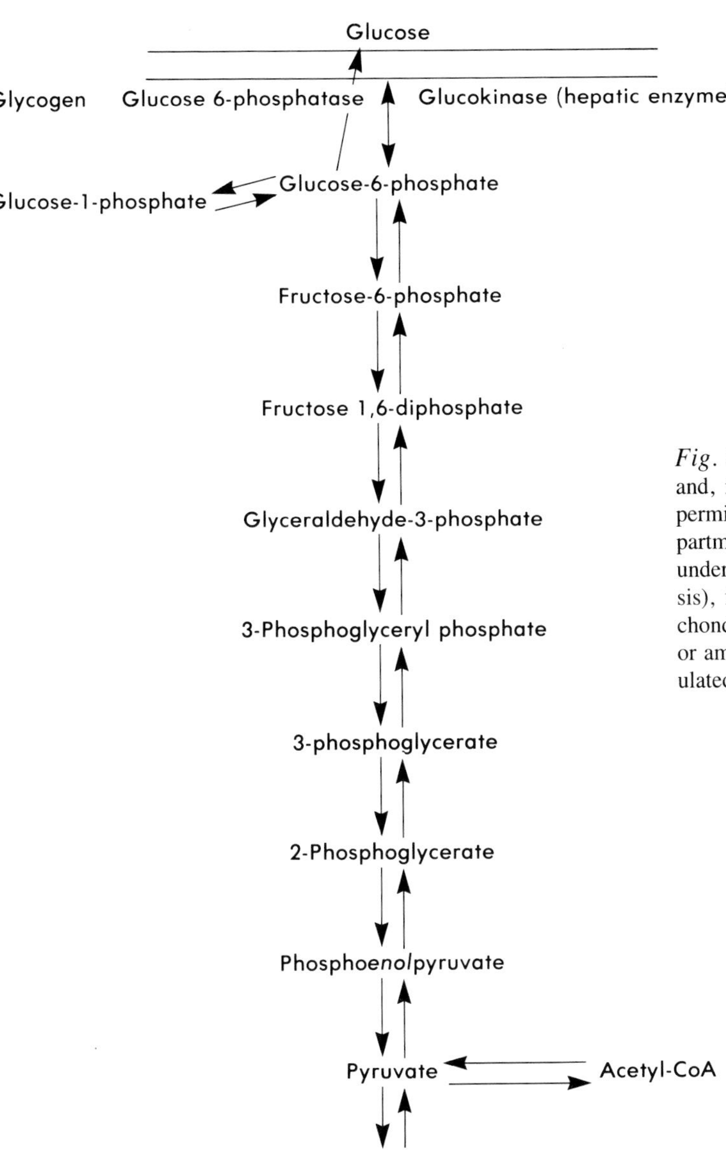

Fig. 24-3 Glycolysis. These reactions are entirely cytoplasmic and, in response to mass action, readily reversible. Reversibility permits glycolysis and gluconeogenesis in the same cellular compartment. Mass action is determined by importation of substrate under the influence of insulin (glycolysis and glycogen synthesis), facilitated exit from the pathway (pyruvate entry into mitochondria for the Kreb's cycle), or the entry of products (lactate or amino acids) that promote gluconeogenesis, an event also regulated by glucagon.

versible such that glucose release from the hepatocyte would be impossible except for another pathway involving glucose-6-phosphatase, which cleaves the phosphate group to allow molecular glucose to diffuse freely from the cell. Glucose exit can come from the reversal of the glycolytic pathway in gluconeogenesis or from glucose-1-phosphate from glycogenolysis. Phosphoglucomutase catalyzes conversion of glucose-1-phosphate to glucose-6-phosphate.[26] Glycolysis is disfavored shortly after feeding. Insulin is elevated, and intracellular cAMP is consequently reduced; therefore glycogen synthetase is not phosphorylated, and glycogen synthesis is facilitated (Fig. 24-3). After proceeding to acetyl-CoA, the carbon atoms of the original hexose can be used to synthesize fatty acids in the cytoplasm, or they may enter the mitochondria to participate in the Kreb's cycle, contributing to the electron chain of oxidative phosphorylation (Fig. 24-4).

Insulin promotes glucose storage as glycogen by reducing cytoplasmic cAMP and facilitates lipid synthesis by inducing phosphofructokinase, the rate-limiting step in glycolysis. Acetyl-CoA rises, and fatty acid synthesis is favored by mass action. Abundant presentation of glucose and insulin, as in the case of parenteral nutrition, can exceed the capacity of the hepatocyte to export the lipids on appropriate carrier proteins. This leads to fatty infiltration of the liver. Glucagon counters the effects of insulin by promoting release of glucose from the hepatocyte. This is accomplished by raising intracellular cAMP, which favors phosphorylation of glycogen and glycogenolysis by means of phosphorylase A. Glucagon also enhances the reverse of glycolysis (i.e., gluconeogenesis) by promoting hepatic transport of amino acids and deamination that produces substrates that by mass action push glycolysis in reverse. Catecholamines also promote release of glucose purely by cAMP mediation to enhance glycogenolysis. Glucose release is therefore facilitated by glycogenolysis and gluconeogenesis. The latter synthesis is aided by the arrival of amino acids, especially alanine, which is deaminated to

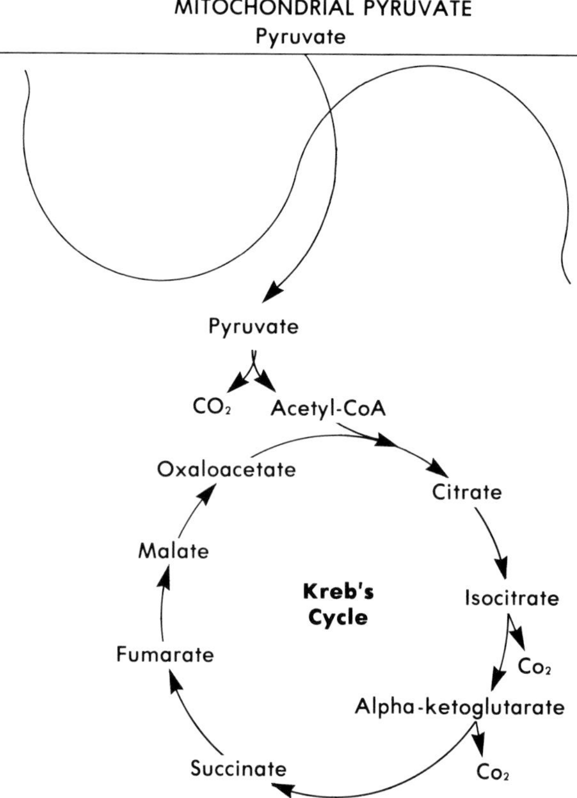

Fig. 24-4 Kreb's cycle. Pyruvate can cross the convoluted double membrane of the mitochondrion where decarboxylation produces acetate, the two-carbon fragment that enters the Kreb's cycle by reacting with oxaloacetate. This cycle generates hydrogen atoms that participate in the oxidative phosphorylation pathways along the cytochrome chain located on the christae of the mitochondrion.

pyruvate. Gluconeogenesis is also supported (through the Cori cycle) by lactate coming to the liver from active muscle engaged in anaerobic metabolism. Lactate enters the gluconeogenic pathway after lactate dehydrogenase catalyzes its conversion to pyruvate.

Lipids

The liver is the major organ of traffic for lipid metabolism. Dietary lipids arrive from the gastrointestinal tract in chylomicrons and from the periphery as high-density lipoproteins. The lipoprotein complexes are processed by the liver in the lysosomal pathway whereby receptors on the sinusoidal aspect of the hepatocytes take up the lipoproteins in specialized depressions in the plasma membrane that are studded with a molecule called clathrin and termed clathrin-coated pits. As receptors are occupied in these pits, the cytoskeleton on the internal aspect of the cell changes to permit an internal pinching off of the pit through endocytosis to form an intracellular vesicle. These vesicles fuse with lysosomes where the acidic lysosomal pH dissociates the receptor and lipoprotein. The receptor recycles to the plasma membrane, and the unbound lipid then becomes available for several fates.

If lipid content in the hepatocyte is high, the dietary fat may be released from the hepatocyte back into the space of Disse in a complex carrier form, i.e., either very low-density lipoprotein (VLDL) or low-density lipoprotein (LDL). If there is a catabolic profile of enzyme availability and mass action is permissive, the lipid is degraded to free fatty acid, then forms fatty acyl-CoA, reacts with carnitine, and is subsequently transported into the mitochondria where the carnitine is recycled and the fatty acid reacts with intra-mitochondral coenzyme A (CoA) for beta oxidation to acetyl-CoA. Acetyl-CoA then enters the pathway of oxidative phosphorylation. Conversely, when metabolic demand calls for lipid synthesis, the acetyl-CoA from carbohydrate or amino acid degradation, which derives from pyruvate diffusing into the mitochondrion, may return to the cytoplasm through the carnitine shuttle. The acetyl group reacts with coenzyme A in the cytoplasm. Alternatively, acetyl-CoA in the mitochondrion reacts with oxaloacetate as the first step in the Kreb's cycle to produce citrate that can exit the mitochondrion to react with the citrate cleavage enzyme in the cytoplasm to regenerate acetyl-CoA (Fig. 24-5). By either route cytoplasmic acetyl-CoA is available to join the acyl carrier protein in the primary reaction of fatty acid synthesis. The acetyl group condenses with malonyl-S-acyl carrier protein to initiate chain elongation, which proceeds by addition of further acetyl groups. The movement of lipid carbons across the compartments of synthesis (cytoplasm) or degradation (mitochondrion) is regulated by mass action effects and insulin, the latter by means of regulation of citrate cleavage enzyme and fatty acid synthetase.[18] Glucagon favors fatty acid degradation and the export of acetoacetate or beta-hydroxy butyrate, which are ketogenic four-carbon molecules.

Synthesized or processed dietary fatty acids that can diffuse out of the mitochondrion without entering the Kreb's cycle in the hepatocyte can react with the hydroxyl groups of glycerol to form triglycerides or diglycerides. The diglycerides may be phosphorylated at the third carbon atom of the three-carbon sugar and ultimately react with choline to form phosphatidyl choline (lecithin), a major lipid for membrane assembly and export into bile. Acetyl-CoA in the cytoplasm may also find its way into cholesterol, a major lipid product of the liver that may be used locally for membranes, exported to the plasma, secreted into the bile directly, or metabolized to bile salts for secretion into bile.

The liver regulates lipid metabolism systemically by release of free fatty acids from the diet or synthesis, diversion of carbohydrate or amino acid carbons to lipids, extraction of lipids from the blood for beta oxidation, and synthesis of lipid carrier proteins.

Amino Acids

The liver receives dietary amino acids after digestion and transports them actively into the cytoplasm so that only a fraction enter the systemic circulation directly. The amino acid pool in the liver may contribute to the synthesis of induced hepatic peptides such as enzymes, plasma proteins, or receptors; or the amino acids may be metabolized to intermediates that by transamination can be converted from one amino acid that is abundant into another that is not appropriately represented in the amino acid pool.

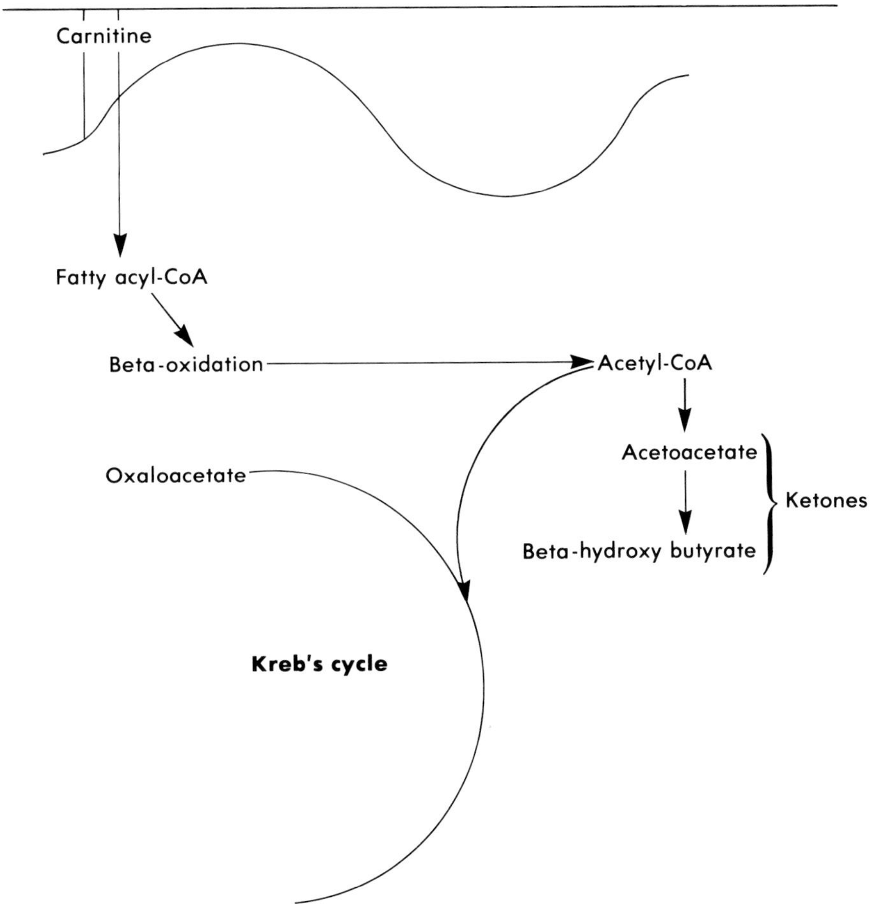

Fig. 24-5 The mitochondrion is the degradative compartment for fatty acids, whereas synthesis occurs in the cytoplasm. Acetyl-CoA from carbohydrate metabolism may leave the double membrane of the mitochondrion as citrate or through the carnitine shuttle to participate in cytoplasmic fatty acid synthesis. However, acetyl-CoA from beta oxidation of lipids does not readily participate in gluconeogenesis.

When the overall pool exceeds synthetic demand, the amino acids can undergo oxidative deamination to pyruvate or various intermediates of the Kreb's cycle where the excess amino acids can contribute to energy generation (Fig. 24-6). The ammonia released from deamination in the liver and elsewhere is metabolized through the ornithine-citrulline cycle to urea. This cycle is principally active in the hepatocyte where 20 to 30 g of urea are produced daily.

Specific Protein Synthesis

The hepatocyte is the principal site for synthesis of most of the plasma proteins other than the immune globulins. Its major product, albumin, should provide approximately one half of the colloidal osmotic pressure of plasma, and that function for this 69,000-dalton protein could be considered its most crucial. However, there is remarkable conservation of the primary sequence of albumin in evolution, which suggests that its structural specificity is of some importance in physiology in addition to its physical property as a globular protein to lend colloidal pressure to intravascular water. Those physiologic properties that require some structural specificity must include binding such substrates as bilirubin, in which case albumin serves as a carrier protein.

The feedback loop to control albumin synthesis is not known, but when amino acid pools are diminished, as in malnutrition or hepatic dysfunction, the plasma albumin levels can fall dramatically. The resulting edema, as seen in kwashiorkor, is partially explained by reduced colloidal osmotic pressure, which hampers reentry of fluid at the distal aspect of the capillary. Albumin levels reflect malnutrition, but the relatively long half-life of this protein makes it inappropriate for sensitive monitoring of visceral protein synthesis.[24] Transferrin or retinol-binding protein, which are hepatic products involved in plasma transport, are better markers for protein malnutrition.

Lipoproteins are major transport products synthesized in the liver and, to a lesser degree, in the intestines (Table 24-1). Of these, chylomicrons carry dietary cholesterol

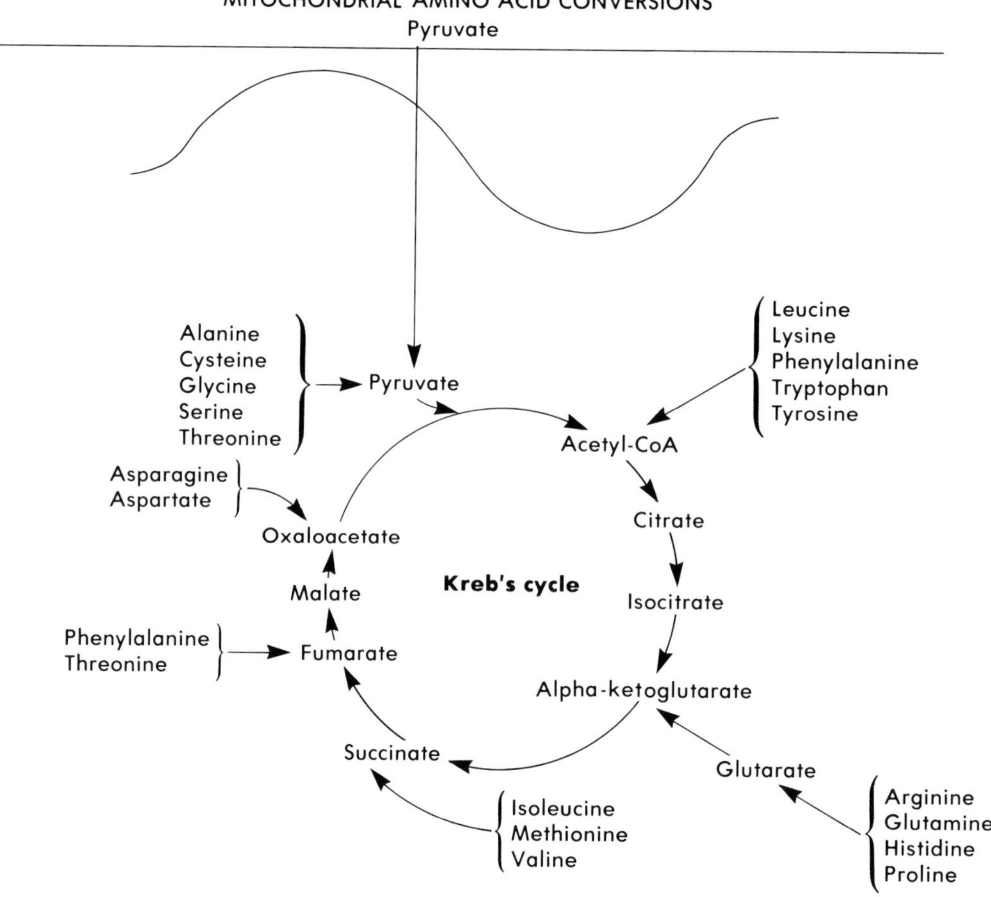

Fig. 24-6 Amino acid interconversion relies on cytoplasmic transamination, whereas metabolism of the carbon skeleton of the amino acid proceeds in the mitochondria. Most intermediates of the Kreb's cycle can readily diffuse from the double convoluted membrane of the mitochondrion to participate in cytoplasmic intermediary metabolism.

Table 24-1 **TYPES OF LIPOPROTEINS SYNTHESIZED BY THE LIVER**

Type	Density (g/cm^3)	Source of Lipids	Destination
Chylomicron	<0.94	Diet	Adipose tissue and liver
VLDL	0.940-1.006	Liver	Adipose tissue
LDL	1.006-1.063	Liver	Peripheral tissue
HDL	1.062-1.21	Peripheral tissues	Liver

triacyl glycerols and other lipids to the liver and to adipose tissue. VLDLs carry triglycerides from their synthetic compartment in the liver to peripheral adipose tissue. LDLs transport cholesterol to peripheral tissues where they play a role in regulating cholesterol synthesis. High-density lipoproteins (HDLs) transport cholesterol and phospholipids back to the liver from the periphery.[26]

The lipid-carrying protein synthesized by the liver is called apolipoprotein, i.e., protein lacking the lipid protein that defines a lipoprotein. The complete lipoprotein unit has a hydrophobic core surrounded by polar head groups that are hydrophilic, and the proteins form a shell around this structure. The lipoprotein is recognized by the appropriate tissue by means of receptors in plasma membrane pits. It is bound and internalized by endocytosis and, as an intracellular vesicle, fuses with lysosomes.[14] Defects in the traffic of lipids can be fatal as in familial hypercholesterolemia in which there is no low-density lipoprotein receptor. Homozygotes with this condition usually succumb to coronary artery disease in childhood.[23]

The components of the coagulation cascade form another major category of hepatic peptides. The hepatocytes synthesize most of the proteins involved in this cascade, with the notable exception of Factor VIII, the antihemophilic factor, which is synthesized in vascular endothelium. Factors II, VII, IX, and X contain a gamma carboxyglutamic acid residue that participates in calcium binding, and the enzymatic carboxylation of this factor requires vitamin K as a cofactor. In cases of incipient hepatic failure associated with alcoholism and the accompanying malnutrition, derangements in coagulation can occur. Restoration of normal balance can often be achieved by giving pharmacologic doses of vitamin K because deficiency of this vitamin is usually more pronounced than the associated impairment of protein synthesis that occurs during malnutrition.

The liver also produces fibrinogen, which is the substrate for thrombin, a serine protease that cleaves fibrinogen to produce the monomer that polymerizes into a clot.[6] In the same manner the liver synthesizes a member of antiplasmins that combat fibrinolysis. A failure of hepatic synthesis leads to an imbalance in these synthetic capabilities that favors fibrinolysis and a clotting picture of disseminated intravascular coagulation.

Lipid Phase Metabolism

Drug Metabolism and Related Functions

Elimination of many drugs depends on their chemical modification, and a large part of that chemical machinery is lodged in the liver. Oxidation, acetylation, sulfation, methylation, hydroxylation, and addition of glucuronide or taurine residues are the major reactions in the armamentarium. The stunning diversity of substrate seems incompatible with the exquisite specificity normally associated with enzymatic catalysis. The fact that the capacity to detoxify twentieth-century drugs by enzymes evolved many millions of years ago is puzzling, unless one recalls that most drugs are derived from alkaloids that are plant products encountered in the diet. In fact, it was inevitable that consumption of plants would require the acquisition of enzyme pathways that could inactivate biologically active molecules absorbed from plant foods. The generosity of substrate acceptance by the active sites of these enzymes is still impressive, and some phenotypic modification of those active sites has been proposed by analogy to the spectrum of chemical recognition used by the immune systems. There is an economy of phenotypic expression of the drug enzyme library in that the capacity to modify a given drug structure is often not detectable unless the cell has been exposed to that structure. Although substrate induction of its metabolizing enzyme is important, the broad induction of many enzymes can be brought about by certain drugs such as barbiturates. These metabolizing enzymes can exist without phenotypic expression for many generations without being induced. This genomic silence permits extensive mutation and proliferation of varied genotypes, all compatible with life. However, the same phenomenon leads to enormous variation in capacity to metabolize certain drugs. For most drugs, a sixfold to tenfold variation in the populace is common.[16]

The chemical modification of drugs in the hepatocyte is localized to the smooth endoplasmic reticulum. The most prominent of the enzyme systems is the cytochrome P_{450} system. The substrate must be lipid soluble to gain access to the enzymes in the tubular system of the reticulum. This requirement segregates the drug-metabolizing activity from water-soluble metabolic intermediates that otherwise could serve as substrates for the enzymes. The products of endogenous metabolism that do participate in the reactions are appropriately lipid soluble and include bilirubin and cholesterol. Some of the products of this fixed membrane system on the smooth endoplasmic reticulum are exported from the hepatocyte into bile as is appropriate for bilirubin, bile acids, and many drugs such as digitoxin or cyclosporine; whereas others leave the hepatocyte in a soluble form for renal excretion.[11]

Bile Formation

Because this topic is covered in depth with respect to bile acids, cholesterol, and bilirubin in other chapters in this book, it will only be briefly discussed here. Bilirubin in the blood arrives at the hepatocyte bound to albumin and is made soluble by addition of glucuronide, a reaction catalyzed by uridine diphosphonucleotide glucuronyl transferase in the smooth endoplasmic reticulum. An intracellular transport molecule, Y protein, receives the insoluble bilirubin at the sinusoidal side of the hepatocyte for delivery to the endoplasmic reticulum; and another transport protein, Z, delivers the soluble bilirubin to the bile canaliculus. Oxidation of cholesterol also transpires in the smooth endoplasmic reticulum to form cholic or deoxycholic acid, and these amphopathic molecules are exported into bile where they form the basis of micellar solubilization. The rate of bile salt synthesis is determined by recirculation of the salts in the enterohepatic circulation, and, curiously, the return of bile salts to the hepatocyte stimulates bile secretion acutely. This fraction of bile flow is called bile salt–dependent bile secretion. With chronic loss of bile salts, as in cases of biliary fistula, the synthetic rate can increase tenfold to partially accommodate the chemical requirements of micelle formation in the small intestine. Thus reduced bile salt recirculation leads to low-volume bile flow, but the concentration of bile salts in that volume may be raised to a level appropriate for micelle formation by increased bile salt synthesis. Synthesized or absorbed cholesterol is released into bile, as is lecithin, to participate in the micellar structure important to fat absorption from the gastrointestinal tract. Finally, immunoglobulin A is processed by a nonlysosomal pathway to receive a protein fragment. This addition forms secretory immunoglobulin A, which is released into bile in large quantities and presumably contributes to immune events in the lumen of the bowel.[1]

The bile canaliculi receive a fluid that is isotonic with respect to anions and cations. The canaliculi have no epithelium other than the hepatocytes themselves. As the canaliculi converge in the portal triads to form the bile ductules, there is an epithelium, but it does little to change the electrolyte composition of bile. However, in the gallbladder, transport of Na^+, K^+ and water leads to substantial concentration of the bile solutes and a sharp rise in calcium. The liver produces 800 to 1000 ml of bile per day, but, owing to the concentrating capacity of the gallbladder, this 40- to 70-ml reservoir often stores 12 hours of bile output awaiting the recognition of feeding and gallbladder contraction under the influence of cholecystokinin.

DERANGED HEPATIC FUNCTION

Despite the enormous latitude of hepatic function and the many mechanisms of compensation and restoration after injury, the hepatocellular mass does eventually fail in stepwise fashion very late in the course of hepatic disease as compensatory mechanisms are exhausted. The various functions decline piecemeal to give a series of derangements that may indicate the nature of the underlying injury, its potential reversibility, and prognosis. Many activities or enzymes can be lost in heritable point mutations, but their deletion is generally compatible with life. Crigler-Najjar syndrome (an autosomal recessive defect in uridine diphosphonucleotide-glucuronyl transferase), the various glycogen storage diseases, and the familial variance in handling certain drugs because of diminished availability of a specific active enzyme[16] all are examples of a genomic defect hampering some specific event. Certain intoxications can foul a specific activity without global hepatic compromise. Examples include cholestatic jaundice caused by various drugs or coumadin blockade of vitamin K–dependent carboxylation in the synthesis of prothrombin and Factors VII, IX, and X.

If scarring reduces blood supply to the hepatic cells or if regeneration of injured cells fails to attain an effective number of functioning units, grades of generalized liver dysfunction are encountered. Child[5] classified hepatic reserve as a measure of liver compromise that correlated with the clinical outcome. Although originally proposed as an index of hepatic function for patients with cirrhosis undergoing portal venous decompression, this classification is useful in determining hepatic reserve in any patient with liver disease. Five straightforward parameters of hepatic function were classified: bilirubin, albumin, ascites, encephalopathy, and nutrition (Table 24-2). The simplicity in this system that categorizes hepatic failure as A, B, or C belies the careful choice of the five parameters. Bilirubin metabolism requires the conjugation/detoxification function of the liver. As bilirubin rises, other P_{450} functions are compromised proportionately. Albumin reflects the synthetic activity of the liver, and, as albumin declines, other plasma proteins such as clotting factors and carrier proteins can be expected to decline also. Ascites is a function of plasma oncotic pressure and the pressure dynamics of lymph formation in the gastrointestinal tract and liver. Encephalopathy reflects problems in hepatic capture of metabolites from the gastrointestinal tract and will be discussed in greater detail below. Nutritional difficulties referred to by Child[5] really center on skeletal muscle wasting as amino acid metabolism fails to provide a pool of amino acids appropriate for the mass action requirements of protein synthesis. If one of these functions such as bilirubin clearance is deranged, similar functions will also be deranged in hepatic microsomes, an example being altered drug metabolism. Thus this sampling of hepatic functions provides representative information for a wide range of hepatic activities and predicts the reserve capacity of the liver to tolerate further insult such as portal venous diversion, resection, or the metabolic demand of operative stress. In progressive liver disorders these same kinds of parameters have prognostic value to assist the surgeon in the appropriate timing of hepatic transplantation.

Table 24-2 **CHILD'S CLASSIFICATION OF HEPATIC RESERVE**

Function	A (Minimal Risk)	B (Moderate Risk)	C (Advanced Risk)
Bilirubin (mg/100 ml)	<2	2-3	>3
Albumin (g/100 ml)	>3.5	3-3.5	<3
Ascites	None	Easily controlled	Poorly controlled
Encephalopathy	None	Minimal	Advanced
Nutrition	Excellent	Good	Poor

Hepatic encephalopathy is an intriguing perturbation in cerebral metabolism and function that occurs because hepatic reserve is incapable of meeting the body's normal metabolic needs. The compromised brain function seen in liver disease can be as subtle as memory loss, as obvious as profound confusion, and as threatening as deep coma. Although the exact pathogenesis remains uncertain, the basic defect appears to be an accumulation of toxic molecules that have not been metabolized by the ailing liver, one candidate being ammonia. This substance is generated by the metabolism of colonic bacteria and by amino acid diversion into gluconeogenesis under the influence of high glucagon levels that are paradoxically further raised by high ammonia levels. The excess ammonia that has not entered the urea cycle in the liver can participate in a variety of reactions in the central nervous system, one being the ability of astrocytes to aid in ammonia's removal by reaction with glutamic acid to form glutamine. However, the ammonia can also react with alpha-ketoglutarate to form glutamic acid, which then receives another ammonia molecule to form glutamine.

Although the degree of encephalopathy does not correlate well with acute changes in plasma ammonia, there is a rough correlation between the development of this problem and the level of glutamine in the cerebrospinal fluid. This correlation may actually be an indirect one caused by the alpha-ketoglutarate depletion and the adenosine triphosphate consumption in the formation of glutamine, thereby resulting in problems with neurotransmission. A role for alpha-ketoglutarate depletion is also suggested by the observation that mental status changes are a function both of absolute amounts of ammonia or glutamine and of the rate of change. A very rapid change is more likely to deplete alpha-ketoglutarate and thereby compromise neurotransmission, whereas chronic hyperammonemia permits accommodation by the alpha-ketoglutarate pool in the central nervous system.[9]

The best example of the sudden presentation of ammonia to the liver in hepatic failure is gastrointestinal bleeding in which an abundant amount of protein is available to the colonic flora for conversion to ammonia. Bleeding into the gastrointestinal tract is dangerous enough, but the danger is amplified when there is an associated encephalopathy. It is for this reason that gastrointestinal bleeding in cirrhotic patients requires treatment with cathartics such as magnesium sulfate ($MgSO_4$) and with agents to suppress the colonic bacterial flora such as neomycin. On a chronic basis, the disaccharide lactulose can also be administered to reduce the availability of ammonia to the central nervous system. Lactulose is not absorbed by the gut but is metabolized by colonic flora to produce lactic, acetic, and formic acids that lower the lumenal pH of the colon to about 5.5. This pH level favors ammonia hydration to the ammonium ion, which is less toxic and cannot participate in the reactions discussed above. This hydration reaction is so prominent that the large intestine becomes a trap for extracellular ammonia accumulating in the colon wall from the general circulation.

Neurotransmission in hepatic failure is also modified by elevated levels of aromatic amino acids, which figure prominently in the physiology of nerve conduction. For example, tryptophan elevation leads to a corresponding marked elevation of its metabolite, serotonin, resulting in profound consequences in cerebral function. In animals the major toxic product of encephalopathy from the gastrointestinal tract is mercaptan (methanethiol), a metabolite of methionine in bacterial metabolism.[9] Mercaptans interfere with the urea cycle and are perhaps pathochemically important in humans, although this remains uncertain. Certainly mercaptans are noteworthy in human liver failure because it is the odor of this compound that is perceptible on the breath of cirrhotics as fetor hepaticus.

Death as a result of hepatic failure follows four specific pathways. First, the sudden subtraction of normal hepatic tissue makes hypoglycemia an immediate hazard. The liver normally delivers 10 g of glucose per hour in fasting conditions, and without this provision fatal hypoglycemia will ensue. This hazard must not be forgotten when massive hepatic resections are performed; the appropriate therapeutic response is intravenous infusion of 10% dextrose. Hepatic failure is also fatal because of the profound coma that occurs in hepatic encephalopathy. There are histologic sequelae in the brain that can render the coma irreversible. Third, hepatic failure patients die from hemorrhage from varices aggravated by insufficient synthesis of clotting factors by the liver. However, the most common mode of death should be titled nutritional. With inadequate amino acid pools, skeletal muscle wasting is profound, leading to respiratory disability that can be compounded by ascites, which further restricts respiratory function through its adverse effects on diaphragmatic excursion. In this advanced state of debility, pneumonia becomes the agent of demise.

Hepatic failure can be treated piecemeal for the many failings of hepatic function, or it can be treated generally by supporting liver regeneration. However, advanced liver failure cannot currently be treated effectively by extracorporeal support as is the case for renal failure. The difficulty in designing a hepatic support is actually quite simple. Renal function is in the aqueous phase across a semipermeable membrane. Hepatic function is largely a lipid phase event that transpires across a membrane of highly specialized living cells. Hepatic transplantation offers the only hope currently available for individuals who have exhaused the last ounce of the remarkable capacity of the liver to respond to metabolic needs.

HEPATIC INJURY AND REGENERATION

The liver may be injured by direct physical violence; anatomic displacement by tumor, granuloma, or abscess; direct hepatocyte toxins such as ethanol, carbon tetrachloride, or endotoxin; viral agents more or less specific to the hepatocyte such as hepatitis B or cytomegalovirus; ischemia or hypoxia; inborn or acquired disorders of metabolism such as glycogen storage disease or fatty infiltration during parenteral nutrition; impedance to venous outflow as in Budd-Chiari syndrome; or noxious events transmitted by the biliary tree as in obstruction or ascending cholangitis. The dominant life-threatening feature of liver injury is a reduction in the available functional hepatocellular mass. This may occur as cellular loss caused by the immediate injury or may be the result of peculiarities of liver scarring as seen in cirrhosis.

After physical injury to the liver, there is an active process of wound healing and scarring similar to that seen elsewhere in the body. Remarkably, however, this process of regeneration faithfully reproduces hepatic cytoarchitecture with sinusoids, hepatic lobules, and proper biliary drainage. In rats a 70% hepatectomy prompts a regenerative event that will restore hepatocellular mass in 3 to 4 weeks. The major hepatotrophic hormone for this process is insulin, and the control mechanism that halts further hepatic growth is not known.[25] However, the parameters for growth control cannot simply be adequate metabolic performance because regeneration proceeds until there is an abundant excess of hepatic tissue, precisely as in the normal situation.

When the hepatocytes are lost as a result of toxins or moderate ischemia or viruses, the dead cells are removed by inflammation, and restoration is accomplished by cell division among adjacent cells in the sinusoidal cords. When sufficient cells are lost, the liver produces regenerative nodules that can become bound down in inflammation and scar. This pattern of nodular cirrhosis may lead to the development of functionally ineffective liver lobules.

The most troublesome pattern of healing is that which follows portal triad inflammation when periportal scarring can limit blood flow into the sinusoids. This portal venous obstruction increases portal venous pressure, which leads to portal systemic flow and variceal dilation of the small venous channels recruited for this diversion. Obstruction to blood flow through the liver can either be postsinusoidal as in the Budd-Chiari syndrome, sinusoidal as in alcoholic cirrhosis, or purely presinusoidal as in the case of schistosomiasis. In the latter condition the function of the hepatocytes is remarkably preserved despite pronounced portal hypertension. That function is gravely compromised when the portal system is acutely decompressed by a surgical portosystemic shunt.

The liver may be generously resected for surgical management of tumor, infection, or trauma. Either the right or left lobe may be resected with impunity if there is no major compromise in hepatic function already. Also, a right lobectomy may be extended to include a portion of the left lobe if necessary without the development of subsequent hepatic failure. Initially patients subjected to varying degrees of hepatic resection will need glucose supplementation, but eventually regeneration of hepatocytes will be sufficient to maintain normal metabolic activities.[3,4,20]

HEPATITIS

The liver may be damaged by a great variety of viral, bacterial, protozoan, or helminthic agents. Fortunately, most of these infectious problems are self-limiting or can be effectively treated medically or by surgical means.

Viral hepatitis, on the other hand, can result in substantial compromise of normal hepatic function and may even be life-threatening. The three forms of hepatitis of greatest interest to surgeons are hepatitis A; hepatitis B; and non-A, non-B hepatitis.

Hepatitis A or infectious hepatitis is caused by a hepatitis A virus (HAV) that is a 27-nm RNA virus. It is transmitted by the fecal-oral route and has an incubation period of approximately 28 days before a syndrome of malaise, anorexia, headache, slight fever, and jaundice develops. Viremia is very brief, which probably explains why needle transmission is almost never seen. However, infective virus is shed in the stools in significant titers for a number of days before the development of symptoms. This asymptomatic infectivity is the most troublesome epidemic-like feature of the disease and requires careful identification of contacts to control epidemic outbreaks. The disease is usually entirely asymptomatic since 50% of American adults have antibody to HAV by age 50. The antibody response to infection is brisk, and lifelong protection is afforded by that response. The disease can be prevented or greatly ameliorated if immune serum globulin (ISG) is given after suspected exposure. The passive immunization does not necessarily prevent viral infection since many individuals will demonstrate lifelong antibody titers to HAV after exposure to virus and administration of ISG. This phenomenon is termed passive-active immunization. Most importantly, ISG is close to 90% effective in protecting exposed individuals from the hepatitis A syndrome. There are now HAV vaccines also available for populations at high risk such as homosexuals, workers in day-care centers, military recruits, and certain foreign travelers.[19]

The virus responsible for hepatitis A damages hepatocytes by lysis in the course of virus replication. A large (5% to 10%) fraction of the liver cells may be infected, and their lysis leads to striking elevations of the transaminases in blood. Mononuclear infiltration congests the liver, and cholestatic jaundice ensues. The bilirubin rarely exceeds 4 mg/100 ml, and the entire syndrome has usually resolved in 3 weeks. During the active illness, patients are advised to rest, maintain a high carbohydrate diet, and avoid hepatotoxins such as alcohol. Full recovery is to be expected in this form of hepatitis with no likelihood of chronic hepatitis. The disease is distinguished from other forms of hepatitis by measuring anti-HAV antibodies acutely when they should not be present and at 3 weeks when the immunoglobulin M levels should be markedly elevated.[28]

Hepatitis B or serum hepatitis differs sharply from the relatively innocent HAV. This 42-nm DNA virus (HBV) not only infects hepatocytes but can join the native DNA in the nucleus to direct hepatocytes in a disastrous syndrome of chronic hepatitis or hepatocellular cancer. The distribution of the virus is wide and intense as exemplified by the facts that 10% of the population in the Far East and Africa carry the virus and there are 500,000 to 1,000,000 new cases of hepatocellular cancer annually in China. The disease is transmitted both by the fecal-oral route and sexual contact. Because of the prolonged viremia, the virus is most readily passed on by needle puncture and blood transfusion. After an incubation period that averages 75 days, an insidious syndrome of malaise, anorexia, and mild jaundice is identified as hepatitis by elevated transaminase, relatively normal alkaline phosphatase, and modest hyperbilirubinemia. The virus replicates in the hepatocyte and is shed in blood and feces. Unlike hepatitis A, the hepatitis may become fulminant with an overall mortality of acute hepatitis B being in the range of 1% to 2%. Of all patients who develop hepatitis B, 10% will go on to develop chronic active hepatitis.

Table 24-3 **ANTIGENIC MARKERS FOR HEPATITIS B**

Marker	Structure	Implication
HBsAg	Envelope protein	Shedding envelope
HBcAg	Core or capsid antigen	Shedding virion
HBeAg	Core antigen	DNA polymerase replicating virus

The infective virion of hepatitis B enters the hepatocyte, which then may shed active virus particles or only envelopes that have an antigenically characteristic protein called HBsAg (hepatitis B surface antigen) (Table 24-3). During the incubation period HBsAg is detectable in serum; during the acute illness another antigen, HBeAg, can also be detected. This antigen is associated with DNA polymerase and is active during viral proliferation. Later in the disease HBeAg disappears, and antibodies to the core antigen, HBcAg, develop. In later convalescence there are antibodies to both core and surface antigens, i.e., anti-HBc and anti-HBs. This circumstance reflects an adequate immune response and lifelong protection. However, the immune response is often imperfect, and a carrier state may develop that is indicated by the persistence of HBsAg and HBcAg. A significant fraction of these carrier patients will have ongoing infection and liver damage, and during the phase of active viral proliferation HBeAg will be detected in the serum, indicating viral DNA polymerase activity.[27] In a prospective Taiwan study the ultimate cause of death in HBsAg-positive or HBsAg-negative men was noted. Among the HBsAg-negative men, 90% had antibody to HBV. The distinguishing factor in the two populations was persistence of viremia. Among the carriers 51% ultimately died of cirrhosis or hepatocellular carcinoma, whereas only 2% of the men in the control group succumbed to these diseases.[2] Failure to clear the virus may be caused by an immune defect in interferon, but the large number of patients with this chronic disease mitigates against some basic immune defect. Rather, the difference between HBsAg positivity or negativity may reflect the susceptibility or random likelihood of HBV latency whereby the HBV-DNA sequence is inserted into hepatocellular DNA.

The treatment of acute HBV hepatitis is supportive, and the management of chronic hepatitis has been disappointing.[7,10,21] There are no effective protocols generally recommended. However, the prevention of HBV disease is quite promising. The HBsAg can be isolated from serum of carriers in the empty viral envelopes that are not themselves infective. The envelopes are treated with pepsin and denatured with urea and formalin in a scheme that inactivates all known viruses to prepare a vaccine. The vaccine is administered acutely, with two boosts at 3 and 6 months to give a 95% antibody response. The vaccine has nearly 100% efficacy. For health care workers exposed by skin puncture, passive immunization with hepatitis B immune globulin (HBIG) plus active immunization with HBV vaccine offers virtually total protection.[13] For elective immunization, health care personnel are screened for anti-HBs, and those who have not already acquired immunity are offered the vaccine. Despite the safety record of HBV vaccine, it is still derived from human plasma, and there is an unscientific fear of transmission of acquired immune deficiency syndrome. This is difficult to imagine with the denaturing process. However, HBV has now been cultured, and the availability of recombinant DNA vaccine products is imminent.[8] Worldwide immunization offers an outstanding potential to eliminate this ghastly untreatable disease. Dissemination of HBV has been greatly curbed by screening blood transfusions for HBsAg and through public education with respect to dangers of needles and certain sexual practices.

After the identification of HBV, it became clear that there were patients who acquired hepatitis from blood transfusion who had never been exposed to HBV.[8] This serum hepatitis is called non-A, non-B hepatitis and represents the greatest infection hazard of blood transfusion today. The obscure name reflects the fact that no antigen or virus has been identified to correlate with the hepatic disease that resembles HBV disease. The danger of subclinical hepatitis from transfusion because of this unidentified agent can be as high as 5%, and among those patients who develop clinically evident hepatitis 50% to 75% will have chronic hepatitis. This disease has a very long incubation period and most frequently is recognized in a patient who was massively transfused and has trouble recovering full vigor some 3 to 4 months after injury or operation. There is no treatment other than supportive care, and prevention of the disease remains a challenge to investigators.

ASSESSMENT OF HEPATIC FUNCTION

The effectiveness of the hepatocellular mass can be assessed by measuring plasma levels of compounds that the liver should either synthesize or modify to facilitate excretion. Prothrombin time and partial thromboplastin time determine the availability of clotting factors synthesized in the liver; fibrinogen can actually be measured directly. Albumin is only produced by the liver, as is the case for carrier proteins such as transferrin. Bilirubin measurements are the standard for assessing the smooth endoplasmic reticulum of hepatocytes and its capacity to solubilize bilirubin by the addition of glucuronide.The water-soluble glucuronide forms the basis for the direct bilirubin value. Insoluble, protein-bound bilirubin reflects the bilirubin not acted on by the liver. When bile flow is impaired because of cholestasis or duct occlusion, both direct and indirect bilirubin values rise as bilirubin glucuronide leaves the hepatocyte into the space of Disse and reenters the circulation. In addition, further conjugation of insoluble bilirubin is disfavored by the mass action abundance of the glucuronide. Gross inadequacy of the liver cell mass can be detected as an elevation in plasma ammonia.

Ongoing damage to hepatocytes can be identified by measuring the levels of circulating intracellular enzymes more or less specific to the liver. Lactate dehydrogenase is the most important catalyst in the Cori cycle where lactate from anaerobic muscle metabolism is converted to pyruvate in the liver for gluconeogenesis. The enzyme is present in a variety of other tissues, but there is a fairly specific hepatic isoenzyme. Amino acid conversion requires a panel of amine transferases such as glutamate pyruvate transaminase or glutamate oxaloacetate transaminase. The enzymes are so abundant in the liver that even modest cell disruption leads to very high circulating transaminase levels.

When bile flow is obstructed, biliary ductules proliferate in the liver. These fragile ducts, looking for a way out of the hepatic substance, release alkaline phosphatase, an enzyme marker for biliary obstruction. High alkaline phosphatase implies biliary obstruction not so much because of hydrostatic damage to the ducts but because of ductular proliferation. Some patients with substantial ductular damage and, consequently, diminished ductular proliferation in ascending cholangitis may show a further rise in alkaline phosphatase after surgically establishing common duct drainage.

When hepatocellular loss is marked, there are physical stigmata that distinguish hepatic disorders from other debilitating processes. Palmar erythema, spider angiomata of the trunk, and xanthelasma are skin signs. Gynecomastia indicates failure of the liver to clear estrogenic steroid hormones in males. The neurologic manifestations may be obvious with confusion and tremor, or the odor of mercaptan may be overwhelming in fetor hepaticus. Any of these findings, plus physical evidence of poor nutrition, strongly supports a diagnosis of hepatic failure.

The structure of the liver can be accurately determined by methods other than laparotomy. Physical assessment by palpation and percussion can give a close estimate of liver span and the presence of gross nodules. Ultrasound examination shows ductal dilation and abscess rather well, whereas computerized tomography can delineate smaller nodules and injuries. Magnetic resonance imaging is a newer technique that offers the possibility of metabolic assessment and topography. Rapid evaluation of hepatocellular function, common duct patency, and cystic duct patency are provided by gamma scintigraphy using the diisopropyl derivative of iminodiacetic acid as the contrast agent. Angiography can be used to evaluate the lobar anatomy when planning a resection. Abnormalities of the ductal system with obstruction are best clarified by percutaneous cholangiography or endoscopic retrograde cholangiopancreatography. The microscopic anatomy of the liver is frequently useful in diagnosing chronic infiltrative processes such as chronic active hepatitis or sarcoidosis, and for this purpose percutaneous liver biopsy is appropriate.

SUMMARY

Zeus punished Prometheus for giving fire to humans by chaining him to a rock where his liver was consumed by a great bird each day for eternity only to regenerate each night. The torture was certainly well considered in that no other organ is critical to life and yet capable of remarkable healing and regeneration. In this chapter the metabolic machinery of the liver has been briefly discussed in terms of the anatomy and physiology of the organ as a gatekeeper of the splanchnic circulation. The functional breadth of the liver is a matter to marvel, but the failure of the liver prods us to seek improvement. However, the function of a destroyed liver can certainly be restored by transplantation, and preterminal hepatic insufficiency can be treated by providing components of hepatic function. The challenge is to so thoroughly understand hepatic function that the therapy of hepatic insufficiency and the prevention of hepatic injuries will be self-evident in the decades ahead.

REFERENCES

1. Alverdy, J., Chi, H.S., and Sheldon, G.F.: The effect of parenteral nutrition on gastrointestinal immunity, Ann. Surg. **202**:681, 1985.
2. Beasley, R.P., et al.: Hepatocellular carcinoma and hepatitis B virus, Lancet **2**:1129, 1981.
3. Blumgart, L.H.: Concepts of liver resections for primary and secondary tumors, Recent Results Cancer Res. **100**:185, 1986.
4. Blumgart, L.H., et al.: Surgical approaches to cholangiocarcinoma at confluence of hepatic ducts, Lancet **1**:66, 1984.
5. Child, C.G.: The liver and portal hypertension, Philadelphia, 1967, W.B. Saunders Co.
6. Collins, J.A.: Blood transfusions and disorders of surgical bleeding. In Sabiston, D.C., editor: Textbook of surgery, Philadelphia, 1986, W.B. Saunders Co.
7. Conn, H.O., Maddrey, W.C., and Soloway, R.D.: The detrimental effects of adrenocorticosteroid therapy in HBsAg-positive chronic active hepatitis, Hepatology **2**:885, 1982.
8. Feinstone, S.M., et al.: Transfusion-associated hepatitis not due to hepatitis A or B, N. Engl. J. Med. **292**:767, 1975.
9. Fraser, C.L., and Arieff, A.I.: Hepatic encephalopathy, N. Engl. J. Med. **313**:865, 1985.
10. Gregory, P.B.: Interferon in chronic hepatitis B, Gastroenterology **90**:237, 1986.
11. Griffeth, L.K., Rosen, G.M., and Raukman, E.J.: Effects of model traumatic injury on hepatic drug metabolism in the rat, Drug Metabol. Dispos. **13**:398, 1985.
12. Guyton, A.C.: Medical physiology, Philadelphia, 1976, W.B. Saunders Co.
13. Jacobson, I.M., and Diensterg, J.L.: Viral hepatitis vaccines, Annu. Rev. Med. **35**:241, 1985.
14. Jones, A.L., and Burwen, S.J.: Hepatic receptors and their ligands, Semin. Liver Dis. **5**:136, 1985.
15. Keller, G.A., et al.: Multiple system organ failure: modulation of hepatocyte protein synthesis by endotoxin activated Kupffer cells, Ann. Surg. **201**:87, 1985.
16. Kupfer A., and Preisig, R.: Inherited defects of hepatic drug metabolism, Semin. Liver Dis. **3**:341, 1983.
17. Langman, J.: Medical embryology, Baltimore, 1963, The Williams & Wilkins Co.
18. Lehninger, A.L.: Biochemistry, New York, 1975, Worth Publishers, Inc.
19. Lemon, S.: Type A viral hepatitis, N. Engl. J. Med. **313**:1059, 1985.
20. Malt, R.A.: Surgery for hepatic neoplasms, N. Engl. J. Med. **313**:1591, 1985.
21. Sagvelli, E., et al.: Effect of immunosuppressive therapy on HBsAg-positive chronic active hepatitis in relation to presence or absence of HBeAg and anti-HBe, Hepatology **3**:690, 1983.
22. Sherlock, S.: Diseases of the liver and biliary system, Oxford, 1975, Blackwell Scientific Publications.
23. Spengel, F.A., and Thompson, G.R.: Receptor mediated low-density lipoprotein catabolism, Klin. Wochenschr. **60**:319, 1982.
24. Starker, P.M., et al.: Serum albumin levels as an index of nutritional support, Surgery **91**:194, 1982.
25. Starzl, T.E., et al.: The effect of diabetes mellitus on portal blood hepatotrophic factors in dogs, Surg. Gynecol. Obstet. **140**:449, 1975.
26. Stryer, L.: Biochemistry, ed. 2, San Francisco, 1981, W.H. Freeman & Co., Publishers.
27. Tiollais, P., Pourcel, C., and Dejean, A.: The hepatitis B virus, Nature **317**:489, 1985.
28. Wollheim, F.A.: Immunoglobulins in the cause of viral hepatitis and in cholestatic and obstructive jaundice, Acta Med. Scand. **183**:473, 1968.

25 Portal Hypertension

Layton F. Rikkers

Portal hypertension is caused by an alteration in splanchnic hemodynamics (usually an increase in resistance to portal venous flow) secondary to a variety of disease processes. In the United States the most common cause is alcoholic cirrhosis. The elevated portal pressure stimulates formation of collaterals between the portal and systemic venous systems. The most important site of collateralization is in the distal esophagus and proximal stomach, where thin-walled submucosal varices may develop. Hemorrhage from these varices is associated with high mortality and constitutes the most significant complication of portal hypertension. Other bothersome sequelae of portal hypertension are ascites, encephalopathy, and hypersplenism.

ANATOMY AND PHYSIOLOGY OF THE HEPATIC CIRCULATION

The liver is served by a dual blood supply from the hepatic artery and the portal vein. The portal vein is the most dorsal component of the hepatoduodenal ligament and is formed behind the pancreas by the confluence of superior mesenteric and splenic veins (Fig. 25-1). The portal vein bifurcates into right and left branches just before entering the substance of the liver. The left gastric or coronary vein drains the lesser curvature of the stomach and enters the portal vein near its origin. This usually minor tributary becomes important in patients with portal hypertension because it is the major collateral joining the high pressure portal venous circulation with the gastric and esophageal varices. The splenic vein travels behind the pancreas for most of its length and is usually joined by the inferior mesenteric vein just before entering the portal vein.

The hepatic artery is one of three major branches of the celiac axis; it travels toward the liver medial to the common bile duct and portal vein in the portal triad. A frequent variation of hepatic arterial anatomy is origination of the right hepatic artery from the superior mesenteric artery, which occurs in approximately 20% of individuals. A replaced right hepatic artery usually lies lateral, rather than medial, to the portal vein and may be inadvertently damaged or ligated during a portacaval shunt procedure.

Total hepatic blood flow averages 1500 ml/min, which represents approximately 25% of the cardiac output. Although the hepatic artery contributes only one third of the blood flow to the liver in healthy individuals, it provides approximately 50% of the oxygen supply. Changes in portal blood flow are caused by vasodilation and vasoconstriction of the splanchnic arterial bed. The hepatic arterioles are also responsive to the usual vasoactive influences, such as catecholamines and sympathetic nervous stimulation, but autoregulated vasodilation of the hepatic arterioles occurs when total hepatic blood flow is decreased in patients with shock or patients who have had surgical portal diversion. The mechanism of this autoregulatory or hepatic arterial "buffer" response is not completely understood. Since the liver plays a major role in homeostasis, it is appropriate that compensatory mechanisms exist to maintain total hepatic blood flow constant.

Many of the hormones secreted into the portal venous circulation are important regulators of hepatic metabolism. In addition, some hormones, particularly insulin, are trophic for the liver and contribute to maintenance of normal liver size and function and capacity for regeneration.

PATHOPHYSIOLOGY OF PORTAL HYPERTENSION

Although portal hypertension is almost always secondary to both increased portal blood flow and increased vascular resistance, its classification is based on the site of abnormal vascular resistance. Obstruction to portal flow can occur at prehepatic, hepatic, or posthepatic locations. An example of prehepatic portal hypertension is portal vein thrombosis, which accounts for approximately 50% of cases of portal hypertension in the pediatric population. Portal hypertension secondary to this cause is accompanied by normal hepatic vascular resistance and development of portal venous collaterals to the liver, which restore some of the lost portal flow. Therefore hepatic function remains normal. Thrombosis of the portal vein is sometimes associated with occlusion of the superior mesenteric and splenic veins, making surgical decompression of the portal venous system impossible. Isolated splenic vein thrombosis, often secondary to pancreatitis, results in left-sided portal hypertension. In individuals with this condition, elevated pressure is present only in the gastrosplenic venous bed and returns to normal following splenectomy. Posthepatic portal hypertension, which causes pressure elevation throughout the sinusoids of the liver and entire portal venous system, is infrequent. An example of posthepatic portal hypertension is hepatic vein thrombosis (Budd-Chiari syndrome), which may develop idiopathically in patients with hypercoagulability.

Intrahepatic portal hypertension can be subclassified into presinusoidal, sinusoidal, and postsinusoidal types.[6] Vascular resistance may be increased at more than one of these levels. For example, cirrhosis, which accounts for 90% of cases of portal hypertension in the United States, is associated with narrowing of hepatic sinusoids secondary to deposition of collagen in Disse's space and distortion of the entire hepatic architecture with varying degrees of increased vascular resistance at the presinusoidal, sinusoidal, and postsinusoidal levels. Whereas portal hypertension secondary to alcoholic cirrhosis is mainly of the sinusoidal type, nonalcoholic cirrhosis frequently has a significant presinusoidal component that contributes to the elevated hepatic vascular resistance. Because cirrhosis is caused by hepatocellular necrosis and subsequent fibrosis, the portal hemodynamic alterations are often accompanied by evidence of liver cell failure. In contrast, patients with pure presinusoidal portal hypertension (e.g., schistosomiasis) have nearly normal hepatocellular function.

Increased portal blood flow alone can occasionally initiate portal hypertension. For example, arteriovenous fistulas in the splanchnic vascular bed and massive splenomegaly, both of which cause increased flow, may result in portal hypertension. However, in most instances the increased flow eventually causes sclerosis of intrahepatic portal venules and a secondary increase in vascular resistance.

Whatever the cause, elevated portal venous pressure is the major stimulus to portal-systemic collateralization.

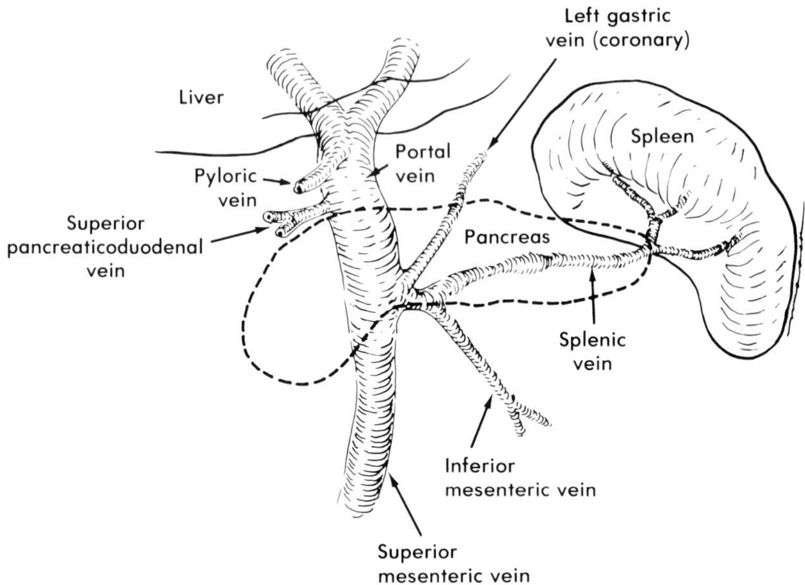

Fig. 25-1 Extrahepatic portal venous circulation. (From Rikkers, L.F.: Portal hypertension. In Goldsmith, H.S., editor: Practice of surgery, vol. 3, General surgery, Thomaston, Conn., 1981, Practice of Surgery, Ltd.)

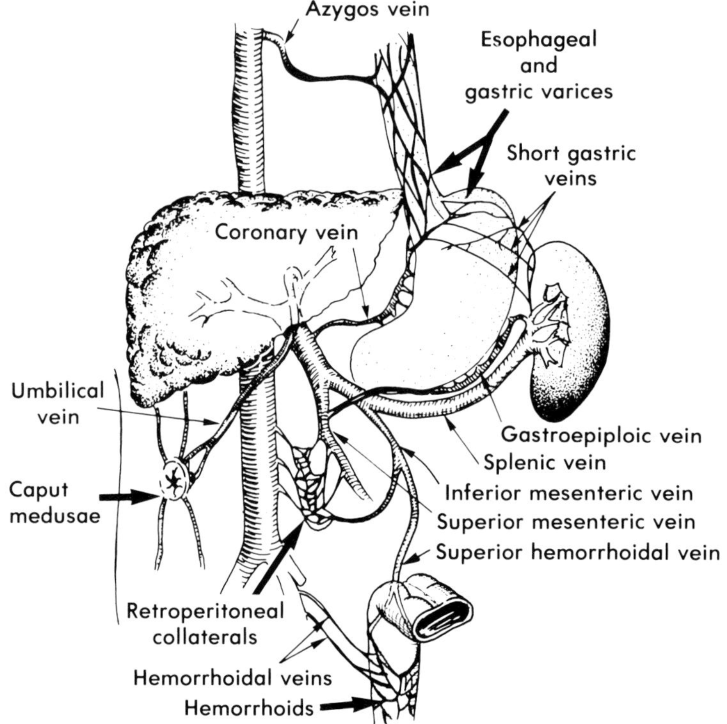

Fig. 25-2 Portal-systemic collateral pathways develop where the portal venous and systemic venous systems are in close apposition *(large arrows).*

Collaterals form in locations where the portal venous and systemic venous circulations are proximate. The major sites of portal-systemic collateralization in patients with portal hypertension are depicted in Fig. 25-2. Clinically, the most important collaterals are the left gastric and right gastric veins; these divert high pressure portal venous blood through gastric and esophageal varices, which can rupture and result in massive upper gastrointestinal hemorrhage.

In experimental models of prehepatic and intrahepatic portal hypertension, development of extensive portal-systemic collaterals returns vascular resistance to normal.[6] However, increased splanchnic blood flow, secondary to elevated cardiac output, results in maintenance of portal hypertension. The cause of the hyperdynamic circulation, which frequently accompanies both experimental and clinical portal hypertension, is not known. Since a large fraction of the increased portal venous flow travels through extrahepatic and intrahepatic shunt pathways, hepatic portal perfusion is usually decreased. Total hepatic blood flow is not decreased to as great a degree as portal flow because of a compensatory increase in hepatic arterial perfusion, which occurs because of the hepatic arterial "buffer" response.

VARICEAL HEMORRHAGE

Esophageal and gastric varices are thin-walled, submucosal veins, which represent part of the portal-systemic collateral network that develops in patients with portal hypertension. Variceal hemorrhage develops in approximately one third of patients with esophagogastric varices and is the most life-threatening complication of portal hypertension. The wide range of reported mortalities (20% to 80%) is mainly caused by the differing degrees of impaired hepatic function in the various populations studied.[17] Whereas variceal hemorrhage frequently results in death in a patient with advanced and decompensated cirrhosis, individuals with prehepatic portal hypertension rarely die of this complication.

Although varices most commonly develop in the esophagus and upper stomach, they may occur at any location within the gastrointestinal tract. However, the site of hemorrhage in over 90% of patients is within 2 cm of the esophagogastric junction. In this location, hydrostatic pressure within the varix probably leads to rupture of the overyling epithelium, which is sometimes only one cell layer thick. Although variceal hemorrhage does not appear to be related to the magnitude of portal pressure, large varices are more likely to bleed than small varices.[14] Other less frequent sites of variceal hemorrhage are within the esophagus and stomach at greater distances from the gastroesophageal junction and in the distal ileum, proximal colon, and rectosigmoid colon. Individuals with portal hypertension and an ileostomy are particularly prone to hemorrhage from varices in the terminal ileum.

Diagnosis of Variceal Hemorrhage

Variceal hemorrhage should be suspected when upper gastrointestinal hemorrhage occurs in a patient with a history of chronic liver disease, alcoholism, or hepatitis. Since bleeding from varices is often massive, the patient frequently has hypotension and hematemesis. However, a history of melena over several days is not uncommon. When the physical examination reveals splenomegaly, dilated abdominal wall veins, and ascites (see the discussion that follows), underlying portal hypertension is likely. Helpful signs that suggest chronic liver disease include jaundice, asterixis, spider angioma, and palmar erythema.

The key procedure in establishing a diagnosis of variceal hemorrhage is upper gastrointestinal endoscopy, which should be accomplished either in the emergency department or soon after admission to the intensive care unit. Hemodynamic stabilization of the patient is essential before endoscopy. Likewise, gastric lavage with a large bore nasogastric tube is helpful in evacuating blood from the stomach before endoscopy. In addition, gastric lavage will determine whether the upper gastrointestinal tract is the site of hemorrhage in the patient who initially has melena or hematochezia, and it may also contribute to control of hemorrhage in a small number of patients. Varices can be established as the cause of bleeding when the person performing the endoscopy observes a bleeding varix or nonbleeding large varices and no other upper gastrointestinal lesions.

Although it has been generally accepted that other lesions, when present, are frequently responsible for upper gastrointestinal hemorrhage in patients with known varices, more recent studies suggest that varices are the cause of bleeding in over 90% of such patients.[5] Since patients with alcoholic cirrhosis are particularly prone to gastritis, Mallory-Weiss tears, and peptic ulceration, even a person skilled in performing endoscopies can have difficulty making the correct diagnosis. Gastritis is present in many patients with varices, and determining which of these two lesions is the cause of the ongoing or recent hemorrhage can be particularly difficult. However, since portal hypertension is probably the major factor underlying life-threatening hemorrhage from both varices and gastritis in patients with varices, they may require the same treatment.[21]

Assessment of Hepatic Hemodynamics

Because the increase in vascular resistance is at the sinusoidal level in patients with alcoholic cirrhosis, the elevated portal pressure can be estimated by wedging a catheter into a hepatic vein. In contrast, individuals with prehepatic or intrahepatic presinusoidal portal hypertension have a normal hepatic venous wedge pressure. The hepatic venous pressure gradient is defined as the hepatic venous wedge pressure minus free hepatic vein pressure. This gradient is determined by percutaneous introduction of a catheter into the femoral or brachial vein and advancement of this catheter into a hepatic vein with recording of pressure while it lies free within the vein and after it has been placed in the wedge position. Portal hypertension is present when this gradient is greater than 5 mm Hg, although variceal hemorrhage seldom develops unless the gradient is greater than 12 mm Hg.[14] Neither the hepatic venous wedge pressure nor the hepatic venous pressure gradient predicts which patients will bleed from varices when the pressure is above 12 mm Hg; therefore, the only usefulness of the measurement is in differentiating presinusoidal from sinusoidal and postsinusoidal portal hypertension.

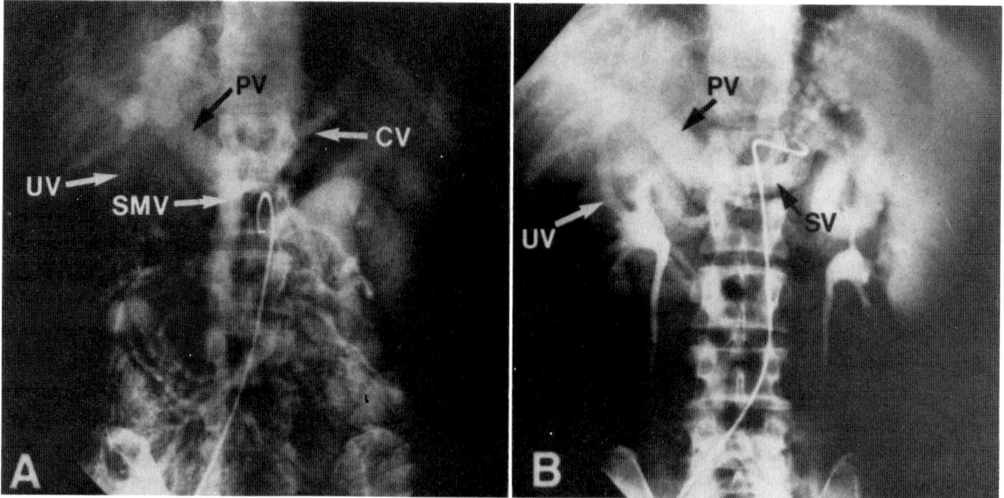

Fig. 25-3 Venous phase films following superior mesenteric (**A**) and splenic (**B**) angiograms in a patient with portal hypertension secondary to alcoholic cirrhosis. *PV*, portal vein; *SMV*, superior mesenteric vein; *UV*, umbilical vein; *CV*, coronary vein; *SV*, splenic vein.

More direct and more invasive methods of measuring portal pressure are by percutaneous and transhepatic puncture of an intrahepatic portal venous radical and by cannulation of the umbilical vein under local anesthesia. These methods may be particularly useful in patients who are suspected of having portal hypertension but who have a normal hepatic venous wedge pressure.

Selective visceral angiography is a useful technique for defining both the anatomy and the hemodynamic status of the portal venous system.[17] Venous phase films following a superior mesenteric arterial injection demonstrate opacification of the superior mesenteric and portal veins in most patients, and the degree of portal venous opacification can be graded to estimate hepatic portal perfusion (Fig. 25-3). The anatomic course and size of the splenic vein can be determined following a selective celiac axis or splenic artery injection. Absence of portal vein visualization following both the superior mesenteric and splenic arterial injections suggests either portal vein thrombosis or spontaneous reversal of portal flow. The latter condition develops when hepatic vascular resistance becomes so elevated that a fraction of hepatic arterial perfusion of the liver is drained by the portal vein rather than by hepatic veins. The diagnosis can be confirmed by observing portal venous opacification following selective injection of contrast material into the hepatic artery. Patients with isolated splenic vein thrombosis have a normal superior mesenteric angiogram but the splenic vein fails to opacify following a splenic arterial injection. Instead, prominent gastric varices and a markedly enlarged left gastroepiploic vein can usually be seen. A preoperative angiographic study is generally completed by injection of contrast material into the left renal vein if it is to be used in a shunting procedure.

The portal venous system and its collaterals can be more accurately defined by introduction of contrast following percutaneous, transhepatic entry into the portal venous system, cannulation of the umbilical vein, or splenoportography, which is accomplished by direct injection of contrast into the spleen after percutaneous puncture of this organ. Since these techniques are more invasive than selective visceral angiography, they are infrequently used in most centers.

Although it would be of potential value to quantify total hepatic blood flow, portal venous blood flow, and the degree of portal-systemic shunting, none of the methods available for clinical use are sufficiently reliable in patients with chronic liver disease to warrant their routine application. Likewise, direct measurement of flows by electromagnetic flowmeters during surgery are of limited value because of the unpredictable effects of surgery and anesthesia on hepatic hemodynamics.

Medical Management of Variceal Hemorrhage

Since the majority of patients who initially have acute variceal hemorrhage are high risks for emergency surgical intervention because of decompensated hepatic function and/or hypotension, in most centers the initial management of these patients is nonoperative. Because variceal hemorrhage is often associated with other complications of chronic liver disease and portal hypertension—such as encephalopathy (see discussion that follows), cirrhosis, and coagulopathies—an appropriately prioritized and coordinated treatment plan for these individuals is essential. The first priority is restoration of circulating blood volume and reversal or prevention of hemorrhagic shock. Large bore intravenous cannulas should be inserted in both upper extremities and, if hypotension is present, an isotonic crystalloid solution should be rapidly infused until type specific blood is available. Blood should be sent to the laboratory for typing and cross-matching of at least 4 units and for determinations of hematocrit, white blood cell count, platelet count, prothrombin time, partial thromboplastin time, serum electrolytes, blood urea nitrogen, and creatinine as a guide for subsequent management. Adequacy of fluid resuscitation should be monitored by urinary output through an indwelling urethral catheter and frequent assessment of vital signs. When the prothrombin time is prolonged, fresh frozen plasma should make up a component of the intravenous fluid volume administered. Although some degree of thrombocytopenia secondary to hypersplenism is frequently present, the platelet count is seldom less than 50,000/mm^3. When more profound thrombocytopenia is present, platelet packs should be administered.

Blood in the gastrointestinal tract is a potent inducer of encephalopathy (see discussion that follows). Therefore a nasogastric tube should be inserted for administration of a cathartic and lactulose if evidence of encephalopathy is present. The nasogastric tube can also be used for gastric lavage before diagnostic endoscopy.

Once hemorrhage has been controlled, attention should be directed to treatment of malnutrition, ascites, and encephalopathy if these are present. In the majority of patients, only modest dietary protein restriction (30 to 60 g) is required. Since most patients accumulate some ascites during resuscitation from a variceal hemorrhage, salt intake should be limited to 1 to 2 g/day. When intravenous hyperalimentation is required, standard solutions diluted to reduce the nitrogen content should be used rather than the unproven, expensive formulations, which are rich in branched chain amino acids.

Vasopressin

Vasopressin lowers portal pressure by constricting the arterioles in the splanchnic circulation and thereby decreasing inflow to the portal venous system. Because vasopressin also causes decreased cardiac output, increased blood pressure, and coronary vasoconstriction, it should not be administered to patients with coronary artery disease.

Administration of vasopressin results in control of active variceal hemorrhage in approximately 50% of patients.[9] It appears to be just as effective when administered through a peripheral vein as when given directly into the superior mesenteric artery.[4] Although the initial dose is usually 0.4 U/min, this may be increased by 0.2 U/min increments to a maximum of 1.0 U/min. Because of the effects of vasopressin on systemic hemodynamics and the coronary circulation, all patients receiving it should be monitored in an intensive care unit.

Balloon Tamponade

Acute variceal hemorrhage may also be controlled by direct compression of upper gastric and esophageal varices by inflatable balloons. Fig. 25-4 is a schematic drawing of the Sengstaken-Blakemore tube, which consists of a three-lumen tube, gastric balloon, and esophageal balloon. In most series, this device successfully controls acute variceal hemorrhage in over 80% of patients.[17] However, unless it is used according to a strict protocol, morbidity and mortality associated with the Sengstaken-Blakemore tube are significant. Complications that may result in death include esophageal perforation secondary to intraesophageal inflation of the gastric balloon, ischemic necrosis of the esophagus, asphyxiation secondary to upper migration of the esophageal balloon, and aspiration. The latter complication occurs frequently and can be avoided by attachment of a nasogastric tube to the Sengstaken-Blakemore tube before insertion and nasotracheal intubation to protect the airway. Since recurrent variceal hemorrhage follows balloon deflation in approximately 20% to 50% of patients, more definitive therapy should be planned for patients who require balloon tamponade.

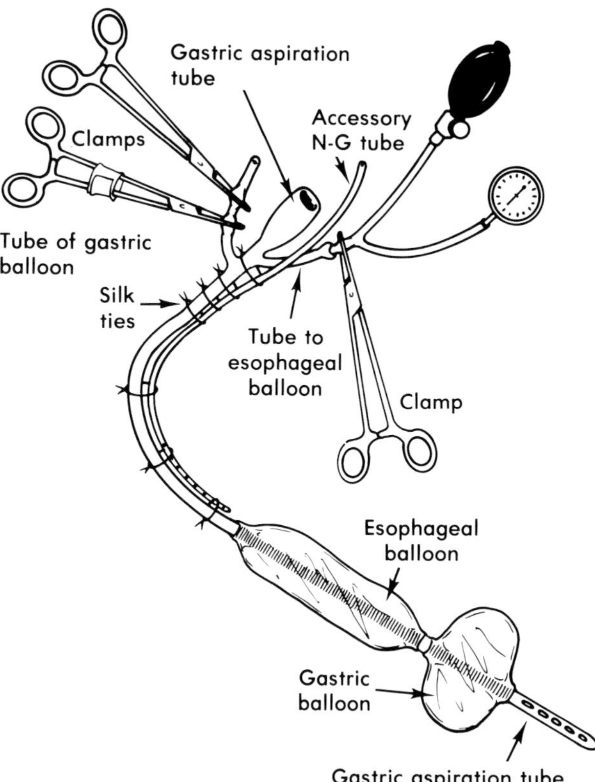

Fig. 25-4 The modified Sengstaken-Blakemore tube has an accessory nasogastric tube attached to prevent aspiration of secretions that accumulate above the esophageal balloon. (From Rikkers, L.F.: Portal hypertension. In Goldsmith, H.S., editor: Practice of surgery, vol. 3, General surgery, Thomaston, Conn., 1981, Practice of Surgery, Ltd.)

Variceal Sclerosis

Esophageal varices may be nonoperatively obliterated either by direct injection of sclerosing agents into the varices through an endoscope or by percutaneous, transhepatic embolization and sclerosis of the coronary vein. Because this latter technique is complicated by a high frequency of recurrent bleeding within the first week, portal vein thrombosis in a significant percentage of patients and intraperitoneal hemorrhage, its use is presently declining.[23] In contrast, endoscopic variceal sclerosis has recently become popular for control of acute variceal hemorrhage and is presently challenging surgery as an alternative method for long-term management of these patients.

Wide application of endoscopic sclerotherapy has occurred in only the past 5 to 10 years. Although several techniques for endoscopic sclerosis have been described, most sclerotherapists now administer intravariceal injections of sclerosing agents (sodium or sodium tetradecyl sulfate) through flexible endoscopes in awake patients. Mortality secondary to the technique has occurred in 1% to 3% of patients in most series and is usually secondary to aspiration pneumonitis, worsening of variceal hemorrhage, or esophageal perforation.[12] More frequent but nonlethal complications have included retrosternal chest pain, esophageal ulceration, and fever.

When applied to the recently or acutely bleeding patient, endoscopic sclerotherapy has resulted in control of hemorrhage in 85% to 95% of patients.[12] Sclerotherapy has been generally unsuccessful in patients who are bleeding from gastric varices. When bleeding is brisk or massive, obtaining temporary control by balloon tamponade before attempting sclerotherapy is preferable. In the few studies that have compared endoscopic sclerotherapy to balloon tamponade or emergency portacaval shunt in the acutely bleeding patient, no differences in short-term survival have been noted.[1,3]

Although endoscopic sclerosis initially was used only in patients with either advanced liver disease or diffuse splanchnic venous thrombosis, it is presently being applied in some centers as a definitive, long-term treatment for all patients who have bleeding from esophageal varices. All four controlled trials that have compared endoscopic sclerotherapy to medical treatment have shown that sclerotherapy repeated at intervals of 3 to 6 months decreased the frequency of recurrent hemorrhage.[12] However, as many as one half to two thirds of patients rebled before complete eradication of varices had been achieved. In two of the four studies, patients undergoing sclerotherapy have lived significantly longer than those receiving medical therapy.

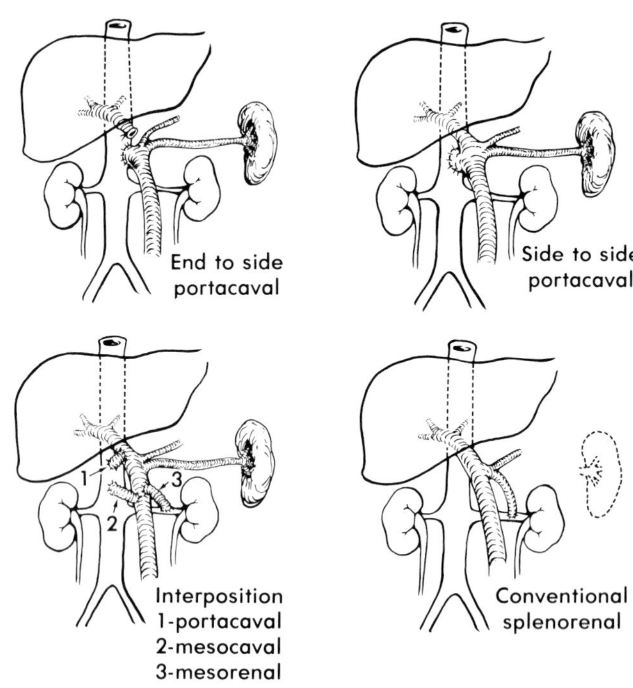

Fig. 25-5 Nonselective shunts decompress the entire portal venous system and divert all portal blood flow away from the liver.

Propranolol

Propranolol has recently been proposed as a pharmacologic means of preventing recurrent hemorrhage in patients who have previously bled from esophagogastric varices. Hemodynamic studies have shown that propranolol, administered in a dose sufficient to decrease the heart rate by 25%, reduces hepatic venous wedge pressure and directly measured portal venous pressure.[2,15] Propranolol's effect on portal pressure is most likely mediated through a reduction in splanchnic blood flow secondary to decreased cardiac output rather than by alteration of resistance in the hepatic vasculature or collateral vessels. Two controlled studies have compared propranolol to medical treatment for patients with cirrhosis who have bled from varices, but only one of these studies has shown a reduction in the frequency of recurrent hemorrhage in the propranolol group.[2,15] Until further studies are completed, propranolol will remain an experimental therapy for the long-term control of variceal hemorrhage.

Surgical Management of Variceal Hemorrhage

Since none of the operative procedures for variceal hemorrhage eliminate the elevated hepatic vascular or portal venous resistance, they do not reverse the abnormal physiologic state. Rather, some of the procedures may have adverse physiologic consequences of their own. Shunt operations decompress either all or a portion of the portal venous circulation. Those procedures that divert all portal blood flow away from the liver are termed *nonselective shunts*, whereas those that preserve some degree of hepatic portal perfusion are called *selective shunts*. All remaining operative procedures for variceal hemorrhage come under the heading of nonshunting operations.

Nonselective Shunts

Nonselective shunts in common use are shown in Fig. 25-5. All of these procedures decompress the entire splanchnic venous system and return portal pressure to normal. Therefore, as long as they remain patent, variceal hemorrhage is prevented. However, an undesirable physiologic consequence of these procedures is the complete diversion of portal blood flow away from the liver, which then becomes dependent on the hepatic artery for its blood supply. Although the hepatic artery may supply sufficient oxygen and nutrients, shunting of hepatotrophic hormones contained in portal blood may result in liver atrophy and eventual hepatic failure. In addition, it has been postulated that some of the nitrogenous compounds absorbed from the intestines are toxic to the brain and may contribute to the syndrome of encephalopathy. Complete portal diversion decreases hepatic extraction of these compounds, which can then be delivered directly to the cerebral circulation.

There are two hemodynamically distinct types of nonselective shunts, the end-to-side portacaval shunt and several varieties of side-to-side portal-systemic shunts. The end-to-side portacaval shunt was the first shunt used clinically and is the prototype against which all other operative procedures for portal hypertension have been compared. This shunt is constructed by division of the portal vein near its bifurcation and anastomosis of its splanchnic end to the inferior vena cava; the hepatic end of the portal vein is oversewn. Because this procedure results in a large cal-

SELECTIVE SHUNTS

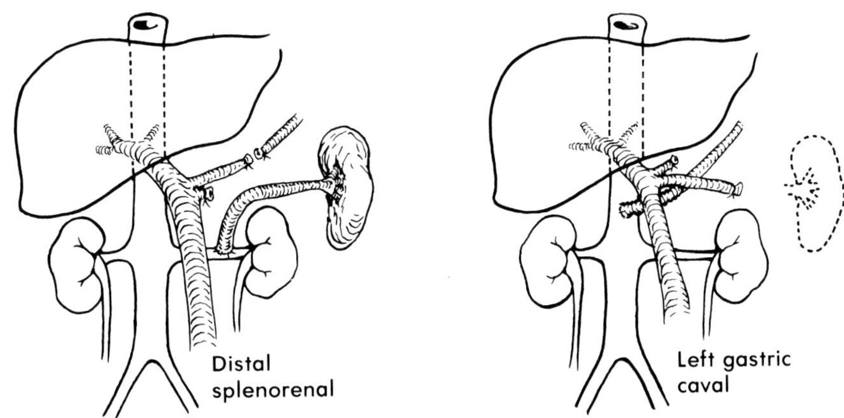

Fig. 25-6 Selective shunts decompress only the gastrosplenic component of the portal venous system and maintain portal hypertension and portal blood flow to the liver.

iber vein-to-vein anastomosis, it reliably prevents recurrent variceal hemorrhage. Since the intrahepatic sinusoidal network does not communicate with the shunt, sinusoidal pressure frequently remains high.

The end-to-side portacaval shunt is the only surgical procedure for variceal hemorrhage that has been compared to standard medical treatment in randomized, controlled studies.[18] Although these trials differed with respect to several minor points, the major findings were similar. First, the portacaval shunt reliably prevented recurrent variceal hemorrhage. In contrast, medical treatment alone was followed by recurrent hemorrhage in over 70% of patients. Second, patients with shunts lived marginally longer than medically treated patients, but in no individual trial was the difference in survival statistically significant. Whereas medically treated patients often died secondary to recurrent hemorrhage, patients with shunts died of progressive hepatic failure. Third, spontaneous and severe encephalopathy frequently occurred following a portacaval shunt. Encephalopathy was rare in patients without shunts except when induced by an upper gastrointestinal hemorrhage.

When the anastomosis of a side-to-side portal-systemic shunt is large enough to maintain long-term patency, it usually diverts the entire portal blood flow from the liver. Because the hepatic limb of the portal vein remains in continuity with the shunt, side-to-side shunts also decompress the hepatic sinusoids. Since hepatic sinusoidal hypertension is a key factor in the production of cirrhotic ascites, side-to-side portal-systemic shunts effectively relieve ascites, as well as prevent recurrent variceal hemorrhage.

The side-to-side portacaval shunt is constructed by direct anastomosis of the portal vein to the inferior vena cava. Because a large shunt can be constructed and a vein-to-vein anastomosis is used, this procedure has the highest long-term patency rate of all the side-to-side portal-systemic shunts.

Interposition grafts can be placed in the portacaval, mesocaval, and mesorenal positions. Most available data indicate that all of these procedures have hemodynamic consequences similar to those of the side-to-side portacaval shunt, i.e., effective portal decompression and complete diversion of portal blood flow. Although these shunts are reportedly easier to construct than the side-to-side portacaval shunt, the shunt thrombosis rate is considerably higher.[22]

The conventional splenorenal shunt procedure combines a proximal splenorenal shunt with splenectomy. Because the smaller, proximal end of the splenic vein is used, shunt occlusion rates have ranged from 10% to 25%.[18] Although splenectomy invariably relieves hypersplenism, thrombocytopenia and leukopenia are rarely of clinical significance in patients with portal hypertension. The only situation when splenectomy should be considered in this setting is when the platelet count is persistently below 30,000/mm^3 and/or the white blood cell count is less than 1200/mm^3, since these levels may lead to life-threatening complications of hemorrhage and sepsis.

Selective Shunts

The only truly selective portal-systemic shunts are the distal splenorenal shunt and the left gastric–vena caval shunt (Fig. 25-6). The latter procedure has been used mainly in patients with nonalcoholic cirrhosis in Japan.[11] Because of its technical difficulty and the necessity of a large diameter left gastric vein, which frequently is not present in patients with alcoholic cirrhosis, this shunt is unlikely to gain popularity in the United States. The distal splenorenal shunt consists of anastomosis of the distal end of the splenic vein to the left renal vein and disconnection of the portal-superior mesenteric venous component of the splanchnic venous circulation from the gastrosplenic component. The objectives of the distal splenorenal shunt are (1) decompression of the gastrosplenic venous circulation, (2) preservation of hepatic portal perfusion, and (3) maintenance of an elevated portal venous pressure. Extensive experience with this procedure has shown that these objectives are achieved at least in the early postoperative period.[26] However, since the high pressure portal venous network is in juxtaposition to the decompressed gastrosplenic venous system, collaterals eventually reform and portal flow to the liver gradually diminishes with time. Evidence has been presented that loss of portal perfusion occurs more rapidly in patients with alcoholic cirrhosis than in individuals with nonalcoholic cirrhosis.[8]

Both controlled and noncontrolled clinical trials have suggested that the frequency of postoperative encephalopathy is less after the distal splenorenal shunt than after nonselective shunts.[7] Encephalopathy rates following the distal splenorenal shunt have ranged from 10% to 15%, whereas the rates following nonselective shunts have ranged from 30% to 50%. Although the low frequency of encephalopathy following the distal splenorenal shunt has been attributed mainly to preservation of hepatic portal perfusion, inhibition of intestinal absorption of cerebral toxins secondary to maintenance of intestinal venous hypertension may also play a role.[19] Since some patients lose hepatic portal perfusion either acutely (portal vein thrombosis) or gradually (continuing collateralization) after the distal splenorenal shunt, this latter mechanism may account for the low frequency of encephalopathy observed in this group.

None of the controlled trials of the distal splenorenal shunt have demonstrated longer survival following this procedure than after nonselective shunts.[7] However, two large noncontrolled experiences have suggested that the distal splenorenal shunt results in longer survival than nonselective shunts in patients with nonalcoholic cirrhosis.[26,28] Because the distal splenorenal shunt decompresses neither the splanchnic viscera nor the hepatic sinusoids, it is ineffective in relieving already present ascites. In fact, approximately 25% of patients develop moderate to severe ascites in the early postoperative period following this procedure.[20] Thus the distal splenorenal shunt should not be used for patients with difficult to control preoperative ascites.

Nonshunting Operations

Nonshunting operations have one or more of the following objectives: (1) decrease of portal venous inflow (e.g., splenectomy), (2) interruption of collateral pathways to varices (e.g., esophagogastric devascularization), or (3) obliteration or elimination of varices (e.g., transthoracic ligation of varices and esophagogastrectomy). Since an elevated portal venous pressure is maintained, a distinct advantage of all of these procedures is that portal blood flow to the liver is preserved. However, elevated portal venous pressure is the stimulus to portal-systemic collateralization, and reformation of varices and recurrent variceal hemorrhage frequently occur.

In patients with cirrhosis, splenectomy alone minimally alters portal pressure and recurrent variceal hemorrhage is frequent. The only setting in which splenectomy reliably prevents future variceal hemorrhage is isolated splenic vein thrombosis without generalized portal hypertension.

The most extensive nonshunting operation is the procedure recently described by Sugiura and Futagawa.[24] The Sugiura procedure consists of splenectomy, proximal gastric devascularization, vagotomy, pyloroplasty through an abdominal incision, and esophageal devascularization and esophageal transection and reanastomosis through a thoracotomy (Fig. 25-7). This procedure has been very effective in preventing variceal hemorrhage in Japanese patients with nonalcoholic cirrhosis. Similar, but less extensive, devascularization procedures have been associated with frequent recurrent hemorrhage when applied to patients with alcoholic cirrhosis.[13] Whether the Sugiura procedure will be more effective in this population remains to be proven.

A simple and rapid method of interrupting esophageal collateral pathways is transabdominal esophageal transec-

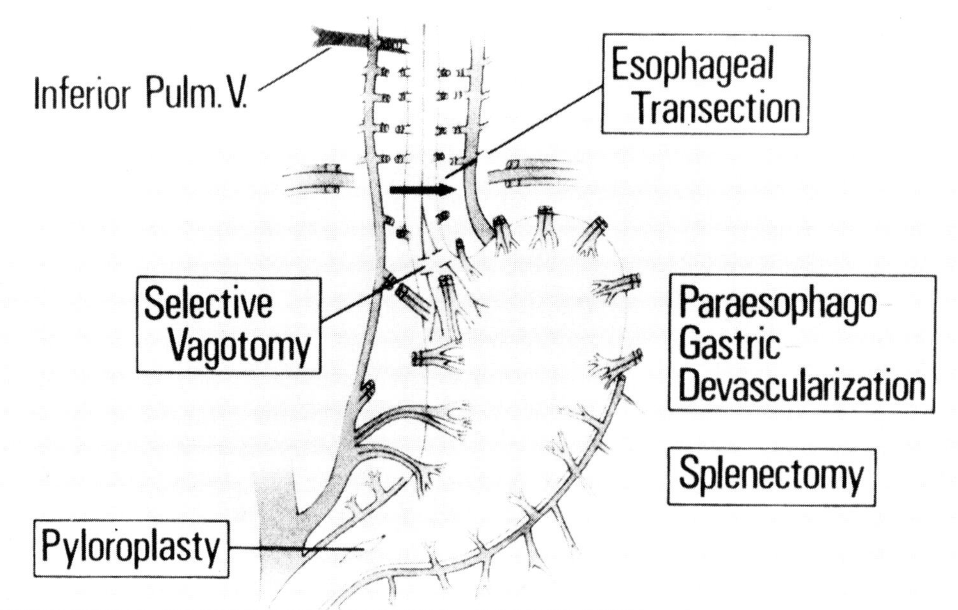

Fig. 25-7 Sugiura procedure. (From Sugiura, M., and Futagawa, S.: Arch. Surg. **112:**1318, 1977. Copyright 1977, American Medical Association.)

tion and reanastomosis with the end-to-end-anastomosis (EEA) stapling instrument combined with ligation of the coronary vein.[25] Since this procedure has been associated with frequent recurrent hemorrhage, it is not recommended as an appropriate option for control of variceal hemorrhage.

Management of Acute Variceal Hemorrhage

Fig. 25-8 is an algorithm for management of the acute variceal bleeder. The sequential application as indicated of intravenous vasopressin infusion, balloon tamponade, and endoscopic variceal sclerosis results in control of acute variceal hemorrhage in over 80% of patients. Emergency surgery is reserved for those few patients who continue to bleed despite aggressive nonoperative treatment. The advantage of this approach is that it allows time before surgery for improvement of hepatic functional reserve, which is the major determinant of early postoperative survival. Hepatic reserve is most easily estimated by Child's classification, which consists of two biochemical indices (serum bilirubin and albumin) and three clinical variables (ascites, encephalopathy, and nutrition) (see Table 24-2). Approximate operative mortality rates for Child's class A, B, and C patients are as follows: up to 5%, 5% to 15%, and 20% to 50%, respectively. It has been shown that a particular Child's class can be significantly improved when an interval of medical management and nutritional support precedes elective surgery.[9]

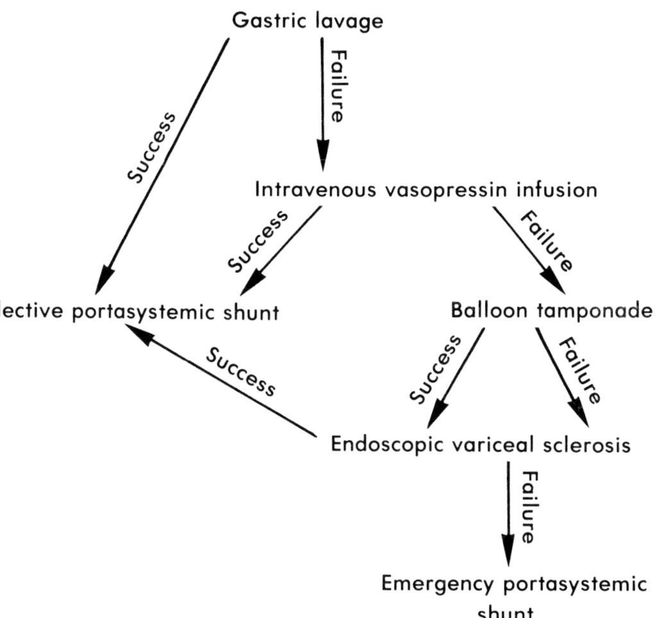

Fig. 25-8 Algorithm for management of acute variceal hemorrhage.

When bleeding persists despite all nonoperative measures, emergency surgery should be expeditiously performed. Although some surgeons prefer a nonshunting operation in this setting, the most reliable way to control persistent, active variceal hemorrhage is portal decompression.

Selection of Operative Procedure

No single surgical procedure is ideal for all patients who hemorrhage from esophagogastric varices.[20] The alternatives include the end-to-side portacaval shunt, one of the side-to-side portal-systemic shunts, the distal splenorenal shunt, and a variety of nonshunting procedures (Table 25-1). The most important factors that should determine selection of the appropriate operation are status of hepatic hemodynamics, clinical circumstances, and experience and skill of the surgeon.

Because it is technically easy to perform and reliably decompresses the portal venous system, the end-to-side portacaval shunt is generally preferred for emergency situations when the patient is actively bleeding at the time of surgery. A side-to-side portal-systemic shunt is preferred for patients with intractable preoperative ascites in addition to variceal hemorrhage. When feasible, a vein-to-vein anastomosis should be selected rather than an interposition synthetic graft, which frequently thromboses in the late postoperative period.

The distal splenorenal shunt is reserved for the majority (approximately two thirds) of patients who have evidence of portal blood flow to the liver on preoperative angiography, compatible anatomy, and absent or easily controlled preoperative ascites. The distal splenorenal shunt may occasionally be performed in the emergency setting when hemorrhage is temporarily controlled by balloon tamponade, allowing time for preoperative angiography.

Either a nonshunting procedure or endoscopic sclerotherapy should be selected for patients with diffuse splanchnic venous thrombosis and no major portal tributaries available for anastomosis. Nonshunting procedures may also be indicated when preoperative angiography reveals excellent hepatic portal perfusion but prior splenectomy makes a distal splenorenal shunt impossible.

Table 25-1 **OPERATIONS FOR PORTAL HYPERTENSION**

Type of Shunt	Portal Perfusion	Encephalopathy	Control of Ascites	Control of Bleeding
End-to-side portacaval shunt	None	Frequent	Fair	Excellent
Side-to-side shunts (many varieties)	None	Frequent	Best	Good
Distal splenorenal shunt	Preserved	Infrequent	Poor	Excellent
Nonshunting procedures	Preserved	Infrequent	Fair	Poor

Effects of Treatment for Variceal Hemorrhage on Survival

Regardless of which treatment is selected, only 40% to 60% of patients with alcoholic cirrhosis will live for 5 years after the onset of variceal hemorrhage. All controlled trials have failed to show a difference in survival between therapies in this population of patients. In fact, when use of the portacaval shunt and endoscopic sclerotherapy have been compared with standard medical treatment, only marginal prolongation of survival has been found.[12,18] The relentless progression of liver disease in patients with alcoholic cirrhosis, often secondary to continued alcoholism, is most likely the main factor determining survival. In studies of large populations, this dominant factor appears to override any potential benefit to survival of the therapy applied. However, it should be emphasized that all controlled studies to the present time have consisted almost exclusively of patients with alcoholic cirrhosis. Noncontrolled studies suggest the long-term survival of patients with nonalcoholic cirrhosis and noncirrhotic portal hypertension may be better following procedures that preserve portal blood flow to the liver (distal splenorenal shunt, nonshunting operations, endoscopic variceal sclerosis). In the United States today the most popular treatments for variceal hemorrhage are the distal splenorenal shunt and endoscopic variceal sclerosis. Although controlled trials are ongoing, these therapies have not yet been compared regarding their relative effects on quality and length of survival.

ASCITES

Although ascites frequently accompanies sinusoidal and postsinusoidal portal hypertension, it seldom develops secondary to pure presinusoidal portal hypertension. Several factors appear to contribute to the pathogenesis of cirrhotic ascites.[27] The initiating factor is probably altered hemodynamics in the hepatic and splanchnic circulations. Elevated hepatic sinusoidal and intestinal capillary pressures result in transudation of fluid into the interstitial space. Since the hepatic sinusoids are more porous than the intestinal capillaries, the liver's interstitial fluid contains a higher protein concentration than the intestinal transudate. When the rate of interstitial fluid formation exceeds the capacity for lymph drainage, ascites accumulates. This third-spacing of extracellular fluid results in a circulating volume deficit, and secondary mechanisms such as aldosterone secretion and redistribution of blood flow within the kidney are set into motion to restore plasma volume. The expansion of plasma volume maintains portal hypertension and results in further ascites formation.

Ascites may cause significant morbidity and even mortality. Ascites is the sine qua non for spontaneous bacterial peritonitis, and development of tense ascites almost always precedes the onset of the hepatorenal syndrome. Both of these complications are associated with high mortality. In addition, ascites often develops before hemorrhage from esophagogastric varices and may contribute to the magnitude of portal pressure in these patients.

Ascites can be effectively managed by simple medical treatment in 95% of patients. The key elements of medical management are dietary salt restriction and diuretic therapy. Dietary salt should initially be limited to 20 to 30 mEq/day. Since secondary hyperaldosteronism is present in the majority of patients with ascites, spironolactone is a rational and physiologic first line diuretic. The combination of salt restriction and spironolactone (a specific aldosterone antagonist that blocks the action of aldosterone to promote sodium excretion and potassium retention) in a dose of 100 to 400 mg/day results in an effective diuresis in approximately two thirds of patients. When this regimen fails, either hydrochlorothiazide or furosemide should be added. Therapy should be carefully monitored with frequent estimations of serum electrolytes, blood urea nitrogen, creatinine, and body weight.

The most effective surgical procedures for the less than 5% of patients with medically intractable ascites are the peritoneovenous shunt and any one of the side-to-side portal-systemic shunts. Since implantation of a peritoneovenous shunt is associated with considerably less morbidity and mortality than construction of a side-to-side portacaval shunt, it is the surgical therapy of choice for most patients with intractable ascites.[16] A side-to-side portal-systemic shunt should be considered only for patients who develop both variceal hemorrhage and intractable ascites.

The peritoneovenous shunt basically functions as a megalymphatic and returns the ascitic fluid to the vascular compartment. The combination of an expanded circulating volume and decreased intra-abdominal pressure results in improved renal perfusion, which is reflected by an increased glomerular filtration rate, urinary volume, and sodium excretion and by decreased plasma renin activity and aldosterone concentration.

Insertion of the peritoneovenous shunt may be done with the patient under local anesthesia (Fig. 25-9). The valve is implanted in the abdominal musculature and the peritoneal tubing is placed within the abdomen through a subcostal incision. The venous tubing is inserted into the internal jugular vein through a small cervical incision after it is brought to the neck through a subcutaneous tunnel. Although the technique of shunt insertion is quite simple, rapid transfusion of ascites into the central venous compartment may result in life-threatening complications. Expansion of the intravascular volume can result in variceal hemorrhage or pulmonary edema or both. As yet unidentified substances within ascitic fluid cause disseminated intravascular coagulation in some patients. Shunt occlusion and sepsis also occur quite frequently. Because of these complications, no trial has yet demonstrated prolongation of survival following this procedure, although ascites is relieved in a high percentage of patients. Therefore this operation should be reserved for patients with truly intractable ascites.

PORTAL-SYSTEMIC ENCEPHALOPATHY

Portal-systemic encephalopathy (PSE) is a psychoneurologic syndrome secondary to hepatocellular dysfunction in combination with portal-systemic shunting. A person with this syndrome may initially have diverse symptoms and signs including changes in the level of consciousness, intellectual deterioration, changes in personality, and the characteristic flapping tremor, which is called asterixis.

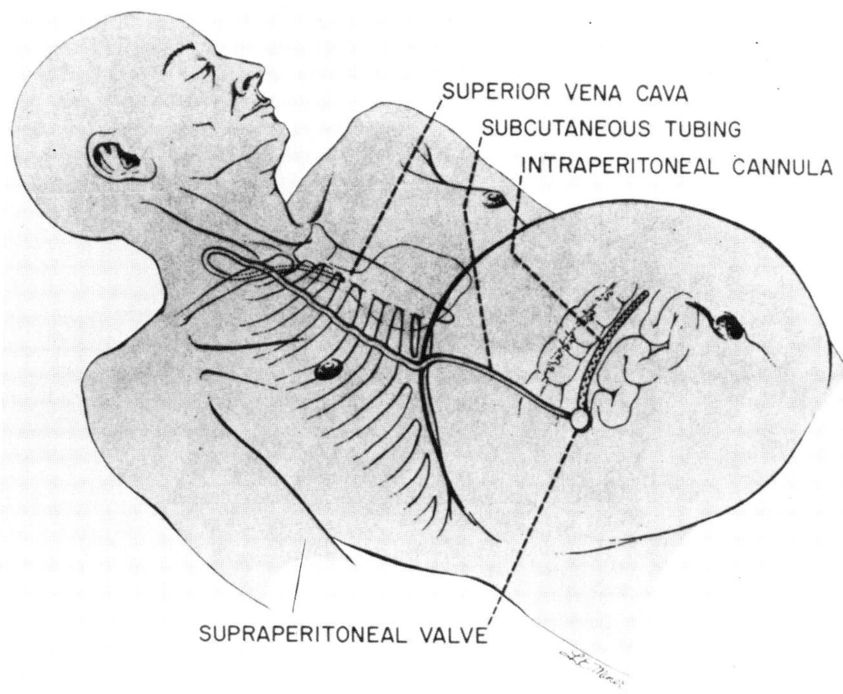

Fig. 25-9 Leveen peritoneovenous shunt transports ascites from the abdomen to the superior vena cava. (From Reinhardt, G.F., and Stanley, M.M.: Surg. Gynecol. Obstet. **145:**420, 1977. By permission of Surgery, Gynecology, and Obstetrics.)

PSE occasionally develops spontaneously in patients with chronic liver disease but most frequently occurs following portal-systemic shunting procedures, especially those that completely divert portal blood flow from the liver. As previously mentioned, PSE develops in approximately 25% to 50% of patients who undergo nonselective shunting procedures.

Although many theories have been advanced, the exact pathogenesis of PSE remains obscure.[10] The key element in most theories is the intestinal absorption of one or more cerebral toxins, which either directly bypass the liver or fail to be inactivated by the liver and thereby gain access to the brain. Leading candidate toxins include ammonia, mercaptans, and gamma-aminobutyric acid (GABA). Another prominent theory is that the altered plasma profile of amino acids present in patients with chronic liver disease may lead to depletion of normal neurotransmitters and accumulation of false neurotransmitters in the brain.

It is uncommon for encephalopathy to develop spontaneously. Rather, one or more of the following factors is usually responsible for inducing an episode of PSE: excess dietary protein, gastrointestinal hemorrhage, infection, metabolic alkalosis, sedatives, azotemia, and constipation. Most of these precipitating factors lead to hyperammonemia, lending support to ammonia as one of the cerebral toxins responsible for the syndrome.

Treatment of encephalopathy should begin with identification and elimination of any precipitating factors that may be present. Blood within the gastrointestinal tract should be removed by catharsis, sedatives should be discontinued, infection should be treated with antibiotics or surgical drainage or both, and dietary protein should be restricted. Patients known to be susceptible to PSE should be chronically treated with stool softeners and mild protein restriction (50 to 60 g of protein per day).

Specific pharmacologic treatment of PSE is indicated for patients who fail to clear their sensorium following removal of all precipitating factors and for individuals with chronic, persistent PSE. Although several drugs have been proposed, only neomycin, a poorly absorbed antibiotic, and lactulose, a nonabsorbable disaccharide, have proved efficacious for the treatment of encephalopathy. Neomycin appears to act by suppressing urease-containing bacteria, which are responsible for production of ammonia, whereas the mechanism of action of lactulose is through colon acidification and induction of a mild catharsis. Acute encephalopathy can be treated equally effectively by neomycin (1.5 g every 6 hours) or lactulose (30 g hourly until mild diarrhea results and then 20 to 30 g three or four times a day or as required to result in two soft bowel movements a day. Lactulose is preferred to neomycin for chronic treatment since neomycin may result in ototoxicity and/or nephrotoxicity. Although intravenous and enteral administration of solutions rich in branched chain amino acids have been proposed for patients with PSE, there is presently no solid evidence that such treatment is beneficial.

SUMMARY

Variceal hemorrhage is the most life-threatening complication of portal hypertension. After an accurate diagnosis has been made by upper gastrointestinal endoscopy, nonoperative treatment should be initiated. Intravenous vasopressin infusion, balloon tamponade, and endoscopic variceal sclerosis either singly or in combination control acute variceal hemorrhage in over 80% of patients and allow time for medical management of the underlying liver disease. Emergency surgery is rarely indicated.

Therapeutic choices for long-term prevention of recurrent variceal hemorrhage include portal-systemic shunt operations, nonshunting surgical procedures, and endoscopic sclerotherapy repeated at intervals. Shunt operations that divert all portal blood flow away from the liver are termed nonselective shunts, whereas those that preserve some degree of hepatic portal perfusion are called selective shunts. The only selective shunt commonly used in the United States is the distal splenorenal shunt. Although all shunt procedures effectively prevent recurrent hemorrhage, the distal splenorenal shunt is preferred because it is less frequently associated with postoperative encephalopathy than nonselective shunts. Nonshunting operations and long-term sclerotherapy are also infrequently complicated by encephalopathy, but these therapies are less effective in preventing recurrent variceal hemorrhage than procedures that decompress varices. There is presently no evidence that any treatment option is superior to the others with respect to survival.

Cirrhotic ascites can be resolved with medical therapy alone in over 95% of patients. The peritoneovenous shunt should be considered for the occasional individual with intractable ascites that persists despite aggressive medical treatment.

Encephalopathy develops in patients with impaired hepatocellular function and some degree of portal-systemic shunting. Although its exact pathogenesis remains obscure, encephalopathy can be effectively treated in most patients by elimination of any precipitating factors and administration of lactulose.

REFERENCES

1. Barsoum, M.S., et al.: Tamponade and injection sclerotherapy in the management of bleeding esophageal varices, Br. J. Surg. **69:**76, 1982.
2. Burroughs, A.K., et al.: Controlled trial of propranolol for the prevention of recurrent variceal hemorrhage in patients with cirrhosis, N. Engl. J. Med. **309:**1539, 1983.
3. Cello, J.P., et al.: Endoscopic sclerotherapy versus portacaval shunt in patients with severe cirrhosis and variceal hemorrhage, N. Engl. J. Med. **311:**1589, 1984.
4. Chojkier, M., et al.: A controlled comparison of continuous intraarterial and intravenous infusions of vasopressin in hemorrhage from esophageal varices, Gastroenterology **77:**540, 1979.
5. Dave, P., Romeu, J., and Messer, J.: Upper gastrointestinal bleeding in patients with portal hypertension: a reappraisal, J. Clin. Gastroenterol. **5:**113, 1983.
6. Groszmann, R.J., and Atterbury, C.E.: The pathophysiology of portal hypertension: a basis for classification, Sem. Liver Dis. **2:**177, 1982.
7. Henderson, J.M., and Warren, W.D.: Current status of the distal splenorenal shunt, Sem. Liver Dis. **3:**251, 1983.
8. Henderson, J.M., et al.: Hemodynamic differences between alcoholic and nonalcoholic cirrhotics following distal splenorenal shunt—effect on survival? Ann. Surg. **198:**325, 1983.
9. Holman, J.M., and Rikkers, L.F.: Success of medical and surgical management of acute variceal hemorrhage, Am. J. Surg. **140:**816, 1980.
10. Hoyumpa, A.M., Jr., et al.: Hepatic encephalopathy, Gastroenterology **76:**184, 1979.
11. Inokuchi, K., et al.: Results of left gastric vena caval shunt for esophageal varices: analysis of one hundred clinical cases, Surgery **78:**628, 1975.
12. Joffe, S.N.: Nonshunting procedures for control of variceal bleeding, Sem. Liver Dis. **3:**235, 1983.
13. Johnson, G., et al.: Hemodynamic changes with cirrhosis of the liver: control of arteriovenous shunts during operation for esophageal varices, Ann. Surg. **163:**692, 1966.
14. Lebrec, D., et al.: Portal hypertension, size of esophageal varices, and risk of gastrointestinal bleeding in alcoholic cirrhosis, Gastroenterology **79:**1139, 1980.
15. Lebrec, D., et al.: A randomized controlled study of propranolol for prevention of recurrent gastrointestinal bleeding in patients with cirrhosis: a final report, Hepatology **4:**355, 1984.
16. LeVeen, H.H., et al.: Peritoneovenous shunting for ascites, Ann. Surg. **180:**580, 1974.
17. Rikkers, L.F.: Portal hypertension. In Goldsmith, H.S., editor: Practice of surgery, vol. 3, General surgery, New York, 1981, Harper & Row Publishers, Inc.
18. Rikkers, L.F.: Operations for management of esophageal variceal hemorrhage (Medical Progress), West. J. Med. **136:**107, 1982.
19. Rikkers, L.F.: Portal hemodynamics, intestinal absorption and postshunt encephalopathy, Surgery **94:**126, 1983.
20. Rikkers, L.F., Soper, N.J., and Cormier, R.A.: Selective operative approach for variceal hemorrhage, Am. J. Surg. **147:**89, 1984.
21. Sarfeh, I.J., et al.: Clinical significance of erosive gastritis in patients with alcoholic liver disease and upper gastrointestinal hemorrhage, Ann. Surg. **194:**149, 1981.
22. Smith, R.B., III, et al.: Dacron interposition shunts for portal hypertension—an analysis of morbidity correlates, Ann. Surg. **192:**9, 1980.
23. Smith-Laing, G., et al.: Role of percutaneous transhepatic obliteration of varices in the management of hemorrhage from gastroesophageal varices, Gastroenterology **80:**1031, 1981.
24. Sugiura, M., and Futagawa, S.: Further evaluation of the Sugiura procedure in the treatment of esophageal varices, Arch. Surg. **112:**1317, 1977.
25. Wanamaker, S.R., Cooperman, M., and Carey, L.C.: Use of the EEA stapling instrument for control of bleeding esophageal varices, Surgery **94:**620, 1983.
26. Warren, W.D., et al.: Ten years portal hypertensive surgery at Emory, Ann. Surg. **195:**530, 1982.
27. Witte, C.L., Witte, M.H., and Dumont, A.E.: Lymph imbalance in the genesis and perpetuation of the ascites syndrome in hepatic cirrhosis, Gastroenterology **78:**1059, 1980.
28. Zeppa, R., et al.: The comparative survival of alcoholics versus nonalcoholics after distal splenorenal shunt, Ann. Surg. **187:**510, 1978.

26

David W. McFadden and Thomas R. Gadacz

Calculous Disease of the Gallbladder and Common Bile Duct

Bile is a complex isosmotic fluid produced by the liver and composed of water, electrolytes, and various organic solutes, including bile salts, cholesterol, phospholipids, and bilirubin. Approximately two thirds of the total bile manufactured daily is formed directly in the hepatic canaliculus and modified downstream by its admixture with ductular bile. The gallbladder stores and concentrates this hepatic bile and delivers it at intervals into the duodenum to facilitate digestion and absorption of fats.[36,45]

Understanding the physiology of bile composition, secretion, and flow is important to the surgeon primarily because of two clinical abnormalities. One is the failure of bile secretion and/or excretion that results in the buildup of normal biliary components in the blood with impaired fat absorption. Discussion of this problem is considered in Chapter 29. Second is the formation of abnormally composed bile that may lead to gallstone formation. This abnormality is the focus of the present chapter.

BILE FORMATION

Canalicular Bile

A 24-hour canalicular bile flow approximates 400 ml/day as measured by the clearance of inert water-soluble substances such as erythritol or mannitol. An important concept that has been documented experimentally is that the basic mechanism responsible for hepatic bile secretion is similar to that responsible for the elaboration of salt and water by other secretory epithelia.[48] An active transport system is the driving force for the secretion of solutes into canalicular bile. This process results in local osmotic gradients, leading to a corresponding passive flow of water.[36] Presently canalicular bile is believed to consist of two major fractions: a bile salt–dependent fraction that results from active secretion of bile salts into the bile canaliculi and a bile salt–independent fraction. Each fraction comprises approximately 50% of total canalicular bile flow.

Bile Salt–Dependent Fraction

The major components of the bile salt–dependent fraction of canalicular bile are bile salts, cholesterol, and phospholipids. In human studies a positive linear relationship has been demonstrated between canalicular bile flow and bile salt output (Fig. 26-1).[7,45] Most of the bile salts secreted into the canalicular bile are the result of an extremely efficient extraction of the bile salts from the portal blood through the enterohepatic circulation, with only a small minority resulting from de novo synthesis by the hepatocytes. The normal bile salt pool size in humans approximates 6 mmol and cycles in the enterohepatic circulation two to three times per meal, so that the average person secretes between 30 to 60 mmol of bile salts daily.[36] The uptake of bile salts by the liver is largely by way of a sodium-coupled transport mechanism[40] and is powered by a sodium-potassium-ATPase. Bile salt uptake is hormonally modulated by intracellular cyclic AMP levels.[45] Little is known about the route and mechanism of bile salt transport to the canaliculus once it enters the hepatocyte. Vesicular transport in the hepatocytes is one suggested mechanism.

The bile salt–dependent secretion of canalicular bile not only accounts for 50% of the canalicular bile secretion but is a major determinant of both phospholipid and cholesterol secretion into bile. Both phospholipid and cholesterol biliary output increase with bile salt–dependent bile flow but in a nonlinear fashion.[36] Other factors in the biliary output of phospholipids and cholesterol include the noncontinuous nature of the enterohepatic circulation, the endogenous supply of phospholipids and cholesterol, and less well elucidated factors. More importantly, these extremely water-insoluble lipids are kept in solution in the aqueous bile by the formation of mixed micelles with bile salts.[1,36] In summary, the primary event, as well as the rate-limiting step, in the formation of the bile salt–dependent fraction of canalicular bile flow is the uptake of bile salts from the sinusoidal blood across the sinusoidal basal membrane of the hepatocyte. This makes possible the concomitant secretion of phospholipid and cholesterol into the canalicular bile.

Bile Salt–Independent Fraction

Theoretically, bile salt–independent canalicular bile secretion is the amount of bile secretion that occurs in the absence of bile salt output. The concentrations of sodium, potassium, chloride, and bicarbonate in hepatic bile are virtually identical to those found in plasma; and it is these inorganic electrolytes that account for the majority of bile osmolality.[45] In fasting human patients with T-tubes in their common bile ducts it has been estimated that this bile salt–independent bile secretion of an electrolyte-rich solution approximates 50% of total canalicular bile production.[7,36] Contributory mechanisms to the formation of this fraction of bile are poorly understood, but sodium transport as mediated by a sodium-potassium-ATPase appears to be implicated. This sodium pump may be the impetus for the hepatocellular uptake of various anions, including chloride and bicarbonate, which is similar to sodium-coupled bile salt transport. It appears that the major physiologic role of bile salt–independent bile formation may be

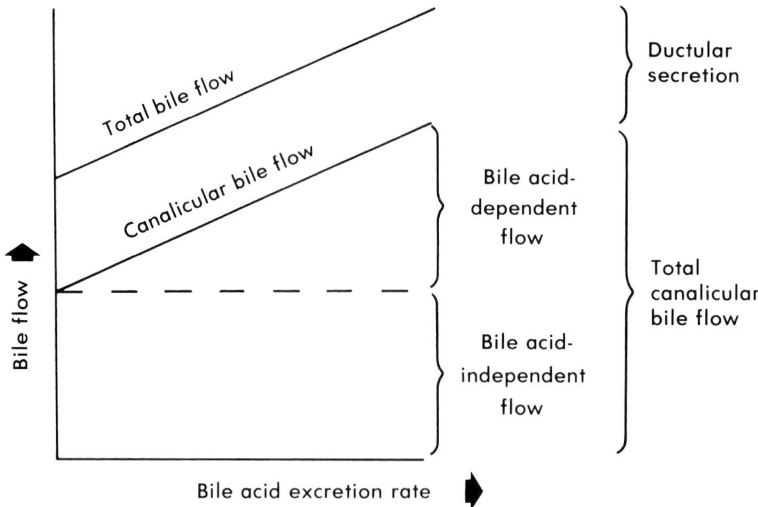

Fig. 26-1 Components of bile flow. Ductular secretion plus canalicular flow accounts for total bile flow. Canalicular flow has bile salt (acid)–dependent and bile salt (acid)–independent components. Bile-dependent canalicular flow varies directly with bile salt (acid) excretion rate. Although the other two components are shown as constant, there is some dependence on bile salt (acid) excretion rate. (Modified from Scharschmidt, B.F.: Bile formation and cholestasis, metabolism and enterohepatic circulation of bile acids, and gallstone formation. In Zakim, D., and Boyer, T.D., editors: Hepatology, Philadelphia, 1982, W.B. Saunders Co.)

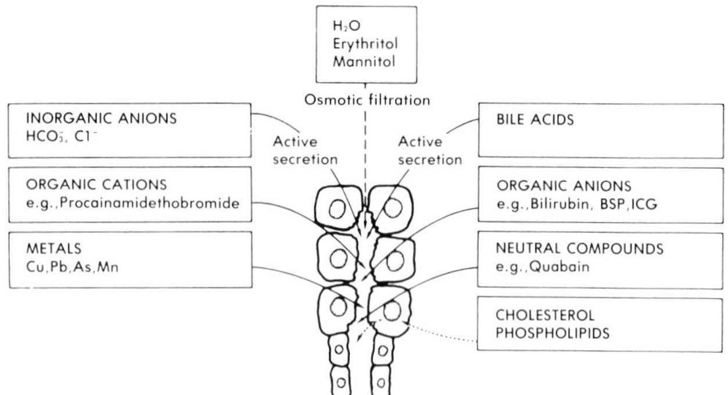

Fig. 26-2 Hepatocellular transport mechanisms that are responsible for the secretion of endogenous and exogenous substances into the bile. (From Paumgartner, G., and Sauerbruch, T.: Clin. Gastroenterol. **12**:3, 1983.)

to dilute and wash out the bile salt–dependent fraction of bile from the canaliculi. The two fractions of canalicular bile flow formation may work together to provide a sufficient bile flow into which a variety of endogenous and exogenous substances may be secreted by the liver (Fig. 26-2).[36]

Ductular Bile

Once it leaves the canaliculus, bile flows through and is modified by ductules and ducts, which secrete a hypertonic fluid composed primarily of water and electrolytes. Approximately one third of total bile produced is ductular bile, which is rich in sodium chloride and sodium bicarbonate presumably because of an active bicarbonate pump and electroneutral sodium chloride pump.[11] The hormonal influence on bile secretion is at its greatest in the ductular system where secretin, cholecystokinin, vasoactive intestinal peptide, and gastrin stimulate an increase in bile secretion through their effects on ductules and ducts. The duct system may also adapt to a primarily absorptive function to further concentrate hepatic bile after cholecystectomy.[36]

Bile Flow

The direction and movement of bile flow within the biliary tract depends on multiple factors. Intrinsic and extrinsic factors all play a part in this complex phenomenon of bile delivery to the gastrointestinal tract. The driving force for canalicular bile flow is the active transport of certain solutes such as bile salts and electrolytes, leading to local osmotic gradients with passive flow of water into the bile canaliculus.[36,42] In addition, the canalicular flow of bile is facilitated by "peristalsis" of the canaliculi. Presumably contractile monofilaments are responsible for these contractions in the canaliculi. Support for these canalicular contractions is based on experimental work in which agents that inhibit microfilament function (i.e., cytochalasins and phalloidin) result in canalicular dilation and cholestasis in laboratory animals.[36,45]

The size of the bile salt pool is also an important determinant of bile flow. The smaller the bile salt load to the hepatocytes, the smaller the amount of bile salt–dependent canalicular bile flow, with a resultant increase in de novo synthesis of bile salts by the hepatocytes. Therefore derangements in the enterohepatic circulation by such diverse factors as terminal ileal disease, portal hypertension, or hepatocellular disease may decrease the amount or availability of bile salts to the hepatocytes and decrease bile flow. It is the bile salt load, not the capacity of the liver for bile salt secretion, that is the rate-limiting factor for bile salt–dependent bile secretion under normal conditions.[36]

Independent of their osmotic properties, bile salts may

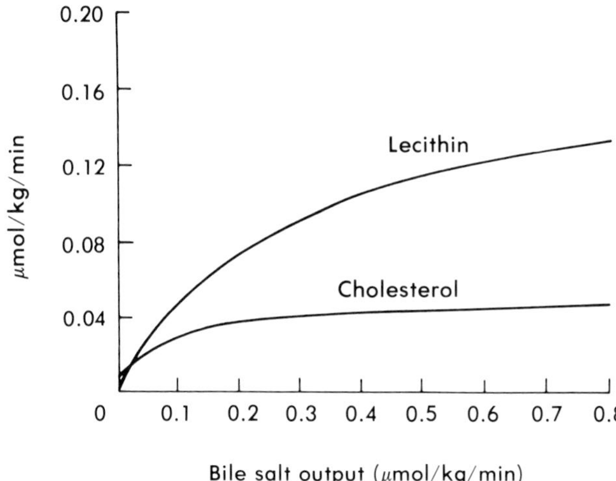

Fig. 26-3 Hyperbolic relationship of lecithin and cholesterol to bile salt output. Al low rates of bile salt secretion (i.e., below 0.16 μmol/kg of body weight per minute) as is observed during fasting, relatively more cholesterol than lecithin is secreted, resulting in cholesterol supersaturation. (Modified from Wagner, C.I., Trotman, B.W., and Soloway, R.D.: J. Clin. Invest. **57**:473, 1976.)

have direct secretory effects as well. The bile salts ursodeoxycholate and 7-keto-lithocholate both stimulate bile flow in the rat, perhaps by stimulation of canalicular bicarbonate secretion.[14] The primary biliary lipids are nonesterified cholesterol and the phospholipid phosphatidyl-choline (lecithin). Biliary output of both of these substances increases curvilinearly with bile salt output so that cholesterol supersaturation generally occurs at low rates of bile acid excretion.[45] Increasing the bile salt load to the liver by the addition of exogenous bile salts to the diet increases the biliary secretion of phospholipids and cholesterol but in a nonlinear fashion, and this results in decreasing the saturation of bile with these substances (Fig. 26-3). Sulfobromophthalein, iodipamide, and various anionic cholerectics (not bilirubin) also stimulate bile flow in human beings. Bile flow is at its lowest during fasting. Bile salts are then largely sequestered in the gallbladder, which minimizes their flux through the enterohepatic circulation and thereby significantly decreases bile salt–dependent canalicular bile formation.

Bile flow within the biliary tract also depends on regional differences in intraluminal pressures.[42] An understanding of the factors that influence intrabiliary pressures is essential in understanding bile flow. The maximum secretory pressure of the liver after manual occlusion of the common bile duct as measured in patients previously subjected to cholecystectomy ranged between 29 and 39 cm of water.[25] In the basal or interprandial state the resistance of the sphincter of Oddi approximates 15 to 17 cm of water with a correspondingly lower pressure in the common bile duct. The common bile duct pressure exceeds resistance to flow from the cystic duct with subsequent entrance of bile into the gallbladder. The secretory rate of bile from the liver is minimal at this time. Once chyme enters the duodenum, hepatic bile secretion increases, and gallbladder contractions begin. Both of these events increase common bile duct pressure. Simultaneously, a decrease in pressure at the sphincter of Oddi occurs, allowing bile free access to the duodenum. Although the significant effects of neurohumoral influences on the gallbladder, common bile duct, and sphincter of Oddi have been well described, their influence on the intrahepatic components of bile flow is less well delineated. Table 26-1 is a compilation of neurohumoral and drug influences on the biliary tract and bile flow.

Table 26-1 **NEURAL, HORMONAL, AND DRUG INFLUENCES ON BILE FLOW**

	C*	D†	GB‡	CBD§	SO‖
Bile salts	↑¶				
Cholecystokinin		↑	↑		↑
Motilin			↑		
Insulin	↑				
Glucagon	↑				
Somatostatin	↓**		↓		
Secretin		↑	↑		↑
Vasoactive intestinal peptide		↑	↓		
Gastrin		↑	↑	↑	↑
Caerulein		↑	↑		↑
Pancreatic polypeptide			↓		
Progesterone			↓		
Estrogens	↓				
Thyroxine	↑				
Corticosteroids	↑				
Vagal input			↑	↑	↑
Sympathetic (alpha)			↑	↑	↑
Sympathetic (beta)			↓	↓	↓
Chlorpromazine	↓				
Phenobarbital	↑				
Iodipamide	↑				
Sulfobromphthalein	↑				
Ampicillin	↑	↑			

*C, Canalicular bile flow.
†D, Ductular bile flow.
‡GB, Gallbladder contraction.
§CBD, Common bile duct.
‖ SO, Sphincter of Oddi contraction.
¶ ↑, Increase flow or contraction.
** ↓, Decrease flow or contraction.

Bile Composition

Water is the solvent or medium for bile. Sodium, potassium, chloride, and bicarbonate concentrations in hepatic bile are essentially equal to those found in plasma, and these inorganic electrolytes account for the majority of bile osmolality. Excretion of these electrolytes is largely responsible for the bile salt–independent aspect of canalicular bile. Mechanisms of hepatic electrolyte transport remain poorly understood. The sodium pump probably is the impetus for the hepatocellular uptake of inorganic anions such as chloride or bicarbonate, although experimental work is contradictory in this field. Sodium-coupled chloride transport by way of a sodium-potassium-ATPase is the best supported mechanism that accounts for isotonic bile (Fig. 26-4). However, evidence of active bicarbonate transport does exist in the isolated rat liver. The movement

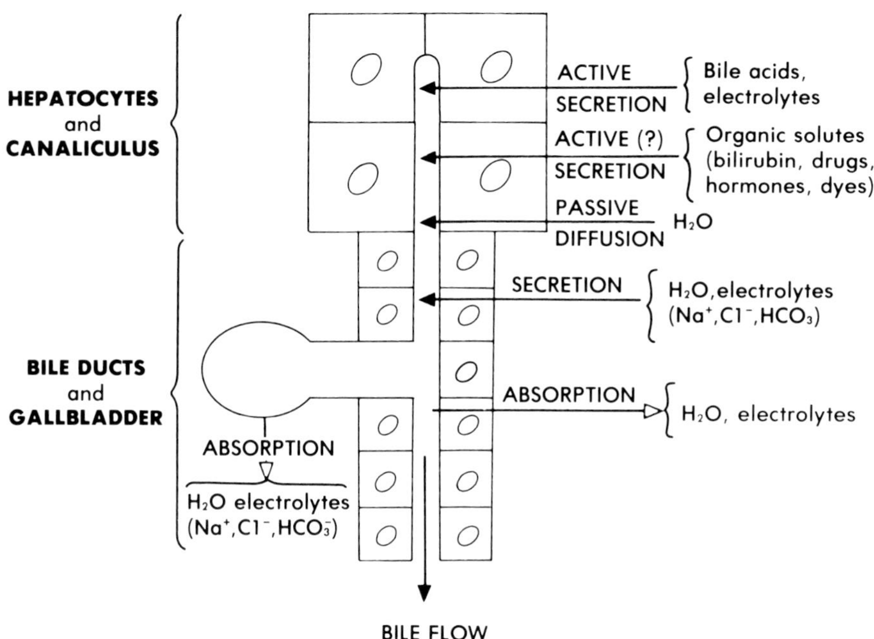

Fig. 26-4 Schematic representation of the formation of bile. Bile secretion begins in the canaliculus with active transport of bile salts (acids), inorganic electrolytes, and possibly other organic solutes. Secretion of these substances is followed passively by water flow into the canaliculus. Bile is concentrated in the gallbladder by the isotonic absorption of water and electrolytes. (From Scharschmidt, B.F.: Bile formation and cholestasis, metabolism and enterohepatic circulation of bile acids, and gallstone formation. In Zakim, D., and Boyer, T.D., editors: Hepatology, Philadelphia, 1982, W.B. Saunders Co.)

of electrolytes from the sinusoid to the canaliculus is also an area of active investigation. Intercellular tight junctions appear permeable to small cations, and it is likely that sodium may enter bile through this paracellular pathway. Potassium and chloride seem to follow this same pathway.[45] The concentration of heavy metals in bile is of great interest because of their well-known toxic effects. The biliary excretion of lead, copper, and manganese appear to be dependent on a saturable transport process. The excretion of other metals such as mercury and arsenic is less efficient and less understood. Active transport systems for digitalis glycosides have also been well described. Protein is a minor component of bile with concentrations ranging from 6 to 300 mg/100 ml. Many of these proteins may represent simple leakage or cellular extrusion; but some, such as immunoglobulin A, are most likely coupled to a special secretory mechanism component. It has been speculated that immunoglobulin A is secreted into the biliary system and functions in the gastrointestinal tract as a local immune defense factor.

Bilirubin and other organic substances account for less than 3% of total biliary solutes by weight. Nevertheless, the hepatic management of bilirubin transport remains an area of intense study. Bilirubin transport is an excellent model for the transport of other organic anions by the liver, including various drugs and dyes. It is also of great clinical interest because hyperbilirubinemia leading to jaundice is probably the most obvious manifestation of cholestasis.[45] Complex interrelations between bile salts and bilirubin excretion exist, and the excretion of bilirubin is certainly enhanced by bile salts.[40] Bilirubin solubility in test solutions is affected by ionic strength, presence of bile salts, pH, calcium, cholesterol, and biliary proteins. In human gallbladder bile, bilirubin concentration rarely exceeds 0.25 mmol/L, accounting for only 1% to 3% of total biliary pigments.[52] These biliary pigments have major clinical importance since they form the components of pigment gallstones, which occur in 20% to 30% of patients with gallstones in the United States.[24]

Numerous reviews[3,52] have documented how scant information is about biliary bilirubin secretion in bilirubin stone formation. Approximately 99% of total biliary bilirubin is conjugated by ester linkages to glucuronic acid; this makes bilirubin soluble in water. Unconjugated bilirubin, like cholesterol, is water insoluble. Consequently, if substantial quantities of unconjugated bilirubin are found in the bile, it can be considered saturated with bilirubin, and pigment stone formation probably results. In patients with increased pigment (bilirubin) stones, substantial amounts of unconjugated bilirubin are found in the bile. The origin of this unconjugated bilirubin is controversial. Its increase can be caused by increased biliary secretion of unconjugated bilirubin or formed by deconjugation of previously conjugated bilirubin. Evidence for the latter is supported by the increased beta glucuronidase activity documented in many pigment stone formers, presumably secondary to bacterial sources.[3] This mechanism is believed to be the primary cause of the increased amount of bilirubin pigment stones found in the Orient. Increased secretion of unconjugated bilirubin is the reason usually given for patients with hemolytic anemias who develop pigment gallstones since pigment gallstones have increased

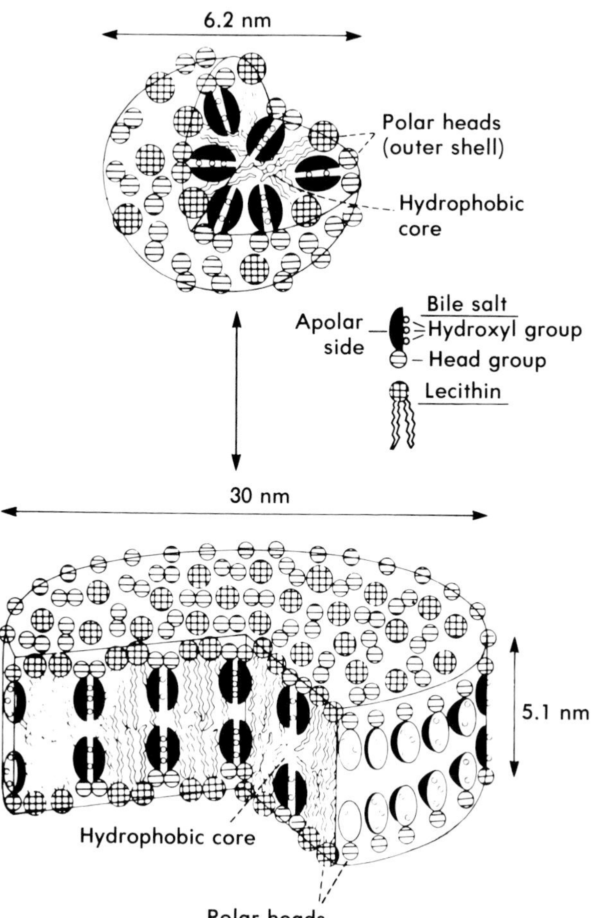

Fig. 26-5 Structure of a mixed micelle. If the solution is bile salt rich, the micelle is sphere shaped; whereas if it is lecithin rich, it is disk shaped. Lecithin-rich micelle is larger and capable of transporting a larger amount of cholesterol. Transition depends on the bile salt/lecithin molar ratio present in native bile. Bile salt molecules in both micellar forms are thought to form pairs (dimers) to avoid contact of the hydroxyl groups *(solid circles)* with the apolar environment of the micellar core. (Modified from Muller, K.: Biochemistry **20:**404, 1981.)

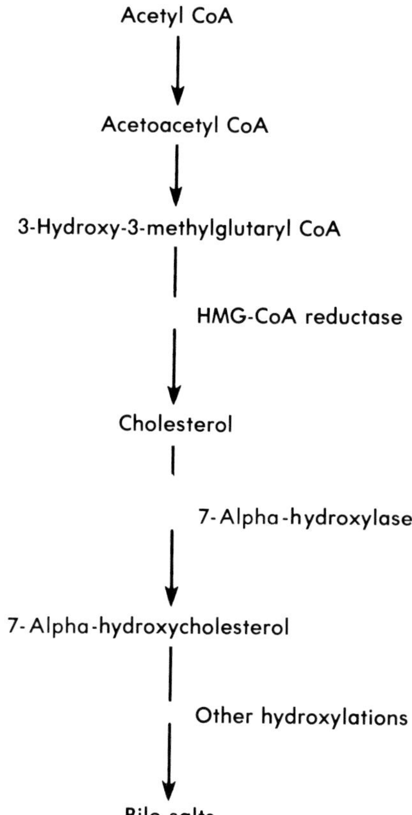

Fig. 26-6 Hepatic synthesis of cholesterol and bile salts. (Reprinted with permission from Postier, R., and Gadacz, T.R.: Hosp. Formulary **15:**608, 1980. Copyright 1980 American Chemical Society.)

production and biliary secretion of total bilirubin. However, increased secretion of unconjugated bilirubin in these patients has not been clearly demonstrated.

Bile is a micellar solution, the predominant solid components of which are bile salts, lecithin, and cholesterol (Fig. 26-5). Both cholesterol and lecithin, the major phospholipid of bile, are insoluble in water. When mixed with bile salts, these three lipids associate into complex aggregates called micelles.[27,38] These micelles allow the lipophilic portions of these three molecules to arrange themselves centrally, with the more peripheral portions being hydrophilic to allow solubility. The bile salts (cholate, chenodeoxycholate, deoxycholate, and lithocholate) compose approximately 60% of the solute content of bile and serve a fundamental solubilizing function for both cholesterol and phospholipids in micelle formation. Lecithin is the second most prominent solute in bile and increases the capacity of the micelles to solubilize more cholesterol.

The major source of biliary cholesterol was formerly thought to be derived from hepatic cholesterol synthesis. Recent studies, however, have shown that a significant proportion of secreted cholesterol is exogenous or dietary in origin.[54] Therefore potential sources for increased cholesterol secretion by the liver into the bile include increased ingestion and absorption of cholesterol, increased hepatic synthesis, mobilization of cholesterol from peripheral tissue pools, and decreased conversion by the liver of cholesterol to bile salts. Hepatic cholesterol synthesis is demonstrated in Fig. 26-6, with 3-hydroxy 3-methyl glutaryl coenzyme-A (HMG CoA) reductase the rate-limiting enzyme in cholesterol synthesis, and cholesterol 7-alpha-hydroxylase the rate-limiting enzyme in the formation of bile salts.[38] Difficulties in assaying this enzymatic system have led to some controversy concerning its role in increased biliary cholesterol secretion. Nevertheless, the incidence of cholesterol cholelithiasis is increased in obesity, in those on a high-caloric diet, and in certain western U.S. Indian tribes because of increased HMG CoA reductase activity and hence increased cholesterol synthesis.[2,38] By lowering serum cholesterol levels, clofibrate therapy also predisposes to cholesterol gallstone formation by increasing hepatic synthesis of cholesterol.[27] Sex factors also affect the regulation of hepatic cholesterol metabolism. Apparently women have an increased hepatic flux of lipoproteins with increased hepatic cholesterol synthesis.[48] Cholesterol secretion by the liver is related in a nonlinear fashion to bile salt secretion, and, if the bile salt pool is low, even normal levels of biliary cholesterol secretion can lead to a bile that is supersaturated with cholesterol. Cholesterol is the predominant (>70%) constituent in pure and mixed cholesterol gallstones, which comprise up to 80% of all gallstones in the western world.[24]

A reduction in phospholipid synthesis or secretion can also result in bile saturated with cholesterol. This putative mechanism for cholesterol saturation of bile has not been thoroughly investigated. Nonetheless, a decrease in the amounts and relative concentrations of phospholipids (lecithin), as well as abnormal patterns of phospholipid secretion, have been reported in patients with gallstones.[5]

Bile salts appear to be the major factor in cholesterol gallstone formation, as well as in its treatment and prevention. The primary bile salts are cholate and chenodeoxycholate (chenate, chenodiol), which are synthesized by the liver. They are secreted into bile as conjugated salts of taurine or glycine. In the proximal small intestine the bile salts are deconjugated by most bacteria to their free (unconjugated) forms. In the distal small intestine the primary bile salts are dehydroxylated to deoxycholate and lithocholate (Fig. 26-7) by anaerobic bacteria. Normally the bile salt pool remains relatively constant, averaging 6 mmol in a 70-kg human. Extremely efficient reabsorption by the distal ileum and selective extraction of bile salts by the hepatocytes from the portal venous blood keep the need for daily hepatic synthesis to a minimum.

Quantitative deficiencies in bile salts lead to saturation of bile with cholesterol. Bile salt deficiency can result from one of several mechanisms. Increased loss of bile salts from the intestine by distal ileal disease or surgical resection, malabsorption, pancreatic insufficiency, or bile salt–binding drugs (cholestyramine) are possible causes of cholesterol saturation of bile. The tremendous capacity of the liver to increase bile salt synthesis in response to loss, however, makes this a relatively unusual cause of cholesterol-saturated bile. An inability to synthesize normal amounts of bile salts has also been postulated. Cholesterol 7-alpha-hydroxylase, the rate-limiting enzyme in bile salt synthesis, has been found to be decreased in certain cholesterol gallstone patients, but the significance of these observations is uncertain since there are technical difficulties in both the assay and interpretation of this enzyme. Patients with the rare disease of cerebrotendinous xanthomatosis who are unable to synthesize normal amounts of bile salts frequently develop cholesterol gallstones. Factors that increase enterohepatic cycling of the bile salt pool could alter the feedback mechanism that regulates bile salt synthesis and thereby could actually reduce the size of this pool. Decreased or absent gallbladder storage of bile, increased gallbladder motility, decreased bowel transit time, and increased proximal small bowel absorption are all theoretic means of suppressing bile salt synthesis.[3] Likewise, a combination of factors can result in cholesterol excess and cholesterol gallstone formation. Such a combined defect occurs in the southwestern U.S. American Indians, especially the Pimas, who apparently have an increased rate of cholesterol secretion and a decrease in bile salt pool.[2,24] In these individuals both cholesterol and lecithin secretory outputs are relatively greater than bile salt secretion. At low rates of bile salt secretion, as occurs after an overnight fast, relatively more cholesterol and fewer bile salts are secreted, resulting in biliary cholesterol saturation. Over 50% of normal subjects have cholesterol-saturated bile after an overnight fast. Finally, exogenous bile salts can also influence cholesterol saturation in bile and have been used both therapeutically and prophylactically to increase the bile salt pool and thus decrease cholesterol saturation.[27] This dissolution therapy will be discussed in detail later.

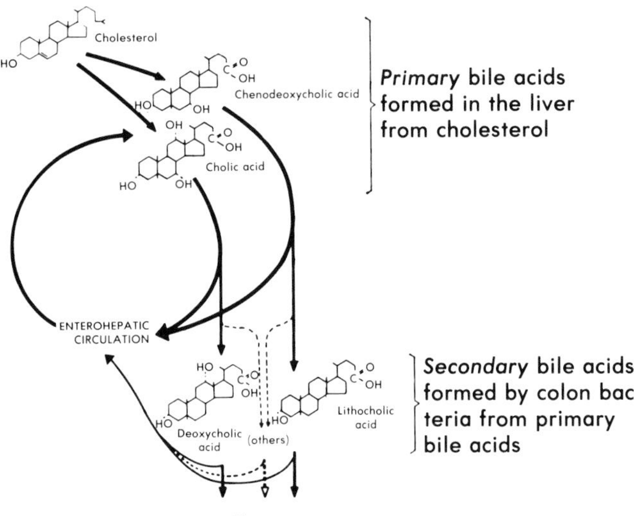

Fig. 26-7 Formation of primary and secondary bile acids from cholesterol and enterohepatic circulation of bile salts. (From Carey, J.B., Jr.: Bile salts and hepatobiliary disease. In Schiff, L., editor: Diseases of the liver, ed. 3, Philadelphia, 1969, J.B. Lippincott Co.)

Over 15 years ago Admirand and Small[1] first described the physiochemical relationship among cholesterol, bile salts, and lecithin as a triangular coordinate plot (Fig. 26-8) that relates a physical state to the chemical composition of lipids in a sample of bile.[5] An excess of cholesterol in relation to bile salts and phospholipids results in either crystal formation or the liquid crystalline phase. Crystallization is probably a prerequisite for cholesterol gallstone formation, but marked saturation has been found in many patients without crystallization.[46] Normal molar ratios of bile salts–to-phospholipids-to-cholesterol are 74:20:6. A potential for crystallization occurs when cholesterol accounts for more than 10% of total biliary lipids (see Fig. 26-3). Subsequent workers have not shown such a well-delineated distinction between normal and lithogenic bile; but the phase diagram, especially as modified by the solubility index,[51] still serves a useful function. Within this system it is possible to assign to any given native bile a cholesterol saturation index as determined by the chemical composition of the bile.[24] Bile may be saturated with cholesterol without crystal formation or cholesterol precipitation. This is called the metastable state. Alternatively, rapid cholesterol precipitation may occur in the labile state. Labile bile is generally turbid without overt crystal or precipitate formation.

Nucleation (nidation) refers to the coalescence of free cholesterol molecules, including other molecules such as proteins, which eventually leads to precipitation and stone formation. The key question in cholesterol gallstone formation is why only a small percentage of patients with saturated bile form cholesterol monohydrate crystals. Cholesterol nucleation can occur by two general mechanisms. Homogenous nucleation is the random coalescence of cholesterol molecules that form a nidus for further cholesterol precipitation. This appears to be most likely in a situation that would occur in very highly saturated bile.[3,15] Heterogenous nucleation is a process in which precipitation occurs around an entity other than a crystal of pure cholesterol. Many different substances may act as nucleating agents to initiate precipitation and propagation of cholesterol from saturated bile. In fact, many cholesterol gallstones have a pigmented center implicating some form of pigment nucleating agent. It is thought that the majority of bilirubin gallstones are formed by heterogeneous nucleation; material such as calcium salts, gallbladder mucosal cells, parasitic fragments and ova, and bacteria have all been suggested.[3] Nucleation promoting factors in gallbladder mucin have also been identified in animal models.[28] In addition, nucleation inhibition differences have been described in normal and abnormal bile.[22,46]

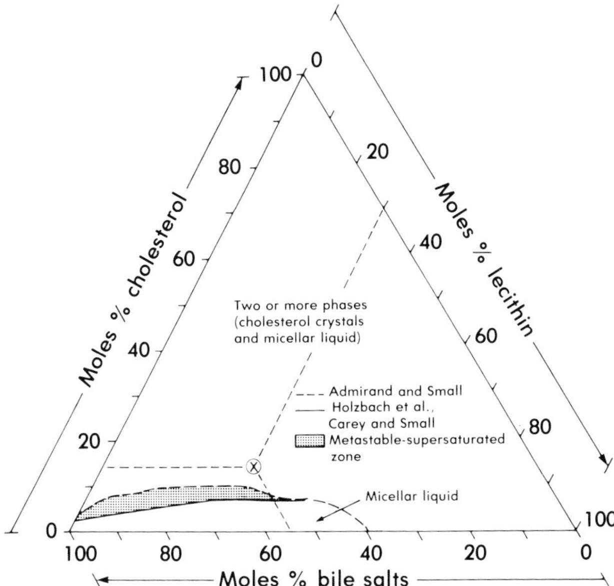

Fig. 26-8 Determination of cholesterol saturation index *(CSI)*. Tricoordinate phase diagram for representing by a single intersecting point *(x)* relative concentrations of cholesterol, lecithin, and bile salt in bile. In this scheme, relative concentration of each lipid is expressed as a percentage of the sum of the molar concentrations of all three. This manipulation permits representation of the relations between three constituents in two dimensions, the water content being invariant at, say, 90% (10% wt/vol solids). In this figure, for example, at point *(x)*, the relative concentration of bile salt from its coordinate is 55% (indicating 55% of the sum of all three lipids), whereas that for lecithin is 30%, and that for cholesterol is 15%. The range of concentrations found consistent with a clear aqueous micellar solution is limited to a small region at the lower left. A solution having the composition represented by point *x*, on the other hand, would initially be visually turbid and contain precipitated forms of cholesterol crystals in addition to bile salt mixed micelles. Last, a solution represented by a point falling in the shaded area below the dashed line would be unstable (i.e., metastable-supersaturated), meaning that by prediction it would be initially clear (micellar). Within a short time, however, various precipitated forms of cholesterol crystals would form, and such a solution would then be visually turbid, similar to all solutions above the dashed line. (From Holzbach, R.T.: Pathogenesis and medical treatment of gallstones. In Sleisenger, M.H., and Fordtran, J.S., editors: Gastrointestinal disease: pathophysiology, diagnosis, management, ed. 3, Philadelphia, 1983, W.B. Saunders Co.)

In summary, there are many ways in which cholesterol can be saturated in the bile. Highly saturated bile is termed labile, and it is in this bile that homogenous nucleation occurs and cholesterol precipitates rapidly and spontaneously. Lower levels of saturation, in which rare spontaneous precipitation of cholesterol occurs, are often termed metastable. It is in this metastable bile that the introduction of extraneous agents may promote heterogeneous crystallization or nucleation.[3] The metastable labile limit[10] is the boundary between these two states and correlates well to the original saturation limit proposed by Admirand and Small.[1,3]

GALLBLADDER

Anatomically the gallbladder is a pear-shaped appendage of the common bile duct with a normal storage capacity of 20 to 40 ml (Fig. 26-9). It is generously supplied with vagal parasympathetic fibers from the hepatic branch

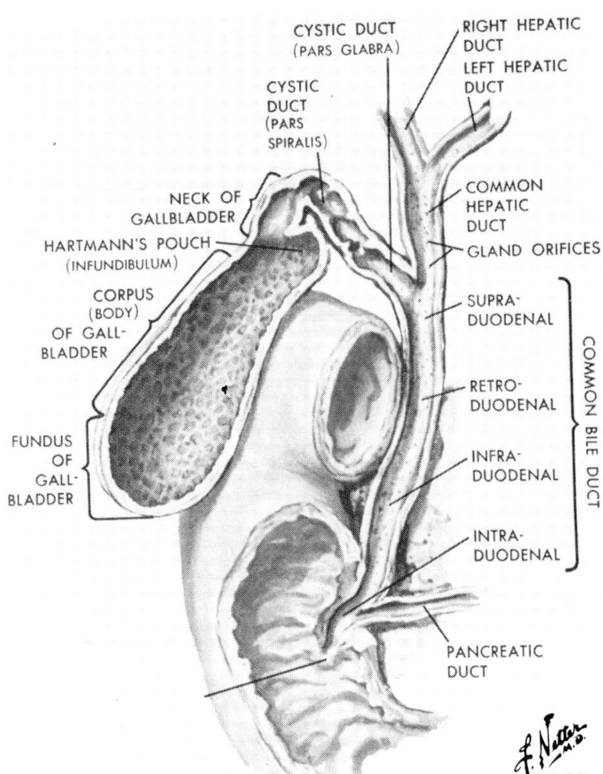

Fig. 26-9 Anatomy of gallbladder. (From Netter, F.H.: CIBA Collection of Medical Illustrations, vol. 3, part III, Indianapolis, Ind., 1964, CIBA Pharmaceutical Co., Division of CIBA-GEIGY Corp.)

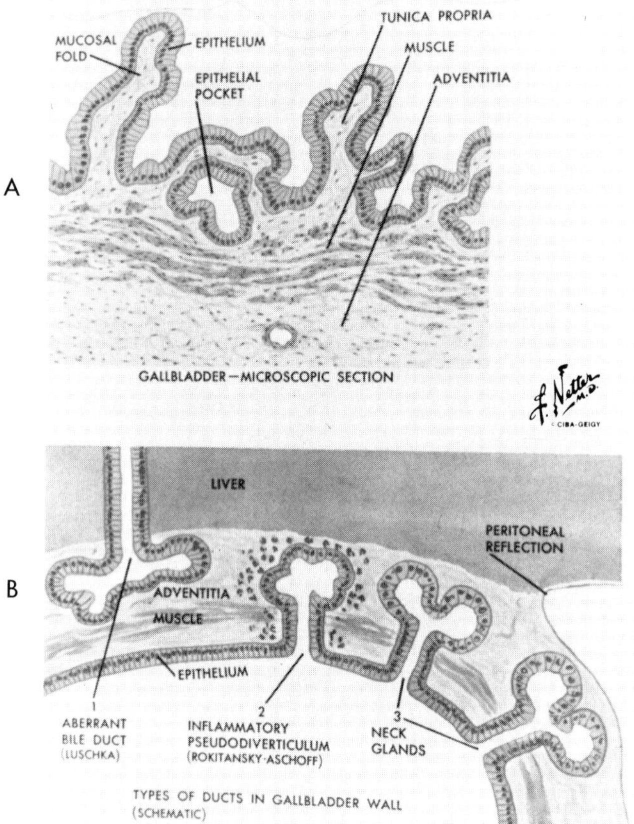

Fig. 26-10 **A,** Microscopic view of gallbladder. **B,** Microscopic view of types of ducts in gallbladder wall. (From Netter, F.H.: CIBA Collection of Medical Illustrations, vol. 3, part III, Indianapolis, Ind., 1964, CIBA Pharmaceutical Co., Division of CIBA-GEIGY Corp.)

of the anterior vagal trunk and numerous branches of the splanchnic sympathetic tree. Histologically, it possesses an inner columnar mucosal layer similar to that seen in the intestine, a thin lamina propria layer, a thin layer of irregularly oriented smooth muscle fibers, the perimuscular connective tissue layer, and a serosa (Fig. 26-10).[42] Its rich, arterial blood supply is from the cystic artery, which is usually a branch of the right hepatic artery, and its less well defined venous drainage leads both to the liver and the portal vein. A wealth of lymphatics is also present within the lamina propria that ultimately drain into the cisterna chyli.

Two significant physiologically interrelated functions are performed by the gallbladder. First, it reabsorbs most of the water and electrolytes from the relatively dilute hepatic bile stored in it at a rate of 15% to 30% of its intraluminal volume per hour. Up to 90% of its total volume may be reabsorbed given a long enough interprandial period.[33] This absorption produces a small volume of dark viscid bile that can contain up to 90% of total body bile salts.[36] Second, during a meal the gallbladder contracts and delivers its contents into the small intestine.[42]

Motor Function

Gallbladder filling is ensured by intraluminal common bile duct pressures high enough to permit free flow from the common hepatic duct into the cystic duct and gallbladder. The interdigestive storage of bile and the digestive release of bile are regulated by complex hormonal and neural systems.

The effect of several hormones on the gallbladder are listed in Table 26-1. Cholecystokinin (CCK) is a heterogeneous polypeptide containing 39 amino acids that is released by the proximal small bowel (i.e., duodenum and proximal jejunum) endocrine and neuronal cells secondary to the presence of fat, peptones, essential amino acids, and magnesium sulfate. Vagal sectioning or the division of the thoracic sympathetics has no obvious effect on this release.[39] The mechanism of action of CCK on the gallbladder apparently involves acinar cell membrane binding, leading to the release of membrane-bound Ca^{++} ions and a concomitant increase in intracellular cyclic GMP, which then leads to gallbladder contraction and evacuation. The polypeptide motilin has also been suggested as an important physiologic modulator of gallbaldder contraction.[45] Gastrin and caerulein (a CCK-like substance) also have demonstrable in vitro and in vivo CCK-like activity. Secretin seems to potentiate the action of CCK in vivo.[42] Pancreatic polypeptide and vasoactive intestinal peptide apparently inhibit gallbladder contraction by stimulation of adenyl cyclase activity in the gallbladder cells, which then promote interdigestive relaxation. Somatostatin also promotes gallbladder relaxation, possibly by inhibiting CCK release from the proximal small bowel intestine.[36,39] The presence of bile salts in the proximal small intestine has been clearly shown to inhibit CCK release.[39]

Parasympathetic stimulation of the gallbladder musculature increases intracystic pressure but is not associated with gallbladder evacuation. Thus the physiologic significance of the vagal innervation of the gallbladder remains uncertain.[42] Vagotomy leads to dilation of the gallbladder with an increase in resting (fasting) volume up to 100%. However, following vagotomy the response of the gallbladder to CCK is unaffected, and emptying is unaltered.[5,45] A maintenance of tone may be the primary function of the parasympathetic innervation. In contrast, the adrenergic innervation of the gallbladder contains both excitatory and inhibitory fibers, with the overall tendency toward an inhibition of gallbladder motility. As with the parasympathetic system, the physiologic significance of this sympathetic innervation is uncertain.[42]

Under physiologic conditions, a meal produces strong gallbladder contractions, leading to bile flow into the duodenum within just a few minutes of its ingestion, presumably modulated by both neural and hormonal mechanisms as previously described. CCK has a major role in stimulating bile flow and gallbladder contraction and inducing relaxation of the sphincter of Oddi. Sustained output of bile and bile salts into the duodenum depends on the bile salt return to the liver and reabsorption through the enterohepatic circulation.[33] Biliary secretion is associated with normal intestinal migratory motor complexes and involves both secretory and motor responses. The fasted (interdigestive phase) small intestine normally demonstrates a cyclic motor complex. Four separate phases have been identified. Phase I is characterized by the near total absence of action potentials. In Phase II there is persistent irregular action potential activity, with Phase III demonstrating large action potentials on every pacesetter potential of that period. Phase IV shows a decline in incidence and intensity of action potentials.[55] The rise in bile secretion into the duodenum during Phase II of the interdigestive motor cycle is predominantly caused by gallbladder contraction with simultaneous relaxation of the sphincter of Oddi. During Phase I of the interdigestive motor cycle minimal amounts of bile enter the duodenum, with the majority entering the gallbladder because of the increased resting tone of the common bile duct and the sphincter of Oddi. The cyclic delivery of bile into the small intestine is not completely determined by the gallbladder, as seen in patients following cholecystectomy who maintain some cyclical biliary delivery, with the bile salt pool residing in the upper small bowel, common bile duct, and branches of the biliary tree during the interdigestive phases.[33]

Normal gallbladder storage and motility may be disturbed under special circumstances and ultimately lead to gallstone formation. In pregnancy the residual volume of the gallbladder increases twofold over normal and is a presumed factor in the increased incidence of cholesterol gallstones in this population of patients. Another factor contributing to cholesterol cholelithiasis is the rise in serum progesterone levels seen in pregnancy during the progesterone peak of the menstrual cycle and in patients taking certain oral contraceptive pills.[5,23,33] All of these conditions have been associated with either impaired gallbladder emptying or an increase in residual (fasting) volume.[8] The risk of cholesterol gallstones may be increased in these patients as a result of the prolonged retention and/or increased concentration of residual bile in the gallbladder. Inadequate mixing or stratification of biliary lipids in bile has likewise been proposed in these conditions because of flaccidity of the gallbladder. Recently, a sizable subgroup of cholesterol gallstone patients has been discovered to possess defective gallbladder emptying independent of clinical presentation, gallstone size, or gallstone number.[37] In these patients, gallbladder emptying may be the primary defect. Defective gallbladder contractility has been shown to appear in the early stages of cholesterol gallstone formation in various animal models.[16]

Although an increase in the fasting volume of the gallbladder is associated with increased stone formation, other factors must influence this process. For example, animals fed a high cholesterol diet demonstrate an increased gallbladder fasting volume but no increase in cholesterol gallstone formation.[27] In this study bile was not supersaturated with cholesterol despite the change in gallbladder volume, indicating that stasis per se does not lead to cholesterol saturation. Thus the role of stasis in gallstone formation needs further clarification.

Gallbladder Absorption and Secretion

With its normal capacity of only 20 to 40 ml, the gallbladder would quickly be filled with bile, which is secreted at volumes approximating 400 to 600 ml/day. Fortunately the gallbladder has an enormous absorptive capacity and within 4 hours can remove up to 90% of the water present in hepatic bile and convert this isotonic solution composed primarily of sodium chloride and sodium bicarbonate to a concentrated solution of impermeable bile salt anions.[45,48]

Table 26-2 **COMPARISON OF HEPATIC AND GALLBLADDER BILE**

	Hepatic Bile	Gallbladder Bile
Percent solids	2%-4%	10%-12%
Na^+ (mEq/L)	140-150	200-300
Cl^- (mEq/L)	90-100	15-50
K^+ (mEq/L)	3.5-5.0	10-25
HCO_3^- (mEq/L)	25-40	10-20
Ca^+ (mEq/L)	2-5	10-20
Bilirubin (mg/100ml)	20-60	200-300
Cholesterol (mg/100 ml)	130-230	400-700
Bile salts (mg/100 ml)	1000-2000	4000-9000

The concentrations of sodium, calcium, and potassium in this altered gallbladder bile double or triple, whereas chloride and bicarbonate anion concentrations decrease (Table 26-2). This absorptive process has been extensively investigated and is largely the result of neutral sodium chloride transport similar to the transport systems described in hepatic biliary secretion and absorption.[17,41] The sodium gradient is maintained by a sodium-potassium-ATPase powering the sodium pump. Also, as in the liver, significant water and ion flow may occur by way of paracellular pathways.[45] This absorption process can be impaired, however, with a resulting gallbladder "secretion." In a variety of in vitro gallbladder preparations from different experimental animals, agents such as exogenous cyclic AMP, prostaglandins (presumably through endogenous cyclic AMP), and various gut peptides, including vasoactive intestinal peptide (VIP) and secretin, have been shown to elicit a net secretory response.[41] The mechanism underlying this observation is probably the result of an inhibition of the normal sodium chloride–coupled transport rather than an actual stimulation of secretion. This secretion may be of physiologic significance since both prostaglandins and VIP–containing nerve fibers have been identified in the gallbladder wall and could play a role in the formation of the "white bile" occasionally noted at operation in the presence of an occluded cystic duct.[41]

Normal human gallbladder mucosa is also capable of absorbing certain amino acids and sugars by specialized transport mechanisms as in the small intestine. A substantial concentration gradient exists for bile salts and bile pigments across the gallbladder wall, which is virtually impermeable to highly charged moieties such as taurocholate, sulfobromophthalein, and iodipamide (Cholografin). Weakly ionized substances such as unconjugated bilirubin and chenodeoxycholate are less well protected from diffusion. In the diseased gallbladder with cholecystitis, though, there is an increased permeability of highly ionized substances and water. The cholecystographic nonvisualization of the gallbladder that is characteristic of inflammatory disease of this organ may be caused by the rapid absorption of iodipamide[41] and not just obstruction of the cystic duct.

Most gastrointestinal mucosa, the gallbladder epithelium included, is injured by direct exposure to high concentrations of bile salts. Under normal conditions, micellar stabilization of the bile salts helps to prevent injury to the gallbladder mucosa from these potentially damaging substances. The high concentration of bile salts in these micelles also decreases the lithogenic index of bile by enhancing cholesterol solubility, especially when the total lipid content is large.[10] Dilute bile (i.e., low concentrations of bile salts), on the other hand, has a decreased ability to solubilize cholesterol. In infected bile bacterial deconjugation of bile salts occurs, resulting in enhanced absorption of these substances by the gallbladder epithelium. Such increased absorption of bile salts decreases the bile salt composition of bile (and thereby the solubility of cholesterol) and has direct injurious effects to the gallbladder mucosa, both of which may contribute to the formation of cholesterol gallstones.

Unconjugated bilirubin is also more rapidly absorbed from the gallbladder than conjugated bilirubin. Absorption appears to be linearly related to the luminal concentration of the pigment. "White bile," which occurs in a chronically obstructed gallbladder, may merely be the product of hydrolyzed conjugated bilirubin with absorption of the free pigment.[35,41] Calcium bilirubinate crystals are more likely to form in concentrated bile (i.e., bile in which the bile salt concentration is high) with its concurrent reduction in pH and increase in the ion product. Thus a high bile concentration is thought to be a contributory factor in the production of pigment stones rather than in the production of cholesterol stones, which are associated with dilute bile.[5]

Pathogenesis of Cholelithiasis

In the preceding discussion an overview of biliary physiology has been presented to speculate on the possible causes of cholelithiasis in order to summarize the documented and putative risk factors for gallstone formation in humans. Most gallstones appear to be primarily composed of cholesterol or pigment, both visually and by chemical analysis (Table 26-3). Two general types of cholesterol stones exist. The large group consists of pale yellow mixed cholesterol stones usually containing more than 70% cholesterol by weight.[24] These stones are generally multiple and range between 0.5 to 2.5 cm in size. They are usually found tightly packed in the gallbladder and faceted. The contiguity of these stones and their uniformity of size may reflect different periods of formation.[24] The smaller subset of cholesterol stones consists of large, pale yellow, solitary, pure cholesterol stones. Pigment stones, on the other hand, have a distinctive brown-to-black color, are generally multiple and irregular, and contain less than 25% cholesterol. They generally contain 60% bile pigment by weight.[24,53] These stones are usually calcium salts of bilirubinate, phosphate, or carbonate. Only 15% to 20% of cholesterol-predominant stones calcify, whereas over 50% of pigment stones are calcified radiographically.

Cholesterol Cholelithiasis

Cholesterol gallstones are more frequent among obese patients,[3,5] probably because overweight individuals have an increased cholesterol synthesis, disproportionately increased biliary secretion of cholesterol, and higher levels of saturated bile. Weight reductions concurrently lead to reductions in bile saturation. High-caloric diets are more common in cholesterol gallstone patients independent of obesity,[44] and the stones presumably result from the increased hepatic cholesterol output. This relationship to caloric intake is not consistent, however, since various mechanisms influence hepatic lipids. In some cases, a low-caloric diet may increase biliary cholesterol saturation by disproportionately lowering bile salt secretion.[3] Dietary cholesterol intake does not singly influence hepatic cholesterol and probably contributes minimally to the development of cholesterol cholelithiasis.[3,5,27] However, diets rich in other lipids such as polyunsaturated fats or low in fiber may increase the cholesterol in bile.[3,48] Demographically there is considerable evidence to suggest higher incidences of cholesterol cholelithiasis among individuals in northern Europe, North America, and South America in contrast to those in the Orient where pigment gallstones are more common.[3] The previously discussed prevalence of cholesterol stones in certain western U.S. Indian tribes is well documented.[2] Finally, familial aggregations of gallstone patients suggest an inherited tendency of cholesterol cholelithiasis as well.[3]

Clofibrate (a serum cholesterol-lowering agent) ingestion is associated with an increased rate of cholelithiasis by its increased mobilization of peripheral tissue cholesterol stores, enhanced biliary cholesterol secretion, and possibly with a reducing effect on hepatic bile salt synthesis.[21] Bile salt sequestrants such as cholestyramine and colestipol are not associated with an increase in cholelithiasis and do not alter hepatic and biliary bile salt composition but may exacerbate the lithogenic tendency in patients with malabsorption or on clofibrate therapy.[3] When fecal losses of bile salts caused by ileal disease, resection, or bypass exceed the hepatic synthetic capacity, bile salt pools decrease, biliary cholesterol saturation increases, and the risk of cholesterol cholelithiasis increases.[5,26] Patients with cystic fibrosis and pancreatic insufficiency have an increased prevalence of cholelithiasis as a result of bile salt malabsorption. Abnormal mucus in these patients that may

Table 26-3 **TYPES OF GALLSTONES**

Characteristics	Cholesterol I	Cholesterol II	Pigment
Incidence	50%-70%	5%-25%	20%-30%
Appearance	Yellow, faceted multiple	Yellow, single	Brown to black
Size	Small (<2.5 cm)	Large	Varies
Composition	Cholesterol >70%	Cholesterol ~ 100%	Cholesterol <10% Bile pigments 50%-70%

promote nucleation, stasis, or gallstone growth has also been suggested as an explanation for this enhanced stone-forming capability.

Aging is also a factor in gallstone formation, although direct evidence supporting this is scant. Bile appears to be more saturated in older patients, especially males, apparently by an increase in biliary cholesterol secretion.[3,5] Estrogens, both endogenous and exogenous, are lithogenic because of an increase in biliary cholesterol saturation,[8] as reflected by larger numbers of females developing cholelithiasis during the childbearing years.[23] Decreases in the proportion of chenodeoxycholate in bile during the female reproductive period with enhanced saturation have been noted that may account for this increase.[3,33] An inhibiting effect on the gallbladder mucosal sodium-potassium-ATPase pump by estrogens has also been detected in these patients.[13] As previously mentioned, progesterones are smooth muscle relaxants that may impair gallbladder emptying and result in biliary stasis. They also impair the gallbladder's response to cholecystokinin.[8] The elevated progesterone levels seen in the second and third trimesters of pregnancy could contribute to gallbladder hypomotility.[8] Gallbladder atony is also seen in diabetes and may favor stasis and the gallstone formation that is commonly observed in this disease.[20] The putative links between cholelithiasis and diabetes and cholelithiasis and pregnancy still warrant further investigation.

Pigment Cholelithiasis

In contrast to the tremendous amount of information available on hepatic metabolism and biliary secretion in patients with cholesterol cholelithiasis, much less is known about the formation of bilirubin gallstones.[5] Two morphologically, clinically, and chemically distinct types of pigment stones occur.[48,52] Brown pigment stones are commonly observed in Oriental subjects and are also similar to those found in the common bile duct in American patients previously subjected to cholecystectomy and who develop recurrent stones months to years following operation. Black pigment stones are seen in patients with hemolytic problems or cirrhosis. The pigment in this second group of stones may be more polymerized prophins or bilirubin.[9] The estimated true proportion of pigment gallstones approaches 20% to 30% of all observed gallstones.[24]

The basic pathologic events underlying pigment gallstone formation are similar to those responsible for the development of cholesterol stones. A change in biliary composition occurs that may result from either a change in the concentration of a normal biliary component, a decrease in solubilizing biliary components, or the presence of foreign compounds.[52] Saturation then occurs with subsequent nidation and gallstone growth. Calcium bilirubinate plays a major role in the formation of the majority of pigment stones. Black and brown pigment stones probably form by different mechanisms,[3,48,53] but in both varieties bilirubinate and ionized calcium complexes usually exceed their solubility product and precipitate as insoluble salts.[52] Surprisingly, no consistent abnormality in bilirubin or related pigment metabolism has been found in the vast majority of patients with pigment stones.[24] Of considerable interest are the well-documented data that the calcium salt of bilirubin in pigment stones is unconjugated, whereas in bile it is almost entirely conjugated.[24,52,53] Factors that increase the concentration of unconjugated bilirubin in bile, a moiety that is highly insoluble, are under investigation. Certainly saturation of bile with unconjugated bilirubin is currently considered a predominate mechanism. Correlations between unconjugated bilirubin excretion and bile salt flow rate are also well documented in patients developing pigment stones.[24] Increased concentrations of less soluble bilirubin complexes such as bilirubin monoglucuronide have likewise been suggested as an etiologic factor. In addition to alterations in bile composition, derangements in gallbladder emptying function (i.e., motility disturbances) with resulting stasis have been implicated in pigment stone formation.[24,47,52] Finally, studies also support the important and probably necessary role of gallbladder mucosal dysfunction, including impaired maintenance of solute concentration, in the pigment lithogenic process.[24,52]

Three distinct clinical settings provide the majority of pigment stones in the western world. Conditions that decrease the life-span of red blood cells, including malaria, hemoglobinopathies, red cell membrane defects, and hemolysis from prosthetic heart valves, are all associated with pigment gallstones.[3] Most studies have been performed in sickle cell disease, which is associated with a nearly 10-fold increase in bilirubin secretion in the bile in which 97% is conjugated. This increased bilirubin load is independent of bile salt secretion rates. The unconjugated bilirubin fraction secretion rate is smaller (9 mg/100 ml) but appears to be dependent on bile salt secretion, which suggests an interaction of this unconjugated fraction with biliary micelles.[24] An increased incidence of pigment stones in patients with hepatic cirrhosis is also well documented. Although less well studied, contributing factors would include a combination of moderately increased biliary unconjugated bilirubin associated with the hypersplenism and resulting mild hemolytic state commonly seen in cirrhotics, decreased hepatic biliary bile salt secretory output, and possible nutritional contributions.[3,24,52] The third clinical setting is that of age, which, like that of cholesterol stones, increases the frequency of pigment stones in the United States without any distinct association with the female sex or obesity.[3,24] Half of these elderly patients with pigment stones have increased concentrations of unconjugated bile or significant hydrolysis of conjugated bilirubin to the unconjugated form or both.[4]

Brown pigment stones occur predominantly in the Orient, although 50% of recurrent common bile duct stones in the United States are also of this variety.[24] The predominant pathogenic feature in the formation of these stones is mechanical dysfunction of the biliary ducts with stasis. The incidence of this type of gallstone is gradually diminishing, especially in urban populations. Normally bile is sterile, but bacterial or parasitic infections of the biliary tract are not uncommon,[3] especially in the Orient where the bile in patients who develop pigment gallstones is usually infected.[4] Bacterial sources, especially *Escherichia coli,* have beta-glucuronidase enzyme activity that increases bile saturation by hydrolyzing bilirubin to the unconjugated water-insoluble form.[3] Other organisms in the biliary tract are also associated with pigmented stones. In many Far Eastern countries, especially Japan, a high incidence of biliary infestation by parasites, predominantly *Ascaris lumbricoides,* is associated with pigment cholelithiasis, choledocholithiasis, and biliary sludge.[24] These parasites generally produce an inflammatory action in the epithelium of the gallbladder and biliary tree, as well as a secondary bacterial infection. Local chemical changes favor the precipitation of calcium salts caused by infection and inflammation of the gallbladder mucosa. Inflammation may also reduce gallbladder motility or distort the hepatic bile ducts, thus contributing to pigment cholelithiasis and choledocholithiasis.[3] Over the past 25 years changes in Oriental hygienic and socioeconomic conditions have resulted in a significant decrease in biliary tract parasitic infections with a decrease in pigment cholelithiasis. Such changes have resulted in a corresponding increase in cholesterol cholelithiasis in the Orient.[24]

Cholecystitis and Cholecystectomy

Biliary colic, chronic cholecystitis, and acute cholecystitis represent the spectrum of gallbladder disease. Biliary colic is discomfort in the right upper quadrant of short duration after a meal caused by obstruction of the cystic duct from a gallstone. It is usually an incomplete obstruction with little inflammatory response. Although called "biliary colic," the pain is not a true colic but a discomfort that gradually increases in severity, reaches a plateau, and then gradually decreases. It does not have the paroxysms of acute pain associated with intestinal obstruction (intestinal colic). Chronic cholecystitis is usually the result of multiple episodes of gallbladder inflammation, which eventually lead to a scarred gallbladder that has lost its functional ability to concentrate bile. As a result, functional studies of the gallbladder with radiocontrast materials show nonvisualization (see p. 441). Such patients usually have dull right upper quadrant discomfort following a meal that often is intermittent and that may last for several hours with little systemic response.

Acute cholecystitis refers to acute inflammation of the gallbladder and is caused by obstruction of the cystic duct by stones in at least 90% of cases. Infection of the gallbladder is probably also an important etiologic component since bacteria of enteric origin may be cultured from gallbladder bile in two thirds or three fourths of patients with acute cholecystitis. In this disorder, a systemic response to the inflammation is common. This is characterized by right upper quadrant pain and tenderness, with a modest-to-moderate increase in temperature. In about 30% of patients a mass is palpable in the right upper quadrant. This mass usually represents omentum and bowel overlying the inflamed gallbladder. About 75% of patients with acute cholecystitis have had previous gallbladder symptoms. Laboratory studies may be abnormal, including a leukocytosis to 15,000 cells/mm and a slight increase in serum alkaline phosphatase, amylase, serum glutamic oxaloacetic transaminase, and serum glutamic pyruvic transaminase. Occasionally the bilirubin may be mildly elevated. A plain abdominal x-ray film is usually of little help in establishing the diagnosis and is more helpful in ruling out other diseases such as a perforated ulcer with free air and a urinary calculous. About 15% of patients will have radiopaque gallstones demonstrable on this x-ray film. Air may occasionally be seen in the gallbladder wall or biliary tract if gas-forming organisms are present or if there is a fistula between the gallbladder and small intestine (cholecystoenteric fistula) from erosion of a gallstone into adjacent bowel that results from adherence of the bowel to the inflamed gallbladder.

The typical presentation of a patient with cholecystitis (acute or chronic) is the right upper quadrant abdominal pain occurring about 1 to 2 hours following a meal. The relationship to food is variable but consistent enough that it is probably caused by the emptying of fat from the stomach into the duodenum, which results in the release of CCK. CCK is a stimulant of gallbladder contraction, and with stones in the gallbladder the increased activity leads to a stone obstructing the cystic duct. The relationship between fat and CCK release and its effects on gallbladder contraction is probably the explanation for the common association of fatty and fried foods and the initiation of gallbladder pain in patients with cholelithiasis. Although acute cholecystitis is the result of cystic duct obstruction by an impacted stone or one attempting to pass from the gallbladder through the cystic duct and into the common duct the majority of the time, it can occur without the presence of gallstones. Acalculous cholecystitis accounts for about 5% of all cases and is found in patients with overwhelming sepsis, prolonged starvation, cystic artery occlusion and prolonged hyperalimentation. The exact pathogenesis of this entity remains to be defined.

The right upper quadrant pain and tenderness that occur with cholecystitis are attributed to distention and inflammation of the gallbladder. Gallbladder pain generally radiates around to the back and between the scapulae. The pain pattern may be short-lived if the stone dislodges itself from obstructing the cystic duct or persistent if the stone becomes impacted. The pain of gallbladder disease is contrasted with the pain associated with pancreatitis, which usually penetrates through to the back. On physical examination the tenderness that occurs in the right upper quadrant may be mild or severe and aggravated on inspiration, in which case it is referred to as Murphy's sign. This latter sign is usually elicited by the examiner when manually indenting the abdominal wall on the right side in the midclavicular line just below the costal margin and having the patient take a deep breath. With inspiration the diaphragm descends, pushing the liver down and anteriorly. With the indentation of the abdominal wall the gallbladder is struck, resulting in sharp pain. Murphy's sign refers to this particular maneuver of elicited pain on inspiration that is localized in the right upper quadrant and usually indicates an impacted stone in the cystic duct. Diffuse discomfort in the entire right upper quadrant is not considered a positive Murphy's sign and is usually more indicative of the resolution of cystic duct obstruction or the presence of liver disease. The position at which the localized tenderness of Murphy's sign is elicited may vary, especially if the patient has a large liver that may extend below the costal margin.

Specific diagnostic evaluation of cholecystitis can be placed in two general categories: patients with acute symptoms and those in whom symptoms have resolved. Those patients with acute symptoms should be evaluated promptly for biliary tract disease since deterioration of their clinical course will generally require an emergency cholecystectomy. This is in contrast to patients with hepatitis and pancreatitis in whom medical support is the preferred treatment. Two studies are extremely helpful in diagnosing biliary tract disease under acute conditions: ultrasound and the radionuclide biliary scan. Both of these studies are relatively noninvasive, rapid, and accurate and have low complication rates. Ultrasound provides information about the gallbladder anatomy, including thickening of the gallbladder wall, and will show the presence of a stone(s), if present, on acoustic shadowing with an accuracy approaching 90%. In a patient with typical symptoms of acute cholecystitis, confirmation of the presence of stones in the gallbladder with ultrasound usually provides sufficient information to justify proceeding with a cholecystectomy. In contrast to ultrasound, technetium-99 radionuclide scanning is a functional test of the gallbladder. This test is performed by injecting technetium intravenously, coupled with various iminodiacetic (IDA) compounds (e.g., 2,6-dimethyl acetanilid [HIDA], para-isopropyl iminodiacetic acid [PIPIDA], 2,6-diisopropyl acetanilid [DISIDA]). The injected radioisotope is excreted by the hepatocytes into bile and concentrated in the gallbladder. Within 5 to 10 minutes of injection the liver is imaged, and shortly afterward the bile ducts and gallbladder are visualized. The visualization of the liver and bile ducts without visualization of the gallbladder is considered an abnormal test. Since ingestion of fat before this test will result in gallbladder contraction and its emptying, it is important that the patient is fasted before the test is begun to prevent a falsely abnormal outcome. Assuming that the test has been performed properly, it is necessary to rely on clinical symptoms for interpretation of nonvisualization of the gallbladder. A symptomatic patient with nonvisualization has acute cholecystitis. Chronic cholecystitis is suggested when symptoms have abated and the gallbladder does not visualize. The various iminodiacetic radionuclide compounds that image the biliary tract are related to the bilirubin level. The technetium HIDA scan will image the biliary tree when the bilirubin is under 6 mg/100 ml. The other compounds will visualize the biliary tree at higher bilirubin levels. In the patient with hyperbilirubinemia it is important to select the appropriate radionuclide material to ensure adequate imaging of the biliary tract. If this is not done, poor visualization of the liver and bile duct will occur and could be misinterpreted. In this circumstance, poor imaging does not indicate complete biliary obstruction but rather parenchymal liver disease.

In patients without active symptoms but with a history suggestive of gallbladder dysfunction and gallstone disease, an oral cholecystogram is an appropriate study to obtain. This study consists of the oral ingestion of an iodinated compound (i.e., iopanoic acid in tablet form) that is administered the evening before the examination. The material is absorbed by the intestine, transported to the liver, secreted into bile, and concentrated by the gallbladder. A plain x-ray film of the right upper quadrant is then obtained to image the gallbladder. The oral cholecystogram combines the advantages of both ultrasound and radionuclide scanning because it shows not only the anatomy of the gallbladder, but also its functional capabilities. A visualized gallbladder without stones is considered normal. The gallbladder can also be visualized with multiple radiolucent defects indicating stones. This finding is interpreted as a functioning gallbladder with gallstones. With no visualization of the gallbladder, several interpretations are possible. It is important to ensure that the patient has ingested all of the tablets and has not had a fatty meal before the x-ray film examination. With poor absorption of the tablets from the intestine or rapid transit, sufficient contrast may not be absorbed, resulting in nonvisualization. This may occur following an acute illness such as gastroenteritis or in a malabsorption disorder such as sprue. In patients with severe liver disease, especially if the bilirubin is greater than 2%, sufficient contrast is not excreted into the bile even though absorbed from the gut to allow visualization of the gallbladder. If the patient has ingested the tablets and absorption from the intestinal tract is normal, transport into bile by hepatocytes is good, and visualization of the gallbladder does not occur, the patient has cholecystitis. An asymptomatic patient without gallbladder visualization has a nonfunctioning gallbladder (chronic cholecystitis). Performed correctly, the oral cholecystogram remains a very reliable test, especially in asymptomatic patients, approaching an accuracy rate of 97%.

The selection of ultrasonography, radionuclide scanning, or oral cholecystography will depend on the clinic presentation of the patient and the resources available to the clinician. Most clinicians prefer a radionuclide scan in the acute case and an oral cholecystogram in the asymptomatic patient. The combination of sonography and radionuclide scanning under acute conditions combines anatomy and function; therefore the tests complement one another.

Patients with acute cholecystitis should be admitted to a general surgical service, resuscitated with intravenous fluids, have concomitant medical problems stabilized, and undergo cholecystectomy at the earliest convenient time once the diagnosis is confirmed with ultrasound or radionuclide study. Additional therapy such as parasympathetic drugs, nasogastric suction, and H_2-receptor antagonists have not been shown to affect the course of the disease. Unless the patient is febrile and has evidence of bacterial infection or is at risk from endocarditis, antibiotics are used only in the periods immediately before, during, and after surgery. Antibiotics for gram-negative organisms that have good tissue penetration are preferred. The main purpose of antibiotics in these patients is to decrease the incidence of a wound infection since cholecystectomy is considered a clean-contaminated case. Observing the patient until symptoms subside or performing cholecystectomy in 6 to 8 weeks during another hospitalization should rarely be necessary. Data exist that refute the practice of delayed operation (i.e., 6 to 8 weeks) if the patient cannot undergo a cholecystectomy within 72 hours of the onset of acute cholecystitis.

In the asymptomatic patient with gallstones discovered incidentally (e.g., on sonogram or plain film of the abdomen obtained for unrelated reasons), the decision to operate should be made on the basis of the likelihood of serious complications or sequelae eventually developing. Generally accepted reasons for cholecystectomy in asymptomatic patients with gallstones include diabetes mellitus, sickle cell disease, a nonopacifying gallbladder on oral cholecystogram, a calcified gallbladder wall, and the presence of large (>2 cm) stones.[50] In the first two instances, cholecystitis is not necessarily more common in these two diseases; but, when it does occur, there is a higher mortality and morbidity, and emergency operation becomes necessary. In patients with diabetes or sickle cell disease, the risks of cholecystectomy are markedly reduced when performed electively and under optimal conditions. A nonfunctioning gallbladder indicates severe gallbladder disease. Calcification of the gallbladder wall is the only significant cancer risk of the biliary tract. Although biliary tract cancer is unusual, the only correlation with the ultimate development of cancer has been a calcified gallbladder wall, not calcified stones. Large stones have the risk of eroding and producing a biliary enteric fistula. When this occurs, these stones can then obstruct the intestine at the ileocecal valve, causing gallstone ileus. In other patients without any of the risk factors, the risks from developing acute cholecystitis and a complication vs. the risk of elective cholecystectomy are almost comparable. It is estimated that on the average a patient who is observed with asymptomatic stones has a life expectancy 2 months greater than the patient with asymptomatic stones who has an elective cholecystectomy.

COMMON BILE DUCT

The common hepatic duct begins at the confluence of the major lobar bile ducts that drain each hepatic lobe. The common hepatic duct then joins with the cystic duct to form the common bile duct. This common bile duct then descends inferiorly and passes behind the first portion of the duodenum and through the substance of the head of the pancreas to enter into the duodenal lumen obliquely through the wall of its second part. In approximately 80% of cases, it forms a common channel with the main pancreatic duct called the ampulla of Vater.[36,42] During most of their passage through the duodenal wall these two structures are enclosed by a complex arrangement of intrinsic circular and longitudinal smooth muscle, i.e., by the sphincter of Oddi (Fig. 26-11). Careful anatomic studies have documented definitively that the sphincter of Oddi's musculature is anatomically and embryologically distinct from the duodenal musculature.[6] The motor activity of the sphincter *vide infra* plays a substantial role in bile delivery to the duodenal lumen.

Motility

In humans the common bile duct demonstrates a well-defined, spontaneous, rhythmic activity in vitro with three to five contractile waves per minute, each lasting 1 to 3 seconds.[42] The significance of these findings in vivo has not been delineated. The common bile duct musculature is

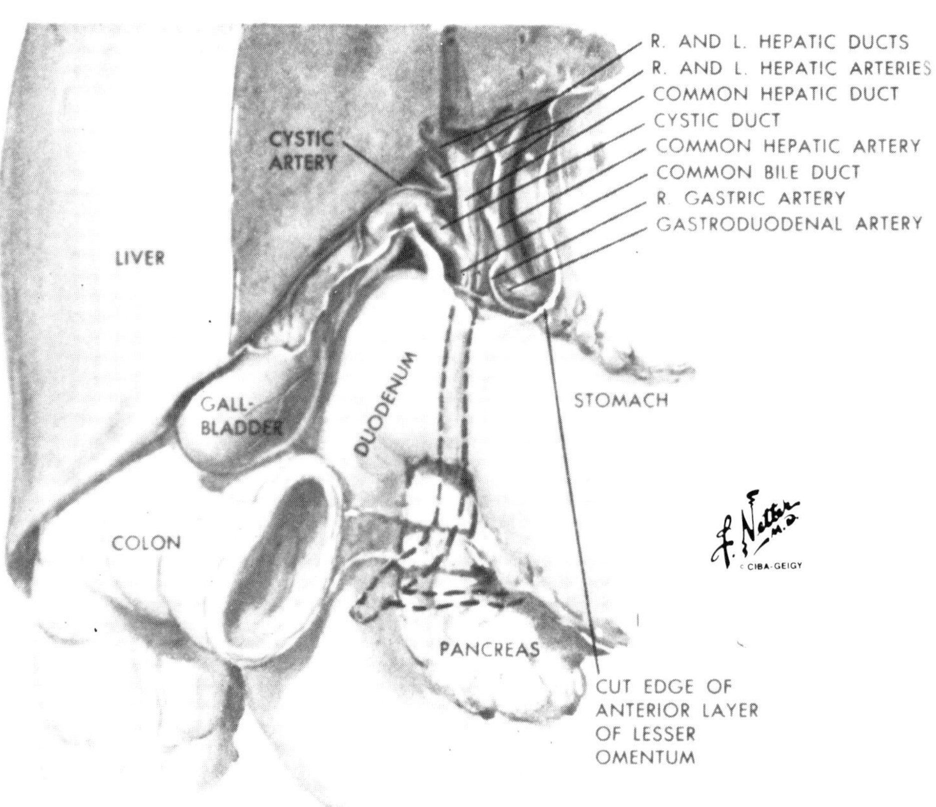

Fig. 26-11 Extrahepatic biliary tract system. (From Netter, F.H.: CIBA Collection of Medical Illustrations, vol. 3, part III, Indianapolis, Ind., 1964, CIBA Pharmaceutical Co., Division of CIBA-GEIGY Corp.)

oriented predominantly in the longitudinal direction and is probably more involved with maintaining tone than intraluminal content propulsion.[30] True peristalsis, as seen in the intestine, is probably not present, nor is it necessary for efficient bile transport. Normally the pressure (11 to 13 cm of water) in the common bile duct is slightly less than the resting pressure or resistance of the sphincter of Oddi, which averages 15 to 17 cm of water. The pressure in the common bile duct exceeds any resistance to flow through the cystic duct so that normally bile enters the gallbladder rather than the duodenum. The efficient delivery of bile into the duodenum necessitates gallbladder contraction and relaxation of the choledochoduodenal junction.[42]

Sphincter of Oddi

Although changes in duodenal activity influence biliary duct pressures, the key factor appears to be the tone of the sphincter of Oddi. In vivo studies have documented the role of choledochoduodenal tone in the regulation of bile flow into the duodenum independent of duodenal motility.[34] Spontaneous rhythmic contraction of the sphincter of Oddi of myogenic origin has also been documented, which may represent a "milking" effect on bile delivery into the duodenum.[42] Cholecystokinin acts directly on the musculature of the sphincter of Oddi as a relaxant and allows duodenal bile delivery.[36] As with the gallbladder, the neural influences on the common bile duct and the sphincter of Oddi are less quantitatively understood and are of questionable physiologic significance (see Table 26-1).

Resting common bile duct, main pancreatic duct, and sphincter of Oddi pressures do not appear to differ significantly between healthy patients and those with gallstones or common bile duct stones or those previously subjected to cholecystectomy, hepatic duct cancer, or chronic pancreatitis.[12] These observations diminish the likelihood of motility or pressure abnormalities as being of any major significance in the pathogenesis of biliary tract lithiasis.

Choledocholithiasis

Common bile duct stones (i.e., choledocholithiasis) can be divided into primary and secondary types. About 15% of patients with gallbladder stones will have simultaneous stones in the common bile duct. These stones are virtually always the same chemically as those in the gallbladder. Primary choledocholithiasis is more difficult to prove and is the subject of much clinical controversy. Generally a 2-year asymptomatic interval after previous cholecystectomy is required before stones found in the common duct can be considered to be primary. The incidence of primary choledocholithiasis varies from 4% to 90%, depending on the criteria used for its identification.[31]

Over 50% of primary common bile duct stones are pigment stones. These are light, soft, crushable yellow or brown stones, often found in association with sludge or debris in other parts of the biliary tree but routinely absent in the gallbladder if this organ has not been previously removed. Primary stones are usually associated with common bile duct dilation, biliary tract infection, advanced patient age, a long history of biliary tract disease, and multiple previous surgical interventions on the biliary tree. Secondary stones in the common duct found in association with primary gallbladder disease and gallstones are rarely associated with biliary tract infection or pathologic changes in biliary tree histology.[31,32] Although controversial, stasis is thought to be a leading factor in primary choledocholithogenesis. Previous operations on the biliary tract or trauma to the sphincter of Oddi may contribute to stasis in the bile ducts since the bile duct dilates following these circumstances. Stasis also occurs with age and seems to correlate with duct dilation and stone formation. The relationship between a motility disorder, stasis, and stone formation is not well defined, but there seem to be several correlations. The stones found in dilated bile ducts are usually pigmented and more frequently occur in elderly patients. Congenital diseases associated with cystic ductular dilation such as Caroli's disease are also associated with primary stone formation.[56]

The role of biliary infection in the genesis of pigment stone formation has been discussed previously. An interrelationship between infection and stasis is thought to promote mucosal inflammatory changes that lead to dilation and extrusion of calcium and abnormal mucus that may act as nidi for stone formation.[43] Periampullary duodenal diverticula are also associated with a high incidence of common bile duct calculous disease,[29] probably because of incompetent choledochoduodenal sphincter function and bacterial contamination. In patients with primary biliary duct stone formation, choledochotomy and T-tube drainage are usually inadequate, and treatment that improves drainage of the duct and reduces biliary stasis such as a choledochoduodenostomy has significantly better results.[29,32,43]

Another method of classifying common duct stones is according to the chemical composition of the stone. This has major therapeutic implications since cholesterol stones are amenable to dissolution and pigment stones cannot be safely dissolved. Following cholecystectomy and common duct exploration, the stones should be saved and incubated in monooctanoin. If the stones dissolve within 5 days, the cholesterol content is sufficiently high (>60%) that any retained common duct stones can be dissolved. Currently, monooctanoin is the preferred compound to dissolve retained cholesterol common duct stones. Monooctanoin is a medium-chain diglyceride and is described in more detail in the following section.

Of the approximately 15% of patients who have choledocholithiasis in combination with cholelithiasis, as many as 50% of them will demonstrate no clinical evidence of common duct disease. Most of the others will experience jaundice, biliary colic, cholangitis (see below), or pancreatitis as a result of obstruction from the stones. Because of the fluctuating nature of the obstruction, serum bilirubin levels are usually less than those seen with malignant disease and rarely exceed 15 mg/100 ml. At initial laparotomy for cholelithiasis, historical suspicions (jaundice, cholangitis, pancreatitis) or physical manifestations (palpable stone, dilated common bile duct, filling defects seen on cholangiography before and during surgery may lead the surgeon to perform a common bile duct exploration with stone removal by means of irrigation, forceps, balloon catheter, or sphincterotomy. The surgically opened common bile duct is usually closed over a soft T-tube to stent the traumatized duct in order to lessen postoperative edema, protect the suture line, and allow postoperative radiologic evaluation and treatment, if necessary, for retained stones.

Cholangitis

Cholangitis usually signifies bacterial infection of an obstructed common bile duct, generally resulting from stones within the duct (i.e., choledocholithiasis), a stricture occluding the diameter of the duct lumen (often resulting from surgical injury), or a neoplasm occluding the duct. Charcot's triad (right upper quadrant pain, jaundice, fever, and chills) is seen in approximately two thirds of these patients. Most of these patients will respond to intravenous broad-spectrum antibiotics unless the duct is virtually totally occluded. In this latter circumstance, the cholangitis becomes suppurative and usually presents with shock and mental status changes in addition to Charcot's triad, warranting urgent resuscitation, antibiotic coverage, and surgical drainage of the duct by means of laparotomy (i.e., choledochotomy). In selected cases, percutaneous or endoscopic drainage of the duct has been successful. If either of these methods is used and the patient does not respond, then adequate drainage must be obtained with a large T-tube placed during surgery.

GALLSTONE DISSOLUTION THERAPY

Numerous compounds and solutions have been used to dissolve gallbladder or common bile duct stones. All of these substances are generally only effective for cholesterol stones. Ether, chloroform, and other organic solvents that are capable of dissolving cholesterol stones are not safe and should no longer be used. Although heparin was also once tried for gallstone dissolution, in vitro studies and in vivo experience has confirmed its ineffectiveness.[19] In contrast, chronic oral therapy with the bile salts chenodeoxycholate (also called chenic and chenodiol) and ursodeoxycholate has been shown to dissolve cholesterol gallbladder stones.[24,38] Such agents often dissolve gallstones in 6 months but not uncommonly require 1 or more years and generally do not prevent the development of gallbladder disease itself. In addition, their use does not necessarily obviate the eventual need for cholecystectomy. In a 2-year controlled clinical trial, only 14% of the patients receiving a high dose (300 mg/day) of chenodeoxycholate had complete dissolution of their stones.[50] Disadvantages of such treatment include the prolonged need for continuous oral therapy and the high reformation rate of new stones once therapy is terminated. In obese patients it may be difficult to achieve a high enough dosage to desaturate bile without the severe side effects of diarrhea from such bile salt treatment. Approximately one fourth of patients receiving this therapy develop transient liver enzyme elevation, and 4% develop significant hepatotoxicity. Since chenodeoxycholate must be concentrated in the gallbladder, a non-functioning gallbladder is a contraindication to treatment. Cholestasis is another contraindication because of its hepatotoxic side effects. Because of the potential irritating effects of these bile salts on the gastric and bowel mucosa, peptic ulcer disease and inflammatory bowel disease are relative contraindications.[38] Patients with underlying liver disease also represent a relative contraindication. The cost of therapy is an additional potential disadvantage. Prolonged treatment is a necessity since 30% to 40% of patients have a recurrence of stone formation within 2 years after the cessation of treatment.[49,50] Although fewer side effects have been reported with ursodeoxycholate than with chenodeoxycholate, the incidence of significant hepatotoxicity with both agents is still a potential problem. Probably dissolution treatment is best reserved currently for elderly patients who are either poor operative risks and compliant, or are at high risk for developing gallbladder disease on the basis of family history or ethnic background.[38] In any event, gallbladder function in these latter patients must be normal, and they should be asymptomatic if such treatment is to be recommended.

Two solutions are in current use for the dissolution of common bile duct stones. These include monooctanoin (Capmul) and sodium cholate. Monooctanoin is the preferred solution for the dissolution of cholesterol common bile duct stones[18,19] because it is safe, effective, and rapid; less experience has been obtained with sodium cholate. Monooctanoin is a medium-chain diglyceride of capric acid and caprylic acid, is an excellent solvent for cholesterol, and is water soluble. For stones that possess greater than 40% by weight cholesterol content, a 90% success rate can be expected with monooctanoin dissolution, generally within 3 to 7 days. The technique of infusion of this substance consists of administering the solution by an infusion pump at 3 to 5 ml/hour into the common bile duct through a previously placed tube (i.e., T-tube) to bathe the retained common bile duct stones. A manometer is placed within the system to prevent the untoward effects of unexpected pressure increases above normal biliary pressures. Increased pressure within the bile duct may result in chills, fever, or abdominal pain. Abdominal cramps may also result from large amounts of monooctanoin emptying into the duodenum. Patients are followed daily with serial liver enzyme determinations, and a cholangiogram through the T-tube is obtained every third or fourth day. If there is no significant change in size or number of stones by the seventh day, the infusion is discontinued.[18,19]

If a stone is low in cholesterol (e.g., pigment stones) or if dissolution is not successful, extraction of stones by the T-tube tract is then recommended. It is important to allow the T-tube tract to mature for at least 6 to 8 weeks. It is well known that approximately 20% of common bile duct stones will be passed spontaneously into the duodenum during this waiting period. For persistent stones that do not pass, extraction is usually performed with a steerable Burhenne or Dormia stone basket under fluoroscopy. Other modifications used to remove stones through the T-tube tract include the use of forceps and a balloon catheter. Stones can be crushed and extracted or pushed through the ampulla of Vater, especially in the case of pigment common bile duct stones.

Another percutaneous technique that can be used to extract stones is choledochoscopy. Percutaneous choledochoscopy can be performed if the T-tube tract is large. The choledochoscope has the advantage of directly visualizing the bile ducts and stones. It has been found useful when large stones impacted in the hepatic ducts can be dislodged under direct visualization. Once dislodgement has occurred, basket extraction can then be used to remove the remaining stones or fragments. Endoscopic papillotomy is yet another technique to rid the common bile duct of retained stones, but it requires a considerable amount of endoscopic expertise. The problems that have been encountered with this procedure include hemorrhage, perforation, and late stricture of the common bile duct. Fragmentation is a newly developed method with the use of contact ultrasound, electrohydraulic lithotripsy, YAG laser, or extracorporeal ultrasound. The main advantage of this approach is the independence of stone composition and the rapidity of fragmentation. The clinical role of these techniques is being explored. Finally, surgical therapy is a highly successful alternative to management of retained common bile duct stones. Common bile duct exploration performed along with choledochoduodenostomy or choledochojejunostomy have been used with good results. For a further discussion of these therapeutic considerations, see Chapter 29.

MALIGNANCY AND CALCULOUS DISEASE

Malignancies involving the gallbladder and biliary tract are uncommon when compared with tumors arising in other portions of the gastrointestinal tract.[1a,13a,21a,51a,55a] Gallbladder cancer is responsible for approximately 4% of all malignant lesions involving the alimentary tract, whereas cancer of the common bile duct has an autopsy incidence of approximately 0.5%. Gallbladder cancer is a disease of the elderly; 75% of patients are over the age 65 years at time of diagnosis. Most patients are women, and histologically most primary tumors are adenocarcinomas. Although the cause of this disorder remains unknown, cholelithiasis has been implicated as an etiologic factor, since as many as 70% to 90% of patients have associated gallstone disease, and the risk of malignant degeneration appears to correlate with the length of time that gallstones have been present. Although malignant tumors of the bile duct are also adenocarcinomas, the relationship between calculous disease and bile duct cancer is less clear. In the Orient a causal relationship has been postulated with biliary parasite infestation such as *Ascaris lumbricoides* and *Clonorchis sinensis* and with the presence of intrahepatic stones. In addition, there appears to be an increased incidence of bile duct carcinoma in patients with inflammatory bile disease, particularly those with ulcerated colitis. Most bile duct malignancies are located in the hepatic or common bile ducts. Like gallbladder cancer, most patients with bile duct malignancies are in the older age group, although they may appear in patients as young as 20 years old.

The signs and symptoms associated with cancer of the gallbladder are similar to those occurring in other types of biliary tract disease. Pain in the right upper quadrant in association with nausea, vomiting, and occasionally weight loss are relatively frequent. At some point in the disease process, jaundice may be encountered in as many as 50% of patients, and the gallbladder is palpable in as many as 25% of patients. Such findings are usually attributed to benign gallbladder disease. It is for this reason that the diagnosis is hardly ever made before surgery. Many of the symptoms associated with gallbladder cancer are also found in patients with bile duct malignancies. However, because of the obstructive nature of biliary tract malignancy, jaundice is more commonly encountered and is often associated with clay-colored stools, diarrhea, and a dark "tea-colored" urine. Because these findings are common to all patients with obstructive jaundice, the diagnosis of bile duct carcinoma is also usually confirmed only at the time of operation.

The treatment of carcinoma of the gallbladder has generally been dismal because of early metastases and extension of the tumor beyond the gallbladder by the time of diagnosis. Even when cholecystectomy in combination with resection of all or part of the right lobe of the liver is attempted as a curative procedure, the overall 5-year survival rate averages no more than 2% to 3%. Obviously, earlier diagnosis and resection when the tumor has been confined to the gallbladder is the only hope of effecting a cure in patients with this devastating tumor.

The outcome in patients with bile duct carcinoma is just as discouraging. The overall 5-year survival rate in patients with this disease approaches 10% to 15%. Like gallbladder cancer, the treatment is surgical, i.e., resection of the affected bile duct. For distal bile duct lesions, this will usually involve a radical pancreaticoduodenectomy (Whipple procedure). For middle common duct or low hepatic duct tumors, bile flow is reestablished with a Roux-en-Y choledochojejunostomy approach in which the proximal duct is anatomosed to a jejunal loop following resection of the involved duct. Tumors at the hilum of the liver, if resectable, provide a more formidable problem in terms of reestablishing bile flow. This circumstance involves a Roux-en-Y hepaticojejunostomy, in which the anastomosis is fashioned between the hilum of the liver and the bowel rather than between individual bile ducts and the intestine.

SUMMARY

A knowledge of the physiology of bile composition, secretion, and flow and their relationships to biliary pathology is crucial if the pathogenesis of calculous disease of the gallbladder and biliary tree is to be properly understood. The complex fluid called bile is produced and modified in the hepatic bile canaliculi in both bile salt–dependent and bile salt–independent fractions and later supplemented by the addition of ductular bile. Bile flow depends on multiple factors, including active transport, peristalsis, and the size of the bile salt pool. The unique interaction between bile salts, phospholipids, and cholesterol into micelles facilitates lipid absorption from the gut. Disproportionate changes in the amounts of any of these substances may lead to saturated bile with lithogenic tendencies. The gallbladder and common bile duct serve as storage vehicles and final modifiers of bile and are often the site of gallstone formation. To manage patients who develop such stones, a variety of dissolution regimens have been used, but, except in the high-risk elderly patient, surgical removal of the gallbladder with exploration of the biliary tree if common duct stones are also present is generally the treatment of choice.

REFERENCES

1. Admirand, W.H., and Small, D.M: The physiochemical basis of cholesterol gallstone formation in man, J. Clin. Invest. **47:**1043, 1968.

1a. Alexander, F., et al.: Biliary carcinoma: a review of 109 cases, Am. J. Surg. **147:**503, 1984.

2. Bennion, L.J., and Grundy, S.M.: Risk factors for the development of cholelithias in man, N. Engl. J. Med. **299:**1161, 1978.

3. Bennion, L.J., et al.: Development of lithogenic bile during puberty in Pima indians, N. Engl. J. Med. **300:**873, 1979.

4. Boonvapisit, S.T., Trotman, B.W., and Ostrow, J.D.: Unconjugated bilirubin and the hydrolysis of conjugated bilirubin in gallbladder bile of patients with cholelithiasis, Gastroenterology **74:**70, 1978.

5. Bouchier, I.A.D.: Biochemistry of gallstone formation, Clin. Gastroenterol. **12:**25, 1983.

6. Boyden, E.A.: The anatomy of the choledochoduodenal junction in man, Surg. Gynecol. Obstet. **104:**641, 1957.

7. Boyer, J.L., and Bloomer, J.R.: Canalicular bile secretion in man: studies utilizing the biliary clearance of (^{14}C) mannitol, J. Clin. Invest. **51:**773, 1974.

8. Braverman, D.Z., Johnson M.L., and Kern, F., Jr.: Effects of pregnancy and contraceptive steroids on gallbladder function, N. Engl. J. Med. **302:**362, 1980.

9. Burnett, W., Dwyer, K.R., and Kennard, C.H.: Black pigment or poly bilirubinate gallstones: composition and formation, Ann. Surg. **193:**331, 1981.

10. Carey, M.C., and Small, D.M.: The physical chemistry of cholesterol solubility in bile: relationship to gallstone formation and dissolution in man, J. Clin. Invest. **61:**998, 1978.

11. Chenderovitch, J.: Secretory function of the rabbit common bile duct, Am. J. Physiol. **223:**695, 1972.

12. Csenoes, A., et al.: Pressure measurements in the biliary and pancreatic duct systems in controls and in patients with gallstones, previous cholecystectomy, or common bile duct stones, Gastroenterology **77:**1203, 1979.

13. Davis, R.A., et al.: Alterations of hepatic Na^+ K^+-ATPase and bile flow by estrogen: effects in liver surface membrane lipid structure and function, Proc. Natl. Acad. Sci. USA **75:**4130, 1978.

13a. Diehl, A.K.: Epidemiology of gallbladder cancer: a synthesis of recent data, J. Natl. Cancer Inst. **65:**1209, 1980.

14. Dumont, M., Erlingee, S., and Lichman, S.: Hypercholeresis induced by ursodeoxycholic acid and 7-ketolithocholic acid in the rat: possible role of bicarbonate transport, Gastroenterology **79:**82, 1980.

15. Evans, D.M., and Wessler, E.L.: Physiochemical considerations in gallstone pathogenesis, Hosp. Pract. **9:**133, 1974.

16. Fridhandler, T.M., Davison, J.S., and Shaffer, E.A.: Defective gallbladder contractility in the ground squirrel and prairie dog during the early stages of cholesterol gallstone formation, Gastroenterology **85:**830, 1983.

17. Frizzell, R.A., Dugas, M., and Schultz, S.G.: Intracellular chloride activities in rabbit gallbladder: direct evidence for a coupled NaCl-influenced process, J. Gen. Physiol. **65:**769, 1975.

18. Gadacz, T.R.: The effect of monooctanoin on retained common duct stones, Surgery **89:**527, 1981.

19. Gadacz, T.R.: Retained common duct stones, In Cameron, J.L., editor: Current surgical therapy 1984-1985, Philadelphia, 1984, B.C. Decker.

20. Grodzki, M., Mazurkiewicz-Rozynska, E., and Czyzyk, A.: Diabetic cholecystopathy, Diabetologia **4:**345, 1968.

21. Grundy, S.M., and Mok, H.Y.I.: Colestipol, clofibrate, and phytosterols in combined therapy of hyperlipidemia, J. Lab. Clin. Med. **89:**354, 1977.

21a. Hamrick, R.E., et al.: Primary carcinoma of the gallbladder, Ann. Surg. **195:**270, 1982.

22. Holen, K.R., et al.: Nucleation time: a key factor in the pathogenesis of cholesterol gallstone disease, Gastroenterology **72:**611, 1979.

23. Honore, L.H.: Cholesterol cholelithiasis in adolescent females, Arch. Surg. **115:**62, 1980.

24. Horbach, R.T.: Pathogenesis and medical treatment of gallstones. In Sleisenger, M.H., and Fordtran J.S., editors: Gastrointestinal disease pathophysiology, diagnosis, management, ed. 3, Philadelphia, 1983, W.B. Saunders Co.

25. Kjellgren, K.: Persistence of symptoms following biliary surgery, Ann. Surg. **152:**1026, 1960.

26. LaMonte, W.W., et al.: Pathogenesis of cholesterol gallstones, Surg. Clin. North Am. **61:**765, 1981.

27. LaMonte, W.W., et al.: Pigment gallstone formation in the cholesterol-fed guinea pig, Hepatology **5:**21, 1985.

28. Lee, S.P., Lamont, J.T., and Carey M.C.: Role of gallbladder mucus hypersecretion in the evolution of cholesterol gallstones: studies in the prairie dog, J. Clin. Invest. **67:**1712, 1981.

29. Lotveit, T., Osnes, M., and Larsen, S.: Recurrent biliary calculi: duodenal diverticula as a predisposing factor, Ann. Surg. **196:**30, 1982.

30. Ludwick, J.R.: Observations on the smooth muscle and contractile activity of the common bile duct, Ann. Surg. **164:**1041, 1966.

31. Lygidcikis, N.J.: Incidence and significance of primary stones of the common bile duct in choledocholithiasis, Surg. Gynecol. Obstet. **157:**434, 1983.

32. Madden, J.L.: Primary common duct stones. In Cameron, J., editor: Current surgical therapy 1984-1985, Philadelphia, 1984, B.C. Decker.

33. Malagelada, J.R.: Gastric, pancreatic, and biliary responses to a meal. In Johnson, L.R., editor: Physiology of the gastrointestinal tract, New York, 1981, Raven Press.

34. Ono, K., et al.: Bile flow mechanisms in man, Arch. Surg. **96:**869, 1968.

35. Ostrow, J.: Absorption by the gallbladder of bile salts, sulfobromophthalein and iodipamide, J. Lab. Clin. Med. **74:**482, 1969.

36. Paumgartner, G., and Sauerbruch, T.: Secretion, composition and flow of bile, Clin. Gástroenterol. **12:**3, 1983.

37. Pomeranz, I.S., and Shaffer, E.A.: Abnormal gallbladder emptying in a subgroup of patients with gallstones, Gastroenterology **88:**787, 1985.

38. Postier, R., and Gadacz, T.R.: Cholecystectomy vs. chenodeoxycholate treatment of gallstones and gallbladder disease, Hosp. Formulary **15:**608, 1980.

39. Rehfield, J.F.: Cholecystokinin, Clin. Gastroenterol. **9:**593, 1980.

40. Reichen, J., and Paumgartner, G.: Uptake of bile acids by perfused rat liver, Annu. J. Physiol. **231:**734, 1976.

41. Rose, R.C.: Absorptive functions of the gallbladder. In Johnson, L.R., editor: Physiology of the gastrointestinal tract, New York, 1981, Raven Press.

42. Ryan J.P.: Motility of the gallbladder and biliary tree. In Johnson, L.R., editor: Physiology of the gastrointestinal tract, New York, 1981, Raven Press.

43. Saharia, P.C., Zuidema, G.D., and Cameron, J.L.: Primary common duct stones, Ann. Surg. **185:**598, 1977.

44. Sarles, H., Hanton, J., and Plancke, N.E.: Diet, cholesterol gallstones, and composition of the bile, Am. J. Dig. Dis. **15:**251, 1970.

45. Scharschmidt, B.F.: Bile formation and gallbladder and bile function. In Sleisenger, M.H., and Fordtran, J.S., editors: Gastro-intestinal disease, ed. 3, Pathophysiology, diagnosis, management, Philadelphia, 1983, W.B. Saunders.

46. Sedaghat, A., and Grundy S.M.: Cholesterol crystals and the formation of cholesterol gallstones, N. Engl. J. Med. **302:**1274, 1980.

47. Soloway, R.D., Trotman, B.W., and Ostrow, J.D.: Pigment gallstones, Gastroenterology **72:**167, 1977.

48. Soloway, R.D., Balistreth, W.F., and Trotman, B.W.: The gallbladder and biliary tract. In Bouchier, I.A.D., editor: Recent advances in gastroenterology 5, Edinburgh, 1984, Churchill Livingstone.

49. Thistle, J.L.: Ursodeoxycholic acid treatment of gallstones, Liver Dis. **3:**146, 1983.

50. Thistle, J.L., et al.: The steering committee and the national cooperative gallstone study group. The natural history of cholelithiasis: the national cooperative gallstone study, Ann. Intern. Med. **101:**171, 1984.

51. Thomas, P.T., and Hofman, A.F.: A simple calculation of the lithogenic index of bile: expressing biliary lipid composition on rectangular coordinates, Gastroenterology **65:**698, 1973.

51a. Tompkins, R.K., et al.: Prognostic factors in bile duct carcinoma: analysis of 96 cases, Ann. Surg. **194:**447, 1981.

52. Trotman, B.W., and Soloway, R.D.: Pigment gallstone disease: summary of the National Institutes of Health-international workshop, Hepatology **2:**879, 1982.
53. Trotman, B.W., et al.: Pigment versus cholesterol cholelithiasis: identification and quantification by infrared spectroscopy, Gastroenterology **72:**495, 1977.
54. Turley, S.D., Anderson, J.M., and Dietschy, J.M.: The contribution of newly synthesized cholesterol to biliary cholesterol in the rat, J. Biol. Chem. **256:**2438, 1981.
55. Vantrappen, G., et al.: The interdigestive motor complex of normal subjects and patients with bacterial overgrowth of the small intestine, J. Clin. Invest. **59:**1158, 1977.
55a. Wanebo, J.H., Castle W.N., and Fechner, R.E.: Is carcinoma of the gallbladder a curable lesion? Ann. Surg. **195:**624, 1982.
56. Witlin, L.T., et al.: Transhepatic decompression of biliary tree in Carolis Disease, Surgery **91:**205, 1982.

27 *Gordon L. Kauffman, Jr.*

Pancreatic Exocrine Function

Pancreatic exocrine function consists of protein synthesis, which occurs in the acinar cell, and bicarbonate production, which occurs in the centroacinar and ductular cells. Although control mechanisms for protein and bicarbonate secretion are quite different, pancreatic disease usually results in a similar reduction in both products.

Much information regarding the processes of pancreatic protein synthesis and bicarbonate production has been derived from experiments conducted in various animal preparations. With respect to information on pancreatic exocrine function, this chapter will mention the experimental model and identify differences in species. When it is available, information derived from human studies will be presented.

HISTORIC CONSIDERATIONS

In the mid-nineteenth century Claude Bernard observed that pancreatic secretion plays a significant role in the digestion and absorption of fats. He noted that fats were emulsified in the lumen of the duodenum only in the portion distal to the entrance of the pancreatic duct. In the late nineteenth century Ivan Pavlov observed that pancreatic secretion was partly controlled by both the vagus nerve and duodenal mucosal acidification. It was also noted that these two stimuli caused the pancreas to secrete fluid of different composition. Vagal nerve stimulation caused the release of a thick, viscous, enzyme-rich fluid, whereas duodenal acidification was associated with high-volume fluid output of very low enzyme concentration. When it was clear that duodenal acidification caused pancreatic stimulation, even in the vagally and sympathetically denervated gland, most investigators believed that reflex neural connections between the duodenum were not involved.

Further experimentation on the acidification of isolated and denervated jejunal segments showed similar pancreatic secretory stimulation. In 1902, at the Physiological Laboratory of University College in London, Bayliss and Starling injected extracts of jejunal mucosal scrapings into the bloodstream, which resulted in the production of a pancreatic secretion. The substance responsible for this observation was named *secretin,* and 3 years later the term *hormone* was suggested for the chemical messengers produced in one organ and released into the blood, then affecting a different target organ. More recently Palade and co-workers were awarded the Nobel Prize in Medicine for their studies on the cellular and subcellular events associated with pancreatic acinar cellular protein synthesis.

ANATOMIC CONSIDERATIONS

Embryology

Formation of the ventral and dorsal endodermal outgrowths, which ultimately form the pancreas, arise from the abdominal foregut in the fourth week of human gestation.[65] The ventral pancreatic bud is initially bilobed and arises from the lateral aspects of the hepatic duct at its entry into the gut tube. The larger dorsal pancreatic bud is a single outgrowth arising from the dorsal aspect of the gut tube, rostral to the hepatic duct. During the fifth week the left lobe of the ventral pancreas disappears, and in the sixth week both dorsal and persisting ventral pancreatic buds have ductal systems that open into the gut tube. The dorsal duct opens directly into the gut lumen, whereas the ventral duct usually opens with the hepatic duct. In the region of the future stomach the gut tube dilates and rotates. This rotation is caused by unequal growth of the original dorsal and ventral borders of the gut tube.

Rotation of the stomach and liver causes the duodenum to be pulled across to the right from its original midline position. As this occurs, the dorsal mesentery of the duodenum, which contains the dorsal pancreas, approaches the dorsal body wall, and the ventral body wall comes into contact with the dorsal pancreas to the right of the midline. During the seventh week of gestation the dorsal and ventral elements of the pancreas fuse in their retroperitoneal position to form a single organ. The duct of the larger dorsal bud is Santorini's duct, which directly enters the lumen in the descending portion of the duodenum. The duct of the ventral bud is Wirsung's duct, which opens into the origin of the hepatic duct, later becoming the common bile duct. In human beings Wirsung's duct is usually the larger and more constant of the two, but Santorini's duct is patent in about 70% of persons.

The pancreas grows rapidly by elongation of the primitive ducts and overgrowth of numerous side branches that arise in groups and assume a lobular arrangement.[19] The columnar epithelium of the main duct takes on a cuboidal configuration in the smaller branches. Acini, the secreting units of the exocrine pancreas, consist of pyramidal cells whose apices are directed toward the lumen of the duct; they begin to appear along the lateral wall and distal ducts in the third month of development (Fig. 27-1). The ducts from which the acini arise are lined by centroacinar cells. Proximal to the centroacinar cells the ducts elongate and form intercalated ducts, which connect to form intralobular ducts lined by columnar epithelium. During the fourth month the lobules enlarge and connective tissue dimin-

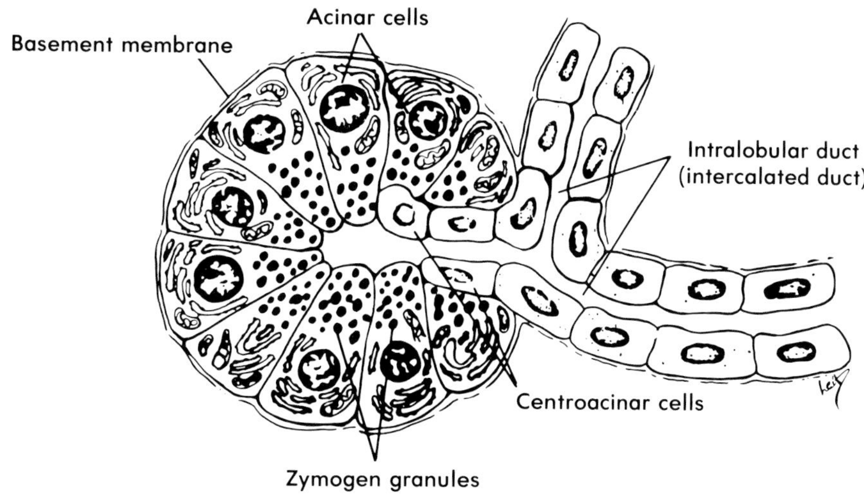

Fig. 27-1 Exocrine acinus of the pancreas.

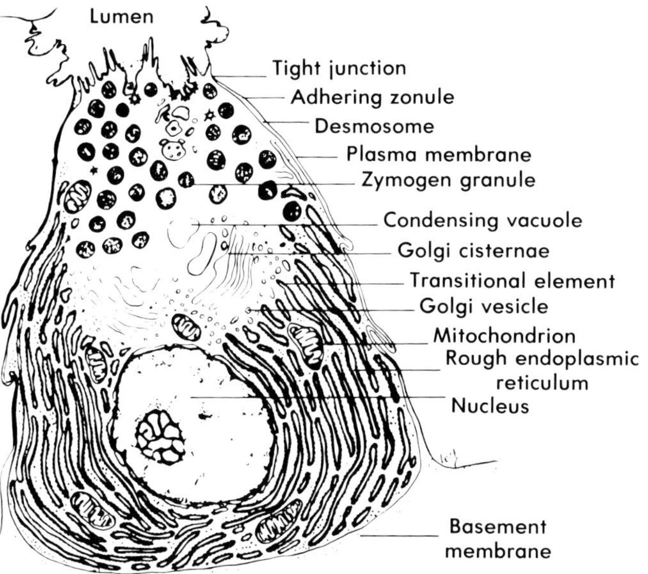

Fig. 27-2 Diagram of pancreatic acinar cell.

ishes, resulting in coalescence and lobe formation. Small granules also appear in the cytoplasm of the acinar cells in the fourth month. These zymogen granules increase in number and accumulate in the apical cytoplasm (Fig. 27-2). Morphologically these acinar cells appear capable of secretion, but no evidence suggests secretory activity during prenatal life.

Gross Anatomy

The pancreas is a solid glandular organ, weighing 70 to 110 g and lying in the retroperitoneum below the left hepatic lobe and posterior to the stomach. It is bordered on the right by the duodenum and on the left by the spleen. The pancreatic head, including the uncinate process, lies within the curvature of and is intimately apposed to the duodenum. The neck, body, and tail of the pancreas extend to the left, crossing the midline, with the tail reaching the root of the splenorenal ligament. The common bile duct and the main pancreatic duct either join (90%) or open separately (10%) into the medial aspect of the second position of the duodenum.[6]

Blood Supply

The major arteries supplying the pancreas are the celiac trunk, situated above the neck of the pancreas, and the superior mesenteric artery, located below the pancreatic neck. Two pancreaticoduodenal arcades, the anterior and posterior, are derived from the union of the anterior and posterior branches of the superior and inferior pancreaticoduodenal arteries and supply the head region. Superior pancreaticoduodenal arteries are branches of the gastroduodenal artery, whereas the inferior pancreaticoduodenal arteries originate from the superior mesenteric artery. The neck and body of the pancreas derive their blood supply from the dorsal pancreatic artery, which may arise from the proximal splenic artery, the celiac trunk, or the superior mesenteric artery; from branches of the dorsal pancreatic artery that enter the posterior surface of the pancreas and pass in the direction of the tail; and from branches of the splenic artery. The tail of the pancreas is supplied primarily by branches of the splenic artery.

A rich vascular anastomotic complex is present in the pancreatic tissue. From the vessels at the exterior of the gland, branches pass internally to form an interlobular plexus, from which a single intralobular artery supplies individual islets of Langerhans as a vascular tuft. From these tufts, blood then passes to the acini. Such a vascular arrangement, with hormone-rich blood from the islets of Langerhans supplying the acini, is considered a *portal system.*[45] This anatomic configuration is consistent with the hypothesis that islet hormones may affect pancreatic exocrine function. Although comprising less than 2% of pancreatic mass, the islets receive 15% to 25% of total pancreatic blood flow.[57]

The functional relationship between pancreatic secretory activity and pancreatic blood flow is poorly understood. No data exist on the effect of a meal on pancreatic blood flow. Several studies suggest that stimulated pancreatic secretory exocrine activity occurs before any measured change in blood flow. Small amounts of intraintestinal hydrochloric acid (HCl) stimulate bicarbonate secretion, whereas significantly larger amounts of HCl are required to increase blood flow.[18] Doses of secretin or cholecystokinin (CCK) that stimulate pancreatic secretion seem to have almost no effect on pancreatic blood flow.[3] These observations suggest that under physiologic conditions pancreatic blood flow is not a limiting factor for exocrine function. Pancreatic blood flow is autoregulated, perhaps by both neural and humoral mechanisms, in order to provide maintenance of blood flow to the pancreas under conditions of mean arterial pressure reduction.[54]

Venous blood from the pancreas directly or indirectly enters the portal vein. Blood from the pancreatic head drains either into the gastroepiploic venous system or directly into the portal vein and drains from the neck, body, and tail into the inferior mesenteric vein or into the splenic vein, which joins with the superior mesenteric vein to form the portal vein.

Nerve Supply

The extrinsic autonomic innervation of the pancreas occurs through both sympathetic and parasympathetic pathways. Afferent *parasympathetic* fibers pass from the pancreas to the inferior ganglion of the vagus nerve, from which fibers travel in the vagus to terminate in the dorsal nucleus of the vagus in the brain.[40] Efferent parasympathetic fibers originate in the dorsal vagal nucleus and are contained in the posterior trunk, which contains fibers from both the anterior and the posterior trunks. These fibers pass through the celiac axis ganglia but do not synapse there. The efferent parasympathetic fibers synapse with cell bodies within the interlobular septa of the pancreas.

Sympathetic innervation of the pancreas originates from the thoracolumbar region.[44] Cell bodies for efferent sympathetic innervation are found in the lateral columns of dorsal segments 5 through 10. The fibers reach the ganglionated dorsal and lumbar sympathetic trunks; they then travel to the prevertebral abdominal sympathetic plexuses, the celiac and superior mesenteric. From these plexuses the sympathetic efferent fibers reach the pancreas along with the arterial supply. Afferent sympathetic fibers originate in the pancreas and reach the dorsal nerve roots by many of the lumbar and greater splanchnic nerves.

Peptidergic neural activity, in which the neurotransmitter is a peptide stored in nerve terminals and released on stimulation to act on a specific local receptor, has been described in the pancreas. Peptidergic neurons are identified by immunofluorescent techniques, using specific antipeptide antibody, and their function s determined by the effect of exogenous administration of the substance on that organ. Vasoactive intestinal polypeptide (VIP) immunoreactivity has been identified in nerves supplying the pancreas.[55] In pigs vagal activity stimulates both pancreatic enzyme and fluid and electrolyte secretion, as well as increased VIP concentration in the pancreatic venous blood. In human beings VIP has a weak secretin-like action, whereas the high doses required to stimulate pancreatic secretion are accompanied by significant side effects.[27] These data suggest that vagally stimulated pancreatic secretion may be mediated in part through VIP-ergic nerves. Nerves containing enkephalin and substance P have also been identified in the pancreas.[55] Exogenous enkephalin administration suppresses pancreatic secretion. The interactions between peptidergic neural activity and other modulating peptides appear to be complex and are not yet fully understood.

Acinus

The functional unit of the exocrine pancreas is the acinus (see Fig. 27-1).[39] Grossly the lobular structure of the pancreas is visible, with the lobules separated by fine connective tissue continuous with that surrounding duct epithelium. Subunits of the lobule are the acini, composed of spheric or short tubular masses of cells. Most cells in the acinus are acinar cells, which form these spherically arranged cellular masses. The smaller centroacinar cells mark the beginning of the ductular system. The lumen draining the acinus is an intercalated duct that communicates with intralobular and interlobular ducts and finally with the main pancreatic duct. The intercalated ducts are lined by centroacinar cells that are smaller than acinar cells. Intralobular and interlobular ducts are striated and lined with low columnar epithelial cells very similar in appearance to centroacinar cells. The synthesis and release of enzymes and bicarbonate, the two major functions of the exocrine pancreas, occur in the acinar cell and duct cells, respectively.

Acinar Cell

Histology

By weight, acinar cells account for more than 80% of the pancreas (see Fig. 27-2). The pyramidal-shaped cells are oriented with their apices, which contain the secretory granules, facing the lumen of the acinus (see Fig. 27-1). The density of these apical zymogen granules may vary as a function of secretory state. The midportion of the acinar cell contains the Golgi complex (apparatus). The basal region, with intense basophilic staining, contains the endoplasmic reticulum. The acinar cell nuclei are located in the basal region. A plasma membrane, which is rather straight basally and laterally but forms microvilli apically, envelops the acinar cell. This cell is designed for the synthesis, packaging, and release of enzymes.

Junctional complexes, a major barrier between duct lumen and pancreatic interstitial space, firmly attach acinar cells to each other and to centroacinar cells. They occur at the apical portion of the lateral plasma membrane and consist of three morphologically defined structures: (1) tight junctions, found near the duct lumen; (2) adhering zonules, where the lateral plasma membranes of two cells are within 200 Ångstrom units (Å) of each other but are not fused; and (3) the zonula adherens, containing desmosomes. These functional complexes are impermeable to macromolecules and secretory proteins (molecular weight, 16,000 to 95,000). Integrity of junctional complexes appears to depend on calcium.

Acinar cells communicate with each other by specialized areas in the lateral plasma membrane called *gap junctions*. At these points the plasma membranes of the adjacent acinar cells are within 20 Å of each other. Freeze-fracture techniques have identified pores between cells with an inner diameter of 200 to 1000 daltons, which permit the movement of small molecules between adjacent acinar cells. The integrity of the gap junction depends on both calcium and intracellular pH.[26,39]

Ultrastructure

The subcellular structure of the acinar cell is highly organized for enzyme synthesis, packaging, and secretion. The most striking feature is the extensive rough endoplasmic reticulum and the accumulation of zymogen granules in the apical cytoplasm. Rough endoplasmic reticulum, consisting of parallel membranous cisterna and interconnecting tubules, which have numerous ribosomes attached to their cytoplasmic surface, primarily is found in the basal cytoplasm. The appearance of the basal cytoplasm is related to the density of the ribonucleoprotein in the basal region. Mitochondria, with cristae and intramitochondrial granules, are situated between the cisternae of the rough endoplasmic reticulum. The nucleus, also found in the basal region of the cell, contains peripherally accumulated chromatin. At intervals around the periphery of the nucleus, the outer and inner nuclear membranes fuse, producing nuclear "pores" approximately 60 nm in diameter. One or more large dense nucleoli may be found within the acinar cell nucleus cells.[26,39]

Cellular Mechanisms of Acinar Cell Protein Synthesis, Packaging, and Release

The processes by which the acinar cell synthesizes, packages, and releases protein products have been defined by combined autoradiographic and cell fractionation techniques.[79] In addition, pulse-chase experiments, in which small pieces of pancreas are incubated in labeled amino acid medium, then in cold amino acid medium, have clearly demonstrated a narrow band of labeled amino acids that move through the secretory machinery of the cell. Radioactivity is highest in the granular endoplasmic reticulum immediately after labeling, in the Golgi apparatus at 10 minutes, in the condensing vacuoles at 40 minutes, and in the zymogen granules at 2 hours (Fig. 27-3).[39,49]

Amino acids required for protein synthesis appear to enter the acinar cell by active transport linked to sodium ion (Na^+) movement down an electrochemical gradient.[4] An amino acid destined to be immediately incorporated into a protein will be picked up by an appropriate transfer ribonucleic acid (tRNA) molecule once it enters the cell. Excess nonactivated amino acids enter an ultracellular pool where they can exchange with other amino acids by the same carrier mechanism.[108]

Proteins for export from the acinar cell are synthesized in ribosomes attached to the cytosolic portion of the rough endoplasmic reticulum.[84] This signal hypothesis has been developed as an explanation for the mechanisms by which a given messenger RNA (mRNA) molecule is translated on a bound or free ribosome. Experimental evidence supports this hypothesis in that mRNA, which is to be translated on membrane-bound ribosomes, contains an initial sequence of cordons that produces a unique sequence of

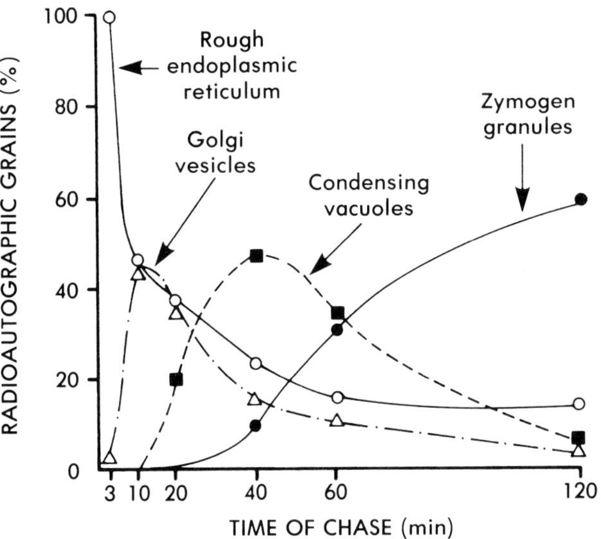

Fig. 27-3 Vectorial movement of secretory proteins in the pancreatic acinar cell derived from pulse-chase experiments using radiolabeled amino acids. (Redrawn from Gorelick, F.S., and Jamieson, J.D.: Structure-function relationships of the pancreas. In Johnson, L.R., editor: Physiology of the gastrointestinal tract, New York, 1981, Raven Press.)

lipophilic amino acids, a terminal extension termed the *signal peptide*. The emergence of the signal peptide from the ribosome allows the ribosome to be attached to the endoplasmic reticulum, thereby producing a common channel between the ribosome and endoplasmic reticulum through which the nascent protein passes into the cisternae.[7,64]

Several modifications of the protein occur during movement from the ribosome to the cisternae of the endoplasmic reticulum. These include both biochemical and tertiary structural changes, which may account for the irreversible segregation of proteins within the rough endoplasmic reticulum. Once in the cisternae, the proteins remain membrane bound within the acinar cell. Secretory proteins move from the cisternae to the Golgi complex within 20 to 30 minutes. Energy derived from adenosine triphosphate (ATP) is required for this intracellular transport, which occurs by transporting vesicles arising from "pinched off" transitional elements of the endoplasmic reticulum.[50] Mature secretory granules then move from the Golgi complex to the apical portion of the acinar cell cytoplasm. Following this, proteins are concentrated in condensing vacuoles, producing mature storage granules where posttranslational modification such as terminal glycosylation or phosphorylation occurs. With appropriate acinar cell stimulation, the contents of these mature vacuoles are released into the lumen by exocytosis. For this process to occur, the zymogen granule membrane must recognize the appropriate fusion position within the plasma membrane of the acinar cell. Following this recognition, fusion and fission of the zymogen granule membrane with the plasmalemma occurs at the site of exocytosis.[20] After discharge of the contents of the zymogen granule, the membrane is thought to be recycled.[66]

Composition of Pancreatic Enzyme Secretion

The major categories of pancreatic enzyme secretion include (1) proteolytic (chymotrypsinogen, trypsinogen, proelastase, procarboxypeptidase A and B), which accounts for nearly 70% of the pancreatic digestive mass,[93] (2) amylolytic (alpha-amylase), (3) lipolytic (lipase, esterase, phophospholipase A, cholesterol esterase), and (4) nucleolytic (ribonuclease, deoxyribonuclease) enzymes. Additional secreted enzymes include co-lipase, trypsin inhibitor, sulfated polyanionic peptidoglycans, and soluble acid lipoproteins.

Under most physiologic conditions the relative concentrations of these enzymes remain constant in the pancreatic juice of each species.[92] Analysis of the enzyme profile in subcellular fractions of pancreatic acinar cells has identified the same ratios of one enzyme to another, as in secreted juice.[52] These observations have supported the theory of "parallel" pancreatic enzyme secretion. However, other studies have shown that one enzyme may be secreted into pancreatic juice preferentially at a higher rate than others, suggesting that in some situations enzyme secretion may not occur in a parallel fashion.[21,87] Thus the composition of proteins in the zymogen granules possibly can be changed by certain stimuli, either through equilibration with specific cytosolic enzymes or from subpopulations of acinar cells that have differing profiles of enzymes within their zymogen granules.

Long-term pancreatic secretory adaptation to change in diet has been rather conclusively proved in the rat.[43] Prolonged feeding of a high-carbohydrate diet produces a significant increase in pancreatic amylase content.[25] Diets high in protein and fat given over a prolonged period cause an elevation of pancreatic trypsinogen and lipase content, respectively.[77,86] It is unknown whether a similar adaptation to diet occurs in human beings.

Centroacinar and Duct Cells

Histology

Centroacinar cells are irregular in shape and are wedged between acinar cells within the acinus (see Fig. 27-1). In histologic sections these cells are distinguished by their pale staining, which is related to the low-density cytoplasm. Cells lining the small ductules, although more regular in shape, are structurally similar to the centroacinar cell. As the ductular system enlarges from the acinus to the main pancreatic duct, the duct cells assume a more columnar appearance.

Ultrastructure

Centroacinar and duct cells, in contrast to acinar cells, have a poorly developed granular endoplasmic reticulum and Golgi complex, no zymogen granules, and few mitochondria.[95] A unique feature of the centioacinar and duct cells is the large nucleus with indentations. The nucleus occupies a large portion of the cell, leaving only a rim of cytoplasm between nucleus and plasma membrane. Infolding of the lateral plasma membrane is more extensive than occurs in the acinar cell. The centroacinar cell possesses a single cilium, which is in contact with the fluid in the acinar lumen. Connections between duct cells and acinar cells or other duct cells are through terminal bars, as described for acinar–acinar cell interaction.

Cellular Mechanisms of Water and Electrolyte Secretion

The ductular elements and centroacinar cells appear to be the primary site of electrolyte secretion, with a contribution from the acinar cell. The following observations support this hypothesis:

1. Alloxan treatment reduces electrolyte secretion with concomitant destruction of ductular elements but not of acinar cells.[41]
2. A copper-free diet with penicillamine supplement[35] or ethionine feeding[1] causes almost total acinar cell atrophy but only partly reduces the maximum electrolyte secretory response to secretin.
3. Carbonic anhydrase, the enzyme necessary for rapid production of bicarbonate (HCO_3^-), has been shown to be present in the centroacinar and ductular cells but not in the acinar cell.[10]
4. Micropuncture experiments demonstrate that HCO_3^- concentration of pancreatic juice increases in the ducts, particularly in the extralobular ducts.[58,97]

Specific ion requirements for pancreatic electrolyte secretion have been identified. Reduction in extracellular Na^+ to a value of ≤80 mM results in a significant reduction in pancreatic secretory rate.[88] Replacement of Na^+ by lithium ion (Li^+) also causes a significant inhibition of pancreatic secretion.[12] Similarly, removal of potassium ion (K^+) from the nutrient solution reduces pancreatic secretion more than 50%, whereas substitution of rubidium for K^+ restores the secretory response to secretin. Chloride (Cl^-) is also required for full pancreatic secretory response to secretin but can be substituted by bromide (Br^-) or iodine (I^-) with little effect on pancreatic secretory function.[13] Finally, HCO_3^- is required for full secretory response to secretin stimulation.[96]

Under conditions of maximum stimulation, HCO_3^- concentration in secreted fluid is fivefold to sixfold greater than in plasma.[97] Also, the electric potential across the duct epithelium is lumen negative relative to the interstitial fluid.[104] Based on these two findings, it has been postulated that the transport of HCO_3^- against an electrochemical gradient is an active process. In contrast, Na^+, K^+, and Cl^- appear to be passively distributed across the duct epithelium. The source of secreted HCO_3^- is thought to be primarily plasma, although metabolically generated CO_2 may also make a minor contribution. Two facts support this hypothesis: (1) the rate of pancreatic secretion is directly related to perfusate (plasma) HCO_3^- concentration, and (2) when carbon-14 (^{14}C)-labeled HCO_3^- is added to perfusate, it appears rapidly in pancreatic juice.[15] Thus researchers have calculated that more than 95% of secreted HCO_3^- is derived from plasma.

Although it is known that specific inhibitors of carbonic anhydrase[29] and of Na^+-K^+ ATPase[85] decrease pancreatic secretion, whether pancreatic HCO_3^- is actively secreted or is secondary to active H^+ transport is unclear. In the former hypothesis carbonic anhydrase catalyzes the formation of carbonic acid (H_2CO_3) from CO_2 and H_2O, which then dissipates to H^+ and HCO_3^-. The HCO_3^- is

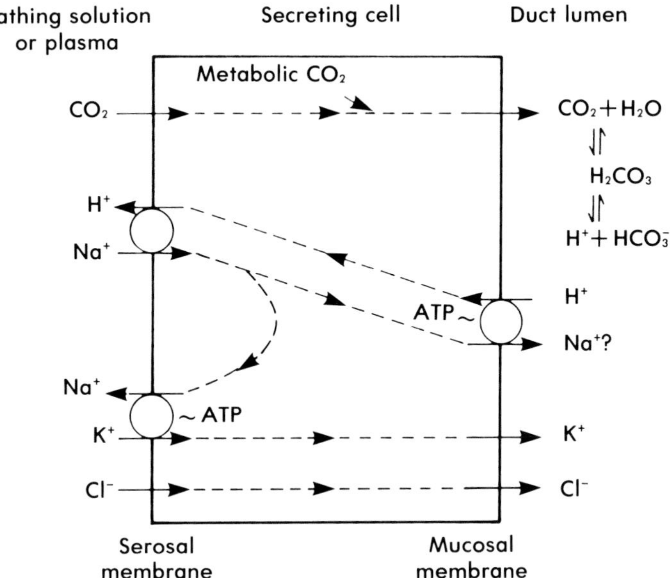

Fig. 27-4 Model for the mechanism of pancreatic electrolyte and fluid secretion. The electrogenic H^+ or OH^- transport is located on the luminal surface. The coupled Na^+ and H^+ exchange at the nutrient (serosal) surface is a secondary active transport process. (Redrawn from Schulz, F.: Electrolyte and fluid secretion in the exocrine pancreas. In Johnson, L.R., editor: Physiology of the gastrointestinal tract, New York, 1981, Raven Press.)

then actively transported into the lumen of the pancreatic ductule. Alternately, HCO_3^- secretion may be related to the active transport of hydrogen ions from lumen into the cell where, with the availability of diffused CO_2, HCO_3^- and H^+ are formed. Hydrogen ions are probably removed by an Na^+ and H^+ coupled transport at the contraluminal portion of the cell membrane. Energy for this active Na^+ and H^+ transport is thought to be derived from an electrochemical Na^+-K^+ ATPase, located also on the contraluminal portion of the cell membrane (Fig. 27-4). Although no electrochemical requirement exists for active Na^+ transport, data suggest that Na^+ is actively transported.[12,85,104] The other ions of significance in pancreatic juice, K^+ and Cl^-, appear to be secreted passively. Others have suggested that Cl^- permeability may affect HCO_3^- transport, perhaps by a related Cl^- and HCO_3^- exchange mechanism. The movement of water is passive, a function of solute movement. Active transport of HCO_3^-, along with Na^+, is accompanied by passive water movement down a concentration gradient. Pancreatic secretion is isosmotic with plasma under all physiologic and most pharmacologic and experimental conditions.

Composition of Pancreatic Water and Electrolyte Secretion

The principal anions in pancreatic juice are HCO_3^- and Cl^-; the cations are Na^+ and K^+. Other ionic constituents include Ca^{++}, Mg^{++}, Zn^{++}, HPO_4^- and $SO_4^=$. As previously noted, pancreatic juice is isosmotic with plasma under most conditions. The two major anions vary reciprocally during secretory stimulation and total 150 mM. The major cation is Na^+, which has a concentration of approximately 160 mM. At low secretory flow rates, the Cl^- concentration is high, and the HCO_3^- low. During stimulation, HCO_3^- concentration exponentially increases, whereas Cl^- exponentially decreases. The rate of secretion has no influence on Na^+ concentration (Fig. 27-5).[8,14]

Three theories have been proposed to explain this pattern of anion secretion. The *unicellular theory* postulates that all cells secrete both HCO_3^- and Cl^- but that the secretory rate of each is a function of degree of stimulation. The *exchange diffusion hypothesis* suggests that the major anion secreted is HCO_3^- but that alone the ductal system HCO_3^- is exchanged for Cl^-; thus a low flow rate would allow more time for HCO_3^- and Cl^- exchange, resulting in a high Cl^- concentration. This hypothesis would also explain the higher HCO_3^- concentration observed at higher flow rates.

The third theory, which has some experimental support, has been termed the *two-component hypothesis*. This suggests that the acinar cell secretes Cl^-, whereas the centroacinar and duct cells secrete HCO_3^-. The anion content of the pancreatic juice is an admixture of the secretion from different types of cells, with HCO_3^- added to a Cl^--rich acinar cell secretion. Micropuncture studies indicate that at high flow rates higher Cl^- concentrations are present in the interlobar ducts, with a progressive decline in Cl^- and rise in HCO_3^- concentrations in samples obtained from sequentially larger ducts (Fig. 27-6). The following observation also supports this hypothesis: rats in which the acinar cells have been destroyed by chronic penicillamine treatment are still able to increase HCO_3^- concentration in secretory fluid during stimulation.

Stimulants and Inhibitors of Pancreatic Protein Secretion

Second Messengers

One of two functionally distinct sequences of intracellular biochemical change is initiated by individual stimu-

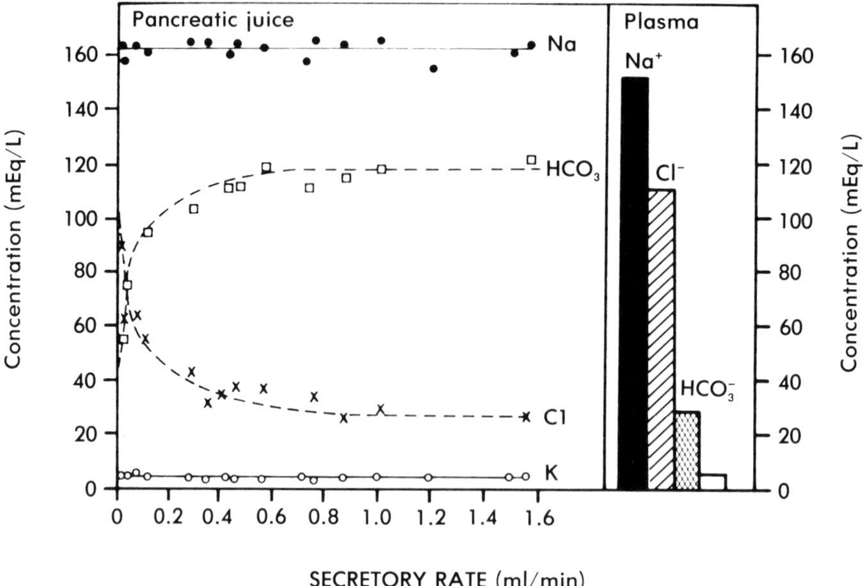

Fig. 27-5 The change in sodium (Na^+), potassium (K^+), chloride (Cl^-), and bicarbonate (HCO_3^-) as a function of secretory rate in the dog. (Redrawn from Bro-Rasmussen, F., Killmann, S.A., and Thaysen, J.H.: Acta Physiol. Scand. **37:**97, 1956.)

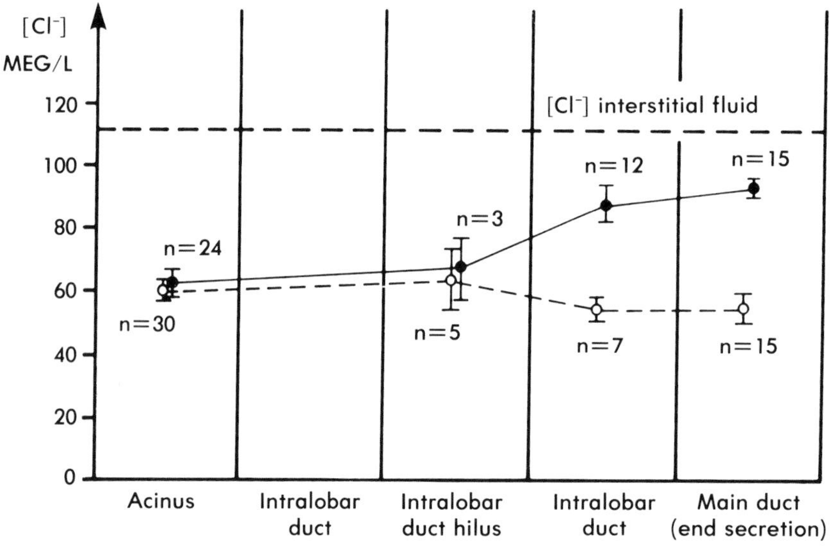

Fig. 27-6 Free flow chloride (Cl^-) concentrations in samples from micropuncture experiments under basal (○) and secretin-stimulated (●) conditions. (Redrawn from Schulz, F.: Electrolyte ⊕ fluid secretion in the exocrine pancreas. In Johnson, L.R., editor: Physiology of the gastrointestinal tract, New York, 1981, Raven Press.)

lants of pancreatic secretion. Certain secretagogues, including CCK, bombesin, and acetylcholine, interact with a specific plasma membrane receptor and cause a rise in cytosolic calcium concentration (Fig. 27-7).[11,113] The mechanism by which this rise in intracellular calcium results in enzyme release is unknown. Following receptor interaction, other secretagogues, including secretin and VIP, produce a rise in cytosolic cyclic adenosine monophosphate (cAMP) by activation of adenylate cyclase and cAMP-dependent protein kinase.[81] The mechanism that causes rises in intracellular cAMP to effect enzyme release is also unknown. Stimulants that act through the calcium pathway do not cause a rise in cAMP. The converse is also true; however, these two independent mechanisms do interact at some yet unidentified step, as evidenced by potentiated responses to combinations of secretory stimulants occurring independent of the second messenger associated with each.[37] The role of cyclic guanylic acid (cGMP) in control of pancreatic secretion is presently unknown.

Neural Stimulants of Pancreatic Secretion

In all species studied, vagal stimulation produces an increase in both pancreatic bicarbonate and enzyme secretion.[46,48,61] Exogenous secretin potentiates this neural re-

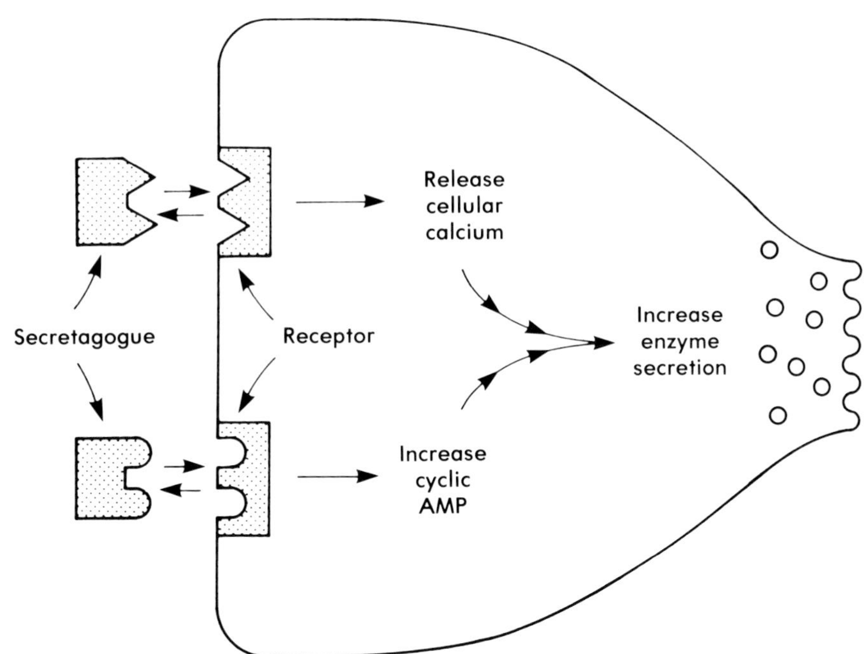

Fig. 27-7 Mechanisms of action of secretagogues on the pancreatic acinar cell. (Redrawn from Gardner, J.D., and Jensen, R.T.: Regulation of pancreatic enzyme secretion in vitro. In Johnson, L.R., editor: Physiology of the gastrointestinal tract, New York, 1981, Raven Press.)

sponse.[47] Cholinergic agents produce rates of bicarbonate and enzyme secretion similar to those obtained during vagal stimulation. Atropine blocks vagal- and cholinergic-stimulated pancreatic secretion, but significant species selectivity exists for volume, bicarbonate, and enzyme secretory inhibition.[46,48,61] In human beings vagal stimulation induced by hypoglycemia augments secretin-stimulated pancreatic protein output. Truncal vagotomy, although reducing bicarbonate response to exogenous stimulants by approximately 25%, does not affect maximum enzyme secretion but does reduce sensitivity to submaximum stimulation.[114]

Splanchnic nerve stimulation is usually associated with inhibition of pancreatic exocrine secretion. The mechanism is thought to be related to intense vasoconstriction and blood flow inhibition; however, splanchnic nerve stimulation has been shown to inhibit pancreatic secretion even when the vasoconstriction has been abolished pharmacologically.[114]

Local neural pathways, probably cholinergically mediated, also appear to play a significant role in pancreatic secretion. The rapidity with which intraduodenal and intrajejunal stimulants produce an increase in pancreatic secretory response has led to the hypothesis that duodenojejunopancreatic neural connections produce a physiologic reflex that significantly facilitates at least the rapid pancreatic response to intraluminal stimulants.[99]

Hormonal Stimulants and Inhibitors

Secretin. Secretin is a polypeptide of 27 amino acids that derives its name from the stimulatory effects it produces on pancreatic bicarbonate secretion. Interestingly, as noted earlier, Bayliss and Starling identified this humoral stimulant of pancreatic secretion in 1902, which not only caused the scientific community to rethink Pavlov's emphasis on an exclusively neural reflex mechanism of pancreatic exocrine secretion, but also ushered in the systematic study of humoral agents and the endocrine system.

Secretin is a strong stimulant of pancreatic bicarbonate and volume output and a relatively weak stimulant of protein output.[22] The whole secretin molecule is required for full biologic activity. The half-life of secretin is about 3 minutes. The intracellular second messenger of secretin-induced pancreatic bicarbonate output is cAMP.[114]

Cholecystokinin. CCK is a polypeptide of 33 amino acids. The biologically active portion of CCK is the C-terminal end, of which the five terminal amino acids are identical to those of the gastrin molecule; thus gastrin produces qualitatively similar effects to those of CCK on pancreatic secretion. CCK is a potent stimulant of enzyme or protein secretion and a weak stimulant of volume and bicarbonate output.[22,103] Seven C-terminal amino acids (CCK-heptapeptide) and sulfation of the tyrosine are required for full biologic activity.[103] The half-life of CCK is 2 to 7 minutes. The intracellular second messenger of CCK-induced protein output is calcium.[114]

Vasoactive Intestinal Polypeptide. VIP is a polypeptide of 28 amino acids and is structurally related to secretin. Qualitatively VIP produces the same effects on pancreatic bicarbonate and volume output but is considerably less potent. VIP-induced pancreatic bicarbonate and volume output is also cAMP mediated.[37]

Bombesin. Bombesin is a polypeptide of 14 amino acids with a molecular structure similar to CCK and gastrin. It therefore stimulates pancreatic enzyme and protein secretion. Some investigators have suggested that the effect of bombesin on pancreatic protein secretion is secondary to bombesin-induced gastrin and CCK release. Although this may play a role in bombesin-induced pancreatic protein output in vivo, bombesin has been shown to have a direct effect on isolated acinar cell preparations in vitro.[37]

PANCREATIC POLYPEPTIDE. Pancreatic polypeptide (PP) consists of 36 amino acids. In general, doses that produce physiologic blood levels, as measured by radioimmunoassay, produce inhibition of secretin-induced bicarbonate and CCK-induced protein output.[105]

SOMATOSTATIN. Somatostatin is a polypeptide of 14 amino acids that inhibits stimulated pancreatic bicarbonate and protein secretion.[16] Somatostatin has also been shown to inhibit intraluminal amino acid and oleate-induced pancreatic protein secretion, suggesting that somatostatin or other mediators may inhibit CCK release.[114]

GLUCAGON. Pancreatic glucagon is a polypeptide of 29 amino acids, 14 of which are similar to secretin. Glucagon inhibits secretin-induced bicarbonate and CCK-induced protein output in dogs and human beings.

Pancreatic Response to a Meal

The total pancreatic secretory response to a meal is a complex interaction between neural and humoral events. This response has been divided into cephalic, gastric, and intestinal phases. Technical experimental constraints make it difficult to provide definitive statements about specific mechanisms regulating pancreatic responses to a meal. Many existing deductions are based on in vivo and in vitro experimental data in animals.

Another obstacle to clarifying the physiologic mechanisms that control stimulation and inhibition of pancreatic exocrine function is the difficulty with which the two major peptide stimulants, secretin and CCK, can be reliably measured in the blood. Reliable and universally accepted specific antibodies to these two peptides, which the radioimmunoassay depends on, have been extremely difficult to produce and use.

In dogs and human beings, pancreatic enzyme secretion in response to a meal represents only 70% to 80% of its maximum secretory capacity. It is presently unknown (1) whether a meal simply does not evoke physiologic mechanisms at a magnitude compatible with maximum pancreatic secretion or (2) whether some neural or humoral mechanism evoked by a meal exerts an inhibitory effect on pancreatic secretory activity.

Cephalic Phase

Visual and olfactory stimuli increase more pancreatic protein than bicarbonate secretion.[78,90] In the dog the cephalic phase of pancreatic enzyme secretion is approximately 25%, and bicarbonate secretion is 10% to 15% of maximum secretory capacity. With background secretin infusion, sham feeding has been shown to increase pancreatic secretion to 50% of CCK-stimulated maximum response in human beings.[24] Gastric antral acidification, which inhibits the cephalic phase of gastrin release, abolishes the cephalic phase of pancreatic secretion, suggesting that in the dog the cephalic phase of pancreatic secretion may be largely caused by gastrin release.[82] In human beings gastrin is also a stimulant of pancreatic enzyme secretion[107]; however, the rapidity with which the pancreas responds to visual and olfactory stimulation, 2 to 4 minutes, suggests that a direct neural component also exists.[80]

Gastric Phase

Several studies have made precise observations leading to the conclusion that the control over pancreatic secretion exerted by the stomach is substantial. The antral release of gastrin, a moderate stimulant of pancreatic enzyme release, has already been discussed. An additional type of gastropancreatic reflux has been described in which distention of either the gastric body or the gastric antrum results in an increase in pancreatic protein output with a lesser effect on bicarbonate secretion.[111,112] The latter antropancreatic reflex is abolished by anticholinergics but not by antral acidification, suggesting that gastrin release is not the mediator of this reflex but rather a true neural cholinergic reflex. Gastric proteolysis releases oligopeptides, which may stimulate the pancreas after they enter the small intestine. The stomach also tightly controls the rate of entry of chyme into the intestine, as well as the size of solid food particles, which in turn determines the rate of release of digestive products.[74] In these various ways the stomach controls the intestinal phase of pancreatic secretion, which is perhaps the most important phase.

Two studies have evaluated meal-stimulated pancreatic secretory activity following an 80% gastrectomy. Meal-stimulated pancreatic secretion was only minimally affected by this surgical procedure, which removes the gastrin-producing cells while greatly disturbing gastric emptying.[60,106] Another study on the effect of gastrin release in relation to the gastric phase of acid secretion demonstrated that distention of innervated canine antral pouches with an alkaline solution increased both pancreatic enzyme secretion and gastrin release, although distention with an acidic solution produced a similar pancreatic secretory response while blocking gastrin release.[23]

Thus one can reasonably conclude that the importance of gastrin as a mediator of the gastric phase of pancreatic secretion, under physiologic conditions, is minimal.

Intestinal Phase

Neural interactions and enteropancreatic reflexes probably account for the earliest pancreatic responses following a meal. Although the denervated pancreas does respond to intestinal stimuli when experimentally transplanted, the magnitude of the protein secretory response following a meal is reduced approximately 50% when compared to the innervated pancreas.[110] Denervation does not interfere with the gland's capacity to secrete protein. Both truncal vagotomy and atropine reduce the pancreatic response to intraluminal oleate and tryptophan by nearly 50%. These observations suggest that innervation is required for full secretory response to intestinal stimulants.

In an attempt to evaluate the relative contribution of the neural and humoral components of this rapid response, a comparison of the latency of protein secretory response was made between instillation of intraluminal stimulants and intraportal administration of CCK. Amylase output was shown to occur within 0.30 to 0.33 minute of intestinal oleate or tryptophan perfusion, whereas 0.59 minute was required for the response to intraportal CCK administration.[99] Atropine or truncal vagotomy increased the latency to intraluminal stimulants by a factor of nearly 10, whereas no effect on the latency to intraportal CCK administration was observed. These observations suggest that the earliest pancreatic response to intestinal perfusion with oleate or tryptophan is neurally mediated. Similar experiments recently have found that the latency of pancreatic bicarbonate output in response to intraduodenal tryptophan was 62 seconds; to oleate, 64 seconds; to intraportal CCK, 28 seconds; and to secretin, 45 seconds.[98] These data suggest that differences may exist in the neural component between stimulated pancreatic enzyme and bicarbonate output.

ACIDIFICATION. In addition to the neural component of postprandial pancreatic secretion, intraduodenal acid, fat, and amino acids stimulate pancreatic secretion by humoral mechanisms. When the duodenum is acidified to a pH ≤4.5, acid load rather than concentration appears to be an important determinant of pancreatic volume and bicarbonate output (Fig. 27-8).[71,76] For equal and titratable acid loads, pancreatic bicarbonate secretion is greater for strong than for weak acids. Pancreatic bicarbonate response to intestinal acidification is also partly a function of the length of intestine acidified.[72] Neutralizing duodenal contents reduces postprandial pancreatic bicarbonate output by about 50%.[2] The threshold pH, above which pancreatic bicarbonate secretion does not occur, is 4.5 in dogs[42] but may be slightly lower in human beings.[30]

These observations suggest that acid entering the duodenum after a meal is a potent stimulus for pancreatic bicarbonate and volume secretion. Following a mixed meal, chyme entering the duodenum may have a pH of 2 to

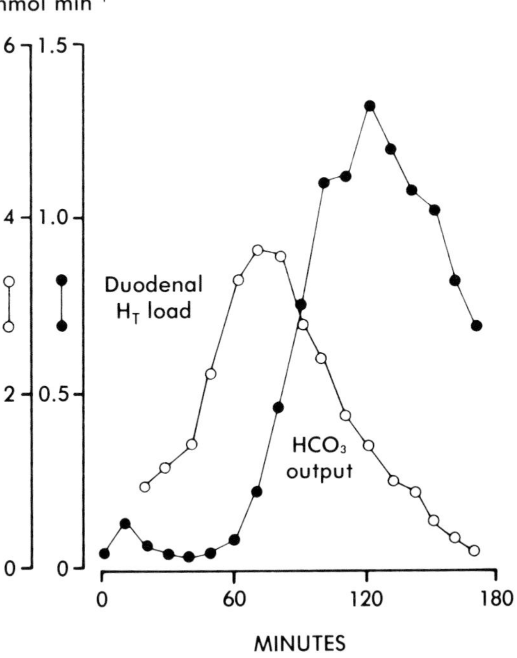

Fig. 27-8 Duodenal acid (H_T) load and pancreatic bicarbonate (HCO_3^-) response to a meal in dogs. (Redrawn from Moore, E.W., Verine, H.J., and Grossman, M.I.: Acta Hepato-Gastroenterol. **26**:30, 1979.)

2.5,[62] which indicates that under physiologic conditions duodenal acidification does contribute to pancreatic bicarbonate and volume secretory response. Pancreatic bicarbonate output following duodenal acidification by a permeable acid (lactic acid) or an impermeable acid (acidified albumin) is not significantly different, suggesting that pancreatic response to intestinal acidification is a function of acid-receptor activation at the intestinal lumen.[101]

One can reasonably conclude that duodenal acidification causes a release of endogenous secretin, which then acts on the pancreas, since primarily bicarbonate and volume output rather than protein output are stimulated.

SECRETIN POTENTIATION. The concentration of secretin in the gastrointestinal mucosa is greatest in the duodenum.[83] Lower concentrations are found distal to the duodenum. Secretin-like immunoreactivity has been found in granular S cells, which are present between the crypts and villi. Although plasma concentration of secretin, as measured by radioimmunoassay, has been shown to increase during intestinal (duodenal) acidification,[56] the data on plasma secretin concentrations following a meal have been inconsis-

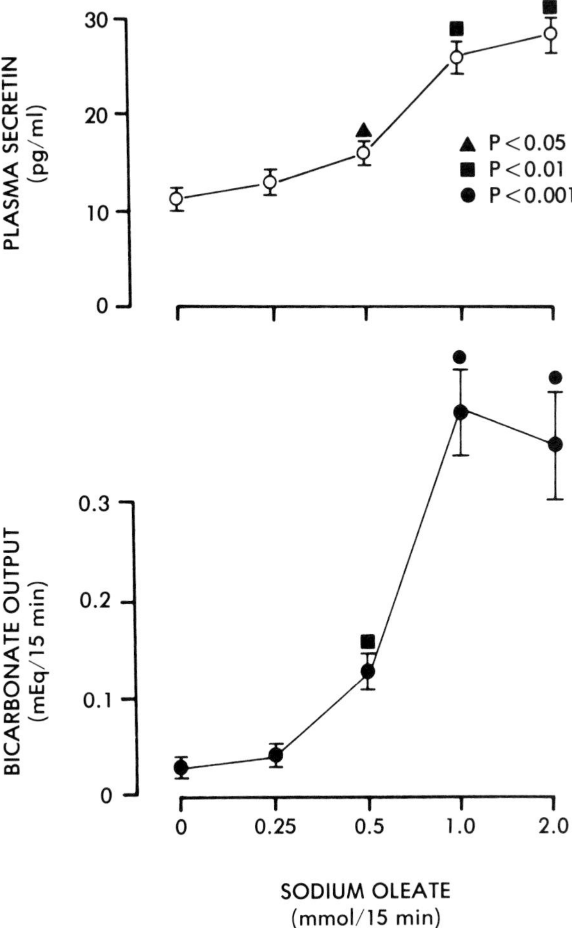

Fig. 27-9 Effect of increasing concentrations of intraduodenal oleate on plasma immunoreactive secretin concentration and pancreatic bicarbonate output in dogs. (Redrawn and reprinted by permission of Elsevier Publishing Co., Inc. from Faichney, A., et al.: Effect of sodium oleate on plasma secretin concentration and pancreatic secretion in dog, Gastroenterology **81**:458, 1981, Copyright 1981 by The American Gastroenterological Association.)

tent. Some investigators[75] have been unable to detect a rise in plasma secretin concentration, whereas others observing a rise have also found it to be smaller than would be expected for the magnitude of pancreatic bicarbonate response (Fig. 27-9).[91] Several explanations may exist for this apparent discrepancy.

First, the magnitude of pancreatic bicarbonate response to a meal is much less than the maximum secretin-stimulated bicarbonate response. Second, during a meal hydrochloric acid secreted by the parietal cells is buffered by weak meal proteins, so the gastric effluent into the duodenum has a pH range of 2 to 4. Thus the secretin response to a meal would not be expected to be as great as the response to duodenal acidification with HCl, a strong acid.

Finally, small increases in plasma secretin concentration following a meal, with a relatively greater pancreatic bicarbonate response than would be expected for that increase, may be explained by the physiologic responses to the administration of more than one stimulatory peptide producing secretory responses that are greater than the sum of the individual responses. This effect has been termed *potentiation*. Potentiation of pancreatic bicarbonate secretion has been shown with CCK and secretin, gastrin and secretin, caerulein and secretin, secretin and L-phenylalanine, but not with secretin and bethanechol.[5]

Additional evidence supports the role of secretin in postprandial pancreatic bicarbonate response. One study found that treatment with antisecretin antiserum reduced bicarbonate output by 80% following a meal in dogs.[17]

These correlations among duodenal acidification, pancreatic bicarbonate secretion, and small changes in plasma secretin concentration suggest that the pancreatic bicarbonate response to a meal is partly mediated by secretin release from the duodenum and proximal small intestine.

FATTY ACIDS. Intraduodenal and intraintestinal products of fat digestion stimulate pancreatic bicarbonate and protein secretion. Intraluminal triglycerides and diglycerides are not stimulants until hydrolyzed.[63] Fatty acids of less than nine carbons do not stimulate pancreatic secretion; those with more than nine carbons, as well as monoglycerides, do stimulate secretion (Fig. 27-10).[67,68] Responses to these stimulatory fatty acids are dose related, being directly related to the length of intestine to which they are exposed and inversely related to the individual rate of absorption from the intestine.[63]

The pancreatic bicarbonate and protein response to intraluminal fatty acids varies and therefore gives few clues as to the mediators. Medium-chain fatty acids stimulate more bicarbonate than protein than do amino acids.[33] Relative secretory rates vary with the intraluminal concentration of an individual fatty acid, as indicated by the observation that pancreatic bicarbonate relative to protein output rises with increasing oleate concentrations. Intraluminal fatty acids possibly stimulate the release of either CCK or secretin, a function of concentration, or the primary mechanism may be CCK release in a milieu that provides for potentiation of interactions with endogenous humoral agents such as secretin. Studies have shown that intrajejunal perfusion with oleate and decanoate augments the pancreatic bicarbonate response to duodenal acidification and potentiates submaximum secretin-stimulated bicarbonate secretion.[32,33] The stimulation of gallbladder contraction by fatty acids suggests that significant amounts of CCK are released under these conditions. Basal plasma CCK concentrations in human beings are low.[9,109] Postprandial plasma CCK concentrations increase significantly, and high concentrations are measured even following instillation of intraduodenal fat.[51]

One study found that intraduodenal oleate produced a

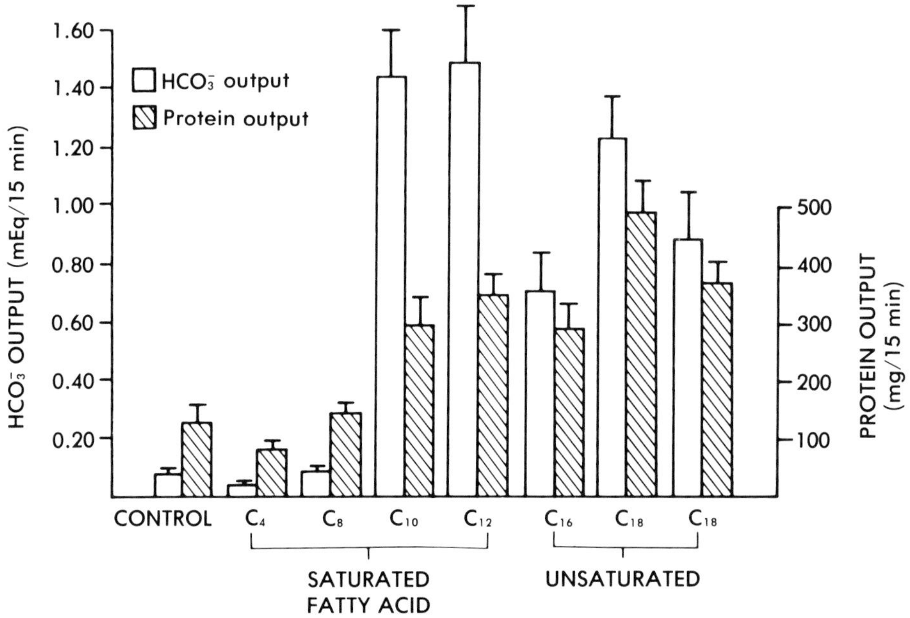

Fig. 27-10 Pancreatic bicarbonate (HCO_3^-) and protein outputs in response to different fatty acids, 80 mM, administered intraduodenally in dogs. (Redrawn from Meyer, J.H.: Release of secretin and cholecystokinin. In Thompson, J.C., editor: Gastrointestinal hormones, Austin, Tex., 1975, University of Austin Press.)

concomitant increase in immunoreactive plasma CCK, pancreatic protein output, and gallbladder pressure in the dog (Fig. 27-11).[36] Truncal vagotomy caused a 45% reduction in pancreatic protein output and completely abolished the gallbladder response but had no effect on the change in immunoreactive plasma CCK. In dogs intraduodenal oleate greatly increases pancreatic volume and bicarbonate secretion and is accompanied by a small but significant increase in plasma secretin concentration.[31] Intravenous lipid administration to dogs does not appear to stimulate the pancreas to secrete bicarbonate or protein (Fig. 27-12).[102]

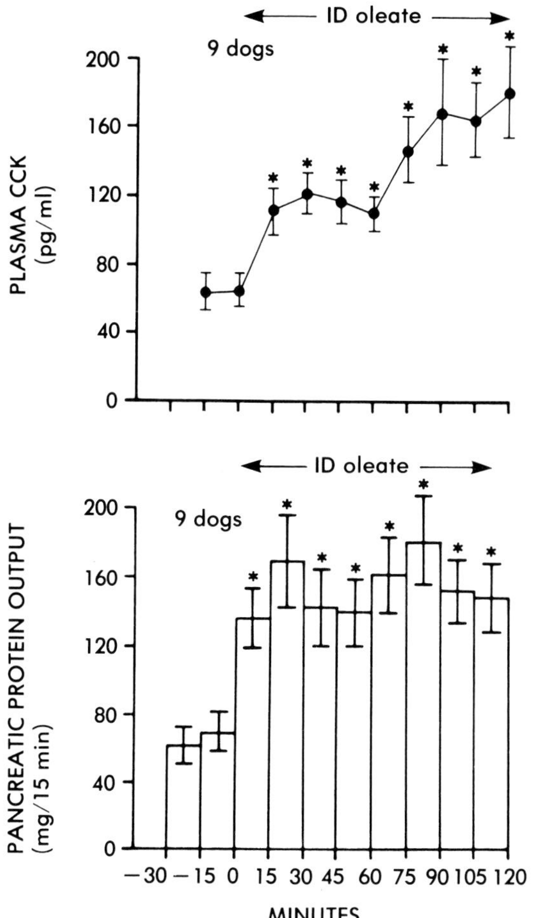

Fig. 27-11 Change in plasma CCK concentration and pancreatic protein output in response to intraduodenal oleate perfusion in dogs. (Redrawn and reprinted by permission of Elsevier Publishing Co., Inc. from Fried, G.M., et al.: Release of cholecystokinin in conscious dogs, Gastroenterology **85:**1113, 1983. Copyright 1983 by The American Gastroenterological Association.)

These observations suggest that intraintestinal fats stimulate the release of both secretin and CCK, which in turn produce responses in pancreatic bicarbonate and protein output.

Amino Acids and Peptides. Intraduodenal and intrajejunal perfusion with products of protein digestion cause the pancreas to secrete fluid that has a high protein concentration of low volume, a response similar to that produced by neural stimulation or exogenous CCK administration.[38,73,107] In the dog the two most potent amino acids that provoke this response are phenylalanine and tryptophan, whereas in human beings they are methionine, valine, and phenylalanine. Protein output is stimulated in the canine pancreas to the same degree by polypeptides, oligopeptides, and individual L-amino acids (Fig. 27-13).[69,70] In human beings trypsin, amylase, and lipase are secreted when neutral amino acids bathe the lumen of the proximal jejunum.[38] In rats diversion of intestinal contents stimulates pancreatic secretion; in this species the presence of trypsin in the lumen apparently inhibits pancreatic secretion, a negative feedback mechanism.[94] This is not the case in dogs[89] and in human beings it is not clear whether such a negative feedback mechanism exists.[53] Large quantities of pancreatic proteases delivered to the duodenum have been shown to suppress pancreatic exocrine output in normal control subjects and patients with chronic pancreatitis.[100]

CCK is found primarily in the jejunal mucosa of dogs, with the duodenal and ileal mucosas having somewhat lower concentrations.[83] In human beings the predominant plasma form of CCK is the octapeptide, which has been shown to increase from 0.5 to 6 femtomoles/ml^{-1} following a mixed meal.[109] Intraduodenal infusion of L-tryptophan and L-phenylalanine is associated with a doubling of plasma CCK-like immunoreactivity. As with secretin, these low concentrations and relatively small increases observed following a meal suggest that the pancreatic en-

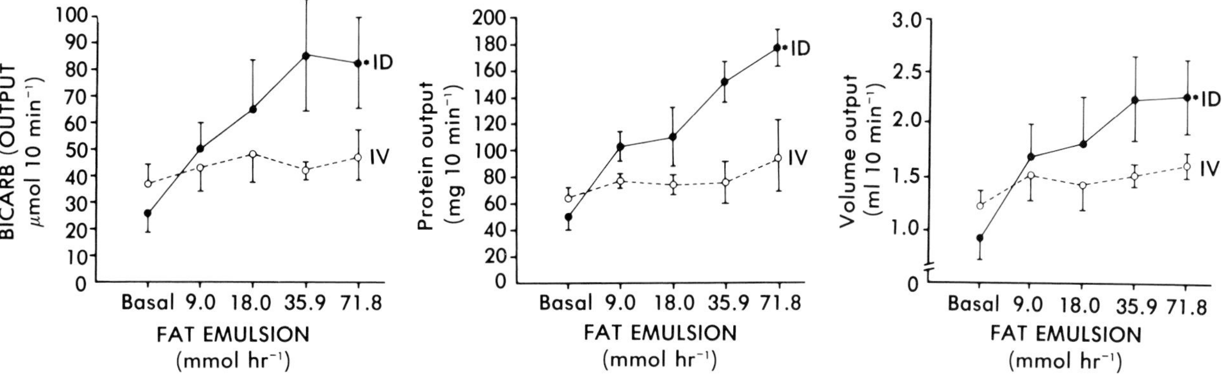

Fig. 27-12 Pancreatic volume, protein, and bicarbonate responses to graded doses of fat emulsion administered intraduodenally *(ID)* or intravenously *(IV)* in dogs. (From Stabile, B.E., et al.: Am. J. Physiol. **246:**G274, 1984.)

zyme secretory response to a meal depends on potentiated interactions between peptides. This has recently been demonstrated in the dog, with intraduodenal perfusion of protein digestive materials potentiating acid-induced bicarbonate but not protein output.[34] As with fats, parenteral administration of amino acid–containing solutions probably does not stimulate pancreatic bicarbonate or protein output in the dog (Fig. 27-14).[102]

SUMMARY. A variety of neural and humoral mechanisms contribute to the intestinal phase of pancreatic exocrine secretion. The early response appears to be primarily neural and cholinergic. Intact vagal-vagal innervation is a prerequisite for full activity. Intraintestinal acid stimulates pancreatic bicarbonate and volume secretion, which is probably mediated in part by secretin release. Intraintestinal fats stimulate both pancreatic bicarbonate and protein secretion, which is most likely mediated partly by secretin and CCK release. Intraintestinal peptides and amino acids stimulate pancreatic protein secretion, which is probably mediated in part by CCK release. Radioimmunoassay studies suggest that the change in plasma concentration of these two peptides is small, implicating potentiated interactions between peptides for realization of full pancreatic secretory activity.

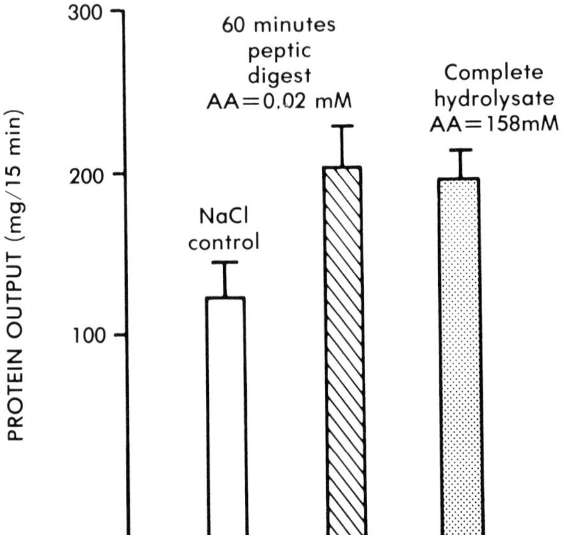

Fig. 27-13 Pancreatic protein responses in dogs to perfused peptic digestive material of 1.75% bovine serum albumin and to an amino acid mixture with a composition similar to a theoretically complete hydrolysate of bovine serum albumin. (Redrawn from Meyer, J.H.: Release of secretin and cholecystokinin. In Thompson, J.C., editor: Gastrointestinal hormones, Austin, Tex., 1975, University of Austin Press.)

PANCREATIC FUNCTION TESTS

Serum Concentrations of Pancreatic Enzymes

The most frequently measured pancreatic enzyme in the blood is amylase. Pancreatic ductal obstruction causes a rise in serum amylase concentration. Amylase may also be derived from the salivary glands, intestine, fallopian tube, breast, and liver. Specific isozymes of amylase provide information regarding the source of serum enzyme elevation. In acute pancreatitis serum amylase may rise rapidly fivefold to ten-fold and return to normal within a few days. Serum lipase also is often elevated in acute pancreatitis. Other conditions that may cause hyperamylasemia include perforated duodenal ulcer, intestinal obstruction, acute mesenteric infarction, and acute cholecystitis. The elevation of the pancreatic isozyme of amylase in a patient with abdominal pain is a very useful indicator for the physician. Unfortunately, in certain conditions such as chronic pancreatitis, serum amylase concentration is usually normal or subnormal.

Urine Concentrations of Pancreatic Enzymes

In acute pancreatitis urinary amylase may be elevated for a longer period than serum amylase and therefore represents a more sensitive test than serum amylase. Urinary clearance of amylase increases in acute pancreatitis. In healthy persons the ratio of amylase clearance to creatinine clearance is less than 5%, whereas in patients with acute pancreatitis it is often significantly higher. Unfortunately the lack of specificity of this test limits its clinical usefulness.

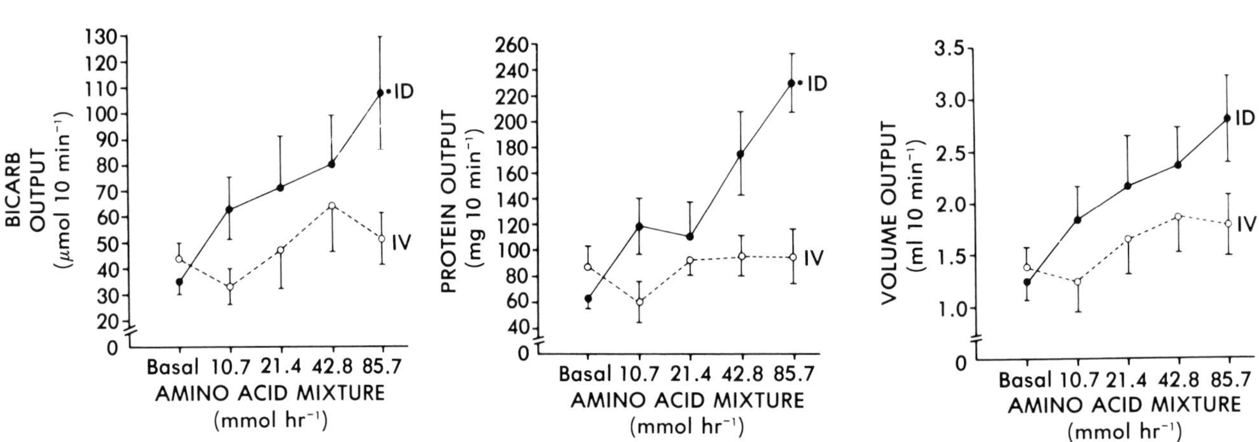

Fig. 27-14 Pancreatic volume, protein, and bicarbonate responses to graded doses of mixed amino acids administered intraduodenally *(ID)* or intravenously *(IV)* in dogs. (From Stabile, B.E., et al.: Am. J. Physiol. **246:**G274, 1984.)

Pancreatic Secretory Tests

Secretin Test

In the secretin test the patient is given secretin (1 U/kg of body weight) intravenously after a nasogastric tube is positioned fluoroscopically in the duodenum. Duodenal drainage fluid is collected for four 20-minute periods after secretin administration. Volume, bicarbonate, and protein concentrations are measured (Table 27-1).[28] Complete ductal obstruction by carcinoma or advanced chronic pancreatitis produces a significant reduction in all parameters. If the duct is partially occluded, the protein concentration may be normal, but the volume may be low. In chronic pancreatitis the volume and protein concentration may be normal, whereas the bicarbonate concentration is low.

Unfortunately, accurate sampling is a difficult problem with this test. Some pancreatic juice may not be sampled, and that sampled may have varying amounts of bilious contamination. Even with this potential for minor error, patients with malabsorption secondary to pancreatic disease will usually have less than 80 mEq/L of bicarbonate in duodenal drainage following secretin administration. The secretin test may be normal or abnormal in patients with acute pancreatitis.

Lundh Test

To conduct the Lundh[59] test, a tube is placed in the very proximal jejunum, and the patient drinks 300 ml of a test meal consisting of corn oil, milk, and dextrose. After the meal, at specific intervals, jejunal aspirates are analyzed for trypsin and perhaps for fats, fatty acids, and bile salts. In healthy persons trypsin output increases two to three times over basal values, and trypsin concentration remains relatively constant. Trypsin concentration that is reduced by more than 90% compared to normal values suggests rather severe pancreatic insufficiency.[59]

Clinical Usefulness of Secretin and Lundh Tests

Clinically the secretin and Lundh tests are infrequently used. Results of both tests may be affected by dilution of pancreatic secretions with meal contents or intestinal juices, autodegradation of secreted enzymes, or partial neutralization or absorption of secreted bicarbonate. Consequently, standard deviation of the mean in "normal" subjects may vary from 25% to 60%, even using dye dilution indicators to correct for volume and direct pancreatic duct cannulation. Also, both these tests are quite insensitive. Pancreatic exocrine secretory tests in 33% to 50% of patients with chronic pancreatitis or carcinoma of the pancreas are within the "normal" range.

Table 27-1 **RESPONSE TO SECRETIN TEST**

Patient	Mean Volume (ml/kg^{-1})	Mean Maximum Bicarbonate Output (mEq/L^{-1})
Normal	3.2	108
Acute pancreatitis	2.4	93
Chronic pancreatitis	2.7	57
Carcinoma of pancreas	1.3	83

Modified from Dreiling, D.: Gut **16:**653, 1977.

Therefore, in the evaluation of the patient with abdominal pain, other tests such as ultrasound, computed tomography, and perhaps endoscopic retrograde cholangiopancreatography are more cost and time effective than the secretin and Lundh tests. Similarly, in patients with pancreatic insufficiency, the condition is usually clinically obvious, and the diagnosis does not depend on these two tests. More than 85% of pancreatic exocrine function must be lost before malabsorption becomes clinically appreciable. By that time both tests are almost universally positive. The physician may even prescribe pancreatic supplements, assuming that the clinical response is indicative of pancreatic insufficiency.

Pancreatic function tests are sufficiently insensitive to establish the diagnosis of chronic pancreatitis or pancreatic cancer in the absence of malabsorption, although they do effectively diagnose pancreatic exocrine insufficiency. In the occasional patient with malabsorption secondary to pancreatic insufficiency, these tests will effectively establish the diagnoses; however, in most cases of pancreatic insufficiency, pancreatic disease is clinically obvious.

SUMMARY

Normal pancreatic exocrine secretion consists of a protein component that includes proteolytic, amylolytic, lipolytic, and nucleolytic enzymes important in the normal digestion of carbohydrates, protein, and fats. A watery, bicarbonate component also is important for the neutralization of acidic chyme that is emptied into the duodenum from the stomach. This secretion is under complex control and includes various neural and humoral mechanisms.

The pancreatic secretory response to a meal has been divided into cephalic (vagal), gastric (through the hormone gastrin), and intestinal phases. The earliest response to a meal appears to be primarily mediated through neural and cholinergic mechanisms and requires an intact vagus nerve for full activity. Antral gastrin release modulates this secretory response through stimulation of pancreatic enzyme output. Following delivery of acidic chyme into the proximal duodenum, pancreatic bicarbonate and volume secretion is elicited and probably is partly mediated by release of the hormone secretin from the duodenal mucosa. Intraintestinal fats stimulate both pancreatic bicarbonate and protein secretion, which is most likely mediated by a combination of secretin and cholecystokinin (CCK) release from the duodenum. Intraintestinal peptides and amino acids stimulate pancreatic protein secretion, probably primarily through CCK release. Since plasma concentrations of secretin and CCK are small in response to a meal, potentiated interactions between these two hormones are implicated in full pancreatic secretory activity.

REFERENCES

1. Almeida, A.L., and Grossman, M.I.: Experimental production of pancreatitis with ethionine, Gastroenterology **20:**554, 1952.
2. Annis, D., and Hallenbeck, G.A.: Effect of excluding pancreatic juice from duodenum on secretory response of pancreas to a meal, Proc. Soc. Exp. Biol. Med. **77:**383, 1951.

3. Aune, S., and Semb, L.S.: The effect of secretin and pancreozymin on pancreatic blood flow in the conscious and anesthetized dog, Acta Physiol. **76**:406, 1969.
4. Begin, N., and Scholefield, P.G.: The uptake of amino acids by mouse pancreas in vitro. 1. General characteristics. Biochem. Biophys. Acta **90**:82, 1964.
5. Beglinger, C., Grossman, M.I., and Solomon, T.E.: Interaction between stimulants of exocrine pancreatic secretion in dogs, Am. J. Physiol. **246**:G173, 1984.
6. Berman, L.G., et al.: A study of the pancreatic duct system in man by the use of vinyl acetate casts of postmorten preparations, Surg. Gynecol. Obstet. **110**:403, 1960.
7. Blobel, G., and Sabatini, D.D.: Controlled proteolysis of nascent polypeptides in rat liver cell fractions. I. Localization of the polypeptides within the ribosome, J. Cell. Biol. **45**:130, 1970.
8. Bro-Rasmussen, F., Killmann, S.A., and Thaysen, J.H.: The composition of pancreatic juice as compared to sweat, parotid saliva, and tears, Acta Physiol. Scand. **37**:97, 1956.
9. Byrnes, D.J., et al.: Radioimmunoassay of cholecystokinin in human plasma, Clin. Chim. Acta **111**:81, 1981.
10. Carter, M.J.: Carbonic anhydrase: isoenzymes, properties, distribution and functional significance, Biol. Rev. **47**:465, 1972.
11. Case, R.M., and Clausen, T.: The relationship between calcium exchange and enzyme secretion in the isolated rat pancreas, J. Physiol. **235**:75, 1973.
12. Case, R.M., and Scratchard, T.: The secretion of alkali metal ions by the perfused cat pancreas as influenced by the composition and osmolality of the external environment and by inhibitors of metabolism and Na^+, K^+-ATPase activity, J. Physiol. **242**:415, 1974.
13. Case, R.M., Harper, A.A., and Scratchard, T.: Ionic requirements for pancreatic secretion, Proc. Int. Anion. Physiol. Sci. XXIV, Washington Abstr. 230, 1968.
14. Case, R.M., Harper, A.A., and Scratchard, T.: The secretion of electrolytes and enzymes by the pancreas of the anesthetized cat, J. Physiol. **201**:335, 1969.
15. Case, R.M., Scratchard, T., and Wynne, R.D.: The origin and secretion of pancreatic juice bicarbonate, J. Physiol. (Lond.) **210**:1, 1970.
16. Chariot, J., et al.: Effects of somatostatin on the external secretion of the pancreas of the rat, Gastroenterology **75**:832, 1978.
17. Chey, W.Y., et al.: Effect of rabbit antisecretin serum on postprandial pancreatic secretion in dogs, Gastroenterology **77**:1268, 1979.
18. Chung, R.S., and Safaie-Shirazi, S.: The effect of secretin on pancreatic blood flow in the awake and anesthetized dog, Proc. Soc. Exp. Biol. Med. **173**:620, 1983.
19. Conklin, J.L.: Cytogenesis of the human fetal pancreas, Am. J. Anat. **111**:181, 1962.
20. Creutz, C.E., Pazoles, C.J., and Pollard, H.B.: Self association of synexin in the presence of calcium, J. Biol. Chem. **254**:553, 1979.
21. Dagorn, J.C., Sohel, J., and Sarles, H.: Now parallel secretion of enzymes in human duodenal juice and pure pancreatic juice collected by endoscopic retrograde catheterization of the papilla, Gastroenterology **73**:42, 1977.
22. Debas, H.T., and Grossman, M.I.: Pure cholecystokinin: pancreatic protein and bicarbonate response, Digestion **9**:464, 1973.
23. Debas, H.T., and Yamagishi, T.: Evidence for pyloropancreatic reflex for pancreatic exocrine secretion, Am. J. Physiol. **234**:E468, 1978.
24. DeFillipi, C., Solomon, T.E., and Valenzuela, J.E.: Pancreatic secretory response to sham feeding in humans, Digestion **23**:217, 1982.
25. Desmuelle, P., Reboud, J.P., and Ben Abdeljlil, A.: Influence of the composition of the diet on the enzyme content of the rat pancreas. In de Reuck, A.U.S., and Cameron, M.P., editors: Ciba Foundation Symposium on the Exocrine Pancreas, Boston, 1962, Little, Brown & Co.
26. Dixon, J.S.: Histology: ultrastructure. In Howat, H.T., and Sarles, H., editors: The exocrine pancreas, London, 1979, W.B. Saunders Co.
27. Domschke, S., et al.: Vasoactive intestinal peptide: a secretin-like partial agonist for pancreatic secretion in man, Gastroenterology **73**:478, 1977.
28. Dreiling, D.: Pancreatic secretory testing in 1974, Gut **16**:653, 1977.
29. Dyck, W.P., Hightower, N.C., and Janowitz, H.D.: Effect of acetazolamide on human pancreatic secretion, Gastroenterology **62**:547, 1972.
30. Fahrenkrug, J., Schaffalitzky de Muckadell, O.B., and Rune, S.J.: pH threshold for release of secretin in normal subjects and in patients with duodenal ulcer and patients with chronic pancreatitis, Scand. J. Gastroenterol. **13**:177, 1978.
31. Faichney, A., et al.: Effect of sodium oleate on plasma secretin concentration and pancreatic secretion in dog, Gastroenterology **81**:458, 1981.
32. Fink, A.S., and Meyer, J.H.: Intraduodenal emulsions of oleic acid augment acid-induced canine pancreatic secretion, Am. J. Physiol. **245** (Gastrointest. Liver Physiol. **8**):G85, 1983.
33. Fink, A.S., Luxenburg, M., and Meyer, J.H.: Regionally perfused fatty acids augment acid-induced canine pancreatic secretion, Am. J. Physiol. **245** (Gastrointest. Liver Physiol. **8**):G78, 1983.
34. Fink, A.S., et al.: Digests of protein augment acid-induced canine pancreatic secretion, Am. J. Physiol. **242** (Gastrointest. Liver Physiol. **5**):G634, 1982.
35. Folsch, U.R., and Creutzfeldt, W.: Pancreatic duct cells in rats: secretory studies in response to secretin, cholecystokinin-pancreozymin, and gastrin in vivo, Gastroenterology **73**:1053, 1977.
36. Fried, G.M., et al.: Release of cholecystokinin in conscious dogs: correlation with simultaneous measurements of gallbladder pressure and pancreatic protein secretion, Gastroenterology **85**:1113, 1983.
37. Gardner, J.D., and Jensen, R.T.: Regulation of pancreatic enzyme secretion in vitro. In Johnson, L.R., editor: Physiology of the gastrointestinal tract, New York, 1981, Raven Press.
38. Go, V.L.W., Hoffman, A.F., and Summerskill, W.H.J.: Pancreozymin bioassay in man based on pancreatic enzyme secretion: potency of specific amino acids and other digestive products, J. Clin. Invest. **49**:1558, 1970.
39. Gorelick, F.S., and Jamieson, J.D.: Structure-function relationships of the pancreas. In Johnson, L.R., editor: Physiology of the gastrointestinal tract, New York, 1981, Raven Press.
40. Govaerts, J.P., and Kiekens, R.: Role of vagal innervation on pancreatic secretion, Surgery **62**:942, 1968.
41. Grossman, M.I., and Ivy, A.C.: Effect of alloxan upon external secretion of the pancreas, Proc. Soc. Exp. Biol. Med. **63**:62, 1946.
42. Grossman, M.I., and Konturek, S.J.: Gastric acid does drive pancreatic bicarbonate secretion, Scand. J. Gastroenterol. **9**:299, 1974.
43. Grossman, M.I., Greengard, H., and Ivy, A.C.: The effect of dietary composition on pancreatic enzymes, Am. J. Physiol. **138**:676, 1943.
44. Harris, P.F.: Anatomy. In Howat, H.T., and Sarles, H., editors: The exocrine pancreas, London, 1979, W.B. Saunders Co.
45. Henderson, J.R., and Daniel, P.M.: A comparative study of the portal vessels connecting the endocrine and exocrine pancreas, with a discussion of some functional implications, Q. J. Exp. Physiol. **64**:267, 1979.
46. Hickson, J.D.: The secretion of pancreatic juice in response to stimulation of the vagus nerves in the pig, J. Physiol. (Lond.) **206**:275, 1970.
47. Hickson, J.D.: The secretory and vascular response to nervous and hormonal stimulation in the pancreas of the pig, J. Physiol. (Lond.) **206**:299, 1970.
48. Holst, J.J., Schaffalitzky de Muckadell, O.B., and Fahrenkrug, J.: Nervous control of pancreatic exocrine secretion in pig, Acta Physiol. Scand. **105**:33, 1979.
49. Jamieson, J.D., and Palade, G.E.: Intracellular transport of secretory proteins in the pancreatic exocrine cell. II. Transport to condensing vacuoles and zymogen granules, J. Cell. Biol. **34**:597, 1967.
50. Jamieson, J.D., and Palade, G.E.: Intracellular transport of secretory proteins in the pancreatic exocrine cell. III. Dissociation of intracellular transport from protein synthesis, J. Cell. Biol. **39**:580, 1968.
51. Jansen, J.B.M.J., and Lamers, C.B.H.W.: Radioimmunoassay of cholecystokinin in human tissue and plasma, Clin. Chim. Acta **131**:305, 1983.

52. Kraehenbuhl, J.P., Rocine, L., and Jamieson, J.D.: Immunocytochemical localization of secretory proteins in bovine pancreatic exocrine cells, J. Cell. Biol. **72:**406, 1977.
53. Krawisz, B.R., et al.: In the absence of nutrients pancreatic-biliary secretions in the jejunum do not exert feedback control of human pancreatic or gastric function, J. Lab. Clin. Med. **95:**13, 1980.
54. Kvietys P.S., et al.: Pancreatic circulation: intrinsic regulation, Am. J. Physiol. **242** (Gastrointest. Liver Physiol. **5**):G596, 1982.
55. Larsson, L.I.: Innervation of the pancreas by substance P, enkephalin, vasoactive intestinal polypeptide and gastrin/CCK immunoreactive nerves, J. Histochem. Cytochem. **27:**1283, 1979.
56. Lee, K.Y., Tai, H.H., and Chey, W.Y.: Plasma secretin and gastrin responses to a meat meal and duodenal acidification in dogs, Am. J. Physiol. **230:**784, 1976.
57. Lifson, N., et al.: Blood flow to the rabbit pancreas with special reference to the islets of Langerhans, Gastroenterology **7:**466, 1980.
58. Lightwood, R., and Reber, H.A.: Micropuncture study of pancreatic secretion in the cat, Gastroenterology **72:**61, 1977.
59. Lundh, G.: Pancreatic exocrine function in neoplastic and inflammatory disease: a simple and reliable new test, Gastroenterology **42:**275, 1962.
60. MacGregor, I., Parent, J., and Meyer, J.H.: Gastric emptying of liquid meals and pancreatic and biliary secretion after subtotal gastrectomy or truncal vagotomy and pyloroplasty in man, Gastroenterology **72:**195, 1977.
61. Magee, D.F., and White, T.T.: Influence of vagal stimulation on secretion of pancreatic juice in pigs, Ann. Surg. **161:**605, 1965.
62. Malagelada, J.R., Go, V.L.W., and Summerskill, W.H.J.: Different gastric, pancreatic, and biliary responses to solid-liquid or homogenized meals, Dig. Dis. Sci. **24:**101, 1979.
63. Malagelada, J.R., et al.: Regulation of pancreatic and gallbladder functions by intraluminal fatty acids and bile acids in man, J. Clin. Invest. **58:**493, 1976.
64. Malkin, L.I., and Rich, A.: Partial resistance of nascent polypeptide chains to proteolytic digestion due to ribosomal shedding, J. Mol. Biol. **26:**329, 1967.
65. McLean, J.M.: Embryology of the pancreas. In Howat, H.T., and Sarles, H., editors: The exocrine pancreas, London, 1979, W.B. Saunders Co.
66. Meldosi, J.: Membranes and membrane surfaces: dynamics of cytoplasmic membranes in pancreatic acinar cells, Philos. Trans. R. Soc. Lond. (Biol.) **268:**39, 1974.
67. Meyer, J.H.: Release of secretin and cholecystokinin. In Thompson, J.C., editor: Gastrointestinal hormones, Austin, 1975, University of Texas Press.
68. Meyer, J.H., and Jones, R.S.: Canine pancreatic responses to intestinally perfused fat and products of fat digestion, Am. J. Physiol. **226:**1178, 1974.
69. Meyer, J.H., and Kelley, G.A.: Canine pancreatic responses to intestinally perfused proteins and protein digests, Am. J. Physiol. **231:**682, 1976.
70. Meyer, J.H., Kelly, G.A., and Jones, R.S.: Canine pancreatic response to intestinally perfused oligopeptides, Am. J. Physiol. **231:**678, 1976.
71. Meyer, J.H., Way, L.W., and Grossman, M.I.: Pancreatic bicarbonate response to various acids in duodenum of the dog, Am. J. Physiol. **219:**964, 1970.
72. Meyer, J.H., Way, L.W., and Grossman, M.I.: Pancreatic response to acidification of various lengths of proximal intestine in the dog, Am. J. Physiol. **219:**971, 1970.
73. Meyer, J.H., et al.: Canine gut receptors mediating pancreatic responses to luminal L-amino acids, Am. J. Physiol. **231:**669, 1976.
74. Meyer, J.H., et al.: Sieving of solid food by the canine stomach and sieving after gastric surgery, Gastroenterology **76:**804, 1979.
75. Miller, T.A., et al.: The effect of fat on secretin release, Ann. Surg. **187:**303, 1978.
76. Moore, E.W., Verine, H.J., and Grossman, M.I.: Pancreatic bicarbonate response to a meal, Acta Hepato-Gastroenterol. **26:**30, 1979.
77. Morisset, J., and Dunnigan, J.: Effects of glucose, amino acids and insulin on adaptation of the exocrine pancreas to diet, Proc. Soc. Exp. Biol. Med. **140:**1308, 1971.
78. Novis, B.H., Bank, S., and Markes, I.M.: The cephalic phase of pancreatic secretion in man, Scand. J. Gastroenterol. **6:**417, 1971.
79. Palade, G.: Intracellular aspects of the process of protein secretion, Science **189:**347, 1975.
80. Pavlov, I.P.: The work of the digestive gland, Lecture VII, London, 1902, Griffin.
81. Peikin, S.R., et al.: Kinetics of amylase release by dispersed acini prepared from guinea pig pancreas, Am. J. Physiol. **235:**E743, 1978.
82. Preshaw, R.M., Cooke, A.R., and Grossman, M.I.: Sham feeding and pancreatic secretion in the dog, Gastroenterology **50:**171, 1966.
83. Rayford, P.L., Miller, T.A., and Thompson, J.C.: Secretin, cholecystokinin and newer gastrointestinal hormones, N. Engl. J. Med. **294:**1093, 1976.
84. Redman, C.M., Siekevitz, P., and Palade, G.E.: Synthesis and transfer of amylase in pigeon pancreatic microsomes, J. Biol. Chem. **241:**1150, 1966.
85. Ridderstap, A.S., and Bonting, S.L.: Na-K-activated adenosine triphosphatase and pancreatic secretion in the dog, Am. J. Physiol. **216:**547, 1969.
86. Robberecht, P., et al.: Rat pancreatic hydrolases from birth to weaning and dietary adaptation after weaning, Am. J. Physiol. **221:**376, 1971.
87. Rothman, S.S.: Trypsin and chymotrypsin secretion from the rabbit pancreas in vitro, Am. J. Physiol. **211:**777, 1966.
88. Rothman, S.S., and Brooks, F.P.: Pancreatic secretion in vitro in "Cl^--free," "CO_2-free" and low Na^+ environment, Am. J. Physiol. **209:**790, 1965.
89. Sale, J.K., et al.: Chronic and acute studies indicating absence of exocrine pancreatic feedback inhibition in dogs, Digestion **15:**540, 1977.
90. Sarles, H., et al.: Cephalic phase of pancreatic secretion in man, Gut **9:**214, 1968.
91. Schaffalitzky de Muckadell, O.B., and Fahrenkrug, J.: Secretion pattern of secretin in man: regulation by gastric acid, Gut **19:**812, 1978.
92. Scheele, G.A., and Palade, G.E.: Studies on the guinea pig pancreas: parallel discharge of exocrine enzyme activities, J. Biol. Chem. **250:**2660, 1975.
93. Scheele, G., Bartelt, D., and Bieger, W.: Characterization of human exocrine pancreatic proteins by two-dimensional isoelectric focusing/sodium dodecyl sulfate gel electrophoresis, Gastroenterology **80:**461, 1981.
94. Schneeman, B.O., and Lyman, R.L.: Factors involved in the intestinal feedback regulation of pancreatic enzyme secretion in the rat, Proc. Soc. Exp. Biol. Med. **148:**897, 1975.
95. Schulz, F.: Electrolyte and fluid secretion in the exocrine pancreas. In Johnson, L.R., editor: Physiology of the gastrointestinal tract, New York, 1981, Raven Press.
96. Schultz, I.: Influence of bicarbonate, CO_2^- and glycodiazine buffer on the secretion of the isolated cat pancreas, Pflugers Arch. **329:**283, 1971.
97. Schulz, I., Yamagata, A., and Weske, M.: Micropuncture studies on the pancreas of the rabbit, Pflugers Arch. **308:**277, 1969.
98. Singer, M.V.: Latency of pancreatic fluid secretory response to intestinal stimulants in the dog, J. Physiol. **339:**75, 1983.
99. Singer, M.V., et al.: Latency of pancreatic enzyme response to intraduodenal stimulants, Am. J. Physiol. **238** (Gastrointest. Liver Physiol. **1**):G23, 1980.
100. Slaff, J., et al.: Protease-specific suppression of pancreatic exocrine secretion, Gastroenterology **87:**44, 1984.
101. Solomon, T.E., Grossman, M.I., and Meyer, J.H.: Pancreatic response to intestinal perfusion with lactic acid or acidified albumin, Am. J. Physiol. **235:**E560, 1978.
102. Stabile, B.E., et al.: Intravenous mixed amino acids and fats do not stimulate exocrine pancreatic secretion, Am. J. Physiol. **246:**G274, 1984.
103. Stening, G.F., and Grossman, M.I.: Gastrin related peptides as stimulants of pancreatic and gastric secretion, Am. J. Physiol. **217:**262, 1969.
104. Swanson, C.H., and Solomon, A.K.: Micropuncture analysis of the cellular mechanisms of electrolyte secretion by the in vitro rabbit pancreas, J. Gen. Physiol. **65:**22, 1975.

105. Taylor, I.L., et al.: Pancreatic polypeptide, metabolism and effect on pancreatic secretion in dogs, Gastroenterology **76:**524, 1979.
106. Thomas, J.W., and Mason, F.E.: The effects of gastric exclusion operations on pancreatic exocrine secretion, Surgery **75:**461, 1974.
107. Valenzuela, J.E., Walsh, J.H., and Isenberg, J.I.: Effect of gastrin on pancreatic enzyme secretion and gallbladder emptying in man, Gastroenterology **71:**409, 1976.
108. van Venrooij, W.J., et al.: Relationship between extracellular amino acids and protein synthesis in vitro in the rat, Eur. J. Biochem. **30:**426, 1972.
109. Walsh, J.H., Lamers, C.B., and Valenzuela, J.E.: Cholecystokinin-octapeptidelike immunoreactivity in human plasma, Gastroenterology **82:**438, 1982.
110. Wang, C.C., and Grossman, M.I.: Physiological determination of release of secretin and pancreozymin from intestine of dogs with transplanted pancreas, Am. J. Physiol. **164:**527, 1951.
111. White, T.T., Lundh, G., and Magee, D.F.: Evidence for existence of a gastro-pancreatic reflex, Am. J. Physiol. **198:**725, 1960.
112. White, T.T., McAlexander, R.A., and Magee, D.F.: The effect of gastric distension on duodenal aspirates in man, Gastroenterology **44:**48, 1965.
113. Williams, J.A., and Chandler, D.: Ca^{++} and pancreatic amylase release, Am. J. Physiol. **228:**1729, 1975.
114. Wormsley, K.G.: Pancreatic secretion: physiological control. In Duthie, H.L., and Wormsley, K.G., editors: Scientific basis of gastroenterology, Edinburgh, 1979, Churchill Livingstone, Inc.

28
James L. Austin and Howard A. Reber

Acute and Chronic Pancreatitis

Pancreatitis is an inflammatory process involving the pancreas and is divided into acute and chronic varieties.[17] Acute pancreatitis is associated with full recovery of exocrine and endocrine function when the inflammation resolves. Chronic pancreatitis is associated with permanent impairment of both exocrine and endocrine function. The development of chronic pancreatitis may be insidious, or it may involve repeated episodes of acute inflammation indistinguishable clinically from acute pancreatitis.

ACUTE PANCREATITIS

Pathology

Acute pancreatitis may result from a variety of causes:

Cholelithiasis	Malnutrition (protein/calorie)
Alcoholism	Hyperlipidemia
Drugs	Duct obstruction
Trauma	Ischemia
Hyperparathyroidism	Idiopathic

However, because the pancreas responds to different insults in a similar way, its gross and histologic appearance in patients with acute pancreatitis from differing causes is frequently the same.[4]

Edema is a prominent feature of acute pancreatitis, and it is characterized during gross inspection by the glassy separation of pancreatic lobules without evidence of hemorrhage. Microscopically, there is variable interlobular inflammatory cell infiltration. The acinar cells show no evidence of necrosis, and blood flow appears to be maintained in the small capillaries and venules. The edema and accompanying inflammation may extend throughout the retroperitoneum and to the surrounding organs. Fat necrosis, a common pathologic finding in acute pancreatitis, appears as raised, whitish-gray areas embedded in normal omentum or mesentery.

Edema is also present when pancreatic necrosis occurs. Microscopically, pancreatic necrosis is accompanied by vascular thromboses. The acinar cells undergo nuclear and cytoplasmic degeneration in association with thrombosis of the nutrient vessels that supply the individual lobules. Adjacent to the healthy lobules, necrotic areas are found along with intense inflammatory reaction and cellular infiltration.

Early in the disease the acinar cell organelles responsible for protein synthesis appear abnormal. However, zymogen granules remain intact until late in the process of acinar cell necrosis. Then pancreatic enzymes appear to be released as the terminal event of acinar cell death.

Pathogenesis

In all forms of acute pancreatitis, it is believed that pancreatic enzymes normally confined to acinar cells or ducts pass instead into the interstitium of the gland.[55] The activated enzymes in the interstitium then destroy the gland by digestion. Because enzymes can be found in the serum and the peripancreatic fluid of patients with acute pancreatitis, they may also account for some of the systemic effects of the disease. However, the severity of the systemic illness and the progression of changes within the gland may be related to factors other than the direct effects of pancreatic enzymes.[31,39] Some pancreatic enzymes can activate humoral systems throughout the body. For example, trypsin generates bradykinin from kallikrein in experimental acute pancreatitis. Complement factors (C3a and C5a) have also been recovered from the serum in significant quantities during acute pancreatitis in both experimental animals and humans; trypsin can also activate many of these factors. Such secondary humoral systems are undoubtedly important in the development and perpetuation of the cardiovascular, pulmonary, and renal complications seen in acute pancreatitis, but their exact role remains to be determined.

Proposed Mechanisms

Acute pancreatitis in humans is most commonly associated with the passage of gallstones through the biliary tract or with prolonged, excessive consumption of alcohol (see list at left). The factors initiating pancreatitis in these situations are unknown, although several mechanisms have been proposed based on clinical and experimental evidence: (1) pancreatic duct obstruction by gallstones; (2) common channel phenomenon; (3) reflux of activated enzymes into the pancreatic duct; and (4) alterations in pancreatic duct permeability. Other etiologic factors of less certain significance include hyperparathyroidism, malnutrition, hyperlipemia, drugs, and ischemia. A discussion of each of these considerations follows.

Pancreatic Duct Obstruction

Even when gallstones are not found obstructing the ampulla, they can be recovered in the stool of 85% to 90% of patients with gallstone associated pancreatitis.[1] Passage of gallstones through the common duct and ampulla could initiate pancreatitis in several ways. Obstruction of the pancreatic duct could occur through impaction of a gallstone at the ampulla. The inflammation resulting there could also cause spasm of the muscular wall of the sphincter of Oddi at the entrance of the common duct into the duodenum. Interestingly, spasm of the sphincter has also been produced in experimental animals following ingestion of alcohol.

The relationship between pancreatic duct obstruction and pancreatitis has not been clearly defined, although duct obstruction does cause physiologic and morphologic alterations in the pancreas.[5] The suggestion has been made that secretion of pancreatic juice against the obstructed duct leads to increased pressure within the ductal system. This pressure could damage the ducts, and pancreatic enzymes could then leak into the pancreatic interstitium. In this regard, prolonged stimulation with secretin against a totally obstructed duct leads to hemorrhagic pancreatitis in dogs.[19] Total obstruction is probably not common clinically, but partial obstruction during secretion is more likely and does cause pancreatic edema in experimental animals.[33]

Most experiments that examine the effect of increased pressure in the pancreatic duct have used forceful retrograde injection into the duct at pressures up to 300 mm Hg. Histologic examination has shown that ducts rupture at these pressures. However, the maximum pressure that is generated by active secretion in an obstructed pancreatic duct is only 20 to 40 mm Hg.[18] Although ductal pressure is probably an important factor to consider in determining the cause of the initiation of acute pancreatitis, duct obstruction may involve other pathogenic factors yet to be identified. Thus further study is clearly needed.

Common Channel

Although the common duct and the pancreatic duct may empty into the duodenum separately, they usually empty into the ampulla of Vater, which then empties into the duodenum. In some patients there may actually be a longer communication between these two ductal systems before they empty into the ampulla. In either circumstance, this "common channel" may be important in two ways as it relates to pancreatitis. First, bile could reflux into the pancreatic duct under pressure and damage it as discussed previously. However, measurement of pancreatic and bile duct pressures during secretory stimulation have shown that pancreatic duct pressure is generally greater than bile duct pressure. Thus if there is reflux of bile into the pancreatic duct, it probably would occur passively and at low pressure. Second, the chemical characteristics of bile when in contact with the pancreatic duct may be important. For example, experimental exposure of the ducts to deconjugated bile salts during low-pressure perfusion resulted in ductal damage and the leakage of large molecules out of the ductal lumen.[35] Since deconjugation of bile salts frequently results from bacterial infection of the bile, reflux of these substances into the pancreatic duct could be an inciting mechanism in patients who develop pancreatitis. Reflux of contrast material into the pancreatic duct has been demonstrated by cholangiography in patients with gallstone pancreatitis. However, reflux also has been shown in patients with gallstone disease without associated pancreatitis. Thus the exact role of biliary-pancreatic duct reflux in the initiation of acute pancreatitis remains to be defined.

Reflux of Activated Pancreatic Enzymes

Enzymes secreted into the pancreatic ducts are inactive and remain so until they are activated in the duodenum. Pancreatitis could result from the reflux of activated pancreatic enzymes from the duodenum back into the pancreatic duct. However, the sphincter of Oddi effectively prevents reflux; furthermore, reflux of duodenal contents into the pancreatic duct has not been demonstrated in humans. Destruction of the ampulla allowing free communication between the duodenum and the pancreatic duct has produced hemorrhagic pancreatitis in experimental animals. However, patients who have had sphincteroplasties do not have an increased incidence of pancreatitis. Thus there are no clinical analogies to suggest that this mechanism is important in human disease.

Duct Permeability

During pancreatic secretion the pancreatic duct normally contains inactive pancreatic enzymes. Because these enzymes are large molecules (e.g., 25,000 to 50,000 daltons), they are contained within the duct lumen. However, experimental exposure of the ducts to a variety of bile salts, to ethanol, or to elevated pressures increases the permeability of the ducts so that pancreatic enzymes may leak into the interstitium. Since perfusion of permeable ducts with activated enzymes has produced pancreatitis in animals, duct permeability may be important in human disease. Its role in the initiation of pancreatitis is under investigation. Present knowledge suggests that duct permeability may be a potentially important component of all of the proposed mechanisms for the development of pancreatitis.[42]

Hyperparathyroidism

Early studies found that the incidence of pancreatitis in patients with hyperparathyroidism was as high as 20%, but more recent reports indicate a lower figure of 1% to 2%.[7] These differences may reflect the present-day earlier recognition of hyperparathyroidism in patients as a result of modern automated laboratory analyses. Thus the disease is diagnosed in most individuals before pancreatitis develops.

The cause of acute pancreatitis in patients with hyperparathyroidism is unknown. Elevated serum concentrations of parathyroid hormone and hypercalcemia have both been implicated, but elevation of serum parathyroid hormone concentrations in experimental animals did not produce pancreatitis.[13,25] Acute pancreatitis has been reported in patients with hypercalcemia from a number of causes other than hyperparathyroidism. In every case, the pancreatitis was resolved with removal of the abnormal parathyroid tissue or reduction of the serum calcium concentration.[7] When evaluating such patients, it is important to exclude other causes of pancreatitis such as alcoholism or gallstone disease. Only then is it reasonable to assume that the pancreatitis will resolve with treatment of the endocrine abnormality.

Malnutrition

Malnutrition has been reported as a cause of chronic pancreatitis in certain tropical countries.[6,38] It is most commonly associated with atrophy of the pancreatic parenchyma, with pancreatic calcifications, and with diabetes mellitus. The specific etiologic factors are unknown but are probably multiple. The pancreas actively synthesizes enzyme protein, and alterations in diet may change the nature of the enzymes produced. Thus chronic malnutrition may alter the composition of the pancreatic secretion and may injure the pancreas in some way. Others have suggested that the ingestion of a specific food in large quantities (e.g., cassava) may be responsible for the chronic pancreatitis.[6,38]

Patients with nutritional pancreatitis experience recurrent episodes of severe abdominal pain during adolescence. The pain subsides after a few years, and relatively long periods free of pain may follow. Then during the patient's late teens or early twenties, diabetes becomes clinically manifest, and the patient again seeks medical care. Characteristic signs and symptoms of diabetes are found, including microangiopathy. At this stage of the disease, abdominal x-ray films reveal pancreatic calcifications in many patients.

Hyperlipemia

Hyperlipemia is an occasional cause of abdominal pain and pancreatitis.[46] It may be primary and caused by one of the familial forms of lipid disorders, most commonly Type V (Fredrickson's classification); or it may be secondary to the ingestion of certain drugs (e.g., estrogen contraceptive agents). In these patients, the course of the pancreatitis generally parallels the elevation of the serum triglycerides. Thus as the lipid concentrations decrease, the abdominal pain and pancreatitis subside.

The mechanism of pancreatitis in hyperlipemia is not known. Experiments in dogs have shown that high concentrations of free fatty acids in the pancreatic microcirculation damaged the pancreas.[44] These fatty acids are thought to damage the capillary endothelium and/or the acinar cell membranes directly. The generation of free radical oxygen molecules may also be involved.

Drugs

Pancreatitis caused by specific drugs is uncommon. Thiazide diuretics, azathioprine, sulfonamides, estrogen contraceptives, and tetracyclines have been most firmly established as causative agents since pancreatitis subsides in a patient after withdrawal of the drug and recurs when the drug is reinstituted.[32,49] The pathogenesis of the pancreatitis in these situations is entirely unknown.

Ischemia

Acute pancreatitis has been described in patients following aortic aneurysm rupture and in other shocklike states.[54] In these patients ultrastructural studies of the pancreas showed that there was an alteration in the cellular synthetic organelles but that the zymogen granules were released only after cell necrosis. These morphologic findings are similar to the ultrastructural changes that occurred in the other experimental models discussed previously.

In hypotensive patients pancreatitis development parallels the failure of other organs sensitive to impaired vascular perfusion. Commonly in patients with ischemia-related acute pancreatitis, renal failure is also present. Although it seems certain that impaired perfusion of the pancreas during shock can cause pancreatitis, the role of ischemia in the pathogenesis of pancreatitis occurring under nonshock conditions remains to be determined.

Multifactoral Origin of Pancreatitis

The pathogenesis of pancreatitis is probably multifactorial. For example, a common channel may predispose some patients to pancreatitis through duct obstruction or reflux of bile. Increase in duct permeability could follow either event. Physical and biochemical changes in acinar cells from a toxin such as ethanol or from ischemia may effect the synthesis, storage, and discharge of pancreatic digestive enzymes and cause pancreatitis in other patients.

The sequential development of pathologic changes after the initiation of acute pancreatitis requires further study. Although the pancreas may continue to secrete enzymes that could cause progressive gland necrosis, there is histologic evidence that the zymogen granules remain in the cells until the disease is far advanced; thus this speculation seems unlikely. Secretory studies in humans during acute pancreatitis indicate that the response to stimulation is impaired. This impairment may continue for several weeks even in the asymptomatic patient. Experimental studies in animals corroborate these findings. Thus the role of secretion in the initiation and progression of pancreatitis remains unclear.

Ischemia may play a role in the conversion of edematous pancreatitis into the necrotizing form since it is known that ischemia itself can produce pancreatitis. Moreover, the necrosis of pancreatic tissue in edematous pancreatitis is associated with small vessel thrombosis. Animal studies have shown that large-vessel occlusion can convert edematous pancreatitis to a form of pancreatitis characterized by hemorrhage and necrosis. With the current state of knowledge, it is uncertain whether vascular thrombosis is the cause or effect of the necrosis.

Pathophysiologic Effects of Pancreatitis

Fluid Sequestration

Patients with acute pancreatitis commonly sequester approximately 2 L of fluid in the abdominal cavity. The most common site of fluid accumulation is in the lesser sac. The spaces posterior to the pancreas and anterior to the kidneys are the next most common sites. However, larger volumes of fluid can be found free-flowing within the abdominal cavity. In the majority of patients with uncomplicated pancreatitis, the fluid is straw colored and without necrotic debris. The fluid becomes blood tinged or "prune-juice colored" in more severe forms.

Fat Necrosis

Fat necrosis is the best example of local and systemic pancreatic enzyme activity occurring in patients with acute pancreatitis.[29] Locally, fat necrosis is found within the intralobular septa of the gland and within the abdominal cavity. Although the fluid sequestered in the abdominal cavity contains a variety of enzymes, only lipase, in combination with colipase, causes necrosis of fat. These necrotic areas are sharply demarcated from the healthy fat in omentum or mesentery and appear as whitish-grey, firm plaques surrounded by healthy tissue. Chemical analyses of these plaques indicate high concentrations of lipase, calcium, and free fatty acids. It is thought that calcium binds with the free fatty acids to form soap.

Fat necrosis is also occasionally found outside the abdominal cavity in the subcutaneous tissue of the lower extremities and in bone marrow. The subcutaneous lesions appear at the time of an episode of acute pancreatitis. Histologically, these areas of fat necrosis are similar to those noted in the abdomen. In patients with subcutaneous fat necrosis, the serum amylase concentrations are usually elevated even though the serum lipase concentrations may be normal. The explanation for this decrease in serum lipase concentration is unknown, although it may be caused by the consumption of lipase in the process of lipolysis. The extent of fat necrosis throughout the body correlates with the severity of the disease, and patients with multiple sites of involvement are less likely to survive. Other evidence of the relationship of these lesions to acute pancreatitis is their disappearance with resolution of the disease or following pancreatectomy.

Peripheral fat necrosis also may occur in the joints where a significant synovitis can develop. Arthrocentesis reveals a cloudy or creamy fluid with elevated concentrations of lipase.

Extrapancreatic Changes

Hypovolemia resulting from fluid sequestration may account for some of the alterations in normal physiology (e.g., oliguria, decreased cardiac output, and hypotension) during acute pancreatitis. However, hypovolemia alone cannot account for all systemic manifestations of the disease.

CARDIOVASCULAR ALTERATIONS. The usual response to fluid sequestration in uncomplicated cases of acute pancreatitis is a compensatory increase in cardiac output. Pulse rate and cardiac contractility both increase in normal patients without pancreatitis in response to mild hypovolemia. However, in severe pancreatitis the myocardial response to hypovolemia may be impaired. In this situation, the pulse rate may increase, but the volume output does not. Even when intravascular volume is restored with intravenous fluid administration, there may be a progressive depression of left ventricular stroke work accompanied by an increasing pulmonary capillary wedge pressure (PCWP).[8] Not only is cardiac output decreased, but tissue perfusion also falls.[11] Interestingly, no histologic changes have been noted in the myocardium of patients who died from acute pancreatitis, and noninvasive tests of the heart such as echocardiography have not demonstrated structural abnormalities.[4]

Changes in Cardiovascular Function During Acute Pancreatitis

- Depressed contractility
- Decreased left ventricular stroke work
- Decreased systemic vascular resistance
- Decreased tissue perfusion
- Electrocardiogram abnormalities
- ST-segment and T-wave changes

Humoral factors from the pancreas may be important in the development of these cardiovascular complications. Bradykinin and other members of the kallikrein system are increased in patients and in experimental animals with acute pancreatitis. These substances are known to alter cardiac and vascular function in ways that could explain the changes that are seen in acute pancreatitis. The effect of pancreatic enzymes on cardiac function has not been studied.

A myocardial depressant factor (MDF) has been isolated from the serum of experimental animals with acute pancreatitis and with hypovolemic shock.[30] The production of MDF in experimental pancreatitis is temporally related to the release of lysosomal enzymes from pancreatic acinar cells. A substance thought to be MDF has been isolated from the serum of patients with hypovolemic shock, but it has not been isolated from patients with pancreatitis. Thus the role of MDF in mediating the cardiovascular alterations associated with pancreatitis remains to be determined.

RENAL ALTERATIONS. Oliguria is common in patients with acute pancreatitis and fluid sequestration. In uncomplicated disease, the urine output increases when intravenous fluid is given. In more severe cases, renal failure may ensue, and oliguria may persist for 3 to 8 days. In the majority of patients with uncomplicated disease, the blood urea nitrogen (BUN) rises to approximately 40 mg/100 ml and the creatinine to approximately 6 mg/100 ml. They promptly return to normal with adequate fluid replacement.[16]

An important feature of renal failure in some patients with acute pancreatitis is that the renal function may be significantly impaired without the patient's having a history of hypotension. In such cases there is microscopic evidence of a membranous glomerulopathy and acute tubular necrosis. Other studies have shown fat emboli in the small arterioles of patients with acute pancreatitis and renal failure. These observations have not been investigated experimentally.

Some investigators have noted *hypertension* during the patient's first 72 hours of acute pancreatitis.[47] The cause is unknown, but in these patients the systemic and renal vascular resistances are both elevated, and the renal plasma flow and the glomerular filtration rate are both decreased. The significance of this observation and the mechanisms responsible for it are unknown.

RESPIRATORY ALTERATIONS. Fifty to sixty percent of patients with acute pancreatitis exhibit arterial hypoxemia with a partial pressure of oxygen (PO_2) of less than 70 mm Hg while breathing room air.[4,36] The majority improves rapidly as the disease resolves, but some patients show a progressive impairment of oxygenation. There may be a significant lag between the appearance of hypoxemia and objective x-ray evidence of pulmonary disease. Sterile pleural effusions are common in patients with pancreatitis, and analysis of this fluid may show a high concentration of amylase. The volume of pleural effusion, however, is not usually sufficient to account for the ventilatory abnormalities.

Ventilation, gas exchange, and pulmonary circulation may all be affected during acute pancreatitis. Ventilation-perfusion mismatching is caused by a reduction in both pulmonary capillary blood flow and alveolar ventilation. The decrease in pulmonary capillary blood flow does not appear to be cardiogenic. A transient increase in pulmonary vascular resistance has been noted on occasion,[18a,33a] but this finding does not account for the decreased capillary flow in the majority of patients.

Ventilatory and Respiratory Changes in Acute Pancreatitis

Decreased ventilation
- ↓ Vital capacity
- ↓ FEV_1/FVC

Decreased efficiency of gas exchange
- ↓ Carbon monoxide diffusing capacity

Decreased oxygen-carrying capacity of hemoglobin

Most patients with acute pancreatitis have ventilatory abnormalities. The vital capacity is decreased approximately 25% and the forced expiratory volume per second (FEV_1) to forced vital capacity (FVC) ratio is reduced to 65% to 80%. The efficiency of the pulmonary gas exchange measured by the carbon monoxide diffusing capacity is also reduced in most patients with pancreatitis by approximately 25%. The oxygen carrying capacity of hemoglobin is impaired but does not appear to be related to decreased 2,3-diphosphoglycerate (2,3-DPG) levels or hemoglobin concentration. Despite these abnormalities, most patients do not require assisted ventilation.

The mechanism of pulmonary injury in acute pancreatitis is unknown.[31] Sepsis may account for respiratory failure in patients with an abscess, but many patients who develop pulmonary dysfunction are not septic, indicating that other causes are clearly involved. High concentrations of pancreatic enzymes in the circulation at the time of acute pancreatitis may also contribute to respiratory failure. Intravenous infusion of trypsin in sheep increases pulmonary lymph flow and pulmonary transvascular protein clearance. Pretreatment of these animals with a trypsin inhibitor (i.e., aprotinin [Trasylol]) prevents the increased pulmonary vascular permeability.[51] Pulmonary leukostasis with capillary sludging also results from trypsin infusion and is inhibited with aprotinin pretreatment.

Free fatty acids in the circulation can cause respiratory failure, and they may be released as a result of lipolytic digestion of fat by lipase in acute pancreatitis. Serum triglycerides are elevated in some patients with pancreatitis, particularly those patients with a history of chronic alcoholism and/or disorders in lipid metabolism. Experiments performed with isolated dog lungs have confirmed the injurious effects of free fatty acids.[26] Furthermore, histologic studies of diseased lungs in pancreatitis patients have demonstrated the presence of fat emboli.[28]

Phospholipase A_2 (PLA_2) has also been recovered from the serum of patients with acute pancreatitis who developed respiratory failure. The magnitude of pulmonary derangement appears to correlate closely with the level of PLA_2 elevation. The proposed mechanism of action of PLA_2 is through the dissolution of pulmonary surfactant. In patients with the highest levels of PLA_2, neither peritoneal lavage nor pancreatectomy alters the course of respiratory failure.

Endocrine Alterations (Table 28-1). Elevated blood glucose concentrations approaching 130 to 200 mg/100 ml occur in 50% to 75% of patients with acute pancreatitis. However, glucosuria occurs in only approximately one third of patients with hyperglycemia. Although blood sugars greater than 200 mg/100 ml are associated with increased mortality rates,[41] death rarely occurs as the result of the hyperglycemia itself. The majority of the patients die from other serious complications of pancreatitis.

Table 28-1 **ENDOCRINE ABNORMALITIES IN ACUTE PANCREATITIS**

Abnormality	Proposed Mechanism
Hyperglycemia (130-200 mg/100 ml) (Returns to normal 18 to 21 days after resolution of pancreatitis)	Serum glucagon concentrations are greater than serum insulin concentrations in the basal and stimulated state
	Elevation of growth hormone
Hypocalcemia (True or ionized fraction)	Hyperglucagonemia Hypercalcitoninemia Hypoalbuminemia Hypomagnesemia Defect in parathyroid metabolism

A number of factors contribute to the hyperglycemia observed in pancreatitis.[4] In general, both serum glucagon and insulin concentrations are elevated in patients with stress. However, serum insulin concentrations are not high enough to prevent hyperglycemia in these patients. In patients with acute pancreatitis the serum glucagon concentrations are much higher, and the insulin concentrations are lower than in patients with stress from other causes. Serum growth hormone and cortisol concentrations are also higher in patients with acute pancreatitis.

Intravenous infusion of arginine or alanine stimulates moderate secretion of both glucagon and insulin in healthy people. Infusion of these secretagogues in patients with acute pancreatitis results in an increase in serum glucagon concentration that is 9 to 10 times greater than normal and 50% greater than that seen in patients with other forms of stress. Likewise, serum insulin concentrations after secretagogue infusion in pancreatitis patients are 2 to 6 times greater than the normal response.

Fasting hyperglycemia, hyperglucagonemia, and the response to alanine and arginine infusion all change during resolution of pancreatitis. During the first 48 to 72 hours after the onset of the disease, there is a significant fasting hyperglycemia along with hyperglucagonemia and hypoinsulinemia. The elevated concentrations of glucagon and glucose usually return to normal within 18 to 21 days of the resolution of pancreatitis, but the hyperglucagonemia may resolve spontaneously and unpredictably. Impairment of insulin secretion with arginine infusion may continue up to a month after resolution of pancreatitis. Thus administration of high concentrations of insulin to these patients to correct the blood glucose levels may be dangerous, and mild hyperglycemia should be tolerated.

Mild hypocalcemia is seen frequently in patients with pancreatitis and a number of factors may be contributory. A significant portion of serum calcium is normally bound to albumin, and hypoalbuminemia is common in acute pancreatitis; thus the serum ionized calcium is often normal in spite of a low total serum calcium. Fat necrosis with sequestration of calcium in soaps may account for the loss of as much as 1 to 2 g of calcium. Yet neither of these explanations accounts for the severe hypocalcemia sometimes seen in pancreatitis.

In patients with acute pancreatitis, parathyroid hormone (PTH) production and release and peripheral activity in response to hypocalcemia are all normal. Patients with true ionized hypocalcemia have elevated serum PTH concentrations.[23] These concentrations, however, decrease as serum ionized calcium returns to normal. Hypocalciuria and decreased tubular reabsorption of phosphate indicate normal action of PTH in the kidney. Infusion of PTH into patients with acute pancreatitis and hypocalcemia results in increased serum calcium and urinary cyclic AMP indicating unimpaired action of PTH on bone.

Serum concentrations of calcitonin are elevated up to six times the normal amount in hypocalcemic patients with pancreatitis. Evidence exists that the increase in serum calcitonin may precede the hypocalcemia.[9] Infusion of glucagon in healthy humans results in increased serum calcitonin concentrations. Thus hyperglucagonemia may account for the hypercalcitoninemia in acute pancreatitis patients. Against this hypothesis is the observation that the infusion of glucagon in patients with acute pancreatitis does not increase serum calcitonin levels further or change serum ionized calcium concentrations.[4]

Finally, hypomagnesemia may also be present in patients with acute pancreatitis, although it is not always seen in conjunction with hypocalcemia. Correction of hypocalcemia may be impossible without also correcting the hypomagnesemia.

Physiologic Basis of Diagnosis

Clinical Appearance

The diagnosis of acute pancreatitis is based on information in the patient's history, physical findings, laboratory studies (Table 28-2), and observation of the clinical course after institution of treatment.[34] In some instances the diagnosis is in doubt, and the patient is sufficiently ill to require performance of a laparotomy to exclude other catastrophic processes.

Clinically, a patient with acute pancreatitis is initially seen with midepigastric or right upper-quadrant pain that radiates to the back. Onset of pain may be related to eating a large meal. The severity of the pain is variable, although in most cases it is significant enough to cause the patient to seek medical care. The pain is unrelenting and is often associated with nausea or vomiting. Low-grade fever is common. In severe cases tachycardia and orthostatic hypotension may reflect significant fluid sequestration in the abdomen.

Physical examination reveals abdominal tenderness and guarding in the upper abdomen, although the entire abdomen may be diffusely tender. This tenderness is a result of peritoneal irritation by intraperitoneal fluid, which may contain pancreatic enzymes and other noxious substances. Bowel sounds are decreased or absent. There may be splinting of respirations and decreased breath sounds over the lung bases. In patients with hemorrhagic pancreatitis, when blood dissects throughout the retroperitoneum, a bluish discoloration in the flanks (Grey Turner's sign) or in the periumbilical area (Cullen's sign) may be seen.

Most patients with acute pancreatitis have an elevated serum amylase concentration.[53] However, other intra-abdominal conditions may also be associated with moderate elevations in serum amylase level, and some of these conditions (e.g., acute cholecystitis, small bowel infarction, and duodenal perforation) can mimic acute pancreatitis. Thus an elevated serum amylase concentration alone will not always distinguish one disorder from the other.

Table 28-2 **LABORATORY DIAGNOSIS OF ACUTE PANCREATITIS**

Enzyme Elevation	Principle*
Serum amylase concentration	Release of enzyme into circulation
Urinary amylase excretion Amylase/creatinine clearance ratio	Increased renal clearance of amylase in acute pancreatitis
Isoamylases	P-amylase specific to pancreas—increased in acute pancreatitis
Serum lipase	Release from acinar cells or ducts into circulation—no renal clearance

*There may be a failure in the elevation of serum enzymes and amylase/creatinine clearance ratio in patients with acute pancreatitis that is superimposed on chronic pancreatitis.

Amylase exists in the form of isoenzymes that are designated as salivary (S) and pancreatic (P). The S-isoamylase is the predominant form in normal serum and constitutes approximately 60% of total serum amylase. The pancreas is the only organ that contains P-isoamylase in concentrations higher than in serum. S-isoamylase is found in the salivary glands, lungs, and prostate gland. In acute pancreatitis the elevated serum amylase is predominantly the P-isoamylase. Thus measurement of the specific pancreatic fraction in patients with suspected acute pancreatitis could increase the specificity of the test. However, isoenzyme measurements in patients with acute illness are usually not practical or cost-effective and therefore have not found wide clinical application.

During acute pancreatitis renal function changes so that there is an increased clearance of amylase by the kidneys when compared with creatinine.[24] Large amounts of P-isoamylase are found in the urine. The renal clearance of amylase does not change when the serum amylase level is increased for other reasons. This increased renal clearance of amylase is the basis for the use of the amylase-creatinine clearance ratio (ACCR) to diagnose pancreatitis. It requires "simultaneously" obtaining urine and blood samples and analyzing them for amylase and creatinine concentrations. For most patients the clearance ratio probably is no better than the determination of the serum and/or urinary amylase in making the diagnosis of acute pancreatitis. It may, however, help to differentiate patients with acute pancreatitis from those with elevated amylase levels from other intra-abdominal diseases. Because the ACCR may be abnormally elevated in other conditions such as diabetic ketoacidosis and thermal burns, its specificity is thereby limited.

Determination of the serum lipase concentration may be more valuable.[53] The major source of lipase is the pan-

Table 28-3 **PARAMETERS FOR PREDICTING SEVERITY OF ACUTE PANCREATITIS ON THE BASIS OF LOCAL AND SYSTEMIC CRITERIA**

Ranson's Criteria	Satiani and Stone
Initial	
Age over 55 years	Oral temperature >39° C
WBCs >16,000	Respiratory distress (Pao_2 <60 mm Hg)
Blood glucose >200 mg/100 ml	Shock requiring extensive resuscitation
Serum LDH >350 IU/L	WBCs >15,000
Serum SGOT >250 Sigma Frankel U/100 ml	Serum calcium <7 mg/100 ml
During initial 48 hrs	
Hematocrit fall >ten percentage points	
BUN rise >5mg/100 ml	
Serum calcium concentration <8mg/100 ml	
HCO_3^- deficit >4 mEq/L	
Pao_2 <60 mm Hg	
Fluid sequestration >6000 ml	

creas, and it is found in very few other tissues; there are no known isoenzymes of this substance. The serum lipase concentration increases at approximately the same time as serum amylase in patients with acute pancreatitis and provides the same sort of information that serum amylase does. Lipase is not excreted in the urine, and its clearance cannot be measured. Until recently, the method of assay has been difficult, but it is now becoming more standardized. It may become a more valuable test to identify patients with acute pancreatitis in the future.

Other pancreatic enzymes (trypsin, elastase, phospholipase A_2, and ribonuclease) have been measured in the serum and body fluids of patients with acute pancreatitis. Although these tests may provide some additional specificity for pancreatitis when the diagnosis is equivocal, they are not widely available in most institutions.

Prediction of Severity

Estimation of the severity of an attack of acute pancreatitis is important for assessment of potential morbidity and mortality. In individuals experiencing more than one attack, there is no correlation between the severity of individual episodes, and each must be evaluated alone. Ranson demonstrated that a number of factors predict the severity of pancreatitis and the likelihood of death.[41] They are listed in Table 28-3. The mortality rate correlated closely with the number of positive factors. Because these factors provide information from a variety of organ systems, they indicate the magnitude of the effect of pancreatitis throughout the body. Nonetheless, Ranson's system has been somewhat cumbersome to use. To indicate the severity of pancreatitis, Satiani and Stone[50] have identified a variety of clinical parameters that can be evaluated more quickly (Table 28-3).

The severity of the systemic effects of pancreatitis correlates also with the pathologic changes in the pancreas. Thus patients with a larger number of Ranson's positive signs (>4) were much more likely to demonstrate necrotizing and hemorrhagic pancreatitis. However, even though patients with fewer than four positive signs were more likely to have only edematous pancreatitis, many still had serious complications, some of which required surgery.

Paracentesis with examination of the peritoneal fluid in patients with acute pancreatitis also identifies the severity of pancreatitis.[40] Hemorrhagic pancreatitis is more likely to be associated with larger volumes of fluid during the initial aspiration (>10 ml free fluid) and with free fluid that is brown, purple, or dark straw in color.

Combined evaluation of the peritoneal fluid, the biochemical abnormalities associated with pancreatic disease, and the clinical appearance gives the best possible initial assessment of the severity of pancreatitis. The character of the peritoneal fluid is a reflection of the peripancreatic inflammatory process, and when abnormal, it indicates extension outside of the gland. Derangements in other organ systems generally indicate severe pathology within the pancreas and the need for aggressive management to minimize complications and the increased incidence of a fatal outcome.

Treatment of Acute Pancreatitis

Medical Treatment

The first goal of nonoperative treatment of acute pancreatitis is to stop or limit the progression of the disease. Other goals are to replace losses from fluid sequestration and to treat any associated organ failure.

To limit the progression of disease, stimulation of the pancreas is avoided. In some cases attempts have been made to inhibit secretion. Nasograstric suction prevents gastric acid from entering the duodenum and thus avoids the release of the duodenal hormone secretin that would result in pancreatic secretion. Fat and protein in the diet are the primary stimuli for cholecystokinin release from the duodenum, so food is withheld. The production of gastric acid can be limited by the use of atropine or cimetidine. However, controlled trials using these agents have failed to show any advantage. Cimetidine may also be used for patients with a history of peptic ulcer disease to minimize the resurgence of active ulcer-related pathology that occasionally occurs in a stressful situation such as pancreatitis.

Efforts to inhibit active pancreatic secretion have involved the use of hormones such as glucagon and somatostatin. Clinical trials with glucagon in patients with acute pancreatitis did not show any improvement in mortality or morbidity.[37] A similar but less complete experience has accumulated with somatostatin.[52a] Thus although the secretory state of the pancreas during the initiation or the progression of pancreatitis may be important, pharmacologic efforts to inhibit secretion have not been effective. This ineffectiveness may relate to a general inability of the pancreas to respond to physiologic stimuli during acute inflammation.

As previously noted, proteolytic enzyme activity may be important in the progression of systemic complications. Thus efforts have been made to limit the activation and action of pancreatic enzymes released during pancreatitis. Trypsin is normally produced when trypsinogen is activated by enterokinase in the duodenum. Trypsin can then activate all of the other pancreatic enzymes. Trypsin is normally inactivated when it combines with serum and tissue antiproteases, but they are rapidly saturated. The degree of antiprotease saturation may be important clinically because the amount of free (active) trypsin in the circulation correlates with the progression of the disease. Free trypsin would then be available to initiate further activation of enzymes and other humoral systems or to produce direct tissue damage. The trypsin inhibitor aprotinin has been used to inactivate any such free trypsin that might be present, but clinical trials in humans have not shown any beneficial effect. The reasons for its failure could be that other enzymes may be activated independent of trypsin and may be responsible for the systemic complications, that proteases may not be all that important in the disease and its complications, or that this inhibitor is not sufficiently potent in inactivating trypsin. On the other hand, some studies have demonstrated limitation of the severity of respiratory failure in animals given aprotinin before the induction of pancreatitis.[51]

Antibiotics have not been proven to be beneficial as a routine treatment measure in acute pancreatitis. Controlled studies of the use of parenteral ampicillin and cephalosporin have not altered either the course of pancreatitis or the number and the severity of its complications.[14,21] However, when an abscess is suspected, broad-spectrum antibiotics should be used as an adjunct to surgical drainage.[15]

The management of acute pancreatitis without surgery demands close follow-up with frequent reexamination of the patient. Fever of 101° to 102° F is common during the early course of the disease and at this stage rarely signals that an abscess is developing. Later in the course of the disease, however, the presence of an abscess may be heralded by return of fever and leukocytosis.

Most patients tolerate uncomplicated episodes of pancreatitis well. Severe cases may require prolonged supportive treatment, and significant morbidity can result from associated malnutrition. Thus parenteral nutrition is useful in this clinical setting, but studies indicate that this form of nutrition by itself does not influence the course of the disease. The same is true for enteral nutrition using elemental diets.

Peritoneal Lavage

Peritoneal fluid aspiration may be of value in assessing the severity of acute pancreatitis. If examination of this fluid suggests a more severe form of the disease, accompanying peritoneal lavage may be useful as adjunctive treatment. To examine the peritoneal fluid, a percutaneous lavage catheter is inserted into the abdomen, and, if present, a sample of fluid is aspirated. In healthy patients, the fluid in the abdominal cavity is scant and clear. In patients with mild acute pancreatitis, a slightly greater volume of a straw-colored fluid is retrieved. In necrotizing and hemorrhagic pancreatitis, greater volumes of fluid that may be bloody or prune juice in color are returned. These latter findings are associated with a worse prognosis.[33]

If a severe form of pancreatitis appears to exist after examination of the fluid, the abdominal cavity may be lavaged with either lactated Ringer's solution or peritoneal dialysis fluid (Dianeal solution). Generally 1 L of fluid at a time is infused into the peritoneal cavity and allowed to remain in the abdomen for 30 to 60 minutes before drainage. This process is repeated multiple times during the subsequent 24 to 36 hours. With therapeutic peritoneal lavage, prompt improvement in cardiovascular and renal function is common.[40] The fluid retrieved from the abdomen contains large concentrations of pancreatic enzymes and vasoactive substances. These substances can alter physiologic functions throughout the body, and their removal may prevent their passage into plasma. Alternatively, peritoneal lavage may act through dialysis across the peritoneal epithelium to remove toxins and proteases from the blood. Early mortality from respiratory and cardiovascular failure has been decreased dramatically by this approach. Unfortunately, late mortality from sepsis is not decreased with use of this therapeutic modality and has continued to be a problem in these critically ill patients. It is in this situation that more aggressive surgical management may prove beneficial.

Surgical Treatment

Generally edematous pancreatitis can be managed medically. If the clinical appearance suggests that the disease has progressed to a necrotic and/or hemorrhagic variety, surgery may be an appropriate treatment option. There are two theoretic reasons for considering pancreatectomy in patients with necrotizing pancreatitis.[43] First, the progress of pancreatic and peripancreatic necrosis would be stopped by removing the gland. Second, the distant cardiovascular, respiratory, and renal effects would be minimized by removing the source of lipolytic and proteolytic enzymes. In practice, however, the value of such an approach has not been demonstrated. In a controlled study from Europe comparing peritoneal lavage and pancreatectomy, pancreatic resection was not shown to be a more effective treatment alternative.[27]

Complications of Acute Pancreatitis

Pseudocysts develop in approximately 2% of patients with acute pancreatitis and should be suspected when recovery from the acute episode is prolonged; an ultrasound or a computed tomography examination confirms their presence. Pancreatic pseudocysts are fluid-filled spaces that probably result from local exudation of fluid during acute inflammation of the pancreas. The enzyme content of the fluid is usually quite high (>1000 IU of amylase/L). The inflammatory reaction in the adjacent organs and tissues results in a fibrous capsule (without an epithelial lining) that matures over a 4- to 6-week period. Major complications of pseudocysts include spontaneous rupture, infection, or hemorrhage. All of these conditions are potentially life threatening. Although many pseudocysts resolve spontaneously following resolution of the acute episode of pancreatitis, a substantial number persist. Because of the complications associated with pseudocysts, the ones that persist should be drained once they have developed a mature capsule. Drainage, when indicated, is usually accomplished by suturing the cyst wall to a defunctionalized loop of intestine (i.e., jejunum) thereby allowing the cyst contents to drain into the gut lumen.

Pancreatic abscess is a complication in approximately 5% of the patients with acute pancreatitis and is invariably fatal if it is not drained. Administration of antibiotics during the course of acute pancreatitis does not decrease the incidence of abscess. As is true in patients with a pancreatic pseudocyst, the presence of abscess is signaled by the persistence of symptoms in a patient with pancreatitis or the return of symptoms after temporary recovery. Drainage of a pancreatic abscess is mandatory, and antibiotics should be administered before the drainage is performed as adjunctive therapy. The organisms cultured from pancreatic abscesses are usually a variety of gram-negative and gram-positive enteric flora. Although a formal operation is usually required to drain the abscess adequately in selected cases percutaneous aspiration has proven successful.[20] In addition, this technique has been used to establish the diagnosis of abscess when the clinical assessment has been uncertain.[20]

Pancreatic ascites is caused by the chronic leakage of fluid from a pseudocyst or from a disrupted pancreatic duct. The clinical syndrome is characterized by ascites and malnutrition and is frequently seen in an alcoholic patient with chronic pancreatitis. The distinction between patients with pancreatic ascites or with cirrhotic ascites is made by finding high concentrations of protein (>2.9 g/100 ml) in the ascitic fluid of the former. The amylase content is also usually quite high. The malnutrition may result from the loss of pancreatic enzymes from the intestine and their sequestration in the abdomen. An endoscopic pancreatogram to demonstrate the site of leakage should be obtained. If the leak is secondary to a pancreatic pseudocyst, surgical drainage should be accomplished. If the leak is caused by a disrupted pancreatic duct, a trial of parenteral nutrition should be undertaken since many of these ducts will close spontaneously. In the event that closure does not occur, surgery should be performed, and the disrupted duct should be drained into a loop of intestine.

CHRONIC PANCREATITIS

Ninety percent of the cases of chronic pancreatitis are a result of chronic alcohol ingestion. The rest are a result of hyperparathyroidism, protein malnutrition, pancreatic duct obstruction, and a variety of less common causes. Gallstone pancreatitis rarely leads to chronic pancreatitis, although attacks may recur until the offending stones are removed. Patients with alcoholic pancreatitis may have repeated episodes of acute pancreatitis with a trend toward progressive destruction of pancreatic parenchyma and loss of function. Usually the patient has consumed alcohol heavily for a considerable time (100 to 200 g/day for 5 to 10 years) before the first episode of pancreatitis. Although pancreatitis may follow binge drinking in an alcoholic patient, overindulgence by the *non*alcoholic person is a distinctly rare cause of acute pancreatitis. Alcoholic patients with ''acute'' pancreatitis when seen initially probably already have substantial destruction of the gland. Calcifications of the pancreas that are visible on an abdominal x-ray film are commonly seen in patients with chronic pancreatitis and are associated clinically with exocrine insufficiency (75%) and glucose intolerance (30%). Thus the term ''chronic'' implies irreversible destruction of tissue and function.

Although severe abdominal pain is the most common initial complaint in patients with chronic pancreatitis, on rare occasions pain may be absent, and the initial complaints may be malabsorption and diabetes (<5%), the results of acinar and islet cell destruction within the pancreas. Morphologic changes of chronic pancreatic damage are evident in up to 50% of alcoholics during autopsy regardless of whether they have exocrine and endocrine deficiency symptomatically during life.

Pathology

Grossly, the pancreas in a patient with chronic pancreatitis is usually firm and fibrotic, smaller than normal, and with rounded edges. Its anteroposterior diameter may be increased, and if the main pancreatic duct is dilated, it may be palpable as a longitudinal ridge on the anterior surface of the gland during autopsy or surgery. In some cases, the inflammatory process may extend to the surrounding organs with duodenal and colonic fibrous strictures resulting in mechanical obstruction. Pseudocysts are also common in patients with alcoholic pancreatitis.

Histologically, intralobular and extralobular fibrosis is distributed randomly throughout the gland. Proteinaceous precipitates, which may later calcify, are found in the small ducts and are responsible for the calcifications seen on x-ray. As the disease progresses, the small pancreatic ducts as well as the main duct may dilate. Intrapancreatic inflammation of neural elements are common in advanced cases and may account for the marked pain that many patients have. As the fibrosis progresses, less functional exocrine and endocrine tissue remains.

Pathogenesis of Chronic Pancreatitis

Alcohol

In humans, at least two modifications in normal pancreatic physiology are induced by chronic alcohol consumption and may play a part in the pathogenesis of chronic pancreatitis.[48] First, there is an increased concentration of protein present in the pancreatic juice, which may promote the precipitation of protein plugs in the small ducts. Second, there is a decreased concentration of citrate, which normally is secreted by the pancreas in parallel with protein. Because citrate is able to dissolve pancreatic stones and to decrease calcite crystal formation, lower concentrations could favor the development of stones.

Citrate is not the only stabilizer of calcium in pancreatic juice. A protein with a molecular weight of 13,500 that is synthesized in the acinar cells may also be important. This pancreatic stone protein is able to prevent the precipitation of calcium carbonate in a supersaturated solution of calcium that mimics the ionic composition of pancreatic juice. In at least two thirds of patients with chronic calcifying pancreatitis from a variety of causes (alcoholic, hereditary, and idiopathic), its concentration in pancreatic juice is much lower than normal. Thus its decreased concentration might play a role in the pathogenesis of chronic pancreatitis.

Recent evidence suggests that the pancreas, like the liver, is able to metabolize ethanol.[10] The possibility of altered metabolism in patients with alcoholic pancreatitis is currently being investigated.

Pancreatic Duct Obstruction

The role of pancreatic duct obstruction in chronic pancreatitis is incompletely defined. Partial and complete obstruction of the main pancreatic duct in experimental animals and in humans results in dilation of the pancreatic duct and progressive atrophy of acinar tissue with replacement of lobules by fibrous tissue. However, there is a histologic difference between alcoholic pancreatitis and that caused by duct obstruction. In the latter the fibrosis is distributed uniformly throughout the gland, whereas in alcoholic pancreatitis the changes are random.

The degree of obstruction is important in the development of both functional and histologic changes.[5] In cats, obstruction of the main pancreatic duct for 12 weeks by more than 75% of the luminal diameter impaired bicarbonate, water, and protein secretion.[38] Lesser degrees of obstruction decreased enzyme secretion, but the ability to produce high concentrations of bicarbonate was retained. The histologic changes correlated well with the secretory changes. Periductal fibrosis and duct dilation were most impressive in cats with greater degrees of obstruction, but some perilobular fibrosis and acinar atrophy were found in all animals. Unrelieved obstruction resulted in progressive secretory impairment and replacement of the gland with fibrous tissue. Although experimental pancreatic duct obstruction leads to pancreatic duct dilation, a dilated duct in a patient with alcoholic chronic pancreatitis may occur without apparent obstruction.

Pancreatic duct obstruction may be more important in the pathogenesis of other forms of chronic pancreatitis (e.g., duct stricture and pancreas divisum). When pancreatitis develops in patients with pancreas divisum, the main duct drains into the duodenum through an abnormally narrow accessory papilla. If the obstruction is relieved before irreversible parenchymal changes occur, chronic pancreatitis may be averted.

Diagnosis

The diagnosis of chronic pancreatitis is usually straightforward, especially in alcoholic patients with diabetes, upper-abdominal pain, and pancreatic calcifications seen on an x-ray film. In some patients the diagnosis is less obvious. In these instances, a computed tomography (CT) scan or ultrasound may demonstrate the firm, dense, constricted pancreas characteristic of chronic pancreatitis. Likewise, endoscopic retrograde cholangiopancreatography (ERCP) may prove helpful in making a diagnosis by demonstrating multiple constrictions and obliterations throughout the pancreatic ductal system. Tests of pancreatic function are sometimes useful in demonstrating altered secretory activity and may provide the only indication of pancreatic disease.

Because the pancreas possesses a large functional reserve, steatorrhea does not occur until approximately 85% of its function has been lost.[12] Then diarrhea and large bulky stools result from the malabsorption. However, tests of pancreatic secretory ability can detect milder functional abnormalities. Several kinds of tests are available. One requires intubation of the duodenum with a gastroduodenal tube for collection of pancreatic juice. Pancreatic secretion is stimulated either by the intravenous administration of cholecystokinin and/or secretin or by the consumption of a standard meal. Duodenal juice is then collected and analyzed for its enzyme and bicarbonate content. In chronic pancreatitis, the volume of juice secreted is low, and usually the concentrations of enzymes and bicarbonate are likewise impaired (Table 28-4). In most institutions where these tests are performed, the hormonal stimulation method is preferred because it is easier to standardize and the results are easier to interpret. However, both tests are somewhat cumbersome to perform.

The other kind of pancreatic function test is simpler to perform because it does not require the placement of a duodenal tube. Bentiromide, a synthetic peptide linked to a para-aminobenzoic acid (PABA), which stimulates pancreatic secretion, is fed to the patient with a standard meal. Chymotrypsin in the pancreatic juice selectively cleaves the bentiromide molecule to liberate PABA. PABA is absorbed and excreted in the urine where it is assayed. Although the test is simple, it is less sensitive than the hormonal stimulation method already described. For this reason, milder degrees of pancreatic insufficiency may be overlooked. Unfortunately, even the most sensitive techniques probably detect only moderately advanced pancreatic insufficiency, i.e., patients with more than 50% loss of function.

The major clinical value of secretory testing is to differentiate pancreatic insufficiency from other causes of malabsorption such as celiac disease. Serial testing may be useful in studying progressive deterioration in an individual patient.

ERCP is more sensitive than function tests in diagnosing chronic pancreatitis, but it also has limitations. In a recent study its sensitivity was evaluated in a group of 200 patients with the disease.[45] It was disappointing that 15% of

Table 28-4 **CHARACTERISTICS OF PANCREATIC JUICE IN HEALTHY PATIENTS AND THOSE WITH CHRONIC PANCREATITIS**

	Volume	$[HCO_3^-]$	HCO_3^- Output†	Lipase Output	Trypsin Output
Healthy patients	3-5 ml/kg/hr*	100-135 mEq/L	15-35 mEq/hr	150 KU/hr	35 KU/hr
Patients with chronic pancreatitis	2 ml/kg/hr	90 mEq/L	10 mEq/hr	25 KU/hr	10 KU/hr

*Expressed as ml/kg bodyweight/hr.

†Output (i.e., the total number of units or milliequivalents) is a reflection of volume *and* concentration.

the patients without pancreatic calcifications had normal ERCP findings. In 7.5% of the patients the study could not be performed for technical reasons. The most significant features of chronic pancreatitis as seen on ERCP included dilation and irregular caliber of the main pancreatic duct and its side branches, variation in the caliber of the side branches, a tortuous main duct in the body and tail of the pancreas, and the presence of ductal stones.

Nonoperative Management

The initial management of chronic pancreatitis is nonoperative and involves the treatment of malabsorption and diabetes and the control of abdominal pain.[3]

Pain

Early in the disease abdominal pain may occur only in association with recurrent episodes of acute pancreatitis. With progression, it occurs more frequently, and each episode lasts longer so that patients may experience pain on a daily basis. Frequently patients consume alcohol in an attempt to relieve the discomfort, and many become addicted to narcotics.

All patients should be advised to stop drinking alcohol, but even if they do, the effect on pain relief is uncertain. Stopping drinking is more likely to be beneficial in those with "early" disease who still have residual pancreatic function. With far-advanced disease where most of the exocrine function has been lost, the relationship between continued drinking and the persistence of pain is less clear. On the other hand, these latter patients are more likely to experience spontaneous pain relief as the disease progresses. This observation provides a clue to the mechanism of pain that appears to be related to the ability of the pancreas to secrete. It also explains why pancreatic enzyme replacement therapy may help to relieve pain in some patients, presumably because such treatment inhibits pancreatic secretion.

Malabsorption

Although many patients limit their oral intake of food because it causes pain, malabsorption also can be an important cause of malnutrition. When malabsorption occurs, carbohydrates continue to be well absorbed, but creatorrhea (undigested meat fibers in stool) and especially steatorrhea may require treatment. Generally patients should be given diets with liberal amounts of carbohydrate (400 g or more) and protein (100 to 150 g) and as much fat as can be tolerated without the production of diarrhea. Even when an optimum treatment regimen has been established, fat malabsorption and steatorrhea will continue, posing no problem as long as diarrhea is controlled and nutrition is adequate. If fat ingestion is aggravating, medium chain triglycerides, which are absorbed directly in the small bowel without pancreatic enzyme action, may be helpful in improving nutritional deficiencies. Vitamin supplements are important in dietary management as well.

The absorption of ingested nutrients may be improved by the oral replacement of pancreatic enzymes, but several problems limit the efficiency of such therapy.[2,3] Chronic alcoholism frequently injures the small bowel mucosa so that intestinal absorption may be impaired. Chronic pancreatitis is associated as well with diminished gastric acid secretion and delayed gastric motility and emptying. Perhaps because of impaired acid neutralization by pancreatic bicarbonate, the duodenal pH is lower than normal after the patient eats. This change is particularly important because lipase is inactivated at low pH.

Sufficient enzyme replacement should be provided to supply 30,000 to 50,000 U of lipase to be taken with each of four meals daily. If diarrhea remains a problem, a reduction in dietary fat may help. In some patients, cimetidine, 300 mg one-half hour before meals, along with the oral enzymes taken with each meal, is effective. This regimen presumably reduces intragastric acid and the intraduodenal destruction of lipase by decreasing acid secretion.

Diabetes

Diabetes is common in patients with chronic pancreatitis. Most patients have glucose intolerance initially and then develop overt diabetes as the disease progresses. Complications such as retinopathy and peripheral vascular disease are less common than in patients with adult-onset diabetes mellitus, but because many patients with chronic pancreatitis are unreliable alcoholics, complications related to insulin therapy are more common. Chronic pancreatitis patients have low basal serum insulin concentrations that do not increase adequately after eating. In contrast, basal serum insulin concentrations are characteristically high in patients with adult-onset diabetes and increase with eating by as much as twofold. Although the islets are relatively well preserved during chronic pancreatitis, they are surrounded by variable amounts of fibrous tissue. This tissue may prevent the hormones (i.e., insulin and glucagon) from entering the lymphatics and capillaries draining the islets.

Because oral agents to lower blood sugar are not often effective in managing diabetes, most patients require insulin therapy. Since insulin reactions are common, mild hyperglycemia and glucosuria should be tolerated.

Surgical Treatment

The major indication for surgical intervention in chronic pancreatitis is to relieve the chronic intractable pain from which many of these patients suffer. Two surgical approaches have been used for this purpose. They include: (1) drainage operations, during which an attempt is made to relieve ductal obstruction; and (2) resection operations, during which diseased pancreatic tissue is removed. Choice of surgical procedure is best made using knowledge of duct anatomy, which may be obtained preoperatively through ERCP or at the time of surgery through operative pancreatography. Even without pancreatography, the presence of large (>0.5 cm) calculi seen on plain abdominal x-ray film reliably indicates a dilated duct system. Because dilated ducts imply obstruction, drainage operations are usually successful when they are present. Pancreatectomy may be indicated when the ducts are not dilated, the disease is confined to one segment of the gland, and the rest of the gland is relatively normal or when a previous drainage procedure has been unsuccessful. Alcoholic patients who have stopped drinking but still have pain are usually the best surgical candidates.

Drainage Procedures

A lateral (longitudinal) pancreatojejunostomy (Puestow procedure) is the most extensive of the drainage procedures and the one most frequently performed (Fig. 28-1). It involves a longitudinal incision in the pancreas through the anterior wall of the main pancreatic duct. A Roux-en-Y limb of jejunum is then sutured to the opened duct along its length so that the pancreatic juice drains directly into the small intestine. Ductal calculi and other debris are also removed.

Theoretically, preoperative exocrine insufficiency might be expected to improve after drainage procedures since pancreatic enzymes, with the obstruction relieved, can empty more easily into the gut. Although improvement might occur in some cases, this result has been impossible to document clinically, and the surgery should never be performed in an attempt to improve malabsorption. There is also no evidence to suggest that functional recovery from parenchymal regeneration occurs after drainage procedures.[2] On the other hand, since the pancreatic juice is diverted from the second portion of the duodenum and enters the small bowel more distally after pancreatojejunostomy, some worsening of the malabsorption might be expected because food would not mix as well with whatever pancreatic enzymes were present. In practice, however, pancreatic drainage procedures of this kind almost never make a clinically significant impact on the degree of malabsorption.

No immediate change in insulin requirement is seen after pancreatojejunostomy. However, in one series of patients followed for 10 years after pancreatojejunostomy, approximately 20% experienced worsening of their diabetes,[52] which was probably a result of the continuing glandular (and islet) destruction with time since the inflammatory process was not arrested by the surgery.

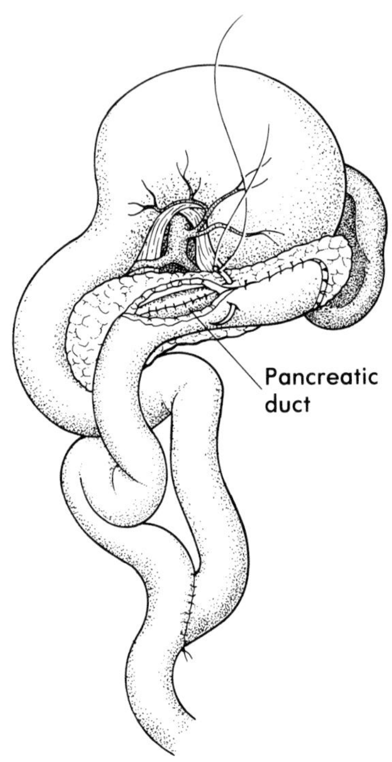

Fig. 28-1 Lateral (longitudinal) pancreatojejunostomy (Puestow procedure) is the most frequently used drainage procedure for chronic pancreatitis. A Roux-en-Y limb of jejunum is sutured to the opened pancreatic duct along its length. (From Way, L.: Current surgical diagnosis and treatment, Los Altos, Calif., 1985, Lange Medical Books.)

Resection Operations

When pancreatic parenchyma is removed, insufficiency is more frequent. Its severity is related to the amount of functional tissue that remains (Fig. 28-2). With distal resections of 40% or less, pancreatic insufficiency is usually no different than it was before surgery. In resections that remove 50% to 80% of the distal pancreas, clinically significant steatorrhea appears anew in at least 20% of the patients. Diabetes mellitus also worsens in 20% to 30% of the patients. In patients undergoing 80% to 95% distal resections, approximately 50% may expect a worsening of both steatorrhea and diabetes. Distal resections, although removing variable amounts of parenchyma, do not alter gastric emptying and the mixing of food with pancreatic juice. Pancreatoduodenectomy (Whipple procedure) (Fig.

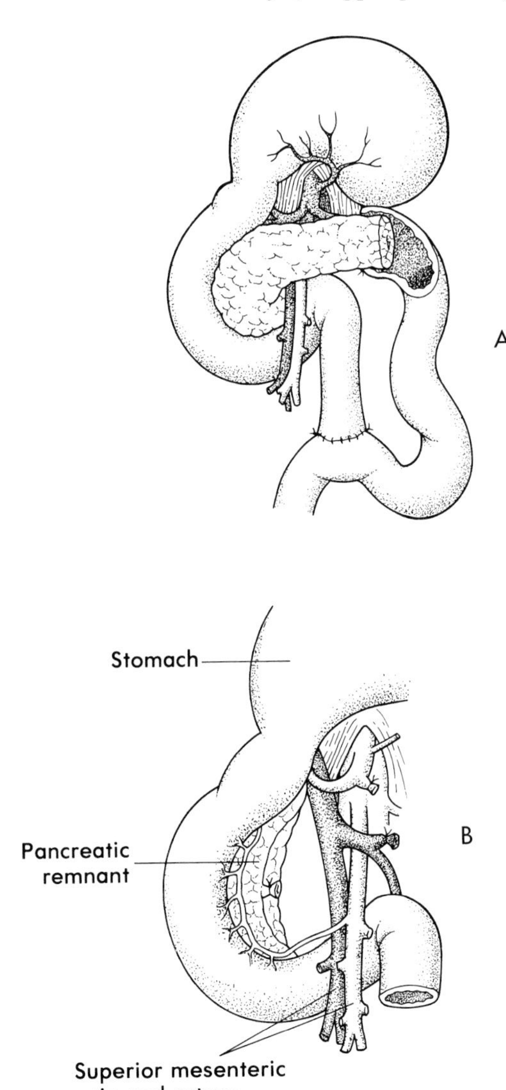

Fig. 28-2 Surgical resection for chronic pancreatitis. **A,** Distal resection of the pancreas with pancreatojejunostomy. **B,** Subtotal pancreatectomy. (From Way, L.: Current surgical diagnosis and treatment, Los Altos, Calif., 1985, Lange Medical Books.)

28-3), on the other hand, significantly alters this relationship. Thus at least 55% of patients experience clinically troublesome steatorrhea after this operation, which involves distal gastrectomy and gastrojejunostomy as well as pancreatic resection. Since at least 50% of the pancreas remains following this procedure, the changes incident to the gastric surgery are probably responsible for much of the malabsorption.

Diabetes after pancreatoduodenectomy is worsened in only approximately 10% of the patients. When total pancreatectomy is performed, all patients require insulin and pancreatic enzyme replacement. Although both diabetes and malabsorption can be managed in these patients, to do so is particularly difficult in irresponsible alcoholics who may be addicted to narcotics. In this group, the mortality associated with poor diabetic control is significant. Thus total pancreatectomy should almost never be performed under these circumstances.

SUMMARY

There are a number of causes of acute pancreatitis. The individual mechanisms have not been clearly established.

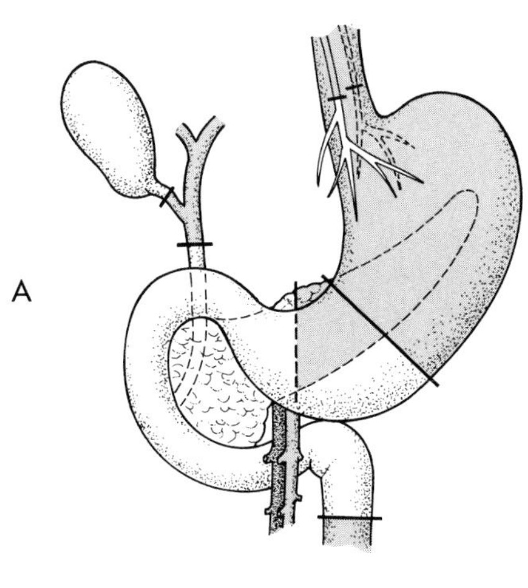

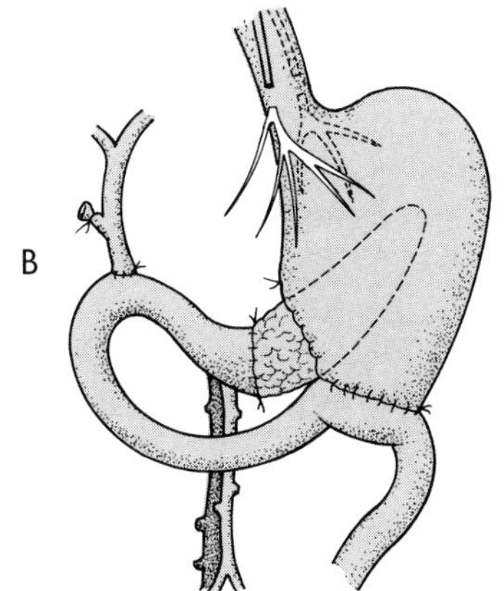

Fig. 28-3 Pancreatoduodenectomy (Whipple procedure). **A,** Preoperative anatomic relationships. **B,** Postoperative reconstruction showing pancreatic, biliary, and gastric anastomoses. A cholecystectomy (if gallstones are present) and bilateral truncal vagotomy are also part of the procedure. In many cases the distal stomach and pylorus can be preserved, and vagotomy is then unnecessary. (From Way, L.: Current surgical diagnosis and treatment, Los Altos, Calif., 1985, Lange Medical Books.)

The systemic manifestations of acute pancreatitis are important in assessing the severity of the disease and in predicting survival in individual patients. Acute pancreatitis usually resolves without altered digestive function or permanent damage to other organ systems affected during the acute disease. Acute pancreatitis generally does not recur if the cause (e.g., gallstones) is removed.

Chronic pancreatitis is associated with permanent damage to the gland. Digestive and endocrine functions are altered according to the degree of glandular damage. Although the cause of the pancreatitis may be removed, there is usually no improvement in either endocrine or exocrine function. In many cases these changes may be progressive. Systemic manifestations of chronic pancreatitis are related to the degree of digestive impairment (e.g., malabsorption), the degree of endocrine impairment (e.g., diabetes mellitus), and/or the inciting cause (e.g., alcoholism). Patients with chronic pancreatitis also may have recurrent episodes of acute pancreatitis.

REFERENCES

1. Acosta J.M., and Ledesma, C.L.: Gallstone migration as a cause of acute pancreatitis, N. Engl. J. Med. **290:**484, 1974.
2. Austin, J., and Reber, H.A.: Pancreatic resection and pancreatic insufficiency. In Condon, R., and DeCosse, J.J., editors: Surgical care II, Philadelphia, 1985, Lea & Febiger.
3. Austin, J., and Reber, H.A.: Chronic pancreatitis. In Rakel, R.E., editor: Conn's current therapy, ed. 38, Philadelphia, 1985, W.B. Saunders Co.
4. Austin, J.L., and Reber, H.A.: The pathologic features of acute pancreatitis. In Howard, J., Jordan, G., and Reber, H.A., editors: Surgical diseases of the pancreas, Philadelphia, 1986, Lea & Febiger.
5. Austin, J., et al.: Effects of partial pancreatic duct obstruction and subsequent drainage on pancreatic function in cats, J. Surg. Res. **28:**426, 1980.
6. Balasegaram, M.: Pancreatitis in the tropics. In Howard, J.M., Jordan, G.J., Jr., and Reber, H.A., editors: Surgical diseases of the pancreas, Philadelphia, 1986, Lea & Febiger.
7. Bess, M.A., Edis, A.J., and VanHeerden, J.A.: Hyperparathyroidism and pancreatitis, JAMA **243:**246, 1980.
8. Bradley, E.L., et al.: Hemodynamic consequences of severe pancreatitis, Ann. Surg. **198:**130, 1983.
9. Canale, D.D., and Donabedian, R.K.: Hypercalcitoninemia in acute pancreatitis, J. Clin. Endocrinol. Metab. **49:**738, 1975.
10. Clemente, F., et al.: Biochemical events in rat pancreatic cells in acute and chronic alcohol intoxications. In Gyr, K.E., Singer, M.V., and Sarles, H., editors: Pancreatitis: concepts and classification, New York, 1984, Elsevier North-Holland, Inc.
11. DiCarlo, V., et al.: Hemodynamic and metabolic impairment in acute pancreatitis, World J. Surg. **5:**329, 1981.
12. DiMagno, E.P., Go, V.L.W., and Summerskill, W.H.J.: Relations between pancreatic enzyme outputs and malabsorption in severe pancreatic insufficiency, N. Engl. J. Med. **288:**813, 1973.
13. Elliott, D.W.: Pancreatitis associated with hyperparathyroidism. In Howard, J.M., Jordan, G.J., Jr., and Reber, H.A., editors: Surgical diseases of the pancreas, Philadelphia, 1986, Lea & Febiger.
14. Finch, W.T., Sawyers, J.L., and Schenker, S.: A prospective study to determine the efficacy of antibiotics in acute pancreatitis, Ann. Surg. **183:**667, 1976.
15. Gerzof, S.G., et al.: Percutaneous drainage of infected pancreatic pseudocysts, Arch. Surg. **119:**888, 1984.
16. Goldstein, D.A., Llach, F., and Massry, S.G.: Acute renal failure in patients with acute pancreatitis, Arch. Intern. Med. **136:**1363, 1976.
17. Gyr, K.D., Singer, M.V., and Sarles, H., editors: Pancreatitis: concepts and classification, Amsterdam, 1984, Excerpta Medica.
18. Hallenbeck, G.A.: Biliary and pancreatic intraductal pressures. In Code, C.F., editor: Handbook of physiology, vol. 2, Baltimore, 1967, The Williams & Wilkins Co.

18a. Halmagyi, D., et al.: Pulmonary hypertension in acute hemorrhagic pancreatitis, Surgery, **76:**637, 1974.
19. Herman, R.E., and Davis, J.H.: The role of incomplete pancreatic duct obstruction in the etiology of pancreatitis, Surgery **48:**318, 1960.
20. Hills, M.C., et al.: The role of percutaneous aspiration in the diagnosis of pancreatic abscess, Am. J. Radiol. **141:**1035, 1983.
21. Howes, R., Zuidema, G.D., and Cameron, J.L.: Evaluation of prophylactic antibiotics in acute pancreatitis, J. Surg. Res. **18:**197, 1975.
22. Imrie, C.W., Allam, B.F., and Ferguson, J.C.: Hypocalcemia of acute pancreatitis: the effect of hypoalbuminemia, Curr. Med. Res. Opin. **4:**101, 1976.
23. Imrie, C.W., et al.: Parathyroid hormone and calcium homeostasis in acute pancreatitis, Br. J. Surg. **65:**717, 1978.
24. Johnson, S.G., Ellis, C.J., and Levitt, M.D.: Mechanisms of increased renal clearance of amylase/creatinine in acute pancreatitis, N. Engl. J. Med. **295:**1214, 1976.
25. Kelly, T.R.: Relationship of hyperparathyroidism to pancreatitis, Arch. Surg. **97:**267, 1968.
26. Kimura, T., et al.: Respiratory failure in acute pancreatitis: a possible role for triglycerides, Ann. Surg. **189:**509, 1979.
27. Kivilaakso, E., et al.: Pancreatic resection versus peritoneal lavation for acute fulminant pancreatitis, Ann. Surg. **199:**426, 1984.
28. Lankisch, P.G., Rahlf, G., and Koop, H.: Pulmonary complications in fatal acute hemorrhagic pancreatitis, Dig. Dis. Sci **28:**111, 1983.
29. Lee, P.C., and Howard, J.M.: Fat necrosis, Surg. Gynecol. Obstet. **148:**785, 1979.
30. Lefer, A.M.: Vascular mediators in ischemia and shock. In Cowley, R.A., and Trump, B.F., editors: Pathophysiology of shock, anoxia, and ischemia, Baltimore, 1982, The Williams & Wilkins Co.
31. Malik, A.B.: Pulmonary edema after pancreatitis: role of humoral factors, Circ. Shock **10:**71, 1983.
32. Mallory, A., and Kern, F.: Drug-induced pancreatitis: a critical review, Gastroenterology **78:**813, 1980.
33. McMahon, M.J., Playforth, M.J., and Pickford, I.R.: A comparative study of methods for the prediction of severity of attacks of acute pancreatitis, Br. J. Surg. **67:**22, 1980.
33a. Miyashiro, A., et al.: Reversible pulmonary hypertension and cardiac failure with chronic recurrent pancreatitis, Chest **71:**669, 1977.
34. Moosa, A.R.: Diagnostic tests and procedures in acute pancreatitis, N. Engl. J. Med. **311:**639, 1984.
35. Mosely, J., and Reber, H.A.: The effect of bile salts on the pancreatic duct mucosa, Br. J. Surg. **67:**59, 1980.
36. Nath, B.J., and Warshaw, A.L.: Pulmonary insufficiency. In Bradley, E.L., editor: Complications of pancreatitis, Philadelphia, 1982, W.B. Saunders Co.
37. Olazabal, A., and Fuller, R.: Failure of glucagon in the treatment of alcoholic pancreatitis, Gastroenterology **74:**489, 1978.
38. Pitchumoni, C.S.: "Tropical" or "Nutritional pancreatitis"—an update. In Gyr, K.F., Singer, M.V., and Sarles, H., editors: Pancreatitis: concepts and classifications, New York, 1984, Elsevier North-Holland, Inc.
39. Popieruitis, A.S., and Thompson, A.G.: The site of bradykinin release in acute experimental pancreatitis, Arch. Surg. **98:**73, 1969.
40. Ranson, J.H.C., and Spencer, F.: The role of peritoneal lavage in severe acute pancreatitis, Ann. Surg. **187:**565, 1978.
41. Ranson, J.H.C., et al.: Prognostic signs and the role of operative management in acute pancreatitis, Surg. Gynecol. Obstet. **139:**69, 1974.
42. Reber, H.A.: Acute pancreatitis: the role of duct permeability. In Gyr, K.F., Singer, M.V., and Sarles, H., editors: Pancreatitis: concepts and classification, Amsterdam, 1984, Excerpta Medica.
43. Reber, H.A., and Smale, B.: Planned operation for acute pancreatitis: the American experience. In Howard, J., Jordan, G., and Reber, H.A., editors: Surgical diseases of the pancreas, Philadelphia, 1986, Lea & Febiger.
44. Saharia, P., et al.: Acute pancreatitis with hyperlipemia: studies with an isolated perfused canine pancreas, Surgery **82:**60, 1972.
45. Sahel, J.: The usefulness of endoscopic retrograde pancreatography for the classification of chronic pancreatitis. In Gyr, K.F., Singer, M.V., and Sarles, H., editors: Pancreatitis: concepts and classification, New York, 1984, Elsevier North-Holland Inc.
46. Sanfey, H., and Cameron, J.L.: Pancreatitis associated with hyperlipemia. In Howard, J.M., Jordan, G.J., Jr., and Reber, H.A., editors: Surgical diseases of the pancreas, Philadelphia, 1986, Lea & Febiger.
47. Sankaran, S., Lucas, C.E., and Walt, A.J.: Transient hypertension with acute pancreatitis, Surg. Gynecol. Obstet. **138:**225, 1974.
48. Sarles, H., Devaux, M.A., and Noel Jorund, M.C.: Action of ethanol on the pancreas. In Gyr, K.F., Singer, M.V., and Sarles, H., editors: Pancreatitis: concepts and classification, New York, 1984, Elsevier North-Holland, Inc.
49. Satake, K., and Nakashima, Y.: Drug-induced pancreatitis. In Howard, J.M., Jordan, G.J., Jr., and Reber, H.A., editors: Surgical diseases of the pancreas, Philadelphia, 1986, Lea & Febiger.
50. Satiani, B., and Stone, H.H.: Predictability of present outcome and future recurrence in acute pancreatitis, Arch. Surg. **114:**711, 1979.
51. Tahamont, M.B., et al.: Increased lung vascular permeability after pancreatitis and trypsin infusion, Am. J. Pathol. **109:**15, 1982.
52. Taylor, R.H., et al.: Ductal drainage or resection for chronic pancreatitis, Am. J. Surg. **141:**28, 1981.
52a. Trapnell, J.E., and Imrie, C.W.: Special studies of therapy in acute pancreatitis. In Howard, J., Jordan, G., and Reber, H.A., editors: Surgical diseases of the pancreas, Philadelphia, 1986, Lea & Febiger.
53. Warshaw, A.L., and Nath, B.J.: Laboratory diagnosis of acute pancreatitis. In Howard, J., Jordan, G., and Reber, H.A., editors: Surgical diseases of the pancreas, Philadelphia, 1986, Lea & Febiger.
54. Warshaw, A.L., and O'Hara, P.J.: Susceptibility of the pancreas to ischemic injury in shock, Am. Surg. **188:**197, 1978.
55. Wedgwood, K., and Reber, H.A.: Acute pancreatitis: the concepts of pathogenesis. In Howard, J., Jordan, G., and Reber, H.A., editors: Surgical diseases of the pancreas, Philadelphia, 1986, Lea & Febiger.

29 *Elvira L. Muller and Henry A. Pitt*

The Jaundiced Patient

Over the past 50 years much has been learned about the metabolism of bilirubin and the pathophysiology of the jaundiced patient. In particular, during the 1970s numerous advances were made that have totally changed the diagnostic approach and management of jaundiced patients. Included among these new and important diagnostic tests were ultrasonography, computed tomography, thin-needle transhepatic cholangiography, endoscopic retrograde cholangiography, and biliary scintigraphy. Several of these diagnostic studies have also led to newer therapeutic options such as percutaneous transhepatic biliary drainage, endoscopic sphincterotomy, and percutaneous or endoscopic balloon dilation or placement of an endoprosthesis. During this same period, advances have also been made in perioperative and operative management that have resulted in improved operative survival. Before discussing in more detail the various diagnostic and therapeutic modalities now available, jaundice will be defined, normal and abnormal bilirubin metabolism discussed, different types of jaundice classified, and the multiple pathophysiologic effects of jaundice explained.

NORMAL BILIRUBIN METABOLISM

Jaundice, or icterus, may be defined as a yellowish staining of the skin, deeper tissues, and excretions with bile pigments. Normally serum bilirubin concentrations range between 0.5 and 1.3 mg/100 ml. Jaundice usually becomes clinically evident at concentrations greater than 2 to 2.5 mg/100 ml. Because bilirubin preferentially concentrates in elastic tissue, the yellow discoloration may first become apparent in the sclerae of the eye.

Approximately 80% to 85% of circulating bilirubin is a product of the destruction of senescent red blood cells by the reticuloendothelial system. The remaining 15% to 20% results from bone marrow destruction of maturing erythroid cells or the turnover of heme and heme products. Circulating bilirubin is primarily unconjugated and is transported to the liver tightly bound to albumin. The liver has a selective capacity to remove unconjugated bilirubin and other organic anions from plasma. Although the exact mechanism is unknown, bilirubin is transferred from plasma to cytoplasmic anion-binding proteins.

Unconjugated bilirubin is water insoluble. The enzyme uridine diphosphate glucuronyl transferase converts unconjugated bilirubin to the conjugated form, bilirubin diglucuronide. After conjugation with glucuronic acid, bilirubin is rapidly extracted into the bile through active transport. Excretion appears to be the rate-limiting step in the metabolism of bilirubin. After excretion, bile flows through the larger biliary ductal collecting system, may or may not be stored in the gallbladder, and enters the intestines. Some of the bilirubin is excreted in the stool. The remainder is converted by intestinal bacteria in the distal small intestine and colon to urobilinogen, which is reabsorbed from the small intestine. Some urobilinogen is excreted by the liver back into the bile, whereas the remainder is excreted in the urine.

Thus normal bilirubin metabolism goes through various steps, including: (1) production, (2) uptake by the hepatocyte, (3) conjugation, (4) excretion into bile ducts, and (5) delivery to the intestine. The steps in this metabolic pathway may be affected by a genetic disorder, hepatocellular disease, or obstruction of the bile-collecting system. The best classification system delineates the cause of jaundice by the point at which the metabolic pathway is affected.

CLASSIFICATION OF JAUNDICE

Numerous terms have been linked with the word jaundice. Among these many "types" of jaundice are acholuric, catarrhal, cholestatic, congenital hemolytic, familial nonhemolytic, hematogenous, hepatocellular, infectious, inogenous, latent, malignant, mechanical, medical, nonobstructive, obstructive, occult, painless, physiologic, surgical, and toxemic. To avoid confusion, however, a classification system based on the normal metabolism of bilirubin seems most appropriate. In this system (Table 29-1), jaundice may result from (1) increased production of bilirubin, (2) impaired uptake of bilirubin by the hepatocyte, (3) impaired conjugation of bilirubin, (4) impaired transport or excretion by the hepatocyte or bile canaliculus, or (5) obstruction of the intrahepatic or extrahepatic bile ducts.

Increased production of bilirubin resulting from hemolysis may be the result of either genetic or acquired disease. Inherited hemolytic anemias or hemolysis incited by sepsis, hemolysins, burns, transfusion reactions, or massive blood transfusions all cause unconjugated hyperbilirubinemia. Impaired uptake of bilirubin by the hepatocyte may occur in some drug reactions such as with flavaspidic acid and in Gilbert's syndrome, the most common cause of familial, unconjugated, nonhemolytic hyperbilirubinemia. Gilbert's syndrome affects approximately 2.5% of the population, but the bilirubin level is rarely greater than 3 mg/100 ml.

Neonatal jaundice is usually the result of immaturity of the hepatic conjugating and transport systems. Neonatal jaundice reaches its peak in 2 to 5 days and disappears in 2 weeks. A total or severe lack of the enzyme uridine diphosphate glucuronyl transferase is seen in the Crigler-Najjar form of familial, nonhemolytic jaundice. In Type I Crigler-Najjar syndrome in which no enzyme is present, the patient usually dies within the first year of life.

Table 29-1 **CLASSIFICATION OF JAUNDICE**

Step in Metabolic Pathway	Alteration	Examples
Bilirubin production	Increased	Hemolysis, extensive hematoma, multiple transfusions
Bilirubin uptake by the hepatocyte	Impaired	Gilbert's disease, drug-induced
Bilirubin conjugation	Impaired	Neonatal jaundice, Crigler-Najjar syndrome
Bilirubin transport or excretion by the hepatocyte or bile canaliculus	Impaired	Hepatitis, cirrhosis, drug-induced, jaundice of pregnancy, benign postoperative jaundice, Dubin-Johnson syndrome, Rotor syndrome
Bile flow through the intrahepatic and extrahepatic ducts	Mechanical obstruction	Tumor, stones, postoperative strictures, primary sclerosing cholangitis

Impairment of bilirubin transport or excretion by the bile canaliculus results in intrahepatic cholestasis, which is also referred to as "medical" jaundice. Impaired bilirubin transport and excretion into the bile canaliculus after conjugation results in increased serum levels of conjugated bilirubin. Hepatitis, either viral, alcoholic, or drug-induced, is the most common cause of intrahepatic cholestasis. Cirrhosis, a diffuse fibrotic process in the liver, usually caused by excessive alcohol intake over many years, may result in hepatocellular failure. Drugs such as estrogens, oral contraceptives, and anabolic steroids may also cause a defect in the excretion of bilirubin. The jaundice of pregnancy is presumably secondary to the high levels of estrogen. Genetic defects in the transfer of bilirubin and other organic anions across the hepatocyte membrane exist in both the Dubin-Johnson and Rotor syndromes. The common causes of extrahepatic or "surgical" jaundice are presented in Table 29-1 and will be discussed more fully in the remainder of this chapter.

PATHOPHYSIOLOGY OF JAUNDICE

Patients who are jaundiced are at increased risk of developing renal failure, bleeding problems, infections, and wound complications and of dying after surgery. Several authors have reported a direct correlation between operative mortality and the degree of jaundice. In one such analysis of 155 patients undergoing operations of the bile duct, Pitt and colleagues[49] reported that mortality was significantly increased ($p < 0.01$) among patients whose bilirubin was greater than 10 mg/100 ml (Table 29-2). In this analysis mortality was 3% for 101 patients with a bilirubin less than 5 mg/100 ml, 9% for 23 patients with a bilirubin between 5 and 10 mg/100 ml, and 23% for 31 patients with a bilirubin greater than 10 mg/100 ml.

The association between jaundice and postoperative renal failure has been known for many years. The reported incidence of postoperative acute renal failure varies considerably. However, in recent series[1,49] 15% to 20% of patients have developed this problem. Moreover, the mortality rate in jaundiced patients developing renal failure is high, ranging from 25% to 80%. Several theories have been proposed to explain the cause of renal failure in jaundiced patients. Among these theories are the possibilities that (1) bile pigments damage renal tubules, (2) renal perfusion is decreased, (3) renal tubules are more sensitive to anoxia and hypotension, and (4) endotoxins cause renal damage. Although multiple factors may be involved, this latter theory is presently the most highly regarded.

Table 29-2 **CORRELATION OF SERUM BILIRUBIN WITH POSTOPERATIVE MORTALITY**

Bilirubin (mg/100 ml)	Patients (No.)	Mortality (%)
<1.5	61	3.3
1.5-5	40	2.5
5-10	23	8.7
10-20	22	18.2*
>20	9	33.3*

Modified from Pitt, H.A., et al.: Am. J. Surg. **141**:66, 1981.
*$p < 0.01$ vs. patients with bilirubin <5 mg/100 ml.

Endotoxin has been found in the peripheral blood of approximately 50% of patients with obstructive jaundice.[8,30] This phenomenon may be the result of a lack of bile salts in the gut lumen that normally prevent absorption of endotoxins and inhibit anaerobic bacterial growth. Moreover, hepatic reticuloendothelial function is also impaired in jaundiced patients[12]; therefore hepatic clearance of endotoxin is also reduced. Endotoxin causes renal vasoconstriction and redistribution of renal blood flow away from the cortex.[8] Endotoxemia also causes several disturbances in coagulation, including activation of complement, macrophages, leukocytes, and platelets.[30] As a result, glomerular and peritubular fibrin is deposited. This factor, in combination with reduced renal cortical blood flow, results in the tubular and cortical necrosis observed in jaundiced patients with renal failure.

The fact that endotoxins play an important role in the renal failure observed in jaundiced patients is further supported by two recent studies in which oral bile salts were given before surgery to jaundiced patients.[8,15] In a study by Evans and associates,[15] two of nine jaundiced patients not receiving oral bile salts before surgery developed acute renal failure. Creatinine clearance in these patients decreased from a mean value of 85 to 55 ml/min. In comparison, none of nine jaundiced patients treated before surgery with oral bile salts developed renal problems. Moreover, mean creatinine clearance increased from 79 to 99 ml/min in the treated patients. The difference between the changes in creatinine clearance in the two groups was statistically significant ($p < 0.01$).

In a study by Cahill[8] 54% of 24 jaundiced patients not given oral bile salts before surgery were found to have systemic endotoxemia, which was associated with renal impairment in two thirds of the cases. In comparison, none of eight jaundiced patients given 500 mg of sodium deoxycholate every 8 hours for 48 hours before surgery had portal or systemic endotoxemia. Moreover, none of these eight patients had evidence of renal impairment ($p < 0.02$). In this study oral bile salt administration did not have any significant effect on small bowel microbial flora, suggesting that a direct effect on the endotoxin molecule may be involved.

Disturbances of blood coagulation are also commonly present in jaundiced patients. The most frequently observed clotting defect in patients with biliary obstruction is prolongation of the prothrombin time. This problem results from impaired vitamin K absorption from the gut and is usually reversible by parenteral administration of this vitamin. Decreased bile levels in the small intestine may also result in diminished absorption of other fat-soluble vitamins and fats and thereby contribute to weight loss and loss of calcium. This latter factor, as well as the above-mentioned increase in circulating endotoxin, may further contribute to clotting abnormalities.

In experimental animals, endotoxin affects Factors XI and XII and causes platelet and direct endothelial damage.[30] Moreover, endotoxin release in jaundiced patients results in a low-grade disseminated intravascular coagulation with increased fibrin degradation products. Hunt and co-workers[29] have shown that patients with circulating endotoxin or increased fibrin degradation product levels before surgery for jaundice are at increased risk for hemorrhagic complications and carry a very poor prognosis. In addition to problems with endotoxemia, cirrhotic patients may have even more complicated clotting abnormalities, including problems with thrombocytopenia secondary to hypersplenism and fibrinolysis.

In addition to renal clotting problems, jaundiced patients are also prone to infectious complications following surgery. Jaundiced patients have a number of defects in cellular and humoral immunity that make them more prone to infection. Several authors have now documented that jaundiced patients have delayed cutaneous hypersensitivity[16,52] and abnormal lymphocyte function.[16,19] As mentioned earlier, patients with jaundice also have impaired hepatic reticuloendothelial function. This myriad of immune defects clearly contributes to the high incidence of infectious complications observed in jaundiced patients.

The presence of bacteria in the bile at the time of surgery has also been associated with an increased incidence of postoperative infective sequelae.[32,46] Among other factors such as advanced age, choledocholithiasis, and recent cholangitis, jaundice has been correlated both with bactibilia and with postoperative infective complications. In a recent analysis of 134 patients undergoing bile duct operations, Pitt, Postier, and Cameron[46] found that 64% of 95 jaundiced patients had bactibilia. In this analysis 86% of patients with benign biliary obstruction had positive bile cultures compared to 46% of those with malignant obstruction.

Other problems that face jaundiced patients are anorexia, weight loss, and resultant malnutrition. Appetite is adversely influenced by the lack of bile salts in the intestinal tract. In addition, patients with pancreatic or periampullary malignant lesions may have partial duodenal obstruction or abnormal gastric emptying, perhaps secondary to tumor infiltration of the celiac nerve plexus. Patients with pancreatic or ampullary tumors may also have pancreatic endocrine and exocrine insufficiency. This latter problem may further compound other nutritional defects that in turn may multiply the immune deficits of the jaundiced patient.

DIAGNOSTIC INVESTIGATIONS

When confronted by a patient with jaundice, the objective of the physician is to identify potentially treatable causes without subjecting the patient to needless risk, discomfort, or expense. In this regard, the most important distinction to be made is whether the jaundice is caused by intrahepatic cholestasis or extrahepatic obstruction. Fortunately, within the past decade a variety of diagnostic modalities for visualizing the biliary tree have been developed that usually permit the distinction between "medical" and "surgical" jaundice to be made rapidly. However, the indiscriminate use of these newer tests may place a patient at added risk and expense. Therefore the following discussion is intended to summarize the advantages and disadvantages of various imaging techniques and to provide a rationale for deciding which tests to use and in what sequence.

Clinical Evaluation

The first and perhaps most important step in the workup of the jaundiced patient is a careful history, physical examination, and review of routine laboratory tests. In this regard, occupation, recent travel, recent exosure to hepatitis, or contact with jaundiced persons may be important. Similarly, any exposure to transfusions, blood tests, tattoos, drug ingestions, hepatotoxins, or dental work should also be noted. Moreover, the patient should be questioned about alcohol consumption. A family history regarding hemolytic or congenital hyperbilirubinemias may be informative. Previous operations on the biliary tract would raise suspicions of residual choledocholithiasis or benign biliary strictures. Hepatitis following transfusion or halothane toxicity may also appear after a surgical procedure.

The rapidity of onset and course of jaundice should be described and may give a clue to the diagnosis. Viral hepatitis might be suspected if the jaundiced patient presented with a rapid onset associated with nausea and anorexia. A history of biliary colic might raise suspicions of choledocholithiasis. Pancreatic cancer, on the other hand, is more likely to present with progressive, painless jaundice and weight loss. The presence of fever, chills, and upper abdominal pain in addition to jaundice (Charcot's triad) is suggestive of cholangitis, which occurs more often in patients with choledocholithiasis than in those with malignant obstruction.

It is also important to determine from the patient the color of the urine and stool. Total obstruction of the biliary tract results in acholic stools, increased bilirubin in the urine, and absence of urine urobilinogen. If bilirubin is present in the urine, levels of conjugated bilirubin are increased. Stools that are silver suggest the presence of blood, which may indicate an ampullary lesion that is both bleeding and obstructing the distal bile duct. Intermittent jaundice may also be indicative of an ampullary tumor or, more likely, a benign process.

On physical examination the abdomen should be carefully palpated. A small liver may be discovered in severe cirrhosis or hepatitis. A tender liver edge may be found in hepatitis, congestive heart failure, or alcoholic hepatitis. A palpable, nontender gallbladder may be noted in pancreatic or ampullary carcinoma (Courvoisier's sign). A tender gallbladder, on the other hand, may be palpated in choledocholithiasis. The signs of cirrhosis (i.e., ascites, spider angiomata, or periumbilical venous enlargement) should also be noted. A test for stool color and stool guaiac should be performed routinely. The presence of occult blood can suggest not only the possibility of an ampullary, pancreatic, or alimentary tract carcinoma but also portal hypertension.

On the basis of clinical findings and routine laboratory tests, experienced clinicians can correctly separate intrahepatic from extrahepatic obstruction with a very high accuracy rate. In a 1973 study, Knill-Jones and colleagues[33] found that computer analysis of clinical history, physical examination, and laboratory data could correctly distinguish between hepatocellular disease and extrahepatic biliary obstruction in 89% of the cases. More recently, O'Connor and associates[43] reported that the respective accuracies in diagnosing extrahepatic obstruction by clinical evaluation, computed tomography, ultrasound, and biliary scintigraphy were 84%, 81%, 78%, and 68%, respectively. This analysis suggests that clinical evaluation is a comparable noninvasive method to detect extrahepatic biliary obstruction. However, although the sensitivity of clinical examination in this study was 95%, the specificity was only 76%. Thus nearly one fourth of patients diagnosed as having extrahepatic obstructive disease will actually have hepatocellular disease. Therefore, although the history and physical examination are vital in evaluating the patient with jaundice, further tests are usually essential.

Biochemical Evaluation

Along with the history and physical examination, biochemical evaluation is part of the initial workup of the jaundiced patient. Hyperbilirubinemia is the sine qua non of jaundice, and the level of bilirubin can indicate the severity of the disease process and be used to follow its progression. Laboratory tests should include serum direct (conjugated) and indirect (unconjugated) bilirubin measurements and alkaline phosphatase, serum transaminase, and amylase determinations. The urine should also be tested for bilirubin and urobilinogen.

Patients with hemolysis have an increase in the indirect (unconjugated) fraction of bilirubin, whereas the direct (conjugated) bilirubin level is normal. The total bilirubin concentration in hemolysis rarely exceeds 4 to 5 mg/100 ml. Bilirubin is absent in the urine of patients with hemolysis since indirect bilirubin is not excreted by the kidney. If hemolysis is suspected, further laboratory tests should include a complete blood count, a blood smear, reticulocyte count, erythrocyte fragility test, and a Coombs' test.

In most cases of hepatic parenchymal disease broad derangements of liver function tests are seen. The concentrations of both conjugated and unconjugated fractions of bilirubin are increased in the serum. With the increased level of conjugated bilirubin, bilirubinuria develops. In patients with acute hepatitis, serum glutamic oxaloacetic transaminase (SGOT) and serum glutamic pyruvic transaminase (SGPT) are markedly elevated. The bilirubin and alkaline phosphatase levels in these patients may also be slightly increased, but the serum amylase is usually normal. As in hepatitis, the serum bilirubin level in patients with cirrhosis will increase in proportion to the degree of parenchymal damage. Serum transaminases are also increased in alcoholic liver disease, with the rise in SGOT usually being much greater than that in SGPT. Additional laboratory tests such as an albumin level and prothrombin time can also be quite helpful in assessing the degree of parenchymal injury since both albumin and prothrombin synthesis occur in the liver.

In extrahepatic obstruction an increase in the fraction of direct bilirubin is seen along with a moderate increase in indirect bilirubin. The highest elevations of bilirubin are usually found in patients with malignant extrahepatic obstruction with concentrations as great as or exceeding 20 mg/100 ml. With malignant obstruction the alkaline phosphatase is also elevated to the same degree. Other liver function tests are usually normal or only slightly elevated, and the amylase concentration is usually normal. Common bile duct stones, on the other hand, rarely cause an increased bilirubin level greater than 10 to 12 mg/100 ml. With choledocholithiasis alkaline phosphatase is also usually elevated to a moderate degree. As a gallstone passes through and momentarily obstructs the ampulla of Vater, serum transaminase levels may transiently increase, sometimes to levels quite high. In this setting, of course, hyperamylasemia may also develop. Serum transaminases may be elevated in cases in which long-standing obstruction results in liver damage or fibrosis.

The alkaline phosphatase is often a more sensitive indicator of obstruction and may be elevated when the bilirubin level is normal. This circumstance occurs most commonly with incomplete or partial obstruction. However, increased levels of alkaline phosphatase activity may also be the result of bone disease. If this possibility is suspected, serum 5′-nucleotidase levels that parallel changes in liver alkaline phosphatase should also be measured to verify that the increase is from a hepatobiliary source.

In most jaundice cases laboratory tests will not provide information regarding the specific cause. The primary goal of examination of bilirubin fractionation is to differentiate parenchymal disease and extrahepatic obstruction from unconjugated hyperbilirubinemia. The proportion of direct and indirect bilirubin usually will not differentiate intrahepatic disease from extrahepatic obstruction. Nevertheless, an experienced clinician can usually accurately differentiate intrahepatic cholestasis from extrahepatic obstruction when allowed to take a history, perform a physical examination, and review routine laboratory data.

Radiologic Evaluation

Abdominal Radiology

The likelihood of a plain abdominal x-ray film providing diagnostic information in the jaundiced patient is low. However, because abdominal x-ray films are safe, always available, performed quickly, and may provide useful information, they should be the first radiographic procedure in all patients in whom biliary tract disease is suspected. The abdominal x-ray films may reveal gallstones, a calcified gallbladder wall, or the outline of a distended gallbladder. Although approximately 15% to 20% of gallstones will be visualized in this manner, cholangiography will still be necessary to determine whether common duct stones are present and to rule out some other cause of jaundice such as hepatic parenchymal disease or an obstructing tumor. Plain x-ray films may also be diagnostic of a spontaneous biliary fistula when air is present in the biliary tree or of emphysematous cholecystitis when air is noted in the gallbladder lumen or wall.

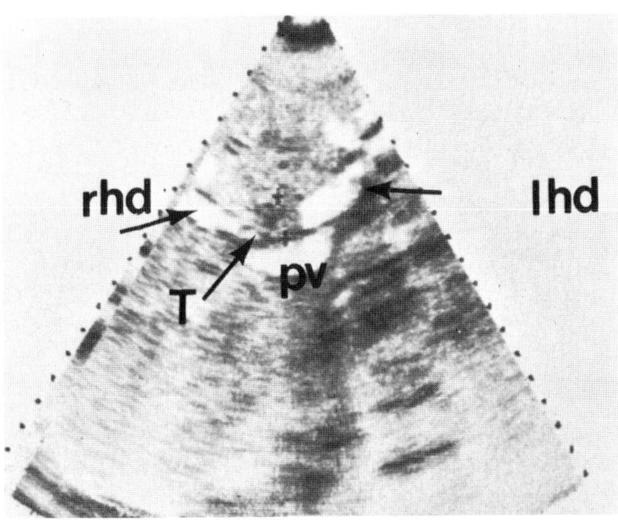

Fig. 29-1 Ultrasonic demonstration of Klatskin tumor *(T)* anterior to portal vein *(pv)* and at the bifurcation of the right *(rhd)* and left *(lhd)* hepatic ducts. (From Pitt, H.A., Roslyn, J.J., and Tompkins, R.K.: Surgical resection of bile duct cancer. Reprinted from Wanebo, H.J., editor: Hepatic and biliary cancer, New York, 1986, by courtesy of Marcel Dekker, Inc.)

Ultrasonography

In the jaundiced patient the first objective of noninvasive radiology is to differentiate hepatocellular disease from extrahepatic biliary obstruction. In this regard, ultrasound has become the initial screening procedure after a plain abdominal x-ray film. Ultrasound is noninvasive, inexpensive, and widely available. Further developments in the technique, including focused transducers and real-time ultrasound that visualizes motion, have enabled imaging of smaller components of the liver and biliary tree.

Of particular value in the patient with jaundice is the high success rate of ultrasound in the identification of bile duct dilation. Most series report that ultrasound will detect dilation of the intrahepatic or proximal extrahepatic bile ducts with at least an 80% accuracy rate.[2,58] The normal intrahepatic duct diameter is less than 4 mm, and biliary ducts of this diameter are not normally seen on ultrasound. Dilated ducts are easily detectable, however, and a dilated biliary tree may even be identified before the onset of clinical jaundice.[64]

Failure of ultrasound to detect dilated ducts usually indicates an intrahepatic source of jaundice. In this setting continued observation or a liver biopsy would then be indicated. However, failure to detect dilated ducts does not entirely rule out extrahepatic obstruction. In intermittent or partial obstruction the intrahepatic biliary tree may not be dilated. Likewise, in long-standing obstruction, especially if there is secondary biliary fibrosis or cirrhosis, dilated ducts may not be seen. In these cases where extrahepatic obstruction is suspected in spite of a negative ultrasound, direct cholangiography, either by means of the transhepatic or endoscopic route, may be necessary.

Because of the high success rate of identifying ductal dilation, ultrasound can usually differentiate hepatocellular disease from extrahepatic causes of jaundice. Taylor, Rosenfield, and Spiro[57] reviewed 275 jaundiced patients and reported that accurate differentiation of intrahepatic vs. extrahepatic obstruction was made in 96% of the cases. Moreover, this degree of accuracy has also been confirmed by others.

In comparison, ultrasound has limited success in identifying the exact cause and precise location of an obstructing lesion (Fig. 29-1). The anatomic level of the obstruction can be estimated in perhaps half of the patients. In addition, the cause of the obstruction is evident in a far lower proportion. This low yield in determining the cause of obstruction is caused by (1) failure to visualize the entire common bile duct, especially the distal third, and (2) inability to detect common duct stones. The distal end of the choledochus is frequently obscured by duodenal or colon gas. Moreover, according to some investigators,[21,26] ultrasound will identify the presence of common bile duct stones in only 10% of patients.

Thomas, Pellegrini, and Way[58] have shown that, of 101 patients initially evaluated by ultrasound, the need for further tests was eliminated in only 25 patients. Thus, although ultrasound is a valuable initial step in the evaluation of the jaundiced patient, further diagnostic studies such as direct cholangiography are usually necessary to identify the cause and exact location of the obstruction.

Computed Tomography

Computed tomography (CT) is another noninvasive technique that has a role similar to ultrasound in the evaluation of the jaundiced patient. As with ultrasound, the primary purpose of the CT scan is to differentiate intrahepatic disease with nondilated ducts from dilated ducts caused by extrahepatic obstruction. Numerous studies have reported that CT is more than 90% accurate in detecting the presence of ductal dilation.[45,58] CT has been reported to have a slightly higher success rate than ultrasound because it provides a better definition of anatomic structures and can use contrast media to enhance delineations (Fig. 29-2, *A*).

Despite agreement regarding the reliability of CT in identifying biliary ductal dilation, the accuracy of CT in determining the site and cause of obstruction is controversial. Gold and associates[21] reported that CT could determine the site of obstruction in 12 of 19 jaundiced patients (62%). Other reports suggest that the cause of bile duct obstruction could be determined by CT in only 30% to 40% of patients.[58] In comparison, Pedrosa, Casanova, and

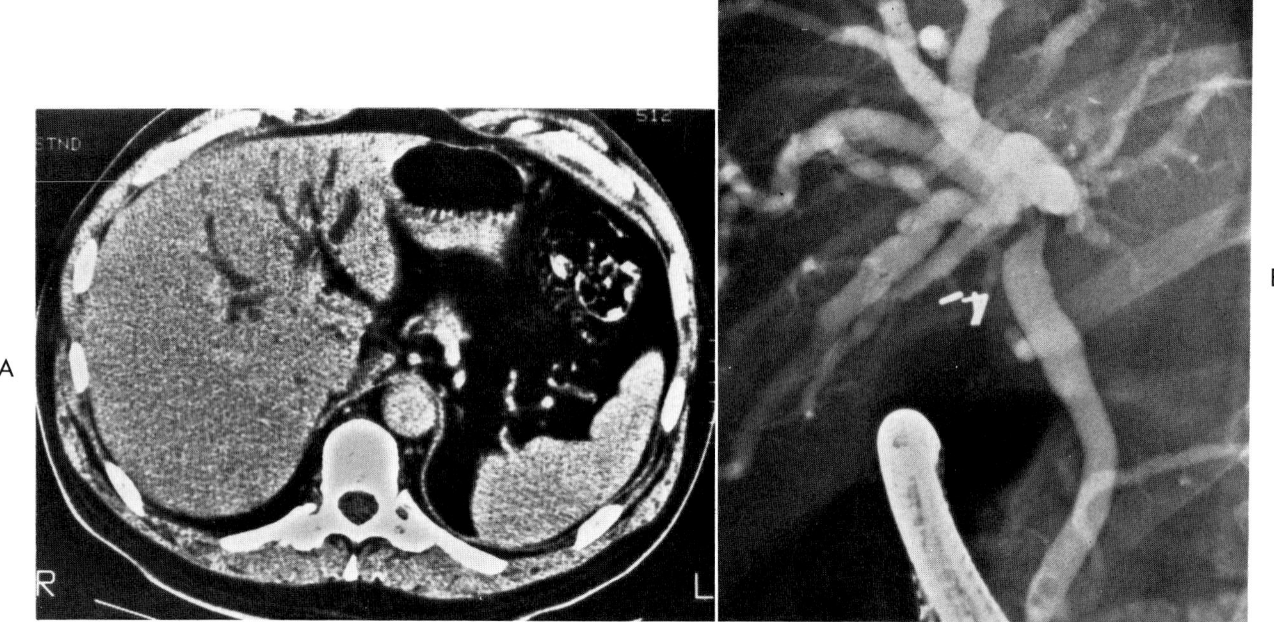

Fig. 29-2 **A,** Computed tomography of a patient demonstrating dilation primarily of the left, but also of the right, hepatic duct. **B,** Endoscopic retrograde cholangiogram in same patient showing a defect in the proximal common hepatic duct secondary to a cholangiocarcinoma.

Table 29-3 **COMPARISON BETWEEN ULTRASONOGRAPHY AND COMPUTED TOMOGRAPHY IN DIAGNOSIS OF THE JAUNDICED PATIENT**

Criterion	Ultrasound	CT
Identifying ductal dilation	80%-85%	>90%
Identifying cause of obstruction	35%-40%	40%-80%
Patient selection	Thin patient	Obese patient, bowel gas present
Other factors	Less expensive, no radiation	More expensive, radiation

Rodriquez[45] showed that the overall accuracy of CT in determining the exact location of obstruction was 97% and that the cause of obstruction could be correctly identified by CT in 94% of the cases.

This wide range of reported accuracy of CT in delineating the cause and anatomic location of an obstructing lesion results primarily from differences in the reported ability of CT to detect obstructing common bile duct stones. CT shows the common bile duct in cross section instead of longitudinally, and small stones in the common bile duct may not be identified. Pedrosa, Casanova, and Rodriquez[45] have reported that calculi were visible in 14 of 17 patients (82%), whereas other radiologists have had greater difficulty in visualizing common bile duct stones.

When compared to ultrasound, CT is more likely to identify the cause and location of extrahepatic biliary obstruction (Table 29-3). In a study of 103 patients Baron and associates[2] showed that CT was slightly more accurate than ultrasound in identifying the presence of biliary obstruction (96% vs. 87%). Moreover, the precise level of obstruction was shown by CT in 88% of patients compared to 60% for ultrasound. In addition, the cause of obstruction was predicted accurately by CT in 70% and by ultrasound in only 38%.

In summary, CT and ultrasound have similar value in the diagnosis of biliary ductal dilation. CT may be the preferred initial screening procedure in obese patients or in those patients with dressings or large amounts of bowel gas. Although most authorities agree that CT is slightly more accurate than ultrasound in detecting the nature and anatomic level of obstruction, ultrasound is generally preferred as the initial screening test because it is less expensive, more widely available, and does not expose the patient to radiation. Again, if either CT or ultrasound shows the presence of dilated ducts, direct cholangiography by either the percutaneous or endoscopic route should be performed since these latter invasive procedures provide needed information regarding the site and cause of the obstructing lesion.[21,58]

Biliary Scintigraphy

^{131}I-rose bengal was the first radioisotope used for visualization of the biliary system. Since 1975, ^{99m}Tc-labeled pyridoxylidene-glutamate and N-substituted iminodiacetic acid (IDA) derivatives have also been introduced. These labeled compounds are rapidly extracted from the blood and excreted into the bile. Early iminodiacetic acid derivatives, such as 2,6-dimethyl acetanilide (HIDA), failed to visualize the biliary system in patients with a bilirubin level greater than 5 mg/100 ml. However, more recently developed compounds such as 2,6-diisopropyl acetanilide (DISIDA) can visualize the ductal system if serum bilirubin levels are as high as 20 to 30 mg/100 ml.

Biliary scintigraphy is the imaging procedure of choice in the initial examination of a patient with suspected acute cholecystitis. This technique may also aid in the localization of hepatobiliary leaks following trauma or surgery. In addition, it provides a method of noninvasively evaluating the patency of a biliary-enteric anastomosis and of studying the kinetics of bile flow in patients suspected of having disorders of biliary motility.

Biliary scintigraphy plays only a limited role in the evaluation of a patient with jaundice. The technique has been shown to be useful in the diagnosis of complete common bile duct obstruction. Any appearance of the nucleotide in the gastrointestinal tract would indicate patency of bile flow into the duodenum. However, other available noninvasive tests such as ultrasound or CT have generally been shown to be more accurate and therefore are preferred.

In a blinded prospective study reported by O'Connor and co-workers,[43] the overall accuracy of biliary scintigraphy in differentiating medical from surgical jaundice was only 68%, compared to 78% for ultrasound and 81% for CT. In a similar study by Matzen and colleagues[35] the biliary scan was again less successful in identifying extrahepatic obstruction when compared to ultrasound or CT. Moreover, the anatomic resolution is much poorer with biliary scintigraphy; and although this method can verify total obstruction of the biliary tract, scintigraphy rarely identifies the exact site and nature of an extrahepatic obstructing lesion.

Intravenous Cholangiography

Intravenous cholangiography (IVC) was introduced in the 1950s and was once the only method available for evaluation of the bile ducts. Intravenous injection of iodipamide results in the rapid excretion of contrast material in bile. The development of other methods of visualizing the biliary tree, however, such as ultrasound, CT, and direct cholangiography have markedly diminished the earlier role of IVC. In comparison to these other methods, IVC has several disadvantages, including faint visualization, allergic reaction to the contrast medium, and nonvisualization in patients with a serum bilirubin level higher than 2 to 3 mg/100 ml.

In a review of 140 patients who had an intravenous cholangiogram performed, Goodman and co-workers[23] reported allergic reactions in two patients and nonvisualization in 10 patients who had an elevated bilirubin concentration. In the remaining 128 patients only 55% had technically adequate intravenous cholangiograms. Among those patients who subsequently had adequate cholangiograms, the diagnostic accuracy for IVC was only 60%, largely because of missed stones. A more recent study by Eubanks and associates[14] reviewed 100 consecutive intravenous cholangiograms and showed that 40% were of limited or no value. Moreover, marginal visualization was subject to interpretation. Therefore these analyses suggest that IVC is frequently nondiagnostic or inaccurate and should rarely be used now that improved noninvasive techniques and direct cholangiography are widely available.

Transhepatic Cholangiography

Transhepatic cholangiography (THC) with the "skinny" (Chiba) needle was introduced by Okuda and colleagues in 1974.[44] Since then, growing experience with this technique and its accompanying high success rate in visualizing the biliary ductal system have made THC the procedure of choice in most patients with extrahepatic obstruction. THC involves passage of a slender, flexible steel needle into an intrahepatic bile duct under radiographic control, followed by injection of contrast medium to outline the bile ducts.

THC is indicated if dilated bile ducts are visualized on ultrasound or CT. If the clinical suspicion of extrahepatic obstruction remains high despite a negative ultrasound or CT scan, THC may also be useful. Gold and co-workers[21] state that THC is successful in differentiating intrahepatic from extrahepatic obstruction in 96% of cases. If failure to visualize the biliary tree after 10 attempts at passing the needle into an intrahepatic duct (which should be easily accomplished if the duct is dilated) is considered evidence of hepatocellular disease, THC can differentiate intrahepatic disease from extrahepatic obstruction with an accuracy of almost 100%.[34]

In addition, THC is highly accurate in defining the site and cause of extrahepatic obstruction. Several studies have confirmed the observation by Gibbons, Griffiths, and Cormack[20] that THC is able to define the site of the obstructing lesion in approximately 95% of patients and the cause of the obstruction in nearly 90% of cases. In a series of 25 patients, Gold and associates[21] reported that THC was 100% successful in establishing both the nature and level of obstruction. THC also provides an anatomic map before a surgical procedure. Recent developments have also combined THC with such therapeutic maneuvers as the insertion of biliary stents or endoprostheses, percutaneous stone extraction, biliary dilation, transhepatic drainage, and the performance of manometric and perfusion studies.

The success rate of entering a bile duct during THC increases with the experience of the radiologist. In patients with dilated intrahepatic ducts, THC is nearly 100% successful. In patients with nondilated bile ducts, the success rate is approximately 70%. Although THC is an invasive procedure, it has an acceptably low complication rate. In a review of 700 patients, Mueller, van Sonnenberg, and Simeone[40] noted a major complication rate of 5% to 6%. The most commonly reported complications include sepsis, bile leak, hemorrhage, and, rarely, death. Even with more frequent passes of the needle (i.e., as many as 15 attempts), no increase in the complication rate has been reported. Thus, in managing most jaundiced patients, the advantages of THC are considered in terms of establishing a diagnosis, determining the site and cause of obstruction, and providing specific anatomic detail to outweigh the relatively low incidence of complications.

Endoscopic Retrograde Cholangiography

Endoscopic retrograde cholangiography (ERC) was first performed in 1968. With a side-viewing duodenoscope the sphincter of Oddi is cannulated under direct vision, and contrast material is injected into the biliary tree. Thus, as with THC, ERC provides direct visualization and gives an anatomic map of the biliary ducts (see Fig. 29-2, *B*). Also like THC, ERC has been shown to be highly accurate in defining the site and cause of extrahepatic obstructive jaundice. In 1974 Vennes, Jacobson, and Silvis[62] reported that, in 60 patients with proven biliary obstruction, the site of obstruction was predicted by ERC in 53 patients (88%), and the correct diagnosis was made in 46 patients (76%). More recently, Thomas, Pellegrini, and Way[58] showed that, of 41 technically adequate ERCs, accurate diagnostic information was found in 86%, partially diagnostic information in 7%, and no diagnostic information in only 7%.

The technique of ERC requires skilled personnel. The success rate of ERC is approximately 85% to 90%[26,34,58] and improves with the experience of the endoscopist. Like THC, the complication and mortality rates of ERC are acceptably low. In a review of 10,000 ERCs, Bilbao and associates[4] reported a complication rate of less than 3% and a mortality rate of less than 0.1%. The two major complications of the procedure are sepsis and acute pancreatitis. Prophylactic antibiotics should be administered before the procedure if biliary obstruction is suspected.

In the jaundiced patient shown to have dilated ducts on ultrasound or CT, direct cholangiography by either THC or ERC is the next procedure to be used. Because THC is less expensive, more widely available, requires less expertise than ERC, and has a higher success rate if dilated ducts are present, it is generally the preferred test (Table 29-4). In cases of total biliary obstruction THC will visualize the proximal biliary tree, whereas ERC will frequently only be able to delineate the anatomy of the distal bile ducts. Thus THC would provide important information about the anatomy of the proximal bile ducts, i.e., the information that is most useful to the surgeon. THC is also the preferred procedure if other percutaneous therapeutic manipulations such as biliary drainage, balloon dilation, or percutaneous placement of an endoprosthesis are necessary for lesions near the hilum. In addition, ERC may be difficult or impossible to perform in patients with ampullary stenosis or in those who have undergone a previous antrectomy and gastroenterostomy.

In several instances, however, ERC would be the preferred procedure (see Table 29-4). Percutaneous THC is contraindicated in patients whose bleeding abnormalities are uncorrectable. In addition, gastric, duodenal, or ampullary abnormalities may be visualized and biopsied during ERC. Moreover, cannulation of the pancreatic duct is often helpful in those patients suspected of having a pancreatic lesion. Similarly, in patients with postcholecystectomy symptoms or sphincter of Oddi dyskinesia, ERC enables visualization and cannulation of the ampulla and manometric pressure recordings. As with THC, therapeutic manipulations such as endoscopic sphincterotomy and stenting may be carried out in conjunction with ERC.

In summary, the method of direct cholangiography that is chosen, either THC or ERC, is individualized in each case. In certain situations such as totally obstructing proximal lesions, THC may be the procedure of choice. On the other hand, when noninvasive studies suggest periampullary or pancreatic pathology, ERC provides additional useful information. Finally, the choice between these two procedures may ultimately be decided by the expertise of the radiologists and endoscopists at an individual institution.

Angiography

In the jaundiced patient with cirrhosis, portal hypertension, and bleeding esophageal varices, angiography is indicated before a shunting procedure. In the evaluation of jaundice from other causes, however, angiography is not a routine investigative procedure. One rare indication for angiography is in the jaundiced patient with active gastrointestinal bleeding who is suspected of having hemobilia. In the opinion of some investigators,[3,65] angiography and venography should be used before surgery to evaluate the resectability of liver tumors, tumors of the hilum, extra-

Table 29-4 **COMPARISON OF TRANSHEPATIC CHOLANGIOGRAPHY AND ENDOSCOPIC RETROGRADE CHOLANGIOGRAPHY**

Criterion	Transhepatic Cholangiography	Endoscopic Retrograde Cholangiography
Success rate	>90% with dilated ducts ~70% with nondilated ducts	80%-90% whether or not ducts are dilated
Identifies the site and cause of obstruction	90%-100%	75%-90%
Complications	5% (range, 3%-10%)	5% (range, 2%-7%)
Mortality	0.2%-0.9%	0.1%-0.2%
Expense	Less	More
Skill required	Less	More
Patient selection	Proximal lesions, surgically distorted gastroduodenal anatomy, failed retrograde cholangiogram	Distal lesions, pancreatic pathology, coagulopathy, ascites, failed transhepatic cholangiogram

hepatic biliary tumors, and tumors in the head of the pancreas. However, in the jaundiced patient who is already at an increased risk of renal failure, the additional dye load given during angiography will further increase the risk of renal problems. Therefore, in our opinion, angiography should be used selectively and only when resection is seriously contemplated. Most patients with hepatobiliary tumors will need an operation to provide a tissue diagnosis and to at least attempt bypass of the obstructing lesion. In most instances resectability can be determined during surgery without the aid of angiography.

Liver Biopsy

The development in the past decade of ultrasound and computed tomography has made percutaneous liver biopsy unnecessary in most cases of jaundice caused by extrahepatic obstruction.[13] However, numerous indications for a liver biopsy remain. If clinical and laboratory data indicate intrahepatic cholestasis and if dilated bile ducts are not present on ultrasound or computed tomography scans, a liver biopsy is usually the next test. Thus a liver biopsy may be a diagnostic aid if all previous diagnostic studies are negative or equivocal or if parenchymal disease is suspected along with extrahepatic obstruction.

A liver biopsy may be useful in establishing the precise diagnosis for the cause of intrahepatic cholestasis, storage disease, unexplained hepatomegaly, and liver infections. Among the cholestatic causes for jaundice in which a liver biopsy may be helpful are hepatitis, cirrhosis, drug-induced cholestasis, and primary biliary cirrhosis. Further indications for percutaneous biopsy of the liver are storage diseases such as amyloidosis and glycogen storage disease and liver infections such as tuberculosis, histoplasmosis, and coccidiomycosis. Serial liver biopsies are also used to follow the course of a disease process such as chronic active hepatitis or the sequelae of viral hepatitis, hemochromatosis, and Wilson's disease.

Liver biopsy is a relatively safe procedure. In reviews of very large series of liver biopsies, mortality rates of 0.01% to 0.02% and a serious complication rate of 0.2% to 0.4% have been reported. The most frequent complications of liver biopsy are hemorrhage and bacteremia. This latter problem occurs most often in patients with chronic bile duct infections. Percutaneous liver biopsy is contraindicated if the patient is uncooperative or if an uncorrectable coagulation defect is present. If the patient has a prolonged prothrombin time or partial thromboplastin time or a diminished platelet count, attempts should be made to correct these abnormalities with vitamin K, fresh frozen plasma, or specific component therapy. If the coagulopathy persists and liver biopsy is essential, laparoscopic or open liver biopsy must be considered.

PATIENT MANAGEMENT

Patients with obstructive jaundice and those with hepatocellular disease severe enough to cause jaundice are prone to develop many secondary problems. As mentioned in the section on pathophysiology of jaundice, these patients are at increased risk for developing renal failure, bleeding problems, infections, and wound complications. Patients with chronic liver disease and cirrhosis may also develop ascites and encephalopathy. Moreover, jaundiced patients are at increased risk for gastrointestinal bleeding, which may be the result of portal hypertension, stress gastritis secondary to biliary or other infections, or increased gastric acid production following Roux-en-Y biliary diversion. In addition to these many problems, pruritis is frequently encountered in jaundiced patients and is often their most distressing problem. The exact cause of this problem remains obscure but is thought to be at least partially related to increased bile salt levels in the skin. In some patients, relief from itching can be obtained by binding bile salts in the intestinal lumen with an agent like cholestyramine and thereby preventing their reabsorption. The fact that various sedatives can also provide relief indicates that increased bile salt levels are not the only mechanism.

In managing patients with severe underlying or secondary liver disease, delicate balances must frequently be achieved: (1) the balance between achieving adequate renal blood flow and urine output and preventing further accumulation of ascites may be extremely difficult; (2) a fine balance is needed to control pruritis without oversedating a patient with borderline encephalopathy; and (3) biliary sepsis must be controlled adequately and at the same time nephrotoxic agents must be avoided. These and other subjects will be discussed in more detail in the subsequent section on preoperative preparation. However, before addressing these fine points of patient management, data will be presented on methods of assessing the risk of complications following biliary manipulations and on newer nonoperative approaches to the treatment of the jaundiced patient.

Assessment of Risk

Once the diagnosis of obstructive jaundice has been established, the next concern of the clinician is an assessment of the patient's operative risk. The outcome of this assessment may determine whether the patient is an operative candidate or should undergo one of the nonoperative options for relief of jaundice. In part, this risk assessment is the same as that for any patient potentially undergoing a major abdominal operation. However, certain considerations such as ongoing biliary sepsis and the presence of biliary cirrhosis are unique to the jaundiced patient.

Among the factors that must be considered when assessing risk are cardiac, pulmonary, and renal function, as well as coagulation, nutritional, and immune parameters. In assessing a patient's cardiopulmonary status, the patient's age, history of a recent myocardial infarction, and the presence of congestive heart failure, significant valvular aortic stenosis, or a disturbance of normal cardiac rhythm have all been correlated with increased operative risk.[22] As discussed in more detail in the section on the pathophysiology of jaundice, it is particularly important to detect mild disturbances in renal function and clotting abnormalities before operative or nonoperative biliary manipulation.

Most patients with benign biliary problems are adequately nourished. However, various degrees of malnutrition are frequently seen in patients with malignant obstruction and in those with chronic liver disease. The various factors leading to anorexia, weight loss, malabsorption, and malnutrition in the jaundiced patient have already been discussed. Quantification of the degree of malnutrition, however, may be important because of direct correlation with postoperative outcome. Thus in jaundiced patients we routinely measure serum albumin and transferrin, triceps skin folds, and perform delayed hypersensitivity skin tests as suggested by Buzby and associates.[7] Calculation of a Prognostic Nutritional Index[7] from these values will give an estimated risk of the likelihood that subsequent complications will occur and aids in identifying those patients who may benefit from preoperative nutritional support.

Those jaundiced patients with severe cholangitis are also at very high risk. Patients with the most severe form of "toxic" cholangitis associated with shock and mental confusion have a significant chance of dying despite appropriate treatment with antibiotics and operative and nonoperative biliary decompression. To further assess the risk of preoperative cholangitis, Pitt, Postier, and Cameron[47] recently analyzed 73 consecutive patients undergoing choledochotomy for common duct stones. Of these patients, 33 had clinical cholangitis, whereas the remaining 40 patients had no fever or chills before surgery. As might be expected, patients with preoperative cholangitis were significantly older and more likely to have jaundice, to have retained common duct stones, to have bactibilia, and to have anaerobes isolated from their bile. Despite these clear differences, however, patients with cholangitis before surgery were not more likely to develop infective sequelae or biliary complications or death following operation. However, patients with preoperative cholangitis were much more likely ($p < 0.001$) to develop an increase in serum creatinine that in turn contributed to a longer ($p < 0.01$) postoperative hospitalization. Undoubtedly, sepsis, jaundice, and underlying renal disease contributed to the renal problems observed in these patients. However, prolonged aminoglycoside therapy may also have played a significant role in the renal problems observed in one third of the cholangitis patients.

Another factor that Schwartz[54] has recently highlighted as an additional risk factor is cirrhosis. Patients with cirrhosis who require operative or nonoperative biliary manipulations for relief of jaundice experience excessive morbidity, usually from bleeding, and mortality. McSherry and Glenn[39] have also documented that cirrhosis is secondary only to cardiovascular disease as a cause of death following surgery for nonmalignant biliary tract disease. Thus the knowledge that a patient with jaundice has cirrhosis may influence perioperative management, short- and long-term results, and even the decision as to whether surgery is justified.

Several authors have demonstrated that mortality following biliary surgery correlates directly with the preoperative serum bilirubin. Explanations for this phenomenon include depressed liver function, vitamin K–dependent coagulation abnormalities, altered immune status, and increased risk of renal failure in jaundiced patients. A serum bilirubin greater than 10 mg/100 ml increases the risk of complications and death following biliary procedures. Although serum bilirubin, by itself, is a good indicator of morbidity and mortality, multiple other factors may be important when assessing risk. In an effort to determine which patients undergoing biliary surgery were at greatest risk, Pitt and co-workers[49] analyzed 15 clinical and laboratory parameters in 155 consequent patients. These authors found that eight factors (see boxed material at left) were associated with an increased risk of death following surgery. In addition, they demonstrated that the number of biliary risk factors present before surgery strongly correlated with postoperative morbidity and mortality (Fig. 29-3). These authors suggested that this risk factor analysis had the potential advantages of being able to be performed in any hospital and providing information on risk within 24 to 48 hours of admission. In their analysis, patients with five or more biliary risk factors were most likely to develop postoperative complications.

Subsequent analyses by Hunt,[29] Blamey and associates,[5] and Dixon and colleagues[11] have also confirmed that a number of these clinical and routine laboratory assessments are important risk factors. In these analyses the most consistent predictors of outcome were shown to be the presence of malignancy, elevated serum bilirubin, hypoalbuminemia, and increased serum creatinine. Hunt and co-workers[30] have likewise shown that endotoxemia in association with increased fibrin degradation products in blood and urine are also important indicators of risk in jaundiced patients. Another test that has been recently suggested by McPherson and associates[38] as a predictor of outcome in

BILIARY RISK FACTORS

Age >60 years	Albumin <3 g/100 ml
Malignant obstruction	Creatinine >1.3 mg/100 ml
Hematocrit <30%	Bilirubin >10 mg/100 ml
White blood cells >10,000/mm³	Alkaline phosphatase greater than three times normal

Modified from Pitt, H.A., et al: Am. J. Surg. **141:**66, 1981.

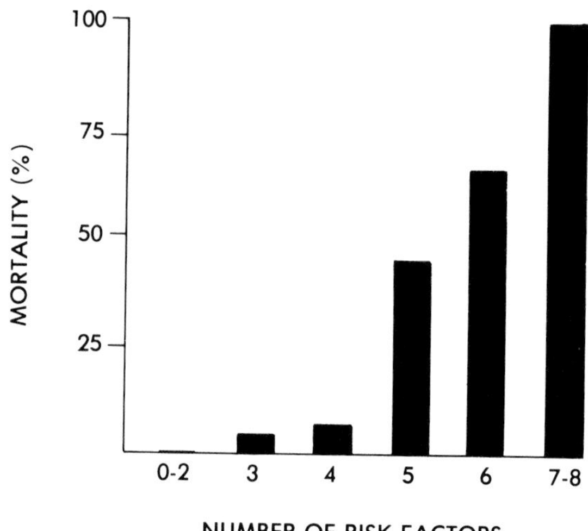

Fig. 29-3 Correlation between mortality and number of risk factors in 155 consecutive patients. (From Pitt, H.A., et al.: Am. J. Surg. **141:**66, 1981.)

jaundiced patients is antipyrine elimination. Antipyrine is an analgesic drug metabolized by the liver. By measuring its disappearance from the blood following oral administration, the magnitude of hepatic dysfunction can be calculated. However, this test and those suggested by Hunt to detect fibrin degradation products are not presently available in most hospitals. Until these tests are more readily available, simple parameters of liver and renal function, measurement of serum albumin, and assessment of the degree of sepsis and the possibility of malignant obstruction should provide extremely useful information about an individual patient's potential risk.

Nonoperative Approach

With the development of thin-needle percutaneous transhepatic cholangiography for diagnosis of the jaundiced patient, percutaneous and endoscopic treatment modalities have also evolved. As recently as the mid-1970s, the only option for decompression of patients with obstructive jaundice was surgery. In the mid-1980s, however, available options in most tertiary referral centers included percutaneous transhepatic tube drainage, endoscopic sphincterotomy, percutaneous or endoscopically placed endoprostheses, and balloon dilation, either by the percutaneous or endoscopic route. Although the relative risks and benefits of percutaneous transhepatic drainage (PTD) and endoscopic sphincterotomy are now clearly established, the late results of endoprosthesis placement and balloon dilation are only now becoming available.

Percutaneous Transhepatic Drainage

This nonoperative technique of biliary decompression was introduced in 1974. Shortly thereafter, numerous authors confirmed that PTD could be performed with little morbidity. As a result, many of these authors recommended that PTD should be used routinely both for palliation of patients with advanced malignant neoplasms and for preoperative preparation of severely jaundiced patients (Fig. 29-4). However, more recent reports by several authors[28,37,52] have cautioned that a significant proportion of patients undergoing PTD are subject to both early and late complications.

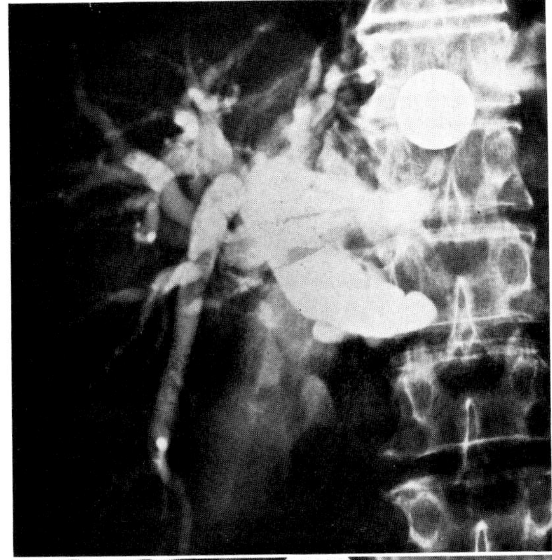

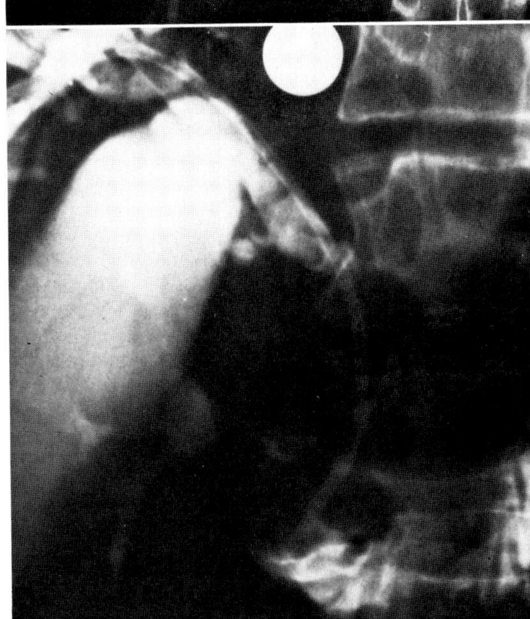

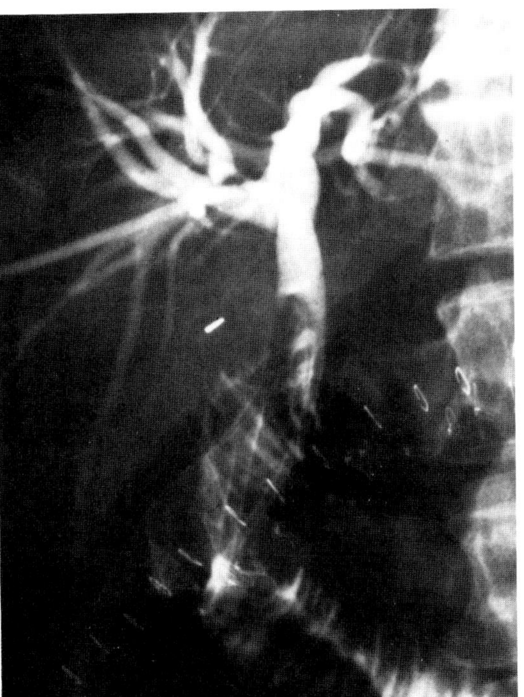

Fig. 29-4 **A,** Transhepatic cholangiogram demonstrating a very dilated common bile duct secondary to cancer of the head of the pancreas. Inferior to the common bile duct is the faint outline of a massively dilated gallbladder. **B,** Percutaneous transhepatic catheter has been placed through the obstructing lesion and into the duodenum of the same patient. **C,** Postoperative tube cholangiogram in the same patient following cholecystectomy and Roux-en-Y choledochojejunostomy. Percutaneously placed stent has been retained and crosses the anastomosis for the performance of postoperative cholangiography. Distal hook of this Ring catheter was cut off at surgery to facilitate catheter removal.

A careful analysis of these more recent studies suggests that major complications occur in 10% to 25% of patients undergoing PTD. The most frequent serious complications include bacteremia, which is seen in 10% to 20% of patients, hemobilia, which occurs in 7% to 15% of patients, and liver abscesses, which develop in 2% to 5% of patients undergoing prolonged drainage. Moreover, 1% to 2% of patients will require an emergency laparotomy following PTD, and the mortality directly related to this radiologic procedure varies between 1% and 2%.

Recent analyses from UCLA[24,56] suggest that both morbidity and mortality following PTD are related to the underlying disease process. In an analysis of 95 patients undergoing PTD over a 4-year period,[24] postprocedure morbidity ($p < 0.05$) and mortality ($p < 0.01$) were significantly greater when PTD was being performed for palliation as opposed to preoperative preparation. Thirty-day hospital mortality in patients undergoing PTD for palliation of end-stage malignancies was 26%, a figure that has recently been substantiated in four other studies from the United States. Moreover, 30-day mortality approached 40% in patients with end-stage malignancies and a bilirubin greater than 20 mg/100 ml. Thus, in patients with advanced malignant neoplasms and severe jaundice, the risks of PTD may outweigh the benefits. Even in these patients, however, PTD may be justified if pruritis is incapacitating and cannot be controlled medically. Further discussion of the role of PTD in preparation of jaundiced patients for surgery will be reviewed in a subsequent section on preoperative preparation.

Endoscopic Sphincterotomy

Endoscopic sphincterotomy (ES) is a technique by which the sphincteric fibers of the sphincter of Oddi are cut endoscopically with a device known as the sphincterotome, thereby allowing stones trapped within the common bile duct to pass into the duodenum. Collective studies[9,18,42,55] from the United States, England, Europe, and Japan all document that ES is a relatively safe and effective procedure. Specific details about the mortality, morbidity, and late complications following ES are presented in Table 29-5. In most series, procedure-related mortality occurs in slightly more than 1% of patients. Major postprocedure morbidity is seen in an average of 8% of patients. These early complications include hemorrhage, pancreatitis, cholangitis (usually because of stone impaction), and duodenal perforation. However, the requirement for emergency surgery for management of a complication following ES occurs on the average in only 1.5% of patients. Clearly morbidity, mortality, and the success of the procedure are related to experience.

Table 29-5 **MORTALITY, MORBIDITY, AND LATE COMPLICATIONS OF ENDOSCOPIC SPHINCTEROTOMY**

Complications	Mean (%)	Range (%)
Mortality	1.1	0.4-1.7
Morbidity		
Major—early	8.2	4.4-8.7
Hemorrhage	2.8	1.8-5
Pancreatitis	2.7	0.6-3.3
Cholangitis/impaction	1.8	0.8-2.3
Duodenal perforation	1	0.2-1.5
Emergency surgery	1.5	0.4-2.4
Unsuccessful procedure	9.8	3.4-14
Late complications		
Gallbladder problems	14.9	14.7-15.2
Recurrent stones	5.9	2.8-20.5
Sphincter stenosis	3	0.8-3.7

Initial reports of late complications following ES suggested that when this procedure was performed with the gallbladder in situ, later gallbladder problems developed in about 15% of patients. More recent reports suggest that this figure may be somewhat high; however, little data are available on the long-term requirements for cholecystectomy in patients who have previously undergone an ES. Of note also is the fact that an average of 6% of patients having previously undergone an endoscopic sphincterotomy will develop recurrent gallstones. Moreover, the incidence of subsequent sphincter stenosis following endoscopic sphincterotomy has averaged 3% in the few available reports. However, as with subsequent gallbladder problems and recurrent stones, long-term data are not yet available.

Most authorities would agree that ES is an appropriate procedure in patients who have previously undergone cholecystectomy and then develop recurrent or primary common duct stones. Even in these patients, however, one wonders whether routine ablation of the sphincter is necessary when most experienced biliary surgeons perform a sphincteroplasty or biliary diversion in less than one half of similar patients. ES may also be an appropriate procedure for very carefully selected patients who have previously undergone cholecystectomy and are now suspected of having stenosis or dyskinesia of the sphincter of Oddi. Only recently have reports been published describing the use of ES in the urgent management of patients with gallstone pancreatitis or cholangitis. Determination of whether ES provides any advantage over surgery in these high-risk patients must await the results of ongoing randomized trials.

Endoprosthesis

In patients with malignant obstruction of the biliary tract, nonoperative intubation with an indwelling tube (such as polyethylene), i.e., endoprosthesis, has been recommended as an alternative to surgery. The largest experience with endoprostheses placed either by the percutaneous or endoscopic routes comes from Europe. Burcharth[6] from Denmark has the largest experience with percutaneous placement of endoprostheses, whereas Hagenmuller[27] has recently reported the collected results of endoprostheses placed by six European endoscopists. A summary of these reports is presented in Table 29-6. The number of patients in these two reports is almost identical, and in each case more than 90% of the patients had malignant obstruction. Burcharth reports that percutaneous placement of an endoprosthesis was successful in 88% of patients vs. 84% for endoscopic placement as reported by Hagenmuller. Moreover, both reported morbidity and mortality are significantly higher and median survival somewhat lower in those patients treated with endoscopic placement of an endoprosthesis when compared with the percutaneous route. Although this sort of analysis may not be fair because of differences in patient population, both reports suggest that placement of an endoprosthesis by either route is not a benign procedure. Of note also is the very short median survival of these patients. Although not specifically reported, it must be assumed that a number of these patients died within 30 days of the placement of an endoprosthesis. It is necessary to obtain such data to compare results with palliative bypass surgery and with palliative placement of biliary drainage catheters.

Bilionasal Drainage

Bilionasal drainage is another biliary endoscopic approach that has been advocated in recent years to provide drainage. This technique has been suggested for (1) decompression of obstructed bile ducts, (2) prevention of stone impaction at the time of endoscopic papillectomy, (3) treatment of a biliocutaneous fistula, (4) dissolution of common duct stones, (5) aspiration of bile for chemical and bacteriologic analysis, and (6) drainage in malignant biliary obstruction. The principle behind this technique is to provide drainage through a long catheter placed within the biliary tree and exiting through the nose. Although this technique may be suitable in a number of temporary situations, the use of bilionasal drainage for more permanent decompression of obstructed ducts seems inappropriate. Moreover, the ability of even experienced endoscopists to place a bilionasal catheter past a proximal obstruction is quite limited (Fig. 29-5). Problems with dislodgement and the small caliber of these catheters have limited their usefulness.

Balloon Dilation

Occasionally strictured or stenosed bile ducts responsible for jaundice can be dilated. Dilation of biliary strictures with a Gruntzig balloon catheter may be performed by either the percutaneous or endoscopic route.[17,63] Several reports of a small number of patients managed in this manner are now beginning to appear in the literature. Although it appears that balloon dilation of biliary strictures is reasonably safe, initial data suggest that this procedure is more likely to be successful in patients who have had a previous biliary-enteric anastomosis. In contrast, balloon dilation of strictured bile ducts that are otherwise in continuity have been quite dismal when compared with surgical results.

Table 29-6 **RESULTS OF PERCUTANEOUSLY AND ENDOSCOPICALLY PLACED ENDOPROSTHESES**

Findings	Percutaneous Endoprostheses Burcharth*	Endoscopic Endoprostheses Hagenmuller†
Malignant	91%	95%
Successful	88%	84%
Complications	17.6%	26.3%
Deaths	1.5%	7.9%
Median survival	3.2 months	2.5 months

*455 patients treated.
†454 patients treated.

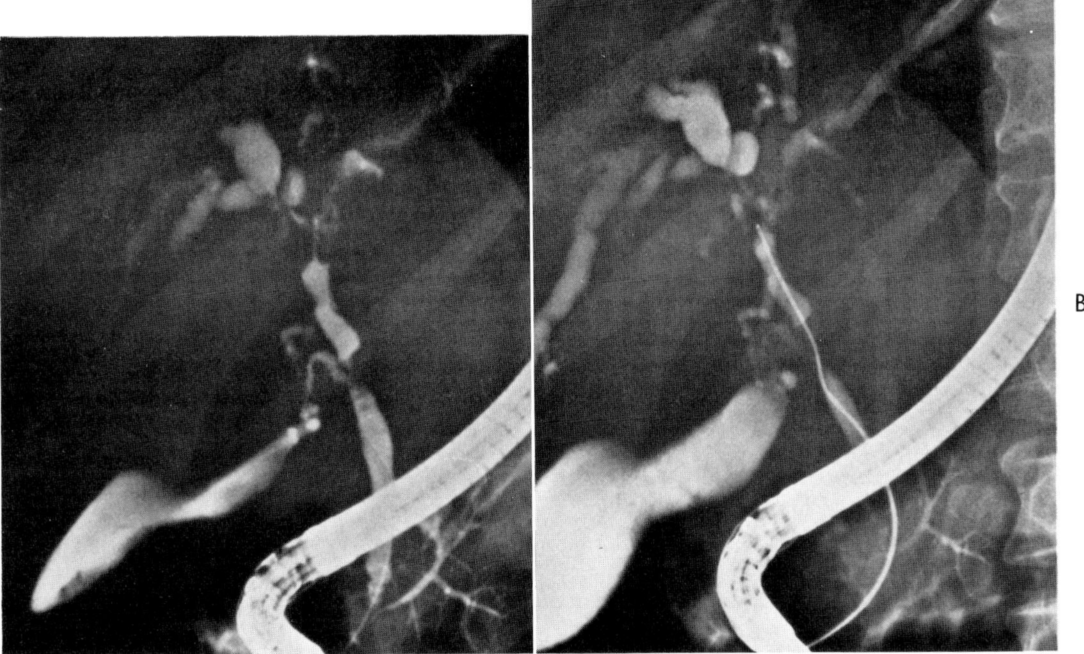

Fig. 29-5 **A,** Endoscopic retrograde cholangiography demonstrates an extensive cholangiocarcinoma involving liver hilum and common hepatic-cystic duct junction. **B,** Attempt to establish nasobiliary drainage in the same patient was unsuccessful because of the difficulty of draining the most proximal hilar lesion.

In analyzing these reports, care must be taken to assess the length of the follow-up period. This factor is extremely important because Pitt and associates[48] have recently reported that less than 50% of all recurrent strictures occurred by 2 years after a previous surgical repair and only 80% of patients with recurrent strictures had become symptomatic by 5 years after their previous operation. Moreover, the criteria that radiologists and endoscopists are using for "successful" ballon dilation allow for multiple procedures to be performed. Since many of these procedures require general anesthesia and some are followed by sepsis and renal problems, the overall hospital stay and cost of balloon dilation may actually be more than that necessary with one successful operation. Nevertheless, balloon dilation probably is appropriate in selected, high-risk patients with complex biliary problems.

Operative Approach

Preoperative Preparation

The preoperative preparation of jaundiced patients is in part the same as that of any patient undergoing a major abdominal operation. However, certain aspects of preoperative preparation such as the management of cholangitis and prevention of renal problems are unique to these patients. In patients with biliary cirrhosis, the special problems of fluid management and intraoperative bleeding must also be anticipated.

General Considerations. Patients with a history of congestive heart failure, most cirrhotics, and those with "toxic" cholangitis all need careful monitoring of their fluid balance. In these patients measurement of central venous pressure and, in many instances, pulmonary capillary wedge pressure will be necessary. As the result of secondary hyperaldosteronism, cirrhotic patients retain both sodium and water. Therefore, to avoid fluid overload the administration of both sodium and fluids to cirrhotic patients needs to be carefully monitored.

On the other hand, jaundiced patients and especially those with cirrhosis and cholangitis are at increased risk of developing renal insufficiency. Therefore maintenance of adequate blood volume is extremely important if renal problems are to be averted. Thus many of the same patients who are at risk for fluid overload are also prone to renal failure, and to avoid difficulties a very fine balance must be maintained. In 1965 Dawson[10] suggested that the liberal use of perioperative mannitol could achieve the goals of maintaining adequate blood volume, causing an osmotic diuresis, and protecting the kidneys. As mentioned earlier in the section on pathophysiology, preoperative treatment with oral bile salts may also be effective in preventing postoperative renal problems.

Patients with obstructive jaundice, cholangitis, or cirrhosis are all prone to excessive intraoperative bleeding. The most common clotting defect in patients with obstructive jaundice is prolongation of the prothrombin time, which is generally reversible by administration of parenteral vitamin K. Patients with severe jaundice and/or cholangitis may also develop disseminated intravascular coagulation, which may require infusion of platelets and fresh frozen plasma. Reversal of disseminated intravascular coagulation, however, requires control of the underlying source of sepsis. In cirrhotic patients clotting abnormalities may be more complicated. Mild degrees of thrombocytopenia usually do not require therapy. However, when thrombocytopenia becomes severe, intraoperative transfusion of platelets may be necessary; splenectomy is rarely indicated in this situation. If a cirrhotic patient with intraoperative or postoperative hemorrhage does not respond to these measures, fibrinolysis should be considered. This diagnosis can be established by demonstrating a shortened clot lysis time and hypofibrinogenemia. Schwartz[54] has recommended the use of the ϵ-aminocaproic acid if fibrinolysis occurs.

Another important consideration in preoperative preparation is the patient's nutrition. Although debate continues about the role of preoperative total parenteral nutrition, our opinion is that those patients who are obviously malnourished clinically and/or anergic on skin testing will benefit by an adequate period of preoperative total parenteral nutrition. However, in managing patients with obstructive jaundice, the very patients who might benefit most from a period of preoperative total parenteral nutrition are also those who might deteriorate with the passage of time because of progression of obstructive jaundice or cholangitis. One option would be to manage these patients with nonoperative biliary decompression while focusing on improvement of nutrition and treatment of sepsis. Present data would suggest, however, that reversal of nutritional and immune deficits in jaundiced patients with underlying malignancies may be extremely difficult and, if conceivably possible, may take up to several months.

Control of Sepsis. The initial management of patients with acute cholangitis secondary to biliary obstruction includes both systemic antibiotics and appropriate fluid and electrolyte replacement. In the rare patient who presents in septic shock and does not respond to initial treatment with fluids, an inotropic agent such as dopamine may also be required. In this setting we have usually also given one or two large doses of steroids. If the patient's condition does not stabilize with this initial management, emergency measures are indicated to achieve biliary decompression. In the past, the only option available to the patient and his physician has been emergency surgery. However, nonoperative options such as percutaneous transhepatic drainage (PTD) and endoscopic papillotomy are now also available in many institutions. In 1978 Nakayama, Ikeda, and Okuda[41] from the Chiba University in Japan reported that 10 of 11 patients with acute cholangitis were successfully managed with PTD. In a more recent analysis from UCLA, Grace and associates[24] demonstrated that the morbidity and mortality were the same when PTD was performed in patients with and without preprocedure cholangitis. Thus, when experienced radiologists are available, percutaneous transhepatic drainage may be an appropriate option for the initial management of septic jaundiced patients. In patients with stones impacted at the ampulla, endoscopic papillotomy may also be considered for treatment of cholangitis. Surprisingly little data have been published on the role of endoscopic sphincterotomy in managing patients with cholangitis, and what data are available suggest that morbidity and mortality are increased in this subpopulation. Hopefully, randomized trials comparing these newer nonoperative options with operative decompression will provide data on the relative merits of these procedures. In the meantime, the availability and expertise of radiologists and endoscopists in an individual institution will probably dictate which procedure is chosen.

In those patients who respond rapidly to initial medical management, operative or nonoperative biliary decompression can be delayed. Before performing invasive diagnostic studies, however, we have generally waited until the patient has been afebrile for at least 48 hours. Even though the incidence of sepsis following transhepatic cholangiography or endoscopic retrograde cholangiography is higher in patients who present with cholangitis, these procedures can still be performed safely in this setting. Once the diagnosis has been established, however, surgery should be undertaken without further delay.

Proper choice of antibiotics is another important consideration in the initial management of patients with cholangitis. In choosing one or more antibiotics for these patients, several factors must be considered. The properties of an antibiotic that are important include: (1) antibacterial spectrum; (2) biliary excretion; (3) blood, liver, and tissue levels; and (4) toxicity. With the plethora of newer antibiotics, several agents or combinations of antibiotics are now available that provide a broad antibacterial spectrum against biliary organisms. For many years, the combination of a penicillin and an aminoglycoside has been recommended to cover the gram-negative aerobes such as *Escherichia coli* and *Klebsiella pneumoniae* and the *Streptococcus fecalis* (enterococcus) that are so frequently isolated from the bile of patients with biliary sepsis. Recent studies by Pitt and associates[49,50] have also suggested that anaerobes, including *Bacteroides fragilis,* are isolated from the bile in elderly patients, those with cholangitis, and those with complex biliary problems. In these situations, anaerobic coverage is also indicated. To achieve this purpose the addition of a newer broad-spectrum penicillin with anaerobic coverage, clindamycin, metronidazole, or cefoxitin might also be considered.

Since severe cholangitis can be life-threatening, treatment with antibiotics with known toxicities can be justified. However, of particular concern is the use of potentially nephrotoxic aminoglycosides in septic, jaundiced patients. Now that newer broad-spectrum penicillins such as piperacillin and mezlocillin and third-generation cephalosporins such as cefoperazone, which have both broad antibacterial spectrum and extremely high biliary excretion, are available, these agents might be considered for treatment of septic jaundiced patients. Determination of whether these newer options are, in fact, less toxic and as efficacious as older regimens, including an aminoglycoside, must await the result of ongoing trials.

Preoperative Drainage. During the 1970s surgical relief of biliary obstruction in severely jaundiced patients was associated with postoperative morbidity in 40% to 60% and mortality in 15% to 20% of patients. During this same period, numerous authors reported that percutaneous transhepatic drainage (PTD) could be performed with little morbidity. For this reason, preoperative PTD was recommended and supported by retrospective and nonrandomized studies. However, more recent reports from several institutions have cautioned that a significant proportion of patients undergoing PTD are subject to both early and late complications.

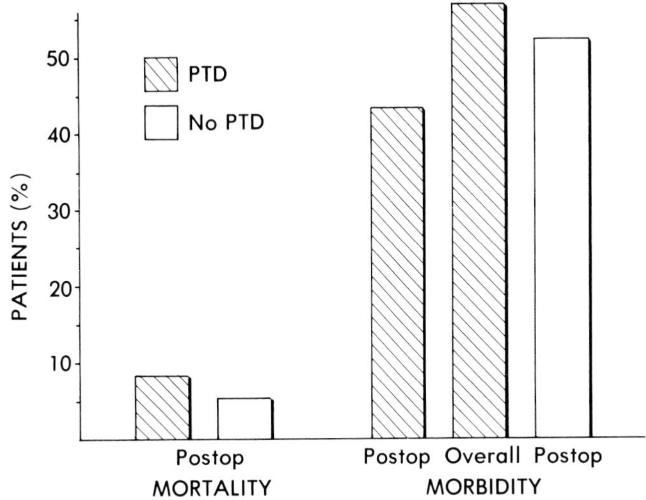

Fig. 29-6 Postoperative mortality and morbidity in a group of 37 patients undergoing preoperative percutaneous transhepatic drainage *(PTD)* vs. 38 patients who went to surgery without undergoing preoperative drainage *(No PTD)*. Overall morbidity in PTD patients represents postoperative plus PTD complications. (From Pitt, H.A., et al.: Ann. Surg. **201:**545, 1985.)

Thus controversy has existed as to what role preoperative biliary drainage should play. To answer this question, three prospective, randomized studies have recently been reported. The first such study was performed by Hatfield and co-workers[28] from South Africa. These investigators failed to demonstrate any advantage in terms of postoperative morbidity or mortality for preoperative PTD. In this study four of 29 drained patients (14%) and four of 28 undrained patients (14%) died. However, five of the eight deaths occurred in patients in whom either PTD could not be performed (one patient) or in whom no surgical procedure was done (five patients). The second prospective, randomized study was done at the Hammersmith Hospital in London by McPherson and colleagues.[37] In this study of 65 patients hospital mortality was actually higher in the drained (32%) than in the undrained (19%) patient ($p > 0.05$). In this study five of 11 deaths in the drained group occurred in patients who never came to operation.

The third study was done at UCLA by Pitt and co-workers.[52] In this study of 75 patients, hospital mortality was 8% among drained patients and 5% in those patients who underwent surgery without preoperative PTD (Fig. 29-6). In both this study and the Hammersmith study, no significant differences in postoperative morbidity were noted between the drained and undrained patients. Moreover, in both of these studies the duration of hospital stay was significantly longer ($p < 0.05$) in the patients who had preoperative biliary tract drainage. Thus, although retrospective analyses suggested that preoperative PTD might be beneficial, prospective, randomized studies have not supported this early enthusiasm. One criticism of each of these prospective studies, however, is that the duration of preoperative drainage (10 to 18 days) may not have been sufficient to reverse the multiple metabolic and immunologic abnormalities associated with severe obstructive jaundice.

Surgical Options

The list of biliary problems that may cause obstructive jaundice is quite long. Among the benign causes are postoperative strictures, common bile duct and intrahepatic stones, congenital problems (such as Caroli's disease and choledochal cysts), chronic pancreatitis, sphincter of Oddi stenosis, primary sclerosing cholangitis, and posttraumatic strictures. The most common malignant cause of biliary obstruction is carcinoma of the pancreas. However, malignant and benign tumors of the biliary tree, ampulla, and duodenum may also present with jaundice and require surgical therapy.

BENIGN LESIONS. The most common benign cause of obstructive jaundice is choledocholithiasis. In the management of these patients at surgery, cholangiography, usually through the cystic duct, is performed before the common duct is opened (choledochotomy). This x-ray film is obtained to define anatomy and to visualize the number and position of the gallstones in the extrahepatic ducts. Generally a vertical choledochotomy is then performed, with the exact location being chosen after consideration of such items as (1) the ductal anatomy, (2) the position and number of stones, and (3) whether a biliary drainage procedure is contemplated. Stones in the distal bile duct may frequently be "milked" out of the choledochotomy incision through gentle finger manipulation. This maneuver is greatly aided by freeing the lateral duodenal sweep of its peritoneal attachments (the so-called Kocher maneuver). A variety of instruments, including stone forceps, irrigating catheters, baskets, and Fogarty biliary catheters, are available for retrieving stones from the ductal system. At this point operative cholangioscopy (choledochoscopy) is routinely performed to visualize the inside of the common duct to ensure that no stones have been missed. If the cholangioscope can be easily passed through the sphincter of Oddi, no further manipulation of the sphincter is required. If not, the sphincter is initially probed with a No. 10 or No. 12 French Red Robinson catheter to ensure patency. If this catheter cannot be passed, a No. 3 Bake's dilator is gently passed through the sphincter. At no time, however, is the sphincter dilated. After the duct has been cleared by cholangioscopy and the sphincter's patency documented, a T-tube is inserted within the duct to provide postoperative biliary drainage while the choledochotomy incision is healing. Completion cholangiography is also routinely performed.

With this routine and with the aid of operative cholangioscopy, transduodenal sphincterotomy (cutting the fibers of the sphincter of Oddi) or sphincteroplasty (suturing the cut edge of these transected fibers) is only rarely necessary. These procedures should probably be reserved for impacted stones that cannot be retrieved by the techniques described earlier in patients with small-caliber bile ducts. Occasionally, anastomosis of the common bile duct to the duodenum (choledochoduodenostomy) will be necessary to provide adequate biliary drainage. We have generally reserved choledochoduodenostomy for elderly patients with large ducts who have multiple common duct stones, twice recurrent stones, or "primary" stones when a motility disorder is suspected or a peri-Vaterian duodenal diverticulum is present. In young patients, the more formidable Roux-en-Y choledochojejunostomy (anastomosis of the common duct to a defunctionalized limb of jejunum) would be performed for the same indications mentioned earlier. In patients with intrahepatic stones with or without congenital or acquired dilation, the Roux-en-Y choledochojejunostomy would be performed high, near the junction of the right and left hepatic ducts. For more details concerning these surgical options, see standard books on operative technique.

Numerous operations have been proposed for the management of patients who sustain operative injury to their biliary system. In addition, considerable controversy continues regarding (1) the best operation to perform, (2) the type of biliary stent (a synthetic prosthesis temporally placed within a repaired biliary duct to prevent postopera-

Table 29-7 **RESULTS OF STRICTURE REPAIR IN 138 PATIENTS MANAGED AT UCLA, 1955-1979**

Period	Number of Patients	Mortality (%)	Good Result (%)
1955-1969	72	4	68
1970-1979	66	0	86*
1955-1979	138	2	77

Modified from Pitt, H.A., Roslyn, J.J., and Tompkins, R.K.: Surgical resection of bile duct cancer. In Wanebo, H.J., editor: Hepatic and biliary cancer, New York, 1986, Marcel Dekker, Inc.
*$p < 0.01$ vs. 1955-1969.

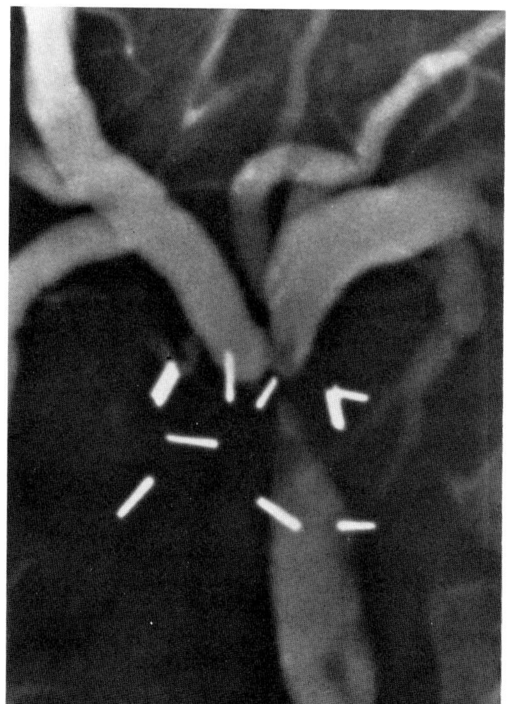

Fig. 29-7 **A,** Transhepatic cholangiogram showing a benign postoperative biliary stricture.

tive stricture formation) to use, and (3) the optimal time for postoperative stenting. Over a 25-year period from 1955 through 1979, 138 patients underwent 172 operations at the UCLA Medical Center for repair of iatrogenic injuries to the bile ducts.[50] The results of surgery in the 72 patients initially managed between 1955 and 1969 and the 66 patients initially managed between 1970 and 1979 are presented in Table 29-7. For the entire 25 years, 77% of 138 patients achieved an excellent or good result following their initial operation, and overall operative mortality was 2%. However, when the periods before and after 1970 were compared, results were found to be significantly better ($p < 0.01$) in the more recent years. Since 1970 an excellent or good result has been achieved following one repair in 86% of patients.

In this series of operative stricture repairs, a number of factors were correlated with a good or poor outcome. Patients less than 30 years of age were significantly more likely ($p < 0.025$) to achieve an excellent or good result. As might be expected, the number of previous repairs was also important. As the number of previous repairs increased, the percentage of patients achieving a good result decreased ($r = -0.96$; $p < 0.05$). Over the 25 years of this study, a number of operations were performed, but the most common operation was a Roux-en-Y choledochojejunosotomy or hepaticojejunostomy (anastomosis of the hepatic ducts to the jejunum). These procedures accounted for 73% of the operations and the best results obtained ($p < 0.01$). Over the 25 years analyzed, various types of stents were used. The best results, however, were obtained with silastic, transhepatic U- or J-tubes (Fig. 29-7). Of 20 patients, 18 (90%) stented with silastic transhepatic tubes achieved an excellent or good result. These results are particularly impressive when it is realized that this type of stenting was generally reserved for the most difficult strictures in the hepatic hilum. In those patients requiring prolonged stenting for 9 to 12 months, the tubes are changed every 3 months to prevent occlusion with biliary "sludge."

In managing patients with choledochal cysts, we prefer total excision over cystenterostomy on the basis of (1) low operative mortality, (2) fewer long-term complications of stone formation and cholangitis, and (3) reduced risk of malignant degeneration in the remaining cyst wall. In those patients in whom excision is not possible because the patient is too ill or the procedure is considered to be too risky, we prefer Roux-en-Y choledochocystojejunostomy (anastomosis of the cyst to a defunctionalized limb of the jejunum).

Detailed discussion of the surgical approach to the multiple other benign causes of biliary obstruction is beyond the scope of this chapter. In brief, we prefer Roux-en-Y hepaticojejunostomy with transhepatic stents for bilateral Caroli's disease and for the initial management of unilateral Caroli's disease. For persistent distal bile duct obstruction secondary to chronic pancreatitis, we prefer Roux-en-Y choledochojejunostomy. Should this problem occur, surgery is indicated when persistent elevation of the alkaline phosphatase is documented and, hopefully, before the patient becomes jaundiced or develops severe biliary cirrhosis. Pitt, Roslyn, and Tompkins[51] have also been advocates of an aggressive surgical approach for primary sclerosing cholangitis. In patients with primary sclerosing cholangitis whose diseases are confined to the distal common bile duct or a predominant stricture at or near the confluence of the hepatic ducts, we prefer a biliary-enteric

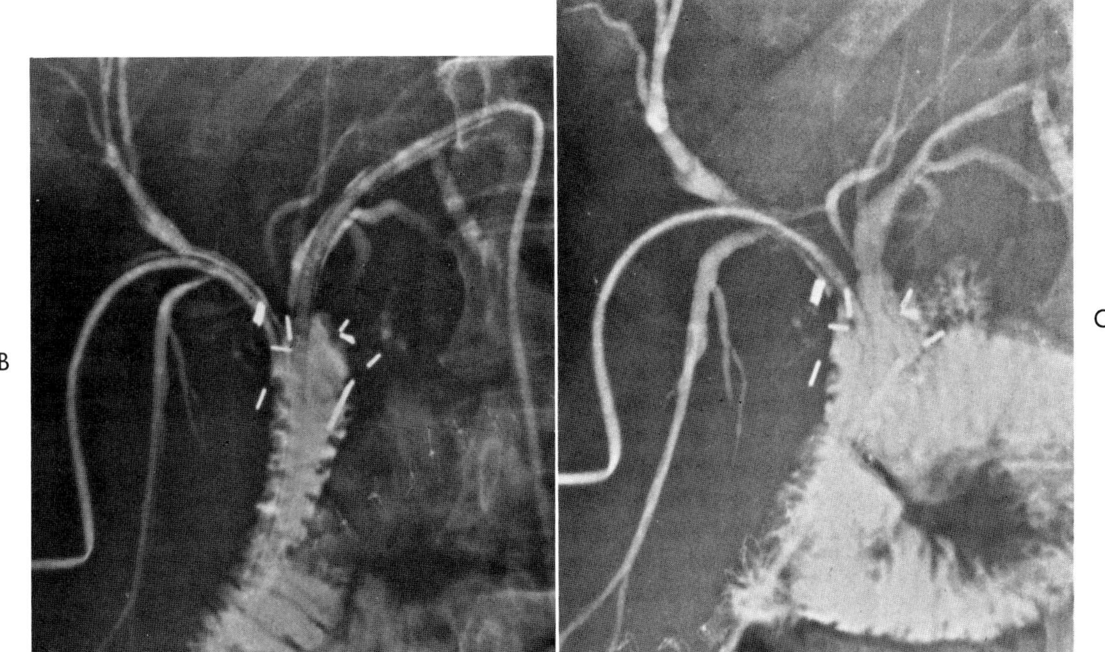

Fig. 29-7, cont'd **B,** Tube cholangiography in the same patient 6 months following bilateral hepaticojejunostomies and placement of bilateral transhepatic stents. **C,** Tube cholangiography performed 9 months after surgery in the same patient. Left transhepatic stent has been removed. Right stent was left in place for an additional 3 months.

anastomosis with or without silastic transhepatic stents, depending on the level of obstruction. For further discussion of the operative management of patients with benign lesions of the bile ducts, see the monograph by Tompkins and Pitt.[59]

MALIGNANT LESIONS. Carcinoma of the pancreas continues to be the most common malignant cause for obstructive jaundice. Operative management in these patients will depend on the extent of disease. If extension to the liver can be documented before surgery, nonoperative management with percutaneous or endoscopic placement of an endoprosthesis is a reasonable approach. Presently trials are under way to compare the morbidity, mortality, and quality of subsequent existence in patients with localized unresectable lesions managed by operative biliary diversion or endoprosthesis. Unless these trials show a definite advantage for the nonoperative approach, we would prefer a palliative surgical bypass because it usually obviates the need for any long-term tubes or requirement for another procedure if an endoprosthesis becomes occluded with biliary "sludge." In performing a palliative bypass, the choice between the gallbladder and the common duct as a site for anastomosis to the jejunum depends on the anatomy of the cystic duct and the local extent of the tumor. If the cystic duct is patent and its entrance to the common bile duct is at least 1.5 cm from the point of obstruction, the gallbladder is used. If these criteria are not met, a Roux-en-Y choledochojejunostomy is performed. The addition of a gastrojejunostomy is individualized but performed in most patients because of the risk of duodenal obstruction that commonly occurs in patients with pancreatic cancer.

If a chance for surgical cure exists, the Whipple procedure (pancreatoduodenectomy) is the procedure of choice. Several recent reports have documented very acceptable rates of morbidity and mortality for pancreatoduodenectomy. Trede[61] from Mannheim, West Germany has recently reported an operative mortality rate of 2.5% in 118 pancreatoduodenectomies performed for cancer and 81 performed for chronic pancreatitis. Similarly, Jones and colleagues[31] from Toronto reported a 5% mortality when pancreatoduodenectomy was performed in 87 patients with periampullary adenocarcinoma. At UCLA Grace and coworkers[25] reported a 6% mortality following 96 pancreatoduodenectomies, 70 of which were performed for periampullary adenocarcinoma. During the last 5 years of this analysis, only one of 45 patients died following surgery, a mortality rate of 2%. With these acceptable mortality rates and because the differentiation between a distal bile duct and a pancreatic carcinoma cannot always be made at the time of surgery, we continue to advocate pancreatoduodenectomy for periampullary tumors causing jaundice.

The number of patients with cholangiocarcinomas referred to the UCLA Medical Center over the past 30 years has increased steadily (Fig. 29-8). Whether this increased number of patients is the result of a maturation of referral patterns or a true increased prevalence of this disease is difficult to know. In managing these patients at surgery, the location and extent of the tumor will dictate therapy. Lesions of the distal bile duct account for only a small percentage of the patients seen at a tertiary referral center. If there is no evidence of distant spread of a distal bile duct tumor, pancreatoduodenectomy is the treatment of choice. If a lesion of the middle third of the duct is localized and can be separated from the hepatic artery and portal vein, resection with hepaticojejunostomy should be performed. With proximal lesions the proximity to the portal vein, hepatic artery, inferior vena cava, and the liver itself precludes curative resection in the majority of patients.

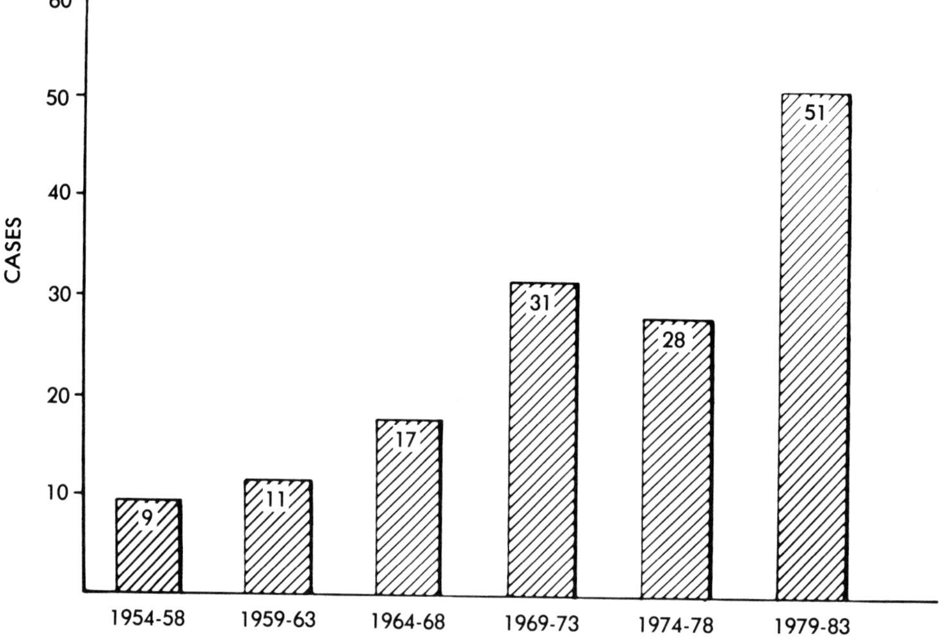

Fig. 29-8 Number of patients with cholangiocarcinoma managed at the UCLA Medical Center for each 5-year period from 1954 through 1983. (From Pitt, H.A., Roslyn, J.J., and Tompkins, R.K.: Surgical resection of bile duct cancer. Reprinted from Wanebo, H.J., editor: Hepatic and biliary cancer, New York, 1986, by courtesy of Marcel Dekker, Inc.)

High operative mortality and no obvious improvement in survival even in patients who have undergone extensive resections have prompted us to reserve these radical operations for specific cases. Thus in many cases the tumor is merely dilated and stented with transhepatic, silastic catheters. Although not yet proven to be efficacious, we have generally recommended postoperative irradiation for hilar tumors that have not been resected.

During Tompkins and associates' 24 years of experience,[60] 50 of 95 patients (53%) underwent resection of their biliary tumor, whereas the remaining 45 patients (47%) underwent a palliative procedure. In Pitt, Roslyn, and Tompkins' most recent 51 patients,[48] there has been a trend away from attempts at curative resection (27%) and a greater emphasis on palliation (73%). Palliative biliary diversion was achieved in five of these individuals (10%) nonoperatively with percutaneous transhepatic drainage. For upper-third lesions, this change in approach has resulted in a reduction in mortality for resection from 23% to 0% and a reduction in mortality for palliation from 16% to 9%.

Postoperative Care

In jaundiced patients who are not septic before surgery, prolonged postoperative administration of antibiotics is unnecessary. However, antibiotics should be continued in patients who remain febrile from cholangitis. In addition, to avoid increased intrabiliary pressures, biliary tubes should be left to gravity drainage in the early postoperative period. Furthermore, a closed drainage system should be used to prevent contamination of bile by hospital-acquired, multiple, resistant organisms. These resistant organisms most likely gain access to the biliary tree through the drainage system rather than as a result of any influence of systemic antibiotic administration.[49]

Another consideration in patients who have undergone Roux-en-Y biliary diversion is the increased gastric acid production that occurs following this procedure. In 1971 McArthur and Longmire[36] reported that 10 of 97 patients had documented peptic ulcer disease following choledochojejunostomy for treatment of benign biliary obstruction. It has been hypothesized that diversion of alkaline bile from the first portion of the duodenum increases the risk of peptic ulceration and resultant bleeding. Subsequent studies in animals and a recent study by Sato and coworkers[53] in human beings have documented increased gastric acid production after choledochojejunostomy. Because of the potential for peptic ulcer disease and upper gastrointestinal hemorrhage in these patients, we have routinely given our jaundiced patients who have undergone Roux-en-Y biliary diversion either antacids or H-2 receptor blockers (e.g., cimetidine) in the early postoperative period. Whether these agents should be continued for a longer period of time following surgery is unknown.

SUMMARY

In recent years tremendous strides have been made in our understanding of bilirubin metabolism and the pathophysiology of jaundice. Numerous advances, including ultrasonography, computed tomography, thin-needle transhepatic cholangiography, endoscopic retrograde cholangiography, and biliary scintigraphy have totally changed the diagnostic approach to the jaundiced patient, making it now possible to determine with greater certainty and clarity the cause of jaundice in a given clinical setting. Such technology has also led to new therapeutic options to treat jaundice, including percutaneous transhepatic biliary drainage, endoscopic sphincterotomy, and percutaneous or endoscopic balloon dilation or placement of an endoprosthesis, obviating the need for direct surgical intervention. Such advances have led to a number of new questions that remain unanswered with regard to managing the jaundiced patient. These questions include: (1) the relative efficacy of endoscopic sphincterotomy vs. surgery for patients with bile duct stones and especially for patients with cholangitis and gallstone pancreatitis, (2) the long-term results of balloon dilation of biliary strictures, (3) the relative efficacy of endoprostheses vs. palliative bypass surgery, and (4) whether prolonged preoperative drainage is ever indicated. Over the past decade, much has also been learned about the immune deficits of the jaundiced patient. However, very little is known about mechanisms to reverse these immune abnormalities, especially in the patient with an underlying malignancy. Moreover, despite improvements in operative mortality, the survival of patients with adenocarcinoma of the pancreas and proximal bile ducts remains dismal. In this regard, future efforts should probably be directed at identifying the causes for cancer in these organs. A breakthrough in this area of research is what is really needed to further reduce the number of jaundiced patients.

REFERENCES

1. Allison, M.E.M., et al.: Renal function and other factors in obstructive jaundice, Br. J. Surg. **66**:392, 1979.
2. Baron, R.L., et al.: A prospective comparison of the evaluation of biliary obstruction using computed tomography and ultrasonography, Radiology **145**:91, 1982.
3. Beazley, R.M., et al.: Clinicopathological aspects of high bile duct cancer: experience with resection and bypass surgical treatments, Ann. Surg. **199**:623, 1984.
4. Bilbao, M.K., et al.: Complications of endoscopic retrograde cholangiopancreatography (ERCP): a study of 10,000 cases, Gastroenterology **70**:314, 1976.
5. Blamey, S.L., et al.: Prediction of risk in biliary surgery, Br. J. Surg. **70**:535, 1983.
6. Burcharth, F.: Results of the percutaneous implantation of endoprostheses. In Classen, M., Geenen, J., and Kawai, K., editors: Nonsurgical biliary drainage, Berlin, 1984, Springer-Verlag.
7. Buzby, G.P., et al.: Prognostic nutritional index in gastrointestinal surgery, Am. J. Surg. **139**:160, 1980.
8. Cahill, C.J.: Prevention of postoperative renal failure in patients with obstructive jaundice—the role of bile salts, Br. J. Surg. **70**:590, 1983.
9. Cotton, P.B., and Vallon, A.G.: British experience with duodenoscopic sphincterotomy for removal of bile duct stones, Br. J. Surg. **68**:373, 1981.
10. Dawson, J.L.: Postoperative renal function in obstructive jaundice: effect of mannitol diuresis, Br. Med. J. **1**:82, 1965.
11. Dixon, J.M., et al.: Factors affecting morbidity and mortality after surgery for obstructive jaundice: a review of 373 patients, Gut **24**:845, 1983.
12. Drivas, G., James, O., and Wardle, E.N.: Study of reticuloendothelial phagocytic capacity in patients with cholestasis, Br. Med. J. **1**:1568, 1976.

13. Edmondson, H.A., Schiff, L., and Schiff, E.R.: Needle biopsy of the liver. In Schiff, L., and Schiff, E.R., editors: Diseases of the liver, Philadelphia, 1982, J.B. Lippincott Co.
14. Eubanks, B., et al.: Current role of intravenous cholangiography, Am. J. Surg. **143**:731, 1982.
15. Evans, H.J.R., et al.: The effect of preoperative bile salt administration on postoperative renal function in patients with obstructive jaundice, Br. J. Surg. **69**:706, 1982.
16. Fortner, J.G., et al.: Immunologic function in patients with carcinoma of the pancreas, Surg. Gynecol. Obstet. **150**:215, 1980.
17. Geenen, J.E.: Balloon dilatation of bile duct strictures. In Classen, M., Geenen, J., and Kawai, K., editors: Nonsurgical biliary drainage, Berlin, 1984, Springer-Verlag.
18. Geenen, J.E., Vennes, J.A., and Silvis, S.E.: Resume of a seminar on endoscopic retrograde sphincterotomy, Gastrointest. Endosc. **27**:31, 1981.
19. Gianni, L., et al.: Bile acid induced inhibition of the lymphoproliferative response to phytohemagglutinin and pokeweed mitogen: an in vitro study, Gastroenterology **78**:231, 1980.
20. Gibbons, C.P., Griffiths, G.J., and Cormack, A.: The role of percutaneous transhepatic cholangiography and grey-scale ultrasound in the investigation and treatment of bile duct obstruction, Br. J. Surg. **70**:494, 1983.
21. Gold, R.P., et al.: Transhepatic cholangiography: the radiological method of choice in suspected obstructive jaundice, Radiology **133**:39, 1979.
22. Goldman, L., et al.: Multifactorial index of cardiac risk in noncardiac surgical procedures, N. Engl. J. Med. **297**:845, 1977.
23. Goodman, M.W., et al.: Is intravenous cholangiography still useful? Gastroenterology **79**:642, 1980.
24. Grace, P.A., et al.: The risks of percutaneous transhepatic drainage in patients with cholangitis, Am. J. Roentgen. **148**:367, 1987.
25. Grace, P.A., et al.: Improved morbidity and mortality following pancreaticoduodenectomy, Am. J. Surg. **151**:141, 1986.
26. Gregg, J.A., and McDonald, D.G.: Endoscopic retrograde cholangiopancreatography and gray-scale abdominal ultrasound in the diagnosis of jaundice, Am. J. Surg. **137**:611, 1979.
27. Hagenmuller, F.: Results of endoscopic bilioduodenal drainage in malignant bile duct stenoses. In Classen, M., Geenen, J., and Kawai, K., editors: Nonsurgical biliary drainage, Berlin, 1984, Springer-Verlag.
28. Hatfield, A.R.W., et al.: Preoperative external biliary drainage in obstructive jaundice: a prospective controlled clinical trial, Lancet **2**:896, 1982.
29. Hunt, D.R.: The identification of risk factors and their application to the management of obstructive jaundice, Aust. N.Z. J. Surg. **50**:476, 1980.
30. Hunt, D.R., et al.: Endotoxemia, disturbance of coagulation, and obstructive jaundice, Am. J. Surg. **144**:325, 1982.
31. Jones, B.A., et al.: Periampullary tumors: which ones should be resected? Am. J. Surg. **149**:46, 1985.
32. Keighley, M.R.B., et al.: Hazards of surgical treatment due to microorganisms in the bile, Surgery **75**:578, 1974.
33. Knill-Jones, R.P., et al.: Use of sequential Bayesian model in diagnosis of jaundice by computer, Br. Med. J. **1**:530, 1973.
34. Matzen, P., et al.: Accuracy of direct cholangiography by endoscopic or transhepatic route in jaundice—a prospective study, Gastroenterology **81**:237, 1981.
35. Matzen, P., et al.: Ultrasonography, computed tomography, and cholescintigraphy in suspected obstructive jaundice—a prospective comparative study, Gastroenterology **84**:1492, 1983.
36. McArthur, M.S., and Longmire, W.P., Jr.: Peptic ulcer disease after choledochojejunostomy, Am. J. Surg. **122**:155, 1971.
37. McPherson, G.A.D., et al.: Preoperative percutaneous transhepatic biliary drainage: the results of a controlled trial, Br. J. Surg. **71**:371, 1984.
38. McPherson, G.A.D., et al.: Antipyrine elimination in patients with obstructive jaundice: a predictor of outcome, Am. J. Surg. **149**:140, 1985.
39. McSherry, C.K., and Glenn, F.: The incidence and causes of death following surgery for nonmalignant biliary tract disease, Ann. Surg. **191**:271, 1980.
40. Mueller, P.R., van Sonnenberg, E., and Simeone, J.F.: Fine-needle transhepatic cholangiography: indications and usefulness, Ann. Intern. Med. **97**:567, 1982.
41. Nakayama, T., Ikeda, A., and Okuda, K.: Percutaneous transhepatic drainage of the biliary tract: technique and results in 104 cases, Gastroenterology **74**:554, 1978.
42. Nakajima, M., et al.: Five years' experience of endoscopic sphincterotomy in Japan: a collective study from 25 centers, Endoscopy **2**:138, 1979.
43. O'Connor, K.W., et al.: A blinded prospective study comparing four current noninvasive approaches in the differential diagnosis of medical vs. surgical jaundice, Gastroenterology **84**:1498, 1983.
44. Okuda, K., et al.: Nonsurgical, percutaneous transhepatic cholangiography: diagnostic significance in medical problems of the liver, Am. J. Dig. Dis. **19**:21, 1974.
45. Pedrosa, C.S., Casanova, R., and Rodriquez, R.: Computed tomography in obstructive jaundice. I. The level of obstruction, Radiology **139**:627, 1981.
46. Pitt, H.A., Postier, R.G., and Cameron, J.L.: Biliary bacteria, Arch. Surg. **117**:445, 1982.
47. Pitt, H.A., Postier, R.G., and Cameron, J.L.: Consequences of preoperative cholangitis and its treatment on the outcome of operation for choledocholithiasis, Surgery **94**:447, 1983.
48. Pitt, H.A., Roslyn, J.J., and Tompkins, R.K.: Surgical resection of bile duct cancer. In Wanebo, H.J., editor: Hepatic and biliary cancer, New York, 1986, Marcel Dekker, Inc.
49. Pitt, H.A., et al.: Factors affecting mortality in biliary tract surgery, Am. J. Surg. **141**:66, 1981.
50. Pitt, H.A., et al.: Factors influencing outcome in patients with postoperative biliary strictures, Am. J. Surg. **144**:14, 1982.
51. Pitt, H.A., et al.: Primary sclerosing cholangitis: results of an aggressive surgical approach, Ann. Surg. **196**:259, 1982.
52. Pitt, H.A., et al.: Does preoperative percutaneous biliary drainage reduce operative risk or increase hospital cost? Ann. Surg. **201**:545, 1985.
53. Sato, T., et al.: Effect of biliary reconstruction procedures on gastric acid secretion, Am. J. Surg. **144**:549, 1982.
54. Schwartz, S.I.: Biliary tract surgery and cirrhosis: a critical combination, Surgery **90**:577, 1981.
55. Siegel, J.H.: Endoscopic papillotomy in the treatment of biliary tract disease: 258 procedures and results, Dig. Dis. Sci. **26**:1057, 1981.
56. Stambuk, E.C., et al.: Percutaneous transhepatic drainage: risks and benefits, Arch. Surg. **118**:1388, 1983.
57. Taylor, K.J.W., Rosenfield, A.T., and Spiro, H.M.: Diagnostic accuracy of gray-scale ultrasonography for the jaundiced patient: a report of 275 cases, Arch. Med. **139**:60, 1979.
58. Thomas, M.J., Pellegrini, C.A., and Way, L.W.: Usefulness of diagnostic tests for biliary obstruction, Am. J. Surg. **144**:102, 1982.
59. Tompkins, R.K., and Pitt, H.A.: Surgical management of benign lesions of the bile ducts, Curr. Probl. Surg. **19**:374, 1982.
60. Tompkins, R.K., et al.: Prognostic factors in bile duct carcinoma, Ann. Surg. **194**:447, 1981.
61. Trede, M.: The surgical treatment of pancreatic carcinoma, Surgery **97**:28, 1985.
62. Vennes, J.A., Jacobson, J.R., and Silvis, S.E.: Endoscopic cholangiography for biliary system diagnosis, Ann. Intern. Med. **80**:61, 1974.
63. Vogel, S.B., et al.: Evaluation of percutaneous transhepatic balloon dilatation of benign biliary strictures in high-risk patients, Am. J. Surg. **149**:73, 1985.
64. Weinstein, D.P., Weinstein, B.J., and Brodmerkel, G.J.: Ultrasonography of biliary tract dilatation without jaundice, Am. J. Radiol. **132**:729, 1979.
65. Williamson, B.W.A., Blumgart, L.H., and McKellar, N.J.: Management of tumors of the liver: combined use of arteriography and venography in the assessment of resectability, especially in hilar tumors, Am. J. Surg. **139**:210, 1980.

30

Barry A. Levine and Charles D. Livingston

Splenic Physiology and Dysfunction

The spleen has been a focus of surgical attention for many centuries. However, only in recent times have the hematologic and immunologic roles of this organ been elucidated. Although surgeons have been in the forefront of much of this research, it has remained primarily the purview of internists and especially hematologists to care for patients with splenic disorders. Only by understanding clearly the pathophysiologic bases underlying diseases of the spleen can surgeons expect to act as partners with their colleagues in determining advisability and timing of splenectomy. It is with this concept in mind that the present chapter is written.

NORMAL PHYSIOLOGY AND ANATOMY OF THE SPLEEN

The spleen is an organ weighing between 75 and 150 g and is located in the left upper quadrant of the abdomen (Fig. 30-1). It is attached by reflections of the peritoneum to the undersurface of the left hemidiaphragm (lienodiaphragmatic ligament), the upper pole of the kidney (lienorenal ligament), and the splenic flexure of the colon (lienocolic ligament). The main arterial blood supply of the spleen is carried by the splenic artery, which after arising from the celiac axis and coursing on top of the pancreas enters the hilum of the organ. In the hilum of the spleen, the artery divides into six to eight segmental branches that supply corresponding segments of the organ. These are end arteries without significant cross flow. Arterial blood also reaches the spleen through the short gastric arteries extending from the greater curvature of the stomach. Venous drainage is through the splenic vein, which joins the inferior mesenteric vein behind the inferior border of the pancreatic tail. This vein continues and joins the superior mesenteric vein to form the portal vein posterior to the head of the pancreas. Short gastric veins also drain the spleen.

The normal spleen holds between 30 to 40 ml of mature red cells and one fourth of the circulating platelets in a reserve pool. Unlike other parts of the reticuloendothelial system, such as the lymph nodes and liver, the spleen possesses intraparenchymal trabeculae, which are made up in part by smooth muscle. This enables the spleen to hold larger quantities of blood and in turn to provide additional blood for the systemic circulation during times of need. Intravenous injection of epinephrine causes contracture of the spleen and release of its contents into the systemic circulation. In contrast, intravenous injection of sodium pentobarbital induces relaxation of the muscular tone of the spleen causing an increase in the amount of blood pooled there. This sequestration of red cells can result in a reduction of as much as 37% of the circulating red blood cell population.

The cellular makeup of the spleen reflects its immunologic function. The sinuses and trabecular spaces contain a large number of phagocytic macrophages. In fact, the spleen contains more macrophages than any other organ of the body including the liver. Splenic white pulp is made up of lymphoid germinal centers containing both B-cell and T-cell lymphocytes. In addition to the population of normal red blood cells, neutrophils and platelets are present in the spleen. Mesenchymal tissue is also present and has the ability to form blood cells in situ when necessary either to compensate for a failing bone marrow or as part of a disease state as occurs in a disorder such as myelofibrosis.

The microanatomy of the spleen has for many years been a mystery and even today continues to spark debate.[11] Blood enters by way of the splenic artery, which divides into trabecular arteries (Fig. 30-2). These arteries subsequently leave the trabeculae and enter the white pulp as central arteries. Central arteries then penetrate the lymphatic substance of the white pulp, sending off arterioles at right angles that either end in the white pulp or continue through it to the marginal zone adjacent to the red pulp. Once the arteriole enters the red pulp, it becomes known as the artery of the pulp and breaks up into further arteriolar branches. Ultimately this blood that is brought to the red pulp by the arteriolar branches is collected in the splenic venous sinuses. Splenic sinuses in turn drain to pulp veins, then into trabecular veins, and finally into the splenic veins. Reticular connective tissue known as splenic cords makes up the tissue between the splenic sinuses within the red pulp.

If the microcirculation of the spleen were completely understood, pathophysiology of the spleen could be better explained. Controversy surrounds the nature of the vascular connection between the terminal arteriolar vessels and the splenic sinuses. One view, known as the open or discontinuous circulation theory, states that arterial vessels terminate within the red pulp and marginal zone by opening directly into the reticular substance of the splenic cords. Blood products then circulate within the reticular substance before flowing out through the wall of the splenic sinus. Another theory suggests a closed circulation in which there is endothelial continuity between the terminal arteriolar vessels and the splenic sinuses. As in many situations in medicine, the truth probably lies somewhere between the two theories. Direct endothelium-lined channels linking terminal arterial vessels and splenic sinuses surely exist, producing a closed circulation. However, in addition, some vessels terminate blindly in the reticular substance of the red pulp, forcing blood products to circulate within the reticular system of the splenic cord before passage through splenic sinuses.

The microvasculature of the spleen allows it to accomplish many functions. Aged or damaged red blood cells entering the reticular substance are recognized and removed. In addition, foreign bodies such as bacteria come in close contact with reticular substance of the splenic cords, undergo phagocytosis, and are engulfed. Red blood cells with membrane defects known as pits are also skillfully removed.

In addition to the recognition and filtering capacity, the splenic tissue also provides certain systemic immunologic functions. Tuftsin, a substance that directs polymorphonuclear leukocytes to engulf bacteria, is produced solely in the spleen. Opsonin, which prepares bacteria for engulfment by polymorphonuclear leukocytes, is also produced in the spleen. A remote effect of the spleen on pulmonary

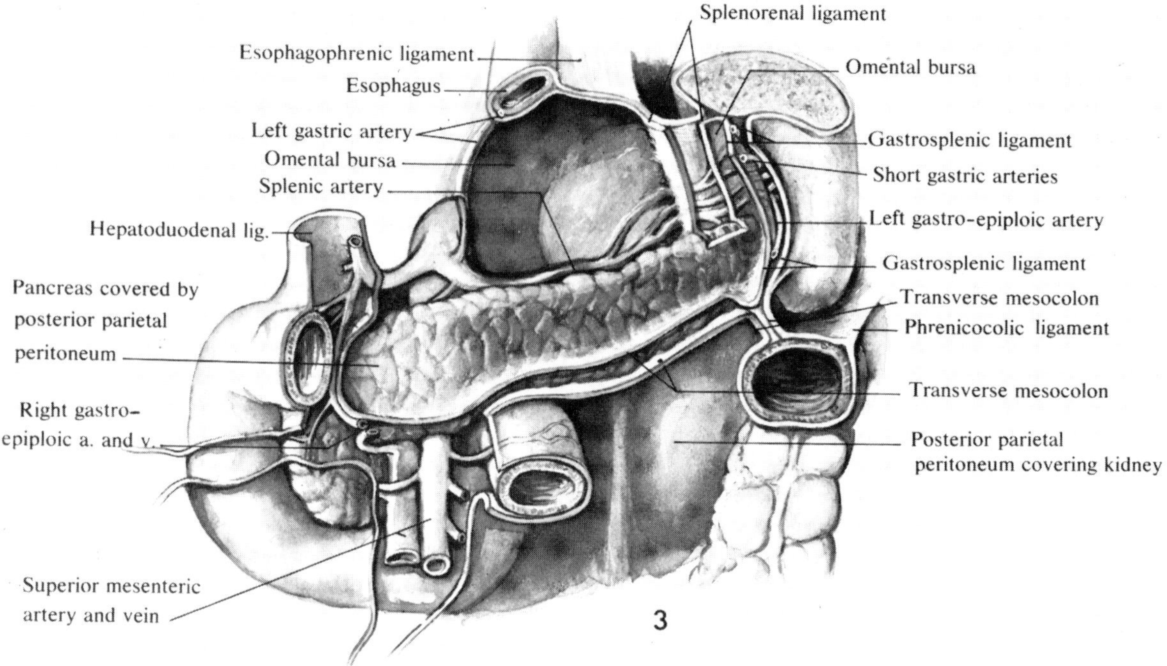

Fig. 30-1 Anatomic relationship of the spleen within the abdominal cavity. (From Healy, J.E.: A synopsis of clinical anatomy, Philadelphia, 1969, W.B. Saunders Co.)

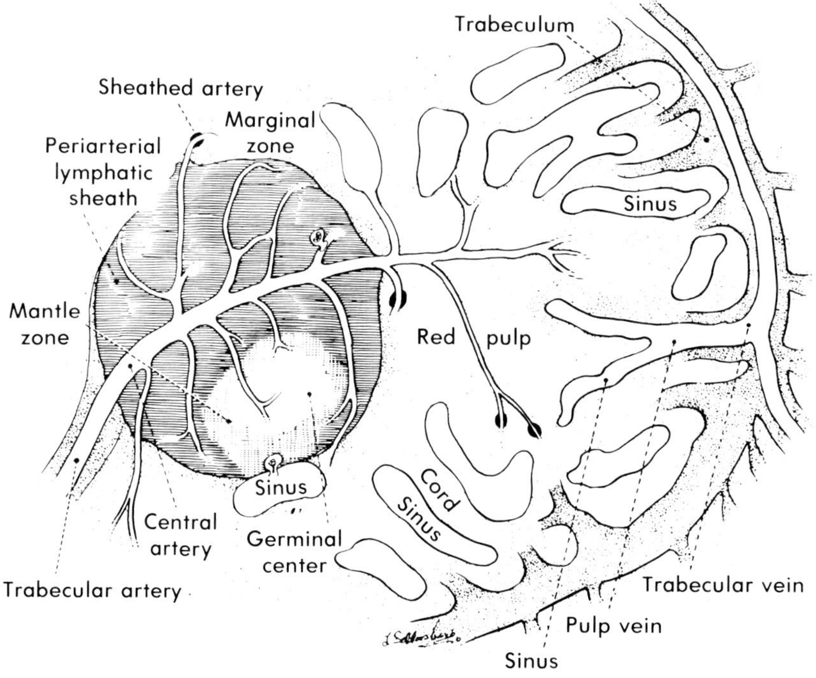

Fig. 30-2 Microanatomy of the spleen. (Reprinted by permission of the publisher from Weiss, L.: The spleen. In Greep, R.O., editor: Histology, New York, Copyright 1966 by Elsevier Science Publishing Co., Inc.)

macrophages has also been demonstrated; however, the factors mediating this have not yet been identified.

PATHOPHYSIOLOGY OF SPLENOMEGALY AND HYPERSPLENISM

The terms splenomegaly and hypersplenism, although sometimes used synonymously, have different meanings. *Splenomegaly* refers strictly to the physical enlargement of the spleen, no matter the cause. *Hypersplenism* is a physiologic term used to define hyperfunction of the spleen's filtering and disposal roles, which results in decreased numbers of circulating formed blood elements.[10] Thus a patient may have splenomegaly without hypersplenism, hypersplenism without splenomegaly, or both in combination.

Even with knowledge of its anatomy and physiology, understanding the role of the spleen in the spectrum of diseases with which it appears to be involved remains a difficult task. In the past the presence or absence of splenomegaly was used as a marker of splenic disease. However, as many as 3% of healthy, young patients have been found to have asymptomatic splenomegaly. In contrast, 93% of patients with idiopathic hypersplenism do not have a palpable spleen. With these facts in mind, attention has turned to understanding the function of the microcirculation and its interaction with the lymphoid and reticular elements of the spleen to explain pathophysiology of disease.[12]

One pathologic entity in which splenomegaly does play a role is hypersplenism secondary to portal hypertension.[18] In this disease process, the elevated portal venous pressure secondary to hepatic disease results in a concomitant increase in pressure within the splenic vein, trabecular veins, and in turn the splenic sinuses. As a result circulation time through the spleen is slowed. Normally 98% to 99% of erythrocytes pass quickly through the spleen by way of the endothelium-lined sinus. However, 1% to 2% enter the cordal system and remain there for periods up to 1 hour.

With elevation of portal pressure and slowing of circulation through the spleen, the time spent by erythrocytes within the cordal system is also increased. It is known that the red blood cell is incapable of oxidative metabolism and depends almost entirely on the anaerobic metabolism of glucose for its energy. The level of glucose within the cordal system is extremely low and predisposes the red blood cell to loss of energy necessary to maintain membrane integrity. Subsequently this leads to early hemolysis.[40] In addition, anaerobic metabolism of the small amount of glucose present within the cordal system results in a decrease in the local pH. This in turn results in an interference with the sodium pump located within the erythrocytic membrane. The inevitable outcome is an accumulation of intracellular sodium with osmotic swelling of the cell. A third deleterious effect of the cordal environment is the presence of a low ambient cholesterol level. The cholesterol of the erythrocyte membrane exists in equilibrium with the surrounding free-serum cholesterol. Therefore when the red cells remain in a region with low cholesterol levels, membrane cholesterol is depleted, causing the red blood cells to change to a spheroidal configuration that is osmotically fragile. As the time spent by erythrocytes within the cordal structure increases, lysis of these deficient red cells increases.

A final factor that increases the disappearance of red cells in splenomegaly is phagocytosis. As the circulation time of red blood cells through the spleen is slowed, the amount of time that fragmented or damaged red blood cells spend in juxtaposition to resident phagocytes is maximized, thus increasing the rate of phagocytosis. In addition, it has been shown that in the presence of splenomegaly there is an accumulation of a greater than normal number of phagocytes in the splenic cords. Platelets and polymorphonuclear leukocytes are trapped and removed by the spleen in a fashion similar to that of red blood cells.

DISEASES INVOLVING THE SPLEEN

A large number of congenital and acquired diseases involve the spleen, and the patient may benefit from its removal. The more common diseases that may necessitate the assistance of a surgeon in treatment will be discussed in the following sections. A summary of those disease states in which splenectomy may be of value is tabulated in Table 30-1.

Congenital Anemias

Congenital anemias exist in which splenectomy as a form of treatment offers lasting benefits.[8,27] These include hereditary spherocytosis, elliptocytosis, and thalassemia.

Spherocytosis

True spherocytosis is a genetically determined, autosomal dominant disease of the red blood cell membrane. It

Table 30-1 **THE ROLE OF SPLENECTOMY IN THE TREATMENT OF DISORDERS AFFECTING THE SPLEEN**

Usually Beneficial	Sometimes Beneficial	Not Beneficial
Spherocytosis	Pyruvate kinase deficiency	Sickle cell disease
Elliptocytosis	Immune hemolytic anemia (warm type)	Glucose 6-phosphate deficiency
Thalassemia	Lymphocytic lymphoma	Immune hemolytic anemia (cold type)
Idiopathic thrombocytopenic purpura	Lymphocytic leukemia	Thrombotic thrombocytopenic purpura
Splenic neutropenia	Myeloid metaplasia	
Hodgkin's disease	Sarcoidosis	
Felty's syndrome		
Gaucher's disease		
Splenic abscess		

is the most common of symptomatic hemolytic anemias. In patients with this disease the red blood cell is smaller, spheroid in shape, and has a thickened cell wall membrane that demonstrates osmotic fragility. Because of the cell's shape and thick, noncompliant cell membrane, passage of the red blood cell through the cordal structure of the spleen is difficult and slowed. Since low levels of glucose are present within the splenic cordal system, a reduction of cellular adenosine triphosphate (ATP) necessary for maintenance of membrane stability is seen. The reduced cellular ATP coupled with the cellular osmotic fragility results in increased lysis of the cell within the spleen.

Normally the bone marrow's ability to compensate for splenic hemolysis is sufficient to maintain an acceptable hematocrit. Superimposed problems such as immune hemolytic anemia may produce a crisis of drastically reduced hematocrit. However, the usual patient with spherocytosis exhibits mild anemia, reticulocytosis, and mild jaundice from the increased bilirubin secondary to red cell breakdown. Cholelithiasis is seen in 30% to 60% of patients and results from oversaturation of bile with bilirubin, yielding bilirubinate stones. Splenomegaly is found in 80%. Diagnosis is usually made by inspection of the peripheral blood smear that shows at least 60% of the red blood cells to be spherocytes. Indications for splenectomy include symptomatic cholelithiasis and inability to maintain the hematocrit over 30% without transfusion. Patients respond favorably to splenectomy because such a procedure removes the filter that extracts the abnormally-shaped red blood cells. Although the majority of red cells postoperatively will still exist as spherocytes, they will enjoy a more normal life-span.

Elliptocytosis

Congenital elliptocytosis is a disease very similar to spherocytosis. In this defect 50% to 90% of red blood cells are ovoid in shape because of an abnormal red blood cell membrane. As in spherocytosis, there is a degree of osmotic fragility. Splenectomy likewise produces a normal red blood cell life-span and should be carried out for the same indications as in spherocytosis.[20]

Thalassemia

Thalassemia appears to be a congenital defect of hemoglobin synthesis. It involves a spectrum of several closely related variants that can be carried as a major (homozygous) or minor (heterozygous) trait. Three basic types, referred to as the alpha, beta, and gamma variants, may be present.[29] These are classified according to abnormalities in the synthesis of one or another polypeptide chain, which compromise the normal human hemoglobin. Red blood cells in patients with thalassemia exhibit an increased proportion of fetal hemoglobin and increased osmotic fragility, both of which render the red blood cell more susceptible to lysis within the spleen. Patients with thalassemia major exhibit symptoms early in childhood. These may include severe anemia, jaundice from increased red blood cell breakdown, poor growth, gallstones (bilirubinate), splenomegaly, and early death. In those patients with thalassemia minor, a milder form of the disease compatible with normal life, mild anemia, jaundice, and splenomegaly are seen. The diagnosis is usually made from the peripheral blood smear that shows hypochromic, microcytic anemia and distorted red blood cells. Diagnosis is confirmed by hemoglobin electrophoresis that demonstrates an elevated level of fetal hemoglobin and diminished levels of normal hemoglobin A. Splenectomy has been shown to reduce the hemolytic process in these patients and to decrease transfusion requirements to maintain an acceptable hematocrit. It is performed only in symptomatic patients who possess an inability to maintain a hematocrit level of at least 30%.

Hereditary Nonspherocytic Hemolytic Anemias

Hereditary nonspherocytic hemolytic anemias, including enzyme deficiencies of pyruvate kinase and glucose 6-phosphate, may also result in increased hemolysis. Patients with pyruvate kinase deficiency frequently have splenomegaly, but those with glucose 6-phosphate deficiency do not. The spleen is a place of increased red cell destruction in only some of the patients with pyruvate kinase deficiency. Therefore splenectomy will not result in uniform improvement. The spleen does not seem to play a role in the anemia of glucose 6-phosphate deficiency; thus splenectomy is not indicated in its treatment.

Sickle Cell Disease

Sickle cell disease, seen mostly in the black population, is a congenital disease of hemoglobin synthesis, resulting in the substitution of hemoglobin A (Hb A) with hemoglobin S (Hb S) within the red blood cell. Sickle cell abnormalities may be clinically expressed as *trait* (heterozygous with Hb S representing 20% to 45% of circulating hemoglobin) or *disease* (homozygous with Hb S representing 76% to 100% of circulating hemoglobin). Hemoglobin F is also present in increased amounts. In the presence of reduced oxygen tension, distortion of the Hb S chain occurs, resulting in sickling of the red blood cells. Patients with sickle cell trait rarely have symptoms or require treatment. Diagnosis is made by noting the characteristic sickling on microscopic examination of the peripheral blood smear and demonstration of 80% Hb S with hemoglobin electrophoresis. In most patients with sickle cell disease (approximately 1% of blacks), the spleen undergoes infarction with subsequent contraction. This has been referred to as autosplenectomy. Splenectomy is thus found to benefit only those few patients in whom sequestration of red blood cells is demonstrated by radiolabeled-chromium–tagged red cell studies. Symptoms, most of which are related to vascular occlusion in various organs, include skin ulceration, joint pain, hematuria, central nervous system manifestations, and abdominal cramping and pain. Treatment for these symptoms is supportive. Survival of those afflicted with sickle disease is rare past the second decade.

Immune Hemolytic Anemia

Immune hemolytic anemia[2] is a disease process that is identified by premature destruction of red blood cells as a result of either antibodies or complement fixation. Classification of hemolytic anemia may be by two methods. The first method is by etiology. Idiopathic cases account for 60% of this type of classification, whereas those that are secondary to underlying events such as lymphoid malignancy, collagen vascular diseases, and drug reactions account for the remainder. The second method of classification depends on the type of antibodies present—warm or cold. This classification has prognostic significance relating to the outcome of the treatment in patients and has therefore gained predominance.

Warm antibody immune hemolytic anemia is caused by the reaction of IgG antibody with the red blood cell surface. This reaction occurs optimally at 37° C. Although this antibody does not fix complement, it does alter the red blood cell membrane, causing spherocytosis. In addition, it has been shown that monocytes and macrophages present within the spleen and liver have a receptor for the FC portion of the IgG molecule that allows the macrophages to recognize, bind, and remove the damaged red blood cells within the substance of the spleen. Therefore removal of red blood cells does not result from direct hemolysis through complement fixation.

Warm antibody immune hemolytic anemia occurs in drug-induced hemolytic states and may be of two types. The first or hapten type results from elaboration of antibody directed to the inciting drug and not to the red blood cell. The combination of antibody and drug hapten has an affinity for the red blood cell surface that results in the destruction of the "innocent bystander" red cell. The second type of drug-induced hemolytic anemia is an autoimmune type in which a drug such as Aldomet causes production of antibodies directly against host red blood cells.

Diagnosis of patients with idiopathic or secondary immune hemolytic anemia of the warm antibody type usually begins with the anemic patient. Clinical splenomegaly is present in 50% of patients. Examination of the peripheral blood smear reveals reticulocytosis and spherocytes. The direct Coombs's test, which detects red cells already coated with antibody or complement, is positive in 90% of the cases. Examination of the bone marrow reveals erythroid hyperplasia.

Intravenous injection of radiolabeled-chromium–tagged red blood cells demonstrates a shortened red cell half-life. A half-life of less than 12 days is hard evidence of a significant hemolytic process. In addition, demonstration by splenic scanning of a chromium-tagged red blood cell accumulation in the splenic region provides evidence of sequestration. These tests help to identify those patients in whom splenectomy may be a successful treatment.

Initially though these patients should be managed with a course of corticosteroids. It has been shown that corticosteroids inhibit the removal of damaged red blood cells by the reticuloendothelial system of both the liver and spleen. As has been noted earlier, splenectomy can be effective in reducing the clearance of antibody-coated red blood cells but tends to be more efficacious in situations of very high antibody concentrations. Splenic removal has been less effective in the form of the disease having lower antibody concentrations because the hepatic portion of the reticuloendothelial system accounts for the majority of red blood cell destruction. In this setting 60% to 80% of patients in whom corticosteroids have been used as the first line of treatment have shown clinical improvement. Initial dosage of prednisone is 60 to 100 mg/day with a median time of response of 7 days. If no response is seen within 3 weeks, further treatment with corticosteroids is ineffective.

In patients with a positive response, steroids should be gradually tapered over 3 to 6 months with careful monitoring of the patient for relapse. In 60% to 70% of patients, a complete remission is seen. However, the 30% to 40% of patients who are either resistant to corticosteroids or suffer a relapse after steroid withdrawal are candidates for splenectomy. Splenectomy has been effective in 50% to 60% of these patients, resulting in either complete relief of hemolysis or a significant reduction in the required dosage of corticosteroids.

Approximately 10% of the patients with warm antibody immune hemolytic anemia will be resistant to both corticosteroids and splenectomy and will require treatment with an immune-suppressive agent such as azathioprine or cyclophosphamide. In this subgroup of patients a 50% to 60% response can be expected. Usually these medications are given in therapeutic dosages for 1 to 3 months and then maintained in lower dosages for 6 to 12 months. In those patients in whom warm-type immune hemolytic anemia is secondary to a drug, removal of the drug from the patient will suffice for treatment.

The second type of immune hemolytic anemia is that involving a cold agglutinin syndrome and thus has been called the cold antibody type of the disease. The disorder is caused by an IgM antibody that fixes complement optimally at 4° C. Affected patients have an extremely high titer of cold agglutinins. In a majority of these patients, hemolysis occurs when low blood temperature is achieved, usually in exposed portions of the body such as the tips of the fingers and toes, the nose, and the ears. When the blood is thus exposed, the complement sequence is triggered and causes a direct red cell lysis. Although the liver and spleen have receptors for the recognition of C3B (the component of the complement sequence involved in this disease) and can bind and ingest these red cells, under most circumstances hemolysis occurs directly as the result of complement fixation triggered by the IgM antibody.

Patients with the cold antibody type of immune hemolytic anemia are usually found in northern climates during the winter. They frequently have combined symptoms of Raynaud's phenomenon or acral cyanosis on exposure to the cold. There are a few patients who have dramatic intravascular hemolysis with resultant hemoglobinuria following exposure to cold. In these patients a direct Coombs's test will be positive for complement components on the red cell and negative for immunoglobulin. The titer of cold agglutinin is usually extremely high.

The treatment of patients with the cold agglutinin type of immune hemolytic anemia is usually supportive with protection from cold exposure. In those patients who cannot be treated conservatively, a trial of an immunosuppressive agent, either cyclophosphamide or azathioprine, can result in a reduction in the cold agglutinin titer and in alleviation of hemolysis. Corticosteroid therapy and splenectomy have been found ineffective in this disorder.

Idiopathic Thrombocytopenic Purpura

Idiopathic thrombocytopenic purpura (ITP)[13] is a disease characterized by low numbers of circulating platelets and a shortened platelet life-span. It occurs predominantly in females, except in patients under 10 years of age in which the incidence in male children is more common. In adult females the peak incidence occurs in the second to third decades. The most common symptoms are purpura and ecchymosis. However, vaginal bleeding, epistaxis, bleeding gums, gastrointestinal hemorrhage, and hematuria are also commonly seen. Rarely cerebral vascular accidents may serve as the initial symptom. In 97% of patients with ITP the spleen is of normal size and not palpable on clinical examination.

The cause of ITP is not known. It has been theorized that an immune mechanism serves to bring about the removal of circulating platelets by the reticuloendothelial system of the spleen. There is a subset of patients with ITP whose onset of the disease seems clearly related to a previous upper respiratory tract infection with either infectious mononucleosis, measles, chicken pox, mumps, or hepatitis. In these patients it is believed that the previous infection stimulates the immunologic system, which results in removal of platelets within the substance of the spleen.

In patients without a prior history of upper respiratory tract infections, only 15% show a satisfactory and permanent response to systemic steroid administration. In contrast, 78% of the patients who initially fail to respond to steroids have favorable permanent results after splenectomy. In patients who are initially treated with splenectomy without prior treatment with steroids, 85% respond with a permanent remission. When these patients are compared to patients in whom steroids are given before surgical splenectomy, a higher incidence of postoperative complications is seen in the steroid surgery group.

In the subset of patients with ITP following an upper respiratory tract infection, a somewhat different picture is seen. In these patients thrombocytopenia is very frequently mild and may be transitory in nature. In patients who have lasting thrombocytopenia, 85% have complete and permanent reversal of thrombocytopenia following splenectomy. In comparison, 64% have complete and permanent recovery following treatment with corticosteroids.

The most common result following splenectomy for idiopathic thrombocytopenia is the rapid return to normal of the number of circulating platelets. In at least 80% of patients the platelet count can be expected to be above 80,000 within 24 hours. In less than 6% of postoperative patients is the platelet count below 20,000 6 days following surgery.

From available evidence it would seem that the best approach in treating patients with idiopathic thrombocytopenic purpura should include an initial, brief trial of corticosteroids. If this is successful, no operative therapy is needed. However, if it is either unsuccessful or if a relapse occurs, then immediate splenectomy should be performed. Permanent response to splenectomy can be expected in 85% to 95% of patients.

Thrombotic Thrombocytopenic Purpura

Thrombotic thrombocytopenic purpura (TTP)[3,13,36] is primarily a disease of the microvasculature. Although its cause is unknown, two theories have been proposed to explain its pathogenesis. The first assumes that disseminated intravascular thrombosis is the primary pathogenic feature of the disease. Initial subintimal deposition of hyaline-like material produces endothelial injury, which in turn triggers platelet deposition and thrombosis. Others have argued that the vascular subintimal deposition is in fact secondary to re-endothelialization of a primary intravascular thrombosis.

The clinical features present in TTP consist of purpura, hemolytic anemia, waxing and waning neurologic deficits, renal disease, and fever.[13] Laboratory findings reveal anemia with leukocytosis, thrombocytopenia, and renal insufficiency with accompanying azotemia. The urinalysis frequently shows proteinuria, hematuria, and granular casts. The peripheral blood smear reveals evidence of fragmentation and destruction of red blood cells. Bone marrow biopsy demonstrates evidence of hyperplasia of erythroid and myeloid components with normal or increased megakaryocytes.

Neurologic manifestations take the form of seizures, coma, or aphasia. Marked fluctuations in neurologic signs are present. The renal manifestations may progress to complete anuria. Pathologic examination of affected tissue reveals occlusion of arterioles and capillaries with a hyaline-like material and mild inflammation with limited areas of infarction. There are subintimal depositions of hyaline material and even aneurysmal dilation of some arterioles.

In the past the outlook for patients with this disease was indeed dismal. Treatment had included antiplatelet agents such as aspirin and dipyridamole, heparin administration, systemic steroids, and splenectomy. The majority of survivors had been treated with both systemic steroids and splenectomy.[3,36] However, recently treatment has changed to include whole blood exchange transfusion and frequent plasmapheresis with reinfusion of fresh frozen plasma. Survival with this regimen has been over 50%. Splenectomy is no longer considered as a treatment modality.

Splenic Neutropenia

Splenic neutropenia is a relatively rare disease of unknown cause, comprising less than 3% of all hematologic diseases involving the spleen. Approximately 70% of patients with this disease demonstrate splenomegaly on physical examination. Because of the splenomegaly it is likely that alterations in the microcirculation of the spleen increase the amount of time spent by neutrophils within the reticular substance of the splenic pulp. Once this occurs cells are less resistant to damage and phagocytosis because of low pH and glucose levels found in these regions. Splenic-derived immunoglobulin may also be a factor in destruction of neutrophils.

Patients with this disease usually have recurrent infections. The white blood cell count may be extremely low, and in as many as 30% to 40% of patients it is below 1000 cells/mm^3. In approximately 15% of patients the platelet count is below 100,000, reflecting increased destruction of platelets by the spleen. In one third of the patients the reticulocyte count is greater than 5% suggesting an element of hypersplenic hemolytic anemia.

Examination of the bone marrow aspirate usually reveals a compensatory hyperplasia of the neutrophilic granulocytes. If platelets and erythrocytes are being destroyed by the spleen, megakaryocytes and erythroid precursors also exhibit hyperplasia within the bone marrow. Over 95% of patients with this disease who undergo splenectomy have a prompt and permanent return of their hematologic parameters and enjoy a full clinical recovery.

Splenic Involvement in Lymphoma and Lymphocytic Leukemia

The spleen may frequently be involved in lymphoma and lymphocytic leukemia.[1] In the past splenectomy was reserved for those patients in whom operative staging was necessary. However, recently it has been appreciated that patients with lymphocytic lymphoma and chronic lymphocytic leukemia may benefit from splenectomy for treatment of anemia, thrombocytopenia, and leukopenia.[1] In these diseases the spleen is infiltrated with neoplastic cells. When this occurs, the normal route of blood flow through the spleen is made circuitous. This is particularly true of the passage of blood elements through the reticular substance of the splenic cords. As the neoplastic infiltration progresses, overall transit time of blood through the splenic pulp is markedly increased. Thus cells spend more time within the confines of the pulp where, because of low glucose levels and pH levels, hemolysis occurs. In addition, the malignant infiltrative process distorts the normal sinus apertures resulting in damage to the cells as they cross. The overall result is anemia, thrombocytopenia, and leukopenia.

Patients who undergo chromium-labeled erythrocyte studies and who demonstrate shortened erythrocyte survival and splenic sequestration have been shown to respond favorably to splenectomy. In these patients an increase in hemoglobin, platelet count, and white blood cell count occur following surgery. It has also been demonstrated that even in patients with negative splenic sequestration studies there is frequently an improvement in anemia following splenectomy, possibly resulting from removal of a splenic-derived antibody important to hemolysis of red cells within the spleen.

Staging of Hodgkin's Lymphoma

Hodgkin's disease[8] is a malignant process of uncertain cause involving the lymphoid system. Spread of the disease is usually by contiguity among the elements of the lymphoid system. Staging is classified according to the extent of the disease and the presence or absence of systemic symptoms. Stage I implies involvement of lymph nodes within one area; Stage II disease involves lymph nodes in two different anatomic areas on the same side of the diaphragm; Stage III involves lymphoid areas on both sides of the diaphragm; and Stage IV disease denotes systemic spread with either bone marrow or hepatic involvement. An A or B subset is applied for the presence or absence of systemic symptoms including fever or loss of 10% or more of body weight.

The basis of treatment for Hodgkin's disease is radiation therapy to localized disease with systemic chemotherapy given to patients with Stage III and IV disease. Modern treatment of Hodgkin's disease demands accurate clinical staging of the patient. Operative staging procedures reveal a surprisingly high incidence of splenic and para-aortic lymph node involvement not appreciated by physical examination or noninvasive testing. It is believed that to effect cure, these areas must be treated.

Staging laparotomy for Hodgkin's disease involves total splenectomy and complete abdominal exploration with wedge and needle biopsies of both lobes of the liver. In addition, abdominal lymph node biopsies are performed in the aortic, mesenteric, splenic, caval, iliac, portal, and celiac regions. Radiopaque markers are placed at the splenic pedicle and in any areas of node excision or tumor mass. Bilateral iliac crest bone marrow biopsy is performed at the same time. It has been shown that approximately 30% of patients undergoing staging laparotomy, regardless of the extent of preoperative evaluation, will have either upgrading or downgrading of their stage because of the operation.[5] The removal of the spleen and its histologic examination can help to minimize diagnostic errors and reduce the amount and location of radiation needed for treatment. Such reduction yields lower complication rates of radiation pneumonitis and nephritis. Therefore patients in whom preoperative evaluation does not establish the stage of disease should undergo a complete staging laparotomy.

Myeloid Metaplasia

Myeloid metaplasia is a disease in which the bone marrow ceases to form blood elements because it is replaced with fibrous tissue. As a result, hematopoietic elements within the liver and spleen begin to produce blood elements, a process termed *extramedullary hematopoiesis*. The significance of myeloid metaplasia as a surgical problem relates to its chronicity. During physical examination most patients are found to have splenomegaly as well as hepatomegaly resulting from the hematopoietic functions that the spleen and liver assume in this disease. Anemia is usually present, and mild thrombocytopenia occurs in approximately one third of patients; however, thrombocytosis can be seen in as many as 20% of patients. Late in this disease the spleen may function in an adverse fashion and lead to severe thrombocytopenia and hemolytic anemia secondary to the hypersplenism. In this circumstance splenectomy may be quite beneficial.

In the past splenectomy was reserved for those patients in whom splenomegaly became clinically symptomatic. However, more recently chromium-tagged red cell testing for both cell survival and splenic sequestration has been used. With these tests patients in whom splenectomy may result in symptomatic improvement and in reduction in both transfusion requirements and bleeding episodes caused by thrombocytopenia have been identified earlier.

Felty's Syndrome

Felty's syndrome[32] describes the clinical association of chronic rheumatoid arthritis, splenomegaly, and leukopenia. It is believed by some that Felty's syndrome is part of a spectrum of diseases including rheumatoid arthritis and lupus erythematosus. Patients with this syndrome may also exhibit anemia, hepatomegaly, susceptibility to infection, and weight loss. Splenomegaly is present in a majority of patients. The basis of the observed neutropenia is thought to be the result of an antibody directed toward the neutrophils that cause their destruction and removal by the spleen. The average white blood cell count is below 2000/mm^3 with a differential count showing a relative neutropenia. Pathologic examination of spleens removed for Felty's syndrome shows weights ranging from 500 to 1400 g. The microscopic appearance is that of chronic passive congestion; no more specific pathologic findings have been identified. In patients with Felty's syndrome who exhibit hypersplenism splenectomy has proved effective in 70% to 80% of cases in correcting the neutropenia.[32] Steroids have an inconsistent effect with no lasting benefit. It is rare for patients to relapse following splenectomy for Felty's syndrome.

Sarcoidosis

Involvement of the spleen in sarcoidosis[4] may produce anemia and thrombocytopenia. Splenomegaly is present in 25% of patients with only 20% of these demonstrating clinical hypersplenism. However, hypersplenism can be present in the absence of splenomegaly, resulting from infiltration of the spleen by sarcoid granulomata. Splenomegaly not associated with sarcoid infiltration also occurs. Anemia and thrombocytopenia result from the entrapment and sequestration of red blood cells and platelets. Splenic phagocytosis of the formed elements of the blood within the spleen also may occur because of congestion with resultant stasis and the accompanying increase in splenic circulation time. An immune mechanism for hemolysis in sarcoid involvement of the spleen has been advocated. However, in most patients with anemia and hypersplenism the direct Coombs's test is negative.

Most patients with splenic sarcoid involvement have known sarcoidosis and are first seen with anemia and thrombocytopenia. Hemoglobin levels below 8 g/100 ml and platelet counts below 100,000 mm^3 are not uncommon. The reticulocyte count is elevated, and neutropenia may be present. Examination of bone marrow aspirates reveals generalized hyperplasia. The most serious clinical manifestation of this disorder is thrombocytopenia with resultant episodes of hemorrhage. Radiolabeled-chromium–tagged red blood cell studies of survival and splenic sequestration are useful in determining those patients in whom splenectomy might improve the anemia. Patients with hemolytic anemia caused by sarcoidosis who have appropriately abnormal chromium-tagged red blood cell studies have benefited from splenectomy.[4] Treatment of sarcoid hypersplenism with steroids has not been successful.

Gaucher's Disease

Gaucher's disease[15] is an inborn error of metabolism in which there is an accumulation of glycolipid cerebrosides in cells of the reticuloendothelial system. Clinically this results in enlargement of the liver and spleen with attendant hypersplenism. The mechanism of the hypersplenism is an infiltration of the spleen by the glycolipids to a level 100 times that normally present. As a result, the normal pathway of blood elements through the spleen is distorted, causing difficult passage for red cells, platelets, and neutrophils. As in other infiltrative disorders of the spleen, passage time of blood is slowed. This results in the increased removal of cells from the circulation; thus thrombocytopenia, anemia, and neutropenia can result.

Half of the patients with Gaucher's disease initially have significant hemorrhage caused by the thrombocytopenia.[15] Others appear only with symptomatic splenomegaly or anemia. Splenomegaly is present in all patients, whereas a characteristically mild, normocytic, and normochromic form of anemia is observed in 80%. Patients with Gaucher's disease who demonstrate thrombocytopenia caused by hypersplenism are uniformly improved following splenectomy. Relapses following splenectomy are extremely rare. Steroids have not been found useful in the treatment of hypersplenism associated with Gaucher's disease.

Splenic Abscess

Splenic abscess[6,14] is a relatively rare clinical entity that most often results in the seeding of the spleen from a remote site of infection.[6] Bowel flora including *E. coli* and *Klebsiella* are frequent offenders. Splenic abscess may also be seeded from other remote sites such as the heart, where *Staphylococcus* is the usual causative organism, and from decubitus ulcers and septic uterine conditions. In patients with suppressed immunologic function, abscess of the spleen may also include opportunistic infections such as nocardiosis and candidiasis.

Tenderness involving the region of the abscess is present in the majority of cases, and most patients demonstrate fever. Physical examination reveals an enlarged, tender mass in the upper left quadrant of the abdomen. Liver-spleen scan or abdominal CAT scan characteristically establishes the diagnosis. Treatment of the disorder is splenectomy and drainage of any associated abscess. Overall mortality of splenic abscess is 60% with over half of the deaths resulting from the underlying illness.[14] Failure to consider the diagnosis and/or late diagnosis are responsible for a significant number of deaths.

Hypersplenism Secondary to Portal Hypertension

Hypersplenism may result from portal hypertension resulting from a variety of causes. Perhaps the most common cause is Laënnec's cirrhosis. However, hypersplenism can also be a consequence of portal hypertension secondary to postnecrotic cirrhosis, primary biliary cirrhosis, schistosomiasis, or hepatic vein thrombosis (Budd-Chiari syndrome). Acute thrombosis of the splenic vein or portal venous system also results in splenomegaly and hypersplenism. The cause of hypersplenism in these diseases is massive congestion of the spleen. With chronic elevation in the splenic venous pressure there is chronic increase in volume of the spleen. As this occurs the trabeculae are thickened and sclerosed. Splenic microcirculation is affected and a greater percentage of central arterioles end within the reticular substance of the splenic cord. Normal circulation of blood through the spleen is altered and becomes more circuitous. As a result, the formed elements of the blood spend an increasing amount of time within the spleen. An increased rate of cellular damage with hemolysis and phagocytosis inevitably follows, causing a mild anemia, thrombocytopenia, and neutropenia.

Patients with hypersplenism caused by elevation of portal pressure have signs and symptoms of the underlying disease. Those with cirrhosis may demonstrate the peripheral stigmata of chronic liver disease, including muscle wasting, gynecomastia, spider angiomata, testicular atrophy, jaundice, and ascites. Eighty percent of patients also demonstrate splenomegaly.

The major life-threatening process in patients with severe cirrhosis is exsanguinating hemorrhage from esophageal varices caused by portal hypertension. Treatment of this disease entity is controversial but includes decompression of the portal system through an operative shunting procedure. The portal-systemic shunt controls the life-threatening esophageal bleeding and relieves hypersplenism in the majority of cases. However, this result is not uniform. In some cases where elevated portal venous pressures have been chronically present, changes including fibrosis of the splenic capsule and trabeculae may have occurred, which can prevent the spleen from returning to normal size. Therefore splenomegaly and the resulting hypersplenism may persist. Fortunately, this is not a frequent problem.

When patients who have undergone portacaval shunt for treatment of bleeding esophageal varices continue to show clinical evidence of hypersplenism, chromium-tagged red cells may demonstrate persistence of reduced red blood cell survival and splenic sequestration. In these patients splenectomy should be used to correct the disorder.

SPLENIC TRAUMA

Splenic injury may result from either penetrating or blunt trauma or operative misadventure. In most large trauma centers splenic injuries caused by blunt trauma usually predominate. Both sudden deceleration and direct application of blunt forces to the upper abdomen and lower chest frequently result in injury to the splenic substance. Indeed, the spleen is the most commonly injured intra-abdominal organ in cases of blunt trauma.

Patients admitted to the emergency department with splenic injury frequently have a history of blunt abdominal trauma either caused by a motor vehicle accident, a fall, or an altercation. Gunshot wounds and stab wounds are also a common cause of splenic injuries in metropolitan emergency rooms. Initial complaints almost always include left upper quadrant pain made worse by deep inspiration. Those with severe splenic wounds may exhibit symptoms of hypotension. However, the majority of patients have stable vital signs initially. Examination of the patient may reveal palpable fractures of the left lower ribs. Left upper quadrant abdominal tenderness and guarding are usually present.

Management of the patient with splenic injury should be identical to that given to any trauma victim (Fig. 30-3). An airway should be established if indicated, and any external bleeding should be controlled with pressure. Large intravenous catheters should be inserted for volume replacement and a urinary catheter used to monitor adequacy of renal perfusion and circulating blood volume. Associated injuries occur in a significant percentage of patients, and efforts should be undertaken to identify and treat them. In patients with penetrating abdominal trauma, along with signs of either significant intra-abdominal blood loss or an acute abdomen, management should include early surgery. In those patients with closed head injury and/or altered mental status resulting from drug intoxication or in those with equivocal abdominal findings, diagnostic peritoneal lavage is highly accurate in identifying intraabdominal bleeding, which is commonly caused by splenic injury.

Management of splenic trauma has recently undergone reevaluation. In the past splenectomy was the treatment of choice for even minor splenic injury. However, recent recognition of the spleen's role in protection against infection has significantly altered management. Sepsis following splenectomy is a clinical entity that affects patients who are devoid of splenic function.[17,30,31,39] This sepsis is often overwhelming, usually involves the lung, and may result in death within 24 to 48 hours of onset. The common causative agents are encapsulated microorganisms—most commonly *Streptococcus pneumoniae, Haemophilus influenzae, Klebsiella pneumoniae,* and *E. coli*. Initially it was believed that only asplenic patients with underlying hematologic diseases were affected. However, recent evidence has shown that even normal patients are at an increased risk for sepsis following splenectomy. It is true that patients with underlying hematologic disorders such as thalassemia have the highest rate of postsplenectomy sepsis—affecting as many as 10% of these patients. However, patients with splenectomy for trauma and no underlying

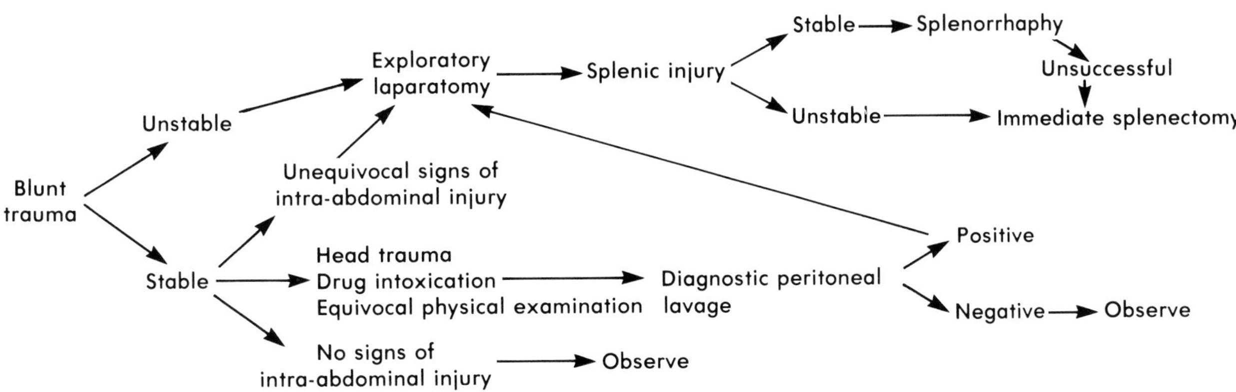

Fig. 30-3 Treatment algorithm for patients suffering blunt trauma to the spleen.

disorder have a rate of sepsis between 0.5% and 1.0%. This is approximately 50 times that expected in the normal population.

With growing clinical recognition of sepsis following splenectomy, further investigation into splenic function has yielded several interesting facts. In addition to the spleen's role as a filter for blood-borne bacteria, it also is the sole site for the production of tuftsin, a substance that directs polymorphonuclear leukocytes to engulf bacteria.[7] It also is an important site of production of immunoglobulin and opsonin, which is necessary in the preparation of bacteria for phagocytosis.[19] A remote effect by the spleen on the function of pulmonary macrophages and their ability to adequately phagocytize bacteria has been described, although the mediating factors have not been identified. Thus with this knowledge of the spleen's role in combating infection, preservation of this organ has become important to surgeons.

Some surgeons have advocated observation as a treatment for selected patients with splenic injury.[16,41] In this approach stable patients with physical examinations suggesting splenic injury undergo scanning of the liver and spleen to confirm the diagnosis. Those with definite injuries are admitted to the intensive care unit for monitoring. Patients who remain stable continue to be observed whereas those requiring moderate amounts of blood transfusion are taken to the operating room for either splenic repair or removal. Opponents of this management scheme warn that a high number of other intra-abdominal injuries will be missed if patients with blunt abdominal trauma are treated by observation.[24]

The majority of surgeons who care for trauma patients elect to subject those individuals with blunt abdominal trauma and evidence of splenic injury to exploratory celiotomy. When a splenic injury is encountered at the time of operation, the management should involve attempted repair. It has been recently shown that in stable patients, repair is frequently successful.[26,33,35,38] Lacerations may be treated with electrocautery or topical hemostatic agents using modalities such as microvascular collagen or omentum. Suture of splenic lacerations has also met with some success. In selected patients partial splenectomy may be indicated. As noted previously, the splenic artery divides into multiple segmental branches as it enters the hilum. This end-arterial supply of the spleen makes segmental resection possible. In those patients in whom a partial splenectomy is contemplated, complete mobilization of the spleen by division of its attachments to the diaphragm, colon, and kidney is necessary to bring the organ up into the wound and thus facilitate examination and repair. In several large series repair has been accomplished in 80% of patients treated for splenic injury. In those patients who are unstable or who have suffered irreparable damage to the spleen, splenectomy should be promptly performed to gain life-saving hemostasis.

Splenic autotransplantation has been suggested as one way to preserve splenic function in patients who require splenectomy for trauma. In animal studies autotransplantation of the spleen into the peritoneal cavity has proved beneficial in reducing the mortality of pulmonary sepsis following splenectomy.* Recently studies in trauma patients undergoing splenectomy have shown that autotransplantation of splenic material into the peritoneal cavity is feasible.[34] Whether this method of splenic preservation will result in a reduction of postsplenectomy sepsis will require a large clinical study. It should be remembered that sepsis following splenectomy in otherwise healthy trauma patients is approximately 1%. Therefore the relative benefits and risks of intraperitoneal implantation of splenic material, particularly in patients with associated injuries, must be compared to its possible benefits. In patients with either severe associated injuries or intraoperative hypotension, splenectomy remains the procedure of choice for management of splenic injuries.

In patients who do require splenectomy for trauma, one method of protection against sepsis following splenectomy is the administration of polyvalent pneumococcal vaccine. *Streptococcus pneumoniae* is the most common causative organism in postsplenectomy sepsis—being responsible for 50% of cases. Although the polyvalent pneumococcal vaccine does not cover all organisms responsible for postsplenectomy sepsis, it does exert a significant protective effect against the most common pathogen.[42]

Prophylactic antibiotics have been suggested as another manner of reducing the incidence of sepsis following splenectomy, particularly in children. Penicillin or ampicillin have been proposed as the drugs of choice. However, major arguments have been made against this method of treatment. First, the causative agents in postsplenectomy sepsis are probably not sensitive to any one antibiotic. Second, since a prolonged period of antibiotic administration would be required in any type of prophylaxis, resistant organisms might be selected out. It has been shown in animal studies that antibiotics delivered within 24 hours after the onset of sepsis following splenectomy are successful in preventing mortality.[23] Therefore it would seem more reasonable to reserve antibiotic administration for high-risk situations such as an upper respiratory tract infection or suspected infection.

SUMMARY

The spleen, although sometimes envisioned as a simple filter, does in fact also possess complicated immunologic properties. Both functions may be adversely affected by genetic inheritance, hematopathology, malignancy, sepsis, portal hypertension, and trauma, leading to severe patient illness. By understanding the physiologic bases of those disorders that affect the spleen and closely cooperating with hematologic colleagues in the management of splenic disease, surgeons can plan their therapy to alleviate some of the more serious aspects of these difficult clinical problems involving this important organ.

---

*References 9, 21, 22, 25, 28, and 37.

REFERENCES

1. Adler, S., et al.: Splenectomy for hematologic depression in lymphocytic lymphoma and leukemia, Cancer **35:**521, 1975.
2. Axelson, J.A., and LoBuglio, A.F.: Immune hemolytic anemia, Med. Clin. North Am. **64:**597, 1980.
3. Bernard, R.P., Bauman, A.W., and Schwartz, S.I.: Splenectomy for thrombotic thrombocytopenic purpura, Ann. Surg. **169:**616, 1969.
4. Bertino, J., and Myerson, R.M.: The role of splenectomy in sarcoidosis, Arch. Intern. Med. **106:**213, 1960.
5. Cannon, W.B., and Nelson, I.S.: Staging of Hodgkin's disease: a surgical perspective, Am. J. Surg. **132:**224, 1976.
6. Chulay, J.D., and Lankerani, M.R.: Splenic abscess: report of 10 cases and review of the literature, Am. J. Med. **61:**513, 1976.
7. Constantopoulos, A., et al.: Defective phagocytosis due to tuftsin deficiency in splenectomized rats, Am. J. Dis. Child. **125:**663, 1973.
8. DeWeese, M.S., and Coller, F.A.: Splenectomy for hematologic disorders, West. J. Surg. **67:**129, 1959.
9. Dickerman, J.D., et al.: The protective effect of intraperitoneal splenic autotransplants in mice exposed to an aerosolized suspension of Type III *Streptococcus pneumoniae,* Blood **54:**354, 1979.
10. Doan, C.A.: Hypersplenism, Bull. N.Y. Acad. Med. **25:**625, 1949.
11. Doan, C.A.: The spleen: its structure and functions, Postgrad. Med. **43:**126, 1968.
12. Doan, C.A., and Wiseman, B.K.: Hypersplenic cytopenic syndromes: a 25-year experience with special reference to splenectomy. In "Proceedings of the Sixth International Congress of the International Society of Hematology," New York, 1958, Grune & Stratton, Inc.
13. Doan, C.A., Bouroncle, B.A., and Wiseman, B.K.: Idiopathic and secondary thrombocytopenic purpura: clinical study and evaluation of 381 cases over a period of 28 years, Ann. Intern. Med. **53:**861, 1960.
14. Gadacz, T., Way, L.W., and Dunphy, J.E.: Changing clinical spectrum of splenic abscess, Am. J. Surg. **128:**182, 1974.
15. Gruenberg, H., and Penner, J.A.: Gaucher's disease: observations on its clinical course, Mich. Med. **74:**323, 1975.
16. King, D.R., et al.: Selective management of injured spleen, Surgery **90:**677, 1981.
17. King, H., and Schumacker, H.B.: Splenic studies: susceptibility to infection after splenectomy performed in infancy, Ann. Surg. **136:**239, 1952.
18. Liebowitz, H.R.: Splenomegaly and hypersplenism: pre- and postportacaval shunt, N.Y. State J. Med. **63:**2631, 1963.
19. Likhite, V.V.: Opsonin and leukophilic globulin in chronically splenectomized rats with and without heterotropic autotransplanted splenic tissue, Nature **253:**742, 1975.
20. Lipton, E.I.: Elliptocytosis with hemolytic anemia: the effects of splenectomy, Pediatrics **15:**67, 1955.
21. Livingston, C.D., Levine, B.A., and Sirinek, K.R.: Protection from pulmonary sepsis afforded by splenic autotransplants, Surg. Forum **33:**31, 1982.
22. Livingston, C.D., Levine, B.A., and Sirinek, K.R.: Intraperitoneal splenic autotransplantations: protection afforded in an epidemic of murine mycoplasmosis, Arch. Surg. **118:**458, 1983.
23. Livingston, C.D., Levine, B.A., and Sirinek, K.R.: Penicillin and natural immunity protect against postsplenectomy sepsis, J. Surg. Res. **34:**332, 1983.
24. Livingston, C.D., et al.: Traumatic splenic injury: its management in a patient population with a high rate of associated injury, Arch. Surg. **117:**670, 1982.
25. Livingston, C.D., et al.: Transplant site affects splenic B and T cell survival and function, Arch. Surg. **120:**89, 1985.
26. Moore, F.A., et al.: Risk of splenic salvage after trauma, Am. J. Surg. **148:**800, 1984.
27. Motulsky, A.G., et al.: Anemia and the spleen, N. Engl. J. Med. **259:**1164 & 1215, 1958.
28. Moxon, E.R., and Schwartz, A.D.: Heterotrophic splenic autotransplantation in the prevention of *Hemophilus influenzae* meningitis and fatal sepsis in Sprague-Dawley rats, Blood **56:**842, 1980.
29. Necheles, T.F., Allen, D.M., and Gerald, P.S.: The many forms of thalassemia: definition and classification of the thalassemia syndromes, Ann. N.Y. Acad. Sci. **165**(art. 1):5, 1969.
30. Oakes, D.D.: Splenic trauma, Curr. Probl. Surg. **18:**346, 1981.
31. O'Neal, B.J., and McDonald, J.C.: The risk of sepsis in the asplenic adult, Ann. Surg. **94:**775, 1981.
32. O'Neal, J., Jr., et al.: The role of splenectomy in Felty's syndrome, Ann. Surg. **167:**81, 1968.
33. Pachter, H.L., Holfstetter, J.R., and Spencer, F.C.: Evolving concepts in splenic surgery, Ann. Surg. **194:**262, 1981.
34. Patel, J., et al.: Preservation of splenic function by autotransplantation of traumatized spleen in man, Surgery **90:**683, 1981.
35. Ratner, M.: Surgical repair of the injured spleen, J. Pediatr. Surg. **12:**1019, 1977.
36. Reynolds, P.M., et al.: Thrombotic thrombocytopenic purpura—remission following splenectomy, Am. J. Med. **61:**439, 1976.
37. Schwartz, A., Dadash-Zadeh, M., and Goldstein, R.: Antibody response to intravenous immunization following splenic autotransplantation in Sprague-Dawley rats, Blood **49:**779, 1977.
38. Sherman, R.: Perspectives in management of trauma to the spleen, J. Trauma **20:**1, 1980.
39. Singer, D.B.: Postsplenectomy sepsis, Perspect. Pediatr. Pathol. **1:**285, 1973.
40. Wennberg, E., and Weiss, L.: The structure of the spleen and hemolysis, Annu. Rev. Med. **20:**29, 1969.
41. Wesson, D.E., et al.: Ruptured spleen—when to operate?, J. Pediatr. Surg. **16:**324, 1981.
42. Winkelstein, J.A., Lambert, G.H., and Swift, A.: Pneumococcal serum 81: opsonizing activity in splenectomized children, J. Pediatr. **87:**430, 1975.

31 Gastrointestinal Hemorrhage

Kenneth R. Sirinek and Barry A. Levine

Acute hemorrhage from the gastrointestinal tract has been recognized by clinicians for over 5000 years.[2] Initial descriptions of sanguinous discharges appear both in ancient Chinese manuscripts and Egyptian papyri. The Ebers papyrus, with its extensive description of symptoms, findings, and complications, recorded hemorrhage as a possible sequela of peptic ulceration. Hippocrates also recognized bleeding from peptic ulceration but unfortunately recommended phlebotomy as appropriate treatment. Further understanding of the clinical significance of gastrointestinal hemorrhage came from the early writings of both Galen and Avicenna. Later significant, but not always correct, contributions included those of Littre, Morgagni, and Ewald. In fact, as late as 1891 Ewald included application of leeches to the abdomen as therapy in such cases.

The modern era of understanding and therapy for gastrointestinal hemorrhage followed developments in several disparate medicine-related fields.[2] Discovery of the ABO blood group system by Landsteiner, coupled with techniques to preserve blood and infuse fluids parenterally, made blood transfusion—and thus successful resuscitation from hemorrhage—a reality. Forty years after Roentgen's discovery of x-rays, Hampton's use of barium contrast studies of the gastrointestinal tract to detect the source of gastrointestinal bleeding revolutionized diagnosis. An even greater delay ensued between the inception of general anesthesia and the first reported series of patients undergoing successful operation to control gastrointestinal bleeding sites. The final major contribution was the refinement of the endoscope, since its clinical introduction over a century ago, into a useful and clinically applicable diagnostic and therapeutic instrument.

Gastrointestinal hemorrhage is a common clinical problem crossing national and socioeconomic boundaries. A recent report indicated that 25,100 patients per year required hospitalization in England and Wales for gastrointestinal hemorrhage from all sources.[2] In the United States such bleeding accounted for 1% to 2% of all medical and surgical hospital admissions during a similar time period.[38] This translates into an estimated 150 hospitalized patients per 100,000 population in the United States, a figure comparable to that seen among the rural populations of Sweden.[12,21] At the lesser end of the scale is an admission rate of only 47 per 100,000 for a defined population from the Oxford region of England.[42] Despite this threefold difference in reported geographic incidences, there appears to be no difference in rate of gastrointestinal hemorrhage when rural and urban areas are compared.[26]

High-risk rates for gastrointestinal bleeding have been correlated with specific aspects of peptic ulcer disease.[26] High-risk categories include patients with blood group O, widows and single persons, persons in stress-producing occupations, and the seasons of fall and spring. Advancing age seems to be a specific risk factor for all patients with gastrointestinal bleeding. Recent studies indicate that almost 50% of such patients are over 60 years of age.[2]

Mortality from gastrointestinal hemorrhage has not declined in the past 40 years, remaining at 8% to 10%.[6] A mortality rate of almost 25% has been reported when only patients with massive bleeding are considered.[40] This unacceptably high rate has persisted in spite of the introduction of blood transfusion, intensive care units, sophisticated monitoring equipment, and new therapeutic modalities. It should be emphasized, however, that these innovations have taken place during an era when the proportion of older people in the patient pool has markedly increased. Thus it would appear that the negative medical aspects of an aging population have offset the beneficial effects of evolving medical technology related to the patient with gastrointestinal hemorrhage.

If further strides at reducing the morbidity and mortality associated with gastrointestinal bleeding are to be made, every clinician must be familiar with the pathophysiologic response to hemorrhage, the various gastrointestinal abnormalities likely to give rise to bleeding, the principles and strategies underlying diagnosis, and the therapeutic approaches based on cause. These components are important in the management of the patient with gastrointestinal hemorrhage and form the basis of this chapter.

PATHOPHYSIOLOGIC ALTERATIONS IN GASTROINTESTINAL HEMORRHAGE

Acute gastrointestinal hemorrhage has usually been described by clinical terms that estimate both the rate of bleeding and volume of blood lost. These descriptors range from minor or trivial, through moderate, and finally to severe or torrential. The magnitude of the pathophysiologic response (see Chapter 8) needed to maintain homeostasis parallels the degree of acute blood loss. Blood loss beyond compensatory mechanisms results in hypovolemic shock and, if untreated, eventually becomes irreversible, leading to death. Thus the term shock, in its most basic definition, connotes a state of inadequate tissue perfusion in which the circulation fails to meet the nutritional and metabolic needs of the cell.

The clinical manifestations of acute gastrointestinal bleeding will depend on the rate of bleeding and the total amount of blood loss and will yield signs and symptoms that correlate with the severity of shock.[15] A progression of organ involvement (skin to kidney to heart and brain) is usually seen. Associated disease such as hypertension or congestive heart failure, as well as the concomitant use of various medications (i.e., antihypertensives, calcium channel blockers) by a given patient may alter the timing and magnitude of this normal physiologic response.

Mild hemorrhagic shock occurs with loss of less than 20% of blood volume. Adrenergic vasoconstriction of blood vessels to the skin and skeletal muscles results in extremities that are pale and cool to palpation. The patient may complain of feeling cold, weak, or lethargic or of being thirsty. Moderate shock represents loss of 20% to 40% of the circulating blood volume. A low urine output signals this stage and is the most sensitive indicator of hypovolemia. In contrast, tachycardia and hypotension may not occur until late and are relatively poor indicators of a compromised vascular compartment. The patient in severe shock has lost more than 40% of his blood volume. A rapid, thready pulse and hypotension now occur in conjunction with either oliguria or anuria. Signs of myocardial ischemia may be apparent on an electrocardiogram. Ischemia to the central nervous system in its earliest stages is usually manifested as agitation and restlessness. In its most severe form the patient may be obtunded.

INITIAL TREATMENT

Initial treatment of the patient with acute gastrointestinal bleeding involves two major components: (1) placement of appropriate monitoring devices, and (2) resuscitation. A large-bore needle should be placed into an available peripheral vein to secure an adequate means to infuse blood and intravenous solutions. A cutdown on a peripheral vein or a central subclavian catheter may be indicated in some patients. Placement of a Swan-Ganz catheter is indicated in certain clinical situations (i.e., elderly patient, associated heart disease). However, in the majority of patients it is not necessary, and its lack should not deter rapid treatment.

Blood should be obtained for hematologic indices, coagulation profile, serum chemistries, hepatic and renal function studies, and for type and crossmatch for 4 to 6 U of packed red cells and fresh frozen plasma. Insertion of a Foley catheter is mandatory to monitor urine output. If the patient is hypotensive, the legs may be elevated, or the patient may be placed in the Trendelenburg position. A nasogastric tube should be placed for decompression of the stomach in order to prevent vomiting and possible aspiration of gastric contents. It also can be an important diagnostic aid in determining whether an upper gastrointestinal cause is the source of hemorrhage (refer to section on diagnosis). If time permits, if the patient is hemodynamically stable, and if facilities are available, the patient should be admitted to an intensive care unit.

Initial intravenous fluid resuscitation should be carried out with either normal saline or lactated Ringer's solution. The rate of fluid infusion will depend on the specific patient's condition and response to therapy. The patient in shock should be given a rapid infusion of at least 1 L or more of fluid. Further therapy will be dictated by the response to this initial therapy as monitored by blood pressure, heart rate, and urine output. In spite of these measures, the patient in shock may require volume expansion with fresh plasma or serum albumin.

When packed red cells are available, their infusion will depend on response to the initial fluid bolus, rate and amount of blood loss, starting hematocrit, and continued or recurrent bleeding. Hemodilution is not an immediate response, and equilibration of the hematocrit may take 6 hours or more. Therefore an admission hematocrit of less than 30% may indicate a significant acute blood loss requiring early transfusion. With continued or recurrent bleeding, the blood bank should be notified to keep ahead of blood use by at least 6 U.

During the initial phase of resuscitation vital signs should be obtained frequently (every 15 minutes). This should include urine output since it is the most sensitive indicator of adequacy of intravascular volume. Pulmonary wedge pressure and cardiac output are additional hemodynamic parameters that are available in patients with Swan-Ganz catheters. Once the patient has responded to emergency therapy, vital signs may be obtained on an hourly basis. A portable chest x-ray film and electrocardiogram should be obtained once the patient has been stabilized.

Further hemodynamic monitoring, nasogastric tube aspiration, and serial hematocrits should continue to diagnose recurrent bleeding. Certainly diagnostic efforts to ascertain the source of hemorrhage may be initiated at this time, beginning—even in the transiently stable patient—with an examination of the upper gastrointestinal tract by means of flexible fiberoptic endoscopy. If bleeding recurs, an emergency operation may be indicated. Special diagnostic and therapeutic measures may be indicated in certain disease states; i.e., placement of a Sengstaken-Blakemore tube in a patient with portal hypertension and bleeding esophageal varices. These considerations will be discussed in subsequent sections of this chapter.

DIAGNOSIS OF GASTROINTESTINAL HEMORRHAGE

Initial investigation to determine the source (see boxed material on p. 512) and the cause of gastrointestinal hemorrhage should begin shortly after the patient has been stabilized and admitted to the hospital. Thus the patient's history, physical examination, and laboratory tests should be an integral part of medical care that is rendered simultaneously with the placement of monitoring equipment and early resuscitation. A sense of urgency should be applied to this workup phase to either identify or eliminate possible serious sequela. The major diagnostic goal during this early stage is to determine whether the bleeding originates from the upper or lower gastrointestinal tract—with the

MAJOR SOURCES OF GASTROINTESTINAL HEMORRHAGE

Inflammatory
- Esophagitis
- Gastritis
- Stress ulcer
- Gastric ulcer
- Duodenal ulcer
- Stomal ulcer
- Regional enteritis
- Ulcerative colitis
- Diverticulitis

Neoplasms
- Adenocarcinoma
- Polyps
- Leiomyoma

Vascular
- Esophageal varices
- Hemangioma
- Angiodysplasia
- Aortointestinal fistula
- Hemorrhoids

Mechanical
- Hiatus hernia
- Mallory-Weiss syndrome
- Diverticulosis

Anomalies
- Duplications
- Meckel's diverticulum

Systemic Disease
- Uremia
- Collagen diseases

Blood Dyscrasias
- Hemophilia
- von Willebrand's disease

Other
- Epistaxis
- Hemoptysis
- Bleeding from oropharyngeal cavity
- Malingering

ligament of Treitz serving as the established boundary between these two segments. The prognostic significance of this determination is that bleeding from the lower gastrointestinal tract is usually intermittent, of smaller volume, and therefore not as acutely life-threatening as that arising from the esophagus, stomach, or duodenum.

History and Physical Examination

Salient features of the patient's illness should be elicited. In this regard a family member may provide important additional information. A history of hematemesis localizes the hemorrhage to a site proximal to the ligament of Treitz, often proximal to the pylorus. Hematemesis refers to the vomiting of blood that may be either bright red or brown and precipitated, in which case it resembles coffee grounds. Melena and hematochezia are less reliable indicators of the bleeding site. Melena is defined as the passage of black, tarry stools and most often occurs from a bleeding site proximal to the jejunum but may accompany more distal lesions. The tarry color is usually attributable to the action of gastric acid on hemoglobin, resulting in the production of acid hematin, although melena can accompany other bleeding lesions throughout the gastrointestinal tract (usually proximal to the ileocecal valve) and is secondary to the effects of bacteria and various digestive enzymes on the intraluminal blood. Hematochezia usually heralds bleeding from the lower gastrointestinal tract, particularly the colon or rectum, but has been occasionally observed in patients with a duodenal ulcer. Hematochezia is defined as the passage of fresh red blood from the rectum.

A history of peptic ulcer disease, addiction to alcohol, or the use of nonsteroidal antiinflammatory drugs suggests an upper gastrointestinal tract bleeding source. Dysphagia may indicate an esophageal lesion, whereas weight loss and anorexia are suggestive of a malignancy. A history of inflammatory bowel disease or prior bouts of diverticulitis in a patient with hematochezia should point to the lower gastrointestinal tract as the site of hemorrhage. If the patient has had a previous bleeding episode, the possibility that the bleeding is from the same lesion is greatly increased.

Physical findings will often indicate the extent of vascular volume depletion rather than lead to specific identification of the anatomic site of hemorrhage. Thus careful evaluation of pulse and blood pressure (both upright and supine) and of skin color and the presence or absence of diaphoresis will give an indication of the magnitude of hemorrhage. The stigmata of certain diseases may also be noted on physical examination and direct one's attention to the possible site of bleeding. For example, the findings of spider angiomas, abdominal venous distention, palmar erythema, jaundice, and muscle wasting are often found in patients with cirrhosis and portal hypertension and suggest that the bleeding may be from esophageal varices. The presence of melanin spots on the oral mucosa, lips, and digits suggests Peutz-Jeghers syndrome and the possibility that the hemorrhage may be caused by the presence of polyps in the small bowel. In any patient with petechiae and ecchymoses, the possibility of a hemorrhagic diathesis must be considered and excluded. Finally a careful examination of the oropharynx and nose should be included in the evaluation of any patient with gastrointestinal bleeding since vomited blood in this circumstance may actually arise from swallowed blood secondary to nasopharyngeal bleeding.

Laboratory Tests

An important early step in the evaluation of a patient with gastrointestinal hemorrhage is determination of the hematocrit. This will provide a baseline against which subsequent determinations can be compared. The initial hematocrit may be normal or decreased, depending on the rate of blood loss and the degree of extracellular fluid shift that has occurred to maintain circulating blood volume. Repeat hematocrit readings at 2- to 4-hour intervals are mandatory to determine the adequacy of blood replacement. A low hematocrit in the face of what was thought to be adequate transfusion therapy indicates continued bleeding.

Other laboratory tests of importance include coagulation studies, a liver function profile, and a determination of blood urea nitrogen (BUN). Coagulation studies, including platelet counts, will provide an assessment of the adequacy of clotting factors since derangements in blood clotting commonly occur following multiple blood transfusions and can actively aggravate the hemorrhage that one is attempting to control. Demonstration of hepatocellular dysfunction may not only aid in diagnosis (e.g., varices in a patient with cirrhosis) but may also indicate the need for replacement therapy (e.g., vitamin K, fibrinogen) to prevent a coagulation problem. In an otherwise normal patient, BUN elevation suggests the presence of bleeding proximal to the ligament of Tretiz. This occurs because the metabolic breakdown products of digested blood that are absorbed in the proximal gut are reflected in the BUN level.

Techniques to Localize the Site and Cause of Bleeding

If a patient has hematemesis, a bleeding site proximal to the ligament of Treitz is virtually assured. In contrast, hematochezia can result from a lesion in the colon or the rapid passage of blood from a bleeding site in the upper gastrointestinal tract, including lesions in the stomach and duodenum. Similarly, melenic stools may result from bleeding lesions throughout the gut from the level of the esophagus to the proximal colon. Although aspiration of gastric contents with a soft nasogastric tube may show blood in the stomach in a patient with melena or hematochezia confirming a proximal site of bleeding, its absence by no means rules out an upper gastrointestinal source. The bleeding may either have stopped before placement of the tube or could be from a site distal to a competent pyloric sphincter. Because of these limitations in diagnosis, special procedures are generally needed to delineate the site and cause of gastrointestinal hemorrhage.[6] These procedures may either localize or exclude various sites as sources of hemorrhage. In addition, they may demonstrate pathologic lesions that are potential but not actual causes of bleeding. These special procedures include: endoscopy, barium contrast radiography, radionuclide imaging, arteriography, and exploratory celiotomy.

Use of any of these special techniques will depend on its availability and assessed accuracy rate at each individual institution. Use of a particular procedure will vary with the clinical presentation of the patient. Endoscopy provides the best help in patients with suspected upper gastrointestinal bleeding, whereas radionuclide scanning and arteriography are commonly used in those patients with presumed distal bleeding sites. The order of use and the timing of these special procedures vary considerably among physicians and surgeons.

Some clinicians believe that the routine use of special diagnostic procedures in suspected upper gastrointestinal bleeding is seldom indicated since 80% to 90% of patients with upper tract hemorrhage stop bleeding spontaneously.[48] They contend that the small advantage gained in terms of localizing the bleeding site is offset by the associated complication rate in using these procedures. Others contend that controlled trials have failed to show any reduction in mortality rates associated with early diagnosis provided by special diagnostic techniques.[13,39] Steer and Silen[48] have cautioned that the lack of merit of these diagnostic maneuvers has not been proven; rather therapeutic improvements or the willingness to use them have lagged behind diagnostic innovations.

In contrast, others advocate a vigorous diagnostic approach to all patients with gastrointestinal tract hemorrhage, particularly those with upper tract bleeding.[37] Clinicians holding this viewpoint argue that the bleeding site should be expeditiously identified because hemorrhage may recur or persist in 25% of patients, whereas early surgical intervention may be required in 10% to 25%.[6] Further, patients requiring an early operation (e.g., a vessel in the base of an ulcer, spurting bleeder) can be identified confidently. With this approach, Palmer[37] was able to demonstrate the bleeding lesion in 93% of his patients. Further justifying early diagnostic intervention, he noted that 40% of his patients who had a prior hemorrhagic episode were bleeding from a different site.[37] Most clinicians stand somewhere between these extremes in management and will individualize the need for special diagnostic approaches for a given patient.[6]

Endoscopy

Panendoscopy of the esophagus, stomach, and duodenum performed with a flexible fiberoptic instrument should be the first diagnostic maneuver in the majority of patients with suspected or proven (i.e., hematemesis) upper gastrointestinal tract hemorrhage. Generally the diagnostic accuracy using this technique will approach 90%.[23,32] An overall complication rate of 0.9% has been recorded for a large series of patients, with about half of them being classified as major (e.g., perforation, aspiration, or bleeding).[18]

The timing of endoscopy remains controversial. Proponents of early endoscopy want to identify those patients who will need immediate surgical intervention.[48] Endoscopy during the active bleeding phase has the advantage of correctly identifying the source in the patient with a possibility of more than one lesion (e.g., gastritis vs. esophageal varices as may occur in the cirrhotic patient with portal hypertension). Such a vigorous diagnostic approach has led to a greater appreciation of the frequency with which acute mucosal lesions cause massive bleeding.[6] These benefits must be weighed against the small but increased risk of aspiration secondary to endoscopy that may occur when it is performed during the acute bleeding phase. Although they recognize this risk, most experienced surgical endoscopists still prefer early endoscopy to plan possible acute, as well as more chronic, therapy.

In most patients with lower intestinal bleeding, anoscopy and proctosigmoidoscopy should be performed following a careful, digital rectal examination. Absence of blood above the rectum in the acutely bleeding patient implicates the anorectal region as the bleeding site. If bleeding is present above the rectum, careful inspection of the colonic mucosa on proctosigmoidoscopy may demonstrate an inflammatory ischemic, or neoplastic lesion that could be responsible for the hemorrhage. If no source of bleeding is found in the rectosigmoid area and the rectum is reasonably free of fecal marterial, fiberoptic colonoscopy may be of value in identifying the bleeding site. On the other hand, if active bleeding is present or the colon is filled with a considerable amount of fecal material, colonoscopy is usually contraindicated because of the obstructed view that exists in such an unprepared bowel.

Barium Contrast Radiography

The accuracy of barium contrast radiography in the diagnosis of acute upper gastrointestinal tract hemorrhage has been reported at only 20% to 50%.[23,32] This figure will probably decline further with the increasing recognition that superficial mucosal lesions are a common source of gastric hemorrhage, coupled with the declining incidence of gastric cancer. Additional limitations of barium studies in the diagnosis of upper tract causes of hemorrhage include the inability to examine a patient in the upright position when actively bleeding, the presence of blood clots in the stomach, and blurred films secondary to movement in an acutely distressed individual.[6] Further, the use of contrast radiography in diagnosing a colonic source of bleeding in lower gastrointestinal hemorrhage has proven to be no better.[48] In fact, the identification of colonic diverticula on barium enema, a lesion not uncommonly found in elderly patients, may lead one to believe falsely that this is the source of hemorrhage, when in fact another cause is present. In addition, the use of barium in both upper and lower gastrointestinal tract examinations may preclude the subsequent use of angiography. Thus rarely, if ever, will barium studies be of value during initial evaluation of a patient with gastrointestinal hemorrhage. Instead, such studies should be reserved to evaluate the patient who has clearly stopped bleeding.

Radionuclide Imaging

Radionuclide imaging with either technetium-99m (^{99m}Tc) sulfur colloid or ^{99m}Tc pertechnetate-labeled red blood cells is an effective noninvasive technique that can identify bleeding when the rate is as low as 0.1 ml/min (Fig. 31-1).[1,53] With ^{99m}Tc sulfur colloid imaging, scans of the abdomen are obtained shortly after intravenous injection of this nuclide to look for its extravasation from the vascular system.[1] Labeling red blood cells with ^{99m}Tc pertechnetate is generally a more sensitive method because the labeled erythrocytes are retained in the vascular compartment for a longer period of time than with ^{99m}Tc sulfur colloid, and thus repeated scanning is permitted for periods as long as 24 to 36 hours after the intravenous injection of ^{99m}Tc. Use of this nuclide permits detection of slow or intermittent bleeding.[53]

The accuracy with both techniques has been quite impressive, and the absence of any associated side effects

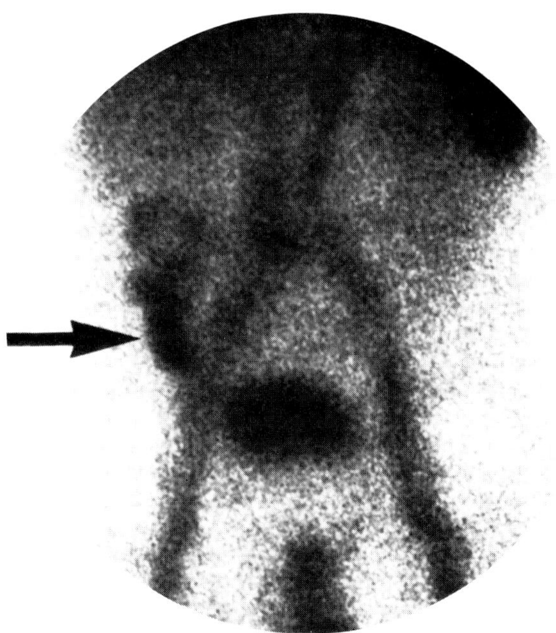

Fig. 31-1 Radionuclide scan using ^{99m}Tc pertechnate-labeled red blood cells. Arrow indicates bleeding site in right colon.

from either of these nuclides has been an especially attractive feature. In anatomic regions of the gastrointestinal tract where endoscopic evaluation is not possible (i.e., small intestine and occasionally large intestine when adequate preparation for colonoscopic examination cannot be obtained), information derived from radionuclide imaging may be of considerable value. In addition, in patients with intermittent bleeding use of this methodology as a screening test for active bleeding should reduce the incidence of negative angiographic studies. The major deficit of radionuclide scanning is that the procedure identifies only a general abdominal region where bleeding exists rather than a specific anatomic site. Imaging with ^{99m}Tc pertechnetate may also prove useful in the demonstration of ectopic gastric mucosa that may be present in a Meckel's diverticulum or enteric duplication cyst.

Angiography

If endoscopic examination of the upper gastrointestinal tract or colon fails to reveal a site of bleeding or if the mucosa cannot be adequately evaluated (e.g., bleeding too rapid, visualization of colonic mucosa obscured by feces and/or blood), selective visceral angiography should be performed, particularly if evidence of massive bleeding exists (e.g., continued hypotension and/or dropping hematocrit in spite of "adequate" blood transfusions). For less pronounced bleeding or hemorrhage that appears intermittent, nuclide scanning should generally precede angiography.

Use of angiography involves catheterization of the celiac and/or mesenteric arterial systems through a percutaneous femoral arterial approach. This technique can demonstrate a bleeding site if the rate of hemorrhage at the time of examination is in excess of 0.5 ml/min.[3,4] If a bleeding site is present, contrast medium escapes from the vasculature into the lumen of the involved segment, which is easily recognized on x-ray films. Arteriography may also be helpful in the demonstration of nonbleeding lesions when abnormal vasculature is present. Examples of such lesions include the vascular blush of a tumor, a vessel displaced by a tumor, an arteriovenous fistula, a visceral aneurysm, or an hemangioma.

Angiography should provide an accurate diagnosis of the cause of bleeding in approximately 75% of patients in whom it is performed.[3] This diagnostic accuracy occurs with a background complication rate of less than 2%.[22] Selective angiography has been particularly valuable in identifying bleeding sites in the small bowel and colon—areas that are notoriously difficult to identify with other diagnostic procedures. Once a site of bleeding is diagnosed, various techniques can be used through the angiographic catheter to stop the hemorrhage. These approaches are described in more detail later in this chapter in the section entitled "Interventional Angiography."

Exploratory Celiotomy

On rare occasions the procedures just discussed will fail to identify the bleeding site, in which case an abdominal exploration may be used as a last-resort diagnostic maneuver. When this becomes necessary, careful evaluation of the entire gastrointestinal tract is mandatory. This will require careful inspection of the serosal surface in the search for an identifiable bleeding lesion. Particular efforts should be used to identify a primary vascular abnormality such as a vascular malformation, fistula, or ectasia since these lesions are usually the responsible culprits. Several ancillary maneuvers have been recommended, including perioperative endoscopy, Doppler probes, injections of various dyes such as methylene blue to detect increased areas of blood flow, and transillumination of the bowel, but their success rates in defining the source of bleeding have been low.[48] Occasionally intraluminal blood will appear to be localized to a specific segment of the intestinal tract, suggesting that the hemorrhage may be originating from that site. Unfortunately, when celiotomy becomes a diagnostic maneuver, its success in identifying the bleeding site has only been modest. More often than not, the operation will prove to be of little benefit, and another hemorrhagic episode will need to occur before the procedures described above are successful in establishing its cause.

ETIOLOGY OF GASTROINTESTINAL HEMORRHAGE

Hemorrhage from the gastrointestinal tract may have many diverse causes. Generally, hemorrhage occurs from an abnormality within the gastrointestinal tract, although a disease process in an adjacent organ with secondary involvement of the stomach or intestine may be the inciting cause. Occasionally a systemic disorder such as a coagulation problem may be the major underlying factor. Eight disease categories leading to hematemesis, melena, and hematochezia are shown in the boxed material on p. 512. No attempt has been made to make this list all inclusive; rather, representative causes have been listed for each major category. When all causes of gastrointestinal bleeding are considered as a whole, upper tract bleeding is much more commonly encountered than that arising from lesions distal to the ligament of Treitz.

Upper Gastrointestinal Tract Bleeding

In a recent collected survey of 2205 patients, 84% of all episodes of acute blood loss from the upper gastrointestinal tract were secondary to six pathologic entities.[16] Most of this blood loss originated from the distal esophagus, stomach, and proximal duodenum. Causes included duodenal ulcer (24%), acute gastritis (20%), gastric ulcer (15%), esophageal varices (14%), esophagitis (6%), and Mallory-Weiss mucosal tears (5%). The National Survey by the American Society of Gastroenterological Endoscopy (ASGE) on Upper Gastrointestinal Hemorrhage involving 2225 patients reported a similar etiologic distribution.[44] In comparison with this large collected series, the local incidence in a defined geographic setting will vary from institution to institution, depending on the population of patients served by a given hospital. Most city/county type hospitals encounter gastritis and esophageal varices as sources of hemorrhage more commonly than community hospitals where peptic ulcer disease is responsible for the majority of bleeding.

Specific Causes of Bleeding

Peptic Ulcer Disease. If one combines the incidence of bleeding from both duodenal and gastric ulcers, peptic ulcer disease will be responsible for hemorrhage in almost 40% of patients. It has been estimated that 25% of hospitalized ulcer patients will have gastrointestinal bleeding if followed for a 10-year period.[6] The frequency of bleeding is directly related to the duration of the disease; however, there appears to be a slightly greater tendency to bleed during the first year of disease than in subsequent years of follow-up. Bleeding may be manifest as hematemesis, melena, and rarely as hematochezia. Melena alone occurs most often in the presence of a competent pyloric sphincter and usually indicates that the ulcer is in the duodenum rather than the stomach. Of ulcer patients with hemorrhage, 70% are men; this percentage rate reflects the fact that men have a higher incidence of ulcers rather than the fact that gender is a disportionate bleeding risk factor. Onset of ulcer disease late in life is associated with a higher incidence of bleeding vs. onset at an early age, with the highest incidence of hemorrhage occurring during the fifth decade of life.[6] However, age per se does not appear to be the most important factor.

There is an increased incidence of bleeding in duodenal ulcer patients with blood group O. Hemorrhage is also more common in postbulbar ulcers, especially when they occur in the older age group. Gastrointestinal hemorrhage is the first sign of peptic ulcer disease in approximately 10% of patients. Melena or hematemesis occurs in about 50% of patients with the Zollinger-Ellison syndrome.[6]

Hematemesis and melena may also occur from recurrent ulceration following any operation originally performed to manage peptic ulcer disease. Bleeding has been found to be the presenting symptom in 40% of patients with recurrent ulcers following partial gastrectomy.[6] Ulceration is always located on the jejunal side of the anastomosis because of the relative inability of small intestinal mucosa to withstand acid-peptic digestion. Barium contrast study is a poor diagnostic examination for this entity, and it is most successfully visualized by endoscopy. The Zollinger-Ellison syndrome is a possible cause not only of the first occurrence of peptic-ulcer disease, but also of recurrent ulcer.[6]

Acute Gastritis. Duodenal ulcer is the most common cause of upper tract bleeding, with gastric ulcer ranking third. In second place are a variety of acute erosive diseases of the stomach, generally referred to as acute gastritis. Histologically, these lesions are usually erosions rather than ulcers since they generally do not penetrate to the level of the muscularis mucosa as is typical of a true ulcer. These lesions may be secondary to various drugs or arise as a result of stress. Drug-induced gastritis generally occurs in patients taking nonsteroidal antiinflammatory agents such as aspirin, indomethacin, and naproxen. Individuals on long-term steroid management may also present with such erosive lesions. Excessive alcohol consumption is likewise associated with erosive gastritis and may be responsible for gastrointestinal hemorrhage distinct from the esophagogastric varices that occur in alcoholic individuals secondary to cirrhosis and portal hypertension. Bleeding from drug-induced erosive gastritis may be minimal or massive. In either case it can generally be managed with aggressive nonoperative therapy by discontinuing the inciting drug and ensuring that acid pH is adequately buffered.

Only rarely will a surgical procedure be necessary to control such bleeding.

Acute stress gastritis (also called stress ulceration) of the stomach and duodenum is a source of gastrointestinal hemorrhage in the acutely ill patient under a variety of clinical circumstances. It must not be confused with acute hemorrhage from chronic peptic ulcer disease that may be exacerbated by the stress of an acute illness. The distinction between gastric erosion and ulceration is histologic and clinically most likely represents progression of the pathologic process through the muscularis mucosa into the capillary-rich submucosa.[47]

The causes and circumstances that result in stress ulcerations are diverse. Although some overlap exists, there appear to be a number of separate clinical situations in which stress ulcers develop, including the following:

1. In the patient sustaining trauma secondary to an operation, an accident, or a violent act who is at risk for stress ulcer formation in the immediate post-trauma period
2. In patients critically ill with sepsis, jaundice, renal failure, or pulmonary failure—usually found in the intensive unit care—who start bleeding from the gastric mucosa at various stages of organ failure
3. In patients suffering from major thermal injury
4. In patients with intracranial disease, trauma, or an operation who develop lesions known as Cushing's ulcer

The onset of the multiple lesions that make up stress ulcerations is insidious, and their development is usually painless. In the patient without a nasogastric tube the bleeding remains undetected until the individual vomits blood or passes a melenic stool. Hemorrhage from acute stress gastritis may occur within the first 24 hours after injury, but the usual onset of bleeding develops at 5 to 10 days after the initial insult. In patients at risk for the development of stress gastritis, prophylactic antacid therapy to neutralize intragastric acidity has dramatically lessened the incidence of bleeding from this entity (see Chapter 16).

Esophagogastric Varices. Bleeding from varices is a manifestation of portal hypertension and accounts for 14% of the patients with gastrointestinal hemorrhage.[16] The bleeding point is usually a tear in the esophageal mucosa within 2 cm of the esophagogastric junction secondary to rupture of a varix. This lesion must be differentiated from a Mallory-Weiss tear in which no varix lies below the mucosal disruption. It must be remembered that patients with varices secondary to portal hypertension frequently may bleed from other upper gastrointestinal sources. Merigan and associates[33] found that varices were responsible for the bleeding in only 53% of patients with cirrhosis. Outstanding features of esophageal bleeding include the magnitude of blood loss that can occur and the high mortality rate associated with such lesions.

Esophagitis and Mallory-Weiss Tears. Esophagitis and Mallory-Weiss tears as causes of upper gastrointestinal hemorrhage are responsible for approximately 10% to 11% of patients who present with upper gastrointestinal tract hemorrhage.[16] Bleeding from esophagitis usually occurs in association with hiatal hernias. Typically such bleeding is slow and usually presents as chronic blood loss. Patients with this problem can usually be managed without surgery as part of a therapeutic program to alleviate the symptoms referable to reflux esophagitis. If the mucosa in the distal esophagus is particularly friable, suture control of the bleeding may become necessary at the same time that an antireflux procedure is performed.

The Mallory-Weiss syndrome represents a tear in the gastric mucosa near the esophagogastric junction. This tear extends in a longitudinal direction and may be several centimeters in length. It often follows a bout of forceful retching and/or vomiting. The mucosal disruption extends through the mucosa and submucosa with usual sparing of the muscularis mucosa. Most of these lesions are confined to the stomach just below the esophagogastric junction. Occasionally, the lesion may straddle the esophagogastric junction, and only rarely does it involve the distal esophagus alone. More than two thirds of patients with this entity will have an associated hiatal hernia. Usually the bleeding from this disorder will stop spontaneously, but occasionally surgical intervention will become necessary, in which case oversewing of the bleeding mucosal edges through a high gastrotomy incision is performed.

Other Sources of Bleeding. The entities described above are responsible for approximately 85% of all episodes of acute blood loss from the upper gastrointestinal tract. The remaining 15% arise from a variety of miscellaneous causes. These include various vascular abnormalities such as telangiectasia and hemangiomas, blood dyscrasias, and tumors such as leiomyomas or leiomyosarcomas that can grow to considerable size in the gastric submucosa and erode into the plexus of veins and arteries supplying blood to the stomach. Occasionally a gastric carcinoma may also erode into an underlying vessel. Usually these neoplastic causes of bleeding are mild. Other sources of upper tract hemorrhage include hematobilia, erosion of a pancreatic pseudocyst into the stomach, and invasion of a pancreatic carcinoma into the third or fourth portion of the duodenum.

Lower Gastrointestinal Tract Bleeding

Bleeding from the small intestine and colon is much less frequent than that arising proximal to the ligament of Treitz. Nonetheless, it can be severe and just as serious and may arise from any site from the ligament of Treitz to the anus.[7] Usually it is occult or signaled by melena or hematochezia. When bleeding arises from the small bowel, a primary neoplasm is the most likely source. These neoplasms may include benign tumors such as leiomyomas and polyps that usually are malignant and such tumors as carcinomas, sarcomas, lymphomas, and occasionally leukemic implants. A number of vascular abnormalities may give rise to small intestinal bleeding and include various types of hemangiomas and telangiectasias. Bleeding is also common in inflammatory bowel diseases involving the jejunum and ileum but is usually intermittent and frequently occult; massive hemorrhage from such a source is distinctly uncommon. Intussusception can be seen in all age groups but is particularly common in childhood and generally occurs before the age of 2. Its presentation as lower intestinal tract bleeding is manifest by the passage of dark clots and occasionally stool that has the consistency and appearance of "currant jelly."[7] A Meckel's diverticulum may also bleed and occasionally is an initial cause of small bowel bleeding in children and young adults. This bleeding occurs because of peptic ulceration of ectopic gastric mucosa that is present in the diverticulum.[41] When such a circumstance arises, an ulcerlike pain in the periumbicial region of the abdomen often precedes bleeding.

Bleeding from colonic sources comprises the vast majority of causes of lower gastrointestinal tract hemorrhage.[8] Although massive hemorrhage is much less common than that observed from lesions proximal to the ligament of Treitz, substantial bleeding can occur from a number of lesions distal to the ileocecal valve. These include diverticular disease of the colon, vascular malformations, and ischemic colitis.[10] Both benign and malignant tumors may also cause bleeding, but this is much more likely to be occult and intermittent.

Diverticular disease of the colon is clearly the most frequent cause of major hemorrhage distal to the ileocecal valve.[5,8] Such bleeding is particularly common in patients over 50 years of age. In a majority of instances diverticular bleeding arises from the right colon, although it may occur anywhere throughout the large intestine. Fortunately it stops spontaneously in most patients, even though recurrent episodes are not infrequent. It must be emphasized that in the evaluation of a patient with lower intestinal bleeding the existence of documented diverticula does not necessarily ensure that bleeding is coming from this source. In fact, other sources of hemorrhage have been identified in as many as 50% of patients with diverticular disease.

Vascular abnormalities of the colon were thought to be infrequent causes of lower intestinal tract bleeding a decade or two ago but now are recognized as being relatively common.[7,8] In fact, arteriovenous malformations of the right colon are the major cause of lower gastrointestinal tract hemorrhage of obscure origin. Most patients with angiodysplastic disorders of the colon are over 60 years of age, and many have associated cardiac disease. For unexplained reasons, an association with aortic stenosis commonly exists.

Another important cause of colonic bleeding that also generally occurs in older patients is ischemic colitis.[10] This entity represents a syndrome of hypoperfusion resulting from decreased intestinal blood flow. The left colon is most often involved. The mucosal ischemia leads to necrosis that then results in hemorrhage. Generally the disease is self-limiting, and, because the full thickness of the intestinal wall is not involved, surgery is usually not indicated. On barium enema a characteristic "thumb printing" sign is noted that represents a combination of muscle spasm, submucosal edema, and minute mucosal ulcerations. On colonoscopic examination, mucosal blebs are commonly seen in the affected colonic segment.

Initially with ulcerative colitis there may be massive bleeding from the lower intestinal tract, but usually the hemorrhage is more modest. Patients with this disorder are generally very sick and have a history of recurrent diarrhea and abdominal pain consistent with the diagnosis. When the friable colonic mucosa is seen on endoscopic evaluation, the explanation for bleeding in this disorder becomes apparent. Generally the marked malnutrition and chronic anemia associated with the colitis will require colonic resection to effect adequate treatment.

Finally, bleeding from the lower intestinal tract may arise from various neoplastic lesions and disorders of the anus and rectum.[34] Usually such bleeding is modest and self-limiting. If blood is not mixed with stool or appears on the toilet paper, it usually indicates a source in the anorectal region such as a hemorrhoid, an anal fissure or ulcer, or proctitis. If blood is mixed with stool, the possibility of a colonic polyp or malignancy becomes more likely. In either case a careful rectal examination and proctosigmoidoscopy should be carried out to determine the specific diagnosis. If these diagnostic maneuvers are unrevealing, barium enema and colonoscopy should be performed.

MANAGEMENT OF GASTROINTESTINAL HEMORRHAGE

In the management of the patient with gastrointestinal hemorrhage, three priorities are paramount. These include resuscitation, identification of the bleeding site, and the use of measures to arrest the bleeding. Principles underlying resuscitation have already been briefly reviewed and are discussed in great detail in Chapter 8. Similarly, diagnostic maneuvers to localize the site of bleeding have been considered. This section will describe the various nonoperative strategies currently used to bring about cessation of bleeding. In the event that such therapeutic modalities are ineffective, an approach to surgical therapy is also described (Fig. 31-2).

Nonoperative Therapy

Gastric Lavage

The placement of a nasogastric tube is both a diagnostic and a therapeutic maneuver. Detection of blood in the gastric aspirate confirms a bleeding site proximal to the ligament of Treitz. The nasogastric tube can also be used to gauge the magnitude, persistence, and/or recurrence of bleeding from the gastrointestinal tract. When blood is detected, every effort should be made to thoroughly aspirate it and remove any clots that may be present in the gastric lumen. The purpose of such aspiration is to prevent gastric distention and thus enhance contraction of the gastric musculature, which will often assist in the arrest of bleeding if it is coming from a gastric source. It will also eliminate the stimulus to secrete acid through gastrin release, which by itself may further irritate the bleeding site. An additional purpose for aspiration is to reduce fibrinolysis at the bleeding site, which can be aggravated by blood remaining in the stomach. To provide for the most efficient aspiration, a large bore nasogastric or orogastric tube (i.e., No. 30 French or larger) is usually necessary. Aspiration is generally best accomplished by using an Ewald tube that is passed through the mouth and into the stomach.

Although no controlled trials are available for comparison with room temperature lavage solutions, traditionally gastric lavage has been performed with ice-cold solutions of saline or water. It remains to be determined, however, whether the temperature is truly that important. Generally the stomach is lavaged with 60-ml aliquots of solution at a

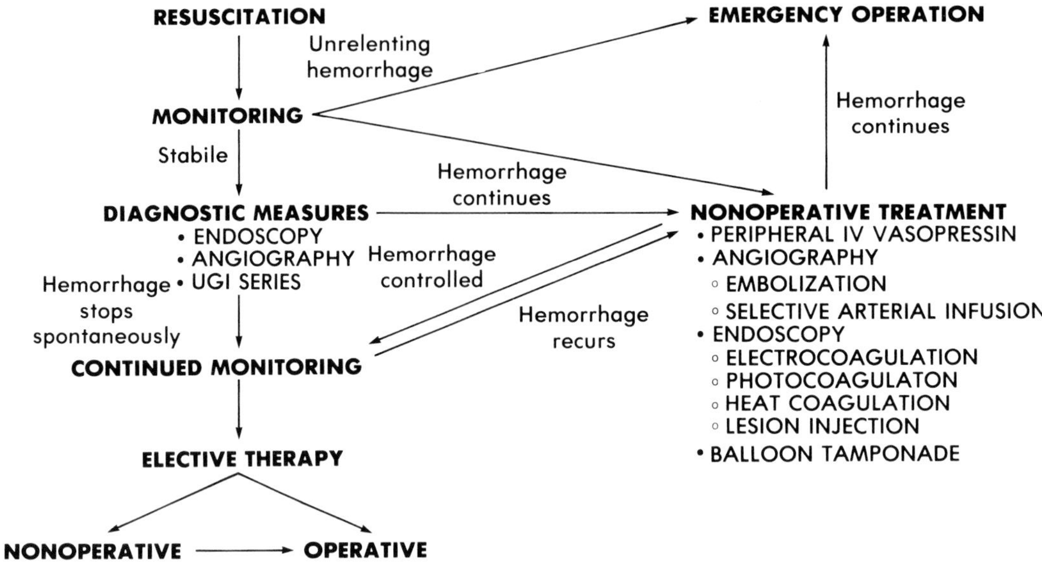

Fig. 31-2 Logical approach to management of patient with acute gastrointestinal hemorrhage.

time. This volume allows adequate fragmentation of clots and aids in the successful evacuation of any blood that may remain in the stomach. With this approach many clinicians have found that active bleeding from upper gastrointestinal sources is often stopped. Palmer[38] reported that bleeding stops for at least a few hours in two thirds of his patients when lavage is properly performed. Opponents of lavage contend that it may precipitate recurrent bleeding by washing off clots, it increases the risk of aspiration of gastric contents, and it is probably of little value since bleeding stops spontaneously in 80% to 90% of patients, irrespective of the therapy used.[48]

Whether lavage is truly a necessary exercise will probably never be a settled issue, but there is no question that it does provide a means of gauging the rate of bleeding and determining whether other therapeutic endeavors (e.g., arteriography) are necessary. In addition, most clinicians agree that it is an appropriate procedure to perform in preparation for emergency endoscopy when continued hemorrhage is present.

Balloon Tamponade

Balloon tamponade was first introduced by Sengstaken and Blakemore[6] in 1950 for the control of bleeding from gastroesophageal varices. The present modification is a triple lumen tube with gastric and esophageal balloons. Endotracheal intubation is a mandatory prerequisite to prevent aspiration. The position of the tube must be verified by x-ray film before balloon inflation to prevent inadvertent inflation of the gastric balloon in the distal esophagus. Once correct positioning has been assured, the gastric balloon should be inflated with 150 to 200 ml of normal saline, and gentle traction applied to maintain compression at the esophagogastric junction. If bleeding persists the esophageal balloon may be inflated with air to 40 to 60 mm Hg pressure. Balloons must be deflated at 24 hours to prevent esophageal necrosis. If bleeding recurs, the balloons may be reinflated for another 12 to 24 hours while plans are being made for some additional therapeutic maneuver. Initial success occurs in about 90% of patients so treated. However, two thirds of these patients will rebleed when the balloons are deflated. This treatment modality should be viewed as a temporizing procedure to prevent a patient from bleeding to death from esophageal varices. Major complications, including aspiration and esophageal rupture, have been reported frequently.

Intravenous Vasopressin

Vasopressin is a cyclic octopeptide, also called antidiuretic hormone, which is synthesized in the hypothalamus and stored in the posterior pituitary gland. Its endogenous release is a physiologic response during shock to preserve the integrity of the intravascular compartment following hemorrhage or severe dehydration. Vasopressin is a potent vasoconstrictor acting at the level of the arterioles and precapillary sphincters. It is this latter property that has prompted the use of exogenously administered vasopressin as a therapeutic drug to arrest hemorrhage from the gastrointestinal tract.

Since its introduction by Kehne, Hughes, and Gompertz in 1956 in patients with bleeding esophageal varices, vasopressin has become an accepted clinical modality for the control of gastrointestinal hemorrhage.[28] In initial reports vasopressin was given as an intravenous bolus of 20 U over a 20-minute period. This method of administration resulted in a myriad of side effects that included hypertension, bradycardia, coronary vasoconstriction, cardiac arrhythmias, water retention, and extremity gangrene.[49] In an attempt to avoid these adverse effects, Nusbaum and colleagues[35,36] recommended selective intraarterial infusion of vasopressin at a decreased dosage for control of both variceal and nonvariceal upper gastrointestinal bleeding. More recent studies have shown that a continuous intravenous infusion of vasopressin is as effective as an intraarterial infusion.[11,24,52] Additional benefits (i.e., ease of administration, universal availability without the need for special equipment and personnel, and avoidance of treatment delay) have made the intravenous route of vasopressin administration the treatment of choice under most circumstances.[52] The greatest efficacy of vasopressin has been recognized in control of bleeding from gastric mucosa, esophageal varices, and colonic lesions.

Although vasopressin has been shown to control gastrointestinal hemorrhage, its efficacy in terms of decreasing morbidity and mortality rates has been questioned.[14] In a placebo-controlled trial Fogel and associates[14] noted that a continuous intravenous infusion of vasopressin (40 U/hr) neither controlled bleeding nor altered the outcome in a group of 60 patients with gastrointestinal hemorrhage. Lack of efficacy occurred in patients with bleeding from both variceal and nonvariceal sites. In contrast, other studies[31,46] have shown a reduction in mortality rates, transfusion requirements, and operating time when this agent is used to control bleeding before surgery. The therapeutic efficacy of these studies vs. that of Fogel's group may be secondary to the higher dosage (60 vs. 40 U/hr) of vasopressin used in the latter studies. Experimental evidence exists that such increased vasopressin dosages result in significant reductions in splanchnic arterial blood flow without compromising either cardiac output or coronary blood flow below those mild reductions seen with extremely small vasopressin dosages.[17]

Present clinical recommendations for vasopressin therapy include administration in the emergency center, the intensive care unit, and the operating room. Once the diagnosis of gastrointestinal bleeding has been made, the patient may be given an initial loading bolus of vasopressin (20 U over 20 minutes) before infusion of large amounts of blood or crystalloid. This will keep the splanchnic circulation vasoconstricted during restoration of the intravascular volume and thereby prevent continued or recurrent hemorrhage from the gastrointestinal tract. This should be followed by a continuous intravenous infusion of vasopressin at 60 U/hour. An initial lower dose is indicated in the older patient with a history of myocardial dysfunction. In contrast, vasopressin should not be given to the angina patient or the individual with a documented history of myocardial infarction.

In patients deemed suitable for vasopressin therapy, treatment is usually continued for at least 24 hours after bleeding has ceased. Vasopressin dosage should then gradually be reduced to prevent hypotension secondary to an expanded intravascular compartment with ensuing vasodilation. If gastrointestinal bleeding recurs, therapy may be restarted, but success is less likely, and other measures will most likely need to be used. Similar dosages of vasopressin have been used intraoperatively without any adverse effects.[46] Reductions in cardiac output may be offset with isoproterenol, but dopamine is contraindicated because of its vasodilatory action—in spite of vasopressin administration—on the splanchnic circulation.[45,51]

Transendoscopic Therapy

In recent years there has been marked enthusiasm for the development of safe and effective endoscopic techniques for the treatment of upper gastrointestinal hemorrhage. Purported advantages of these techniques include treatment under direct vision as the diagnosis is made and prevention of an emergency operation with its attendant morbidity and mortality. These techniques include topical application of hemostatic agents, thermocoagulation, electrocoagulation, and laser photocoagulation. In addition, transendoscopic sclerotherapy of bleeding esophageal varices has gained considerable popularity.

Cyanoacrylate tissue adhesives have been applied as an aerosol to a bleeding surface by means of an endoscopic catheter.[43] Other topical agents have included fibrinogen, thrombin, and an iron powder-oil mixture that is held in place by an externally placed electromagnet.[43] In addition, an electrically heated thermal probe can be passed through an endoscope and pressed against a bleeding lesion. Current instruments remain crude and may cause full-thickness tissue injury.

Radiofrequency electric current has been used for coagulation for the past 60 years. Electrocoagulation is performed by intermittent bursts of energy with resultant tissue desiccation.[43] The bipolar technique is purported to have the theoretic advantage of less deep tissue injury. In contrast, the monopolar electrode has the advantage of superficial deposition of energy during tissue desiccation by spark jumping. This fulguration can coagulate larger-caliber vessels better than the methods in which the electrodes are in contact with the tissue. Use of this technique has been associated with a success rate of 95% without significant complications.[43]

The word LASER is an acronym for *l*ight *a*mplification by *s*timulated *e*mission of *r*adiation. The laser is a device that produces an intense beam of radiation of precise wavelength in the optical region of the spectrum. Laser photocoagulation has been accomplished with both argon and Neodymium-YAG lasers. The Neodymium-YAG laser has been more effective because of its greater tissue penetration. However, the risk of tissue damage is also increased. Reports to date have shown that both lasers have a 60% to 90% success rate in halting acute upper gastrointestinal hemorrhage.[43]

Finally, a variety of sclerosing agents have been used to halt bleeding from esophagogastric varices. Success has varied from 75% to over 90%.[20,25,50] A variety of sclerosing agents have been used, but the one most popular in this country is a 5% solution of sodium morrhuate. Through an endoscope the sclerosing agent is usually injected directly into a varix or adjacent to it.

Interventional Angiography

Localization of gastrointestinal bleeding sites and the control of bleeding with intraarterial vasopressin or transcatheter embolization are new applications of selective visceral angiography. In most circumstances endoscopy should precede angiography since endoscopic localization of the bleeding site should facilitate the angiographic procedure. On the other hand, barium contrast studies are rarely helpful and should be withheld in the acutely bleeding patient.

Arteriography is routinely performed using the femoral route and standard Seldinger techniques. For lower esophageal and gastric lesions the left gastric artery is selectively catheterized. Duodenal bleeding requires a celiac arteriogram followed by selective studies of the gastroduodenal and pancreaticoduodenal arteries. Superior mesenteric arteriography is obtained for small bowel lesions and suspected right colon sites. Superior and inferior mesenteric arteriograms are obtained for a suspected colonic bleeding site. Once the site of bleeding has been demonstrated by extravasation of contrast media into the gastric or intestinal lumen, treatment may be instituted with either intraarterial vasopressin or by transcatheter vessel occlusion.

Vasopressin is infused at a rate of 0.2 U/minute for 20 minutes followed by a repeat arteriogram.[27] If bleeding persists, the dosage of vasopressin is increased to 0.4 U/minute for 20 minutes and once again is followed by a repeat angiogram. If bleeding still persists, vasopressin infusion should be abandoned as a method of therapy, and transcatheter occlusion should be considered. For those in whom bleeding is controlled, vasopressin is usually infused at the dosage at which cessation of bleeding occurred for 12 to 24 hours. The dosage is then halved over two

A

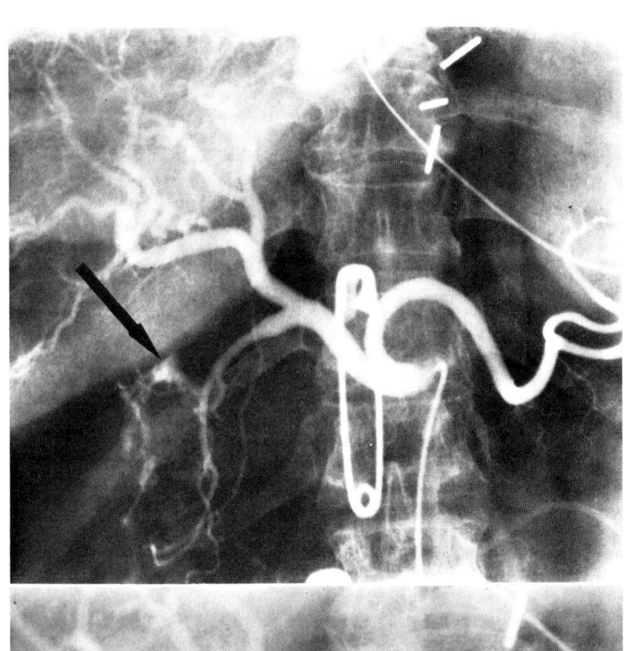

B

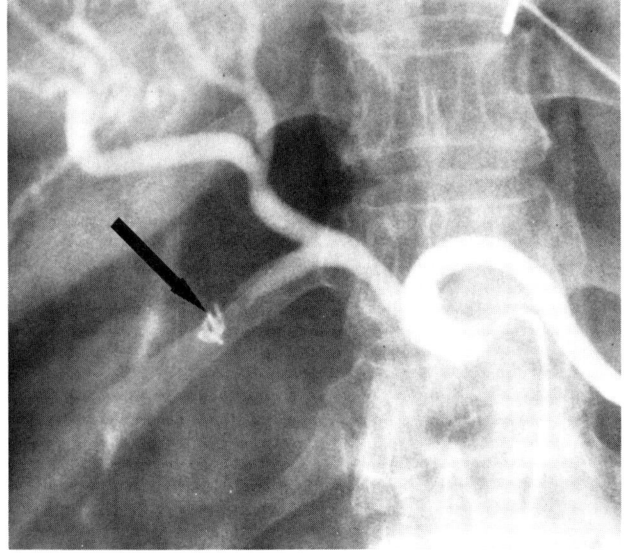

Fig. 31-3 Selective celiac arteriogram showing extravasation *(arrow)* from posterior-superior pancreatoduodenal artery **(A)** and control of bleeding site by transcatheter embolization of coil *(arrow)* in gastroduodenal artery **(B).**

subsequent 12-hour treatment periods. The catheter is kept patent with a saline infusion for another 24-hour period. If bleeding recurs, transcatheter occlusion is considered; if not, the catheter is removed.[27]

Transcatheter occlusion of a bleeding vessel is most commonly accomplished using combinations of autologous blood clot or Gelfoam. Isobutyl-w-cyanoacrylate and Ivalon, a compressible plastic foam of polyvinyl alcohol have also been used to create permanent occlusion. More recently, detachable small balloons and coils attached to angiographic catheters have been introduced for the control of hemorrhage. The embolization procedure is performed through the arteriography catheter. Repeat angiograms are obtained to document successful thrombosis and control of the bleeding site (Fig. 31-3).[27]

Hemorrhage from the distal esophagus can be demonstrated by selective left gastric arteriography and successfully controlled by selective intraarterial vasopressin administration in the majority of patients.[27] Therapeutic success includes control of bleeding from esophagitis, Mallory-Weiss tears, tumors, and endoscopic trauma. Mucosal hemorrhage secondary to gastritis or superficial erosions can be controlled in 84% of patients, whereas bleeding from a gastric ulcer can be stopped with infusion of vasopressin into the left gastric artery in about two thirds of patients.[27] In contrast, hemorrhage from a duodenal ulcer can be controlled with vasopressin infusion in only 50% of patients. The dual blood supply of the duodenum (celiac axis and superior mesenteric artery) is probably responsible for this failure rate. The other half require transcatheter embolization of the pancreatoduodenal artery.

Infusion of vasopressin into the superior mesenteric artery decreases portal venous pressure 25% to 35% and stop variceal bleeding in slightly over half of patients.[27] Percutaneous transhepatic portal vein catheterization followed by transcatheter occlusion of the coronary vein is another successful treatment modality but has a significantly higher complication rate.[27] Infusion of vasopressin into the superior mesenteric artery can also successfully control hemorrhage from small bowel tumors, vascular malformations, and diverticula and angiodysplasia of the right colon. Intraarterial vasopressin successfully controls acute colorectal bleeding in as many as 90% of patients.[27] Recurrent bleeding occurs in about 25% of these patients within 24 hours. Lower gastrointestinal bleeding requires cannulation of the inferior mesenteric artery, if it is patent. Left colon lesions are less responsive to this mode of therapy and may require earlier surgical intervention.

Surgical Therapy

To optimize the clinical management of patients with gastrointestinal hemorrhage, consultation between medical and surgical gastroenterologists should occur soon after admission. This combined initial approach should identify those patients needing only medical therapy. In addition, such cooperation will minimize the chances of unnecessary delays, with the attendant increased risks, for patients requiring emergency surgical treatment. Accepted guidelines for triage of this latter group remain controversial, but a working classification should be established for each institution.

Classic indications for emergency surgical intervention routinely include persistent hypotension or shock in spite of adequate resuscitative measures and significant recurrent bleeding during maximum medical therapy. Additional criteria are the requirements for more than 6 U of blood during the first 24 hours of treatment or for 3 U/24 hours to maintain stable hemodynamic indices. For upper gastrointestinal hemorrhage, identification of a bleeding vessel at time of endoscopy as an indication for surgical intervention has received more recent attention in part because of the more universal use of that procedure during the acute bleeding phase. The source of bleeding, age of patient, associated critical illness, and availability of blood products are additional mitigating circumstances that may modify the therapeutic approach.

The proportion of patients requiring emergency surgical treatment for gastrointestinal bleeding varies among published series and ranges between 12% to 35%.[44] This variability is most likely secondary both to differing patient populations and to reported incidences of specific causes from a particular institution. The National American Society of Gastroenterological Endoscopy Survey on Upper Gastrointestinal Bleeding contains data from 277 physicians across the nation, reflecting an unbiased sampling. Silverstein and associates[44] reported that 15.6% of patients underwent surgery with an overall surgical mortality rate of 24%. Of the operations, 85% were emergency procedures with a 30% mortality vs. a death rate of 10% for elective operations. This compares to an overall series mortality rate of 11% and to an 8.5% mortality rate for those receiving only medical therapy. Mortality rates also varied widely for major diagnostic categories.

Specific Surgical Therapy

Before surgery the patient should be brought to the best possible hemodynamic state. A secure intravenous route for continued blood and fluid replacement must be established as necessary; a urinary catheter should be placed to monitor the adequacy of hydration; and in many patients, particularly the elderly, a Swan-Ganz catheter is also of value. Four to six units of crossmatched packed red blood cells and fresh frozen plasma should be on hand, with more available on demand. A nasogastric tube should be in place in order to empty gastric contents before induction of general anesthesia. At operation all the contents of the abdomen must be carefully explored in a systematic fashion.

Upper Gastrointestinal Tract. Hematemesis and/or blood in the nasogastric aspirate implicates a site proximal to the ligament of Treitz, even though the specific source of upper gastrointestinal bleeding may not have been localized before surgery. Absence of signs of portal hypertension should then direct attention to the stomach and duodenum as the most common sites of bleeding. Some lesions (i.e., gastric cancer, leiomyoma) are readily apparent. Others (i.e., duodenal ulcer) may be identified only after careful palpation.

Superficial lesions of the stomach or duodenum may be missed and require direct inspection of the gastroduodenal mucosa. A generous (usually approximately 6 cm) longitudinal antropyloroduodenotomy is made anteriorly to explore for such bleeding sites. Clotted and unclotted blood should be removed. Sponges should be placed distally in the duodenum to prevent reflux of previously shed blood. If a bleeding ulcer is found in the posterior duodenal bulb, it can usually be controlled by suture ligation followed by closure of the incision in a transverse fashion (Heineke-Mikulicz pyloroplasty). To ensure continued control of hemorrhage after surgery, suture ligation of the gastroduodenal artery both superior and inferior to the duodenal bulb is often added. Finally a truncal vagotomy is accomplished.

If a bleeding site is not found, a separate vertical gastrotomy is then made and extended to within a few centimeters of the gastroesophageal junction. Division of the short gastric vessels may be necessary to facilitate thorough examination of the proximal stomach. When all of these procedures fail to demonstrate the origin of bleeding, attention should be directed to the duodenum for evidence of a postbulbar ulcer, diverticulum, or neoplasm. If the bleeding has stopped without identification of a specific lesion, further surgery should cease; a gastrectomy or another ulcer operation are contraindicated. The pyloroduodenotomy and gastrotomy should be closed longitudinally, and the patient observed for recurrent hemorrhage. This latter group should comprise a very small minority of patients. With the extensive use of endoscopy and arteriography, the bleeding site should be documented before surgery to allow for the planning of an appropriate surgical approach.

Specific entities

Esophageal lesions. Nonvariceal esophageal bleeding is rarely a cause for an emergency operation. Blood loss is usually on a chronic basis and can be treated either medically or by elective surgery once the site and cause have been established. If an emergency operation is required, it is often associated with a high mortality rate, primarily because of the occurrence of such lesions in an older age group of patients. Only 10% of patients with the Mallory-Weiss syndrome will require surgical intervention for persistent or recurrent bleeding. The surgical procedure includes proximal gastrotomy with suture ligation of the offending submucosal bleeding site. Postoperative rebleeding has been reported in 10% of such treated patients with surgical mortality as high as 10%.[29]

Variceal hemorrhage. Treatment of the patient with acute variceal hemorrhage remains a therapeutic dilemma. In a recent study of 85 consecutive patients with endoscopically proven, clinically significant, variceal hemorrhage a 42% 6-week mortality for those treated medically was reported.[19] One third of the patients experienced rebleeding within 6 weeks. It was therefore concluded that any substantial improvement in long-term survival must result from a decrease in early mortality.[19]

Intravenous infusion of vasopressin with adjunctive use of balloon tamponade, transhepatic embolization, and sclerotherapy should control the acute episode of variceal bleeding in 75% to 90% of patients.[31] Emergency portasystemic shunts for persistent bleeding have reported surgical mortality rates as high as 50%.[19] More recently emergency, side-to-side portacaval shunts have been performed with a 30-day mortality of 24%.[30] This is in contrast to a 3.5% mortality when the same operation is performed on an elective basis.[30]

Duodenal ulcer. Hemorrhage from a duodenal ulcer remains the most frequent cause of massive upper gastrointestinal bleeding.[44] Although there is no consensus among surgeons regarding the best operation for such lesions, the choice should be tailored to the physiologic reserve of the patient. High-risk patients should undergo a procedure that is both effective in controlling the bleeding and that can be performed expeditiously. Oversewing of the bleeding point, combined with truncal vagotomy and pyloroplasty, is an appropriate therapeutic choice in this setting. More latitude for choice of surgery exists in the low-risk patient. In this latter group the mortality for a vagotomy and gastric resection is similar to that for vagotomy and pyloroplasty.[29]

Overall surgical mortality rates, inclusive of both emergency and elective patients, range between 5% and 10% and show a direct correlation with age of the patient and the volume of blood transfused. Recurrent hemorrhage has been found less in vagotomy and partial gastrectomy patients (5%) than in patients undergoing vagotomy and pyloroplasty (10%).[29] Multiple organ failure is responsible for two thirds of the deaths for both groups of patients.[44]

Hemorrhage from a recurrent ulcer (stomal) is usually not massive. In a series of 117 patients only 4% required an emergency operation.[29] For high-risk patients, oversewing the bleeding point with revagotomy is the procedure of choice. Revagotomy (usually by means of a transthoracic route) and resection are optimum treatments for most healthy surgical candidates under nonemergency conditions.

Stress ulceration. The therapy of choice for stress ulceration is prevention. Once bleeding has started, an emergency operation is required in about 10% of these patients.[29] A variety of surgical strategies have been recommended, including vagotomy and pyloroplasty, gastrectomy, total gastrectomy, and gastric devascularization.[29] The surgical mortality for all of these procedures has been similar, ranging from 30% to 50%.

Lower Gastrointestinal Tract. The need for surgical management of a source of bleeding distal to the ligament of Treitz will depend on the underlying cause and whether nonsurgical approaches such as angiography have been successful in bringing about its cessation. If an underlying malignancy is a possible responsible cause, exploratory celiotomy should be performed, and resection of the involved intestine in combination with lymph node drainage routes carried out. Even if hemorrhage is successfully arrested with nonsurgical maneuvers, demonstration of a small intestinal source would generally require surgery since the exact cause cannot be discerned in most instances and the possibility of a small bowel neoplasm must always be entertained. Again, a local resection in continuity with lymphatic drainage routes is appropriate. If other sources of small bowel bleeding, such as a Meckel's diverticulum, various duplications, and congenital arteriovenous malformations are likely sources and bleeding can be arrested without surgery, a conservative approach is usually indicated, and surgical therapy reserved for those patients who may develop recurrent hemorrhage. If a colonic polyp is the responsible bleeding source, it generally should be removed since the likelihood of recurrent bleeding is high and the possibility of an underlying malignancy is always present. Under most circumstances such polyps can be removed by endoscopic colonoscopy. Bleeding is not uncommonly observed in patients with inflammatory bowel disease, but it usually is modest and can be managed with conservative therapy. In the event that severe bleeding occurs from ulcerative colitis, subtotal or total colectomy is almost always indicated. In contrast, bleeding from Crohn's disease of a recurrent nature can generally be controlled by limited intestinal resection.

Management of colonic bleeding from either diverticulosis or an arteriovenous malformation has been the subject of considerable controversy.[8] Most surgeons recommend a conservative approach if nonsurgical maneuvers can control such bleeding and reserve surgery for those individuals in whom recurrent hemorrhage becomes a problem. Generally segmental resection of the bleeding site is adequate treatment in this group of patients. Recently a more aggressive stance has been taken with respect to angiodysplastic abnormalities because the natural history of this disorder is one of recurrent bleeding. Thus, Boley, Brant, and Frank[8] recommend that the demonstration of a vascular malformation on angiography, with or without evidence of active bleeding, warrants colonic resection. This is generally accomplished as an elective procedure if active bleeding can be controlled. Since virtually all of these abnormalities are limited to the right colon, resection of that portion of the intestine is carried out.

Occasionally massive hemorrhage from the colon will occur in which all attempts at diagnostic localization prove unrewarding. In this circumstance total abdominal colectomy becomes necessary as a lifesaving maneuver.

OCCULT HEMORRHAGE

The term occult gastrointestinal bleeding encompasses a spectrum of clinical definitions. To the majority of clinicians occult bleeding means intermittent, chronic, slow blood loss from the gastrointestinal tract. To others the term means anemia coupled with a positive test for blood in the stool. Finally occult bleeding has been defined in terms of continued blood loss from an undetermined site in spite of exhaustion of available diagnostic modalities.

Chronic blood loss from the gastrointestinal tract may occur without producing specific symptomatology. The patient may present with a history of melena or intermittent episodes of a small amount of bright red blood per rectum. Additional vague symptoms of weakness and chronic fatigue may be the only reason for seeking medical advice. Demonstration of a microcytic, hypochromic anemia without known blood loss from another source in these patients warrants a thorough examination of the gastrointestinal tract.

Although the barium contrast upper gastrointestinal series may detect a potentially responsible lesion, there is no proof that that particular entity is the cause of bleeding. In Palmer's series of 1400 patients 59% had another nonbleeding lesion found during the course of evaluation.[38] Therefore esophagogastroduodenoscopy should be performed in all patients with occult bleeding. The source of bleeding is found in as many as 40% of patients who undergo upper endoscopy for workup of iron deficiency anemia and/or melena. A double-contrast barium enema, anoscopy, proctosigmoidoscopy, and colonoscopy should be obtained to identify potential colorectal sources of bleeding. In contrast to its general lack of usefulness for acute gastrointestinal bleeding, colonoscopy has found the source of bleeding in 30% to 40% of patients with chronic blood loss.[9] The majority of lesions found have included polyps, vascular malformations, and superficial ulcerations.

Selective visceral angiography has been quite useful in patients with occult bleeding. The bleeding site has been identified in approximately 50% of patients,[9] and in another 25% to 30% of these patients the angiograms have demonstrated a highly suspicious lesion. As already noted, radionuclide imaging with labeled red blood cells is a noninvasive technique that may prove helpful in identifying the source of hemorrhage but is less specific in demonstrating the actual anatomic site. Further, the use of exploratory celiotomy to diagnose the site of occult gastrointestinal bleeding has been generally unsuccessful. In one series the use of intraoperative endoscopy at the time of celiotomy increased the diagnostic yield to 80% in a group of patients subjected to this diagnostic maneuver,[9] although this has not been a uniform experience.[48]

In the face of all of these diagnostic modalities, a group of patients will continue to carry the diagnosis of occult gastrointestinal bleeding. Care must be taken to ensure proper follow-up for these individuals. Serial blood counts should be obtained to assess the degree of anemia and to indicate any episodes of acute bleeding superimposed on the chronic anemia. The patient and/or family must be instructed to look for recurrent symptoms, the presence of melena, and to routinely test the stool for occult blood. The last important factor is to ensure continuity of care to prevent the patient from being lost to follow-up.

SUMMARY

Hemorrhage from the gastrointestinal tract is responsible for approximately 1% to 2% of all hospital admissions. Hemorrhage originating from a source proximal to the ligament of Treitz is referred to as upper gastrointestinal tract hemorrhage, whereas hemorrhage distal to this anatomic boundary is termed lower gastrointestinal tract hemorrhage. Common causes of upper tract hemorrhage include duodenal ulcer, acute gastritis, gastric ulcer, esophageal varices, esophagitis, and Mallory-Weiss mucosal tears. Common causes of lower tract hemorrhage include diverticulosis, angiodysplastic lesions of the colon, ischemic colitis, and various neoplastic and inflammatory lesions of the small and large intestine. In the management of any patient with gastrointestinal tract hemorrhage, three priorities are paramount. These include resuscitation, identification of the underlying bleeding site, and the use of appropriate measures to stop the bleeding. Hematemesis virtually always implicates a source of bleeding proximal to the ligament of Treitz, whereas melena and hematochezia are less reliable indicators of the underlying bleeding site. Endoscopy provides the best help in locating the site of bleeding in patients with suspected upper gastrointestinal hemorrhage, whereas radionuclide scanning and arteriography are commonly used when a distal bleeding site is presumed. With the availability of various endoscopic and angiographic techniques to control bleeding, the vast majority of patients with gastrointestinal hemorrhage can be managed without surgery. In those patients requiring surgical management the type of procedure will be determined by the underlying cause. For a bleeding peptic ulcer, for example, surgical management may require vagotomy and partial gastrectomy, whereas an angiodysplastic lesion of the colon will usually necessitate a right colectomy. In a small percentage of patients, the source of gastrointestinal bleeding will remain occult in spite of vigorous diagnostic investigation. In this group of patients careful follow-up is mandatory. Continued surveillance of the gastrointestinal tract with various endoscopic maneuvers, barium contrast studies, and, on occasion, radionuclide scanning and/or angiography to search for sources of unexplained anemia will identify the underlying cause in a majority of these individuals.

REFERENCES

1. Alavi, A.: Detection of gastrointestinal bleeding with ^{99m}Te-Sulfur colloid, Semin. Nucl. Med. **12:**126, 1982.
2. Allan, R.N.: History, epidemiology, mortality. In Dykes, P.W., and Keighley, M.R.B., editors: Gastrointestinal Haemorrhage, Boston, 1981, Wright PSG.
3. Baum, S.: Angiography and the gastrointestinal bleeder, Radiology **143:**569, 1982.
4. Baum, S., et al.: The operative radiographic demonstration of intraabdominal bleeding from undetermined sites by percutaneous selective celiac and superior mesenteric arteriography, Surgery **58:**797, 1965.
5. Behringer, G.E., and Albright, N.L.: Diverticular disease of the colon: a frequent cause of massive rectal bleeding, Am. J. Surg. **125:**419, 1973.
6. Bogoch, A.: Hematemesis and melena. Part I. Etiology and medical aspects. In Bockus, H.L., editor: Gastroenterology, vol 1, Philadelphia, 1974, W.B. Saunders Co.
7. Boley, S.J., Sammartano, R., and Adams, A.: The nature and etiology of vascular ectasias of the colon, Gastroenterology **72:**650, 1977.
8. Boley, S.J., Brant, L.J., and Frank, M.S.: Severe lower intestinal bleeding: diagnosis and treatment. In Torsoli, A., editor: Gastrointestinal emergencies, Clinics in Gastroenterology, Philadelphia, 1981, W.B. Saunders Co.
9. Bowden, T.A., et al.: Occult gastrointestinal bleeding: locating the cause, Am. Surg. **46:**80, 1980.
10. Bray, S.J., et al.: Lower intestinal bleeding in the elderly, Am. J. Surg. **137:**57, 1979.
11. Chojkier, M., et al.: A controlled comparison of continuous intraarterial and intravenous infusion of vasopressin in hemorrhage from esophageal varices, Gastroenterology **77:**540, 1979.
12. Cytler, J.A., and Mendeloff, A.I.: Upper gastrointestinal bleeding: nature and magnitude of the problem in the U.S. Dig. Dis. Sci. **26**(suppl):90, 1981.
13. Dronffield, M.W., et al.: A prospective randomised trial of endoscopy and radiology in acute upper-gastrointestinal-tract bleeding, Lancet **1:**1167, 1977.
14. Fogel, M.R., et al.: Continuous intravenous vasopressin in active upper gastrointestinal bleeding: a placebo-controlled trial, Ann. Intern. Med. **96:**565, 1982.
15. Gann, D.S., and Amaral, J.F.: Pathophysiology of trauma and shock. In Zuidema, G.D., Rutherford, R.D., and Ballinger, W.F., editors: The management of trauma, Philadelphia, 1985, W.B. Saunders Co.

16. Gardner, B., and Richardson, J.D.: Gastrointestinal bleeding. In Polk, H.C., Stone, H.H., and Gardner, B., editors: Basic surgery, Norwalk, CT, 1983, Appleton-Century-Crofts.
17. Gaskill, H.V., Sirinek, K.R., and Levine, B.A.: Hemodynamic effects of vasopressin: can larger doses be safely given? Arch. Surg. **118:**434, 1983.
18. Gilbert, D.A., Silverstein, F.E., and Tedesco, F.J.: National ASGE surgery on upper gastrointestinal bleeding: complications of endoscopy, Dig. Dis. Sci. 26(suppl):55, 1981.
19. Graham, D.Y., and Smith, J.L.: The course of patients after variceal hemorrhage, Gastroenterology **80:**800, 1981.
20. Hennessy, T.P.J., Stephens, R.B., and Keane, F.B.: Acute and chronic management of varices by injection sclerotherapy, Surg. Gynecol. Obstet. **154:**375, 1982.
21. Herner, B., Kallgard, B., and Lauritzen, A.: Haematemesis and melena from a limited reception area during a 5-year period, Acta Med. Scand. **177:**483, 1965.
22. Hessel, S.J., Adams, D.F., and Abrams, H.L.: Complications of angiography, Radiology **138:**273, 1981.
23. Hoare, A.M.: Comparative study between endoscopy and radiology in acute upper gastrointestinal hemorrhage, Br. Med. J. **1:**27, 1975.
24. Johnson, W.C., et al.: Control of bleeding varices by vasopressin: A prospective randomized study, Ann. Surg. **186:**369, 1977.
25. Johnston, G.W., and Rodgers, H.W.: A review of 15 years' experience in the use of sclerotherapy in the control of acute haemorrhage for oesophageal varices, Br. J. Surg. **60:**797, 1973.
26. Johnston, S.J., et al.: Epidemiology and course of gastrointestinal haemorrhage in north-east Scotland, Br. Med. J. **3:**655, 1973.
27. Kadir, S., and Athanasoulis, C.A.: Angiographic management of gastrointestinal bleeding, Ann. Rev. Med. **30:**41, 1979.
28. Kehne, J.H., Hughes, F.A., and Gompertz, M.L.: The use of surgical pituitrin in the control of esophageal varix bleeding, Surgery **39:**917, 1956.
29. Larson, D.E., and Farnell, M.B.: Upper gastrointestinal hemorrhage, Mayo Clin. Proc. **58:**371, 1983.
30. Levine, B.A., and Sirinek, K.R.: Direct portacaval anastomosis-safe and effective in patients with previous abdominal operations, Am. J. Surg. **152:**721, 1986.
31. Levine, B.A., Gaskill, H.V., and Sirinek, K.R.: Portosystemic shunting remains procedure of choice for control of variceal hemorrhage, Arch. Surg. **120:**296, 1985.
32. McGinn, F.P., et al.: A prospective comparative trial between early endoscopy and radiology in acute upper gastrointestinal haemorrhage, Gut **16:**707, 1975.
33. Merigan, T.C., et al.: Gastrointestinal bleeding with cirrhosis: A study of 172 episodes in 158 patients, N. Engl. J. Med. **263:**579, 1980.
34. Moody, F.G.: Rectal bleeding, N. Engl. J. Med. **290:**839, 1974.
35. Nusbaum, M., et al.: Pharmacologic control of portal hypertension, Surgery **62:**299, 1967.
36. Nusbaum, M., et al.: Clinical experience with selective intra-arterial infusion of vasopressin in the control of gastrointestinal bleeding from arterial sources, Am. J. Surg. **123:**165, 1972.
37. Palmer, E.D.: Upper gastrointestinal hemorrhage, Springfield, Ill., 1970, Charles C Thomas, Publisher.
38. Palmer, E.D.: Upper gastrointestinal hemorrhage. JAMA **231:**853, 1975.
39. Peterson, W.L., et al.: Routine early endoscopy in upper-gastrointestinal-tract bleeding: a randomized controlled trial, N. Engl. J. Med. **304:**925, 1981.
40. Rahn, N.H., et al.: Diagnostic and interventional angiography in acute gastrointestinal hemorrhage, Radiology **143:**361, 1982.
41. Rutherford, R.B., and Akers, D.R.: Meckel's diverticulum: a review of 148 patients with special reference to the pattern of bleeding and to mesodiverticular vascular bands, Surgery **59:**618, 1966.
42. Schiller, K.F.R., Truelove, A.C., and William, D.G.: Haematemesis and melena with special reference to factors influencing the outcome, Br. Med. J. **2:**7, 1970.
43. Silverstein, F.E., Gilbert, D.A., and Auth, D.C.: Endoscopy hemostasis using laser photocoagulation and electrocoagulation, Dig. Dis. Sci. **26**(suppl):31, 1981.
44. Silverstein, F.E., et al.: The national ASGE survey on upper gastrointestinal bleeding. I. Study design and baseline data, Gastrointestinal Endoscopy **27:**73, 1981.
45. Sirinek, K.R., and Thomford, N.R.: Isoproterenol in offsetting adverse effects of vasopressin in cirrhotic patients, Am. J. Surg. **129:**130, 1975.
46. Sirinek, K.R., Martin, E.W., and Thomford, N.R.: Peripheral vasopressin provides safe and adequate control of portal hypertension during shunt operations, Am. J. Surg. **131:**103, 1976.
47. Skillman, J.J., and Silen, W.: Stress ulceration in the acutely ill, Ann. Rev. Med. **27:**9, 1976.
48. Steer, M.L., and Silen, W.: Diagnostic procedures in gastrointestinal hemorrhage, N. Engl. J. Med. **309:**646, 1983.
49. Swan, K.G., Hobson, R.W., and Kerr, J.C.: Experimental observations and clinical recommendations on vasopressin for control of gastrointestinal hemorrhage, Am. Surg. **43:**545, 1977.
50. Terblanche, J., et al.: Acute bleeding varices: a five-year prospective evaluation of tamponade and sclerotherapy, Ann. Surg. **194:**521, 1981.
51. Teterick, C.E., et al.: The portal hypertensive effect of dopamine, J. Surg. Res. **22:**671, 1977.
52. Thomford, N.R., and Sirinek, K.R.: Intravenous vasopressin in patients with portal hypertension, J. Surg. Res. **18:**113, 1975.
53. Winzelberg, G.G., et al.: Detection of gastrointestinal bleeding with ^{99m}Tc-labeled red blood cells, Semin. Nucl. Med. **12:**139, 1982.

32

Stuart I. Myers and Thomas A. Miller

Acute Abdominal Pain: Physiology of the Acute Abdomen

The term "acute abdomen" refers to the sudden unexpected onset of acute abdominal pain, usually accompanied by other symptoms such as nausea, vomiting, anorexia, and abdominal distention. Such pain may be secondary to many etiologic possibilities, all of which can present clinically in a variety of ways, depending on the underlying anatomic focus of disease, the duration of the pathophysiologic process, and the specific pathology involved. Accurate diagnosis of the cause of an acute abdomen depends on the physician's understanding of the embryology, anatomy, neurophysiology, and natural history of each potential specific etiology. The goal of this chapter is to examine the physiologic derangements responsible for the development of the acute abdomen and how much knowledge aids in its diagnosis and treatment.

EMBRYOLOGY OF ABDOMINAL VISCERA

Acute abdominal pain can originate from virtually any intraabdominal structure, and at times even from extraabdominal sources. Thus diagnosis of the underlying disease process responsible for the development of an acute abdomen requires accurate knowledge of the embryology of these abdominal structures and extraabdominal organs such as the heart, lungs, and esophagus.

Development of the Heart, Lungs, and Diaphragm

The vascular system of the human embryo starts to develop between 3 and 4 weeks of gestation. The original cardiogenic plexus that will form the heart is located anterior to the prochordal and the neural plates. As the central nervous system grows rapidly in the cephalic direction, it extends over the central cardiogenic area. The heart tubes come to lie in a new area ventral to the foregut as it descends into the pericardial cavity. At the beginning of the fourth week, the partitioning into chambers and the ingrowth to the heart of the autonomic nerves begin (Fig. 32-1).[5,12,17] The central tendon of the diaphragm (as well as part of the liver) originates from the septum transversum. However, this does not separate the pericardial cavity from the abdominal contents because the lateral aspects of the pericardioperitoneal canals remain open and connect the cavities. These canals are vitally important to the growing lung buds and eventually contain most of the lung growth and become the primitive pleural cavities. The caudal expansion of the pericardioperitoneal canals is limited by the pleuroperitoneal fold that originates from the cranial ligament of the original mesonephros. This fold expands in an anterior and medial direction and by the seventh week fuses with the mesentery of the esophagus and the septum transversum to form the diaphragm. Invading myoblasts from the body wall contribute to the development of the muscle of the diaphragm. These myoblasts are derived from the third through the fifth cervical segments, and their innervation (i.e., phrenic nerve) remains as the central diaphragm descends from the original position in the neck to its adult position. The peripheral portion of the diaphragm, formed from the body wall, retains its inner-

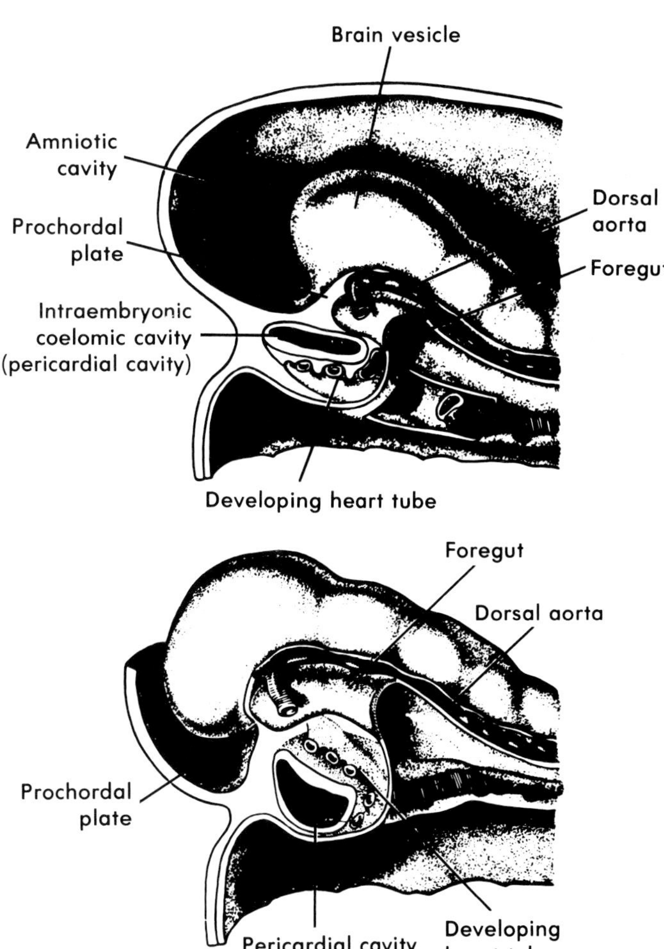

Fig. 32-1 Result of the rapid growth of the brain vesicles on the position of the pericardial cavity and the developing heart tube. Initially the angiogenetic cell clusters and the pericardial cavity are located in front of the prochordal plate. As a result of the rotation along a transverse axis through the prochordal plate, the cardiogenic plexus finally comes to lie dorsal to the pericardial cavity. (From Langman, J.: Medical embryology, ed. 2, Baltimore, 1969, The Williams and Wilkins Co.)

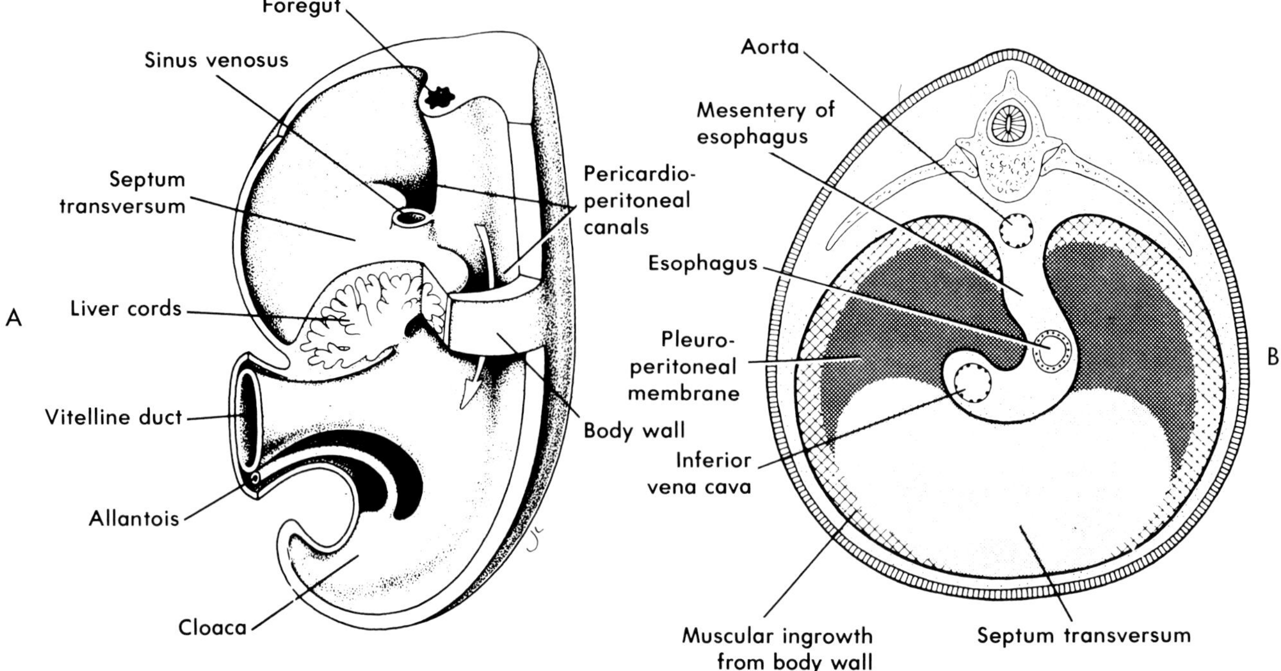

Fig. 32-2 **A,** Model of a portion of an embryo of approximately 5 weeks. Parts of the body wall and the septum transversum have been removed to show the pericardioperitoneal canals. Note the size and thickness of the septum transversum and the liver cords penetrating the mesenchyme. **B,** Schematic representation of the definitive diaphragm, indicating the origin of the various components. (From Langman, J.: Medical embryology, ed. 2, Baltimore, 1969, The Williams and Wilkins Co.)

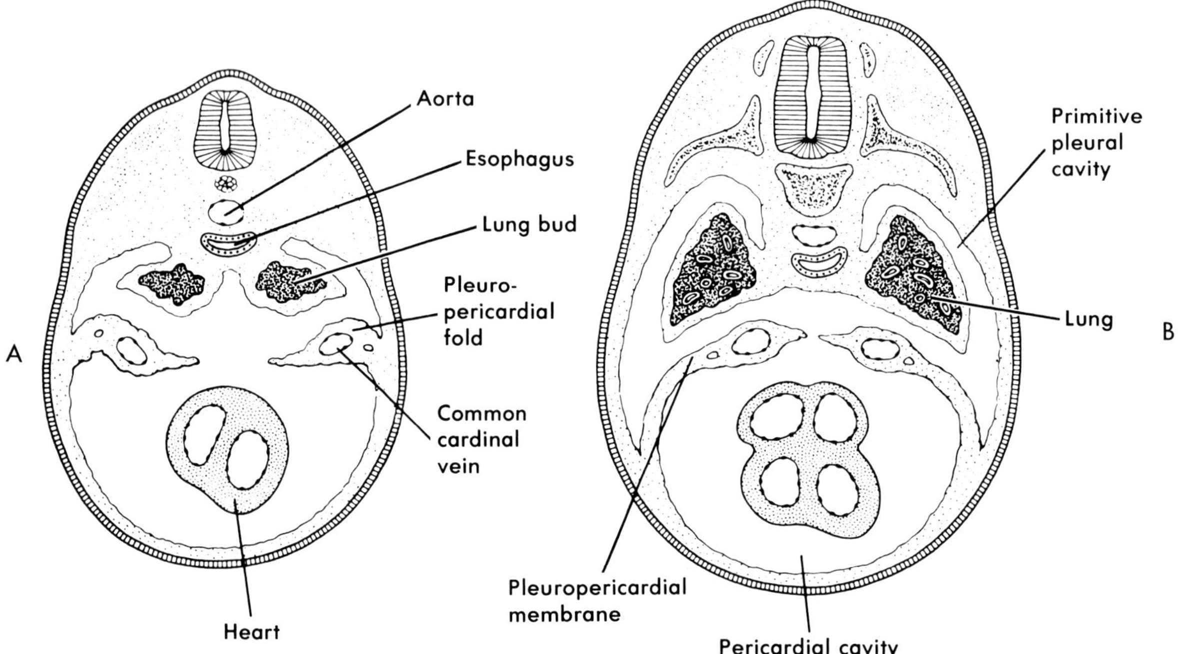

Fig. 32-3 Schematic drawings at two successive stages of development showing the transformation of the pericardioperitoneal canals into the primitive pleural cavities and the formation of the pleuropericardial membranes. **A,** Note the relationship of the common cardinal vein to the pleuropericardial ridge. **B,** As a result of the expansion of the pericardioperitoneal canals, the mesenchyme of the body wall is split into the pleuropericardial membranes and the definitive body wall. (From Langman, J.: Medical embryology, ed. 2, Baltimore, 1969, The Williams and Wilkins Co.)

vation by the lower seven intercostal nerves that supply the adjacent body wall (Figs. 32-2 and 32-3).[5,12,17]

Development of the Gut

The gut begins to develop during the fourth week of gestation. The primitive gut is derived from both the endoderm (which gives rise to most of the epithelium and glands) and the mesoderm (which gives rise to muscular and fibrous parts surrounding the endodermal lining). The epithelium of the primitive mouth and anus is derived from surface ectoderm and develops separately from the primitive gut tube. Because of this circumstance, the ectodermal and endodermal elements of these two regions develop separate blood supplies, lymphatic drainage systems, and neural innervations. The gut tube is comprised of a foregut, midgut, and hindgut. Each of these regions has its own blood supply and nervous innervation and retains these distinctions throughout development and into adulthood.

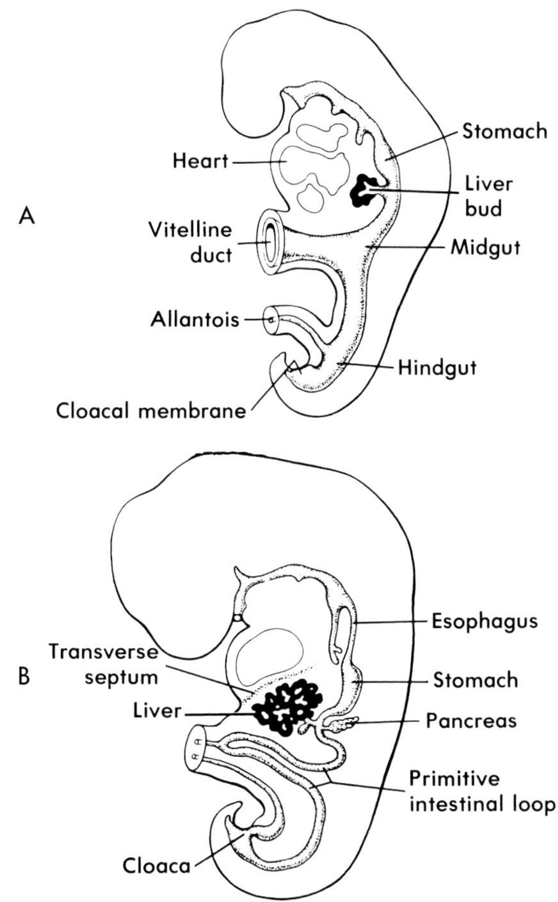

Fig. 32-4 **A,** Drawing of a 3-mm embryo (approximately 25 days) to show the primitive gastrointestinal tract. Note the formation of the hepatic diverticulum. The hepatic diverticulum is formed by the entodermal epithelial lining of the terminal part of the foregut. **B,** Drawing of a 5-mm embryo (approximately 32 days). The epithelial liver cords penetrate the mesenchyme of the transverse septum. Note the primary intestinal loop. (From Langman, J.: Medical embryology, ed. 2, Baltimore, 1969, The Williams and Wilkins Co.)

Foregut

The foregut extends from the pharynx to the duodenum at the level of entrance of the common bile duct. Caudal to the primitive pharynx and respiratory tract is the narrow esophagus, which widens to form the stomach and duodenum. During formation, the stomach rotates around its longitudinal axis in a 90-degree clockwise fashion that results in its left side facing anteriorly and its right side facing posteriorly. The left vagus nerve thus becomes anterior, and the right vagus becomes posterior in its location. The posterior portion of the stomach also grows more than the anterior portion during this rotation, which gives rise to the greater and lesser curvatures. Of further note, the duodenum takes on its U-shaped loop configuration during this rotation and rotates to the right to assume its retroperitoneal location. The liver bud develops as a ventral outgrowth of endoderm and grows into the septum transversum to form the liver and the various components of the biliary tract. The pancreas develops as separate ventral and dorsal buds that arise from endoderm distal to the liver bud. The ventral pancreatic bud develops into the major portion of the pancreatic head; whereas the dorsal bud develops into the dorsal pancreas, which consists of the superior pancreatic head, the uncinate process, and the pancreatic body and tail. Although not actually part of the foregut, the spleen develops from mesenchymal cells derived from the stomach mesentery and obtains a similar blood supply to the foregut, i.e., the celiac artery (Figs. 32-4 to 32-6).[5,12,17]

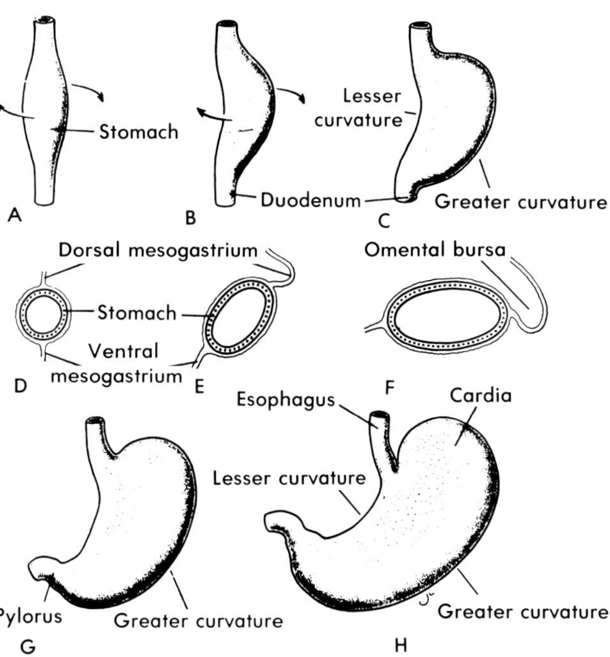

Fig. 32-5 Schematic representation of the positional changes of the stomach. **A, B,** and **C,** rotation of the stomach along its longitudinal axis as seen from anterior; **D, E,** and **F,** in transverse section the effect of rotation on the peritoneal attachments; **G** and **H,** rotation of the stomach around the anteroposterior axis (seen from anterior). (From Langman, J.: Medical embryology, ed. 2, Baltimore, 1969, The Williams and Wilkins Co.)

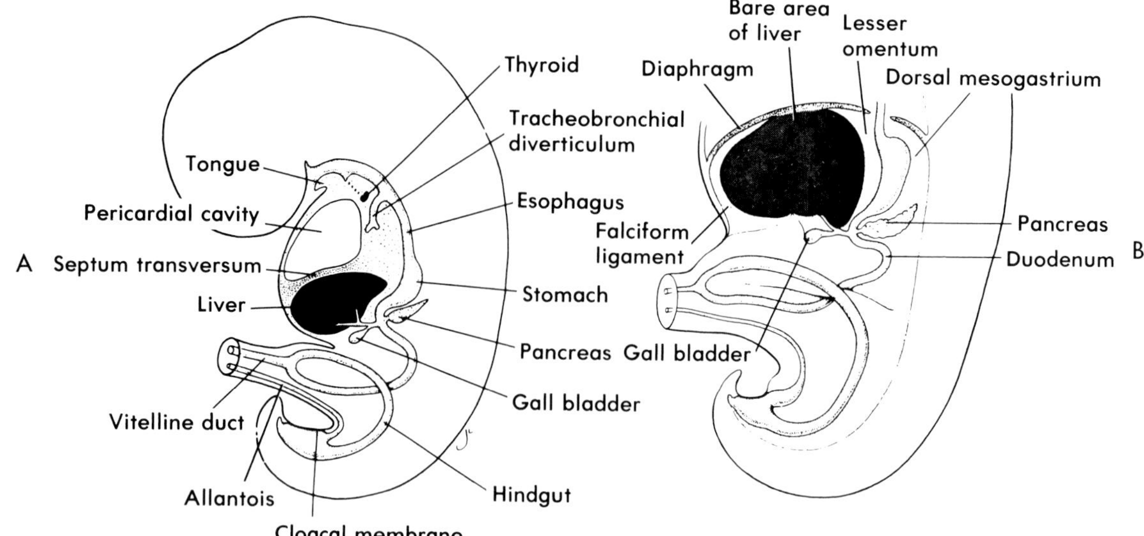

Fig. 32-6 **A.** Drawing of a 9-mm embryo (approximately 36 days). The liver expands caudally into the abdominal cavity. Note condensation of mesenchyme in the area between the liver and the pericardial cavity, foreshadowing the formation of the diaphragm. **B,** Drawing of a slightly older embryo. Note falciform ligament extending between liver and anterior abdominal wall, lesser omentum between liver and anterior abdominal wall, and lesser omentum between liver and foregut (stomach and duodenum). The liver is entirely surrounded by peritoneum, except in its contact area with the diaphragm. This area is known as the bare area of the liver. (From Langman, J.: Medical embryology, ed. 2, Baltimore, 1969, The Williams and Wilkins Co.)

Midgut

The midgut can be separated into cranial and caudal portions. The cranial portion includes the duodenum distal to the entrance of the common bile duct, all of the jejunum, and the proximal part of the ileum. The caudal portion includes the distal ileum, appendix, ascending colon, and the proximal two thirds of the transverse colon. The apex of the midgut is represented by the vitelline or omphalomesenteric duct. This duct, when patent in the adult, persists of a Meckel's diverticulum. The midgut greatly elongates during its development, forming the primary intestinal loop. The cranial portion elongates much more than the caudal portion. This elongation causes a physiologic herniation during the sixth week of gestation as the abdominal cavity temporarily becomes too small to adequately contain the primary intestinal loop. At this stage of development, the primary intestinal loop also rotates 270 degrees in a counterclockwise direction around the axis of the superior mesenteric artery from which it derives its blood supply. After the third month the greatly elongated small intestinal loops and colon begin to return to the abdominal cavity, which by now has also developed to an adequate size to accommodate these structures. The jejunum returns first and lies normally on the left side, whereas the cecum enters last, lying in the right upper quadrant at first and then descending into its permanent position in the right lower quadrant (Fig. 32-7).[5,12,17]

Hindgut

The hindgut extends from the origin of the distal one third of the transverse colon to the cloacal swelling. The cloacal membrane represents the contact area between the surface ectoderm and endoderm of the cloaca. The hindgut is at first connected to the cloaca as is the allantois. As further development occurs, a urorectal septum forms in the angle between the allantois and the hindgut, dividing the cloaca into its two portions: an anterior urogenital sinus and a posterior anorectal canal. Thus the cloacal membrane also divides into two distinct areas, an anal membrane and a urogenital membrane separated by the perineum. The anal membrane forms on the bottom of the proctoderm and becomes surrounded by mesenchymal swellings that develop into the anal glands. By the ninth week, the anal membrane ruptures, forming an open communication between the hindgut and the outside of the body. The upper part of the anorectal canal develops from the hindgut and its endoderm and is supplied by the artery of the hindgut, the inferior mesenteric artery. The lower portion of the anorectal canal forms from the surface ectoderm and is supplied by its vascular supply, the internal iliac artery (Fig. 32-8).[5,12,17]

Development of Mesenteries

Initially during development, the foregut, midgut, and hindgut are in contact with the posterior abdominal wall. At the 8-mm embryo stage this mesenchymal bridge becomes membranous, forming the dorsal mesentery. The divisions of this mesentery derive their names from the organs to which they are attached. These divisions are the dorsal mesogastrium in the area of the stomach, the mesoduodenum in the area of the duodenum, and the dorsal mesocolon in the area of the colon. The dorsal mesentery of the primary intestinal loop is termed the mesentery

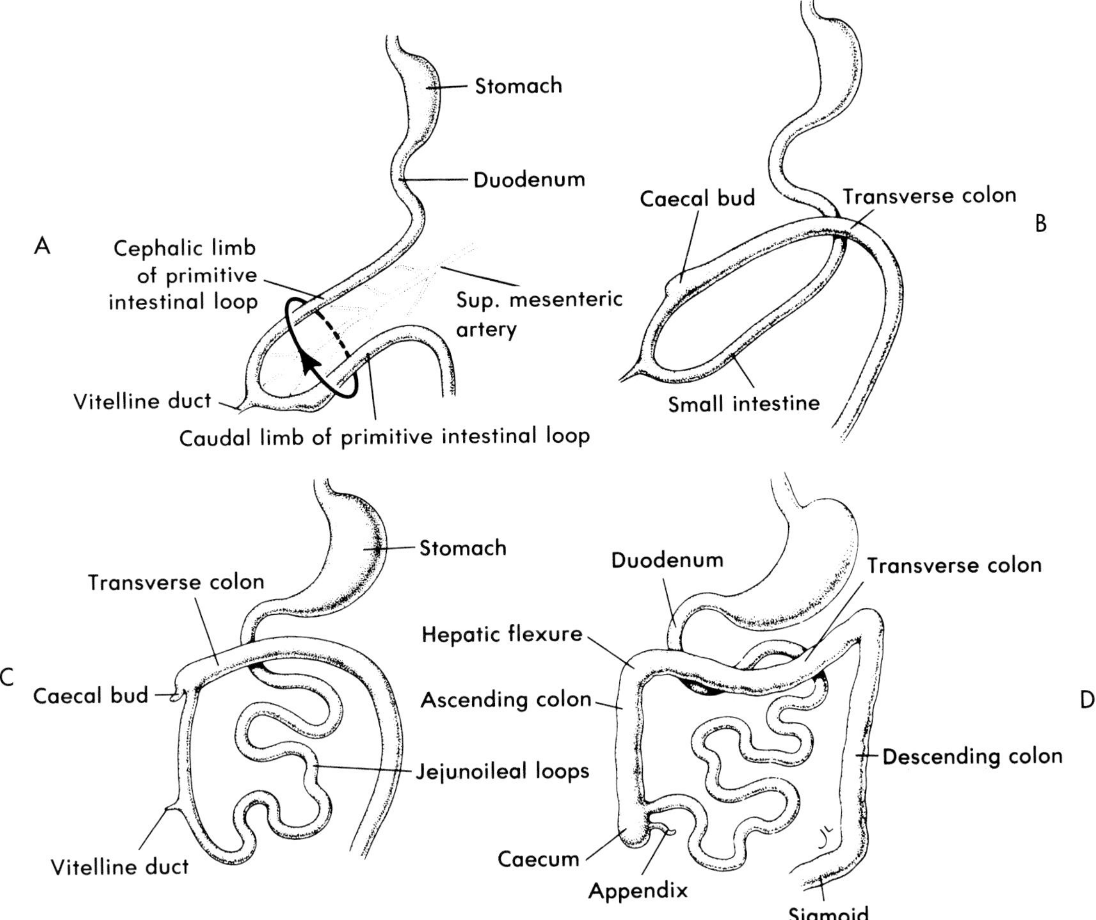

Fig. 32-7 **A,** Schematic drawing of the primitive intestinal loop before rotation (lateral view). The superior mesenteric artery forms the axis of the loop. Arrow indicates the direction of the anticlockwise rotation. **B,** Similar view as in **A,** showing the primitive intestinal loop after 180-degree anticlockwise rotation. The transverse colon passes in front of the duodenum. **C,** Anterior view of the intestinal loops after 270-degree anticlockwise rotation. Note the coiling of the small intestinal loops and the position of the caecal bud in the right upper quadrant of the abdomen. **D,** Similar view as in **C,** with the intestinal loops in the final position. Caecum and appendix are located in the right lower quadrant of the abdomen. (From Langman, J.: Medical embryology, ed. 2, Baltimore, 1969, The Williams and Wilkins Co.)

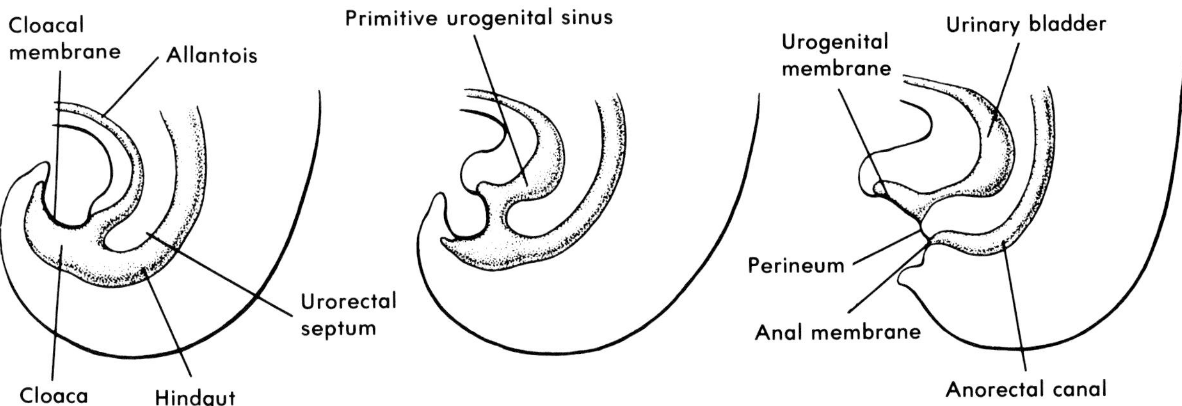

Fig. 32-8 Drawings of the cloacal region in embryos at successive stages of development. Note route of descent followed by the urorectal septum (from figure on left to figure on right) and the formation of the anorectal canal and the perineum. (From Langman, J.: Medical embryology, ed. 2, Baltimore, 1969, The Williams and Wilkins Co.)

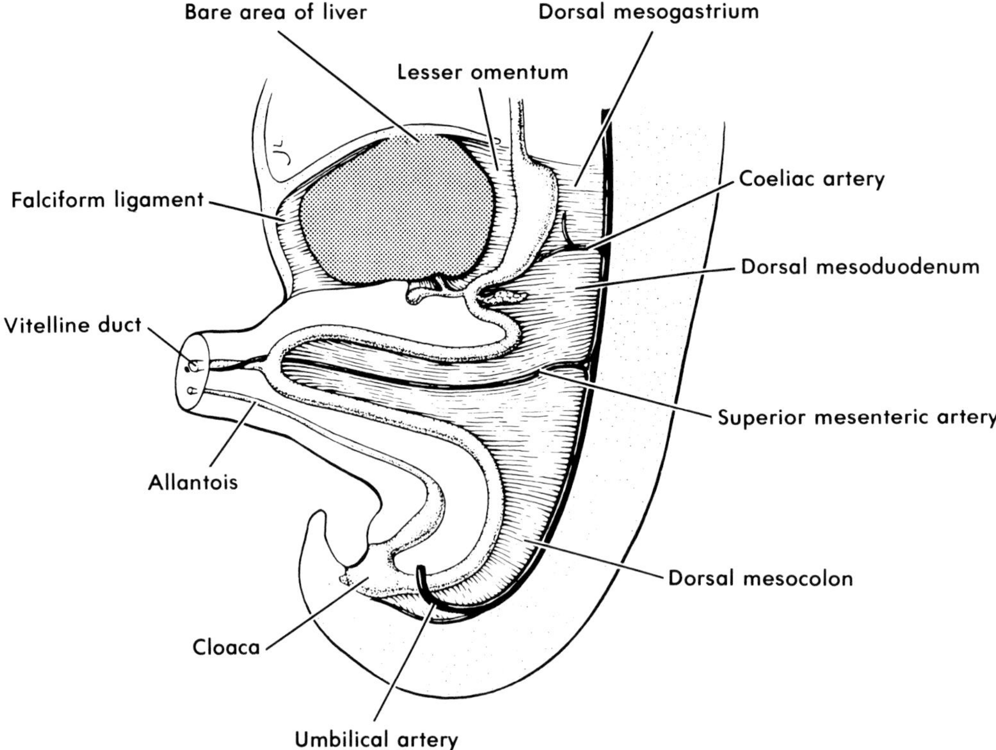

Fig 32-9 Schematic drawing showing the primitive dorsal and ventral mesenteries. Note how the liver is connected to the ventral abdominal wall and to the stomach by the falciform ligament and lesser omentum, respectively. The superior mesenteric artery runs through the mesentery proper and continues toward the yolk sac as the vitelline artery. (From Langman, J.: Medical embryology, ed. 2, Baltimore, 1969, The Williams and Wilkins Co.)

proper. Throughout development the mesentery serves as the conduit through which traverses the arterial blood supply, venous and lymphatic drainage routes, and neural pathways that supply the gut. In spite of rotational changes that take place in the gut and the ultimate fixation of the duodenum and ascending and descending portions of the colon to the retroperitoneum, the neural pathways and the vascular supply and drainage routes remain within the dorsal mesentery, originating as midline structures.

The permanent retroperitoneal position of the duodenum results from the rotational changes in the stomach and duodenum already described, as well as pressure effects attendant to the enlarging pancreas. The duodenum and pancreas become pressed against the dorsal body wall. The mesoduodenum fuses with the adjacent somatic peritoneum; and both structures disappear, as most of the duodenum becomes fixed in the retroperitoneum, except the proximal duodenum, which remains intraperitoneal and attached to a dorsal mesoduodenum. In similar fashion the ascending and descending colons assume their adult positions in the peritoneal cavity, with their mesenteries becoming adherent to the adjacent somatic peritoneum with subsequent fusion and fixation of these structures to the retroperitoneum The cecum and appendix do not fix and are free intraperitoneal structures. The transverse colon retains its mesentery and covers the duodenum with an additional peritoneal layer that later fuses with the greater omentum.

The peritoneum is composed of continuous visceral and parietal layers. Although both layers are derived from mesoderm, each develops separately. The visceral layer is derived from splanchnic mesoderm originating from the gut tube, and its blood supply is through visceral vessels. In contrast, the parietal layer is derived from somatic mesoderm originating from the lining on the inside of the body cavity, and its blood supply is through blood vessels of the body wall. Similarly, the nerve supply to each layer differs. The visceral layer is supplied by autonomic nerves (i.e., sympathetic and parasympathetic), and the parietal by somatic innervation (i.e., spinal nerves). The pathways involving the sensation of pain differ from each layer and differ in quality as well. Visceral pain is dull, crampy, and aching; whereas parietal pain is sharp, often severe, and persistent (Figs. 32-9 and 32-10).[5,12,17]

Development of the Urogenital Tract

Development of the urogenital tract is equally complex and begins as a growth of intermediate mesoderm parallel to the dorsal mesentery that forms the rudimentary pronephric glomeruli and pronephric ducts. These glomeruli evolve in the thorax and are replaced by development of mesonephric glomeruli that lie between T8 and L4 vertebrae. The degeneration of the pronephric glomeruli is accompanied by a degeneration of the proximal pronephric duct. The remaining pronephric duct is called the mesonephric duct. The mesonephros itself only functions for

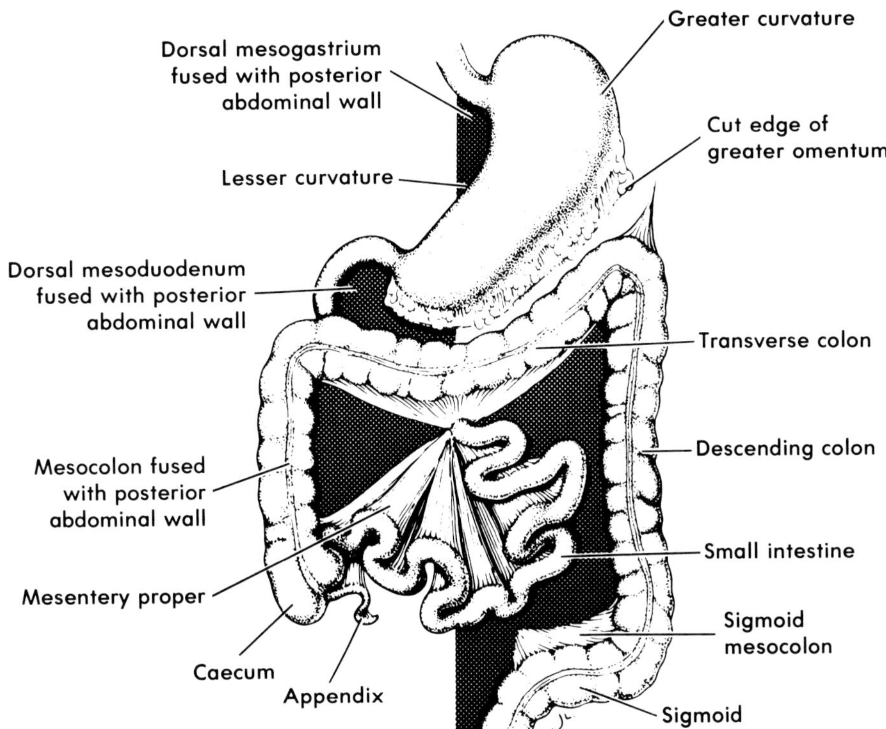

Fig. 32-10 Frontal view of the intestinal loops after removal of the greater omentum. The cross-hatched areas indicate the parts of the dorsal mesentery that fuse with the posterior abdominal wall. Note the line of attachment of the mesentery proper. (From Langman, J.: Medical embryology, ed. 2, Baltimore, 1969, The Williams and Wilkins Co.)

months 2 and 3 of gestation and is replaced by the metanephros. The ureteric bud arises from the caudal end of the mesonephric duct and grows into the intermediate mesoderm, which begins to develop the metanephric cap. The metanephric cap develops the glomerular capsule, the convoluted tubules, and the loop of Henle. The ureteric cap develops the major and minor calyces, collecting tubules, renal pelvis, and ureters. The forming kidneys initially develop in the pelvis but later ascend to take their adult positions. When the ascent is complete, they are then innervated by autonomic nerves (Figs. 32-11 through 32-15).[5,12,17]

The genital ridges appear in the fourth week and lie between the mesonephros and dorsal mesentery along the midline. These ridges are the earliest gonads and are formed from coelomic epithelium and mesenchyma. The germ cells appear in the yolk sac at the sixth week of development and migrate to the genital ridges. The germ cells either form the male testis or the female ovary. The testis comes to lie 10 segments below its level of origin in the second month as the body elongates and is thus a shift in position in relation to the body wall. The testis remains in close proximity to the inguinal canal until the seventh month when it descends through the inguinal ring into the scrotum. The testis retains its original blood supply from the aorta. The female ovary descends less than the testis, but it still descends to a level below the pelvic rim.

The male and female embryos develop two pairs of genital ducts during the sixth week of development, the Wolffian ducts and the müllerian ducts. The müllerian ducts arise from the coelomic epithelium from the urogenital ridge and cranially open in the coelomic cavity with a funnel-like structure that forms the abdominal ostia of the fallopian tube and the remainder of the fallopian tube. Caudally the müllerian duct runs lateral to the mesonephric duct and crosses the midline to fuse with the müllerian duct from the opposite side and forms a septum that fuses and forms the uterovaginal canal. The caudal portion of the fused müllerian ducts continues to grow caudally to the wall of the urogenital sinus. The wolffian ducts open on either side of the ureterovaginal canal into the urogenital sinus. In the male the wolffian duct forms the ductus deferens, and the müllerian duct disappears. In the female the müllerian ducts continue development to form the oviducts and uterus, and part of the vagina.

Embryologic Basis of Abdominal Pain

Knowledge of the embryologic development of structures within the abdomen can add greatly in the anatomic localization of abdominal pain. Since the normal embryologic development of abdominal viscera proceeds with bilateral midline sensory innervation, pain arising from such viscera is usually described as being in the abdominal midline. The position of pain in the midline is determined by the embryologic origin of the viscera involved. An epigastric location of abdominal pain is typical of a foregut origin. Umbilical midline pain is more typical of pain arising from the midgut. Hypogastric (i.e., lower abdominal) midline pain is more indicative of an origin from hindgut structures. Finally, pain arising in the pelvis is more typi-

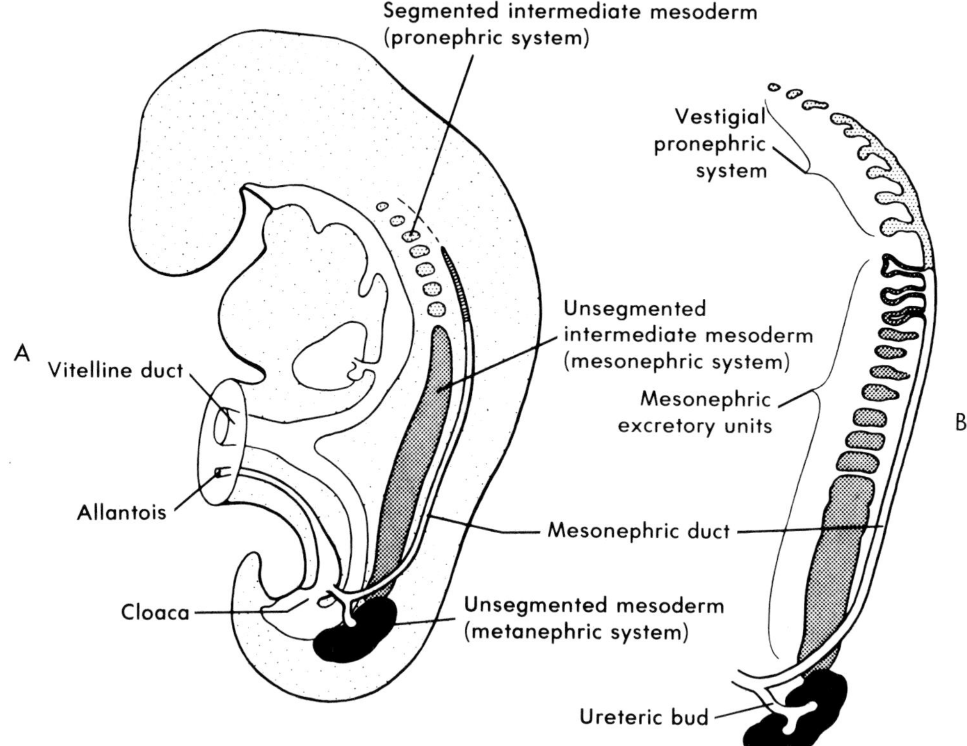

Fig. 32-11 **A,** Schematic diagram showing the relation of the intermediate mesoderm of the pronephric, mesonephric, and metanephric systems. In the cervical and upper thoracic regions the intermediate mesoderm is segmented; in the lower thoracic, lumbar, and sacral regions it forms a solid, unsegmented mass of tissue, the nephrogenic cord. Note the longitudinal collecting duct, initially formed by the pronephros but later taken over by the mesonephros. **B,** Schematic representation of the excretory tubules of the pronephric and mesonephric systems in a 5-week-old embryo. The ureteric bud penetrates the metanephric tissue. Note the remnant of the pronephric excretory tubules and longitudinal collecting duct. (From Langman, J.: Medical embryology, ed. 2, Baltimore, 1969, The Williams and Wilkins Co.)

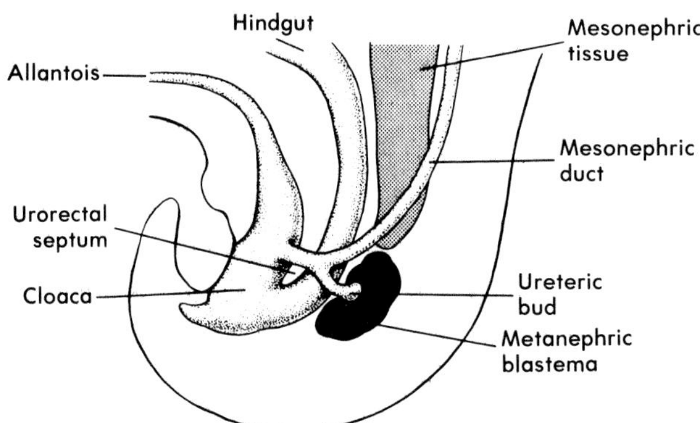

Fig. 32-12 Schematic drawing to show the relationship of the hindgut and cloaca at the end of the fifth week. The ureteric bud begins to penetrate the metanephric blastema. Note the urorectal septum, which will grow in caudal direction to divide the cloaca into the urogenital sinus and anorectal canal. (From Langman, J.: Medical embryology, ed. 2, Baltimore, 1969, The Williams and Wilkins Co.)

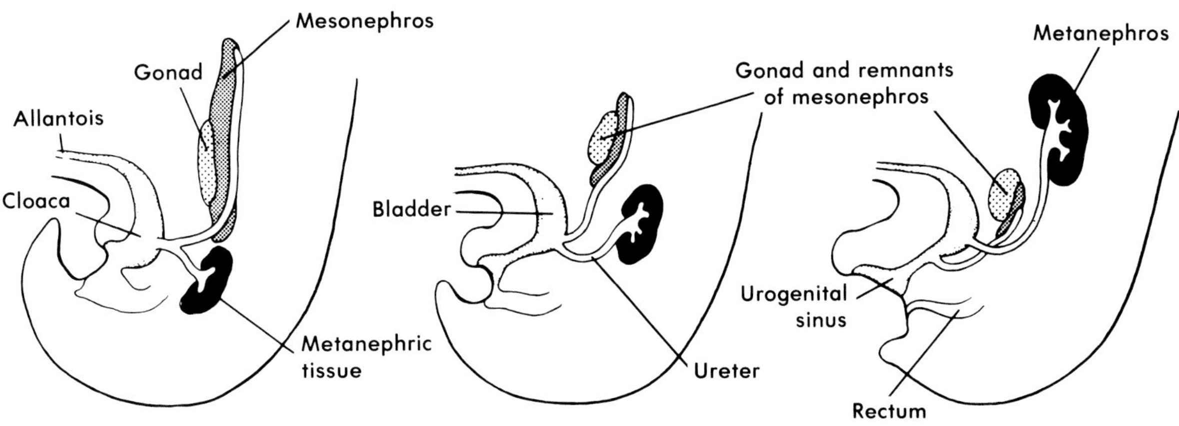

Fig. 32-13 Ascent of the kidney. Note the change in position between the metanephros and mesonephric system. The mesonephric system degenerates almost entirely, and only a few remnants persist in close contact with the gonad. In both the male and female embryo the gonad descends from its original level to a much lower position. (From Langman, J.: Medical embryology, ed. 2, Baltimore, 1969, The Williams and Wilkins Co.)

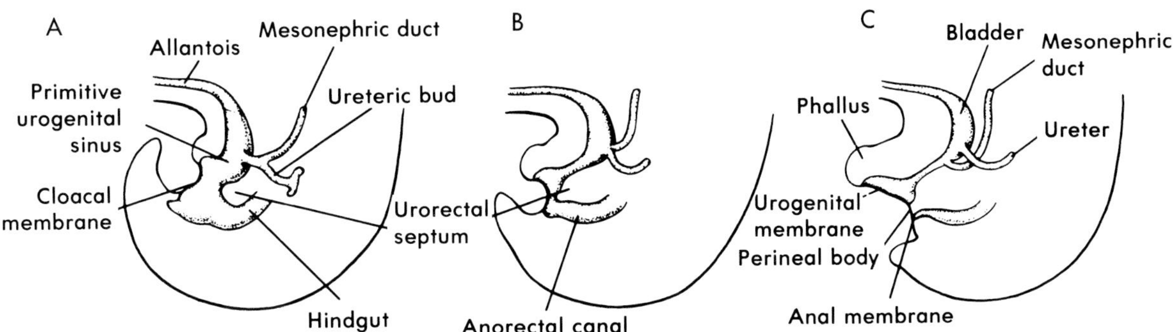

Fig. 32-14 Diagrams showing the division of the cloaca into the urogenital sinus and anorectal canal. Note that the mesonephric duct is gradually absorbed into the wall of the urogenital sinus and that the ureters enter separately. **A,** End of fifth week. **B,** 7 weeks; **C,** 8 weeks. (From Langman, J.: Medical embryology, ed. 2, Baltimore, 1969, The Williams and Wilkins Co.)

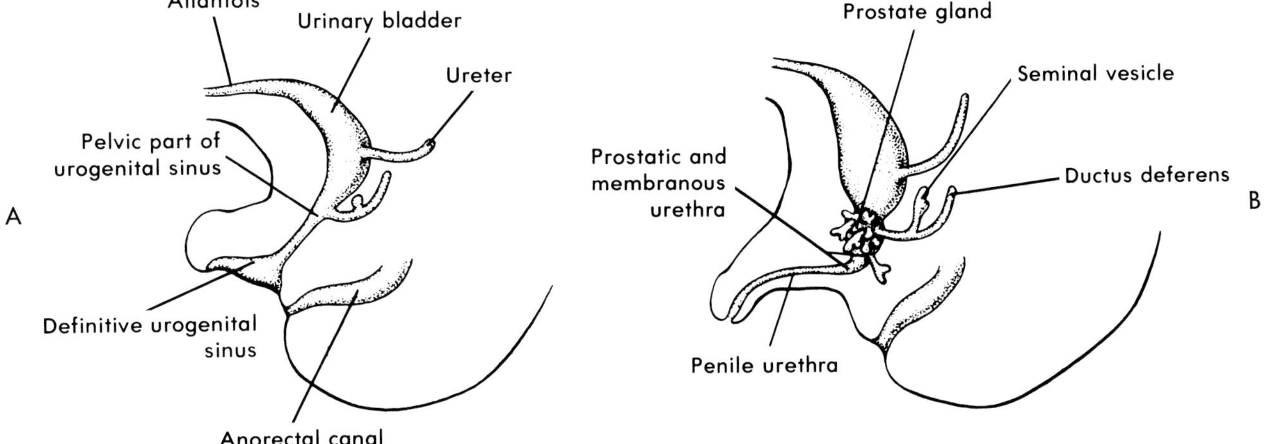

Fig. 32-15 **A,** Development of the urogenital sinus into the urinary bladder, the pelvic part of the urogenital sinus, and the definitive urogenital sinus. **B,** In the male, the urogenital sinus develops into the prostatic, membranous, and penile portions of the urethra. The prostate gland is formed by outbuddings of the urethra, whereas the seminal vesicles are formed by an outbudding of the ductus deferens. (From Langman, J.: Medical embryology, ed. 2, Baltimore, 1969, The Williams and Wilkins Co.)

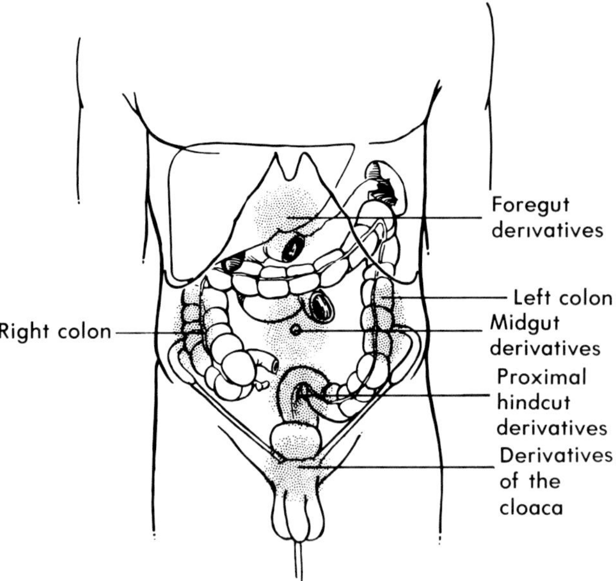

Fig. 32-16 Visceral pain from most parts of the gastrointestinal tract is felt in the midline at four levels that are related to the four embryologic divisions of the tract. The exception is visceral pain from the right or left side of the colon that may be felt in the right or left flank, respectively. (From Currie, D.J.: Abdominal pain, New York, 1979, Hemisphere Publishing Co.)

cal of disease originating from structures derived from the cloaca (Fig. 32-16).

PHYSIOLOGY OF PAIN MEDIATION[1,3,10]

Anatomic Pathways

For the sensation of abdominal pain to occur, receptors for pain known as nociceptors must be activated by some damaging stimulus. When this occurs, such nociceptive input is transmitted from the site of origin to the central nervous system through small, thinly myelinated or unmyelinated fibers termed the A-delta and C-neuronal fibers, respectively. The A-delta fibers are rapidly transmitting and give the sensation of a sharp, pricking, well-localized type of pain. These fibers, measuring 3 to 4 μm in diameter, are distributed principally to muscle and skin and are primarily involved with the transmission of somatic pain through spinal nerves. In contrast, the C-fibers are more slowly transmitting and give rise to the sensation of a dull, sickening, poorly localized type of pain that is more gradual in its onset and of longer duration. These fibers are located in the walls of hollow viscera and in the capsule of solid organs; they are also found in muscle, periosteum, and parietal peritoneum. These fibers are primarily involved in the transmission of visceral pain through autonomic nervous system. Much of the gastrointestinal tract is also innervated by branches of the vagus nerve. Despite the fact that 90% of these fibers are sensory, they do not appear to be involved with the mediation of pain, since the ability to feel pain arising from abdominal viscera is unaltered following vagotomy. Most of the afferent input from the vagus nerves appears to be concerned with modulation and regulation of gastrointestinal motility and secretion.

The neural pathways responsible for pain mediation differ, depending on whether the pain is derived from the abdominal wall or originates in the intraabdominal viscera. The anterior and lateral abdominal walls are supplied by nerves arising from spinal segments T7 through L1; the posterior abdominal wall by L2 through L5. Pain arising from the abdominal wall is transmitted to the spinal cord through the spinal nerves (Fig. 32-17). Because such pain fibers enter the spinal cord on the same side from which the focus of pain arises, it is perceived as originating on that side (i.e., right or left). Further, such pain is additionally localized to the area of the abdomen from which it originates (e.g., right upper abdomen vs. right lower abdomen). In contrast, pain arising from intraabdominal viscera is generally felt in the midline because sensory input from such viscera generally enters the spinal cord on both sides. As previously noted, the embryologic derivation of these viscera will determine whether this pain is perceived in the epigastrium, the periumbilical region, the hypogastrium, or the pelvis. The innervation of the gut depends on its embryologic origin. In general, the initial position of each structure (e.g., diaphragm, foregut) determines its segmental afferent innervation that remains with that structure even though its anatomic location may change during later development in utero. Afferent nerves innervate viscera as part of the plexus that is located around the arterial supply to that viscus. Thus foregut structures (including

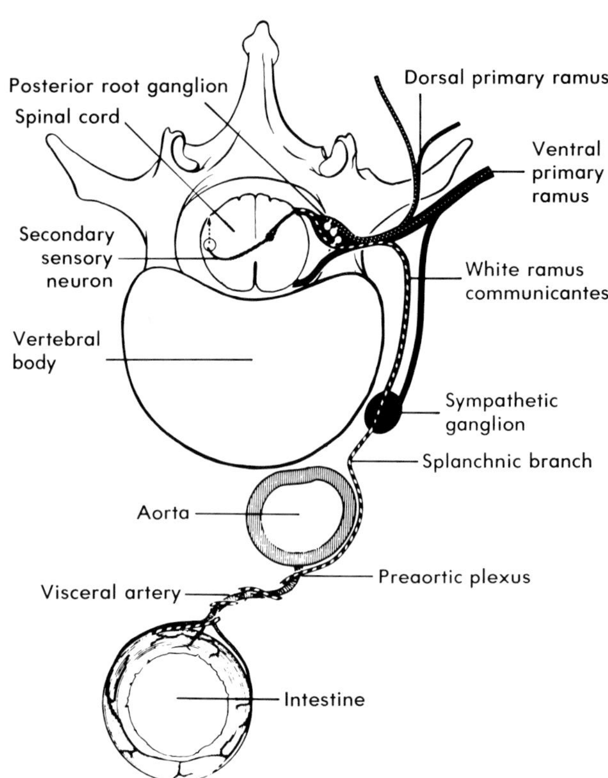

Fig. 32-17 Pathways of the peripheral processes of the cells of a typical posterior root ganglion. Some pass through the spinal nerve to the skin or other somatic structures with the dorsal or ventral primary rami. Others supply the viscera through the white rami communicantes, sympathetic ganglia and trunk, and preaortic plexus to reach a viscus such as the intestine by traveling with its artery. (From Currie, D.J.: Abdominal pain, New York, 1979, Hemisphere Publishing Co.)

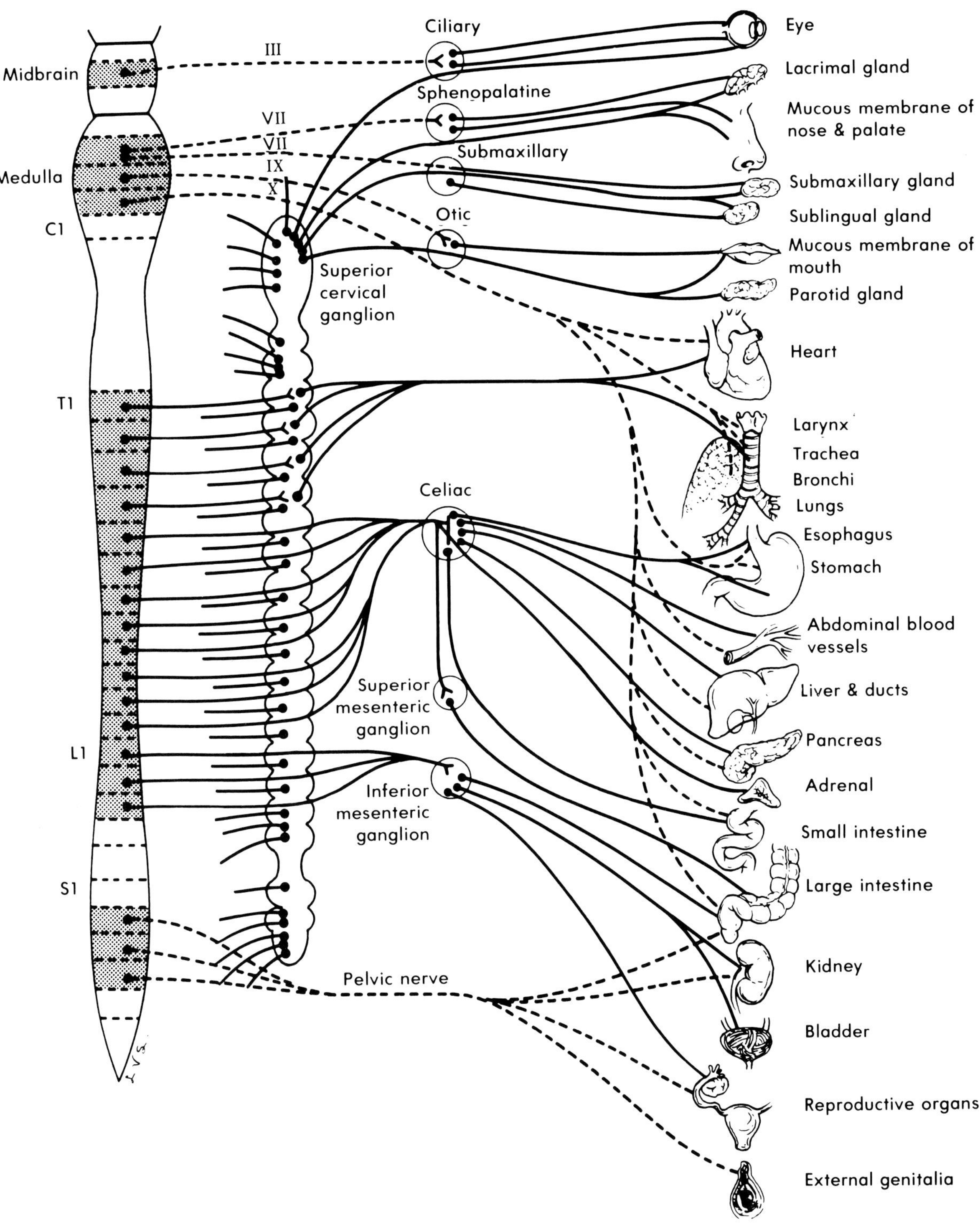

Fig. 32-18 Diagram of autonomic nervous system. The visceral afferent fibers mediating pain travel with the sympathetic nerves, except for those from the pelvic organs, which follow the parasympathetics of the pelvic nerve. Sympathetics are represented here by solid lines; parasympathetics by dashed lines. (From Way, L.W.: Abdominal pain and the acute abdomen. In Sleisenger, M.H., and Fordtran, J.S., editors: Gastrointestinal disease: pathophysiology, diagnosis, management, ed. 3, Philadelphia, 1983, W.B. Saunders Co.)

the spleen) derive their arterial supply from the celiac artery. Sensory innervation is derived from nerves originating from the celiac plexus. Pain sensation is mediated by the greater splanchnic nerves (T5 to T9 spinal cord level). The arterial supply to the midgut is the superior mesenteric artery and its branches. Afferent sensory input is from the lesser and least splanchnic nerves (T10 to T12 spinal levels). The pancreas is interesting, since it develops at the border of the foregut and midgut and derives arterial and afferent innervation from both the celiac and superior mesenteric arteries and plexus. The hindgut receives separate arterial and afferent supply proximally and distally. The proximal hindgut is supplied by the inferior mesenteric artery and the nerve fibers from the interior mesenteric plexus (T12 to L1 spinal cord levels). The distal hindgut receives its blood supply from the paired internal iliac arteries and its nerve branches, the lowest splanchnic nerve (T11 to L1 spinal segments), and the hypogastric plexus (S3 to S5 spinal segments). These nerve branches form the pelvic plexus, which arborizes distally with branches of the internal iliac artery (Fig. 32-18).

Sensory innervation of the genitourinary structures is also important to a proper understanding of the presentation of acute abdominal pain. The kidneys, ureter, vault of bladder, and gonads are supplied by visceral afferent nerves entering the spinal cord at T10 to L2. The sensory supply of the kidney, ureter, and gonads is from T10 to L1. The vault of the bladder derives its afferent nerve supply from T11 to L2 through the hypogastric plexus. The base of the bladder, ovary, uterine cervix and upper vagina are cloacal structues and receive their blood supply from the internal iliac arteries and their afferent nerve supply from the hypogastric and plevic plexuses. The rest of the uterus is supplied solely by the hypogastric plexus (T12 to L1) (Fig. 32-18).

Whether pain fibers are derived from visceral structures or the abdominal wall, they enter the spinal cord through the posterior nerve root (see Fig. 32-17). They then bifurcate and ascend or descend a distance of one to three spinal segments, forming part of what is termed the tract of Lissauer. The ganglion cells of these neurons have been separated histologically by Rexed[21] (on the basis of longitudinal arrangement of the neurons into columns and their underlying cytoarchitecture) into ten lamina designated by I to X. Rexed laminae I, II, and III represent those neurons that terminate in the marginal zone and substantia gelatinosa; laminae IV, V, and VI in the nucleus proprius; and laminae VII and VIII in the nucleus intermedius. The A-delta fibers from mechanoreceptors (tactile sensation) and heat nociceptors and the C-fibers from polymodal nociceptors synapse in the marginal zone, the substantia gelatinosa (laminae I, II, and III), and the laminae V with second-order neurons. These second-order neurons are either relay

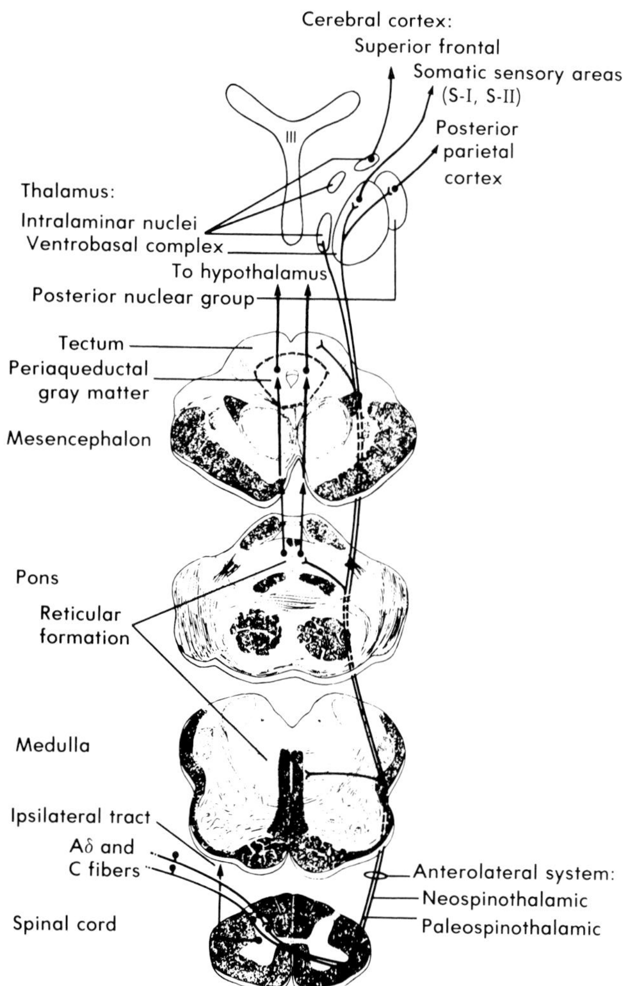

Fig. 32-19 The anterolateral system of spinothalamic, spinoreticular, and spinotectal fibers conveys information about pain to several regions of the brain stem and diencephalon. (Reprinted by permission of the publisher from Kandel, E.R., and Schwartz, J.H., editors: Principles of neuronal science, ed. 2, New York, Copyright 1985 by Elsevier Science Publishing Co.)

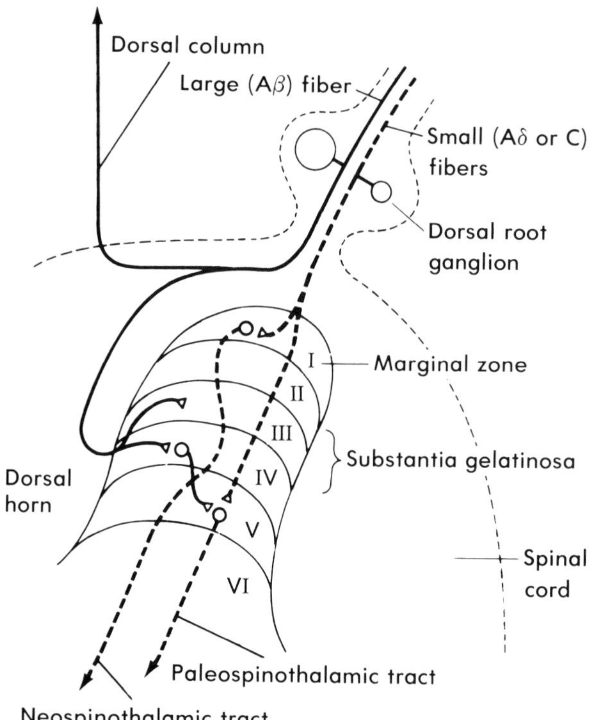

Fig. 32-20 Schematic drawing of dorsal horn of the spinal cord illustrating that nociceptive neurons, the axons of which form the ascending anterolateral system, are found in laminas I and V of the dorsal horn. Neurons in the marginal layer (lamina I) receive input primarily from small A and C fibers, but there is greater convergence of large- and small-fiber input on nociceptive neurons in lamina V. This difference is reflected in the electrophysiology of these cells. Many nociceptive neurons in the marginal layer do not respond to nonpainful touch stimuli, whereas those in the deeper layers display a wider dynamic range. (Reprinted by permission of the publisher from Kandel, E.R., and Schwartz, J.H., editors: Principles of neuronal science, ed. 2, New York, Copyright 1985 by Elsevier Science Publishing Co.)

cells that project axons that ultimately decussate in the anterolateral fasiculus to the brainstem and thalamus or interneurons that transmit pain information to other neurons or relay cells. The axons of the relay cells ascend in the anterolateral system, which is comprised of the neospinothalamic tract (i.e., lateral spinothalamic tract) and the paleospinothalamic tract. The neospinothalamic tract (a more recent phylogenetic development) contains the axons from Rexed Lamina I and project directly to the thalamus (Figs. 32-19 and 32-20).[1,10,21]

The neospinothalamic tract is an oligosynaptic pathway that has few synapses with long intersynaptic distances and is rapidly conducting, topographically located, and responsible for accurate spatial localization of the pain stimulus. The neospinothalamic pathway travels supraspinally in such a fashion that it maps somatotopically on the posteroventral nuclei of the thalamus and from there to the postcentral cortex. Smaller branches from these regions also pass to the retricular nuclei of the brainstem. The paleospinothalamic tract (or spinorecticulothalamic tract) is phylogenetically older, and its relay cells reside in the deeper layers of the dorsal horn, primarily Rexed lamina V. This pathway is medial to the neospinothalamic tract, is slowly conducting, and does not have somatotopic organization. Fibers within this tract travel in a supraspinal direction to the reticular activating system and to the intralaminar nuclei of the thalamus. From the thalamus there is a diffuse arborization to the limbic system, cerebral cortex, and basal ganglia. This anterolateral system of nerve tracts is primarily crossed, but it has a small and very significant component of uncrossed fibers as well (Fig. 32-21).*

The complex interactions of the afferent fibers just described can lead to the transmission of pain impulses or occasionally the inhibition of this transmission. Melzack and Wall[15] suggested a gate control theory to explain this interaction. This theory proposed that the thick fibers within the substantia gelatinosa may actually exert a negative feedback effect (inhibitory) on the transmission of the thin fibers. Thus, when excited, the thin fibers that ordinarily cause stimulation on the first transmission or "T" cells and the transmission of pain impulses, could at times have their effects overridden by the thick fibers as if these latter fibers were acting as a gate. Complicating this potential interaction is the additional influence of the higher centers of the brain, which also can exert their influence by changing the threshold to pain impulse transmission through a positive or negative feedback effect.[1,10,15] The gate theory was proposed before the current understanding of the presence of many neuroactive substances described below was known and is presently being debated as an acceptable explanation for the mediation of pain. Whether such a gate does in fact exist remains to be established.

*References 1, 2, 7, 10, 21, and 23.

Role of Neuroactive Agents in Mediating Pain

The classical pain pathways of nociception have been further complicated in complexity by the discovery of many neurogenic substances within the peripheral nervous system, spinal cord, and supraspinal nervous system that are now known to interact with neural impulses to both augment and inhibit transmission. Over the past 10 years, an increasing number of these substances has been identified in various animal species. A comprehensive discussion of these agents and the experimental evidence implicating their role in nociception are beyond the scope of this chapter. Only those agents thought to be important in the mediation of abdominal pain will be discussed. These include the endogenous opioid system, substance P, and the monoamines.

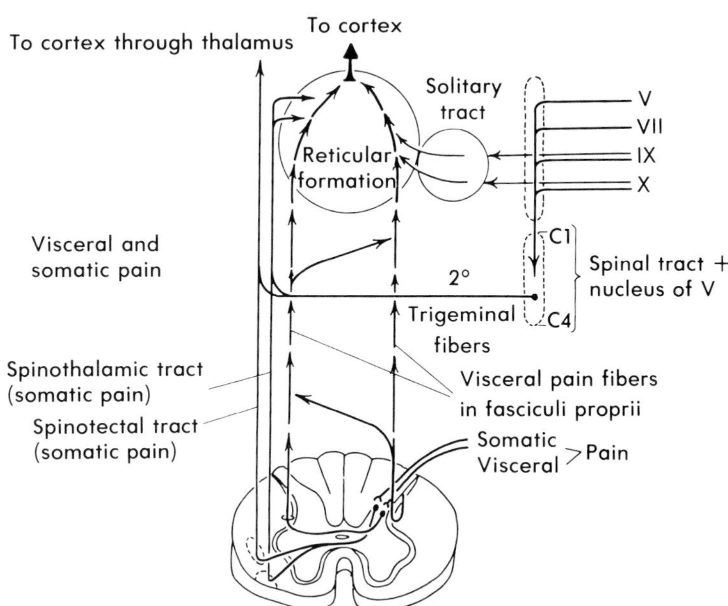

Fig. 32-21 Schematic representation of the transmission of visceral and somatic pain from its site of origin to the brain. (From Pansky, B., and Allen, D.J.: Review of neuroscience, New York, 1980, MacMillan Publishing Co.)

Three major families of endogenous opioids have been described, each being derived from a different precursor molecule that contains the classic enkephalin sequence (Tyr-Gly-Gly-Phe), which indicates that it is indeed an opioid peptide.[1,10,22] The first family is the beta-endorphin/corticotrophin family, which has propiomelanocortin as its precursor. This precursor contains one opioid peptide sequence from which the beta-endorphins, corticotrophins, and melanotropins are derived. The beta-endorphins are located primarily in the hypothalamus, have a limited axonal distribution, and are thought not to have activity in endogenous nociception. The second family is the enkephalin group, which is derived from the precursor molecule proenkephalin. Proenkephalin contains seven copies of the opioid sequence, six having a Met-enkephalin core and the other a Leu-enkephalin core (from which enkephalin is derived). The enkephalins are found in the spinal cord, amygdala, caudate, periductal grey, locus ceruleus, nucleus raphe magnus, and the thalamic periventricular nuclei of the brain. The third family is the dynorphin/neoendorphin family, derived from the precursor, prodynorphin. Prodynorphin has three opioid sequences that have a Leu-enkephalin core that gives rise to the dynorphins and neoendorphins. These substances are distributed within the spinal cord, amygdala, caudate, periaqueductal grey, locus ceruleus, and the magnocellular neurosecretory nuclei of the hypothalamus.

Experimental studies have found a variety of subtypes of the enkephalins and dynorphins. These subtypes possess differences in amino acid structure and sequence. In addition, they have been shown pharmacologically to have different states of enzymatic degradation. Thus, within each opioid family, different subtypes could be located in different areas of the nervous system that could conceivably modify neural transmission by speed and duration of action. The complexity of the opioid system is further demonstrated by the discovery of subtypes of the opioid receptors themselves. Such receptors have been classified as Mu, kappa, delta, and sigma. The mu receptor is the one most identified with opioid agonists and antagonists. However, the distribution of the receptors in the nervous system is not uniform. Kappa receptors are most prevalent in the spinal cord, whereas mu and delta receptors are most prevalent in the supraspinal nervous system. Mu receptors are more prevalent than the delta variety in those areas of the brain most involved with nociception (i.e., the thalamus, the raphe nuclei, and the periductal grey). Thus the distribution of the subclasses of receptor sites could influence nociception at any level of the nervous system concerned with this action. The pharmacologic manipulation of these various families of opioid peptides and the subclasses of receptor sites could have major implications in the treatment and manipulation of nociception in the future.[1,10,16,19]

Substance P comprises the next major group of neuroactive substances. Substance P has been shown to increase both vascular permeability and bronchial smooth muscle contraction and has been found in primary afferent nerves involved in nociception in animal studies.[9] Patients with familial dysautonomia, a disease in which severe diminished pain and temperature threshold sensitivity exists, have depleted levels of substance P in the substantia gelatinosa.[18] Further, the effects of substance P seem to be blocked by exogenous morphine.[8] Taken together, these findings suggest that substance P is involved in nociception.

The third major family of neuroactive substances is the monoamines. The monoamines exert their effects both in the spinal cord and supraspinally. The action of the level of the dorsal horns of the spinal cord seems to be inhibition of those neurons excited by the nociceptive pathway. This antinociceptive effect appears to be initiated supraspinally and mediated through descending pathways to the level of the dorsal root nuclei. Serotonin is one of these monoamine substances.[20] It is located in serotoninergic cell bodies in the raphe magnus that give rise to pathways that descend in the dorsolateral white matter to the dorsal root, where they terminate in the Rexed laminae and exert their inhibitory effects on those neurons esponsible for nociception. Norepinephrine has been found to modify nociception at the level of the dorsal root nuclei.[26] The other effect of the monoamines has been suggested by studies that have shown an inhibition of morphine analgesia by monoamine depletion through reserpine pretreatment, destruction of the raphe magnus, and interruption of the descending dorsolateral columns of the spinal cord. Thus the monoamines could influence nociception through several mechanisms.

The foregoing discussion emphasizes that the sensation of pain (abdominal or otherwise) is the expression of complex interactions between the anatomic divisions of the nervous system and the biologic interaction of various neurogenic agents at all levels of the spinal and supraspinal nervous system.

TYPES OF ABDOMINAL PAIN*

Visceral Pain (Figs. 32-17 and 32-18)

A previously noted, sensory receptors within the wall of the abdominal viscus and its derivatives are responsible for the type of pain referred to as visceral pain. The major forces that give rise to this type of pain are related to changes in geometry such as stretching or sudden distention as may occur in the wall of the gut, resulting in increased tension on the wall of the particular viscus affected. For those viscera that are hollow, these pain fibers are located within the muscular wall; in organs such as the liver, spleen, and kidneys, which are solid in consistency, the nerve endings of these pain fibers are located in their respective capsules and result in pain from stretching of the capsule as may occur from parenchymal swelling in a condition such as hepatitis.

Those factors thought to be directly responsible for the development of visceral pain include inflammation and ischemia. Inflammation, either chemically or bacterially induced, is thought to lower the pain threshold for a given stimulus and thereby sensitizes the nerve endings of pain fibers. The exact mechanism responsible for this remains unknown but may be related to the release of various vas-

*References 5, 6, 13, 14, 24, and 25.

oactive substances such as bradykinin, histamine, serotonin, and prostaglandins. Ischemia also causes visceral pain. Again the mechanism is not clear, but possible routes of mediation include the accumulation of acidic metabolic end products, the release of various vasoactive substances, and the lowering of the pain threshold to various other stimuli. Both spasm and overdistention of a hollow viscus presumably cause pain from the resultant decrease in normal blood flow to the muscle of the viscus wall. The ischemia then sets into motion the stimulation of nerve endings of pain fibers through the proposed mechanisms already noted. An example of spasm of a hollow viscus would be the ureter during attempted passage of a ureteral calculus. An example of overdistention of a hollow viscus is that which occurs during intestinal obstruction.

The mediation of visceral pain is transported from visceral structures through the autonomic nervous system. The major route is through sympathetic nerves, except for those of the middle and upper esophagus and pelvic organs, which follow parasympathetic pathways. The cell bodies for these afferent nerves are located in the dorsal routes of the spinal cord and the homologous cranial nerve ganglia. Further transmission of pain then occurs through the various pathways of the spinal cord already described, being ultimately received in the cerebral cortex. Such pain is perceived as being dull, aching, or cramping. Depending on the region of the gastrointestinal tract from which it arises, it is perceived in the abdominal midline in the epigastrium (foregut structures); periumbilical region (midgut structures); lower abdomen (hindgut structures), the latter also being referred to as the hypogastrium; or the pelvis (cloacal structures).

Visceral pain always indicates the earliest manifestation of intraabdominal disease but does not necessarily indicate that surgical intervention will be required for treatment. A patient often has visceral pain from the disordered motility secondary to food poisoning or a viral gastroenteritis, but usually the diagnosis is sufficiently obvious that any surgical considerations are clearly unwarranted. It is when visceral pain becomes supplanted by somatic pain, as is caused by other disease processes, that surgical intervention becomes a likely possibility.

Somatic Pain (Fig. 32-17)

Somatic pain (also referred to as parietal pain) is the type of pain that arises from irritation of the parietal peritoneum. It is mediated mainly by spinal nerve fibers that innervate the abdominal wall. Like those pain fibers mediating visceral pain through sympathetic pathways, these fibers also enter the spinal cord through the dorsal route ganglia and travel to the cerebral cortex for interpretation through the previously described pathways in the spinal cord. In contrast to visceral pain, which is perceived in one of three regions of the abdomen (i.e., epigastric, periumbilical, hypogastric), somatic pain is more localized and is perceived as arising from one of four quadrants of the abdominal wall, i.e., the right upper quadrant, right lower quadrant, left upper quadrant, or left lower quadrant. Thus, in determining the source of the pain, one must be familiar with those organs that normally reside in each of these quadrants. For example, the right lower quadrant includes the appendix, the cecum, the ascending colon, the distal ileum, and, in the case of a female, the right fallopian tube and ovary. In contrast to visceral pain where a change in geometry is responsible for the stimulation of nerve endings, somatic pain arises in response to acute changes in pH or temperature, as may occur in bacterial or chemical inflammation. In addition, somatic pain may arise in response to a sudden increase in pressure as may occur in an incision. Somatic pain is perceived as being sharp and pricking and is often constant.

Referred Pain

Referred pain is the phenomenon that occurs when pain is perceived in an area of the body other than the site of its origin. The pain usually arises in a deep structure; is superficial in its distant presenting location; and is often intense, sharp, and localized in the distant site. It occurs because of the existence of shared central pathways for afferent neurons arising from different sites. For example, visceral pain fibers synapsing in the spinal cord with pain fibers from the skin, may give rise to a painful sensation in the skin itself as though it originated there even though the source of the pain was actually from some visceral structure. An example of this would be a ruptured spleen that results in irritation of the left hemidiaphragm (supplied by cervical nerves 3, 4, and 5) being perceived as arising in the left shoulder, also supplied by the same nerve roots. Other common areas of referred pain that may present on the surface of the body are shown in Figs. 32-22 and 32-23. Being aware of such referred pain patterns can often

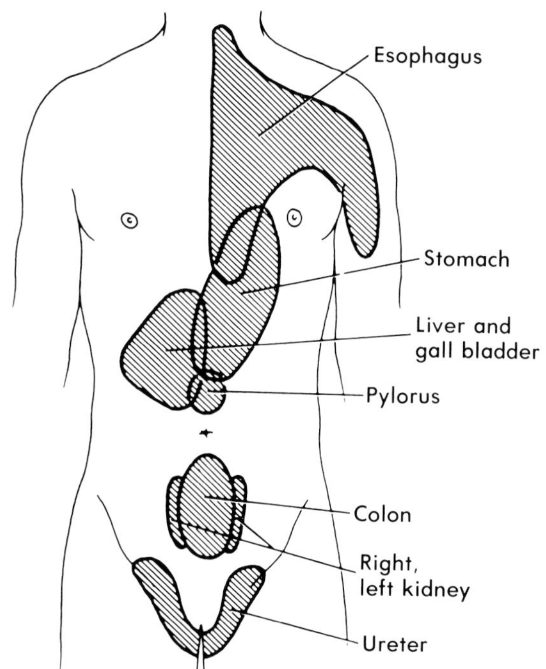

Fig. 32-22 Anterior areas of visceral referred pain. (From Cheung, L.Y., and Ballinger, W.F.: Manifestations and diagnosis of gastrointestinal diseases. In Hardy, J.D., editor: Hardy's textbook of surgery, Philadelphia, 1983, J.B. Lippincott Co.)

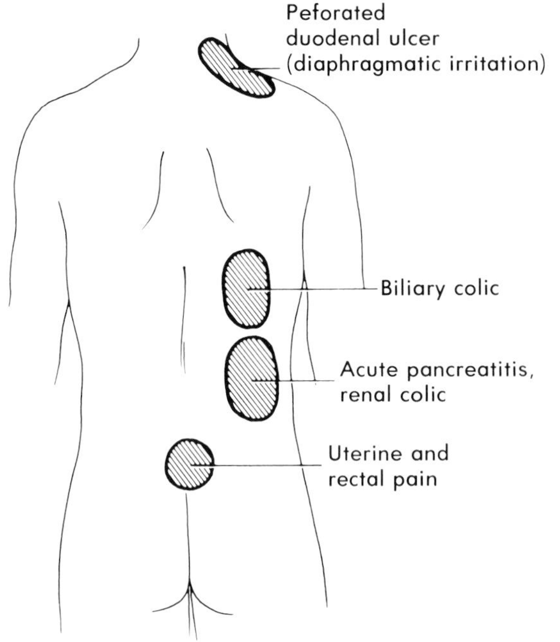

Fig. 32-23 Posterior areas of visceral referred pain. (From Cheung, L.Y., and Ballinger, W.F.: Manifestations and diagnosis of gastrointestinal diseases. In Hardy, J.D., editor: Hardy's textbook of surgery, Philadelphia, 1983, J.B. Lippincott Co.)

assist in the diagnosis of intraabdominal pathology when other evidence of disease is lacking.

EVALUATION OF THE PATIENT WITH ABDOMINAL PAIN*

In any patient who presents with the acute onset of abdominal pain, an orderly and systematic approach to diagnosis must be undertaken to determine whether surgical intervention is required. The more intense and severe the pain is, the more likely surgery is indicated. Usually a thoughtfully conducted history and physical examination in combination with appropriate laboratory studies provide the necessary information relevant to diagnosis and the assurance as to whether surgery is indicated. The types of disease processes that may be responsible for the onset of acute abdominal pain are summarized below.

History

A careful history is absolutely mandatory in determining the characteristics of the pain and the likelihood of a given diagnosis. The *character* and *onset* of the pain are particularly imortant in this regard. Colicky pain usually indicates some type of obstructive process and represents disordered motility. This type of pain is associated with

*References 5, 6, 11, 13, 14, and 24.

CLASSIFICATION OF CAUSES OF ABDOMINAL PAIN ACCORDING TO RATE OF DEVELOPMENT OF THE PAIN

Sudden Onset (Instantaneous)
Perforated ulcer
Rupture of abscess or hematoma
Rupture of esophagus
Ruptured ectopic pregnancy
Infarct of abdominal organ, heart, or lung
Spontaneous pneumothorax
Ruptured or dissecting aortic aneurysm

Rapid Onset (Minutes)
Peforated viscus
Strangulated viscus (strangulated obstruction, torsion)
High small intestinal obstruction
Pancreatitis
Acute cholecystitis; biliary colic
Mesenteric infarction
Ureteral or renal colic
Ectopic pregnancy
Pneumonitis
Peptic ulcer
Diverticulitis
Appendicitis (less commonly than gradual onset)

Gradual Onset (Hours)
Appendicitis
Strangulated hernia
Low mechanical small bowel obstruction
Cholecystitis
Pancreatitis
Duodenal ulcer
Gastritis
Gastric ulcer
Mesenteric lymphadenitis
Terminal ileitis (regional enteritis; Crohn's disease)
Meckel's diverticulitis
Sigmoid diverticulitis
Ulcerative colitis
Perforated tumor (usually of the colon or stomach)
Intraabdominal abscess
Ectopic pregnancy before rupture
Threatening abortion
Ureteral colic
Cystitis or pyelitis
Salpingitis (PID)
Prostatitis
Urinary retention
Mesenteric cyst
Small bowel tumor or infarct

From Way, L.W.: Abdominal pain and the acute abdomen. In Sleisenger, M.H., and Fordtran, J.S., editors: Gastrointestinal disease: pathophysiology, diagnosis, management, ed. 3, Philadelphia, 1983, W.B. Saunders Co.

intestinal obstruction, the passage of a ureteral calculus, and acute cholecystitis. It signifies hyperperistalsis of smooth muscle in its attempt to push fluid pass the obstruction. Between such colicky episodes, the pain greatly lessens or subsides entirely. The more intense the pain, the more noxious the stimulus of pain usually is. Thus, when a viscus has perforated or a major arterial vessel has become occluded, the pain may be excruciating in nature. Such pain is usually persistent and unrelenting. Similarly, pain associated with some infectious process (e.g., appendicitis, intraabdominal abscess) is also usually sustained and may even become more severe with time. Clues to the underlying cause of pain may also be indicated by the type of onset. Pancreatitis is often gradual and no uncommonly follows an alcoholic binge. In contrast, a perforated hollow viscus such as occurs with a peptic ulcer or a ruptured abdominal aortic aneurysm produces the sudden onset of pain that frequently is associated with the sensation of impending doom.

The *location* of pain is also helpful in establishing the underlying diagnosis. This is particularly true with somatic pain that is produced by irritation of the parietal peritoneum. An understanding of referred pain and the patterns by which a given intraabdominal disease process may express itself is frequently of great help in pinpointing the underlying cause. Thus unexplained back pain may actually represent disease in the pancreas or biliary tract. Of equal importance is the *duration* of pain. The longer the duration, the more likely a surgical problem exists. This is particularly true if the pain has existed for longer than 5 or 6 hours.

In addition to pain, associated factors that may give clues to its underlying cause include a history of previous intraabdominal disease. Thus the development of acute pain in the patient who has been taking H_2-receptor blockers for control of peptic ulcer disease suggests that it may be related to an aggravation of that process. Similarly a previous diagnosis of gallstones by ultrasonography or cholecystography indicates the possibility that the present pain problem may be associated with acute cholecystitis. Although vomiting suggests some obstructive process, it is also commonly encountered with other intraabdominal processes, making it a less specific diagnostic aid.

Physical Examination

The overall appearance of the patient often gives valuable clues concerning the severity of the intraabdominal process. The magnitude of the pain is often reflected in the facial expression as is the body habitus. A relative immobility or unwillingness to change postural positions suggests an underlying peritonitis. Similarly flexion of the hips with the knees drawn up to maintain comfort suggests tension on the abdominal wall and the presence of peritoneal irritation. Finally, any restriction of diaphragmatic excursion with respiration also suggests peritoneal irritation.

Actual examination of the abdomen will give more specific information. Any localized or generalized distention should be noted, since this may indicate peritonitis or the presence of intestinal obstruction. Similarly sites where hernias are likely to occur should be examined, since incarceration may be the cause of the pain. Particularly important in evaluating the abdomen is auscultation and careful palpation. In the presence of peritonitis, bowel sounds are routinely diminished and often absent. In contrast, hyperperistalsis with high-pitched bowel sounds suggests some type of intestinal obstruction. Palpation is especially helpful and will not only reveal areas of tenderness, but also the extent, if present, of muscle rigidity. Tenderness usually suggests peritoneal irritation, and the area where this is most maximal suggests the anatomic point of underlying disease. In eliciting the presence or absence of tenderness, it is important to emphasize that palpation should be gently performed and that the palpation should begin at that portion of the abdomen most removed from the point of suspected disease. Rigidity (also called guarding) represents a protective mechanism on the part of the abdominal musculature to limit peritoneal irritation from the underlying intraabdominal disease process. Its presence generally indicates underlying peritoneal irritation even though its absence does not exclude that possibility. In patients with a perforated abdominal viscus, rigidity is often diffuse, giving rise to what is known as a "board-like" abdomen. In this circumstance not only is the abdomen rigid in palpation throughout, but diffuse tenderness is also observed that is usually quite severe.

Rebound tenderness is another manifestation of peritoneal irritation and generally parallels the extent of tenderness. It is usually elicited by deeply palpating the tender area and then quickly releasing the examining hand. On release, sudden, immediate pain results. More gentle ways of demonstrating rebound tenderness include light percussion over the area in question and jarring the abdomen by either shaking the patient's bed or asking him to cough. With both of these latter maneuvers, the inflammatory focus within the abdomen irritates the adjacent parietal peritoneum and causes localized pain, thereby stimulating the rebound phenomenon.

In any patient who comes to the physician with acute abdominal pain, several other maneuvers are also appropriate to complete the examination. These include a rectal examination and also a pelvic examination in the case of a female patient. The pliability of the rectal walls allows careful examination of the entire lower pelvis through gentle palpation to determine the presence or absence of pain, masses, or unusual swellings that could represent a pelvic appendicitis. Similarly, a pelvic examination in the woman will not only further aid in obtaining such information, but is also helpful in determining the presence or absence of ovarian, fallopian tube, or uterine disease as a possible explanation for the abdominal pain.

Two special maneuvers that may prove helpful diagnostically are the *psoas sign* and the *obturator sign*. The psoas sign is elicited by stretching the peritoneum over the psoas muscle by extension of the thigh at the hip (Fig. 32-24). If an infection involving the psoas sheath exists, as may occur with a psoas abscess or a pelvic or retrocecal appendix, pain is elicited in this maneuver. The obturator sign is performed by internally rotating the thigh and

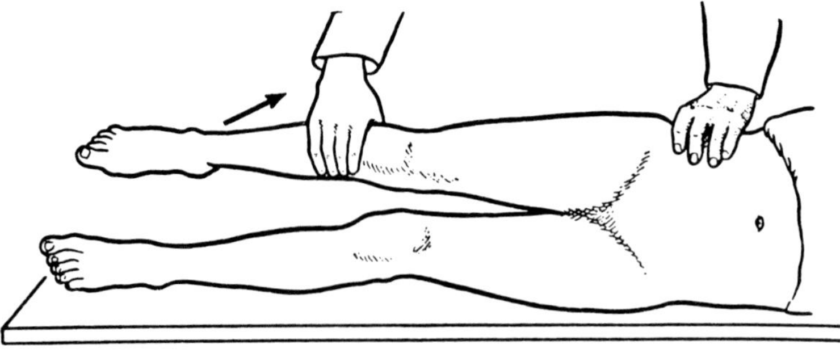

Fig. 32-24 Method of performing the iliopsoas test. (From Silen, W.: Cope's early diagnosis of the acute abdomen, ed. 15, New York, 1979, Oxford University Press.)

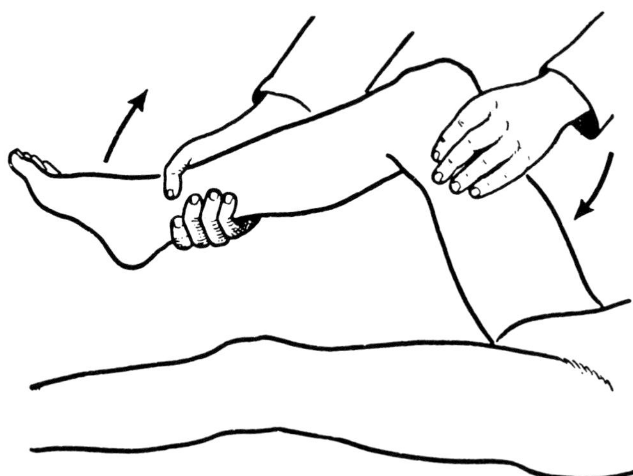

Fig. 32-25 Method of performing the obturator test. (From Silen, W.: Cope's early diagnosis of the acute abdomen, ed. 15, New York, 1979, Oxford University, Press.)

thereby stretching the obturator fascia, (Fig. 32-25). Again, if inflammation is present involving the obturator fascia, as may occur with appendicitis, pain will be elicited by this maneuver.

Occasionally the skin may be exquisitely sensitive to gentle touch in the dermatone corresponding to that innervated by the same nerve roots supplying an area of parietal peritoneum that is being irritated by an intraabdominal inflammatory process. Such hypersensitivity is termed *hyperesthesia*. Although not commonly present, hyperesthesia is also a clue to the underlying source of abdominal disease.

Laboratory Tests

In any patient developing acute abdominal pain, adequate evaluation should include a number of laboratory tests. A complete white blood cell count with differential is often helpful in determining whether a bacterial or viral infection is responsible for the underlying abdominal disease. The hematocrit is less helpful but may indicate evidence of anemia or hemoconcentration from accompanying dehydration. Urinalysis may demonstrate pyuria or hematuria, in which case a renal cause of abdominal pain is suggested. Occasionally an inflamed appendix overlying the ureter will reveal similar abnormalities. Liver function studies and amylase determinations in the serum will often assist in determining whether the underlying source of disease resides in the pancreas, liver, or biliary tree.

Radiologic studies may also be of help in defining the underlying diagnosis. An upright film of the abdomen, for example, may demonstrate free air under the diaphragm, indicating a perforated viscus or air/fluid levels suggestive of intestinal obstruction. Since pneumonia may masquerade as a cause of upper abdominal pain, the chest x-ray film is also helpful in excluding an underlying pneumonic process. In patients in whom the history and physical are suggstive of biliary tract or pancreatic disease, abdominal ultrasound is often of value. This may reveal the presence of acute cholecystitis (with or without gallstones), pancreatitis, a pseudocyst of the pancreas, or some other unsuspected inflammatory process. Similarly ultrasound may demonstrate an unsuspected abdominal aortic aneurysm. Although barium contrast studies are usually not indicated in the workup of patients with acute abdominal pain, occasionally such information will be helfpul, particularly if intestinal obstruction is present, in excluding a large bowel obstruction or defining more accurately the source of small bowel obstruction. Obviously, each patient needs to be individualized, and careful judgment rendered in the choice of tests ordered.

APPENDICITIS: PROTOTYPE OF ABDOMINAL PAIN[5,6,11,24]

Among the various intraabdominal pathologic processes that may be responsible for the acute development of abdominal pain, appendicitis is clearly the most common. For this reason, a discussion of its clinical presentation is appropriate and highlights in practical terms the pain patterns that occur when a particular intraabdominal organ is diseased and the accompanying physical findings that may be expected.

Appendicitis is basically an obstructive process in which the appendiceal lumen, usually at its opening into the cecum, is obstructed by a fecalith, mucous plug, tumor, or some foreign body. Because the epithelial surface distal to this obstruction continues to maintain its normal secretory processes, the accumulated intraluminal fluid that would ordinarily be discharged into the cecal lumen now results in appendiceal distention. The resultant stretch in the appendiceal wall triggers pain receptors that are carried by visceral afferent nerves to the spinal cord. Such painful information is then transported through the spinothalamic tracts of the spinal cord to the patient's cerebral cortex for interpretation. Because the appendix is a midgut structure, this visceral stimulation presents itself as a periumbilical pain, which is usually colicky in nature, coincident with attempts of the appendiceal musculature to overcome the obstructive process. Accompanying this development of periumbilical pain is a reflex ileus that is nearly always manifested by the feeling of anorexia and often is associated with nausea and vomiting. As the pathologic process within the appendiceal wall persists, invasion by microorganisms with secondary inflammation eventually results, with a gradual onset of a low-grade fever and an accompanying leukocytosis. At this point in the pathologic process, the obstruction may still be reversible, particularly if caused by a mucous plug or a small fecalith, which may be dislodged by the continuing muscular contractions of the appendix. If this circumstance does not supervene, however, the inflammation progresses further, resulting in edema of the appendiceal wall to involve the whole organ distal to the site of obstruction. When this occurs, the neighboring parietal peritoneum becomes irritated, and its stimulation leads to a change in the character of the pain, which now moves from the periumbilical region to become localized in the right lower quadrant. Accompanying this localization, the pain becomes much more pronounced and constant.

In addition to this sequence of events, important physical findings now become evident that are generally not present when only the visceral expression of pain is manifested. Thus the patient now has tenderness on palpation of the right lower quadrant with evidence of abdominal rigidity (guarding) and rebound tenderness, all manifestations of peritoneal irritation. In some patients, hyperesthesia may also be present. The point of maximum tenderness in appendicitis is usually at an anatomic location known as McBurney's point, a site two thirds of the distance from the umbilicus to the right anterior superior iliac spine. Usually by this point in the disease, nausea is much more pronounced, vomiting is frequently present, and clear evidence of fever and leukocytosis can generally be demonstrated. Bowel sounds are also diminished and may be absent entirely. Thus the derivation of the appendix as a midgut structure and its anatomic location in the right lower abdomen make the clinical presentation of this disease entirely consistent with what one would expect.

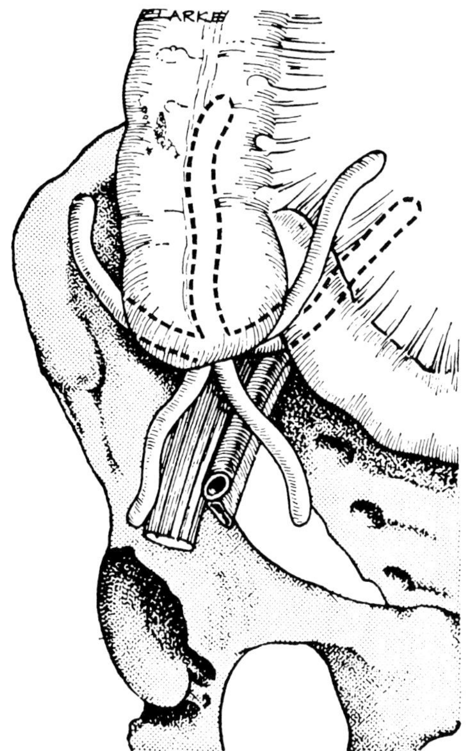

Fig. 32-26 Various possible positions of the appendix. (From Silen, W.: Cope's early diagnosis of the acute abdomen, ed. 15, New York, 1979, Oxford University Press.)

Although the clinical presentation described above is typical of the majority of cases of appendicitis, it cannot be emphasized too strongly that no evaluation of abdominal pain is complete without a rectal examination, and if the patient is a female a pelvic examination. Not only do these examinations help to rule out another cause for the abdominal pain that may simulate appendicitis such as a tubo-ovarian abscess from pelvic inflammatory disease; but occasionally the appendix, which is normally anteriorly displaced, resides in a retrocecal location or is located more posteriorly along the pelvic brim (Fig. 32-26). In either of these situations the physical manifestations of disease in the right lower quadrant may be less pronounced or not present at all, thus suggesting another cause for the abdominal pain. A rectal and pelvic examination may be especially helpful in this setting by revealing tenderness on palpation of the right rectal or vaginal walls. Other diagnostic maneuvers that may further secure the diagnosis include the demonstration of a positive psoas sign and/or obturator sign (see Figs. 32-24 and 32-25). Another complicating factor in the presentation of appendicitis is its occurrence during pregnancy. As the uterus increases in size from the developing fetus, the cecum and appendix move superiorly to the right upper quadrant. Thus the diagnosis of appendicitis must be entertained when a pregnant patient complains of right upper quadrant pain.[5]

The ultimate outcome of appendicitis, if left untreated, is perforation. This may take the form of a generalized peritonitis if the inflammation involving the appendix has not been contained by the surrounding omentum. If protection by the omentum has occurred, the peritonitis is usually greatly modified and may remain localized to the right lower quadrant or ultimately develop into an appendeceal abscess. The cause of the perforation is probably multifactoral in origin and includes the local pressure effects from the increasing intraluminal pressure, local tissue ischemia from the obstructing lesion (particularly if induced by a fecalith), and the build-up of acid metabolites from the resultant anaerobic metabolism and cellular death that results when the obstructed appendix impedes the venous and lymphatic drainage that ultimately supervenes from the increased intraluminal pressure. Under most circumstances perforation can be expected to occur within 36 to 48 hours following the onset of appendicitis. For this reason surgical intervention with appendectomy should be undertaken once the diagnosis has been made.

PAIN PATTERNS ARISING FROM INTRAABDOMINAL VISCERA[4,5,6,11,24]

This section will describe the common types of pain arising from intraabdominal disease and the pathways responsible for this pain. Tables 32-1 and 32-2 summarize the descriptions of pain and the sequential innervation for the various viscera involved.

Esophagus

Although the esophagus is primarily an intrathoracic organ, its distal portion resides within the abdomen so that an understanding of pain patterns arising from this organ is mandatory if the cause of acute abdominal pain is to be correctly diagnosed. Sensory afferent pain fibers from the esophagus are derived from the upper six thoracic segments of the spinal cord. Visceral pain is mostly a result of distention of the esophagus and is felt anteriorly from the suprasternal notch to the epigastrium. Somatic pain is usually caused by inflammation or neoplastic infiltration of the esophagus and radiates to the back. If the pain stimulus is severe, reflex spinal arcs are excited, leading to regional muscle contraction that can then result in restriction of inspiration, severe chest pain (resembling angina), tachypnea, and shortness of breath. Additional pain can be felt in the distribution of the cervical sympathetics (e.g., face, jaw, neck, arms). The usual esophageal pain is a deep thoracic pain at the level of the pathologic lesion. Thus a disease process developing in the upper esophagus generally produces pain in the neck, whereas disease in the lower esophagus is commonly felt in the region of the lower sternum or xiphoid process, but may also occur in the epigastrium.

Common presentations of esophageal pain are seen with *pyrosis,* spasm, structure, and spontaneous rupture. Pyrosis is a common disorder most frequently caused by regurgitated gastric contents. Acid with bile is a stronger stimulus for this pain than acid alone. Lower esophageal sphincter tone that normally prevents pyrosis is decreased by large meals, air swallowing, and physical exertion. Pyrosis is increased by bending forward, stooping, tight clothing, and in the obese. Dysphagia associated with pyrosis implies a concomitant stricture. Esophageal *spasm* is

Table 32-1 **SENSORY INNERVATION OF THE VISCERA**

	Viscera	Artery	Nerve Plexus	Primary Pain	Referred Pain
Heart	Heart	Coronaries	Cardiac	Central chest	Shoulder, arm, neck
Esophagus	Esophagus	From aorta	Esophageal	Central chest	Midline back
Foregut	Stomach, pancreas, liver, gallbladder, proximal duodenum	Celiac	Celiac	Midepigastrium	—
Midgut	Distal duodenum, jejunum, ileum, ascending and transverse colon	Superior mesenteric	Superior mesenteric	Umbilicus	—
Proximal hindgut	Descending and sigmoid colon	Inferior mesenteric	Inferior mesenteric	Hypogastrium	—
Gonads	Testis, ovary	Gonadal	Renal	Gonad	Umbilicus
Proximal urinary	Kidney, ureter	Renal	Renal	Costomuscular, loin	Groin, scrotum labia
Bladder, body of uterus	Bladder, body of uterus	Internal iliacs	Hypogastric	Hypogastrium	Groins
Cloaca	Rectum, upper anus, cervix, upper vagina, base of bladder, prostate	Internal iliacs	Pelvic	Midpelvis	Midsacrum

From Currie, D.J.: Abdominal pain, New York, 1979, Hemisphere Publishing Co.

a motility disorder that has symptoms of intermittent pain and dysphagia. This pain is increased by cold liquids, gastroesophageal reflux, and stress. The motility of the lower half of the esophagus has been shown to have increased tertiary contractions with abnormal (decreased) peristalsis. Severe pain is accompanied by diffuse muscle spasm and the distribution of pain described above. *Stricture* of the esophagus can be benign or malignant. The presentation and evolution of symptoms range from pain with swallowing to steady severe thoracic and back pain. The several presentations depend on the underlying disease process. Spontaneous *rupture* usually follows vomiting after a large meal or alcoholic binge. The patient presents with sudden severe thoracic pain, usually in the region of the xiphosternum (since most ruptures occur in the lower esophagus), and shock.

Occasionally the diagnosis of retrosternal pain, often indicative of esophageal disease, can be confused with myocardial ischemia (i.e., angina). Reflux esophagitis and hiatal hernia can both mimic the pain of myocardial ischemia. In distinguishing between these possibilities and a true cardiac origin of the pain, it should be remembered that reflux-induced pain from the esophagus is usually relieved by antacids and food, whereas myocardial pain is not.

Stomach and Duodenum

The afferent nerves to the stomach and duodenum that mediate pain arise from spinal cord segments T5 through T9 and travel through the greater splanchnic nerves and the celiac plexus. Visceral pain is felt in the midepigastrium, and this is by far the most common presentation. Somatic pain is also felt in the midepigastrium; but, if it arises from the stomach, it may also be experienced in the left upper quadrant. Somatic pain is usually secondary to spread of the inflammatory or neoplastic infiltrate process outside the serosa of the stomach or duodenum. Referred pain is quite rare.

The vagus nerves also are involved with sensory innervation to the stomach. However, any decrease in the pain of acid-peptic disease following vagotomy is not caused by an interruption of direct pain pathways but rather by a diminution in gastric acid secretion. Under normal conditions the gastric sensory afferents are not usually responsive to acid and bile, and pinching the normal gastric mucosa does not lead to pain. However, congestion and inflammation in the mucosa, as seen in ulcer disease or gastritis, can decrease the threshold to these noxious stimuli.

The most common conditions leading to gastric and duodenal pain are acid-peptic disease and its complications, gastritis, postgastrectomy syndromes, neoplasia, gastric volvulus, and a strangulated paraesohageal hiatal hernia. The peptic ulcer pain can arise from the stomach, duodenum, lower esophagus, or at the site of the previously fashioned gastrojejunostomy. This pain can be decreased by neutralizing gastric acid secretion. Severe disease will also involve pain arising from smooth muscle contraction of the surrounding viscus. Duodenal ulcers can cause burning or gnawing superficial pain. This pain characteristically has times of severity associated with increasing levels of acid bathing the ulcer. The pain increases 2 to 3 hours after meals and at bedtime. It is decreased by

Table 32-2 **SEGMENTAL INNERVATION OF WALLS OF BODY CAVITIES AND PREDOMINANT SENSORY INNERVATION OF VISCERA**

	Cervical 2 3 4 5 6 7 8	Thoracic 1 2 3 4 5 6 7 8 9 10 11 12	Lumbar 1 2 3 4 5	Sacral 1 2 3 4 5
PARIETES				
Central diaphragm	3 — 5			
Thoracic walls		1 — 12		
Anterior and lateral abdominal walls		5 —	1	
Posterior abdominal wall			1 — 4	
Pelvic walls				1 — 5
VISCERA				
Heart		1 — 6		
Esophagus		1 — 6		
Thoracic aorta		3 — 12		
Derivatives of foregut		5 — 9		
Testis, ovary		10–11		
Derivatives of midgut		10—	1	
Kidney, ureter		10—	1	
Vault of bladder		11 —	2	
Derivatives of proximal hindgut		12—	1	
Body of uterus		12—	1	
Abdominal aorta			1 — 4	
Derivatives of cloaca				3–4

From Currie, D.J.: Abdominal Pain. New York, 1979, Hemisphere Publishing Co.

food and antacids fairly promptly. The symptoms also seem to be worse in the fall and spring, for reasons not entirely defined. The pain of a penetrating duodenal ulcer is secondary to the posterior penetration of the ulcer and its surrounding inflammation. It presents as a constant, deep, dull aching back pain that may or may not occur with the more typical epigastric pain usually seen in duodenal ulcer disease.

Perforation of an ulcer (usually duodenal) presents with sudden, severe diffuse abdominal pain caused by the spread of chemical irritants throughout the peritoneal cavity. This pain is associated with guarding, often diffuse (giving rise to a boardlike abdomen) and rebound tenderness, both findings associated with peritonitis. In contrast, pain is not a hallmark of hemorrhage as the blood tends to buffer the ulcer. Gastritis can present with pain similar to peptic ulcer disease but is usually decreased less easily by antacids and is more steady in character. The pain of postgastrectomy syndromes is associated with the size of the gastric pouch, the presence of an afferent loop syndrome, dumping, alkaline reflux, gastritis, and obstruction. The mechanisms of pain are similar to those described above.

Liver

The liver capsule is sensitive to stretch and inflammation, in contrast to the parenchyma of the liver itself which is not sensitive to pain. The surrounding peritoneum can also respond to inflammation or growth of the liver. Pain arising from the right lobe of the liver and surrounding peritoneum travels by way of afferent nerves involving the sixth through twelfth thoracic segments, whereas those involving the left lobe are mediated through nerves reaching the sixth and seventh thoracic segments, in both cases reaching the spinal cord through the greater splanchnic nerves and the celiac ganglia. Afferent pain fibers from the surrounding peritoneum also travel by way of the phrenic nerves. Pain from an expanding liver capsule can often be felt as right upper quadrant pain that may be increased with breathing. Common disorders with these symptoms are hepatitis, congestive hepatomegaly, and an expanding hematoma.

Spleen

The parenchyma of the spleen, like the liver, is insensitive to pain. The splenic capsule, however, is sensitive to stretching, and the surrounding parietal peritoneum is sensitive to inflammation and blood. When present, visceral pain of the spleen is felt as a dull vague epigastric pain, but this is generally not common. Somatic pain of the surrounding peritoneum is common and is usually stimulated by blood from rupture of an injured spleen. The pain is commonly referred to the top of the left shoulder. Sudden sharp left upper quadrant pain can be caused by splenic rupture or splenic infarction. Splenic infarcts are not common but have two broad causes. The first is emboli which can emanate from the heart during myocardial infarction or atrial fibrillation, endocarditis, or aneurysm formation. The second broad category is hematologic. Etiologies in this group result in splenic arterial thromboses and are most commonly represented by sickle cell disease, leukemia and polycythemia vera. Massive splenomegaly can cause a dull aching left upper quadrant pain by traction on the peritoneal attachments of the spleen.

Gallbladder and Bile Ducts

The spectrum of gallstone disease can produce all of the types of pain previously described for the stomach, duodenum, liver, or spleen. The gallbladder and bile ducts arise from the foregut, and pain is transmitted to the spinal cord through the greater splanchnic nerves (T5-T9) and the celiac plexus. The pain sensaton mediated by the paired splanchnic nerves is interpreted by the brain as arising in the abdominal midline (epigastric region) and is called biliary colic. Uncomplicated biliary colic is not really a "colic" but a steady, dull, deep visceral pain arising in the upper epigastrium. This visceral presentation can be caused by distention of the gallbladder with stones, cystic duct obstruction, or distal obstruction of the common bile duct. Severe biliary colic can be associated with pain radiating to the back and pain on contraction of the lower intercostal muscles. The pain caused by intercostal contraction is felt as a tightness or constricting sensation and can mimic the pain orginating from myocardial ischemia.

Acute inflammation of the gallbladder changes the midline deep visceral pain of biliary colic to a more severe somatic pain involving the right upper quadrant. If the inflammation spreads to the serosa and involves the peritoneum, the parietal peritoneal irritation can cause pain referred to the inferior angle of the scapula; diaphragmatic irritation can cause pain referred to the right shoulder. In as many as 10% of patients presenting with acute cholecystitis, both a right upper and left upper quadrant pain may be present. One patient out of 25 will present with left upper quadrant pain only. As the inflammation progresses, the pain generally becomes localized to the right upper quadrant, and its severity relates to both somatic and visceral components. As the inflammation becomes further advanced, the upper abdominal and lower thoracic muscles become rigid and tender. This acute progressive inflammation can further progress to gangrene and perforation of the gallbladder, leading to the formation of a paracholecystic abscess or diffuse peritonitis.

Pancreas

Sensory innervation of the pancreas is similar to that of the gallbladder, with sensory afferent pain fibers arising from the greater splanchnic nerves (T5-T9) and the celiac plexus. Visceral pain and somatic pain present in the midepigastrium. Referred pain presents in the back at the level of the first lumber vertebra.

Visceral pancreatic pain is not common but can be classically demonstrated during pancreatic duct injection during retrograde endoscopic examination. This pain is constant, midline, and midepigastric. Abdominal pain is not present early in the course of the pancreatic cancer. Unfortunately, visceral pain tends to be mild to moderate, resulting in delayed diagnosis. Later in the disease process, visceral pain can evolve and is caused by pancreatic duct obstruction. The local spread of tumor can infiltrate surrounding perineural tissue, and the pain can spread.

Somatic pain is much more common with diseases of the pancreas and is produced in states of inflammation (e.g., acute pancreatitis). The sensory afferent fibers for somatic pain are carried in the first lumber nerve. This nerve does not have good localization to the anterior abdominal wall; for this reason the pain of acute pancreatitis commonly presents as back pain without signs of anterior wall peritoneal irritation (anterior abdominal wall muscle rigidity or tenderness). The back pain is referred and originates from stimulation of the posterior parietal peritoneum.

Small Intestine

The sensory innervation of the small intestine is that of the midgut and consists of visceral afferent fibers from T10 to L1 splanchnic nerves through the superior mesenteric ganglion. Visceral pain commonly emanates from mechanical obstruction and is located in the midline at the level of the umbilicus. Midgut somatic pain involves local parietal peritoneal stimulation. The pain is felt locally at the site of stimulation and is associated with surrounding muscle contraction or guarding. Common causes for midgut somatic pain are ischemia, inflammation, tumor infiltration, and traction on the mesentery. Referred pain from the midgut is quite rare.

Mechanical small bowel obstruction presents as crampy periumbilical pain with obstipation, abdominal distention, and nausea and vomiting. Distention of the bowel causes this visceral presentation of abdominal pain. The lower the level of obstruction, the greater the distention that will be seen. The higher the level of obstruction, the earlier nausea and vomiting will be seen. If the obstruction evolves into ischemic, gangrenous, or inflamed bowel, the components described for somatic small bowel pain come into play.

Intestinal ischemia can be acute or chronic. Acute intestinal ischemia can be caused by an arterial embolus or in situ thrombosis distal to a narrowed visceral artery. The pain produced is a sharp steady pain and is thought to be caused by acid-metabolite accumulation or anoxia in the ischemic tissue. Progression of the ischemia leads to edema and hemorrhage into the bowel wall that can become transmural, resulting in watery or bloody diarrhea. The presentation of sudden vascular occlusion of the small bowel is acute abdominal pain followed by watery or bloody diarrhea and shock. This syndrome is most commonly seen with occlusion of the superior mesenteric artery and only rarely with the celiac artery. Intestinal ischemia can occur as a result of mechanical small bowel obstruction and can have signs and symptoms of both processes.

Large Bowel and Rectum

Like the appendix, which has already been discussed, the proximal large bowel (including the cecum, ascending colon, and most of the transverse colon) is derived embryologically from the midgut and has a vascular and sensory supply similar to the other midgut structures. Visceral pain presents as periumbilical pain that can include the right side of the abdomen when distention of the cecum is such that traction on the mesentery occurs. Similar to the small bowel, somatic pain presents over sites of inflammation, obstruction, tumor infiltration, or ischemia; referred pain is rare.

The distal large bowel, from the splenic flexure (to include the distal transverse colon) to the distal sigmoid, develops from the hindgut. The vascular supply is from the inferior mesenteric artery, and the neural innervation is from nerve segments T12 to L1 and the inferior mesenteric plexus. Visceral pain is felt in the suprapubic area in the midline. Left-sided pain can be caused by traction of the mesentery by distention of the left colon, either lower left-sided pain from distention in the descending colon or in the upper left quadrant from distention of the splenic flexure. The sigmoid colon is attached to peritoneum proximally and distally so distention is felt in the midline as visceral pain above the pubis.

The pathologic entities most commonly affecting the distal colon are carcinoma, diverticular disease, colitis, and ischemia. These disease entities can present with simple visceral pain or complex variations of visceral and somatic pain. Carcinoma is usually and unfortunately insidious in its growth and becomes symptomatic only when it causes partial or complete obstruction. Symptoms can range from obstipation, diarrhea, or complete colonic obstruction. Diverticulosis is associated with a variety of complications, including bleeding, obstruction, and inflammation that may result in perforation or abscess formation. Mild obstruction will be perceived as visceral pain; in contrast, hemorrhage is painless unless it causes diarrhea and cramping. Inflammation and infection will localize somatic pain to the anatomic area involved, which is most commonly the left lower quadrant. Ischemia will cause symptoms as mentioned in the above section. Colitis and/or an irritable colon present generally with two regions of pain: the left lower quadrant and the hypogastric area. The pain is crampy in nature and associated with diarrhea.

The rectum develops from the cloaca and is thus quite different in its sensory and vascular supply from that of hindgut structures. The arterial supply is the internal iliac arteries, and the afferent sensory nerve supply is from the pelvic splanchnic nerves (S3 and S4) and the pelvic plexuses. Visceral and somatic rectal pain is appreciated centrally in the pelvis and can be referred to the midsacral region in the midline.

Abdominal Aorta and Iliac Arteries

Pain from these retroperitoneal structures is unusual. The sensory afferent visceral nerves that mediate pain arise from the lumbar nerves (L1 to L4), and somatic pain is perceived in the back at this level. Referred pain is unusual. Pathologic processes of the aorta and iliac arteries that cause painful symptoms are acute occlusion of these vessels and aneurysmal dilation and rupture. Acute occlusion presents with pain from the level of the occlusion distally that can be accompanied by pallor, pain, pulselessness, paresthesias, and paralysis of the extremities. Acute occlusion also presents with abdominal or back pain at the level of occlusion. Aneurysmal dilation can cause compression and erosion of the surrounding viscera, which would present as visceral or somatic pain of these structures. Erosion of the aneurysm into a viscus can lead to hemorrhage as well.

Female Pelvic Viscera

The sensory innervation of the uterus and the fallopian tubes originates between segments T12 and L1 of the spinal cord. These spinal roots send fibers to the lumbar sympathetic ganglia, periaortic plexus, and inferiorly to the hypogastric plexus and the bilateral plevic plexuses. The afferent nerves branch with the hypogastric artery to send branches to the fallopian tubes and uterus. Visceral pain localizes in the midline of the suprapubic area. Severe visceral pain from the uterus can radiate to the groins (L1) or, as in pregnancy, the inner thighs (L2). Somatic pain is felt in the localized anatomic area experiencing the peritoneal irritation. Ectopic pregnancy, salpingitis, and spontaneous incomplete abortions can cause severe somatic pelvic pain.

The sensory innervation of the cervix is from pelvic splanchnic nerves (i.e., spinal segments S3 and S4) and the pelvic plexus. Visceral pain is felt centrally in the pelvis as is somatic pain. Severe pain can radiate to the midsacral region in the midline. The sensory innervation of the ovaries is from the T10 and T11 spinal segments because of their embryologic development high in the posterior abdominal cavity. Visceral pain may be periumbilical, whereas direct somatic pain is felt locally at the area of pathology. Ovulation and its bleeding can cause severe abdominal pain, which is usually short-lived, and not lasting more than 24 hours. Torsion of the ovary and functional or neoplastic cysts of this organ can all present with acute abdominal pain.

Genitourinary System

The genitourinary system is made up of the kidneys, bladder, ureter, urethra, and in the male, the prostate and testes. Each anatomic division will be described separately.

The urinary bladder receives sensory afferent nerves from the thoracic and lumbar nerves (T11 to L2 to the vault), the hypogastric plexus (to the base), and the pudendal nerves. The urinary bladder develops from the cloaca and is supplied by the hypogastric artery. Visceral pain is felt in the hypogastrium and somatic pain in the suprapubic area. Referred pain is felt in the groins. Pain from the bladder is commonly from distention. Pain from such distention can emanate from several sources: the bladder itself, through its visceral and somatic afferent nerves; and through traction on the parietal peritoneum. Bladder pain is most commonly sensed in the suprapubic area, but also is felt in the back and the upper lumbar regions. Inflammatory processes involving the urinary bladder are common causes of abdominal pain.

The base of the bladder, prostate, and urethra receive sensory innervation from the pelvic splanchnic nerves (S3 and S4) and the pelvic plexuses. Visceral pain is felt in the central pelvis as is somatic pain. Referred pain is felt in the midsacral region of the back and the distal end of the urethra. Inflammation of the base of the bladder or urethra is a common cause of pain that is felt at the tip of the urethra on urination. Common associated findings with this pain are urgency, frequency, and dysuria.

The testes have a similar sensory innervation to that of the ovary, since both structures develop medial to the kidney and are supplied by thoracic splanchnic nerves T10 and T11 and the renal plexus. Visceral pain is felt in the groin and lower abdomen, and when severe, is associated with nausea, vomiting, and weakness. Somatic pain is also felt over the gonads, and referred pain is felt in the umbilical region.

The kidney, renal pelvis, and upper ureter are innervated by the thoracic, least and lumbar splanchnic nerves, and the renal plexus. Visceral pain is felt in the costomuscular region (angle between the twelfth rib and the lateral border of the erector spinae muscles). Somatic pain localizes over the site of irritation; referred pain is rare for these structures. The lower ureter receives the same sensory innervation as the aforementioned structures. Visceral pain caused by obstruction of the lower ureter can also be felt in the costomuscular region but is commonly perceived in the scrotum as well. Somatic pain is localized in the lower abdominal quadrant ipsilateral to the irritation. Pain may be referred to the groin, scrotum, or in the female the labia.

The most common pathologic causes of acute pain are urinary calculi, infections, or neoplasia. Slow, insidious obstruction may not cause discomfort, but rapid obstruction will cause severe renal colic. Renal colic is thought to be from distention of the ureter and renal pelvis and not from muscular contraction. This pain can last for considerable periods of time, often up to 6 hours. The pain is constant and will subside only with relief of the obstruction or following administration of some analgesic. When ureteral obstruction presents on the right side, the associated pain can be easily confused with acute cholecystitis or appendicitis.

SOURCES OF ABDOMINAL PAIN NOT ARISING FROM INTRAABDOMINAL PATHOLOGY

Although intraabdominal lesions are responsible for the development of the acute abdomen in most cases, the acute onset of abdominal pain may also arise from other sources. Any pneumonic process involving the pleura can present at times as abdominal pain. Usually this pain presents in the upper abdomen and is more commonly encountered when the lower lobes of the lung or lower thoracic cage is the site of pathology.[5] Diseases that may present in this fashion include pneumonia, pulmonary emboli, and pneumothoraces. Similarly, various cariac disorders occasionally present as abdominal pain, particularly in the region of the upper epigastrium or left upper quadrant. Examples include both acute and chronic pericarditis and myocardial ischemia, especially if the left ventricle is involved.

Although most intraabdominal lesions ultimately present

physical findings affecting various portions of the abdominal wall, it must not be forgotten that pathology within the abdominal wall itself may be responsible for the onset of acute abdominal pain. In this regard, the most common abdominal wall lesions found are hernias. Such hernias are generally painful and are usually easily demonstrable because of their associated mass effect and the fact that pain arises where hernias are usually located. Further, the pain of reducible hernias tends to be relieved when they are reduced, but incarcerated (nonreducible) and strangulated (incarcerated hernias in which the blood supply to the hernial contents is compromised) hernias produce constant symptoms. Because the contents of incarcerated and strangulated hernias involve intraperitoneal structures, they not infrequently present with symptoms referable to both the abdominal wall and intraabdominal pathology. Inguinal hernias cause symptoms in the groins, whereas epigastric hernias cause symptoms (often vague) of the upper midline. Periumbilical hernias cause symptoms around the umbilicus and spigelian hernias at the lateral border of the junction of the middle and lower thirds of the rectus muscle. The rectus muscle itself can also present with acute pain caused by intramuscular hemorrhage induced by anticoagulation or strenuous muscle effort. This condition often produces a painful mass in the lower left or right quadrants, depending on the size of the resulting hematoma.

An important part of the differential diagnosis of acute abdominal pain is any infection that involves the posterior root ganglia and nerves. The most common infections responsible for this are herpes zoster (reactivation of chicken pox virus) and syphillis. Herpes zoster can be caused by malnutrition, trauma, leukemia, neoplasia, and immunosuppression. The pain arises in the dermatomes (area of skin supplied with afferent nerve fibers by a single posterior spinal root) infected with the virus and often is excruciating. Tabes dorsalis denotes a condition in which there is degeneration of the posterior root ganglia and/or axons in the posterior columns of the spinal cord following infection with syphillis, usually 5 to 20 years earlier. This disease, although presently rare, can present with shooting abdominal pains at any level of the abdomen, usually associated with other neurologic deficits.

Although the aforementioned conditions are the more common nonintraabdominal sources responsible for abdominal pain, a wide variety of other lesions can also present as an acute abdomen, even though rare. Thus the astute physician must bear in mind the possibility of these lesions in the workup of any patient who develops the acute onset of abdominal pain. Among these various disorders are diabetic ketoacidosis, hyperparathyroidism, lead intoxication, hemachromatosis, acute porphyria, epilepsy, essential hyperlipemia, drug addiction, primary peritonitis, and any number of wide assortment of psychiatric disorders.

ACUTE ABDOMINAL PATHOLOGY AND CHEST PAIN

In addition to the abdominal pain presentations just enumerated, it must be emphasized that intraabdominal disease may on occasion present primarily as chest pain suggestive of a cardiac cause. This is particularly true of biliary colic, which can present with upper epigastric midline or chest pain. Associated pain in the right upper quadrant or referred pain to the right inferior angle of the scapula that occurs with gallbladder disease but not with ischemic heart disease will help differentiate these diagnoses. When biliary pain is limited to the chest or upper epigastrium, a careful evaluation must be made of the patient's cardiovascular system. Abscess formation or inflammation in the subphrenic spaces can also prsent with chest pain, although the pain in these situations (usually perceived in the right or left lateral chest) is more atypical than the usual pain presentation with cardiac ischemia.

Studies have shown that one in four patients admitted to the hospital with chest pain will have a problem referable to the gastrointestinal tract. Also, one patient in five evaluated for biliary tract disease will have myocardial pathology as the cause. Thus one must carefully consider the possible roots of sensory innervation to distinguish among those structures that could serve as the source for abdominal pain.

SUMMARY

The term "acute abdomen" is the designation used to denote the clinical condition characterized by the acute onset of abdominal pain, usually in association with other findings such as nausea and vomiting, anorexia, and abdominal distention. A wide variety of intraabdominal and extraabdominal pathologic lesions may be responsible for this condition, many of which have the potential of being life-threatening conditions. For this reason the underlying diagnosis must be promptly made, and appropriate treatment measures instituted. To accomplish this in the most judicious fashion, the treating physician must obtain an accurate data base and be able to extrapolate these data within a fund of knowledge encompassing the anatomy, the embryology, the neurophysiology, and the natural history of each potential cause. This data base derives from the initial history and physical examination, supported by various laboratory tests and radiologic studies. The differential diagnosis of the acute abdomen can be challenging, even to the most astute physician, but is ultimately successful when approached from this frame of reference.

REFERENCES

1. Adams, R.D., and Victor, M.: Principles of neurology, New York, 1985, McGraw-Hill Book Co.
2. Beal, J.M., and Raffensperger, J.G.: Diagnosis of acute abdominal disease, Philadelphia, 1979, Lea and Febiger.
3. Budd, K.: Pain, London, 1982, Update Publication.
4. Capps, J.A., and Coleman, G.H.: An experimental and clinical study of pain in the pleura, pericardium, and peritoneum, New York, 1932, MacMillan Publishing Co.
5. Currie, D.J.: Abdominal pain, New York, 1979, Hemisphere Publishing Corp.
6. de Domball, F.T.: Diagnosis of acute abdominal pain, New York, 1981, Churchill Livingstone.
7. Harrington-Kiff, J.G.: Pain, London, 1982, Update Publication.
8. Husobuchi, Y.: Elevated CSF level of substance P in arachanoiditis is reduced by systemic administration of morphine, Pain **1**(suppl):S257, 1981.
9. Jessell, T.M.: Fifty years of substance P, Nature **295:**551, 1982.
10. Kandel, E.R., and Schwartz, J.H.: Principles of neuroscience, Ed. 2, New York, 1985, Elsevier Science Publishing Co., Inc.

11. Kirkpatrick, J.R.: The acute abdomen—diagnosis and management, Baltimore, 1984, The Williams and Wilkins Co.
12. Langman, J.: Medical embryology, ed. 2, Baltimore, 1969, The Williams and Wilkins Co.
13. MacBride, C.M.: Signs and symtpoms, ed. 5, Philadelphia, 1970, J.B. Lippincott Co.
14. Mackenzie, J.: Symptoms and their interpretation, London, 1909, Shaw and Sons.
15. Melzack, R., and Wall, P.D.: Pain mechanisms, Science **150:**971, 1965.
16. Ninkovic, M., et al.: The distribution of multiple opiate receptors in bovine brain, Brain Res. **214:**163, 1981.
17. Patten, B.M.: Human embryology, ed. 2, New York, 1953, McGraw-Hill Book Co.
18. Pearson, J., Brandeis, L., and Cuello, A.C.: Depletion of substance P–containing axons in substantia gelatinosa of patients with diminished pain sensitivity, Nature **295:**61, 1982.
19. Rance, M.J.: Multiple opiate receptors—their occurrence and significance. In Bullingham, R.E.S., editor: Opiate analgesia—anesthesiology, vol I, London, 1983, W.B. Saunders Co.
20. Reddy, S.V.R., and Yatish, T.C.: Spinal noradrenergic terminal system mediates antinociception, Brain Res. **189:**391, 1980.
21. Rexed, B.: A cytotectonic atlas of the spinal cord in the cat, L. Comp. Neuro. **100:**297, 1954.
22. Rossier, J.: Opioid peptides have found their roots, Nature **298:**221, 1982.
23. Ruch, T.C.: The pathophysiology of pain. In Ruch, T.C., and Patton, H.D., editors: Physiology and biophysics: the brain and neural function, Philadelphia, 1979, W.B. Saunders Co.
24. Silen, W.: Cope's early diagnosis of the acute abdomen, ed. 15, New York, 1979, Oxford University Press.
25. Sinclair, D.C., Weddell, G., and Feindel, W.H.: Referred pain and associated phenomena, Brain **71:**184, 1948.
26. Svelt, W.H.: Neuropeptides and monoaminergic neurotransmitters: their relation to pain, J. Royal Soc. Med. **73:**482, 1980.

33 Physiology of Respiration

Christopher W. Bryan-Brown

The processes by which the body is able to supply tissues with oxygen and enough blood flow to remove carbon dioxide that has been produced during cellular metabolism are governed by feedback mechanisms relating supply to demand. The oxygen and carbon dioxide exchange at the cellular level is termed *"internal" respiration*. The gas exchange occurring between the cardiorespiratory system and the atmosphere is referred to as *"external" respiration*. How well the external respiration is able to respond to changes in cellular metabolism determines the constancy of the internal environment.

RELATIONSHIP BETWEEN INTERNAL AND EXTERNAL RESPIRATION

The coupling of internal and external respiration[51] gives rise to a series of phenomena that need to be taken into account in any consideration of human ventilation (i.e., the movement of air by the lungs into a position where an exchange of oxygen between air and blood and carbon dioxide between blood and air can occur). For example, when a tissue increases its metabolic activity, there is an increased oxygen consumption and carbon dioxide production. Local vasodilation will provide the tissue with a greater supply of oxygen and ability to remove carbon dioxide that has been produced. Total oxygen and carbon dioxide transport are then augmented by increases in both heart rate and stroke volume. The greater cardiac output leads to more efficient use of the pulmonary microvasculature for gas exchange and corresponding increases in both respiratory rate and tidal volume to maintain the body's acid/base status and oxygenation of the arterial blood (see boxed material at right).

Muscle metabolism provides a typical model demonstrating the coupling that exists between internal and external respiration. The high energy phosphate needed for muscle contraction is mostly derived in the mitochondria from the oxidation of either carbohydrates or fat through the tricarboxylic acid cycle. Decarboxylation of glucose generates carbon dioxide in almost equimolar proportion to oxygen use. If fat is the substrate, less carbon dioxide is generated for each mole of oxygen used. The relationship between the amount of carbon dioxide produced and oxygen consumed under a given set of metabolic conditions is described by the respiratory quotient (RQ). If the main source of energy is derived from carbohydrates, the RQ is 1, whereas use of fat results in an RQ of 0.7. Usually there is a mixture of substrates, and the RQ is about 0.8 to 0.9.

> **RESPONSE TO INCREASED INTERNAL RESPIRATION**
>
> **Circulation**
> Sympathetic tone ↑ resulting in
> - Cardiac output ↑
> - Blood flow redistribution
>   - *From* systems with low oxygen requirements (skin, resting muscle, splanchnic circulation)
>   - *To* systems with high oxygen requirements (brain, heart)
>
> Local vasodilation caused by
> - P_{CO_2} ↑ pH ↓
> - Metabolites (e.g., adenosine)
>
> Venous return ↑
>
> **Respiratory Drive**
> Chemoregulation by
> - Carotid body sensors (Pa_{O_2} ↓, Pa_{CO_2} ↑, pH ↓)
> - Central nervous system – medulla (pH ↓, Pa_{CO_2} ↑)
>
> Neuroregulation by respiratory centers: medulla and pons
> - Pulmonary reflexes
> - Other reflex control mechanisms (coughing, swallowing, vomiting)
> - Voluntary control mechanisms (speech, breath-holding)
> - ↑ neural traffic

Although muscle usually has enough food supply (glycogen) when exercise begins to support its contractile function, limited stores of oxygen and creatine phosphate, which regenerate adenosine triphosphate, soon need replacement. Local vasodilation takes place as the oxygen tension falls and is augmented by such factors as the buildup of hydrogen ion (H^+), potassium, and adenosine diphosphate from tissue catabolism, as well as an elevation of muscle temperature and neural activity resulting from the increased metabolic expenditure. The local increase in blood flow adds to an already rising cardiac output by increasing venous return. Oxygen availability to the active muscle is now greater, and more carbon dioxide elimination can take place. If the new work load is maintained and is moderate, a steady state is reached so that internal and external respiration are in equilibrium.

Glycolysis occurring in the cytoplasm is one of the main

pathways for supplying the tricarboxylic acid cycle with acetyl-coenzyme A. The process reduces nicotine adenine dinucleotide (NAD) as 1,3-diphosphoglycerate is produced. As long as there is enough oxygen present to provide for full mitochondrial function, a "shuttle" mechanism across the mitochondrial membrane reoxidizes the NAD in the cytoplasm. If the work load of the muscle is increased above the point at which the oxygen supply can meet this need, anaerobic oxidation of the cytoplasmic NAD by pyruvate is used as a supplemental pathway eventuating in the production of lactate. As this "anaerobic threshold" is exceeded, lactate builds up in the cells, the tissue is able to perform less work, and eventually an equilibrium is reached by a reduction in energy expenditure. Lactic acid production generates carbon dioxide on an almost equimolar basis through buffering of hydrogen ion by intracellular bicarbonate (HCO_3^-), which breaks down to carbon dioxide and water. Carbon dioxide then diffuses into the blood to be excreted in the alveoli of the lung. As lactate concentration increases, HCO_3^- concentration decreases within the cell. This should result in a reciprocal exchange of extracellular HCO_3^- for intracellular lactate across the cell membrane, dependent on the transfer rates of these two ions. When moderate work below the anaerobic threshold ceases, oxygen uptake within muscle cells begins to decrease over 5 minutes or so to the resting level. During this recovery time, the oxygen "debt" created at the beginning of exercise before the steady state was reached is paid back. If lactate was produced, the length of the recovery phase becomes dependent on the concentration of this substance generated during the work period.

Wasserman[51] has described three phases in the coupling of extrinsic to intrinsic respiration when a work load is placed on the body. Phase I is a period of up to 20 seconds from the beginning of exercise. The volume of ventilation each minute and the cardiac output are increased. In this initial phase the arteriovenous oxygen content difference is unchanged, so that gas exchange is increased without a change in the RQ. These findings appear to be a response to a sudden increase in pulmonary blood flow. If cardiac output were increased without a concomitant rise in metabolic rate, a steady state would be reached with a higher venous oxygen content, and equilibrium would be restored. Phase II begins when the RQ begins to fall, which is the first sign of increased oxygen use and carbon dioxide production in the tissues. There is a 25% to 35% lag in carbon dioxide kinetics, as compared to oxygen, because of its greater solubility in tissues. This buffering of carbon dioxide output is therefore seen as a transient depression in RQ, especially for work below the anaerobic threshold. Gas exchange increases until Phase III, when, provided the energy expenditure is below the anaerobic threshold, a steady state is reached. Tissue gas exchange is now equal to pulmonary gas exchange. This takes about 3 minutes for oxygen and 4 minutes for carbon dioxide in the normal individual. When the exercise stops, the RQ will rise above the resting level because carbon dioxide stores accumulated during Phase II are released at a faster rate than oxygen is being taken up to pay off the oxygen debt.

Some practical correlations arise from this transport system. The anaerobic threshold work rate is primarily controlled by the cardiovascular system, and lactic acidosis becomes more severe with each increment of work load above this level. The status of the circulation depends largely on myocardial performance and the adequacy of circulating blood volume. The capacity to meet the demands of an increased metabolic rate will therefore be less in untrained, nonathletic individuals, those with heart disease,[52] and in older adults.[24] Greater work loads can be sustained longer with increasing hemoglobin levels in the blood, even to above normal levels.[57] Conversely, anemia will limit maximum oxygen uptake in the lung. Further, a high inspired oxygen tension will increase blood oxygen content, and in a steady state cardiac output will decrease while oxygen transport remains constant.[35] Hypovolemia, particularly in association with a low red cell mass secondary to hemorrhage, leads to a very poor prognosis in the resuscitation of patients in circulatory shock.[43] When correction of blood volume and hemoglobin deficits are made, the prognosis improves dramatically.[22,41] If hypovolemia is present in a patient, it is probable that, during a time of increased metabolic demand, the peripheral circulatory response may not be able to meet tissue requirements because of the lack of an adequate circulating volume. This circumstance may not necessarily be obvious from traditional hemodynamic monitoring.[40] Another likely deficit caused by hypovolemia is the inability of the body to maximally use the pulmonary microcirculation for gas exchange. This lack of recruitment of the pulmonary circulation as cardiac output increases to compensate for the hypovolemia may be partly responsible for the elevated pulmonary vascular resistance seen with inadequate or late resuscitation. Hypovolemia not only appears to predispose the shock patient to acute respiratory failure,[42] but it also diminishes the likelihood of a favorable outcome.[13] In chronic obstructive lung disease, the recruitment of the pulmonary circulation with greater blood flow is also limited. Most available vessels are likely to be recruited before the needs of an extra metabolic load arise. This is seen as an absence of Phase I and a prolonged Phase II as described earlier.[31] This limitation adversely affects gas exchange in the lungs, preventing maximal oxygen uptake and thereby limiting the response to increased metabolic demands.

Finally, if the patient is not in a stable resting state, large variations in external respiration may occur, often without corresponding changes in the metabolic rate. Excitement, concern, or discomfort may increase the cardiac output out of proportion to the "resting" energy expenditure, causing a hemodynamic increase in pulmonary gas exchange. The intensive care unit is a place where interactions and artifacts frequently give rise to both real and apparently increased energy expenditures.[14,55]

The Control of Ventilation

Under normal physiologic conditions the demands of internal respiration are met by corresponding and appropriate changes in external respiration to ensure oxygen delivery to the body's tissues (see boxed material on p. 551). In tissues with increased metabolic requirements a redistribution of blood flow from less active tissues occurs that is brought about by changes in the sympathetic tone of arterioles with corresponding autoregulation. An overall increase in blood flow (cardiac output) ensues, and alveolar ventilation accordingly increases by the matching of the increased blood flow through the lungs to maintain arterial blood gases within the very narrow limits of normal. In healthy subjects, every liter of blood perfusing the lungs is most efficiently matched by 0.8 L of alveolar ventilation ($\dot{V}_A/\dot{Q}$ ratio). About 5% to 6% of alveolar ventilation is involved in gas exchange unless the oxygen saturation of the venous blood is reduced below normal, in which case a greater percentage of ventilation becomes involved in this process.

The control of breathing resides in the respiratory nuclei of the medulla of the brain. Respiratory drive is defined as the rate of respiratory motor neural discharge during the inspiratory phase of ventilation.[10] This drive is modulated by neurosensory mechanisms that are activated by changes in arterial blood gases, pulmonary stretch receptors, the tension and stretch of respiratory muscles, and the position of the costovertebral joints. In addition, the normal rhythmic discharge of the respiratory center can be overridden by higher centers in the brain to coordinate breathing with such activities as coughing, sneezing, swallowing, vomiting, and speech. The function of the respiratory center can also be modified by pharmacologic agents, physical respiratory restraints, and various disease states.

Chemoregulation

The chemical control of respiratory drive has both peripheral and central elements.[3,6,17] The major peripheral elements are to be found in the carotid bodies, which, although having a mass of only a few milligrams, possess the highest blood flow of any organ in the body (about 2000 ml/100 g of tissue per minute). Despite the very low arteriovenous difference in blood vessels supplying this organ, relative to its size the carotid body has a very high metabolic rate, and oxygen transport is far in excess of that needed for the maintenance of cellular function. Functionally this structure has evolved into a very responsive sensing organ, showing increasing activity with hypercarbia, low arterial pH, and hypoxia. Other receptors found in the ascending arch of the aorta also respond to hypoxia and hypercarbia but may be depressed by increased hydrogen ion concentration. The relative importance of these receptors in the control of breathing in humans is uncertain, but they may be of relevance following bilateral carotid endarterectomy.

The carotid body tissue is innervated by the carotid sinus branch of the glossopharyngeal nerve. There also is innervation from the sympathetic nervous system. Sympathetic and parasympathetic efferent nerve fibers synapse with ganglion cells within the carotid body that seem to be there for the control of blood flow through the carotid sinus tissue. This neural control could have an overriding effect on the sensory function of the organ. Since the effects of the three stimuli (i.e., increased carbon dioxide, decreased oxygen, and decreased pH) appear to be in some degree additive, a unified theory of action has been tentatively proposed; i.e., all stimuli result in an increased hydrogen ion (H^+), and this is the trigger mechanism for neural activity (see boxed material on p. 551).[32] The ventilatory response has been demonstrated to be almost linearly related to carbon dioxide tension.[39] This holds true for carbon dioxide tensions from 20 to 60 mm Hg. Ventilation also increases linearly over a hydrogen ion concentration range of 20 to 60 nEq/L (i.e., pH 7.22 to 7.7). The ventilatory response to hypoxia appears to follow hemoglobin saturation with oxygen. As the hemoglobin is desaturated, the drive for more ventilation increases. Thus hypoxia in terms of oxygen tension gives rise to a hyperbolic respiratory response. Ventilation starts increasing markedly below a Po_2 of 60 mm Hg.[53] Initial studies demonstrating this were very puzzling, particularly since the stimulus of hypoxia had no relation to hemoglobin concentration or oxygen content of arterial blood. Later studies have shown that there is a cytochrome A_3 found in the carotid body that has a very low affinity for oxygen, being about half saturated at a Po_2 of 100 mm Hg. A further decrease in respiratory drive by about 8% occurs when the oxygen tension has risen to 500 mm Hg. At this level there is no further decrease in ventilation, and the cytochrome is fully saturated.[26]

The central chemoreceptor mechanism lies in the ventral surface of the medulla, sensing changes in the carbon dioxide tension from corresponding changes in the H^+ concentration of the cerebrospinal fluid (CSF). Experimental evidence to support this has shown that CSF with varying H^+ concentrations and constant carbon dioxide tension results in a rise in ventilatory drive as the H^+ increases. Whether the H^+ is increased by elevating the carbon dioxide or reducing the HCO_3^-, the response is still the same.[15] This central chemoreceptor has a slower response time than the peripheral receptors and is to some extent governed by changes in the CSF production, local blood flow, and metabolic rate of surrounding tissues. In contrast to peripheral receptors, hypoxia is not a central respiratory stimulant. The absence of carotid body function as a result of neurologic damage or carotid endarterectomy diminishes the response to changes in arterial carbon dioxide only minimally. However, the same individual is unable to compensate for hypoxia, which, if severe, may produce a depressant effect on the central mechanism.

Although the central chemoreceptor area on the medulla is actually sensitive to H^+, it is effectively sensitive to changes in carbon dioxide. This is because the blood-brain barrier is relatively impermeable to H^+ and HCO_3^-. During metabolic acidosis there is a decrease in carbon dioxide tension brought about by the effect of H^+ excess on the peripheral and central chemoreceptors resulting from the induced hyperventilation. Since this condition is one of reduced bicarbonate, the reduction in carbon dioxide tension results in a partial restoration of a normal CSF pH. Thus the hyperventilation in response to metabolic acidosis is mainly mediated by the effect of H^+ on the peripheral chemoreceptor mechanism. In severe metabolic acidosis it may be dangerous to correct the base deficit with large doses of sodium bicarbonate.[37] The restoration of a more normal systemic hydrogen ion concentration with sodium bicarbonate results in the elevation of arterial carbon dioxide tension. Since the bicarbonate does not readily diffuse in and the hydrogen ion out of the CSF, the increased carbon dioxide tension can lead to a decrease in central nervous system pH sufficient to produce a life-threatening decrease in respiratory function.[37] The clinical relevance of this phenomenon is that in any circumstance but an acute base deficit, the correction of acid/base imbalance with sodium bicarbonate should be made in well-spaced, small increments so there is not an opportunity for sudden, sharp elevations in carbon dioxide tension.

Another phenomenon of clinical relevance may arise during mechanical hyperventilation, whether therapeutic or accidental. Passive hyperventilation reduces carbon dioxide tension, which in turn will result in a gradual reduction of CSF HCO_3^-. Experimental work has shown that bicarbonate production is reduced sufficiently to return the CSF pH almost to normal in 6 hours in the dog and in only a moderately longer time in humans. The effect of hypocarbia is to reduce cerebral blood flow and respiratory drive. Because it reduces cerebral blood flow, it is frequently used clinically in the management of increased intracranial pressure. When the partial pressure of carbon dioxide (Pco_2) is acutely reduced below 23 mm Hg, no further reduction in the cerebral blood flow takes place because metabolic acidosis appears to supervene. When such a patient is returned to spontaneous ventilation, the CSF pH will begin to fall below normal as the carbon dioxide tension rises because there is a reduced bicarbonate. This may result in increased cerebral blood flow. In the patient with marginal cerebral dynamics, the possibility of an unwanted increase in intracranial pressure arises. Following prolonged hyperventilation, if the patient has normal pulmonary function, the carbon dioxide tension will rise slowly because the restoration of CSF HCO_3^- is a gradual process and may take up to 24 hours.[8] This becomes a problem in the patient with chronic respiratory failure with an elevated Pco_2. During the treatment of the respiratory failure, if the patient is mechanically hyperventilated to a normal Pco_2 and the CSF HCO_3^- has returned to normal, attempts made to wean the patient from the ventilator result in increased respiratory drive. This can quickly exhaust the patient if there is inadequate pulmonary function to maintain a normal Pco_2. The consequence is that acute is added to chronic respiratory failure.

When a condition of chronic hypercarbia is being corrected by mechanical ventilation, acetazolamide has been suggested as an appropriate therapy to maintain the HCO_3^- of the CSF. By its inhibition of carbonic anhydrase, it reduces the rate of breakdown of carbonic acid. This may prevent the cerebral deficits from occurring in a patient who has chronic respiratory failure and is then ventilated to a normal carbon dioxide tension. Because of this central effect, acetazolamide sometimes is used as a mild respiratory stimulant.

Neuroregulation

Control of ventilation by the central nervous system resides in the medulla and pons. These respiratory centers are not discrete nuclei but are found in and in relation to the reticular formation. Traditionally the brainstem centers are described as being *medullary*, *apneustic* (found in the lower pons), and *pneumotaxic* (found in the upper pons).[3,32] The medullary center consists of loci containing inspiratory neurons and other loci containing expiratory neurons. The interaction of these neurons through negative feedback loops gives rise to rhythmicity of breathing. As neural traffic increases through the brainstem, the activity of this respiratory center increases as an apparently nonspecific response. The *apneustic* center has been found by experimental brain section in animals. When the section is made midpons, the animal takes on a gasping type of respiration, which is sometimes seen following a pontine hemorrhage in humans. The *pneumotaxic* center overrides the respiratory rate and inhibits inspiratory activity when the lungs are inflated. The inspiratory output of these respiratory centers is referred to as the respiratory drive. The input that modulates the activity of the respiratory centers comes from the chemoreceptors already described, various other receptors in the lung and other organs, and from various centers within other parts of the brain. The limbic system controls the respiratory changes produced by emotion. The cerebral cortex controls the changes in ventilation required for such functions as voluntary breath-holding, speech, and pulmonary function testing. Other portions of the brain will override the normal respiratory pattern for such actions as swallowing, vomiting, coughing, and sneezing.

In addition to the chemoreceptor mechanism that has already been described, within the lung itself there are stretch receptors that are the sensory arm of the Hering-Breuer reflex, which is thought to control the magnitude of inspiratory volume and initiate the process of expiration. This reflex was originally described in the cat, where it is transmitted through the vagus nerve. As the lungs are stretched, expiratory drive increases. If the vagi of the cat are sectioned, apnea occurs. This reflex is not thought to play an active part in the control of ventilation in adult humans during normal tidal breathing, but it may be important in states of ventilatory dysfunction. In human beings, position sense from the costovertebral joints and stretch receptors within the intercostal muscles and diaphragm plays a far greater role in determining expiratory drive than the Hering-Breuer reflex. These receptors are also responsible for much of the feeling of dyspnea that occurs when a subject is trying to breathe past a respiratory obstruction. In addition, there are receptors within the lung that react to chemical irritants, dust, and the inspiration of cold gas. The reflexes triggered by these receptors include an increase in ventilatory rate, bronchoconstriction, and bronchorrhea. A specialized receptor, called the J receptor, appears to control the distribution of the pulmonary circulation and possibly bronchial tone in relation to hypoxia and hypercarbia. The J receptor also seems sensitive to changes in the interstitial fluid volume of the lung and may be responsible in part for the dyspnea seen in congestive cardiac failure and other pulmonary interstitial conditions. In the carotid sinuses and the aorta, pressure receptors are present that reflexly cause hypoventilation as the blood pressure rises and hyperventilation when it falls below normal levels.

Oxygen Delivery to Tissues

The delivery of oxygen to tissues from blood and the uptake of carbon dioxide by the blood from tissues occur through a process of diffusion that is governed by the gas tension gradients that exist between cells of a given tissue and the erythrocytes within circulating blood. To understand this relationship, it must be remembered that most of the oxygen in blood (i.e., 98%) is in chemical equilibrium with hemoglobin, to which it is loosely and reversibly bound. Because of the nature of this oxyhemoglobin binding as described by the oxyhemoglobin dissociation curve (Fig. 33-1), hemoglobin remains relatively saturated until the oxygen tension decreases below 50 mm Hg. At this point large amounts of oxygen dissociate from hemoglobin for a relatively small decrement in oxygen tension, so the gradient between blood and tissue falls slowly, enhancing oxygen delivery. Carbon dioxide entering the blood from tissues further enhances this delivery. As the carbon dioxide diffuses into the red cells, it is converted to carbonic acid by carbonic anhydrase, which does not normally exist in significant amounts in the plasma. The effect of the hydrogen ion created is to shift the oxyhemoglobin dissociation curve to the right, which allows more oxygen to be released without a corresponding fall in oxygen tension. The carbon dioxide also combines with hemoglobin to form carbamino compounds, which shifts the curve further to the right. The bicarbonate produced from the breakdown of carbonic acid in the red cell diffuses out, to be balanced by chloride diffusing in, thereby maintaining the Gibbs-Donnan relationship. The chloride makes a minor shift of

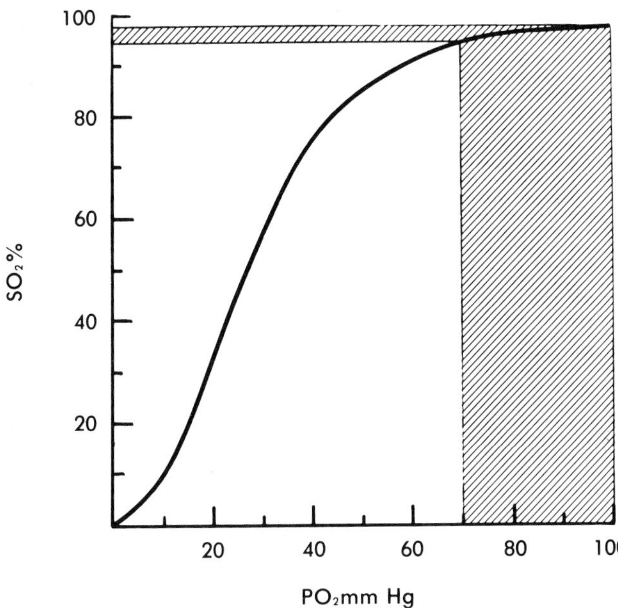

Fig. 33-1 Standard oxyhemoglobin dissociation curve showing the reduction of 3% in saturation (SO_2) when the oxygen tension (PO_2) drops from normal to 70 mm Hg. Since further reductions in PO_2 will produce proportionally greater desaturation of hemoglobin, at least 70 mm Hg is regarded as desirable in critically ill patients.

the oxyhemoglobin dissociation curve to the right to release more oxygen. Deoxyhemoglobin has a greater affinity for carbon dioxide than oxyhemoglobin and is a weaker acid; thus it acts as a further carbon dioxide and hydrogen ion sink, such that, if the RQ is 0.7, there is no difference in pH between arterial and venous blood. These processes are reversed in the lung where the high oxygen tension aids in the release of carbon dioxide, which, in turn, increases the affinity of hemoglobin for oxygen.

Clinical Correlation

The brainstem respiratory centers are exquisitely sensitive to even small doses of morphine,[54] and, although the respiratory depression caused by narcotic analgesics is of great concern when dealing with the surgical patient, many other drugs and combinations of drugs act on both the chemoreceptor system and the central respiratory regulatory system. The major effect of opiates is to reduce the respiratory drive in response to carbon dioxide and to some degree that which results from hypoxia.[18] Recently it has been shown that halothane reduces the sensitivity of the peripheral chemoregulatory reflex pathways to hypoxia.[25] Thus, through the administration of drugs used during anesthesia and the postoperative period, it is quite possible to remove protective reflexes that normally maintain ventilation.[23] The normal response of a subject to overcome respiratory obstruction or additional inspirations and expiratory resistance is to increase respiratory drive. If the effector system (i.e., the respiratory muscles) can respond, there will be a maintenance of alveolar ventilation.[33] The increase in respiratory drive as a result of an incremental increase in carbon dioxide tension under most circumstances will remain approximately the same. Therefore, if an extrinsic resistance puts a greater work load on a ventilatory system that is already unable to respond because of disease, the carbon dioxide level will tend to remain at an increased tension and will be further exacerbated if there is respiratory obstruction. If the carbon dioxide tension remains high as a result of this respiratory failure, CSF bicarbonate will increase, and respiratory drive will tend to decrease so that the subject remains comfortable at this higher level. If the respiratory center is then depressed pharmacologically, the subject will be able to tolerate higher and higher carbon dioxide tensions and may eventually succumb to hypoventilation.[7]

Because the ventilatory drive under a given set of circumstances tends to be similar for any stimulus, marginal patients often show great improvement in ventilation after such maneuvers as administering a bronchodilator, removing an endotracheal tube (which is often a covert form of respiratory obstruction), or discontinuing respiratory support being given through mechanical ventilators having an inspiratory valve with excessive resistance. Anything that makes it physically easier for the patient to breathe will tend to increase the efficiency of his respiratory drive. These considerations are of particular concern in the surgical patient in the immediate postoperative period when the residual effects of muscle relaxants and anesthetic agents may adversely affect ventilation that is already compromised to some degree by the restrictive effects of a thoracoabdominal operation. Thus the initial doses of analgesic drugs to limit pain need to be administered carefully, and their potentially negative effect on respiration closely observed. In patients who have concomitant respiratory disease, this exhortation is even more important.

PULMONARY FUNCTION AND ITS ASSESSMENT

A diminution in pulmonary function is one of the plaguing problems encountered in patients after thoracic and upper abdominal operations. Thus both surgeons and anesthesiologists should have a working knowledge of pulmonary assessment, so that those individuals who will need extra attention and the provision of respiratory therapy following surgery can be detected before serious pulmonary dysfunction supervenes. It has been long known, for example, that patients may have a vital capacity reduced to 20% of normal by an operation like cholecystectomy.[9,12,27] This is approximately the minimum volume that is required to produce a properly expulsive cough. Without an effective coughing mechanism, secretions within the trachea and upper airways cannot be adequately cleared. In a patient already compromised by restrictive pulmonary disease, it is imperative to provide some means of ensuring proper expectoration. This may take the form of exercises to improve vital capacity and/or regional analgesic techniques for the amelioration of the immediate postoperative pain, since much of the reduced ventilatory function following surgery appears to be pain related.

The simplest way to assess pulmonary function following surgery in order to prevent postoperative problems is to acquire an estimate of exercise tolerance. Limitation of normal activity caused by breathlessness may be secondary to both pulmonary and cardiac disease, and in patients with this problem both causes must be evaluated. Assuming that a cardiac cause has been excluded, the lungs can basically fail in one of two ways: there may be either a failure of ventilation, in which case alveolar gas exchange with the atmosphere is limited; or there may be parenchymal disease of the lung, which limits gas exchange between the alveolus and the pulmonary microvascular circulation. As a generalization, inadequate ventilation is represented by a higher than normal arterial PCO_2, and parenchymal lung disease by a decreased PO_2. Sometimes exercise is required to demonstrate the deficiency in gas exchange. An outline of pulmonary assessment appears in the discussion that follows; for a more detailed consideration of pulmonary dysfunction and pulmonary function testing is contained in references 11, 30, 50, and 56.

Blood Gases

Arterial blood gases are used as primary assessment for pulmonary function. Respiratory failure is frequently defined in terms of elevated carbon dioxide and depressed oxygen tension. Carbon dioxide is carried in the blood in physical solution, as bicarbonate and by forming carbamino compounds with proteins (particularly hemoglobin). Although there may be variations in content related to acid/base balance and changes in the hemoglobin affinity for carbon dioxide as a result of saturation with oxygen, the relationship of carbon dioxide tension to content can be considered roughly linear in the normal range of clinical practice.

Carbon dioxide tension in the arterial blood ($PaCO_2$) is normally around 40 mm Hg at sea level. A normal resting adult produces approximately 200 ml of carbon dioxide per minute from cellular metabolism. The alveolar ventilation is about 3.5 L/min. The resulting dilution of carbon dioxide with fresh alveolar gas produces a 5.7% mixture that, with the water-saturated conditions of the alveolus, is approximately 40 mm Hg. If the alveolar ventilation is halved, the amount of carbon dioxide removed will be reduced until the alveolar concentration has doubled. In normal humans this process has a time constant of approximately 20 minutes because a buildup of carbon dioxide in the body stores has to occur before the tension will rise in the circulation. If, on the other hand, ventilation is doubled, the washout of the alveoli occurs within a few minutes; and, although full equilibrium will not be achieved until body stores of carbon dioxide have been reduced, a time constant of less than 5 minutes is usual, and $PaCO_2$ is within the clinical range of accuracy of the final measurement in less than 10 minutes.[32] For steady-state conditions, the $PaCO_2$ may be considered inversely proportional to the alveolar ventilation. This is particularly useful in assessing the ventilatory needs of a patient on mechanical support. Since the ratio of dead space ventilation to total ventilation does not change much over the normal range of tidal volume (see discussion under lung volumes), total ventilation is therefore also inversely proportional to the $PaCO_2$.

The relationship of oxygen tension to the amount of oxygen content of the blood is more complex since normally, as previously noted, more than 98% of the oxygen is carried in combination with hemoglobin in the arterial blood. Although in the healthy adult breathing air at sea level the arterial oxygen tension PaO_2 tension is around 100 mm Hg, the oxygen content of the arterial blood is not significantly diminished for most clinical purposes until the PaO_2 drops below 70 mm Hg. This is because of the nature of hemoglobin affinity for oxygen, as described by the oxyhemoglobin dissociation curve (see Fig. 33-1). If the circulation is intact, most tissues will continue to function by extracting more oxygen from the hemoglobin molecules until about half are used, at which point increased needs are met by greater blood flow. The most sensitive organ to oxygen deprivation is the heart. The oxygen extraction by the myocardium is between 45% to 50% of that delivered. This gives a PO_2 in the coronary sinus of around 23 to 27 mm Hg, so that the heart is operating very near the anaerobic threshold at all times.[5] A reduction in arterial saturation of as little as 5% may require the heart to increase myocardial blood flow. For the treatment of myocardial ischemia, even small amounts of additional oxygen therefore become crucial in maintaining cardiac work and may prevent further ischemic damage. In hypoxic states, as long as the PaO_2 is maintained at 70 mm Hg or above, the hypoxemia is considered mild. Below 60 mm Hg, the hypoxemia is considered severe because of the hemodynamic adjustment needed to maintain oxygen delivery. If the patient is also anemic, the adverse physiologic effects of arterial hypoxemia will be even more severe because of the concomitant reduction in oxygen content.

The $PACO_2$ and alveolar oxygen PAO_2 tensions are approximately complementary; although it must be remembered that the carbon dioxide output during cellular metabolism is usually slightly lower than the oxygen uptake (RQ $= \dot{V}CO_2/\dot{V}O_2$). The PAO_2 plus the $PACO_2$ approximately equals the inspired oxygen tension (PIO_2). Thus at sea level where the PIO_2 is around 150 mm Hg, any reduction of ventilation will increase $PACO_2$ and therefore cause arterial hypoxemia. A very small increment of oxygen in the inspired gas will correct this hypoxemia since it will increase the oxygen fraction in the alveolus without altering the concentration of carbon dioxide. For this reason, after general anesthesia postoperative patients should be given oxygen-enriched air to breathe until the residual effects of muscle relaxants and narcotics, which cause respiratory depression, have worn off. Likewise, in patients with hypoxemia caused by ventilation/perfusion inequalities and diffusion impairments, the condition may be corrected by a modest elevation of the inspired oxygen concentration. In contrast, the hypoxemia produced by a true shunt is only minimally altered by the administration of extra oxygen. Nevertheless, the patient who has arterial hypoxemia as a result of a shunt should not be deprived of additional oxygen, since even a marginal increase in arterial oxygen tension resulting from the additional oxygen that is dissolved in the blood passing through aerated alveoli may be beneficial. It must be emphasized, however, that, when managing a patient with a pulmonary shunt, the best way to improve oxygenation is to reduce the shunt if possible by reexpanding collapsed lung or reducing pulmonary edema.

Although increasing the dissolved oxygen content of the arterial blood from 0.3 to 2 ml/100 ml can be achieved by administering 100% oxygen to an air-breathing patient, the benefits of doing so are debatable. The incremental increase in oxygen is small, and pulmonary oxygen toxicity becomes a problem. The additional oxygen carried in the arterial blood is equivalent to that which would be carried by raising the hemoglobin concentration by a little over 1 g/100 ml. As previously noted, when half the oxygen is removed from the hemoglobin, most tissues are very near the anaerobic threshold. The additional dissolved oxygen is therefore like an increase of about 2 g of hemoglobin, which is being provided without any increase in viscosity. Certainly the administration of oxygen (in high concentrations if necessary) as a first-aid maneuver to support patients whose internal respiration is compromised by hypoxia is likely to be beneficial. In myocardial ischemia and cardiogenic shock, for example, additional inspired oxygen improves myocardial performance and diminishes myocardial hypoxic changes.[5] Used indiscriminately, though, high concentrations of oxygen are likely to have detrimental effects. Pulmonary oxygen toxicity can produce acute respiratory distress and causes lung damage in as little as 2 days. Absorption atelectasis is another possible danger of high inspired oxygen concentrations.

Since oxygen delivery depends on cardiac output and arterial oxygen content, and the latter basically depends on the hemoglobin concentration and an adequate oxygen tension to saturate the hemoglobin, mixed venous oxygen has been viewed as a means of assessing the adequacy of oxygen delivery in meeting the needs of internal respiration. The mixed venous oxygen tension ($P\bar{v}O_2$) is normally around 40 mm Hg, and the mixed venous oxygen saturation ($S\bar{v}O_2$) approximates 70% to 75%. Except in extreme anemia and conditions of peripheral shunting such as septic shock, the $P\bar{v}O_2$ is considered to reflect tissue oxygenation and therefore the adequacy of oxygen delivery. On a moment-to-moment basis, the $S\bar{v}O_2$ is a reflection of cardiac output and can be monitored by placement of a fiberoptic catheter (Swan-Ganz) in the pulmonary artery. As cardiac output falls, the needs of internal respiration are met by increased extraction so the arteriovenous oxygen content difference ($C[a-\bar{v}]O_2$) increases, and the $S\bar{v}O_2$ falls.

Lung Volumes

The volume of air in the lungs following maximum inspiration is referred to as the total lung capacity (TLC). This is conventionally divided into residual volume (RV), which is the volume of air remaining in the lungs after a maximum expiration, and the vital capacity (VC), which is equal to the maximum volume of air exhaled after a maximum inspiration (Fig. 33-2). In a young man with healthy lungs, the RV is approximately 20% of the TLC.

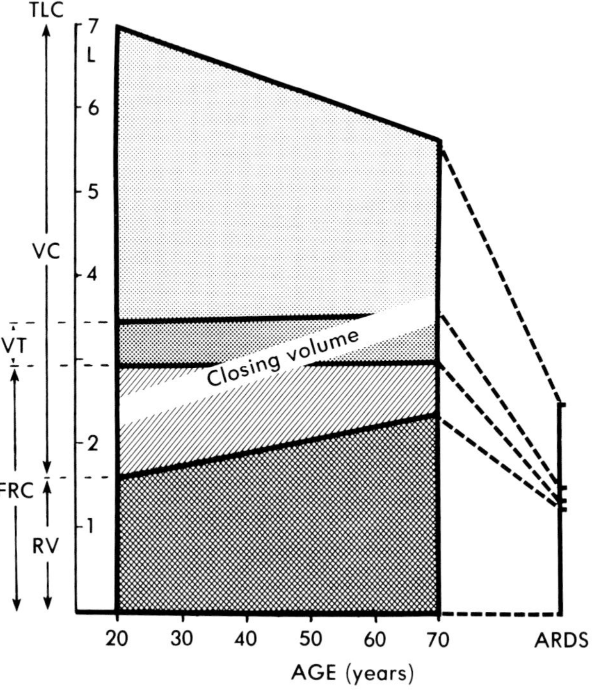

Fig. 33-2 Typical lung volumes of healthy supine 70-kg man. Note that in the midforties, closing volume begins to exceed functional residual capacity *(FRC)*. In addition, total lung capacity *(TLC)* and vital capacity *(VC)* decline with age, and residual volume *(RV)* increases. FRC does not change. An example of severe acute respiratory distress syndrome *(ARDS)* shows that all lung volumes are reduced, including tidal volume *(VT)*. (Modified from Pontoppidan, H., Geffin, B., and Lowenstein, E.: N. Engl. J. Med. 287: 690, 1972.)

The VC can be measured directly with a spirometer, whereas measurement of the RV requires a somewhat more complicated technique such as nitrogen washout or equilibration with a known volume of an inert insoluble gas such as helium. Whole-body plethysmography may also be used to obtain this measurement.

The tidal volume (TV) is the volume of air normally inspired and exhaled during quiet respiration. In the average adult it varies between 500 and 800 ml. The functional residual capacity (FRC) is defined as the volume of air remaining in the lung at the resting end-tidal volume expiratory position. This resting position of the lung is maintained by two forces. These include (1) the intrinsic elasticity of the lung that tends to make the volume smaller, and (2) the chest wall and tone of the respiratory muscles, which keep the lungs expanded. FRC will therefore be reduced if the lungs become stiffer or, if the forces that keep the chest wall expanded decrease because of muscular relaxation or splinting from pain.

During normal ventilation because of gravitational forces and the fact that air rises, the apices of the lungs are more expanded than the bases. (The lung at FRC has a density of about 0.3 g/ml.) The alveolar ventilation at the apices is less than at the lung bases as is the ratio of ventilation to perfusion. Thus the person who breathes room air has a relative increase in nitrogen concentration in the upper regions of the lung.[56] If an air-breathing subject takes a vital capacity breath of 100% oxygen and slowly exhales to residual volume through a nitrogen meter, he is performing a single-breath nitrogen washout test (Fig. 33-3).[56] Under normal circumstances the initial part of the expiration is 100% oxygen, which rises to a plateau as a mixture of alveolar and dead space gas is being measured. The plateau occurs when alveolar gas is being exhaled. As the person approaches residual volume, there is a point at which the airways of the dependent parts of the lung are no longer contributing to the expired gas and most of the expired gas is now coming from the apices. A sudden increase in nitrogen concentration is seen. This point is known as the "closing volume" (CV). In a healthy young man this does not appear until 90% of the vital capacity has been exhaled, and in some individuals it is not even detectable. If the CV exceeds the FRC, part of the respiratory cycle is being conducted with "closed" airways in the inferior portions of the lung, and arterial hypoxia is produced. Under normal circumstances in a healthy young man, the FRC is 30% to 35% greater than the CV. FRC is reduced, however, in the supine position. This reduction is mostly a result of elevation of the diaphragm from pressure of the abdominal contents and partly related to an increase in the central blood volume. Thus in the supine posture the majority of patients are going to have a CV greater than the FRC, producing a setup for atelectasis in the postoperative period if the patient remains bedridden.

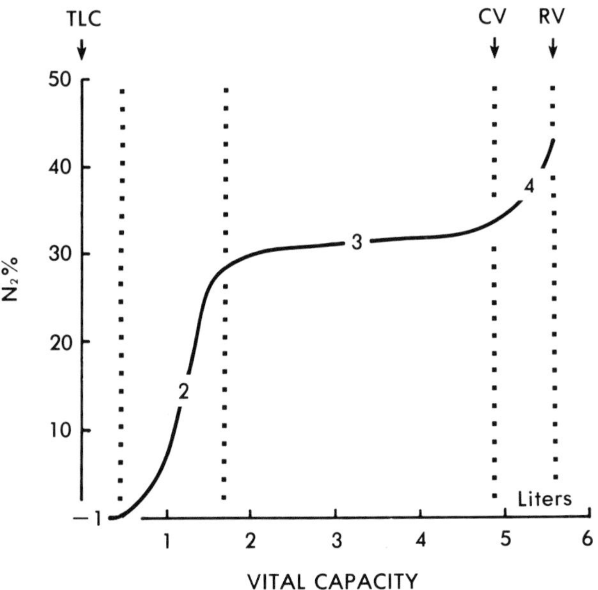

Fig. 33-3 Single-breath nitrogen *(N_2)* washout test (see text). Phase 1 represents pure oxygen being expired (dead space); Phase 2, mixed dead space and alveolar gas; Phase 3, alveolar gas; and the junction between Phases 3 and 4, the closing volume. The steeper and more uneven the gradient for Phase 3, the poorer the mixing of gases in the lung (*TLC,* total lung capacity; *CV,* closing volume; *RV,* residual volume).

As the lungs age, there is a decrease in the TLC and an increase in the RV so that the VC is decreased. In the mature adult, the FRC does not change, but the CV increases. In healthy, older individuals the CV may be as high as 40% of the VC and therefore will exceed the FRC. This accounts for the relative hypoxia seen in resting elderly patients and also indicates the reason for the increased susceptibility for deterioration in pulmonary function observed in these individuals following operation if they are left lying on their backs in bed.[36]

With the advent of bronchospirometry, measurement of independent lung volumes became possible. Using this technique, a normal adult subject laying supine was noted to lose over 0.5 L of FRC. If the subject is turned into the full lateral position, the upper lung takes on a functional residual capacity that is at least as large as that in the upright position, whereas the lower lung is no smaller than when the patient is supine.[47] This information has provided a scientific basis for maneuvers such as turning patients fully every 2 hours, having them do exercises to expand the lungs, and getting them out of bed to maintain alveolar ventilation. In the acute respiratory distress syndrome when the lungs become very stiff and the lung volumes become contracted, even the TLC may be below the CV, and maneuvers such as positive end-expiratory pressure become necessary to maintain gas exchange (see Chapter 35).

Measurement of VC is the major test for determination of pulmonary restriction. In the normal-sized man, a VC that is 50% or less of normal is considered to represent a severe deficit and indicates a high likelihood of postoperative respiratory morbidity. Causes of decreased vital capacity include a reduction of the chest bellows effect from obesity, kyphoscoliosis, or other chest wall deformities; and decreased compliance as a result of conditions that lead to pulmonary edema such as chronic heart failure, pneumonia, or chronic pulmonary fibrosis. Conditions that actually reduce the alveolar ventilation such as postoperative splinting caused by chest pain also decrease VC. Thus a knowledge of the preoperative VC is extremely helpful in determining who may require postoperative ventilatory support and how long such support may be needed. For example, in weaning a patient from mechanical ventilatory support, a VC of 15 ml/kg has been found to be a reasonable minimum requirement.[21] This is about 20% of the normal VC and is safe only in the expectation that the patient will subsequently improve his pulmonary status.

FRC is also markedly reduced following major abdominal surgery and in patients with sepsis or who have sustained severe trauma. An FRC less than 70% of normal is almost always associated with pulmonary arteriovenous admixture (i.e., shunting) and in the critical trauma patient has been associated with progressive development of acute respiratory distress syndrome.[29,38]

Ventilation/Perfusion

For every liter of blood flowing through the lungs, there needs to be 0.8 L of alveolar ventilation to promote the most economic gas exchange. The mismatching of ventilation to perfusion gives rise to the development of dead space when ventilation is relatively increased over arterial perfusion and a shunt effect in regions of lung where circulation predominates over ventilation. In the healthy young subject the ventilation-perfusion ratio throughout the lung is very close to 1. When ventilation and perfusion are mismatched, the initial effect will be a lowering of the oxygen tension and a rise in the carbon dioxide tension in the arterial blood. This will trigger a chemoreceptor response, and ventilation will increase, thereby lowering the carbon dioxide tension toward normal. The dynamics of normal oxygen uptake from the alveolus require that the hemoglobin become saturated within the lung. There is not an equivalent mechanism for compensating for hypoxemia occurring in some parts of the lung by hyperventilating others; therefore, when the lung continues to be afflicted with mismatching ventilation and perfusion, hypoxemia will be only minimally corrected by hyperventilation. When the effort to maintain a normal arterial carbon dioxide tension becomes excessive, the patient may convert from someone whose oxygen tension is only slightly below normal to someone who develops hypercarbia and hypoxemia because of the loss of respiratory drive. This is seen in chronic obstructive lung disease when the Type A ("pink puffer") patient turns into the Type B ("blue bloater") patient and then goes on to progressive respiratory failure. In dry climates the Type A emphysematous patient may experience a progressive loss of alveolar diffusing capacity and stiffening lungs and eventually die of respiratory failure. In moister climates bronchitis and emphysema often coexist, and the Type A patient converts to Type B. An emphysematous person may demonstrate severe arterial hypoxemia if blood gases are obtained during exercise.

Ideally ventilation-perfusion mismatching is demonstrable by a multiple gas infusion technique, which not only gives true shunt and true dead-space measurements but also quantifies the amount of ventilation ($\dot{V}$) and perfusion ($\dot{Q}$) for any given $\dot{V}/\dot{Q}$ ratio.[49] The practical realities of the clinical world make it impossible to obtain this sort of information routinely. Thus, in measuring dead space, both anatomic dead space (that derived from air in the bronchial tubes in which no gas exchanges take place) and physiologic dead space (that portion of the wasted ventilation caused by mismatched ventilation to perfusion) are considered as if they were both true dead space, even though true dead space is really only anatomic dead space.[56] This is demonstrated in the Enghoff modification of the Bohr equation:

$$V_D/V_T = Pa_{CO_2} - P\bar{E}_{CO_2}/Pa_{CO_2}$$

where V_D is dead space; V_T is tidal volume; Pa_{CO_2} is arterial carbon dioxide tension; and $P\bar{E}_{CO_2}$ is mixed-expired carbon dioxide tension. Under normal circumstances the dead-space fraction is approximately one third of the tidal volume, and the alveolar ventilation represents two thirds. If V_D/V_T increases (e.g., to two thirds the tidal volume), the total ventilation has to be doubled to maintain normal arterial carbon dioxide tension. It is important to remember this ratio when patients are recovering from respiratory failure and are being weaned from mechanical ventilation. A V_D/V_T ratio greater than 0.6 is likely to be excessive for successful weaning to be accomplished.[21]

The arteriovenous admixture (shunt) is usually assessed by the shunt equation:

$$\dot{Q}_{PS}/\dot{Q}_T = Cc_{O_2} - Ca_{O_2}/Cc_{O_2} - C\bar{v}_{O_2}$$

where $\dot{Q}_{PS}$ is physiologic shunt; $\dot{Q}_T$ is cardiac output; Cc_{O_2} is calculated-end pulmonary capillary oxygen content; Ca_{O_2} is arterial oxygen content; and $C\bar{v}_{O_2}$ is mixed venous oxygen content. Physiologic shunting is much like the physiologic dead space in that both the true shunt and the contribution of ventilation-perfusion mismatch in hyperperfused regions of lung are treated together as one. Various methods of trying to derive the same information from the alveolar-arterial oxygen gradient $P(A\text{-}a)_{O_2}$ and the arterial tension/inspired fraction oxygen ratio (Pa_{O_2}/F_{IO_2}) may have some value in sequential monitoring of an individual patient, but they may tend to give a very poor idea of the absolute shunt because there is an assumed fixed contribution from the mixed venous oxygen content. Thus the $\dot{Q}_{PS}/\dot{Q}_T$ ratio has been used to follow lung function, particularly in critically ill patients requiring ventilatory support, even though the values tend to increase for reasons other than pulmonary pathology in low cardiac output states, hypovolemia, and with inspired oxygen fractions (F_{IO_2}) greater than 50%.

Pulmonary Compliance

Compliance is the term used to describe the distensibility of the lungs. Its unit of measurement is milliliters per centimeters of water and describes the increase in lung volume in milliliters associated with any corresponding change in pulmonary distending pressure. Compliance is usually measured at the FRC; sometimes it is necessary to generate a compliance curve that shows the compliance at various lung volumes in order to determine the true distensibility of the lungs (Fig. 33-4). Compliance is less below the CV and as the lung becomes fully distended approaching the TLC. When the CV is in excess of the FRC, compliance is found to increase at a higher lung volume than the FRC. Measurement of maximum compliance has been particularly useful in defining the optimal amount of positive end-expiratory pressure that will give the most effi-

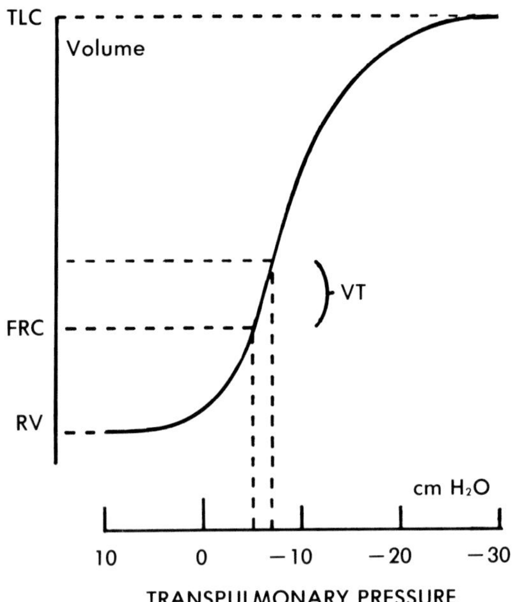

Fig. 33-4 Compliance curve of lungs showing pressure-volume relationship. The lung has less compliance as it nears the residual volume *(RV)* or total lung capacity *(TLC)*. Compliance is greatest at the normal functional residual capacity *(FRC)*, so that the region of tidal volume (VT) is the most efficient for gas exchange. When the FRC is decreased, positive end-expiratory pressure may increase compliance as the FRC is normalized. FRC is at a transpulmonary pressure of −5 because the pressure is measured between the airways and pleura. Normally, V_T is achieved by dropping the intrapleural pressure 2 to 3 cm of water.

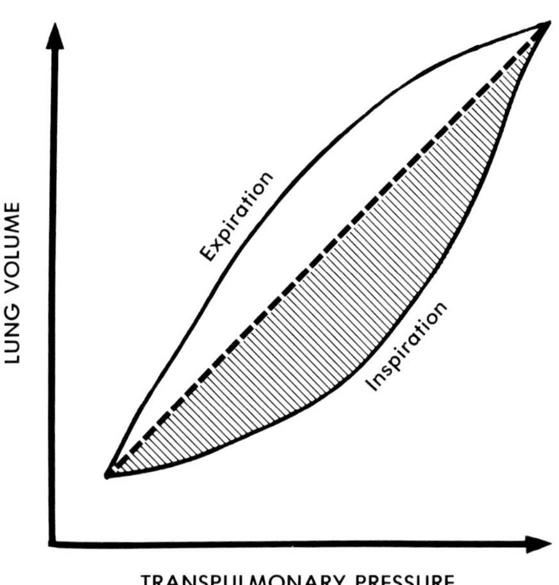

Fig. 33-5 Pressure-volume loop of the lungs. The broken line represents the static compliance curve, whereas the shaded area represents the extra work needed to fill the lung because of airway resistance and frictional forces.

cient gas transfer for the least impedance of the circulation in patients being treated for acute respiratory failure (see Chapter 35).[46]

In pulmonary function testing, the compliance is obtained from measurement of the esophageal pressure in the upright position. This is accomplished by a balloon catheter placed in the middle third of the esophagus. As the subject breathes in, intrathoracic pressure drops. The amount of decrease in intrathoracic pressure is the distending pressure of the lungs. Part of the work of breathing is overcoming the elastic forces within the lungs. These forces are created by a relatively fixed resistance to the deformation of elastic and fibrous elements within the lung parenchyma and are also secondary to other variables such as interstitial edema and surface tension forces acting within the air sacs. The rest of the work of breathing is divided between movement of the chest wall and intra-abdominal pressure upon descent of the diaphragm and airway resistance within the trachea and bronchial tubes.

During a forced maximal inspiration, the fall in intrathoracic pressure is instantaneously greater than that expected from overcoming compliance of the lung. This dynamic information is the basis of the pressure-flow loop that is able to define the work of breathing caused by airway resistance (Fig. 33-5).[33] Thus, during inflation of the lung, portions of the lung with low airway resistance inflate early. At the end of inspiration, portions of relatively low resistance and high compliance tend to deflate, whereas other portions of relatively low compliance and high resistance tend to inflate. This is particularly seen in patients with obstructive pulmonary disease on mechanical ventilation. The peak inspiratory pressure is often much higher than the end-expiratory pressure (Fig. 33-6); i.e., when air flow into the lung has ceased, redistribution of gas within the lung lowers the pressure, enabling a true compliance measurement. For physiologic purposes this circumstance is considered to take place in 4 seconds, but for most clinical purposes, a 2-second inflation is deemed adequate. Accordingly, the peak inspiratory pressure is used to calculate the dynamic compliance.

Under clinical circumstances the intrathoracic or esophageal pressure is not measured routinely. Instead the total compliance is measured, which includes both pulmonary compliance and the compliance of the chest wall and abdominal contents. Normally at FRC, the total compliance is half the lung compliance. The normal adult lung compliance is around 200 ml/cm of water, whereas the total compliance is around 100 ml/cm of water. Stated another way, half the compliant resistance to breathing is the result of the compliance of the chest wall and intra-abdominal pressure. For practical purposes it is acceptable to assume in patients with acute pulmonary disease that, on a moment-to-moment basis, the compliance of the lung will be relatively variable; whereas the compliance of the chest wall and abdomen will be relatively constant, so that total compliance will show changes in pulmonary function. Thus the difference between dynamic and true compliance is an index of airway resistance.

The original observations of von Neergaard[48] on the compliance of the lung resulted in the hypothesis that the alveolar surface of the lung was covered with a thin layer of water and that this layer of water was covered with a surface active agent that reduced surface tension, called surfactant. He postulated that, as the lung volume de-

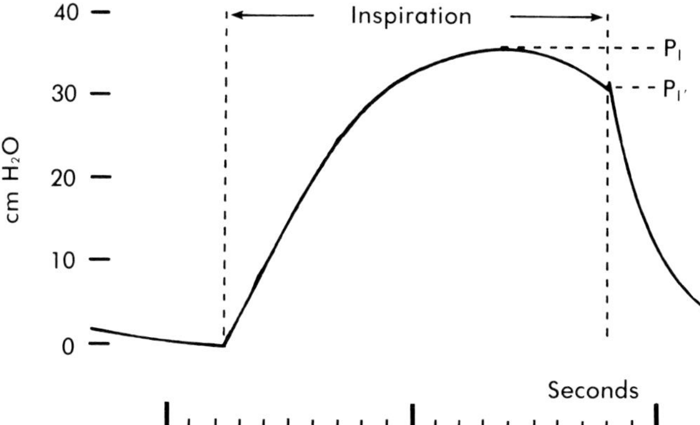

Fig. 33-6 Pressure tracing from a volume ventilator, with a sine-wave delivery, slowing gas delivery at the end of inspiration (Emerson). Note how the inspiratory pressure falls from the peak (P_I) to an end-inspiratory level ($P_{I'}$) as gas is being distributed to higher, resistance units in the lung. $P_{I'}$ gives a more accurate estimate of static compliance.

creased, the diameter of the water-lined alveoli also decreased. Excessive surface tension forces did not collapse the alveolus because the surfactant layer was increasingly concentrated on the now smaller surface area.

In support of this theory lipid substances capable of reducing surface tension have been found in the lung. The major surfactant identified in lung washings has been dipalmitoyl lecithin. At the edges of alveolar surfaces, specialized cells (Type II pneumocytes) secrete both this and other phospholipid surfactants. Although this theory sounds attractive, the thin layer of water lining the alveolus has never been demonstrated in mammalian lung. A more mechanically attractive theory has recently been put forward by Hills[19] who has reasoned that the alveolar surfaces in the lung could be "waterproofed" by surfactant. This would cause any fluid within the alveolus to collect in the corners where surface tension would both tend to push fluid out of the alveolus into the interstitium and provide the forces to alter lung compliance.[20] The absence of adequate dipalmitoyl lecithin in the lungs gives rise to conditions of low compliance and pulmonary collapse such as are seen in both the infant and adult respiratory distress syndromes. Surfactant production is decreased in prematurity and in stress situations such as septic shock and is also seen in oxygen toxicity. Modulation of surfactant production appears to be partially under prostaglandin-E control.

Forced Expiration

Analysis of the FVC can give valuable information about both obstructive and restrictive pulmonary dysfunction. This vital capacity measurement is divided into various timed volumes, which are often compared as percentages of the FVC. The FCV that is exhaled during the first second is referred to as the FEV_1. Normally, the ratio of FEV_1/FVC is around 80% to 85%. Within 3 seconds (FEV_3), almost all the FVC is exhaled; the normal ratio of FEV_3/FVC is nearly 100%. Low ratios of FEV_1/FVC are indicative of obstructive airway disease. When this ratio is less than 65%, it generally represents moderate-to-severe obstruction. In contrast, higher than normal ratios are indicative of restrictive lung disease. Forced expiration testing can be done quite simply and with a portable apparatus by the bedside. Such testing is useful for following the progress of patients being prepared for surgery who have chronic obstructive pulmonary disease and for judging the effectiveness of bronchodilator therapy.

Another flow measurement that may prove useful clinically is the peak expiratory flow. This determination can be easily measured with a flowmeter, which gives the maximum flow rate sustained for 10 ms during a forced expiration. In a healthy adult subject, this measurement is expected to be between 400 to 700 L/min. Moderate-to-severe obstructive lung disease is indicated by flow rates less than 200. Again, this measurement is a simple way to test the effectiveness of respiratory therapy maneuvers and bronchodilators.

A further test to determine the capacity of the lungs to ventilate is the maximum voluntary ventilation (MVV). This is the volume of air exchanged in a specified period, usually 12 seconds, during repetitive maximal respiratory effort. The result is then converted to liters per minute. A healthy young man can usually produce an MVV of 200 L/min. The MVV is a useful test to follow the progress of patients with pulmonary restriction, particularly that caused by muscular weakness, who are trying to improve their ventilatory capacity. Unfortunately, repetition within a reasonable period of time is often too wearing on the patient with chronic respiratory failure who may tire excessively; therefore meaningful comparisons from one test to the next are not possible.

Diffusing Capacity

The uptake of any gas from the lung into the pulmonary circulation depends on a variety of factors. The effectiveness of alveolar ventilation determines whether fresh gas will be delivered to the area where diffusion takes place; the size of the alveolus influences the distance across which the fresh gas has to diffuse; and the surface area of the alveolus and the thickness of the tissue between the alveolus and the blood determine the efficiency of gas transfer. Further, there has to be a partial pressure gradient between the alveolus and the circulation so that the rate of gas exchange will be proportional to the gradient between the mixed venous blood and the alveolar gas. In addition, the uptake of gas in the blood may be augmented by various chemical reactions that will maintain the gradient such as the combination of oxygen with hemoglobin. Finally, the rate of this reaction may be greatly altered during extremes of arterial hypoxemia and anemia and thus may define the limit of how much gas is removed from the lungs by the circulation.

Although one of the prime concerns of maintaining normal pulmonary physiology is to ensure the transfer of oxygen across the alveolar-capillary membrane, this gas is unsuitable to establish the efficiency of diffusing capacity. Variable amounts of it occur in the mixed venous blood, and, as the blood traverses the pulmonary microcirculation, the oxygen tension increases. Thus, to test diffusing capacity, a low concentration of carbon monoxide is used. Carbon monoxide has the advantage of being approximately the same molecular weight as oxygen, combines very quickly and efficiently with hemoglobin and thereby provides a constant gradient between the alveolus and the microcirculation, and over a moderate period of time has a negligibly small venous tension. The largest variable, which will adversely affect this test, is a maldistribution of ventilation-perfusion caused by peripheral airway disease. This test depends only partially on the surface area and thickness of the area of the membrane available for diffusion, and changes in the alveolar-capillary interface make little difference in the diffusing capacity. The carbon monoxide diffusing capacity is around 40 ml/min/mm Hg in a normal man, and is considered mildly abnormal with a 20% reduction and severely abnormal when this capacity is halved.[30]

Respiratory Drive

The factors that control how forcefully a patient can breathe are the neural output of the respiratory center, the conduction of that output to the respiratory muscles, and the corresponding strength of the respiratory muscles. A potentially useful clinical measurement of this force is the occluded inspiratory pressure (sometimes miscalled inspiratory "force"). The airway is occluded at the end of expiration, and the pressure generated when the patient tries to take the next breath is measured. Since this measurement is determined at FRC and there is no change in pulmonary volume, restriction resistance to airflow and the elastic forces within the lung itself have no effect on its value.

When a patient is recovering from acute respiratory failure and is being weaned from ventilatory support, the probability of the weaning being successful is related to the patient having a maximum inspiratory pressure greater than -25 cm of water.[21] To determine this pressure, the airway is occluded for a period of 150 ms at the end of expiration, and the negative pressure created in the airway in the first 100 ms (called the $P_{0.01}$) is measured. The occlusion should occur during a breath when it is unanticipated by the subject, since the reaction to increased respiratory drive because of the occlusion becomes influential after 150 ms.[28] Since the variables that affect $P_{0.01}$ are not fully understood and are related to lung volume and chemoreceptor activity, this measurement remains a research tool and has not yet been subjected to widespread clinical evaluation.[50]

POSTOPERATIVE RESPIRATORY MORBIDITY

Pulmonary complications have long been recognized as a leading cause of postoperative morbidity and mortality. Maneuvers such as nasogastric intubation have been demonstrated to exacerbate the problem by allowing gastric reflux and the potential for aspiration of acidic contents and pathogenic bacteria into the lung, but the main contributing factor appears to be the type of operation performed, with thoracic and abdominal operations being especially noteworthy for the development of postoperative pulmonary dysfunction. The greatest limitation in pulmonary function occurs in patients subjected to upper abdominal surgery, and a large part of this problem appears to be related to the incisional pain.[44] Vertical and midline incisions appear to cause more of a problem than muscle-cutting subcostal incisions.[2] In comparison, thoracic incisions are less troublesome, and lower abdominal surgery is relatively well tolerated. Nonthoracoabdominal surgery seems to have very little adverse influence on respiratory function.

In patients developing pulmonary dysfunction following thoracoabdominal operations, there is generally a marked reduction in FVC and FRC. The reduction in FVC is immediate following surgery and is primarily pain related, whereas the reduction in FRC tends to develop more slowly over the ensuing 12 to 18 hours and may be related to pulmonary changes arising from the restriction caused by pain and perhaps some stress phenomena related to surgery itself.[12] If the FRC can be kept above 60% of normal, postoperative morbidity seems to be markedly reduced.[27] The FRC can be increased and pulmonary problems reduced during the postoperative period with the institution of adequate analgesia,[1] and it is also markedly increased when patients are mobilized early after operation.

The type of anesthesia used also seems to influence the development of postoperative pulmonary problems. Segmental epidural anesthesia has been found to be very effective in maintaining adequate respiratory function after surgery and in allowing the early mobilization of patients. In one study patients receiving epidural anesthesia were able to be mobilized immediately after surgery and were discharged from the hospital on an average of 3 days earlier than their counterpart controls who received intramuscular narcotic analgesia.[34] Despite the superior pain relief provided by epidural local anesthetics, one problem frequently encountered in patients receiving this form of analgesia is severe postural hypotension. In a comparison of conventional narcotic postoperative pain relief with that from epidural use of local anesthetics and narcotics, it was shown that epidural narcotic analgesia, although not as effective at promoting a return of pulmonary function as local anesthetics, enabled patients to be mobilized without postural hypotension.[4] Although it is recognized that many regional techniques of anesthesia may be superior to generalized narcotic analgesia for their ability to provide postoperative pain relief and not depress respiratory drive, it should be noted that, if extensive intercostal nerve blocks or epidural anesthesia are used, there may be a reduction of FVC and the ability to cough effectively following surgery because of muscular weakness, thereby defeating their potentially advantageous effects.

Considerable improvements in respiratory function following surgery have been found by simple maneuvers such as the blocking of a few intercostal nerves during thoracotomy and the infiltration of abdominal wounds with long-acting local anesthetics at the time of laparotomy. The provision of adequate pain relief without respiratory depression also has led to a new look at the use of narcotic analgesics. Such methods as continuous intravenous infusion with these agents and patient-controlled analgesia can maintain a minimum level of analgesia and thus prevent the depressant peak in the painful trough of intermittent intramuscular or intravenous injections administered according to a specific order.[45] Another approach has been to give long-acting analgesics such as methadone in a large dose at the beginning of surgery. The aim of this therapy is to have the drug at an analgesic but not overly depressant level and in the beta phase of elimination by the end of the operation (see Chapter 11). The patient will then remain analgesic for many hours, enhancing the opportunity for early mobilization and the provision of more comfortable chest physiotherapy.[16]

The patient who has diminished pulmonary function before surgery offers a greater challenge for both intraoperative and postoperative management because there is a smaller margin of safety as a result of the dimunition in pulmonary reserve and patient is more prone to respiratory failure if narcotic analgesics are used. A proper physiologic preoperative assessment of such patients with the use of the modalities outlined elsewhere in this chapter and the formulation of a plan on the basis of this information to manage postoperative pain will do much to diminish postoperative respiratory morbidity.

SUMMARY

The supply of oxygen is controlled and distributed to meet regional needs of the body by circulatory and ventilatory adjustments. If the supply begins to fail, these adjustments direct the oxygen to regions of greatest oxygen use. Ventilation is primarily governed by $Paco_2$ and pH. Hypoxic tissues can turn to anaerobic metabolism, but this source of energy is quickly insufficient. There is a lag in venous blood-gas values seen with changes in oxygen uptake. These values can give misleading information about tissue exchange when the respiratory gas exchange is measured. In the clinical situation respiratory function can be evaluated with arterial blood gases and various measurements of pulmonary function. Avoiding postoperative pulmonary morbidity is best performed by maneuvers that keep the lungs expanded, allow coughing and, if possible, avoid nasogastric and endotracheal tubes. Pain relief is a great aid to improved ventilation.

REFERENCES

1. Alexander, J.I., et al.: The role of airway closure in postoperative hypoxemia, Br. J. Anaesth. **5**:34, 1973.
2. Ali, J., and Khan, T.A.: The comparative effects of muscle transection and median upper abdominal incision on postoperative pulmonary function, Surg. Gynecol. Obstet. **148**:863, 1979.
3. Berger, A.J., Mitchell, R.A., and Severinghaus, J.W.: Regulation of respiration. N. Engl. J. Med. **297**:92, 1977.
4. Bromage, P.R., Camporesi, E., and Chestnut, D: Epidural narcotics for postoperative analgesia, Anesth. Analg. **59**:473, 1980.
5. Bryan-Brown, C.W.: Gas transport and delivery. In Shoemaker, W.C., Thompson W.L., and Holbrook, editors: Textbook of critical care, Philadelphia, 1984, W.B. Saunders Co.
6. Cherniak, N.S.: The clinical assessment of the chemical regulation of ventilation, Chest **70**:274, 1976.
7. Cherniak, N.S., and Altose, M.D.: Respiratory responses to ventilatory loading. In Hornbein, T.F., editor: Lung biology in health and disease, vol. 17 (II), New York, 1981, Marcel Dekker, Inc.
8. Christensen, M.S.: Acid-base changes in cerebrospinal fluid and blood, and blood volume changes following prolonged hyperventilation in man, Br. J. Anaesth. **46**:348, 1974.
9. Churchill, E.D., and McNeil, D.: The reduction of vital capacity following operation, Surg. Gynecol. Obstet. **44**:483, 1927.
10. Clark, F.J., and von Euler, C.: On the regulation of depth and rate of breathing, J. Physiol. **222**:267, 1972.
11. Cotes, J.E.: Lung function: assessment and application in medicine (ed. 4), Oxford, 1981, Blackwell Scientific Publications.
12. Craig, D.B.: Postoperative recovery of lung function, Anesth. Analg. **60**:46, 1981.
13. Czer, L.S.C., Appel, P., and Shoemaker, W.C.: Pathogenesis of respiratory failure (ARDS) after hemorrhage and trauma. II. Cardiorespiratory patterns after development of ARDS, Crit. Care Med. **8**:513, 1980.
14. Damask, M.C., et al.: Artifacts in measurement of resting energy expenditure, Crit. Care Med. **11**:750, 1983.
15. Fencl, V., Vale, J.R., and Broch, J.R.: Respiration and cerebral blood flow in metabolic acidosis and alkalosis in humans, J. Appl. Physiol. **27**:67, 1979.
16. Gourlay, G.K., Willis, R.J., and Wilson, R.P.: Postoperative pain control with methadone; influences of supplementary methadone doses and blood concentration-response relationships, Anesthesiology **61**:19, 1984.
17. Hedemark, L.L., and Kronenberg, R.S.: Chemical regulation of respiration: normal variations and abnormal responses, Chest **82**:488, 1982.
18. Hickey, R.F., and Severinghaus, J.W.: Regulation of breathing: drug effects. In Hornbein, T.F., editor: Lung biology in health and disease, vol. 17(II), New York, 1981, Marcel Dekker, Inc.
19. Hills, B.A.: What is the true role of surfactant in the lung? Thorax **36**:1, 1981.
20. Hills, B.A., and Bryan-Brown, C.W.: Role of surfactant in the lung and other organs, Crit. Care Med. **11**:951, 1983.
21. Hodgkin, J.E., Bowser, M.A., and Burton, G.G.: Respirator weaning, Crit. Care Med. **2**:96, 1974.
22. Hopkins, J.A., et al.: Clinical trial of an emergency resuscitation algorithm, Crit. Care Med. **11**:621, 1983.
23. Hornbein, T.F.: To breathe or not to breathe (editorial), Anesthesiology **61**:119, 1984.
24. Horvath, S.M., and Borgia, J.F.: Cardiopulmonary gas transport and aging, Am. Rev. Respir. Dis. **129**(suppl.):68, 1984.
25. Knill, R.L., and Clement, J.L.: Site of selective action of halothane on the peripheral chemoreflex pathway in humans, Anesthesiology **61**:121, 1984.
26. Kronenberg, R., et al.: Comparison of three methods for quantitating respiratory response to hypoxia in man, Respir. Physiol. **16**:109, 1972.
27. Meyers, J.R., et al.: Changes in functional residual capacity of the lung after operation, Arch. Surg. **110**:576, 1975.
28. Milic-Emili, J., Whitelaw, W.A., and Durenne, J.P.: Occlusion pressure—a simple measure of the respiratory center's output, N. Engl. J. Med. **293**:1029, 1975.
29. Monaco, V., et al.: Pulmonary venous admixture in injured patients, J. Trauma **12**:15, 1972.
30. Morris, A.H., et al.: Clinical pulmonary function testing: a manual for uniform laboratory procedures, ed. 2, Salt Lake City, 1984, Intermountain Thoracic Society.
31. Nery L.E., et al.: Ventilatory and gas exchange mechanics in chronic obstructive lung disease, J. Appl. Physiol. **53**:1594, 1982.
32. Nunn, J.F.: Applied respiratory physiology, ed. 2, Boston, 1977, Butterworth Publishers.
33. Nunn, J.F., and Ezi-Ashi, T.I.: The respiratory effects of resistance to breathing in anesthetized man, Anesthesiology **22**:174, 1961.
34. Pflug, A.E., et al.: The effects of postoperative epidural analgesia on pulmonary therapy and pulmonary complications, Anesthesiology **41**:8, 1974.
35. Plewes, J.L., and Farhi L.E.: Peripheral circulatory response to acute hyperoxia, Undersea Biomed. Res. **10**:123, 1983.
36. Pontoppidan, H., Geffin, B., and Lowenstein, E.: Acute respiratory failure in the adult (Part I), N. Engl. J. Med. **287**:690, 1972.
37. Posner, J.B., and Plum, F.: Spinal fluid pH and neurologic symptoms in systemic acidosis, N. Engl. J. Med. **277**:605, 1967.
38. Powers, S.R., Jr., et al.: Studies of pulmonary insufficiency in nonthoracic trauma, J. Trauma **12**:1, 1972.
39. Read, D.J.C.: A clinical method for assessidng the ventilatory response to carbon dioxide, Aust. Ann. Med. **16**:20, 1967.
40. Shippy, C.R., Appel, P.L., and Shoemaker, W.C.: Reliability of clinical monitoring to assess blood volume in critically ill patients, Crit. Care Med. **12**:107, 1984.
41. Shoemaker, W.C., and Hopkins, J.A.: Clinical aspects of resuscitation with and without an algorithm: relative importance of various decisions, Crit. Care Med. **11**:630, 1983.

42. Shoemaker, W.C., et al.: Pathogenesis of respiratory failure (ARDS) after hemorrhage and trauma. I. Cardiorespiratory patterns preceding the development of ARDS, Crit. Care Med. **8**:504, 1980.
43. Shoemaker, W.C., et al.: Clinical trial of an algorithm for prediction in acute circulatory failure, Crit. Care Med. **10**:390, 1982.
44. Stanley, T.H., Allen, S., and Bryan-Brown, C.W.: Management of pain and pain related problems in the critically ill patient, In Shoemaker, W.C., editor: Critical care—State of the art, vol. 6, Fullerton, 1985, Society of Critical Care Medicine.
45. Stapleton, J.F., Austin, K.L., and Mather, L.E.: A pharmacokinetic approach to postoperative pain: continuous intravenous pethidine, Anaesth. Int. Care **7**:25, 1979.
46. Suter, P.M., Fairley, H.B., and Isenberg, M.D.: Optimum end expiratory airway pressure in patients with acute respiratory failure, N. Engl. J. Med. **292**:284, 1975.
47. Svanberg, L.: Influence of posture on lung volumes, ventilation, and circulation in normals, Scand. J. Clin. Lab. Invest. **9**(suppl):25, 1957.
48. von Neergaard, K.: Neue Auffasungen über einen Grundbegriff der Atemtechnik. Die Retractionskraft der Lunge, abhängig von der Oberflächenspannung in der Alveolen, Z. Ges. Exp. Med. 1929, **66**:373, 1929. (Translated by West, J.B., editor: Translations in respiratory physiology, Stroudsburg, 1975, Dowden Hutchinson & Ross.)
49. Wagner, P.D., et al.: Continuous distribution of ventilation-perfusion ratios in normal subjects breathing air and 100% O_2, J. Clin. Invest. **54**:54, 1974.
50. Wanner, A.: Interpretation of pulmonary function tests. In Sackner, M.A., editor: Lung biology in health and disease, vol. 16(I) New York, 1979, Marcel Dekker, Inc.
51. Wasserman, K.: Coupling of external to internal respiration, Am. Rev. Respir. Dis. **129**(suppl):21, 1984.
52. Wasserman, K., and Whipp, B.J.: Exercise physiology in health and disease, Am. Rev. Respir. Dis. **112**:219, 1975.
53. Weil, J.V., et al.: Hypoxic ventilatory drive in normal man, J. Clin. Invest. **49**:1061, 1970.
54. Weil, J.V., McCullough, R.E., and Klin, J.S.: Diminished ventilatory response to hypoxia and hypercapnia after morphine in normal man, N. Engl. J. Med. **292**:1103, 1975.
55. Weissman, C., et al.: Effect of routine intensive care interactions on metabolic rate, Chest **86**:815, 1984.
56. West, J.B.: Respiratory physiology—the essentials, ed. 3, Baltimore, 1985, The Williams & Wilkens Co.
57. Woodson, R.D.: Hemoglobin concentration and exercise capacity, Am. Rev. Respir. Dis. **129**(suppl.):72, 1974.

34 Martin J. Tobin and David R. Dantzker

Ventilatory Support: Who, When, and How?

Although in 1543 Vesalius demonstrated the feasibility of positive-pressure ventilation by inflating an animal's lungs with a bellows,[157] negative-pressure ventilators were initially preferred in humans because of the difficulty of connecting the airway to a ventilatory apparatus. These tank respirators or iron lungs came into use at the end of the nineteenth century and were the mainstay of mechanical ventilation for the first 40 to 50 years of this century. During the 1940s anesthesiologists provided positive-pressure ventilation to patients undergoing surgery by manually compressing a rubber bag filled with oxygen and anesthetic gases. It was not until the Scandinavian polio epidemic of 1952 that the advantages of positive-pressure ventilators over negative-pressure ventilators were recognized; 87% of the patients treated with tank ventilators died compared to 25% of the patients treated with positive-pressure ventilation. Over the same period improved laryngoscope design simplified tracheal intubation, and the advances made in pulmonary physiology during World War II set the scene for further development and application of positive-pressure ventilators. During the last 20 to 30 years significant changes have occurred in ventilator design, modes of ventilation, and monitoring techniques. Probably more than any other technologic advance, mechanical ventilators have been associated with the proliferation of intensive care units. (Abbreviations used extensively in this chapter are defined in the box at right.)

ABBREVIATIONS

ABG	Arterial blood gas
A-C	Assist-control
CMV	Controlled mechanical ventilation
CO_2	Carbon dioxide
CPAP	Continuous positive airway pressure
CPPB	Continuous positive-pressure breathing
CPPV	Continuous positive-pressure ventilation
EPAP	Expiratory positive airway pressure
FIO_2	Fractional inspired oxygen concentration
FRC	Functional residual capacity
HCO_3^-	Bicarbonate
HFJV	High-frequency jet ventilation
HFO	High-frequency oscillator
HFPPV	High-frequency positive-pressure ventilation
HFV	High-frequency ventilation
ICP	Intracranial pressure
I:E ratio	Inspiratory to expiratory time ratio
IFR	Inspiratory flow rate
IMV	Intermittent mandatory ventilation
IPPV	Intermittent positive-pressure ventilation
MIP	Maximum inspiratory pressure
MVV	Maximum voluntary ventilation
O_2	Oxygen
PEEP	Positive end-expiratory pressure
SIMV	Synchronized intermittent mandatory ventilation
$\dot{V}A$	Alveolar ventilation
$\dot{V}A/\dot{Q}$	Ventilation to perfusion ratio
VCO_2	CO_2 production
$\dot{V}D$	Dead-space ventilation
VD/VT	Dead-space tidal-volume ratio
$\dot{V}E$	Minute ventilation
VT	Tidal volume

INDICATIONS FOR VENTILATORY SUPPORT

It is important to remember that the indications for mechanical ventilation are not necessarily the same as those for tracheal intubation. The major indication for mechanical ventilation is acute respiratory failure of which there are two basic causes: ventilatory pump failure causing an inadequate minute ventilation ($\dot{V}E$) and inefficient pulmonary gas exchange (see the boxed material on p. 566). The major goal of mechanical ventilation is to reverse these processes with the minimum risk cost in complications to the patient.

Ventilatory Pump Failure

Inadequate $\dot{V}E$ leads to hypercapnia since $PaCO_2$ is determined by alveolar ventilation ($\dot{V}A$):

$$PaCO_2 \simeq \frac{CO_2 \text{ production}}{\dot{V}A}$$

$\dot{V}A$ is a theoretical term representing that portion of $\dot{V}E$ distributed to gas-exchanging lung units. The remainder of $\dot{V}E$ from the standpoint of gas exchange is "wasted" and considered as dead-space ventilation ($\dot{V}D$), thus the equation:

$$\dot{V}A = \dot{V}E - \dot{V}D$$

$\dot{V}A$ may be decreased as a result of either an inadequate $\dot{V}E$ (hypoventilation) or an increase in $\dot{V}D$ (ventilation to perfusion ($\dot{V}A/\dot{Q}$) inequality). Calculation of the alveolar-arterial PO_2 gradient is clinically useful in differentiating the two processes (see Chapter 33). The alveolar-arterial PO_2 gradient will be normal in pure alveolar hypoventilation and increased in diseases of the lung parenchyma that lead to $\dot{V}A/\dot{Q}$ inequality (Table 34-1).

Hypoventilation may result from reduced respiratory center drive, mechanical defects in the chest wall, or respiratory muscle failure. The clinical importance of altera-

INDICATIONS FOR MECHANICAL VENTILATION

Ventilatory for Pump Failure
1. Reduced respiratory center drive
2. Mechanical defects of the chest wall
3. Respiratory muscle fatigue

Inefficient Pulmonary Gas Exchange
1. Reduction in functional residual capacity (FRC)
2. Ventilation-perfusion mismatch
3. Shunt

Table 34-1 **DIFFERENTIAL DIAGNOSIS OF VENTILATORY PUMP FAILURE AND FAILURE OF GAS EXCHANGE**

	Ventilatory Pump Failure	Failure of Gas Exchange
$Paco_2$	Increased	Usually normal or decreased; sometimes increased
Pao_2	Decreased	Decreased
Alveolar-arterial Po_2 gradient	Normal if pure alveolar hypoventilation	Markedly increased

tions in respiratory drive indices has not been explored in critically ill patients, although starvation has been demonstrated to decrease the hypoxic ventilatory response. Although apnea is an obvious indication for mechanical ventilation, periodic apneas of Cheyne-Stokes respiration should be excluded since this abnormal breathing pattern does not often lead to respiratory failure. Certain acute conditions predispose to a reduction in respiratory drive such as drug overdose, general anesthesia, cerebrovascular accident, and head injury; a decision based on clinical and available laboratory information needs to be made regarding institution of mechanical ventilation in these situations.

Abnormalities in the chest wall are an uncommon cause of ventilatory failure. These may be developmental in nature, as in kyphoscoliosis or obesity, or the result of trauma such as flail chest. Because instability of the rib cage with associated paradoxical respiration and *pendelluft* was considered a major determinant of morbidity in flail chest, surgical fixation was initially employed. In 1956 internal pneumatic splintage was ushered in by Avery, Morch, and Benson,[9] and the addition of positive end-expiratory pressure (PEEP) was later considered important in stabilizing the rib cage.[39] More recent studies indicate that conservative management is preferable and mechanical ventilation should be reserved for patients having the same indications as with any other cause of acute respiratory failure.[126,137,155] The basic tenet of this approach is that pulmonary dysfunction is caused by the underlying parenchymal injury resulting from pulmonary contusion and not related to paradoxic motion of the rib cage.

The importance of respiratory muscle dysfunction and fatigue as a factor in the development of ventilatory failure has long been underestimated, and its clinical importance is still incompletely understood.[127] Fatigue may be defined as the acute loss of ability of a muscle to continue to generate a required force during muscle contraction. This may lead to hypoventilation and inadequate lung expansion with consequent atelectasis and pneumonia. Predisposing conditions to respiratory muscle fatigue include generalized neuromuscular diseases, disorders in which greater energy demands increase work of breathing, and disease states associated with reduced energy supplies such as anemia, reduced cardiac output, or malnutrition. Respiratory muscle dysfunction may be a more common occurrence in the postoperative state than previously realized, particularly following abdominal surgery. Laboratory measurements useful in assessing respiratory muscle strength include maximum inspiratory pressure (MIP) and maximum voluntary ventilation (MVV), although these parameters have been evaluated in the context of weaning rather than when mechanical ventilation is instituted.[132] However, it is often difficult to obtain accurate values in critically ill patients. Respiratory muscle fatigue can often be detected clinically by observing the pattern of abdominal and chest wall motion. The diaphragm is the principal inspiratory muscle in the supine patient, and the outward motion of the abdomen during inspiration is the clinical marker of diaphragmatic breathing. Respiratory alternans (the alternation of diaphragmatic and accessory muscle activation) followed by abdominal paradox (the inward motion of the abdomen during inspiration) has been described as preceding respiratory failure resulting from respiratory muscle fatigue.[31]

Rest is the only known treatment of muscle fatigue, and for the respiratory muscles this means artificial ventilation. Rochester, Braun, and Laine[128] demonstrated that artificial ventilation in patients with pulmonary disease reduced diaphragmatic electromyogram activity to about 10% of the value during spontaneous respiration. The optimal duration of the rest period is unclear, although complete recovery from clinically important fatigue may take as long as 24 hours. Mechanical ventilation will also be associated with a reduction in the oxygen cost of breathing. Normally the respiratory muscles account for less than 5% of the total oxygen consumption, compared to 25% in patients being weaned from mechanical ventilation[62] or even more when the work of breathing is increased resulting from obstruction or decreased compliance. In this situation the increased oxygen demands by the respiratory muscles may deprive other body tissues of oxygen and may represent the source of lactic acid in patients with decreased cardiac output. If cardiac output is low or oxygen demands high, there may be insufficient oxygen for the muscles themselves. In an experimental model of cardiogenic shock in dogs, Aubier, Trippenbach, and Roussos[8] found that all of the animals died of ventilatory failure resulting from respiratory muscle fatigue. Despite similar levels of cardiac output, a second group of animals who were mechanically ventilated survived probably because of the reduced oxygen cost of breathing.

In patients with underlying lung disease hypercapnia results from increasing $\dot{V}A/\dot{Q}$ inequality despite increases in $\dot{V}E$. Since dead-space ventilation often increases to greater than 50%, patients must increase $\dot{V}E$ sufficient to maintain a $\dot{V}A$ appropriate for the carbon dioxide production

($\dot{V}CO_2$). Most often, patients are able to accomplish this and may even have a low $PaCO_2$ if accompanying hypoxemia further drives the respiratory center. However, if the degree of lung disease progresses beyond the ability to increase $\dot{V}E$ or if complications such as fatigue, sedation, or postoperative pain limit the ventilatory response, hypercapnia will develop.

The decision to increase ventilation by the institution of mechanical ventilation in these situations should not be based on a single PCO_2 value. Previous arterial blood gas (ABG) results are helpful because they reflect the patient's course and response to conservative therapy. Consideration of the blood pH is essential to distinguish acute from chronic ventilatory failure since patients compensate for long-standing elevation in PCO_2 by retaining bicarbonate (HCO_3^-) and achieving a near normal pH. In acute respiratory acidosis an increase in $PaCO_2$ of 1 mm Hg is associated with a decrease in pH of 0.008 units, whereas the same increase in $PaCO_2$ in chronic respiratory acidosis results in a fall in pH of only 0.003 units. The pH and PCO_2 values must be considered within the clinical setting because there is no threshold value at which mechanical ventilation should be instituted. As a rule of thumb, many clinicians consider a pH value below 7.3 an indication for mechanical ventilation, and in one study of complications during mechanical ventilation, morbidity and mortality were increased in patients with pH values below 7.3.[165]

Inefficient Pulmonary Gas Exchange

Inefficient pulmonary gas exchange resulting in hypoxemia is usually the result of right-to-left shunting or $\dot{V}A/Q$ mismatch (see Table 34-1). In contrast to hypercapnic acidosis, hypoxemia is a less well-defined indication for mechanical ventilation (because it can often be corrected by more conservative therapeutic modalities such as supplemental oxygen delivered by nasal cannula or face mask).

In the setting of $\dot{V}A/\dot{Q}$ inequality, a common cause of abnormal gas exchange in patients with acute or chronic airway obstruction or diffuse infiltrative lung disease, the effect of mechanical ventilation is variable. Most often the matching of ventilation and perfusion is unaffected, although occasionally it may be improved or even worsened.[41] Because oxygenation can usually be improved by increasing the fraction of inspired oxygen (FIO_2), the major indication for mechanical ventilation in these patients is to maintain sufficient $\dot{V}E$ to prevent hypercapnia. Conversely, the presence of a shunt, as seen in conditions such as cardiac or noncardiogenic pulmonary edema, diffuse atelectasis, and lung contusion, is more amenable to direct treatment with mechanical ventilation. In addition, the increase in FIO_2 required to oxygenate adequately the patient with a significant intrapulmonary shunt commonly reaches levels that by themselves are likely to induce lung damage. In this setting mechanical ventilation is mainly beneficial by increasing functional residual capacity (FRC) and thus recruiting previously collapsed or fluid-filled lung units. The degree to which lung volume can be increased depends on the increase in mean airway pressure. This in turn can be manipulated by the size of the tidal volume (V_T) or the addition of positive end-expiratory pressure (PEEP) as will be discussed later.

Table 34-2 **CLASSIFICATION OF MECHANICAL VENTILATORS**

Type	Tracheal Intubation Required	Predictable Tidal Volume	Easy to Employ
Negative-pressure ventilator	−	−	−
Positive-pressure ventilators			
Pressure-cycled	+	−	−
Volume-cycled	+	+	+
Time-cycled	+	+	+
High-frequency ventilation	+/−	−	−

SELECTION OF MECHANICAL VENTILATOR

Ventilators are best classified according to the method by which pressure is applied to achieve lung inflation (Table 34-2).

Negative-Pressure Ventilators

Negative-pressure ventilators attempt to duplicate spontaneous breathing. The entire body or the chest and upper abdomen is placed within an "iron-lung" or tank respirator, and the head and neck protrude to the atmosphere. Subatmospheric pressure is intermittently applied around the body, creating a pressure gradient that promotes air entry into the lungs. $\dot{V}E$ can be altered by changing the negative pressure or the respiratory rate. Although this ventilator type is of more historical than practical interest, there are still patients afflicted by poliomyelitis during the epidemic of the early 1950s who use such ventilators either continuously or periodically. In addition to the tank respirator, the modified cuirass ventilator is occasionally used, consisting of a rigid shell placed around the rib cage with an attached hose connecting the inner surface to an electric pump or modified vacuum cleaner that is intermittently activated. Negative-pressure ventilators have many disadvantages: they can only be applied in the control mode, and adequate ventilation is unlikely in the presence of reduced lung compliance or increased airway resistance. In addition, it is difficult to deliver adequate nursing care to such patients without removing them from the tank.

Positive-Pressure Ventilators

Almost all of the present mechanical ventilators employ the principle of intermittent positive-pressure ventilation (IPPV), which produces lung inflation by generating and applying positive pressure to the airways. Formerly positive-pressure ventilators were operated by a wheel-and-piston or rotary-drive mechanism, so-called single-circuit ventilators. Power from a motor turns a wheel to which is attached a connecting rod, which in turn is attached to the shaft of the piston. Forward movement of the piston produces a sine wave pattern of airflow; variations in inspiratory waveform have generally been overemphasized and are rarely of clinical concern. Currently many ventilators have double circuits, in which the driving power circuit is separated from the patient circuit. External pneumatic pressure, generated in a manner similar to single-circuit

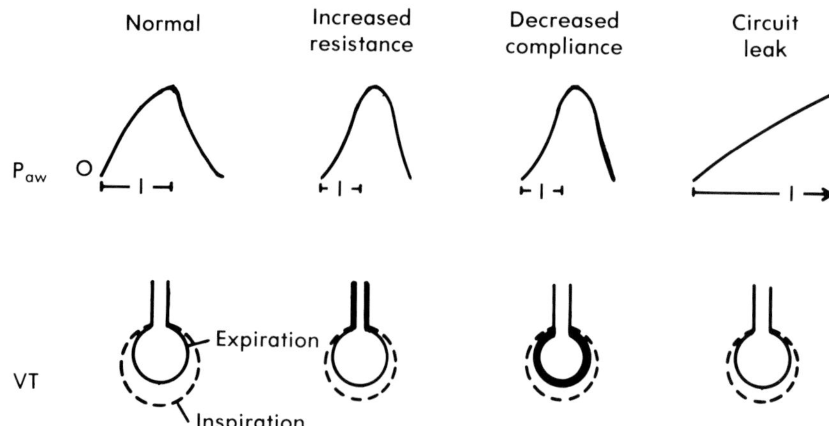

Fig. 34-1 Airway pressure and lung volume change during mechanical ventilation with a pressure-cycled ventilator in patients with normal lung function, increased airway resistance, and decreased compliance, and with ventilator malfunction due to a circuit leak (P_{aw}, Airway pressure; *VT*, tidal volume; *I*, inspiration). (From Tobin, M.J., and Dantzker, D.R.: Mechanical ventilation and weaning. In Dantzker, D.R., editor: Cardiopulmonary critical care, Orlando, 1986, Grune & Stratton, Inc.)

ventilators, compresses a bellows in the patient circuit that delivers inspiratory gas to the patient. Positive-pressure ventilators are classified according to their cycling mechanism: pressure-cycled, volume-cycled, or time-cycled. High-frequency ventilation employs a variety of these cycling mechanisms.

Pressure-cycled Ventilators

Pressure-cycled ventilators allow gas to flow into the lungs until a present airway pressure is reached. When this pressure limit is achieved, an exhalation valve opens allowing exhalation to ensue unless inflation hold is employed. The delivered volume varies with changes in airway resistance, lung compliance, and the integrity of the ventilator circuit (Fig. 34-1). Airway obstruction will result in a low tidal volume (VT) and premature cycling of the ventilator. The same problem arises in a hyperventilating patient who exhales while the ventilator is in the inspiratory phase and reaches the pressure limit prematurely. Most pressure-cycled machines cannot generate airway pressures above 40 to 50 cm H_2O and do not achieve adequate ventilation in patients with low lung compliance. Additionally, most lack a system to deliver controlled concentrations of oxygen and a means to apply positive end-expiratory pressure (PEEP). Significant alterations in the inspiratory time signify problems with this ventilator system. A reduction in inspiratory time may result from airway obstruction or a kink in the ventilator tubing, whereas indefinite prolongation of inspiration indicates a leak in the circuit, since the cycling pressure is not reached. An advantage of these ventilators is that they operate from a pressurized gas source and are immune to electrical power failure. Their many limitations have restricted the use of pressure-cycled ventilators to intermittent positive-pressure breathing (IPPB) therapy or ventilation of comatose patients with normal lungs.

Time-cycled Ventilators

Time-cycled ventilators allow gas to flow to the patient until a preset inspiratory time is achieved. Desired VT is attained by adjusting inspiratory time and flow rate or by setting the VE and respiratory rate. Since these ventilators are capable of generating high airway pressure, they are used interchangeably with volume-cycled ventilators in critically ill patients. Examples of time-cycled ventilators include the Siemens Servo 900 and the Monaghan 225 fluidic ventilator; although the former ventilator is dependent on an electrical power source, the latter can operate from a pressurized gas source.

Volume-cycled Ventilators

Volume-cycled ventilators are currently the most widely used mechanical ventilators. Gas flows to the patient until a preset volume is delivered into the ventilator circuit, even if a very high airway pressure must be generated. To minimize the risk of barotrauma a safety (''pop-off'') pressure limit is set and when exceeded the excess volume is vented to the atmosphere (Fig. 34-2). The presence of a leak in the circuit is detected by monitoring exhaled volume, which will be less than the volume delivered by the ventilator. Volume-cycled ventilators are commonly assumed to guarantee delivery of a predetermined volume to the patient. As the delivered volume is distributed between the patient and the ventilator circuit, a reduction in lung compliance will decrease the volume delivered to the patient and increase the volume of gas compressed within the circuit. This may go undetected because the total volume of gas measured by the spirometer on the expiratory limb of the circuit may show no change.

High-frequency Ventilation

In 1967 Borg, Eriksson, and Sjostrand,[22] reasoning that the ventilation achieved by a lower VT and rapid respiratory rate would reduce the complications of barotrauma and cardiac depression, developed the technique of high-frequency positive-pressure ventilations (HFPPV). Today three mechanical systems are capable of delivering high-frequency ventilation (HFV) (Table 34-3): high-frequency positive-pressure ventilation (HFPPV), high-frequency jet ventilation (HFJV), and high-frequency oscillation (HFO).

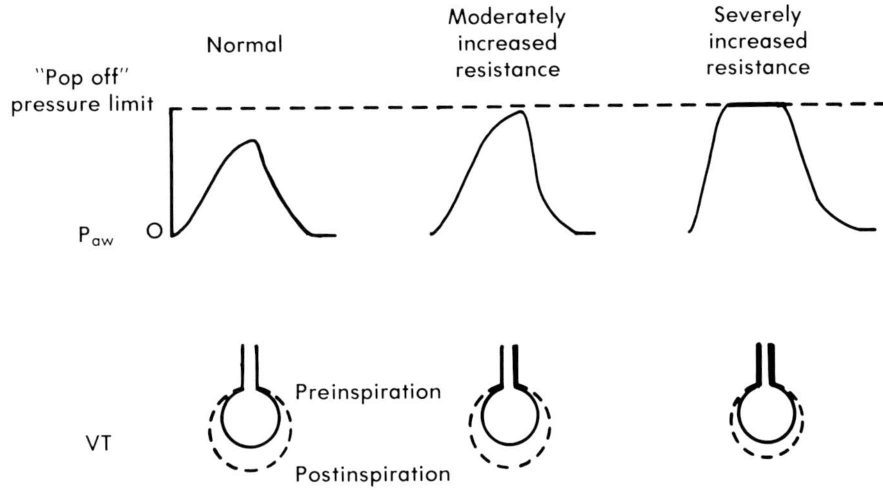

Fig. 34-2 Airway pressure and lung volume change during mechanical ventilation with a volume-cycled ventilator in patients with normal lung function and moderately and severely increased airway resistance. (*P_{aw}*, airway pressure; *VT*, tidal volume). (From Tobin, M.J., and Dantzker, D.R.: Mechanical ventilation and weaning. In Dantzker D.R., editor: Cardiopulmonary critical care, Orlando, 1986, Grune & Stratton, Inc.)

Table 34-3 **HIGH-FREQUENCY VENTILATION**

Type*	Ventilator Rate/Min	Bulk Gas Flow	Gas Entrainment
HFPPV	60-100	+	−
HFJV	60-200	+	+
HFO	600-3000	−	−

*HFPPV, High-frequency positive-pressure ventilation; HFVJ, high-frequency jet ventilation; HFO, high-frequency oscillation.

HFPPV employs a time-cycled, volume-controlled ventilator that delivers a VT usually approaching that of calculated VD, i.e., 60 to 100 ml/cycle. Gas is insufflated using a pneumatic valve principle without external air entrainment. HFJV delivers gas through a small catheter, either a 14- or 16-gauge intracath within the trachea, or a similar bore channel incorporated into the wall of the endotracheal tube opening at its tip. The gas is delivered under high pressure (10 to 60 psi) at frequencies of 60 to 200 cycles per minute. Unlike HFPPV, HFJV entrains humidified gas through the Bernoulli principle, thus enhancing delivered VT. Both HFPPV and HFJV use a compressed gas source and an on-off valve with variable frequency and insufflation time, and require a circuit in which compressible volume and tubing compliance is virtually eliminated. The systems generally remain open to allow continuous egress of gas at high volumes from the lungs. HFO differs from the other techniques in that it moves a volume of gas to and fro in the airway without bulk flow at rates of 10 to 50 Hz (600 to 3000 cycles per minute). Oxygen is added through a bias flow system as required by metabolic rate, and carbon dioxide is removed by an absorber or bypass circuit.

Although several investigators testify to the benefits of HFV, there are no convincing data to state that HFV is indicated in any specific clinical situation, and it must be considered an experimental form of therapy. Although the reduction in peak airway pressure during HFV might decrease the risk of barotrauma, there are no published data to support this speculation. Reduction in peak airway pressure may also be responsible for the reports[27] of successful application of HFV in bronchopleural fistula, a challenging problem in the ventilator-dependent patient. Large portions of the delivered VT escape through the fistula, and attempts to compensate by increasing VT or inspiratory airway pressure usually compound the problem. Lowering the VT and peak airway pressure with HFV may be critical in reducing the magnitude of the air leak and improving $\dot{V}A$. Similarly improved management of tracheoesophageal fistulae is a potential indication for HFV. Mean airway pressure is reduced with HFPPV, thereby reducing the unfavorable effects of mechanical ventilation on cardiac output.[141] In contrast, a PEEP of 5 to 8 cm H_2O is generated by HFJV, so that mean airway pressure may be higher with HFJV than with conventional ventilators.[69] In the only published controlled comparison of HFJV and conventional ventilation in humans, peak airway pressure was lower with HFJV, but mean airway pressure and arterial oxygen and carbon dioxide tensions were similar.[135] HFV has been extensively employed for ventilatory support during laryngoscopy, bronchoscopy, and microlaryngeal and tracheal surgery.[22] Because this ventilator technique may be employed through an uncuffed endotracheal tube or without a tube, cuff trauma to the trachea might be reduced and aspiration might be minimized or prevented by the high-velocity egress of expiratory gas.[69]

Cessation of spontaneous respiration with HFV, possibly caused by the stimulation of muscle spindle or stretch receptors, has been described by Borg, Eriksson, and Sjostrand[22] and postulated as an advantage during thoracoabdominal surgery and as a facilitator in weaning patients who breathe out of phase with the ventilator. Other investigators have noted that spontaneous respiration continues during HFV. Perhaps one of the more attractive features of HFJV is its application in patients with a predictably difficult intubation.[141] A catheter is percutaneously inserted through the cricothyroid membrane, which allows oxygen administration and ventilation by jet insufflation.

A similar system can be adapted when endotracheal tubes are changed in unstable patients by the use of a shortened nasogastric tube as a guiding stylet, through which jet ventilation is delivered.

Several problems exist with HFV. It is more difficult to predict the effect of selected ventilator settings on gas exchange with HFV than with conventional mechanical ventilation, predisposing to initial hypocapnia or hypercapnia. Catheter kinking and obstruction may occur with HFJV. A satisfactory system to humidify rapidly flowing gases remains to be developed.[140] Current methods for monitoring mechanical ventilation are not relevant to HFV; the small VT cannot be measured by conventional equipment, and system pressures may be inaccurate because technology for transducing pressure is inadequate. Restriction of exhalation during HFJV dramatically increases airway pressure because of the high minute volumes delivered. A similar problem may occur during application of HFJV in patients who do not have an endotracheal tube and who intentionally or reflexly close their larynx. Displacement of the insufflating jet catheter may produce rapid insufflation of the gastrointestinal tract with resulting tension pneumoperitoneum.[141] Inadequate experience has been obtained with HFV to know if the technique itself contributes to lung injury.

VENTILATOR MODES

A confusing array of acronyms clouds any discussion of mechanical ventilator modes and settings (Fig. 34-3). Ventilator modes differ from each other in the amount of spontaneous respiration performed by the patient.

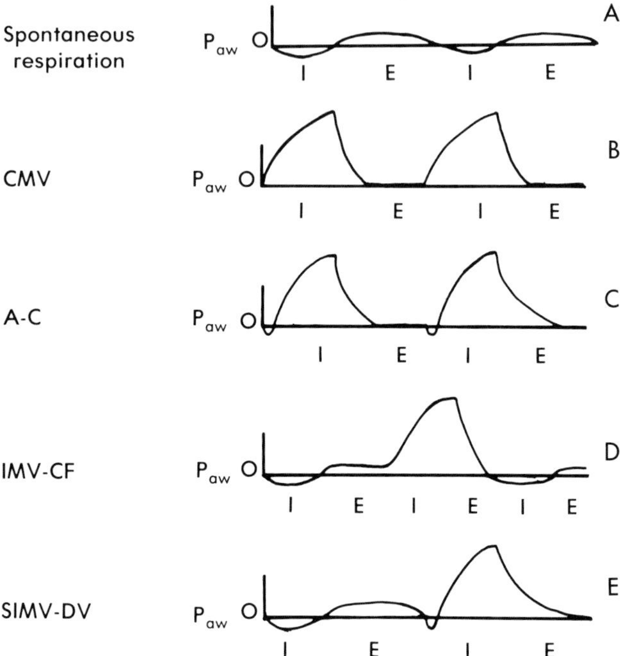

Fig. 34-3 Airway pressure during various modes of ventilation. (*CMV,* controlled mechanical ventilation; *AC,* assist control; *IMV - CF,* intermittent mandatory ventilation delivered by a continuous flow circuit; *SIMV - DV,* synchronized intermittent mandatory ventilation delivered by a demand valve circuit.) (From Tobin, M.J., and Dantzker, D.R.: Mechanical ventilation and weaning. In Dantzker D.R., editor: Cardiopulmonary critical care, Orlando, 1986, Grune & Stratton, Inc.)

Spontaneous Respiration

With certain ventilators the patient can breathe spontaneously through the ventilator circuit when the ventilator rate is set to zero. Through use of the ventilator circuit, positive airway pressure may also be applied during spontaneous breathing. Although such ventilator circuits are attractive in the ease of transition from mechanical ventilation to spontaneous breathing, there is considerable variation in circuit resistance with different ventilator designs and associated significant increases in the work of breathing, compared to breathing on a T-tube circuit.

Controlled Mechanical Ventilation

During controlled mechanical ventilation (CMV) (see Fig. 34-3, *B*), the ventilator delivers a preset number of breaths per minute of a preset volume. The patient cannot trigger additional breaths, as in the case of assist-control (A-C) mode, or achieve successful spontaneous respiration, as in the case of intermittent mandatory ventilation. However, the use of CMV does not prevent the patient from attempting to breathe spontaneously, which results in an asynchronous ventilatory pattern since the ventilator will not respond to the patient's effort. This leads to patient apprehension and air hunger. Because of these disadvantages CMV is restricted to patients who are apneic as a result of brain damage, sedation, or muscle paralysis. In the past CMV was advocated in patients with flail chests where spontaneous breathing was considered deleterious *(vide supra)*. Properly functioning ventilator alarms are crucial to the safe employment of CMV.

Assist-Control Ventilation

In the assist-control (A-C) mode the ventilator delivers a breath either when triggered by the patient's inspiratory effort (see Fig. 34-3, *C*) or independently if such an effort does not occur within a preselected time period. All breaths are delivered under positive pressure by the machine, but unlike CMV the preset rate can be exceeded by the patient's triggering effort. If the patient's spontaneous rate falls below the preset "back-up" rate, controlled ventilation is provided until the patient's spontaneous rate exceeds the "back-up" rate. Clinical experience with A-C indicates that it is a considerable improvement over CMV, but there are no published controlled studies comparing the effect of the two modes of mechanical ventilation. Particular attention must be paid to proper adjustment of the sensitivity of the patient-triggering mechanism. The ventilator may autocycle if it is too sensitive, but a very large negative pressure may be required for triggering when the ventilator is overly insensitive, which is likely to occur when the patient is receiving PEEP.

Intermittent Mandatory Ventilation

Intermittent mandatory ventilation (IMV) was initiated as a new mode of mechanical ventilation in 1971,[89] but an identical unnamed mode of ventilation had been available for almost two decades with the Engstrom ventilator.[19,57] IMV differs from other modes of ventilation in that the patient can breathe spontaneously but in addition receives periodic positive-pressure breaths at a preset volume and rate from the ventilator (see Fig. 34-3, *D* and *E*). Initially this was accomplished by connecting the patient's endotracheal tube to two parallel ventilatory circuits, a conventional ventilator and a side-arm with a reservoir bag, that share a common source of oxygen (Fig. 34-4). When the ventilator delivers a breath, the positive pressure in the circuit closes the one-way valve of the side-arm system and the mushroom valve on the expiratory tubing, thus ensuring delivery of the volume to the patient. On completion of the inspiration, positive pressure is no longer transmitted from the ventilator to the expiratory valve, which opens and permits the exhaled volume to exit through the expiratory tubing. During a spontaneous breath, the generated negative pressure in the expiratory and inspiratory tubing respectively cause the expiratory valve to inflate occluding the expiratory tubing and cause the one-way valve to open allowing inhalation of gas from the side-arm and reservoir bag. Without a reservoir bag the peak flow rate of the system, limited by the maximum flow generated by the hospital's source of compressed air and oxygen, may be insufficient to meet the patient's peak inspiratory flow rate, so that the resulting excessive reduction in the patient's air-way pressure will cause an increase in the work of breathing. During spontaneous expiration, the increase in tubing pressure causes the expiratory valve to open and the side-arm one-way valve to close.

Proponents of IMV have suggested several advantages of this mode of ventilation but have provided little factual support. IMV is believed to prevent the patient from "fighting" the ventilator, reduce muscle paralysis and the need for sedation, reduce the likelihood of respiratory alkalemia, improve cardiac output, improve alveolar ventilation and matching of ventilation and perfusion,[49] reduce oxygen consumption,[51] reduce muscle fatigue and paradoxical breathing,[3] and achieve more rapid weaning from the ventilator.[50] The available supporting evidence is minimal and mainly derived from comparisons of IMV and CMV. Because CMV is rarely employed anymore, a comparison between A-C and IMV would be more meaningful, but such information is scant. Recently two preliminary studies have noted little difference in the risk of respiratory alkalemia with A-C compared to IMV, even in patients with head injury.[40,82] The pH was slightly lower in the IMV patients, but this was because of increased carbon dioxide production as a result of spontaneous breathing.

It has been reported that persistence of spontaneous breathing during IMV reduces the detrimental effects of positive-pressure ventilation on cardiac function.[53,90] Other investigators have observed little or no difference in cardiac output when IMV was compared to A-C[80] or CMV.[163] These results are inconclusive, but IMV might be of value in individual patients who demonstrate significant hemodynamic deterioration during positive-pressure ventilation, provided that they are not adversely affected by the associated increased work of breathing. Because diaphragmatic motion differs during spontaneous breathing and mechanical ventilation,[65] it has been proposed that interspersion of spontaneous breaths between ventilator-delivered breaths would achieve a more normal matching of ventilation and perfusion.[48,111] There is no existing evidence to support this speculation because ventilation-perfusion profiles have never been assessed in patients receiving IMV.

Downs and associates[52] noted a lower oxygen consumption during IMV compared to CMV, but the opposite has been observed by other investigators[62] and by the same investigators in another study.[130] In a preliminary investigation Rodriguez, Lefrak, and Sinks[129] compared A-C and IMV and noted an increase in oxygen consumption of 98 cc/min during IMV, probably consequent to the increased oxygen cost of breathing by the respiratory muscles. Maintaining spontaneous breathing activity during the period of mechanical ventilation has been suggested as a means of exercising the respiratory muscles, thus preserving muscle tone and diminishing muscle dysfunction during wean-

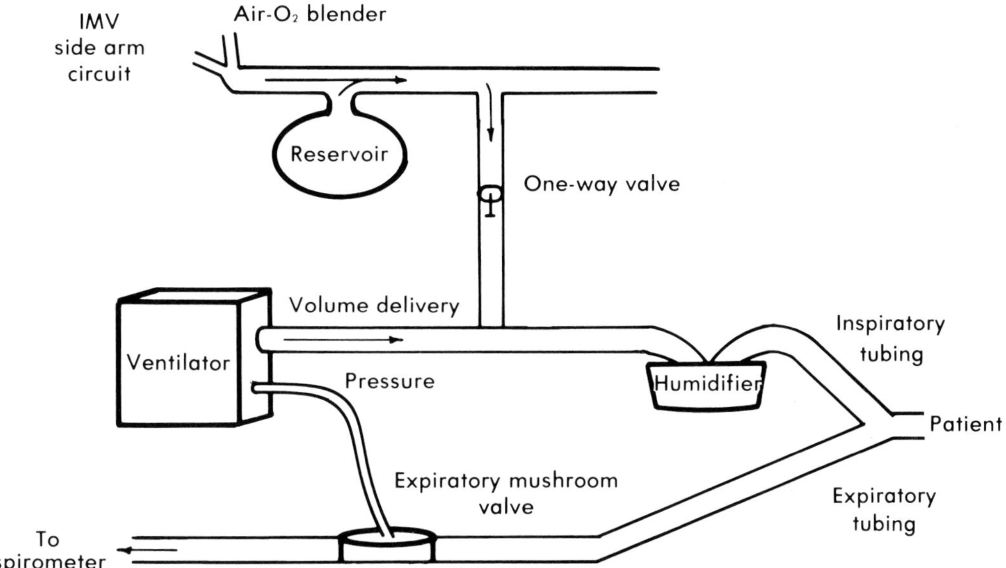

Fig. 34-4 Delivery of intermittent mandatory ventilation by continuous flow circuit. See text for details. (From Tobin, M.J., and Dantzker, D.R.: Mechanical ventilation and weaning. In Dantzker, D.R., editor: Cardiopulmonary critical care, Orlando, 1986, Grune & Stratton, Inc.)

ing.[52] However, evidence that respiratory muscle dysfunction is a consequence of prolonged mechanical ventilation or that IMV will prevent this is lacking.

In one study[103] ventilator-induced barotrauma was less with IMV compared to CMV despite employment of higher peak airway pressure and PEEP with the former ventilator mode. The beneficial effect may be related to fewer ventilator-induced peak airway pressures and the absence of bucking on the ventilator with IMV.

In patients who can sustain spontaneous respiration but have hypoxemia caused by reduced sighing (e.g., during general anesthesia), intermittent lung distention rather than continuous artifical ventilation is the appropriate therapy. Conceptually the former (i.e., intermittent lung distention) is one of the most attractive indications for IMV because it can be used as an intermittent sighing technique to maintain lung distention independently of the need for mechanical ventilation to maintain pH homeostasis.

Several potential disadvantages exist with IMV. Adaptation of mechanical ventilators designed to deliver A-C and CMV requires the addition of a separate side-arm circuit (see Fig. 34-4). The extra tubing has been faulted as increasing the cost and risk of disconnection,[115] and the continuous gas flow has been considered wasteful. Incorrect assembly with reversal of unidirectional valves prohibits inhalation from the side-arm and facilitates the escape of ventilator-delivered volume into the side-arm. Respiratory monitoring is compromised by the addition of a continuous flow circuit because the high gas flows contaminate the patient's exhaled gas, making it difficult to monitor V_T, $\dot{V}_E$, or expired carbon dioxide concentration; Weled, Winfrey, and Downs[162] have described a monitoring system to circumvent this problem. Shortly after the introduction of IMV, Sahn and Lakshminarayan[131] questioned whether delivery of a mandated breath coinciding with a patient's spontaneous inspiration might result in overdistention of the lung and predispose it to rupture. This is an extremely unlikely possibility because the achieved lung volume is likely to be less than a sigh, which has long been employed during mechanical ventilation without adverse consequence.

Subsequently synchronized IMV (SIMV) (see Fig. 34-3, *E*) was introduced to circumvent this problem of "stacking," economize on gas supply, and improve respiratory monitoring and alarm capacity. SIMV is achieved by incorporating a demand valve that senses either a fall in airway pressure (Bennett MA-2, Siemens Servo) or the generation of gas flow (Bourns Bear), causing the valve to open and deliver fresh gas flow during spontaneous inspiration. In a comparison of IMV and SIMV in experimental animals no difference was observed in intrapleural pressure or cardiopulmonary function except for a slight increase in peak and mean airway pressure with IMV.[74] Unfortunately, ventilators incorporating SIMV demand-valve circuits and technologically advanced monitoring systems proliferated before adequate assessment of their limitations. It has now been repeatedly demonstrated that the excessive reduction in airway pressure required to activate the demand valve combined with the inadequate delivery of instantaneous gas flow may cause a twofold or greater increase in the work of breathing[70,71] and oxygen consumption.[75] As the distance between the demand-valve pressure sensor and the patient increases, the volume of tubing that must be decompressed before sensor activation increases with further increase in the work of breathing. Modeling studies with the Bennett MA-2 ventilator indicate that up to 23 cm H_2O change in airway pressure may be necessary to open the demand valve in the presence of a shortened inspiratory time.[112] Such demand-valve gas delivery systems are dependent on the maximum flow rate that is available from the hospital source, usually 75 to 125 L/min, but a patient's peak inspiratory flow rate may exceed 200 L/min. The consequent pressure drop during inspiration is equivalent to breathing against an occluded airway causing air hunger and discomfort and increasing the work of breathing. Incorporation of a reservoir bag into the system provides both a volume and pressure reservoir to match more closely the patient's peak inspiratory flow rate and thus minimize the work of breathing.

Further problems with these newer ventilators are likely to be unraveled with time. Only recently has it been discovered that the number of ventilator-delivered breaths by the Bennett MA2 + 2 may differ significantly from the preset rate when employed in the SIMV mode.[56] This may result in a reduction of 25% to 60% of mechanically delivered breaths. The cause is unknown but thought to be related to the manner in which the patient's breathing pattern interacts with the machine cycle time. This has gone undetected probably because the electronic rate counter on the machine indicates the sum of the patient's spontaneous rate and the mandatory breaths from the ventilator. Thus a reduction in the machine-delivered breaths can only be detected by visually and aurally differentiating the origin of each breath at the bedside and counting the number of ventilator-delivered breaths. A final problem concerning the use of IMV in patients with marked ventilatory limitation is that unexpected alterations in the required level of ventilatory support, as with the sudden development of a mucous plug, will be unavailable.

Independent Lung Ventilation

In a small number of patients with asymmetric lung disease the response to conventional mechanical ventilation may be disappointing, particularly if administration of PEEP is a critical factor. If there are marked differences in compliance between the lungs, most of the ventilator-delivered volume will tend to go to the good lung with consequent risk of barotrauma, but the stiff lung will receive an inadequate volume. Selective intubation of each mainstem bronchus using a double-lumen endotracheal tube and application of independent mechanical ventilation has been attempted in this situation. The endotracheal tube lumina may be connected to separate ventilators and various techniques used to synchronize them.[26] The circuit of a single ventilator may be modified so the lungs are synchronously ventilated,[121] or separate ventilators have been employed without any attempt at synchronization.[77] Employment of independent lung ventilation is rarely necessary.

In summary, mechanical ventilation is delivered to the vast majority of patients in the A-C or IMV modes. Although certain advantages may be derived with either A-C or IMV in individual patients, there is generally little to choose between the two modes of ventilation. Of greater importance is optimal selection of the ventilator settings.

VENTILATOR SETTINGS

The initial ventilator settings are estimated on the basis of the patient's clinical condition and are generally altered after obtaining an arterial blood gas (ABG) or other laboratory information. Several adjustments may be necessary before achieving satisfactory settings, and repeated assessment of these settings is desirable as the patient's condition changes. Although a large variety of variables concerning ventilation is encountered, only three of these can be set independently, and these in turn determine the balance of the variables, e.g., V_T rate and inspiratory flow rate or $\dot{V}_E$ rate and inspiration to expiration ratio.

Inspired Oxygen Fraction

Initially the inspired oxygen fraction (FIO_2) is deliberately set at a high value, often 1.0, to ensure adequate oxygenation. After a 20-minute period an ABG sample is obtained and the FIO_2 adjusted according to the patient's PaO_2. Although many predictive equations have been created to aid in the selection of a proper FIO_2 none are sufficiently accurate to substitute for a trial-and-error approach. Generally a PaO_2 of 60 to 90 mm Hg is sought because this achieves near maximal oxygen saturation. Rarely a deliberately high PaO_2 is desirable. Administration of a high FIO_2 to patients with carbon monoxide intoxication helps by displacing carbon monoxide from hemoglobin and improving oxygen supply to the tissues. High PaO_2 levels may aid in the elimination of nitrogen from a pneumothorax, but this is not as important in patients on a mechanical ventilator as is rapid insertion of a chest tube. Whether a high PaO_2 aids in the resolution of an air embolus is unknown, but it is a reasonable approach in patients who cannot be placed in a hyperbaric oxygen chamber. When therapeutic hyperventilation is employed in patients with brain injury, the resulting vasoconstriction causes a low tissue PO_2 that in turn may benefit from seeking a deliberately high PaO_2, although this is an unproven speculation.

The response to a change in the FIO_2 depends on the underlying pathophysiology, as a shunt responds less well to increased FIO_2 than hypoventilation or $\dot{V}A/\dot{Q}$ mismatch. At high levels of shunt PaO_2 increases little as FIO_2 is augmented, but even the small increase in PaO_2 will significantly increase arterial oxygen content and enhance oxygen delivery[43] but at the risk of increasing potential oxygen toxicity. Supply of oxygen to the tissues depends not only on PaO_2 but also on hemoglobin concentration and cardiac output, both of which should be optimized in patients with hypoxemia.

Administration of a high FIO_2 causes a number of disturbances, including ciliary dysfunction, tracheobronchitis, impaired alveolar macrophage function, and parenchymal injury resembling the adult respiratory distress syndrome (ARDS). The onset of oxygen toxicity is difficult to determine because patients requiring high FIO_2 for prolonged periods often have pulmonary disease resembling that expected with oxygen toxicity. Prolonged exposure to an FIO_2 of 1 is clearly toxic, whereas an FIO_2 of 0.5 is generally considered safe for several weeks, although this recommendation is not based on solid clinical or experimental data. For an FIO_2 between 0.5 and 1 the duration of safe exposure before the onset of toxicity in humans is unknown. But it is clear that there is more to fear from severe hypoxemia than the potential for oxygen toxicity.

Tidal Volume

In spontaneously breathing subjects tidal volume (VT) and respiratory rate are normally adjusted to achieve a $\dot{V}E$ that is least costly to the average force developed by the respiratory muscles. During unhindered breathing, normal VT is 380 cc, with a range of 200 to 550 cc.[153] Tidal volume is fairly constant from breath to breath, but intermittent sighs or yawns, arbitrarily defined as at least three times normal VT occur three to four times/hour in healthy young subjects and up to 12 times/hour in old healthy subjects. Obviously these standards of normal ventilation are unlikely to apply in acute respiratory failure.

In a classic study performed in 1959, Mead and Collier[106] demonstrated that animals mechanically ventilated with normal VT, but without deep breaths developed a drop in lung compliance. This has been repeatedly conformed in healthy subjects breathing spontaneously[61] or receiving mechanical ventilation.[14,55] Reduction in lung compliance with consequent hypoxemia was reversed by active or passive deep breaths and attributed to progressive alveolar collapse. These early investigations were generally confined to patients receiving general anesthesia, and intermittent hyperinflation was recommended in such patients even when spontaneous respiration was adequate in terms of carbon dioxide elimination.[15] Subsequently manufacturers included an automatic sighing feature on mechanical ventilators.

More recent studies have suggested that incorporation of a sighing mechanism during mechanical ventilation provides little benefit. Housley, Louzada, and Becklake[78] found that three signs given over 1 minute to nine patients on prolonged mechanical ventilation produced no significant change in lung compliance or arterial oxygenation. The mode of mechanical ventilation or the usual VT was not stated, and the sigh volume varied from 1.13 to 3.7 times the preceding VT. Levine, Gilbert, and Auchincloss[96] studied 10 patients receiving mechanical ventilation in the A-C mode with a preset VT of 400 to 500 cc. Employment of five sighs set at double the control VT and spaced over a 20-minute period resulted in no change in PaO_2. Although these studies suffer from some methodologic problems, they suggest that conscious patients may not benefit from periodic hyperinflations in the same manner as patients receiving general anesthesia.

In the early 1970s the therapeutic approach to lung volume alterations was reexamined in the light of the developing concepts of small airway disease and closing volume. Closing volume, the lung volume at which small airways especially in the lung bases begin to close, is normally less than the end-expiratory level, i.e., functional residual capacity (FRC). Thus small airways remain patent throughout the respiratory cycle. A reduction in FRC, a common accompaniment of general anesthesia, may cause the FRC to fall below the closing volume and lead to airway closure during some portion of the breath with resultant hypoxemia. With this in mind, Visick, Fairley, and Hickey[158] believed that mechanical ventilation with a large VT would be more likely to exceed closing volume for a greater portion of the breath and found that a VT of 15 cc/kg produced a significant improvement in lung compliance and alveolar arterial oxygen gradient compared to using a VT of 5 cc/kg. In a further study comparing ventilator-delivered volumes of 5 and 10 cc/kg, Weenig and associates[160] observed no difference in alveolar-arterial oxygen gradient between the two delivered volumes when FRC exceeded closing volume but noted a significant reduction in the gradient when closing volume was increased. Additional studies by Cheney,[28] Burnham, Martin, and Cheney,[25] and Cheney and Martin[29] comparing various VT with PEEP in an oleic acid model of lung injury demonstrated that improvement in PaO_2 with increasing VT or PEEP was directly related to the mean airway pressure independent of the method employed, thus suggesting that an increase in FRC is the mechanism for the improvement in gas exchange with employment of high VT. Although PaO_2 increased with increasing VT, the benefit was offset by a similar reduction in cardiac output.

As a result of these studies, a VT of 10 to 15 cc/kg without intermittent sighs is commonly recommended during mechanical ventilation. Although a high VT may be desirable in patients with infiltrative lung disease and reduced lung compliance, in the hope of improving the PaO_2 consequent to increases in mean airway pressure a lower VT may be preferable in patients with normal lungs or with increased lung compliance such as emphysema; however, these hypotheses have never been tested. An additional disadvantage of selecting a high VT is that it may alter respiratory center drive and respiratory muscle proprioception and adversely influence subsequent weaning from the ventilator.

When the VT is set, it is important to remember that part of the volume expands the connecting tubing and is not delivered to the patient. Today tubing compliance in most ventilator circuits is 2 to 3 cc/cm H_2O peak pressure and varies with tubing length, diameter, and structure. With fall in pressure the tubing contracts, and because this volume is measured as exhaled volume by the spirometer placed on the expiratory limb of the circuit, the reduction in delivered volume to the patient may go unnoticed.

Respiratory Frequency

Choosing the number of breaths delivered by the ventilator depends on the employed mode of mechanical ventilation. With CMV the rate is chosen on the basis of the selected VT so that the resulting $\dot{V}E$ is likely to achieve a satisfactory $PaCO_2$, i.e., the normal range (35 to 45 mm Hg) in patients with sudden acute respiratory acidosis or a higher value (see the section on weaning failure) in patients with acute-on-chronic respiratory acidosis. If IMV is employed, it is probably best initially to set the ventilator at a rate close to that being employed by the patient at the preselected VT; subsequently the ventilator rate can be reduced if desired, depending on clinical and laboratory assessment. If hypoventilation with respiratory acidosis is present, a higher back-up rate will be required. The IMV rate should be lower than the patient's overall rate if hyperventilation independent of chemoreceptor stimulation is present. With A-C the backup rate should be set dependent on the patient's needs. This can be higher than the spontaneous rate if an increase in $\dot{V}E$ is required. If the patient's spontaneous rate is adequate, the back-up rate should be set at 2 to 4 breaths below this value to prevent serious hypoventilation if the patient fails to trigger the machine.

Inspiratory Flow Rate

Depending on the individual ventilator, the inspiratory flow rate (IFR) may be independently adjusted or determined by altering VT, rate, and the inspiratory to expiratory time (I:E) ratio. Although a wide range is available, an IFR of approximately 60 L/min is most commonly employed. Increasing IFR during mechanical ventilation of normal lungs causes maldistribution of ventilation with a consequent increase in the alveolar-arterial PO_2 gradient,[17] venous admixture[63] and dead space to VT ratio (VD/VT),[58] and reduced dynamic lung compliance.[10] In contrast, these indices improve during mechanical ventilation of patients with chronic airway obstruction as IFR is increased from 40 to 100 L/min.[32] This beneficial effect is probably the result of a reduction in the I:E ratio accompanying the faster IFR with prolongation of expiration allowing air trapping regions to empty more completely. No benefit was observed with faster IFRs in patients with respiratory failure of other causes. Increasing the IFR is likely to result in a higher peak intrathoracic pressure, although the mean airway pressure may be lessened.[33] Although little adjustment in IFR is necessary in most patients, fine tuning is occasionally required to achieve optimal gas exchange with the least hemodynamic embarrassment. Also, altering the IFR may increase the comfort of some patients who are restless while receiving mechanical ventilation.

Inspiration-Expiration Pattern

The inspiration to expiration (I:E) ratio may be adjusted directly on some time-cycled ventilators, whereas it is indirectly determined by regulating VT, frequency, and IFR on volume-cycled ventilators. Inflation hold, a setting available on many ventilators, provides a short pause at end-inspiration. This modality has been advocated as a means to allow compensation for differences in time-constants between obstructed and unobstructed lung regions.[97] Most experience has been obtained in the management of infantile respiratory distress syndrome where it has been successfully employed, but it has been less enthusiastically received in the adult arena. Instead, a short I:E ratio of about 1:2 is usually sought to minimize gas trapping and mean intrathoracic pressure.

Peak Airway Pressure

In contrast to pressure-cycled ventilators where peak airway pressure is the primary regulator of ventilator-delivered volume, peak airway pressure is indirectly determined by VT, IFR, lung compliance, and airway resistance with volume-cycled ventilators. Theoretically these ventilators deliver a preset VT irrespective of the pressure required but an adjustable "pop-off" pressure limit is usually selected to prevent the development of excessive pressure with consequent risk of barotrauma.

Positive End-Expiratory Pressure

No area of ventilator therapy has aroused so much controversy as positive end-expiratory pressure (PEEP), as testified by the voluminous literature that has accumulated on this topic. A detailed review of PEEP is beyond the scope of this chapter, and selective aspects can only be considered. Application of positive pressure during exhalation was first employed by Barach[11] in 1935 and was shown to be particularly valuable in the prevention of hypoxemia in World War II pilots flying airplanes with nonpressurized cabins. At altitudes of 40,000 to 50,000 feet inspiration of pure oxygen did not prevent hypoxemia, and a pressurized oxygen delivery source was employed. Over the following 20 years this therapeutic principle remained dormant until its resurrection by Ashbaugh and associates[7] in the management of adult respiratory disease syndrome (ARDS). Since then it has received a reputation as a panacea for all respiratory ills.

Patients with diffuse infiltrative lung disease usually have profound hypoxemia associated with reduced lung volumes (measured as FRC), resulting predominantly in an increased shunt. The low FRC places the end-expiratory level of the patient's tidal breath on the low flat portion of the pressure-volume curve of the lung. Similar to increasing V_T, the increased mean airway pressure consequent to the application of PEEP raises the FRC, allowing subsequent inspiration to occur on the steep portion of the curve. This increase in FRC with PEEP occurs because of the recruitment of collapsed alveoli or an increase in the end-expiratory volume of fluid-filled alveoli and thus a reduction in the shunt. Claims that PEEP may actually reduce the extravascular water content of the lung have not been supported by experimental data, although a redistribution of the water from the alveolar to the interstitial compartment may take place as a result of the increase in FRC. Under certain experimental circumstances lung water content can actually be shown to increase as PEEP is applied.

Further increase in FRC by additional PEEP will cause the lung volume to reach the upper flat portion of the pressure-volume curve with deleterious effects on cardiac output and gas exchange and risk of barotrauma. This is particularly a problem when lung compliance is normal or increased as in emphysema. Although PEEP is not ordinarily used in this setting, the combination of a rapid respiratory rate and shortened expiratory time may lead to the unwitting institution of PEEP resulting from a failure of adequate emptying of obstructed lung units ("auto PEEP").[101] Likewise, hyperexpansion of normal regions of the lung may occur as a consequence of the use of PEEP in unilateral lung disease.

Since there is no general consensus as to the goals of PEEP therapy, it is difficult to evaluate its effect in published studies or state the indications for its use. In patients with diffuse lung disease PEEP generally improves arterial oxygenation. This is beneficial because it ameliorates life-threatening hypoxemia and decreases exposure to a potentially toxic FI_{O_2}. Some physicians consider no other applications of PEEP and strive for satisfactory arterial oxygenation (usually oxygen saturation of 90%) with the least level of PEEP. Others believe that PEEP modifies the natural course of lung disease and, with the notion that PEEP has a prophylactic effect against developing lung injury, employ it in patients who achieve a satisfactory Pa_{O_2} with low FI_{O_2}. Prevention of ARDS with prophylactic PEEP has been reported by three groups of investigators,[134,156,161] but these studies are flawed by imprecise criteria for defining ARDS. In a recent controlled study of 92 patients with precise criteria for defining the risk of ARDS and its development, Pepe, Hudson, and Carrico[113] found that 8 cm H_2O PEEP applied at an average of 2.4 hours after risk onset failed to prevent the development of ARDS.

In patients with established lung disease employment of very high levels of PEEP have been recommended to achieve a shunt of 15% or less.[68] Using this goal in a multicentered, uncontrolled study of 28 patients with acute respiratory insufficiency, Kirby and associates[90] employed up to 43 cm H_2O PEEP and observed a survival rate of 17 out of 28 patients (61% with only one death directly caused by respiratory failure) compared to the usually reported survival of 40% to 50%.[64] These results have never been corroborated, and "super" PEEP has never been studied in a prospective, controlled manner. This level of PEEP is associated with profound hemodynamic depression, and administration of fluids and pressors is necessary to diminish the fall in cardiac output. The demonstrable risks of such supportive therapy outweigh the theoretical benefits of "super" PEEP therapy, unless subsequent studies show that PEEP has beneficial effects beyond the observed improvement in pulmonary gas exchange (see the description on the hemodynamic effects of PEEP).

Despite the lack of concrete data regarding the benefits of PEEP, some guidelines of its application should be followed when it is considered necessary therapy. A number of acronyms (Fig. 34-5) are applied, depending on the cir-

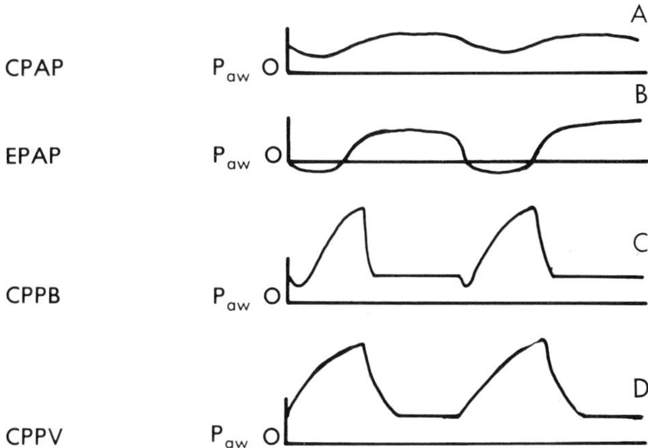

Fig. 34-5 Airway pressure tracings of positive pressure delivered during expiration. (*CPAP*, continuous positive airway pressure; *EPAP*, expiratory positive airway pressure; *CPPB*, continuous positive pressure breathing; *CPPV*, continuous positive pressure ventilation.) (From Tobin, M.J., and Dantzker, D.R.: Mechanical ventilation and weaning. In Dantzker, D.R., editor: Orlando, 1986, Grune & Stratton, Inc.)

cuit involved in the generation of PEEP and whether PEEP is combined with spontaneous breathing or mechanical ventilation. The term *PEEP* only implies that airway pressure is positive at completion of expiration and provides no information on airway pressure during inspiration. In spontaneously breathing patients, whether intubated or not, PEEP can be used in two ways: continuous positive airway pressure (CPAP) or expiratory positive airway pressure (EPAP) (Fig. 34-6). During CPAP (see Fig. 34-5, *A*), airway pressure remains positive during inspiration and expiration, although there is the usual small pressure drop during inspiration compared to expiration. During EPAP (see Fig. 34-5, *B*), airway pressure returns to or drops below atmospheric level during inspiration; the extent of the excursion depends on the preselected level of PEEP.

Changes in airway pressure during use of PEEP in patients being ventilated in the A-C mode will depend on whether the machine is PEEP-compensated, because then the patient generates a sub-PEEP pressure rather than a subatmospheric pressure to trigger the ventilator. With a PEEP-compensated machine airway pressure is maintained continuously above atmospheric pressure and so is labeled continuous positive-pressure breathing (CPPB) (see Fig. 34-5, *C*). If mechanical ventilation is used in the CMV mode, airway pressure is continuously elevated, never falling below the set level, and is designated continuous positive-pressure ventilation (CPPV) (see Fig. 34-5, *D*). During IMV when delivered with PEEP, the patient receives CPPV during the ventilator-delivered breaths and CPAP during spontaneous breathing; however, the form of CPAP differs significantly, depending on the circuit used in its delivery (Fig. 34-7). If a demand-valve apparatus is employed, as in many of the currently available ventilators, an inspiratory effort with a considerable drop in airway pressure is necessary to open the demand valve. At that point the delivered bulk flow may be less than the patient's peak inspiratory flow rate, with consequent depressurization of the system and a further drop in inspiratory airway pressure and increase in the work of breathing. Such problems are obviated with a continuous flow circuit. These differences are of more than academic interest, especially in spontaneously breathing patients or those being ventilated in the IMV mode. The need to develop a subatmospheric breath increases the work of breathing and may result in fatigue of the respiratory muscles, thus worsening the underlying problem. The higher the PEEP, the more likely this is to occur because the pressure change is greater and at high lung volumes the respiratory muscles begin contracting at a shorter length, thus decreasing their efficiency and making them more prone to fatigue.

Consideration must also be given to the type of valve that generates PEEP; threshold valves are preferable to flow-resistance valves (Fig. 34-8). A threshold valve provides a predictable constant expiratory pressure regardless of the respiratory rate or inspiratory flow rate, whereas a flow-resistance valve generates a pressure that is directly proportional to the flow of gas. When a flow-resistance valve is combined with a low flow rate and prolonged expiratory time, the airway pressure will gradually fall to atmospheric level, thus providing "expiratory retard"

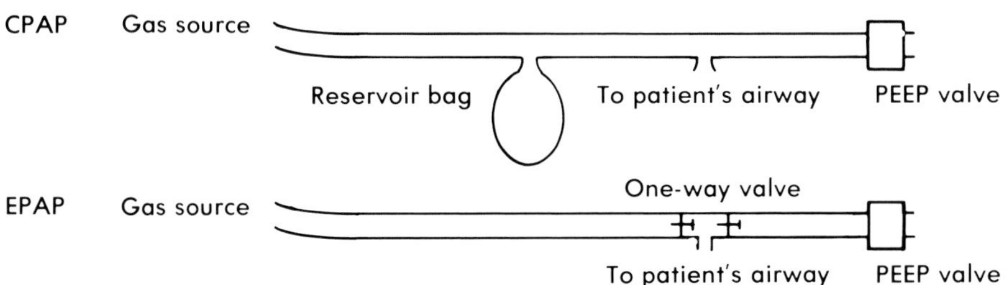

Fig. 34-6 Circuit for delivery of continuous positive airway pressure *(CPAP)* and expiratory positive airway pressure *(EPAP)*. (From Tobin, M.J., and Dantzker, D.R.: Mechanical ventilation and weaning. In Dantzker, D.R., editor: Cardiopulmonary critical care, Orlando, 1986, Grune & Stratton, Inc.)

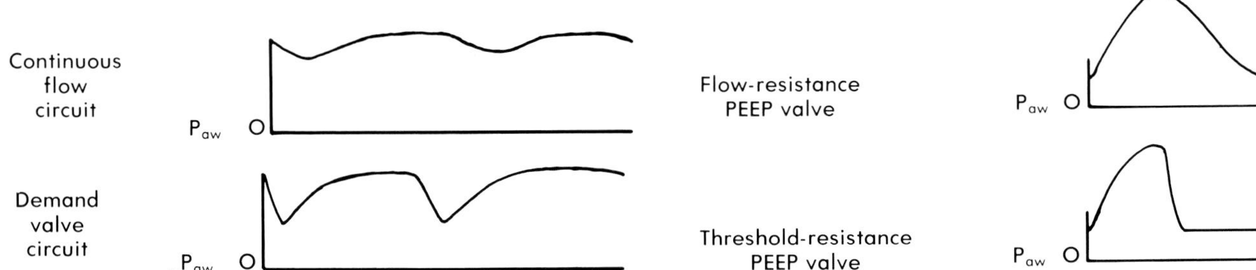

Fig. 34-7 Airway pressure during delivery of continuous positive airway pressure (CPAP) by a continuous flow and demand valve circuits. (From Tobin, M.J., and Dantzker, D.R.: Mechanical ventilation and weaning. In Dantzker, D.R., editor: Cardiopulmonary critical care, Orlando, 1986, Grune & Stratton, Inc.)

Fig. 34-8 Airway pressure during delivery of positive end-expiratory pressure *(PEEP)* by flow-resistance and threshold-resistance valves. (From Tobin, M.J., and Dantzker, D.R.: Mechanical ventilation and weaning. In Dantzker, D.R., editor: Cardiopulmonary critical care, Orlando, 1986, Grune & Stratton, Inc.)

rather than PEEP. Conversely, high expiratory flow rates generate dangerously high PEEP levels. Contrary to manufacturers' statements, few PEEP valves are pure threshold resistors, and most have additional flow-resistance properties. Occasionally clinicians increase the source flow of gas to a breathing circuit to minimize the drop in airway pressure during inspiration, but when this higher flow rate traverses a PEEP valve with flow-resistance properties,the level of PEEP is further increased.

When PEEP is being instituted, it should be done in a systematic manner[79]: (1) ensure that PEEP is the only variable being changed; (2) employ stepwise increments of 3 to 5 cm H_2O; (3) minimize the time interval between changes, e.g., 20 minutes to increase the likelihood that the response reflects the action of PEEP rather than change in the patient's underlying condition; a beneficial response is usually demonstrable within 10 min,[92] although the response is sometimes slower[4,94]; (4) make appropriate evaluations of the response to each change. Many suggestions have been made to determine the optimal level of PEEP, but none have been demonstrated as clearly superior. Also, since there is no uniform, verifiable method of judging the adequacy of tissue oxygenation, the totality of the effect must be evaluated. As a general rule, best PEEP is achieved when the FIO_2 can be reduced to an acceptable level without compromising oxygen delivery.

A similar methodical approach should be employed at the time PEEP is being reduced or discontinued, because abrupt cessation may produce hypoxemia that takes hours or days to reverse or requires the reinstitution of PEEP at a higher level than before its suspension,[99] a response that is observed in one third of PEEP reductions. A systematic approach has been developed to achieve a 90% rate of successful PEEP reduction.[159] Patient criteria include a stable ($\geq$ 12 hours), nonseptic patient who shows resolution or substantial improvement in the disease process initially requiring PEEP and who achieves a PaO_2 of $>$ 80 on an FIO_2 of 0.40 or less. Baseline PaO_2 is measured, PEEP is reduced by 5 cm H_2O, PaO_2 measurement is repeated after 3 minutes and PEEP is returned to the previous level until the PaO_2 measurement is available. If PaO_2 falls by less than 20% of the baseline value, there is a 90% likelihood of successful PEEP reduction, whereas reinstituion of PEEP at 3 minutes in a patient failing the test returns PaO_2 to the baseline level.

In patients receiving PEEP observation of the pressure monitor during the inspiratory phase often reveals a fall in airway pressure. This should not be interpreted as a fall in the positive-pressure gradient against the lung because the fall in pleural pressure balances the fall in airway pressure and transpulmonary pressure remains unchanged. Because transpulmonary pressure is responsible for alteration in lung volume, there is no change in the PEEP effect.

In the belief that glottic closure during talking, coughing, and swallowing is partly responsible for the normal level of FRC, some physicians recommend employment of small levels of PEEP, e.g., 5 cm H_2O, in all intubated patients. Studies in newborn infants have shown that some require active maintenance of FRC, which is accomplished by either increasing expiratory resistance in the upper airway or the persistence of inspiratory muscle activity into expiration. However, the extension of this phenomenon to all patients is premature, especially because even small levels of PEEP may have detrimental consequences and since studies in adults have revealed conflicting results.[108,124]

PEEP has a number of adverse effects, many of which are extensions of those observed with mechanical ventilation in general, and will be reviewed in a later section of this chapter.

VENTILATOR CIRCUIT

Employment of different modes of mechanical ventilation has aroused considerable debate and controversy, but surprisingly little attention has been paid to the ideal functioning of the equipment.

Although optimal plumbing of the equipment may be of little significance during CMV or A-C, it becomes critical during spontaneous breathing or IMV. Important factors include the resistance of the endotracheal tube, equipment dead space, resistance of the inspiratory circuit and humidifier, circuit compliance and gas compression volume, resistance of the expiratory circuit, competence and resistance of the unidirectional valve, and separation of the patient circuit. Marked differences in performance of the systems in different ventilators have a considerable influence on the work of breathing and patient tolerance of the circuit.

The endotracheal tube produces varying degrees of resistance primarily depending on its internal diameter and the flow rates encountered. Sullivan et al.[46,148] calculated the following resistances for endotracheal tubes of different sizes using two flow rates.

	Tube Resistance (cm H_2O/L/sec)	
Tube Size	Flow Rate (0.5 L/sec)	Flow Rate (1 L/sec)
6	11.5	20.2
7	5.9	9.9
8	3.7	6.1

Because normal airway resistance is usually less than 2 cm H_2O/L/sec, spontaneous breathing through an endotracheal tube imposes a significant flow-resistive load. This resistance is further increased by 40% if the tube is not optimally positioned and maximally straight.[73] Obviously obstruction of the tube resulting from poor pulmonary toilet will aggravate the situation. Similarly the humidifier may present a considerable flow resistance to spontaneous breathing because all the inhaled gas must flow through a relatively small hole in a column that is submerged 2 to 3 cm below the water surface.[119] At a flow rate of 120 L/min that mimics the peak inspiratory flow rate of a tachypneic patient, a pressure drop of 11 cm H_2O was recorded with the widely used Bennett humidifier. If such a humidifier is incorporated into a spontaneous breathing circuit, the underwater valve in the tower should be removed. Gas passing through the humidifier is heated, and during subsequent cooling in the inspiratory tubing, condensation with "rain out" occurs. If the resulting accumulation of water is not drained from the tubing, further resistance to breathing results.

In a continuous-flow IMV setup (see Fig. 34-4) a one-way valve (IMV valve) is inserted to prevent rebreathing of exhaled gas. If this valve is incompetent, it will permit exhaled gas to enter the inspiratory circuit and thus increase dead space. Furthermore, part of the ventilator-delivered breath will exit through this valve and thus reduce the volume delivered to the patient. The valve should have a low resistance to minimize the amount of work required to open it. A continuous gas flow and reservoir helps by preventing a significant drop in airway pressure during inspiration.

The construction of the expiratory limb of the circuit may also lead to significant increases in the work of breathing, particularly when PEEP is employed. Positive airway pressure during exhalation may be generated by threshold-resistance or flow-resistance valves (see Fig. 34-8). Ideally a threshold-resistance valve should be used because this provides a constant expiratory pressure irrespective of the respiratory rate or flow rate. In contrast, flow-resistance valves provide retarded expiration, and expiratory airway pressure will return to atmospheric level if expiratory time permits. With high flow rates, a flow-resistance valve causes an increase in PEEP above that expected.

COMPLICATIONS OF MECHANICAL VENTILATION

The successful management of crtically ill patients with mechanical ventilation has resulted in a new group of iatrogenic diseases. Almost every ventilator patient develops some complication, usually of an inconsequential nature but sometimes lethal.[165] These complications are listed below and discussed and summarized in the sections that follow:

1. Complications related to endotracheal and tracheostomy tubes
2. Infection
3. Barotrauma
4. Hemodynamic impairment
5. Renal impairment
6. Hepatic impairment
7. Increased intracranial pressure

Complications of Endotracheal and Tracheostomy Tubes

A large number of complications have been described in association with intubation, varying in type as to whether a nasal or oral endotracheal tube has been used or a tracheostomy has been performed. Almost two thirds of all intubations performed in intensive care units are associated with some complication.[143,144] The placement of an endotracheal tube may be complicated by tooth avulsion (oral tube), nasal bleeding (nasal tube), retropharyngeal or hypopharyngeal perforation, vocal cord hematoma, pulmonary aspiration (8% to 19%), arrhythmias (30% to 60%), and cardiac arrest (<1%).[143] During the time that the tube is in place, laryngeal injury with posterior glottic ulceration (50% to 100%), laryngeal hematoma (5% to 10%), or subglottic stenosis may occur, but most of these lesions heal spontaneously and severe sequelae are uncommon. The cuff may cause tracheal mucosal ulcers (15%), tracheal dilation (2% to 5%), or rarely tracheoesophageal fistula or tracheal rupture. Additional problems of intubation include kinking or disconnection of the tube, herniation of the cuff over the tip of the tube, paranasal complications of sinusitis and otitis with nasal tubes, and pulmonary aspiration. During extubation, stridor caused by laryngeal edema occurs in less than 1% of patients. Problems continue after extubation and include hoarseness (80% to 100%), laryngeal granuloma (3%), laryngeal stenosis (0.5%), laryngeal incompetence with aspiration (22% to 35%), tracheal stenosis, and tracheomalacia (usually mild).

Complications with tracheostomy are generally greater than with endotracheal intubation. The operation may be complicated by subcutaneous or mediastinal emphysema (13%), hemorrhage (5% to 10%), pneumothorax (5%), or other visceral injury. While the tube is in place, problems include stomal infection and bleeding (>30%), tracheoarterial fistula (<1%), and cuff complications similar to those with an endotracheal tube. Decannulation may be difficult in 6% of patients because of the combination of a tight stoma and the creation of a stiff flange by the deflated cuff. Following decannulation, asymptomatic and symptomatic stomal-site tracheal stenosis may be observed (16% and 8%, respectively), but tracheal stenosis at the cuff site is much less frequent. Other rare complications include tracheal granuloma, tracheal dilation, and tracheomalacia.

To minimize the risk of complications intubation should ideally be performed under controlled conditions with all the necessary equipment and medication at hand. Only tubes with a high-volume, low-pressure cuff should be employed, and once in place the lowest cuff pressure to seal the airway should be used. Proper equipment[35] should be available to monitor cuff pressure several times a day. If the period of mechanical ventilation is longer than expected, the question of replacing an endotracheal tube with a tracheostomy arises. With increasing acceptance of prolonged endotracheal intubation the indications for a tracheostomy have become less clearly defined. Management should be individualized, and a tracheostomy should not be performed only because an endotracheal tube has been in place a certain number of days. Endotracheal tubes are satisfactorily tolerated for up to 3 weeks, but if mechanical ventilation is likely to be required for longer periods of time, tracheostomy should be considered early in the course because of ease of long-term airway maintenance. No prospective study has examined the rate of complications with endotracheal intubation extending beyond 3 weeks.

Infection

Mechanically ventilated patients are particularly susceptible to infection, partly because of the adverse effects of ventilator management and also because of the severity of the underlying disease that precipitated ventilator therapy. Various aspects of ventilator management contribute to the development of pneumonia. The endotracheal or tracheostomy tube bypasses the natural defenses of the upper airway and provide a direct conduit for transmission of organisms to the lower airways. Mucociliary transport is depressed by the tube cuff, high FIO_2, and employment of a suction catheter. Macrophage and neutrophil function are also depressed by a high FIO_2. Pulmonary aspiration still occurs despite the presence of an airway tube. Respiratory therapy equipment, a major cause of nosocomial pneumonia in the 1960s, is an uncommon culprit today. Formerly this type of pneumonia resulted from contamination of mainsteam nebulizers, which generated microaerosols containing large numbers of gram-negative bacilli. Today most ventilators employ humidifying cascades that do not generate aerosols and so are rarely a direct cause of pneumonia. However, the tubing and condensate of a ventilator circuit is inevitably contaminated by organisms from the patient's own respiratory tract.[37] Studies indicate that if reasonable care is taken of the ventilator circuit, the tubing need be changed only every 48 hours.[36]

Development of pneumonia is an ominous occurrence because of its high mortality rate; 50% of patients admitted to intensive care units with pneumonia die compared to 4% of patients without pneumonia.[146] Part of this gloomy outcome results from the notorious difficulty in identifying which organisms are responsible for a lower respiratory tract infection,[152] because there is a general consensus that antibiotic therapy is more satisfactory when the infecting organism is known. Conventional bacteriologic methods usually provide misleading information because of the high rate of airway colonization, which occurs in 75% to 100% of patients in intensive care units with a primary respiratory diagnosis. Routine culture of secretions aspirated through an endotracheal tube, with the inevitable recovery of a potpourri of potential pathogens, is unhelpful and may result in serious patient mismanagement. Blood cultures are valuable when positive, but negative results are more common despite severe pneumonia. Quantitative cultures of samples obtained from the lower airways by a fiberoptic bronchoscope, employing the plugged telescoping catheter brush technique, probably provide the least misleading information and may be used when accurate bacteriologic diagnosis is considered necessary.

Barotrauma

The reported incidence of pulmonary barotrauma varies from 0.5%[38] to 40%[21] of mechanically ventilated patients and is diagnosed by the presence of pneumomediastinum, subpleural air cysts, subcutaneous emphysema, pneumothorax, or pneumoperitoneum. The likely sequence of events in the development of interstitial emphysema was described in 1944[100] by Macklin and Macklin, who applied gas under pressure to the trachea of cats. Development of a high-pressure gradient between the alveolus and the adjacent vascular sheet causes the overdistended alveolus to rupture, forcing gas into the interstitial tissue of the underlying perivascular sheath. The gas may dissect centrally along the pulmonary vessels to the mediastinum and rupture into the pericardium either through an area of weakness where the perivascular sheaths join the pericardial collagenous tissue at the point of continuity between the parietal and visceral pleura, or through a pericardial window. The gas may also dissect along the perivascular sheath to the periphery and form subpleural air cysts.[2] A pneumothorax results when gas ruptures through the mediastinal pleura into the pleural space or by rupture of a subpleural cyst. Further gas dissection into the fascial planes of the neck and upper torso results in subcutaneous emphysema. The gas may also progress down through the loosely packed periesophageal areolar tissue into the retroperitoneal space and rupture into the peritoneal cavity, mimicking perforation of an intra-abdominal viscus. A greater hazard is rupture into a bronchial vein with transport to the left heart and the resultant systemic air embolism.

Predisposing risk factors for barotrauma include the presence of underlying lung disease, especially chronic obstructive pulmonary disease (COPD)[93] and aspiration pneumonia[45] or other forms of ARDS.[114] Younger patients appear to have a higher incidence,[114,165] but the reason is unknown. The introduction of volume-cycled ventilators was associated with an increased incidence in one study compared to pressure-cycled ventilators (7% and 0.25%, respectively), as a result of the higher airway pressures with the former.[145] Although an increase in regional lung volume is the primary determinant of alveolar rupture, the increase in regional lung volume is associated with an increase in airway pressure. The increase in airway pressure is more easily measured. Peak airway pressure rather than the level of PEEP is the more important risk factor.[114] In a recent study no patient whose peak airway pressure was less than 60 cm H_2O developed barotrauma, whereas barotrauma occurred in 43% of patients with pressures in excess of 70 cm H_2O. The risk with PEEP was less clearly demonstrable, but the rate of barotrauma increased as PEEP was increased above 8 cm H_2O; other investigators have not documented an increase in barotrauma with PEEP.[38,93] Selection of V_T is important because employment of high V_T, e.g., 22 cc/kg, in the past[21] was associated with an excessive incidence of barotrauma. Additionally, the incidence should be less with a threshold valve rather than a flow-resistance PEEP valve. Intravascular volume status may be important because pneumothorax is more common in the presence of volume depletion.[95] Presumably optimal intravascular volume expands the perivascular sheaths surrounding alveoli and reduces the pressure gradient responsible for alveolar rupture.

Subcutaneous emphysema is rarely of consequence in itself. The risk of a subsequent pneumothorax in mechanically ventilated patients with mediastinal or subcutaneous emphysema has not been defined, although all patients with subpleural air cysts have developed a pneumothorax if positive-pressure ventilation is continued.[2] Pneumothoraces developing in mechanically ventilated patients may be devastating because 60% to 90% are under tension.[2] A thoracostomy tray should be kept at the bedside if such an eventuality is anticipated, and in one series[165] this precaution prevented an increase in mortality in patients developing pneumothoraces. The presence of a pneumopericardium in adults is rarely of any hemodynamic consequence,[81] but infants who develop tamponade experience a very high mortality.[31] In infants needle aspiration of their air frequently results in complications; insertion of a pericardial tube under direct vision is preferable.

A bronchopleural fistula is present following insertion of a chest tube if air continues to leak for longer than 24 hours.[116] The consequences of this complication include failure of lung reexpansion, loss of V_T and PEEP with worsening gas exchange, pleural infection, and unwanted cycling of the ventilator as chest-tube suction pressure may be transmitted to the airway and trigger the machine. Bronchopleural fistula poses a difficult management problem in mechanically ventilated patients, and several therapeutic approaches have been attempted.[120] Mechanical ventilation should be discontinued if possible or the least number of ventilator-delivered breaths compatible with adequate gas exchange should be employed to minimize the bronchopleural pressure gradient. In this situation IMV is likely to be advantageous, although this suggestion is unsupported by scientific data. Reduction in delivered VT should be attempted and chest-tube suction applied at the lowest satisfactory level or discontinued. PEEP should probably be avoided. Several aggressive approaches have been attempted with questionable success including application of PEEP to the chest tube, occlusion of the chest tube during part of the ventilator cycle, independent ventilation of the two lungs, and direct surgical repair. The recent application of high-frequency ventilation appears more satisfactory but has yet to be investigated in a controlled fashion.

Hemodynamic Effects

Reduction in cardiac output is a well-recognized consequence of mechanical ventilation, particularly when PEEP or a high VT is employed. Decreased venous return is the major mechanism, although this may go unnoticed because positive-pressure ventilation increases all intrathoracic pressures, including central venous pressure and pulmonary capillary wedge pressure as clinical measurement of these indices is referenced to atmospheric pressure. Cardiac performance, however, depends on transmural pressures (intracardiac minus intrapleural pressure), which are often reduced despite elevations of the same indices referenced to atmospheric pressure. In addition, pulmonary vascular resistance is elevated as the increase in lung volume stretches the intra-alveolar vessels, reducing their lumina and increasing the resistance to flow. This increase in right ventricular afterload may result in a shift of the interventricular septum to the left with consequent reduction in left ventricular compliance. Earlier suggestions of a reduction in myocardial contractility appear to be unfounded. If not directly measured, this decrease in cardiac output may go unnoticed because it is often associated with a reduction in the shunt causing an increase in PaO_2 and may thus be considered beneficial by the misinformed.[42] The hemodynamic response depends on the patient's fluid status, and any reduction in cardiac output consequent to an increase in pleural pressure can be countered by an increase in the intravascular fluid volume, but only at the expense of an increase in microvascular pressures. Aggravation of hypoxemia with an increase in shunt may also occur in patients with a patent foramen ovale because elevation in pulmonary vascular resistance favors flow through the intracardiac route.

Renal Effects

Alterations in renal function with reduced urine volume and sodium excretion have been described in mechanically ventilated patients.[138] Again, reduction in venous return and decreased cardiac output causing alterations in renal blood flow appears to be the predominant mechanism.[18] Sympathetic nervous system activation and release of antidiuretic hormone (ADH) and renin attempt to compensate for the alterations in arterial pressure and are no longer considered directly responsible for the decrease in urine volume or free-water clearance.[18] Similar mechanisms are presumably responsible for the alterations in renal function with PEEP.

Hepatic Effects

Mechanically ventilated patients often display evidence of hepatic dysfunction of diverse etiology. This usually reflects severity of the underlying systemic disease, but the splanchnic effects of positive-pressure ventilation may be a contributing factor. PEEP increases the resistance to hepatic venous outflow[85] and to bile flow at the choledochoduodenal junction,[86] probably as a consequence of vascular engorgement of the mucosal lining of the intramural common bile duct. Sulfobromophthalein sodium excretion, used as an index of hepatic function, is markedly impaired during positive-pressive ventilation.[87]

Cerebral Effects

Patients sustaining a severe head injury frequently have a coexisting lung injury requiring mechanical ventilation. Application of PEEP causes an increase in intracranial pressure (ICP) secondary to increased pleural pressure, which elevates superior vena caval pressure and thus reduces cerebral venous outflow.[98] This may aggravate the neurologic disorder as cerebral perfusion pressure represents the difference between mean arterial pressure and ICP. Because mean arterial pressure is also reduced by mechanical ventilation and PEEP, the potential for cerebral hypoperfusion is considerable.

The effect of mechanical ventilation and PEEP on ICP is significantly influenced by lung compliance as the increase in pleural pressure with positive-pressure ventilation is buffered by stiff lungs.[83] Continuous monitoring of ICP is valuable in such patients, especially if combined with some measure of cerebral compliance determined by the ICP response to the introduction of 1 ml of saline into the ventricular system. In patients with normal lung compliance an increase in ICP with PEEP is observed only in patients with reduced cerebral compliance.[23] If PEEP is considered necessary despite an increase in ICP, cerebral perfusion pressure may be enhanced by tilting the head of the bed to a 30-degree angle to facilitate cerebral venous outflow, and arterial pressure may be increased by volume loading and pressors. However, the value of such measures has not been adequately assessed. Coughing and bucking on the ventilator should be minimized because the resulting increase in intrathoracic pressure elevates the ICP. PEEP should not be abruptly reduced or discontinued in such patients because this provokes a further increase in ICP,[1,23] probably brought on by the resulting rise in systemic arterial pressure which causes a transient increase in ICP in patients with altered cerebral blood flow autoregulation and reduced cerebral compliance.

Deliberate hyperventilation is commonly employed in patients sustaining severe head injury because lowering $PaCO_2$ to 25 to 30 mm Hg constricts cerebral vessels and lowers ICP. The benefit is diminished after 24 to 48 hours. Patients with cerebrovascular accidents show no benefit.

WEANING

All patients requiring mechanical ventilation have had an episode of respiratory failure; therefore discontinuation of the ventilator is approached with caution. Abrupt cessation of mechanical ventilation and extubation is possible in the majority of postoperative patients, but others with underlying lung disease or recovering from acute respiratory failure require a more gradual approach to the period of transition from mechanical ventilation to spontaneous breathing; this is referred to as weaning. During the process of weaning, separate consideration should be given to the patient's ability to sustain spontaneous breathing after discontinuation of the mechanical ventilator and the ability to protect the airways without a tracheal tube. The rate of weaning failure will depend on the patient population and the aggressiveness of the physician's approach, however, inability to tolerate discontinuation of mechanical ventilation or reintubation has been reported in as many as 17% to 19% of some mechanically ventilated patients.[76,132,149]

Because of the hazards associated with continuation of mechanical ventilation, discontinuation of mechanical ventilation and extubation should be considered as soon as there is significant resolution of the illness precipitating ventilator therapy and a successful outcome is considered likely. When such as stage has been reached, quantifiable physiologic measurements are obtained to help with predicting the likelihood of success.

Weaning Parameters

The patient's clinical status should be stable, and abnormal laboratory indices of a reversible nature should be corrected prior to assessment for weaning. Particular attention should be paid to normalization of any electrolyte imbalance that might exist, especially the presence of metabolic alkalosis. Weaning should rarely be attempted in a hemodynamically unstable patient. The level of consciousness is helpful in reflecting recovery of respiratory center drive in patients with drug overdose or neurologic insult. Not surprisingly, the same considerations used when initiating mechanical ventilation are reassessed when weaning is contemplated—the gas-exchange function of the lung and the rerserve of the ventilatory pump relative to requirements (see the boxed material below).

PARAMETERS USED TO PREDICT WEANING SUCCESS

GAS EXCHANGE
Pa_{O_2} of $\geq$60 mm Hg on FI_{O_2} of $\leq$0.35
Alveolar-arterial P_{O_2} gradient of <350 mm Hg
Pa_{O_2}/FI_{O_2} ratio of >200

VENTILATORY PUMP
Vital capacity of >10-15 ml/kg body weight
Maximum negative inspiratory pressure < −30 cm H_2O
Minute ventilation ($\dot{V}_E$) <10 L/min
Maximum voluntary ventilation >2x resting $\dot{V}_E$

Gas Exchange

No single index of oxygenation is universally accepted to prohibit weaning, and a number of different criteria have been proposed. Suggested criteria to progress with weaning include Pa_{O_2} of $\geq$60 mm Hg on an FI_{O_2} of $\leq$0.35,[149] alveolar-arterial P_{O_2} gradient of <350 mm Hg while inhaling an FI_{O_2} of 1.0,[118] or a Pa_{O_2}/FI_{O_2} ratio of >200.[117]

Ventilatory Pump

The reserve capacity of the ventilatory pump is generally assessed by measuring vital capacity, maximum inspiratory pressure, $\dot{V}_E$, and its relationship to maximum voluntary ventilation. These indices are attractive in that they can be obtained at the bedside with simple equipment. However, difficulty in obtaining measurements in uncooperative patients limits the predictive power of a value that is considered inadequate. A vital capacity of 10 cc/kg[16] or more[59] has been suggested as a prerequisite for sustaining spontaneous ventilation. This value is approximately twice the predicted V_T.[125] In a recent prospective study of 47 patients who were weaned and extubated (with follow-up to $\geq$48 hours) Tahvanainen, Salmenpera, and Nikki[149] found that a vital capacity of 10 cc/kg was falsely positive in 18% (predicted success but actual failure) and falsely negative in 50% of patients (predicted failure but actual success). Similarly, in a prospective study of 33 postoperative patients taking sustained spontaneous respiration with a pH of >7.35 as end point, Milbern and associates[107] found that a vital capacity of 15 cc/kg was falsely positive in 15% and falsely negative in 63% of patients.

Maximum inspiratory pressure (MIP), a valuable indicator of neuromuscular performance,[20] is widely used as a predictor of weaning success. This is measured using an aneroid manometer connected to the endotracheal tube, while the maximum negative pressure during a forceful inspiration from FRC is recorded. In a prospective study of 100 patients Sahn and Lakshminarayan[132] found that all patients who generated a MIP of −30 cm H_2O or lower were successfully extubated but all those with a MIP less negative than −20 cm H_2O were unable to sustain spontaneous respiration. In a recent prospective reevaluation of MIP, which used sustained spontaneous respiration for $\geq$48 hours postextubation as an end point, a MIP of −30 cm H_2O was found to be falsely negative in 100% and falsely positive in 26% of patients.[149] The reason for these disappointing findings may be partly because measurement of MIP alone does not take into account lung compliance. A MIP of −30 cm H_2O carries very different connotations in a patient with ARDS with a low compliance compared to a patient with emphysema with a high lung compliance because a much larger fraction of this MIP will be required to sustain spontaneous respiration in the ARDS patient. A rough measure of respiratory compliance can be obtained by selecting the inflation hold setting and noting the relationship between the resulting plateau in airway pressure, displayed on the ventilator manometer, and the V_T delivered by the ventilator.

Measurement of spontaneous $\dot{V}_E$ and maximum voluntary ventilation (MVV) will indicate the proportion of the patient's ventilatory capacity required to maintain a given level of $PaCO_2$ and also indicate the amount of reserve available for further respiratory demands. A resting $\dot{V}E$ of 10 L/min or less with the capability of doubling this value during maximal ventilatory effort is commonly employed as a weaning parameter. In the study of Sahn, and Lakshminarayan, and Petty[132] the combination of these two indices had a high discriminating value (similar to that of MIP) in predicting the likelihood of successful weaning. In the recent study of Tahvanainen, Salmenpera, and Nikki[149] both indices proved to be poor predictors. An increased spontaneous $\dot{V}E$ indicates an increased demand on the ventilatory pump, which may be caused by increased carbon dioxide production or increased VD/VT ratio. A VD/VT greater than 0.6 has been suggested to preclude successful weaning,[118] but again several patients with such values have been successfully extubated.[149,151] However, it should be clear that because of the predictable onset of muscle fatigue, a patient requiring a high $\dot{V}E$ (≥50% to 60% of MVV) on the ventilator to maintain an acceptable $PaCO_2$ will be unable to prevent the development of hypercapnia when he is removed from the ventilator.

The limitations of these weaning criteria are obvious in that many ambulatory patients with chronic obstructive pulmonary disease do not meet the criteria and yet lead a reasonable, if limited, life-style. In the study of Tahvanainen, Salmenpera, and Nikki[149] 63% of the patients successfully extubated did not fulfill the traditional criteria. Proponents of IMV[107] believe that these criteria prolong the period of weaning and advocate the use of arterial blood gases (ABGs), continuing to lower the number of ventilator-delivered breaths so long as arterial pH remains above 7.35. While assessment of pulmonary factors is of obvious importance, in one study[149] a reduction in urinary output was a more reliable predictor of weaning success (presumably as an indirect reflection of tissue oxygenation) than assessment of pulmonary function.

Methods of Discontinuing Mechanical Ventilation

Abrupt

Many patients who require brief periods of mechanical ventilation can resume and sustain spontaneous respiration with little difficulty. Before extubation these patients should be assessed while breathing spontaneously. Before commencing such a trial, the procedure should be explained to the patient, who is conventionally seated in an upright position. The patient may breathe spontaneously through a T-tube circuit (Fig. 34-9) or through the ventilator circuit as most current ventilators allow. Although breathing through the ventilator circuit reduces the financial cost by obviating the need for a T-tube setup, the work of breathing is considerably higher with the former technique. Certain design characteristics are important if a T-tube system is employed. In order to meet the patient's peak inspiratory flow rate, the gas source flow to the inspiratory limb should be at least twice that of the patient's spontaneous $\dot{V}E$,[44] and an extension piece, usually about 12 inches in length, should be added on the expiratory side to prevent entrainment of room air. The patient's general clinical status should be followed closely by a physician or nurse with specific measurements at 5 minute intervals of

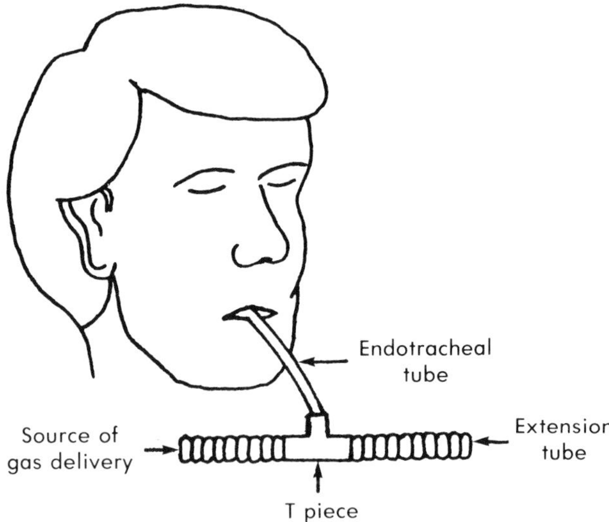

Fig. 34-9 T-tube circuit. Patient's endotracheal tube is attached to a T-piece that connects a gas delivery tube and an extension tube. This allows precise control over the fractional inspired O_2 (FIO_2) concentration, provided that the patient's peak inspiratory flow rate is less than that of the gas delivery source. As the patient's peak inspiratory flow rate increases, room air is entrained, and the FIO_2 is lowered. Addition of sufficient extension tubings circumvents this problem.

the respiratory rate, heart rate, blood pressure, and rib cage-abdominal motion; if the measurements are judged satisfactory, the trial should be continued for 20 to 30 minutes at which time an ABG is obtained. If the vital signs deteriorate during this process, the patient should be reconnected to the ventilator and a more gradual approach to wearning will be required. During this transition from mechanical ventilation to spontaneous breathing (while still intubated), the patient is likely to experience an increase in respiratory rate, a fall in VT, and a modest worsening of ABGs.

If the ABGs at the end of 20 to 30 minutes are judged adequate and vital signs remain stable, the patient can be immediately extubated. Should significant acidosis (pH 7.30 to 7.35, depending on the baseline value) develop, mechanical ventilation should be resumed and any reversible problems should be identified and corrected, or if none are found, a more gradual weaning approach adopted. If the patient's condition is borderline, the trial may be prolonged for up to 1 to 2 hours, but prolonged T-tube trials should be avoided.

Gradual T-tube Wean

With this approach sessions of spontaneous respiration of increasing duration are interspersed between periods of mechanical ventilation. Various approaches can be used such as allowing the patient to breathe spontaneously for 3 to 5 minutes every 30 minutes, gradually increasing the periods off the ventilator until a 30 minute period is reached at which time an ABG is obtained. If the patient's condition is satisfactory, the period of spontaneous respiration may be extended for up to 2 hours, at which time another ABG is obtained and extubation considered. If the patient is unable to sustain satisfactory spontaneous respiration, mechanical ventilation is resumed. The time required to rest fatigued respiratory muscles is unknown, but currently it seems wise to use a period of at least 10 hours.

Intermittent Mandatory Ventilation

Although now used as a primary mode of mechanical ventilation, IMV was introduced as a weaning technique with claims that it was more efficient, safer, and superior to traditional weaning techniques.[52] IMV may be initiated after a period of mechanical ventilation delivered in the A-C mode, or the patient may have been ventilated in the IMV mode throughout. When the patient is considered ready for weaning, the IMV rate should be reduced in steps, usually 1 to 3 breaths per minute at each step, and an ABG obtained after 30 minutes or more at that setting. If the pH remains above 7.30[51] or 7.35,[107] the IMV rate is reduced in further steps until a rate of zero is reached. Thus weaning is guided by the pH response to stepwise reductions in the number of mechanically-delivered breaths, and predictions based on physiologic measurements are not employed.

An advantage of IMV as a weaning technique is that it is performed without changing the breathing circuit, unlike the repeated manipulations required when a T-tube system is used. This is a bonus with a continuous-flow IMV circuit, but with the ubiquitous incorporation of demand valves in current ventilator designs, spontaneous breathing through the ventilator circuit may result in a twofold or larger increase in the work of breathing (see Fig. 34-7). IMV weaning sometimes leads to a false sense of security because there may be a tendency to monitor the patient's clinical status less closely since the patient is considered safe while attached to the mechanical ventilator in contrast to a T-tube. When IMV is employed, problems may arise with the expired volume alarm setup. The alarm is set below the patient's spontaneous V_T to avoid unnecessary signaling. However, at this low setting the alarm may not signal failure of the ventilator to deliver a mechanical breath and unheralded hypoventilation ensues.

IMV and traditional techniques of weaning have been compared in two prospective and one retrospective studies. Hastings and associates[72] studied 18 patients undergoing cardiac surgery randomized to weaning by a T-tube or IMV at 4 inflations per minute, with both groups receiving CPAP 5 cm H_2O. There was no significant difference in the duration of weaning until extubation in the two groups; unfortunately, the authors did not state the steps taken in reducing the IMV rate. No significant difference was noted in Pa_{O_2}, Pa_{CO_2}, cardiac index, shunt, oxygen consumption, or carbon dioxide production in the two groups of patients, but V_D/V_T improved in the T-tube group. In another prospective study of cardiac surgery patients, Prakash, Meij, and Van Der Borden[122] compared weaning using a trial of spontaneous breathing versus IMV with 4 to 5 inflations per minute. They observed no significant difference in the response of cardiopulmonary physiologic indices, but the study was not designed to assess the duration of weaning with the two techniques. Only speculation can be made on the extrapolation of these findings to patients requiring mechanical ventilations for reasons other than cardiac surgery. Indeed, many "high-risk" patients with major thoracic[123] or abdominal surgery[136] can be extubated after a very brief period of mechanical ventilation. In a retrospective analysis of patients requiring mechanical ventilation for various indications, Schachter, Tucker, and Beck[133] noted no differences in the duration of mechanical ventilation or hospital stay in patients receiving IMV versus A-C or CMV.

Weaning Failure

Failure to wean most often results from incomplete resolution of the illness precipitating mechanical ventilation or development of new problems. In patients with significant underlying lung disease the physician must also guard against setting goals that the patient's intrinsic lung function can never meet. Frequently more than one factor is responsible for the lack of success. If weaning failure results from hypoxemia even though the patient fulfilled satisfactory oxygenation criteria before the trial, it usually indicates the persistence of alveolar instability. A further weaning trial using PEEP may be helpful,[60,88] although it is unlikely that extubation will be possible until further healing takes place, and a slightly longer period of mechanical ventilation may be most prudent.

Impaired ventilatory pump performance may be a result of reduced respiratory center drive, excessive demands on the respiratory system, or impaired respiratory muscle function. Respiratory center output may be depressed by metabolic disturbance, pharmacologic agents, sleep deprivation, or neurologic structual damage. An elevated serum HCO_3^-, a common finding in mechanically ventilated patients, is caused by nasogastric suction, diuretics, and antacid administration. If HCO_3^- is elevated so that a metabolic alkalosis develops, this will cause a reduction in respiratory center drive.[147] Significant respiratory center depression may also be a result of malnutrition[47] or more rarely of endocrine disturbance such as myxedema.[164] Although respiratory center output may be reduced by a number of factors, pharmacologic stimulation of the respiratory centers using doxapram, nikethamide, or medroxyprogesterone is rarely beneficial in the patient experiencing difficulty in weaning, although the value of these drugs in this setting has never been formally examined.

Excessive demands on the ventilatory pump may be caused by high ventilatory requirements or excessive work of breathing. Normal subjects can maintain a $\dot{V}_E$ as high as 50% to 60% of the MVV, and this level is referred to as maximum sustained ventilation. A similar relationship is observed in chronic obstructive pulmonary disease (COPD),[127] but there is less firm evidence regarding the degree of reserve in patients with acute respiratory failure. An increased baseline $\dot{V}_E$ with eucapnia or hypercapnia, may be the result of increased carbon dioxide production or increased V_D/V_T. Carbon dioxide production may be increased with hypermetabolism of fever or increased intake of carbohydrate.[34] Formerly it was considered that a V_D/V_T above 0.6 incurs an excessive ventilatory demand with inevitable respiratory failure, but experience indicates otherwise. However, increases in V_D/D_T above this level can only be met by tremendous increases in $\dot{V}_E$ with consequent reduction in ventilatory reserve.

Placing a patient with COPD with compensated hypercapnia on a ventilator and reducing the Pa_{CO_2} to the normal range will result in renal excretion of HCO_3^- to bring pH into the normal range. When weaning is attempted and the patient adopts his usual level of ventilation with resulting increase in Pa_{CO_2}, acute respiratory acidosis will develop because inadequate HCO_3^- is available for buffering action. This may lead to severe dyspnea necessitating reinstitution of mechanical ventilation. A better approach in these patients is to allow a gradual increase in Pa_{CO_2} and thus permit normal renal compensation to take place. Ventilation becomes more efficient at high Pa_{CO_2} levels since each breath excretes a larger amount of carbon dioxide than is achieved at a lower Pa_{CO_2}, and the patient eventually reaches a level of compensated hypercapnia appropriate to his ventilatory ability. It is not unusual for chronic hypercapnic patients to have a further deterioration in pulmonary function during hospital admission. However, following discharge the degree of abnormality commonly returns slowly toward the original baseline.

The work of breathing may be further increased by unnecessary resistive or elastic loads imposed on the respiratory system. Flow resistance to breathing can be minimized by special consideration to the diameter, length, and support of the endotracheal tube, the circuit employed for spontaneous respiration, and the presence of reversible airway obstruction. Increased elastic loading on the respiratory system may be the result of bandages, obesity, ascites, or peritoneal dialysis.

Increasing attention is currently being focused on the role of the respiratory muscle dysfunction as a cause of weaning failure. This may result from excessive demands or impaired energy supplies. Demand on the respiratory muscles increases as the ventilatory requirements and work of breathing increase. A similar situation occurs with less excessive demands if the patient has primary muscle disease or pharmacologic-induced dysfunction as with recent administration of pancuronium, aminoglycosides, or other medications.[4] Recently phrenic nerve injury or dysfunction consequent to employment of cardioplegic solutions during open heart surgery has been observed. Whether prolonged mechanical ventilation results in muscle atrophy remains to be explored, but the current tendency to employ large V_T may alter chest-wall stretch-receptor function and interfere with respiratory muscle performance when spontaneous respiration is resumed.[139]

Inadequate energy supplies cause impaired respiratory muscle performance. Malnutrition may have a number of deleterious effects: diaphragmatic muscle mass is reduced with decreases in both diaphragmatic thickness and area,[5] respiratory muscle strength and MVV may be reduced to less than 50% of normal,[6] respiratory center drive is decreased,[47] and cellular defense mechanisms and surfactant production may be impaired. Severe malnutrition is commonly observed in mechanically ventilated patients,[54] and retrospective studies suggest that malnutrition may prolong the period of mechanical ventilation and contribute to weaning failure.[12,105] The value of nutritional support in enhancing respiratory muscle function and improving weaning success has not been prospectively examined. Associated hypophosphatemia, hypokalemia, and hypomagnesemia also impair muscle performance and may precipitate respiratory failure.[110] Reduced oxygen delivery to the respiratory muscles as a result of hypoxemia[84] or decreased cardiac output[8] predisposes to respiratory muscle failure. Discontinuation of mechanical ventilation markedly increases oxygen consumption by the respiratory muscles and may outstrip oxygen supply and impair oxygen delivery to other vital organs. Treatment of respiratory muscle dysfunction is currently limited to rest (by mechanical ventilation), increasing energy supplies through nutritional support and enhanced oxygen delivery, and minimizing imposed load. The duration of mechanical ventilation necessary to reverse respiratory muscle fatigue is unknown, but in a recent study of patients with *chronic* respiratory failure, mechanical ventilation for 4 to 10 hours/day increased respiratory muscle strength and MVV.[102] The value of aminophylline administration to improve diaphragmatic contractility and endurance[109] and employment of respiratory muscle training exercises[13] remain to be explored in this setting.

Discontinuation of mechanical ventilation in patients with normal left ventricular function results in an increased cardiac output. In contrast, hemodynamic deterioration may develop following discontinuation of mechanical ventilation in patients with a failing left ventricle, not only as a result of improved venous return with consequent increase in preload, but also because the decrease in intrathoracic pressure may increase left ventricular afterload resulting from increased transmural pressure.[104] Successful weaning may be very difficult in such patients, and pharmacologic manipulation may be required to substitute for the beneficial effects of mechanical ventilation.

Even when these causes of weaning failure are considered and management optimized, some patients will continue to remain dependent on mechanical ventilation. This situation calls for a trial of some unusual approaches such as encouraging the patient to ambulate while supporting ventilation with a self-inflating bag[131] or using a cuirass negative-pressure ventilator custom-fitted to the patient's thoracic cage.[44] If the need for mechanical ventilation is the major reason preventing hospital discharge, home ventilator therapy should be considered.[142]

Extubation

In a patient able to breathe spontaneously extubation may be deferred if the patient is considered unable to protect his airways against aspiration or has inadequate expulsive forces for clearance of secretions, or if there is insecurity regarding the patient's ability to sustain ventilation without fatigue. Unlike the weaning procedure, there are no documented parameters that predict successful airway protection following extubation.

Absence of a gag reflex when a tongue blade is vigorously rubbed against the posterior oropharynx is often considered a contraindication to extubation. However, a gag reflex may be absent in about 20% of normal subjects, and aspiration pneumonia still occurs when it is present.[91] Ability to cough is important because the accompanying expulsive forces can normally clear the airways down to the level of the medium-sized bronchi. Although the presence of a tracheal tube prevents normal glottic closure during coughing, it does not impair the ability to develop normal maximal cough pressures of about 80 cm H_2O.[67] In addition to assessment of MIP and vital capacity, maximal expiratory pressure can be measured during an expiratory effort against an occluded airway following a maximal inspiration to total lung capacity. These indices reflect the forces available for successful coughing but cannot be measured in obtunded patients, who pose the greatest dilemma in assessing ability to tolerate extubation. Assessment should also be made of the patient's cough response to irritation of the airways with a suction catheter. Added caution with respect to extubation is necessary in patients with copious airway secretions.

Following extubation there is normally a reduction in $\dot{V}_E$ caused by a decrease in V_T with no change in respiratory rate.[154] The risk of laryngeal incompetence and aspiration is considerable after extubation, being observed in 50% of patients in the immediate postextubation period and decreasing to less than 5% after 8 hours.[24] Up to 20% of mechanically ventilated patients require reintubation, which poses an additional hazard in critically ill patients. Although Tahvanainen, Salmenpera, and Nikki[149] noted that such an event did not appear to affect the patient's outcome, this may be related to the fact that intubations were performed by anesthesiologists, who have a much lower rate of complications.[150]

SUMMARY

Mechanical ventilation has become a mainstay in the management of critically ill patients. The indications for mechanical ventilation consist of disorders causing ventilatory pump failure or inefficient gas exchange. Volume-cycled machines are usually employed in various modes and the ventilator setting adjusted in accordance with the patient's physiologic response. Particular attention should be paid to the ventilator circuit because it may cause significant increases in the work of breathing. A large variety of complications may develop, and clinical and physiologic assessment is continuously required. As soon as the illness precipitating the need for mechanical ventilation has resolved, ventilator support should be discontinued in order to minimize the risk of associated complications.

REFERENCES

1. Aidinis, S.J., Lafferty, J., and Shapiro, H.M.: Intracranial responses to PEEP, Anesthesiology **45**:275, 1976.
2. Albelda, S.M., et al.: Ventilator-induced subpleural air cysts: clinical, radiographic, and pathologic significance, Am. Rev. Respir. Dis. **127**:360, 1983.
3. Andersen, J.B., et al.: Respiratory thoracoabdominal coordination and muscle fatigue in acute respiratory failure, Am. Rev. Respir. Dis. **117**(suppl.):89, 1978.
4. Argov, Z., and Mastaglia, F.L.: Disorders of neuromuscular transmission caused by drugs, N. Engl. J. Med. **301**:409, 1979.
5. Arora, N.S., and Rochester, D.F.: Effect of body weight and muscularity on human diaphragm muscle mass, thickness, and area, J. Appl. Physiol. **52**:64, 1982.
6. Arora, N.S., and Rochester, D.F.: Respiratory muscle strength and maximal voluntary ventilation in undernourished patients, Am. Rev. Respir. Dis. **126**:5, 1982.
7. Ashbaugh, D.G., et al.: Acute respiratory distress in adults, Lancet **ii**:319, 1967.
8. Aubier, M., Trippenbach, T., and Roussos, C.: Respiratory muscle fatigue during cardiogenic shock, J. Appl. Physiol. **51**:499, 1981.
9. Avery, E.E., Morch, E.T., and Benson, D.W.: Critically crushed chests: a new method of treatment with continuous mechanical hyperventilation to produce alkalotic apnea and internal pneumatic stabilization, J. Thorac. Surg. **32**:291, 1956.
10. Baker, A.B., et al.: Effects of varying inspiratory flow waveform and time in intermittent positive-pressure ventilation, Br. J. Anaesth. **49**:1207, 1977.
11. Barach, A.L.: The use of helium in the treatment of asthma and obstructive lesions, Ann. Intern. Med. **9**:739, 1935.
12. Bassili, H.R., and Deitil, M.: Nutritional support in long-term intensive care with special reference to ventilator patients, Can. Anaesth. Soc. J. **28**:17, 1981.
13. Belman, M.J.: Respiratory failure treated by ventilatory muscle training (VMT): a report of two cases, Eur. J. Respir. Dis. **62**:391, 1981.
14. Bendixen, H.H., Hedley-Whyte, J., and Laver, M.B.: Impaired oxygenation in surgical patients during general anesthesia with controlled ventilation, N. Engl. J. Med. **269**:991, 1963.
15. Bendixen, H.H., et al.: Atelectasis and shunting during spontaneous ventilation in anesthetized patients, Anesthesiology **25**:297, 1964.
16. Bendixen, H.H., et al.: Respiratory care, St. Louis, 1965, The C.V. Mosby Co.
17. Bergman, N.A.: Effect of different pressure breathing patterns on alveolar-arterial gradients in dogs, J. Appl. Physiol. **18**:1049, 1963.
18. Berry, A.: Respiratory support and renal function, Anesthesiology **55**:655, 1981.
19. Bjork, V.O., and Engstrom, C.G.: The treatment of ventilatory insufficiency after pulmonary resection with tracheostomy and prolonged artificial ventilation, J. Thorac. Cardiovasc. Surg. **30**:356, 1955.
20. Black, L.F., and Hyatt, R.E.: Maximal static respiratory pressures in generalized neuromuscular disease, Am. Rev. Resp. Dis. **103**:641, 1971.
21. Bone, R.C., Francis, P.B., and Pierce, A.K.: Pulmonary barotrauma complicating positive end-expiratory pressure (abstract), Am. Rev. Resp. Dis. **111**:921, 1975.
22. Borg, U., Eriksson, I., and Sjostrand, U.: High-frequency positive-pressure ventilation (HFPPV): a review based upon its use during branchoscopy and for laryngoscopy and microlaryngeal surgery under general anesthesia, Anesth. Analg. **59**:594, 1980.
23. Burchiel, K.J., Steege, T.D., and Wyler, A.R.: Intracranial pressure changes in brain-injured patients requiring positive end-expiratory pressure ventilation, Neurosurgery **8**:443, 1981.
24. Burgess, G.E., et al.: Laryngeal competence after tracheal extubation, Anesthesiology **51**:73, 1979.
25. Burnham, S.C., Martin, W.E., and Cheney, F.W.: The effects of various tidal volumes on gas exchange in pulmonary edema, Anesthesiology **37**:27, 1972.
26. Carlon, G.C., et al.: Criteria for selective positive end-expiratory pressure and independent synchronized ventilation of each lung, Chest **74**:501, 1978.
27. Carlon, G.C., et al.: High-frequency positive-pressure ventilation in management of a patient with bronchopleural fistula, Anesthesiology **52**:160, 1980.
28. Cheney, F.W.: The effects of tidal-volume change with positive end-expiratory pressure in pulmonary edema, Anesthesiology **37**:600, 1972.
29. Cheney, F.W., and Martin, W.E.: Effects of continuous positive-pressure ventilation on gas exchange in acute pulmonary edema, J. Appl. Physiol. **30**:378, 1971.
30. Cohen, D.J., Baumgart, S., and Stephenson, L.W.: Pneumopericardium in neonates: is it PEEP or is it PIP? Ann. Thorac. Surg. **35**:179, 1983.
31. Cohen, C.A., et al.: Clinical manifestations of inspiratory muscle fatigue, Am. J. Med. **73**:308, 1982.
32. Connors, A.F., McCaffree, D.R., and Gray, B.A.: Effect of inspiratory flow rate on gas exchange during mechanical ventilation, Am. Rev. Respir. Dis. **124**:537, 1981.
33. Cournand, A., et al.: Physiological studies of the effects of intermittent positive-pressure breathing on cardiac output in man, Am. J. Physiol. **152**:162, 1948.
34. Covelli, H.D., et al.: Respiratory failure precipitated by high carbohydrate loads, Ann. Intern. Med. **95**:579, 1981.

35. Cox, P.M., and Schatz, M.E.: Respiratory therapy, pressure measurements in endotracheal cuffs: a common error, Chest **65:**84, 1974.
36. Craven, D.E., et al.: Contamination of mechanical ventilators with tubing changes every 24 or 48 hours, N. Engl. J. Med. **306:**1505, 1982.
37. Craven, D.E., et al.: Contaminated medication nebulizers in mechanical ventilator circuits, Am. J. Med. **77:**834, 1984.
38. Cullen, D.J., and Caldera, D.L.: The incidence of ventilator-induced pulmonary barotrauma in critically ill patients, Anesthesiology **50:**185, 1979.
39. Cullen, P., et al.: Treatment of flail chest: use of intermittent mandatory ventilation and positive end expiratory pressure, Arch. Surg. **110:**1099, 1975.
40. Culpepper, J., et al.: Effect of ventilator mode on tendency to respiratory alkalosis (abstract), Am. Rev. Respir. Dis. **127:**104, 1983.
41. Dantzker, D.R.: Gas exchange in the adult respiratory distress syndrome, Clin. Chest Med. **3:**57, 1982.
42. Dantzker, D.R., Lynch, J.P., and Weg, J.G.: Depression of cardiac output is a mechanism of shunt reduction in the therapy of acute respiratory failure, Chest **77:**636, 1980.
43. Dantzker, D.R., et al.: Gas exchange alterations associated with weaning from mechanical ventilation following coronary artery bypass grafting, Chest **82:**674, 1982.
44. Dean, S.E., and Keenan, R.L.: Spontaneous breathing with a T-piece circuit: minimum fresh gas/minute volume ratio which prevents rebreathing, Anesthesiology **56:**449, 1982.
45. deLatorre, F., et al.: Incidence of pneumothorax and pneumomediastinum in patients with aspiration pneumonia requiring ventilatory support, Chest **72:**141, 1977.
46. Demers, R.R., Sullivan, M.J., and Paliotta, J.: Airflow resistances of endotracheal tubes, JAMA **237:**1362, 1977.
47. Doekel, R.C., et al.: Clinical semistarvation: depression of hypoxic ventilatory response, N. Engl. J. Med. **295:**358, 1976.
48. Downs, J.B.: Ventilatory patterns and modes of ventilation in acute respiratory failure, Respir. Care **28:**586, 1983.
49. Downs, J.B., and Douglas, M.E.: Intermittent mandatory ventilation: why the controversy? Crit. Care Med. **9:**622, 1981.
50. Downs, J.B., Block, A.J., and Vennum, K.B.: Intermittent mandatory ventilation in the treatment of patients with chronic obstructive pulmonary disease, Anesth. Analg. **53:**437, 1974.
51. Downs, J.B., Perkins, H.M., and Modell, J.H.: Intermittent mandatory ventilation: an evaluation, Arch. Surg. **109:**519, 1974.
52. Downs, J.B., et al.: Intermittent mandatory ventilation: a new approach to weaning patients from mechanical ventilators, Chest **64:**331, 1973.
53. Downs, J.B., et al.: Ventilatory pattern, intrapleural pressure and cardiac output, Anesth. Analg. **56:**88, 1977.
54. Driver, A.G., and LeBrun, M.: Iatrogenic malnutrition in patients receiving ventilatory support, JAMA **244:**2195, 1980.
55. Egbert, L.D., Laver, M.B., and Bendixen, H.H.: Intermittent deep breaths and compliance during anesthesia in man. Anesthesiology **24:**57, 1963. In Engstrom, C.G.: The clinical application of prolonged controlled ventilation, Acta Anesthesiol. Scand. **13** (suppl.):1, 1963.
56. Evans, R.N., and Bakow, E.D.: Causes of CO_2 retention in COPD patients breathing supplemental oxygen, Respir. Care **29:**167, 1984.
57. Fairley, H.B.: Critique on intermittent mandatory ventilation, Int. Anesthesiol. Clin. **18:**179, 1980.
58. Fairley, H.B., and Blenkarn, G.D.: Effect on pulmonary gas exchange in variations in inspiratory flow rate during intermittent positive-pressure ventilation, Br. J. Anaesth. **38:**320, 1966.
59. Feeley, T.W., and Hedley-Whyte, J.: Weaning from controlled ventilation and supplemental oxygen, N. Engl. J. Med. **292:**903, 1975.
60. Feeley, T.W., et al.: Positive end-expiratory pressure in weaning patients from controlled ventilation: a prospective randomized trial, Lancet **ii:**725, 1975.
61. Ferris, B.G., and Pollard, D.S.: Effect of deep and quiet breathing on pulmonary compliance in man, J. Clin. Invest. **39:**143, 1960.
62. Field, S., Kelly, S.M., and Macklem, P.T.: The oxygen cost of breathing in patients with cardiorespiratory disease, Am. Rev. Respir. Dis. **126:**9, 1982.
63. Finlay, W.E.I., et al.: The effects of variations in inspiratory: expiratory ratio on cardiorespiratory function during controlled ventilation normo-, hypo-, and hypervolaemic dogs, Br. J. Anaesth. **42:**935, 1970.
64. Fowler, A.A., et al.: Adult respiratory distress syndrome: risk with common predispositions, Ann. Intern. Med. **98:**593, 1983.
65. Froese, A.B., and Bryan, A.C.: Effects on anesthesia and paralysis on diaphragmatic mechanics in man, Anesthesiology **41:**242, 1974.
66. Fulkerson, W.J., et al.: Life-threatening hypoventilation in kyphoscoliosis: successful treatment with a molded body brace-ventilator, Am. Rev. Respir. Dis. **129:**185, 1984.
67. Gal, I.J.: Effects of endotracheal intubation on normal cough performance, Anesthesiology **52:**324, 1980.
68. Gallagher, T.J., Civetta, J.M., and Kirby, R.R.: Terminology update: optimal PEEP, Crit. Care Med. **6:**323, 1978.
69. Gallagher, T.J., Klain, M.M., and Carlon, G.C.: Present status of high-frequency ventilation, Crit. Care Med. **10:**613, 1982.
70. Gherini, S., Peters, R.M., and Virgilio, R.W.: Mechanical work on the lungs and work of breathing with positive end-expiratory pressure and continuous positive airway pressure, Chest **76:**251, 1979.
71. Gibney, R.T.N., Wilson, R.S., and Pontoppidan, H.: Comparison of work of breathing on high gas flow and demand valve continuous positive airway pressure systems, Chest **82:**692, 1982.
72. Hastings, P.R., et al.: Cardiorespiratory dynamics during weaning with IMV versus spontaneous ventilation in good-risk cardiac-surgery patients, Anesthesiology **53:**429, 1980.
73. Haynes, M.S., Cornelius, D.B., and Johnson, R.L.: The contribution of endotracheal tube resistance to total pulmonary resistance and the work of breathing (abstract), Am. Rev. Respir. Dis. **119:**127, 1979.
74. Heenan, T.J., et al.: Intermittent mandatory ventilation; is synchronization important?, Chest **77:**598, 1980.
75. Henry, W.C., West, G.A., and Wilson, R.S.: A comparison of the oxygen cost of breathing between a continuous-flow CPAP system and a demand-flow CPAP system, Respir. Care **28:**1273, 1983.
76. Hilberman, M., et al.: An analysis of potential physiological predictors of respiratory adequacy following cardiac surgery, J. Thorac. Cardiovasc. Surg. **71:**711, 1976.
77. Hillman, K.M., and Barber, J.D.: Asynchronous independent lung ventilation (AILV), Crit. Care Med. **8:**390, 1980.
78. Housley, E., Louzada, N., and Becklake, M.R.: To sigh or not to sigh, Am. Rev. Respir. Dis. **101:**611, 1970.
79. Hudson, L.D.: Ventilatory management of patients with adult respiratory distress syndrome, Sem. Respir. Med. **2:**128, 1981.
80. Hudson, L.D., et al.: Comparison of assisted ventilation and PEEP with IMV and CPAP in ARDS patients (abstract), Am. Rev. Respir. Dis. **117:**129, 1978.
81. Hurd, T.E., Novak, R., and Gallagher, J.: Tension pneumopericardium: a complication of mechanical ventilation, Crit. Care Med. **12:**200, 1984.
82. Hurlow, R.S., et al.: Does IMV correct respiratory alkalosis in patients on AMV? (abstract), Chest **82:**211, 1982.
83. Huseby, J.S., Paulin, E.G., and Butler, J.: Effect of positive end-expiratory pressure on intracranial pressure in dogs, J. Appl. Physiol. **44:**25, 1978.
84. Jardim, J., et al.: The failing inspiratory muscles under normoxic and hypoxic conditions, Am. Rev. Respir. Dis. **124:**274, 1981.
85. Johnson, E.E., and Hedley-Whyte, J.: Continuous positive-pressure ventilation and portal flow in dogs with pulmonary edema, J. Appl. Physiol. **33:**385, 1972.
86. Johnson, E.E., and Hedley-Whyte, J.: Continuous positive-pressure ventilation and choledochoduodenal flow resistance, J. Appl. Physiol. **39:**937, 1975.
87. Johnson, E.E., Hedley-Whyte, J., and Hall, S.V.: End-expiratory pressure ventilation and sulfobromophthalein sodium excretion in dogs, J. Appl. Physiol. **43:**714, 1977.
88. Khan, F.A., et al.: Positive airway pressure in patients receiving intermittent mandatory ventilation at zero rate: the role of weaning of chronic obstructive pulmonary disease. Chest **84:**436, 1983.
89. Kirby, R.R., et al.: A new pediatric volume ventilator, Anesth. Analg. **50:**533, 1971.
90. Kirby, R.R., et al.: High-level positive end-expiratory pressure (PEEP) in acute respiratory insufficiency, Chest **67:**156, 1975.

91. Kulig, K., Rumack, B.H., and Rosen, P.: Gag reflex in assessing level of consciousness (letter), Lancet **i**:565, 1982.
92. Kumar, A., et al.: Continuous positive-pressure ventilation in acute respiratory failure, N. Engl. J. Med. **283**:1430, 1970.
93. Kumar, A., et al.: Pulmonary barotrauma during mechanical ventilation, Crit. Care Med. **1**:181, 1973.
94. Lamy, M., et al.: Pathologic features and mechanisms of hypoxemia in adult respiratory distress syndrome, Am. Rev. Respir. Dis. **114**:267, 1976.
95. Lenaghan, R., Silva, Y.J., and Walt, A.J.: Hemodynamic alterations associated with expansion rupture of the lung, Arch. Surg. **99**:339, 1969.
96. Levine, M., Gilbert, R., and Auchincloss, J.H.: A comparison of the effects of sighs, large tidal volumes, and positive end-expiratory pressure in assisted ventilation, Scand. J. Respir. Dis. **53**:101, 1972.
97. Lindahl, S.: Influence of an end-inspiratory pause on pulmonary ventilation, gas distribution, and lung perfusion during artificial ventilation, Crit. Care Med. **7**:540, 1979.
98. Luce, J.M., et al.: Mechanism by which positive end-expiratory pressure increases cerebrospinal fluid pressure in dogs, J. Appl. Physiol. **52**:231, 1982.
99. Luterman, A., et al.: Withdrawal from positive end-expiratory pressure, Surgery **83**:328, 1978.
100. Macklin, M.T., and Macklin, C.C.: Malignant interstitial emphysema of the lungs and mediastinum as an important occult complication in many respiratory diseases and other conditions: an interpretation of the clinical literature in the light of laboratory experiment, Medicine **23**:281, 1944.
101. Marini, J.J.: Occult positive end-expiratory pressure in mechanically ventilated patients with airflow obstruction, Am. Rev. Respir. Dis. **126**:166, 1982.
102. Marino, W., and Braun, N.M.T.: Reversal of the clinical sequelae of respiratory muscle fatigue by intermittent mechanical ventilation, Am. Rev. Respir. Dis. 1982:125 (Suppl), 85 (abstract).
103. Mathru, M., Rao, T.L., and Venus, B.: Ventilator-induced barotrauma in controlled mechanical ventilation versus intermittent mandatory ventilation, Crit. Care Med. **11**:359, 1983.
104. Mathru, M., et al.: Hemodynamic response to changes in ventilatory patterns in patients with normal and poor left ventricular reserve, Crit. Care Med. **10**:423, 1982.
105. Mattar, J.A., Velasco, I.T., and Esgaib, A.S.: Parenteral nutrition (PN) as a useful method of weaning patients from mechanical ventilation (abstract), JPEN **2**:250, 1978.
106. Mead, J., and Collier, C.: Relation of volume history of lungs to respiratory mechanics in anesthetized dogs, J. Appl. Physiol. **14**:669, 1959.
107. Milbern, S.M., et al.: Evaluation of criteria for discontinuing mechanical ventilation support, Arch. Surg. **113**:1441, 1978.
108. Milbern, S.M., et al.: Physiological CPAP: fact or fiction (abstract), Crit. Care Med. **6**:97, 1978.
109. Murciano, D., et al.: Effects of the theophylline on diaphragmatic strength and fatigue in patients with chronic obstructive pulmonary disease, N. Engl. J. Med. **311**:349, 1984.
110. Newman, J.H., Neff, T.A., and Ziporin, P.: Acute respiratory failure associated with hypophosphatemia, N. Engl. J. Med. **296**:1101, 1977.
111. Nunn, J.F.: The distribution of inspired gas during thoracic surgery, Ann. R. Coll. Surg. Engl. **28**:223, 1961.
112. Op't Holt, T.B., et al.: Comparison of changes in airway pressure during continuous positive airway pressure (CPAP) between demand-valve and continuous-flow devices, Respir. Care **27**:1200, 1982.
113. Pepe, P.E., Hudson, L.D., and Carrico, C.J.: Early application of positive end-expiratory pressure in patients at risk for the adult respiratory distress syndrome, N. Engl. J. Med. **311**:281, 1984.
114. Petersen, G.W., and Horst, B.: Incidence of pulmonary barotrauma in a medical ICU, Crit. Care Med. **11**:67, 1983.
115. Petty, T.L.: Intermittent mandatory ventilation—reconsidered, Crit. Care Med. **9**:620, 1981.
116. Pierson, D.J.: Persistent bronchopleural air leak during mechanical ventilation: a review, Respir. Care **27**:408, 1982.
117. Pierson, D.J.: Weaning from mechanical ventilation in acute respiratory failure: concepts, indications, and techniques, Resp. Care **28**:646, 1983.
118. Pontoppidan, H., Laver, M.B., and Geffin, B.: Acute respiratory failure in the surgical patient. In Welch, C.E., editor: Advances in surgery, vol. 4, Chicago, 1970, Year Book Medical Publishers.
119. Poulton, T.J., and Downs, J.B.: Humidification of rapidly flowing gas, Crit. Care Med. **9**:59, 1981.
120. Powner, D.J., and Grenvik, A.: Ventilatory management of life-threatening bronchopleural fistulae, Crit. Care Med. **9**:54, 1981.
121. Powner, D.J., Eross, B., and Grenvik, A.: Differential lung ventilation with PEEP in the treatment of pneumonia, Crit. Care Med. **5**:170, 1977.
122. Prakash, O., Meij, S., and Van Der Borden, B.: Spontaneous ventilation test versus intermittent mandatory ventilation: an approach to weaning after coronary bypass surgery, Chest **81**:403, 1982.
123. Prakash, O., et al.: Criteria for early extubation after intracardiac surgery in adults, Anesth. Analg. **56**:703, 1977.
124. Quan, S.F., Falltrick, R.T., and Schlobohm, R.M.: Extubation from ambient or expiratory positive airway pressure in adults, Anesthesiology **55**:53, 1981.
125. Radford, E.P., Ferris, B.G., and Kriete, B.C.: Clinical use of a nomogram to estimate proper ventilation during artificial respiration, N. Engl. J. Med. **251**:874, 1954.
126. Richardson, J.D., Adams, L., and Flint, L.M.: Selective management of flail chest and pulmonary contusion, Ann. Surg. **196**:481, 1982.
127. Rochester, D.F., and Arora, N.S.: Respiratory muscle failure, Med. Clin. North Am. **67**:573, 1983.
128. Rochester, D.F., Braun, N.M., and Laine, S.: Diaphragmatic energy expenditure in chronic respiratory failure: the effect of assisted ventilation with body respirators, Am. J. Med. **63**:223, 1977.
129. Rodriguez, R.J., Lefrak, S.S., and Sinks, D.E.: Physiological effects of intermittent mandatory ventilation (abstract), Am. Rev. Respir. Dis. **115**:157, 1977.
130. Ruiz, B.C., et al.: Intermittent mandatory ventilation and assisted mechanical ventilation: a comparison, Presented at the annual meeting of the American Society of Anesthesiologists, New Orleans, Oct. 17, 1977.
131. Sahn, S.A., and Lakshminarayan, S.: Bedside criteria for discontinuation of mechanical ventilation, Chest **63**:1002, 1973.
132. Sahn, S.A., Lakshminarayan, S., and Petty, T.L.: Weaning from mechanical ventilation, JAMA **235**:2208, 1976.
133. Schachter, E.N., Tucker, D., and Beck, G.J.: Does intermittent mandatory ventilation accelerate weaning? JAMA **246**:1210, 1981.
134. Schmidt, G.B., et al.: Continuous positive airway pressure in the prophylaxis of the adult respiratory distress syndrome, Surg. Gynecol. Obstet. **143**:613, 1976.
135. Schuster, D.P., Klain, N.M., and Snyder, J.V.: Comparison of high-frequency jet ventilation to conventional ventilation during severe acute respiratory failure in humans, Crit. Care Med. **10**:625, 1982.
136. Shackford, S.R., Virgilio, R.W., and Peters, R.M.: Early extubation versus prophylactic ventilation in the high-risk patient: a comparison of postoperative management in the prevention of respiratory complications, Anesth. Analg. **60**:76, 1981.
137. Shackford, S.R., Virgilio, R.W., and Peters, R.M.: Selective use of ventilator therapy in flail chest injury, J. Thorac. Cardiovasc. Surg. **81**:194, 1981.
138. Sladen, A., Laver, M.B., and Pontoppidan, H.: Pulmonary complications and water retention in prolonged mechanical ventilation, N. Engl. J. Med. **279**:448, 1968.
139. Smith, A.C., Spalding, J.M.K., and Watson, W.E.: Ventilation volume as a stimulus to spontaneous ventilation after prolonged artificial ventilation, J. Physiol. **160**:22, 1962.
140. Smith, R.B.: Humidification during high-frequency ventilation, Respir. Care **27**:1371, 1982.
141. Snyder, J.V., et al.: Mechanical ventilation: physiology and application, Curr. Probl. Surg. **21**:8, 1984.
142. Splaingard, M.L., et al.: Home positive-pressure ventilation: twenty years experience, Chest **84**:376, 1983.

143. Stauffer, J.L., and Silvestri, R.C.: Complications of endotracheal intubation, tracheostomy, and artificial airways, Respir. Care **27**:417, 1982.
144. Stauffer, J.L., Olson, D.E., and Petty, T.L.: Complications and consequences of endotracheal intubation and tracheotomy: a prospective study of 150 critically ill adult patients, Am. J. Med. **70**:65-76, 1981.
145. Steier, M., et al.: Pneumothorax complicating continuous ventilatory support, J. Thorac. Cardiovasc. Surg. **67**:17, 1974.
146. Stevens, R.M., et al.: Pneumonia in an intensive care unit: a 30-month experience, Arch. Intern. Med. **134**:106, 1974.
147. Stone, D.F.: Respiration in man during metabolic alkalosis, J. Appl. Physiol. **17**:33, 1962.
148. Sullivan, M., Paliotta, J., and Saklad, M.: Endotracheal tube as a factor in measurement of respiratory mechanics, J. Appl. Physiol. **41**:590, 1976.
149. Tahvanainen, J., Salmenpera, M., and Nikki, P.: Extubation criteria after weaning from intermittent mandatory ventilation and continuous positive airway pressure, Crit. Care Med. **11**:702, 1983.
150. Taryle, D.A., et al.: Emergency room intubations—complications and survival, Chest **75**:541, 1979.
151. Teres, D., Roizen, M.F., and Bushnell, L.S.: Successful weaning from controlled ventilation despite high dead-space-to-tidal-volume ratio, Anesthesiology **39**:656, 1973.
152. Tobin, M.J., and Grenvik, A.: Nosocomial lung infection and its diagnosis, Crit. Care Med. **12**:191, 1984.
153. Tobin, M.J., et al.: Breathing patterns. I. Normal subjects, Chest **84**:202, 1983.
154. Tobin, M.J., et al.: Influence of the endotracheal tube on breathing pattern during weaning from mechanical ventilation (abstract), Am. Rev. Respir. Dis. **129**:106, 1984.
155. Trinkle, J.K., et al.: Management of flail chest without mechanical ventilation, Ann. Thorac. Surg. **19**:355, 1975.
156. Valdes, M.E., et al.: Continuous positive airway pressure in prophylaxis of adult respiratory distress syndrome in trauma patients, Surg. Forum **29**:187, 1978.
157. Vesalius, A.: Pulmonis motuum, de humani corporis fabrica libri septem oporinus, Basel 658, 1543.
158. Visick, W.D., Fairlev, H.B., and Hickey, R.F.: The effects of tidal volume and end-expiratory pressure on pulmonary gas exchange during anesthesia, Anesthesiology **39**:285, 1973.
159. Weaver, L.J., Hudson, L.D., and Carrico, C.J.: Prospective analysis of PEEP reduction (abstract), Chest **78**:544, 1980.
160. Weenig, C.S., et al.: Relationship of preoperative closing volume to functional residual capacity and alveolar-arterial oxygen difference during anesthesia with controlled ventilation, Anesthesiology **41**:3, 1974.
161. Weigelt, J.A., Mitchell, R.A., and Snyder, W.H.: Early positive end-expiratory pressure in the adult respiratory distress syndrome, Arch. Surg. **114**:497, 1979.
162. Weled, B.J., Winfrey, D., and Downs, J.B.: Measuring exhaled volume with continuous positive airway pressure and intermittent mandatory ventilation. techniques and rationale, Chest **76**:166, 1979.
163. Zarins, C.K., et al: Does spontaneous ventilation with IMV protect from PEEP-induced cardiac output depression? J. Surg. Res. **22**:299, 1977.
164. Zwillich, C.W., et al.: Ventilatory control in myxedema and hypothyroidism, N. Engl. J. Med. **292**:662, 1975.
165. Zwillich, C.W., et al.: Complications of assisted ventilation: a prospective study of 354 consecutive episodes, Am. J. Med. **57**:161, 1974.

35 *J. David Richardson*

Common Pulmonary Derangements and Respiratory Failure

The understanding of pulmonary derangements is of critical importance for the surgeon involved in the care of seriously ill patients of any type. Discussion of pulmonary dysfunction in the surgical patient must be limited in scope because of the myriad abnormalities that affect the lung. This chapter will focus on the functional anatomy and physiology of the lung, respiratory failure (particularly adult respiratory distress syndrome), and other topics of pulmonary physiology commonly encountered by surgeons.

FUNCTIONAL ANATOMY OF THE LUNG

The trachea and major airways act as conduits for the passage of air into the lungs where gas exchange actually occurs. However, the trachea and major bronchi are not merely passive conduits through which air passes. They perform an important function in the protection of the lungs from inhaled particles. The mucociliary action of the major airways is one of the first barriers in the lung's defense mechanism. The trachea branches into the mainstem bronchi, and subsequently the airways undergo 22 to 25 subdivisions with the last 8 to 10 sequential divisions occurring within the lung parenchyma. The terminal bronchioles are present at about the sixteenth division and are the most distal airways to have continuous mucosal lining. Respiratory bronchioles with partial mucosal lining alternating with alveoli are distal to the terminal bronchioles. The alveolar ducts are next in succession and eventually terminate in the alveolar sacs. These successive branchings of the airways provide a huge surface area for potential gas exchange. There are approximately 300 million alveoli with a surface area of 7 m^2 in the adult lung.[61]

The mucosa consists of an epithelial lining, basement membrane, and lamina propria. Pseudostratified columnar epithelium lines the large airways and consists of ciliated cells and goblet cells. The goblet cells secrete mucus, and the ciliated cells actively propel particulate matter proximally toward the trachea. Each ciliated cell contains approximately 200 cilia that are capable of 1000 beats per minute. It is estimated that the mucus produced by the goblet cells is propelled along with entrapped particles toward the mouth at a rate of 10 to 20 mm/min. This provides the first barrier in the lungs' defense system for particles that have reached the tracheobronchial tree. Other goblet cells are present in the respiratory mucosa and produce immunologically active substances such as immunoglobulin A (IgA). There are numerous speculations about the potential role of this immunoglobulin in lung defense, but the exact function is not known.

The next line of host defense in the lung consists of the alveolar macrophage. The origin of the pulmonary macrophage is from both the interstitial tissue of the alveolar wall and from within the alveolus itself. The pulmonary macrophage apparently arises from a pleuripotential cell such as a circulating monocyte and differentiates into a mature macrophage or remains dormant until needed for macrophage differentiation. Pulmonary macrophages actively engulf bacteria and inert particles. They are endowed with an elaborate enzyme system that allows them to engulf and to complete intracellular killing of engulfed microorganisms. In experimental systems the alveolar macrophages are capable of engulfing and killing 95% of aerosolized bacteria within 4 hours of exposure to the organism.[43]

In addition to macrophages there are four other major cellular components of the alveolar wall: two types of epithelial cells, fibroblasts, and endothelial cells. The two types of epithelial cells lining the alveoli are referred to as Type I and Type II pneumocytes. The Type I cells are thin in shape and cover most of the alveolar surface. Electron microscopic studies demonstrate few intracellular organelles, and Type I cells appear to be relatively inert. The thin layer and low metabolic activity suggest that these cells have adapted to yield maximum oxygen exchange with a minimum of caloric expenditure.[62]

Type II pneumocytes are cuboidal in shape, are fewer in number and cover less surface area than Type I epithelium, have an abundance of intracellular organelles, and are metabolically active. The Type II cell has at least two critical functions. The first is production of a surfactant that is a lipoprotein containing large amounts of saturated lecithins. Lipoprotein is a surface-active compound that stabilizes the surface tension existing between the air-tissue interface in the lung. The surfactant has an extremely short half-life and thus must be constantly produced by the Type II cells. These cells apparently are able to store surfactant in organelles and release this substance as needed, providing the cell is not injured by a process such as the adult respiratory distress syndrome (ARDS). The second function of Type II pneumocytes is a replicative one since they alone have the ability to regenerate after a lung injury such as ARDS. In the pathologic condition of ARDS, necrosis of Type I cells rapidly occurs, and only Type II cells are seen until the reparative process is well under way (see the section on ARDS). Type II cells appear to have the potential of regenerating new Type I cells.

Fibroblasts are the fourth cellular element located within the alveolar wall. They are thought to produce the connective tissue stroma that provides the architectural framework for the lung. These cells are relatively inert during periods of normal lung function, but they may be activated by a number of stimuli, resulting in severe fibrosis in cases of idiopathic pulmonary fibrosis and ARDS.

The fifth cellular component is the endothelial cell, which lines the extensive alveolar-capillary membrane. These cells are water permeable but do not readily permit passage of macromolecules under ordinary circumstances. The metabolic role of the endothelial cells is continuing to be elucidated, but it is known that these cells secrete prostaglandins and have the potential to deactivate many bioactive compounds such as histamine and serotonin.

NORMAL FUNCTION OF THE LUNG

Ventilation

The force that moves air into or out of the lung is the pressure relationship between the alveoli and the atmosphere. Changes in alveolar pressure are primarily dictated by inspiratory and expiratory muscle activity. When alveolar pressure is greater than atmospheric pressure, the air is expelled and the lungs deflated. Conversely, a fall in alveolar pressure below that of atmospheric pressure assures a movement of air into the alveoli, and the lungs expand. Thus the pressure relationships dictate flow, although flow can be modified by resistance changes within the airway system. Muscular activity by the intercostal muscles and diaphragm cause enlargement of the thoracic cage and a decrease in intrapleural pressure. The rapidity and degree of inspiratory effort will largely determine the rate of flow and volume of air delivered to the alveoli. During normal quiet ventilation, expiration occurs passively until the static recoil pressure of the lung that is imparted by the active inspiratory phase of ventilation is negated by the outward recoil pressure of the chest wall. At this point the intra-alveolar pressure should equal atmospheric pressure, and expiration ceases until voluntary contraction of expiratory muscles occurs resulting in an increased intrapleural and hence increased intra-alveolar pressure, which results in an active expiratory effort.

Tests of Ventilation

There are myriad tests of ventilation, and a discussion of many of them is beyond the scope of this chapter. I will only consider some of the more common and clinically useful tests of lung function. The simplest and most informative test of ventilation relies on forced expiration. The forced expiratory volume (FEV) is that volume of gas that can be exhaled over a unit of time (usually 1 second: FEV_1). The forced vital capacity (FVC) represents the total volume of gas that can be exhaled after a full inspiration. The relationship between the FEV_1 and the FVC can be useful in determining normal lung dynamics or an obstructive or restrictive pattern (Table 35-1). The values shown in Table 35-1 indicate that a normal 70 kg person exhales about 80% of a roughly 5 L vital capacity in 1 second. Patients with either obstructive or restrictive pulmonary diseases will have a decreased forced vital capacity, but the relationship of the FEV_1 to the FVC will vary greatly. In obstructive lung disease, the percent of exhaled gas in 1 second will be relatively low; in a restrictive pattern, the percent exhaled within 1 second will be relatively high.

Table 35-1 **RELATIONSHIP OF FORCED EXPIRATION PATTERNS TO PULMONARY DISEASE**

	FEV_1 (L)	FVC (L)	Percent
Normal	4	5	80
Obstructive	1.4	3.3	39
Restrictive	3	3.3	90

Disease processes that increase airway resistance have a dramatic effect on the forced expiratory volume. Causes of increased airway resistance include asthma, chemical irritants, cigarette smoke, chronic bronchitis with structural changes in the airway, and airway obstruction secondary to a foreign body or retained bronchial secretions. Patients with chronic obstructive lung disease secondary to chronic bronchitis or emphysema have several factors that affect pulmonary function and the delayed FEV_1/FVC. The mucosal lining of the airways may be thickened, and that, combined with excessive secretions, leads to increased pulmonary resistance to air flow. Actual destruction of lung tissue may occur with a decrease in the number of small airways of the terminal bronchioles and secondary increased resistance. Additionally, even though the lung volume may be greatly increased with emphysema, there is a loss of normal elastic recoil of the lung. As alveolar walls lose structural integrity, there is a tendency for collapse of the smaller airways because of a loss of support from the lung parenchyma. All of these factors tend to increase airway resistance and thus act as an obstruction to normal gas flow within the airway.

Restrictive lung disease usually occurs because of interstitial fibrosis. The total volume of the lung is reduced, but the elastic recoil pressure of the lung is high, and therefore the FEV_1/FVC will be high. In the clinical situation there is a great deal of overlap between obstructive and restrictive disorders, and mixed patterns of lung disease are extremely common. Thus these illustrations represent an oversimplification of the disease process involved.

Compliance of the lung is represented by an expression that defines a change in volume for a given change in pressure. This change in volume will be greatly affected by changes in small airways that produce increased resistance. This concept of decreased compliance or stiff lungs will be discussed extensively in the section on ARDS.

Certain terms are necessary to understand the concept of ventilation. The first of these terms is *total ventilation*. Total ventilation represents the additive effects of *alveolar ventilation* and *total dead-space ventilation*. It must be remembered that when gas is taken into the lungs, only a portion goes to the alveoli to participate in gas exchange at the alveolar-capillary membrane. The volume of gas that goes to the alveoli is called *alveolar ventilation*. A certain amount of gas will fill the conducting airways and is designated *anatomic dead-space ventilation*. There may also be a portion of gas that goes to alveoli that are not perfused and therefore cannot participate in gas exchange; such alveolar gas is referred to as *physiologic dead space*.

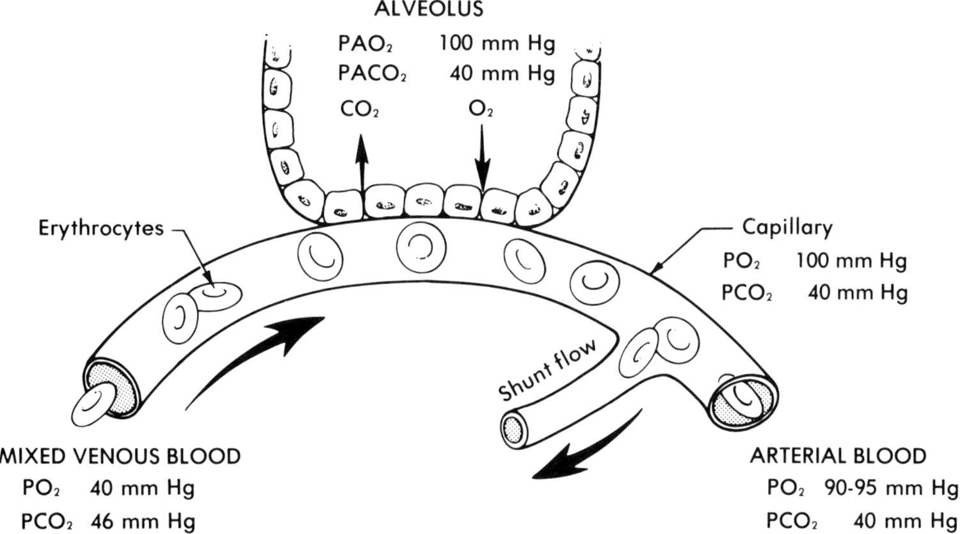

Fig. 35-1 Relationship between driving pressures for oxygen *(O_2)* and carbon dioxide *(CO_2)* exchange at alveolar-capillary membranes.

The elimination of carbon dioxide is directly related to alveolar ventilation but may not be directly related to total ventilation since an increase in dead space must cause an increase in total ventilation if the alveolar ventilation is to remain constant. Therefore simple determination of minute ventilation will not necessarily provide accurate information about the adequacy of alveolar ventilation. However, the effectiveness of alveolar ventilation can be simply determined by measurement of arterial partial pressure of carbon dioxide (P_{CO_2}) and increases or decreases in P_{CO_2} reflect hypoventilation or hyperventilation, respectively, at the alveolar level.

The body has an elaborate system for the maintenance of P_{CO_2} within a narrow normal range by alterations as needed in the alveolar ventilation. An increase in P_{CO_2} causes an increased diffusion of carbon dioxide into the cerebrospinal fluid (CSF) resulting in a decrease in CSF pH. This decrease in CSF pH stimulates ventilation through central chemoreceptor neurons located in the medulla. Conversely, a decrease in P_{CO_2} increases the pH and depresses respiration by the same mechanism. Diaphragmatic excursion accounts for muscular activity necessary for adequate ventilation during quiet resting ventilation. As the minute ventilation increases, accessory muscles of respiration, including abdominal and intercostal musculature, must be used.

Exchange of Oxygen and Carbon Dioxide

The exchange of oxygen and carbon dioxide is the principal function of the lungs and requires a coordinated effort of the individual components of the respiratory cycle to proceed smoothly. Respiratory muscle function, nondiseased airways, alveoli, and normal pulmonary vasculature must be present if the gases and blood are to reach the critical point of gas exchange at the alveolar-capillary level. Fig. 35-1 illustrates the pressure relationships between the alveolar and blood interface that allow gas exchange. The oxygen tissue tension is approximately 40 mm Hg and that of the alveoli is 100 mm Hg, allowing a 60 mm Hg gradient for adequate gas exchange. Carbon dioxide is approximately 25 times more soluble than oxygen. Thus the gradient difference between arterial carbon dioxide (40 mm Hg) and venous carbon dioxide (46 mm Hg) permits adequate carbon dioxide uptake by tissues and exchange at the alveolus.

The oxygen requirements for resting human adults is approximately 150 to 250 cc/min. The volume of oxygen carried in the blood is dependent on the concentration of hemoglobin, and the partial pressure of oxygen (P_{O_2}) with 1 g of hemoglobin binding is about 1.34 cc of oxygen. About 98% of oxygen is transported as oxyhemoglobin, and only a small amount of oxygen or carbon dioxide is carried in a simple solution. The oxygen-carrying capacity is therefore markedly affected in cases of severe anemia in which the hemoglobin concentration is greatly reduced. Therefore 15 g of hemoglobin that is 97% saturated will transport 20 volumes percent of oxygen, whereas 7.5 g of hemoglobin of equal saturation will carry only 10 volumes percent of oxygen. The transport of oxygen will also be affected by the oxyhemoglobin desaturation curve (see Chapter 25 on physiology of respiration for more detailed discussion). The P_{O_2}, for example, at 50% saturation (P_{50}) at a temperature of 37.5° C and a plasma pH of 7.4 is 26.5 mm Hg. Increasing the percent saturation from approximately 50% to 90% will result in a marked increase in P_{O_2} (i.e., the steep portion of the oxyhemoglobin saturation curve). However, once the saturation reaches about 90%, there will be a relatively small incremental change in P_{O_2} because of the flatness of the curve at this point. Increases in temperature and decreases in plasma pH result in a shift of this curve to the right with a greater degree of oxygen in solution. The chemical intermediary that is present within the red blood cell and is responsible for oxygen transport appears to be 2,3-diphosphoglyceric acid (2,3-DPG). Oxygen forms a bond with this substance, allowing much more oxygen to be transported by erythrocytes than would be carried dissolved in a simple solution. This bond between oxygen and 2,3-DPG is not stable, and the oxygen can be released or "off-loaded" from the molecule under conditions such as decreased pH. The storage of blood results in a marked decrease in the concentration of 2,3-DPG and a decrease in the P_{50}.

Hypoxemia

Hypoxemia is rarely caused by abnormalities in oxygen-diffusing ability, although such an abnormality may be a cofactor with other mechanisms. The common causes of hypoxemia are alveolar hypoventilation, ventilation-perfusion ($\dot{V}A/\dot{Q}$) mismatching, or an increase in the intrapulmonary shunts.

The alveolar-arterial gradient (A-aDO_2) may be useful in determining the oxygen exchange across the lung. Ordinarily the A-aDO_2 is less than 20 mm Hg with this difference resulting from the 5% of cardiac output that normally shunts across the lung without being oxygenated. The A-aDO_2 may be calculated after breathing 100% oxygen for 20 minutes and is useful in determining the cause of hypoxemia.

The causes of alveolar hypoventilation are indicated in the boxed material at left. In alveolar hypoventilation that results in hypoxemia, the hypoxemia is caused by a direct decrease in the PO_2 in the alveoli and therefore must be reflected in a decreased PO_2 at the arterial level. Thus there is no abnormality of oxygen exchange across the lung, and the A-aDO_2 will be normal in alveolar hypoventilation (Table 35-2). In ventilation-perfusion mismatching, the capillary blood is directed to alveoli that are being ventilated where the $\dot{V}A/\dot{Q}$ ratio is less than 1. Thus the blood from low ventilation areas will have a PO_2 that is less than normal. As the amount of ventilation-perfusion inequality increases, there is a greater likelihood that hypoxemia will result. In this situation increasing the inspired oxygen content (FIO_2) will increase the PO_2, since the alveoli are being ventilated. In fact, raising the FIO_2 to higher levels will result in an A-aDO_2 that is nearly normal.

Shunting of blood represents a different situation since blood perfuses the capillaries of alveoli that are not ventilated. Therefore there is no potential for oxygen transport in this situation, and increases in FIO_2 do not produce concomitant increases in PO_2. In fact, if the shunt fraction increases to greater than 30%, the rise in FIO_2 to 1.0 will have virtually no effect. The shunt fraction can be calculated by the formula:

$$\frac{Qs}{Qt} = \frac{O_2 \text{ Content capillary} - \text{Arterial } O_2 \text{ content}}{O_2 \text{ Content capillary} - \text{Mixed venous } O_2 \text{ content}}$$

(where Qs is the shunt flow, and QT is the total flow)

The arterial oxygen content and mixed venous oxygen content can be calculated from measurements of the partial pressure and percent saturation of the arterial and mixed venous blood obtained from a pulmonary artery catheter. The capillary oxygen content is more difficult to ascertain accurately since its measurement is based on the assumption that either the arterial-venous difference for oxygen is fixed or that the partial pressure of oxygen at the arterial

CAUSES OF ALVEOLAR HYPOVENTILATION

Thoracic Wall and Neuromuscular Abnormalities
- Trauma
- Kyphoscoliosis
- Obesity
- Guillain-Barré syndrome
- Myasthenia gravis
- Neuromuscular blockade (such as curare)
- Poliomyelitis (anterior horn cell disease)
- Bilateral diaphragmatic paralysis
- Severe malnutrition (muscular atrophy)
- Myxedema
- Pleural restrictive disease
- Upper airway obstruction

Central Respiratory Depression
- Idiopathic hypoventilation
- Sleep apnea syndrome
- Pickwickian syndrome
- Central nervous system altering drugs (opiates, sedatives, anesthetics)
- Central nervous system trauma } Medulla abnormality
- Central nervous system infections } Medulla abnormality
- Stroke

Table 35-2 **EVALUATION OF HYPOXEMIA**

Causes of Hypoxemia	Pathologic Process	PCO_2 Level	Response of PO_2 to Increased FIO_2	A-aDO_2
Alveolar hypoventilation	Decreased PAO_2 and subsequent PO_2	Elevated	Rises	Normal (<20 mm Hg; PAO_2 >500 mm Hg $FIO_2 = 1.0$)
Ventilation-perfusion mismatching	Higher percentage of pulmonary blood flow perfusing portions of lung with ventilation-perfusion ratio <1. Lower percentage of fully oxygenated blood and resultant hypoxemia	Normal or decreased	Rises	Near normal with high FIO_2 (PAO_2 >500 mm Hg if $FIO_2 = 1.0$)
Shunting	Blood perfusing capillary bed of unventilated alveoli	Normal or decreased	No change	Marked difference that increases as percentage of blood increases

and capillary level is 100% saturated. Neither of these assumptions is likely to be true with respiratory failure, and thus formulas used to calculate shunt fraction may introduce error. Therefore if the patient has a major shunt, there will be relatively little effect from increasing the FIO_2. Likewise, both $\dot{V}A/Q$ abnormalities and shunts may be present in the same patient, and the relative contribution of each is difficult to determine without very sophisticated techniques that are not clinically practical.

CLINICAL DISORDERS OF THE LUNG

Acute Respiratory Failure

There is no uniform definition of respiratory failure that would be applicable to all patients since age, presence of chronic pulmonary disease, and inspired oxygen concentration all greatly affect the patient's blood gas status. For this discussion I will define acute respiratory failure as acute dyspnea, partial pressure of oxygen (PO_2) of less than 50 mm Hg while breathing room air, partial pressure of carbon dioxide (PCO_2) greater than 50 mm Hg, and a decreased arterial pH (<7.35). Not all patients will have all of these findings, but two are usually present and hypoxemia is the most important of these.[5]

CAUSES OF ACUTE RESPIRATORY FAILURE

Brain
- Stroke
- Bulbar poliomyelitis
- Drug overdose (such as narcotics)
- Central alveolar hypoventilation
- Anesthetic depression
- Cerebral edema
- Myxedema

Spinal Cord
- Guillain-Barré syndrome
- Spinal cord trauma
- Poliomyelitis
- Amyotrophic lateral sclerosis

Neuromuscular System
- Myasthenia gravis
- Tetanus
- Curare-like agents
- Neuromuscular-blocking antibiotics
- Botulism
- Organophosphate insecticides
- Peripheral neuritis
- Multiple sclerosis
- Severe depletion—K^+, Mg^+, PO_4

Thorax and Pleura
- Muscular dystrophy
- Massive obesity
- Kyphoscoliosis
- Flail chest
- Rheumatoid spondylitis
- Pneumothorax
- Pleural effusion

Upper Airway
- Sleep apnea (obstruction)
- Tonsillar hypertrophy
- Vocal cord paralysis
- Tracheal obstruction
- Epiglottitis
- Laryngeal edema

Cardiovascular
- Cardiogenic pulmonary edema
- Pulmonary embolism
- Uremia

Lower Airway and Alveoli
- Aspiration
- Smoke inhalation
- Severe asthma
- Chronic obstructive lung disease
- ARDS
- Pulmonary fibrosis
- Cystic fibrosis
- Bilateral pneumonia
- Atelectasis
- Pulmonary contusion
- Fat embolism syndrome
- Near drowning
- Radiation injury
- Pancreatitis
- Microembolization

Respiratory failure has been divided into Types I and II. Type I patients have hypoxemia with a normal or low PCO_2. This type of failure is more common in patients with adult respiratory distress syndrome and usually is accompanied by poor lung compliance. Type II patients have both hypoxemia and hypercapnia. These conditions usually result from chronic obstructive lung disease or central nervous system defects resulting in alveolar hypoventilation.

The causes of acute respiratory failure may range from defects in the brain or spinal cord to the level of the alveolus. The myriad causes of acute respiratory failure are shown in the boxed material at left. The Type I pattern of respiratory failure is of greater clinical importance to surgeons than Type II, and the problem of adult respiratory distress syndrome will be discussed in detail.

Adult Respiratory Distress Syndrome

The adult respiratory distress syndrome (ARDS) was described in 1967 by Ashbaugh and associates[3] in 12 adult patients with the clinical features of dyspnea, hypoxemia, decreased pulmonary compliance, and diffuse alveolar infiltrates that resembled pulmonary edema even though there was no prior history of lung disease or congestive heart failure. The term ARDS was derived because Ashbaugh and associates believed that a defect in surfactant metabolism in adults similar to that seen in premature infants might be responsible for the abnormalities observed. Although decreased surfactant levels have been measured in bronchopulmonary lavage fluid from patients with ARDS, it is believed that these changes are secondary rather than primary factors in its cause. Moore and associates[33] described the clinical behavior of pulmonary insufficiency following shock and trauma and began to identify many factors that were thought to be contributory, including fluid overload, massive blood transfusion, thromboembolism, fat embolism, and aspiration.

The critical role of sepsis in the cause of ARDS was defined by Fulton and Jones[16] in an evaluation of injured patients at the University of Louisville. In a study of 399 high-risk trauma patients, ARDS developed in 44 patients. Sepsis was present in 40 of the 44 patients and appeared to be the primary causative factor along with a history of shock, direct chest injury, and several of the factors previously noted. The important role of sepsis, which is often occult at the time pulmonary insufficiency develops, was confirmed by Walker and Eiseman.[58] Thus a hallmark of prevention or control of ARDS is prevention and/or treatment of sepsis, even though this has been an elusive goal.

It appears that ARDS represents a final common pathway to a variety of noxious stimuli or injuries to the lung. Potential causes of ARDS include:

- Air embolism
- Aspiration
- Burns
- Cardiopulmonary bypass
- Drug overdose
- Disseminated intravascular coagulation (DIC)
- Eclampsia
- Fat embolism syndrome
- Near drowning
- Oxygen toxicity
- Pancreatitis
- Pulmonary contusion
- Sepsis
- Smoke inhalation
- Trauma

Some common features of ARDS are frequently used to describe symptoms in a variety of syndromes that in part may be related to ARDS, including shock lung, wet lung, Da Nang lung, noncardiogenic pulmonary edema, capillary leak syndrome, pulmonary contusion, congestive atelectasis, and adult hyaline membrane disease. ARDS is a clinical syndrome, and thus clinical criteria must be used for diagnosis since there is no single laboratory test that can be equated with the condition. Diagnostic criteria may vary slightly from one clinical series to another but generally include the following[37,39]:

1. History of an event resulting in respiratory failure
2. Exclusion of pulmonary or cardiac disease as the primary cause of the respiratory failure
3. Respiratory distress as manifested by dyspnea, hypoxemia, and tachypnea
4. Diffuse pulmonary infiltrates on chest radiograph
5. PO_2 less than 50 mm Hg with fractional inspired oxygen concentration greater than 0.6, reduced pulmonary compliance, increased shunt fraction, and increased dead-space ventilation

Several studies have refined the risk factors thought to contribute to ARDS. Fowler and associates[11] prospectively followed 936 patients with a variety of conditions thought to predispose to ARDS, including sepsis, cardiopulmonary bypass, multiple transfusions, pulmonary contusion, pelvic fracture, severe pneumonia, disseminated intravascular coagulation, and aspiration of gastric contents. The incidence of ARDS for those with a single risk factor was 5.8%, but the addition of multiple factors increased the risk of ARDS to 24.6%. The lowest risk factor was cardiopulmonary bypass whereas sepsis was the highest. A study by Pepe and associates[37] in Seattle confirmed the additive effect of multiple risk factors on the likelihood of the development of ARDS.

Pathology of ARDS

One of the reasons commonly given for inclusion of a variety of insults in the definition of ARDS is that the lung seems to respond to diverse injuries in a remarkably constant pathologic nature.[6] However, the simplistic approach that ARDS merely represents noncardiac pulmonary edema or capillary leak is probably not realistic in light of the complex pathologic process that occurs.[20] The pathologic phases of ARDS are listed below and illustrated in Figs. 35-2 to 35-6:

1. Phase 1 (Early-reversible)
   Interstitial edema
   Fibrin deposition in pulmonary microvasculature
   ± Alveolar edema
   Grossly heavy, edematous, ± hemorrhagic
2. Phase 2 (Early progressive)
   Perialveolar hyaline membranes
   Capillary congestion
   Interstitial edema
3. Phase 3 (Late progressive)
   Decreased congestion and edema
   Perialveolar interstitial fibrosis
   Increased Type II pneumocytes
   Decreased number of capillaries
4. Phase 4 (Resolving)
   Gradually improving architecture
   Decreased fibrosis

The Type I alveolar-lining cell is more prone to injury than the Type II cuboidal cell, and the Type I cells rapidly undergo necrosis. In the earliest phase of ARDS, alveolar and interstitial edema are present. There is active deposition of fibrin, platelets, and leukocytes. The second phase is characterized by hyaline membranes rich in eosinophilic-staining material, which surrounds the alveolar ducts. This phase usually occurs 4 to 5 days after the in-

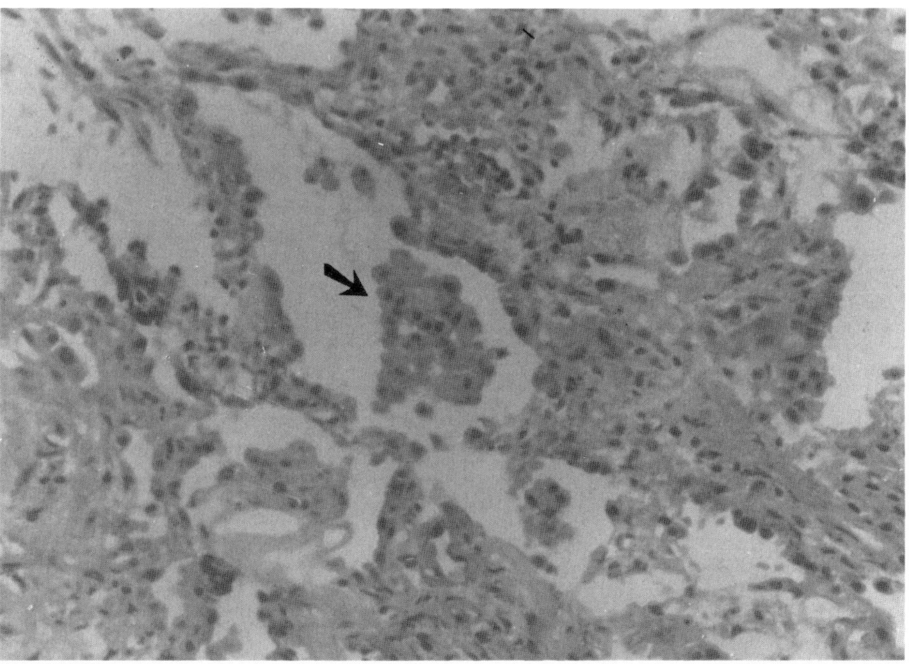

Fig. 35-2 Early phase of ARDS characterized by thickened alveoli and sloughing of pneumocytes into alveolus *(arrow)*.

citing event that produced ARDS. The late progressive phase is characterized by increased interstitial fibrosis and an increase in Type II pneumocytes. These Type II cells proliferate, resulting in a thickened alveolar septum. Superinfection with bacteria or fungi may also occur, further complicating the pathologic condition. The final phase will lead either to further fibrosis and eventual death or to gradual resolution of the process, presumably resulting from the action of scavenger alveolar macrophages. Interstitial and intra-alveolar fibrosis centered primarily around the alveolar ducts appears to be the major long-term consequence of ARDS. These changes occur rapidly, and increased collagen contact was noted in the lungs of all patients who survived more than 12 days.

Parallels have been drawn between idiopathic pulmonary fibrosis and ARDS. Each is characterized by acute alveolar injury manifested by interstitial inflammation, hemorrhage, and edema, followed by a proliferative phase

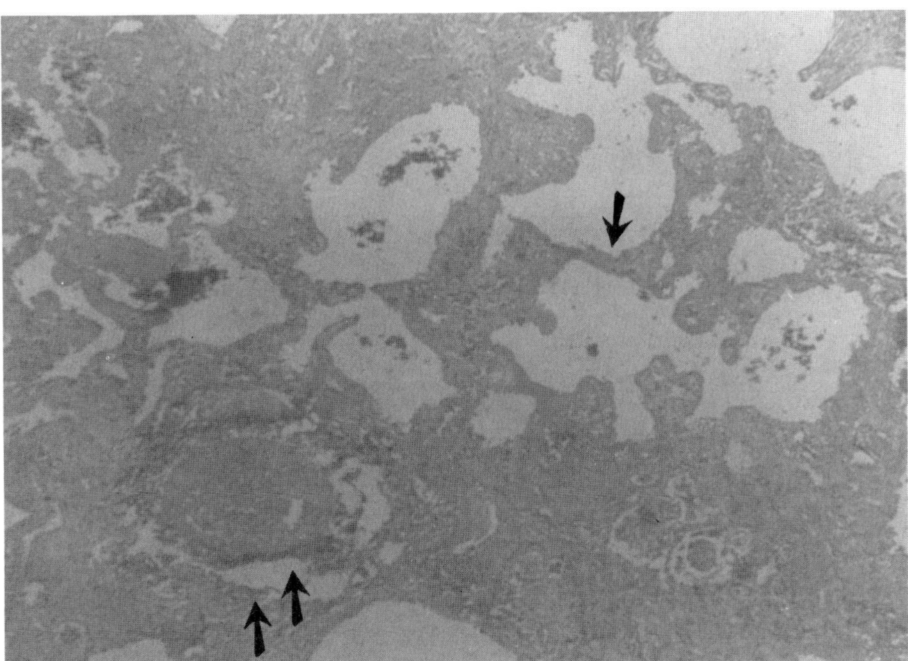

Fig. 35-3 Hyaline membranes *(single arrow)* noted around alveoli, but alveoli are still distinguishable histologically. Vessel thrombosis *(double arrow)* contributes to increased pulmonary artery pressure.

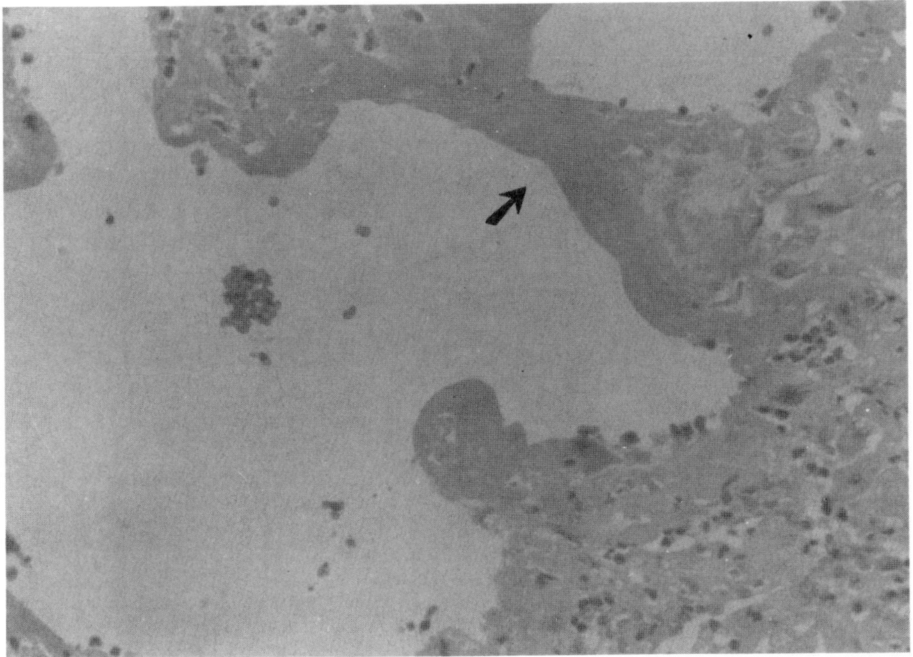

Fig. 35-4 A close view of changes in hyaline membrane *(arrow)* around alveolar wall.

with an increase in Type II pneumocytes culminating in the eventual loss of the alveolar structure and subsequent fibrosis. A variety of mechanisms has been implicated as potential mediators of the fibrotic response even though the exact cause is uncertain. It is known that alveolar macrophages are capable of stimulating fibroblast proliferation and may act to increase pulmonary fibrosis. Whether they initiate the fibrosis in ARDS remains to be defined.

Pathophysiology of ARDS

The initial inciting event in the production of ARDS is believed to occur from a capillary leak presumably resulting from damage to the pulmonary capillary endothelium[1,54] as previously discussed. Potential causes of the capillary endothelial injury are shown below:

1. Direct injury
   Toxins (gases, inhalants)

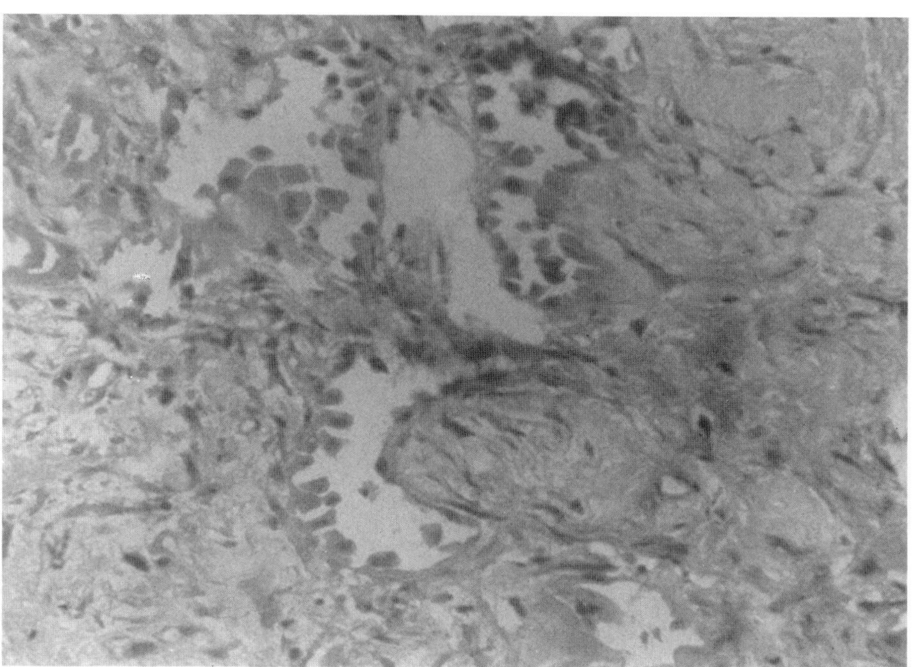

Fig. 35-5 Later stages of ARDS reveal alveolar wall nearly destroyed, walls markedly thickened, and loss of capillaries.

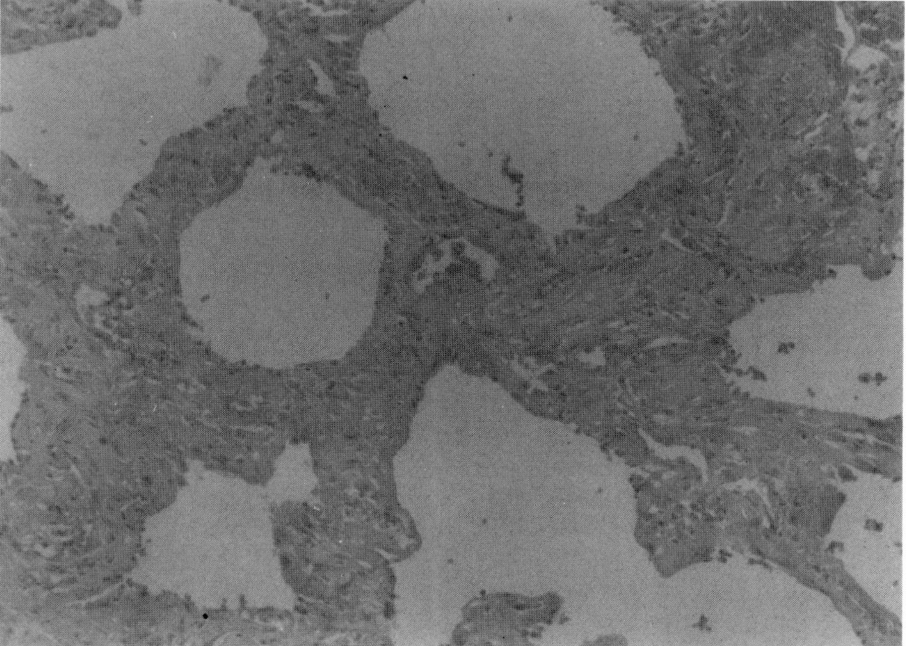

Fig. 35-6 Low-power view of resolving ARDS with marked thickening of airways but resolution of hyaline membranes.

Acid aspiration
Oxygen toxicity
2. Granulocyte injury
Oxygen-free radicals (complement-mediated)
Proteolytic enzymes
Platelet activating factor
Arachidonic acid metabolites
3. Arachidonic acid pathway
Leukotriene
Thromboxane
Prostaglandin
4. By-product of coagulation
Fibrin
Fibrin degradation products

Protein-rich fluid leaks into the interstitium and Starling's forces (see discussion) result in accumulation of edematous fluid. Eventually alveolar edema occurs as the tension in the alveolar wall is overcome. Surfactant abnormalities then develop, and widespread alveolar collapse occurs with a resultant noncompliant or stiff lung. Profound hypoxemia then develops as a result of shunting and ventilation-perfusion mismatch. Presumably the shunt occurs because of blood flow through areas of severe alveolar edema and collapse. Noncompliant lungs are clinically reflected by the high-peak pressures required to deliver an adequate tidal volume. The combination of interstitial and alveolar edema along with the active bronchoconstriction induced by arachidonic acid metabolites is the most likely cause for the loss of lung compliance.

Lung volumes are also decreased with ARDS. The mechanisms responsible for decreased lung volume might include fluid-filled alveoli, atelectasis, compression of alveoli by interstitial edema, and surfactant abnormalities with resultant increased surface tension.

Although the specific causes of ARDS are unknown, intense investigation has yielded much information about the potential physiologic mechanisms responsible for this disorder (or as the case may be, this group of disorders). One of the observations that led to a current theory on the pathogenesis of ARDS was made in the late 1960s on dialysis patients.[21] It was noted that patients developed severe leukopenia while undergoing hemodialysis. It was initially supposed that the leukocytes were trapped on the cellophane membrane of the dialyzer; however, it was later observed that many of these patients had a marked decrease in Po_2 at the time the leukocyte count decreased. A search for the mechanism of this sequence of events prompted a series of laboratory experiments in which sheep plasma exposed to a hemodialyzer was reinfused into the animals. These animals developed both sudden profound leukopenia and pulmonary dysfunction. Examination of fresh lung specimens from these sheep disclosed that the pulmonary vasculature was filled with leukocytes, particularly granulocytes and monocytes, such as were depleted from the blood.[19]

The use of the sheep lymph fistula model[52] produced much of the physiologic framework for the current theories on the pathogenesis of ARDS. It was observed in such experimental preparations that the infusion of activated complement components resulted in pulmonary artery hypertension, profound neutropenia, arterial hypoxemia, and increased pulmonary lymph flow, suggesting a capillary leak. Furthermore, if the animals were rendered granulocytopenic before the infusion of activated complement, its effects could be obviated.

Role of Neutrophil in ARDS. Numerous morphologic and histopathologic studies have disclosed the presence of neutrophils in the pulmonary microvasculature of patients with ARDS and in laboratory animals under various experimental conditions including pancreatitis, endotoxin infusion, infusion of live bacteria, and particulate microembolization.[54] Creation of the same experimental design in animals that are rendered neutropenic produces none of the sequelae noted in intact animals. Furthermore, bronchopulmonary lavage in patients with ARDS has resulted in the retrieval of fluid that is rich in elastase and oxidants (presumably released from neutrophils), which are known to be directly toxic to the lung.

There is a variety of mechanisms through which neutrophilic injury to the lung can occur:[10,45,63]

1. Oxygen-free radicals, which are toxic metabolites derived from molecular oxygen and include superoxide anions, hydrogen peroxide, singlet oxygen ion, and the hydroxy radical, are believed to be injurious to the lung. Furthermore, all of these oxygen by-products are capable of being produced by enzyme systems present in neutrophils. Studies of cultured lung endothelial cells exposed to granulocytes and activated complement show direct cellular injury. Accumulating evidence suggests that "free radical scavengers" such as superoxide dismutase and catalase may ameliorate some of these effects.

2. Proteases released by neutrophils may activate complement, Hageman factor, and plasminogen in the blood, producing both direct pulmonary injury and activating other deleterious pathways that produce pulmonary endothelial damage.

3. Neutrophils release various metabolites of arachidonic acid including prostaglandins, thromboxanes, and leukotrienes. These substances may promote vasoconstriction, alter capillary permeability, and act as chemoattractants for other neutrophils.

4. Neutrophils also release platelet activating factor, which promotes platelet and neutrophil agglutination and increased vascular permeability. Furthermore, normal lung defense mechanisms such as alpha-1-antitrypsin, are permanently deactivated by the superoxide radical and high concentrations of oxygen.

The current hypothesis regarding the pathogenesis of ARDS is that some noxious stimulus (e.g., sepsis, multiple transfusions, or aspiration) triggers by complement activation or activation of the coagulation pathway a cascade of events that results in leukoagglutination, capillary leak, and creation of a fibrin network (Fig. 35-7).[18] The complement component responsible for leukoagglutination is C5a. This polypeptide of 12,000 dalton molecular weight is the activated form of C5. C5a causes granulocytes to become marginated along the pulmonary capillary endothelium. Neutropenic animals and animals genetically deficient in C5 do not develop an alveolar-capillary leak. These granulocytes respond by release of the oxygen-free radical, hydrogen peroxide, and proteolytic enzymes that injure the lung further. This injury recruits more neutrophils, which

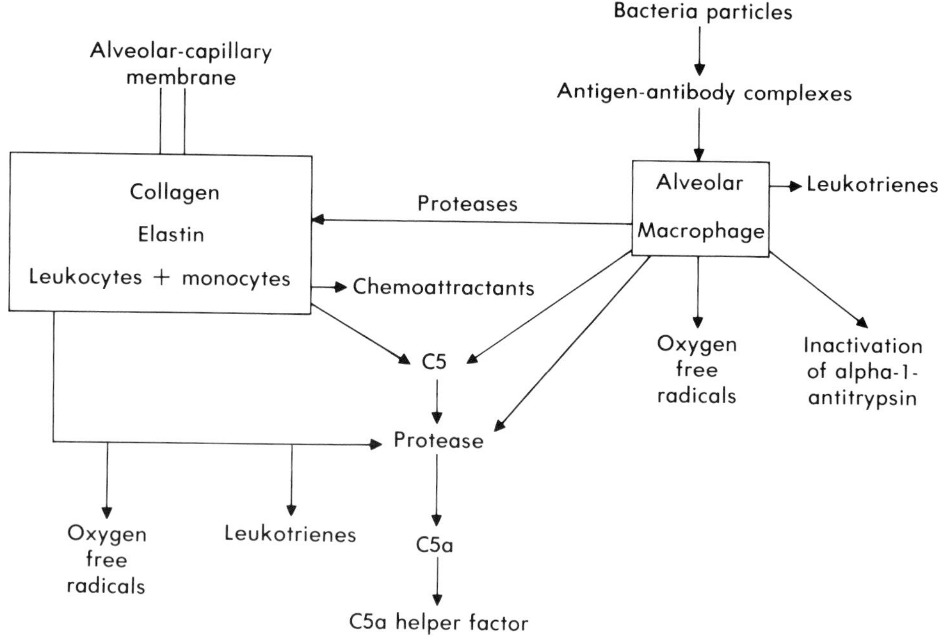

Fig. 35-7 Mechanism of complement-induced injury.

leads to a vicious cycle of further complement activation, production of arachidonic acid metabolites, and even greater direct lung injury. Eventually fibrosis will result from this chain of events as observed pathologically in patients with ARDS.

The presumed pivotal role for the granulocyte and the persistent observation of leukoagglutination in various ARDS models have suggested a potential beneficial role for corticosteroid therapy to prevent or treat this disorder. Unquestionably the role of corticosteroids in the treatment or prevention of ARDS is controversial. Those who argue for their use cite several experimental studies that provide some scientific rationale[19]:

1. Direct protection by methylprednisolone of endothelium that is exposed to granulocytes or endotoxin
2. Decreased production by granulocytes of superoxide radicals and hydrogen peroxide with steroid treatment
3. Inhibition of translocation of leukocytes into the pulmonary vasculature by high-dose methylprednisolone
4. Decreased leukoaggregation in the presence of high doses of methylprednisolone

Role of Coagulation Injury in ARDS. It seems clear that the coagulation system is also inolved in ARDS. Whether this involvement is a primary or secondary event is not well understood. It has been known for a number of years that patients with ARDS have a high incidence of pulmonary vascular occlusion as measured angiographically.[7] Furthermore, both an increased platelet consumption and increased platelet sequestration in the lung are noted in patients with ARDS. A variety of experiments conducted primarily by Malik and associates[26] indicated that complement, neutrophils, fibrin, and fibrin degradation products are essential components for the development of ARDS following microembolization. Platelets do not appear pivotal in the genesis of ARDS but are believed to release serotonin and other arachidonic acid metabolites that increase the pulmonary hypertension, which is a frequently observed event in patients with ARDS. The observation that heparin and fibrinogen depletion did not block the ARDS picture in experimental animals shows that not every portion of the coagulation system is equally important in inciting the chain of events that lead to ARDS. Additionally, certain coagulation products may produce direct lung injury. Manwaring, Thorning, and Curreri[28] showed that the infusion of thrombin and "antigen D" (one of the fibrin degradation products) causes an increased capillary permeability with hypoxemia.

In the normal animal the reticuloendothelial system (RES) plays a major role in the clearance of both aggregates and products of fibrin degradation (FDP). Saba and associates[44] elucidated the role of fibronectin as an important component of this critical RES function. Fibronectin is a protein of 450,000 molecular weight that is located on platelet membranes and throughout the RES. Fibronectin appears to function as an opsonin to aid in the removal of aggregates and FDP. It has been observed that patients with ARDS or a predisposition to this syndrome have a depletion of fibronectin. Since fibronectin can be infused in cryoprecipitate, it was hoped that this material might be beneficial in the treatment of ARDS. Although there was an intitial wave of enthusiasm for the therapeutic effects of fibronectin, clinical confirmation of its use has not been forthcoming.

Role of Arachidonic Acid Metabolite Injury in ARDS. Arachidonic acid is found in endothelial cells throughout the body and acts as a precursor to a number of pathways of potential importance in ARDS[48] (Fig. 35-8). Arachidonic acid may be converted through the cyclooxygenase pathway to prostaglandins or thromboxanes or through the lipoxygenase pathway to the leukotrienes.

Arachidonic acid metabolites may be released by neutrophils, platelets, and pulmonary endothelium. Throm-

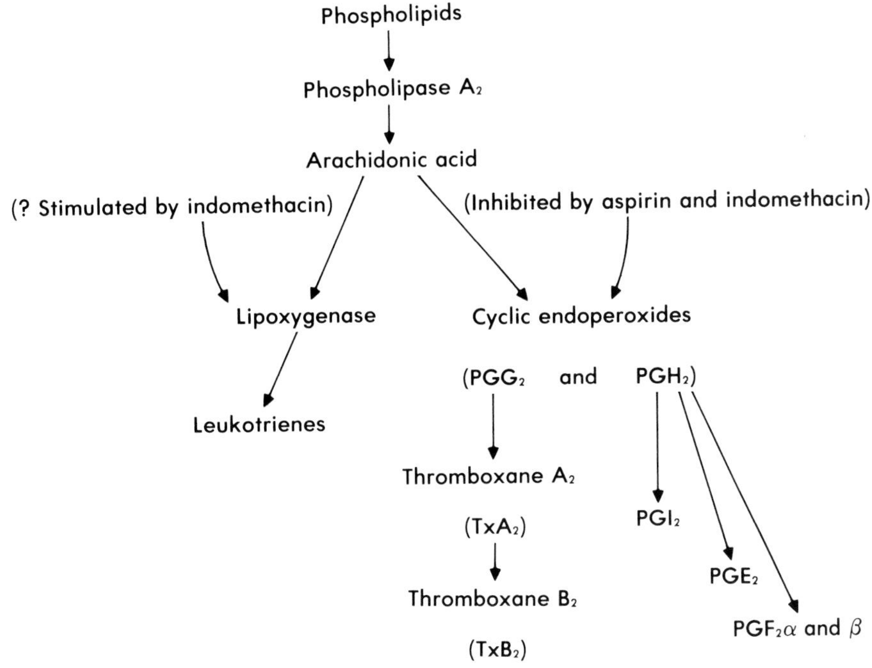

Fig. 35-8 Arachidonic acid metabolism.

boxanes appear to be potent pulmonary vasoconstrictors and bronchoconstrictors and lead to increased pulmonary vascular permeability, all of which are seen in ARDS. Increased pulmonary vascular resistance is observed in patients with ARDS and most laboratory models under experimental conditions that simulate this syndrome. Vasoconstriction is produced by several arachidonic acid metabolites, including prostaglandins E_2, F_2, H_2, and by thromboxane A_2. There is a two-phase response to infuse endotoxin in experimental animals. In the first phase an acute rise in pulmonary vascular resistance begins approximately 1 hour following infusion and can be blocked by thromboxane synthetase inhibitors; this suggests that the first phase is mediated by arachidonic acid metabolites. The second phase begins within 3 to 5 hours following endotoxin challenge and does not respond to arachidonic acid inhibitors, which suggests that this effect is not related to thromboxane.

A key to the understanding of all prostaglandin function is that for each action mediated by a prostaglandin there apparently is an opposite or antagonistic function mediated by another prostaglandin.[31] The lung is no exception, and prostaglandin E_1 and I_2 (prostacyclin) have favorable properties that counteract the deleterious effects of thromboxane. Prostacyclin (PGI_2) has powerful vasodilating properties and acts as an antagonist to platelet and neutrophil aggregation. The search for possible clinical applications of prostacyclin or for agents such as thromboxane that alter deleterious prostaglandins continues. Although a number of interesting observations have been made in the laboratory, none have yet had any widespread clinical use in the treatment of ARDS.

There has been increased interest recently in other arachidonic acid metabolites such as leukotrienes. Much of the work on the leukotrienes has been done by Samuelsson[46] of the Karolinska Institute in Stockholm, who shared the 1982 Nobel Prize for Physiology and Medicine. Work with pure leukotrienes has shown a variety of biologic effects, some of which are summarized below:

1. *Pulmonary effects* (leukotrienes C_4, D_4, E_4)
   a. Potent bronchoconstrictors
   b. Direct action on peripheral airways
2. *Microvascular effects* (leukotrienes C_4, D_4)
   a. Arteriolar vasoconstrictor
   b. Leakage of macromolecules
   c. Direct action on vessel wall (does not require histamine, prostaglandin, or granulocytes)
3. *Effects on leukocytes* (leukotriene B_4)
   a. Increased leukocyte adhesion to small vessel endothelium
   b. Increased interstitial leukocytes (? potential mediator of migration of leukocytes from blood to areas of inflammation)
   c. Activated neutrophils causing aggregation, degranulation, and superoxide production

Leukotrienes C_4, D_4 and E_4 (all containing cysteine) appear to act directly on the postcapillary venule wall to increase pulmonary vascular permeability. They are potent bronchoconstrictors and vasoconstrictors in humans. Additionally, leukotriene B_4 appears to have direct stimulating effects on leukocytes that produce agglutination, degranulation, and release of free-oxygen radicals, which have been implicated with lung injury as previously discussed.

Therapy of ARDS

There is no direct treatment for ARDS, although control of sepsis, especially with drainage of abscesses, adequate debridement of devitalized tissue, and treatment of peritonitis are all goals. The primary goal for treating ARDS is appropriate respiratory support. Prevention of iatrogenic complications by maintaining a proper fluid balance to minimize fluid flux into the lung during the capillary leak phase, prevention of nosocomial infections, and the maintenance of adequate nutrition are all keys to successful management. Maintenance of adequate oxygenation is the prime therapeutic goal in ARDS. The hypoxemia is generally poorly responsive to increasing FIO_2, and mechanical ventilation is required. Given the potential for additive pulmonary injury caused by oxygen toxicity, the FIO_2 should be kept as low as possible and still be consistent with ensuring adequate tissue oxygenation. Generally this level of arterial oxygenation approximates an oxyhemoglobin saturation of 90% with a PO_2 of approximately 60 mm Hg.

Peters[38] has described the following potentially lifesaving steps to assist the surgeon caring for a patient with ARDS:

1. Determine the adequacy of alveolar ventilation. If the patient has a PCO_2 that is elevated or even normal, ventilatory support is needed. A normal PCO_2 in the face of hypoxemia indicates inappropriate alveolar ventilation.
2. Establish maintenance of cardiac output as a first priority of therapy. Factors controlling cardiac output are (a) preload filling pressure, (b) afterload vascular resistance, and (c) contractility of the myocardium. The most common cause of decreased cardiac output in surgical patients is inadequate preload as a result of hypovolemia. Additionally, maintaining an adequate cardiac output has a direct effect on the oxygen available for tissue demands. Table 35-3 shows the effect of variations in caridac output and PO_2 on available oxygen. The importance of maintaining an adequate cardiac output in the face of low PO_2 is well demonstrated.
3. Limit FIO_2 to as low a level as possible to prevent further oxygen toxicity (below 0.4 to 0.5, if possible).
4. Institute positive end-expiratory pressure (PEEP) or continuous positive airway pressure (CPAP) if the shunt fraction is above 20% (see Chapter 34).
5. Suspect pneumothorax if peak inspiratory pressures suddenly increase, and institute rapid treatment.
6. Mobilize the patient.

By increasing functional residual capacity (FRC), the use of PEEP tends to improve oxygenation greatly in ARDS patients, permitting a lower FIO_2 to accomplish the same acceptable level of tissue oxygenation. This increase in FRC is apparently the result of prevention of airway closure and recruitment of unventilated alveoli. The ventilation of previously collapsed but perfused alveoli decreases shunting and improves hypoxemia. This increase in FRC may increase static lung compliance as well. There are many controversies about the use of PEEP that are beyond the scope of this chapter but have been excellently reviewed.[23,60] Although it is clear that PEEP improves oxygenation, its effect on the clinical course of ARDS is less certain. In fact, it has not been uniformly accepted that PEEP actually improves survival.[51] Pepe, Hudson, and Carrico[36] have reported a randomized trial of prophylactic PEEP in patients at high risk for the development of ARDS. Unfortunately, this study did not confirm the efficacy of "early PEEP" in the amelioration or prevention of ARDS. For a more detailed discussion of PEEP, the reader is referred to Chapter 34.

TABLE 35-3 **EFFECTS OF CARDIAC OUTPUT AND PO_2 ON OXYGEN AVAILABILITY**

Cardiac Output (L/min)	PO_2	Available Oxygen (cc/min)
5	60	900
5	40	750
4	60	720
4	40	600

Prichard[40] suggested several possible mechanisms to decrease lung extravascular fluid volume: (1) decrease of transvascular hydrostatic gradient; (2) increase in colloid oncotic pressure; (3) reversal of endothelial injury; and (4) increase of pulmonary lymphatic clearance. Careful attention to fluid balance with monitoring of the left-sided filling pressure of the heart may decrease the net fluid flux into the lung. Thus the goal is to assure adequate filling of the left ventricle without elevating the pulmonary capillary wedge pressure (PCWP). If the PCWP is elevated, judicious diuretics may ameliorate some of the fluid flux into the lung. Low dose dopamine (4 to 10 mg/kg) may aid in promoting a diuretic response without deterioration of cardiac dynamics. There has been a great deal of interest in the use of colloid to raise colloid osmotic pressure and circumvent the pulmonary edema seen in patients with ARDS. However, the ability to maintain normal colloid osmotic pressure during the capillary leakage phase is virtually impossible since there is a rapid movement of macromolecules from the pulmonary vascular to interstitial spaces. The value of blood or colloid-containing fluids is that better filling pressures can be maintained with less volume requirements than if crystalloid solutions alone are infused.

Attempts to alter endothelial injury have focused on two primary fields of investigation: the use of high-dose corticosteroid therapy and the use of agents to alter arachidonic acid metabolism.[22] The theoretic advantages of corticosteroids include inhibition of leukoagglutination, protection against lysosomal enzyme release, and inhibition of phospholipase that is the initial step in arachidonic acid metabolism. Although the empiric use of high-dose steroids for the treatment of ARDS is practiced in many centers, there are no data to justify this practice. There is an assumption that such steroid treatment has few side effects, but experimental laboratory studies demonstrated that a single dose of methylprednisolone markedly depressed the ability of both healthy and injured animals to clear aerolized bacteria from their lungs.[43] Given the propensity for ARDS patients to develop nosocomial pneumonia, I believe the empiric use of steroids is not justified.

A recent randomized trial from Dallas[59] included 81 acutely ill patients requiring mechanical ventilation and judged to be at high risk for the development of ARDS. Sodium methylprednisolone succinate (30 mg/hour) was used in about half the patients and placebo in the remainder. There was no difference in the number of patients who developed ARDS; however, there was a higher incidence of infectious complications in the steroid treated group. Ashbaugh and Maier[2] believe that sodium methylprednisolone succinate is useful in preventing pulmonary fibrosis that occurs with ARDS. In ten consecutive patients who were not responding to conventional treatment, lung biopsies were performed and pulmonary fibrosis documented. High-dose methylprednisolone (125 mg every 6 hours) therapy was initiated and continued until oxygenation began to improve. Eight of these patients survived. These two studies illustrate the difficulty in defining the proper role for steroid therapy because the studies compared different patient groups and used greatly different doses of methylprednisolone. Further studies are needed to properly define the role steroids play in the treatment of ARDS.

There has been considerable discussion about the inhibition of various products of arachidonic acid metabolism in the treatment of ARDS. It has been shown that aspirin and indomethacin block the cyclo-oxygenase pathway. However, there is an inhibitory effect on both thromboxane and prostacyclin that could potentially negate any specific effects of such therapy. Additionally, some studies suggest that indomethacin stimulates the lipoxygenase pathway. The mechanism for such a phenomenon might rest in the shunting of arachidonic acid from the blocked cyclo-oxygenase pathway to the lipoxygenase system. Other drugs that inhibit the cyclo-oxygenase pathway include ibuprofen and meclofenamate. Additionally, experimental studies using various thromboxane synthetase inhibitors such as dazoxiben, have been reported. This area will continue to be refined but has not reached the stage of clinical use for ARDS.

Smoke Inhalation and Pulmonary Dysfunction Following Burns

Abnormalities in the airways and lungs are common problems following burn injury. The abnormalities may include smoke inhalation (with or without any surface burn), direct thermal injury to the airway, and alterations in pulmonary function as a result of the burn wound.

A critical element of smoke inhalation is the nature of the chemical injury induced by the substance under combustion. Many models of experimental smoke inhalation using wood or charcoal as the source of smoke failed to produce the lethal inhalational injury often observed in patients.[53] It is now clear that much of the lethality of smoke inhalation results from combustion of plastic and synthetic material that release aldehydes and organic acids that are direct toxins to the upper and lower airways. Chlorine, ammonia, and sulfur compounds may also be by-products of combustion and result in the formation of potent acids and bases causing further airway injury. Direct injury to the major airways and a marked increase in bronchial blood flow may lead to formation of severe edema,[34] which is manifested in increased airway resistance. Bronchoconstriction may occur as a direct result of toxins on the airways or through a mediator such as the leukotrienes. Clinically this phase is marked by wheezing that may be severe. An increase in dead-space ventilation is also observed. Ventilation-perfusion abnormalities occur as a result of alveolar collapse from bronchospasm and peribronchiolar edema. Many patients with severe burn injury have frothy edematous fluid evident in their major airways and alveoli. The source of this edematous fluid may be direct alveolar injury with an increase in lung water or may be caused by retrograde flow of the severe mucosal edema of the bronchi. Studies in humans have tended to confirm the latter as the cause of the severe edema that is observed clinically.

Some authors have included smoke inhalation as a cause of ARDS.[36] It is clear that there is a prompt migration of neutrophils into the bronchial mucosa following such inhalation. This process is probably related to complement activation that triggers the cascade of physiologic consequences described in the previous section on ARDS.

Direct pulmonary or upper airway burns are probably a lesser cause of airway and/or lung injury than is commonly believed. Burns occurring in a closed space, particularly if associated with facial burns and burns of the nasal hairs, must be suspected of producing direct thermal injury. Direct thermal burns are usually confined to the upper airway since the oropharynx and the nasopharynx quickly dissipate heat. Thus direct upper airway injury with edema and the potential for airway obstruction are of major concern after such thermal injuries. Furthermore, the patient must be closely observed for progressive swelling that continues throughout the first 24 to 36 hours after injury. The need for high-volume fluid resuscitation to treat a major cutaneous burn undoubtedly worsens the edema and increases the potential for obstruction. Although the presence of carbonaceous sputum or the observation of soot in the airways leads to a high index of suspicion for direct thermal injury to the airway, these findings correlate poorly with the need for intubation.

Determinations of carbon monoxide levels should be obtained in such burn patients. Direct observation of the color of the arterial blood is necessary because a bright red color may be an early indicator of high carbon monoxide levels in the blood.Carbon monoxide preferentially binds with the hemoglobin molecule (CO-Hgb) instead of oxygen and interferes with the ability of hemoglobin to offload oxygen at the cellular level. When levels of CO-Hgb are in the 20% to 40% range, the symptoms may be difficult to recognize but usually include nonspecific central nervous system manifestations. Coma and even death (from severe cerebral hypoxia) are likely to occur with CO-Hgb levels in the range of 40% to 50% and greater than 60%, respectively.[9]

Demling[9] noted a number of pulmonary effects that may result from the burn wound. Particularly, thromboxane A_2 is released from burn tissue and, as discussed in the section on ARDS, has a number of potentially deleterious consequences, including bronchoconstriction with increased airway resistance and decreased compliance and vasoconstriction with resultant pulmonary artery hypertension.

There is no specific therapy for smoke inhalation at this time. Ventilatory support will usually be promptly required in severe cases. The ventilatory therapy should be aimed at providing appropriate levels of oxygenation with the least possible FIO_2 and PEEP to avoid oxygen toxicity and barotrauma. Unfortunately, many smoke inhalation patients require high levels of inspired oxygen and PEEP. Nosocomial pneumonias are common, and aseptic technique should be practiced when providing ventilatory therapy.

Pulmonary Contusion

Pulmonary contusion represents a direct injury to the lung causing localized alveolar flooding with erythrocytes. Pulmonary contusion has been acknowledged as an entity since World War II when "traumatic wet lung" was recognized as a clinical syndrome. Clinicians have always believed that fluid administration had an adverse effect on pulmonary contusion. In the decade between 1965 to 1975, enormous strides were made in the recognition of pulmonary contusion as a distinct entity, and the ability to produce effective laboratory models contributed greatly to the understanding of this problem. Although pulmonary contusion is often included among the causes of ARDS, it appears to have a different pathologic mechanism than the neutrophil-induced capillary leak phenomenon now thought to be the hallmark of ARDS.

A number of studies by Fulton and Peter[13–15] provide much of the understanding of the physiology of pulmonary contusion. Fulton and Peter developed a model of experimental contusion and found that the Po_2 was a progressive change that worsened over the first 24 hours after injury. Histologic studies of the lung taken immediately after injury showed only interstitial hemorrhage with little or no edema present. Two hours after injury there was significant edema present with a marked thickening of alveolar walls but no appreciable cellular infiltration. By 24 hours there was loss of normal alveolar architecture and profuse round cell infiltration.

Physiologic studies using a model of severe lung injury showed decreased blood flow and an increase in pulmonary vascular resistance in the injured lung. Consequently, there was a marked increase in blood flow in the noncontused lung. These changes were also progressive. Furthermore, it was noted that surfactant was decreased between 24 and 48 hours with a decreased compliance and worsening of lung mechanics.[35] The infusion of saline with or without blood produced a further fall in Po_2. When saline was rapidly infused, a marked rise in pulmonary artery pressure occurred with a shift of blood flow to the opposite lung and a subsequent increase in edema of the noncontused lung. Increased lung water was noted in both the contused and noncontused lungs.

Richardson and associates[42] and Trinkle and associates[55] developed a less severe injury model that produced an isolated contusion to study the effects of various manipulations on more limited injury. They noted that the administration of fluid caused an increase in the zone of edema surrounding the central area of contusion. The greater the volume of fluid given and the more rapid its rate of administration, the more severe was the injury produced. In studies of combined pulmonary contusion and shock, colloid did not prevent lung edema but did provide a more efficient resuscitation in terms of restoring hemodynamic parameters with less lung water produced in the area of contusion. Mehtylprednisolone was the only agent studied that decreased the extent of the pulmonary contusion.

These studies led to a series of clinical recommendations that seem valuable in the care of patients with pulmonary contusions and flail chest[41]: (1) judicious use of crystalloid solutions, avoiding unnecessary administration of sodium-containing solutions and the raising of pulmonary vascular pressure above physiologic limits; (2) liberal use of blood for resuscitation—this is done not to increase colloid osmotic pressure but to limit the amount of crystalloid required for resuscitation; (3) use of intravenous diuretics (usually 20 mg furosemide) for patients who receive excessive crystalloid resuscitation; and (4) avoid use of corticosteroids in this clinical setting because, although methylprednisolone limits the size of the contusion experimentally, there is concern about its effect on lung defenses.

One of the most controversial areas in surgical physiology concerns the debate of the appropriate use of crystalloid versus colloid solutions for the resuscitation of injured patients. A brief attempt to summarize the pros and cons of this discussion is in order for the neophyte in surgical physiology. To understand the issues concerning crystalloid and colloid, it is important to understand some basic precepts of capillary physiology. In 1896, Starling reported his observations on the absorption of fluids from connective tissue spaces into small vessels. Starling hypothesized that fluid flux was predicated by the equation:

$$\text{Net fluid flux} = K\,(\Delta P - \Delta\pi)$$

where K is the permeability of the membrane of the vessel wall; ΔP is the hydrostatic pressure gradient; and $\Delta\pi$ is the protein osmotic gradient across the wall.

If at least a portion of the deleterious effects of many noxious insults on lung (e.g., ARDS resulting from sepsis, pulmonary contusion, smoke inhalation, or aspiration injury) was caused by the net movement of fluid into the lung, then attempts were made to modify factors shown in the Starling equation. The three factors that could be altered were wall permeability, hydrostatic pressure gradient, and osmotic pressure gradient. There are few, if any, known methods to correct wall permeability abnormalities in the clinical setting, so attempts focused on means to affect hydrostatic and osmotic pressure gradients. One potential method to alter osmotic pressure in a way that would limit fluid movement into the lung was to infuse albumin solution in an attempt to raise the colloid osmotic pressure within the vascular system. Proponents[25,50] of this approach believed that the lung was better protected from edema formation with a colloid resuscitation and that hydrostatic pressure was less likely to be elevated.

Unfortunately, in many situations that are deleterious to the lung (e.g., ARDS and smoke inhalation), there is an alveolar-capillary leak; and if the pores in the capillary are large enough to allow protein and solute to cross the vessel wall, the osmotic pressure gradient, $\Delta\pi$, disappears. If this occurs, then

$$\text{Net fluid flux} = K\,\Delta P$$

where K is membrane permeability and ΔP is pressure gradient. Since this is a common occurrence in many of the important problems affecting the lung, it obviates most of the potential value of colloid infusion. In fact, since colloid may be sequestered in the connective tissue pores, it may actually promote a net fluid accumulation outside the vessel. This fact plus the high cost of colloid-containing solutions makes their use in conditions that result in alveolar-capillary leak undesirable.

Clinical trials[57] have shown that when overinfusion is avoided (and thus alter the ΔP), even large volumes of balanced salt solutions (crystalloids) are well tolerated.

Pulmonary Embolism

The etiology and clinical findings associated with pulmonary embolism are generally well recognized. The physiologic consequences of pulmonary embolism are manifested through several mechanisms. The occlusion of pulmonary arteries by clots leads to alveoli that are ventilated but not perfused, resulting in wasted ventilation or increased dead-space ventilation. Initially there is a reflex airway constriction that tends to limit ventilation to unperfused areas, but within 24 hours this reflex appears relatively unimportant in limiting ventilation-perfusion imbalance. The redistribution of blood flow from unperfused areas leads to a relative overperfusion of other alveoli, further increasing the ventilation-perfusion mismatch. Surfactant production is impaired after 24 hours, leading to local atelectasis and edema that may result in congestive atelectasis that grossly resembles pulmonary infarction. Pulmonary infarction is actually an unusual event, probably occurring in less than 10% of cases of pulmonary embolism caused by the lungs' dual blood supply.

It also appears that pulmonary embolism initiates a humoral-reflex mechanism that causes generalized pulmonary vasoconstriction. The cause of this vasoconstrictive mechanism is not precisely understood and a variety of medications has been implicated. Serotonin, bradykinin, and prostaglandins have been incriminated as the substances that cause generalized pulmonary vasoconstriction and that further heighten ventilation-perfusion imbalance. Hypoxemia without carbon dioxide retention is commonly seen following pulmonary embolus. There is an increase in the physiologic shunt and dead-space ventilation. Experimental embolism studies suggest that most cases of hypoxemia are the result of ventilation-perfusion inequity. Thus the addition of supplemental oxygen generally results in rapid improvement in hypoxemia (as opposed to a large shunt where addition of oxygen fails to improve hypoxemia).

The pulmonary vascular bed has a large capacitance with a number of vascular beds that are unused under normal circumstances. These vascular beds may be ''recruited'' under conditions of vascular occlusion by pulmonary embolus. Thus about 50% of the vasculature of the lung must be occluded before pulmonary hypertension occurs. The development of a major embolus may lead to an increase in pulmonary artery pressure. If this pressure is high and sustained, right ventricular failure may result, although this event is certainly not the usual case.

Studies on patients with pulmonary emboli have documented the consequences of these physiologic events.[47] Abnormalities noted in patients with pulmonary emboli include the following:

1. Hyperventilation: 83% of patients had a minute ventilation of greater than 8 L.
2. Pulmonary restriction: Over 80% of patients had a decreased vital capacity. Possible mechanisms might include chest splinting because of pleural pain or decreased lung compliance on the basis of surfactant loss and congestive atelectasis.
3. Bronchoconstriction: A decrease in the forced expiratory volume over a unit of time (FEV_1) and in maximum mid-expiratory flow rate may occur as a reflex mechanism or through the release of substances such as those discussed in the section on ARDS.
4. Hypoxemia: This appears to be secondary to ventilation-perfusion inequality.
5. Pulmonary hypertension: This occurs to a variable degree depending on the extent of the pulmonary embolism.

Atelectasis

Atelectasis is derived from a Greek term meaning ''airless'' and refers to a loss of volume of the lung (either lobar, segmental, or subsegmental). The term may be confusing because a number of mechanisms of atelectasis have been proposed[12] and are outlined as follows:

1. Absorption atelectasis occurs following obstruction of a major bronchus or multiple secondary bronchi with subsequent resorption of the air in the distal lung. This type of atelectasis is of major concern to the surgeon because the obstructing agent may be a mucous plug, foreign body, or tumor.
2. Passive atelectasis refers to a condition resulting from a space-occupying condition in the thorax such as a pneumothorax or hydrothorax.
3. Compression atelectasis follows a space-occupying lesion within the lung parenchyma such as might result from a tumor or emphysematous bulla. In both the passive and compression types of atelectasis, the lung being compressed may be completely normal initially.
4. Adhesive atelectasis occurs in the presence of patent bronchi and presumably is secondary to surfactant abnormalities. It is seen in association with pneumonia and other inflammatory conditions of the lung.
5. Cicatrization atelectasis refers to an airless condition of the lung associated with pulmonary fibrosis.

Atelectasis secondary to bronchial obstruction by tumor or foreign body may be associated with a variety of symptoms such as secondary pneumonia or wheezing, depending on the location and degree of obstruction involved. In some patients significant bronchial obstruction does not cause atelectasis because the lobe may continue to be ventilated by the passage of air from nonobstructed segments into the obstructed portion through interlobar communications. This phenomenon is referred to as *collateral ventilation* and explains why atelectasis may not be apparent even when a tumor or foreign body results in near total bronchial obstruction. Therefore the absence of atelectasis on a chest radiograph does not rule out the possibility of a central obstructing lesion in the bronchus.

The pathophysiology of atelectasis may be related to three major factors, each of which contributes to bronchial obstruction in the postoperative patient: (1) a decrease in the cough or expulsion mechanism from the bronchus; (2) changes in bronchial secretions leading to tenacious adherent sputum; and (3) a reduction of bronchial caliber, which may occur as a result of direct airway trauma caused by conditions such as intubation, edema, or inflammation.

Many classic studies on the incidence of atelectasis were published in the 1940s and 1950s and may no longer be applicable to patients because today greater emphasis is placed on pulmonary care. Atelectasis occurred in 10% of thoracic and upper abdominal procedures reported by Moersch in 1943[32] but in only 4% of nonabdominal operations. Kurzweg[24] studied the incidence of postoperative pulmonary complications and found that on the average they occur in 2.5% to 3% of all operations. However, complications were much higher in abdominal operations, particularly upper abdominal procedures, occurring in 10% to 20% and 20% to 30%, respectively. Atelectasis involving smaller airways (''microatelectasis''), which may not be diagnosed by chest radiography, is presumably present even more frequently.

The clinical examination should be adequate for early diagnosis of atelectasis in most patients. Bronchial breathing or moist rales occurring most commonly at the lung bases is the hallmark of the clinical condition. A chest radiograph need not be routinely obtained in the typical patient with postoperative atelectasis. Atelectasis may be manifested by tachypnea, fever, and tachycardia, but these are late signs. The cause of the fever is presumably infection secondary to bacterial proliferation in the atelectatic area of the lung. Shields[49] demonstrated in 1949 that intravenously administered bacteria tend to localize at the site of atelectasis. Collapse of the lung also interferes with the lung's host defenses and does not permit adequate macrophage function in engulfing bacteria.

Successful treatment of atelectasis depends on prompt mobilization of bronchial secretions by deep breathing, coughing, and nasotracheal suctioning if necessary. In patients with major areas of collapse that involve an entire segment or lobe of the lung or in patients in which effective nasotracheal suctioning cannot be performed, therapeutic bronchoscopy is indicated to remove secretions and mucous plugs. Increased mobilization of the patient is helpful when possible. Pain medication should be judiciously used to help avoid splinting to alleviate postoperative pain without producing harmful respiratory depression. Through the years mechanical means of pushing air into the lungs, such as intermittent positive pressure breathing, have fallen into disrepute because of their ineffectiveness, their cost, and the risk of nosocomial infection.

Pneumonia

Pneumonia is one of the most common pulmonary derangements affecting surgical patients. Postoperative pneumonia may be initiated by atelectasis or acquired as a nosocomial infection in patients treated by endotracheal intubation or tracheostomy and mechanical ventilation. In a patient hospitalized for community-acquired pneumonia, the typical signs of infection—productive cough, purulent sputum, fever, and rales—are usually present. Leukocytosis is the rule, and an infiltrate is generally present on the chest radiograph. The diagnosis of pneumonia in a postoperative patient is occasionally somewhat more difficult because the classic signs may be absent or altered by other conditions occurring in the postoperative state. A report from the University of Louisville School of Medicine[29] has used the following criteria for the diagnosis of postoperative pneumonia:

1. New postoperative infiltrate seen on chest x-ray film
2. A temperature of at least 38° C for at least 24 hours
3. Purulent sputum production and/or cultured pathogens
4. Antibiotic therapy deemed to be needed to treat the pulmonary process

Although these specific criteria may be challenged, it is important to define the clinical parameters necessary to make a diagnosis before effective study of this condition can be undertaken. With the criteria outlined above, which my associates and I hoped would eliminate those patients with atelectasis, the incidence of pneumonia was 1.3% of all operated cases over a 7-year period. This rate compares with an incidence of 0.75% of all surgical patients reported by the National Nosocomial Infection Study[8] but is much lower than the 17% reported by Garibaldi and associates.[17] However, the latter study did not require culture evidence of pneumonia and undoubtedly included many patients with atelectasis.

The mortality rate for patients with postoperative pneumonia is high (from 15% to 50%) with the specific rate dependent on the diagnostic criteria. Certain risk factors are predictors of a poor outcome including: (1) gram-negative pneumonitis, particularly *Pseudomonas;* (2) signs of remote organ failure; (3) bilateral pneumonia; (4) emergency operation preceding pneumonia; (5) positive blood culture; (6) postoperative peritonitis; and (7) pneumonia acquired while receiving mechanical ventilation. It is postulated that several of these risk factors, including positive blood culture, the development of bilateral pneumonia, and the occurrence of multiple organ failure, represent a breakdown of host defense mechanisms and thus ensure a high mortality.

Further analysis of patients with postoperative pneumonia indicate that the following three etiologic mechanisms are involved: (1) postatelectasis (as discussed in the previous section); (2) postaspirations; and (3) following the introduction of mechanical ventilation for hypoxemia.

Aspiration is a major risk factor for the development of pneumonia in surgical patients. The following list indicates various conditions that predispose to aspiration.

1. Alteration of consciousness
   Head injury
   Stroke, seizure, coma
   Alcohol intoxication
   Drug overdose
   Cardiac arrest
   General anesthesia
   Oversedation
2. Derangements of swallowing mechanism and esophageal function
   Tracheostomy
   Laryngeal lesions (e.g., carcinoma, ulcers)
   Pseudobulbar palsy
   Esophageal obstruction (e.g., cancer, benign stricture)
   Incompetent lower esophageal sphincter (with or without hiatus hernia)
   Achalasia

Zenker's or epiphrenic diverticulum
Tracheoesophageal fistula
Nasogastric intubation
3. Defective cough reflex
Post local anesthesia of larynx and trachea
Neuromuscular disorders

Drugs that alter the state of consciousness such as general anesthesia and postoperative pain medications are particularly important to surgeons. Likewise, alcohol intoxication, substance abuse, and head injuries are frequently encountered in patients who suffer traumatic injuries. A variety of disorders of swallowing and esophageal function is commonly seen by surgeons and and may predispose the patients to aspiration. The treatment of pneumonia will depend in large part on which of the three etiologic mechanisms mentioned previously is responsible for the pulmonary infection. If the pneumonia occurs as a consequence of atelectasis, then vigorous pulmonary toilet with nasotracheal suction and/or therapeutic bronchoscopy as indicated will usually result in a prompt resolution of the process. Antibiotics specific to the pathogen cultured should be instituted, but mechanical treatment to eliminate the source of bronchial obstruction seems the most important part of the treatment regimen.

The treatment of aspiration pneumonia is more conventional. A variety of specific treatment recommendations for pneumonia following aspiration includes the following:

1. Bronchopulmonary lavage to remove acid and/or particulate matter from the airways
2. Corticosteroids to obviate the inflammatory response produced by the low pH in the tracheobronchial tree
3. Empiric use of antibiotics (to cover a broad spectrum or narrow spectrum such as oral cavity flora)
4. Selective use of antibiotics (based on organisms seen on Gram's stain of aspirated material or on culture results)

There is no one protocol for the treatment of aspiration that has been proven with randomized trials to be more effective than other treatment modalities. At the University of Louisville School of Medicine, I use the following guidelines in the management of aspiration:

1. Heavy emphasis is placed on preventing aspiration.
2. If aspiration has been observed or is thought to have occurred, liberal use is made of therapeutic bronchoscopy.
3. Corticosteroids are not used for the treatment of aspiration.
4. Cultures are obtained but antibiotics are not used until clinical and radiologic evidence of pneumonitis exists.

Bronchoscopy has little if any role in the removal of acid from the tracheobronchial tree since acid absorption through mucosa is almost instantaneous, but bronchoscopy is useful in the removal of particulate matter that may be a nidus for the development of infection. My associates and I have avoided corticosteroids because of their deleterious effects on pulmonary host defenses as noted previously in this chapter.

One final type of pneumonia that is seen with increasing frequency in surgical patients is that occurring in the immunocompromised patient. The causative agents for pneumonia in immunosuppressed patients are rarely encountered in community-acquired pneumonia. Etiologic agents are bacterial (either gram-negative or gram-positive organisms or *Mycobacterium*), fungal (including *Aspergillus, Cryptococcus, Candida,* or *Nocardia*) and protozoan *(Pneumocystis),* or viral (e.g., cytomegalovirus or herpes). When the patient with alterations in immune status develops pneumonia, vigorous diagnostic techniques must often be used to obtain adequate specimens for special staining, culture, and light microscopy and even electron microscopy to aid in establishing a diagnosis. Reliance on simple sputum cytology is often not adequate in this clinical setting, and a biopsy of involved lung parenchyma may be mandatory despite the critical nature of the patient's illness. The means of obtaining a biopsy of affected lung will depend in large measure on the skill and experience of the physician obtaining the specimen. Acceptable techniques include percutaneous needle biopsy, transbronchial biopsy, and open lung biopsy. Empiric treatment often is necessary in these desperately ill patients and initially must be based on the likelihood of the patient's having a specific diagnosis.[30] Patients with acquired immune deficiency syndrome (AIDS) tend to have a high incidence of infection caused by *Pneumocystis, Legionella,* and *Mycoplasma.* Patients with defects in cellular immunity not related to AIDS have the additional risks of gram-negative or gram-positive bacterial pneumonias and eventually may need empiric coverage. The neutropenic patient has a higher risk of *Pseudomonas* infection in addition to those previously mentioned and may require empiric treatment with carbenicillin or piperacillin.

Pneumothorax

Pneumothorax occurs when air escapes from the pulmonary parenchyma and causes the lung to collapse away from the chest wall. In simple or closed pneumothorax, this condition is not progressive, the mediastinal structures are not shifted, and the opposite lung is not compressed. In contrast, a tension pneumothorax is caused by the progressive accumulation of air within the thoracic cavity, leading to a shift in the cardiomediastinal structures with possible compression of the contralateral lung. Tension pneumothorax results from a one-way valve phenomenon in which air enters the thoracic cavity from an opening in the pulmonary parenchyma or the chest wall. Air enters the pleural space during inspiration but cannot escape during expiration. The increased pleural pressure decreases venous return to the heart by kinking or distorting the low pressure vena cava and/or by direct pressure on the cava. Hypotension and complete circulatory collapse may occur within minutes if the condition is not promptly treated.

Pneumothorax may occur with a variety of conditions:

1. Trauma
Blunt
Penetrating
2. Iatrogenic
Nerve blocks
Subclavian catheters
3. Barotrauma
Mechanical ventilation
Positive end-expiratory pressure

4. Rupture of abnormal pulmonary parenchyma
   Congenital bleb
   Pneumatocele
   Emphysematous bulla
   Catamenial (?)
5. Idiopathic

Both penetrating and blunt trauma commonly result in a pneumothorax. Blunt trauma may be associated with a pneumothorax caused by laceration of the lung from a rib fracture. However, a pneumothorax may also occur in the absence of rib fractures because of the sudden compression of the chest wall against a closed glottis. This rapid increase in the intrathoracic pressure leads to a disruption of the alveoli and to a subsequent pneumothorax. A pneumothorax may also result from barotrauma in which the increased pressure on the airway (usually from positive-pressure mechanical ventilation and PEEP) results in a "blow-out" type of alveolar injury with secondary air leak.

Pneumothorax may occur because of disease or abnormality in the underlying lung tissue. Spontaneous pneumothorax often results from apical blebs that appear to be congenital in nature. Likewise, acquired conditions such as bulbous emphysema or pneumatocele following staphylococcal pneumonia result in a thinning of the pulmonary parenchyma that may leak air and result in a pneumothorax.

The type of physiologic defect produced in the lung by a simple pneumothorax is a restrictive one. The degree of restriction and secondary respiratory compromise is determined by the degree of pneumothorax. In relatively mild cases (<30% pneumothorax), the degree of physiologic insult may be mild. However, an increase in the degree of pneumothorax or bilateral pneumothoraces may result in more serious respiratory compromise.

It is important in estimating the degree of pneumothorax to remember that the lung is a three-dimensional cylinder rather than a two-dimensional structure as seen on chest radiograph. If only the loss in diameter on the chest radiograph is considered, then the decrease from 20 cm to 16 cm is considered to be a 20% pneumothorax. If, however, the lung is regarded as a sphere, then the volume loss with such a change in diameter is much greater. The volume may be determined by $V = \pi r^3$; thus the diameter reduction from 20 to 16 cm causes a radius change from 10 to 8 cm. This decrease results in a net volume loss of 50% rather than the 20% calculated by simple measurement of diameter loss.

Treatment of a pneumothorax will vary depending on its cause, the degree of clinical embarrassment produced, and associated factors. A small simple pneumothorax resulting from blunt trauma or arising spontaneously may be safely observed and may resolve without treatment. Large degrees of collapse should be treated. Aspiration is occasionally successful if a continuing air leak is not present. If the patient is moderately symptomatic, has bilateral pneumothoraces, or will require positive-pressure ventilation (for surgery or mechanical ventilation), then a thoracostomy tube should be inserted and connected to an underwater seal to produce a negative pressure and aid in lung reexpansion.

Flail Chest

Flail chest is defined as the paradoxic motion of a segment of chest wall such that the flail area is depressed with inspiration (and its negative intrathoracic pressure) and is moved outward during expiration (Fig. 35-9). A flail chest occurs when a group of ribs are fractured in more than one area or when there is a costochondral separation and a lateral rib fracture. The physiologic abnormalities resulting from flail chest have been controversial. It was once believed that the lung functioned as a bellows and that the loss of chest wall rigidity because of a flail chest caused a "to-and-fro" movement of air from one hemithorax to another rather than the normal effective exchange of air. The concept of to-and-fro motion was termed *pendelluft*. The concept was demonstrated invalid in a series of studies by Maloney.[27] The hypoxemia associated with flail chest probably has two origins: (1) there is associated damage to the underlying lung in the form of pulmonary contusion (see the previous section on pulmonary contusion); and (2) the loss of mechanical stability and flail motion may lead to a loss of lung volume. Considerable recent clinical experience suggests that pulmonary contusion is the primary mode that renders the patient hypoxemic.

Treatment of flail chest has gone through several historic phases. Initial attempts to treat flail chest relied on external mechanical stabilization through a traction device or by tapes or belts. The introduction of the piston-driven ventilator led to the development of internal pneumatic stabilization[4] in which the patient's respiratory drive was eliminated by rendering the patient alkalotic and allowing the ventilator to "stabilize" the flail segment. The patient was generally maintained on mechanical ventilation until the flail segment stabilized. Unfortunately, this method of

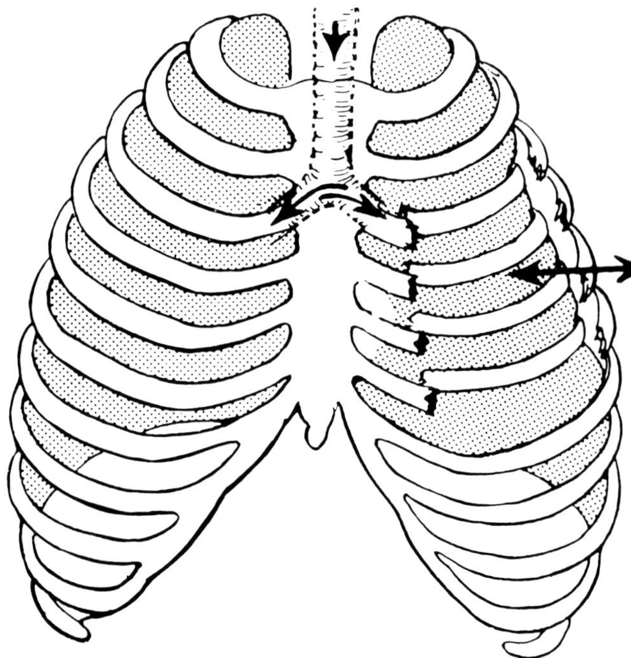

Fig. 35-9 Fracture of chest wall in two locations is necessary for development of flail chest. Classical concept of altered mechanics causing "to-and-fro" movement of air between major bronchi *(double arrow)* has largely been dispelled.

treatment was associated with continued high mortality secondary to complications of therapy such as nosocomial pneumonia, tracheostomy and endotracheal tube complications, and electrolyte disorders.

Recently there has been a trend toward selective managment of flail chest[41,56] depending on the degree of hypoxemia produced and the extent of the flail segment. The basic tenets of this treatment include: (1) avoidance of overresuscitation with crystalloid infusion, which may worsen a pulmonary contusion; (2) vigorous pulmonary toilet to control secretions and prevent atelectasis; and (3) selective use of endotracheal intubation and early extubation and weaning from mechanical ventilation based on physiologic parameters rather than chest wall instability. Large series involving many patients have shown that this is a safe and effective method of treating patients with flail chest.

PULMONARY AND MEDIASTINAL NEOPLASIA

Tumors of the Lung

A variety of neoplastic disorders may affect the lung. Clinically they may manifest themselves with symptomatology similar to other pulmonary disorders, including wheezing, coughing, hemoptysis, pain, or at times an unexplained pneumonia caused by a pneumonitis distal to the site of the tumor. Occasionally a patient may be totally symptom-free; and an unexplained solitary pulmonary nodule, called a coin lesion, is identified on a chest x-ray film that has been obtained for an entirely different reason. Such nodules are sharply circumscribed, are localized in the peripheral lungs, are 5 cm or less in diameter, and may or may not demonstrate calcification. At least half of these lesions turn out to be malignant; and the larger their size, the more likely a malignancy is present. For this reason all solitary pulmonary nodules must be considered malignant until proven otherwise.[8b] Unfortunately, routine studies such as bronchoscopy, sputum sample analysis, and even transthoracic biopsy are usually nondiagnostic. Consequently, the majority of patients who have such lesions initially will need to undergo exploratory thoracotomy to confirm the diagnosis. If the lesion is benign, a wedge resection of the lung is generally adequate management. In contrast, malignant lesions should be treated with a formal lobectomy or pneumonectomy to enhance the chances of cure. In fact, compared with other presentations of pulmonary cancer, an undiagnosed pulmonary nodule is usually the only stage of bronchogenic cancer in which a good-to-excellent change for cure can be expected.

Of the various kinds of benign neoplasms that may affect the bronchopulmonary tree, hamartomas (mixed tumors) are the most common.[35a] Other types include fibrous mesotheliomas, various xanthomatous, and inflammatory pseudotumors and other rare lesions such as lipomas and myoblastomas. Benign tumors are generally slow growing and often first present with bronchial obstruction, pneumonitis, or hemoptysis. Such tumors account for only 1% to 2% of all pulmonary neoplasms and surgical excision consisting of ennucleation or wedge resection offers an excellent prognosis.

Malignancies are the most frequently encountered neoplasms of the lung; and, of the various types encountered, bronchogenic carcinoma is responsible for as many as 93% of them.[8a] Presently this is the most common malignancy in men (and is becoming a frequently diagnosed tumor in women) and is clearly associated with cigarette smoking and probably atmospheric pollution as well. Most carcinomas arise from the bronchial epithelium and typically involve the upper lobes of the lung (63%). The various cell types with their growth characteristics and frequency of occurrence are shown in Table 35-4.

Most patients who develop carcinoma of the lung have a long history of sustained cigarette smoking. Typical symptoms associated with carcinoma include cough, wheezing, hemoptysis, and occasionally fever, all caused by pneumonitis distal to the site of the tumor. Pain is a relatively late symptom and generally indicates chest wall extension. Weight loss is usually not seen until the cancer is quite advanced. If the tumor involves the thoracic or superior pulmonary sulcus at the root of the neck, a *Pancoast's syndrome* may result. This includes involvement of the brachial plexus, the sympathetic ganglia at the base of

Table 35-4 **CELL TYPES AND CHARACTERISTICS OF CARCINOMA OF LUNG**

Type of Carcinoma	Percent	Sex	Growth Characteristics
Epidermoid	50	75% in men	Occurs in major bronchi, causing distal atelectasis, tends to spread by lymphatics
Undifferentiated large cell	20	38% in women	Located more peripheral from hilus of lung, spreads by lymphatics and bloodstream
Small cell (oat cell)	9	80% in men	Very cellular and largely extrabronchial, causing little or no atelectasis, early lymphatic and hematogenous spread
Adenocarcinoma	20	30% in women	Majority occur in periphery of lung, metastasize by bloodstream
Bronchiolar or alveolar cell	1	—	Occurs as a diffuse, patchy pneumonia and as a slow-growing, well-circumscribed local lesion

From Richardson, J.D.: Hemoptysis. In Polk, H.C., Jr., Stone, H.H., and Gardner, B., editors: Basic surgery, ed. 3, Norwalk, Conn. 1987, Appleton-Century-Crofts.

the neck, Horner's syndrome (ptosis miosis, enophthalmos, and decreased sweating on the involved side), and frequently destruction of ribs and vertebrae and loss of strength in the upper arm of the affected side.

As many as 20% of patients will present with symptoms remote from the lung, indicating metastatic disease. Typical sites of metastasis include the liver and brain. Other extrapulmonary manifestations are related to various humoral agents that may be secreted by the tumor. An ACTH-like substance elaborated by oat cell carcinoma may closely mimic Cushing's syndrome. In addition, a parathormone-like substance produced by some squamous cell carcinomas simulates clinical findings typical of primary hyperparathyroidism. An inappropriate ADH syndrome may also occur, manifested by water retention and symptoms of hyponatremia. Although the exact mechanism responsible for this condition remains to be determined, pulmonary osteoarthropathy is frequently associated with carcinoma of the lung. This condition is different from arthritis because the bones rather than the joints are tender, and x-ray films of the fingers demonstrate a fine linear deposition of calcium along the periosteum. Clubbing of the fingers also occurs in patients developing carcinoma of the lung, the mechanism again remaining yet undefined.

Because of the relatively poor prognosis that exists in patients who develop carcinoma of the lung, care must be taken to ensure its resectability and to prevent an unnecessary thoracotomy. The absolute and relative signs of inoperability are summarized in Table 35-5. In determining such information, CT scanning is often helpful in assessing mediastinal nodes. If mediastinal adenopathy is present, mediastinoscopy should be performed to determine the presence of metastases. This technique involves an incision above the suprasternal notch through which a fiberoptic mediastinoscope is introduced into the superior mediastinum, enabling identification of lymph nodes and the ability to biopsy them. This technique is especially useful in diagnosing central lesions in which tissue samples for malignancy prove positive in about 65% of cases. It is, however, less suitable for more peripheral lesions.

When first diagnosed, more than 50% of patients will have inoperable carcinoma of the lung. Another 25%, when explored, will be discovered to have nonresectable lesions because of neoplastic extension into the mediastinum or carina. Of those patients actually amenable to surgical excision, only about 8% (or two of the initial 100 patients) will live for 5 years. The type of surgical procedure performed will relate to the nature and extent of the tumor and may range from a segmental resection to a total pneumonectomy.

Of those tumors found to be surgically resectable, a malignant solitary pulmonary nodule without lymph node involvement is generally associated with a 50% 5-year survival rate. Squamous cell carcinoma without node metastases treated by lobectomy or pneumonectomy yield 30% to 35% 5-year survival rates. If nodal involvement is present in either of these circumstances, the 5-year survival rate drops to 10% or less. For those tumors that are histologically adenocarcinomas or undifferentiated large cell cancers, the survival rate is even more dismal.

A particular circumstance that continues to remain controversial with respect to treatment involves that patient who is believed to be surgically resectable in other respects but has positive mediastinal lymph nodes.[35b] Although some investigators recommend surgical treatment combined with radiography for squamous cell carcinoma,[21a] the generally dismal outcome in the experience of most surgeons has suggested that radiotherapy alone is the treatment of choice for this stage of the disease.[7a] Radiation therapy may also be of value in the prevention of hemoptysis or bronchial obstruction by reducing the tumor mass in patients who have unresectable lesions.

The role of multiple drug chemotherapy in the management of bronchogenic carcinoma remains to be clearly defined. Recent experience in the treatment of oat cell carcinoma has been extremely encouraging, resulting in an objective response rate (i.e., measurable decrease in tumor size) in as many as one third of patients so treated.[18a] With such therapy, patients who normally would have succumbed from their disease in less than 6 months are now

Table 35-5 **SIGNS OF INOPERABILITY IN LUNG CANCER**

Absolute Signs of Inoperability		Relative Signs of Inoperability	
Lymphatic metastasis	Cervical nodes, axillary nodes	Lymphatic spread	May be removed at surgery (e.g., mediastinal nodes
Hematogenous metastasis	Brain, liver, bones, kidney, adrenals	Phrenic nerve paralysis	May be excised with tumor
Direct extension	Pleura—effusion, with malignant cells, esophagus, aorta, widened carina at bronchoscopy	Pericardial extension	May be excised with tumor
Small-cell undifferentiated carcinoma		Chest-wall extension	Superior sulcus (Pancoast) tumor, may be resected after preoperative irradiation
Superior vena cava syndrome			

From Richardson, J.D.: Hemoptysis. In Polk, H.C., Jr., Stone, H.H., and Gardner, B., editors: Basic surgery, ed. 3, Norwalk, Conn. 1987, Appleton-Century-Crofts.

surviving as long as 2 years or more. Whether similar success rates will be demonstrated with other types of carcinomas must await further study.

Although the preceding has centered around bronchogenic carcinoma, other malignancies, collectively known as the bronchial adenomas, may also affect the lungs. The two most common types are carcinoid (85%) and cyclindromas (12%), also called the adenoid cystic type. These tumors are generally located in the walls of the major bronchi. When examined bronchoscopically, usually only a small amount of the tumor is visible, with a much larger portion of it extending outside of the bronchus, a situation known as the *iceberg effect*. Of these two types, the cyclidromas are usually more aggressive and tend to invade adjacent tissues and metastasize to nodes more frequently. Treatment of both types will depend on their size and location. Accordingly, procedures that have been used in their treatment range from sleeve resection of the bronchus for very small lesions to lobectomy or pneumonectomy for larger lesions. As many as 90% of patients with these tumors are cured after surgical resection, with the carcinoid type of lesion being more favorable in this regard.

Tumors of the Mediastinum

In addition to tumors directly involving the pulmonary parenchyma, a number of neoplastic conditions may also arise in the mediastinum.[49a] These tumors are generally asymptomatic, except when they grow large enough to cause compression of an adjacent structure. They usually first come to the attention of a physician when noted on a routine chest film. The particular source of the tumor in a given patient will depend on the particular mediastinal compartment in which the tumor arises. As an example, the anterior mediastinum contains the thyroid gland, the thymus, and the pericardium; accordingly, tumors arising in this location develop from these structures. A summary of the types of tumors arising in various portions of the mediastinum is detailed in the boxed material below.

COMMON MEDIASTINAL TUMORS

Anterior Mediastinal Compartment
- Parathyroid adenomas
- Thyroid tumors, goiters, and cysts
- Thymic tumors and cysts
- Teratomas
- Pericardial cysts

Superior Mediastinal Compartment
- Thyroid tumors
- Parathyroid adenomas
- Bronchogenic cysts
- Lymphomas

Middle Mediastinal Compartment
- Lymphatic tumors
- Lymphomas
- Bronchogenic cysts

Posterior Mediastinal Compartment
- Neurogenic tumors
- Neurilemomas
- Ganglioneuromas
- Gastroenteric cysts

Because a malignant process must always be considered when a mediastinal tumor is diagnosed, surgical excision is the treatment of choice. For virtually all benign lesions and for most malignant processes, complete cure can be expected with such surgical approach.

SUMMARY

This chapter has dealt with some basic physiologic mechanisms involved in the pulmonary derangements commonly encountered in surgical patients. The lung seems to have a limited number of ways of reacting to injury, and thus a variety of noxious stimuli tends to produce abnormalities of the lung that behave similarly. Many of these abnormalities have been included in a discussion on the adult respiratory distress syndrome. It seems clear that for surgical patients sepsis is the most common provocation of ARDS.

The physiology and basic principles of treatment of a number of other commonly encountered disorders such as smoke inhalation, pulmonary contusion, atelectasis, pneumonia, pneumothorax, flail chest and pulmonary neoplasms are also discussed. A thorough understanding of the basic physiologic mechanisms underlying these common problems is crucial for any surgeon who deals with critically ill patients.

REFERENCES

1. Anderson, R.R., et al.: Documentation of pulmonary capillary permeability in the adult respiratory distress syndrome accompanying human sepsis, Am. Rev. Respir. Dis. **119:**869, 1979.
2. Ashbaugh, D.G., and Maier, R.V.: Idiopathic pulmonary fibrosis in adult respiratory distress syndrome, Arch. Surg. **120:**530, 1985.
3. Ashbaugh, D.G., et al.: Acute respiratory distress in adults, Lancet **2:**319, 1967.
4. Avery, E.E., Morch, E.T., and Benson, D.W.: Critically crushed chests: a new method of treatment with continuous mechanical hypoventilation to produce alkalotic apnea and internal pneumatic stabilization, J. Thorac. Surg. **32:**301, 1956.
5. Balk, R., and Bone, R.C.: Classification of acute respiratory failure, Med. Clin. North Am. **67:** 551, 1983.
6. Blaisdell, F.W.: Pathophysiology of the respiratory distress syndrome, Arch. Surg. **108:** 44, 1974.
7. Bone, R.C., Francis, P.B., and Pierce, A.K.: Intravascular coagulation associated with adult respiratory distress syndrome, Am. J. Med. **61:**585, 1976.

7a. Byfield, J.E.: Radiation therapy, local tumor control, and prognosis in bronchogenic carcinoma: current status and future prospects, Am. J. Surg. **143:**675, 1982.

8. Centers for Disease Control: National nosocomial infection study report, 1976, annual summary, Atlanta, 1978, Centers for Disease Control.

8a. Chung, C.K., et al.: Carcinoma of the lung: evaluation of histological grade and factors influencing prognosis, Ann. Thorac. Surg. **33:**599, 1982.

8b. Dedrick, C.G.: The solitary pulmonary nodule and staging of lung cancer, Clin. Chest Med. **5:**345, 1984.

9. Demling, R.H.: Early pulmonary abnormalities from smoke inhalation, JAMA **251:**771, 1984.
10. Fantone, J.C., Kunkel, S.L., and Ward, P.A.: Chemotactic mediators in neutrophil-dependent lung injury, Annu. Rev. Physiol. **44:**283, 1983.
11. Fowler, A.A., et al.: Adult respiratory distress syndrome: risk with common predispositions, Ann. Intern. Med. **98:**593, 1983.
12. Fraser, R.G., and Pare, J.A.P.: Diagnosis and diseases of the chest, Philadelphia, 1978, W.B. Saunders Co.
13. Fulton, R.L., and Peter, E.T.: The progressive nature of pulmonary contusion, Surgery **67:**499, 1970.

14. Fulton, R.L., and Peter, E.T.: Physiologic effect of fluid therapy after pulmonary contusion, Am. J. Surg. **126:**773, 1973.
15. Fulton, R.L., and Peter, E.T.: Compositional and histologic effects of fluid therapy following pulmonary contusion, J. Trauma. **14:**783, 1974.
16. Fulton, R.L., and Jones, C.E.: The cause of posttraumatic pulmonary insufficiency in man, Surg. Gynecol. Obstet. **140:**179, 1975.
17. Garibaldi, R.A., et al.: Risk factors for postoperative pneumonia, Am. J. Med. **70:**677, 1981.
18. Hosea, J., et al.: Role of complement activation in a model of adult respiratory distress syndrome, J. Clin. Invest. **66:**375, 1980.
18a. Ihde, D.C.: Current status of therapy for small cell carcinoma of the lung, Cancer **54:**2722, 1984.
19. Jacob, H.S.: Complement-mediated leucoagglutination - a mechanism of tissue damage during extracorporeal perfusions, myocardial infarction, and in shock;, Q.J. Med. **207:**289, 1983.
20. Jones, J.G., Minty, B.D., and Royston, D.: The physiology of leaky lungs, Br. J. Anaesth. **54:**705, 1982.
21. Kaplow, L.S., and Goffinet, J.A.: Profound neutropenia during the early phase of hemodialysis, JAMA **203:**1135, 1968.
21a. Kirsh, M.D., Rotman, H., and Argenta, L.: Carcinoma of the lung—results of treatment over 10 years, Ann. Thorac. Surg. **21:**371, 1976.
22. Kopolovic, R., et al.: Effects of ibuprofen on a porcine model of acute respiratory failure, J. Surg. Res. **36:**300, 1984.
23. Kuckelt, W., et al.: Effect of PEEP on gas exchange, pulmonary mechanics, and hemodynamics in adult respiratory distress syndrome (ARDS), Intensive Care Med. **7:**177, 1981.
24. Kurzweg, F.T.: Pulmonary complications following upper abdominal surgery, Am. Surg. **19:** 967, 1953.
25. Lutz, P.L., et al.: Pulmonary edema related to changes in colloid oncotic and pulmonary artery wedge pressure in patients after acute myocardial infarction, Circulation **51:**350, 1975.
26. Malik, A.B., et al.: Role of blood components in mediating lung vascular injury after pulmonary vascular thrombosis, Chest **83:**215, 1983.
27. Maloney, J.V., Schmutzer, K.J., and Raschke, E.: Paradoxical respiration and 'pendelluft', J. Thorac. Cardiovasc. Surg. **41:**291, 1961.
28. Manwaring, O., Thorning, D., and Curreri, P.W.: Mechanism of acute pulmonary dysfunction produced by fibrinogen degradation products, Surgery **84:**85, 1978.
29. Martin, L.F., et al.: Postoperative pneumonia, Arch. Surg. **119:**379, 1984.
30. Masur, H., Shelhamer, J., and Parillo, J.E.: The management of pneumonia in immunocompromised patients, JAMA **253:**1769, 1985.
31. Miller, T.A.: Protective effects of prostaglandins against gastric mucosal damage: current knowledge and proposed mechanisms, Am. J. Physiol. **245:**G601, 1983.
32. Moersch, H.J.: Bronchoscopy in treatment of postoperative atelectasis, Surg. Gynecol. Obstet. **77:**435, 1943.
33. Moore, F.D., et al.: Posttraumatic pulmonary insufficiency, Philadelphia, 1969, W.B. Saunders Co.
34. Moylan, J.A., and Alexander, L.G.: Diagnosis and treatment of inhalation injury, World J. Surg. **2:**185, 1978.
35. Nichols, R.T., Pearce, H.J., and Greenfield, L.J.: Effects of experimental pulmonary contusion on respiratory exchange and lung mechanics, Arch. Surg. **96:**723, 1968.
35a. Oldham, H.N., Jr.: Benign tumors of the lung and bronchus, Surg. Clin. North Am. **60:**825, 1980.
35b. Pearson, F.G., et al.: Significance of positive superior mediastinal nodes identified at mediastinoscopy in patients with resectable cancer of the lung, J. Thorac. Cardiovasc. Surg. **83:**1, 1982.
36. Pepe, P.E., Hudson, L.D., and Carrico, J.C.: Early application of positive end-expiratory pressure in patients at risk for adult respiratory distress syndrome, N. Engl. J. Med. **311:**281, 1984.
37. Pepe, P.E., et al.: Clinical predictors of the adult respiratory distress syndrome, Am. J. Surg. **144:**924, 1982.
38. Peters, R.M.: Lifesaving measures in acute respiratory distress syndrome, Arch. Surg. **138:**368, 1979.
39. Petty, T.L., and Fowler, A.A.: Another look at ARDS, Chest **82:**98, 1982.
40. Prichard, J.S.: Edema of the lung: Springfield, Ill., 1982, Charles C Thomas, Publisher.
41. Richardson, J.D., Adams, A., and Flint, L.M.: Selective management of flail chest and pulmonary contusion, Ann. Surg. **196:**103, 1982.
42. Richardson, J.D., et al.: Pulmonary contusion and hemolyse—crystalloid versus colloid replacement, J. Surg. Res. **16:**330, 1974.
43. Richardson, J.D., et al.: Lung bacterial clearance following pulmonary contusion, Surgery **86:**730, 1979.
44. Saba, T.M., et al.: Cryoprecipitate reversal of opsonic surface binding glycoprotein deficiency in septic surgical and trauma patients, Science **201:**622, 1978.
45. Sacks, T., et al.: Oxygen radicals mediate endothelial cell damage by complement-stimulated granulocytes, J. Clin. Invest. **61:**1161, 1978.
46. Samuelsson, B.: Leukotrienes: mediators of immediate hypersensitivity reactions and inflammation, Science **220:**568, 1983.
47. Sasahara, A.A., et al.: Clinical and physiologic studies in pulmonary thromboembolism, Am. J. Cardiol. **20:**10, 1967.
48. Seale, J.P.: Prostaglandins, slow-reacting substances (leukotrienes) and the lung, Aust. N.Z. J. Med. **11:**550, 1981.
49. Shields, R.T.: Pathogenesis of postoperative pulmonary atelectasis, Arch. Surg. **58:**489, 1949.
49a. Silverman, N.A., and Sabiston, D.C., Jr.: Mediastinal masses, Surg. Clin. North Am. **60:**757, 1980.
50. Skillman, J.J., Restall, D.S., and Salzman, E.W.: Randomized trial of albumin versus electrolyte solutions during abdominal aortic operations, Surgery **78:**291, 1975.
51. Springer, R.R., and Stevens, P.M.: The influence of PEEP on survival of patients in respiratory failure: a retrospective analysis, Am. J. Med. **66:**196, 1979.
52. Staub, N.C., et al.: Preparation of chronic lung lymph fistulas in sheep, J. Surg. Res. **19:**351, 1975.
53. Stephenson, S.F., et al.: The pathophysiology of smoke inhalation injury, Ann. Surg. **182:**652, 1975.
54. Stevens, J.H., and Raffin, T.A.: Adult respiratory distress syndrome—etiology and mechanisms, Postgrad. Med. J. **60:**505, 1984.
55. Trinkle, J.K., et al.: Pulmonary contusion, pathogenesis and effect of various resuscitative measures, Ann. Thorac. Surg. **16:**569, 1973.
56. Trinkle, J.K., et al.: Management of flail chest without mechanical ventilation, Ann. Thorac. Surg. **19:**355, 1975.
57. Virgilio, R.W., et al.: Crystalloid versus colloid resuscitation: is one better?, Surgery **85:**129, 1979.
58. Walker, L., and Eiseman, B.: The changing patterns of posttraumatic respiratory distress syndrome, Ann. Surg. **181:**693, 1975.
59. Weigelt, J.A., et al.: Early steroid therapy for respiratory failure, Arch. Surg. **120:**536, 1985.
60. Weisman, I.M., Rinaldo, J.E., and Rogers, R.M.: Positive end-expiratory pressure in adult respiratory failure, N. Engl. J. Med. **307:**1381, 1982.
61. West, J.B.: Pulmonary pathophysiology; Baltimore, 1982, Williams & Wilkins.
62. Whitcomb, M.E.: The lung—normal and diseased, St. Louis, 1982, The C.V. Mosby Co.
63. Wong, C., Flynn, J., and Demling, R.H.: Role of oxygen radicals in endotoxin-induced lung injury, Arch. Surg. **119:**77, 1984.

36

Gary L. Pellom and Andrew S. Wechsler

Normal Cardiac Function

As a component of the cardiovascular system, the heart is responsible for maintaining adequate blood flow to meet the metabolic needs of the body. This is accomplished by the integration of neural, metabolic, anatomic, and physiologic subsystems that combine to form the intact, functioning human heart. An understanding of cardiac function must consider each of these factors since a knowledge of only one, or even several, without an appreciation of the others gives an incomplete picture of the physiologic mechanisms responsible for this function. In discussing cardiac physiology, it is appropriate to begin with the molecular events underlying contraction and relaxation, in order to provide the basis for understanding the performance of the intact organ.

MOLECULAR MECHANISMS IN CONTRACTION AND RELAXATION

The basis of cardiac function is the relationship between the contractile proteins actin and myosin. The nature of this relationship determines to a large extent the characteristics of activation and relaxation in individual muscle cells and in the intact heart. As in skeletal muscle, the functional unit of cardiac muscle is the sarcomere. The sarcomere is composed principally of four proteins. These are the previously mentioned contractile proteins actin and myosin and a regulatory complex consisting of tropomyosin and troponin. In electron micrographs, the sarcomere appears as an arrangement of thick and thin filaments. This arrangement is shown schematically in Fig. 36-1. The thick filament exists as an aggregate of myosin molecules. Myosin consists of a pair of heavy, coiled polypeptide chains, each of which is attached to a globular head region. These head regions project from the axial core of the myosin aggregate and form cross-bridges to the thin filament (Fig. 36-2). The thin filament is made up of actin in association with troponin and tropomyosin. Actin is a globular molecule that polymerizes to form a double-stranded alpha helical filament. Actin filaments attach to the Z line of the sarcomere and project inward as the thin filament. Here they interact to various degrees with the thick filament. This interaction is regulated by troponin and tropomyosin.

Tropomyosin spans the length of the thin filament, and the troponin complex is normally located at every seventh actin site.[3] Troponin consists of several subgroups that are responsible for binding calcium ions and for regulating the formation of attachments between actin and the myosin by way of the cross-bridges.[29] In the resting state, tropomyosin blocks binding sites on actin so that cross-bridge interaction is prevented. The presence of calcium bound to the troponin complex leads to a conformational change in tropomyosin, such that the actin-myosin association is no longer blocked.

The head region of myosin is the enzymatically active portion of the molecule.[18] Adenosine triphosphate (ATP) binds here and is hydrolyzed to adenosine diphosphate (ADP) and phosphorus (P). In this form, the affinity of myosin for actin is enhanced, such that if calcium is present an actin-myosin complex is formed. As the hydrolysis products are released from the complex, the myosin head undergoes a conformational change that displaces the actin filament relative to the myosin. In this manner, force generation and shortening are accomplished. The addition of ATP to the actin-myosin complex results in dissociation of the filaments. The ATP is once again hydrolyzed, and the process repeats.[2]

Force generation during activation depends to a large extent on the number of cross-bridge attachments that are formed.[13] This number is a function of the degree of filament overlap and the level of calcium present. The rate of shortening is a measure of the ATPase activity of myosin.[24] It has been established that myosin exists in several forms that are distinguished by the composition of their heavy chains.[22] These various forms differ in their ATPase kinetics and thus in their rate of fiber shortening.[28] The composition of the myosin subunits is genetically determined; however, it has been shown to change in response to such hormones as thyroxin and to chronic elevations in mechanical loading of the muscle.[12,21]

Excitation-Contraction Coupling

Myocardial contraction is initiated following a rise in cytosolic calcium. During the plateau phase of the cardiac action potential, a small number of calcium ions enter the muscle cell through slow channels. These ions do not significantly alter myoplasmic [Ca^{++}], but they do cause release of calcium stores from the sarcoplasmic reticulum.[5] This release significantly elevates myoplasmic [Ca^{++}]. Calcium is now available to bind to troponin, and muscle activation occurs. This process, in which calcium entry triggers intracellular calcium release and muscle activation, is called excitation-contraction coupling (Fig. 36-3).

It is interesting to note the amplification of the effects of calcium in this process. The small number of ions entering the cell through the slow channel causes the release of intracellular stores that raises the myoplasmic [Ca^{++}] from a resting value of 10^{-7} M to 10^{-5} M.[2] In turn, each calcium ion that binds to troponin activates seven actin binding sites. This two-step amplification illustrates the exquisite sensitivity of the muscle cell to calcium.

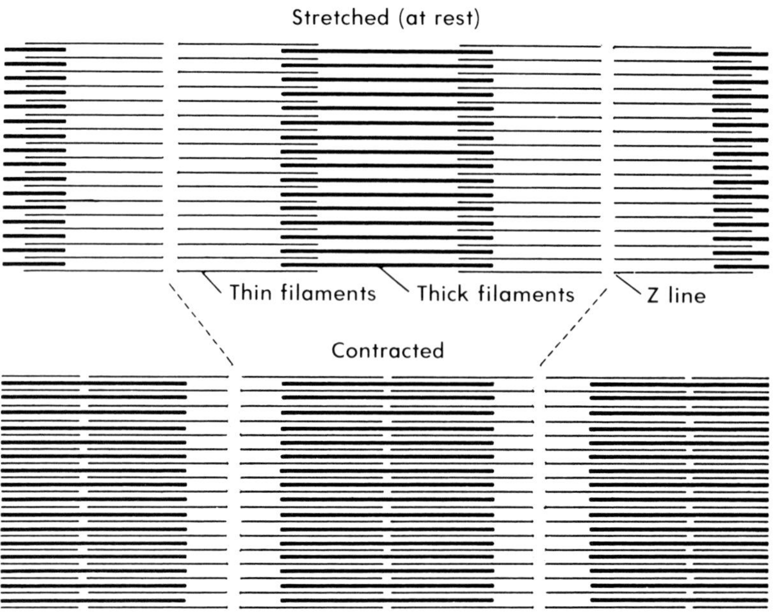

Fig. 36-1 Schematic diagram showing the pattern of thick and thin filaments of one sarcomere. Degree of filament overlap varies with the phase of contraction. (From Murray, J., and Weber, A.: Sci. Am. **230**[2]:58, 1974.)

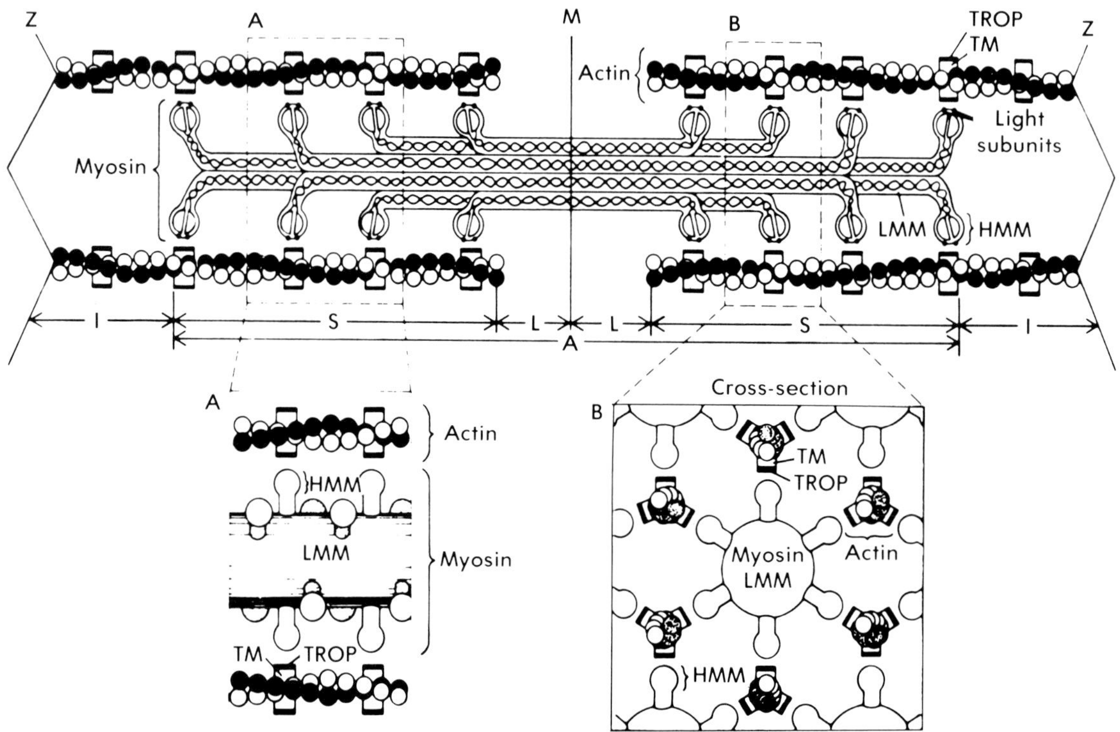

Fig. 36-2 More detailed representation of filament structure. Helical tails of the myosin molecules form a rigid, rodlike structure. Globular heads project from this toward the actin filament. *A* and *B*, Three-dimensional relationships. Each myosin is seen to interact with six actin filaments *(B)*. Note steric hindrance provided by troponin *(TROP)* and tropomyosin *(TM)*. (From Sodeman, W.A., Jr., and Sodeman, T.M., editors: Sodeman's pathologic physiology, ed. 6, Philadelphia, 1979, W.B. Saunders Co.)

Muscle relaxation depends on the presence of adequate levels of ATP, which act to dissociate the actin-myosin complexes and provide energy for the restoration of myoplasmic [Ca^{++}] to resting levels. The latter is accomplished primarily by a calcium-activated ATPase in the membrane of the sarcoplasmic reticulum. In addition, smaller amounts of calcium are extruded from the cell through a $Na^+ - Ca^{++}$ exchange mechanism that operates secondary to the $Na^+ - K^+$ ATPase of the sarcolemma[13] and is not voltage dependent, as are the slow channels.

MECHANICS OF ISOLATED MUSCLE

Much of what is known about the nature of cardiac function has been learned from studies of isolated muscle. Under these conditions, it is possible to finely control the loading of the muscle while making accurate measurements of force development and shortening characteristics. From these studies, three factors have arisen that determine the behavior of isolated muscle. These are muscle preload, afterload, and contractile state.[25]

Preload is defined as the distending force, or load, that is placed on a muscle before contraction. The preload and the distensibility of the muscle are the determinants of the initial length of the muscle before contraction. The load encountered by the muscle after activation is defined as the afterload. The magnitude of the afterload determines the nature of the subsequent contraction. If the muscle is able to generate a force equivalent to the afterload, then shortening occurs. Such a contraction is termed isotonic, since the force developed by the muscle is equal to the load and therefore remains constant during shortening. If the muscle is unable to generate force equal to the load, no external shortening occurs and the contraction is said to be isometric. Contractility refers to the intrinsic ability of the muscle to contract independently of loading conditions. This meaning will become clearer as the characteristics of muscle activation are explained.

Isotonic contractions are useful for studying the shortening characteristics of isolated muscle. From these studies, several fundamental principles of cardiac muscle mechanics have been developed. The first of these defines the relationship between afterload and shortening. As the afterload is increased, the extent of muscle shortening and the velocity of shortening decrease.[25] This effect is shown in isolated cat papillary muscle in Fig. 36-4, *A* and *B*.

Cardiac muscle exhibits length-dependent properties: the length of the muscle before contraction affects the nature of the contraction. As initial muscle length is increased, there is an increase in both the extent and the velocity of shortening (Fig. 36-5). A third property of cardiac muscle

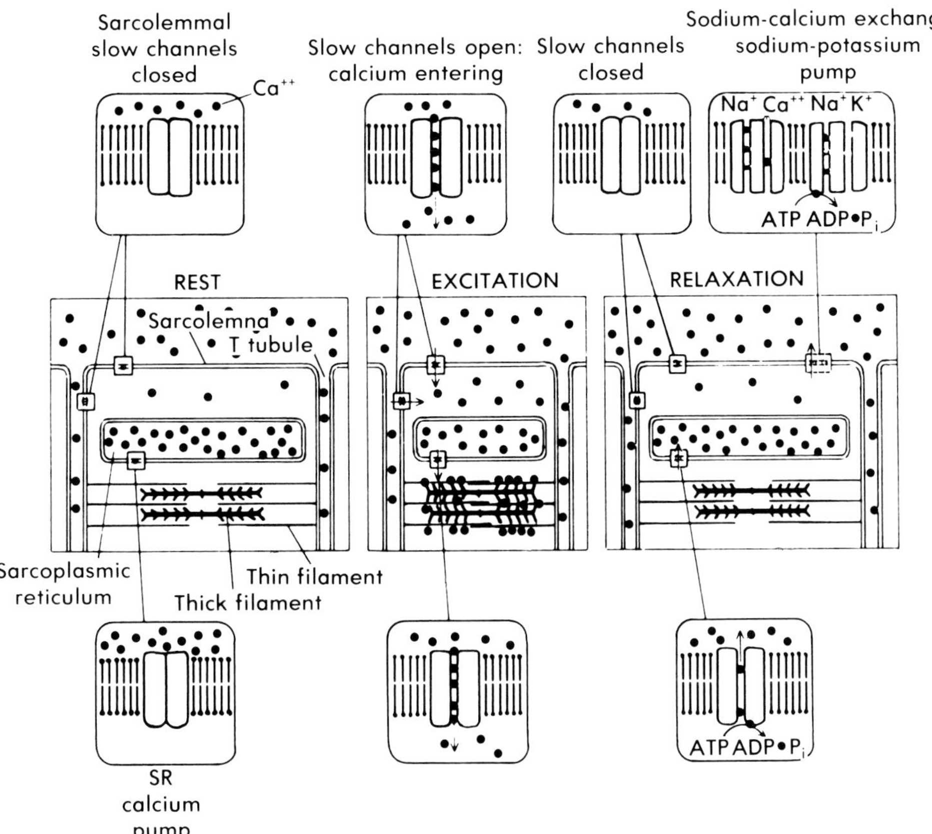

Fig. 36-3 Representation of the transmembrane calcium movements during a contraction cycle. At rest, calcium concentration in the sarcoplasm is low compared with the extracellular space and the interior of the sarcoplasmic reticulum. Slow channel is closed, and Ca^{++} pumps are inactive. During excitation, the slow channel opens, allowing a small number of extracellular Ca^{++} ions to enter the cell. This entry triggers a release of Ca^{++} from the sarcoplasmic reticulum, and contraction proceeds. Relaxation is accomplished by the active restoration of resting gradients. (From Katz, A.M., and Smith, V.E.: Hosp. Pract. **19**[1]:69, 1984.)

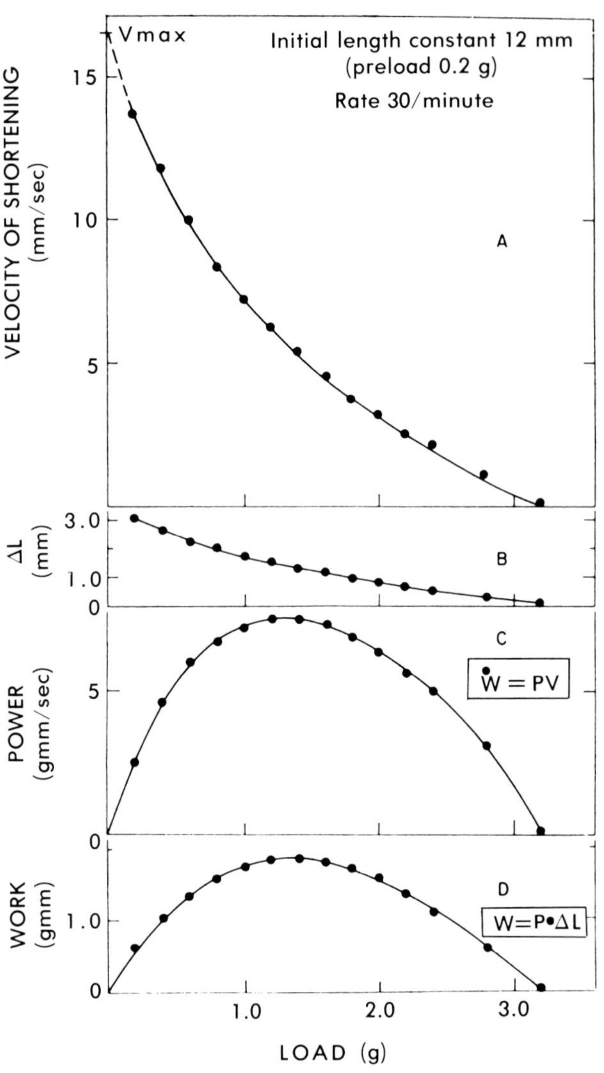

Fig. 36-4 Force-velocity relations for isolated cat papillary muscle. **A,** Velocity of the isotonic contraction is seen to be a decreasing function of load. Extrapolation of the velocity at 0 load *(dashed line)* provides an estimate of Vmax. **B,** Extent of shortening also decreases with increasing load. **C** and **D,** Concomitant effects of increasing load on power and work. (From Sonnenblick, E.H.: Fed. Proc. **21**[suppl. 12]:975, 1962.)

involves the response of the muscle to inotropic agents. Positive inotropes enhance the contractility of the muscle, as defined by an increase in the rate and extent of shortening generated from a given preload. Fig. 36-6 shows the effects of a positive inotrope on the velocity *(A)* and extent *(B)* of shortening. A unique feature of the force-velocity relationship is that it allows an estimation of the contractile state of the muscle. Theoretically, the velocity of muscle shortening at zero load should be determined only by the kinetics of the actin-myosin association. Since any muscle contraction is necessarily loaded to some extent by the preload, the velocity of shortening at zero load (Vmax) can be obtained only by extrapolation of the force-velocity curve to zero load. For the relationship shown in Fig. 36-6, the addition of norepinephrine resulted in an increase in the extrapolated value of Vmax. In contrast, Fig. 36-5 demonstrates the required load independence of contractility as suggested by the stable estimates of Vmax.[25]

Isometric contractions provide a convenient means to study force development in isolated muscle. When a muscle is stimulated to contract isometrically, the amount of force (tension) developed depends only on the length before contraction and the inotropic state of the muscle. Variations in afterload are not a factor since by definition the magnitude of the afterload always exceeds the force-generating capability of the muscle. Increasing the initial

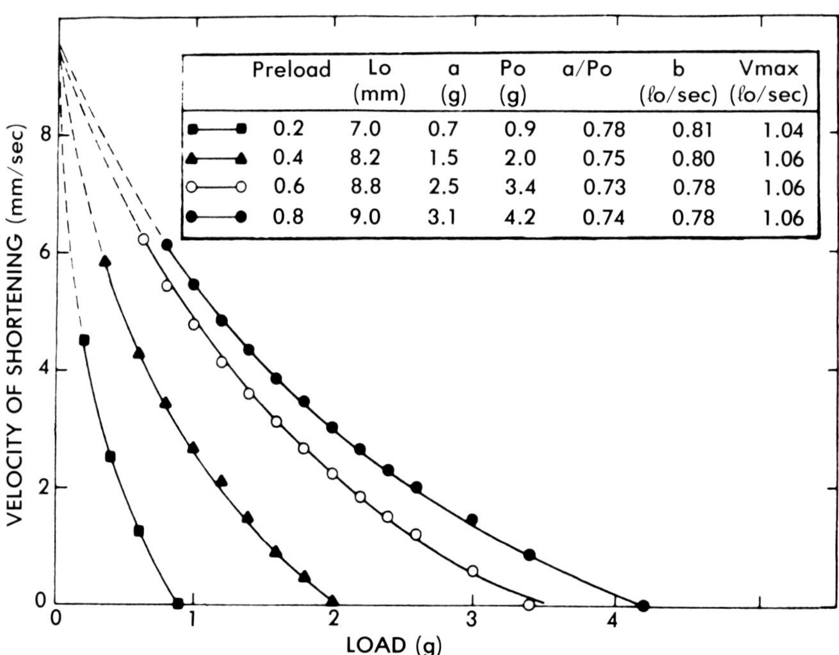

Preload	Lo (mm)	a (g)	Po (g)	a/Po	b (ℓo/sec)	Vmax (ℓo/sec)
■—■ 0.2	7.0	0.7	0.9	0.78	0.81	1.04
▲—▲ 0.4	8.2	1.5	2.0	0.75	0.80	1.06
○—○ 0.6	8.8	2.5	3.4	0.73	0.78	1.06
●—● 0.8	9.0	3.1	4.2	0.74	0.78	1.06

Fig. 36-5 Effects of varied preload on the force-velocity relations of cat papillary muscle. As the preload is increased, the velocity of shortening increases. However, the maximum velocity (*V*max) does not change. (From Sonnenblick, E.H.: Fed. Proc. **21**[suppl. 12]:975, 1962.)

length of the muscle at a given contractile state results in an increase in the level of resting tension borne by the muscle (Fig. 36-7). As the length of the muscle increases, the peak force generated from any given length also increases (Fig. 36-7), as does the rate of force development *(dF/dt)*. The addition of Ca^{++} has the effect of a positive inotrope on the isometric preparation. Specifically, resting tension is unaffected, but the peak force, time to peak force, and *dF/dt* are enhanced.

When a muscle fiber is distended, a point is reached at which force development is maximum. The length at this point is termed Lmax. Further increases in muscle length beyond Lmax result in a reduction in the amount of developed tension.[2] This and other length-dependent properties of the muscle can be explained in part by relating the various muscle lengths to the degree of overlap in the thick and thin filaments of the sarcomere (Fig. 36-8). At rest, sarcomere length, defined as the distance between adjacent Z lines, averages 1.8 μm. As the muscle is lengthened, sarcomere length increases. More importantly, there is an increase in the degree of overlap between the chemically active portions of the thick and thin filaments. Since the potential for the formation of force-generating cross-bridges is increasing, there is a concomitant increase in the amount of force developed. The length of the sarcomere at Lmax averages 2.2 μm.[2] At this distance, the thick and thin filaments are arranged such that all myosin heads lie adjacent to actin filaments. In this state, the probability of interaction between the filaments is greatest; hence, force generation is greatest. With the application of large forces, cardiac muscle can be distended beyond Lmax. Little

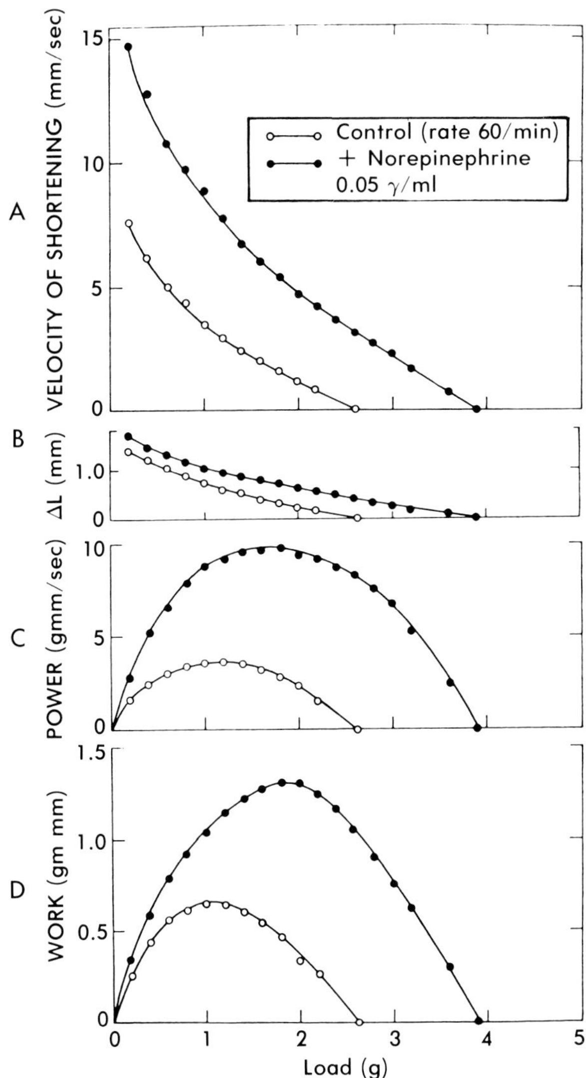

Fig. 36-6 **A,** Application of norepinephrine causes an increase in the velocity of shortening and *V*max. **B,** Amount of muscle shortening is also increased at any shortening load. **C** and **D** show concomitant effects of load on power and work. (From Sonnenblick, E.H.: Fed. Proc. **21**[suppl. 12]:975, 1962.)

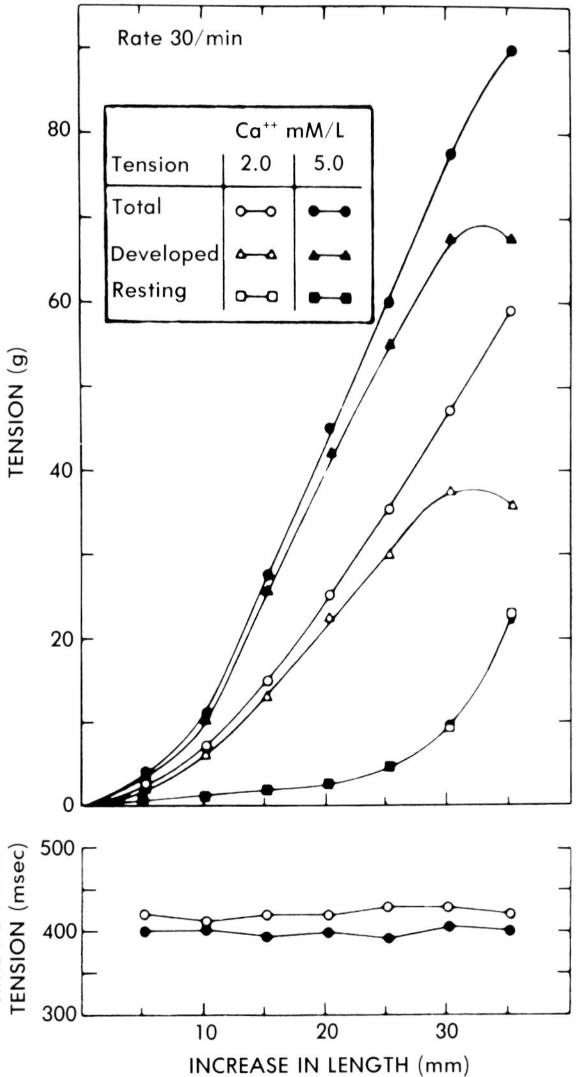

Fig. 36-7 When a muscle contracts isometrically, the amount of tension that is developed depends on the length and inotropic state of the muscle. In this figure the upward exponential curve *(squares)* represents the resting tension existing in the muscle as it is stretched to increasing lengths. Developed tension *(open triangles)* generated during isometric contraction from each length increases as the muscle is stretched. Addition of calcium does not affect the resting length tension curve but does cause an upward displacement of developed tension. Total tension is equal to the sum of developed and resting tension. (From Braunwald, E., editor: Heart disease, ed. 2, Philadelphia, 1984, W.B. Saunders Co.)

change occurs in the amount of filament overlap, even though active tension declines sharply. This decline has been attributed to damage of the myocyte as a result of the large deformations produced by this loading force.[26] This relationship explains why overdistention of the heart (excessive filling) results in deterioration of cardiac function.

Examination of the resting force-length relationship reveals a nonlinear relationship between applied force and deformation.[8] This behavior is illustrated in the resting length-tension curves of Figs. 36-7 and 36-8. At the lower ranges of preload, a given increment in applied force results in a relatively large degree of fiber deformation. In the upper range, the same increment in applied force results in a smaller deformation. This behavior is a manifestation of the mechanical properties of the tissue. The significance of this property will become evident when filling of the intact heart is discussed.

FUNCTION OF THE INTACT HEART

The heart is composed of a complex array of muscle fibers that are arranged to form the various cardiac chambers. Each of these fibers operates under the same basic principles as those that have been established for isolated muscle, namely, a dependence on preload, afterload, and contractility. Each of these factors finds its analog at the organ level, and together they determine the ability of the intact heart to establish and maintain the circulation of blood in the body.

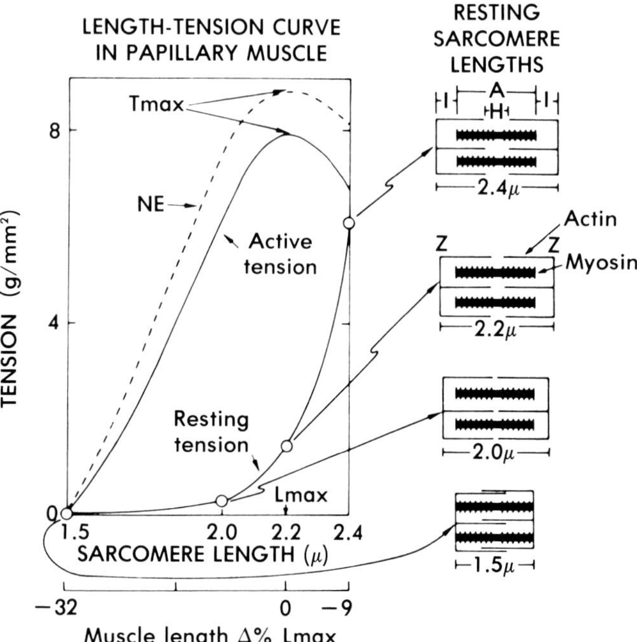

Fig. 36-8 Representation of the relationship between active tension, resting tension, and filament overlap in the feline right ventricle. These relationships form the basis of the Frank-Starling principle as seen in the intact heart. Note that the degree of active tension that is developed depends on the extent of filament overlap. Maximum active tension is developed at a sarcomere length of 2.2 μm (*L*max), which also corresponds to the optimum length for filament interaction. (From Sodeman, W.A., Jr., and Sodeman, T.M., editors: Sodeman's pathologic physiology, ed. 6, Philadelphia, 1979, W.B. Saunders Co.)

Wall Forces

The force relationships that govern the function of muscle fibers in the intact heart are determined by chamber pressures and geometries. At any point in the cardiac cycle, the pressure within a given chamber exerts a load on the wall of the chamber. This load (in dynes) is equivalent to the product of the pressure (dynes/cm^2) and the area over which the pressure acts (cm^2). In accordance with Newton's law of motion, this load must be precisely balanced by opposing forces in the wall. These forces, normalized to the areas over which they act, are known as wall stresses.[23] Fig. 36-9 shows the chamber pressure acting on a section of the wall of the left ventricle and the two principal resultant forces. Assuming an ellipsoidal representation for the left ventricle, application of the Laplace relationship results in the following expression for the meridional (σ_1) and equatorial (σ_2) components of stress:

$$\frac{\sigma_1}{R_1} + \frac{\sigma_2}{R_2} = \frac{P}{h} \quad (1)$$

where R_1 and R_2 represent the principal radii of curvature for the ellipsoid; P is the ventricular pressure; and h is the wall thickness. A number of expressions are available for independent solutions of σ_1 and σ_2 based on ventricular dimensions and pressure. These expressions and their limitations have been recently reviewed.[32]

An alternative method of conceptualizing force considers only the net force existing in the wall, rather than the normalized force.[11] The net wall force at any level may be calculated by imagining that the ventricle has been transected by a plane (Fig. 36-10). The force necessary to hold the ventricle intact, then, is the net force acting in the wall at that level. This force is equal to the product of the ven-

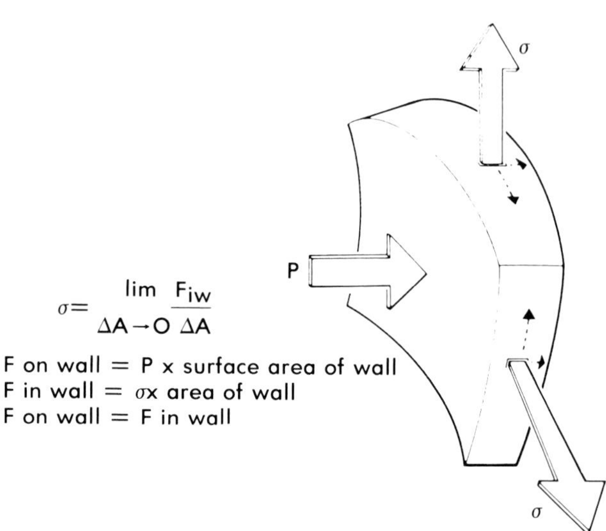

Fig. 36-9 Section removed from the wall of the left ventricle is acted on by a force equal to the product of the chamber pressure multiplied by the area over which it acts. For this element to be in equilibrium, opposing forces exist in the wall, which precisely balance this load. These forces are called wall stresses. This figure shows the loading pressure and the two principal resultant forces. (From Sandler, H., et al.: Fed. Proc. **28**[4]:1344, 1969.)

tricular pressure and the area of the chamber included in the plane. For a sphere, this force is constant at any level. For an ellipsoid, the net force depends on the plane of the section. If the section is made normal to the long axis of the ventricle, then the pressure × area product is equivalent to the net force in the meridional direction. The magnitude of this force decreases as the plane of section is moved toward the poles of the ellipse, since chamber area is decreasing.[31] Wall thickness also decreases toward the poles[20]; therefore, stresses and deformation tend to remain uniform. If the plane of section is considered in the long axis, the pressure × area product approximates the equatorial component of wall force. Fig. 36-11 shows pressure, equatorial wall stress, and net wall force for the left ventricle during one cardiac cycle.

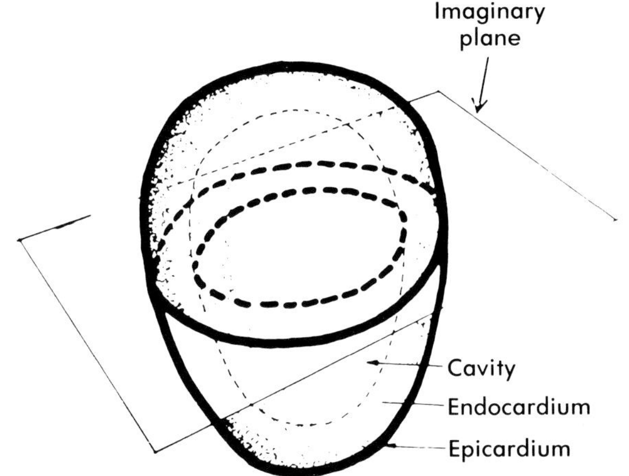

Fig. 36-10 Net wall force concept considers that the ventricle is divided by an imaginary plane located at the level of interest. Net wall force is simply the force necessary to hold the ventricle together at the given level. It is equal to the ventricular pressure multiplied by the area of the chamber involved in the plane. (From Hefner, L.L., et al.: Relation between mural force and pressure in the left ventricle of the dog, Circ. Res. **11**:654, 1962. By permission of the American Heart Association.)

Ventricular Geometry and the Cardiac Cycle

Efforts to quantify ventricular function often begin with the adoption of simplified geometric models. The normal left ventricle has been represented as an ellipsoidal shell, a sphere, or a cylinder, with various degrees of success. Even during the dynamic events of filling and ejection, accurate determinations of ventricular dimensions can be obtained with the appropriate use of these models. The elliptical model of left ventricular geometry is often used because it accurately represents the configuration of the left ventricle throughout the cardiac cycle.[20,23] In this model, the left ventricle is considered as a general ellipse axisymmetric about its major axis, having a finite but varying wall thickness. The base-to-apex (major) axis is consistently greater than the transverse (minor) axis. The thickness of the ventricular wall is maximum in the equatorial minor axis plane and tapers to a minimum value at the poles of the ellipse.[20] During the cardiac cycle, muscle shortening produces variations in ventricular dimensions, with the resultant generation of pressures and volume displacements. Fig. 36-12 illustrates left ventricular chamber dimensions and pressure for several beats. The complex anatomy, configuration, and contraction pattern of the right ventricle have precluded efforts to model this chamber accurately with simple geometric reference figures. Accordingly, the remainder of this section describes the pattern of hemodynamic events in both chambers, with the inclusion of dimensional information for the left ventricle.

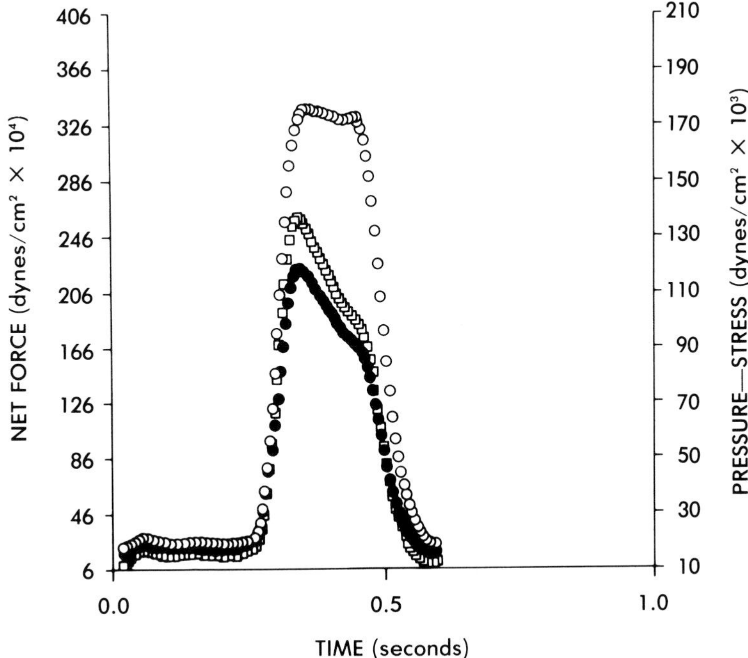

Fig. 36-11 Left ventricular pressure and wall forces for one cardiac cycle in the canine heart. Shown here are pressure *(open circles)*, equatorial wall stress *(open squares)*, and net wall force *(closed circles)*. Note the fall in stress and wall force as the ventricle unloads itself during ejection.

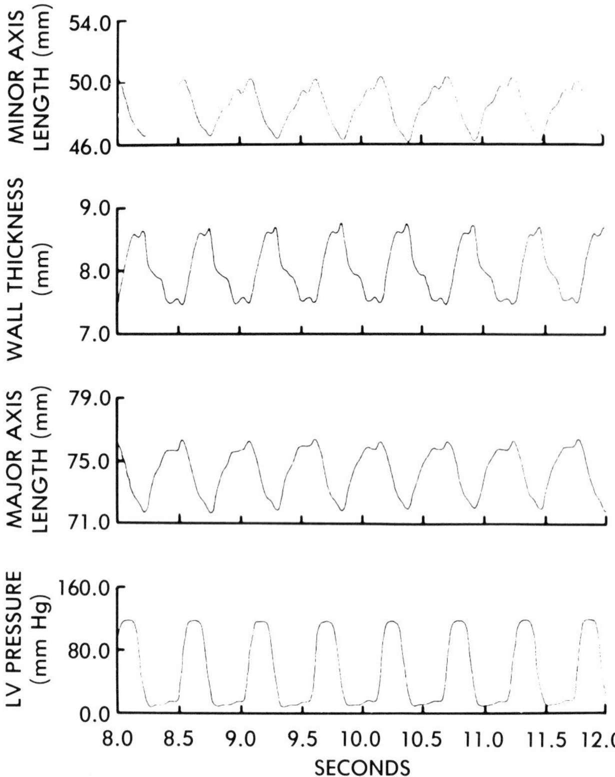

Fig. 36-12 Left ventricular chamber dimensions and pressure in the conscious dog.

The cardiac cycle can be thought of as beginning with atrial contraction, as indicated by the P wave of the electrocardiogram (Fig 36-13). Atrial contraction provides a final, active increment in ventricular filling before systole. With the onset of the QRS complex, the period of isovolumic ventricular contraction begins. This marks the beginning of ventricular systole. As ventricular pressures rise above atrial pressures, the atrioventricular valves close. The vibrations generated by the abrupt closure of these valves are responsible for the first heart sound. In the left ventricle, the minor axis dimension shortens, the major axis lengthens, and the thickness of the ventricular wall increases,[20] resulting in an ellipsization of the chamber. During this period, there is a rapid rise in the rate of pressure generation *(dP/dt)*. This parameter reaches a maximum value at the onset of the ejection phase. Ejection begins when pressure within each of the ventricles rises above the pressures in their respective outflow tracts. The higher ventricular pressures result in an opening of the semilunar valves, and the phase of rapid ejection ensues. Rapid ejection is followed by reduced ejection as pressures in the ventricles and great arteries fall.

In left ventricular ejection, the minor and major axes shorten, and the wall becomes thicker, resulting in a decrease in internal chamber volume. In the canine heart the major axis, minor axis, and wall thickness changes account, respectively, for 9%, 47%, and 44% of volume output during systolic ejection.[20] In the right ventricle, contraction occurs in a peristaltic wave moving from the sinus region toward the conus.[16] As ventricular and arterial pressures fall, flows in the great vessels reverse. This point marks the end of systole and the beginning of the first

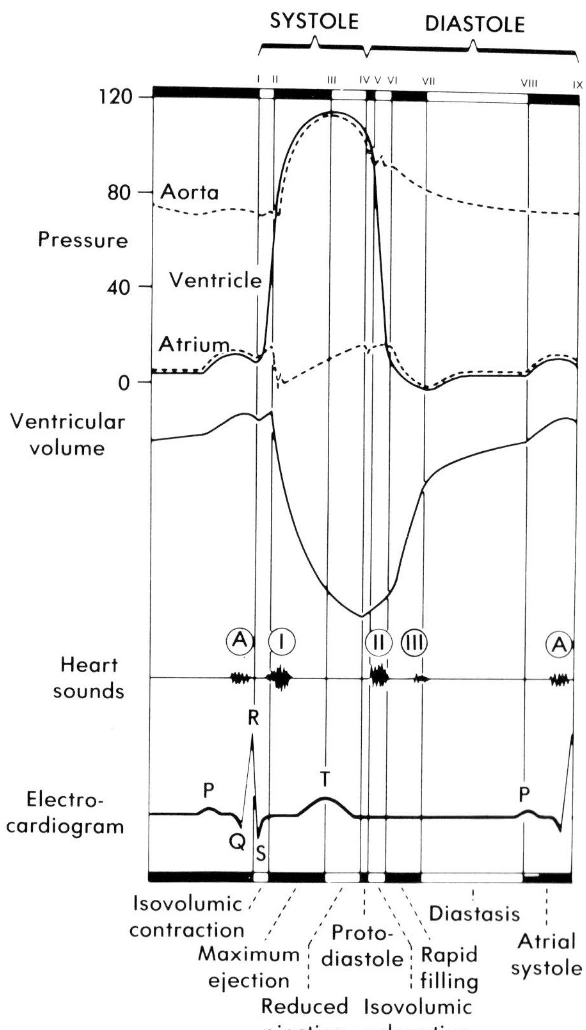

Fig. 36-13 Phases of the cardiac cycle. Shown are left ventricular pressure and volume and the correlation of these measurements to left atrial and aortic pressures, heart sounds, and the electrocardiogram. *(A)* represents the atrial sound, *(I)* the first heart sound, *(II)* the second heart sound, and *(III)* the third heart sound. (From Katz, A.M.: Physiology of the heart, New York, 1977, Raven Press.)

phase of diastole, known as protodiastole. Protodiastole ends with the closure of the semilunar valves, which produces the second heart sound. Such closure is also marked by the incisura of the arterial pressure tracing. Protodiastole is followed by the period of isovolumic relaxation. During this period, the geometric patterns observed during isovolumic contraction generally are reversed, and the peak fall in *dP/dt* occurs. Ventricular pressures fall until they are less than pressures in the atria. The atrioventricular valves open, and diastolic filling begins.

Diastolic filling is composed of several phases. The first of these is the rapid filling phase, during which rapid volume expansion occurs. This phase is sometimes associated with an audible third heart sound. As the ventricles become full, the rate of filling shows and the period of diastasis is approached. During diastole, the left ventricle becomes more spherical as the minor axis dimension increases with respect to the major axis, and the wall becomes thinner.[20] The end of diastole is marked by atrial systole and the generation of the fourth heart sound.

Diastolic Behavior

Relaxation

Diastole represents the period of relaxation and filling in the cardiac cycle. During relaxation, the ion fluxes that occurred during the process of excitation-contraction coupling are reversed, and the contractile proteins assume their resting configurations. In the filling phases of diastole, the relaxed sarcomeres lengthen as the ventricles distend with blood and the initial muscle length for the next beat is determined. Relaxation is often thought of as a passive event since pressures and flows are rapidly falling; however, it is a period of considerable metabolic activity, requiring the presence of ATP initially to dissociate the actin-myosin complexes and later to provide the energy for the active transport, which restores the resting ion gradients. In order for relaxation to occur, sarcoplasmic [Ca^{++}] must be reduced to a level such that Ca^{++} dissociates from the troponin complex. This activity is accomplished by pumps in the membrane of the sarcoplasmic reticulum and to a lesser extent by transport mechanisms in the sarcolemma.[13]

The common feature of these transport processes is the requirement for ATP. In light of this, abnormalities of relaxation have been explained in part on the basis of reduced ATP availability in the injured or diseased heart.[9] An additional role has been suggested for ATP in the relaxation process. Adding ATP to a cell that has normal levels of ATP results in an enhancement of the uptake of Ca^{++} by the sarcoplasmic reticulum. Thus ATP may act in a regulatory manner in controlling Ca^{++} transport. Slight reductions in cellular levels as a result of moderate degrees of energy deprivation could result in impaired relaxation, even though sufficient levels are available to saturate the primary transport mechanisms.[13]

Filling

The importance of the filling events of diastole as determinants of cardiac function was first noted by Frank in the late nineteenth century. Frank observed a direct relationship between end diastolic volume and the force of contraction in the isolated frog heart.[6] Later, Starling made similar observations in the mammalian heart. This work culminated in the concept of the Frank-Starling relationship, which was simply stated as "the energy of contraction, however measured, is a function of the length of the muscle fiber."[27]

In the intact heart, diastolic filling determines the length of the muscle fibers before contraction and therefore influences the force of contraction. The nature and extent of this filling, in turn, are influenced by a number of factors; among these are the level of filling pressure, the material properties of the myocardium, the geometry of the chamber, and such external forces as pericardial and pleural pressures.[9]

Within any of the cardiac chambers, the filling pressure produces distending forces within the wall of the chamber. These forces are a function of the magnitude of the pressure and the size and shape of the chamber. The resulting distention produced by a given increment of force is governed by the material properties of the myocardium. Because these forces act to determine the length of the muscle fibers before contraction, they may be considered analogs to the preload previously described for isolated muscle.

The "material properties" of the myocardium refer specifically to the elastic and viscous characteristics of the muscle. An elastic material deforms when acted on by an external force and recovers from the deformation when the force is removed. For a substance with linear elastic properties, deformation *(e)* is related to the force *(f)* as:

$$f = E\,(e) \tag{2}$$

where *E*, the slope of the relationship, is known as the coefficient of elasticity or Young's modulus.[17] An increase in *E* reflects an increase in the stiffness of the material. In a viscoelastic material, force is a function of both deformation and the rate of deformation. Heart muscle is known to possess both elastic and viscous properties.[19] The analysis of these properties and their influence on diastolic filling is complicated by the fact that the elastic properties, and possibly the viscous properties, are nonlinear entities.[19]

When a force is applied along the long axis of an isolated papillary muscle, the deformation of the muscle will obey the following relationship, assuming that the rate of deformation is small so that viscous effects are not important[8]:

$$F = \alpha\,[e^{\beta(x-x^*)} - 1] \tag{3}$$

where x is the muscle length, x^* is the resting muscle length, and α and β are elastic constants analogous to the coefficient of elasticity of Equation 2. *F* is the fiber stress. Stress is an expression of normalized force, here equal to the applied force divided by the cross-sectional area of the muscle specimen. This nonlinear elasticity of heart muscle is the principal factor affecting the relationship between diastolic pressure and volume in the intact left ventricle.[7] Fig. 36-14 shows the pressure-volume curve obtained by slowly filling a canine heart with saline. Several important points are apparent from this illustration. First, even though the ventricle is composed of muscle that displays exponential elastic behavior, the relationship between pressure and volume is not truly exponential. It is approximately linear in the lower pressure ranges and approaches exponentiality in the upper pressure ranges. Second, the elastic nature of the myocardium resists deformation above a filling pressure of about 20 mm Hg. The significance of the second factor is that the increasing stiffness of the cardiac muscle prevents overextension of the individual sarcomeres, permitting the heart to function on the ascending limb of the Frank-Starling relationship, where increased volume results in increased output.

Systolic Function

The peak force that can be generated at a given contractile state and end diastolic volume is attained in the isovolumically contracting heart.[30] As the end diastolic volume is raised, the peak developed force increases in a linear fashion (Fig. 36-15). This behavior demonstrates the

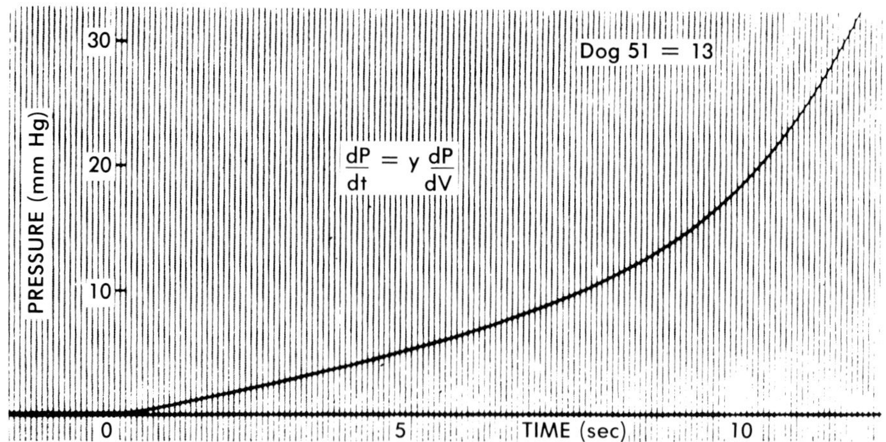

Fig. 36-14 Relationship between pressure and volume (expressed as time of infusion of volume at a constant rate) in the isolated, arrested canine heart. The relationship is approximately linear in the lower pressure ranges and becomes exponential in the upper range. The increasing instantaneous slope of the pressure-volume curve reflects the increase in chamber stiffness that occurs as the ventricle is filled. (From Diamond, G., et al.: Diastolic pressure-volume relationship in the canine left ventricle, Circ. Res. **29:**267, 1971. By permission of the American Heart Association.)

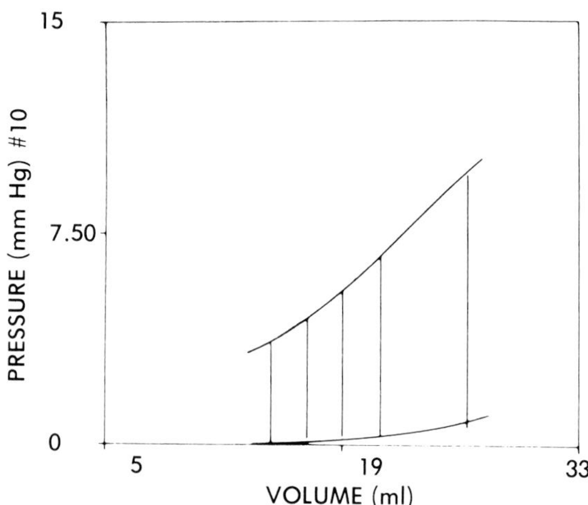

Fig. 36-15 Development of pressure in the isovolumically contracting canine left ventricle. As resting volume is increased, the peak generated pressure increases. Line connecting the peak pressures defines the limit of force generation for the contracting ventricle. (From Strauer, B.E., editor: The heart in hypertension, Heidelberg, 1981, Springer-Verlag.)

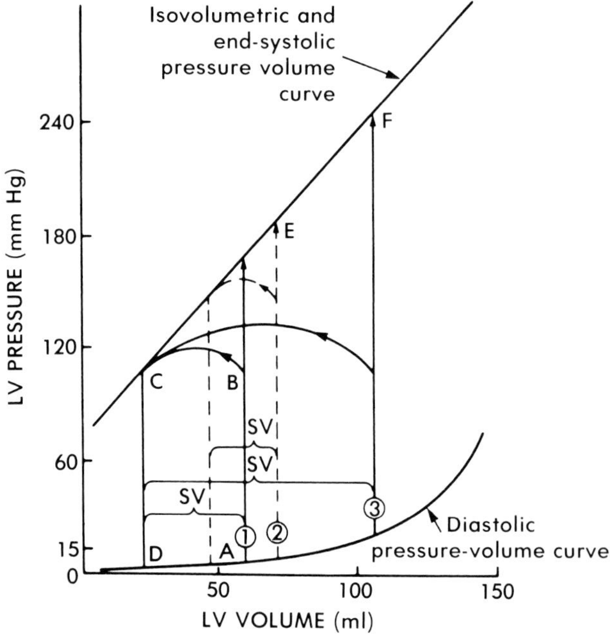

Fig. 36-16 Schematic diagram of the pressure-volume loops for several beats under various loading conditions. Contraction 1 is considered control, contraction 3 shows the effects of increased preload, and contraction 2 shows the effects of increased afterload on stroke volume *(SV)* and pressure generation. Points *E* and *F* represent the peak pressures that could be generated if the ventricle were to contract isovolumically from preloads at points 2 and 3, respectively. Note that points *E* and *F* define the limit for shortening in the ejecting heart. See text for further details. (From Braunwald, E., editor: Heart disease, ed. 2, Philadelphia, 1984, W.B. Saunders Co.)

operation of the Frank-Starling relationship in the intact ventricle, where force generation is an increasing function of fiber length, expressed here as end diastolic volume. The line that results from relating peak force to initial volume defines the limit of force generation for the ventricle. When the ventricle is permitted to eject, this line also defines the limit of systolic shortening.[30]

Fig. 36-16 depicts the pressure-volume relationships for an ejecting ventricle under changing conditions of preload and afterload. Contraction 1, originating from end-diastolic volume *A*, contracts isovolumically to point *B*. At point *B*, the ventricular pressure just exceeds aortic pressure, and ejection begins. During ejection (points *B* to *C*), the force sustained by the muscle fibers in the wall of the ventricle represents the afterload. Ejection continues until a point is reached at which muscle force is maximum for a given volume (point *C*). This point contracts the isovolumic pressure-volume line and represents the end of systolic shortening. When preload is altered as in contraction 3, there is a change in stroke volume, but the extent of fiber shortening does not change. Contraction 3 still proceeds to point *C*. Increasing the afterload by augmenting aortic pressure (contraction 2) results in both decreased stroke volume and a change in the extent of fiber shortening. Thus the degree of fiber shortening in the ejecting heart is determined by the instantaneous load borne by the muscle, not by alterations in loading before contraction.[30] The ability of the ventricle to generate force is influenced by the contractile state of the muscle. A change in contractility is represented by a change in the peak force.

Electrical Activity

Electrically excitable tissues communicate within themselves and with other structures through the generation of action potentials. Within the heart there are certain cells that generate spontaneous action potentials, which propagate and serve as a stimulus to initiate contraction. This property is referred to as automaticity. A second property, intrinsic to the electrical activity of the heart, is conductivity. Conductivity describes the low-resistance intercellular connections that permit any depolarization to be spread throughout the mass of the heart.

Under normal circumstances, contraction of the heart is initiated by action potentials generated in the sinoatrial (SA) node. This structure, located at the junction of the right atrium and the superior vena cava, has the highest rate of intrinsic pacemaker activity found in the heart. Action potentials generated here spread slowly over the right and left atria, with resultant atrial contractions. Excitation moves to the cardiac ventricles through the atrioventricular (AV) node. In contrast to the atria, impulse conduction through this structure is extremely slow. This delay permits the completion of atrial contraction before ventricular activation. Having passed through the AV node, the wave of excitation enters the bundle of His, a structure located in the subendocardium of the right surface of the interventricular septum. The His bundle then divides into right- and left-sided branches, which ramify in the fibers of the Purkinje system. The Purkinje system extends over the subendocardial surfaces of both ventricles. Its electrical activity is characterized by a high conduction velocity, which permits near-simultaneous activation of the ventricles.

Many factors affect the nature of pacemaker activity and excitation in the heart. These include neural, hormonal, physiochemical, and pathologic influences. These influences often exert their effects by alterations of events occurring at the cellular level, specifically by inducing changes in the transmembrane electrical potential and ion movement. Transmembrane electrical potential *(Vm)* in cardiac cells comes about as a result of an unequal distribution of ions across the cell membrane. In cardiac cells, as in most other cells of the body, the internal potassium concentration is high and the internal sodium concentration is low. The contribution of each of these ions to the net charge on the membrane can be estimated from the Nernst equation.[4] For an unspecified ion X:

$$E = \frac{58}{Z} \log \frac{[\mathrm{X\ out}]}{[\mathrm{X\ in}]} \tag{4}$$

where E is the equilibrilum potential resulting solely from ion X, and Z is the charge number of the ion. If the membrane is permeable only to X, then V_m equals E. When more than one ion is involved, V_m becomes a weighted average of the equilibrium potential of each ion. The weighting factors depend on the relative conductance of each ion. Conductance *(g)* is the reciprocal of resistance and is an expression of the ease with which an ion can cross the cell membrane. Thus, in general terms, for a cell permeable to ions A, B, C, Vm could be approximated from the equation

$$Vm = \frac{gA}{gA + gB + gC} E_A + \frac{gB}{gA + gB + gC} E_B + \frac{gC}{gA + gB + gC} E_C \tag{5}$$

in the case of cardiac tissue, the major ions involved in transmembrane flux are Na^+, K^+, and Ca^{++}, such that

$$Vm = \frac{g\mathrm{Na}}{g\mathrm{Na} + g\mathrm{K} + g\mathrm{Ca}} E_{\mathrm{Na}} + \frac{g\mathrm{K}}{g\mathrm{Na} + g\mathrm{K} + g\mathrm{Ca}} E_{\mathrm{K}} + \frac{g\mathrm{Ca}}{g\mathrm{Na} + g\mathrm{K} + g\mathrm{Ca}} E_{\mathrm{Ca}} \tag{6}$$

In the quiescent cardiac cell, K^+ permeability greatly exceeds Na^+ and Ca^{++} permeability—or, in terms of conductances, gK greatly exceeds gCa and gNa. Given this fact, Equation 6 then reduces to the Nernst equation for K^+, and the resting V_m equals or approaches E_K.

Action potentials in cardiac tissue result from changes in the relative conductances of the principal ions Na^+, K^+, and Ca^{++}. Ion concentrations across the membrane actually change very little. The arrival of an action potential causes a rise in the resting V_m toward threshold value for the particular cell. Once threshold is achieved, a complex pattern of conductance changes ensues. Cardiac muscle cells and cells of the Purkinje system have a high relative gK at rest. Membrane potential is -80 to -90 mV, and threshold is approximately -60 mV. When cardiac muscle cells are stimulated, gNa becomes markedly elevated in what is known as Phase 0 of the action potential (Figs. 36-17 and 36-18). Sodium ions are now better able to cross the membrane. Note that this movement is favored by both chemical and electrical gradients, so it occurs quite rapidly. The net inward movement of positive charge causes depolarization of the cell; Vm moves toward and then past 0 mV. As the cell depolarizes, gNa falls, completing Phase 0. Phase 1 is characterized by a rapid fall in Vm thought to be the result of a transient increase in membrane permeability to chloride (Cl^-). Phase 2 is the plateau phase of the action potential. This is brought about by a slow inward Ca^{++} and Na^+ current balanced by an outward K^+ current. Repolarization occurs in Phase 3 and is a result of a further increase in gK combined with an inactivation of the slow inward current of Phase 2.

There are striking differences between action potentials seen in the nodal structures and those just described (Fig. 36-17). Recordings from cells of the SA node reveal a less negative resting potential, a decreased rate of Phase 0 depolarization, no plateau, and a reduced rate of Phase 3 depolarization. Perhaps most significant is the behavior that nodal tissue displays in Phase 4. During this phase, Vm is not constant but moves steadily toward threshold.

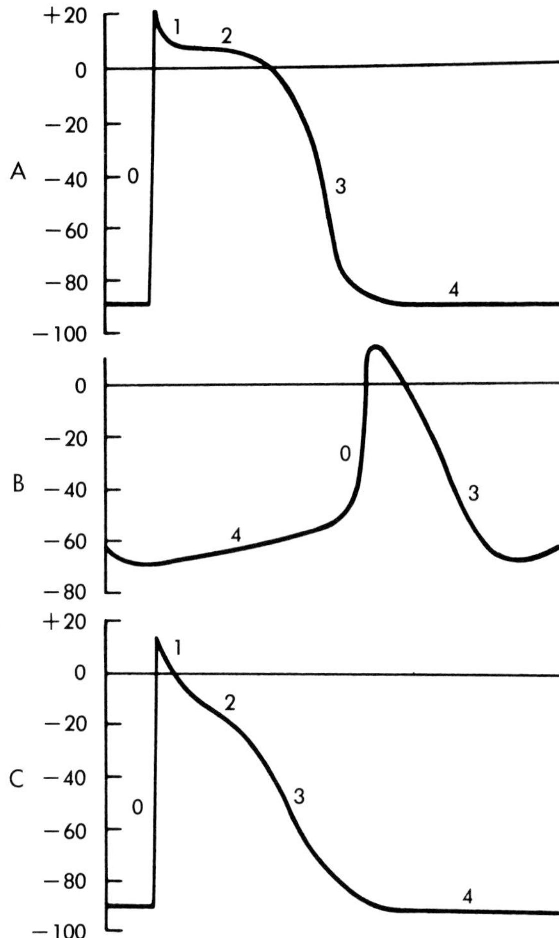

Fig. 36-17 Action potentials seen in various cardiac tissues: ventricular muscle cell, **A,** sinoatrial node, **B,** and atrial muscle, **C.** Time base for **B** is half that of **A** and **C.** (From Berne, R.M., and Levy, M.N., editors: Physiology, St. Louis, 1983, The C.V. Mosby Co.)

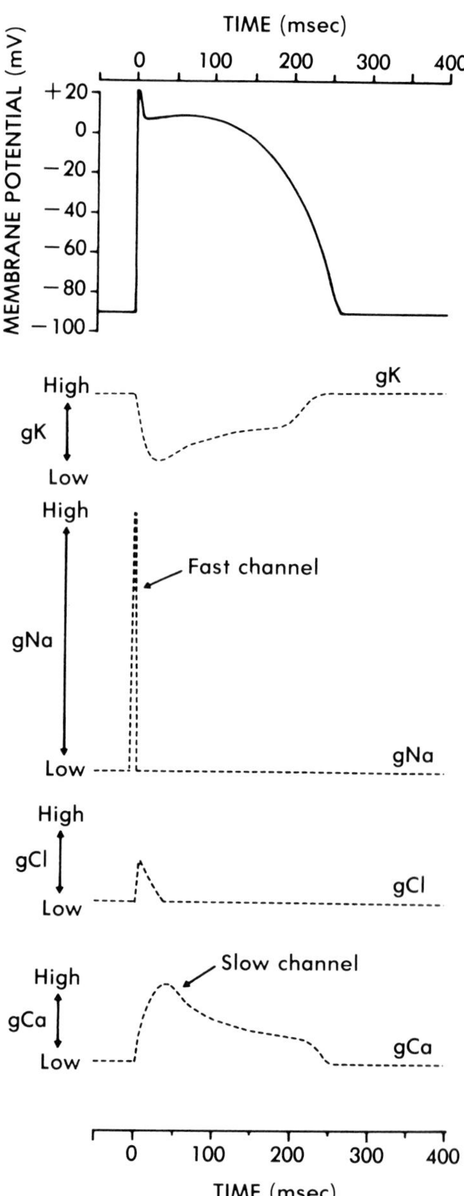

Fig. 36-18 Conductance changes seen within a Purkinje fiber. Typical action potential is shown at the top, with the accompanying changes in conductance for potassium *(gK),* sodium *(gNa),* chloride *(gCl),* and calcium *(gCa).* (From Katz, A.M.: Physiology of the heart, New York, 1977, Raven Press.)

The basis for this behavior is believed to be a time-dependent decrease in the outward K^+ movement in the presence of a small, steady, inward movement of Ca^{++}. The loss of the K^+ current disrupts the balance of charge and results in membrane depolarization. When the membrane potential reaches threshold, an action potential is generated. In this manner, nodal tissue serves as a pace generator for the heart. The rate of pacemaker activity depends upon the minimum Phase 4 V_m, the rate of depolarization, and the threshold potential. These factors are under neural and hormonal controls that act to vary the heart rate (Fig. 36-19). For example, increased vagal activity results in the release of acetylcholine at the SA node. This has the effect of increasing *g*K, which hyperpolarizes the membrane and slows the heart rate. Conversely, catecholamines can increase the inward Phase 4 Ca^{++} current, which would increase both the rate of depolarization and the heart rate (see the following discussion on neural control).

Neural Control

The sympathetic and parasympathetic divisions of the autonomic nervous system act in concert to regulate cardiac function. Sympathetic effects are excitatory and are mediated through nerve fibers distributed to the atria, ventricles, and nodal tissue. Parasympathetic influences are generally inhibitory and act predominantly on atrial and nodal tissues.

The terminal regions of the sympathetic fibers synthesize and store norepinephrine, which is released as a result of nerve stimulation. Norepinephrine acts on beta-adrenergic receptors imbedded in the membrane of the cardiac cell. Beta receptors in the myocardium are of two types, beta 1 and beta 2. Beta 1 receptors are distributed exclusively to the ventricles, and their activation results in an increase in ventricular contractility.[10]

The mechanism of action is thought to involve increases in the level of cyclic AMP, which in turn promotes the phosphorylation and activation of calcium channels in the

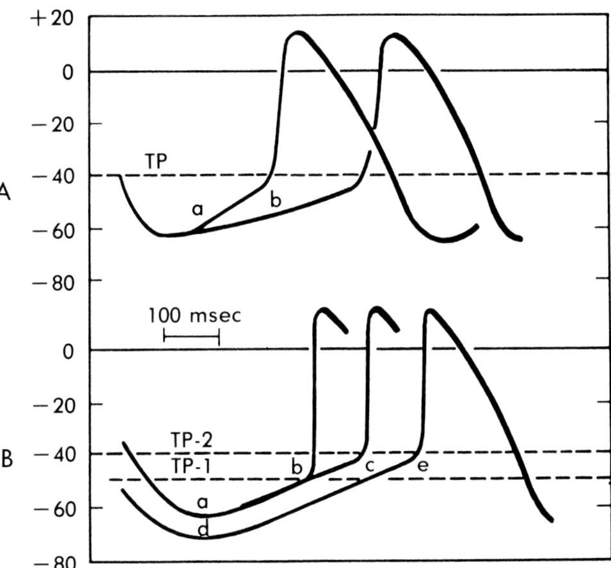

Fig. 36-19 Altering rate of pacemaker activity. **A,** Rate of firing is slowed by a decrease in the rate of phase 4 depolarization. Threshold potential *(TP)* is not changed. **B,** Changing threshold at a given rate of phase 4 depolarization can alter heart rate by changing the time required to reach TP (tracings a-b and a-c). Hyperpolarization can also influence rate (tracings a-e). (From Berne, R.M., and Levy, M.N., editors: Physiology, St. Louis, 1983, The C.V. Mosby Co.)

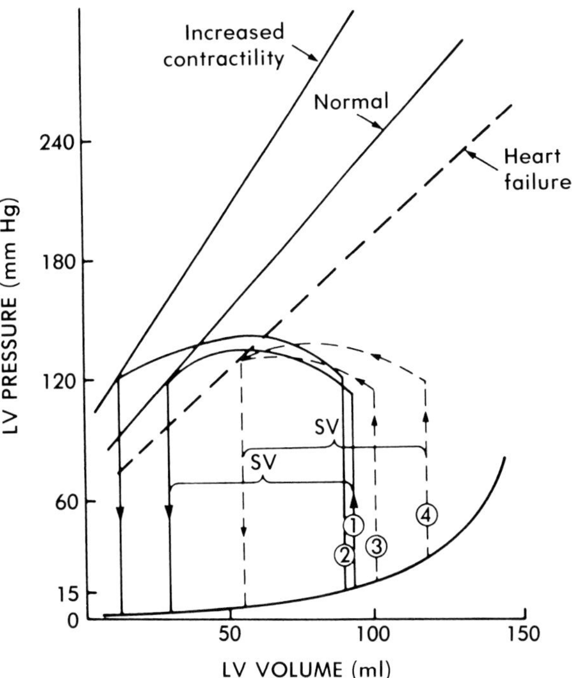

Fig. 36-20 Conceptual pressure-volume loops for hearts at three contractile states. Note the effect of the contractile state on the stroke volume *(SV)* generated from similar preloads at points *1, 2,* and *3.* During heart failure, SV may be decreased despite a slightly larger end-diastolic volume at a comparable level of aortic pressure (see contraction 3). If end-diastolic volume is further increased, SV may be restored (see contraction 4). (From Braunwald, E., editor: Heart disease, ed. 2, Philadelphia, 1984, W.B. Saunders Co.)

membrane. The net effect of beta 1 stimulation is an increase in calcium influx, which causes an increase in the contractile state of the muscle.[28] Beta 2 receptors are found in the atria. The activation of these receptors results in an increased heart rate through their positive chronotropic effects. The stimulus for activation of beta 2 receptors differs from that of beta 1 types in that beta 2 receptors are sensitive to epinephrine as well as norepinephrine.

Parasympathetic effects are mediated by fibers of the vagus nerve that are distributed to the atria and, to a lesser extent, to the ventricles. Activation of these fibers results in a release of acetylcholine, which causes a depression of cardiac function characterized by a reduction in heart rate and atrial contractility. Ventricular contractility is affected to a lesser extent.[14] The diminution in ventricular function seen during vagal stimulation can be explained in part by reduced ventricular filling, which occurs secondarily to the fall in atrial contractility.[2] Acetylcholine produces its negative chronotropic effects by hyperpolarizing the nodal tissue. Hyperpolarization is a consequence of the increase in potassium permeability caused by the application of acetylcholine. Acetylcholine also binds to muscarinic receptors on the sympathetic nerve fibers. Activation of the muscarinic receptors results in reduced catecholamine release during sympathetic stimulation. Thus the inhibitory influences of parasympathetic activity are more pronounced when sympathetic activity is high.[14]

In recent years, an increasing emphasis on neural control of heart function has been evolving. Trauma, anesthesia, and anxiety all evoke major alterations in cardiovascular function and may be the precipitants of arrhythmias or cardiac dysfunction.

Heart Failure

Contraction 3 in Fig. 36-20 represents a decreased contractile state, as might be seen in conditions of heart failure. Failure occurs when the heart can no longer pump blood commensurate with the needs of the body. This condition can occur as a result of depression in the intrinsic contractility of the muscle or as a result of the imposition of increased loading conditions on ventricular ejection.[1] The heart can compensate in several ways. Contractile state can increase with endogenous catecholamine release. Also, muscle preload can be augmented by the increased filling pressure that often accompanies the reduced pumping ability of the failing ventricle. Hypertrophy and/or chamber dilation also can occur.

Associated with these compensatory mechanisms are certain detrimental factors that may contribute to the eventual failure of the heart. Increased preload results in an increased level of wall stress throughout diastole. Wall stress has been shown to be related to myocardial oxygen consumption[15]; therefore, incorporation of this mechanism necessarily increases the flow requirements of the myocardium. As chamber enlargement occurs, several aspects of active force relations are affected. From the net wall force concept developed earlier, it is simple to see how an increase in chamber size results in a decrease in the efficiency of the ventricular contraction. Recall that wall force *(F)* is equal to the product of chamber pressure *(P)* and area *(A)*. Rearranged, this gives $P = F/A$. The generation of a given pressure within the large ventricle (larger *A*) then requires the existence of a greater wall force. A second aspect of chamber enlargement concerns the unloading of the ventricle during systole. In a normal heart, the muscle load (stress) peaks soon after the onset of ejection and then declines through the remainder of systole (see Fig. 36-11). This occurs because the chamber size decreases more than the pressure increases, resulting in a partial unloading of the ventricle. To generate a given stroke volume, the enlarged heart undergoes a smaller degree of systolic shortening. It therefore unloads itself less than would a smaller heart ejecting the same volume. Worsened ejection resulting from prolonged high wall tension creates an afterload mismatch in the coupling of the heart of the periphery. Vasodilator therapy normalizes this loading of the heart and thereby facilitates ejection. At the same time, smaller volumes and wall tension decrease myocardial oxygen consumption.

SUMMARY

For many years, the complexity of the cardiovascular system prevented the systematic study of its properties. Although that complexity remains, several basic principles by which the heart functions have been determined. These principles include the dependence of myocardial performance on preload, afterload, and contractility. Preload is defined as the distending force, or load, that is placed on cardiac muscle before contraction. The preload and the distensibility of the muscle are the determinants of the initial length of the muscle before contraction. The load encountered by cardiac muscle after activation is defined as the afterload. The magnitude of the afterload determines the nature of the subsequent contraction. Contractility refers to the intrinsic ability of cardiac muscle to contract, independent of loading conditions. Heart failure occurs when the heart can no longer pump blood commensurate with the needs of the body. This condition can occur as a result of depression in the intrinsic contractility of cardiac muscle or as a result of the imposition of increased loading conditions on ventricular ejection. Understanding the interplay among these various parameters and how their imbalance can be corrected or lessened, both medically and surgically, underlies the rationale for treatment in patients with cardiac dysfunction.

REFERENCES

1. Braunwald, E.: Pathophysiology of heart failure. In Braunwald, E., editor: Heart disease, Philadelphia, 1984, W.B. Saunders Co.
2. Braunwald, E., Sonnenblick, E.H., and Ross, J.: Contraction of the normal heart. In Braunwald, E., editor: Heart disease, Philadelphia, 1984, W.B. Saunders Co.
3. Bremel, R.D., and Weber, A.M.: Cooperation with actin filament in vertebrate skeletal muscle, Nature (New Biol.) **238:**97, 1972.
4. DeVoe, R.D., and Maloney, P.C.: Principles of cell homeostasis. In Mountcastle, V.B., editor: Medical physiology ed. 14, 1980, St. Louis, The C.V. Mosby Co.
5. Fabiato, A., and Fabiato, F.: Calcium and cardiac excitation-contraction coupling, Annu. Rev. Physiol. **41:**473, 1979.
6. Frank, O.: On the dynamics of cardiac muscle, Am. Heart J. **58**(2):282, 1959.
7. Glantz, S.A.: Computing indices of diastolic stiffness has been counterproductive, Fed. Proc. **39:**162, 1980.
8. Glantz, S.A., and Kernoff, R.S.: Muscle stiffness determined from canine left ventricular pressure-volume curves, Circ. Res. **37:**787, 1975.
9. Grossman, W., and Barry, W.H.: Diastolic pressure-volume relations in the diseased heart, Fed. Proc. **39:**148, 1980.
10. Hedberg, A., Minneman, K.P., and Molinoff, P.B.: Differential distribution of beta-1 and beta-2 adrenergic receptors in cat and guinea-pig heart, J. Pharmacol. Exp. Ther. **213:**503, 1980.
11. Hefner, L.L., et al.: Relation between mural force and pressure in the left ventricle of the dog, Circ. Res. **11:**654, 1962.
12. Hoh, J.F.Y., McGrath, P.A., and Hale, P.T.: Electrophoretic analysis of multiple forms of rat cardiac myosin: effects of hypophysectomy and thyroid replacement, J. Mol. Cell. Cardiol. **10:**1053, 1978.
13. Katz, A.M., and Smith, V.E.: Relaxation abnormalities. I. Mechanisms, Hosp. Pract. **19**(1):69, 1984.
14. Levy, M.N., and Martin, P.J.: Neural control of the heart. In Berne, R.M., editor: Handbook of physiology, section 2, the cardiovascular system, vol. 1, the heart, Bethesda, Md., 1979, American Physiological Society.
15. McDonald, R.H., Jr., Taylor, R.R., and Gingolani, H.E.: Measurement of myocardial-developed tension and its relation to oxygen consumption, Am. J. Physiol. **211:**667, 1966.
16. Meier, G.D., et al.: Contractile function in canine right ventricle, Am. J. Physiol. **239**(8):H794, 1980.
17. Mirsky, I., and Pasipoularides, A.: Elastic properties of normal and hypertrophied cardiac muscle, Fed. Proc. **39:**156, 1980.
18. Morkin, E.: Contractile proteins of the heart, Hosp. Pract. **18**(6):97, 1983.
19. Pouleur, H., et al.: Diastolic viscous properties of the intact canine left ventricle, Circ. Res. **45:**410, 1979.
20. Rankin, J.S., et al.: The three-dimensional dynamic geometry of the left ventricle in the conscious dog, Circ. Res. **39**(3):304, 1976.
21. Rupp, H.: The adaptive changes in the isoenzyme pattern of myosin from hypertrophied rat myocardium as a result of pressure overload and physical training, Basic Res. Cardiol. **76:**79, 1981.
22. Samuel, J.L., et al.: Distribution of myosin isozymes within single cardiac cells: an immunohistochemical study, Circ. Res. **52:**200, 1983.
23. Sandler, H., and Ghista, D.N.: Mechanical and dynamic implications of dimensional measurements of the left ventricle, Fed. Proc. **28**(4):829, 1981.
24. Schwartz, K., et al.: Myosin isoenzymic distribution correlates with speed of myocardial contraction, J. Mol. Cell. Cardiol. **13:**1071, 1981.
25. Sonneblick, E.H.: Implications of muscle mechanics in the heart, Fed. Proc. **21:**975, 1962.
26. Sonnenblick, E.H., et al.: Redefinition of the ultrastructural basis of the cardiac length-tension relations, Circulation **48**(suppl. 4):65, 1973.
27. Starling, E.H.: The Linacre lecture on the law of the heart, London, 1918, Longmans, Green & Co.
28. van Breeman, C., Aaronson, P., and Loutzenhiser, R.: Na-Ca interactions in mammalian smooth muscle, Pharmacol. Rev. **30:**167, 1979.
29. Weber, A., and Murray, J.M.: Molecular control mechanisms in muscle contraction, Physiol. Rev. **53:**612, 1973.
30. Weber, K.T., and Janicki, J.S.: The heart as a muscle-pump system and the concept of heart failure, Am. Heart J. **98**(3)371, 1979.
31. Weber, K.T., et al.: Contractile mechanics and the interaction of the right and left ventricles, Am. J. Cardiol. **47:**686, 1981.
32. Yin, F.C.P.: Ventricular wall stress, Circ. Res. **49**(4):829, 1981.

37

John W. Brown and Daniel H. Raess

Cardiac Failure and Resuscitation

Heart failure is not a disease but a "pathophysiological state in which an abnormality of cardiac function is responsible for failure of the heart to pump blood at a rate commensurate with the requirements of the metabolizing tissues."[3] It is the syndrome that may accompany any form of cardiac disease and commonly occurs in the clinical settings of severe trauma, sepsis, all forms of congenital and acquired heart disease, and during both cardiac and noncardiac major surgical procedures. It occurs when the heart is unable to pump blood at the increased flow rate needed to provide for the increased oxygen demands of the body during periods of stress. Cardiac failure subsequent to acute myocardial infarction and following cardiac surgical procedures has been studied intently over the past several years; these studies form much of the basis of our current understanding of the pathophysiology of cardiac failure. The ability to determine and quantitate cardiac performance is important to surgeons from the standpoint of assessment of operative risk and the management of the surgical patient preoperatively, intraoperatively, and postoperatively.

The purpose of this chapter is to define cardiac failure and the deviation from normal physiology that it produces. The underlying mechanism by which many disease states cause the heart to fail will be outlined, as well as the methods currently available to diagnose and quantitate the degree of cardiac failure and the rationale for their use. Emergency cardiac resuscitation using electrical, pharmacologic, and mechanical maneuvers will be analyzed for their physiologic effects. Finally, the immediate care of the patient following a successful resuscitation will be reviewed in light of current physiologic concepts.

EPIDEMIOLOGY OF HEART FAILURE

Little has been written about the incidence of heart failure, and virtually all studies before the Framingham study were hampered by the absence of uniform diagnostic criteria defining what heart failure is. It is generally accepted that a strong correlation exists between heart failure and advancing age; 80% of patients admitted to the hospital with failing hearts are older than 60 years.[11] The estimated prevalence of heart failure for 1983 in the United States was 2.3 million patients and the estimated incidence of new cases for that same year was 400,000.[8] Overt heart disease and age are the principal determinants of the incidence of heart failure, and nearly 90% of patients with this problem have systemic hypertension or coronary artery disease or both as the primary risk factors (Fig. 37-1). Diabetes, renal disease, obesity, and smoking are also positive risk factors for heart failure but are far less important than age, hypertension, and coronary disease.[11]

NEW YORK HEART ASSOCIATION FUNCTIONAL CLASSIFICATION OF HEART FAILURE

Class I	No limitation of physical activity.
Class II	Slight limitation of physical activity because of dyspnea, palpitations, fatigue, or angina.
Class III	Marked limitation of physical activity. Less than ordinary activity produces symptoms.
Class IV	Symptoms present at rest. With any physical activity, increased discomfort is experienced.

After it is first diagnosed, the prognosis of heart failure is grim and is directly related to the degree of myocardial dysfunction as defined by the New York Heart Association Functional Classification (see the boxed material above). The 5-year survival rate for all patients with heart failure is less than 50% and for patients with marked left ventricular dysfunction (i.e., class IV of the functional classification), the 1-year mortality is greater than 50%.[11]

CAUSES OF HEART FAILURE

Heart failure is a common clinical syndrome in which the heart is unable to maintain adequate blood flow to meet metabolic demands. The pathophysiologic factors that lead to its development vary considerably. Some of the major factors are: pressure overload, volume overload, loss of muscle, decreased myocardial contractility, and restricted cardiac filling. The most common cause is pressure overload from systemic hypertension. All types of left ventricular outflow obstruction (e.g., aortic stenosis) may also cause pressure overload. Causes of such overload in the right heart (i.e., right ventricle) include pulmonary hypertension or pulmonary embolus. Volume overload can be caused by numerous conditions such as aortic or mitral regurgitation, anemia, arteriovenous fistula, and cirrhosis in which the excess blood volume is caused by secondary hyperaldosteronism. Volume overload may be selective as is seen in atrial septal defect with a large left-to-right shunt. In this situation, the right ventricle is volume overloaded, but the left ventricle is unaffected. Prolonged pressure and/or volume overload lead to intrinsic changes in myocardial contractility that are commonly irreversible.[17]

Loss of cardiac muscle is a common pathophysiologic pathway leading to heart failure and is best exemplified by the patient with coronary artery disease following myocardial infarction. The loss of muscle and contractile function produces a pressure and/or volume overload on the remaining normal muscle and can lead to the same irrevers-

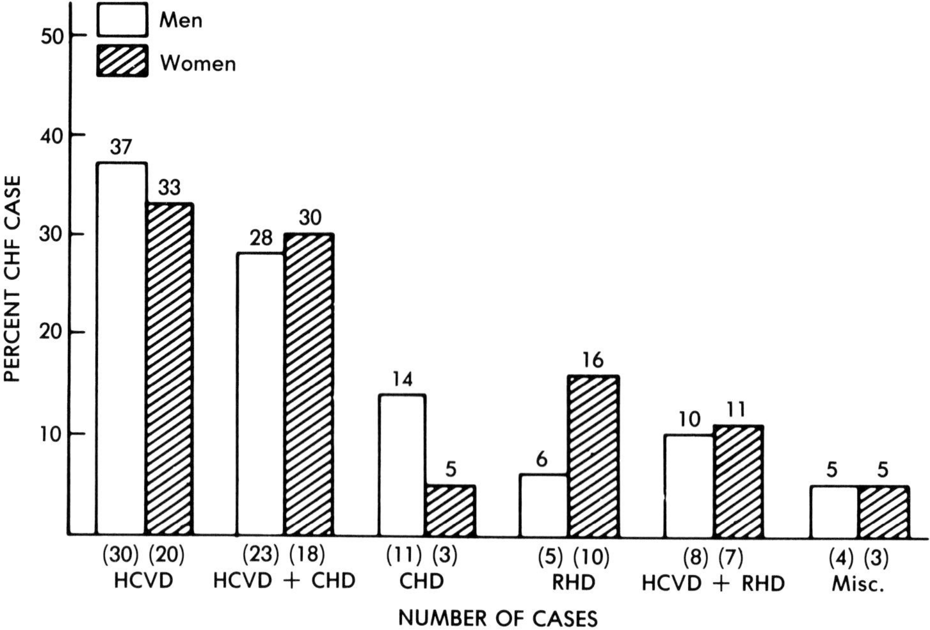

Fig. 37-1 Etiology of congestive heart failure (CHF) (16 year follow-up results) for men and women 30 to 60 years of age at entry into the Framingham study. The number at the top of each bar for a particular type of heart disease is the percentage of men or women with that diagnosis. The numbers in the parentheses are the actual numbers of subjects in the study with the indicated diagnosis. *CHD,* Coronary heart disease; *HCVD,* hypertensive cardiovascular disease; *RHD,* rheumatic heart disease; *Misc,* miscellaneous.[15] (From McKee, P.A., et al.: Reprinted by permission of N. Engl. J. Med. **285:**1441, 1971.)

ible changes seen with primary pressure or volume overload. A loss of 40% or more of the myocardium generally results in death from cardiogenic shock. This latter condition is characterized by the following hemodynamic parameters: (1) a peak systolic blood pressure of less than 90 mm Hg or 30 mm Hg below previous basal levels; (2) a cardiac index of less than 2.0 L/min/m^2; and (3) a pulmonary capillary wedge mean pressure of greater than 20 mm Hg. The common clinical features accompanying these parameters include: (1) urine output of less than 0.5 ml/kg/hour; (2) peripheral vasoconstriction (i.e., cool, clammy skin); and (3) confusion, coma, agitation, or lethargy.

Decreased contractility of the myocardium is seen in states of myocardial ischemia, pressure and volume overload, and in association with various cardiomyopathies. Restricted filling of the heart is encountered during pericardial tamponade and constrictive pericarditis and in conditions producing a stiff, noncompliant ventricle that resists filling (i.e., hypertrophic cardiomyopathies, hypertension, and aortic stenosis).

Common clinical causes of heart failure are coronary artery disease, hypertension, valvular heart disease, cardiomyopathy, congenital heart disease, and pulmonary hypertension. In the United States, coronary artery disease comprises 60% to 70% of patients with Class IV heart failure.[17] Systemic hypertension is becoming a less common cause because of earlier recognition and institution of appropriate pharmacologic therapy. Similarly, valvular and congenital heart disease are becoming less important causes of heart failure because of earlier diagnosis and the availability of surgical procedures to correct or manage these conditions at an earlier stage of disease than existed as recently as a decade ago. Cardiomyopathies are a frequent cause of end stage heart failure. Although some of these disorders are presumed to be postviral in etiology, the majority are idiopathic.

The most common cause of failure of the right ventricle is failure of the left ventricle, even though a number of clinical conditions primarily affect the right ventricle and can lead to cardiac failure. These latter conditions include mitral stenosis, emphysema and other forms of chronic lung disease, pulmonary emboli, and idiopathic pulmonary hypertension.

Although it is beyond the scope of this chapter to comprehensively discuss the sequence of pathophysiologic events leading to heart failure with each disease that is capable of causing it, a more detailed discussion of the mechanisms by which cardiac failure develops in patients with ischemic coronary artery disease is appropriate since this condition is by far the most common cause of the failing heart in the United States. Those factors contributing to failure in patients with coronary artery disease are listed in the boxed material on p. 627, top left. Ischemia is a particularly important factor because ischemic muscle loses its ability to contract and thus regional wall motion and resultant cardiac function may be markedly depressed. In many situations, the restoration of blood flow by coronary bypass or angioplasty may improve regional wall motion in the ischemic region and prevent further progression of contractile dysfunction. Not uncommonly though, chronic ischemia leads to permanent and irreversible regional wall motion abnormalities.[17]

PATHOPHYSIOLOGY OF HEART FAILURE IN CORONARY ARTERY DISEASE

- Ischemia
- Acute myocardial infarction
  - Loss of critical muscle mass
  - Mechanical complications
    - Papillary muscle rupture/dysfunction
    - Rupture of the interventricular septum
    - Rupture of the free ventricular wall/septal junction
    - Ventricular aneurysm

Myocardial infarction and subsequent scar formation lead to a permanent reduction in pumping ability and functional reserve because of the reduction in the number of contractile elements. If the infarction exceeds 40% of the total left ventricular mass, cardiogenic shock and death usually ensue despite aggressive resuscitation efforts.[17] With infarctions of less severe magnitude, resuscitative efforts are much more commonly successful and should be aimed at preservation of the ischemic and vulnerable peri-infarction zone.

Profound heart failure and shock following lesser degrees of myocardial damage may occur because of a mechanical complication of an infarction as summarized in the boxed material above. Papillary muscle dysfunction and/or rupture cause varying degrees of mitral regurgitation and most commonly result from an inferior infarction. In addition to the cardiac dysfunction resulting from the infarcted tissue, mitral regurgitation causes volume overload and further reduces cardiac function. Left ventricular aneurysm formation, which not uncommonly occurs following a large anterior infarction, further contributes to ventricular dysfunction in a number of ways. The aneurysm's paradoxic systolic expansion reduces forward stroke volume by trapping blood in that portion of the ventricle in which the aneurysm is located. Further, as the aneurysm matures and becomes fibrotic, it reduces the compliance characteristics of the ventricle and thereby increases the end diastolic volume and pressure, which then reduce myocardial blood flow and increase the wall stress on the remaining normal muscle.[17] Finally, myocardial infarction infrequently results in ventricular septal rupture, leading to an acquired ventricular septal defect and a left-to-right shunt. The increased volume overload resulting from the shunt may precipitate acute and severe heart failure.

Most of the entities discussed previously lead to a reduction in cardiac output, which is the principal manifestation of the failing heart. However, several entities increase cardiac output and cause high output failure; these include fever, pain, and anemia. Although less common, these causes should be considered in patients whose ventricular reserve is reduced and in whom the usual etiologies of cardiac failure have been excluded.

Precipitating Events in Heart Failure

Many patients with varying forms of compensated heart failure and decreased cardiac reserve have minimal symptoms at rest. Only when they encounter stressful situations do symptoms of overt failure develop. Some of the common events that precipitate cardiac failure in patients with coronary artery disease are shown in the boxed material above. Interruption of preoperative medical therapy is a common cause of overt heart failure. Cardiac glycosides, afterload reducing agents, diuretic therapy, and beta blockers are frequently discontinued before many surgical procedures and are not restarted until the patient can tolerate an oral diet. Fluid overload in the form of blood, blood products, and crystalloid solutions may precipitate overt cardiac failure in patients with reduced cardiac reserve by increasing preload. Similarly, surgical or systemic infection increases demands on the heart and can stress a compromised myocardium as can postoperative anemia in a setting of reduced ventricular reserve. Tachyarrhythmias can markedly worsen a diseased heart by decreasing diastolic filling time and increasing myocardial oxygen consumption. Finally, the development of unrelated illnesses or a second form of heart disease can provoke worsening heart failure. An example of this would be a patient with valvular heart disease who develops coronary artery disease and the resultant ischemia to the myocardium. In short, any factor that changes preload, afterload, heart rate, or contractility (singly or in combination) may cause marginally compensated individuals to lapse into overt failure. Nonmyocardial factors that may contribute to the development of heart failure are shown in the boxed material on p. 628, top left.

EVENTS THAT PRECIPITATE HEART FAILURE

- Interruption of preoperative medical treatment
  - Cardiac glycosides
  - Diuretics
  - Beta blockers
  - Nitrates
  - Afterload reducers
- Anemia
- Fluid, salt, and dietary excesses
- Surgical or systemic infections
- Surgical, physical, environmental and emotional stresses
- Cardiac arrhythmias
- Pulmonary embolism
- Unrelated illnesses

Myocardial Contractility in Heart Failure

In many circumstances, the intrinsic and irreversible reduction in myocardial contractility leads to heart failure, irrespective of the underlying cause. The boxed material on p. 628, bottom left, lists the more important mechanical and biochemical changes in the myocardium that have been noted in animal models of heart failure. Mechanical alterations include a decreased velocity and force of shortening of myocardial contractile elements without a significant change in elastic properties or passive length-tension relationships. During myocardial ischemia, filling pressures become severely elevated, and the fraction of the end-diastolic left ventricular volume that is ejected during systole (i.e., the ejection fraction) falls. The ventricle becomes stiff and cannot relax to fill.[17] The patient may have

NONMYOCARDIAL FACTORS CONTRIBUTING TO HEART FAILURE

Acidosis, hypoxemia
Arrhythmias and conduction disturbances
- Tachyarrhythmias
- Bradyarrhythmias
- Bundle-branch block, heart block
- Atrioventricular dissociation

Cardiovascular depressant drugs
- Antiarrhythmics (disopyramide, lidocaine, quinidine, and procainamide in high doses)
- Barbiturates, anesthetic agents
- Antihypertensive drugs
- Narcotics/tranquilizers in high doses
- Propranolol
- Vasodilators (alpha-blocking agents, nitrates, nitroprusside)

Circulating toxic substances
Fever
Hypovolemia
- Inadequate fluid/salt intake
- Excessive sweating, vomiting, diarrhea
- Blood loss
- Diuretics and sodium restriction
- Excessive postcapillary vasoconstriction (sympathomimetic drugs, reflex sympathetic stimulation)

Pain, vasovagal reactions
Miscellaneous conditions
- Pneumothorax, hemothorax
- Cardiac tamponade
- Pulmonary embolus

From Strobeck, J.E.: Cardiogenic shock, Heart Failure 1:13-35, 1985, by permission of the American Heart Association.

MYOCARDIAL MECHANICAL AND BIOCHEMICAL CHANGES OCCURRING IN HEART FAILURE

Mechanical Alterations of the Myocardium
- Decrease in velocity of shortening
- Decrease in force development
- Decrease in maximum rate of force development

Biochemical Alterations of the Myocardium
- Decrease in actomyosin ATPase activity
- Increase in collagen
- Decrease in myocardial norepinephrine
- Decrease in synthesis of norepinephrine
- Decrease in function of sarcoplasmic reticulum

From Spann, J.F., Jr., et al.: Contractile state of cardiac muscle obtained from cats with experimentally produced ventricular hypertrophy and heart failure, Circ. Res. **21**:341-354, 1967. Reprinted by permission of American Heart Association, Inc.

dyspnea, angina, and pulmonary congestion; and a gallop rhythm may be heard on auscultation of the heart. Despite these clinical presentations, the heart may be normal or nearly normal in size on chest x-ray film.

A number of biochemical alterations have been linked to cardiac failure. To date, no single biochemical derangement has been shown to be consistently associated with a reduction in intrinsic contractility, but changes in actinomysin ATPase activity and isoenzyme shifts have been implicated as playing important roles.[17]

COMPENSATORY MECHANISMS THAT MAY OVERSHOOT

Increase in preload
Increase in systemic vascular resistance
Excessive rise in heart rate
Increase in circulating catecholamines
Activation of renin-angiotensin system

Compensatory Mechanisms in Heart Failure

Numerous compensatory mechanisms occur in heart failure (see the boxed material above). They include: (1) an increased preload caused by the enhanced salt and water retention secondary to activation of the renin-angiotensin-aldosterone system; (2) an increase in heart rate from elevated circulating catecholamines; and (3) an increase in systemic vascular resistance.[17] These mechanisms occur to maintain cardiovascular function in the face of decreased intrinsic cardiac contractility. Despite their compensatory function, they all have the potential for overshooting and producing deleterious effects in cardiac function. A thorough understanding of these overshoot mechanisms and the ability to measure them form much of the current therapeutic approach to managing heart failure.

In heart failure the decreased cardiac output and accompanying renal hypoperfusion cause retention of salt and water by activation of the renin-angiotensin-aldosterone system, which can lead to an excessive preload. Initially, the increase in preload is effective in increasing cardiac output through the Frank-Starling mechanism. As preload increases further, however, it leads to congestive symptoms (e.g., dyspnea) without any further improvement in cardiac performance. These considerations are discussed in greater detail in Chapter 40.

In the normal heart an increase in heart rate can greatly increase cardiac output to considerably high levels. The increased heart rate seen in patients with heart failure occurs because of an increase in circulating catecholamines released from the adrenal medulla. The excessive tachycardia (>100) can have serious deleterious effects because it increases myocardial oxygen demand in the frequent situation in which coronary artery perfusion is severely compromised. Another potentially deleterious effect of increased heart rate is the decrease in diastolic filling time accompanying the tachycardia. Decreased filling time is particularly deleterious to cardiac output in the thick, stiff, noncompliant, hypertrophied heart seen in the clinical setting of systemic hypertension, aortic stenosis, and hypertrophic cardiomyopathy. Thus an excessive heart rate in the clinical setting of heart failure can increase demand at the same time that it decreases supply of oxygen to the myocardium.

Another compensatory mechanism seen in heart failure is an incrase in systemic vascular resistance. In the face of a decreased cardiac output, systemic vascular resistance increases afterload by reflex neurohumeral mechanisms to

Table 37-1 **HEMODYNAMIC MEASUREMENTS**

Parameter	Measurement	Normal Range
Systemic arterial blood pressure (BP)	Direct	120/80 mm Hg (systolic/diastolic) 95 mm Hg (mean)
Pulmonary arterial pressure (PAP)	Direct (through Swan-Ganz catheter)	20/10 mm Hg (systolic/diastolic) 13 mm Hg (mean)
Heart rate (HR)	Direct	80 ± 10 beats/min
Pulmonary capillary wedge pressure (PCWP)	Direct (through Swan-Ganz catheter)	10 ± 2 mm Hg
Central venous pressure (CVP)	Direct	2 ± 2 mm Hg
Cardiac index (CI)	Direct	3.0 ± 0.5 L/min/m^2
Stroke volume index (SVI)	[(CI/HR) × 1000]	40 ± 7 ml/min/m^2
Systemic vascular resistance index (SVRI)	[(BP − CVP)/CI × 80]	1700-2600 dynes × sec × cm^{-5} × m^2
Pulmonary vascular resistance index (PVRI)	[(PAP − PCWP)/CI × 80]	45-225 dynes × sec × cm^{-5} × m^2
Oxygen consumption (Vo_2)	(CI) × (a − vo_2)*	100-170 ml/min/m^2
Oxygen delivery	(CI) × (Cao_2) × 10*	520-720 ml/min/m^2
Oxygen extraction	(Cao_2 − Cvo_2)/Cao_2*	22%-30%

*a − vo_2, Arteriovenous oxygen difference; Cao_2, capillary arterial oxygen; Cvo_2, capillary venous oxygen.

maintain an adequate perfusion pressure to vital organs. The peripheral circulation is normally under the fine control of circulating and neuronally released moieties that can act directly or indirectly to alter vascular tone. These moieties include renin, angiotensin II, and arginine vasopressin. Angiotensin II plays a particularly important role in vascular tone and is known to be a potent vasoconstrictor. It promotes the release of catecholamines from the adrenal glands and also causes release of aldosterone. This latter substance increases preload by causing salt and water retention, the effects of which have already been discussed. Arginine vasopressin is also a vasoconstrictor and increases afterload by increasing systemic vascular resistance.[7] Although these hormones and enzymes may transiently increase cardiac output, they eventually contribute a further burden to the failing myocardium already operating inefficiently under an afterload stress.

HEMODYNAMIC MONITORING

A thorough understanding of the pathophysiology of heart failure and the compensatory mechanisms that can aggravate it is needed if effective therapy is to be prescribed. Such therapy cannot be provided unless data are available indicating the status of cardiac function. Although not a substitute for careful clinical evaluation, continuous bedside invasive hemodynamic monitoring has greatly aided our ability to make cardiovascular assessments and therapeutic decisions. The Swan-Ganz catheter has proved especially valuable in monitoring cardiac function; it allows measurement of stroke volume and cardiac output and the calculation of systemic and pulmonary vascular resistance. Total body oxygen delivery, extraction, and use can also be calculated. Normal ranges for these values are given in Table 37-1.

Cardiac output can be measured quickly and reproducibly with the Swan-Ganz catheter. A thermister at the tip of the catheter records the changes in pulmonary artery blood temperature produced by injection of a bolus of cold 5% dextrose solution. Cardiac output is then calculated from this temperature change using a small digital computer. A cardiac index of less than 2 L/minute/m^2 indicates a seriously depressed cardiac output. Cardiac index is obtained by dividing the patient's measured cardiac output by the total body surface area and is a useful way of "indexing" the cardiac output to the size of the systemic circulation.

The other major parameter measured by the Swan-Ganz catheter is the filling pressure of both the right and left ventricles. The proximal part of the standard triple lumen Swan-Ganz catheter allows measurement of right atrial pressure (i.e., right ventricular filling pressure) whereas the distal part, which is in the pulmonary artery, provides a means of measuring pulmonary capillary wedge pressure when the balloon is inflated. This latter measurement reflects pulmonary venous and left atrial pressures. This pressure measurement is a very useful index of left ventricular filling pressure and reflects intravascular volume and myocardial contractility, as well as left ventricular compliance and the diastolic filling period. Thus knowledge of this pressure provides a basis for planning specific therapy and the adequacy of that therapy. For example, in studies of ventricular function following acute myocardial infarction, maximum cardiac output is generally achieved with a pulmonary capillary wedge pressure between 14 and 18 mm Hg and a pulmonary artery and diastolic pressure of 20 to 24 mm Hg.[22] Raising filling pressures above these levels does not improve cardiac output and significantly increases the risk of pulmonary edema.

THERAPY OF HEART FAILURE

The primary goal in treatment of heart failure of any cause is to rapidly restore adequate tissue perfusion to meet existing metabolic demands. Therapy should be directed at the primary factor or factors causing the failure (see Table 37-2). In the 1970s the standard approach to cardiac failure was the use of inotropic and vasoconstrictor drugs to increase cardiac output and maintain systemic pressure. These approaches to heart failure frequently increased myocardial oxygen demands and exacerbated the ischemic cardiac damage. Understanding these consequences has led to the development of newer pharmacologic agents, the use of circulatory assist devices, and a more aggressive surgical approach to patients in cardiogenic shock.[22] The surgical treatment of the failing heart is described in Chapter 40.

The therapeutic approach to a given patient will require repeated evaluation of his clinical and hemodynamic status. A marked reduction in blood pressure and central pulses may rapidly produce irreversible cerebral and myocardial damage and should be treated aggressively. In this circumstance, the patient should be placed in the supine position with legs elevated to increase venous return. Inotropic vasoconstrictor drugs such as epinephrine, norepinephrine, or dopamine should be administered intravenously while the patient is being clinically evaluated and appropriate monitoring catheters are being inserted. The minimum dose of inotropic or vasopressor agent should be used until an accurate blood pressure can be obtained. A list of inotropic and vasopressor agents and indications for their use is given in Table 37-3.

Electrocardiographic monitoring should be done to detect rate, conduction, and rhythm alterations. If acute hemodynamic deterioration caused by ventricular tachycardia or atrial fibrillation with rapid ventricular response occurs, electrocardioversion should be carried out. Antiarrhythmic drugs can be employed when the hemodynamic status is not seriously compromised or following cardioversion to prevent recurrence of ventricular rate and rhythm dysfunction. Severe bradycardia associated with hypotension and caused by excess vagotonia is treated with atropine. In patients with bradycardia unresponsive to atropine, a transvenous ventricular pacemaker may be needed to restore adequate cardiac output.

Pain and anxiety, which increase myocardial oxygen demands, are treated with morphine—4 to 8 mg every 30 minutes until pain is relieved or until toxic side effects are observed. Morphine is also useful in lowering peripheral and pulmonary vascular resistance and in reducing pulmonary edema. The pharmacologic approach to heart failure depends on the degree of cardiac impairment. It may range from minimal treatment with diuretic therapy in patients with dyspnea on exertion to the use of combinations of inotropic and vasodilator drugs in patients in cardiogenic shock.

Vasodilator Therapy

Many patients with mild heart failure and most surgical patients postoperatively have elevated systemic vascular resistance secondary to release of endogenous catecholamines. Hemodynamic assessment quantitates the degree of excessive afterload. Vasodilator therapy is a useful approach in managing these patients if hypotension is not a problem and preload is elevated. Clinically available vasodilators and their primary peripheral site of action in heart failure are shown in the boxed material below. The dose of vasodilator needs to be titrated carefully in order to avoid hypotension (systolic pressure <90 mm Hg). It should be noted that vasodilators have no inotropic action and exert their effects solely by decreasing preload and afterload. They increase capillary flow and decrease capillary hydrostatic pressure and thereby decrease myocardial oxygen demand. These agents are of particular benefit in

Table 37-2 **THERAPY FOR HEART FAILURE**

Cardiac Factor	Therapy
Increased preload	Salt restriction Diuretics Venodilators
Increased afterload	Arteriolar dilators
Decreased contractility	Digitalis and other inotropic agents
Increased heart rate	Improvement of left ventricular performance (?) Beta blockers

PRIMARY PERIPHERAL SITE OF ACTION OF VASODILATORS IN HEART FAILURE

Venous	Venous and Arterial	Arterial
Nitrates	Nitroprusside	Phentolamine
	Prazosin	Hydralazine
	Trimazosin	Minoxidil
	Captopril*	Dopamine
	Teprotide*	Amrinone
	Calcium blockers	
	Pirbuterol	
	Dobutamine	
	Dopamine analogs	

*Angiotension inhibition per se produces anteriolar dilation, but these agents also increase bradykinin, a potent vasodilator.

Table 37-3 **CLINICAL INDICATIONS FOR INOTROPES IN ADULTS***

Agent	Cardiac Index	Heart Rate	Vascular Tone	Urine Output	Central Venous Pressure	Combination Agent(s)
Isoproterenol (Isuprel)	<2.4 L/min/m^2	<110	Constricted	<30 ml/hr	≥15 mm Hg	Dopamine, epinephrine
Dopamine	Any	Any	Any	<30 ml/hr	12-15 mm Hg	Dobutamine, nitroprusside, isuprel
Dobutamine	<2.4 L/min/m^2	No >130	Constricted	Any	≥15 mm Hg	Dopamine, epinephrine
Norepinephrine	<2.4 L/min/m^2	Any	Dilated	<30 ml/hr	≥15 mm Hg	Regitine
Epinephrine	<2.4 L/min/m^2	No >130	Constricted	Any	≥15 mm Hg	Nitroprusside, dobutamine
Amrinone	<2.4 L/min/m^2	Any	Constricted	Any	≥15 mm Hg	Dopamine

*Clinical variables favorable for use of specific inotropes, i.e., isuprel is best used in patients with cardiac index <2.4, heart rate <110, constricted vascular tone, low urine output (<30 ml/hour), and venous pressure of 15 or above.[4]

patients with heart failure associated with valvular aortic or mitral regurgitation.

The long-term prognosis of patients in heart failure treated with vasodilator therapy has not yet been shown to be favorably altered.[22] However, vasodilators have a major role in the management of acute heart failure after myocardial infarction and following cardiac surgery.

Catecholamine Therapy

If a patient's cardiac index following optimization of preload, afterload, and heart rate is less than 2.5 L/minute/m^2, an inotropic agent should be considered (see Table 37-3).[4] Most of the cardiovascular effects of these drugs are mediated through alpha- and beta-receptors in the heart and blood vessels; also their effects are dose related. Many catecholamines are nonselective in their effects, thus affecting all vascular beds. Some (including dopamine, dobutamine, and amrinone) are selective, however, and more favorably increase blood flow to the heart, brain, and kidney. Catecholamines are known to increase myocardial oxygen demand, but this potentially deleterious effect is offset by the rise in perfusion pressure and the decrease in ventricular chamber size associated with the improved contractility that occurs following treatment with these drugs.

Inotropic agents remain the mainstay of therapy for acute heart failure in the surgical patient. Amrinone, a newer, more selective inotropic agent, is a phosphodiesterase inhibitor and leads to intracellular accumulation of 3′5′ cAMP.[22] Because it augments myocardial contractility and reduces peripheral vascular resistance without causing an increase in heart rate, amrinone is almost the perfect inotrope and has already found usefulness in many clinical situations.

CARDIAC RESUSCITATION

Kouwenhoven is recognized as the modern day father of cardiopulmonary resuscitation. His experiments combining artificial respiration, sternal compression, and electrical defibrillation in laboratory animals, and eventually in humans, established the principles for the technique that has been taught to a large segment of the American population in an effort to prevent the estimated 1000 daily prehospital deaths from cardiac arrest in the United States.[10] Historically, sternal compression and artificial respiration as possible treatment modalities for cardiac arrest were suggested as early as 1786. Toward the end of the nineteenth century, there were occasional reports of successful resuscitative efforts.[9,10,12] For the next 50 years emergency thoracotomy and open cardiac resuscitation were the standard practice for cardiac arrest. In 1947 internal defibrillation was first reported.[1] It was not until the 1960s, however, that the combination of external cardiac massage, artificial respiration, and external defibrillation allowed cardiac resuscitative efforts to move out of the operating room and into the general population.[25] In 1963 the American Heart Association established a committee to study and evaluate cardiopulmonary resuscitation. Ten years later a National Conference on Standards for Cardiopulmonary Resuscitation and Emergency Cardiac Care was cosponsored by the American Heart Association, the National Science Foundation, and the National Research Council. The standards derived from this conference was published in 1974; widespread instruction and implementation of both basic and advanced life support techniques were recommended to ensure delivery of effective cardiopulmonary resuscitation and emergency care to the entire population.[16] Updated standards and guidelines were published in 1980.[21]

The goal of cardiopulmonary resuscitation (CPR) is to support the metabolic requirements of vital organs by providing artificial circulation of oxygenated blood and to restore the ability of the heart to maintain an adequate cardiac output. For didactic purposes, CPR has been divided into both basic and advanced life support techniques (Fig. 37-2). Safar has included a third category of prolonged life support in which cerebral resuscitation and postresuscitative intensive therapy are instituted.[19] According to the American Heart Association, advanced life support to occur when special equipment of any kind or drug therapy is used in the resuscitative efforts.

Because of the swift onset of irreversible brain injury when cessation of normal circulation has exceeded 5 minutes, time is of the essence in the initiation of supportive measures. Lengthy diagnostic maneuvers are postponed until treatment with cardiopulmonary resuscitation is begun. Any patient with unexpected loss of consciousness and/or loss of femoral or carotid pulsations may be assumed to have sustained a cardiac arrest. Additional findings such as loss of heart sounds, pupillary dilation, and loss of spontaneous respirations are supportive signs. Although it would seem intuitively obvious when to begin CPR on an electrocardiographically monitored patient, it should be remembered that a normal-appearing electrocardiogram may persist even during electromechanical dissociation of the arrested heart. In this circumstance, additional circulatory support must be provided immediately. The basic technique during any arrest involves airway control, supportive ventilation, and supportive circulation (Fig. 37-2).

Before artificial ventilatory support can be established, the airway must be established quickly and reliably. The tongue must be moved from the back of the throat to open the airway. The head is tilted backward, thus extending the neck and lifting the chin forward. If suction is available, the pharynx is cleared of secretions, and if possible, an oropharyngeal airway is inserted. Manual removal of obstructing material should be accomplished if no suction is available. Similarly, if placement of an oropharyngeal airway is not possible, the patient's nose is occluded and mouth-to-mouth ventilation is begun. Since the oxygen concentration of expired air is only 17 mm Hg, breathing should be replaced by a tight-fitting mask connected to a nonrebreathing bag delivering 100% oxygen as soon as possible. If available, a cuffed endotracheal tube provides the most reliable airway security, but it requires trained personnel and additional equipment for its placement. Endotracheal intubation should be accomplished only after initial oxygenation attempts have been accomplished. If two rescuers are in attendance, external massage may be established as soon as an unobstructed airway is present. During this maneuver, the patient should be placed on a firm surface. The lower third of the sternum is depressed

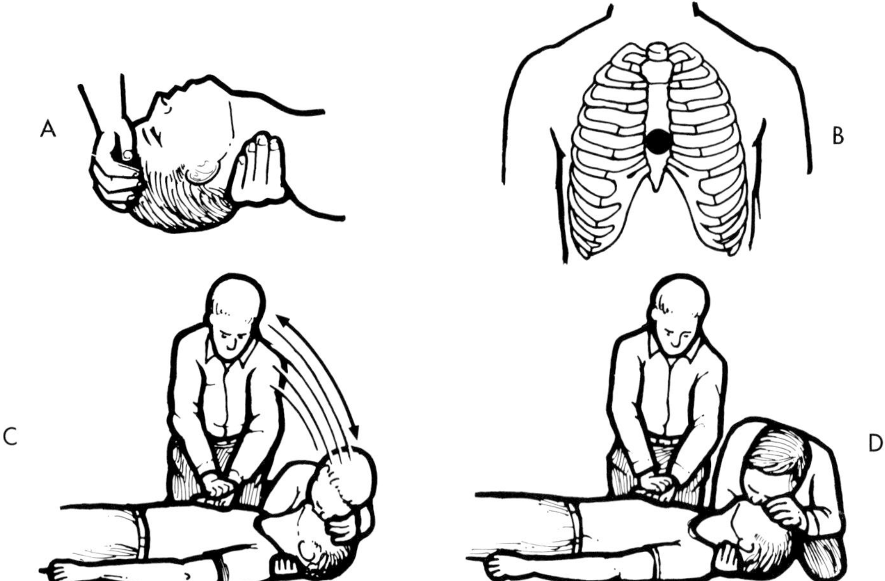

Fig. 37-2 The ABC's of resuscitation. *Airway*—tilt head backward and gently lift neck; clear oropharyngeal secretions **A.** *Breathing*—after 5 quick breaths, check for pulse. If present, continue 12 breaths per minute. *Circulation*—if no pulse is present, begin sternal compression with 4 to 5 cm excursions **(B).** If one rescuer is in attendance, compress 80 times minute with two quick breaths after every 15 compressions **(C).** With two rescuers, interpose one lung inflation after every fifth sternal compression delivered at 60 compressions per minute **(D).**

4 to 5 cm toward the spine at a minimum rate of 60 times/minute. With the two-rescuer technique, one respiration is given after every fifth sternal compression. Using the single-rescuer technique, cardiac compressions are begun after several quick lung inflations, and then after every 15 sternal compressions two inflations are given. Since 60 compressions/minute are needed to artificially maintain circulation, the compressions in the single-operator technique are delivered at a rate of 80/minute to make up for the lack of compressions during lung inflation (see Fig. 37-2).

Should external massage prove inadequate, open chest massage should be considered in the hospitalized patient. Critically low organ blood flow during external compression has led to new interest in open chest cardiac massage since better organ perfusion has been consistently demonstrated with this technique. To employ this procedure, the heart is exposed through an incision in the interspace between the left fourth and fifth ribs anterolaterally. The pericardium is opened anteriorly to the phrenic nerve and the heart is grasped between both palms and forcefully compressed. When performed by experienced personnel, this technique is of proven benefit and should be known by every surgeon.

Once adequate basic life support is being administered, definitive treatment of underlying etiologic factors responsible for the cardiac arrest, as well as return and maintenance of spontaneous cardiac output, is the next priority. A central venous catheter is inserted to ensure delivery of therapeutic agents. Electrocardiographic monitoring is begun. Ventricular fibrillation should be treated with electrical countershock. To do this, external electrodes are positioned on the chest wall over the base and apex of the heart. Two to four hundred joules of direct current are applied. For internal defibrillation when the chest has been opened, smaller hand-held paddles are used and require energy levels of between five and twenty joules. Proper positioning of the paddles and good electrical coupling with the skin are important in external defibrillation. It is also important when beginning defibrillation attempts to correct the pH and electrolyte balance of the patient. In the in-hospital situation, an arterial line not only will allow arterial pressure monitoring, but also will provide ready access to the arterial blood for pH, electrolyte, and blood gas determinations. Unless acidosis can be at least partially corrected, restoration of cardiac activity will be temporary at best. Although empiric administration of bicarbonate may be required, potentially lethal side effects of overzealous administration of sodium bicarbonate include decreased cerebral blood flow, increased plasma osmolality, and increased oxygen-hemoglobin association.[2] It is presently recommended that a single dose of 50 mEq of sodium bicarbonate be given initially; subsequent doses are determined from the calculated base deficit derived from arterial blood sampling, frequently necessary to obtain as often as every 5 to 10 minutes. In the presence of a reasonable pH, normal oxygenation, and a functioning defibrillator, defibrillation should be possible. A weak spontaneous fibrillation may be converted to a more vigorous pattern by administration of 5 to 10 ml of 1:10,000 dilution of epinephrine through a central vein or by intracardiac injection if no other option is available.

Numerous myocardial stimulants are available for the treatment of myocardial depression. Besides epinephrine, calcium chloride, isoproterenol, dopamine, dobutamine, and norepinephrine may all be helpful in efforts to improve cardiac contractility. The presence of myocardial irritability, premature ventricular contractions, and ventricular tachycardia should be aggressively treated. To treat these rhythm disturbances, lidocaine hydrochloride is administered in a bolus of 1 mg/kg followed by a constant infusion of 1 to 4 mg/kg/minute. In patients refractory to lidocaine, procainamide, quinidine, or bretylium may be administered. If documented potassium levels are less than 3.5 mEq/100 ml, administration of potassium chloride may be needed to prevent further problems with myocardial irritability known to be aggravated by hypokalemia. A sudden ventricular arrythmia secondary to myocardial ischemia may result in sudden death. Thus continued rhythm aberrations after resuscitation should prompt electrophysiologic investigation of the arrhythmia by programmed electrical stimulation. Control of the irritable focus (usually a reentrant focus in endocardial scar tissue) can usually be achieved medically but may require surgical ablation. This latter procedure is usually accomplished at the time of a coronary bypass procedure or in conjunction with a ventricular aneurysm resection. Occasionally, complete heart block may occur following cardiopulmonary arrest. This conduction abnormality is commonly encountered in patients with severe coronary artery disease, many of whom have also sustained a myocardial infarction. In this situation, direct pacing of the myocardium is performed by placing a percutaneous transthoracic electrode into the myocardium or preferably through an intravenous balloon-tipped, flow-directed catheter, which can be positioned in most instances without fluoroscopic control. It should be emphasized that pacing may not achieve effective cardiac output if acidosis, hypoxia, or electrolyte imbalance have not been corrected.

Physiology of CPR

Although it is clear that external cardiac massage can successfully resuscitate patients who have sustained cardiac arrest and maintain both cerebral and coronary perfusion, the actual mechanism whereby manual compression of the chest accomplishes this feat remains to be determined. In recent experiments using dogs, dynamic coronary flow decreased to zero or negative values during compression. Antegrade coronary flow occurred primarily during noncompression periods and seemed to be related to the diastolic aortic perfusion pressure.[13,23] Stroke volume and coronary blood flow in this canine preparation were maximized with manual compression when performed with moderate force and brief duration. Increasing the rate of compression increased total cardiac output, without compromising total coronary flow. This study indicated that direct cardiac compression could prove to be a major determinant of the magnitude of stroke volume during manual external cardiac massage.[13,23]

Other investigators have proposed that blood flow occurs not by direct cardiac compression but rather by an intrathoracic pressure mechanism. This alternative hypothesis suggests that increasing intrathoracic pressure during external compression forces blood from the thoracic vessels into the systemic circulation.[18,24] In this hypothesis, the heart acts as a passive conduit and not as a pump. Support for this hypothesis has been provided by Criley and associates,[5] who observed that repetitive coughing in patients sustaining cardiac arrest in the cardiac catheterization laboratory maintained blood flow without external compression. Further work by this group emphasized the passive role of the heart and the closure of venous valves at the thoracic inlet during compression. Two dimensional echocardiography also documented static mitral and aortic valve opening and chamber size during external chest compression.

Regardless of the basic mechanism of CPR techniques, it is beneficial to increase the systemic venous pressure either by leg elevation, volume administration, abdominal binding, or venoconstriction. Proponents of the thoracic pump theory hypothesize that high-pressure ventilation simultaneous with chest wall compression may improve systemic arterial blood flow. Whether this latter contention will be borne out clinically remains to be defined.

Postresuscitative Care

Care of the postresuscitation patient should focus on two basic considerations: (1) recurrence of the cardiac arrest and (2) multiple organ system damage. Survivors of cardiac arrest have a notorious probability of sustaining a second arrest within 48 hours of successful resuscitation from the first arrest. Second, blood flow to multiple organs may be severely compromised during the arrest, resulting in physiologic derangements that may adversely affect the patient during the early postresuscitation period.

Since the majority of patients who have cardiopulmonary arrest have coronary artery disease, it is important to establish the presence or absence of a myocardial infarction following resuscitation. Thus continuous electrocardiogram monitoring should be done, and daily myocardial isoenzyme determinations should be obtained. To accomplish this, the patient should be placed in a specialized cardiac care unit; such a setting will permit both continuous electrocardiogram and arterial pressure monitoring, the latter being an index of the effectiveness of cardiac output. Occasionally, elevations in cardiac enzymes, commonly observed in infarction, may be difficult to interpret following vigorous cardiac massage, since resuscitation itself may alter such enzyme levels. In this situation, Davidson and associates[6] noted that resuscitation and electrical defibrillation did not adversely influence the findings of technetium pyrophosphate scanning in patients with myocardial infarction, making this technique potentially useful in diagnosing infarction when electrocardiogram and enzyme evidence are confusing.

If hypoperfusion is a problem following resuscitation, a flow-directed Swan-Ganz catheter should be placed in the pulmonary artery for determination of filling pressures, cardiac output, and peripheral resistance. Central volumes should be optimized and pulmonary capillary wedge pressure maintained in the range of 14 to 18 mm Hg. Cardiac output determinations may be accomplished by the thermodilution method, and inotropic medication may be administered and afterload reducing measures undertaken to maintain a cardiac index of at least 2.5 L/minute/m^2. Should severe hemodynamic instability continue despite optimal pharmacologic support, consideration should be given to mechanical support of the failing circulation, such as intra-aortic balloon counterpulsation. Frequently used to provide diastolic pressure augmentation and decrease left ventricular afterload, the balloon pump is very effective in the postarrest situation, particularly in patients with severe coronary artery disease.

Mechanical ventilation should be instituted after resuscitation to maintain normal pH and blood gas levels. Supplemental oxygen should initially be administered as a fraction of inspired oxygen of 100%, and the patient weaned as rapidly as possible to 50% to prevent potential oxygen toxicity problems. Mechanical ventilation should continue until it is obvious that the patient can generate spontaneously a tidal volume and forced vital capacity that would maintain adequate blood gases when weaned from the respirator. General supportive measures such as nasogastric suction and urinary catheter drainage should also be accomplished. Chest x-ray examinations should be followed serially to prevent the insidious development of pneumonia or other pulmonary problems. Appropriate laboratory studies, including hematocrit, electrolytes, and serum albumin, should be determined every 2 or 3 days to aid in the optimization of adequate fluid balance. Finally, hypothermia, with its inherent increase in peripheral vascular resistance, should be avoided.

Postresuscitation encephalopathy is frequently a problem following survival after a cardiac arrest and should assume a prominent role in treatment. Efforts should be employed in all comatose patients to prevent extremes in blood pressure. Mechanical control of the ventilation, as well as neuromuscular blocking agents, generally facilitate control of arterial pressure.[19] Moderately controlled hyperventilation is recommended to counteract any cerebral acidosis and to decrease the intracerebral pressure. Corticosteroid administration and intravascular volume depletion by diuretic therapy are adjuncts to hyperventilation in controlling intracerebral pressure. Barbiturate loading and prolonged immobilization, with controlled ventilation have also been found useful in decreasing postischemic brain damage. Should profound neurologic symptoms persist, serial neurologic examinations need to be performed and the magnitude of central nervous system dysfunction documented with electroencephalography.[19]

Renal function should be closely monitored in the postresuscitation period. Proper management of the body's fluid compartments needs to be a high priority. Specifically, the brain and lung should be closely monitored to prevent cerebral or pulmonary edema. Should either of these problems become evident, fluids need to be restricted and diuretics administered. If renal failure becomes obvious in the immediate resuscitation period, volume limitation and exclusion of potassium from all intravenous solutions need to be assured. If hyperkalemia is still a problem, sodium polystyrene sulfonate (Kayexalate) instillation into the gut to bind potassium may prove helpful. If these conservative methods do not result in control of the potassium level, peritoneal dialysis should be instituted by placing a Tenckoff catheter into the abdominal cavity. The majority of adult patients will tolerate 1 to 2 L of peritoneal dialysis fluid without significant hemodynamic changes. However, prolonged dialysis in these hemodynamically unstable patients is generally associated with significant mortality.[14]

It is estimated that approximately 40% of prehospital resuscitation patients may survive. In-hospital resuscitative efforts vary in their survivorship, depending on the patient's prearrest condition. Induced fibrillation in the cardiac catheterization laboratory is almost uniformly successfully treated. In contrast, ventricular fibrillation in the elderly, septic surgical patient undergoing shock is obviously low.

SUMMARY

Heart failure is the physiologic state in which the heart is unable to meet the demands of the systemic circulation and metabolizing tissues. The etiologic factors responsible for such failure are numerous and range from chronic pressure or volume overload as a result of valvular heart disease or systemic hypertension to direct loss of myocardial contractile elements and their replacement with noncontractile scar caused by ischemic heart disease. These many disease processes usually result in irreversible changes in the myocardium, adversely affecting both systolic and diastolic function. Compensatory physiologic mechanisms attempting to maintain an adequate circulatory state result in many of the symptoms of heart failure on a chronic basis. Control of the "overshoot" of these neurohumoral compensatory mechanisms remains the mainstay of therapy of heart failure. More intensive manipulation of contractility and the preload and afterload status of the heart are useful in more decompensated individuals and in patients who have depressed function after surgical stress. Invasive monitoring with the Swan-Ganz catheter is required to follow filling pressures and cardiac output and to calculate the systemic vascular resistance.

Millions of lay persons have been trained in the basic life support techniques of cardiopulmonary resuscitation (CPR). The efficacy of closed chest compression with mouth-to-mouth ventilation in salvaging patients with cardiac arrest until professional help can be obtained have moved resuscitative efforts from the hospital to the world of the common man. Once trained personnel become available, advanced techniques using defibrillation, endotracheal intubation, and appropriate pharmacologic therapy are used as needed. Postresuscitative therapy centers on prevention of another arrest, correction of arrest-related metabolic aberrations, and protection of the cerebral circulation. New CPR methods are evolving that may save even more lives and provide still better support in the postresuscitative state.

REFERENCES

1. Beck, C.S., and Pritchard, L.H.: Ventricular fibrillation abolished by electric shock, JAMA **135**:985, 1947.
2. Bishop, W., and Weisfeld, M.L.: Sodium bicarbonate administration during cardiac arrest, JAMA **235**:506, 1976.
3. Braunwald, E.: Preface. In Braunwald, E., editor: Congestive heart failure: current research and clinical applications, New York, 1982, Grune & Stratton.
4. Copeland, J.D.: Perioperative uses of inotropic drugs. In Utley, J.R., editor: Perioperative cardiac dysfunction, vol. 3, Baltimore, 1985, Williams & Wilkins.

5. Criley, J.M., et al.: Cough induced cardiac compression: self administered form of cardiopulmonary resuscitation, JAMA **36:**1246, 1976.
6. Davidson R., et al.: Technetium-99m stannous pyrophosphate myocardial scintigraphy after cardiopulmonary resuscitation and cardioversion, Circulation **60:**252, 1979.
7. Francis, G.S.: Neurohumoral mechanisms in congestive heart failure, Am. J. Cardiol. **55:**15A, 1985.
8. Gibson, T.C., White, K.L., and Klainer, L.M.: The prevalence of congestive heart failure in two rural communities, J. Chronic Dis. **19:**141, 1966.
9. Jude, J.R., Kouwenhoven, W.B., and Knickerbocker, G.G.: Cardiac arrest: report of application of external cardiac massage in 118 patients, JAMA **178:**1063, 1961.
10. Jude, J.R., Balooki, H., and Nagel, E.L.: Cardiac resuscitation in the operating room, Ann. Surg. **171:**948, 1970.
11. Kannel, W.B., et al.: Role of blood pressure in the development of congestive heart failure, N. Engl. J. Med. **287:**781, 1972.
12. Keen, W.W.: Case of total laryngectomy and a case of abdominal hysterectomy in both of which massage of the heart for chloroform collapse was employed, with notes of 25 other cases of cardiac massage, Therapy CAZ, **28:**217, 1904.
13. Maier, G.W., et al.: The physiology of external cardiac massage: high impulse cardiopulmonary resuscitation, Circulation **70**(1):8, 1984.
14. Mattor, J.A., et al.: Cardiac arrest in the critically ill. II. Hyperosmolar states following cardiac arrest, Am. J. Med. **56:**162, 1974.
15. McKee, P.A., et al.: The natural history of congestive heart failure: the Framingham study, N. Engl. J. Med. **285:**1441, 1971.
16. Oldham, H.N.: Cardiopulmonary arrest and resuscitation. In Sabiston, D.C., and Spencer, F.C., editors: Gibbon's surgery of the chest, Philadelphia, 1983, W.B. Saunders Co.
17. Parmley, W.W.: Pathophysiology of congestive heart failure, Am. J. Cardiol. **55:**9A, 1985.
18. Rudikoff, M.T., et al.: Mechanism of blood flow during cardiopulmonary resuscitation, Circulation **61:**345, 1980.
19. Safar, P.: Cardiopulmonary cerebral resuscitation, Stovavger, Norway, 1981, Asmund S. Laerdo.
20. Spann, J.F., Jr., et al.: Contractile state of cardiac muscle obtained from cats with experimentally produced ventricular hypertrophy and heart failure, Circ. Res. **21:**341, 1967.
21. Standards and guidelines for cardiopulmonary resuscitation and emergency cardiac care, JAMA **244:**453, 1980.
22. Strobeck, J.E.: Cardiogenic shock, Heart Failure **1:**13, 1985.
23. Voohees, W.D., Babbs, C.F., and Tucker, W.A.: Regional blood flow during cardiopulmonary resuscitation in dogs, Crit. Care Med. **8:**134, 1980.
24. Weisfeldt, M.L., Chandra, N., and Tsitlik, J.: Increased intra-thoracic pressure—not direct heart compression—causes the rise in intrathoracic vascular pressure during CPR in dogs and pigs, Crit. Care Med. **9:**377, 1981.
25. Zoll, P.M., et al.: The effects of external currents on the heart. Control of cardiac rhythm and induction and termination of cardiac arrhythmias, Circulation **14:**145, 1956.

38 Assisted Circulation

O. Howard Frazier and Rolando Colon

Low cardiac output is an altered physiologic state that results from many diseases of the myocardium and may necessitate mechanical circulatory assistance. Whatever its origin, low cardiac output is usually accompanied by varying degrees of dysfunction of the kidneys, brain, or lungs or by failure of these vital organs. Such failure manifests clinically as oliguria or anuria; as paresis, paralysis, or sensorium changes caused by decreased cerebral blood flow; or as hypoventilation, ventilation-perfusion imbalances, or alveolar-capillary blocks in pulmonary gas exchange. Other failure states (i.e., hepatic or hematologic shortcomings) may coexist and may affect any of the 5000 enzyme systems and metabolic pathways of the liver, the quantity and quality of circulating hemoglobin, and coagulation factor integrity. These failure states may also cause generalized mitochondrial dysplasia and disrupt the critical processes of oxidative phosphorylation and cytochrome function in all organ systems.[24]

A wide variety of etiologic factors may be involved in producing a low cardiac output state, but all share an adverse effect on myocardial function resulting in depressed cardiac performance and inadequate oxygen delivery to tissues. The triggering mechanisms may differ, however, and include blood loss resulting from a vascular injury, third-space sequestration from pancreatitis, or endotoxemia from an intraabdominal abscess. These mechanisms may lead to such diverse consequences as myocardial depression caused by hypoxia, acidosis, or calcium shifts; inadequate filling pressures; arrhythmias; changes in afterload; inadequacies in preload; systemic and pulmonary vasoconstriction or vasodilation; and variations in capillary permeability.

As these variables have become appreciated and their effects on cardiac function more fully understood, support of the failing circulation has left the realm of fantasy and become a realistic option for many critically ill patients. As investigative work continues in all areas of mechanical assistance and clinical experience increases, many patients who previously would have died of their low cardiac output state can now be supported until their myocardial function recovers sufficiently to sustain a meaningful life or until they can undergo cardiac transplantation.

HISTORIC PERSPECTIVE

The heart is one of the simplest organs in the body, but it is absolutely essential to survival since it functions as a pump to transport substances to and from the tissues. Despite the early attempts of LeGallois[43] in 1812 to replace the heart, surgeons for many years considered this organ untouchable. The development of a clinical system of extracorporeal circulation in the early 1950s provided the basis for surgical procedures on the open heart.[25] Extracorporeal oxygenation and support of the circulation became established with the introduction of safer, more reliable oxygenators. In 1956 Kolff[37] designed a coil-type membrane oxygenator for clinical use, and in 1962 Cooley, Beall, and Grondin[13] designed an economic, disposable bubble oxygenator.

With these developments and with the rising importance of heart disease as a cause of death in the United States, scientists became interested in creating an artificial heart that would provide a functional substitute for the natural heart. In 1958 Kusserow[40] described an intra-abdominal pump for partial replacement of the right heart. Later he and Clapp[41] developed a pump that was attached to the back of a dog to assist the left heart. As early as 1958, Akutsu and Kolff[1] reported total replacement of the natural heart in a dog. This animal was supported 5½ hours by an air-driven reciprocating pump. In commenting on the artificial heart, Kolff defined it as "a mechanical prosthetic heart which completely substitutes for the natural heart, anatomically and physiologically."

Because of this early successful work, researchers believed that mechanical support of the heart was a very straightforward problem and that clinical use of the total artificial heart would soon be implemented. Despite this initial success, the full limitations of biomaterials, geometric design, and driving and power systems were not adequately appreciated. Improvements in the various types of pumps led to increased survival of the experimental animals receiving them.[2,55] In 1969 the feasibility of short-term support with a pneumatically driven artificial heart in human beings was demonstrated by Cooley and associates,[14] who supported a patient for 64 hours with an artificial heart fabricated from Dacron reticular fabric. The patient's own heart had not allowed weaning from cardiopulmonary bypass.

While attempts were in progress to develop a total artificial heart, various heart assist devices were also being tested. These systems were less complex than the total artificial heart, and the surgery necessary to implant them was generally less invasive. In 1971 Bernhard and associates[7] reported that either right or left ventricular bypass was possible in calves for periods of 85 to 170 days, respectively; they also reported on 16 calves that survived from 7 to 42 days with a simultaneous biventricular bypass. In the same year, Akutsu's group (Takagi and associates)[77] reported 2-month survival in a calf with a series-type left-sided heart assist device. Little was done clinically at this time, however, because these devices required a pneumatic power source, and materials failure, hemolysis, and thrombosis remained serious problems. Al-

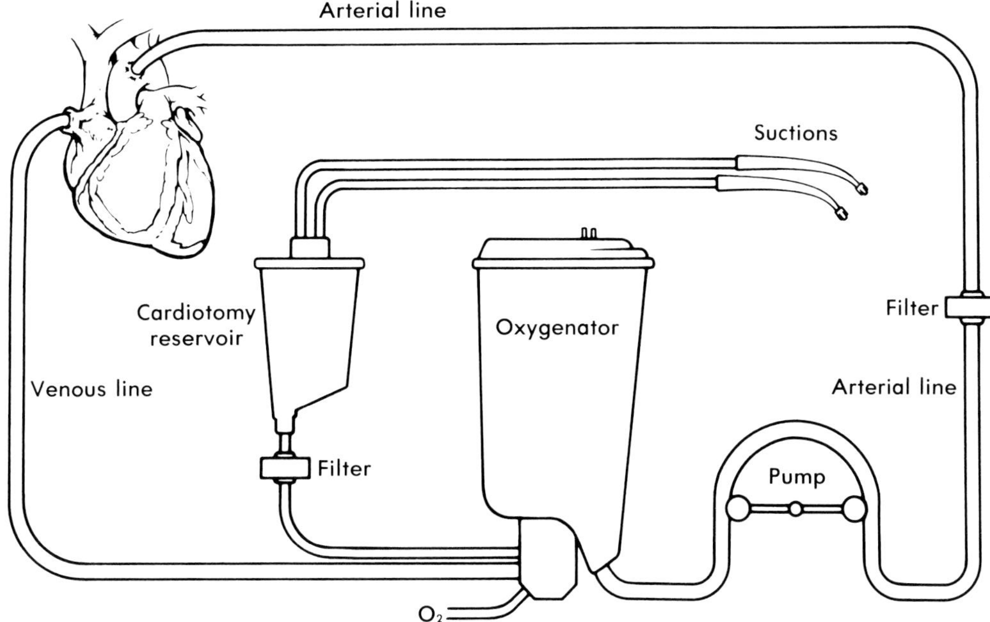

Fig. 38-1 Cardiopulmonary bypass (CPB) circuit.

though DeBakey[18] reported two successful cases in which bypass-type left-sided heart assist devices were used clinically for 4 to 10 days, and although Kantrowitz, Krakauer, and Sherman[35] demonstrated the clinical use of a series-type left-sided heart assist device to support the failing circulation after cardiac surgery, clinical application by other investigators was almost nonexistent.

As the 1970s unfolded, however, clinical use of assist devices increased. This was especially true of the intra-aortic balloon pump (IABP), which has remained an important modality in the treatment of low cardiac output to the present. Developed in 1961 by Kolff's group (Moulopoulos and associates),[49] this assist device is based on the principle of counterpulsation. Kantrowitz and co-workers[36] first demonstrated its potential clinical use in 1967. Clinical application of the IABP, as well as other approaches to the failing circulation, has been championed by other investigators, including Norman in Houston (1975),[50] Bernhard and associates in Boston (1976),[8] Navratil (Thoma and associates) in Vienna (1977),[79] Senning with Turina and Bosio in Zurich (1977),[80] and Pierce and colleagues in Hershey (1977).[62] By the end of the 1970s, the ability to assist the failing circulation had become an established clinical reality; at present such assistance is an important modality throughout the world in supporting patients who otherwise would die of a low cardiac output state.

CARDIOPULMONARY BYPASS

The prototype of assisted circulation is the extracorporeal heart-lung machine, or cardiopulmonary bypass (CPB) circuit. Its development more than 30 years ago has made possible modern cardiac surgery and has paved the way for the development of other assist devices to support the circulation when a diseased heart is no longer capable of maintaining an adequate cardiac output. Thus a discussion of assisted circulation would not be complete without a brief consideration of CPB and understanding of how it works physiologically.

Because open heart surgery requires a quiet, blood-free operative field, the function of the patient's heart and lungs must be curtailed during surgery and assumed by a CPB circuit. The physiologic goal of CPB is to maintain adequate blood flow and mean arterial pressure and thus allow optimum end-organ perfusion during elective cardiac arrest. Blood flow of 40 to 60 ml/kg of body weight/minute can provide a cardiac index of approximately 2.5 L/minute/m^2, which is normal for an anesthetized adult.

All CPB circuits have a venous reservoir, a gas-exchange device (oxygenator), a blood pump, a heart exchanger, blood filters, and a bubble trap (Fig. 38-1). Venous blood is drained into the oxygenator by means of passive flow, which depends on the central venous pressure and on the oxygenator's position being lower than the operating table. Once the blood has traversed the oxygenator, it passes through the blood pump and is returned to the patient's body. An arterial heat exchanger, which controls the temperature of the blood, is usually located between the blood pump and the aortic cannula or may be incorporated in the oxygenator. Before returning to the body, the blood passes through a bubble trap, which ensures that no air is accidentally injected into the patient.

Suction devices are necessary to remove excess blood from the operative field and to decompress the heart. Usually, two suction pumps are used, each connected to an individual pump head. Suctioned blood goes to a cardiotomy reservoir, where it is filtered to remove platelet-leukocyte aggregates and fibrin before the blood enters the oxygenator. A blood filter is also frequently present between the arterial pump and the patient.

Oxygenator

By providing contact between a broad film of blood and a suitable gas mixture, the oxygenator serves as an artificial lung, which oxygenates the venous blood and removes carbon dioxide. The two main types of oxygenators are bubble and membrane. *Bubble oxygenators* create a large blood-gas surface, injecting oxygen directly into the blood. Direct injection of oxygen into the blood creates a foaming action, consisting of gas bubbles forced to the surface by the hydrostatic pressure exerted by the blood. An antifoaming agent is used to remove these bubbles before the blood is returned to the patient. *Membrane oxygenators* interpose a gas-permeable membrane between the oxygenating gas and the blood. Gas transfer depends on the permeability of the particular membrane to the individual gases and the pressure gradient of these gases across the membrane.

Much controversy exists over which type of oxygenator is better. Advocates of membrane oxygenators claim these devices minimize trauma to platelets and erythrocytes.[9,27,71,82,88] Controlled experiments in laboratory animals, however, suggest that blood trauma is a function of pump time rather than of the type of oxygenator used.[76] Others suggest that a better hemodynamic response occurs with use of membrane oxygenators.[44] Although one oxygenator probably has no significant advantage over the other for most cardiac procedures, for open heart surgery when the pump time is expected to be prolonged, the membrane oxygenator apparently is the more appropriate choice.

Blood Pump

The pump component of the CPB circuit provides for blood flow through the unit and maintains artificial systemic circulation and end-organ perfusion during cardiac arrest. Blood pumps provide either kinetic or positive displacement. *Kinetic pumps* propel the blood through a rotating impeller, which creates a centrifugal force that drives the blood out of the pump into the system. *Positive-displacement pumps* are further subdivided into those in which blood inside a tube is displaced by the compressive action of a rotating member *(rotary pumps)* and those in which the blood is propelled from a cavity by the reciprocating action of a piston or diaphragm *(reciprocating pumps)*.

Most current CPB pumps are rotary models of the roller type. In these devices a roller advances over a blood-containing collapsible tube, propelling the blood column ahead of the roller and out of the pump. No direct contact occurs between the blood and the roller itself, and no valves are necessary. These features probably account for the blood components undergoing minimum trauma. In contrast to the body's own physiologic system, roller pumps provide nonpulsatile perfusion. Although the merits of pulsatile and nonpulsatile flow have been debated,[28,86,87] most cardiac procedures employ nonpulsatile flow with acceptable results.

Surgical Considerations

Cannulation Techniques

Venous return is diverted into the CPB circuit through cannulas in the vena cava, right atrium, or femoral vein, depending on the type of cardiac procedure. Double-caval cannulas provide the best decompression of the venous system but fail to remove blood that enters the right atrium from the coronary sinus and the thebesian veins.[4] Systemic venous return can also be diverted to the circuit by a single large-caliber cannula, which is introduced into the right atrium and the inferior vena cava through the right atrial appendage. The choice of cannula depends on the type of surgical procedure.

Femoral vein cannulation for femoro-femoral bypass is indicated when the patient has had previous open heart procedures resulting in extensive adhesions. Surgery on the ascending aorta and aortic arch also requires cannulation of the femoral vessels.

Arterial cannulation for delivery of oxygenated blood is done through a major artery, usually the ascending aorta itself. The femoral artery may be cannulated if the patient has had previous open heart surgery, as already mentioned, or in procedures that involve the ascending aorta and the aortic arch.

Prevention of Cardiac Distention

Decompression of the heart, particularly of the left ventricle, is accomplished by placing a pump in the left atrium through the right superior pulmonary vein or the apex of the left ventricle. Excess blood in the pericardium or in the operative field is removed with additional suction devices and is returned to the circuit, thus minimizing blood loss. These additional suction devices are responsible for most of the blood trauma previously attributed to the oxygenator.[72]

Prevention of Air Embolism

To prevent systemic or coronary air embolization, intracardiac air must be removed before CPB is terminated. Air can be present in the pulmonary veins, left atrium, or left ventricle. During the restoration of left ventricular function, air is aspirated from the ascending aorta by a suction needle connected to a roller pump. The patient is placed in Trendelenburg's position, and a 19-gauge needle is inserted repeatedly into the left ventricular cavity, removing air that may be trapped within the multiple recesses of the endocardial surface. Manual inflation of the lungs by the anesthesiologist forces blood from the pulmonary veins into the left atrium and helps evacuate air from the pulmonary vasculature.

Systemic Responses

CPB results in several hemodynamic changes that directly affect patient management. An initial decrease in blood pressure is attributed to hemodilution,[63] hypothermia, or relative hypovolemia. This period of initial hypotension is followed by an increase in systemic vascular resistance, which is believed to be caused by the release of endogenous catecholamines and the activation of the renin-angiotensin system.[16,63] This increased vascular resistance may render the patient hypertensive, and intraoperative vasodilator therapy may be necessary to reduce the left ventricular afterload before CPB is discontinued. Reported hypotension after rapid reinfusion of bronchial venous drainage is attributed to the release of vasodilator prostaglandins, which are produced by the lungs during isolation from the circulation.[42] Cerebral blood flow, based on flow velocity through the middle cerebral artery, is increased during CPB; this increase is attributed to hemodilution rather than to cerebral autoregulatory mechanisms.[45]

Fluid shifts during and after CPB have been adequately described but are still not well understood. An increase in extracellular water is accompanied by a decrease in the red blood cell mass, which persists during the early postoperative period, mainly in patients who received crystalloid priming solution.[12] A decrease in sodium excretion is accompanied by a marked increase in potassium excretion, which accounts for the extensive potassium replacement required by these patients.[12,57] The glomerular filtration rate is enhanced, probably because of the increase in extracellular volume that occurs during the first 2 postoperative days.

During CPB the lungs are neither ventilated nor perfused. Pulmonary changes include a loss of surfactant, swelling of pneumocytes, alveolar septal edema, and areas of hemorrhage and leukocyte sequestration.[67,75]

Alterations in host-defense mechanisms and in the complement system during CPB are a major concern in the prevention of postoperative infections. A reduction in the opsonic capacity of the host-defense system is attributed to reduced levels of the third component of complement (C3) and the hemolytic activity of complement. This reduction is believed to result from hemodilution and complement consumption.[83] Other studies have shown a decrease in the proliferative responses of lymphocytes.[84] Hypothermia has been found to inhibit mobilization of leukocytes from the bone marrow; this is thought to be the source of the neutrophilia seen during CPB.[64]

Overall, CPB can maintain the body in a nearly normal hemodynamic state and acid/base balance, permitting cardiac surgeons to perform complex procedures in a motionless, bloodless field.

INTRAAORTIC BALLOON PUMP

The intraaortic balloon pump (IAPB) is widely used for the circulatory support of patients with postoperative left ventricular failure, cardiogenic shock after acute myocar-

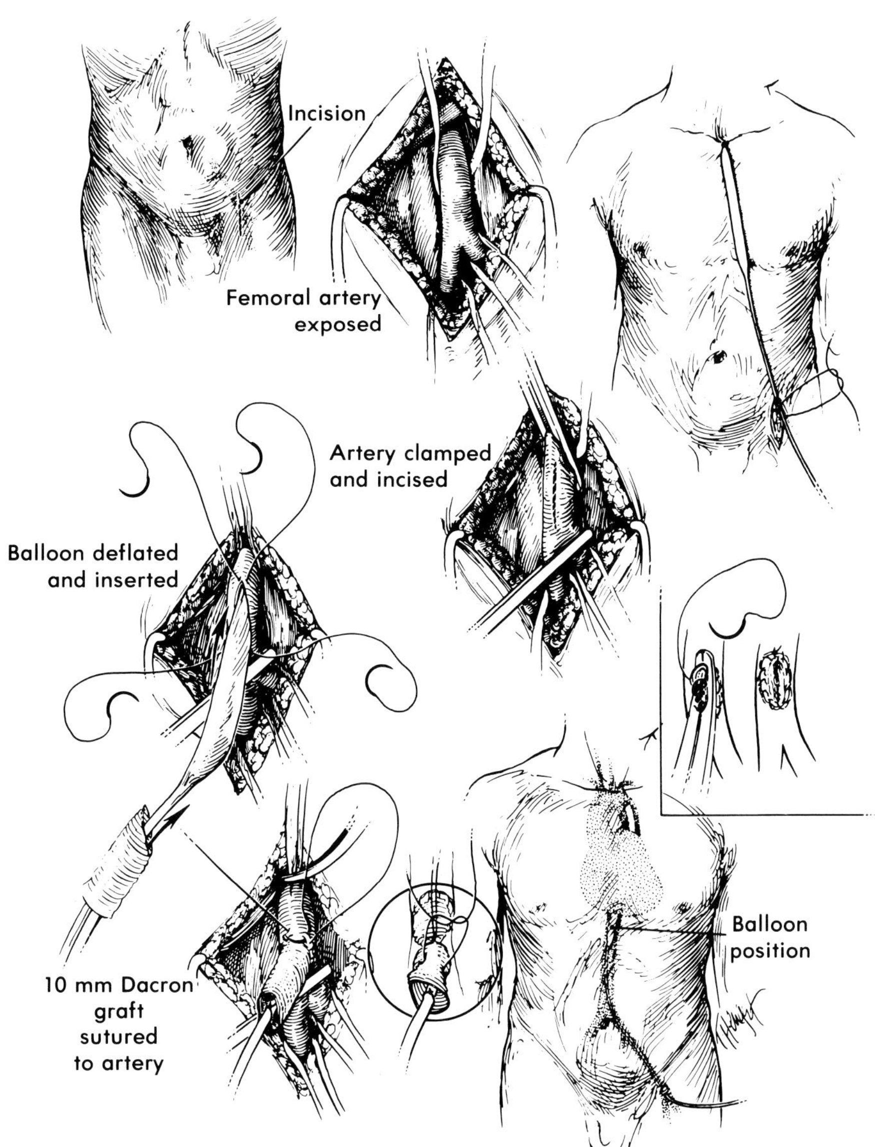

Fig. 38-2 Intraaortic balloon pump (IABP) placement, using the technique of transfemoral insertion.

dial infarction, unstable angina refractory to medical treatment, or recurrent myocardial ischemia after acute myocardial infarction.[11,20,38,69]

The IABP is an intravascular volume-displacement device that augments the patient's existing circulation. Balloon inflation and deflation is precisely synchronized with the cardiac cycle. Inflation is initiated during diastole after the aortic valve closes, and deflation is synchronized with systole. The balloon and cable are constructed of antithrombogenic, biocompatible materials and are inserted via the right or left common femoral artery through a short segment of prosthetic vascular graft, which is anastomosed to the artery to allow temporary vascular access (Fig. 38-2).[21] The cable is attached to a portable pneumatic-drive console, and the balloon is positioned in the descending thoracic aorta, distal to the origin of the left subclavian artery and above the origins of the renal arteries.

Transthoracic Approach

In some patients neither femoral artery is suitable for balloon insertion because of extensive atherosclerotic aortoiliac disease, tortuosity, or small vessels. When these circumstances exist, the transthoracic approach is used.[26,81] To obviate the need for general anesthesia and repeat sternotomy for balloon removal after using the transthoracic route, some investigators have advocated sewing a woven graft to the aorta and introducing the balloon through this graft, much the same as in the transfemoral approach. Removal is then accomplished under local anesthesia by simply exposing the graft, withdrawing the balloon, and ligating the graft.[39,47,65,78] This approach, however, increases the risk of graft infection, thromboembolism, and graft-aorta disruption.[56]

With the transthoracic approach a purse-string suture is placed on the right lateral aspect of the ascending aorta to facilitate balloon insertion. A stab incision is made in the center of the area encompassed by the purse-string suture, and the device is advanced to the appropriate position in the descending thoracic aorta (Fig. 38-3). The balloon is attached to the pump console, vented, and filled with helium. Pumping is initiated by the same method used for transfemoral insertion. Hemostasis is achieved at the aortotomy site by tightening the purse-string suture about the catheter. The catheter is secured with the ends of the suture and is brought out through the inferior aspect of the incision. In postoperative patients who require transthoracic insertion, the sternum is left open and only the skin is closed; the sternum is later closed in a delayed fashion.[22] This technique reduces compression of an acutely dilated heart and decreases the amount of surgical manipulation required at the time of balloon removal. After being weaned from the balloon, the patient is returned to the operating room, the sternotomy is reopened, and the mediastinum is explored. The thrombus is removed, and surgical hemostasis is carefully obtained.

Percutaneous Femoral Approach

Under selected circumstances, the balloon may be inserted percutaneously through the femoral artery.[10] This technique has been useful in the recovery room when it is necessary to use the balloon rapidly. Generally the percutaneous approach is not practical in the operating room because it is technically quick and easy to expose the femoral artery surgically and insert the balloon directly. In addition, the low cardiac output encountered in the operating room frequently obscures the femoral artery pulse, which must be exactly located if the percutaneous route is used.

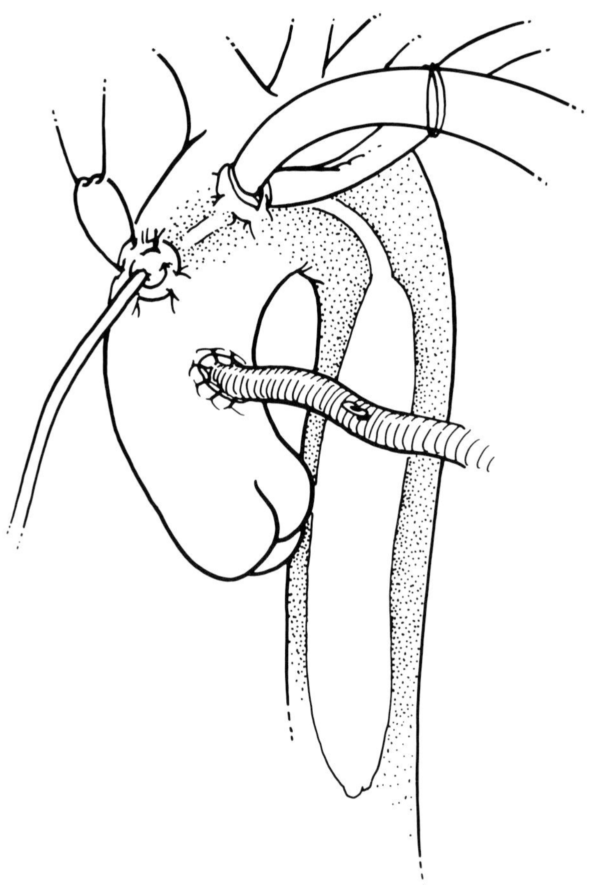

Fig. 38-3 Technique of transthoracic insertion of IABP. In this diagram the heart has been intentionally deleted to better demonstrate the IABP insertion site in the ascending aorta of a patient undergoing aortocoronary bypass grafting.

Hemodynamic Effects

Once the balloon has been inserted, its actuation results in a reduction of left ventricular outflow impedance during systole, phase-shifting of the peak arterial pressure contour into diastole, and augmentation of the stroke volume and cardiac output (500 to 800 ml/minute).[31] Balloon pumping also causes marked increases in coronary perfusion pressures during diastole; reductions in left ventricular volumes and filling pressures; and decreases in left ventricular chamber radii, wall tensions, and oxygen consumption.[70,74,85] Myocardial oxygen supply/demand ratios are increased.[30,61] Right-sided heart performance is improved by balloon-induced decreases in left-sided heart filling pressures.[29]

From a physiologic standpoint, IABP actuation results in alternating hemodynamic effects that cannot be replicated with pharmacologic agents. The first effect, diastolic augmentation, is the result of rapid displacement of aortic blood volume at end systole. This volume displacement,

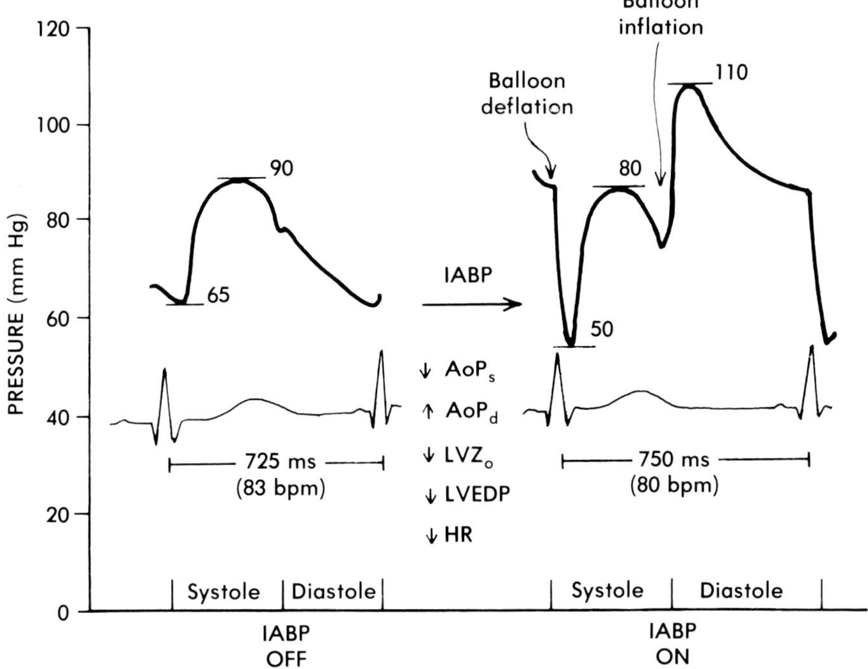

Fig. 38-4 Arterial blood pressure tracing and ECG with and without IABP support. Balloon actuation decreases the heart rate *(HR)* and systolic aortic pressure *(AoP_s)* while it increases diastolic aortic pressure *(AoP_d)*. *LVZ_o*, Left ventricular impedance; *LVEDP*, left ventricular end-diastolic pressure; *ms*, milliseconds; *bpm*, beats per minute; *pressure*, arterial blood pressure in mm Hg.

which results from inflation of the balloon in the descending thoracic aorta, increases diastolic perfusion pressures to the coronary arteries and peripheral circulation. Myocardial and tissue perfusion is enhanced without increases in myocardial work or ejection impedance because balloon inflation is timed to begin after closure of the aortic valve.

The second effect, a reduction in left ventricular ejection impedance or "unloading," is caused by rapid deflation of the balloon at end diastole. The resultant reduction in the aortic blood volume produces a marked decrease in intra-aortic pressure, and as systole begins, aortic pressure and impedance are lowered. The reduction in left ventricular ejection impedance increases the ejection fraction and reduces developed wall tension; stroke volume and cardiac output both increase (Fig. 38-4).

IABP actuation also:

1. Decreases the heart rate and systolic aortic pressure (afterload) and thus myocardial oxygen consumption
2. Increases the diastolic aortic pressure (increasing the diastolic gradient for coronary and systemic perfusion), stroke volume index, and cardiac index
3. Decreases the mean pulmonary capillary wedge pressure, which can be equated with the left atrial and left ventricular end-diastolic pressures (preload)
4. Decreases the total pulmonary vascular resistance

The decrease in pulmonary vascular resistance affects the right side of the heart by decreasing the systolic pulmonary artery pressure (afterload) and the mean right atrial pressure, which can be equated with the right ventricular end-diastolic pressure (preload). The indices for left and right ventricular systolic work per minute are essentially unchanged. These effects decrease the myocardial oxygen demand, increase all the indices of myocardial oxygen supply, and enhance cardiac performance.

The foregoing benefits are more pronounced when IABP actuation is initiated in the presence of a reduced coronary blood flow. In such cases counterpulsation may actually increase myocardial oxygen consumption, presumably by improving the oxygen supply to previously underperfused areas of myocardium. This is particularly important in attempting to limit a myocardial infarction. Other possible benefits include reflex reductions in systemic vascular resistance, which may contribute to the decrease in left ventricular afterload, and the opening of potential coronary collateral channels.

Indications for Use

Precardiotomy, intracardiotomy, and postcardiotomy low output states and postinfarction cardiogenic shock unresponsive to intensive medical management are the main indications for IABP counterpulsation. In a substantial proportion of patients with these problems, the hemodynamic abnormalities can be reversed, depending on the severity of the deficits. Balloon counterpulsation also helps stabilize the condition of many critically ill patients so that emergency coronary arteriography and left ventricular angiography can be performed with reasonable safety. Determination of the need for emergency revascularization, infarctectomy, mitral valve replacement, or repair of ruptured interventricular septa during continued IABP support is extremely helpful. The striking reversal of preinfarction anginal pain and ST-segment abnormalities with balloon counterpulsation provides clinical and electrocardiographic (ECG) confirmation of the IABP's instanta-

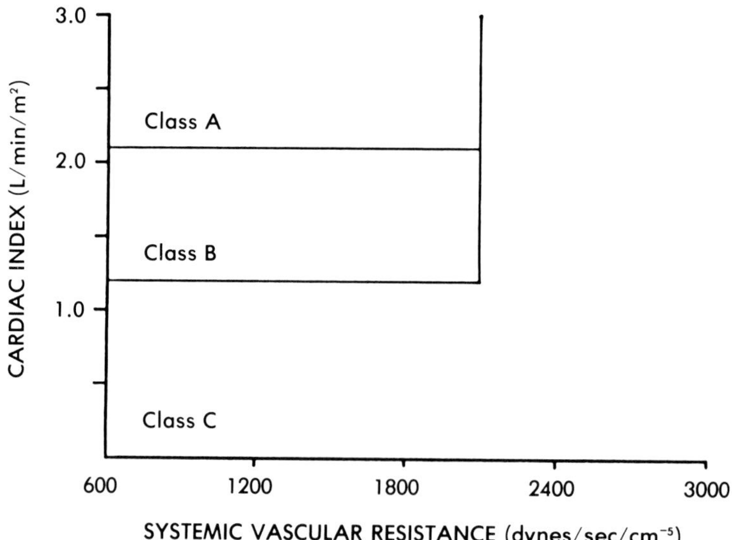

Fig. 38-5 The Texas Heart Institute's scheme for classifying IABP patients. Cardiac index (CI) is plotted against systemic vascular resistance (SVR). Class A: CI ($L/min/m^2$) >2.1 and SVR ($dynes/sec/cm^{-5}$) <2100; Class B: CI = 2.1 to 1.2 and SVR <2100; Class C: CI <1.2 and SVR >2100.

neous effects. Its urgent and emergency use as a means of stabilizing patients with refractory, life-threatening ventricular dysrhythmias and as an adjunct in resuscitating patients from cardiac arrest is well recognized.

Postoperative Care and Complications

To assess the immediate postoperative progress of patients who have undergone IABP counterpulsation, a system of scoring based on plotting systemic vascular resistance against the cardiac index has been developed (Fig. 38-5).[53] This is a simple yet accurate method of evaluating a patient's cardiovascular status. Patients who remain in Class A during the first 8 hours postoperatively invariably survive from a cardiac standpoint. On the other hand, patients who remain in Class C for the first 8 hours invariably expire. Pharmacologic manipulation can be used to reduce systemic vascular resistance when appropriate and to elevate the cardiac output with inotropic agents or digitalis as the situation requires.

Few complications of IABP have been reported.[33] Lower limb ischemia can occur, however, and aortic dissection has been noted.[27] To correct ischemia, the balloon should be removed as quickly as possible, and a Fogarty catheter thrombectomy and angioplasty should be performed. If the balloon cannot be removed, a femoro-femoral crossover graft may be used to supply the involved artery distal to the site of balloon insertion.

Texas Heart Institute Series

From 1972 to 1984, 1169 patients whom we treated underwent IABP support at the Texas Heart Institute in Houston. Ninety percent (1052) of these were surgical (postcardiotomy) patients, whereas the remaining 10% (117) suffered from postinfarction cardiogenic shock. The average duration of IABP support was 59.5 hours for survivors, in contrast to 16.9 hours for nonsurvivors. The average duration of support was 44 hours for surgical patients and 65 hours for medical patients. The methods of insertion are summarized in Table 38-1. Fifty-eight percent of the postcardiotomy patients were weaned from IABP support, whereas only 44% of the patients with postinfarction cardiogenic shock were weaned (Table 38-2). In our center, the average age was 57 years old, with the youngest patient a 6-year-old male and the oldest an 81-year-old female.

In our experience, the IABP has been a safe and reliable method of mechanical cardiac support. Insertion is generally easy and rapid, and the device effectively increases the oxygen supply and decreases the oxygen demand of the myocardium while concomitantly improving the cardiac output. When this technique has been used to support the failing heart, the survival rate has consistently remained between 55% and 60%.[3,48]

LEFT VENTRICULAR ASSIST DEVICE

The left ventricular assist device (LVAD) is a more effective form of cardiac assist than the IABP. In contrast to intravascular in-series volume-displacement devices, which augment the existing circulation, LVADs are extravascular, volume-capturing devices designed to augment or replace the existing circulation and provide advanced forms of mechanical circulatory support. These blood pumps are constructed of biocompatible materials and may be interposed between the left ventricular apex and the thoracic or abdominal aorta or between the left atrium and the aorta. Inlet and outlet valves impart unidirectional flow, and the devices are actuated with external pneumatic-drive consoles.[52]

The timing of LVAD filling and ejection, or prosthetic diastole and systole, can be precisely synchronized with the cardiac cycle in this advanced method. The central and peripheral aortic pressure is modified or phase-shifted in synchrony with the heart. In this respect, LVADs are sim-

Table 38-1 **METHOD OF INTRAAORTIC BALLOON PUMP (IABP) INSERTION (TEXAS HEART INSTITUTE, 1972-1984)**

		Femoral Approach		
	Transthoracic Approach	Surgical	Percutaneous	Total
Male	125	693	90	908
Weaned	67	426	51	544
Unweaned	58	267	39	364
Female	56	186	19	261
Weaned	20	91	10	121
Unweaned	36	95	9	140
Total				
Weaned	87	517	61	665
Unweaned	94	362	48	504
TOTAL PATIENTS	181	879	109	1169

Table 38-2 **MEDICAL VS. SURGICAL IABP INSERTIONS (TEXAS HEART INSTITUTE, 1972-1984)**

	Medical	Surgical	Total
Male	94	814	908
Weaned	42	502	544
Unweaned	52	312	364
Female	23	238	261
Weaned	10	111	121
Unweaned	13	127	140
Total			
Weaned	52	613	665
Unweaned	65	439	504
TOTAL PATIENTS	117	1052	1169

ilar to IABPs but are more profound and invasive. Unlike IABPs, which optimally depend on an intact ECG signal, LVADs can be actuated asynchronously, independent of an intact ECG signal. Thus LVADs combine (1) the concept of synchronous and asynchronous diversion of the cardiac output by partial or total capture of the stroke volume from the left ventricle or the left atrium and (2) the concept of synchronous counterpulsation/diastolic augmentation.

Hemodynamic Effects

Actuation of the LVAD results in:

1. A profound reduction in left ventricular outflow impedance during systole (or diastole) to such an extent that the aortic valve does not open and the device captures all available cardiac output
2. Complete phase-shifting of the peak arterial pressure contour into diastole (counterpulsation/diastolic augmentation)
3. Augmentation of the stroke volume and cardiac output (through the pump) up to 6 L/minute in human beings.[5,6,51,54,58]

In addition, the LVAD produces proportionate major increases in coronary perfusion pressures during diastole; marked reductions in left ventricular volumes and filling pressures; and profound decreases in the left ventricular radius, wall tension, and oxygen consumption. As with the IABP, but to a far greater extent, myocardial oxygen supply is increased, but demand is reduced, and right-sided heart performance is proportionately improved by LVAD-induced decreases in left-sided heart filling pressures.[17,59]

Clinical Effectiveness

A clear understanding of the LVAD's clinical effectiveness is best gained by viewing the biologic left ventricle and the prosthetic left ventricle as two pumps that are connected in series when synchronously actuated and in series-parallel when asynchronously actuated. Each pump has its own pressure-volume relationship, stroke volume, output, and stroke work. The net effect of LVAD actuation can be predicted as the result of an integrated biologic-prosthetic in-series or series-parallel pump system.

This system's approach can be further demonstrated if left-sided heart failure is viewed as a reduction in contractility accompanied by decreased forward flow. This failure to generate pressure and displace volume can extend over a wide spectrum of states, ranging from compensated to decompensated. Biologic left ventricular performance can be assessed on the basis of the ejection fraction (the ratio of stroke volume to end-diastolic volume). Within limits, the stroke volume can be enhanced by augmenting the filling volume (Frank-Starling response) or by augmenting myocardial contractility with catecholamines or digitalis.[59] Reductions in ejection impedance produce elevated ejection fractions and stroke volumes, whereas increases in ejection impedance have the opposite effect.[68]

Biologic left ventricular function is greatly influenced by either synchronous or asynchronous LVAD actuation, and complete capture of the cardiac output can be achieved without opening the biologic aortic valve. During periods of ventricular fibrillation or standstill, the systemic, pulmonary, and coronary circulations are completely supported by the LVAD.

Myocardial oxygen consumption is principally determined by four hemodynamic variables: (1) peak developed wall tension, which is governed by systolic pressure and cardiac size; (2) contractile state; (3) heart rate; and (4) external stroke work.[73] When the low impedance of the LVAD during biologic systole is substituted for left ventricular outflow (aortic) impedance, peak systolic left ven-

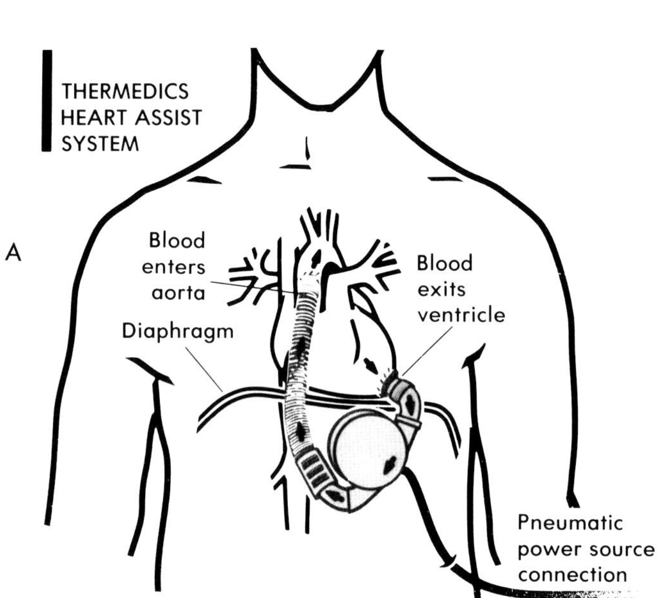

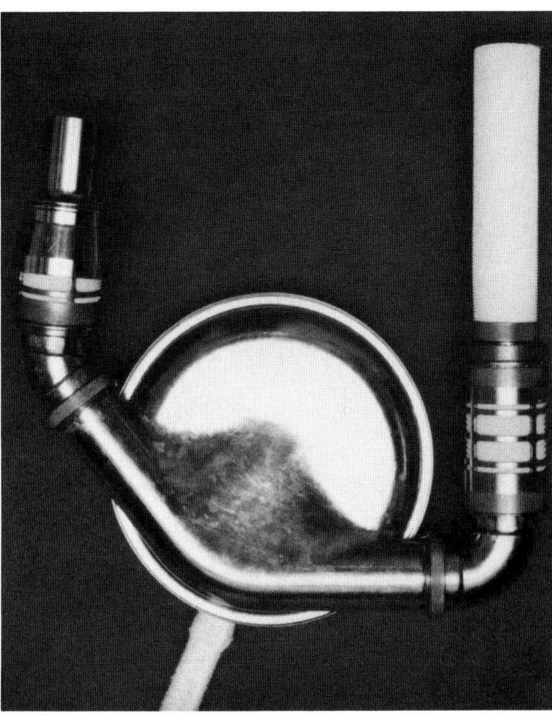

Fig. 38-6 **A,** Schematic diagram of the left ventricular assist system. **B,** Left ventricular assist device (LVAD) manufactured by Thermedics, Inc., Woburn, Mass.

tricular pressure is greatly reduced, and myocardial oxygen consumption is correspondingly decreased. Left ventricular chamber size, external work, and heart rate are also reduced. Moreover, during biologic diastole, LVAD ejection produces an increase in both systemic and coronary blood flow.[74]

The LVAD's effectiveness primarily results from its ability to reduce left ventricular ejection impedance during biologic systole and eject blood during biologic diastole. In reducing impedance, LVAD actuation can be compared with vasodilator (nitroprusside) therapy and IABP actuation, both of which cause lesser reductions in left ventricular impedance. Vasodilator therapy, intraaortic balloon pumping, and LVAD actuation are all escalating methods of achieving moderate-to-profound reductions in afterload.

The LVAD that we use at the Texas Heart Institute consists of a pulsatile pusher-plate pump that fills by means of a conduit from the left ventricular apex and ejects blood through a 22 mm woven Dacron graft into the ascending aorta. Rotatable joints are attached to the inlet and outlet portions to accommodate anatomic variations and to contain 25 mm porcine xenograft valves. All metallic components except the pusher plate are fabricated from a titanium alloy, and the blood-contacting surfaces are textured to promote deposition of a pseudoneointima. The maximum stroke volume is 90 ml (Fig. 38-6).

Indications for Use and Complications

The decision to use the LVAD is primarily based on the inability to wean a patient from CPB after optimum pharmacologic support and IABP use. One of the complications of LVAD implantation is hemorrhage, which is related to the coagulopathy induced by prolonged extracorporeal bypass. Another problem is that implantation of the device is a major surgical procedure, requiring as much as an additional hour of CPB time.

According to our experience, recovery of ventricular function is virtually ensured in patients who survive 48 hours of LVAD support. Thus most instances of cardiac failure could probably be corrected with an LVAD. When studied for potential cardiac transplantation, adults with terminal cardiomyopathies have generally shown reversible pulmonary vascular changes. Most patients exhibit right ventricular hypertrophy, which is probably related to pumping against the elevated resistance resulting from chronic left ventricular failure. Accordingly, simple unloading of the left ventricle should be adequate for chronic support. In addition to greatly simplifying internal powering of the device, this would allow the patient to remain untethered and to undergo rehabilitation. Further, simplicity of implantation of a left-sided heart assist device is important for long-term survival. Several investigators[46,60,66] have obtained improved results by using left-atrial-to-aortic blood flow. This is simpler and less invasive than the LVAD technique and may ultimately prove to be the procedure of choice in supporting the left side of the heart.

TOTAL ARTIFICIAL HEART

Although the ultimate cardiac assist device is the totally implantable artificial heart (TAH), the problems associated with its development have been considerable. The design of a TAH requires not only a knowledge of cardiac anatomy and physiology and techniques of implantation but also a thorough understanding of mechanical engineering, particularly fluid dynamics. The TAH must be able to maintain circulation during normal daily activity yet be

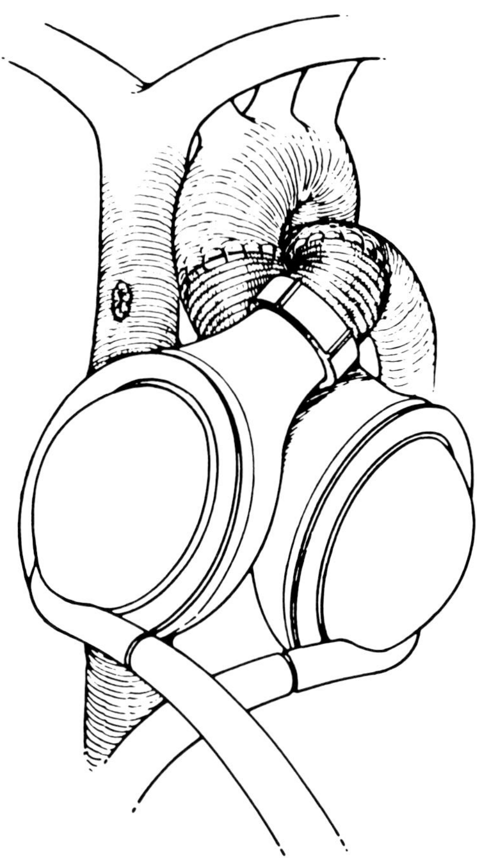

Fig. 38-7 Human total artificial heart (TAH). Left ventricle is attached to the snap-on connection on the left atrium and is then attached to the aorta. Right ventricle is attached to the right atrial and pulmonary artery cuffs.

flexible enough to augment cardiac output during periods of increased activity.

The TAH consists of a power source, an engine, an actuator, and a pump, which includes the bladder, valves, and vascular connections (Fig. 38-7). Hemodynamic control of the entire system is necessary. Artificial hearts currently under development consist of an energy source and two pumps designed to replace the right and left ventricles of the diseased heart. The biologic atria are retained and are attached to the inlet port of each prosthetic ventricle. The outflow tracts of the prosthetic ventricles are sutured to the pulmonary artery and the aorta. The TAH is anatomically more restricted than the LVAD because of the proximity of the inflow and outflow orifices, which must be aligned with the atria and the great arteries. Energy from the power source collapses the bladders within the pumping chambers, ejecting blood into the outlet conduit and the thoracic aorta.

Artificial hearts are currently powered by external pneumatic units, whose power lines are passed percutaneously to the TAH. The Food and Drug Administration has granted approval to power the pneumatic heart for 3-hour periods with an over-the-shoulder battery pack.[19] To make such a device practical, a TAH with an implantable energy converter is being designed.

Probably more than 50,000 patients per year could be candidates for artificial circulatory support devices. This large number precludes the use of external pneumatic power. The TAH must allow patients in a predominantly productive age group (40 to 60 years) to return, as much as possible, to their previous activities.

Indications for Use

Although the TAH is now available for long-term implantation, we prefer to use it as a temporary means of maintaining the circulation until a suitable donor is found for subsequent cardiac transplantation. In three patients in whom we have implanted TAHs, the devices have functioned satisfactorily from a mechanical standpoint. In each case the objective was to use the device as a preliminary measure until conventional cardiac transplantation could be performed. In the first patient, the TAH supported the circulation for 64 hours before cardiac transplantation.[14] The second patient was supported for 54 hours,[15] and the third patient was supported by the TAH for 30 days before undergoing transplantation. At that time the third patient had a normal renal function and was a better candidate for transplantation than at the moment of TAH implantation.

This experience reveals the feasibility of staged cardiac replacement and encourages further development of cardiac prostheses. The TAH's use as a bridge to transplantation appears to be limited more by transplantation immunology than by problems related to temporary mechanical support of the circulation. Prolonged use of the TAH in its current form may jeopardize a patient's ability to undergo successful transplantation because of an increased risk of infection.

At this time, transplantation is a more appropriate method of cardiac substitution, particularly since the introduction of the immunosuppressive agent cyclosporine.[34] A decrease in the incidence of infection and rejection during the postoperative period has been noted, particularly when Prednisone has been combined with cyclosporine, allowing earlier hospital discharge and a decrease in the overall costs associated with transplantation.

VENTRICULAR ASSIST SYSTEM

Long-term implantable ventricular assist systems (VASs) are potentially useful in patients with end-stage cardiac disease in whom the underlying pathophysiologic processes are established and irreversible. As shown in Fig. 38-8, the VAS consists of five major subsystems: (1) an implantable pusher-plate blood pump, (2) an electric-mechanical energy converter, (3) an implantable control unit with batteries, (4) a volume compensation unit, and (5) an external monitoring unit with batteries and a battery charger. For such a blood pump to be clinically useful, it must provide flow rates of 10 L/minute or greater, maintain pumping rates up to 120 beats/minute, generate the mean arterial pressures of 120 mm Hg or greater, and maintain mean filling pressures of 15 mm Hg or less.

Researchers at the Texas Heart Institute in Houston have designed a pump that meets these criteria.[23,31] The pump's major components (see Fig. 38-8) are a rigid outer housing with inlet and outlet ports, a pusher-plate-actuated pumping diaphragm, and valved inlet and outlet conduits. The cylindric pump chamber measures 10.8 cm in diameter and 4.2 cm in height, weighs 270 g, and has a volume dis-

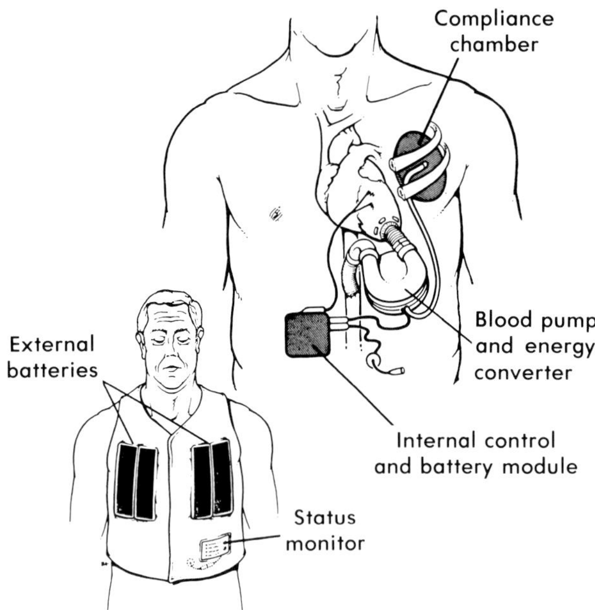

Fig. 38-8 The Texas Heart Institute (THI)/Gould ventricular assist system (VAS), which is being developed for ultimate clinical use in human beings.

placement of 186 ml. The maximum stroke volume is 90 ml, with a pusher-plate excursion of 1.52 cm. The pump diaphragm is 0.08 cm thick and is fabricated from Biomer, a linear-segmented polyurethane.

In experimental animals this VAS has been responsive to varying physiologic demands because of its simple, reliable, autoregulated control modes, which are ECG synchronous and computer controlled. The system is physiologically and anatomically biocompatible with the body and blood and is nonthrombogenic and nonhemolytic, necessitating only minimum anticoagulation. It can provide up to 10 hours of external power with inexpensive, rechargeable batteries and more than 30 minutes of tether-free operation at pump outputs of 7 L/minute with internal, rechargeable batteries. Clinical use of such systems in treating refractory postcardiotomy low cardiac output and in providing a bridge to cardiac transplantation is imminent.

SUMMARY

The prototype of assisted circulation is the extracorporeal heart-lung machine, or cardiopulmonary bypass (CPB) circuit. Its development more than 3 decades ago has made possible modern cardiac surgery and has paved the way for developing other assist devices for the failing circulation when the diseased heart is no longer capable of maintaining an adequate cardiac output. Among methods of assisted circulation currently employed clinically, the most successful short-term ventricular assist device is the intra-aortic balloon pump (IABP), which is generally used initially in cases of cardiac failure. The IABP instantaneously benefits the circulatory system by decreasing the systolic arterial pressure (afterload), left ventricular end-diastolic pressure (preload), mean left atrial and pulmonary capillary wedge pressures, and heart rate while increasing the diastolic perfusion pressure and cardiac output without increasing the mean arterial pressure.

Left ventricular assist devices (LVADs) are more hemodynamically effective than IABPs during profound left ventricular failure because they can capture the total cardiac output, augment and increase systemic coronary perfusion, and function in the absence of an intact ECG signal, as well as during ventricular fibrillation or standstill. If support can be maintained, ventricular recovery can occur even in the severely depressed myocardium.

Electrically actuated devices that offer increasingly longer durability and reliability could be useful in several clinical areas. Possible candidates would include patients with advanced ischemic or idiopathic cardiomyopathies refractory to surgical or medical management, as well as patients who are refractory to or dependent on pharmacologic, IABP, or short-term LVAD support. Long-term assistance also appears feasible as a primary method of treating intraoperative or postinfarction myocardial failure and as a bridge to cardiac transplantation. Whereas the total artificial heart can maintain the entire circulation satisfactorily, its major benefit resides in its ability to support the failing circulation until a cardiac transplant can be performed.

Mechanical cardiac assist devices have proved effective in both augmenting and capturing cardiac output in patients who require short-term cardiac assistance. The need remains for a reliable long-term support system. Experimental studies are promising, however, and should eventually produce a device that can benefit patients who need partial or total long-term support.

REFERENCES

1. Akutsu, T., and Kolff, W.J.: Permanent substitutes for valves and hearts, Trans. Am. Soc. Artif. Intern. Organs **4**:230, 1958.
2. Akutsu, T., et al.: A sac type of artificial heart inside the chest of dogs, J. Thorac. Cardiovasc. Surg. **47**:512, 1964.
3. Bedderman, C., et al.: Intraaortic balloon pumping in women: effects of balloon size on survival, Thorac. Cardiovasc. Surg. **28**:428, 1980.
4. Bennet, E.V., et al.: Comparison of flow differences among venous cannulas, Ann. Thorac. Surg. **36**(1):59, 1983.
5. Berger, R.L., et al.: Successful use of a left ventricular assist device in cardiogenic shock from massive postoperative myocardial infarction, J. Thorac. Cardiovasc. Surg. **78**:626, 1979.
6. Berger, R.L., et al.: Successful use of a paracorporeal left ventricular assist device in man, JAMA **243**(1):46, 1980.
7. Bernhard, W.F., et al.: Biventricular bypass: physiologic studies during induced ventricular failure and fibrillation, J. Thorac. Cardiovasc. Surg. **62**:859, 1971.
8. Bernhard, W.F., et al.: A left ventricular aortic blood pump for circulatory support in postoperative patients with acute left ventricular failure. In Unger, F., editor: Assisted circulation, Berlin, 1979, Springer-Verlag.
9. Boers, M., et al.: Two membrane oxygenators and a bubbler: a clinical comparison, Ann. Thorac. Surg. **35**(4):455, 1983.
10. Bregman, D., et al.: Percutaneous intraaortic balloon insertion, Am. J. Cardiol. **46**:261, 1980.
11. Buckley, M.J., et al.: Hemodynamic evaluation of IABP in man, Circulation **41**(suppl. II):11, 1970.
12. Cohn, L.H., Angell, W.W., and Shumway, N.E.: Body fluid shifts after cardiopulmonary bypass. I. Effects of congestive heart and hemodilution, J. Thorac. Cardiovasc. Surg. **62**(3):423, 1971.
13. Cooley, D.A., Beall, A.C., Jr., and Grondin, P.: Open heart surgery using disposable oxygenators. Scientific exhibit, American College

of Surgeons, 48th Annual Clinic Congress, Atlantic City, N.J., 1962.
14. Cooley, D.A., et al.: First human implantation of cardiac prosthesis for staged total replacement of the heart, Trans. Am. Soc. Artif. Intern. Organs **15:**252, 1969.
15. Cooley, D.A., et al.: Total artificial heart in two-staged cardiac transplantation, Cardiovasc. Dis. Bull. Tex. Heart Inst. **8**(3):305, 1981.
16. Cooper, T.J., et al.: Factors relating to the development of hypertension after cardiopulmonary bypass, Br. Heart J. **54**(1):91, 1985.
17. Daly, B.D.T., et al.: Right ventricular effects of left ventricular unloading with an abdominal left ventricular assist device in the calf, Physiologist **17**(3):205, 1974.
18. DeBakey, M.E.: Left ventricular bypass pump for cardiac assistance: clinical experience, Am. J. Cardiol. **27:**3, 1971.
19. DeVries, W.C., et al.: Clinical use of the total artificial heart, N. Engl. J. Med. **310**(5):273, 1984.
20. Dunkman, W.B., et al.: Clinical and hemodynamic results of IABP and surgery for cardiogenic shock, Circulation **46:**465, 1972.
21. Frazier, O.H.: Cardiopulmonary assistance. In Cooley, D.A., editor: Techniques in cardiac surgery. ed. 2, Philadelphia, 1984, W.B. Saunders Co.
22. Frazier, O.H., et al.: Morbidity in balloon counterpulsation: transfemoral versus transthoracic insertion, Trans. Am. Soc. Artif. Intern. Organs **30:**108, 1984.
23. Fuqua, J.M., et al.: Development and evaluation of electrically-actuated abdominal left ventricular assist systems for long-term use, J. Thorac. Cardiovasc. Surg. **81:**718, 1981.
24. Gibbon, J.H., Jr.: Artificial maintenance of circulation during experimental occlusion of the pulmonary artery, Arch. Surg. **34:**1105, 1937.
25. Gibbon, J.H., Jr.: Application of a mechanical heart and lung apparatus to cardiac surgery, Minn. Med. **37:**171, 1954.
26. Gueldner, T.L., and Lawrence, G.H.: Intraaortic balloon assist through cannulation of the ascending aorta. Ann. Thorac. Surg. **19**(1):88, 1975.
27. Hessel, E.A., et al: Membrane vs. bubble oxygenator for cardiac operations: a prospective randomized study, J. Thorac. Cardiovasc. Surg. **80**(1):111, 1980.
28. Hickey, P.R., Buckley, M.J., and Philbin, D.M.: Pulsatile and nonpulsatile cardiopulmonary bypass: review of a counterproductive controversy, Ann. Thorac. Surg. **36**(6):720, 1983.
29. Holub, D.A., et al.: Changes in right ventricular function associated with intraaortic balloon pumping (IABP) in the cardiogenic shock patient, Clin. Res. **25:**553A, 1977.
30. Igo, S.R., et al.: Determinants of induced subendocardial ischemia as reflected by DPTI/TTI ratios, in occluded and nonoccluded zones of bovine left ventricle, Physiologist **17:**253, 1974.
31. Igo, S.R., et al.: Intraaortic balloon pumping: theory and practice—experience with 325 patients, Artif. Organs **2**(3):249, 1978.
32. Igo, S.R., et al.: Theoretic design considerations and physiologic performance criteria for an improved intracorporeal (abdominal) electrically-actuated long-term left ventricular assist device (E-type ALVAD) or partial artificial heart, Cardiovasc. Dis. Bull. Tex. Heart Inst. **5:**172, 1978.
33. Isner, J.M., et al.: Complications of the intraaortic balloon counterpulsation device: clinical and morphologic observations in 45 necropsy patients, Am. J. Cardiol. **45:**260, 1980.
34. Kahan, B.D.: Cyclosporin A: a new advance in transplantation, Tex. Heart Inst. J. **9**(3):253, 1982.
35. Kantrowitz, A., Krakauer, J., and Sherman, J.L.: A permanent mechanical auxiliary ventricle, J. Cardiovasc. Surg. **9:**1, 1968.
36. Kantrowitz, A., et al.: Initial clinical experience with intraaortic balloon pumping in cardiogenic shock, JAMA **203**(2):135, 1968.
37. Kolff, W.J.: Disposable membrane oxygenator (heart-lung machine) and its use in experimental surgery, Cleve. Clin. Q. **23:**69, 1956.
38. Kramer, J.S., et al.: Clinical management ancillary to phase-shift balloon pumping in cardiogenic shock: preliminary comments, Am. J. Cardiol. **27:**123, 1979.
39. Krause, A.H., Bigelow, J.C., and Page, U.S.: Transthoracic intraaortic balloon cannulation to avoid repeat sternotomy for removal, Ann. Thorac. Surg. **21:**562, 1976.
40. Kusserow, B.K.: A permanently indwelling intracorporeal blood pump to substitute for cardiac function, Trans. Am. Soc. Artif. Intern. Organs **4:**227, 1958.
41. Kusserow, B.K., and Clapp, J.F., III: Partial substitution of ventricular function over extended periods by a mechanical pump, Trans. Am. Soc. Artif. Intern. Organs **7:**332, 1961.
42. Lajos, T.Z., Venditti, J., and Vennuto, R.: Hemodynamic consequences of bronchial flow during cardiopulmonary bypass, J. Thorac. Cardiovasc. Surg. **89**(6):934, 1985.
43. LeGallois, J.J.C.: Experiences sur le principe de la vie, Paris, 1812. (Translated by J.G. Nancrede and N.C. Nancrede, Philadelphia, 1813.)
44. Liddicoat, J.E., et al.: Membrane vs. bubble oxygenator: a clinical comparison, Ann. Surg. **181**(5):747, 1975.
45. Lundar, T., et al.: Cerebral perfusion during nonpulsatile cardiopulmonary bypass, Ann. Thorac. Surg. **40**(2):144, 1985.
46. Magovern, G.J.: Long-term left heart assist using the centrifugal pump without anticoagulation. Paper presented at New Developments in the Partial Mechanical Support of the Failing Heart, University of Maryland School of Medicine, Baltimore, Sept. 23, 1983.
47. McCabe, J.C., et al.: Complications of intraaortic balloon insertion and counter-pulsation, Circulation **57**(4):769, 1978.
48. McGee, M.G., et al.: Retrospective analyses of the need for mechanical circulatory support (intraaortic balloon pump/abdominal left ventricular assist device or partial artificial heart) after cardiopulmonary bypass: a 44-month study of 14,168 patients, Am. J. Cardiol. **46:**135, 1980.
49. Moulopoulos, S.D., Topaz, S., and Kolff, W.J.: Extracorporeal assistance to the circulation and intraaortic balloon pumping, Trans. Am. Soc. Artif. Intern. Organs **8:**85, 1962.
50. Norman, J.C.: An intracorporeal (abdominal) left ventricular assist device (ALVAD). XXX. Clinical readiness and initial trials in man, Cardiovasc. Dis. Bull. Tex. Heart Inst. **3**(3):249, 1976.
51. Norman, J.C.: Partial artificial hearts: mechanical cloning of the ventricle, Artif. Organs **2**(3):235, 1978.
52. Norman, J.C., et al.: An intracorporeal (abdominal) left ventricular assist device: initial clinical trials, Arch. Surg. **112:**1442, 1977.
53. Norman, J.C., et al.: Prognostic indices for survival during postcardiotomy intraaortic balloon pumping: methods of scoring and classification, with implications for left ventricular assist device utilization, J. Thorac. Cardiovasc. Surg. **74**(5):709, 1977.
54. Norman, J.C, et al.: Total support of the circulation of a patient with post-cardiotomy stone heart syndrome by a partial artificial heart (ALVAD) for 5 days followed by heart and kidney transplantation, Lancet **1:**1125, 1978.
55. Nose, Y., et al.: Elimination of some problems encountered in total replacement of the heart with an intrathoracic mechanical pump: venous return, Trans. Am. Soc. Artif. Intern. Organs **12:**301, 1966.
56. Nunez, L., et al.: Transthoracic cannulation for balloon pumping in a "crowded aorta," Ann. Thorac. Surg. **30:**400, 1980.
57. Pacifico, A.D., Digerness, S., and Kirklin, J.W.: Acute alterations of bodily composition after open cardiac operations, Circulation **41:**331, 1970.
58. Pae, W.E., and Pierce, W.S.: Mechanical left ventricular assistance: current devices, future prospects. In Moran, J.M., and Michaelis, L.L., editors: Surgery for the complications of myocardial infarction, New York, 1980, Grune & Stratton, Inc.
59. Patterson, S., and Starling, E.H.: On the mechanical factors which determine the output of the ventricles, J. Physiol. **48:**357, 1914.
60. Pennock, J.L., Wisman, C.B., and Pierce, W.S.: Mechanical support of the circulation prior to cardiac transplantation, Heart Transplant. **1**(4):299, 1982.
61. Philips, P.A., and Miyamoto, A.M.: Application of the supply-demand ratio for the early detection of subendocardial ischemia. In Norman, J.C., editor: Coronary artery medicine and surgery: concepts and controversies, New York, 1975, Appleton-Century-Crofts.
62. Pierce, W.S., et al.: Prolonged mechanical support of the left ventricle, Circulation **58** (suppl. I):133, 1978.
63. Putman, E.A., and Manners, J.M.: Vascular resistance during cardiopulmonary bypass: its effect on vascular performance in the immediate post bypass: period, Anesthesia **38**(7):635, 1983.

64. Quiroga, M.M., et al.: The effect of body temperature on leukocyte kinetics during cardiopulmonary bypass, J. Thorac. Cardiovasc. Surg. **90**(1):91, 1985.
65. Roe, B.B., and Chatterjee, K.: Transthoracic cannulation for balloon pumping: report of a patient undergoing closed chest decannulation, Ann. Thorac. Surg. **21**:568, 1976.
66. Rose, D.M., et al.: Long-term survival with partial left heart bypass following perioperative myocardial infarction and shock, J. Thorac. Cardiovasc. Surg. **83**(4):483, 1982.
67. Royston, D., et al.: The effect of surgery with cardiopulmonary bypass on alveolar-capillary barrier function in human beings, Ann. Thorac. Surg. **40**(2):139, 1985.
68. Sarnoff, S.J.: Myocardial contractility as described by ventricular function curves: observations on Starling's law of the heart, Phys. Rev. **35**:107, 1955.
69. Scheidt, S., et al.: Intraaortic balloon counterpulsation in cardiogenic shock: report of a cooperative clinical trial, N. Engl. J. Med. **288**(19):979, 1973.
70. Schelbert, H.R., Covell, J.W., and Burns, J.W.: Observations on factors affecting local forces in the left ventricular wall during acute myocardial ischemia, Circ. Res. **29**:306, 1971.
71. Siderys, H., et al.: A comparison of membrane and bubble oxygenation as used in cardiopulmonary bypass patients, J. Thorac. Cardiovasc. Surg. **68**(5):708, 1975.
72. Solis, R.T.: Blood filtration during cardiopulmonary bypass, J. Extra-Corporeal Tech. **6**:64, 1974.
73. Sonnenblick, E.H., Ross, J., Jr., and Braunwald, E.: Oxygen consumption of the heart: newer concepts of its multifactorial determination, Am. J. Cardiol. **22**:328, 1968.
74. Spotnitz, H.M., Covell, J.W., and Ross, J.: Left ventricular mechanics and oxygen consumption during arterial counter-pulsation, Am. J. Physiol. **217**:1352, 1969.
75. Svennevig, J.L., et al.: Should the lungs be ventilated during cardiopulmonary bypass? Clinical, hemodynamic, and metabolic changes in patients undergoing elective coronary artery surgery, Ann. Thorac. Surg. **37**(4):295, 1984.
76. Tabak, C., Eugene, J., and Stemmer, E.A.: Erythrocyte survival following extracorporeal circulation: a question of membrane vs. bubble oxygenators, J. Thorac. Cardiovasc. Surg. **81**(1):30, 1981.
77. Takagi, H., et al.: Pathophysiologic studies on prolonged continuous pumping of series-type left heart assist device in calves, Trans. Am. Soc. Artif. Intern. Organs **17**:189, 1971.
78. Tchervendov, C.I., and Salerno, T.A.: Preliminary experience with a new technique of insertion and removal of the intraaortic balloon pump into the ascending aorta (letter to the editor), J. Thorac. Cardiovasc. Surg. **87**:475, 1984.
79. Thoma, M., et al.: Drive technology of mechanical circulation support systems—consequences from clinical experience, Med.-Markt, Acta Medicotech. **5**:150, 1977.
80. Turina, M., Bosio, R., and Senning, A.: Clinical application of paracorporeal, uni and biventricular artificial heart, Trans. Am. Soc. Artif. Intern. Organs **25**:625, 1978.
81. Ugorji, C.C., et al.: Transascending aortic intraaortic balloon insertion with delayed sternal closure: a retrospective analysis, Cardiovasc. Dis. Bull. Tex. Heart Inst. **7**(3):307, 1980.
82. VanDenDungen, J.J.A.M., et al.: Clinical study of blood trauma during perfusion with membrane and bubble oxygenators, J. Thorac. Cardiovasc. Surg. **83**(1):108, 1982.
83. Van Velzen-Blad, H., et al.: Cardiopulmonary bypass and host defense functions in human beings. I. Serum levels and role of immunoglobulins and complement in phagocytosis, Ann. Thorac. Surg. **39**(3):207, 1985.
84. Van Velzen-Blad, H., et al.: Cardiopulmonary bypass and host defense functions in human beings. II. Lymphocyte function, Ann. Thorac. Surg. **39**(3):212, 1985.
85. Weber, K.T., and Janicki, J.S.: Intraaortic balloon counter-pulsation: a review of physiological principles, clinical results and device safety, Ann. Thorac. Surg. **17**:602, 1974.
86. Wesolowski, S.A., Fisher, J.H., and Welch, C.S.: Perfusion of pulmonary circulation by non-pulsatile flow, Surgery **33**:370, 1953.
87. Wesolowski, S.A., Sauvage, L.R., and Pinc, R.D.: Extracorporeal circulation: the role of the pulse in maintenance of the systemic circulation during heart lung bypass, Surgery **37**:663, 1955.
88. Wright, J.S., et al.: Some advantages of the membrane oxygenator for open-heart surgery, J. Thorac. Cardiovasc. Surg. **69**(6):884, 1975.

39 *Edward L. Bove*

Congenital Heart Lesions

The surgical treatment of congenital heart defects has progressed at a rapid rate since its beginning nearly a half century ago. Numerous technical achievements have been made possible by advances in many fields. Precise knowledge of anatomy and physiology, detailed noninvasive diagnostic capabilities, better perfusion and myocardial preservation techniques, and improved neonatal intensive care have all played major roles in allowing the management of congenital heart disease to progress to the extent that it has. Nearly all congenital heart defects are now amenable to surgical repair. This chapter will discuss the pathophysiology underlying a few of the cardiac defects more commonly encountered by the pediatric cardiac surgeon and the physiologic rationale behind their treatment.

ADJUSTMENTS IN THE CIRCULATION AFTER BIRTH

Although it is beyond the scope of this presentation to discuss in detail the physiology of the intrauterine circulation and its adaptation to extrauterine life, a brief description is included to aid in the understanding of the topics to follow.

Oxygen-enriched placental blood returns to the fetus through the umbilical vein and then passes through the liver. It then joins the inferior vena caval return and enters the right atrium. Much of this blood passes across the patent foramen ovale by preferential streaming into the left atrium, left ventricle, and ascending aorta, where it is distributed to the brain and coronary circulations (Fig. 39-1). Superior vena cava return is directed across the right atrium, tricuspid valve, and right ventricle to be ejected into the pulmonary artery. Nearly all this blood passes across the patent ductus arteriosus into the descending aorta. Because the ductus is nonrestrictive, both ventricles essentially function as a unit and eject blood against the same overall resistance. However, systemic vascular resistance is very low because of the placental circulation, and pulmonary vascular resistance is high in the nonaerated fetal lung, resulting in less than 10% of the fetal cardiac output going to the lungs.

At birth the placenta is eliminated from the circulation, resulting in an abrupt rise in systemic vascular resistance. Expansion of the lungs leads to a fall in pulmonary vascular resistance. As arterial and alveolar partial pressure of oxygen (Po_2) increase, pulmonary vascular resistance falls further and pulmonary blood flow rises, resulting in an increase in left atrial pressure and functional closure of the flap valve of the foramen ovale. The increase in arterial Po_2 also causes constriction of the smooth muscle in the wall of the ductus arteriosus, closing the duct and completing the separation of the two circulations. Pulmonary vascular resistance falls to adult levels within 2 to 4 weeks in the term infant.

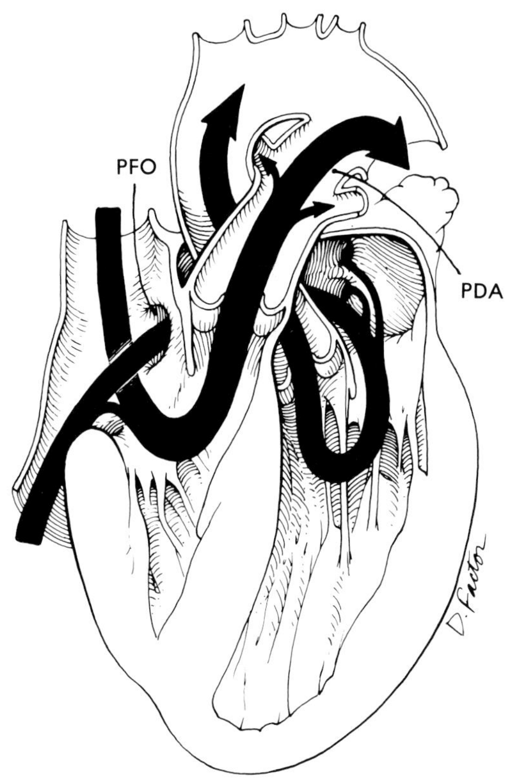

Fig. 39-1 Course of the intracardiac circulation before birth. Most inferior vena cava blood passes across the patent foramen ovale *(PFO)* to the left atrium. The superior vena cava return is directed predominantly across the patent ductus arteriosus *(PDA)*.

CONGESTIVE HEART FAILURE

Simply defined, congestive heart failure is the failure of myocardial oxygen supply to meet oxygen demand. The classic findings of congestive heart failure in infants include tachypnea, tachycardia, diaphoresis, and hepatomegaly. Peripheral edema and rales are not typically noted in infants. The newborn myocardium is already functioning at maximal stroke volume and can only increase cardiac output by increasing heart rate. Further, the newborn myocardium has a reduced density of contractile elements. For these reasons, the already stressed neonate with limited cardiac reserve is easily susceptible to congestive heart failure. Congenital heart disease typically results in congestive heart failure in two ways: volume overload or pressure overload.

Volume overload occurs with either a large communication between the systemic and pulmonary circulations or

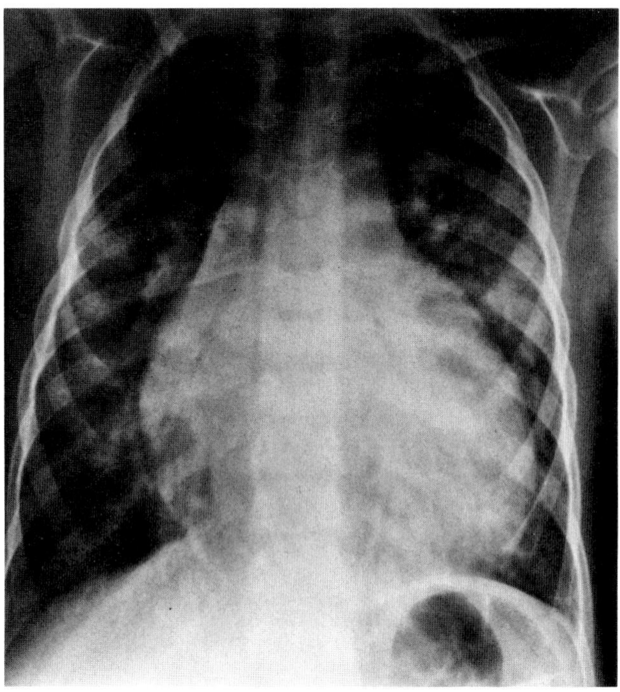

Fig. 39-2 Chest x-ray film of a patient with an atrial septal defect. There is cardiomegaly and an increase in pulmonary vascular markings secondary to the large left-to-right shunt.

valvar regurgitant lesions (Fig 39-2). When a left-to-right shunt occurs, the volume of shunted blood is dependent on the relative resistances of the two vascular beds. As the pulmonary vascular resistance falls over the first few weeks of life, pulmonary blood flow may increase dramatically, producing a large volume overload of the left ventricle. Because this shunt is dependent on a falling pulmonary vascular resistance, congestive failure from volume overload is not usually seen until 2 or 3 weeks of age.

Pressure overload results from an obstruction to ventricular emptying. This obstruction is usually located at the level of the semilunar (pulmonary or aortic) valve but may be seen with subvalvar or supravalvar blockage. When the ventricle can no longer eject an adequate blood volume through the obstruction, pulmonary and systemic venous congestion with congestive heart failure results.

Cyanosis

Cyanosis is a blue discoloration of the skin and mucous membranes caused by the presence of at least 5 g/100 ml of unsaturated circulating hemoglobin. When noted in infancy, the administration of 100% oxygen is a reliable test to establish the presence of intracardiac shunting secondary to congenital heart disease. If the Po_2 in the right radial artery rises above 250 mm Hg, cyanotic heart disease is virtually eliminated. Although values less than 250 mm Hg are not certain indicators of cardiac disease, a Po_2 below 100 mm Hg generally indicates a cardiac problem.

Cyanosis resulting from congenital heart disease may be caused by decreased pulmonary blood flow with intracardiac right-to-left shunting or by abnormalities of intracardiac mixing. When cyanosis is caused by decreased pulmonary blood flow, two conditions are necessary: obstruction to flow into the lungs and an intracardiac communication between the two circulations proximal to the obstruction. The obstruction may be located anywhere between the systemic venous atrium (tricuspid atresia) and the branch pulmonary arteries (tetralogy of Fallot). Resistance to flow through the obstruction is equal to or greater than that through the communication, allowing desaturated blood to enter the systemic circulation directly.

Cyanosis may also occur secondary to inadequate mixing of the blood between the systemic and pulmonary circulations. This situation is classically seen in transposition-type physiology. Although total systemic and pulmonary blood flow may be normal or increased, the effective flow is reduced. That is, the amount of desaturated blood actually reaching the lungs and the amount of fully saturated blood reaching the body is decreased. This condition is discussed more fully later in this chapter.

Finally, common mixing occurs when desaturated and saturated blood freely mix, allowing some desaturated blood to reach the body. This can occur at atrial (common atrium), ventricular (common or single ventricle), or great vessel level (truncus arteriosus).

OBSTRUCTIVE LESIONS

Coarctation of the Aorta

Coarctation is a narrowing in the thoracic aorta most commonly located just distal to the left subclavian artery opposite the insertion of the ductus arteriosus or ligamentum arteriosum (Fig. 39-3, *A*). Obstruction to left ventricular emptying results in a pressure overload of the ventricle, which may lead to congestive heart failure. In infancy associated defects often dictate the hemodynamic condition. When the ductus arteriosus is patent, blood may flow from the pulmonary artery across the duct into the descending aorta (Fig. 39-3, *B*). In this situation, differential cyanosis will be present with desaturated blood perfusing the lower extremities and saturated blood perfusing the upper body. Approximately 20% of patients have an associated ventricular septal defect. The impedance to left ventricular emptying imposed by the coarctation increases the left-to-right shunt and results in severe congestive heart failure from combined pressure and volume overload. Other obstructive lesions in the left heart may also be seen with coarctation, most commonly aortic stenosis secondary to a bicuspid aortic valve.

When coarctation results in congestive heart failure in infancy, nonoperative treatment carries a high mortality. Most patients with coarctation, however, are asymptomatic, and the defect is not found until after infancy. The discovery of upper-extremity hypertension with diminished or absent femoral pulses typically leads to the diagnosis. Flow murmurs over the back and palpable pulsations in the subscapular area from prominent collaterals may be present. All extremity pulses must be carefully palpated. A decrease in the left arm pulse may indicate involvement of the origin of the left subclavian artery in the coarctation. Plain chest x-ray films may show dilation of the aorta proximal and distal to the narrowed segment ("3" sign) and notching of the ribs secondary to enlarged intercostal arteries. Aortography is generally recommended to accu-

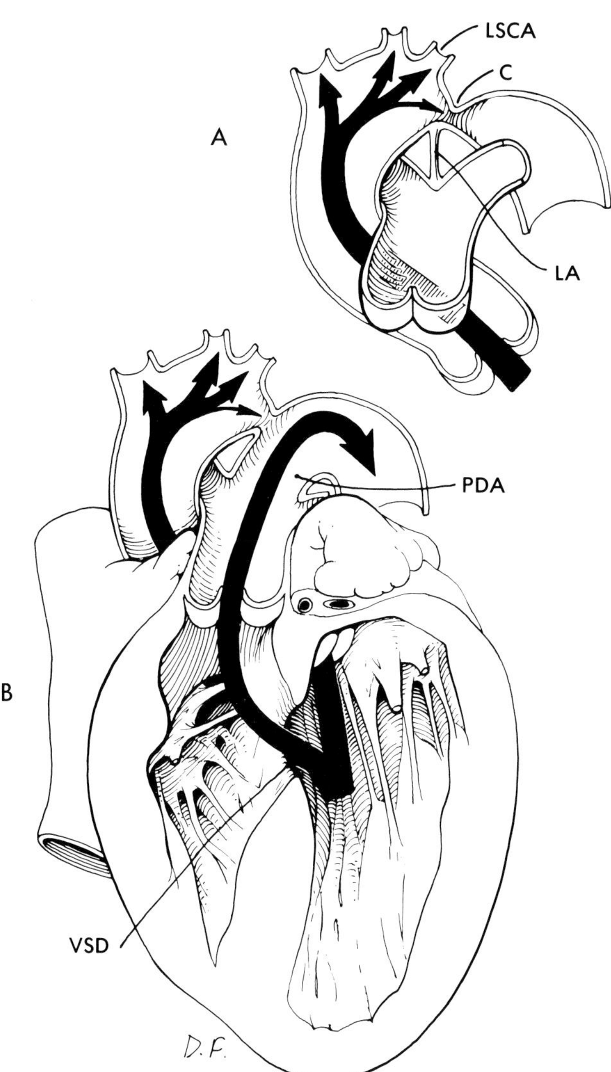

Fig. 39-3 Hemodynamic abnormalities in coarctation of the aorta. **A,** Pathophysiology in the older child or adult. **B,** In infancy a patent ductus arteriosus allows blood flow to the descending aorta from the right ventricle. *LSCA,* left subclavian artery; *C,* coarctation; *LA,* ligamentum arteriosum; *PDA,* patent ductus arteriosus; *VSD,* ventricular septal defect.

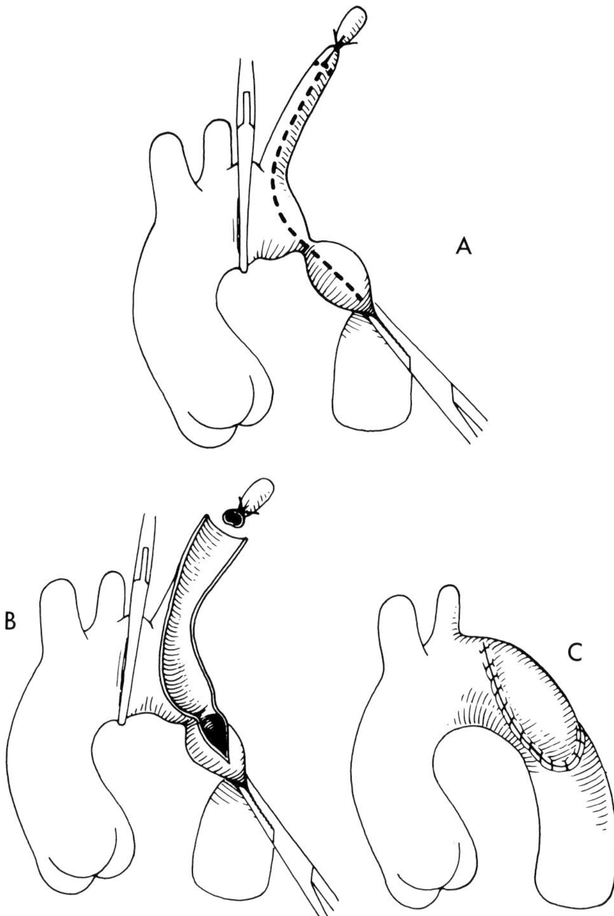

Fig. 39-4 Repair of coarctation using the subclavian angioplasty technique. **A,** Left subclavian artery is mobilized and divided distally. **B,** Longitudinal incision through the artery and adjacent aorta is made. This incision must extend distally beyond the coarctation until normal aorta is reached. **C,** Completed repair.

rately define the anatomy of the coarctation before surgical repair. In rare cases the coarctation may be in an unusual location.

The exact cause of hypertension in coarctation remains obscure. The etiology in older patients is apparently more than just obstruction, as relief of coarctation in adulthood does not result in the restoration of normal blood pressure in every case. It seems certain that in these cases a renal mechanism is in part responsible. In a classic experiment performed by Scott and Bahnson, coarctation was surgically created in dogs. The resultant hypertension was relieved by removal of one kidney and transplantation of the other above the level of the coarctation. When abnormal plasma renin activity is unmasked by volume depletion, abnormally high renin-angiotensin activity has been found in patients with coarctation.[35]

Virtually all patients with hemodynamically significant coarctation of the aorta should undergo operative repair. The ideal age for repair in the symptomatic child is not well defined but is probably between the ages of 3 and 5 years. Early operation increases the risk of recoarctation with growth of the aorta, whereas delaying repair beyond childhood increases the chance of persistent hypertension.[8] The presence of congestive heart failure in infancy dictates operative intervention regardless of age or size.

The classic surgical technique remains resection of the narrowed segment with end-to-end anastomosis. However, recurrent narrowing at the suture line remains a problem with this technique, particularly when repair is done in infancy. Additionally, exercise-induced upper extremity hypertension with significant arm-to-leg gradients have been found in some children with end-to-end repairs.[19] This is most probably caused by the inelasticity of the circumferential suture line, which becomes a relative obstruction when velocity of flow is increased. To avoid a circumferential suture line, some groups have advocated a patch angioplasty technique using prosthetic material.[38]

The best method available to relieve coarctation is the subclavian angioplasty procedure, first reported by Waldhausen and Nahrwald in 1966 (Fig. 39-4). Originally advocated in infants, its application is being expanded for older patients as well. This technique uses the left subclavian artery as an onlay patch and avoids both a restrictive circumferential anastomosis and foreign material. Further, a viable arterial patch is ideally suited for growth.

Aortic Stenosis

The most common cause of obstruction to left ventricular ejection is aortic stenosis. The obstruction is typically located at the level of the valve but may be subvalvar or supravalvar (Fig. 39-5). Valvar aortic stenosis is usually caused by a bicuspid aortic valve with varying degrees of fusion of the commissures, although fused tricuspid valves may also be found. A dome shaped unicusp valve may result in significant obstruction in infancy. Subvalvar aortic stenosis may be discrete or diffuse. In the discrete form, a fibrous membrane is found just below the aortic valve leaflets. The diffuse form is seen in obstructive cardiomyopathies such as idiopathic hypertrophic subaortic stenosis or muscular tunnel-type subvalvar hypoplasia. In supravalvar stenosis, the obstruction is most commonly caused by an hourglass deformity of the ascending aorta just above the valve.

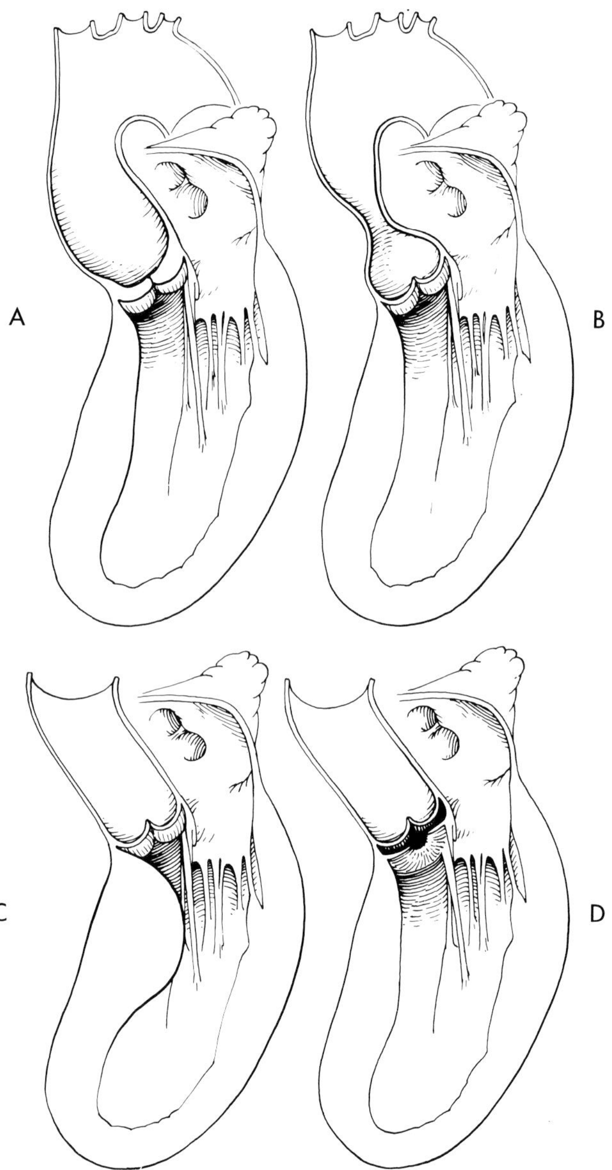

Fig. 39-5 Anatomic types of left ventricular outflow tract obstruction. **A,** Valvar stenosis secondary to a bicuspid aortic valve. Note the poststenotic dilation of the ascending aorta. **B,** Hourglass narrowing of the ascending aorta resulting in supravalvar stenosis. **C,** Subvalvar stenosis resulting from diffuse hypertrophy of the ventricular septum or **D,** from a discrete suboaortic membrane.

Valvar aortic stenosis may present at any age. In infancy severe stenosis may cause congestive heart failure.[40] However, in most children, an asymptomatic heart murmur is detected on physical examination beyond the neonatal period. When symptoms are present in childhood, exertional dyspnea, syncope, and angina pectoris are the usual manifestations. Syncope is caused by the inability of the left ventricle to maintain adequate cerebral blood flow through a narrow, fixed orifice valve during exercise. Angina pectoris, although rare in childhood, may be seen when pressure overload results in significant left ventricular hypertrophy and myocardial blood flow does not adequately perfuse the thickened, hypertensive ventricular muscle.

Indications for operation in patients with valvar aortic stenosis include syncope, congestive heart failure, or angina with a significant left ventricular outflow tract gradient. A significant gradient is usually considered to be at least 50 mm Hg unless cardiac output is greatly depressed. The timing of operative intervention in the asymptomatic child with moderate or severe obstruction is less well defined. Electrocardiographic changes indicating left ventricular strain or ischemia, either at rest or induced during exercise, are considered definite indications. Severe gradients of greater than 70 mm Hg are best treated surgically, even in the absence of symptoms or electrocardiographic changes.

Relief of valvar aortic stenosis is accomplished by direct incision of fused commissures. The incision is stopped 1 to 2 mm from the anulus to avoid detaching all leaflet support and creating significant aortic regurgitation. In a true bicuspid valve, rudimentary commissures must not be incised or a flail leaflet will result. Although satisfactory reduction of the gradient can usually be accomplished, it may be difficult to provide complete relief of obstruction in all cases.[1] Certain bicuspid valves may not lend themselves to valvotomy and may remain obstructive despite lack of commissural fusion. Valve replacement, often combined with techniques to enlarge a small aortic anulus, may be necessary in these unusual situations.[26]

Operation for subvalvar stenosis is recommended for the same indication as in valvar obstruction. However, the required gradient may be somewhat less for discrete subvalvar stenoses because resection of the membrane is more often curative.[42] Many patients with untreated discrete subvalvar stenosis will develop progressive aortic regurgitation secondary to turbulence beneath the valve. Early resection of the membrane may prevent this complication. Diffuse, muscular left ventricular outflow tract obstruction is more difficult to relieve. Transaortic resection of hypertrophied septal muscle or bypass of the obstruction by insertion of a valved conduit from the left ventricular apex to the aorta is usually needed.[9,34]

LEFT-TO-RIGHT SHUNTS

Atrial Septal Defect

Atrial septal defect (ASD) accounts for approximately 10% of all congenital cardiac lesions. The defect in the septum allows blood to flow from the left to the right atrium, producing a volume overload of the right ventricle and pulmonary circulation. The shunt is directed from left to right because of the greater diastolic compliance and lower diastolic pressure in the right-sided chambers. Moderate-sized defects result in pulmonary blood flow from one and one-half to three times the systemic flow, whereas in large defects the pulmonary to systemic flow ratio exceeds 3 to 1. In most cases, pulmonary artery pressure and systemic blood flow remain normal.

ASDs usually occur as isolated lesions and tend to remain asymptomatic until early adult life.[15] When present, symptoms are often nonspecific and consist of fatigue or mild dyspnea on exertion. In the presence of a large left-to-right shunt, overt congestive heart failure can occur at any age. Most commonly, however, near normal activity is maintained until the third or fourth decade when symptoms of congestive failure become manifest.

Any chronic left-to-right shunt may eventually produce changes of pulmonary vascular occlusive disease. Although these changes occur more frequently and earlier in life with defects that cause both an increase in pulmonary blood flow and pressure, uncomplicated ASDs may result in irreversible pulmonary occlusive changes. This problem is discussed more fully in the following section about ventricular septal defects.

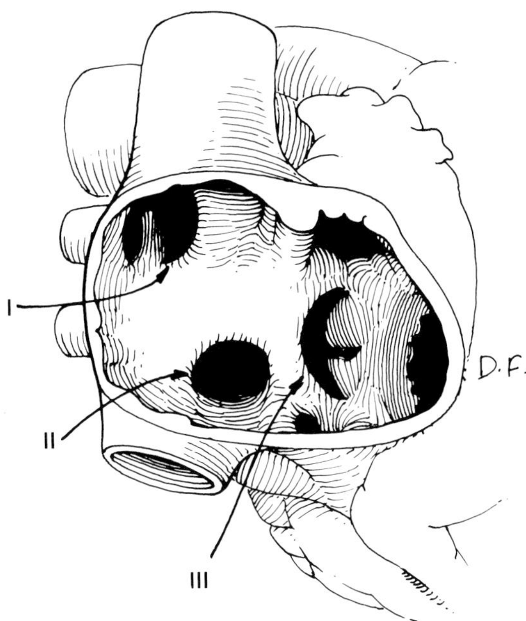

Fig. 39-6 Location of the three common types of atrial septal defect. The sinus venous defect is shown with anomalous drainage of the right upper lobe pulmonary vein *(I)*. The ostium secundum defect is in the midportion of the septum *(II)*. The ostium primum defect is located in the base of the septum with its inferior edge formed by the continuity of the tricuspid and mitral valves *(III)*. Note the cleftlike anomaly in the anterior leaflet of the mitral valve visible through the defect.

The majority of ASDs occur in the center of the atrial septum and are referred to as ostium secundum defects (Fig. 39-6). In approximately 5% to 10% of patients, the defect is located high in the atrial wall, where the superior vena cava joins the right atrium. These defects are known as sinus venosus ASDs and are almost always associated with drainage of the right upper lobe pulmonary veins to the right atrium or superior vena cava. About 5% of patients have another variety of defect called an ostium primum ASD. These defects, which are located low in the septum, are part of a more complex anomaly referred to as endocardial cushion defect. In its simplest form, the ostium primum atrial defect is associated with a cleft in the anterior leaflet of the mitral valve. Mitral regurgitation may be present and can be severe.

Any ASD in which pulmonary blood flow is at least one and one-half times the systemic flow should be closed. Operative correction prevents the long-term complications of congestive heart failure and pulmonary vascular occlusive disease. Studies on patients not having surgery indicated that life expectancy is significantly reduced to the fourth or fifth decade of life. Further, some patients may develop pulmonary vascular occlusive disease with marked elevations of pulmonary vascular resistance and reversal of shunt flow in adult life. Because most children will be asymptomatic, elective repair is advised before school age. This type of ASD should be repaired in adults of any age because excellent results have also been reported in this group.[24,43]

The technique of repair involves suture closure during cardiopulmonary bypass in the majority of patients. Through an incision in the right atrium the anatomy is easily exposed. In large defects a patch of pericardium or dacron may be necessary to avoid tension on the edges of the repair. In sinus venosus defects with partial anomalous pulmonary venous return, closure is achieved by modifying the patch to redirect the pulmonary veins to the left atrium. Ostium primum ASDs must also be repaired with a patch because no lower rim of atrial septum is present. The lower edge of this defect is the junction of mitral and tricuspid valves on the crest of the ventricular septum. If significant mitral regurgitation is present preoperatively, the valve should be carefully studied at the time of operation and a valvuloplasty performed.[30]

Ventricular Septal Defect

Excluding bicuspid aortic valve, ventricular septal defect (VSD) is the most common congenital structural cardiac anomaly. It accounts for 20% to 25% of all cardiac lesions and is estimated to occur in 2 of 1000 liveborn infants. The hemodynamics, symptoms, and treatment depend on the size of the VSD and on the magnitude of the shunt. With a small VSD, right ventricular pressure remains normal, the pulmonary to systemic flow ratio (Q_p/Q_s) is less than 1.5 to 1, and symptoms are usually absent. Moderate-sized defects have right ventricular pressure up to half of systemic levels and a Q_p/Q_s up to 2.5 to 1 or 3 to 1. Some degree of congestive heart failure is often present, but growth is usually normal. A large VSD is present when the Q_p/Q_s exceeds 3 to 1. Right ventricular pressure usually exceeds one-half that of the left ventricle but may be normal where pulmonary vascular resistance is low. Severe congestive failure with poor growth is often found.

Approximately 50% of VSDs discovered in infancy will undergo spontaneous reduction in size or complete closure. Thus all defects are initially managed medically if symptoms of congestive heart failure are present. Small VSDs usually do not require treatment and nearly all will close. Spontaneous closure becomes less likely with larger defects but may still occur.

In response to the increasing pulmonary blood flow seen with moderate and large VSDs, pulmonary arteriolar resistance rises, and pulmonary artery pressure may also become elevated. A sustained increase in pulmonary artery flow and pressure can lead to early development of pulmonary vascular occlusive disease. Irreversible changes in resistance may become apparent by 2 years of age with an isolated large VSD. These changes have been classified by Heath and Edwards[25a] on a histologic level. The early changes in the small pulmonary arteries and arterioles of medial hypertrophy (Grade I) and intimal proliferation (Grade II) are considered reversible. More advanced changes consisting of intimal fibrosis (Grade III) and progressive dilation lesions with eventual arterial necrosis (Grades IV through VI) are irreversible.

Cardiac catheterization documents the magnitude of the shunt, right ventricular and pulmonary artery pressure, and pulmonary vascular resistance. Left ventricular cineangiography, in addition to two-dimensional echocardiography, delineates the location and number of VSDs. Associated defects, including coarctation, aortic stenosis, patent ductus arteriosus, and pulmonary stenosis, are common and must be identified.

Most VSDs are single and are located high in the membranous portion of the ventricular septum, just beneath the aortic valve. These defects are classified by their relationship to structures in the right ventricle.[29] The typical, high VSD, referred to as an infundibular defect, can be found beneath the anteroseptal commissure of the tricuspid valve (Fig. 39-7). Inlet VSDs are located more inferiorly beneath the septal leaflet of the tricuspid valve, and subarterial defects occur high in the septum immediately below the pulmonary valve. When a VSD extends to the anulus of the tricuspid valve, it is referred to as perimembranous; otherwise, it is a muscular defect. VSDs may be single or multiple. Muscular defects occurring in the heavily trabeculated portion of the septum are more likely to be multiple.

The indications for surgery depend on the hemodynamic situation and presence of symptoms. With moderate and large VSDs, persistent severe congestive heart failure (often with failure to thrive) despite medical management is an operative indication. When heart failure is well controlled medically, the primary factor influencing the decision to operate is the pulmonary arterial pressure and the pulmonary vascular resistance (PVR). These should be assessed by 12 months of age. If the pulmonary arterial pressure is greater than one half of systemic levels by this age, prompt surgical intervention should be carried out to prevent progressive changes in PVR. Moderate defects with minimal symptoms and normal pulmonary artery pressure and resistance may continue to be observed because late spontaneous closure may still occur. If they do not close by 3 to 5 years of age, operative therapy is indicated.

If the PVR is found to be severely elevated above two thirds the systemic resistance, VSD closure is contraindicated. When the resistance reaches this level, pulmonary resistance will often progress further and eventually exceed that of the systemic circulation. Reversal of flow through the defect then occurs (Eisenmenger's syndrome), and cyanosis results. Closure of the VSD in this situation would result in right-sided heart failure and shortened life expectancy.

The optimal surgical treatment of VSDs consists of primary closure in most situations.[2,37] In infants deep hypothermia with reduced flow on cardipulmonary bypass is used to facilitate exposure and reduce operative risk.[4] The operative approach for the majority of defects is through the right atrium and tricuspid valve. A patch of dacron is sutured to the right ventricular side of the defect edge; care is used not to injure the conduction tissue, which must be precisely located for each VSD.[33] In complex lesions, the AV node and bundle of His may be identified with endocardial mapping. Subpulmonary defects are best closed through the pulmonary artery or right ventricle. Muscular defects may require a left ventriculotomy for proper exposure. In each case, initial exposure through the tricuspid valve allows the surgeon to plan the best approach.

Complete repair in infancy may not be advisable in all

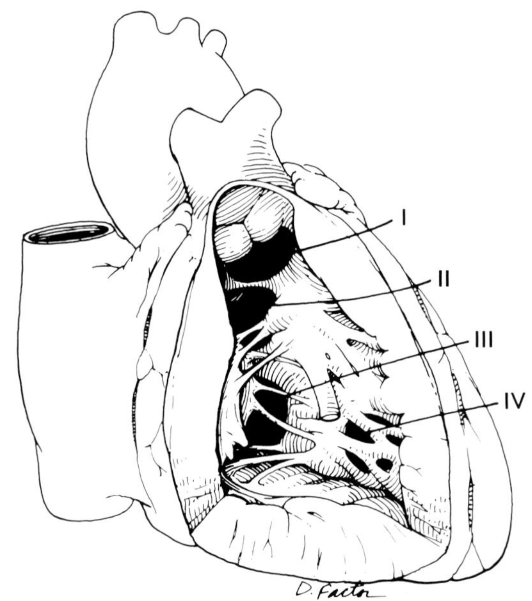

Fig. 39-7 Location of the common types of ventricular septal defect. Subarterial defects *(I)* are located in the infundibular portion of the septum, beneath the pulmonary valve. In the most common type, perimembranous infundibular *(II)*, part of the defect edge is formed by the tricuspid valve. Inlet defects *(III)* are found more inferiorly beneath the septal leaflet of the tricuspid valve. Muscular defects *(IV)* are remote from the valve anulus.

cases. When multiple defects are found, for example, palliation with pulmonary artery banding is usually indicated. By constricting the main pulmonary artery, the resistance to flow into the lungs is markedly increased, reducing the magnitude of the left-to-right shunt and controlling congestive heart failure. Further, the pulmonary vascular bed is protected against the development of pulmonary vascular occlusive disease, allowing complete repair to be done at less risk when the patient is older.

Patent Ductus Arteriosus

Patent ductus arteriosus (PDA) is the most common cause of left-to-right shunting at the great artery level. Since aortic pressure is greater than pulmonary artery pressure throughout all phases of the cardiac cycle, shunting occurs in both systole and diastole. This gives rise to the typical continuous or machinery-like murmur. Additionally, the diastolic runoff into the low resistance pulmonary circulation results in a wide pulse pressure and bounding arterial pulses. A large PDA may allow substantial left-to-right shunting and significant heart failure. Pulmonary artery pressure and resistance may be elevated as described in the previous section, resulting in eventual pulmonary vascular occlusive disease.

The anatomy of the duct is quite constant. Its aortic end originates just distal to the left subclavian artery and it enters the pulmonary artery bifurcation or proximal left pulmonary artery.

Any duct that remains patent beyond infancy should be closed. Elective closure is usually recommended in early childhood.[41] A large PDA in a patient with heart failure and pulmonary hypertension should be closed immediately. Small PDAs may be complicated by bacterial endarteritis, aneurysm formation, or calcification. Closure prevents these complications.

The operative approach is through a left thoracotomy. Exposure of the duct is easily accomplished after opening the mediastinal pleura. Care must be taken to avoid injury to the recurrent laryngeal nerve. Closure of the duct may be done by simple ligation, usually over a length of duct or by division and suture.

RIGHT-TO-LEFT SHUNTS

Tricuspid Atresia

Tricuspid atresia is an uncommon defect in which the tricuspid valve is completely absent. The atrial septal defect that is invariably present shunts all vena cava blood directly to the left atrium. The degree of cyanosis is dependent on the amount of pulmonary blood flow. When no communication between left and right ventricles is present, the ductus arteriosus is the sole source of flow to the lungs (Fig. 39-8, *A*). These patients are deeply cyanotic in early infancy, and the emergent administration of a prostaglandin infusion may be necessary.[20] Prostaglandins of the E-type relax the smooth muscle in the wall of the duct and are used to maintain ductal patency before palliative surgery.

In some cases a ventricular septal defect allows blood flow from the left ventricle directly to the hypoplastic right ventricle and then to the pulmonary circuit (Fig. 39-8, *B*). Depending on the size of this communication, cyanosis may be mild. However, these septal defects often undergo spontaneous reduction in size, thus decreasing pulmonary blood flow as the child grows. Less commonly, the aorta

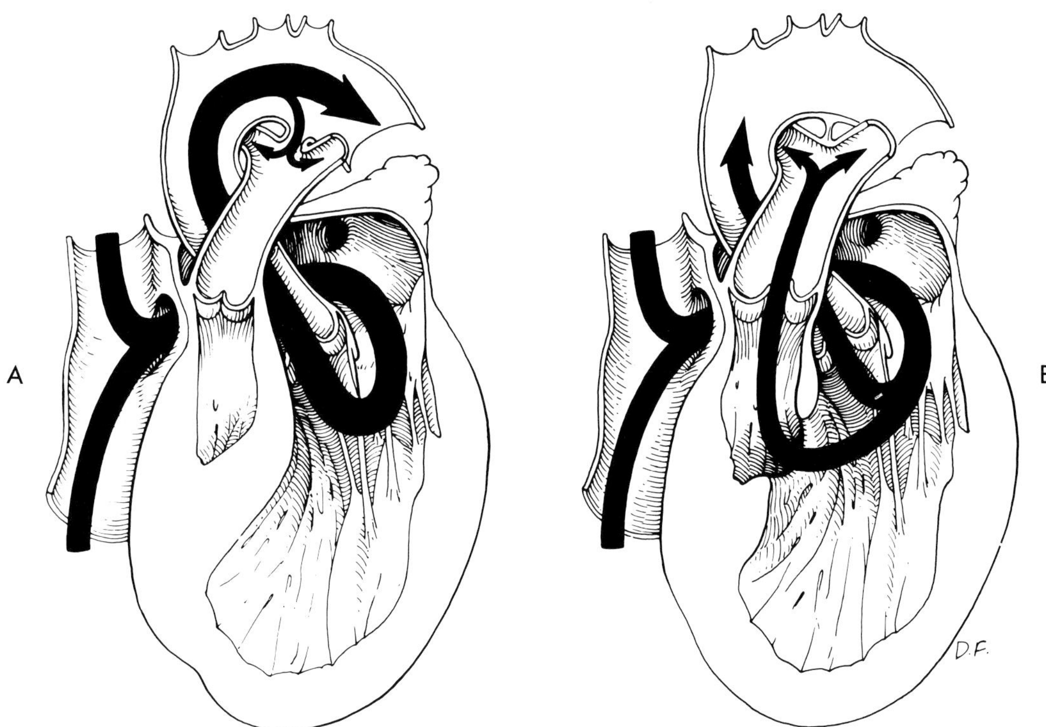

Fig. 39-8 **A,** Tricuspid atresia with normally related great vessels and without a ventricular septal defect. Pulmonary blood flow is duct dependent. **B,** When a septal defect is present, forward flow across the pulmonary valve can occur.

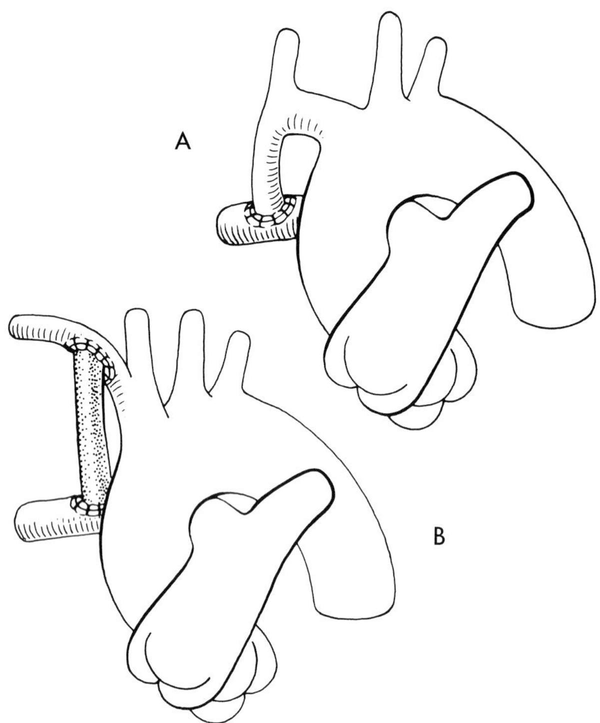

Fig. 39-9 **A,** Standard Blalock-Taussig anastomosis between the right subclavian and pulmonary arteries. **B,** Modification of the procedure with an interposition polytetraflouroethylene graft.

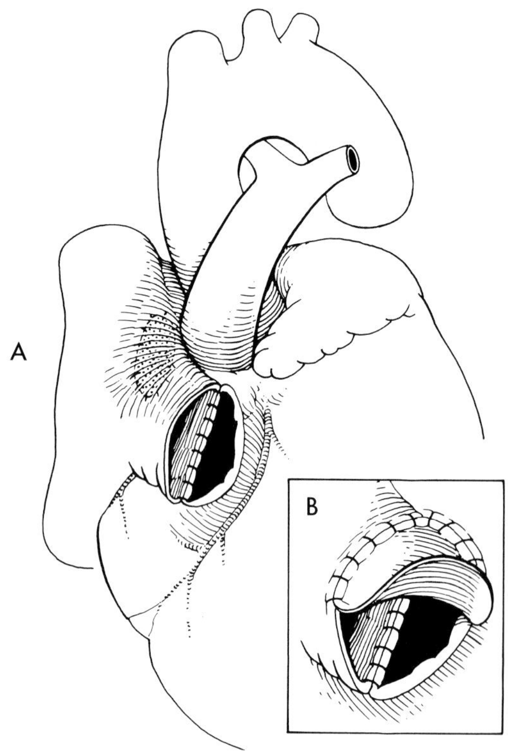

Fig. 39-10 **A,** Fontan procedure for tricuspid atresia. When the great vessels are normally related, a direct connection can be made between the right atrium and hypoplastic right ventricle. **B,** This anastomosis is enlarged with a pericardial patch to ensure a wide communication. The atrial septal defect is closed with a patch.

and pulmonary artery are transposed and the pulmonary artery receives the direct output of the left ventricle, resulting in an increase in pulmonary blood flow and pressure.

The initial surgical treatment of tricuspid atresia with decreased pulmonary blood flow is aimed at increasing this flow by a systemic artery–to–pulmonary artery shunt.[16,18] The Blalock-Taussig procedure in which the subclavian artery is anastomosed end-to-side to the pulmonary artery is the most commonly used operation (Fig. 39-9, *A*).[11] This procedure provides a source of pulmonary blood flow with minimum risk of increasing pulmonary vascular resistance or causing congestive heart failure.[3] The standard Blalock-Taussig shunt may not be suitable in all situations, particularly in neonates with small subclavian or pulmonary arteries. Flow through the shunt may be poor with inadequate relief of cyanosis. Modification of the procedure with an interposition graft of polytetrafluoroethylene between the sides of the subclavian and pulmonary arteries has been used in these cases (Fig. 39-9, *B*).[13,17] A relatively large graft (5 or 6 mm) is used even in infants since flow is limited by the smaller-sized native vessels. With growth of the subclavian and pulmonary arteries, flow can potentially increase and maintain effective palliation. Other shunt procedures are used much less commonly today. They include the Waterston (ascending aorta to right pulmonary artery), Potts (descending aorta to left pulmonary artery), and Glenn (superior vena cava to right pulmonary artery) anastomoses.

The most satisfactory form of treatment for tricuspid atresia was first reported in 1971 by Fontan and Baudet.[20a] This procedure is most commonly done by direct connection of the right atrium to the pulmonary artery or hypoplastic right ventricle (Fig. 39-10). The atrial septal defect is closed, thus separating systemic and pulmonary blood flow. All systemic venous blood perfuses the lungs directly, often without an intervening ventricular pump. In most cases, the insertion of a prosthetic valve is avoided. This procedure restores normal systemic oxygenation and eliminates left ventricular volume overload. Although the early results with this procedure have been most gratifying, long-term follow-up is lacking.[21,39] Specifically, the late effects of chronic venous hypertension and lack of pulsatile pulmonary blood flow are unknown.

Tetralogy of Fallot

The most common congenital heart defect resulting in cyanosis is tetralogy of Fallot. In this abnormality, obstruction to pulmonary blood flow occurs at the level of the right ventricular outflow tract, usually secondary to a combination of infundibular and pulmonary valvar stenoses (Fig. 39-11). The basic anatomic defect is anterior and superior displacement of the infundibular (outlet) portion of the ventricular septum. This obstructs right ventricular outflow and results in a large malalignment ventricular septal defect (Fig. 39-12). Overriding of the aorta above the VSD and right ventricular hypertrophy (secondary to obstruction) complete the tetrad.

The clinical status of patients with tetralogy of Fallot is dependent on the severity of the right ventricular outflow tract obstruction. In its severest form, pulmonary atresia

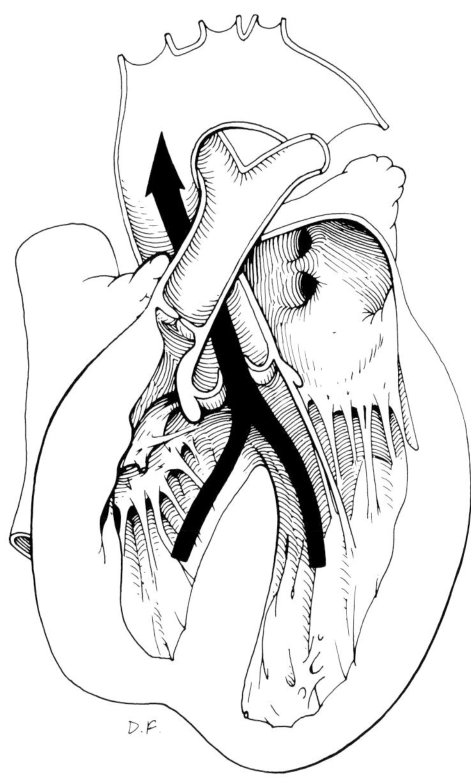

Fig. 39-11 Typical anatomy in tetralogy of Fallot. The large ventricular septal defect with overriding of the aorta is shown. The right ventricular outflow tract obstruction results in desaturated blood crossing the ventricular septal defect directly into the aorta.

may be present with duct dependent pulmonary blood flow. More commonly, infundibular obstruction coexists with varying degrees of pulmonary valve hypoplasia, resulting in moderate cyanosis. Patients with tetralogy of Fallot may have hypercyanotic or "tet" spells. These occur when the dynamic portion of the obstruction is transiently worsened secondary to increased contractility of the muscle in the right ventricular outflow tract. Pulmonary blood flow is dramatically reduced with an increase in the right-to-left shunt across the VSD.

Complete repair can be done in nearly all patients with tetralogy of Fallot. Only in rare cases with marked hypoplasia of the pulmonary arteries is complete repair impossible. Elective repair may be done any time after infancy.[14,27] When significant cyanosis occurs before 1 year of age, some surgeons recommend complete repair at that time. Most, however, would prefer palliation with the Blalock-Taussig shunt, postponing complete repair until the age of 3 or 4 years. Specific contraindications to repair in infancy include significant hypoplasia of the pulmonary arteries and the origin of the anterior descending coronary artery from the right coronary artery. Since relief of the obstruction in the latter situation may require the insertion of a valve-bearing conduit, repair is best postponed until the patient reaches the age of 5 or 6 years.

Complete repair includes relief of right ventricular outflow tract obstruction and closure of the VSD. Relief of the obstruction is governed by the individual anatomy. Whenever possible, pulmonary valve function should be

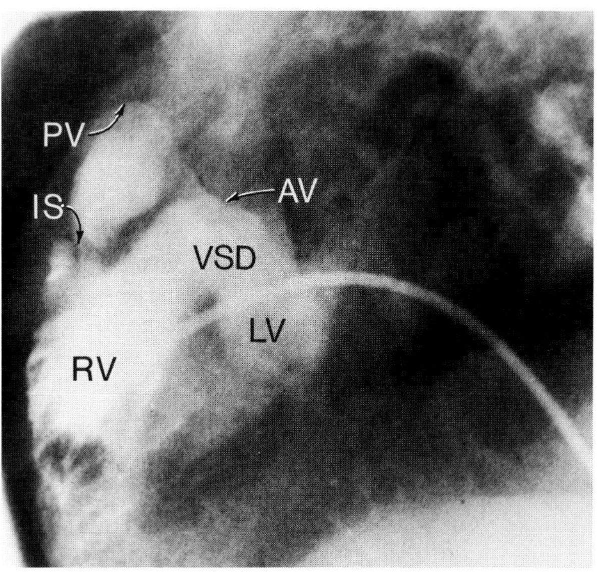

Fig. 39-12 Cineangiogram from a patient with tetralogy of Fallot. *PV,* pulmonary valve; *AV,* aortic valve; *IS,* infundibular stenosis; *VSD,* ventricular septal defect; *RV,* right ventricle; *LV,* left ventricle.

preserved and resection of right ventricular muscle minimized.[12] This is best accomplished by a limited incision in the right ventricular outflow tract and release of obstructing muscle bundles. If pulmonary valvar stenosis is present, a commissurotomy is performed. The incision is closed with a patch to widen the right ventricular infundibular diameter. The patch is confined to the subanular position unless the pulmonary valve anulus is hypoplastic.[10] In this situation, the patch must be extended across the valve ring. The ventricular septal defect is closed with a patch taking sutures on the right ventricular side of the septum. Care must be taken when suturing along the inferior rim of the defect to avoid injuring the conduction tissue. Exposure of the VSD is nearly always possible through the tricuspid valve. This allows the surgeon to minimize the right ventricular incision, confining it to only the length necessary to relieve the outflow tract obstruction.

The operative mortality for repair of tetralogy of Fallot is 5% or less. Symptomatic results are excellent, although patients must be followed up for the development of late ventricular dysfunction and arrhythmias.[22,23]

INADEQUATE MIXING

Transposition of the Great Arteries

In transposition of the great arteries (TGA), two separate independent circulations—systemic and pulmonary—are present. In the simplest form of TGA, the aorta arises from the right ventricle and receives the desaturated systemic venous return and the pulmonary artery arises from the left ventricle and receives oxygenated pulmonary venous blood (Fig. 39-13). Some exchange of blood between the two circulations (mixing) must be present to sustain life. This most commonly occurs by means of an interatrial communication allowing saturated blood to pass from the left to the right atrium and then to the right ventricle and aorta. An equal amount of desaturated blood must pass from right to left atrium to reach the pulmonary circulation. The adequacy of this mixing determines the amount of saturated venous blood reaching the aorta (effective systemic blood flow) and desaturated venous blood reaching the pulmonary artery (effective pulmonary blood flow) and thus the clinical status of the infant.

Even with adequate intracardiac mixing, the newborn with TGA is noticeably cyanotic. Quite often the interatrial defect is restrictive, and profound cyanosis is detected within hours of birth. Arterial Po_2 may be below 25 to 30 mm Hg, and progressive acidosis over the first days of life can occur. The clinical presentation is also influenced by the presence of associated lesions. In approximately 10% of cases, a large ventricular septal defect or hemodynamically significant pulmonary stenosis is present. When only the ventricular septal defect is present, cyanosis is lessened because mixing occurs at both the atrial and ventricular levels. However, since total pulmonary blood flow is elevated further, severe congestive heart failure usually results. If pulmonary stenosis is also present, volume overload is reduced, tending to lessen the effect of the ventricular septal defect. When pulmonary stenosis is particularly severe, with or without a ventricular septal defect, total pulmonary blood flow may be reduced below normal and cyanosis worsened. Finally, communication between the two circulations may also occur from a patent ductus arteriosus. Similar to the situation with a large ventricular septal defect, both effective and total pulmonary blood flow are increased, improving oxygenation but resulting in congestive heart failure.

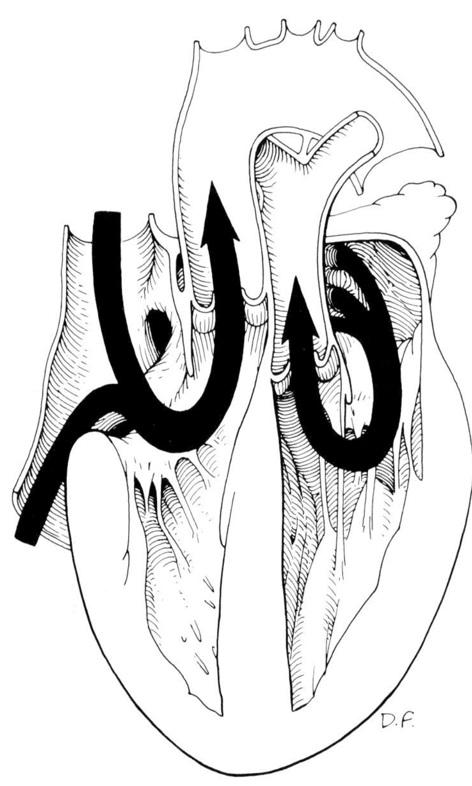

Fig. 39-13 Anatomy of transposition of the great arteries. The aorta arises from the right ventricle, and the pulmonary artery from the left ventricle.

The initial treatment of an infant with TGA is aimed at improving the intracardiac mixing by enlarging the atrial septal defect. This is performed in the cardiac catheterization laboratory after the diagnosis is established. The procedure, known as balloon atrial septostomy and originated by William Rashkind in 1966, involves passage of a balloon-tipped catheter from the right to the left atrium across the foramen ovale. Once the catheter tip is positioned in the left atrium, the balloon is inflated and the catheter forcibly withdrawn to tear a portion of the atrial septum. This procedure is repeated two or three times to ensure a wide patency in the septum. Prompt improvement in arterial oxygenation is usually noted immediately following the septostomy. When balloon atrial septostomy is unsuccessful or is performed on children older than 1 to 2 months where the thickness of the septum will not lend itself to balloon atrial septostomy, enlargement of the septal defect by an operative procedure devised by Blalock and Hanlon in 1950 may be indicated. The procedure does not require cardiopulmonary bypass and is done by removing a portion of atrial septum from the interatrial groove above the right pulmonary veins.

A few neonates may continue to have unsatisfactory oxygenation even with a large atrial septal defect.[31] The poor mixing in these cases may be caused by failure of the pulmonary vascular resistance to fall to its normally low levels after birth. The diastolic compliance of the two ventricles remains about equal, and no mixing of blood between the two sides occurs. When this is coupled with closure of the ductus arteriosus, effective pulmonary blood flow may be very poor. This situation may be temporarily treated with the administration of a prostaglandin infusion, maintaining ductal patency and allowing mixing at the great vessel level.[6,28] This restores satisfactory oxygenation for a few days until pulmonary vascular resistance falls.

When TGA is associated with a large ventricular septal defect, significant congestive heart failure and pulmonary hypertension may be apparent very early in life. Banding of the main pulmonary artery to reduce pulmonary blood flow and pressure may be indicated. This procedure, however, invariably results in a drop in arterial Po^2 because pulmonary blood flow is reduced by the band. An adequate interatrial communication is mandatory. Where significant pulmonary hypertension is present, treatment should be done before 3 months of age or pulmonary vascular occlusive disease may result. If severe pulmonary stenosis is present and pulmonary blood flow and pressure are below normal, a systemic artery–to–pulmonary artery shunt (Blalock-Taussig) may be performed.

Correction of TGA may be performed at the atrial, ventricular, or great vessel level, depending on the exact anatomy and associated defects. Most commonly, physiologic correction is achieved at the atrial level by redirecting venous inflow. This technique was first successfully performed by Senning in 1959 and revised by Mustard in 1964. Mustard's procedure involves complete removal of the atrial septum followed by the placement of a "baffle" (usually pericardium) to repartition the atria (Fig. 39-14). Vena cava blood drains behind the baffle to the mitral valve, left ventricle, and pulmonary artery, and the pulmonary veins drain to the tricuspid valve and then to the systemic circulation through the right ventricle. In the Senning procedure, very little prosthetic material is used because redirection of venous inflow is done using the patient's own atrial tissue. Although more difficult to perform, Senning's operation may allow better growth and function of the atrial chambers. The operative mortality for both procedures is low (<5%), even in infancy, and long-term results are good.[5] Significant technical complications such as obstruction to caval (usually superior vena cava) or pulmonary venous flow have been largely overcome and are now uncommon.[44] Troublesome atrial arrhythmias continue to be a problem, but their incidence has also been reduced with current surgical techniques designed to avoid injury to the SA node (and its artery) and the AV node.

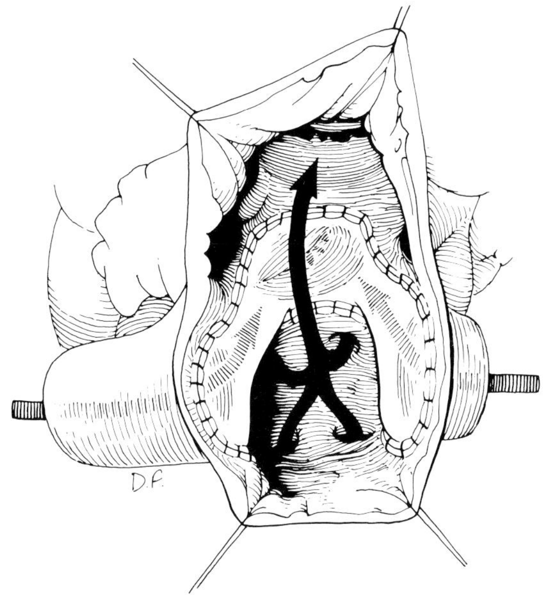

Fig. 39-14 Appearance of the atrial baffle in the Mustard procedure. Superior and inferior vena cava blood passes behind the patch to the mitral valve. The pulmonary venous blood passes over the patch to the tricuspid valve.

The major long-term difficulty with either the Mustard or Senning procedure is the possible failure of the right ventricle to perform at systemic workloads for long periods of time.[7] Late congestive heart failure, often with tricuspid insufficiency, has been recognized in a small percentage of children. Careful studies of right ventricular function late after repairs have shown impaired performance even in asymptomatic patients. The exact cause remains unclear. Most children, however, enjoy excellent long-term results after Mustard or Senning operations.

The arterial repair of TGA has the benefit of restoring the left ventricle as the systemic pump.[25] Although early operative mortality was quite high, current techniques have reduced the risk to acceptable levels. In addition to the aorta and pulmonary artery being relocated, the coronary arteries must be transferred to the posterior great vessel (neo-aorta) (Fig. 39-15). Successful performance of this procedure seems to require that the left ventricle be prepared to pump against systemic resistance. Patients with TGA and a large ventricular septal defect retain high pressure in the left ventricle and are ideal candidates for arterial repair. Banding of the pulmonary artery to raise left ventricular pressure in patients with TGA and intact ventricular septum has been advocated to prepare the left ventricle for an arterial switch procedure.[45] When arterial repair is done within the first month of life, however, preliminary banding is unnecessary.

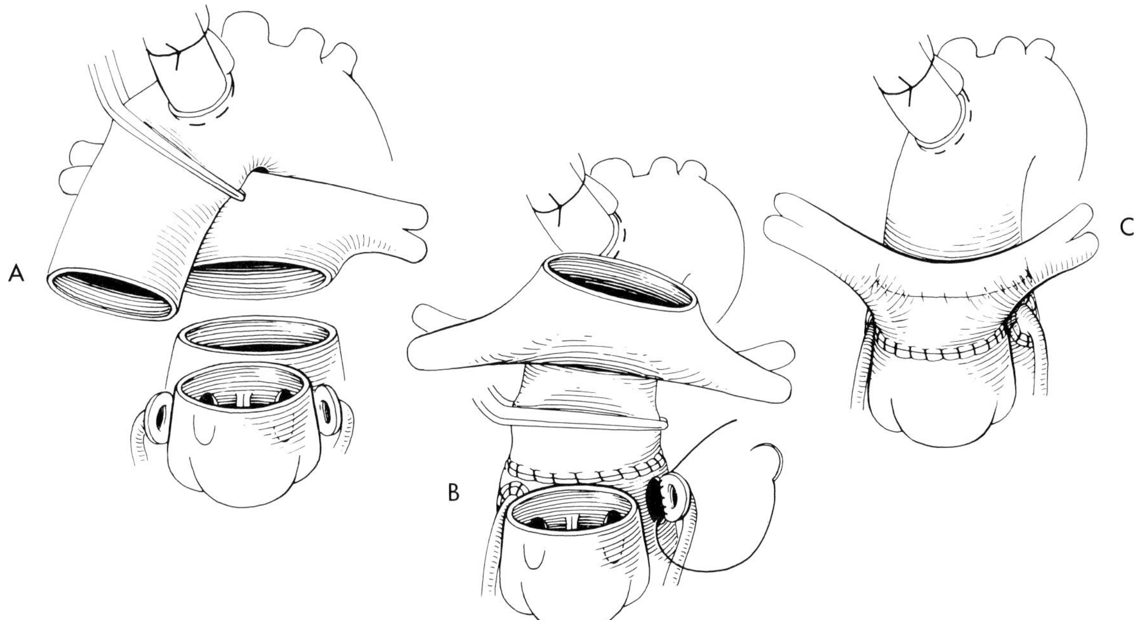

Fig. 39-15 Steps in the performance of the arterial switch procedure. **A,** The pulmonary artery is transsected just proximal to its bifurcation. The aorta is transsected at the same level. The coronaries are removed with wide buttons of adjacent aorta. **B,** The distal aorta is brought behind the pulmonary artery confluence and anastomosed to the proximal pulmonary artery. The coronary arteries are then relocated to the new aorta. **C,** The right ventricular outflow tract is reconstructed by anastomosing the distal pulmonary artery confluence to the proximal aorta.

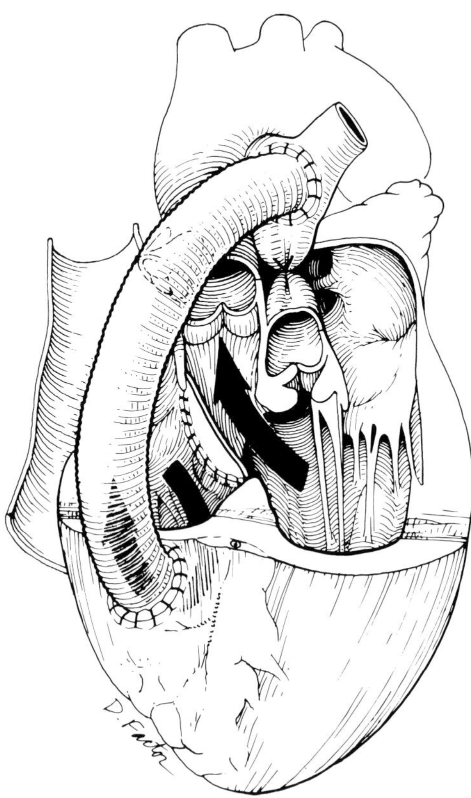

Fig. 39-16 Repair of transposition of the great arteries with ventricular septal defect and pulmonary stenosis. The defect is patched to place both great vessels in continuity with the left ventricle. The pulmonary artery is ligated proximally. The right ventricle is then connected to the distal pulmonary artery with a valved conduit.

In those patients with TGA, large ventricular septal defect, and left ventricular outflow tract obstruction (pulmonary stenosis), repair can be carried out at both the ventricular and great vessel levels. The ventricular septal defect is closed in a way that diverts left ventricular blood through the defect into the aorta (Fig. 39-16). The main pulmonary artery is ligated and the right ventricle then connected to the pulmonary artery bifurcation with a valved extracardiac conduit. The left ventricle is restored as the systemic pump, and the coronary arteries do not require relocation.[32]

SUMMARY

Successful surgical treatment of most forms of congenital heart disease is now possible. However, the surgeon must be knowledgeable in more than just cardiac anatomy to achieve this success. In particular, a thorough understanding of cardiac physiology in infants and children is essential so that a well-conceived treatment plan can be devised even for the most complex of anomalies. In some cases, one or more palliative procedures may be necessary, either because no definitive repair is ultimately possible or because it is best postponed until the patient is older. These procedures must provide satisfactory immediate palliation and, in addition, ensure that ultimate repair can be performed with the lowest possible risk.

Early corrective surgery, now routinely performed for many defects, is expected to significantly reduce the associated complications of congenital heart disease. The elimination of pulmonary vascular disease, chronic cyanosis, and long-standing congestive heart failure are only a few examples of the advantages of early correction. However, examining the benefits of surgical repair in light of the late results is increasingly important. The development of ventricular dysfunction or electrophysiologic abnormalities are examples of potentially serious consequences that may detract from an apparent early success. In some cases, a number of late studies have led to alterations in surgical technique designed to better maintain excellent long-term functional results. These evaluations will serve as a stimulus for cardiac surgeons to continue to strive for improvement in the treatment of congenital heart disease.

SUGGESTED READINGS

1. Keith, J.D., Rowe, R.D., and Vlad, P., editors: Heart disease in infancy and childhood, ed. 3, New York, 1978, Macmillan, Inc.
2. Rudolf, A.M., editor; Congential diseases of the heart, Chicago, 1974, Year Book Medical Publishers, Inc.
3. Stark, J., and de Leval, M., editors: Surgery for congenital heart defects, London, 1983, Grune & Stratton, Inc.

REFERENCES

1. Ankeney, J.L., Tzeng, T.S., and Liebman, J.: Surgical therapy for congenital aortic valvular stenosis, J. Thorac. Cardiovasc. Surg. **85**:41, 1983.
2. Arciniegas, E., et al.: Surgical closure of ventricular septal defect during the first twelve months of life, J. Thorac. Cardiovasc. Surg. **80**:921, 1980.
3. Arciniegas, E .: et al.: Results of the Mustard operation for dextrotransposition of the great arteries, J. Thorac. Cardiovasc. Surg. **81**:580, 1981.
4. Arciniegas, E., et al.: Classic shunting operations for congenital cyanotic heart defects, J. Thorac. Cardiovasc. Surg. **84**:88, 1982.
5. Barratt-Boyes, B.G., et al.: Repair of ventricular septal defect in the first two years of life using profound hypothermia-circulatory arrest techniques, Ann. Surg. **184:** 376, 1976.
6. Benson, L.N., et al.: Role of prostaglandin E_1 infusion in the management of transposition of the great arteries, Am. J. Cardiol. **44**:691, 1979.
7. Benson, L.N., et al.: Assessment of right ventricular function during supine bicycle exercise after Mustard's operation, Circulation **65**:1052, 1981.
8. Bergdahl, L., Bjork, V.O., and Jonasson, R.: Surgical correction of coarctation of the aorta, J. Thorac. Cardiovasc. Surg. **85**:532, 1983.
9. Bjornstad, P.G., et al.: Aortoventriculoplasty for tunnel subaortic stenosis and other obstructions of the left ventricular outflow tract, Circulation **60**:59, 1979.
10. Blackstone, E.H., Kirklin, J.W., and Pacifico, A.D.: Decision-making in repair of tetralogy of Fallot based on intraoperative measurements of pulmonary arterial outflow tract, J. Thorac. Cardiovasc. Surg. **77**:526, 1979.
11. Blalock, A., and Taussig, H.B.: The surgical treatment of malformations of the heart, JAMA **128**:189, 1945.
12. Bove, E.L., et al.: The influence of pulmonary insufficiency on ventricular function following repair of tetralogy of Fallot, J. Thorac. Cardiovasc. Surg. **85**:691, 1983.
13. Bove, E.L., et al.: Subclavian-pulmonary artery shunts with polytetrafluoroethylene interposition grafts, Ann. Thorac. Surg. **37**:88, 1984.
14. Castaneda, A.R., et al.: Repair of tetralogy of Fallot in infancy, J. Thorac. Cardiovasc. Surg. **74:** 372, 1977.
15. Craig, R.J., and Selzer, A.: Natural history and prognosis of atrial septal defect, Circulation **37**:805, 1968.
16. de Brux, J.L., et al.: Tricuspid atresia, J. Thorac. Cardiovasc. Surg. **48**:378, 1978.
17. de Leval, M.R., et al.: Modified Blalock-Taussig shunt, J. Thorac. Cardiovasc. Surg. **81**:112, 1981.

18. Dick, M., Fyler, D.C., and Nadas, A.S.: Tricuspid atresia: clinical course in 101 patients, Am. J. Cardiol. **36:**327, 1975.
19. Freed, M.D., et al.: Exercise-induced hypertension after surgical repair of coarctation of the aorta, Am. J. Cardiol. **43:**253, 1979.
20. Freed, M.D., et al.: Prostaglandin E_1 in infants with ductus arteriosus–dependent congenital heart disease, Circulation **64:**899, 1981.
20a. Fontan, F., and Baudet, S.: Surgical repair of tricuspid atresia, Thorax **26:**240, 1971.
21. Fontan, F., et al.: Repair of tricuspid atresia in 100 patients, J. Thorac. Cardiovasc. Surg. **85:**647, 1983.
22. Fuster, V., et al.: Long-term evaluation (12 to 22 years) of open heart surgery for tetralogy of Fallot, Am. J. Cardiol. **46:**635, 1980.
23. Garson, A., et al.: Status of the adult and adolescent after repair of tetralogy of Fallot, Circulation **59:**1232, 1979.
24. Hairston, P., et al.: The adult atrial septal defect: results of surgical repair, Ann. Surg. **179:**799, 1974.
25. Jatene, A.D., et al.: Anatomic correction of transposition of the great vessels, J. Thorac. Cardiovasc. Surg. **72:**364, 1976.
25a. Heath, D., and Edwards, J.E.: The pathology of hypertensive pulmonary vascular disease: a description of six grades of structural changes in the pulmonary arteries with special reference to congenital cardiac septal defects, Circulation **18:**533, 1958.
26. Jones, M., Barnhart, G.R., and Morrow, A.G.: Late results after operations for left ventricular outflow tract obstruction, Am. J. Cardiol. **50:**569, 1982.
27. Kirklin, J.W., et al.: Routine primary repair vs. two-stage repair of tetralogy of Fallot, Circulation **60:**373, 1979.
28. Lang, P., et al.: Use of prostaglandin E_1 in infants with d-transposition of the great arteries and intact ventricular septum, Am. J. Cardiol. **44:**76, 1979.
29. Lincoln, C., et al.: Transatrial repair of ventricular septal defects with reference to their anatomic classification, J. Thorac. Cardiovasc. Surg. **74:**183, 1977.
30. Losay, J., et al.: Repair of atrial septal defect primum, J. Thorac. Cardiovasc. Surg. **75:**248, 1978.
31. Mair, D.D., and Ritter, D.F.: Factors influencing systemic arterial oxygen saturation in complete transposition of the great arteries, Am. J. Cardiol. **31:**742, 1973.
32. Marcelletti, C., et al.: The Rastelli operation for transposition of the great arteries, J. Thorac. Cardiovasc. Surg. **72:**427, 1976.
33. Milo, S., et al.: Surgical anatomy and atrioventricular conduction tissues of hearts with isolated ventricular septal defects, **79:**244, 1980.
34. Norman, J.C., Nihill, M.R., and Cooley, D.A.: Valved apico-aortic composite conduits for left ventricular outflow tract obstructions, Am. J. Cardiol. **45:**1265, 1980.
35. Parker, F.B., et al.: Preoperative and postoperative renin levels in coarctation of the aorta, Circulation **66:**513, 1982.
36. Quaegebeur, J.M., Rohmer, J., and Brom, A.G.: Revival of the Senning operation in the treatment of transposition of the great arteries, Thorax **32:**517, 1977.
37. Rizzoli, G., et al.: Incremental risk factors in hospital mortality rate after repair of ventricular septal defect, J. Thorac. Cardiovasc. Surg. **80:**494, 1980.
38. Sade, R.M., Taylor, R.M., and Chariker, E.P.: Aortoplasty compared with resection for coarctation of the aorta in young children, Ann. Thorac. Surg. **28:**346, 1979.
39. Sanders, S.P., et al.: Clinical and hemodynamic results of the Fontan operation for tricuspid atresia, Am. J. Cardiol. **49:**1733, 1982.
40. Sandor, C.G.S., et al.: Long-term follow-up of patients after valvotomy for congenital valvular aortic stenosis in children, J. Thorac. Cardiovasc. Surg. **80:**171, 1980.
41. Saw, H.S., et al.: A guideline to the management of patent ductus arteriosus in infants and children, Aust. N.Z. J. Surg. **48:**378, 1978.
42. Shem-Tov, A., et al.: Clinical presentation and natural history of mild discrete subaortic stenosis, Circulation **66:**509, 1982.
43. St. John Sutton, M.G., Tajik, A.J., and McGoon, D.C.: Atrial septal defect in patients ages 60 years or older: operative results and long-term postoperative follow-up, Circulation **64:**402, 1981.
44. Trusler, G.A., et al.: Current results with the Mustard operation in isolated transposition of the great arteries, J. Thorac. Cardiovasc. Surg. **80:**381, 1980.
45. Yacoub, M., et al.: Clinical and hemodynamic results of the two-stage anatomic correction of simple transposition of the great arteries, Circulation **62**(suppl. I):I190, 1980.

40 *William E. Walker*
Acquired Cardiac Disorders

Cardiovascular physiology is in many ways easier to understand than that of other body systems, since it involves the principles of fluid dynamics, well known to all students of general physical sciences. The essential end-result of cardiovascular function is cellular homeostasis, which requires an adequate flow of blood through tissues. This blood flow allows the transfer of various substances, including oxygen, nutrients, hormones, and drugs from blood to the cells of all of the body systems and the simultaneous removal of the end-products of metabolism.

CARDIOVASCULAR SYSTEM

The cardiovascular system includes a pump, the heart, and an array of blood vessels that carry blood from the heart to the tissues and subsequently return it to the heart following the exchange processes that occur in the various capillary beds. Large arteries function mainly as conduits to the periphery. The important function of the arterioles is to change their diameter; this affects both the arterial blood pressure and the relative amount of blood flow to different vascular beds. The veins and venules not only carry blood back to the heart from the periphery but also can modify the amount of this return by changing their diameter. Control of the entire system is regulated at at least four levels: local neural reflexes, the central nervous system, the endocrine system, and finally direct local influences through a principle of flow known as "autoregulation."

Normal circulatory function requires an adequate availability of blood for the heart to pump (sometimes referred to as "venous return" and analogous to "preload" in muscle mechanics), a frequency of cardiac contraction within an acceptable range, an adequate strength of cardiac contraction (sometimes referred to as "myocardial contractility"), and a level of peripheral resistance or, more accurately, input impedance, since the flow is pulsatile rather than steady, analogous to "afterload" in muscle mechanics, within limits adequate to produce a "normal" arterial blood pressure necessary for perfusion of vital structures but not so high as to put undue strain on the heart or damage the arterial system.

Although normal atrial systole augments the cardiac output, it is not essential to an adequate level of circulatory function as demonstrated by patients with atrial fibrillation; thus "cardiac" function connotes ventricular function in virtually every clinical instance. Acquired disorders of cardiac function therefore are limited to intrinsic cardiac or extrinsic conditions producing abnormal ventricular loading, and the frequency of or strength of cardiac contraction. Although right ventricular failure has specific causes, clinical implications, and remedies, the vast majority of cases of "cardiac" failure relate to failure of left ventricular function.

This chapter outlines the common types of cardiovascular pathology, their associated physiologic defects, and the rationale behind their surgical treatment. The reader should bear in mind that each disorder disturbs the cardiovascular system by affecting the cardiac rate, cardiac pump function, or cardiac loading alone or in various combinations. Understanding the physiologic basis of these derangements allows the physician to evaluate optimally the clinical situation and predict most accurately the response to surgical therapy.

Cardiopulmonary Bypass[15,24,34,35]

Although "open-heart" surgery began in Minneapolis with the cross-circulation procedures of Lillihei, the development of effective cardiopulmonary bypass by Gibbon in Philadelphia was the essential step in making such procedures safe and commonplace. This apparatus draws venous blood from the right side of the heart, allows gas-exchange in an extracorporeal oxygenator, and pumps the resulting blood back into the arterial side of the circulation.

Cardiopulmonary bypass has three important attributes: it allows the surgeon to operate on a motionless heart emptied of blood; it maintains circulation to the rest of the body while the heart is stopped; and it provides for an autotransfusion system where spilt blood is recovered and returned to the patient through the oxygenator. Because of mechanical limitations of the system, a relatively low systemic blood flow (equivalent of "cardiac output") and mean arterial blood pressure are maintained on bypass, averaging 50 ml/kg/min and 40 to 60 mm Hg, respectively. Much has been made of the fact that arterial blood flow from the pump is nonpulsatile, but various attempts at producing pulsatile blood flow have failed to effect significant clinical benefits in patients.

Three additional facets of routine cardiopulmonary bypass contribute to postoperative physiologic derangements: anticoagulation, hemodilution and hypothermia. The coagulability of blood must be obviated completely to avoid thrombosis of blood in the oxygenator, plastic bypass circuitry, and reservoir, as well as thrombosis of blood left lying occasionally in the pericardium or pleural space. The anticoagulation is established by the adminstration of heparin (3 mg/kg) just before the establishment of bypass; the level of anticoagulation can be monitored by the activated clotting time, and additional doses of heparin given as necessary. When the procedure is complete and the cannulae have been removed from the aorta and right atrium, the heparin is reversed with protamine, 1.5 to 2 mg for each milligram of heparin. Despite this reversal of heparin, bleeding tends to be pronounced, caused by a combination of platelet loss and dysfunction, sequestration of some essential clotting factors in the bypass circuitry, and possible continuing hypothermia. The platelet count, prothrombin time, and partial thromboplastin time are all abnormal in the immediate postoperative period, but specific blood component therapy is not required unless bleeding is profuse. The diffuse capillary "ooze" present before the chest is closed in many patients is unimportant in itself since it will stop in a few hours; its importance is the fact that it can mask the origin of significant bleeding from a small artery or vein. Such bleeding may not stop with time and may necessitate a reexploration of the patient.

The pump apparatus is primed with 1500 to 2000 ml of lactated Ringer's solution, and, when this is mixed with the patient's blood, considerable hemodilution occurs. This electrolyte priming reduces the need for blood transfusion with its associated infectious and immunologic hazards. The hemodilution itself is helpful because it reduces the blood's viscosity and thereby promotes effective tissue blood flow, threatened both by hypothermia and by the nonpulsatile, low-pressure flow described above. As the operation proceeds, the patient may "take up" fluid from the circulating prime as edema, and more electrolyte solution is added to the prime to compensate for this. Finally, at the end of bypass, all of the prime in the bypass apparatus is returned to the patient, further increasing the electrolyte and water load. The end-result of all of this is that the patient tends to accumulate fluid both during the pump run and in the immediate postoperative period and this fluid must be dealt with or significant pulmonary edema, ascites, or peripheral edema may ensue and contribute to postoperative morbidity.

Moderate hypothermia (28° C) is used for most routine cardiac procedures, both to assist in keeping the heart cold during its arrest and to reduce tissue metabolic rates and thereby diminish the need for oxygen and substrate delivery. In the unlikely event of mechanical failure of some part of the bypass apparatus, even this level of hypothermia affords a considerably longer safe period for repair of the equipment. Normothermia is used for very short procedures such as single coronary bypass grafting or closure of atrial septal defects. More profound hypothermia (20° to 25° C) is used for very long procedures or those in whom obligatory cerebral ischemia is required, e.g., in those patients undergoing repair of aortic arch lesions. Cooling and rewarming are effected by use of the heat exchanger on the oxygenator, which works efficiently. The use of hypothermia contributes to the physiologic insult of cardiopulmonary bypass of producing redistributions of blood flow during cooling and rewarming, allowing for the possibility of reperfusion injury and acidosis. In addition, either cooling or rewarming can produce increased capillary permeability, leading to significant tissue edema and later to the need for excretion of the acquired extra fluid. In spite of rewarming on the pump, the hypothermia tends to recur following cessation of bypass, depressing cardiovascular function and contributing to the postbypass coagulopathy described above. It should be noted in passing that partial cardiopulmonary bypass is an excellent, controlled mode of rewarming for patients with accidental hypothermia or for those with significant hypothermia following resuscitation from major trauma.

One additional point of significance that merits emphasis about cardiopulmonary bypass is that the morbidity and mortality inherent in the technique, unrelated to the heart itself, are related exponentially to the time on bypass. The old axiom about the patient starting to die when he is put on the pump has more than a little truth to it. The cardiac surgeon cannot afford to be slow.

Myocardial Protection[8,16,17,32]

Of all the technical modifications that have been made in the actual conduct of cardiac surgery since the inception of cardiopulmonary bypass, none has affected morbidity and mortality as much as the widespread acceptance, approximately 10 years ago, of the need for careful myocardial protection during the obligatory period of ischemic cardiac arrest.

The essential step in the development of clinical myocardial protection was the technique that has come to be known as "cold cardioplegia"; i.e., when the aorta is cross-clamped to render the heart ischemic, a volume (usually 500 or 1000 ml) of cold (4° C), hyperkalemic (20 to 30 mEq/L) balanced salt solution is infused rapidly into the aortic root. Asystolic cardiac arrest ensues within a few seconds, and the myocardium is cooled uniformly. The effects of these two maneuvers (rapid arrest and cooling) are to retain maximal amounts of energy substrates in the myocardial cells for the maintenance of viability during ischemia and to reduce the metabolic rate significantly, thus using up less energy substrate. Systemic hypothermia contributes also, since inevitably some blood remains within the heart and the colder this is, the less rapid will be the tendency of the myocardial temperature to drift back towards normal.

The adoption of this technique reduced dramatically the mortality of any procedure requiring a period of "warm" ischemic arrest longer than about 30 minutes. This result is demonstrated best by the reduction in mortality of single valve replacement from 15% to 20% before cold cardioplegia to 1% to 2% after its routine use at most centers. Coronary bypass procedures were affected much less, since the old technique involved multiple, short periods (about 10 minutes) of warm arrest with normal perfusion between. This latter technique seems to work almost as well as a longer period of arrest protected by cold cardioplegia but is more time-consuming.

Although the two simple ideas of rapid cardiac arrest with potassium and profound myocardial cooling produced a dramatic improvement in the results of cardiac surgery, there has been considerable subsequent discussion of how to optimize the technique. Whether or not secondary administration of the cardioplegic solution at intervals during the arrest period and whether or not cold blood should be used as the cardioplegic solution continue to be tested. Other research has dealt with the addition of certain components to the cardioplegia solution such as magnesium, calcium-channel blockers, beta-blockers, vasodilators, and energy-related substrates such as glutamate. The difficulty in determining the possible benefit of these extra components is that the results are so good without any of these maneuvers that it has been hard to show any difference in patients, although results of animal experiments have been reported supporting each. These has been a growing recognition that the early reperfusion period on termination of arrest may be as important as the period of actual ischemia in affecting outcome, and the addition of free-radical scavengers to the infusate and postischemic energy substrate enhancement have shown considerable promise in this regard.

One other important aspect of myocardial protection must be mentioned, i.e., that the heart must be kept empty during the arrest period not only to prevent its rewarming but also to prevent cardiac chamber distention. The ventricles are highly sensitive to overdistention, and irrecoverable injury may occur rapidly; thus its occurrence constitutes an emergency requiring immediate attention. The situation is seen most often with cardiac asystole or ventricular fibrillation when there is aortic valve insufficiency, but other mechanisms can produce overdistention.

Although future investigative efforts may bring significant advances in the cardioplegic technique, the fact remains that iatrogenic myocardial injury is not a feature of current cardiac procedures unless the surgeon errs, with the exception of those few patients who have severe, preoperative left ventricular failure caused by acute myocardial infarction, or long-standing valvular dysfunction. It should not be forgotten, however, that this ischemic arrest period should be as short as possible without sacrificing the accuracy of the technical procedure.

Ischemic Heart Disease*

Atheromatous occlusive disease can affect virtually any major artery, but it has a certain predilection for the coronary arteries among others. Coronary artery occlusive disease produces a wide variety of clinical syndromes, but the combination of these syndromes is the major cause of morbidity and mortality in advanced societies. Accepted predisposing factors include cigarette smoking; hypertension; a history of the disease in young, male family members; diabetes mellitus; congenital hyperlipidemias; and chronic renal failure. Longitudinal epidemiologic studies of the disease such as the Framingham study have confirmed these associations but have now tended to discredit other factors such as uncomplicated obesity and a stressful lifestyle. It is unknown whether lifetime eating habits and regular exercise affect the development of the disease in later life; there is somewhat circumstantial evidence that they may. It can be said with certainty, however, at least in 1987, that there is little significant information suggesting that either dietary modification or exercise therapy has life-prolonging effects after the onset of symptoms.

A distinction in terminology should be made between ischemic heart disease, which has connotations of myocardial cellular dysfunction caused by ischemia (acute or chronic), and coronary artery occlusive disease, which may or may not produce myocardial ischemia. Approximately 99% of ischemic heart disease is produced by coronary artery occlusive disease, the remaining few cases being the result of coronary spasm (Prinzmetal's "variant" angina), coronary embolism, trauma, and occasionally collagen vascular diseases. The great majority of morbidity and mortality associated with coronary artery occlusive disease is caused by myocardial infarction; thus the therapeutic mechanisms prolonging life relate both to the prophylaxis and optimal management of acute myocardial infarction.

*References 6,7,18,20,29,37.

CLINICAL SYNDROMES IN ISCHEMIC HEART DISEASE

Asymptomatic
Sudden death syndrome
Chronic stable angina
Unstable angina
Acute myocardial infarction
Ventricular aneurysm
Chronic ischemic cardiomyopathy

Common clinical syndromes that are seen in patients with ischemic heart disease are listed in the boxed material above.

It is clear that a significant number of instances of myocardial ischemia, both those that are temporary and those that produce infarction, are "silent" or asymptomatic; i.e., patients either have strongly positive stress tests without symptoms in the presence of significant occlusive disease or present with clearly documented old myocardial infarctions, never having had chest pain. It is thought that approximately 30% of temporary ischemia and myocardial infarction is "silent."

Angina is a "crushing" precordial pain that may radiate into either arm or up into the neck but usually not through to the back and is produced regularly as the heart responds to the increased demands of exercise, emotion, cold, or eating a meal. The attacks last only a few minutes and resolve either spontaneously or in response to vasodilator therapy (sublingual nitroglycerin). Angina becomes "unstable" when it lasts longer, comes on with minimal stimulus, becomes more frequent, or becomes refractory to therapy. Unstable angina is a marker for early myocardial infarction and demands more urgent assessment and management than stable angina.

The management of patients with ischemic heart disease is predicated on an estimate of individual prognosis. Whereas in the past surgery was indicated because of intractable angina, this is now less common with the effective pharmacologic regimes available today; in most instances angina can be controlled adequately by a combination of vasodilators, beta-blockers, and calcium channel blockers such as nifedipine. The prognosis of any patient is related primarily to two factors: the extent and severity of the blockages of the coronary arteries and the function of the left ventricle; this latter consideration in most cases refers to whether or not the patient has had one or more prior myocardial infarctions.

Myocardial Infarction

Myocardial infarction is segmental myocardial necrosis produced by sudden occlusion of a major coronary artery. This occlusion is caused in 99% of instances by the super-

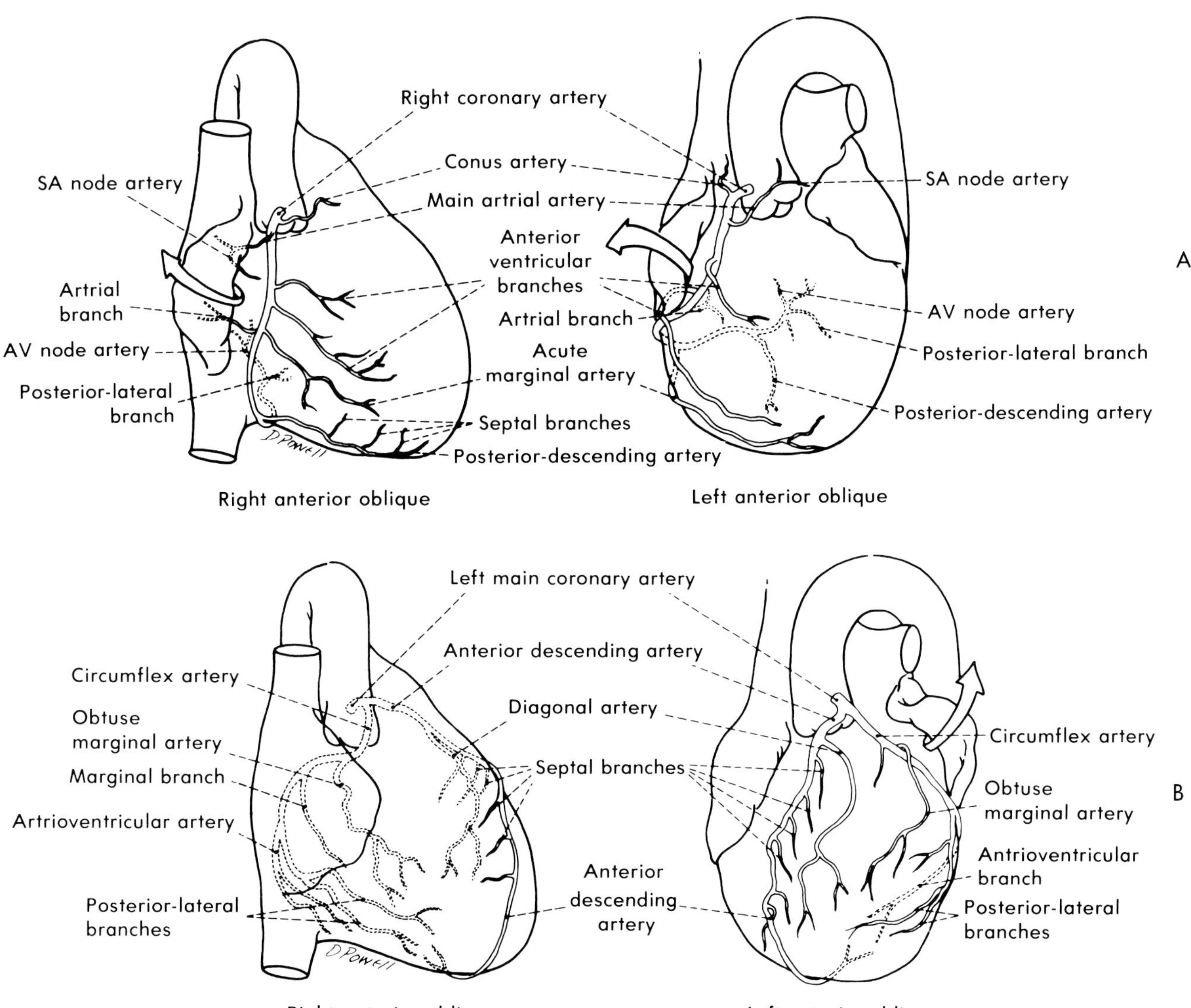

Fig. 40-1 **A,** Diagram of the right coronary arterial circulation in the right anterior oblique and left anterior oblique projections. **B,** Diagram of the left coronary arterial circulation in the right anterior oblique and left anterior oblique projections. (From Peter, R.H.: Coronary arteriography. In Sabiston, D.C., Jr., and Spencer, F.C., editors: Gibbon's surgery of the chest, ed. 4, Philadelphia, 1983, W.B. Saunders Co.)

imposition of an intravascular thrombosis at the site of a preexisting atheromatous plaque; this plaque usually, but not always, has already produced significant stenosis and the secondary development of collateral circulation to the myocardial segment supplied by the artery in question. The remaining 1% comprises conditions such as coronary spasm, embolism, and trauma. Thus a second pathologic process (thormbosis) produces myocardial infarction; the atheromatous plaque alone does not produce infarction; and the vast majority of patients with coronary artery occlusive disease will do well long-term, as long as myocardial infarction does not occur. Most myocardial infarctions involve the left ventricular myocardium, but occasionally occlusion of the right coronary artery may produce predominant right ventricular infarction, the treatment of which may be different (Fig. 40-1).

The significant early complications of myocardial infarction include malignant ventricular dysrhythmias; heart block; cardiogenic shock; and a group of problems, sometimes referred to as "disruptive myonecrosis," in which the infarcted myocardium actually ruptures, producing mitral insufficiency if the papillary muslce is involved, pericardial tamponade if the free wall is involved, or a ventricular septal defect with acute left-ro-right shunt if the interventricular septum is involved. Surgical therapy should be considered for all of these patients, since their outlook otherwise is very poor.

Late complications of myocardial infarction necessitating surgery include ventricular aneurysm, which is a saccular expansion of the infarction scar producing angina, congestive failure, dysrhythmias, and peripheral thromboembolism. Such aneurysms usually occur in anterior infarctions caused by occlusion of the left anterior descending artery proximal to its major diagonal and septal branches and perhaps in instances where there has been development of a collateral circulation.

Evaluation and Management

The workup of an otherwise healthy patient with typical angina, especially if "unstable," is now clear—early cardiac catheterization/coronary angiography, and consequent myocardial revascularization if indicated. If the symptoms are less clear or if there is only some strong marker of the disease, there are several levels of noninvasive tests available, each with its own degree of sensitivity and specificity.

There is thus a hierarchy of tests available for the evaluation of patients who may have coronary artery occlusive disease, as shown in the boxed material below.

Little reliance is now placed on a negative "resting" test, and stress tests are routine for asymptomatic patients, those with atypical chest pain, and occasionally those with angina. A positive stress test mandates left heart catheterization and coronary arteriography.

TESTS FOR ISCHEMIC HEART DISEASE

- Resting electrocardiogram
- Echocardiogram
- Resting MUGA*
- Exercise electrocardiogram
- Exercise thallium⁺
- Exercise MUGA
- PET‡ Scan with stress
- Cardiac catheterization

*MUGA, multiple uptake gated acquisition, is a radionuclide left ventriculogram; ejection fraction can be calculated with this technique.

⁺The exercise thallium test assays ischemic nonperfusion and subsequent reperfusion.

‡PET, positron emission tomography, a sensitive new test for measuring reduced perfusion during ischemia; a useful stressing agent is IV Persantine, a powerful coronary vasodilator.

Although there has been some controversy in the past, most enlightened groups dealing with large numbers of patients now recommend surgical revascularization to all patients with left main coronary stenosis, to those with significant disease in all three major coronary systems (left anterior descending, circumflex, and right), and to many of those with severe disease in two systems, especially after a myocardial infarction. Percutaneous transluminal coronary angioplasty (PTCA) is performed routinely on those with single-vessel disease, on some of those with double-vessel disease, especially in the absence of prior myocardial infarction, and even in some centers on those with disease of all three major systems.

Myocardial Revascularization

The essential factor permitting rational and directed repair of stenotic coronary arteries was selective coronary angiography developed by Sones at the Cleveland Clinic in 1958. Since the prognosis of ischemic heart disease is related not to the severity of symptoms, but to the extent of the coronary occlusive disease and functional state of the left ventricle, the use of coronary angiography to delineate the amount of disease present was critical in the assessment of future risks in the various subsets of patients (Fig. 40-2).

Although surgeons had been interested in operations for ischemic heart disease for over 50 years since such pi-

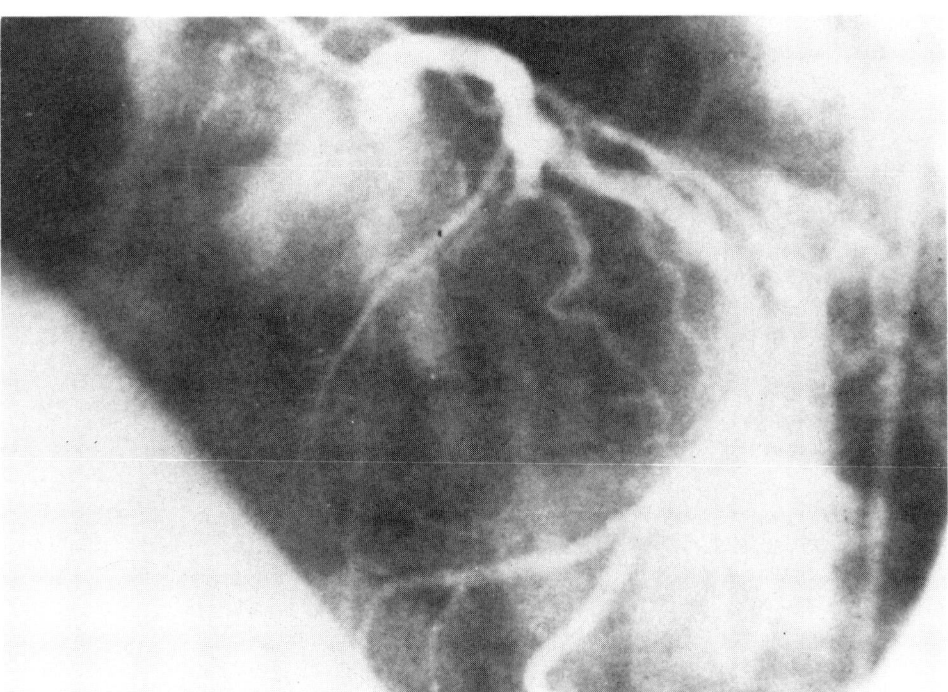

Fig. 40-2 Left anterior oblique view of coronary arteriogram following left coronary injection. Left anterior descending artery shows total occlusion with no collateral flow. Diagonal artery also has tight stenosis. (Reproduced with permission from Sellinger, S.L., et al.: Coronary bypass surgery in evolving acute myocardial infarction. In Roberts, A.J., editor: Difficult problems in adult cardiac surgery. Chicago, Copyright © 1985 by Year Book Medical Publishers, Inc.)

oneers as O'Shaughnessy and Beck attempted to induce collaterals to the myocardium across the pericardial space, it was not until 1967 that Favaloro,[7] again at the Cleveland Clinic, began the procedures that we now know as coronary bypass grafting. In the years preceding this, surgeons had attempted local repair of stenotic coronary arteries, and in retrospect it is unclear why the bypass principle, which was then available for larger peripheral arteries, had not been applied before. Suffice it to say that surgeons of the time, when asked, say they did not think the technique would work in such small vessels.

Coronary artery bypass grafting has become routine, with between 150,000 and 200,000 procedures carried out annually in the United States. Although in the past cardiac surgery tended to be limited to large centers and university hospitals, it is now clear that equally good or better results of coronary artery surgery can be obtained in "community" hospitals, as long as there is a high level of expertise in the various members of the surgical team. It is true, however, that there is a relationship between surgical mortality and number of procedures performed in a given institution; this was shown in the results of a Veterans' Administration study, in which there was an unacceptable surgical mortality rate in some of the participating hospitals which contributed very few patients. The risk of elective coronary grafting in the past few years has been in the order of 1%, although the mortality rate is now rising because of the willingness of cardiologists and surgeons to

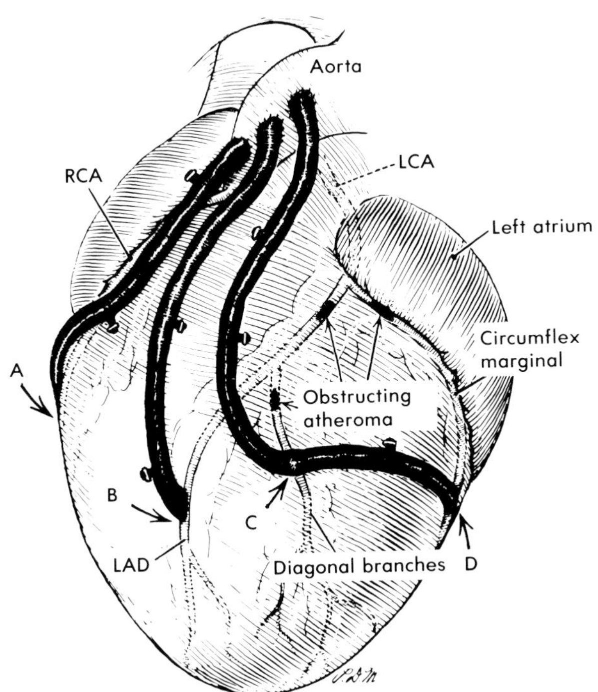

Fig. 40-3 Diagrammatic representation of quadruple coronary bypass graft operation using a saphenous vein showing sequential anastomatic graft from left circumflex marginal to left anterior descending *(LAD)* diagonal *(D* to *C) LAD* graft *(B)*, and right coronary artery *(RCA)* graft *(A)*. *LCA*, left coronary artery. (From Cohn, L.H.: Surgical techniques of emergency coronary revascularization. In Cohn, L.H., editor: The treatment of acute myocardial ischemia—an integrated medical/surgical approach, Mount Kisco, N.Y., 1979, Futura Publishing Co., Inc.)

submit older and more complicated patients to the procedure. Because of this, the comparison of survival statistics between different institutions has become extraordinarily difficult.

Two graft conduits comprise the vast majority of those used: the greater saphenous vein (Fig. 40-3) and internal mammary artery. Patency rates for these two conduits at 5 years have been 80% to 90% for the vein and 95% to 100% for the artery. This discrepancy in patency rates widens after about 10 years, when the veins begin to fail because of proliferative medial fibrosis and occasionally fatty plaques not unlike atheroma; whereas the mammary artery does not seem to be affected much be its translocation and maintains its lack of occlusive vascular disease even with the passage of time. Although both of these conduits have always been available and the increased patency rate of the mammary artery well known for some time, it is only recently that a study by Loop and associates[18] of Cleveland has suggested that long-term survival was improved by the use of the mammary artery. Because graft patency rates are related to the size and quality of the coronary artery grafted, it had always been assumed that the increased mammary patency related only to small coronary arteries, which are less important as effectors of survival. Most vein patency results were obtained before the advent of widespread use of antiplatelet agents such as aspirin and dipyridamole (Persantine), and it is possible that these drugs invalidate the apparent superiority of the mammary artery.

When mammary arteries and greater saphenous veins have not been available for whatever reason, surgeons have used the cephalic vein from the arm, the lesser saphenous vein, homograft veins, and even grafts of polytetrafluoroethylene. Although the letter two techniques have a great attraction because of simplicity, results with such conduits have clearly not been as satisfactory, with patency rates in the order of 50%.

Long-term results of the bypass graft procedures have been highly satisfactory for most groups of patients, at least up to ten years following surgery, with average survival rates being essentially "normal" at 90% and 80% for 5 and 10 years, respectively. These survival rates compare to 50% and 35% for patients with triple-vessel disease at 5 to 10 years with drug therapy alone and constitute the logical basis for recommending the operation. Whether or not the rampant, totally uncontrolled use of percutaneous transluminal coronary angioplasty (Figs. 40-4 and 40-5) by today's cardiologists and such projected techniques as laser angioscopy by the cardiologists of tomorrow will affect survival at all is unknown, and the fact remains that bypass surgery is the conservative approach to those with significant occlusive disease of their coronary arteries.

As more and more patients have survived long periods following successful bypass surgery, the need for second and even third bypass procedures has arisen, either because of progression of native coronary disease or because of degeneration of vein grafts. Although redo operations are harder for the surgeon, the results in otherwise satisfactory candidates have generally approximated those in patients on whom surgery is performed for the first time, with the exception of a slightly increased surgical mortal-

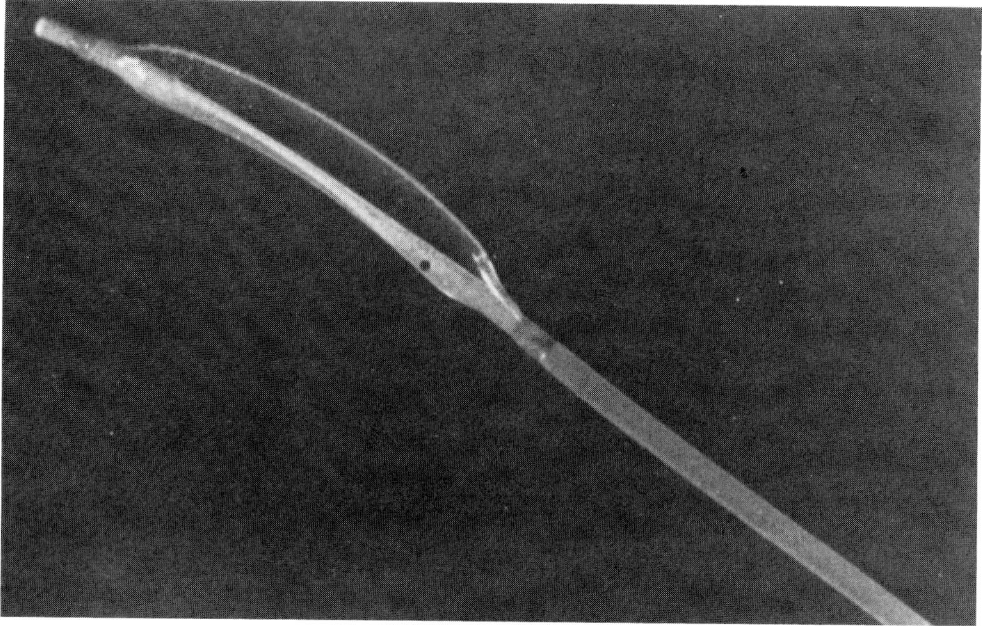

Fig. 40-4 USCI Gruntzig Dilaca coronary dilation catheter. The inflated balloon diameter varies from 2 to 3.7 mm. The balloon length is 12 mm. The catheter shaft size is No. 4 F with a length of 20 cm. (Reproduced with permission from Dorris, G., et al.: Percutaneous transluminal coronary angioplasty and its relationship to coronary artery bypass graft surgery. In Roberts, A.J., editor: Coronary artery surgery—application of new technologies, Chicago, Copyright © 1983 by Year Book Medical Publishers, Inc.)

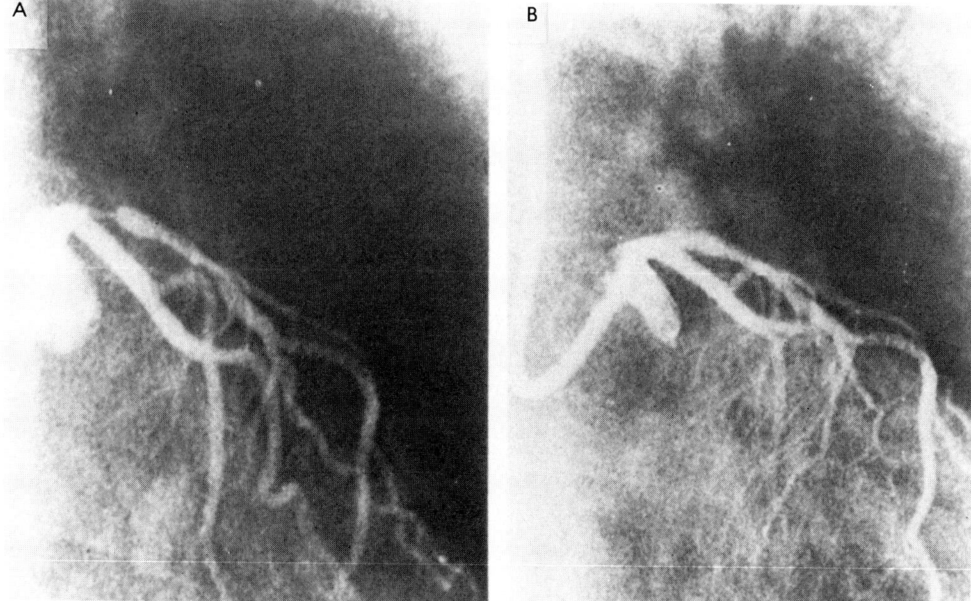

Fig. 40-5 **A,** Preangioplasty and **B,** postangioplasty coronary arteriograms obtained during a successful coronary dilation of a left anterior descending artery stenosis using a percutanous transluminal coronary angioplasty approach. (Reproduced with permission from Dorris, G., et al.: Percutaneous transluminal coronary angioplasty and its relationship to coronary artery bypass graft surgery. In Roberts, A.J., editors: Coronary artery surgery—application of new technologies, Chicago, Copyright © 1983 by Year Book Medical Publishers, Inc.)

ity. For whatever reason, the prediction that an ever-increasing number of patients would be returning for redo coronary bypasses has not come true, and this number has been fairly constant over the past few years. Such observations suggest that surgical techniques have indeed improved over the two decades that the procedure has been performed; this consideration, together with other factors such as antiplatelet agents and better drug therapy, may avoid large numbers of redo procedures in the future.

Emergency coronary bypass procedures are used universally for uncontrollable unstable angina, with results similar to elective procedures; but the use of routine emergency bypass in the first few hours of myocardial infarction has not gained widespread acceptance in spite of the excellent results reported from Spokane, Wash. and Des Moines, Iowa, for over 10 years. The survival rates reported from these two centers are vastly superior to those of medical treatment of myocardial infarction, and it is unclear whether cardiologists in other centers fail to refer patients for emergency bypass surgery out of ignorance, doubt over the veracity of the reported results, blind conservatism, or simply a mercenary reluctance to give up the patient's care.

Cardiac Replacement

Otherwise healthy patients with end-stage heart disease from atherosclerosis, like those with idiopathic cardiomyopathy, become candidates for cardiac replacement when no other treatment will suffice. Until now, cardiac transplantation has been much more successful than the permanent artificial heart, with rates of survival of 80% and 50% or better at 1 and 5 years, respectively. The use of cyclosporine as an immunosuppressive agents has lessened markedly the infectious complications and cost of the procedure. It is often a difficult decision in patients with severe heart disease whether or not to try some lesser procedure first, because of the difficulties of converting to a transplant should the first procedure not meet with success, although temporary artificial heart support can alleviate this problem somewhat. Apart from the cost, the limiting factor in transplantation so far has been donor availability. It remains to be seen whether the permanent artificial heart will have a useful role in the future.

SURGERY FOR CARDIAC DYSRHYTHMIAS*

Although most clinical texts on cardiology deal with disorders of cardiac "rhythm" rather than cardiac "rate," depression of cardiac output relates much more to the latter than to the former. The normal frequency of cardiac contraction in healthy persons in sinus rhythm can vary from 50 to 90 times per minute, depending largely on the state of physical conditioning, whereas those with superior athletic conditioning can have resting heart rates even lower.

In patients whose cardiovascular systems are otherwise normal, alterations of cardiac rate between 40 and 150 beats per minute can be asymptomatic, but symptoms will generally occur with exercise at these heart rates extremes or if there is other cardiovascular pathology. It is an apparent paradox that the management of myocardial ischemia in patients with normal heart rates includes beta-blockers to reduce the heart rate, but in those with slow heart rates management includes the implantation of a pacemaker to increase the heart rate.

Bradycardias

Types

The common causes of symptomatic bradycardia are:

1. Sick sinus syndrome
2. Congenital heart block
3. Acquired heart block
4. Iatrogenic heart block
5. Atrial fibrillation
6. Bradycardia-tachycardia syndrome

Complete heart block may be congenital and is generally asymptomatic and benign as long as the child's heart is otherwise structurally normal. Pacemakers may be required to allow maximal exercise during adolescence or young adulthood. Acquired heart block occurs most often in the elderly, usually in the presence of ischemic heart disease, but occasionally without it. The condition produces significant symptoms at rest or with minimal exercise and is one of the prominent causes of syncope ("Stokes-Adams attacks"); it also can cause sudden death by degeneration of the rhythm into asystole as a result of loss of the ventricular escape beats or ventricular fibrillation.

Patients with acute inferior myocardial infarction caused occlusion of the right coronary artery have a marked tendency for heart block. This is because the atrioventricular nodal artery is a branch of the right coronary at the crux of the heart and its occlusion or decompression produces ischemia and consequent dysfunction of the atrioventricular node. Patients with various grades of incomplete heart block in the context of inferior myocardial infarction are candidates for prophylactic temporary pacemakers, placed percutaneously through a subclavian or jugular vein. Swan-Ganz catheters with pacemaker electrodes incorporated are also available and may be placed in this situation. The heart block of acute myocardial infarction usually resolves, but permanent pacemaking is required if it does not.

Postoperative heart block is seen occasionally in patients undergoing repair of septal defects, valve replacement, or complex intra-atrial repair of congenital heart disease. Because this heart block may not occur immediately, temporary pacing wires are always placed in these patients at the time of surgery so that external pacing may be introduced rapidly if required. Even those patients who have a permanent pacemaker implanted at the time of cardiac surgery require temporary lead placement for easy manipulation of the heart rate in the immediate postoperative period.

The sick sinus syndrome denotes chronic sinus bradycardia, usually regular but occasionally irregular, which occurs in older patients with or without ischemic heart disease. With heart rates in the range of 30 to 40 beats per minute, the symptoms are essentially the same as those of complete heart block, although sudden death is much less likely. This syndrome now commonly requires permanent pacemaking; its use is perhaps more common than in cases of complete heart block.

---

*References 9,10,19,23,26, and 36.

Occasionally, patients with chronic atrial fibrillation have significant bradycardia requiring a pacemaker. Their bradycardia is not resolved by stopping the digoxin therapy, which they almost always are receiving, although it must be ascertained that they do not merely have digitalis toxicity before placing a pacemaker.

The final group requiring pacemaker therapy is that with the bradycardia-tachycardia syndrome. In these patients episodes of supraventricular tachycardia require digoxin prophylaxis, but for some reason in this group digoxin therapy produces profound, symptomatic bradycardia. To make possible the administration of digoxin doses sufficient to prophylax the tachycardia, a pacemaker must be placed.

Pacemaker Management Techniques

Permanent pacemakers were introduced approximately 30 years ago and were originally large and heavy; they were placed in the left chest through a formal thoracotomy, and pacing leads were sutured to the ventricular myocardium. The batteries were relatively short-lived, requiring replacement every year or two, and the lead systems were undependable. Current pacemakers approach the size and weight of a silver dollar, last up to 10 years on their lithium batteries, and have thoroughly dependable lead systems.

Two different methods of use are available: epicardial and endocardial. The epicardial approach uses a subxiphoid access to the pericardium, the lead is screwed into the undersurface of the right ventricle, and the battery box implanted subcutaneously in the left upper abdominal quadrant (Fig. 40-6). The technique is highly dependable, but requires general anesthesia for lead placement. The battery box may be replaced using local anesthesia. The endocardial approach uses a catheter system placed through the cephalic, subclavian, or either jugular vein, with the catheter tip being advanced and impacted into the apex of the right ventricle (see Fig. 40-6). The battery box is implanted in a subcutaneous pocket inferior to the clavicle. This approach is more time-consuming, less dependable, and has the potential hazard of perforating the right ventricle; but it requires only local anesthesia.

A wide selection of pacemakers that vary greatly in their levels of sophistication is now available. All are now of the "demand" type that fire only when they do not sense a QRS complex, and many can be programmed for such modalities as rate, size of electrical impulse, and sensing level after they have been implanted. There has also been a trend toward dual-chamber pacemakers that pace the atria and ventricles sequentially and to pacemakers that sense changes in the native sinus rate (e.g., in response to exercise) and change the rate of ventricular firing accordingly. These sophisticated systems are expensive and unnecessary in the vast majority of pacemaker candidates but can occasionally be beneficial in those with exercise intolerance or congestive cardiac failure.

Supraventricular Tachycardias

Recurrent episodes of supraventricular tachycardia can be caused by reentry of cardiac excitation impulses through an anomalous muscle bundle, the bundle of Kent, connecting the atrial and ventricular myocardia, which are normally electrically separate (Fig. 40-7). This is known as Wolff-Parkinson-White syndrome and is characterized electrocardiographically by the presence of a short PR interval and small "delta" waves at the beginning of the QRS complex. This bundle can occur anywhere in the atrioventricular groove or junction of the atrial and ventricular septa and can be mapped by the cardiologist in the laboratory. It is a relatively easy procedure for the surgeon

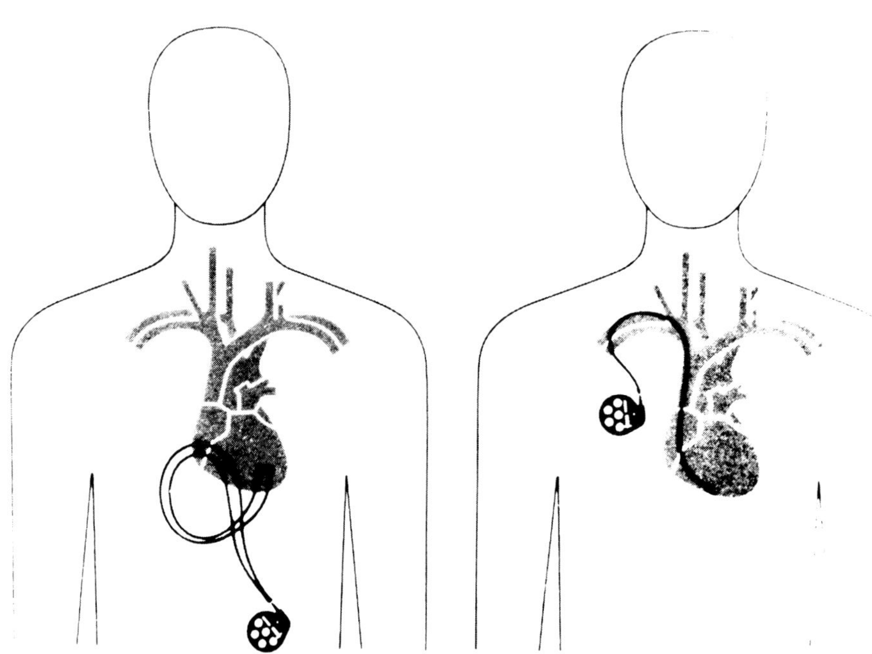

Fig. 40-6 Schematic representation of electrode configuration for permanent epicardial pacing *(left)* and perivenous endocardial pacing *(right)*. (Courtesy Medtronic Corporation.)

to divide the bundle with the use of cardiopulmonary bypass and ECG control, thus relieving the patient not only of real morbidity and potential mortality, but also obviating the need for lifelong antidysrhythmic drugs and their significant side effects. This treatment modality was introduced at Duke University in 1968, and the technique has now been extended to other mechanisms of tachycardia such as concealed accessory connections, nodal and atrial tachycardia, and even refractory atrial fibrillation. There is now also a place for cryoablation of some of these anomalous electrical pathways and other supraventricular tachycardia-producing phenomena; indeed not only can the surgeon do this in the operating room, but the cardiologist can cryoablate certain areas of the heart in the laboratory.

Ventricular Tachycardia

This dysrhythmia produces morbidity and mortality by rate-induced depression of cardiac output and be degeneration into ventricular fibrillation. Most patients with sustained ventricular tachycardia have significant ischemic heart disease and usually have had one or more myocardial infarctions, although the condition may be idiopathic or related to other forms of structural heart disease. Significant ventricular tachycardia is thought to occur in more than 5% of patients surviving myocardial infarction, and thus the problem is not as uncommon as might be supposed. It is estimated that about one third of patients with ventricular tachycardia cannot be controlled by the variety of antidysrhythmic drugs available today; these individuals are candidates for surgical therapy.

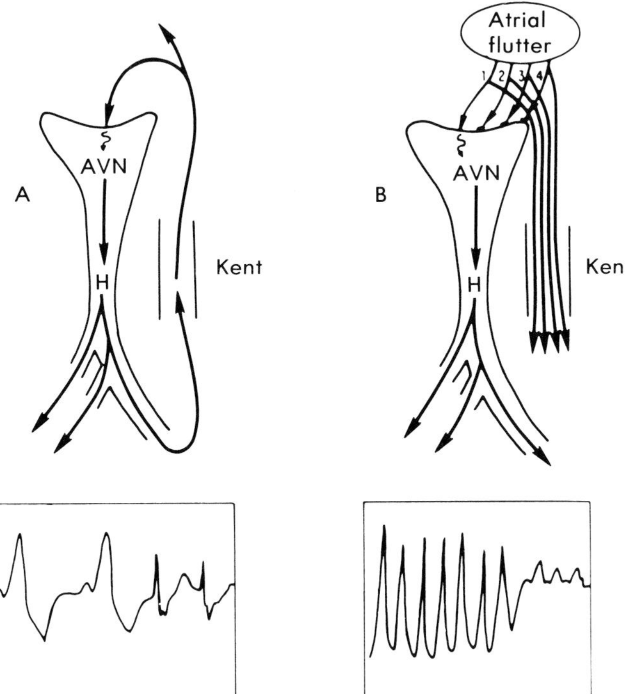

Fig. 40-7 Two tachycardias found in Wolff-Parkinson-White syndrome patients are shown. **A,** Reentry type. The wise QRS of preexcitation changes to a narrow QRS during the reentry tachycardia (*box*). **B,** Fast ventricular response during atrial flutter. The rhythm strip shows the rapid ventricular response progressing to ventricular fibrillation (*box*). (From Sealy, W.C., and Selle, J.G.: Surgical treatment of supraventricular arrhythmias. In Roberts, A.J., and Conti, C.R., editors: Current surgery of the heart, Philadelphia, 1987, J.B. Lippincott Co.)

Although coronary bypass surgery, resection of ventricular aneurysms, and valve replacement may relieve the patient of ventricular tachycardia, there has been a growing awareness of the need for a "directed" surgical approach. In this procedure the cardiologist accompanies the surgeon to the operating room, assisting in the accurate location of the area of the heart producing the dysrhythmia. This is accomplished by inducing ventricular tachycardia electrically and "mapping" the various areas of the epicardium and endocardium. The area in question often comprises subendocardial scar tissue; it is relatively easy to resect it locally or to try to isolate it electrically by an encircling incision. If the area involves vital structures such as the mitral apparatus, membranous septum, or aortic annulus, local cryoablation may be substituted.

Following these maneuvers, other needed procedures such as valve replacement and coronary bypass are performed. The risk of surgery is similar to that of other major cardiac procedures and relates prominently to the degree of left ventricular dysfunction present before surgery. Approximately 75% of survivors have either relief of their tachycardia without further drug therapy or a significant reduction in their drug requirements, and it seems that this form of treatment may be applicable to an ever-increasing group of patients in the future.

Implantable Defibrillator

Patients with chronic, recurrent ventricular fibrillation ("sudden death syndrome") are now candidates for implantation of an electronic device that senses the dysrhythmias and delivers an electric shock to reverse it. The device is similar in size to the original pacemakers, is implanted through power to sustain many cardioversions over a period of several-years. This is an expensive mode of therapy, but it may be worthwhile for certain high-risk individuals or for those proven unresponsive to pharmacologic or other surgical control.

VALVULAR HEART DISEASE*

The four major cardiac valves guard the inlets and outlets of the right and left ventricles, stopping the backward flow of blood through these areas in systole and diastole, respectively. The inlet valves, "tricuspid" on the right and "mitral" on the left, are both supported by muscles, the papillary muscles, the tendons (chordae tendineae) of which insert into the free edges of the valve leaflets; systolic contraction of the papillary muscles supports the atrioventricular valves and prevents their prolapse into the atria. The outlet or semilunar valves, "aortic" on the left and "pulmonary" on the right, each have three leaflets, the edges of which appose to each other during diastole, thereby preventing regurgitation from the outlet vessels to the ventricles.

In the absence of other diseases of the heart and pulmonary vascular system, the right-sided valves are not essential; and cardiac function, although far from normal, can sustain acceptable outputs after the loss, from disease

*References 1,2,4,5,11,14,17,21,30, and 31.

or at surgery, of one or both of the tricuspid and pulmonary valves. In the presence of an elevated pulmonary vascular resistance or other cause of pulmonary hypertension, however, the loss of right-sided valve function will require surgical restoration of valvular competence for acceptable levels of cardiac function.

Valvular dysfunction consists either of obstruction to blood flow through the valve, usually termed "stenosis," (e.g., mitral stenosis), or of regurgitation of blood through the valve during that part of the cardiac cycle when the valve should be closed, normally termed "insufficiency" or "regurgitation" (e.g., mitral insufficiency or regurgitation). Stenosis of the outflow valve increases afterload on the ventricle, whereas insufficiency of either inflow or outflow valve increases preload.

The vast majority of clinically important valvular dysfunctions comprise problems with the left-sided valves. Acquired diseases of the right-sided valves are very uncommon and for practical purposes are restricted to insufficiency of the tricuspid valve caused by chronic right ventricular overload from left-sided cardiac disease or to acute or subacute bacterial endocarditis. Tricuspid valve stenosis can occur in rheumatic heart disease, and the peculiar association of pulmonary valve stenosis with the carcinoid syndrome is widely known but clinically rare.

Types

Mitral Stenosis

When rheumatic fever and its associated pancarditis were common before the advent of antibiotics, mitral stenosis was the most important clinical valvular heart disease, and even today in underdeveloped countries it continues to be prevalent. The healing response to the immune-related endocarditis produced fibrosis not only of the valve leaflets but also of the chordae tendineae, normally over a period of many years after the acute illness. This restricts valve motion, and, in addition, fusion of the valve commissures occurs, reducing further the effective valve orifice. The consequent reduction in effort-induced increases in cardiac output and in pulmonary hypertension lead to a clinical picture of chronic dyspnea and exercise intolerance, which if untreated progresses to dyspnea at rest and paroxysmal noctural dyspnea. Atrial fibrillation intervenes commonly, worsening the functional deficit, and sets up the possibility of mural thrombus formation and subsequent thromboembolism from the left atrium.

The management of mitral stenosis depends purely on the degree of symptomatology; i.e., when the patient has

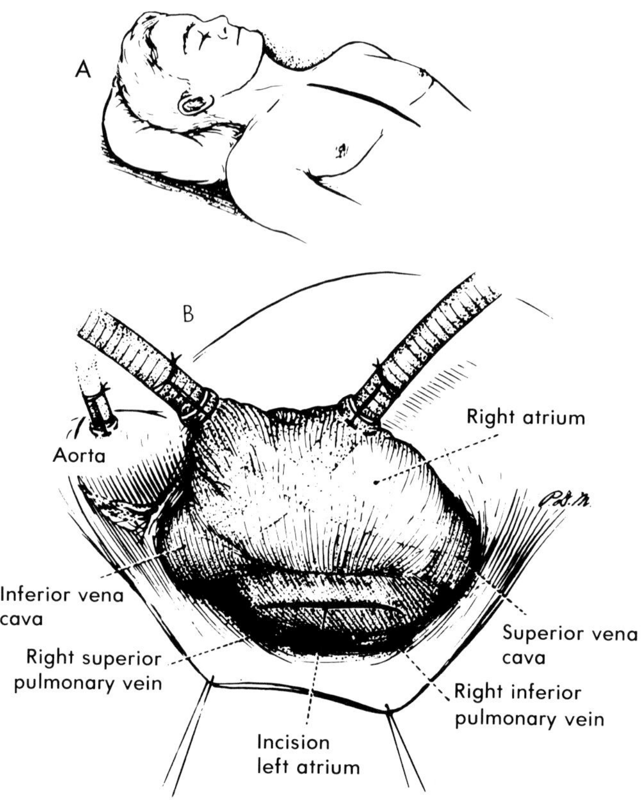

Fig 40-8 **A,** Median sternotomy incision. **B,** Cannulation technics for cardiopulmonary bypass and incision used to open the left atrium. (From DiSesa, V.J., Collins, J.J., Jr., and Cohn, L.H.: Mitral valve replacement with the porcine bioprosthesis. In Ionescu, M.I., and Cohn, L.H., editors: Mitral valve disease, London, 1985, Butterworth and Co.)

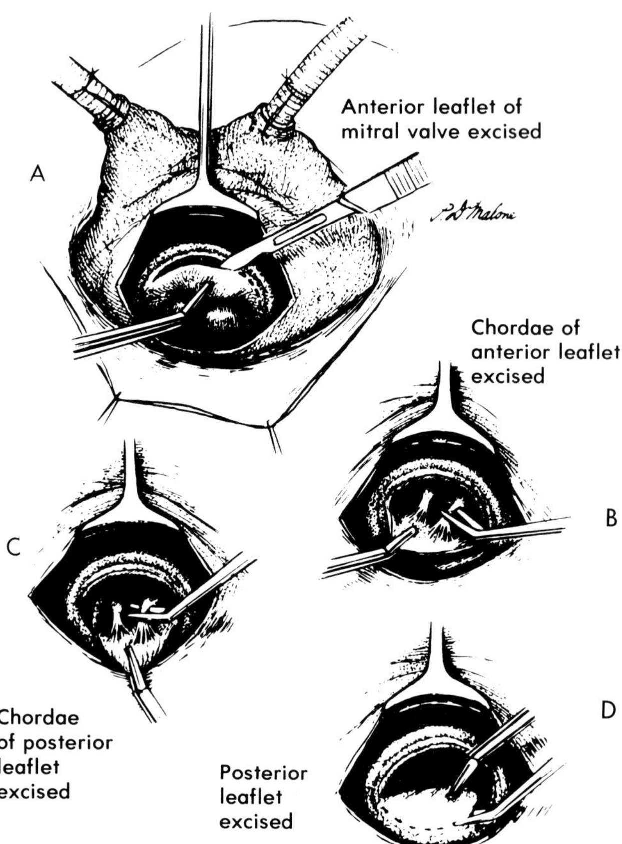

Fig. 40-9 **A,** Left atrium opened. The anterior leaflet of the mitral valve is being incised. **B,** Chordae to the anterior leaflet are exposed and cut. **C,** Chordae to the posterior leaflet are exposed and cut. **D,** Posterior mitral leaflet is excised. (From DiSesa, V.J., Collins, J.J., Jr., and Cohn, L.H.: Mitral valve replacement with the porcine bioprosthesis. In Ionescu, M.I., and Cohn, L.H., editors: Mitral valve disease, London, 1985, Butterworth and Co.)

sufficient symptoms, investigation and surgery are undertaken. Unlike other valve lesions, moderate mitral stenosis can be tolerated well over long periods, without the development of irreversible cardiac damage. Cardiac catheterization shows a depressed cardiac output and a pressure gradient across the mitral valve. With these two measurements, the mitral valve area may be calculated. With significant disease this area is reduced from its norm of 4 to 6 cm^2 to approximately 1 cm^2 or less.

In spite of the description of successful repair of mitral stenosis by Sir Henry Souttar in 1925, it was not until 1950 that Harken and Bailey in this country and Brock in England popularized the surgical treatment. For the next two decades, large numbers of patients underwent "closed" mitral valvotomy, with the valve being dilated by an instrument inserted either through the left atrial appendage or the apex of the left ventricle. This approach worked well in most instances, attended by low mortality, but the stenosis tended to recur and require reoperation at a median time of about 10 years. Valvotomy is now performed "open" with cardiopulmonary bypass; the commissures are split, and the subvalvular apparatus is mobilized as necessary. If the valve is also insufficient, a not uncommon occurrence with advanced mitral stenosis, or if it is heavily calcified or otherwise irreparable, it is replaced with a prosthetic valve (Figs. 40-8 to 40-11).

There has been recent interest in dilating mitral valves with balloon catheters at the time of cardiac catheterization; it is as yet unknown whether this works as well as surgical repair. It is also unclear whether open mitral valvotomy gives much better results than the closed technique; but valvotomy performed relatively early in the clinical course provides more opportunity for repair and probably less morbidity in the subsequent years, compared to postponement of the operation for a few years and the need of a valve replacement at that time.

Mitral Insufficiency

Rheumatic disease, bacterial endocarditis, myxomatous degeneration, left ventricular dilation from cardiomyopathy or aortic valve disease, and ischemic heart disease are all causes of clinical mitral insufficiency. Signficant acute mitral insufficiency from bacterial endocarditis or from a ruptured papillary muscle in the context of acute myocardial infarction constitutes a surgical emergency, and immediate replacement of the mitral valve is undertaken. The results of this procedure vary with the patient's overall

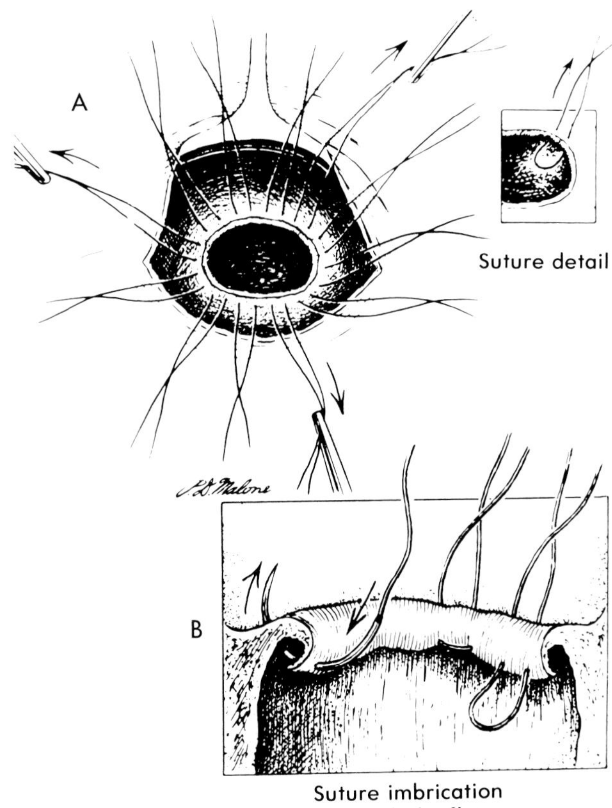

Fig. 40-10 **A,** Mattress suture technic—ventricle to atrium. **B,** Imbrication of fragile leaflet tissue. (From DiSesa, V.J., Collins, J.J. Jr., and Cohn, L.H.: Mitral valve replacement with the porcine bioprosthesis. In Ionescu, M.I., and Cohn, L.H., editors: Mitral valve disease, London, 1985, Butterworth and Co.)

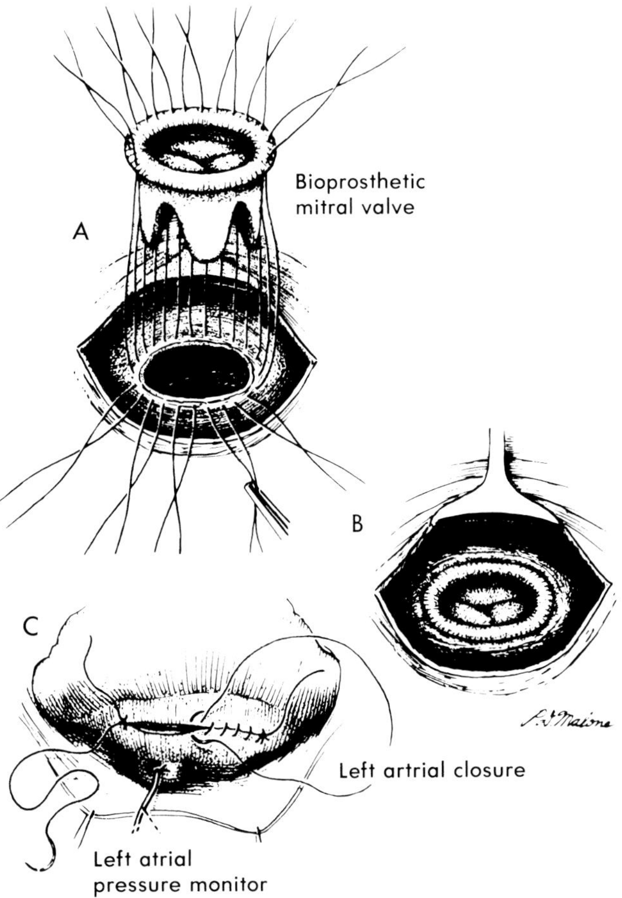

Fig. 40-11 **A,** Seating of the valve. **B,** Valve tied to place. **C,** Left atrial incision is closed, and a pressure monitor catheter is inserted through the right superior pulmonary vein into the left atrium. (From DiSesa, V.J., Collins, J.J., Jr., and Cohn, L.H.: Mitral valve replacement with the procine bioprosthesis. In Ionescu, M.I., and Cohn, L.H., editors: Mitral valve disease, London, 1985, Butterworth and Co.)

condition and are generally better in those individuals with endocarditis than in those with ruptured papillary muscles who tend to have other cardiac damage and usually require coronary bypass in addition to mitral valve replacement.

Most patients with mitral insufficiency have congestive cardiac failure, and the decision to undertake surgery depends on their symptoms, their rate of progression, and the results of cardiac catheterization. Modest mitral insufficiency is tolerated well for long periods, and many of these patients have a slow progression of their disease. If symptoms are serious or rapidly progressive, especially if cardiac catheterization shows left ventricular dysfunction or significant coronary disease, surgery is recommended.

Some insufficient mitral valves can be repaired, obviating the need for valve replacement with its consequent morbidity and mortality, and the work of Carpentier[4] in Paris must be recognized in this context. It seems that surgeons in this country do not see as many patients with early, repairable mitral insufficiency as does Carpentier, but the fact remains that repair is applicable to a significant number of patients who in the past were subjected to valve replacement. Repair can involve resection of a redundant leaflet, narrowing of a dilated annulus, shortening or lengthening of chordae tendineae, and even transfer of functioning leaflet tissue from one leaflet to the other. The reported results of these maneuvers have been satisfactory in general, but the actual value of repair vs. replacement is not yet known.

The results of mitral valve replacement vary according to the patient's underlying pathology; isolated replacement in a young person with rheumatic disease or myxomatous degeneration should have a mortality of no more than 1% to 2%, but surgery in older patients with ischemic heart disease can carry mortalities as high as 20%. Replacement of the mitral valve for insufficiency increases the afterload on the left ventricle, and in fact the ejection fraction can fall after satisfactory surgery. This is not a reason to avoid surgery, except in the presence of severe left ventricular dysfunction, since the trade-off is a reduced preload. Patients with mitral insufficiency should be followed carefully for the development of left ventricular dysfunction, so that this problem does not arise.

Aortic Stenosis

A biscuspid aortic valve is the most common congenital cardiac defect, and patients with this disorder can develop calcific aortic stenosis in later life. Other causes include idiopathic calcification of a tricuspid valve and rheumatic disease. Many patients with significant aortic stenosis are asymptomatic, but effort dyspnea, angina in the absense of coronary disease, and syncope are the common symptoms. Syncope is an ominous symptom, and in its presence urgent investigation and surgery are undertaken. There is a significant incidence of sudden death in patients with aortic stenosis, particularly in those with syncope.

Although the diagnosis is usually clear from clinical and noninvasive studies, cardiac catheterization is undertaken to delineate the status of left ventricular function and the coronary arteries. Aortic stenosis is the one valvular heart disease in which surgery is undertaken in the asymptomatic or virtually asymptomatic patient because of incipient left ventricular dysfunction; even in the absence of symptoms, irreversible damage to the left ventricle may occur, precluding an optimal surgical result. Repair of acquired aortic stenosis is not feasible, and prosthetic replacement is required. As in mitral stenosis, there has been recent interest in balloon dilation of the aortic valve, but this is clearly on shakier theoretic grounds than in the mitral valve, since surgical dilation does not work.

Because of the marked left ventricular hypertrophy present in aortic stenosis, great care must be paid to intraoperative myocardial protection, especially when coronary artery stenosis is a complicating factor. The results of aortic valve replacement are good, even in the presence of coronary disease and extreme old age—many patients in their eighth decade, and even some who are older, are candidates. The mortality rate varies from 1% to 5%, depending on the clinical circumstances.

Aortic Insufficiency

Insufficiency of the aortic valve is produced by rheumatic disease, annuloaortic ectasia, aortic dissection, bacterial endocarditis, idiopathic degeneration with or without calcification, collagen vascular diseases, and in the past syphilis. Symptoms are mainly effort intolerance and dyspnea, but occasionally angina occurs without obvious coronary disease. The degree of aortic regurgitation can be inferred accurately from the width of the pulse pressure, but cardiac catheterization can be useful, especially if there is some question of the presence of coronary artery disease.

As in mitral insufficiency, mild aortic insufficiency is tolerated well with only moderate ventricular dilation and elevation of preload; but, if severe aortic regurgitation is left untreated, the left ventricular dilation and dysfunction become only partly reversible. Also, as in the mitral valve, acute aortic insufficiency from endocarditis, trauma, or any other reason is a surgical emergency demanding immediate surgery. The clue to the acuteness of the situation is the combination of profound regurgitation and a small left ventricle.

Isolated aortic valve replacement for insufficiency gives highly satisfactory results, with mortality in the 1% to 5% range, depending on the circumstances. If the cause is complex, such as aortic dissection, the results are less satisfactory, primarily from causes unrelated to the valve itself.

Choice of a Prosthesis and Long-Term Outlook

Although there appears to be a bewildering array of valve prostheses available, there are in fact two major categories and relatively small differences between the members of each category. The first category comprises "tissue" valves, which are either actual porcine aortic valves (Hancock, Carpentier, or Angell), or valves constructed of bovine pericardium (Ionescu). The second category comprises various types of "mechanical" valves made of plastic, metal, and pyrolytic carbon; these include ball-in-cage (Starr), tilting-disk (Bjork, Lillihei), and most recently hinged bi-leaflet (St. Jude).

The choice between the two categories is clear. The mechanical valves are durable, but thrombogenic even with the required chronic anticoagulation with dicumarol. Patients with mechanical prostheses in the aortic and mitral positions have major thromboembolic complications at rates of as high as 2% and 5% per year, respectively. These rates assume the presence of normal anticoagulation; if the patient is not compliant for any reason, major prosthetic thrombosis requiring valve re-replacement supervenes rapidly in most instances. On the other hand, tissue valves are largely free of thromboembolism without anticoagulation, with the exception of mitral valve replacement, which is associated with chronic atrial fibrillation; but their drawback is that they have a finite life span due to calcification and fibrosis. This degeneration is accelerated in children or in others with active calcium metabolism such as those with chronic renal failure. Excluding these latter groups, the median useful lifetime of tissue valves is in the range of 10 to 15 years, and at this time a new valve must be substituted. Although the incidence of thromboembolism is very low with tissue valves, it is worthwhile to maintain these patients on aspirin and dipyridamole. There is now also accepted evidence that the addition of dypyridamole to dicumarol is useful in those individuals with mechanical prostheses.

Examples of groups who are candidates for the two categories of valves are: (1) mechanical valve—a young person with long life expectancy needing an aortic valve who can remember to take dicumarol and who lives close to the "prothrombin time laboratory" for control of dicumarol, and (2) tissue valve—a forgetful old person with short life expectancy, who requires a mitral valve is in sinus rhythm and who is geographically distant from the laboratory. The tissue valve is also appropriate for the young woman who wishes to have children—the complications of anticoagulant therapy during labor and delivery outweigh the need for a future re-replacement. Most patients do not fall so neatly into one of the groups, and some compromise must be reached. The choice between valves within the two categories largely belongs to the surgeon, although there is now a marked shift toward the St. Jude valve as the mechanical prosthesis of choice because of its excellent hemodynamics and putative lower rate of thromboembolism.

Patients with valve prostheses have an annual mortality rate of about twice the age-adjusted norm of 2%, but clearly this depends on the clinical situation and the presence or absence of concomitant disease. Although the old adage about major organ transplantation substituting one disease for another is equally true for valve replacement, especially mechanical valves, the fact remains that valve replacement is a highly satisfactory procedure.

PERICARDIAL DISEASE[3,27]

The fibrous pericardial sac that contains the heart is not normally thought of as a significant factor in cardiovascular physiology, but two specific pericardial conditions concern the surgeon: pericardial effusion with tamponade and chronic constrictive pericarditis. Pericardial tamponade is defined as significant compression of the heart by pericardial fluid; not only are the great veins and atria compressed, reducing venous return to the ventricles, but also, importantly, the ventricles do not fill optimally during diastole, and cardiac output is depressed in spite of "normal" systolic function.

Pericardial effusions are not uncommon, occurring for example in patients with acute viral pericarditis, myocardial infarction, and congestive cardiac failure, but only rarely in these conditions do the effusions reach the magnitude requiring surgical intervention. In those with chronic uremic pericarditis and malignant pericardial involvement, usually from direct spread of bronchogenic carcinoma, expansion of the effusion to the point of tamponade is seen often. In these two situations the effusion is usually bloody and commonly exacerbated rapidly by bleeding.

The accumulation of liquid or clotted blood within the pericardium can produce tamponade following cardiac surgery, but this should be virtually unknown with proper postoperative drainage techniques. Penetrating cardiac trauma and, rarely, blunt trauma also produce pericardial tamponade; and since the pericardium is normal in these patients, a relatively small volume of blood (as little as 200 ml) may produce the tamponade; in those with tamponade from chronic pericardial disease, the volume is normally much greater, up to 1 L or more of fluid. Trauma from within the heart in the form of a perforating transvenous pacemaker lead or central venous pressure/Swan-Ganz catheter can produce unsuspected tamponade and should be considered in any patient becoming hypotensive in the presence of one of these devices.

The classic triad of physical signs of pericardial tamponade (i.e., arterial hypotension, increased jugular venous pressure, and "muffled" heart sounds) is usually present and often accompanied by facial cyanosis from high venous pressure. Pulsus "paradoxus," a noticeable drop in arterial blood pressure with inspiration, is usually an exaggeration of the normal response to ventilation and is more prominent in those subjected to positive pressure ventilation.

Since the management of patients with pericardial tamponade depends on an assessment of how "tight" the effusion is, it is essential that answering this question should be approached logically. The degree of arterial hypotension and elevation of venous pressure are related to the severity of the tamponade, and in those individuals with only moderate degrees of tamponade a good clinical test is to observe the patient's response to a Valsalva maneuver; i.e., if palpable radial pulses are not lost with a Valsalva, the situation is not critical. It is also useful to test the response to a rapid infusion of intravenous fluid—patients with only moderate tamponade will usually show a significant rise in arterial blood pressure. The presence of supraventricular dysrhythmias, in particular intermittent sinus arrest, is a sign of significant tamponade and incipient cir-

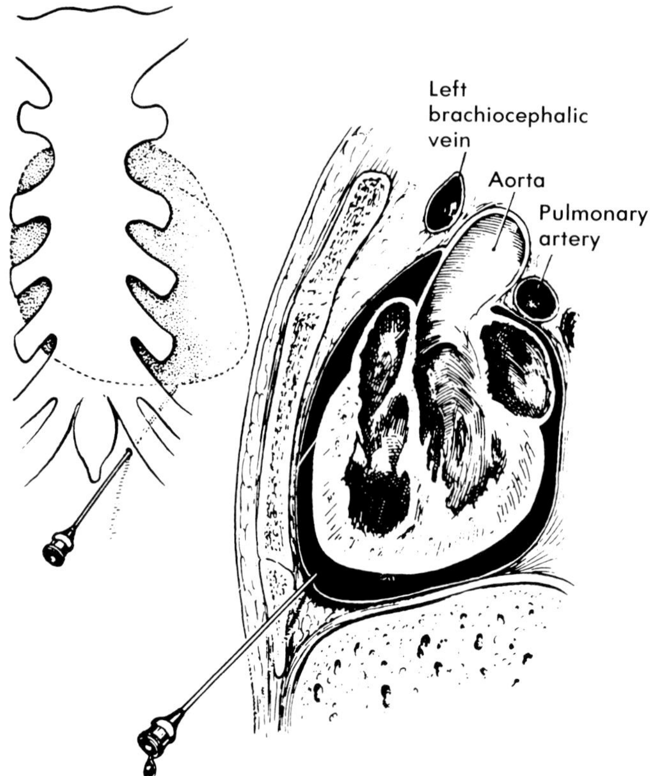

Fig. 40-12 For pericardiocentesis, a 16-gauge plastic-sheathed needle is introduced beneath the costal margin and passed through the properitoneal fat and into the pericardial cavity through the tendinous part of the diaphragm. (From Edwards, E.A., Malone, P.D., and Collins, J.J., Jr.: Operative management of the thorax, Philadelphia, 1972, Lea & Febiger.)

culatory failure. The diagnosis of tamponade is usually easy in the presence of trauma, uremia, or thoracic cancer but may be more difficult in other conditions.

Fluid drainage may be accomplished either percutaneously by needle pericardiocentesis or catheter placement (Fig. 40-12) or surgically by a subxiphoid pericardial window. In the situation of traumatic hemopericardium, a sternotomy or thoracotomy will be required. It should not be forgotten that intravenous volume expansion will improve the situation in many of these patients. The gravity of the situation will dictate the need for percutaneous or surgical decompression; patients in whom circulatory arrest seems imminent should have temporary percutaneous decompression. Pericardiocentesis should not be undertaken lightly in the presence of only modest tamponade, however, since the heart may be punctured and the situation worsened; I have seen patients die from this sequence of events.

It is a fundamental principle of management of tamponade that endotracheal intubation should be avoided except as a last resort, since positive pressure ventilation frequently causes cardiac arrest in those with significant tamponade; for this reason the patient in the operating room should be prepped and draped before induction of anesthesia and intubation so that rapid decompression may be achieved if necessary.

It used to be thought that a formal pericardectomy was necessary in patients with uremic or malignant pericardial tamponade, but it is now clear that a generous subxiphoid window will suffice—I have never seen a patient require a second exploration following this conservative surgical technique. Some cardiologists have advocated percutaneous drainage with instillation of corticosteroids in those with uremia. I have not found this technique satisfactory, probably because of an inherent inability of the method to drain the pericardium completely, thereby preventing apposition of the visceral and parietal pericardia with consequent loss of the pericardial space so that fluid can not reaccumulate.

Chronic constrictive pericarditis is produced in response to such chronic infections as tuberculosis and histoplasmosis, collagen vascular diseases, acute purulent pericarditis, and occasionally after what appear to be uncomplicated cardiac surgery or myocardial infarction with Dressler's syndrome (fever, pericardial friction rub and pain, and often pericardial effusion). The scarring can be severe with obliteration of the pericardial space, thickening of the pericardium to 1 inch or more, and severe fibrosis and calcification with calcific deposits growing into the myocardium. The massive pericardial thickening obstructs venous return and produces diastolic cardiac dysfunction, giving physical signs similar to severe "congestive" cardiac failure with elevated venous pressure, edema, ascites, and hepatomegaly. For this reason the diagnosis can be obscured, especially if calcification is not apparent on the chest X-ray film, but cardiac catherization will usually show small ventricular cavities, equalization of atrial pressures, and the typical "dip and plateau" pattern of diastolic ventricular pressure.

Surgical management of chronic constrictive pericarditis can be difficult and dangerous and is often facilitated by cardiopulmonary bypass. Careful attention must be paid to freeing the atria and venae cavae, as well as the ventricles, with recognition of the fact that the visceral pericardial layer may be as important as the parietal layer. This visceral pericardectomy is complicated by the occasional "invasion" of the ventricular myocardium itself by calcific deposits.

CARDIAC TUMORS[12,13,22,28]

Primary tumors of the heart are rare, with an approximate ratio of 3:1 between benign and malignant neoplasms. Between one third and one half of all cardiac tumors in most series are benign myxomas, 90% of which occur in the atria and a large majority in the left atrium. All kinds of malignant tumors have been described as originating in the heart, but the majority comprise either rhabdomyosarcomas or angiosarcomas. Clinically important metastatic disease of the heart is even less common; metastatic melanoma is recognized occasionally, but cardiac metastases virtually never merit surgical intervention.

Atrial myxomas usually appear either as "mitral" stenosis or as peripheral arterial embolism—the myxomatous embolus can usually be identified at the time of peripheral embolectomy, and for this reason arterial emboli recovered at surgery should be examined histologically with care. The diagnosis of atrial myxomas and other cardiac tumors can often be made definitively by 2-D echocardiography. Although there continues to be some discussion as to whether atrial myxomas constitute true neoplasms or are some form of anomalous thrombotic process, the fact remains that they can recur, and the surgical principle in their removal is to excise them in continuity with the atrial wall from which they are derived, often the interatrial septum in the area of the foramen ovale.

Surgical excision of malignant primary cardiac tumors is undertaken occasionally, but the tumors are difficult to excise completely, and the prognosis is generally hopeless.

INTENSIVE CARDIAC CARE[25,33]

Nowhere in cardiovascular medicine and surgery is the application of physiologic principles more appropriate and useful than in the intensive care unit, and surgeons can take pride in the fact that every important part of modern cardiac care, including preload augmentation and reduction, afterload reduction, control of both tachycardia and bradycardia, mechanical ventilation, pharmocologic inotropic support, and the use of mechanical support devices such as the intra-aortic balloon pump, with the exception of the Swan-Ganz catheter, originated not in the coronary care unit but in the cardiac surgical intensive care unit. In addition, the two essential mechanisms of cardiac resuscitation, external defibrillation and external cardiac massage, were developed on the surgical service of the Johns Hopkins Hospital.

Although in the past the two major clinical presentations of severe cardiac compromise, cardiogenic shock and acute left ventricular failure with pulmonary edema, were thought to represent different pathophysiologic mechanisms, it is clear that the two are essentially the same; i.e., afterload augmentation in the first will convert it into the latter, and preload reduction in the latter will convert it into the former. Management of either of the above or what cardiac surgeons have called "postoperative low cardiac output syndrome," demands careful attention to heart rate, loading conditions, and judicious inotropic support, including mechanical devices.

Although surgeons traditionally used central venous pressure as a measure of preload and clinical signs of vasoconstriction or vasodilation as measures of afterload, these were inexact at best, and the use of the Swan-Ganz catheter in the management of patients with acute left ventricular failure must be recognized. The fact remains, however, that this level of monitoring is one of the most overused techniques in current medical practice, and has perhaps the highest cost:benefit ratio of any procedure used.

The pulmonary artery catheter affords reasonably accurate measurement of cardiac output by thermodilution and thereby the straightforward calculation of peripheral resistance, i.e., mean arterial pressure/cardiac output. Some would recommend subtracting some measure of venous pressure from the mean arterial pressure, but, since the left ventricle "sees" the resistance of the whole circulatory system, and not just that of the arteries and arterioles, it would seem purer to use total resistance by analogy to the input resistance of an electrical circuit. Since the flow of blood from the left ventricle is pulsatile and not steady, true afterload is in fact the aortic input impedance (i.e., pulsatile aortic pressure/pulsatile aortic flow); but at present the clinical calculation of impedance is impractical, and resistance is a reasonable approximation.

In most clinical situations measurement of "pulmonary capillary wedge pressure"—the pulmonary artery pressure distal to a balloon occluding the proximal pulmonary artery—is very close to left ventricular end-diastolic pressure, the usual clinical parameter of left ventricular preload.

Armed thus with preload and afterload and a reasonable measure of left ventricular contractile function, i.e., the cardiac output produced at the measured preload, one can begin to optimize the first two and augment the last as indicated. The vast majority of patients who are hypotensive following cardiac surgery are hypovolemic, and replacement of crystalloid solution and packed red cells will be both a therapeutic and a diagnostic modality. Wedge pressures of 0 to 5 mm Hg are considered low, 5 to 15 mm Hg considered intermediate, and over 15 mm Hg high. High wedge pressures with low cardiac output (less than 2.5 L/min/cm^2 of body surface area) usually indicate a need for inotropic support. Dobutamine, dopamine, epinephrine, and isoproterenol infusions are used to augment contractile function, and the recent addition of amrinone can be helpful in some patients. Epinephrine and isoproterenol infusions may produce unacceptable increases in afterload and heart rate respectively, and these may necessitate the use of other drugs or mechanical support.

Hypotension is rarely caused by low afterload, although this does occur, but it may be complicated by high afterload, thereby reducing further the cardiac output. In this situation the judicious use of afterload reducing agents such as nitroglycerin and nitroprusside may augment cardiac output without reducing blood pressure significantly. Although normal resistance is inversely proportional to body size, normal afterload is represented by an input resistance of 900 to 1300 dynes·sec·cm^{-5} (pressure/flow = dynes·$cm^{-2}/cm^3 \cdot sec^{-1}$).

One of the more difficult judgments to make in managing cardiac surgical patients is whether or not to treat an abnormal preload, afterload, or cardiac output in a patient who seems to be doing well clinically, i.e., in a patient with normal skin color and temperature, no sweating, good urine output, and clear mentation. The best advice is that one should treat the whole patient rather than just one of his hemodynamic parameters.

It is obvious that a patient with left ventricular failure can have any one of many combinations of these parameters, and that primary manipulations directed towards one parameter may have adverse effects on others, requiring secondary therapy. The beneficial effects of mechanical ventilation in patients with circulatory failure can hardly be overemphasized, especially in the presence of any degree of pulmonary edema. Last, derangements of heart rate should be reversed—optimal cardiac function in these patients is seen usually at heart rates of 90 to 120 beats per minute.

Postoperative cardiac surgical patients can have complex hemodynamic derangements, but, if the operation is performed properly and the myocardium protected during the ischemic arrest period, by far the most common derangement should be a low preload from hypovolemia. An adequate intravascular volume is the cornerstone of postoperative cardiac care.

SUMMARY

Normal circulatory function requires an adequate availability of blood for the heart to pump, a frequency of cardiac contraction within an acceptable range, an adequate strength of cardiac contraction, and a level of peripheral resistance that ensures satisfactory peripheral perfusion but is not so high as to put undue strain on the heart itself. Aberrations in any of these parameters can disturb normal cardiac function with the development of disease states that may affect cardiac rate, cardiac pump function, cardiac loading, or various combinations of these activities. Of the acquired cardiac disorders that may develop, atherosclerotic disease of the coronary arteries is clearly most common, with valvular disease being second in frequency. Less commonly encountered disorders include rhythm abnormalities, pericardial disease, and cardiac neoplasms. Each of these acquired lesions can now be surgically managed with an acceptable morbidity and mortality. Directly contributing to this success is not only a properly performed operation with adequate myocardial protection during the ischemic arrest period, but also the tremendous strides in knowledge concerning normal cardiac physiology and its various pathophysiologic states that have been obtained over the last several decades, resulting in vast improvements in perioperative care. The magnitude of such advances becomes apparent when it is realized that, although postoperative cardiac surgical patients can have complex hemodynamic aberrations, the most common derangement presently encountered is a low preload from hypovolemia that can be successfully managed in most cases by ensuring an adequate intravascular volume.

SUGGESTED READINGS

Kirklin, J.W., Barrett-Boyes, B.G.: Cardiac surgery, New York, 1986, John Wiley & Sons, Inc.

Roberts, A.J.: Difficult problems in adults cardiac surgery, Chicago, 1985, Year Book Medical Publishers, Inc.

Sabiston, D.C., and Spencer, F.C.: Gibbon's surgery of the chest, ed. 4, Philadelphia, 1983, W.B. Saunders Co.

REFERENCES

1. Bailey, C.P.: The surgical treatment of mitral stenosis, Dis. Chest. **15**:377, 1949.
2. Baker, C., Brock, R.C., and Campbell, M.: Valvulotomy for mitral stenosis, Br. Med. J. **1**:1283, 1950.
3. Blalock, A., and Burwell, C.S.: Chronic pericardial disease, Surg. Gynecol. Obstet. **73**:433, 1941.
4. Carpentier, A., et al.: Reconstructive surgery of mitral incompetence: ten-year appraisal, J. Thorac. Cardiovasc. Surg. **79**:338, 1980.
5. Cohn, L.H., and Gallucci, V.: Cardiac bioprostheses. New York, 1982, Yorke Medical Books.
6. Copeland, J.G., and Goldman, S.: Improving results with coronary artery bypass grafting, Philadelphia, 1986, Hanley and Belfus, Inc.
7. Favaloro, R.G.: Saphenous vein graft in the surgical treatment of coronary artery disease, J. Thorac. Cardiovasc. Surg. **58**:178, 1969.
8. Gay, W.A., and Ebert, P.A.: Functional, metabolic, and morphologic effects of potassium-induced cardioplegia, Surgery **74**:284, 1973.
9. Guiraudon, G.M., et al.: Encircling endocardial ventriculotomy: a new treatment for life-threatening ventricular tachycardia, Ann. Thorac. Surg. **26**:438, 1977.
10. Harken, A.H., Josephson, M.E., and Horowitz, L.N.: Surgical endocardial resection for the treatment of malignant ventricular tachycardia, Ann. Surg. **190**:456, 1979.
11. Harken, D.W., et al.: The surgical treatment of mitral stenosis, N. Engl. J. Med. **239**:801, 1948.
12. Harvey, W.P.: Clinical aspects of cardiac tumors, Am. J. Cardiol. **21**:328, 1968.
13. Heath, D.: Pathology of cardiac tumors. Am. J. Cardiol. **21**:315, 1968.
14. Hufnagel, C.A., Harvey, W.P.: The surgical correction of aortic regurgitation, Bull. Georgetown Univ. Med. Center **6**:60, 1953.
15. Ionescu, M.I.: Techniques in extracorporeal circulation, ed. 2, London, 1981, Butterworth Publishers.
16. Kirklin, J.W., Conti, V.R., and Blackstone, E.H.: Prevention of myocardial damage during cardiac operations, N. Engl. J. Med. **301**:135, 1979.
17. Lefrak, E.A., and Starr, A.: Cardiac valve prostheses, New York, 1979, Appleton-Century-Crofts.
18. Loop, F.D., et al.: Influence of the internal mammary graft on 10-year survival and other cardiac events, N. Engl. J. Med. **314**:1, 1986.

19. Lowe, J.L., and Sabiston, D.C.: The surgical management of cardiac arrhythmias, J. Cardiovasc. Surg. **1:**1, 1986.
20. Lytle, B.W., et al.: Fifteen hundred coronary reoperations: results and determinants of early and late survival, J. Thorac. Cardiovasc. Surg. **93:**847, 1987.
21. Matloff, J.M.: Cardiac valve replacement, Boston, 1985, Martinus Nijhoff Publishing.
22. McAllister, H.A., and Fenoglio, J.J.: Tumors of the cardiovascular system. In Atlas of tumor pathology, Washington, 1978, AFIP.
23. Phibbs, B., et al.: Indications for pacing in the treatment of bradycardia, JAMA **252:**1307, 1984.
24. Reed, C.C., and Stafford, T.B.: Cardiopulmonary bypass, ed. 2, Houston, 1985, Texas Medical Press.
25. Roe, B.B.: Perioperative management in cardiothoracic surgery, Boston, 1981, Little, Brown & Co., Inc.
26. Sealy, W.C., Anderson, R.W., and Gallagher, J.J.: Surgical treatment of supraventricular tachyarrhythmias, J. Thorac. Cardiovasc. Surg. **73:**511, 1977.
27. Shabetai, R.: The pericardium. New York, 1981, Grune & Stratton, Inc.
28. Silverman, N.A.: Primary cardiac tumors, Ann. Surg. **191:**127, 1980.
29. Sones, F.M., and Shirley, E.K.: Cine coronary angiography, Mod. Con. Cardiovasc. Dis. **31:**735, 1962.
30. Souttar, H.S.: The surgical treatment of mitral stenosis, Br. Med. J. **2:**603, 1925.
31. Starr, A., and Edwards, M.L.: Mitral replacement: clinical experience with a ball-valve prosthesis, Ann. Surg. **154:**726, 1961.
32. Stiles, Q.R., and Kirklin, J.W.: Myocardial preservation, J. Thorac. Cardiovasc. Surg. **82:**870, 1981.
33. Utley, J.R.: Perioperative heart dysfunction. Baltimore, 1985, The Williams and Wilkins, Co.
34. Utley, J.R.: Pathophysiology and techniques of cardiopulmonary bypass, vol. 1. Baltimore, 1982, The Williams and Wilkins Co.
35. Utley, J.R.: Pathophysiology and techniques of cardiopulmonary bypass, vol. 2, Baltimore, 1983, The Williams and Wilkins Co.
36. Weirich, W.L., Gott, V.L., and Lillihei, C.V.: Treatment of complete heart block by the combined use of myocardial electrode and an artificial pacemaker, Surg. Forum **8:**360, 1958.
37. Wheatley, D.J.: Surgery of coronary artery disease, St. Louis, 1986, The C.V. Mosby Co.

41 Physiology of Urine Formation

Alan S. Tonnesen and Edward J. Weinman

The kidneys subserve three major functions. First, the kidney maintains fluid and electrolyte homeostasis, which is considered briefly in this chapter and is discussed more fully in Chapter 2. Second, the kidney functions as an endocrine organ; it produces the active metabolite of vitamin D and erythropoietin and also serves as both a target organ and an organ of catabolism for various peptide hormones. Third, the kidney is an organ of excretion for certain intermediate and end products of metabolism and for several drugs. Given the central role of the kidney in metabolic processes, it is not surprising that renal failure is characterized by protean clinical manifestations.

OVERVIEW OF FLUID AND ELECTROLYTE HOMEOSTASIS

In normal individuals remarkable constancy exists in the total amount of fluid, electrolytes, and solutes in the body as a whole as well as in the individual compartments within the body. This constant internal environment is maintained by rapid adjustments in the rates of excretion of solutes and waste material in response to wide variations in the rates of intake and body metabolism. The amount and composition of the fluid in the cells differ from those of the extracellular fluid. The ionic composition and volume of the cells are maintained by specific ion pumps and channels in the cellular membranes. Although critical to survival of the organism, these transport processes are not considered further in this chapter except as they pertain to vectorial transport of fluids and solutes by the kidney.

The kidney in normal persons is the major organ of regulation for control of fluid and electrolyte balance. Its ability to accomplish this is manifested by variations in intake of several orders of magnitude resulting in no change in the amount of fluid or electrolytes in the body and no alteration in the composition of either the fluid or cellular compartments of the body.[6,46,47] This concept is illustrated schematically in Fig. 41-1. In an individual ingesting or receiving 100 mEq of sodium daily, the 24-hour urinary excretion is also 100 mEq. When such an individual decreases the intake of sodium to 10 mEq or increases it to 200 or more mEq daily, a rapid adjustment in excretion occurs so that input and output are matched. The transient net gains or losses of sodium in normal individuals are clinically insignificant. Unlike sodium, water is lost and gained from the body by nonrenal routes. Nonetheless, the major adjustments to altered intake of water are mediated by alterations in the rate of urinary excretion. The same general schema holds for other electrolytes. General as well as specific mechanisms modulate the renal response to alterations in intake and permit maintenance of overall balance.

The operation of such feedback systems involves sensor and effector mechanisms. Many processes exist for detecting changes in the amount or composition of fluid compartments of the body. Sensors for alterations in the extracelluar fluid volume, for example, are located within the heart, great blood vessels, and central nervous system and experimentally also appear to exist in the liver, gastrointestinal tract, and within the kidney itself. Perturbations in volume or composition of the extracellular fluid result in changes in the levels of systemic and locally produced hormones and nerve traffic to the kidney, which affects the renal transport of fluid and electrolytes. As discussed later, the renal response is modulated in specific subsegments of the nephron that are responsive to these stimuli. Renal mechanisms regulate the rates of absorption and secretion of specific solutes and water. Mechanisms that affect the rates of transport of several electrolytes, nonelectrolytes, and water simultaneously have also been identified.

RENAL PHYSIOLOGY

Renal Blood Flow

The kidneys account for 0.5% of the total body mass, but receive 20% to 25% of the total cardiac output. This high rate of blood flow in relation to renal mass is necessary to support glomerular filtration but far exceeds the normal metabolic needs of the kidney. The distribution of blood flow within the kidney roughly parallels the distribution of glomerular filtration, being highest in the superficial cortex and diminishing progressively toward the medulla.[49]

Anatomy

The renal artery (or arteries, if multiple) enters the kidney at the hilum (Fig. 41-2). The main renal artery divides into branches, forming interlobar arteries. At the level of the corticomedullary junction, the interlobar arteries divide to form the arcuate arteries, which travel parallel to the renal surface. The interlobular arteries arise from the ar-

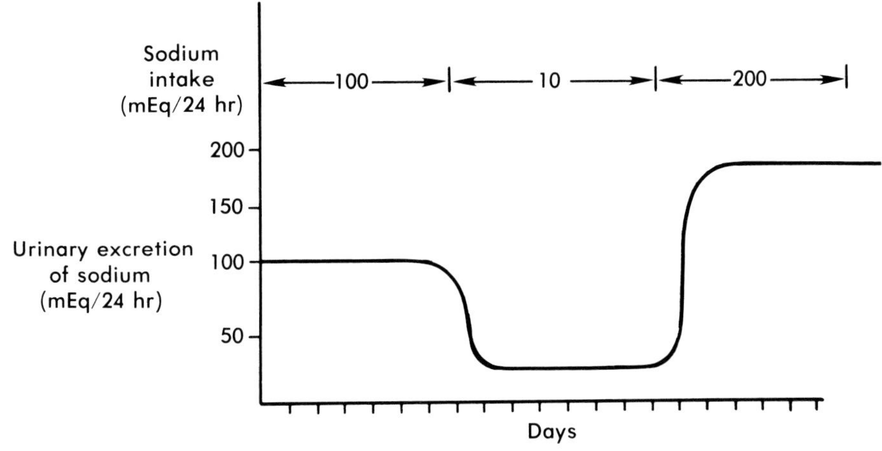

Fig. 41-1 Influence of sodium intake on urinary excretion of sodium.

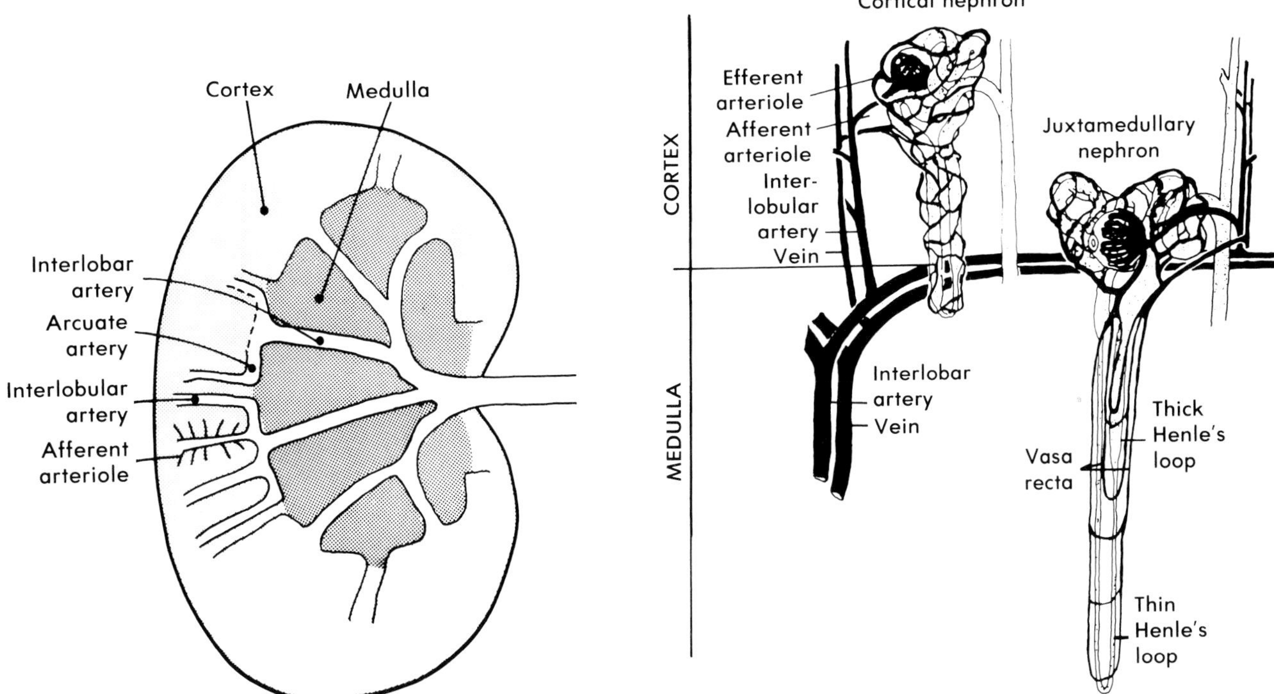

Fig. 41-2 Schematic representation of the major arterial renal vasculature.

Fig. 41-3 Schematic comparison of the postglomerular vasculature of the superficial and juxtamedullary nephrons. Note the vasa recta arising from the juxtamedullary efferent arteriole. The density of the vasculature becomes progressively less as it descends into the medulla. (Modified from Pitts, R.F.: Physiology of the kidney and body fluids, Chicago, 1974, Year Book Medical Publishers, Inc.)

cuate arteries and subsequently divide into the afferent arterioles. These arterioles break up into the glomerular capillary tufts, reunite to form the efferent arteriole, and as they surround the renal tubules, become the peritubular capillaries (Fig. 41-3). Juxtamedullary efferent arterioles divide into vasa recta. The vasa recta descend in parallel with Henle's loops and form an anastomosing system that becomes progressively less dense from the outer to the inner medulla. The peritubular capillaries and vasa recta empty into the interlobular veins. These drain to the arcuate veins, which finally join to form the renal veins.[49]

Distribution of Plasma Flow

Renal blood flow manifests the property of *autoregulation* (Fig. 41-4), which describes the constancy of blood flow in the face of changes in mean arterial pressure ranging from 70 to 180 mm Hg. The mechanism of autoregulation has not been totally clarified. The myogenic theory postulates that in response to an increase in pressure, the afferent arteriole vasoconstricts. Thus the resistance in the afferent arteriole increases and blood flow is held constant. Others have suggested that the tubuloglomerular feedback mechanism (see later discussion on glomerular filtration) and renal nerves are necessary for complete and efficient autoregulation.

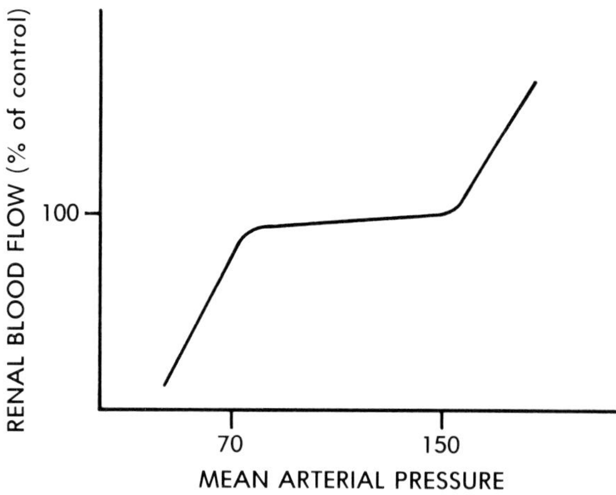

Fig. 41-4 Autoregulation of renal blood flow. As the mean systemic arterial pressure varies over wide ranges, the renal blood flow remains relatively constant.

Plasma flow to the cortex averages 2.0 ml/g of tissue/minute and accounts for approximately 90% of the total renal plasma flow. The outer medulla receives about 1.0 ml/g of tissue/minute and accounts for about 9% of the total renal plasma flow. Blood flow to the inner medulla accounts for only about 1% of total renal plasma flow.[30,35,38] The relative distribution of blood flow between the cortex and medulla is under metabolic control and may vary under different conditions. During water diuresis renal blood flow increases, but a relatively greater increase occurs in flow to the outer medulla as compared to the cortex. Increased sodium intake tends to elevate outer cortical blood flow, with less influence on inner cortical flow. The mechanisms controlling the intrarenal distribution of blood flow are not completely clarified but may include the sympathetic nervous system, the renin-angiotensin system, prostaglandins, and antidiuretic hormone (ADH).

Physiologic Significance of Blood Flow Alterations and Distribution

Alterations in renal blood flow may play a role in overall fluid and electrolyte metabolism by the kidney.[35] The rate of glomerular filtration depends on plasma flow. Alterations in the ratio between the glomerular filtration rate and the renal plasma flow (i.e., the filtration fraction) may affect the rates of water and solute absorption in the proximal convoluted tubule. Alterations in blood flow may be a contributing factor in the concentration-dilution function of the kidney. At least under experimental circumstances, however, changes in blood flow can be dissociated from alterations in renal function.

Alterations in the distribution of blood flow between the outer and inner zones of the kidney have also been postulated as factors in the renal excretion of electrolytes. Some have suggested that the long-looped juxtamedullary nephrons are "sodium-retaining" nephrons, whereas those on the cortex absorb less sodium. Thus sodium excretion in the urine could be affected by the distribution of blood flow through greater or lesser perfusion of salt-retaining or salt-wasting nephrons. Despite some support for this hypothesis, considerable evidence also suggests that alterations in the distribution of blood flow are not the sole or major mechanism subserving sodium and water balance.

Glomerular Filtration

The initial process of urine formation is the generation of an ultrafiltrate of plasma across the glomerular capillaries.

Anatomy

Blood enters the glomerular capillaries from the afferent arteriole. The glomerular capillary endothelial cell is the initial barrier. Fenestrae between the endothelial cells are approximately 6.1 nm in size, indicating that this potential route of diffusion or convection could seive only formed elements of blood, not dissolved proteins or electrolytes. The glomerular capillary basement membrane lies adjacent to the endothelial cells. This membrane, which is produced by the mesangial cells of the glomerulus, is composed of glycoproteins with fixed negative charges. This charge serves to retard the passage of proteins. In addition, the glomerular capillary membrane behaves as if pierced with pores of fixed molecular dimensions. The estimated size of these pores is of such magnitude as to exclude large-sized proteins but not small solutes.

Thus the basement membrane excludes macromolecules on the basis of both charge and size. The glomerular capillary basement membrane abuts the processes of the visceral epithelial cells, the podocytes. The physical space between the podocytes is large. The podocytes, however, are also lined by negative charges and thus serve to retard the passage of negatively charged proteins into the proximal tubule.

Filtration Barrier

Because of the anatomic features just outlined, the glomerular capillary filtration apparatus acts as a very efficient semipermeable membrane system that effectively excludes passage of molecules with a radius greater than 38 to 44 angstroms (Å) while allowing ready passage of molecules less than 20 Å.[8] Functionally, endothelial fenestrae appear to permit passage of molecules at least as large as 6.1 nm in radius. The basement membrane excludes molecules greater than 6.1 nm, partially retards passage of those with a radius of 5.2 nm, and is freely permeable to molecules with a radius of 3.0 nm. The foot processes block passage of molecules with radii as small a 3.0 nm. It is important to note that these dimensions do not correspond to clearly identifiable structural pores, but rather reflect the functional characteristics of the filtration barrier.

Glomerular Dynamics

An understanding of the process of glomerular filtration can be appreciated by considering the components of the modified Starling equation:

$$SNGFR = k_f\,[(HP_{gc} - HP_t) - (OC_{gc} - OC_t)]$$

SNGFR is the filtration rate of a single nephron. K_f is the permeability coefficient, which is equivalent to the product

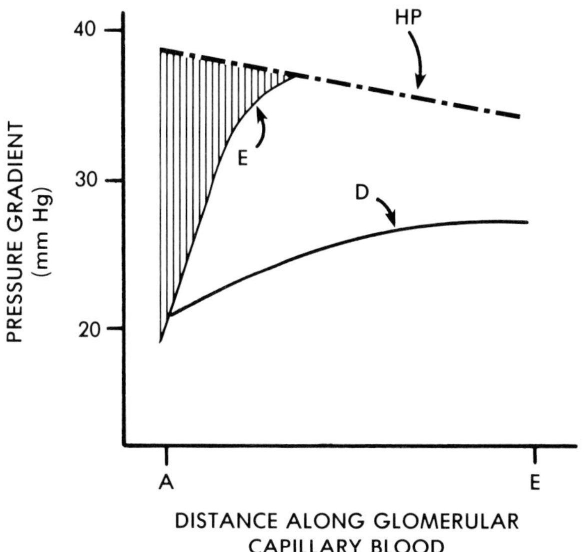

Fig. 41-5 Effect of glomerular plasma flow on the mean ultrafiltration pressure gradient. *A* represents the afferent arteriolar end of the glomerular capillary bed, whereas *E* represents the efferent arteriolar end. The *HP* line is the hydrostatic pressure gradient, i.e., the difference between glomerular hydrostatic pressure and the pressure in the early proximal tubule. Curves *E* on the graph and *D* represent the rise in colloid osmotic pressure as plasma passes from *A* to *E*. The vertically shaded area limited by curve *E* on the graph and *HP* is proportional to the mean ultrafiltration gradient during states of low flow, when filtration equilibrium exists. The area limited by curves *D* and *HP*, which is obviously much larger, represents the gradient during high glomerular plasma flow, when filtration disequilibrium exists. Thus high glomerular plasma flow maintains a higher mean ultrafiltration pressure gradient, supporting a higher glomerular filtration rate. (Modified from Maddox, D.A., and Brenner, B.M.: Annu. Rev. Med. **28:**91, 1977.)

of the hydraulic conductivity of the glomerular capillary membranes and the surface area available for filtration. HP_{gc} is the hydrostatic pressure in the glomerular capillary bed, and HP_t is the hydrostatic pressure in the most proximal regions of the proximal tubule (i.e., Bowman's space). OC_{gc} is the oncotic pressure in plasma perfusing the glomerular capillary apparatus, and OC_t is the oncotic pressure of the tubular filtrate. Normally, OC_{gc} is equal to 22 to 25 mm Hg at the arteriolar end of the glomerular capillary bed, and OC_t is essentially zero.

The net ultrafiltration pressure gradient is equal to the mean hydrostatic pressure gradient minus the mean oncotic pressure gradient as the plasma traverses the glomerular capillary from the afferent to the efferent arteriole (Fig. 41-5).[34] The hydrostatic pressure in the proximal tubule remains relatively constant. The glomerular capillary pressure drops only a few millimeters of mercury as it traverses the capillary bed. As a result, the hydrostatic gradient from capillary to Bowman's space is relatively constant from the afferent to the efferent end of the arteriole. By contrast, however, the oncotic pressure in the glomerular capillary rises as water is removed from the capillary space. The concentration of protein and thus the oncotic pressure is higher in the efferent as compared to the afferent arteriole. The oncotic pressure in the tubular fluid is zero.

The net ultrafiltration pressure gradient at any point along the glomerular capillary is equal to the difference between the hydrostatic pressure gradient and the oncotic pressure gradient (see Fig. 41-5). The net ultrafiltration pressure is greatest at the afferent arteriolar end of the glomerulus and becomes progressively lower as the oncotic pressure rises. Filtration can proceed until the oncotic pressure in the glomerular capillary becomes equal to the hydrostatic pressure gradient. The net pressure for ultrafiltration across the entire glomerulus thus is determined by the geometric mean of the difference between the hydrostatic pressure gradient curve and the oncotic pressure gradient curve (see Fig. 41-5).

Glomerular plasma flow does not appear at first to be represented in the Starling equation. Glomerular plasma flow is a critical determinant of the glomerular filtration rate, however, and determines both the hydrostatic and the oncotic pressure gradients. A consideration of the effects of extreme examples gives an indication of the importance of glomerular plasma flow in determining the rate of filtration.

As illustrated in curve E of Fig. 41-5, the efferent arteriole may be considered as nearly closed. In this circumstance a net pressure gradient for ultrafiltration exists at the afferent arteriolar end of the capillary, and filtration proceeds. Initially the net gradient for ultrafiltration is high, but as the macromolecules in the glomerular capillary plasma are rapidly concentrated by loss of filtered water, the oncotic pressure rises to a level that ultimately equals the hydrostatic pressure gradient. Filtration equilibrium is thus attained, and the entire potential surface area for filtration is not used. If the efferent arteriole is now released momentarily and a fresh bolus of plasma is allowed to enter, ultrafiltration will occur and continue until the ultrafiltration pressure gradient is again reduced to zero.

By extrapolating to normal conditions, one can thus appreciate that the total rate of filtration (the glomerular filtrate rate) will depend highly on plasma flow rate. This dependency derives from progressive displacement of the equilibrium pressure point toward the efferent end of the capillaries. In other words, with no change in hydraulic conductivity, increases in the rate of glomerular capillary blood flow recruit greater areas of the capillary for filtration.

In contrast to the previous circumstance, an alternative situation exists in which glomerular plasma flow is high, as shown by curve D in Fig. 41-5. If the rate of plasma flow is high enough that filtration equilibrium is not obtained by the efferent end of the glomerulus, the entire filtering surface area is used for ultrafiltration, and the rate of filtration depends less on glomerular plasma flow. As Fig. 41-5 indicates, the areas between the hydrostatic pressure gradient curve and the oncotic pressure gradient curve are greatly different in states of low and high plasma flow. The shaded areas between the two curves represent the total ultrafiltration pressure gradient acting to cause filtration across the glomerular capillary bed. Thus the higher the glomerular capillary plasma flow, (1) the lower is the oncotic pressure gradient resisting filtration, (2) the higher the hydrostatic pressure gradient favoring filtration, and (3) the larger the surface area exposed to pressures that favor filtration.

Regulation of Glomerular Filtration Rate

Although the determinants of the glomerular filtration rate (GFR) are well described, the factors regulating the rates of filtration are still incompletely understood. The two major factors are the glomerular plasma flow and the hydraulic permeability of the filtration barrier. Each of these variables may be affected independently by disease conditions, hormones, and drugs. The rate of glomerular filtration exhibits two interesting phenomena: autoregulation and tubuloglomerular feedback regulation. Autoregulation of the GFR rate is similar to that observed for renal blood flow. As blood pressure changes over wide ranges, the GFR remains constant.

The phenomenon of tubuloglomerular feedback regulation of GFR is manifest by decreases in the rate of glomerular filtration associated with increases in the rate of flow of tubular fluid through Henle's loop.[20,25] A reduction in the glomerular capillary blood flow and a decrease in hydraulic conductivity account for the reduction in filtration. The tubuloglomerular feedback loop operates more efficiently to reduce glomerular filtration when tubular fluid flow increases than to increase filtration in response to reductions in tubular flow. The exact signal initiating the response is still controversial. The transport of chloride or sodium or the osmolality of the tubular fluid at a distal nephron site may be the triggering stimulus. It has also been proposed that this triggering step is transduced through the renin-angiotensin system to cause alterations in the rate of renal plasma flow. This occurs by presumably altering the tone of the afferent arteriole or by altering the surface area for filtration through a direct effect on the mesangial cells of the glomerulus.

Glomerular Ultrafiltrate

The process of filtration results in the formation of an ultrafiltrate of plasma. This is a solution containing no formed elements and having a greatly reduced protein content. The electrolyte composition of the ultrafiltrate, however, is not identical to plasma. Because of the differences in protein content in the glomerular capillary blood as compared to that in Bowman's space, a separation of charge occurs. Anions and cations will distribute asymmetrically across this membrane to achieve electrochemical equilibrium. Thus the concentration of anions such as chloride are higher and the concentration of cations such as sodium are lower in the fluid of Bowman's space as compared to that of the capillary blood.

Tubular Function

The kidney filters approximately 144 L of fluid daily. The renal tubules reabsorb back into the bloodstream vast quantities of this filtrate so as to match the rate of urinary excretion with the rate of fluid intake into the body. In addition, the kidney directly adds certain substances and drugs into the tubular fluid for ultimate excretion. The composition and volume of the glomerular filtrate is progressively altered as it is transported down the length of the nephron.

Physiology of Renal Transport Mechanisms

Renal tubular cells are polar cells with one side facing the tubular fluid (the luminal or apical membrane) and one side facing the interstitium of the kidney and the peritubular capillaries (the basolateral membrane) (Fig. 41-6).

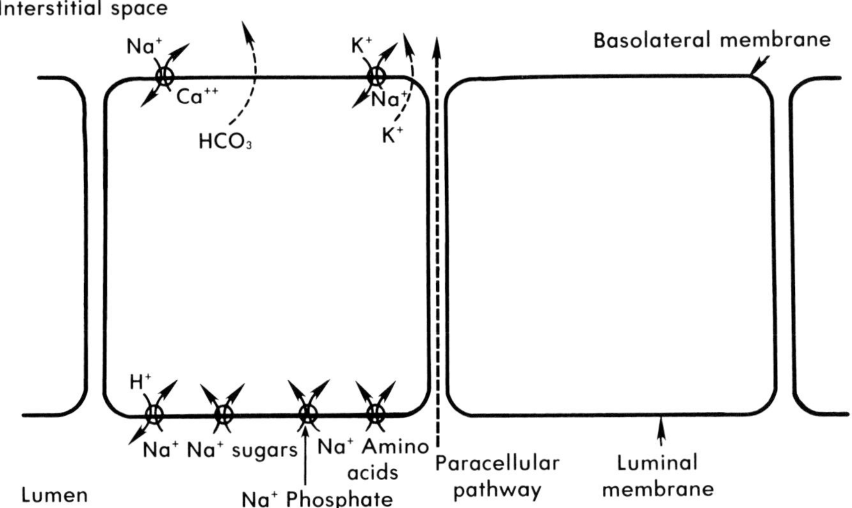

Fig. 41-6 Schematic representation of renal tubular cells. Not all mediated and passive transport pathways are illustrated. Sodium-dependent co-transport systems for sugars, phosphate, and amino acids and the counter-transport system for sodium and hydrogen ions in the luminal membrane are shown. Sodium-potassium adenosine triphophatase (Na^+-K^+ ATPase) and sodium-calcium exchange are illustrated in the basolateral membrane. The interrupted line shows passive diffusion pathways for bicarbonate and potassium across the basolateral membrane and for water and some solutes between the cells (the paracellular pathway).

Vectorial transport in either the absorptive or secretory direction involves the operation of specific transport proteins and ion channels in the given membranes and the permeability properties of the tubule itself. The specialized nature of each nephron segment derives from differences in the types of proteins in the membranes and differences in permeability.

Despite these regional differences, it is worth considering some general factors that account for vectorial transport.[51] First, some transport processes are capable of displacing substances across membranes against an electrochemical gradient, a process known as active transport. These processes require the expenditure of metabolic energy. If the transport process directly requires hydrolysis of high-energy compounds, it is termed *primary active transport*. The best example of such a transport process is the sodium-potassium adenosine triphosphatase Na^+-K^+ ATPase enzyme pump located in almost all cells of the body, including the basolateral membrane of renal tubule cells. This protein subserves both an enzymatic role (i.e., hydrolysis of ATP) and a transport function. Na^+-K^+ ATPase translocates three sodium molecules out of the cell in exchange for two potassium molecules into the cell. Thus the pump is electrogenic and results in displacement of charge. Because of the action of Na^+-K^+ ATPase, the concentration of potassium inside the cell is considerably higher than that of plasma. Conversely, the concentration of sodium is lower. The basolateral membrane of renal tubular cells is more permeable to potassium than to sodium. Intracellular potassium diffuses out of the cell down its electrochemical gradient and renders the inside of the cell electronegative.

The electrochemical gradients generated across the membranes of the cells can also be harnessed for the transport of other solutes. This process ultimately requires metabolic energy, but by itself the process does not result in hydrolysis of high-energy compounds. Such a process, if it involves a specific transport protein (i.e., mediated transport), is designated as *secondary active transport*. The operation of this type of mechanism can be illustrated by the reabsorption of glucose and the secretion of protons in the proximal convoluted tubule. The luminal membrane of the proximal convoluted tubule contains a transport protein with affinity for sodium and glucose. Both sodium and glucose must be on the carrier protein for the transporter to be active. The energy for the translocation of sodium and glucose from the lumen into the renal cell derives from the electrochemical gradient for sodium across the luminal membrane. Thus glucose transport can be described as a sodium-dependent co-transport system and is a secondary active transport process. The sodium entering the cell through this mechanism is removed across the basolateral membrane by the Na^+-K^+ ATPase pump. The glucose is metabolized or exits across the basolateral membrane into the blood. Several other co-transport systems analogous to that of glucose but involving different transport proteins have been described in the brush border membrane of the proximal tubule.[51] Examples include the sodium-dependent phosphate and amino acid transporters that mediate the reabsorption of these solutes from the lumen.

The electrochemical gradient for sodium can also be used for sodium-dependent counter-transport systems. In the proximal tubule, hydrogen ion (H^+) generated by the cell exchanges for sodium in the lumen. This sodium-proton counter exchanger is also a secondary active transport process. Another well described counter-transport system is the sodium-calcium counter-transporter. This transport protein is probably located in the basolateral membrane of the cell.

In addition to cation transport systems, anion exchange transport systems have been identified in various segments of the nephron and appear to be located in the brush border and basolateral membranes. These transport systems are important in the renal excretion of organic metabolites such as urate and oxalate. An organic base transport system has also been identified. In distal nephron segments, a H^+-ATPase has been located, which is important in the renal excretion of acid. Finally, membranes of renal tubule cells also have finite passive permeabilities to electrolytes and nonelectrolytes. The movement of electrolytes and nonelectrolytes by diffusion is governed by electrochemical driving forces and the permeability of the membrane to the solute.

The presence of and the factors controlling the activity of specific transport proteins, whether primary pumps, co- or counter-transporters, or ion channels in specific nephron segments, are areas of great investigational interest and research and are considered in greater detail in textbooks of renal physiology. The location of specific transport proteins is segregated in specific nephron segments, a finding that permits specialization of function along the length of the nephron. In addition, the amount and activity of these transport proteins is under metabolic control.

Thus, in the final analysis, input to the kidney from peripheral sensors or drugs alters the rates of transport within cells of the renal tubules directly by changing the activity or amount of the transporters or indirectly by altering critical electrochemical gradients across the cell membranes. It is important to note, however, that in certain nephron segments, particularly the proximal tubule, fluid and electrolytes can "back-leak" from the interstitium into the lumen through a paracellular pathway between the cells. In such "leaky" epithelia the rates of back-leak may have important effects on the net rates of transport.

Absorptive and Secretory Functions of Renal Tubules

Several organizational levels of renal tubules exist. The nephron can be subdivided into subsegments, each of which differs in morphology, function, and response to drugs, hormones, and other stimuli. This is termed *axial heterogeneity*. Differences also may exist in the function of anatomically similar segments in superficial nephrons as compared to juxtamedullary nephrons, which has been termed *internephronal heterogeneity*. Although internephronal heterogeneity may be of some physiologic importance, it is useful to view the kidney as a single nephron, as illustrated in Fig. 41-7. As glomerular filtrate courses along the nephron, its composition and volume are progressively altered by the presence of the transport processes in the cells of the subsegment, the relative concentration gradients across the membranes of the cells, and the paracellular pathways. Each nephron segment receives

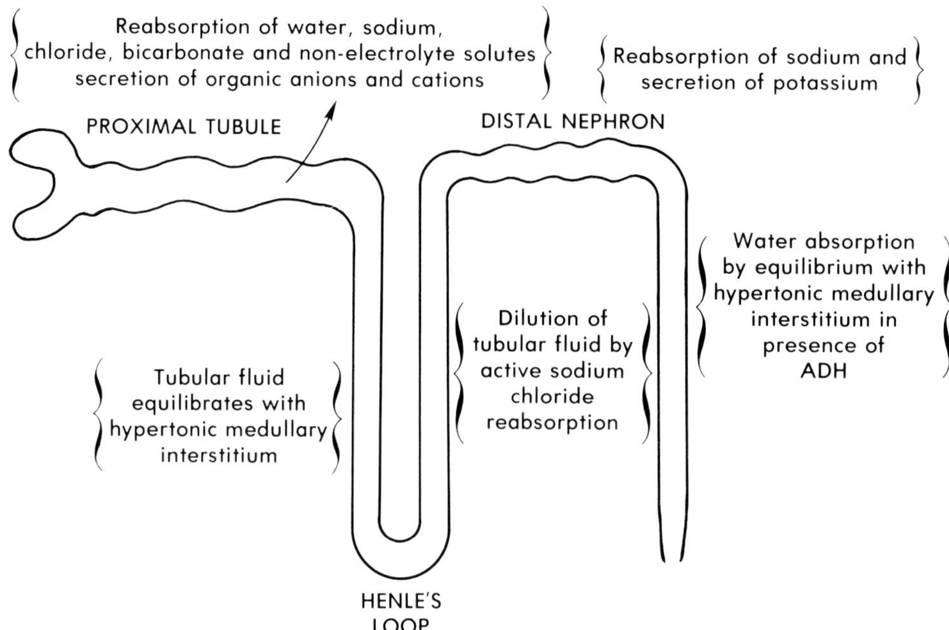

Fig. 41-7 Stylized nephron illustrating the major anatomic divisions and the major fluid and electrolyte transport functions of each division.

tubular fluid different in composition from that in the preceding segment.[27]

Proximal Convoluted Tubule. The proximal convoluted tubule reabsorbs approximately 60% of filtered sodium and water. The osmolality of the fluid in the proximal tubule is nearly isotonic to plasma. Sodium is reabsorbed by the sodium-dependent co-transport and counter-transport processes described earlier and by the diffusion of sodium into the cell. The sodium entering the cell ultimately is removed from the cell by the Na^+-K^+ ATPase pump in the basolateral membrane. Some of the sodium pumped into the interstitium leaks back into the lumen through the paracellular pathway. In the process of flow along the proximal tubule, most of the filtered glucose, amino acids, and bicarbonate is reabsorbed. A significant amount of phosphate is also reabsorbed. Thus, the glomerular filtrate is rendered free of glucose, amino acid, and bicarbonate by the end of the proximal tubule. As bicarbonate is removed, the chloride concentration rises, creating conditions for chloride to diffuse out of the lumen through the paracellular pathway.

The proximal convoluted tubule is a water-permeable segment. As sodium and solutes are removed by transport systems, the luminal fluid becomes hypotonic relative to that of the interstitial space. It is also believed that the effective osmolality of the ions in the interstitial space exceeds that of the tubular fluid. Water therefore rapidly equilibrates across the proximal tubule by moving through the paracellular pathway. Given the high permeability to water in the proximal tubule, the luminal fluid is maintained nearly iso-osmolar.

The proximal convoluted tubule also adds substances to the tubular fluid. Organic anions and bases are removed from blood and translocated into the cells by specific transport proteins in the basolateral membrane. Once inside the cell, these anions and cations can gain access to the tubule fluid by passive or mediated mechanisms across the luminal membrane. Proximal tubule cells also produce ammonia (NH_3), which can diffuse into the lumen, undergo protonation to NH_4^+, and thereby become "trapped" in the tubular fluid.

Thin Limbs of Henle's Loop. In contrast to the proximal tubule, the thin limbs perform little in the way of mediated transport. The descending limb segment of Henle's loop is highly water permeable but impermeable to electrolytes and solutes. The osmolality of the interstitium is progressively higher from the cortex to the tip of the papilla. With the lack of transport systems, the low premeability to solutes, and the high permeability to water in the descending limb, the tubular fluid is progressively concentrated as it equilibrates with the hypertonic interstitium. Thus, at the bend of the Henle's loop, the tubular fluid volume is considerably reduced and its concentration of solutes increased as water is abstracted. In human beings osmolality at the tip of Henle's loop can be as high as 1200 mOsm/kg of water. The water permeability of the ascending limb, unlike that of the descending limb, is low, whereas the permeability to urea and sodium are higher. As a result sodium diffuses down its concentration gradient from the lumen into the interstitium, whereas urea enters the tubular fluid. The net result is a progressive dilution of fluid in the thin ascending limb.[29]

Thick Ascending Limb of Henle's Loop. The properties of the thick ascending limb are strikingly different from that of the thin limbs of Henle's loop. The thick ascending limb is impermeable to water. The luminal membranes of the thick ascending limb's cells contain a transporter for sodium chloride. As fluid moves up this nephron segment, the tubular fluid is progressively diluted as sodium is removed by this secondary active transport process. Fluid

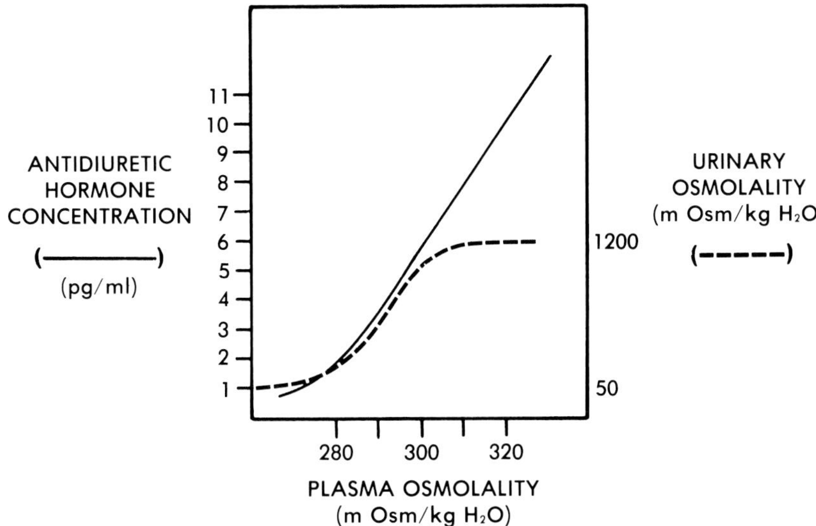

Fig. 41-8 Relationship between extracellular fluid osmolality (represented by plasma osmolality) and antidiuretic hormone (ADH) concentration and urine osmolality. As plasma osmolality rises, ADH levels rise. As the ADH level rises, the urine osmolality increases to its maximum value of about 1200 mOsm/kg of water. Despite further elevations of ADH concentration, urine osmolality does not rise higher.

exiting the thick ascending limb is reduced in osmolality to less than that of plasma. This fluid is hypotonic regardless of the osmolality of the excreted urine. The absorbed sodium chloride is partly retained in the interstitium of the medulla and is critically important in the renal handling of water. The thick ascending limb also reabsorbs calcium and magnesium.

Distal Nephron Segments. Several anatomic and functional subsegments are included in the term *distal nephron*. Considered as a whole, however, this segment finely regulates the composition and volume of the excreted urine. The proximal tubule subserves bulk reabsorption, whereas the distal nephron is responsible for regulation of urinary volume and composition. The distal nephron continues to reabsorb sodium from the filtrate. In addition, the distal nephron (specifically the cortical collecting tubule) secretes potassium. Almost all the potassium that appears in the urine derives from secretion in the distal tubule. The absorption of sodium and the secretion of potassium are influenced by aldosterone. The distal nephron also reabsorbs calcium and, in the absence of parathyroid hormone, phosphate. Hydrogen ions are secreted in the distal portion of the nephron, probably by an H^+-ATPase located in the luminal membrane. Water permeability remains very low in the distal convoluted tubule and the tubular fluid remains hypotonic. The osmolality of the distal tubular fluid is largely caused by urea. The cortical collecting duct epithelium is relatively impermeable to urea, and in the absence of ADH, to water. The presence of ADH renders the cortical collecting duct permeable to water. ADH also increases the water permeability of the medullary collecting duct. Urea permeability in the medullary collecting duct is greater than that of the cortical portion and increases in response to ADH. These considerations are important in understanding the mechanisms involved in the concentration and dilution of urine.

Renal Modulation of Fluid and Electrolyte Homeostasis

Water. In normal human beings excreting a maximmally concentrated urine, approximately 500 ml/day are required to excrete obligatory solutes. The normal kidney is also able to generate approximately 20 L of solute-free water. In other words, a normal individual could ingest or receive up to 20 L of water daily, excrete all of it, and not alter the volume or composition of any water compartment in the body. The development of maximum urinary dilution and concentration depends on precise interactions between almost every nephron segment. This integrated system is disrupted by several renal diseases and drugs and results in an early loss of maximum concentrating and diluting ability. Under such conditions the range of fluid intake that can be accommodated may be severely restricted, and the intake of water may have to be adjusted to conform to the regulatory range of the kidney.

Concentration of the urine depends critically on the presence of ADH. Arginine vasopressin is the mammalian ADH. ADH is produced in the supraoptic nucleus of the hypothalamus and translocated to the posterior pituitary gland for storage and release. The regulation of the ADH release is normally under control of the osmolality of the immediate extracellular fluid enviroment near the osmole receptors in the supraoptic and paraventricular nuclei of the hypothalamus.[45] The range of regulation is narrow, and the gain of the system is high (Fig. 41-8). ADH secretion is almost completely suppressed when plasma osmolality is less than 280 mOsm/kg of water and becomes greatest when osmolality exceeds 290 mOsm/kg of water.

Although the osmolality of the plasma is the major determinant of ADH release, it is important to note that ADH release can occur in response to nonosmolar stimuli. Both depletion of the intravascular volume and hypotension can result in release of ADH directly and in a resetting of the relationship between osmolality and plasma ADH concentration so that ADH is released at lower osmolalities. Depletion of intravascular volume by 8% to 15% is sufficient to stimulate ADH release despite normal plasma osmolality. Similarly, hypotension will cause ADH release despite a normal osmolality of the plasma and a normal intravascular volume. Finally, a variety of other stimuli, which have been loosely called "stressful," (e.g., pain, nausea, and vomiting) will cause ADH release in the presence of normal plasma osmolality, volume status, and blood pressure. Although several drugs, including narcotics, have been implicated in stimulating ADH release, it appears that this is not a primary pharmacologic effect. If the drug causes hypotension, nausea, or anxiety, ADH is released. If these side effects are avoided, no change in plasma ADH level occurs.

ADH binds to specific receptors on the basolateral membrane of the collecting duct cells. Adenylate cyclase is then activated and cyclic adenosine monophosphate (cAMP) produced. Cyclic AMP activates protein phosphatases, which through additional metabolic steps results in a change in the water permeability of the cells of the collecting duct. The increase in the water permeability of the collecting duct allows the fluid within the lumen to come into osmotic equilibrium with the hypertonic medullary interstitium. ADH also alters the urea permeability of the medullary collecting ducts. In addition to its effects on water permeability, ADH increases the rate of sodium chloride transport in the thick ascending limb of Henle's loop and may also decrease plasma flow to the medulla of the kidney. These actions tend to increase the tonicity of and limit the removal of solute from the interstitium and also to enhance the formation of a concentrated urine when distal tubule fluid equilibrates with interstitial fluid. The maximum tonicity of the urine that can be achieved thus depends on a normal response by distal tubule cells to ADH and the tonicity of the medullary interstitial fluid. The tonicity of the interstitial fluid in turn depends on the delivery of filtrate to the thick ascending limb of Henle's loop, the reabsorption of sodium chloride in the thick ascending limb, and by the diffusion to urea out of the collecting ducts.

Water and electrolyte balance are also under the control of the renin-angiotensin-aldosterone system. Renin, an enzyme produced by the kidney, is the rate-limiting step in this system. Its release is stimulated by an intrarenal baroreceptor mechanism, by beta-adrenergic stimulation, and by changes in the delivery of sodium or chloride to the distal nephron. Prostaglandins and calcium also appear to be important in the mechanism underlying its release. Once released, renin causes the conversion of angiotensinogen, a precursor protein produced in the liver, to angiotensin I (AI). A second enzyme, angiotensin-converting enzyme, which is found in all vascular beds, then catalyzes the conversion of AI to angiotensin II (AII), the most active product of the system. AII causes vasoconstriction, elicits the production of aldosterone by the adrenal cortex, stimulates water ingestion (thirst), and has important interactions with the sympathetic nervous system as well as inhibiting further renin release.

Aldosterone production and release by the adrenal cortex are also enhanced by hyperkalemia and negative sodium balance. Further, adrenocorticotropic hormone (ACTH) may play a permissive role in its production. The predominant action of aldosterone is to stimulate the reabsorption of sodium and secretion of potassium by the distal nephron; it thus minimizes the amount of sodium that is excreted in the urine.

As a whole, the renin-angiotensin-aldosterone system is activated by states of inadequate circulating plasma volume or extracellular fluid volume and abnormalities in their composition. It responds by enhancing electrolyte reabsorption and fluid intake and by causing vasoconstriction.[4] (For additional discussion of this system, see Chapters 2 and 45.)

Sodium. Approximately 20,000 mEq of sodium are filtered by the kidneys each day. The kidney is the sole organ of excretion of sodium in normal individuals, and the urinary excretion of sodium matches the dietary intake. In an average healthy person sodium ingestion ranges from 50 to 250 mEq/day. Thus the urinary excretion of sodium is less than 1% of the filtered load. Sixty percent of filtered sodium is reabsorbed in the proximal convoluted tubule. Sodium is also reabsorbed in the thick ascending limb of Henle's loop and in the distal nephron. In the distal nephron aldosterone enhances the rate of sodium reabsorption. Various organs sense the intake of sodium. The rates of absorption at multiple sites within the kidney can be altered by many mechanisms. In addition to stimuli generated outside the kidney, the kidney is capable of directly altering its own rates of reabsorption when the intake of sodium varies.

In an individual with normal renal function the urine can be rendered almost free of sodium. In conditions of excess intake of sodium, the kidney is capable of excreting all this cation, at least up to intakes of several hundred milliequivalents per day. These renal adjustments in the rates of reabsorption of sodium occur in many nephron segments. In the proximal convoluted tubule the rate of sodium reabsorption is increased in states of depletion and decreased in states of expansion in the extracellular fluid volume. These altered rates of transport are mediated by changes in the concentrations of circulating factors, local factors generated by the kidney, renal nerve traffic, and renal hemodynamic factors. Collectively these stimuli affect the rate of sodium and water transport out of the lumen of the proximal tubule and the rate of back-leak through the paracellular pathway.

It has been demonstrated, however, that changes in the rates of reabsorption in the proximal tubule alone do not necessarily result in changes in the urinary excretion of sodium; this is because of the capacity of downstream nephron segments to compensate and independently adjust their rates of sodium reabsorption. Thus the response to a change in the extracellular fluid volume also must involve a change in the rates of sodium reabsorption in Henle's loop and in distal nephron segments. In response to a volume challenge or an increase in sodium intake, for example, the rate of aldosterone secretion is reduced; this factor decreases the rates of sodium reabsorption in the distal nephron. Similarly, sodium depletion results in increased rates of reabsorption in Henle's loop and in the distal nephron segments. The response to alterations in sodium intake are thus integrated over a range of sodium intakes by many mechanisms acting on several subsegments of the nephron. Drugs, disease states of the kidney, and clinical conditions engendering the development of substances that directly or indirectly affect the tubular reabsorption of sodium may limit the kidney's ability to regulate the rates of sodium excretion.[28,46,47]

POTASSIUM. Unlike with sodium, the urine cannot be rendered free of potassium. Despite this, the range of potassium intakes that can be tolerated is quite large. The renal response to rapid alterations in potassium intake are slower than that for sodium. In human beings rates of potassium ingestion and excretion can be increased progressively with no change in the plasma or tissue concentration of potassium as long as such step increases in intake occur over several days. Sudden and large increases in potassium intake can overwhelm both the capacity of the kidney to excrete the load and the ability of other tissues to sequester potassium.

Filtered potassium is reabsorbed in the proximal convoluted tubule. The major regulatory site for potassium excretion is the distal nephron. In this segment potassium is taken up across the basolateral membrane into the cell by the operation of the Na^+-K^+ ATPase pump. The potassium content of the cells of the distal tubule is above electrochemical equilibrium. A finite permeability of the luminal membrane to potassium permits potassium to diffuse out of the cell into the lumen. The process across the luminal membrane is passive and governed by the prevailing electrochemical gradients from cell to lumen.

The major determinant for potassium secretion appears to be the concentration of potassium in the luminal fluid. When luminal flow is high, the secreted potassium is rapidly diluted and the gradient for potassium secretion maintained. In states of low flow the cell-to-lumen potassium concentration gradient is rapidly decreased and the absolute rate of secretion diminished. Thus flow rate past the distal tubule is a major factor influencing the urinary secretion and excretion of potassium. Another factor is the electric potential difference from the cell to the lumen of the distal tubule. The lumen's negative potential difference is generated by the tubular reabsorption of sodium. The greater the rate of sodium reabsorption, the more negative is the voltage in the lumen. The link between sodium and potassium transport therefore derives not from the presence of a counter-transport process, but rather from electrochemical coupling.

Aldosterone increases the rate of potassium secretion by several mechanisns.[54] It increases the permeability of the luminal membrane to potassium; enhances the rate of sodium reabsorption, rendering the tubule lumen more electroengative; and increases the activity of the Na^+-K^+ ATPase pump. The rate of aldosterone secretion is influenced by the renin-angiotensin system and by the plasma concentration of potassium. Sodium depletion can stimulate the renal production of renin, which ultimately results in stimulation of aldosterone secretion. The generated aldosterone thus serves a role in sodium conservation. Increases in dietary intake of potassium can directly increase the secretion of aldosterone. The aldosterone serves to increase urinary excretion of potassium.

It is important to note that aldosterone is not the only factor affecting potassium metabolism. In addition to urinary excretion, potassium is taken up and released by other tissues of the body. Although those nonrenal mechanisms can help modulate the plasma concentrations of potassium, they do not serve to eliminate potassium from the body. The renal excretion of potassium may be affected by kidney diseases, various hormones, and therapeutic drugs.[18,24,53]

BICARBONATE. The metabolism of food results in the generation of approximately 1 mEq of H^+/kg body weight/day of nonvolatile acid. This acid must be excreted by the kidney. The kidney filters approximately 3500 mEq of bicarbonate, which must be reabsorbed. Although the overall body production of acid is only 70 mEq/day in a 70 Kg individual, the kidney must secrete 3500 plus 70 mEq/day to reabsorb filtered bicarbonate and dispose of metabolic acid. The bulk of filtered bicarbonate is absorbed in the proximal tubule by a process linked to the secretion of protons in the lumen. Sodium ions and protons undergo counter-exchange in this nephron segment. The secreted protons combine with filtered bicarbonate and, under the influence of carbonic anhydrase, are converted to carbon dioxide and water. The carbon dioxide readily crosses the luminal membrane into the cell. Within the cell, carbon dioxide is hydrated to carbonic acid (catalyzed by carbonic anhydrase), which dissociates into a hydrogen ion and a bicarbonate ion. This bicarbonate exits through the basolateral membrane and is returned to the blood. The hydrogen ion is then secreted into the luminal fluid.

The rate of reabsorption of bicarbonate in the proximal tubule is influenced by several factors. In general, when the rates of sodium reabsorption are enhanced or inhibited in the proximal tubule, parallel changes occur in the capacity for bicarbonate reabsorption. Systemic acid-base conditions and potassium balance also affect the rates of bicarbonate reabsorption. Bicarbonate that escapes reabsorption in the proximal tubule can be reabsorbed in more distal nephron sites by a proton pump that requires ATP. The capacity of the distal nephron for bicarbonate reabsorption, however, is limited. The net result of these processes is to reclaim filtered bicarbonate but not to dispose of metabolic acid.[11]

NONVOLATILE ACIDS. Nonvolative acids are excreted by two processes. First, hydrogen ions that are secreted into the lumen are buffered by the conversion of Na_2HPO_4 to NaH_2PO_4, a process known as the *formation of titratable acid*. Approximately 30 mEq of acid are eliminated by this mechanism each day, and the amount is relatively fixed. Second, nonvolatile acid excretion occurs through the renal production of ammonia, (NH_3) from the metabolism of glutamine. NH_3 is a gas that diffuses into both the lumen and the peritubular capillary blood. In the lumen NH_3 is protonated to NH_4^+ and in this state is trapped in the lumen because of the lower permeability of the ionized species. This process is known as *nonionic diffusion trapping*. In response to acidosis, an increase in the rate of renal NH_3 production is the major mechanism for eliminating fixed acid from the body. Bones and other tissues can act as temporary buffers, but ultimately excretion by the kidney is required.[36,50]

CALCIUM AND MAGNESIUM. Calcium is reabsorbed in the proximal tuble, Henle's loop, and in certain subsegments of the distal nephron. Magnesium, on the other hand, is reabsorbed predominantly in the Henle's loop. Acutely and chronically, the reabsorption of calcium and probably magnesium are affected by parathyroid hormone (PTH). The absolute rates of excretion of these substances, however, depend on the balance between delivery to the kidney and the renal transport mechanisms. In states of PTH excess, for example, the absolute rates of calcium absorption by the kidney are increased despite the absolute rates of excretion also being increased. Kidney diseases and drugs such as diuretics can influence the renal excretion of calcium.[13,15,31]

PHOSPHATE. Filtered phosphate is reabsorbed by a sodium-dependent mechanism in the proximal tubule. In the presence of permissive amounts of PTH, phosphate rejected from the proximal tubule cannot be reabsorbed in more distal nephron segments. The rate of phosphate reabsorption in the proximal tubule is influenced by PTH and vitamin D. PTH, through specific receptors in the proximal tubule and the generation of cAMP, inhibits the tubular reabsorption of phosphate and is a major regulating factor. Increases in the ingestion of phosphate transiently reduce the plasma concentration of ionized calcium and result in the release of PTH. PTH causes a phosphaturia and a normalization of the serum concentrations of phosphate and ionized calcium. Other hormones, including corticosteroids, glucagon, and insulin, can affect handling of phosphate by the kidney. In addition, abnormalities in phosphate metabolism are intimately involved in the genesis of the multifactorial systemic manifestations of advanced renal disease. Hypophosphatemia also affects renal function and can result in a decreased rate of reabsorption of bicarbonate and calcium.[13,31]

OTHER METABOLITES. The kidneys also excrete a variety of metabolic waste products and drugs. Well-described organic-acid and organic-base secretory systems are present in the kidney. In general, organic compounds are taken up at the antiluminal border of the cell and secreted into the lumen. Some of these substances such as urate are also reabsorbed by the kidney. Thus urate undergoes bidirectional tubular transport. The excretion of organic compounds is complex and influenced by kidney disease, drugs, and hormones.

Tubular Function in Renal Disease

The ability of the kidney to regulate rates of excretion and contribute to overall body homeostasis may be affected by several factors. Drugs and disease conditions may selectively alter one or another specific transport process. Diffuse parenchymal disease is often characterized by many abnormalities. Compensating mechanisms may provide a margin of reserve, which blunts the clinical expression of the abnormality. For example, even when up to 90% of renal function is destroyed, the serum concentrations of calcium, phosphate, and potassium may be normal. With additional damage, abnormalities in plasma concentrations of these substances become evident. Under such circumstances intake must be matched to output to maintain homeostasis. One characteristic of renal disease is the loss of the kidney's ability to regulate water and sodium balance, resulting in the excretion of relatively fixed amounts of solutes. Intake that exceeds the kidney's ability to excrete will result in increases in body water and solutes, whereas limitations in intake may result in states of depletion.[9]

CLINICAL ASSESSMENT OF RENAL FUNCTION

Urinalysis

The urinalysis has long been used as a screening test for renal or systemic disease.[19] Typical tests that are components of the urinalysis include measurement of urinary glucose, protein, pH, and specific gravity, as well as microscopic examination. The use of the urinalysis in the diagnosis of specific disease conditions is a critical part of the preoperative evaluation of patients and in following patients in the postsurgical period.[22]

Urine Osmolality and Specific Gravity

The term *specific gravity* refers to the weight of a fixed volume of solution expressed as a multiple of the weight of the same volume of pure water. The addition of physiologic solutes to water generally increases its density and thus its specific gravity. Unfortunately, the relationship between the concentration of solute in the solution (i.e., osmolality) and the specific gravity depends heavily on the nature of the solute. For example, a small amount of protein greatly increases specific gravity but changes osmolality very little. Osmolality is thus a far more useful measure of urinary concentration than specific gravity. The potential differences that may exist in a given patient between urinary osmolality and urinary specific gravity are important to remember since specific gravity measurements are often used in clinical medicine as an index of the kidneys' concentrating ability. The specific gravity of a voided urine specimen, for example, may indicate a value representative of normal renal concentrating ability (e.g., 1.018), when in fact the urinary osmolality is the same as in plasma. (See prior discussion on water regulation and the following section on urine osmolality and urine flow rate.)

Urinary pH

Urinary pH varies greatly from 4.4 to 8.0 and reflects the need of the body to excrete acid or base to maintain plasma pH at 7.4. A persistently alkaline urine ($pH > 7$) is seen in metabolic alkalosis and may indicate urinary tract infection with a urea-splitting organism. A relatively alkaline urine is found in patients with renal tubular acidosis, a condition caused by incomplete reabsorption of bicarbonate or insufficient secretion of hydrogen ion. A discussion of these complex disorders is beyond the scope of this chapter.

Proteinuria

By definition, proteinuria refers to excretion of more than 100 mg of protein in 24 hours. A small amount of protein, especially of low molecular weight, is filtered by the glomerulus, but the bulk of it is reabsorbed in the proximal tubule. When found in the urine, protein usually reflects glomerular disease but may also indicate renal tubular defects, polycystic kidneys, infection, hypertension, or renal vein thrombosis. The molecular weight of the protein is often helpful in distinguishing its etiology. Urinary protein of large molecular weight (> 55,000 daltons) generally indicates glomerular basement membrane injury (glomerulonephritis), whereas low-molecular-weight urinary protein indicates renal tubular injury (acute tubular necrosis, infection). In many glomerular diseases the excretion of larger proteins increases dramatically. When protein excretion exceeds 3.5 g/24 hours, the diagnosis of nephrotic syndrome is made. Many etiologies of nephrotic syndrome exist and are considered in detail in Chapter 43.

Glycosuria

Glycosuria occurs when the amount of glucose filtered exceeds the capacity of the proximal tubular reabsorption mechanism. Thus glycosuria occurs in the presence of elevated glucose levels (e.g., > 180 mg/100 ml), an elevated GFR, or a reduction in tubular transport function secondary to disease or drugs. Glycosuria in the absence of high exogenous carbohydrate loads and stress usually means that a patient has diabetes mellitus. The two common tests for urine glucose are *copper reduction*, which detects many substances other than glucose, and *glucose oxidase*, which is much more specific. False-positive glucose oxidase results may be seen if the specimen is contaminated with hydrogen peroxide or hypochlorites, and false-negative results may occur in the presence of L-dopa or aspirin.

Urinary Sediment

Microscopic examination of the urinary sediment can give important information regarding the level within the urinary tract at which disease is active. The presence of casts containing cellular elements implies parenchymal renal disease, whereas free red blood cells can arise at any level. Likewise, white blood cell casts indicate inflammatory renal disease, and casts composed of epithelial cells are associated with tubular damage.

Various types of urinary crystals may also be important aids to diagnosis of disease. Crystals of calcium oxalate or calcium phosphate may mean that the patient has hypercalcemia or calcium-containing renal calculi. Uric acid crystals reflect hyperuricosuria and uric acid stone formation and may indicate that the patient has gout or other diseases associated with hyperuricemia. Similarly, cystine crystals indicate that the patient probably has cystinuria since such crystals are almost never found in the urine under normal conditions. Finally, triple-phosphate crystals indicate the presence of urinary tract stones produced by infection with urea-splitting organisms. For greatest clinical value, such determinations should be obtained before administration of diuretics.

Renal Function Tests

Tests of renal function can be classified as those predominantly related to (1) renal blood flow, (2) GFR, and (3) tubular transport function.[22]

Renal Blood Flow

Clinical measurement of renal blood flow is indirect, and methodologic problems hamper the interpretation of data. The most frequently used method is the clearance measurement of substances that are actively secreted into the urine and whose clearance is limited primarily by renal plasma flow. *p*-Aminohippuric acid (PAH) is such a substance. Approximately 85% to 95% of PAH is cleared from plasma in one passage through the kidney under normal circumstances. Renal plasma flow is equal to the clearance of any substance divided by its extraction ratio. The calculation of the extraction ratio requires the measurement of the concentration of the substance in the renal venous plasma. Clearance of a substance such as PAH will not be higher than the renal plasma flow. It must be emphasized, however, that a reduction in PAH clearance may be caused by a decrease in tubular secretory function, which results in a lowered extraction ratio, as well as by a reduction in renal plasma flow. Because of the nonspecificity of such clearance techniques, they are not widely used today in the clinical setting.

Renal blood flow can also be estimated by various radiologic methods, including angiography and scans of the kidney using radioisotopes.[1] Although useful in experimental studies, determination of the rates of renal blood flow with these techniques is not usually employed clinically. Rather, the clinical use of measuring renal blood flow by nuclear scanning or angiography is to determine (1) the patency of the vascular tree in suspected cases of renovascular catastrophies and renal transplants and (2) the relative as opposed to the absolute differences in blood flow between the kidneys.

Glomerular Filtration Rate

The GFR is often estimated by measuring the clearance of creatinine. The plasma creatinine concentration is typically used alone to evaluate renal filtration function. The plasma creatinine level indicates the balance between creatinine excretion by the kidney and creatinine production by muscle. The total excretion of creatinine is proportional to the muscle mass of the body, and derangements in muscle mass must be considered in interpreting the serum concentration of creatinine. Although a serum creatinine concentration of 1.2 or 1.4 mg/100 ml may be consistent with a normal GFR in a muscular young male, a similar plasma value in an elderly, inactive female may indicate a 50% to 75% reduction in GFR. The use of serum creatinine is also limited by the requirement for a steady state. If the GFR is unstable, changes in serum concentration of creatinine will lag behind by 1 to 2 days.

The clearance of creatinine is the result of both filtration and secretion, which results in an overestimate of the true GFR by as much as 30%. The overestimation increases as GFR falls and the serum creatinine concentration rises. Thus creatinine clearance represents the maximum likely GFR. Despite these shortcomings and the difficulties in obtaining quantitative collections of urine, the safety and simplicity of measuring creatinine clearance warrant its use for estimating GFR. For more accurate estimation of the GFR, measurement of inulin clearance can be employed.

Inulin is a carbohydrate that is filtered but not metabolized, secreted, or reabsorbed. Its clearance rate is considered to be the best measurement of true GFR.

Tubular Transport Function

Fractional Rates of Solute Excretion. Tests of tubular function include determinations of the fractional rates of excretion of a solute, the concentration of the solute in the urine, and the urinary osmolality. The term *fractional excretion* is defined as the ratio of the amount of a substance filtered at the glomerulus that is excreted in the urine; this is expressed as a percentage. The fractional excretion rate can be calculated as the clearance of a substance divided by the clearance of a glomerular filtration marker. Thus the fractional excretion (FE) of a solute (s) is calculated from the following expression:

$$FE_s(\%) = \frac{C_s}{C_{cr}} \times 100 = \frac{(U_s \times \dot{V}) \div P_s}{(U_{cr} \times \dot{V}) \div P_{cr}} \times 100 = \frac{U_s / P_s}{U_{cr} / P_{cr}} \times 100$$

where C is the clearance; U_s and P_s are the urine and ultrafiltrable plasma concentrations of the solute; U_{cr} and P_{cr} are the urine and plasma concentrations of the glomerular filtration marker, creatinine (cr); and $\dot{V}$ is the urine flow rate.

Normal fractional rates of excretion for the major solutes of plasma have been determined. For example, in normal human beings the FE of urate is approximately 7% to 10% of the filtered load. In patients with tubular defects in the absorption of urate or in individuals receiving a drug that inhibits the absorption of urate, the FE of urate rises. The FE of any solute can be determined to evaluate tubular function. Since urate and phosphate are handled predominantly in the proximal convoluted tubule, calculation of the FE of these two substances can be used to reflect transport activity in this nephron segment.

A frequently used clinical test is the determination of the fractional rate of sodium excretion.[21,41] In normal individuals the FE of sodium is less than 1%. The FE of sodium increases when sodium is ingested, when diuretics are administered, or when renal tubular disease is present. In a patient with signs of fluid overload, a low FE rate of sodium is inappropriate. In a patient with normal hydration or in a patient who is volume depleted, a FE of sodium greater than 1% is inappropriate and may indicate renal tubular disease or administration of diuretics.

The measurement of urine sodium concentration alone is of less value than the determination of the fractional rate of excretion. The urinary sodium concentration is determined not only by the degree of sodium reabsorption but also by the degree of urinary dilution. Thus the excretion of 100 mEq of sodium in a liter of urine results in sodium concentration of 100 mEq/L. The excretion of the same 100 mEq in 3000 ml of urine results in a concentration of only 33 mEq/L. In the presence of the same absolute and fractional rates of excretions of sodium, the sodium concentration can vary threefold.

Urine Osmolality and Urine Flow Rate. The measurement of the osmolality of urine is useful when interpreted together with the clinical condition of the patient. Since urinary concentration depends on the integrated function of multiple nephron segments, determination of the urine osmolality is a relatively sensitive test of tubular function. When urine osmolality should be elevated, such as in hyperosmolality of the plasma, hypovolemia, or hypotension, the findings of an iso-osmolar urine suggests that the kidney is incapable of producing a concentrated urine. The finding of a high urine osmolality conversely suggests that integration of nephron function is relatively intact.

The measurement of urine output is probably the most frequently performed renal function test. As a single measure of renal function, however, the urine flow rate is not a very specific test. Patients with severe renal failure may have normal urine flow rates. The urine flow rate depends on the intake or administration of water, the concentration of ADH, the tonicity of the medullary interstitium, the response of the kidney to ADH, the glomerular filtration rate, and the tubular reabsorption of sodium. Given the number of factors that can influence the measured urine flow rate, this determination is not usually of clinical value as a measure of tubular function. However, quantitative measurement of the urine output is of value in specific clinical situations.

CLINICAL CORRELATIONS

Effects of Anesthesia and Surgery on Renal Function

Physicians have recognized since the beginning of this century that anesthetics can influence renal function. Most studies involving currently used anesthetics have been performed on human beings, but exact mechanisms by which the observed changes are produced have not been clarified. Despite this lack of information, total renal blood flow, as measured by PAH clearance, falls by 20% to 40% during anesthesia with potent inhalation anesthetics or during balanced anesthesia with nitrous oxide, narcotics, and muscle relaxants. These changes occur in the absence of major changes in blood pressure. The same anesthetics generally cause a somewhat lesser reduction (20% to 30%) in GFR. The effects of anesthesia on blood flow and GFR are increased as the depth of anesthesia is increased. Vigorous hydration before the induction of anesthesia blunts but does not totally prevent the changes in blood flow and GFR. With deeper levels of anesthesia, hydration has no effect on the decrease in blood flow and filtration rate. Subarachnoid and epidural anesthesia have few direct effects on renal plasma flow and GFR.

In response to anesthesia, the urine flow rate decreases even more than either the GFR or the rate of renal plasma flow. The decrease in urine flow rate is usually accompanied by a modest increase in urine osmolality, although urine osmolalities greater than 700 to 800 mOsm/kg of water are unusual. The effects of inhalation anesthesia and regional anesthesia on the urine flow rate appear to be similar.

The mechanisms responsible for the changes in renal function following induction of anesthesia are unclear. It has been demonstrated that well-conducted general anesthesia is not associated with significant elevations in plasma renin activity or in the plasma concentration of vasopressin. Almost all the modern general anesthetics and the regional blocks tend to cause a reduction in sympathetic nerve activity and in catecholamine concentrations.

Methoxyflurane has been reported to be an indirect renal toxin and results in renal injury.[37] The toxicity of this agent is caused by the generation of inorganic fluoride from the metabolism of methoxyflurane; the typical patient has polyuria that is resistant to therapy with vasopressin. The only other anesthetic that releases significant amounts of fluoride is *enflurane*. Only very prolonged and deep anesthesia with this agent, however, has resulted in fluoride levels which are associated with changes in renal function.[12] Aside from these two agents, no other general anesthetics are associated with direct renal toxicity. The observed changes in renal function following anesthesia are not usually associated with morphologic changes. These functional changes are rapidly reversed when the anesthetic state is discontinued.

When surgery is performed during the anesthetic state, several additional changes in renal function occur. Renal plasma flow and GFR may decrease further, and ADH release is greatly stimulated. ADH concentrations often increase to levels that are supramaximum for urinary concentration. The effect of surgery on ADH concentrations may be blunted somewhat by increasing the depth of anesthesia. In addition, following the surgical stimulus, stimulation of the sympathetic nervous system and of renin release may occur. When surgery is performed, the changes in renal plasma flow and GFR persist into the immediate postoperative period. The degree and the duration of renal function depression increases roughly in proportion to the magnitude of the surgical procedure performed. The factors responsible for this persistent suppression of renal function have not been well clarified.

Alterations in Renal Function in Response to Systemic Diseases

Besides primary diseases of the kidney, renal function may be altered by systemic diseases as well. The renal response to depletion of the extracellular fluid volume, regardless of etiology, in patients with normal renal function is a decrease in the urinary excretion of sodium and water. This response reflects the influence of normal homeostatic mechanisms that attempt to maintain the fluid volume of the body. Diseases characterized by external losses of fluid and electrolytes or blood, as well as clinical conditions characterized by no external loss but rather by a sequestration of fluids within the body (as in patients with pancreatitis, in whom fluid is lost from the vascular to the interstitial space), may initiate this response. In patients with diseases such as cirrhosis or heart failure, in whom total body fluid may be increased although the "effective" circulating volume is decreased, this response is also triggered.

In all of these conditions body sensors detect a state of volume depletion and initiate a series of stimuli that result in sodium and water avidity by the kidney. This response is adaptive in the cases of sequestration and internal shifts but may be maladaptive in a patient with congestive heart failure. The characteristics of conditions in which a decreased effective circulating volume occurs are:

1. A decrease in the GFR and a rise in the serum concentration of blood urea nitrogen (BUN) and creatinine
2. A rise in the BUN/creatinine ratio in plasma
3. A low urinary concentration of sodium, usually less than 20 mEq/L, on a spot sample of urine
4. A rise in urine osmolality to greater than 800 mOsm/kg of water
5. Fractional excretion of sodium less than 1%

The administration of diuretics; the presence of high rates of excretion of nonelectrolyte osmoles such as glucose, mannitol, or urea; or renal disease may render these urine indices of volume depletion nondiagnostic. In the absence of these confounding variables, the urinary indices reflect the intact nature of the renal response to loss of effective circulating volume. If a patient, who by other criteria is volume depleted, manifests inappropriately high rates of excretion of sodium (>40 mEq/L on a spot sample of urine or a fractional excretion of sodium >1%) in the absence of a diuretic or high osmolar loads, the possibility of acute or chronic renal injury must be considered. As a clinical rule, urinary excretion of sodium or preferably the fractional excretion of sodium and the urine osmolality, should be obtained immediately when assessment of fluid balance is required. For maximum clinical value, such determinations should be obtained before administration of diuretics.

In patients who by other criteria appear to have expansion of the extracellular fluid volume, but whose urinary excretion of sodium is low and urinary osmolality is high, the physician must consider that the kidney may be sensing effective circulating volume as being inadequate. In such a patient central hemodynamic monitoring may indicate that the central volume is appropriate or overexpanded and that the renal response reflects hormonal or nervous override of normal volume regulatory mechanisms. Hemodynamic monitoring may also indicate that the central volume is depleted, despite the apparent presence of fluid excess by other criteria. Under such circumstances the renal response is appropriate.

Liver Disease and the Kidney

Patients with advanced liver failure, and especially those with hepatic cirrhosis, develop a characteristic type of renal dysfunction termed *hepatorenal syndrome (HRS)*. This syndrome consists of renal dysfunction characterized by a reduction in GFR, severe sodium retention (urine Na usually <10 mEq/L), and severe oliguria. Hepatic coma, ascites, relative hypotension, and jaundice are frequently present. Further, the severity of these abnormalities does not correlate well with the degree of renal dysfunction. Small amounts of protein are found in the urine, and hyaline and granular cases are typical in HRS patients. Impaired renal concentrating ability usually occurs although the urine osmolality is often modestly elevated. The most characteristic abnormality is the extremely low concentrations of sodium found in the urine. This has been attributed primarily to a reduction in distal delivery of sodium to the tubules because of reduced filtration and enhanced proximal reabsorption.

One of the most prominent and consistent findings in patients with HRS is an alteration in renal blood flow. In patients with cirrhosis and HRS angiography reveals severe attenuation of interlobar arteries, with loss of visualization of arcuate and interlobular arteries.[1] The constriction may be segmental, giving a beaded appearance. The nephrogram is diminished, with a loss of the normal distinction between cortex and medulla. The arterial washout phase is prolonged, and the renal vein rarely visualizes. Xenon scans reflect a labile diminution in flow, which affects the superficial cortex to a greater degree than the juxtamedullary region. This renal vasoconstriction is not reversed by alpha-adrenergic blockade. Autopsy reveals no evidence of this vasoconstriction. Of further interest, kidneys from patients with HRS have been successfully transplanted with no vasoconstrictive problems following transplantation.

The GFR is severely reduced in HRS. Consequently, serum creatinine is usually in the range of 4 to 6 mg/100 ml. The reduction in GFR appears to be functional and is probably related to the severe abnormalities in renal blood flow and its distribution, since most investigators do not report any characteristic pathologic abnormality of kidneys at autopsy or following biopsy in patients with HRS. Although glomerular sclerosis has been found in some patients, it does not correlate with the degree of renal dysfunction.

Although ADH, PTH, the kallikrein-kinin system, natriuretic hormone, vasoactive intestinal peptide, and prostaglandins have all been proposed as possibly playing a role in the pathogenesis of this syndrome, the renin-angiotensin-aldosterone system has received the most attention in studies of HRS. Cirrhotic patients without HRS have elevated plasma renin activity and aldosterone concentrations. Whereas renin levels correlate inversely with sodium excretion, aldosterone levels do not.[43] It seems unlikely that elevated aldosterone levels are primarily responsible for the profound sodium retention found in HRS patients since sodium excretion can be dissociated from plasma aldosterone levels by various experimental manipulations in these patients.[5,16,17,48]

Much debate has surrounded the role of disturbances in extracellular and plasma fluid volumes and the distribution of cardiac output in HRS patients. The concept of "effective circulating blood volume" has been invoked to explain the apparent paradox of an increased extracellular fluid volume seen in these patients associated with renal responses usually found in states of volume depletion. Volume expansion by intravenous infusion of fluid, by body immersion in water, or by reinfusion of ascitic fluid will usually cause an increase in GFR and sodium excretion. Unfortunately, in the case of administration of intravenous fluids, the net sodium and water balance are positive. The relative hypovolemia has been explained by splanchnic pooling, a reduction in colloid osmotic pressure secondary to hypoalbuminemia, and an increase in vascular capacitance secondary to systemic vasodilation. Since some patients do not respond to these factors, this proposed concept to account for the findings in HRS cannot entirely explain the observed abnormalities. An alternate proposal suggests that sodium and water retention are the primary events that cause the expanded extracellular fluid volume and vasodilation. This hypothesis, however, fails to explain why some patients *do* respond to augmentation of their intravascular volume with diuresis. Thus no adequate explanation exists at present for the abnormalities.

Bilirubin per se does not cause the renal functional abnormalities seen in HRS, but bile salts do induce vasodilation, hypotension, and sodium retention when administered chronically. In contrast, acute bile duct ligation in dogs, which induces bile stasis within the liver, has been reported to cause an increase in GFR and sodium excretion.[2]

A final hypothesis to explain HRS speculates that the deranged liver performance in cirrhotic patients permits the passage of endotoxin produced in the gut into the systemic circulation. The endotoxin then produces the characteristic hemodynamic and renal functional changes.[42] It has been further postulated that jaundiced patients without cirrhosis may be at risk for increased endotoxin absorption because of a deficiency of bile acids in the lumen of the gut. Currently available data are only suggestive, and no studies have shown that low levels of endotoxin can produce the entire spectrum of observed clinical abnormalities.

The treatment of HRS has been unsuccessful unless hepatic function improves. It is critical to maintain intravascular volume throughout any illness in patients with preexisting liver disease. Since systemic hemodynamics are often abnormal in patients with cirrhosis, invasive monitoring is frequently required. The choice of fluid for maintenance of intravascular volume remains controversial. In some patients establishment of a peritoneovenous shunt will restore intravascular volume, diminish the volume of ascites, and improve renal function. Crystalloid infusion alone rarely causes more than a transient improvement and uniformly results in accumulation of massive amounts of edema and ascitic fluid. Protein-containing solutions produce a more lasting response, but no data show that these improve survival. The use of vasodilators and vasopressors in these patients is also controversial. When hypotension is clearly present, some patients will have improvement in their urine output when dopamine is used to restore normotension. As with fluid resuscitation, however, little evidence suggests that survival is improved. Although dialysis will support life in patients with HRS, it is often difficult to remove significant amounts of fluid without producing severe hypotension. Thus, unless the liver itself improves, treatment of the associated renal dysfunction in HRS patients is rarely effectual.[40]

Abnormalities in Urine Volume

Oliguria

Oliguria may be defined as a urine flow rate that is reduced below the level capable of excreting obligatory solutes. Osmolar excretion is calculated by multiplying the urine flow rate by the urine osmolality. The daily osmolar load averages 12 mOsm/kg body weight/day, which is equivalent to an osmolar excretion rate of 0.5 mOsm/kg/hour. Since each milliliter of urine is capable of excreting 1 mOsm (maximum urinary concentration, approximately

1000 mOsm/L of water), it is unlikely that osmolar excretion is adequate if the urine output is less than 0.5 ml/kg/hour.

Oliguria or a low osmolar excretion suggests that GFR is reduced. However, the presence of a "normal" urine output is no guarantee that the GFR is normal. In healthy persons the kidney normally reabsorbs 98% to 99% of the glomerular filtrate. Any reduction in the efficiency of the concentrating mechanism will result in excretion of a larger fraction of the glomerular filtrate. For example, if the fractional excretion of filtrate rose to 10%, a GFR of 10 ml/minute (10% of normal) would result in a urine output of 1 ml/minute, or 60 ml/hour. Thus, although the presence of oliguria indicates that renal function is impaired, the absence of oliguria provides no assurance that function is not impaired. Since the excretion of catabolic products primarily depends on glomerular filtration, most chemical and clinical abnormalities of oliguric renal failure can be observed in patients despite the presence of a "normal" urine output.

Polyuria

Polyuria is defined literally as a large volume of urine.[3] Generally this implies that the urine output exceeds the flow rate required to maintain a balance of fluid within body compartments; if allowed to persist, this will result in a depletion of extracellular fluid volume. The clinical recognition of an excessive urinary output, or polyuric state, is occasionally difficult. A urine output greater than 300 ml/hour suggests the diagnosis of polyuria. One must recognize, however, that it is appropriate for the body to excrete fluid administered in excess of body needs.

"True" polyuria results from two primary mechanisms, each of which evolves from the known physiology of the kidney. The first is an *osmotic diuresis*. This form of diuresis results when the proximal tubule fails to reabsorb the bulk of the filtered solute. This may be caused by tubular epithelial disease, an overload or saturation of reabsorptive mechanisms, or nonabsorbable, osmotically active substances. Osmotic diuretics increase medullary blood flow, which reduces the solute concentration in the medullary interstitium. Whereas approximately 50% of the volume entering the descending limb is normally reabsorbed, less than 10% may be reabsorbed during an osmotic diuresis. In the distal nephron segments the absolute amount of sodium chloride that is reabsorbed probably increases, but the ability to compensate for proximal defects is limited. In the collecting duct, water reabsorption is limited by the lack of a hypertonic medullary interstitium. The presence or absence of ADH becomes less important in these circumstances. During osmotic diuresis the urine will approach iso-osmolality.

An osmotic diuresis is frequently encountered in surgical patients. Hyperglycemia will saturate the reabsorptive capacity of the proximal tubule when the blood sugar approaches 180 to 300 mg/100 ml. The administration of mannitol or urea represents therapeutic attempts at attaining an osmotic diuresis. Fluid and electrolyte resuscitation following injury and in the perioperative period results in positive water and electrolyte balance. During recovery the hormonal mechanisms mediating this retention abate, and the excess will be excreted. Radiocontrast agents employed in various radiologic procedures typically have osmolalities higher than 1000 mOsm/kg of water and routinely produce an osmotic diuresis. With damage to the proximal tubule, sodium reabsorption is depressed, and an osmotic diuresis may ensue.

The second example of a "true" polyuria is seen in the patient undergoing *water diuresis*. In contrast to an osmotic diuresis, in which the urinary osmolality is relatively isotonic, water diuresis results in production of a very dilute urine (urinary osmolality of 50 to 100 mOsm/kg water). A water diuresis may result either from a lack of ADH or from an inability of the collecting duct to respond normally to ADH. Low ADH concentrations are normally seen in the presence of hypoosmolality of the extracellular fluid. A pathologic lack of ADH (diabetes insipidus) may be seen in patients with hypothalamic and pituitary lesions and following surgery on the pituitary gland and hypothalamus.[39] In the normal kidney with a GFR of 100 ml/minute, 60 to 70 ml/minute will be reabsorbed by the proximal tubule. Half of the remaining fluid, or 15 to 20 ml/minute, will be reabsorbed in Henle's loop, If no further reabsorption occurs, as in the case of diabetes insipidus, as much as 15 ml/minute (or 900 ml/hour) could be excreted as urine. Urine flow rates of this magnitude are not usually observed, however, since diabetes insipidus rapidly results in hypovolemia, a reduction in GFR, and an increase in the percentage of electrolytes and fluid reabsorbed in the proximal tubule.

Thus a urine output in excess of 900 ml/hour suggests that mechanisms other than or in addition to diabetes insipidus are present. These considerations are especially important in the management of patients following head trauma and pituitary or brain surgery.[44]

Use of Diuretics

The major diuretics in use in the in-hospital situation are the osmotic diuretics and the high-ceiling loop diuretics. *Osmotic diuretics,* such as mannitol, are filtered by the glomeruli and act as a nonreabsorbable solute in the proximal tubule.[52] Mannitol obligates water relative to sodium such that vigorous administration of mannitol will result in hypernatremia. It is also important to remember that the kidney is the sole route of excretion of mannitol. Systemic administration of mannitol to a patient whose GFR is reduced may result in a failure to obtain a diuresis and, more importantly, the retention of unwanted osmoles in the plasma.

The major clinical uses of agents such as mannitol may be (1) the purposeful reduction in the extracellular fluid volume in patients with cerebral edema, (2) the initiation of an increase in the urine flow rate in patients with specific types of drug overdoses, and (3) the preparation of some patients for procedures that may be associated with renal injury. The third use derives from experimental observations that high urine flow rates may protect the kidney from some types of acute renal injury.[14,33] The translation of these animal observations to the clinical domain, however, must be made with great caution.

The *loop-acting diuretics* operate from the luminal side of the tubule and appear to inhibit a sodium chloride co-transport system in the luminal membrane of Henle's loop. They gain access to tubular fluid by the organic anion secretory system and, depending on the degree of binding to plasma proteins, by filtration. The diuretic response depends on the delivery of sodium chloride to the thick ascending limb of Henle's loop. Failure to observe a diuretic response thus may derive from failure of the drug to be secreted, such as in patients with renal disease, in patients with retention of organic anions that compete for the secretory site, or in circumstances when a greatly enhanced rate of sodium reabsorption in the proximal convoluted tubule and reduced delivery of filtrate to the thick ascending limb occur. The dose-response relationship of the loop-acting diuretics is such that relative degrees of impaired rates of secretion (and thus the diuretic response) may be overcome by administration of higher doses of the drug.

The major indication for potent loop-acting diuretics is to reduce the extracellular fluid volume.[7,23] If administered in excess or inappropriately, the loop-acting diuretics can cause depletion of the extracellular fluid volume, hypokalemia, and alkalosis. The attendant depletion of the extracellular fluid volume results in increased rates of fluid and electrolyte transport in the proximal tubule, a decrease in delivery of filtrate to the Henle's loop, and thus a partial internal brake on the unmodified effect of diuretics to deplete the extracellular fluid volume. Such protection, however, is only relative, is often incomplete, and depends on the operation of normal homeostatic mechanisms. In the clinical use of these drugs, such defense mechanisms cannot always be documented as being present, and the drugs must be used with caution. Frequent monitoring of the state of hydration of the patient is required. If, in addition to the diuretic, sodium and fluids are administered to match the urinary output, or if the patient has internal sources of fluids that can be mobilized (edema, effusions), the extracellular fluid volume will tend to be sustained and the delivery of filtrate to the site of diuretic action and the distal nephron maintained. This may result in high rates of potassium excretion and hypokalemia.

It has been suggested that diuretics may be of value in maintaining renal function in conditions where acute renal injury is likely to occur.[14,33] As with mannitol, experimental data indicate that pretreatment with loop diuretics may be of value.[33] In clinical circumstances, however, the injurious event or toxin usually occurs before diuretics are administered. Perhaps the most widely disputed issue as it pertains to the surgical patient is the use of diuretics in the oliguric patient with suspected acute renal failure. Before diuretics are used, the etiology of the oliguria must be evaluated. If such an evaluation results in the diagnosis of acute renal injury (vasomotor nephropathy or acute tubular necrosis), controversial recommendations exist on the use of diuretics. Most studies suggest that neither the degree nor the duration of acute renal failure is altered by the use of loop-acting diuretics.[10,26] Some studies indicate a worsening degree of renal injury. Nonetheless, a finite number of oliguric patients with acute renal injury will respond to diuretic administration by converting from an oliguric to a nonoliguric form of acute renal failure. Although diuretics do not alter the course or outcome, it is easier to manage patients with polyuric acute renal failure than those who are oliguric.

To date, no clinical or laboratory signs are available to indicate which patients would be responsive to diuretics. As a practical and pragmatic approach, it is recommended that oliguric patients be thoroughly evaluated. If acute renal failure is the most probable diagnosis and the patient is normally hydrated, 200 to 400 mg of furosemide can be administered as a single intravenous bolus. If no response is obtained, further diuretic administration should be halted. In a patient who is severely overloaded with fluid and unresponsive to diuretics, dialysis or continuous ultrafiltration may be required to remove the excess fluid.[23,32]

SUMMARY

The kidney is responsible for maintenance of fluid and electrolyte balance; participates in several endocrinologic systems, including regulation of vitamin D homeostasis, the renin-angiotensin system, erythropoietin production, and catabolism of peptide hormones; and serves as the execretory route for endogenously produced and exogenously administered substances. In maintaining fluid and electrolyte balance, the kidney responds to several hormones, including aldosterone, parathyroid hormone, and antidiuretic hormone, to alter excretion in a way designed to adjust output to match intake.

Fluids and electrolytes are regulated by the production of a large volume of plasma ultrafiltrate through glomerular filtration, from which varying components are reabsorbed by the renal tubular system before excretion. In addition, several specific secretory transport processes exist that accelerate excretion of a variety of substances. The proximal renal tubule reabsorbs about 60% of the filtered sodium and water in isotonic ratios and removes almost all the bicarbonate, glucose, and amino acids. It also adds several organic acids and bases to the tubular fluid. Henle's loop and its associated vascular bundles set the stage for the production of concentrated and diluted urine. The descending limb performs little active transport, whereas the thick ascending limb is very active in reabsorbing sodium from the filtrate before its entry into the distal nephron. The distal nephron segments finely regulate the composition of the excreted urine in terms of sodium, potassium, hydrogen ions, and water concentration.

The clinical assessment of renal function is closely related to an understanding of renal physiology and consists of examination of the formed elements in the urine as well as of the chemical composition of the urine. Specific tests of renal blood flow, glomerular filtration, and tubular transport can also be evaluated. Many systemic diseases, as well as anesthesia, drugs, surgery, and various bodily insults, can greatly alter renal function, with the potential for permanent renal damage. Only by clearly appreciating the dynamics of normal kidney physiology can the physician appropriately recognize derangements in renal function and thus initiate judicious treatment before irreversible injury ensues.

REFERENCES

1. Adams D.R., Hollenberg, N.K., and Abrams, H.L.: Angiography of renal failure. In Griffith, J.H., editor: Radiology of renal failure, Philadelphia, 1976, W.B. Saunders Co.
2. Bailey, M.E.: Endotoxin, bile salts and renal function in obstructiive jaundice, Br. J. Surg. **63:** 774, 1976.
3. Baylis, P.H., Gaskill, M.B., and Robertson, G.L.: Vasopressin secretion in primary polydipsia and cranial diabetes insipidus, Q. J. Med. **50:**345, 1981.
4. Berliner, R.W.: Mechanisms of urine concentration, Kidney Int. **22:**201, 1982.
5. Better, O.S., and Schrier, R.W.: Disturbed volume homeostasis in patients with cirrhosis of the liver, Kidney Int. **23:**303, 1983.
6. Bonventre, J.V., and Leaf, A.: Sodium homeostasis: steady states without a set point, Kidney Int. **21:**880, 1982.
7. Brater, D.C.: Determinants of response to loop diuretics, Fed. Proc. **42:**1694, 1983.
8. Brenner, B.M., and Hostetter, T.H.: Mechanisms of glomerular barrier function, Contrib. Nephrol. **26:**9, 1981.
9. Bricker, N.S., and Fine, L.G.: The renal response to progressive nephron loss. In Brenner, B.M., and Rector, F.C., editors: The kidney, ed. 2, Philadelphia, 1981, W.B. Saunders Co.
10. Brown, C.B., Ogg, C.S., and Cameron, J.S.: High dose furosemide in acute renal failure: a controlled trial, Clin. Nephrol. **15:**90, 1981.
11. Chan, Y.L., Biagi, B., and Giebisch, G.: Control mechanisms of bicarbonate transport across the rat proximal convoluted tubule, Am. J. Physiol. **242:**F532, 1982.
12. Cousins, M.J., et al.: Metabolism and renal effects of enflurane in man, Anesthesiology **44:**44;, 1976.
13. Dennis, V.W., Stead, W.W., and Myers, J.L.: Renal handling of phosphate and calcium, Ann. Rev. Physiol. **41:**257, 1979.
14. de Torrente, A., et al.: Effects of furosemide and acetylcholine in nonepinephrine-induced acute renal failure, Am. J. Physiol. **4:**131, 1978.
15. Dirks, J.H.: The kidney and magnesium regulation, Kidney Int. **23:**771, 1983.
16. Epstein, M.: Deranged sodium homeostasis in cirrhosis, Gastroenterology **76:**622, 1979.
17. Epstein, M.: Determinants of abnormal renal sodium handling in cirrhosis: a reappraisal, Scan. J. Clin. Lab. Invest. **40:**689, 1980.
18. Giebisch, G.: Newer aspects of renal tubular potassium transport, Contrib. Nephrol. **21:**106, 1980.
19. Graff, S.L.: A handbook of routine urinalysis, Philadelphia, 1982, J.B. Lippincott Co.
20. Haberle, D.A., and von Baeyer, H.: Characteristics of glomerulotubular balance, Am. J. Physiol. **244:**F355, 1983.
21. Harrington, J.T., and Cohen, J.J.: Measurement of urinary electrolytes—indications and limitations, N. Engl. J. Med. **293:**1241, 1975.
22. Haycock, G.B.: Old and new tests of renal function, J. Clin. Pathol. **34:**1276, 1981.
23. Heidenreich, O., Greven, J., and Weintze, K.: Diuretic agents: actions on a molecular level, Clin. Exp. Hypertens. (A) **5:**177, 1983.
24. Jamison, R.L., Work, J., and Schafer, J.A.: New pathways for potassium transport in the kidney, An. J. Physiol. **242:**F297, 1982.
25. Kiil, F.: Mechanisms of glomerulo-tubular balance: the whole kidney approach, Renal Physiol. **5:**209, 1982.
26. Kleinknecht, D., Ganeval, D., and Gonzales-Duque, L.A.: Furosemide in acute oliguric renal failure: a controlled trial, Nephron **17:**51, 1976.
27. Knepper, M., and Burg, M.: Organization of nephron function, Am. J. Physiol. **244:**F579, 1983.
28. Knox, F.G., et al.: Role of hydrostatic and oncotic pressures in renal sodium reabsorption, Circ. Res. **52:**491, 1983.
29. Kokko, J.P.: Transport characteristics in the thin limbs of Henle, Kidney Int. **22:**449, 1982.
30. Ladefoged, J., and Munch, O.: Distribution of blood flow in the kidney. In Fisher, J.W., editor: Kidney hormomes, London, 1971, Academic Press.
31. Lang, F.: Renal handling of calcium and phosphate, Klin. Wochenschr. **58:**985, 1980.
32. Lant, A.F.: Modern diuretics and the kidney, J. Clin. Pathol. **34:**1267, 1981.
33. Levinsky, N.G., Bernard, D.B., and Johnson, P.A.: Enhancement of recovery of acute renal failure. In Brenner, B.M., and Stern, J.M., editors: Acute renal failure: contemporary issues in nephrology, vol. 6, New York, Churchill Livingstone, Inc.
34. Maddox, D.A., and Brenner, B.M.: Glomerular filtration of fluid and macromolecules: the renal response to injury, Annu. Rev. Med. **28:**91, 1977.
35. Maher, J.F.: Pathophysiology of renal hemodynamics, Nephron **27:**215, 1981.
36. Masora, E.J.: An overview of hydrogen ion regulation, Arch. Intern. Med. **142:**1019, 1982.
37. Mazze, R.I., Trudell, J.R., and Cousins, M.J.: Methoxyflurane metabolism and renal dysfunction: clinical correlation in man, Anesthesiology **35:**247, 1971.
38. Navar, L.G., et al.: Intrinsic control of renal hemodynamics, Fed. Proc. **41:**3022, 1982.
39. Notman, D.D., Mortek, M.A., and Moses, A.M.: Permanent diabetes insipidus following head trauma: observations in ten patients and an approach to diagnosis, J. Trauma **20:**599, 1980.
40. Papper, S.: Hepatorenal syndrome, Contrib. Nephrol. **23:**55, 1980.
41. Pru, C., and Kjellstrand, C.M.: The clinical usefulness of ther FeNa test in acute renal failure: a critical analysis, Proc. Dial. Transplant. Forum **10:**240, 1980.
42. Richman, A.V., Gerber, L.I., and Balis, J.U.: Peritubular capillaries: a major target site of endotoxin-induced vascular injury in the primate kidney, Lab. Invest. **43:**327, 1980.
43. Rosoff, L., Jr., et al.: Renal hemodynamics and the renin-angiotensin system in cirrhosis: relationship to sodium retention, Dig. Dis. Sci. **24:**25, 1979.
44. Schrier, R.W., and Szatalowicz V.L.: Disorders of water metabolism, Contrib. Nephrol. **21:**48, 1980.
45. Schrier, R.W., Berl, T., and Anderson, R.J.: Osmotic and nonosmotic control of vasopressin release, Am. J. Physiol. **236:**F321, 1979.
46. Seely, J., and Levy, M.: Control of extracellular fluid volume. In Brenner, B.M., and Rector, F.C., editors: The kidney, ed. 2, Philadelphia, 1981, W.B. Saunders Co.
47. Skorecki, K.L., and Brenner, B.M.: Body fluid homeostasis in man: a contemporary overview, Am. J. Med. **70:**77, 1981.
48. Skorecki, K.L., and Brenner, B.M.: Body fluid hemeostasis in congestive heart failure and cirrhosis with ascites, Am. J. Med. **72:**323, 1982.
49. Thurau, K., and Levine, D.Z.: The renal circulation. In Rouiller, C., and Muller A.F., editors: The kidney: morphology, biochemistry, physiology, New York, 1971, Academic Press, Inc.
50. Warnock, D., and Rector, F.C.: Renal acidification mechanisms. In Brenner, B.M., and Rector F.C., editors: The kidney, ed. 2, Philadelphia; 1981, W.B. Saunders Co.
51. Warnock, D.G., and Eveloff, J.: NaCl Entry mechanisms in the luminal membrane of the renal tubule, Am. J. Physiol. **242:**F561, 1982.
52. Warren, S.E., and Blantz, R.C.: Mannitol, Arch. Intern. Med. **141:**493, 1981.
53. Wright, F.S.: Potassium transport by successive segments of the mammalian nephron, Fed. Proc. **40:**2398, 1981.
54. Young, D.B., and Paulsen, A.W.: Interrelated effects of aldosterone and plasma postassium on potassium excretion, Am. J. Physiol. **244:**F28, 1983.

42 *Joseph N. Corriere, Jr.*

Obstruction of the Urinary Tract

Obstructive diseases of the urinary tract can be congenital or acquired, occur at any level in the organ system, and be found at all ages and in both sexes. Most patients eventually develop signs or symptoms related to the disease process causing the obstruction, the obstructed urinary tract organs per se, or renal failure symptoms secondary to progressive loss of functioning renal tissue. With the more liberal use of noninvasive diagnostic imaging modalities such as ultrasound, as well as the routine use of laboratory studies, more and more totally asymptomatic patients with obstructive uropathy are being discovered, even in the prenatal period. Fortunately, most obstructive problems are reversible if discovered at an early stage, so a high index of suspicion of their presence can help prevent needless morbidity and mortality. In the following discussion, an emphasis will be placed on the physiologic derangements in renal function and the function of the renal collecting system that occur during both the urinary obstruction and the reparative process after the obstruction has been relieved.

Incidence

Because of the variety of lesions that can cause obstructive uropathy, it is difficult to give a true overall incidence of this disease process. One has to go back to Campbell's pioneering work cataloging pediatric urologic disorders to get a sense of the problem in children, where it is the most common renal collecting system disorder that requires surgical correction.[3] In an autopsy study of 15,919 patients 15 years old or younger, he found 316 to have hydronephrosis, an incidence of 1.99%. The majority of the patients, 256 (81%), were less than 1 year old, and 148 (57.8%) of these infants were males. Only 14 (4.4%) were between the ages of 3 and 10 years, and 11 (3.5%) were between 11 and 15 years of age. Campbell found over half of the hydronephroses to be bilateral and over 80% of the lesions to have their origin above the level of the bladder.

A concomitant series of 512 children whose diseases were recognized clinically rather than at autopsy had a less skewed age distribution. Only 114 (22.3%) were less than 1 year of age, 124 (24.2%) were between 1 and 2 years of age, and 234 (45.7%) were between the ages of 3 and 10 years. Forty children (7.8%) were between the ages of 11 and 15 years. However, as with the autopsy series, over 80% of the lesions were secondary to supravesical disorders. The screening of patients with both prenatal and postnatal ultrasound is changing these figures because asymptomatic hydronephrotic kidneys are being found more and more frequently and being operated on earlier and earlier.

During middle age, pelvic disease in women and ureteral calculus disease in both sexes account for most cases of obstructed ureters. Indeed, the prevalence of calculi causing renal colic or hematuria and acute or chronic hydroureteronephrosis is about 5% in women and 10% in men in the United States.[13] Later in life, bladder outlet obstruction, specifically benign prostatic hyperplasia, will cause voiding symptoms in approximately 50% of men over the age of 60, and about 10% of men over 40 years of age will eventually need a prostatectomy.[15]

NORMAL FUNCTION

Renal Pelvic and Ureteral Function

The collecting system of the upper urinary tract, the renal pelvis and ureter, is composed of intermingled, smooth muscle layers arranged in a helical fashion. The function of this unit is to convey urine from the kidney to the bladder. Ureteral contractions follow stimulation by a bolus of urine entering the pelvis and a cell-to-cell propagation of action potentials. Neurotransmission is thought to occur by diffusion rather than any direct neuromuscular synapses.[26]

It is difficult to know if a true pacemaker exists in the renal pelvis.[9] Resection of any part of the collecting system does not seem to disturb the function of the unit. Urine flows continuously from the collecting ducts into the calyces. The bulk of this urine flows into the upper ureter, and then a pelvic contraction begins active contraction and propagation of a bolus of urine toward the bladder. Normal resting pressure in the renal pelvis is about 6.5 mm Hg. During acute obstruction, as from a ureteral calculus, this will rise to 50 to 70 mm Hg. During chronic obstruction, the mean intrapelvic pressures are about 21 mm Hg.[18] This suggests that pelvic pressures decrease in time after acute obstruction has remained elevated.

As the urine bolus enters the ureter, the ureteral walls coapt and move the bolus toward the bladder. A pressure of about 20 mm Hg is generated in the normal ureter during a contraction. This can rise to 110 mm Hg during a brisk diuresis.[22] The ureter enters the bladder at an oblique angle and then enters a submucosal tunnel. This mechanism produces a flap valve effect, which prevents urine in the bladder from refluxing back into the ureter.

Bladder Function

The main functions of the urinary bladder are to serve as a storage area for urine produced by the kidneys and to act as an efficient voiding mechanism. Because of its unique ureterovesical junction, the bladder protects the upper-urinary tract and renal parenchyma from the high pressures of voiding and straining and prevents bacteria from ascending to the kidney.

The bladder and its outlet are innervated by the parasympathetic, sympathetic, and somatic nervous systems. The parasympathetic nerves from spinal cord segments S2 to S4 are carried to the bladder and posterior urethra by the pelvic nerves. The sympathetic nerves from spinal cord segments T10 to L2 are carried to this same area by the hypogastric nerves. The somatic sensory and motor nerves from spinal cord segments S2 to S4 are carried to the striated muscles of the pelvic floor by the internal pudendal nerves. Also, afferent sensory nerves from the bladder and urethra carry proprioception, pain, and temperature in the pelvic nerves and, to some extent, in the hypogastric nerves.[19]

The bladder is composed of a meshwork of smooth muscle fibers, which continue past the bladder neck into the proximal urethra. As the bladder fills with urine, these fibers lengthen and increase their intramural tension. This increased tension is transmitted to the bladder and urethra, which increases the intravesical, bladder neck, and intraurethral pressure. During filling, the intravesical pressure stays below 15 cm of water, whereas the maximum intraurethral pressure is usually above 100 cm of water. While the bladder fills, afferent stimulation signals the brain of the distention. This sensation can be normally suppressed by the cerebral cortex until volitional voiding is desired.

Immediately before voiding, the striated muscles of the pelvic floor relax and then parasympathetic stimuli cause the smooth muscle of the bladder to contract. Intravesical pressure rises to 70 to 100 cm of water, the bladder neck is pulled open, the urethral closure mechanism shortens, and the intraurethral pressure falls to less than 5 cm of water. When intravesical pressure exceeds intraurethral pressure, voiding occurs.[5]

The role of the sympathetic fibers is less clear. They may be important in the maintenance of continence and not in the act of micturition. Contraction of the bladder neck and urethra by alpha-receptors and relaxation of the bladder body by beta-receptors are probably important only in the promotion of urine storage.[19]

TYPES OF LESIONS

Obstructing lesions of the urinary tract are best divided into intrinsic diseases of the organ system and extrinsic diseases that secondarily cause urinary tract obstruction (Fig. 42-1). Obviously, the bulk of the congenital disorders are found in children, commonly in the neonatal period or infancy, whereas renal and ureteral calculi are the most common causes of obstructive uropathy in young and middle-aged adults. Benign prostatic hyperplasia and urethral strictures are seen in males in later life, which is also the time when genitourinary tract tumors occur and can cause urinary tract obstruction. Ureteral strictures are usu-

COMMON CAUSES OF URINARY OBSTRUCTION

Intrinsic Diseases of the Urinary Tract

Congenital Disorders
Ureteropelvic junction lesions
Primary megaureter
Ectopic ureter
Ectopic ureterocele
Neuropathic bladder disease
Urethral valves
Detrusor sphincter dyssynergia
Ureteral dysplasia (prune belly syndrome)

Metabolic and Inflammatory Disorders
Urinary calculi
Blood clots
Fungus balls
Sloughed papillae (papillary necrosis)
Renal, ureteral, or vesical tuberculosis
Urethral strictures
Prostatic inflammatory diseases
Meatal stenosis
Foreign body

Neoplastic Disorders
Benign prostatic hyperplasia
Renal pelvic and ureteral tumors
Bladder tumors
Prostatic tumors
Urethral tumors

Traumatic Disorders
Ureteral stricture (postsurgical)
Urethral stricture

Extrinsic Obstruction of the Ureter

Vascular Lesions
Accessory vessels
Aortic, iliac aneurysms
Ovarian vein syndrome
Circumcaval (retrocaval) ureter

Pelvic and Retroperitoneal Masses
Pregnancy
Enlarged uterus—benign, malignant disorders
Hydrometrocolpos
Ovarian lesions
Embryologic remnants (cysts of Gartner's duct)
Pelvic and retroperitoneal tumors, primary and metastatic
Pelvic lipomatosis
Lymphocele
Uterine prolapse

Inflammatory Diseases
Retroperitoneal fibrosis
Retroperitoneal abscess
Retroperitoneal hemorrhage
Tubo-ovarian abscess; pelvic inflammatory disease
Appendiceal or diverticular abscess
Endometriosis
Granulomatous (Crohn's) disease of the bowel

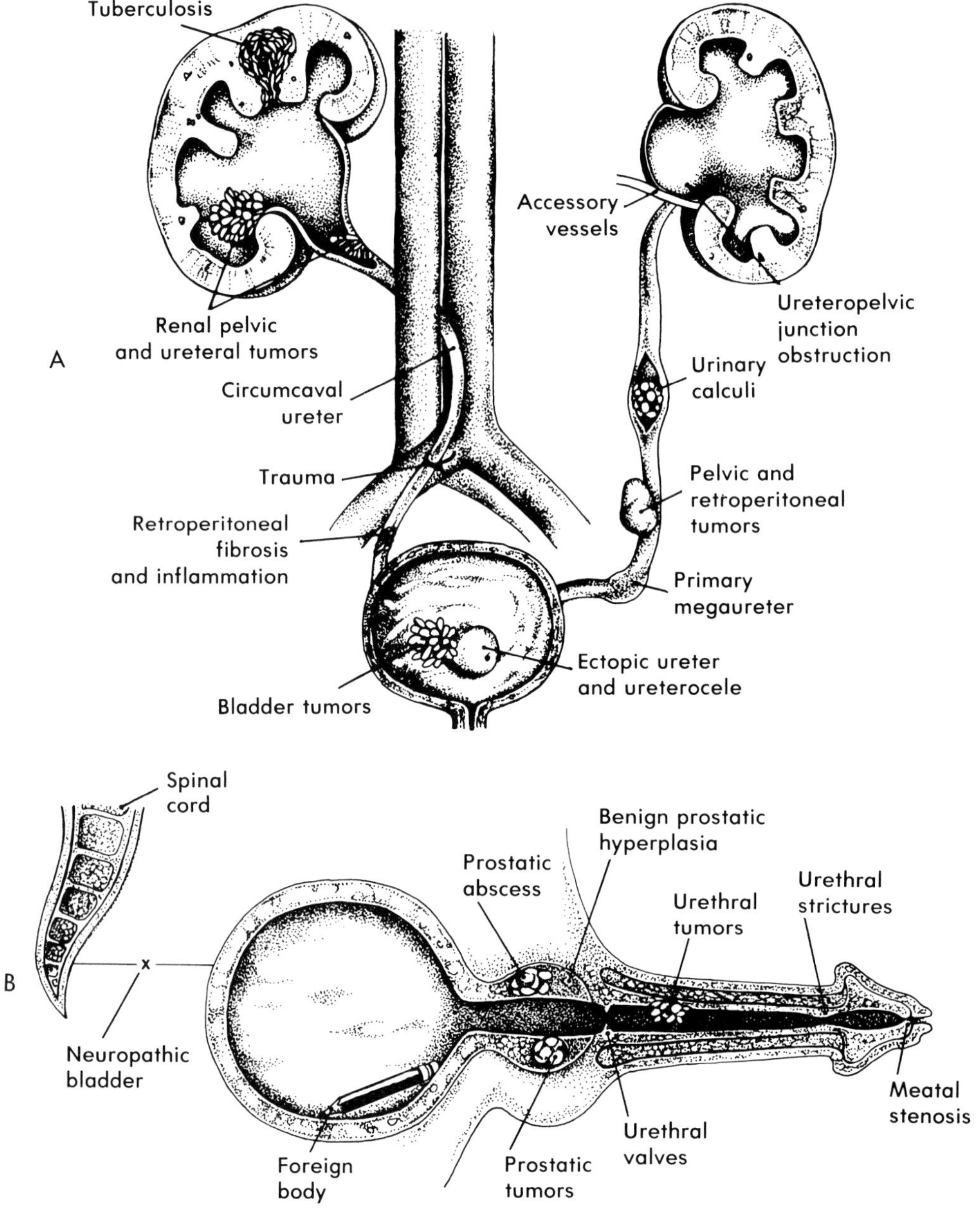

Fig. 42-1 **A,** Causes of upper urinary tract obstruction. **B,** Causes of lower urinary tract obstruction.

ally caused by surgical trauma or tuberculosis. Virtually any retroperitoneal or pelvic neoplastic or inflammatory process can secondarily involve and obstruct the ureters. The more common problems encountered are shown in the boxed material above.

CLINICAL PRESENTATION

Obstruction of the upper urinary tract is usually accompanied by flank pain. This discomfort is caused by distention of the collecting system and renal capsule and quickly dissipates when the obstruction is relieved. The pain is usually caused by acute obstructions, not chronic problems. If the obstruction occurs in the upper portion of the ureter, the pain may radiate into the ipsilateral testicle in the male. If low in the ureter, near the bladder, the pain may be felt in the ipsilateral scrotum, labia, or inner aspect of the thigh. This is known as referred pain and is related to the common nerve supply shared by the urinary and genital systems.

Afferent nerve terminals exist in the renal capsule and parenchyma, and the epithelium and smooth muscle of the renal pelvis and ureter. The sympathetic nerve supply is mainly from the celiac ganglia and aortic plexus. Preganglionic fibers are received through the lesser and least splanchnic nerves from the T6 through L1 ganglia. The hypogastric plexus receives impulses from the bladder (S2 through S4), whereas the pudendal nerve supplies the urethra.

Visceral pain travels to the lateral spinothalamic tract up the cord to the premotor cortex of the frontal lobes. The

T10 through T12 and L1 segments are the visceral afferents for the kidney and ureter but also serve the margin of the diaphragm, large bowel, ovary, tube and uterus, appendix, duodenum, small bowel, gallbladder, pancreas, testes, spleen, and abdominal aorta. The afferent somatic nerves of these segments are also represented in this area.

This common segment innervation is present because of normal intrauterine organ migration. During development the kidney arises in the lower lumbar and sacral regions and ascends to its final flank position while the gonads and genital ducts develop high in the abdomen and descend approximately 10 segments below this level of origin to eventually descend into the scrotum.

Referred pain is through a viscerosomatic reflex arc. The afferent fiber enters the cord to form a synapse with a cell in the lateral horn of the gray matter. This cell's preganglionic fiber connects with a sympathetic ganglion whose postganglionic fiber connects to a peripheral spinal nerve. This connection to peripheral nerves accounts for the hyperesthesia or pain referred from visceral pathologic conditions to dermatomes innervated by somatic nerves originating at the same cord levels. The genitofemoral and ilioinguinal nerves are the usual pathways for referred pain to the groin and upper inner thighs.

Although classically described as colicky pain caused by contraction and relaxation of the ureter, the discomfort may be constant in nature. The patient is restless and cannot get into a comfortable position. Frequency and urgency may be seen if the obstructing lesion is near the bladder and irritating that organ. Commonly, reflex nausea and vomiting may be present, and if the obstructed renal unit is infected, bacteremia, fever, and chills may develop. Usually urine volume is not noticeably changed when only one kidney is totally obstructed. Anuria will occur with bilateral obstruction or in the patient who has a solitary obstructed kidney.

When acute ureteral obstruction occurs, hematuria may be seen and is usually secondary to damage of the transitional epithelium of the upper urinary tract by the offending lesion, usually a calculus. When chronic obstruction is present, it is common for veins in the submucosa of the renal pelvis to become quite large and thin walled. Minimal trauma to these chronically distended renal units may cause these veins to rupture and blood will be present in the urine. This is a particularly common first sign of a dilated collecting system structure in children.

Chronic obstruction of the upper urinary tract is usually virtually asymptomatic. Vague abdominal complaints may be elicited, especially after a large fluid intake. If obstruction is of a long-standing bilateral nature, symptoms of chronic renal failure, namely, polyuria and polydipsia, as well as fatigue, may be present.

Patients with infravesical obstruction will usually have all of the symptoms of prostatism—frequency, urgency, hesitancy, nocturia, a slow intermittent urinary stream, and perhaps (overflow) urinary incontinence. Some patients will have complete urinary retention. Hematuria may be present because of rupture of distended mucosal veins in the bladder, urethra, or prostate, and if the patient has an infected lower urinary tract, dysuria will be a common complaint. Patients with neuropathic bladder disease will usually mimic the patient with bladder neck obstruction but will also have complaints relative to their primary neurologic problem.

EXAMINATION AND DIAGNOSTIC STUDIES

Physical Examination

Patients who have obstructed renal units may have tenderness in the costovertebral angle or in the abdomen at the level of the obstructing lesion. Infected, septic patients may be febrile. A tender mass in the flank may indicate a long-standing obstructing kidney, and a midline suprapubic mass may indicate a distended bladder. Children with the prune belly syndrome do not have the anterior abdominal muscles but have bilateral undescended testicles and chronic hydronephrosis.

A large, smooth prostate on rectal examination in an elderly male will suggest benign prostatic hyperplasia. A nodular prostate at any age suggests a neoplasm of that organ. Bowel or pelvic organ lesions may be palpated on rectal or vaginal examination as may masses extrinsic to these organ systems. The external sphincter tone should be noted in patients suspected of having neurologic disorders. Finally, inspection of the urethral meatus for stenosis should not be overlooked.

Laboratory Evaluation

A urinalysis will be helpful in the diagnosis of bilateral obstructive uropathy, for concentrating ability is lost in the course of this disease process. White blood cells and bacteria may be found if infection is present. Urinary tract infections should be confirmed by a urine culture. Hematuria may be seen.

Serum chemistries, especially a blood urea nitrogen and creatinine, are necessary to monitor renal function. Serum electrolytes should be measured, especially in the azotemic patient. A creatinine clearance may be necessary to help plan and follow therapeutic measures that will be instituted. If a carcinoma of the prostate is suspected, an acid phosphatase level should be determined. In patients with suspected urothelial tumors, a cytologic evaluation of urine may be helpful. Stone chemistries eventually may be needed if the patient is found to have a urinary tract calculus.

Imaging Studies

Radiographic studies with contrast agents are the most useful tests to determine the level of urinary tract obstruction and to obtain diagnostic information about the cause of the obstruction. In the patient with normal or near normal renal function, the first procedure ordered should be an intravenous urogram (IVU). Most of the time, this study will be sufficient to diagnose upper tract lesions, but retrograde or antegrade pyelograms may be needed if the kidney is poorly functioning. In the child, a voiding cystourethrogram, in conjunction with the IVU, will usually be all that is required.

Although good quality urograms are possible even in the face of moderate azotemia,[23] the diabetic patient with severely compromised renal function may develop a further reduction in function with iodonated contrast materials.[24] In these situations, as well as in the neonate who has poor renal function because of age, ultrasound evaluation may be a better first choice study or at least it should be used to corroborate the diagnosis.

The renal scan is also used in children, but it does not give fine anatomic detail. Its use in conjunction with a diuretic can evaluate the physiologic function of a dilated upper tract by determining emptying time of the renal pelvis.[14] Computed tomography may also be useful, especially in complicated cases of intrinsic or extrinsic upper tract disease. Finally, if a urethral stricture is suspected, a retrograde urethrogram is the appropriate study to perform to delineate the problem. If a bowel lesion is under consideration, barium studies of the gastrointestinal tract should also be obtained.

Diseases of the bladder and urethra in the adult are best diagnosed by cystoscopy and panendoscopy. Up to 40% of the time, the cystogram phase of an IVU will demonstrate supposed abnormalities that are not actually present or will be interpreted as normal even though a lesion is present in the bladder. Biopsies of bladder lesions and the sampling of individual kidney urine for cytologic analysis are also easily accomplished through a cystoscope.

Urodynamic Studies

If contractility or voiding dynamics of the bladder are thought to be abnormal, physiologic testing of this organ should be performed. By measuring the rate and volume of urine flow, a voiding flow rate can be calculated. By filling the bladder through a urethral catheter and measuring bladder sensation and the intravesical pressure at various volumes and then seeing if the detrusor contracts (a cystometrogram), a reasonable indication of bladder function is obtained. Rarely, electromyographic study of the external urethral sphincter and urethral pressure profilometry are necessary in patients with complicated symptoms.[8]

As mentioned previously, a renal isotope drainage study in conjunction with a diuretic challenge can give a good indication of the presence of obstruction in a dilated upper urinary tract.[14] In the patient with a complicated problem, pressure and flow measurements through a percutaneous intrarenal pelvic catheter are necessary for proper diagnosis.[29]

CONSEQUENCES OF OBSTRUCTION ON RENAL FUNCTION

To gain an understanding of the effects of obstructive uropathy on the urinary tract, it is best to consider the organ system as a closed space with an opening for fluid to enter at one end and a relief valve at the other end. Despite obstruction occurring in the system, fluid continues to enter the space. Because of this, the collecting system must dilate to accept the increased volume. Although leaks may develop to relieve the inevitable increase in pressure, the final outcome, because the kidneys are enclosed by a fairly indistensible capsule, is compression and destruction of the renal parenchyma, a phenomenon called hydronephrosis (Fig. 42-2).

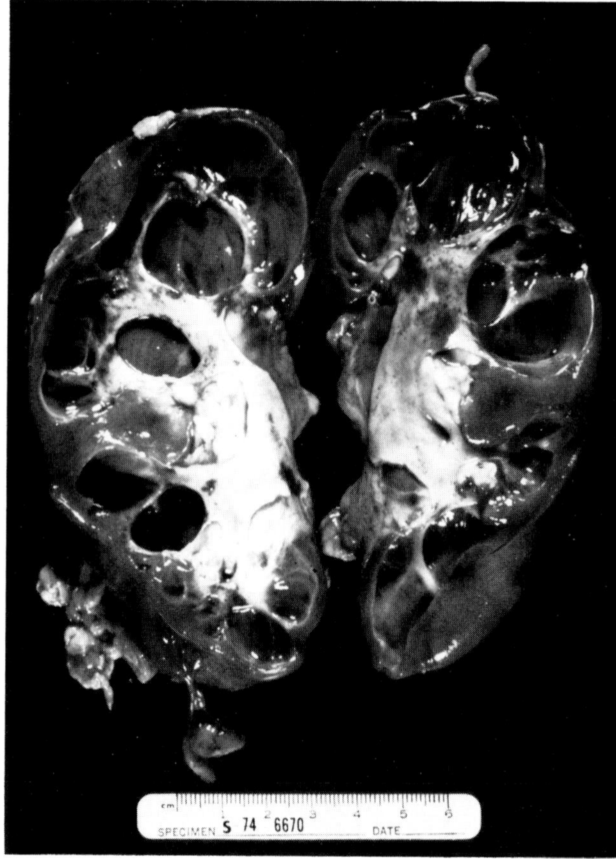

Fig. 42-2 Hydronephrosis with renal parenchymal thinning.

Three major mechanisms lead to renal parenchymal damage in urinary tract obstruction: (1) the pressure effect on the kidney, (2) ischemia, and (3) concomitant pyelonephritis. As the hydronephrosis progresses, the parenchyma is compressed. The renal papillae take the brunt of the pressure, but eventually the cortex is obliterated as well. The total renal blood flow decreases in time, and the transmission of increased intratubular pressure to the surrounding vasculature decreases postglomerular blood flow. Pressure is also exerted on the vasa recta and eventually on the preglomerular vessels, especially the interlobar, arcuate, and interlobular arteries. Secondary renal infection is promoted by obstruction and is so common that obstructive uropathy should always be looked for in the patient with an unexplained urinary tract infection, especially if fever, chills, and flank pain are prominent complaints.

The sequence of renal dysfunction that results from obstruction follows[7]:

1. Loss of concentrating ability
2. Reduced ability to excrete acid
3. Decreased glomerular filtration
4. Decreased renal blood flow after initial increase
5. Decreased sodium and water reabsorption

Since the first damage occurs in the medulla of the kidney, it follows that tubular function would be affected initially. In all ages the first defect seen is an inability of the organ to concentrate urine. Exogenous vasopressin will not correct the lesion, which is caused by a decrease in the corticopapillary interstitial osmotic gradient. The reduced ability to excrete acid and the subsequent inability to reduce the urinary pH are probably caused by damage to the collecting ducts. Some investigators believe this pH effect is only seen when glomerular filtration decreases, whereas others believe it is secondary to a decrease in the total number of nephrons.

The reduction in glomerular filtration rate (GFR) is dependent on the degree and duration of obstruction and whether the obstruction is unilateral aor bilateral.[21] The peritubular capillary pressure and interstitial pressure rises that occur with obstruction will reduce GFR within 20 minutes of unilateral obstruction, and the permeability of the tubular walls will increase. This leaky fluid is removed through the renal lymphatics.[10]

In contrast to these findings, renal blood flow (RBF) will increase to about 50% of normal within the first 1 to 2 hours after obstruction. This is most likely caused by release of a vasodilating prostaglandin.[6] This increase in flow seems limited to the renal cortex and falls within 6 hours of the occlusion to approximately 30% of normal because of a progressive increase in the resistance of the afferent arterioles.

Although initially the decrease in GFR allows for a more complete absorption of sodium, with prolonged obstruction, urinary sodium concentration is increased, urinary osmolality is decreased, and a dilute urine is excreted. This is caused by impaired salt and water reabsorption rather than by hyperfiltration by undamaged nephrons.[28]

The effects of bilateral renal obstruction are surprisingly less severe than those of unilateral renal obstruction. Intratubular pressure rises higher in bilateral obstruction but declines in a few hours. Similarly, glomerular capillary pressure increases more rapidly with bilateral occlusion but falls to normal, not below normal as with unilateral obstruction. It appears that afferent arteriolar resistance does not increase as much in this situation. The reason for these differences is unclear. A possible explanation is that when both kidneys are blocked, the composition of the circulating blood—increased amounts of plasma potassium, phosphate, creatinine, urea, and total solutes, as well as other normally eliminated substances—may relax vascular smooth muscle.[12] It should be noted that serum sodium does not change in serum concentration during bilateral renal obstruction.

Postobstructive Diuresis

In some patients with azotemia, an osmotic diuresis of a varying intensity may ensue after relief of obstruction. It is more marked after an acute, complete blockage or an acute blockage superimposed on a chronic, partial obstruction. The mechanism of this diuresis is the sudden increase in GFR, which allows a rapid large delivery of sodium to the tubules with decreased reabsorption in the proximal and probably the distal tubules.[11]

It should be stressed that this phenomenon does not happen in the presence of a normal kidney, and most patients who have their obstructive uropathy relieved either have no significant natriuresis or have a physiologic diuresis that results in release of pathologically retained sodium and a reduction of total body sodium to normal. Most of the time this diuresis is gone within 72 hours.[17]

Renal Recovery after Relief of the Obstruction

After removal of a unilateral obstruction, GFR rapidly returns to normal. Glomerular capillary pressure rises and then falls a few hours after relief of the obstruction.[4] Renal blood flow remains low after the relief. Both of these effects are attributed to a persistent elevation in afferent arteriolar resistance. Because of these effects, urine osmolality and the reabsorption of sodium and water remain impaired. The speed and amount of return to normal function will depend on the magnitude of permanent damage sustained by the nephron units.

Release of bilateral renal obstruction produces similar effects except in patients who develop postobstructive diuresis. In these patients, the sodium balance is usually restored in 3 days, but the concentrating defect may persist for a longer period.

Therapeutic Considerations

In the unilateral obstructed kidney, tube drainage and repair of the obstructing lesion are all that are necessary to obtain maximum recovery because total renal function in the patient is at a level sufficient for normal body function. However, in the azotemic patient with bilateral obstruction, close observation must begin immediately after relief of the obstruction to prevent vascular collapse from a massive diuresis. An intravenous solution of one-half normal saline should be started. After the urine is removed from the distended collecting system, cultured, measured, and discarded, careful monitoring of the urine output is initiated. A milliliter-for-milliliter replacement of the output should be infused. Sometimes the output is massive and the infusion rate must be adjusted hourly.

After 72 hours, the effect should be over. If large volumes of urine are still forthcoming, the patient may be overhydrated. The infusion should then be cut back to about 50% of the output and, when the urine output is less than a few liters a day or the patient can keep up with the output by oral intake, the intravenous therapy may be discontinued. If the azotemia persists, prolonged drainage by tube or temporary diversion may be necessary to return the renal function to a level sufficient to allow surgical repair of the obstructing lesion.

CONSEQUENCES OF OBSTRUCTION ON THE UPPER TRACT

When obstruction of the ureter occurs, action potentials and contractions increase. The baseline pressure rises to approximately 70 mm Hg in a few hours, and the ureter eventually becomes an open fluid-filled space. The walls are unable to coapt even though action potentials still occur.[1] Eventually, however, they cease, and the hydraulic pressure falls to normal as the ureter dilates, sometimes to gigantic proportions, to accommodate its increased fluid load.

Postobstructive Recovery

The postobstructed dilated ureter has a decreased ability to develop intraluminal pressures required for urine transport. Despite muscle hypertrophy and increased contractility, the increase in ureteral diameter changes the thickness/radius ratio in the Laplace relationship. Removal of the obstructing lesion and prolonged drainage many times will be all that is needed to return the ureter to normal function. However, if the side walls cannot coapt, ureteral motility may not be sufficient to propel a bolus of urine from the kidney to the bladder. Tapering the ureter by surgical removal of a strip of muscle to decrease its circumference often will improve its performance. The tapered ureter can then coapt its walls more easily and generate higher intraluminal pressures.[27]

CONSEQUENCES OF OBSTRUCTION ON BLADDER FUNCTION

The detrusor of the urinary bladder supplies a limited amount of contractile energy during voiding. It is essentially myogenic, and the amount of energy increases with bladder filling, reaching a maximum at 250 to 450 ml. The muscle fibers of the detrusor probably follow Starling's law and are more efficient when lengthened up to a point where they then begin to decompensate.[20]

During infravesical outlet obstruction, bladder outlet resistance increases, which decreases the voiding flow rate but does not affect the power or total energy of the detrusor. A higher voiding pressure develops by passive adaptation. Voiding pressures of well over 100 cm of water develop. As obstruction progresses, more energy is needed for one void. Because available energy is limited, the voided volumes decrease and residual urine develops when the need exceeds the energy supply.

The detrusor develops large endoscopically visible muscle bundles known as trabeculae. The smooth muscle cells do not really hypertrophy or develop hyperplasia; instead, a massive connective tissue buildup occurs between the muscle bundles.[2] The bladder becomes stiffer and less malleable, tending to reduce detrusor strength. Eventually, the bladder may fail to contract at all and the patient will develop urinary retention.

The effects of obstruction on the upper urinary tract as discussed earlier obviously may develop with infravesical obstruction. At times, the vesicoureteral junctions become distorted by the bladder pathologic conditions and vesicoureteral reflux develops. When this occurs, the high intravesical pressure of voiding may be transmitted to the kidneys and ureters, accelerating the destructive process to these organs. Vesicoureteral reflux also allows bacteria in the bladder to infect the kidneys.

Postobstructive Recovery of the Bladder

The tissue changes in the bladder wall with partial urethral obstruction, namely, thickening of the musculature and the increase in intracellular connective tissue, seem to be reversible if the duration of obstruction does not exceed 8 weeks.[16] In severe or prolonged obstruction, permanent morphologic and functional damage will occur. At times, the bladder is so damaged it is unable to contract at all. Most of the time, however, even if bladder recovery is not complete, adequate detrusor contractions will be possible to empty the bladder in an efficient manner.

In the patient who has had severe obstruction, tube drainage, either with a urethral or suprapubic catheter, may be necessary for days, weeks, or even months to see recovery of detrusor function. Although the drug bethanechol chloride will increase bladder muscle contractility, it is ineffective in this clinical setting because it causes the musculature of the neck, as well as the body, of the bladder to contract and, in effect, cancels out the benefit of the drug.[25]

SUMMARY

Urinary tract obstruction is a fairly common problem seen at all ages and in both sexes. Mild obstructions may have minimum or no effects on renal function or urine transport and storage and need little or no therapy. Indeed, anatomic dilation of the collecting system does not of itself mean pathologic physiology—all that dilates is not obstructed. On the other hand, sudden total blockage or silent chronic occlusion may lead to acute or chronic renal failure and be life threatening.

Imaging and physiologic studies are now quite refined and, for the most part, exacting in determining the site of obstruction and its significance. Unfortunately, other than improving drainage and awaiting self-repair, there is little to offer in terms of treatment to the urinary tract that has been damaged by the process. We are able, however, to understand what damage has been done and how to support the organism in lieu of normal renal and collecting system function while awaiting recovery.

REFERENCES

1. Backlund, L.: Experimental studies on pressure and contractility in the ureter, Acta Physiol. Scand. **59** (suppl. 212):1, 1963.
2. Barnard, R.J., Dixon, J.S., and Gosling, J.A.: A clinical and morphological evaluation of the trabeculated urinary bladder, Prog. Clin. Biol. Res. **78:**285, 1981.
3. Campbell, M.: Urinary obstruction. In Campbell, M.: Clinical pediatric urology, Philadelphia, 1951, W.B. Saunders Co.
4. Dal Canton, A., et al.: Effects of 24 hour unilateral ureteral obstruction on glomerular hemodynamics in rat kidney, Kidney Int. **15:**457, 1979.
5. Drach, G.W., Gleason, D.M., and Bottaccini, M.R.: New techniques for the evaluation of bladder function, Urol. Clin. North Am. **6:**541, 1979.
6. Gaudio, K.M., et al.: Renal perfusion and intratubular pressure during ureteral occlusion in the rat, Am. J. Physiol. **238:**F205, 1980.
7. Gillenwater, J.Y., et al.: Renal function one week after release of chronic unilateral hydronephrosis in man, Kidney Int. **7:**179, 1975.
8. Gleason, D.M., Bottaccini, M.R., and Drach, G.W.: Urodynamics, J. Urol. **115:**356, 1976.
9. Gosling, J.A., and Dixon, J.S.: Species variation in the location of upper urinary tract pacemaker cells, Invest. Urol. **11:**418, 1974.
10. Heney, N.M., O'Morchoe, P.J., and O'Morchoe, C.C.C.: The renal lymphatic system during obstructed urine flow, J. Urol. **106:**455, 1971.
11. Howards, S.S.: Post-obstructive diuresis: a misunderstood phenomenon, J. Urol. **110:**537, 1973.
12. Jaenike, J.R.: The renal functional defect of postobstructive nephropathy. The effects of bilateral ureteral obstruction in the rat, J. Clin. Invest. **51:**2999, 1972.
13. Johnson, C.M., et al.: Renal stone epidemiology: a 25 year study in Rochester, Minnesota, Kidney Int. **16:**624, 1979.
14. Koff, S.A.: Ureteropelvic junction obstruction: role of newer diagnostic methods, J. Urol. **127:**898, 1982.
15. Lytton, B., Emery, J.M., and Harvard, B.M.: The incidence of benign prostatic obstruction, J. Urol. **99:**639, 1968.
16. Magasi, P., Csontai, A., and Ruszinko, B.: Beitrage zur blasenwamtre-generation, Z. Urol. Nephrol. **62:**209, 1969.
17. McDougal, W.S., and Wright, F.S.: Defect in proximal and distal sodium transport in postobstructive diuresis, Kidney Int. **2:**304, 1972.

18. Michaelson, G.: Percutaneous puncture of the renal pelvis intrapelvic pressure and the concentrating capacity of the kidney in hydronephrosis, Acta Med. Scan. Suppl. **559:**1, 1974.
19. Raezer, D.M., et al.: Autonomic innervation of canine urinary bladder. Cholinergic and adrenergic contributions and interaction of sympathetic and parasympathetic nervous systems in bladder function, Urology **2:**211, 1973.
20. Schafer, W.: Detrusor as the energy source of micturition. In Hinman, F., Jr., editor: Benign prostatic hypertrophy, New York, 1983, Springer-Verlag.
21. Suki, W., et al.: Patterns of nephron perfusion in acute and chronic hydronephrosis, J. Clin. Invest. **45:**122, 1966.
22. Swenson, O., Fischer, J.H., and Smyth, B.T.: Studies of normal and abnormal peristalsis, Med. J. Aust. **146:**805, 1959.
23. Talner, L.B.: Urographic contrast media in uremia, Radiol. Clin. North Am. **10:**421, 1972.
24. Van Zee, B.E., et al.: Renal injury associated with intravenous pyelography in non-diabetic and diabetic patients, Ann. Int. Med. **89:**51, 1978.
25. Wein, A.J. et al.: The effect of oral bethanechol chloride on the cystometrogram of the normal male adult, J. Urol. **120:**330, 1978.
26. Weiss, R.M.: Ureteral function, Urology **12:**114, 1978.
27. Weiss, R.M.: Clinical correlations of ureteral physiology, Am. J. Kidney Dis. **2:**409, 1983.
28. Wilson, D.R.: Micropuncture study of chronic obstructive nephropathy before and after release of obstruction, Kidney Int. **2:**119, 1972.
29. Wolk, F.N., and Whitaker, R.H.: Late followup of dynamic evaluation of upper urinary tract obstruction, J. Urol. **128:**346, 1982.

43 Renal Failure

Marc I. Lorber

The outlook of patients suffering with renal failure, regardless of etiology, has changed dramatically since the early 1960s. Before that time the uremic patient was subjected to a progressive downhill course requiring severe protein and salt restriction, ultimately resulting in coma and uremic death. During the World War II German occupation of the Netherlands, William Kolff developed the forerunner of the modern hemodialysis machine.[5] It was not until 1960, however, that long-term maintenance of patients on hemodialysis became a realistic possibility.[20] As maintenance hemodialysis became more commonplace, the ultimate goal of renal replacement therapy by transplantation enjoyed parallel success with the introduction of effective prophylactic immunosuppression.[50] The feasibility of maintenance hemodialysis and renal transplantation thus altered the outlook for patients suffering from renal failure and has had a major impact on physicians' ability to manage patients with various surgical problems in whom renal function is severely compromised or absent entirely.

NORMAL RENAL FUNCTION

The physiology of urine formation and excretion has been detailed in Chapter 41, but the salient features as they relate to renal failure merit reemphasis. Each human kidney contains approximately 1 million nephrons that collectively respond to the metabolic alterations and fluid and electrolyte changes in the body to achieve internal homeostasis (Fig. 43-1). Extracellular fluid volume regulation is initiated as blood passing through the afferent renal arteriole is subjected to glomerular filtration. A fraction of the water and accompanying dissolved solute is separated from the formed cellular elements and macromolecules in the blood. The glomerular filtrate generally excludes substances with molecular weights greater than 70,000 daltons, whereas small-molecular-weight substances (less than 15,000 daltons) are uniformly included. Middle-range molecules are filtered in a more selective fashion.

The glomerular filtration mechanism maintains a relatively high hydrostatic pressure because of the unique anatomy of the glomerulus placing the glomerular capillary bed between two arteriolar structures. Renal blood flow is regulated primarily at the arteriolar level, and the glomerular filtration rate (GFR) relates directly to renal blood flow. The fraction of renal blood flow represented by GFR has been termed the *filtration fraction*. Renal blood flow normally approximates 25% of cardiac output. Therefore, if the normal renal blood flow is 600 ml/minute/kidney and GFR is approximately 120 ml/minute, the normal filtration fraction is 0.2.

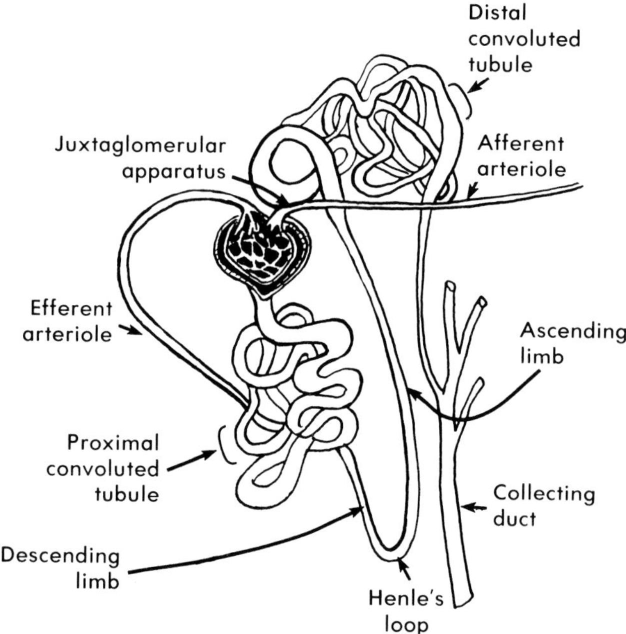

Fig. 43-1 Anatomy of an isolated nephron. Each nephron functions as an independent filtration unit in production of the final urinary product, reflecting excesses of water, electrolytes, metabolic by-products, as well as various other toxins. The human kidney normally contains 1 million nephrons.

The GFR can be measured directly using micropuncture techniques; however, its estimation using the concept of solute clearance is employed more often in the clinical setting, as shown by the relationship:

$$\text{Clearance} = \frac{\text{Urine concentration} \times \text{Urine volume}}{\text{Plasma concentration}}$$

Clearance of a particular substance can be used to predict GFR accurately only if the substance is neither secreted nor reabsorbed by the renal tubular system. Inulin represents such a substance, and inulin clearance has become the standard for estimation of GFR. The clinical setting would be more conveniently served if an endogenously produced substance could be used. Clearance of creatinine, a by-product of skeletal muscle metabolism, closely parallels the value obtained using inulin clearance. Thus, for most clinical purposes, creatinine clearance (CrCl) is measured to estimate GFR.

Approximately 80% of available solids and water present in the glomerular filtrate are reabsorbed in the proximal renal tubule. The proximal tubular filtrate maintains an isosmotic relationship with the blood; however, the process of reabsorption may also require energy expenditure (active transport). Although some substances such as glucose are absorbed very efficiently by the proximal tubule, other substances are reabsorbed partially (e.g., sodium) or not at all (e.g., creatinine). The process is further complicated by the active and passive secretion of certain substances. The countercurrent exchange mechanism found within the renal medulla enhances the reabsorption of solute and water as the filtrate traverses Henle's loop. The ascending limb of Henle's loop represents an additional site of active electrolyte and thereby passive water reabsorption. The energy-dependent processes whereby chloride and sodium reabsorption occur are crucial for maintenance of normal tubular function.

By the time the distal convoluted tubule is encountered, approximately 90% of the glomerular filtrate has been reabsorbed. The final reabsorption processes are controlled hormonally by aldosterone and antidiuretic hormone (ADH). Aldosterone mediates active chloride reabsorption and thus sodium exchange for potassium and hydrogen ion. ADH regulates additional water reabsorption by its modulating effects on collecting duct and distal tubular permeability. Thus the final urinary product reflects excesses of water, electrolytes, and metabolic by-products, as well as products of drug metabolism and other potentially toxic substances.

RENAL DYSFUNCTION

Abnormal renal function impacts on surgical practice in several different settings, including (1) acute renal failure in acutely injured or critically ill patients recovering from major surgery, (2) chronic renal dysfunction in patients suffering from various surgical disorders unrelated to their renal disease, (3) angioaccess for hemodialysis, and (4) surgical care of patients with chronic renal failure by renal transplantation. Therefore the surgeon caring for patients with renal dysfunction should be well versed in the consequences of altered renal physiology and the resultant effects on the body's homeostasis.

Renal disease can involve alterations in glomerular function alone, tubular function alone, or both in combination (Table 43-1). Glomerular dysfunction can result in two basic pathophysiologic abnormalities: (1) diminished glomerular filtration and (2) increased glomerular capillary permeability. Thus patients with renal insufficiency can manifest diminished filtration by reduced clearance of metabolic by-products and reduced urinary volume. When such a pure glomerular lesion results in reduction of glomerular blood flow, as might occur in acute glomerulonephritis, the kidney remains able to concentrate the urinary filtrate, but dilute urinary excretion may not be possible. Further, the increased permeability of the glomerular capillaries results in a diminution of the normal barrier to macromolecules. Large amounts of protein losses occur, whereas glomerular filtration and blood flow—as measured by clearance—are unaffected. Persistent proteinuria with hypoproteinemia and negative nitrogen balance, as observed in the nephrotic syndrome, leads to a cascade of events, including reduction of relative blood volume, activation of the renin-angiotensin-aldosterone system, sodium retention, stimulation of ADH secretion, and water retention with resultant peripheral edema. When glomerular injury is severe, permanent loss of function with the associated irreversible morphologic changes of glomerular thrombosis or necrosis is observed.

Acute renal tubular injury, as has been associated with aminoglycoside nephrotoxicity, can be localized to particular anatomic regions. The site of injury can often be determined by the results of specific clinical measurements. Proximal tubular injury, for example, can affect renal regulation of substances that are normally reabsorbed at that level of the nephron. Therefore, since essentially all the glucose and protein present in the glomerular filtrate are normally reabsorbed in the proximal renal tubule, urinary excretion of those substances in the absence of other demonstrable pathology suggests a proximal tubular injury. Similarly, injury to transport mechanisms located in the ascending limb of Henle's loop results in abnormal handling of monovalent anions and cations, including chloride, sodium, potassium, and hydrogen. Perhaps more imporantly, damage to these energy-dependent ion exchange mechanisms cause altered renal medullary osmolarity with impairment of the concentrating ability of the kidney. Finally, alterations in responsiveness to the sodium-conserving influence of aldosterone and to the effects of ADH on water reabsorption in the distal tubule result in an inability to excrete an adequately concentrated urinary product. In this latter circumstance, however, one must remember that insufficient hormonal stimulation (i.e., ADH in diabetes insipidus) or end-organ insensitivity to appropriate hormone levels may also adversely affect the kidney's ability to concentrate urine.

Although isolated renal tubular damage to a specific anatomic region is possible, one must also recognize that it is more common to observe a condition that results from a combination of insults causing global tubular damage. Further, because renal tubular cells are metabolically very active and cellular turnover is high, these cells are capable of regeneration following injury. Thus renal failure resulting from tubular damage can be completely reversible. This is in direct contrast to glomerular pathology, which frequently progresses and leads to irreversible renal failure.

PATIENT WITH ACUTE RENAL FAILURE

Despite improved technology allowing effective substitution of lost renal function in critically ill patients through dialysis, acute renal failure (ARF) continues to be associated with mortality rates in excess of 70%.[2,28,56] Naturally those figures reflect more directly the complexity and severity of clinical conditions treated in intensive care units; however, it seems clear that uremic problems accompanying ARF require special attention, particularly when complications such as infection, poor nutrition, and multiorgan dysfunction occur.

Types of Acute Renal Dysfunction

Prerenal Azotemia

Acute renal dysfunction has characteristically been classified as prerenal, renal, or postrenal according to the etiologic nature of the precipitating event. Prerenal failure or azotemia (elevated blood urea nitrogen [BUN] and serum

Table 43-1 **COMMON ETIOLOGIES OF ACUTE RENAL DYSFUNCTION**

Diagnosis	Primary Level of Injury	Clinical Manifestations	Preventive or Therapeutic Measures
Prerenal azotemia	Pantubular	Volume contraction, oliguria	Volume repletion
Acute tubular necrosis	Pantubular	Oliguria, polyuria, anuria, isosthenuria, uremia	Volume repletion, avoidance of hypotension
Acute pigment load Hemolysis Rhabdomyolysis	Proximal Tubule	Hemoglobinuria, myoglobinuria	Urinary alkalinization, hydration, forced osmotic diuresis
Drug-induced nephrotoxicity			
Aminoglycosides	Proximal tubule, secondary immune response	Nonoliguric uremia	Adequate hydration, monitoring of circulating drug levels, avoidance of other nephrotoxins
Cephalosporins	Pantubular	Nonoliguric uremia	Adequate hydration, avoidance of other nephrotoxins
Other antimicrobials	Tubular, secondary immune response	Nonoliguric uremia	Adequate hydration, avoidance of other nephrotoxins
Cyclosporine	Probably afferent arteriole	Oliguric or nonoliguric uremia	Monitor circulating drug levels, avoidance of excessive doses
Nonsteroidal anti-inflammatory drugs	Inhibition of autoregulation with decreased renal blood flow	Usually oliguric uremia	Avoidance of setting off other nephrotoxins or renal insufficiency
Radiographic contrast agents	Pantubular	Usually oliguric uremia	Monitoring of volume of agents, hydration, avoidance of concomitant nephrotoxins
Chemotherapeutic agents	Pantubular	Usually oliguric uremia	Hydration, urinary alkalinization, forced diuresis, monitoring of drug levels
Organic solvents/metals	Pantubular/glomerular	Nonoliguric or oliguric uremia	Hydration, forced diuresis, chelating agents
Hyperuricemia	Pantubular	Hyperuricemia, oliguria, renal calculi, polyuria, natriuresis	Uric acid control, hydration, urinary alkalinization, correction of underlying disorders
Hypercalcemia	Distal tubule	Reduced concentrating ability, nephrocalcinosis	Hydration, forced diuresis, mithramycin for acute crisis
Hyperoxaluria	Pantubular	Reduced concentrating ability, renal calculi, nephrocalcinosis	Elimination of oxalate-rich foods from diet, hydration, oxalate-binding agents
Nephrotic syndrome	Glomerular	Polyuria, proteinuria, peripheral edema	Generalized support, protein repletion, hydration
Acute glomerulonephritis	Glomerular	Hypertension, proteinuria, hematuria, nephrotic urinary sediment	Antibiotics for potential causative infections, generalized supportive care
Urinary obstruction	Urinary collecting system, prostate, urethra	Oliguria, collecting system, dilation	Correction of underlying abnormality

creatinine concentrations) indicates a condition that has resulted in diminshed renal blood flow, usually because of decreased effective circulatory volume, and thereby altered renal function. Among the many potential etiologic factors, acute hemorrhage, dehydration, "third-space" gastrointestinal losses, sepsis and resultant peripheral vasodilation, peritonitis, cardiac failure, renal artery injury or embolization, and pancreatitis represent some of the more common considerations.

The underlying mechanism in each of these situations is renal hypoperfusion and/or ischemia. Reduction of arterial volume or pressure results in afferent arteriolar dilation with concomitant increases in vasomotor tone at the efferent renal arteriole.[6] This vasomotor process of renal autoregulation allows maintenance of GFR at the expense of blood delivery to the peritubular regions. Reduction of the mean arterial pressure below 80 to 90 mm Hg precipitates, through hormonal and autonomic responses, a progressive fall in renal blood flow. This situation is reversible and not associated with actual renal pathology if diagnosed and treated early, thus the term *prerenal azotemia.* When sustained, however, this situation can result in intense global renal vasoconstriction as attempts to maintain GFR become less successful. The resultant cellular hypoxia, often termed *vasomotor nephropathy,* represents the final common pathway leading to true ARF.[9,18] Once sustained tubular damage occurs, filtrate back-leak, intraluminal obstruction from cellular swelling, persistent vasoconstriction, and alterations in glomerular permeability create a cycle that results in clearly evident renal failure. Histolog

Table 43-2 **DIAGNOSTIC INDICES IN ACUTE RENAL FAILURE**

Index	Normal Value	Prerenal Azotemia	Acute Tubular Necrosis	Obstruction
Urinary volume	≥ 0.5 ml/kg	≤ 0.5 ml/kg	Variable	Variably diminished
Urinary specific gravity	1.003-1.025	≥ 1.020	1.010	Variable
Urinary sodium	Variable	< 20 mEq/L	> 40 mEq/L	> 40 mEq/L
Urinary fractional sodium excretion	< 1%	< 1%	> 3%	> 3%
Creatinine clearance	100-120 ml/min	Normal to mild reduction	Progressive reduction	Variable
Serum creatinine	0.6-1.3 mg/dl	Mild elevation	Progressive elevation	Variable elevation
Blood urea nitrogen (BUN)	10-20 mg/dl	Elevation	Progressive elevation	Variable
BUN/creatinine ratio	10:1	> 20:1	Variable	Variable

ically, the injury appears as a tubular cell insult, thus the term *acute tubular necrosis (ATN)*, which has become a frequently used clinical designation.

Postrenal Azotemia

Renal dysfunction resulting from urinary obstruction is known as postrenal azotemia. Obstruction can occur at any level of the urinary collecting system. Renal calculi, blood clots, tumors, and papillary necrosis represent a few of the more common intrinsic upper urinary tract findings leading to this condition. External retroperitoneal abnormalities, including retroperitoneal fibrosis, neoplasia, massive retroperitoneal hemorrhage, or rarely massive intraperitoneal hemorrhage or ascites leading to elevated intraabdominal pressure, can also result in postrenal azotemia by obstructing normal urinary flow through the ureters. Accidental surgical ligation of a ureter may also be a cause. Lower urinary tract abnormalities that can result in postrenal azotemia include bladder calculi, blood clots, prostatic hypertrophy, and carcinoma. Finally, retroperitoneal urinary extravasation, as may occur from an injury to the urinary tract such as a gunshot wound, can mimic postrenal azotemia because the urinary product becomes reabsorbed rather than excreted. As with prerenal azotemia, the postrenal form is not associated with actual renal pathology unless the cause of obstruction is sustained and not relieved.

Renal Azotemia

Specific abnormalities of the kidneys that develop acutely can result in overt ARF. The most frequently observed abnormalities encountered by the surgeon include ATN, pigment nephropathy from free myoglobin or hemoglobin, direct nephrotoxicity from drugs or radiographic contrast materials, and acute interstitial nephritis from infection.

ATN represents the end stage of ischemic insult, as discussed earlier. The point at which an ischemic injury ceases to be prerenal marks the development of obvious tubular injury and renal failure. ATN is generally considered a reversible injury; however, when ischemia is severe and prolonged, acute cortical necrosis and irreversible renal failure result.

Extensive trauma can cause hemolysis and muscle destruction. The resultant hemoglobinuric or myoglobinuric renal failure occurs because of accumulation of pigment casts in the proximal tubular lumen and accumulation of breakdown products in the tubular cells.[19] This gives rise to intense vasoconstriction as well as proximal tubular obstruction, thereby preventing glomerular filtration. Radiographic contrast agents similarly are directly toxic to renal tubular cells and also induce intense renal vasoconstriction.[10,39]

The mechanisms underlying drug toxicity to the kidney vary depending on the particular drug. The aminoglycoside antibiotics represent a typical group of drugs that exert toxicity through renal vasoconstriction, alterations in glomerular capillary permeability, and direct tubular cell disruption.[4,27]

Finally, acute interstitial nephritis or glomerular nephritis can result following induction of immune responses in the kidney to various drugs or microorganisms.[6]

Diagnosis

Critically ill patients are extremely vulnerable to alterations in intravascular volume and renal perfusion that can result in acute renal injury. The most direct clinical determinations that allow assessment of renal perfusion include measurements of urinary volume, urinary specific gravity, electrolyte excretion, examination of the urinary sediment, and serum determinations of creatinine and BUN (Table 43-2). Adjunctive information regarding the status of cardiac and respiratory function, as well as direct central hemodynamic measurements, have become indispensable tools in the management of complicated illnesses.

The measurement of urinary output over time provides an important direct determination of the adequacy of renal perfusion. The minimum hourly urinary excretion should approximate 0.5 ml/kg of body weight. In the absence of urinary obstruction and cardiac pump failure and assuming that the kidney is otherwise intact, urine production below that rate implies an inadequate circulating blood volume. Although a decrease in urine output is frequently seen in renal disease, it is important to remember that oliguria does not necessarily accompany significant renal injury. Direct nephrotoxic injury from various sources results in nonoliguric renal failure in 25% to 50% of patients.[53]

The intact nephron is capable of concentrating the urine to approximately 1300 mOsm/L (specific gravity, 1.040). This is slightly more than a fourfold increase over the normal plasma osmolarity, which is approximately 300 mOsm/L (specific gravity, 1.010). Thus the prerenal azotemia that occurs when circulating blood volume is decreased, resulting in oliguria and an increase in urinary concentration, can often be differentiated from the azotemia induced by a renal tubular injury (i.e., ATN), in which the urinary concentrating ability of the kidney is diminished, as determined by measurement of urine specific gravity. Determination of urinary osmolarity and specific gravity may be misleading in critically ill patients since these measurements can be altered by significant proteinuria, glycosuria, and the use of radiographic contrast materials, mannitol, furosemide, or other osmotically active drugs or metabolites.

Among alternate methods developed to assist in the differentiation of true ARF from prerenal azotemia, the calculation of fractional sodium excretion (FENa) has proved to be discriminating and effective.[38] FENa represents the percentage of sodium in the initial glomerular filtrate that is excreted in the urine. The calculation requires simultaneous determinations of plasma sodium (PNa) and creatinine clearance (CrCl) with similar urinary determinations. FENa is calculated by dividing the product of urinary sodium (UNa) and total urinary volume (V) by the total sodium filtered as follows:

$$\text{FENa}\ (\%) = \frac{(\text{UNa})\ (\text{V})}{(\text{PNa})(\text{CrCl})}$$

Normally the FENa represents less than 1% of the filtered sodium load. Patients with ARF tend to excrete larger quantities of sodium despite oliguria, whereas patients with prerenal azotemia conserve urinary sodium. FENa, however, is also limited in its clinical usefulness because values are frequently 1% in acute glomerulonephritis. Finally, this calculation becomes less accurate when considering nonoliguric situations, such as high-output renal failure.

Examination of the urine and urinary sediment frequently yields additional important information. Hemoglobin from hemolysis and myoglobin from rhabdomyolysis can be readily identified. Proteinuria can be screened using urinary dipstick evaluation. Prerenal azotemia is frequently associated with small amounts (1+, 2+), whereas heavier proteinuria suggests intrinsic renal injury. The urinary sediment can assist in the differentiation of infection, as well as primary renal disorders. Prerenal azotemia is associated with occasional fine granular and hyaline casts, whereas ATN is characterized by large numbers of tubular epithelial cells, epithelial cell casts, and coarse granular casts. Red blood cells and red cell casts frequently suggest acute glomerulonephritis.

Creatinine, a normal end product of creatine phosphate metabolism in muscle, is a substance that is primarily filtered, but not reabsorbed, by the nephron. Its clearance has already been discussed as an estimate of GFR. If one assumes that muscle mass remains constant, daily creatinine production also remains constant, averaging 10 to 20 mg/kg/day. The normal serum creatinine is 0.6 to 1.3 mg/100 ml in the patient with normal renal function. Patients suffering abnormal renal function therefore sustain elevation in serum creatinine as urinary clearance diminishes. Total renal failure is associated with a serum creatinine rise at an average rate of 1 to 2 mg/100 ml/day.

Similarly, BUN directly reflects adequacy of renal function. The incremental daily rise in BUN approximates 20 to 25 mg/day in the complete absence of glomerular filtration. However, since urea production is less constant than creatinine, BUN determination is much less discriminating in distinguishing prerenal from renal azotemia. The BUN/creatinine ratio is much more useful in this regard. A ratio in excess of 20:1 frequently signifies prerenal azotemia, whereas a ratio of 10:1 or less might indicate intrinsic renal disease.

Prevention

The kidneys are relatively well protected from ischemic insult because of their normally high blood flow. The metabolic, hormonal, and hemodynamic alterations associated with critical illness, however, greatly increase their vulnerability to various forms of injury. The high mortality that frequently accompanies ARF should serve as appropriate warning that the emphasis should be on prevention. Thus important aspects of prevention should be initiated during the period of preoperative evaluation and preparation.

Radiographic studies employing hyperosmotic contrast agents, vigorous bowel preparation, and restricted fluid intake can result in significant dehydration and increased susceptibility to ARF. Similarly, endogenous intravascular fluid losses associated with the third-space phenomenon in patients with pancreatitis, bowel obstruction, peritonitis, and so on may result in severe intravascular dehydration, as can fever, fistulous drainage, vomiting, and diarrhea. All these states of severe volume loss and dehydration make the kidneys vulnerable to the development of ARF.

The history and physical examination therefore can provide indispensible data to the clinician in determining patients at risk. Preexisting illnesses that can increase the incidence of ARF include hypertension, diabetes mellitus, and renal insufficiency. Symptoms or signs suggesting urinary obstruction, such as decreased urinary stream, incomplete bladder emptying, and urinary urgency or frequency, should be fully evaluated before elective surgery. Abnormal laboratory studies indicating renal problems or dehydration demand complete investigation. Except in life-threatening situations, no patient should undergo major surgical intervention without having electrolyte disturbances and associated dehydration corrected first.

Often the accepted approach is to begin intravenous fluid therapy the evening before surgery. This is particularly important when the patient has been subjected to an extensive preoperative evaluation, has been receiving acute or chronic diuretic therapy, or may otherwise be suspected of having mild dehydration. Selected patients, including the elderly, those with preexisting cardiac disease, and those determined to be at increased risk, should undergo preoperative preparation to optimize volume status. This is generally best accomplished with central venous cannulation, or ideally with right-sided heart catheterization with a Swan-Ganz catheter, 12 to 24 hours before planned surgery. Cardiac filling pressures and output can thereby be maximized and renal perfusion optimized.

The intraoperative management of patients undergoing major procedures demands communication and cooperation between the anesthesiologist and surgeon. Hypovolemia or the peripheral vasodilation of anesthesia with resultant renal vasoconstriction should be minimized. The catecholamine discharge associated with operative trauma alone can have deleterious effects on renal blood flow. Diminished renal perfusion can result from anesthetic-related myocardial depression, myocardial ischemia, or cardiac arrhythmia. Hemorrhage, or else spasm from reperfusion following major vascular occlusion, can result in renal hypoperfusion and acute renal injury.

Direct renal injury can result from the use of nephrotoxic medications. The nephrotoxicity associated with the aminoglycoside antibiotics is well known. Penicillins, cephalosporins, and sulfonamides can precipitate acute interstitial nephritis. Inhibitors of prostaglandin biosynthesis, such as aspirin and nonsteroidal anti-inflammatory agents,[8] affect glomerular autoregulation and can prevent intrarenal vasodilation and resultant hypoperfusion injury. Narcotics, such as morphine and meperidine, diminish GFR, and various anesthetic agents stimulate ADH release, thereby diminishing urinary output. Vasoactive amines with alpha-adrenergic activity mediate renal vasoconstriction and can precipitate renal ischemia. The nonpulsatile flow during cardiopulmonary bypass can also contribute to ARF. Thus a good understanding and judicious use of necessary but toxic drugs and appropriate use of technology required during complex surgical procedures must be supplemented with good surgical technique to minimize the incidence of serious renal insult.

Management

Despite preventive measures, the surgeon will frequently be faced with a situation likely to result in ARF. Accumulating evidence suggests that nonoliguric renal failure is prognostically preferable to the oliguric form of ARF.[42] Because fluid overload and serious electrolyte abnormalities are less often encountered in nonoliguric renal failure, dialysis can often be avoided. Further, without the need for fluid restriction it becomes less difficult to prevent severe nutritional deficits. These considerations have suggested that attempts to convert oliguric to nonoliguric ARF might be desirable. Although controversy continues, experimental and clinical evidence suggests that the conversion of oliguric ARF to nonoliguric ARF is sometimes possible.[3,48] In practical terms this controversy has provided a rational clinical approach to the patient who develops acute oliguria. Depending on the clinical situation, a test challenge with fluids, diuretics, or a combination of both can influence and perhaps modify the degree of renal injury. A favorable response would suggest less severe injury, at least some preservation of function, and the necessity for continued volume repletion. A poor response would alternately indicate the need to change the management approach to prevent the additional sequelae of ARF.

Fluid and Electrolytes

Measures to prevent acute volume overload should accompany the diagnosis of oliguric ARF. Total daily fluid intake is restricted to the sum of urinary output and approximate insensible loss. The sodium chloride load should be estimated for each patient, with insensible loss replaced with 5% dextrose solution and urinary output with 0.45% saline. Without the usual compensatory capacity of the kidneys, it is essential to monitor fluid status closely because hyponatremia (sodium, 120 mEq/L) from too much free water or hypernatremia from too little free water can result in neurologic abnormalities (see Chapter 2).

Oliguric ARF requires careful monitoring of serum potassium. Acute hyperkalemia is particularly troublesome in the critically ill, catabolic patient. Serum potassium levels approaching 6.0 mEq/L require urgent therapy, especially when associated with muscle weakness, electrocardiographic changes, or a rapid rate of rise. Immediate temporizing maneuvers should include intravenous administration of sodium bicarbonate (45 mEq) or glucose (25 g, 50% solution) and insulin (10 to 15 units, regular) to redistribute potassium into cells. This should be followed by attempts to remove potassium from the body, for example, using an ion exchange resin such as sodium polystyrene sulfonate (Kayexalate). Kayexalate, when administered into the intestinal tract, exerts its hypokalemic influence through cationic exchange. Kayexalate is constipating, however, and it is advisable to concomitantly administer sorbitol to promote catharsis. Although kayexalate can be administered orally or by enema, it is more effective and complications such as acute colonic perforation are fewer following oral administration.

Largely because of the loss of renal acid/base regulatory capacity, acidosis and less frequently alkalosis become major management considerations in renal failure. The setting of ARF is often associated with requirements for parenteral nutrition, a catabolic state, intestinal bicarbonate losses, and lactic acidosis or ketoacidosis. Although sodium bicarbonate administration can alleviate the metabolic acidosis, volume is frequently rate limiting, and dialysis support may become necessary. The restriction of protein also can slow the rate of metabolic acid accumulation; however, this maneuver may not be advisable for the critically ill patient who is already severely protein depleted.

Hypocalcemia, hypermagnesemia, and hyperphosphatemia also complicate management in patients with ARF. Because seriously ill patients are often hypoalbuminemic, ionized calcium can be normal even when total serum calcium levels are greatly reduced. This effect can be measured directly or estimated using the knowledge that total calcium is reduced approximately 0.8 mg/100 ml for every 1.0 mg/dl reduction in serum albumin. Phosphate binders, usually aluminum hydroxide, are generally employed to control hyperphosphatemia. Calcium and phosphate abnormalities should be corrected simultaneously to avoid exceeding a calcium phosphate product of 70, the level above which injury to the cardiac conducting system, central nervous system, vascular endothelium, and kidneys has been described.[21,52]

Uremic Problems

The symptomatic manifestation of renal failure is called *uremia*. The toxic complications associated with uremia are outlined in Table 43-3. Although thought to be caused primarily by middle-molecular-weight nitrogenous metab-

Table 43-3 **TOXIC COMPLICATIONS OF UREMIA**

Toxicity	Pathophysiology	Systemic Manifestations
Cardiac	Metabolic acidosis, calcium, oxalate deposition ? Circulating toxins Aseptic inflammation	Decreased myocardial contractility, myocardial calcifications, heart failure, pericarditis
Central nervous system	? Circulating toxins Metabolic acidosis	Lethargy, headaches, tremor, seizures, coma
Coagulation	Platelet dysfunction	Hemorrhagic diathesis
Dermatologic	? Tissue deposition of toxins ? Melanin deposition	Pruritus, hyperpigmentation
Endocrine	Generalized reduction in hormone levels, end-organ hyporesponsiveness, abnormal hormonal metabolism	Glucose intolerance, sexual dysfunction, hypothyroidism
Gastrointestinal	Enhanced vagal tone, metabolic acidosis	Nausea, vomiting, diarrhea, anorexia
Peripheral nervous system	? Circulating neurotoxins ? Guanidines	Peripheral neuropathy
Pulmonary	Hypervolemia, metabolic acidosis, capillary leak	Pulmonary edema, cardiac failure, Kussmaul respiration

Table 43-4 **INTERVENTIONAL THERAPY FOR RENAL FAILURE**

Method	Advantages	Disadvantages
Hemodialysis	Rapid, efficient, and widely available; treatment is intermittent; acute or chronic setting	Requires high-flow vascular access; requires sophisticated equipment and personnel; large fluid and electrolyte shifts; hemodynamic instability; anticoagulation needed
Peritoneal dialysis	Slow, gradual dialysis; no anticoagulation needed; minimum equipment and technical support; acute or chronic setting	Less predictable fluid removal; less efficient; risk of peritonitis; requires suitable peritoneal membrane
Continuous hemofiltration	Continuous dialysis; very efficient fluid removal; minimum equipment; acute setting	Less efficient than hemodialysis; anticoagulation needed; requires sophisticated personnel
Renal transplantation	Restoration of physiologic renal function; improved quality of life	Risks of rejection, infection, and other complications of systemic immunosuppression

olites (500 to 10,000 daltons), the BUN remains the best gauge of impending uremic symptomatology. When renal function deteriorates below 10% of normal or BUN exceeds 100 mg/dl, uremic symptoms generally become apparent. Common complaints such as muscle or abdominal cramping, nausea, vomiting, and diarrhea can be largely ascribed to alterations in autonomic tone resulting from progressive metabolic acidosis. Acidosis also can precipitate development of Kussmaul respiration, depression in cardiac contractility, glucose intolerance, central nervous system depression, and encephalopathy. The etiology of uremic pericarditis remains controversial; however, aseptic inflammation describes the characteristic histopathology. Deposition of uncleared metabolites into tissues can produce severe pruritus. Also, as discussed later in this chapter, platelet function abnormalities of uremia result in development of a hemorrhagic diathesis. The potential risks of therapy (dialysis) must be weighed against the consequences of delay when initiation of dialysis is considered. Generally, early institution of therapy for critically ill patients is sensible because fluid and electrolyte balance are frequently labile, and the nutritional requirements for these individuals can be more effectively addressed.

Use of Dialysis

The widespread availability of dialysis support has dramatically altered therapeutic options for patients suffering from ARF. The initial critical decisions regarding institution of dialysis are those of timing and methodology. Acute renal dysfunction with severe fluid overload, acidosis, and hyperkalemia with associated multiorgan system dysfunction can present formidable management dilemmas. Additional indications for emergency dialysis include acute toxin loads that are dialyzable, including methanol, ethylene glycol, and salicylates. Similarly, uremic complications such as encephalopathy, pericarditis, and bleeding caused by platelet dysfunction are at least partly reversible with dialysis. Aggressive initiation of dialysis is frequently advisable to facilitate nutritional support and obviate metabolic complications in severely ill catabolic patients. The types of dialysis available are discussed in the following sections and summarized in Table 43-4 in terms of their relative advantages and disadvantages.

Hemodialysis

Hemodialysis remains the mainstay in therapy for ARF. The principles of osmotic diffusion are put into practice as toxic solutes are removed. Concentration gradient, molecular size, and degree of protein binding represent primary considerations. Clearance is generally greater for small-molecular-weight molecules that are not protein bound and lower for larger molecules, as well as those with high degrees of protein binding. Ten to 15 hours of dialysis per week is generally required to achieve the equivalent clearance of toxic materials that would result if 10% renal function was present. Fluid removal can also be accomplished with dialysis because of the hydrostatic pressure gradient across the membrane interface between the blood and dialysate. The quantity of fluid removal can be manipulated by altering the magnitude of the pressure gradient across the membrane in relation to the fixed ultrafiltration coefficient of the particular dialyzer being used.

Because hemodialysis is accomplished extracorporeally in adults, and flow must generally exceed 200 ml/minute, specialized vascular access is necessary. Until recent years acute hemodialysis was generally performed through externalized arteriovenous shunts. the refinement in technology allowing *single-needle dialysis* has dramatically altered the approach to vascular access in the setting of ARF. Hemodialysis can now readily be accomplished through central venous catheterization using one of several specially designed catheters. This approach has effectively eliminated the requirement for creation of formal vascular access in the acute setting and has been quite safe and effective. Complications are limited to those associated with subclavian vein catheterization and include primarily hemothorax, pneumothorax, and the later risk of catheter sepsis. The safety and efficiency of this approach has been examined, and very low rates of complications and technical difficulties have been documented.[55] Single-needle dialysis technique can also be accomplished by femoral vein cannulation. Many clinicians consider this latter approach less desirable because of requirements for frequent insertion and removal of catheters, the higher incidence of bleeding complications, and the increased risk of infection associated with groin cannulation.

Peritoneal Dialysis

The peritoneum as a dialysis membrane was initially suggested in 1926 by Rosenak and Siwon.[44] Although effective, the technique was associated with unacceptably high morbidity and mortality. Peritoneal dialysis has waxed and waned in popularity over the years, but it remains an effective and in many ways advantageous technique for renal substitution. The installation of sterile dialysate into the peritoneal cavity is straightforward, and well-designed catheters that maximize efficiency and minimize morbidity are now available. Solutes are removed by the concentration gradient between the dialysate and those present in the interfacing capillary bed, depending on molecular charge and size. Fluid is removed by creating an osmotic gradient, usually by the addition of hypertonic glucose to the dialysate. This results in water movement into the peritoneal cavity, which can then be readily drained externally through the catheter.

Urea clearances of 20 to 30 ml/minute can be achieved using peritoneal dialysis, and uremic symptomatology can be prevented. Peritoneal dialysis is considerably less stressful hemodynamically, accomplishes dialysis in a slower, more continuous fashion with less dramatic electrolyte flux, and requires less specialized personnel and equipment when compared to hemodialysis. It is frequently too inefficient for application to highly catabolic patients with acute electrolyte abnormalities or fluid overload, and peritonitis is a significant risk. It can, however, maintain metabolic status once acute emergency situations are overcome.

Continuous Hemofiltration

A more recent adaptation of hemodialysis that allows less rapid, continuous solute filtration with flexibility in management of fluid balance is continuous hemofiltration.[30-32] The hemofilter is an extracorporeal device with semipermeable capillary tubes, which allows selective filtration of fluid and solutes (Fig. 43-2). The ultrafiltration coefficient is high, thereby allowing large volumes of ultrafiltration at relatively low pressures. Volumes in excess of 500 ml/hour can generally be removed at normal arterial pressure. Solutes are removed somewhat more slowly than by hemodialysis; however, the rate is generally adequate to maintain patients who are otherwise metabolically stable. The pore size of the capillary tubes in the hemofilter allows passage of molecules less than approximately 10,000 daltons, and solute clearances rarely exceed 20 to 25 ml/minute.

Continuous hemofiltration requires a minimum of equipment; however, highly skilled nursing care is essential. The filter is driven by arterial pressure, usually across a standard external arteriovenous (AV) shunt. The AV pressure gradient provides flow across the hollow fibers that permits diffusion, and the filtrate is drained through a side port while nonfiltered material returns directly to the venous circulation. The ultrafiltration rate is generally maintained at approximately 500 ml/hour; however, volumes approaching 30 L/day can be achieved if necessary. Replacement fluid is then composed of appropriate electrolytes such as sodium, chloride, bicarbonate, calcium, magnesium, and so on. It addition, glucose and amino acid solutions of appropriate composition are included to support nutritional requirements. Volume replacement is determined by the patient's hemodynamic status and is easily regulated according to hourly needs.[31]

Critically ill patients suffering from associated ARF typically require a minimum of 40 kcal/kg energy and 1 g/kg protein to achieve adequate nutritional support.[1,37] These nutritional requirements are easily adminstered using continuous hemofiltration to control fluid balance. Thus in selected patients, depending on their size and the degree of their catabolic state, continuous hemofiltration can offer an ideal method of support.

PATIENT WITH CHRONIC RENAL FAILURE

Acute renal failure, if diagnosed early and treated aggressively, is usually reversible and results in no permanent impairment in kidney function. In contrast, chronic renal failure (CRF) represents a substantial and permanent loss of nephron function that, depending on its magnitude, can severely alter the body's ability to maintain homeostasis. All the causes that typically give rise to ARF may also result in CRF. In addition, abnormal immunologic processes, infection, metabolic derangements, systemic diseases (e.g., diabetes, hypertension), congenital abnormalities, neoplasia, and trauma may lead to CRF.

As the population of CRF patients has increased in size, primarily because of improved methods for long-term patient management using dialysis and transplantation, it has

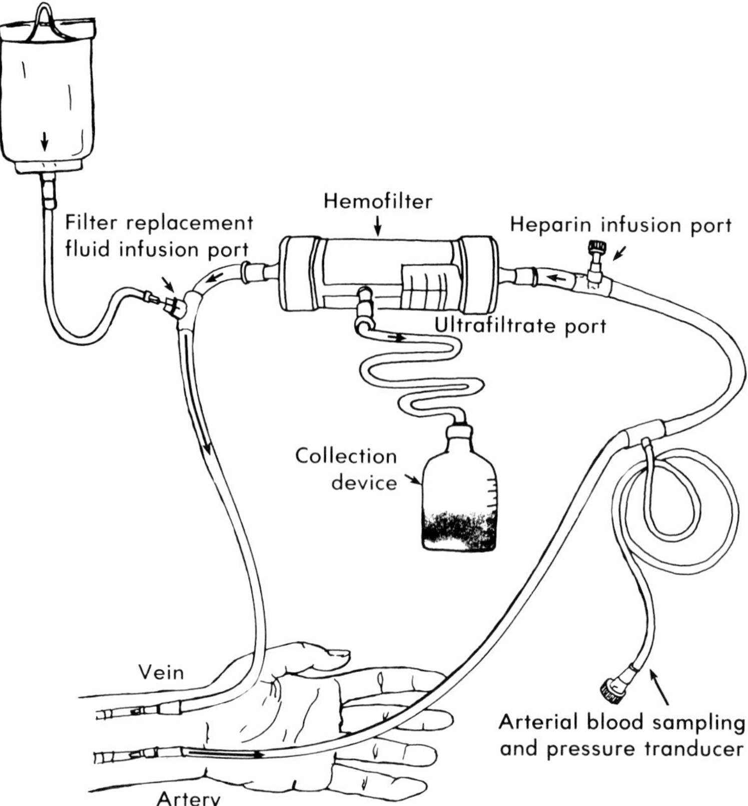

Fig. 43-2 Continuous hemofiltration provides a mechanism allowing large volumes to undergo ultrafiltration across the normal arteriovenous pressure gradient. The large volume of ultrafiltrate can readily be replaced using a formula individualized for specific patient requirements. Replacement fluid generally consists of appropriate electrolytes, glucose, amino acids, and so on needed to maintain homeostasis and to meet nutritional needs.

become apparent that certain unique problems must be addressed when surgical diseases are considered. Procedures for hemodialysis and peritoneal dialysis access are common; however CRF is also associated with several surgical diseases that require operative intervention. Poor nutrition, chronic anemia, coagulopathy, fluid and electrolyte disturbances, endocrinologic derangements, cardiovascular diseases, and alterations in host defense are among the sequelae of CRF that demand scrutiny. Cooperation and teamwork among members of the surgery, nephrology, and anesthesiology teams have fostered the development of effective strategies that provide optimum management, including surgical intervention with acceptably low morbidity and mortality for this high-risk patient population.

Vascular Access for Hemodialysis

Maintenance hemodialysis is usually accomplished using a surgically created internal AV fistula or a subcutaneous AV shunt of prosthetic material. The versatility of the radiocephalic AV fistula first described in 1966 by Brescia and associates[7] has been well documented. Long-term patency rates have been good, infection rates low, and overall satisfaction acceptably high.[16,22,43] Other sites where endogenous AV fistulas can be surgically created to provide effective dialysis access include the median cubital vein and brachial artery at the elbow and the cephalic vein and brachial artery in the mid-upper arm (Fig. 43-3). The major disadvantage of the surgically created AV fistula is that several weeks of maturation are necessary before sufficient venous dilation occurs to allow adequate flow for dialysis. The endogenous AV fistula, however, remains the hemodialysis access of choice for most situations.

Frequently, venous access difficulties or time contraints mitigate against the creation of an endogenous AV fistula. Experience with various methods for creation of external AV shunts have been unrewarding, so use of the subcutaneous AV shunt has become common. Although there was enthusiasm for the bovine heterograft,[14] most surgeons currently favor the subcutaneous, AV shunt using expanded polytetrafluoroethylene (PTFE). The requirements for placement include only an artery and vein that are in proximity and amenable to vascular anastomosis. Comparison of patency rates indicate that PTFE shunts are less durable than primary AV fistulas; however, 60% to 80% figures at 2 years postoperatively have been frequently reported.[24,54]

Secondary Hyperparathyroidism

The abnormalities of calcium and phosphorus metabolism that result in abnormal parathyroid hormone production and chief cell hyperplasia represent an additional surgical disease peculiar to the CRF patient population

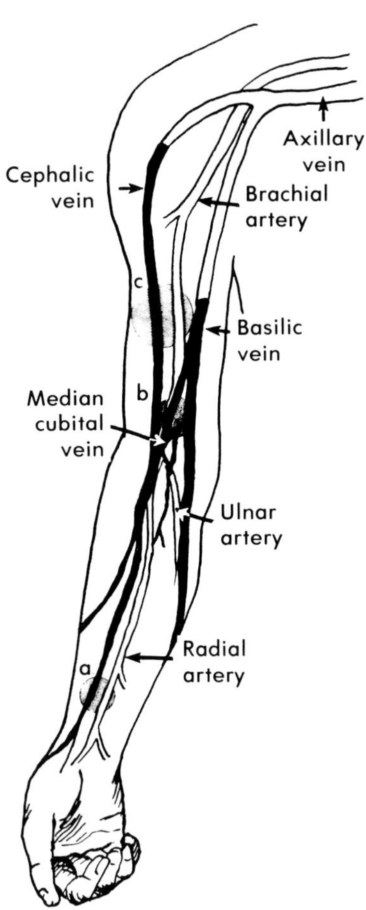

Fig. 43-3 Potential sites for creation of endogenous arteriovenous (AV) fistula for hemodialysis. The most frequently used AV fistula is created by joining the radial artery and cephalic vein at the wrist *(a)*. Other potentially suitable anastomoses include the brachial artery and medial cubital vein at the elbow *(b)* and the brachial artery and cephalic vein at the mid-upper arm *(c)*.

(see Chapter 55). Depending on the criteria used, sequelae from secondary hyperparathyroidism have been estimated in 10% to 45% of patients undergoing chronic hemodialysis. Fortunately, severe problems, including bone pain, pathologic fractures, metastatic calcifications, intractable pruritus, marked fatigue, and muscle weakness, occur in only a minority of patients; however, dramatic improvement has been documented following parathyroidectomy.[12]

Other Surgical Diseases

Patients suffering from CRF are certainly not protected from developing surgical illness unrelated to their renal dysfunction. Although they develop and require care for the entire spectrum of disease problems, CRF patients develop some diseases at rates above those of the age-matched population without renal failure. Pericardial abnormalities, including pericarditis and tamponade, represent complications of uremia that can be minimized by effective dialysis. Such complications can be life-threatening, and severe cases may require pericardiectomy. Similarly, major cardiac valvular and atherosclerotic disease can be treated in the CRF population with acceptable operative results.

Uremic gastrointestinal disturbances have been well documented; again, however, most are easily controlled with adequate dialysis. Peptic ulcer disease has been reported to occur more often among dialysis and transplant patients, possibly related to the gastric damaging effects of urea and steroids, the latter being a common component of the immunosuppression regimen in transplantation. Nonetheless, the association between corticosteroids and gastric ulceration remains a controversial issue. Finally, cytomegaloviral-induced ulceration of the gastrointestinal tract can complicate the clinical course of patients following transplantation.

Perioperative Care

An important, recurrent theme characterizing the requirements for successful management and therapy of surgical disease cannot be overemphasized when considering the care of the CRF patient: *attention to detail*. The lack of normal renal autoregulatory mechanisms greatly diminishes the margin for error, and seemingly minor indiscretions in management can become life-threatening clinical dilemmas. Initial evaluation of these patients therefore must ensure that respiratory and cardiovascular function is acceptable; previously undetected abnormalities that could adversely affect outcome must also be identified and corrected. Other preoperative measures, such as bowel preparation, should proceed as for the patient without renal failure. Ensuring that the patient is adequately dialyzed during the preoperative period is especially important. Optimization of cardiovascular and pulmonary function requires appropriate fluid balance. Adequate removal of uremic ''toxins,'' normalization of electrolyte balance, and correction of severe anemia are crucial. Finally, in the elective setting, a period of vigorous nutritional supplementation can be extremely beneficial.

Another important aspect of the preoperative management program is timing and frequency of dialysis. When possible, it is advisable to avoid dialysis during the early postoperative period. Dialysis should therfore be planned for the day immediately preceding proposed surgery. Usual guidelines dictate a 4- to 5-hour hemodialysis or a 12-hour peritoneal dialysis session. Alternatively, patients maintained by chronic ambulatory peritoneal dialysis (CAPD) generally continue to receive dialysis until called to the operating room, at which time the peritoneal cavity is simply drained. Because electrolyte fluxes, particularly potassium, can be a major difficulty during anesthesia, surgery should not be performed before confirming preoperative optimization of serum levels. Most patients tolerate transient postdialysis hypokalemia well; thus potassium supplements are usually not administered unless hypokalemic symptomatology, such as a cardiac arrhythmia, develops. The efficacy of preoperative dialysis using a low-potassium dialysis bath becomes problematic, however, when a patient requires digitalis therapy. In that situation, care must be taken to avoid hypokalemia because of the increased incidence of digitalis toxicity associated with potassium depeletion.

The hemorrhagic diathesis associated with renal failure was first recognized in the eighteenth century. Attempts to understand the nature of uremic bleeding were initiated in the mid-1950s, and recent advances allowing improved understanding of platelet biochemistry and physiology have begun to clarify many important issues.[15] Abnormal availability of platelet-membrane phospholipid ("platelet factor 3") has been associated with renal failure, and decreased platelet adhesiveness and defective platelet-platelet interaction were found to characterize the uremic coagulopathy.[13,41,46] Bleeding time was improved by dialysis, and several dialyzable agents, including urea, guanidine succinate, and phenols, were hypothesized as etiologic agents.[17,41] As experience mounted, it became clear that dialysis alone was insufficient to reverse uremic coagulopathy, and attention was redirected to abnormalities in platelet-membrane phospholipid.

A series of observations have indicated that in addition to abnormalities in arachidonic acid metabolism, the factor VIII–von Willebrand's complex has been implicated in the pathogenesis of the hemostatic defect in renal failure.[35,45] Initial experiences indicated that transfusion with cryoprecipitate, and more recently with the synthetic ADH analog, 1-deamino-8-D-arginine vasopressin (DDAVP), which causes the release of von Willebrand's factor multimers from endothelial cells, will normalize the bleeding time in uremic patients.[23,35] This has been an important observation for surgeons because the ability to control abnormal uremic bleeding reduces the risk associated with operative intervention.

The mainstay of therapy for the uremic hemorrhagic diathesis continues to be adequate dialysis since well-dialyzed patients have a significantly reduced incidence of peri- and postoperative bleeding complications. The surgeon must be extremely careful to ensure complete intraoperative hemostasis. When problems arise and "surgical" bleeding is controlled, cryoprecipitate (10 units) of DDAVP (0.3 μg/kg) should be administered. Although the duration of action of these agents varies, they can be repeatedly administered with the expectation of reversing uremic hemorrhage.

Anemia is a universal finding associated with CRF. Studies have widely documented that chronically anemic patients tolerate induction of anesthesia and subsequent surgical procedures. Most often, preoperative red cell transfusions are seriously contemplated when the hematocrit falls below 20% to 25%; they are considered mandatory when the hematocrit is less than 15%. The surgeon must be aware of the preoperative levels since the anemic patient tolerates unexpected blood loss with a diminished margin for error.

Evidence documenting compromised host defenses in CRF continues to accumulate.[28] The increased incidence of septic complications may be diminished by a good dialysis program; however, prophylactic perioperative antibiotics seem appropriate. The usual approach has been to administer broad-spectrum antibiotics with antistaphylococcal activity beginning preoperatively and continuing for 24 to 48 hours following surgery. Additional measures include meticulous aseptic technique, as well as frequent examination of operative wounds with early and aggressive drainage when infection occurs.

The safe conduct of anesthesia and anesthetic management in the patient with renal failure requires the same careful thought and attention to detail as is appropriate for any patient. Again, it should be emphasized that the margin for error is greatly diminished when considering patients with CRF. Volume status, electrolyte management, and hemodynamic considerations demand careful attention and precise regulation. Although transfusion is usually not a prerequisite to induction of anesthesia, red cell replacement must be ensured. Many drugs are metabolized abnormally by the patient with renal failure, and agents must be chosen carefully. Dosage schedules also require appropriate alterations. Finally, anesthetic agents, particularly those used for neuromuscular blockade, present unique management challenges in CRF patients. Pancuronium and D-tubocurarine have been particularly problematic because of their effects on intracellular electrolyte balance, most importantly the tendency toward release of intracellular potassium and resulting hyperkalemia. Fortunately, newer agents used for neuromuscular blockade are safer and less problematic when considering anesthesia for CRF.

Following surgery, CRF patients require strict attention to fluid and electrolyte replacement. Parameters other than urinary output must be employed to estimate volume replacement. Operative blood loss can be combined with the physical examination to estimate replacement therapy. It is also necessary to estimate third space volume losses and losses from drains and fistulas when considering postoperative fluid managment. Frequently, when major surgery is performed, monitoring of central venous pressure or preferably pulmonary artery pressures become indispensable in the postoperative care of CRF patients.

Electrolyte disturbances can occur rapidly when caring for the postoperative CRF patient. Surgical trauma with resultant tissue damage, transfusion of banked blood, and the tendency toward acidosis all favor release of intracellular potassium stores and hyperkalemia. CRF patients therefore require close and frequent monitoring to determine the need for early dialysis. The timing of postoperative dialysis is critical since one must frequently choose an appropriate compromise between volume and electrolyte status and the increased risk of bleeding from requisite anticoagulation during dialysis. When one also considers the possibility of uremic coagulopathy further complicating this decision, the necessity for careful attention to detail during the entire perioperative period becomes obvious.

SELECTION OF CANDIDATES FOR RENAL TRANSPLANTATION

The safety and success of renal transplantation is well documented and now widely accepted worldwide. Kidney transplantation, when applied to appropriate end-stage renal disease (ESRD) patients, offers the greatest opportunity for full rehabilitation and return to productive life. Advances in the immunogenetics of the HLA system, improved patient management techniques, and the advent of new approaches to immunosuppression have all made important contributions. It is hoped that cyclosporine represents the first of many immunosuppressive agents that exert their activity selectively. The specificity of cyclosporine for helper T lymphocytes has allowed significant reduction in morbidity and mortality while improving the overall success of clinical renal transplantation.[11,25]

PRETRANSPLANT EVALUATION

General
History and physical examination
Nutritional assessment
Detailed psychosocial evaluation
Complete hematologic evaluation
Chest roentgenogram
Electrocardiogram

Gastrointestinal Evaluation
Upper gastrointestinal contrast study (selected patients)
Lower gastrointestinal contrast study (selected patients)

Biliary Evaluation
Ultrasound or oral cholecystogram

Cardiovascular Evaluation
Coronary angiography
(all diabetic patients; otherwise as indicated)

Urologic Evaluation
Urinalysis with urine culture
Voiding cystourethrogram
Cystoscopy when indicated

Immunologic Evaluation
Tissue typing
Immune profile to determine responder status
Transfusion history
Cytomegalovirus titer

Who among the ESRD population are appropriate candidates for renal transplantation? Although most individuals suffering ESRD are possible transplant candidates, several important issues must be considered. Medical and psychosocial factors have a major impact on an individual's ability to achieve successful transplantation and rehabilitation from ESRD. The pretransplant evaluation must therefore be designed to identify those factors that could ultimately prove detrimental to a successful outcome (see boxed material above).

Before the widespread use of cyclosporine, consensus dictated that transplantation should be reserved for ESRD patients in younger age-groups. Renal transplantation was considered contraindicated for patients older than 50 to 55 years. Recent experience using cyclosporine immunosuppression for the older patient suggested a 10% decrement in 1-year graft survival when compared to the general recipient population. Patient survival at 1 year was acceptable (94%); however, when actuarial figures at 4 years were considered, patient survival was somewhat lower (82%). Deaths in this age group, however, were usually unrelated to immunosuppression or complications of immunosuppressive therapy.[26] Thus age restriction should not be considered absolute, and renal transplantation can be offered to older patients with acceptable expectation for success.

Although most renal diseases that result in renal failure have not been recurrent following transplantation, this possibility should be considered in some settings. Among the various forms of glomerulonephritis, the membranoproliferative, rapidly progressive, and focal sclerosing variants have been reported to recur in more often in transplanted organs.[33] Reports suggesting recurrent glomerulonephritis also have rarely implicated immunoglobulin A nephritis, glomerulonephritis associated with systemic disease, (e.g., Henoch-Schönlein purpura), and membranous glomerulonephritis. Among other systemic diseases associated with renal failure, including systemic lupus erythematosus, scleroderma, sickle cell disease, amyloidosis, Fabry's disease, and cystinosis, the general experience indicates that transplantation can be successfully performed.[49] The associated problems that these patients manifest, however, place them at higher-than-average risk. Primary oxalosis, a rare autosomal recessive disorder of glyoxalate metabolism, has been associated with a very high incidence of recurrent renal failure because of oxalate deposition in the transplanted organ.[47]

Diabetes mellitus is perhaps the most common systemic disorder for which kidney transplantation has been performed. When considering the Type I population of diabetic patients, nephropathy has been estimated to occur in 15 patients/1 million population/year in the United States.[29] This group has represented a challenging patient population with many serious associated medical problems. Although diabetic patients represent a group at increased risk, primarily because of associated vascular and microvascular complications, successful transplantation is frequently preformed. Long-term studies have now followed diabetic patients after renal transplantation. Three-year actuarial graft survival under cyclosporine immunosuppression has been reported at 80%.[40] Biopsy data have substantiated that changes consistent with diabetic glomerulopathy occur in almost all diabetic renal transplant recipients;[36] however, deterioration in renal function has not been well documented. The diabetic patient therefore has benefited from renal transplantation, but associated risks primarily caused by complications of vascular and microvascular disease result in increased morbidity and mortality.

Absolute contraindications to renal transplantation are few but include irreversible central nervous system disease, severe liver insufficiency, infection, malignancy, or advanced systemic disease. As already discussed, several contributing factors can provide relative contraindications to renal transplantation. Patients are selected for transplantation after detailed evaluation of individual medical and psychosocial considerations in an attempt to optimize ultimate rehabilitation.

A complete medical profile of potential renal transplant recipients is critical to the pretransplant evaluation (see boxed material at left). The history, physical examination, laboratory results, specific organ system, and immunologic examinations provide important prognostic data. A clinical psychologist or social worker provides information ensuring that potential financial and social difficulties may be anticipated and addressed. The pretransplant evaluation frequently identifies abnormalities better handled before initiation of immunosuppressive therapy. Any necessary dental work should be completed before transplantation. Surgical procedures, including cholecystectomy for galltones, have increased in importance with the widespread use of cyclosporine because of the agent's hepatoxic side effects and its recent association with development of biliary calculous disease.[34] Also, procedures such as splenectomy for hypersplenism and parathyroidectomy for symptomatic secondary hyperparathyroidism should be performed. Similarly, infectious diseases should be treated and their resolution ensured before transplantation. Careful attention to these pretransplant details can pay tremendous dividends in the form of reduced posttransplant morbidity and mortality.

Particularly since the introduction of cyclosporine, the results following renal transplantion in the management of ESRD have been gratifying. Patients can now be offered transplantation as a therapeutic option with confidence. Studies have documented four-year allograft and patient survival under cyclosporine therapy exceeding 70% and 90%, respectively, for recipients of primary cadaveric allografts. Similarly, analysis has shown that recipients of grafts from haploidentically related donors who were stimulatory in the mixed lymphocyte reaction had a 90% graft and 98% patient survival at 4 years. These improved results have been underscored by the gratifying observation that 89% of patients successfully transplanted were considered vocationally rehabilitated.[26]

SUMMARY

The widespread application of maintenance dialysis and renal transplantation has dramatically improved the outlook for patients suffering from renal failure. This also has impacted substantially on surgical diseases, because patients can now be effectively managed in the presence of severely compromised or absent renal function. Abnormal renal function and physicians' ability to manage its sequelae affects surgical practice in various settings: acute renal failure (ARF) that complicates the clinical course of injured or critically ill patients postoperatively, chronic renal failure (CRF) in patients requiring surgery for operative disorders unrelated to their renal disease, angioaccess for hemodialysis, and renal transplantation.

ARF has been classified according to the etiology of the precipitating events into prerenal azotemia and failure, intrinsic renal failure, and postrenal or obstructive forms. Largely because of associated complications, including infection, poor nutrition, and multiorgan dysfunction, ARF continues to result in high mortality rates exceeding 70%. Clinical indices such as measurements of urinary volume, urinary specific gravity, electrolyte excretion, examination of the urinary sediment, and serum determinations of blood urea nitrogen and creatinine allow the clinician to assess renal function accurately. The high mortality associated with the development of ARF emphasizes the necessity of preventive measures, including ensurance of adequate hydration, optimum cardiac performance, identification of structural genitourinary abnormalities, and judicious use of potentially nephrotoxic medications.

When faced with a situation likely to result in ARF, the surgeon must be prepared to provide effective management strategies to minimize adverse sequelae. Fluid and electrolyte balance, acid-base regulation, and avoidance of uremic complications are all essential. The methodology to be used, as well as the timing in initiating interventive support for the ARF patient, are extremely important. Hemodialysis remains the mainstay in support of patients suffering severe ARF; however, peritoneal dialysis or the more recently developed technique of continuous hemofiltration have specialized applications.

Patients with CRF continue to increase in numbers, primarily as the result of improved long-term management using dialysis and transplantation. Surgery for hemodialysis and peritoneal dialysis access, parathyroidectomy for secondary hyperparathyroidism, pericardiectomy for uremic pericarditis, gastrointestinal disorders, and the general spectrum of surgical diseases require strict attention to detail. The ability of the surgery, anesthesiology, and nephrology teams to cooperate closely during the preoperative, operative, and postoperative periods is essential to the successful outcome for this complex patient population.

Finally, for the patient with end-stage renal disease, renal transplantation has increasingly grown as the therapy of choice. Advances in immunosuppressive regimens have elevated the posttransplant prognosis such that patients can be offered this modality with confidence not only for a high degree of technical success, but also for an excellent chance of vocational rehabilitation.

REFERENCES

1. Abel, R.M.: Nutritional support in the patient with acute renal failure, J. Am. Coll. Nutr. **2**:33, 1983.
2. Abl, A.M., Buckley, M.I., and Austen, W.G.: Etiology, incidence, and prognosis of renal failure following cardiac operations, J. Thorac. Cardiovasc. Surg. **71**:323, 1976.
3. Anderson, R.J., Linus, S.L., and Bernz, A.S.: Nonoliguric renal failure, N. Engl. J. Med. **296**:1134, 1977.
4. Bennett, W.M., Luft, F., and Porter, G.A.: Pathogenesis of renal failure due to amino glycoside and contrast media, Am. J. Med. **69**:767, 1980.
5. Billingham, R.E.: Dedication: proceedings of the Sixth International Congress of the Transplantation Society Transplant. Proc. **9**:37, 1977.
6. Brenner, B.M., Dworkin, L.D., and Ichikawa, I.: Glomerular ultrafiltration. In Brenner, B.M., and Rector, F.C., editors: The kidney, Philadelphia, 1986, W.B. Saunders Co.
7. Brescia, M.J., et al.: Chronic hemodialysis using venipuncture and a surgically created arteriovenous fistula, N. Engl. J. Med. **275**:1089, 1966.
8. Brezin, J.H., et al.: Reversible renal failure and nephrotic syndrome associated with nonsteroidal anti-inflammatory drugs, N. Engl. J. Med. **301**:1271, 1979.
9. Brezis, M., Rosen, S., and Epstein, F.H.: Acute renal failure. In Brenner, B.M., and Rector, F.C., editors: The kidney, Philadelphia, 1986, W.B. Saunders Co.
10. Byrd, L., and Sherman, R.L.: Radiocontrast-induced acute renal failure: a clinical and pathophysiologic review, Medicine (Baltimore) **58**:270, 1979.
11. Calne, R.Y., et al.: Cyclosporine A in patients receiving renal allografts from cadaver donors, Lancet **2**:1323, 1978.
12. Campbell, D.A., Dafoe, D.C., and Swartz, R.D.: Medical and surgical management of secondary hyperparathyroidism. In Thompson, N.W., and Vinik, A.I., editors: Endocrine surgery update, New York, 1983, Grune & Stratton, Inc.
13. Castaldi, P.A., Rozenberg, M.C., and Stewart, J.H.: The bleeding disorder of uremia: a qualitative platelet defect, Lancet **2**:66, 1966.
14. Chinitz, J.L., et al.: Self sealing prosthesis for arteriovenous fistula in man, Trans. Am. Soc. Artif. Intern. Organs **18**:452, 1972.
15. Deykin, D.: Uremic bleeding, Kidney Int. **24**:698, 1972.
16. Ehrenfeld, W.K.: Surgical techniques for hemodialysis access. In Barker, W.F., editor: Peripheral arterial disease, Philadelphia, 1975, W.B. Saunders Co.
17. Eknoyan, G., et al.: Platelet function in renal failure, N. Engl. J. Med. **280**:677, 1969.

18. Flamenbaum, W.: Pathophysiology of acute renal failure. In Solez, K., and Whelton A., editors: Acute renal failure, New York, 1984, Marcel Dekker, Inc.
19. Flamenbaum, W., et al.: Acute renal failure associated with myoglobinuria and hemoglobinuria. In Brenner, B.M., and Lazarus, J.M., editors: Acute renal failure, Philadelphia, 1983, W.B. Saunders Co.
20. Graham, W.B.: Historical aspects of hemodialysis, Transplant. Proc. **9**:49, 1977.
21. Hanley, D.A., and Sherwood, L.M.: Secondary hyperparathyroidism in renal failure, Med. Clin. North Am. **62**:1319, 1978.
22. Ishihara, A.M.: The current state of the art for vascular access in hemodialysis, Contemp. Cont. Dial., September 1980, p. 29.
23. Janson, P.A., et al.: Treatment of the bleeding tendency in uremia with cryoprecipitate, N. Engl. J. Med. **303**:1318, 1980.
24. Jenkins, A.M., Buist, T.A.S., and Glover, S.D.: Medium term follow-up of 40 autogenous vein and forty polytetrafluoroethylene grafts for vascular access, Surgery **88**:667, 1980.
25. Kahan, B.D., editor: Proceedings of the First International Congress on Cyclosporine, Transplant. Proc. **15** (suppl. 4), 1983.
26. Kahan, B.D., et al.: Impact of cyclosporine on renal transplant practice at the University of Texas Medical School at Houston, Am. J. Kidney Dis. **5**:288, 1985.
27. Kaloyanides, G.J., and Pastoriza-Munoz, E.: Aminoglycoside nephrotoxicity, Kidney Int. **18**:571, 1980.
28. Kasishe, B.L., and Kjellstrand, C.M.: Perioperative management of patients with chronic renal failure and postoperative renal failure, Urol. Clin. North. Am. **10**:35, 1983.
29. Knowles, H.C.: Magnitude of the renal failure problem in diabetic patients, Kidney Int. **6**:2, 1974.
30. Kramer, P., et al.: Intensive care potential of continuous arteriovenous hemofiltration, Trans. Am. Soc. Artif. Intern. Organs **28**:28, 1982.
31. Kramer, P., et al.: Management of anuric intensive care patients with arteriovenous hemofiltration, Int. J. Artif. Organs **3**:225, 1980.
32. Kramer, P., et al.: Continuous arteriovenous haemofiltration: a new kidney replacement therapy, Proc. Eur. Dial. Transplant Assoc. **18**:743, 1981.
33. Kreis, H.: Transplanted kidney: natural history. In Hamburger, J., et al., editors: Renal transplantation, Baltimore, 1981, Williams & Wilkins.
34. Lorber, M.I., et al.: Hepatobiliary and pancreatic complications of cyclosporine therapy in 466 renal transplant recipients, Transplantation **43**:35, 1987.
35. Mannucci, P.M., et al.: Deamino-8-D-arginine vasopression shortens the bleeding time in uremia, N. Engl. J. Med. **308**:8, 1983.
36. Mauer, S.M., et al.: Development of diabetic vascular lesions in normal kidneys transplanted into patients with diabetes mellitus, N. Engl. J. Med. **295**:916, 1976.
37. Mault, J.R., et al.: Starvation: a major contributor to mortality in acute renal failure, Trans. Am. Soc. Artif. Intern. Organs **29**:390, 1983.
38. Miller, T.R., et al.: Urinary diagnostic indices in acute renal failure, Ann. Intern. Med. **89**:47, 1978.
39. Mudge, G.H.: Nephrotoxicity of urographic radiocontrast drugs, Kidney Int. **18**:540, 1980.
40. Najarian, J.S., et al.: A single institution, randomized, prospective trial of cyclosporine versus azothioprine, antilymphocyte globulin for immunosuppression in renal allograft recipients, Ann. Surg. **201**:142, 1985.
41. Rabiner, S.F., and Hrodek, O.: Platelet factor 3 in normal subjects and patients with renal failure, J. Clin. Invest. **47**:901, 1968.
42. Rasmussen, H.H., and Ibels, L.S.: Acute renal failure: multivariant analysis of causes and risk factors, Am. J. Med. **73**:211, 1982.
43. Rohn, M.S., et al.: Arteriovenous fistulas for long-term dialysis, Arch. Surg. **113**:153, 1978.
44. Rosenak, S., and Siwon, P.: Experimentelle untersuchungen ueber die peritoneale assucheidung harnpflichtigen substanzen aus dem blute, Mitt a d Gronzgeb D. Med. U Chir. **39**:391, 1926.
45. Ruggeri, Z.M., et al.: Multivein composition of factor VIII/von Willebrand factor following administration of DDAVP: implications for pathophysiology and therapy of von Willebrand's disease subtypes, Blood **59**:1272, 1982
46. Salzman, E.W., and Neri, L.L.: Adhesiveness of blood platelets in uremia, Thromb. Diath. Haemorh. **15**:84, 1966.
47. Scheinman, J.I., Najarian, J.S., and Mauer, S.M.: Successful strategies for renal transplantation in primary oxalosis, Kidney Int. **25**:804, 1984.
48. Schrier, R.W.: Acute renal failure, Kidney Int. **15**:205, 1979.
49. Sreepada, T.K.: Hemodialysis and transplantation in systemic diseases. In Friedman, E., editor: Renal failure, New York, 1978, John Wiley & Sons, Inc.
50. Starzl, T.E.: Experience in renal transplantation, Philadelphia, 1964, W.B. Saunders Co.
51. Stewart, J.H., and Castaldi, P.A.: Uraemic bleeding: a reversible platelet defect corrected by dialysis, Q. J. Med. **36**:409, 1967.
52. Sutton, R.A.L., and Dirks, J.H.: Calcium and magnesium: renal handling and disorders of metabolism. In Brenner, B.M., and Rector, F.C., editors: The kidney, Philadelphia, 1986, W.B. Saunders Co.
53. Swartz, R.D.: Interventive support for acute renal failure in the critically ill patient. In Bartlett, R.H., Whitehouse, W.M., and Turcotte, J.G., editors: Life support systems in intensive care, Chicago, 1984, Year Book Medical Publishers, Inc.
54. Tellis, V.A., et al.: Expanded polytetrafluoroethylene graft fistula for chronic hemodialysis, Ann. Surg. **189**:101, 1979.
55. Vanholden, R., et al.: Complications of subclavian vein catheter hemodialysis: a five year prospective study—257 consecutive patients, Int. J. Artif. Organs **5**:297, 1982.
56. Wilkins, R.G., and Faraghen, E.B.: Acute renal failure in an intensive care unit: incidence, prediction, and outcome, Anesthesia **38**:628, 1983.

44 George S. Benson

Neurogenic Bladder and Urinary Diversion

Urinary continence and micturition are processes that are controlled by complex neurologic mechanisms. When normal neurologic control is lost, a variety of lower urinary tract syndromes, which are collectively known as *neurogenic bladder disease,* may be produced. Because these syndromes are commonly encountered in the practice of surgery, a familiarity with their pathophysiology is mandatory if urinary tract complications are to be prevented. This chapter summarizes the anatomy and physiology of normal urinary continence and micturition and provides a classification of neurogenic bladder disease to aid in diagnosis and management. In addition, several important aspects of normal lower urinary tract function are poorly understood and controversial. These controversies, particularly as they relate to the clinical management of neurogenic bladder disease, will also be discussed.

ANATOMY AND PHYSIOLOGY OF CONTINENCE AND MICTURITION

Anatomy of the Bladder and Its Outlet

Embryologically and anatomically the urinary bladder can be divided into the detrusor and trigone. Contrary to classical thinking, the detrusor musculature is not composed of outer and inner longitudinal and middle circular muscle layers, but rather is composed of a meshwork of smooth muscle fibers, many of which run at right angles to each other.[43] In the region of the bladder neck, muscle bundles arch toward and away from the bladder outlet in such a manner that, with contraction of the detrusor musculature, the bladder neck is pulled up and open. The ureters enter the bladder posteriorly near the superior portion of the trigone and course through submucosal "tunnels" to the level of the ureteral orifices. The length of the submucosal "tunnel" is an important factor in the prevention of vesicoureteral reflux during bladder contraction.

Functionally, the bladder is better divided into body and base than into detrusor and trigone.[33] The base is defined as that part of the bladder circumferentially distal to the level of the ureteral orifices and the body as that part proximal to the ureteral orifices. Neuroanatomically and neuropharmacologically, all portions of the bladder base differ from the bladder body; these differences will be discussed in the following paragraphs.

A solid body of clinical data convincingly demonstrates that a continence mechanism exists in the area of the bladder neck and proximal urethra in both the male and the female.[39] The existence of an anatomic sphincter composed of annular fibers in the area of the bladder neck was denied by Clark in 1883,[11] and over the past century, most investigators have reiterated Clark's observation. However, many anatomic studies done by careful investigators present remarkably conflicting results concerning the anatomy of the bladder neck and proximal urethra.

Those advocates of the "no anatomic sphincter" position differ among themselves on the muscular anatomy of the bladder neck. Woodburne concluded that the "muscle in this region does not constitute a sphincter of annular fibers." The "arching muscle fascicles which arch toward and then away from the urethral opening and do not encircle it" were viewed by him as "an opening mechanism rather than a sphincter."[43] The closure properties of this region were postulated to be secondary to its high concentration of elastic tissue. Common to most of the "no anatomic sphincter" descriptions is the belief that at least part of the urethral musculature is a direct continuation of the detrusor. Thus Woodburne states that in the human, "its (bladder) internal longitudinal fascicles are traceable directly downward into the submucosal layer of the urethra."[43] According to Tanagho and Smith, "the proximal urethra of the male and the whole urethra in the female consist of two muscular layers, (1) an inner longitudinal coat (a direct continuation of the inner longitudinal coat of the bladder); and (2) an outer circular coat of oblique fibers that are the direct continuation of the outer longitudinal coat of the bladder." The sphincter mechanism, according to these investigators, "is achieved by the oblique and circular fibers around the urethra. Because of their special arrangement, these muscle fibers are occlusive in the passive relaxed state and they do not hinder the active opening of the bladder neck during voiding."[38]

Another viewpoint concerning the muscular anatomy of the bladder neck is that a definite sphincteric muscle completely encircling the bladder neck does exist. Gosling has reported that, at least in the male, the "bladder neck smooth muscle is histologically and histochemically different from that which comprises the detrusor" and that "a complete circular collar" is present, which also surrounds the preprostatic portion of the urethra.[18]

In the male, but not in the female, a second continence mechanism is present in the area of the membranous urethra (that part of the urethra traversing the striated musculature of the pelvic floor) (Fig. 44-1).[39] The membranous urethra contains not only smooth muscle but also elastic tissue. In addition, periurethral striated muscle extending from the bladder neck to the level of the membranous urethra has been recognized for years. The issue of whether this periurethral striated muscle forms part of the complex musculature of the perineum or whether this intrinsic

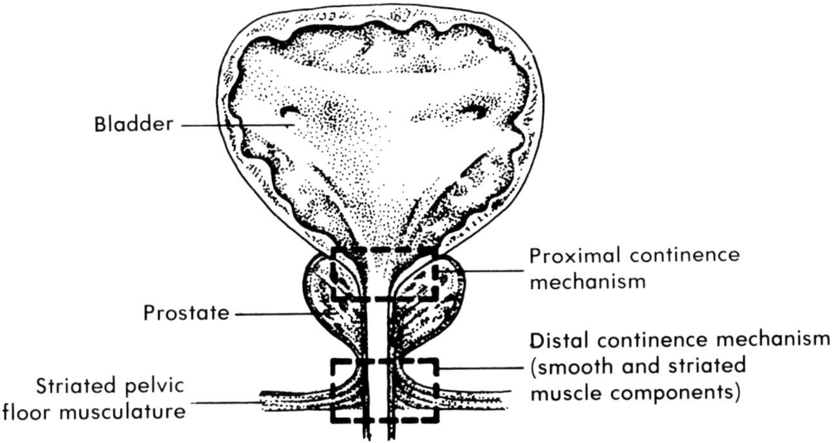

Fig. 44-1 Proximal and distal continence mechanisms in the male.

striated musculature is anatomically separate from the external striated musculature of the pelvic floor has not been resolved.[19]

Innervation of the Bladder and Its Outlet

The bladder and its outlet are innervated by the two divisions of the autonomic nervous system (parasympathetic and sympathetic) and by the somatic nervous system.[41] The terms parasympathetic and sympathetic should not be confused with the terms adrenergic and cholinergic. Parasympathetic and sympathetic are anatomic terms that signify the location of the cell bodies of autonomic nerves. Parasympathetic nerves originate in the craniosacral portions and sympathetic nerves in the thoracolumbar portion of the spinal cord. Cholinergic and adrenergic are physiologic terms that indicate the type of neurotransmitter released at nerve terminals. The neurotransmitter released by cholinergic nerves is by definition acetylcholine, whereas the adrenergic neurotransmitter is a catecholamine. Cholinergic nerves include somatic motor neurons, preganglionic autonomic fibers, and postganglionic parasympathetic fibers. Postganglionic sympathetic fibers are, in general, adrenergic in nature, and the catecholamine responsible for neurotransmission in the lower urinary tract is norepinephrine.

The primary motor nerve supply to the bladder is carried through the pelvic nerve, a parasympathetic nerve derived from sacral segments S2 to S4. Classically, micturition has been viewed as a relatively simple spinal reflex. Bladder distention stimulates afferent fibers that are also carried in the pelvic nerve. These sensory fibers enter the cord through the posterior sacral roots and synapse with the pelvic nerve nuclei in the intermediolateral portion of the cord. Preganglionic efferent fibers then exit the cord in the ventral nerve roots and are carried to peripheral ganglia in the pelvic nerve. In the ganglia these preganglionic fibers then synapse with postganglionic cholinergic fibers, which innervate the bladder and urethra. This spinal micturition reflex is controlled, by both facilitation and inhibition, by descending central nervous system pathways (Fig. 44-2).

An alternative explanation and denial that micturition is accomplished by a segmental sacral reflex has been forwarded by DeGroat and Bradley.[6,8] According to these investigators, sensory afferent fibers carried in the pelvic nerve do not synapse with efferent nerve cell bodies in the spinal cord but are carried directly to the pons where they synapse in a pontine micturition center. Nerve fibers then descend in the cord and, according to DeGroat, synapse with pelvic nerve cell bodies in the sacral spinal cord (Fig.

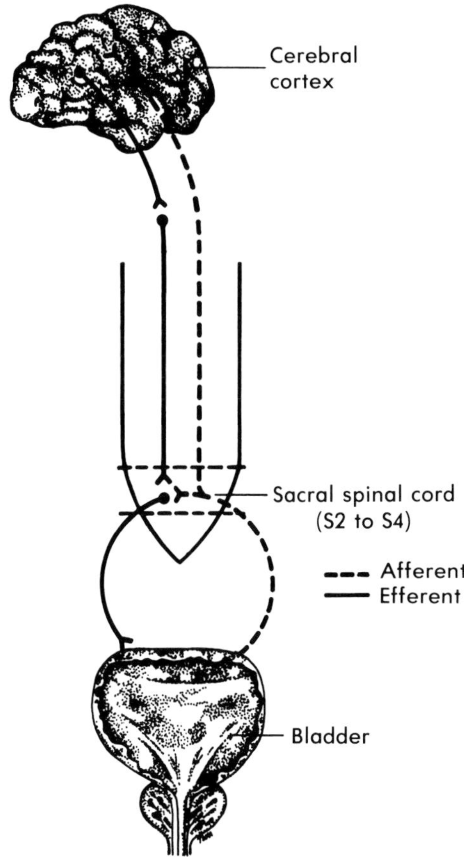

Fig. 44-2 Bladder innervation (sacral spinal reflex hypothesis). Bladder distention results in increased afferent activity in the pelvic nerve. These sensory fibers synapse with parasympathetic nerves in the sacral spinal cord, and efferent impulses (also carried in the pelvic nerve) result in bladder contraction. This spinal reflex is modulated by descending tracts in the spinal cord.

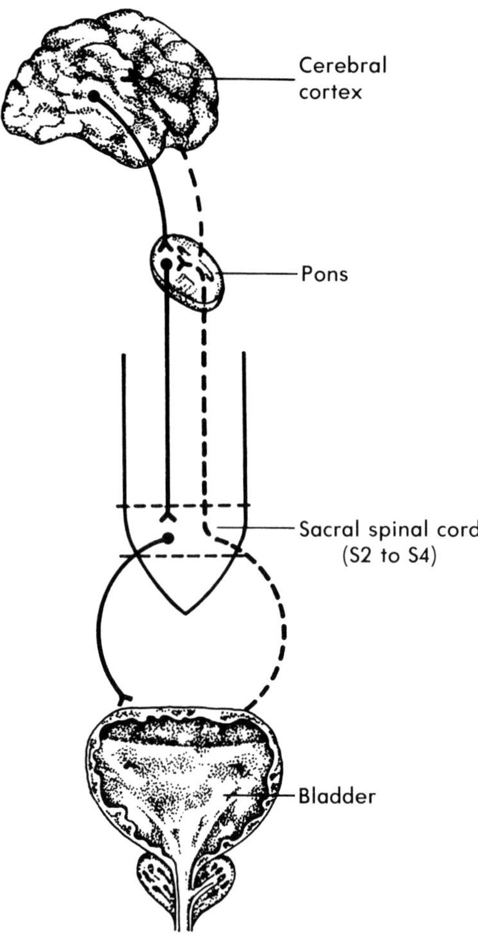

Fig. 44-3 Bladder innervation (pontine micturition center hypothesis). Bladder distention results in increased afferent activity in the pelvic nerve. These sensory fibers ascend in the spinal cord to finally synapse with nerves in the pons. Stimuli are then carried in nerve tracts from the pons to again synapse with parasympathetic nerves in the sacral spinal cord.

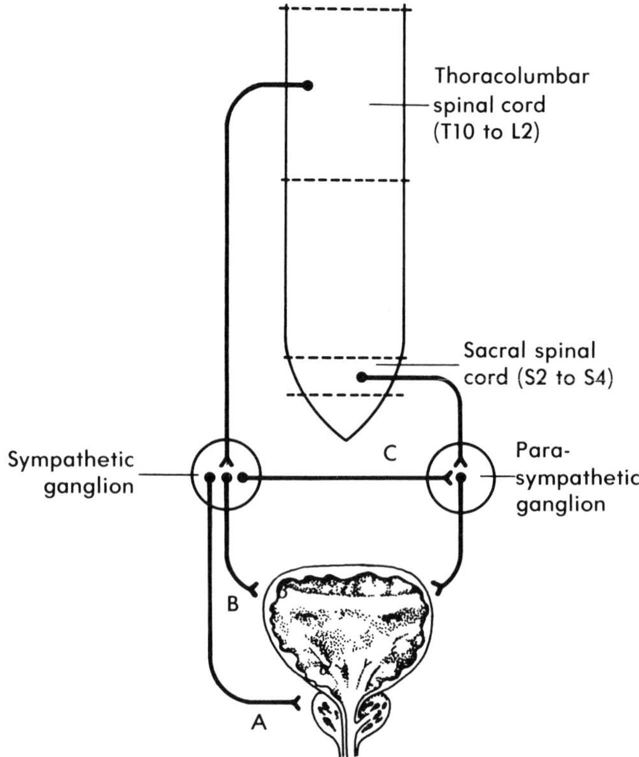

Fig. 44-4 Sympathetic innervation of the lower urinary tract. **A,** Alpha-adrenergic receptor stimulation of the bladder base and urethra; **B,** beta-adrenergic receptor stimulation of the bladder body; **C,** alpha-adrenergic receptor-mediated inhibition of parasympathetic ganglionic transmission.

44-3). Thus the peripheral parasympathetic pathways controlling bladder function are the same in both the sacral reflex arc and the pontine micturition schemes, and both viewpoints incorporate cerebral control of micturition. The spinal cord organization of the micturition reflex is, however, significantly different.

Acetycholinesterase-positive (presumptive cholinergic) nerves have been identified by light microscopy in all areas of the bladder. In vitro bladder muscle strips respond by contracting when stimulated with acetylcholine; this contraction with acetylcholine stimulation is blocked by pretreating the muscle strips with cholinergic muscarinic receptor-blocking agents (atropine, propahtheline).[3] This evidence supports the contention that the parasympathetic neurotransmitter responsible for bladder contraction is acetylcholine and that voiding is therefore a cholinergically mediated event. In vivo stimulation of the pelvic nerve also causes bladder contraction. Unlike the in vitro situation, however, the bladder contraction cannot be completely abolished with pretreating the experimental animal with atropine. This relative atropine resistance of the urinary bladder has led to the hypothesis that at least part of the parasympathetic bladder innervation is noncholinergic.[41]Several putative neurotransmitters, including vasoactive intestinal polypeptide (VIP), enkephalin, adenosine triphosphate, and others, are currently being investigated.

The bladder and its outlet are also innervated by the sympathetic division of the autonomic nervous system. Preganglionic sympathetic nerves arise from the thoracolumbar portion of the spinal cord (T10 to L2). These preganglionic fibers synapse in ganglia located near the spinal cord (paravertebral ganglia), between the paravertebral ganglia and end organ (preganglia), or near or within the end organ (peripheral ganglia). Postganglionic sympathetic fibers then innervate the end organ itself. In addition, sympathetic neurons synapse with parasympathetic ganglia, and adrenergic stimulation has been demonstrated to slow neurotransmission through parasympathetic ganglia[12] (Fig. 44-4).

Morphologically, the various regions of the bladder and its outlet vary remarkably with respect to their adrenergic innervation. The bladder base and urethra are densely innervated by adrenergic fibers, whereas adrenergic fibers in the bladder body are sparse. In addition, muscle bath and radioligand binding studies have demonstrated that the bladder base and urethra have a high concentration of alpha-adrenergic receptors and a low concentration of beta-adrenergic receptors. Conversely, the bladder body contains more beta-receptors than alpha-receptors.[27] In the lower urinary tract, stimulation of alpha-adrenergic receptors causes smooth muscle contraction, whereas stimulation of beta receptors causes relaxation.[33] With sympathetic nerve stimulation, the bladder base and urethra contract (through alpha-receptors) and the bladder body relaxes (through beta-receptors). These actions are veiwed as promoting urine storage.

As previously discussed, the anatomy of the striated musculature in the area of the membranous urethra is not well understood. The innervation of the musculature in this region is equally controversial. The nerve supply to the entire perineal striated musculature is generally thought to be somatic in nature. These fibers originate in the sacral cord (S2 to S4) and are carried in the pudendal nerve. Several researchers believe that the portion of the pelvic floor striated musculature that is located periurethrally (intrinsic striated musculature) is anatomically separate from the extrinsic striated musculature of the perineum. Furthermore, evidence has been presented that this intrinsic striated musculature, or urethral striated sphincter, is not innervated by the pudendal nerve but rather by autonomic nerves coming form the pelvic plexus.[13]

Micturition and Continence (a simplified scheme)

Although our understanding of normal lower urinary tract anatomy and physiology is far from complete, a relatively simple approach to patient care, integrating consistent basic science findings and clinical observations, enables the physician to rationally treat most patients with neurogenic bladder disease.

The lower urinary tract has two primary functions: urine emptying (micturition) and urine storage (continence). Micturition is primarily a parasympathetically mediated event. Afferent impulses signaling bladder distension synapse with efferent fibers that exit from the sacral spinal cord. Conscious cerebral control over the micturition reflex occurs through pathways that facilitate or inhibit the micturition reflex (either sacral or pontine). Efferent stimuli (primarily cholinergic) cause the bladder to contract. With bladder contraction, the bladder base is pulled up and open, and when intravesical pressure exceeds the intraurethral pressure, micturition occurs.

Under normal circumstances, continence requires the absence of uninhibited bladder contractions. In females the only continence mechanism, or "continence zone," is located in the area of the bladder neck and proximal urethra. The bladder neck and proximal urethra are thought to remain closed by two mechanisms: (1) the inherent elasticity of the tissue and (2) contraction of the smooth muscle in this area (mediated through alpha-adrenergic receptors). In the male two "continence zones" are present. The proximal continence area is composed of the bladder neck and proximal urethra. The second or distal continence mechanism is located near the area of the membranous urethra. This distal continence mechanism is also thought to be dependent on the inherent elasticity and alpha-receptor–mediated contraction of the smooth muscle of the urethra. The importance of the striated musculature of the pelvic floor in helping to maintain passive continence is controversial. In normal micturition, however, the pelvic floor musculature reflexly relaxes just before detrusor contraction. In some pathologic states, contraction of the pelvic floor striated musculature with detrusor contraction can cause functional obstruction or urine flow in the area of the membranous urethra.[7]

DIAGNOSIS AND CLASSIFICATION OF NEUROGENIC BLADDER DISEASE

Diagnosis

Symptoms

Patients afflicted with neurogenic bladder disease may have a variety of symptoms. In fact, many patients with neurogenic bladder disease are incorrectly diagnosed because their initial symptoms so closely mimic other types of urologic disease. For instance, hesitancy, straining to void, decrease in the force and caliber of the urinary stream, and urinary retention are symptoms not only of bladder outlet obstruction (secondary to urethral stricture, benign prostatic hyperplasia, or prostatic carcinoma) but also of some types of neurogenic bladder disease. Dysuria and fever are symptoms not only of uncomplicated infections in otherwise normal patients but also of infection complicated by lower urinary tract dysfunction. In general, patients with neurogenic bladder disease are more prone to infection than the general population. Urinary urgency can occur secondary to bladder outlet obstruction, but it also can be seen when normal cortical function is lost and uninhibited contractions occur. Severe urgency can lead to urgency incontinence, which should be differentiated from stress incontinence and from overflow incontinence secondary to urinary retention.

History

In patients who have any of these symptoms, a diagnosis of neurogenic bladder disease should at least be entertained. Does the patient have a history of cerebrovascular disease, disk disease, diabetes mellitus, multiple sclerosis, or back or pelvic trauma or surgery? Does the patient have any neurologic symptoms, weakness, paresthesias, blurred vision, tremor? Since sacral segments S2 to S4 innervate the rectum and penis as well as the bladder, a history of constipation, fecal incontinence, and impotence should be ascertained. A careful history of medications taken by the patient should also be obtained. Many drugs, including antihistamines, antidepressants, and over-the-counter cold remedies, have anticholinergic or sympathomimetic side effects and can significantly alter lower urinary tract function.

Physical Examination

A complete physical examination should be performed with special attention directed to the urologic and neurologic systems. Palpation of the abdomen may reveal masses (hydronephrotic kidneys or a distended bladder). A rectal examination in males to evaluate the prostate gland and rectal sphincter tone is mandatory. Females should undergo a pelvic examination to exclude pelvic masses, cystocele, or a urethral diverticulum.

A neurologic examination should include an evaluation of sensation of the perineal or saddle area, which is supplied by sacral segments S2 to S4. The bulbocavernosus reflex is often helpful in determining the status of the afferent and efferent limbs of the sacral reflex. This reflex is elicited by squeezing the glans penis or clitoris and determining the presence of an immediate contraction of the external anal sphincter, which can be felt with an examining finger in the rectum. Although this reflex cannot be elicited in all neurologically intact individuals and it does not directly test bladder innervation, the presence of a bulbocavernosus reflex is indicative that at least some reflex activity through the sacral spinal cord is intact.

Laboratory, Radiologic, and Urodynamic Evaluation

Any patient with suspected neurogenic bladder disease must have a urinalysis and urine culture to rule out infection and a serum creatinine to estimate renal function. Determination of the blood sugar to screen for diabetes and a serologic screening test for syphilis may be required. An excretory urogram is usually necessary to evaluate any ureteral or renal changes secondary to bladder dysfunction or vesicoureteral reflux. Specifically, hydronephrosis, urinary tract stones, and renal scarring secondary to pyelonephritis can be evaluated with this study. A voiding cystourethrogram is often required to rule out vesicoureteral reflux, particularly in children with congenital neurologic defects such as myelodyslasia. In addition, various neurologic studies may be necessary to exclude specific neurologic lesions. Head or spine computerized tomographic scans, myelograms, and electromyograms are often indicated in these patients to confirm or exclude suspected neurologic disease.

The diagnosis and management of most patients with neurogenic bladder disease is usually dictated by the results of urodynamic studies. Objective measurements of lower urinary tract function are extremely helpful; the extent of the urodynamic evaluation necessary to adequately manage patients with neurogenic bladder disease is, however, controversial.[23,29]

The cystometrogram is the most useful study in objectively assessing lower urinary tract dysfunction. For this study the patient is asked to empty his or her bladder and then a catheter is inserted and residual urine volume measured. Water or carbon dioxide is then instilled into the patient's bladder at a given rate and the intravesical pressure recorded as the bladder is filled (Fig. 44-5).

Bladders in normal individuals demonstrate accomodation; that is, intravesical pressure increases little with relatively large increments in volume. In addition to residual urine volume, the bladder capacity can be estimated. Although bladder capacity varies greatly from patient to patient, the bladder capacity of most individuals falls in the 300 to 500 ml range. The presence or absence of bladder sensation and the presence of uninhibited bladder contractions and normal detrusor contractions can be ascertained. Although a variety of classifications for neurogenic bladder disease exist, most of them depend heavily on the findings of the cystometrogram to categorize types of bladder dysfunction.

The cystometrogram can be performed simultaneously with other studies to yield additional information. Normally, pelvic floor striated muscle electromyographic activity diminishes just before the onset of a bladder contraction. When functional obstruction at the level of the membranous urethra is suspected (detrusor-striated sphincter dyssynergia), a combined cystometrogram and pelvic

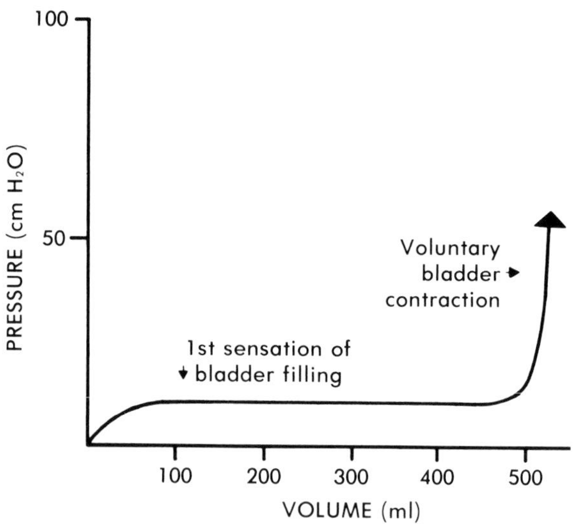

Fig. 44-5 Normal cystometrogram.

floor electromyogram can be performed. An increase in electromyographic activity during bladder contraction is characteristic of this lesion (Fig. 44-6).

Determination of the voiding flow rate is helpful to rule out obstruction. Maximum voiding flow rates are related to the voided volume; nomograms exist for the interpretation of results into normal or obstructed patterns.[36] The voiding flow rate can be performed simultaneously with other parameters of lower urinary tract function. For example, the recording of urine flow rate, intravesical pressure, and pelvic floor electromyographic activity can be obtained simultaneously with a fluoroscopically monitored voiding cystourethrogram. Combined studies such as these may give additional diagnostic information in difficult clinical situations.

The bethanechol supersensitivity test is occasionally helpful in determining the integrity of bladder innervation. This test is based on the principle that denervated smooth muscle becomes supersensitive to neurotransmitters.[25] The cystometrogram is performed and the intravesical pressure at 100 ml of volume recorded. Bethanechol chloride (0.35 mg/kg), a muscarinic cholinergic receptor agonist, is then injected subcutaneously. Repeat cystometrograms are done at 15 minutes, 30 minutes, and 45 minutes following the injection of bethanechol. The intravesical pressure during these subsequent cystometrograms at 100 ml volume is again recorded. An increase of 15 cm of water over the preinjection value is considered positive. Although this test is used primarily to determine the intactness of the motor innervation to the bladder, the bethanechol supersensitivity test has also been reported to be positive in cases of patients with only sensory neuropathy.[22] Several clinical entities that cause false-positive results (notably cystitis) limit the usefulness of this study.[30] Other diagnostic studies have been developed in an attempt to measure the integrity of bladder innervation. Sacral latency times can be measured by a stimulating electrode placed on the penis and a recording electrode placed on the external anal spincter. This study measures the conduction time of nerve impulses carried through the afferent pudendal nerve, sacral cord, and motor pudendal nerve. Like the clinically useful bul-

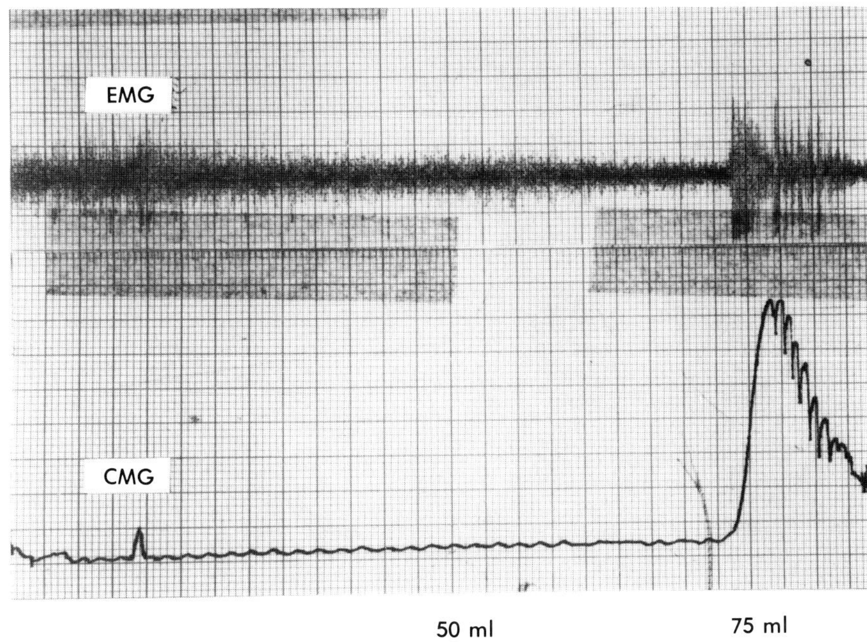

Fig. 44-6 Combined cystometrogram *(CMG)* and pelvic floor striated muscle electromyogram *(EMG)* in patient with detrusor-striated sphincter dyssynergia. (Note increase in electromyographic activity at time of bladder contraction.)

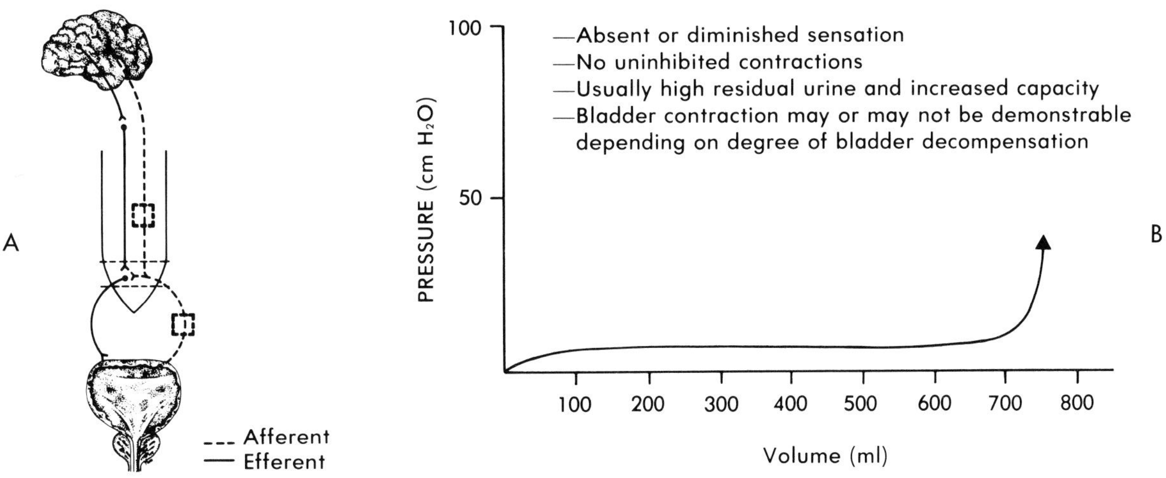

Fig. 44-7 Sensory neurogenic bladder. **A,** Site of lesion indicated by box. **B,** Cystometrogram.

bocavernosus reflex, it does not directly test bladder innervation but does give some information concerning the integrity of the sacral spinal cord.

Classification of Neurogenic Bladder Disease

Numerous schemes exist for the classification of neurogenic bladder disease.[40] The Lapides classification is one of the oldest and simplest and the one familiar to most physicians.[24] Although many patients do not fit exactly into one of the categories of the Lapides classification, this scheme nevertheless provides an excellent framework for understanding many of the principles of neurogenic bladder disease.

The Lapides classification is based primarily on the cystometrogram. This scheme categorizes patients as having neurologic disease that affects (1) sensory nerves to the bladder, (2) motor nerves to the bladder, (3) both motor and sensory nerves to the bladder, (4) descending and ascending spinal cord tracts, or (5) the cerebral cortex.

Sensory Neurogenic Bladder (Fig. 44-7)

If only the peripheral sensory nerves from the bladder or the sensory components of the ascending spinal cord tracts are interrupted, the patient will not be aware of bladder filling and may initially have painless urinary retention and overflow incontinence. One might anticipate that the cystometrogram would be normal except for the absence of bladder sensation. This is usually not the case, however. Typically, the patient with sensory neurogenic bladder disease voids infrequently and with time develops a large bladder capacity. With over-distention, the bladder loses its ability to effectively contract and empty. The cystometrogram commonly demonstrates a large residual urine volume, a large bladder capacity, absent or reduced sensation, no uninhibited bladder contractions; frequently, no detrusor activity can be demonstrated. By far the most common cause of sensory neurogenic bladder disease is diabetes mellitus. Any diabetic patient with voiding symptoms or recurrent urinary tract infections should be evaluated for sensory neurogenic bladder disease. This is particularly important in older diabetic males with signs and symptoms of outlet obstruction from benign prostatic hyperplasia. Other diseases (multiple sclerosis, pernicious anemia, and central nervous system syphilis) can selectively damage the sensory innervation of the bladder and may also occur with sensory neurogenic bladder disease.

Motor Neurogenic Bladder (Fig. 44-8)

This uncommon lesion occurs with diseases that damage only the parasympathetic motor supply to the bladder. As both the motor and sensory nerves to the bladder are carried in the pelvic nerve, injury to the pelvic nerves by surgery or trauma usually does not result in a pure motor neurogenic bladder. Patients with motor neurogenic bladder disease typically have acute painful urinary retention. After the bladder is emptied, a cystometrogram is usually normal except for the inability of the patient to initiate a detrusor contraction. Sensation is intact and uninhibited detrusor contractions are absent.

Motor neurogenic bladder disease is occasionally seen with a herniated lumbar disk and may be associated with viral illnesses such as herpes zoster, mononucleosis, and infection with cytomegalovirus.[31] Another cause of acute painful urinary retention, particularly in young women, is psychogenic urinary retention.[2] This entity can be very difficult to differentiate from motor neurogenic bladder disease. Usually, extensive neurologic and urodynamic studies including bethanechol supersensitivity testing are necessary to rule out significant underlying pathologic conditions. Psychogenic urinary retention should be a diagnosis of exclusion and should be made only after the viral diseases mentioned earlier and multiple sclerosis have been excluded.

Autonomous Neurogenic Bladder (Fig. 44-9)

If both the motor and sensory components of the parasympathetic bladder innervation are disrupted, the bladder is effectively denervated. Patients usually have urinary retention, and overflow incontinence may occur. The patient may void to some extent by abdominal straining, but effective bladder emptying is rarely achieved. The cystometrogram typically demonstrates a high residual urine volume, large bladder capacity, a lack of sensation, and no uninhibited or voluntary detrusor contractions. Voiding flow rates in patients with autonomous neurogenic bladders usually demonstrate a low maximum sustained flow rate and an intermittent stream.

Any lesion affecting the sacral spinal cord, cauda equina, or pelvic nerves may produce this lesion. Trauma to the sacral portion of the spinal cord or cauda equina and congenital lesions such as myelomeningocele result in autonomous neurogenic bladders. In addition, patients who have undergone extensive pelvic surgery such as abdominoperineal resections for colon cancer are at significant risk to develop this lesion.

Reflex Neurogenic Bladder (Fig. 44-10)

According to the Lapides classification, which is based on the concept of a spinal reflex arc, reflex neurogenic bladder disease is seen in patients who have complete spinal cord lesions above the level of S2. When the ascending and descending spinal cord tracts are interrupted, the patient will exhibit uncontrolled and uninhibited reflex-mediated bladder contractions secondary to bladder filling. Since reflex voiding cannot be inhibited by higher centers, patients with reflex neurogenic bladder disease usually have incontinence. A cystometrogram will demonstrate a complete lack of sensation and uninhibited bladder contractions (usually at low bladder volumes).

When considering DeGroat's hypothesis of a pontine (rather than a sacral) micturition center, the pathophysiology of this lesion is somewhat more difficult to comprehend. DeGroat has demonstrated, however, that kittens re-

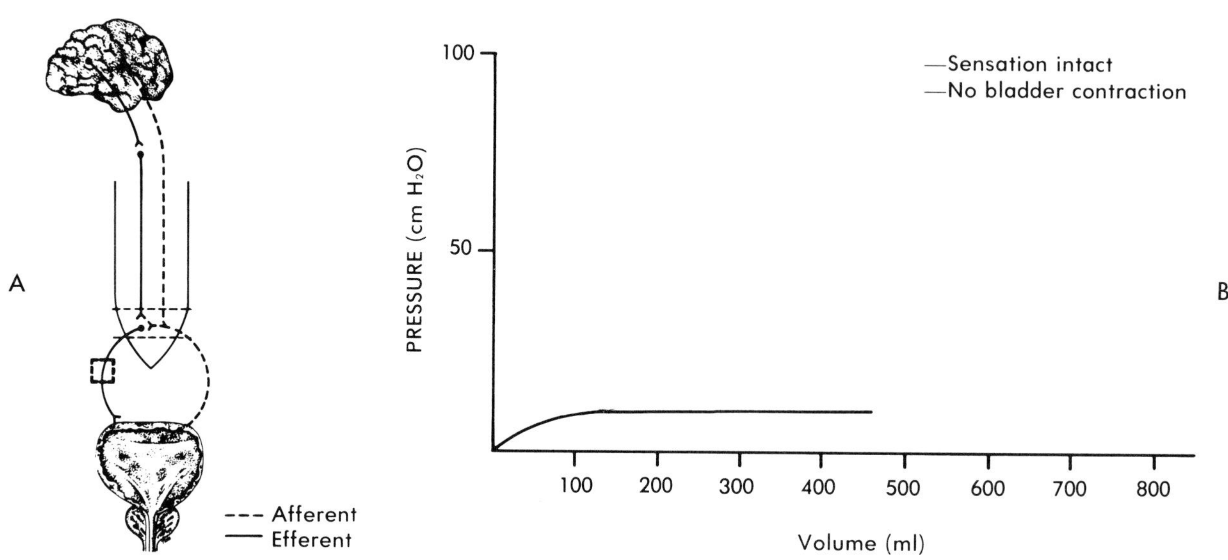

Fig. 44-8 Motor neurogenic bladder. **A,** Site of lesion indicated by box. **B,** Cystometrogram.

flexly void through a sacral spinal reflex. With maturation of the animal, however, voiding occurs through the pontine micturition center rather than through a simple sacral spinal reflex. With interruption of the ascending and descending spinal cord tracts, it is hypothesized that the infantile or sacral reflex again becomes operational.

Patients with reflex neurogenic bladder disease usually empty their bladders unless detrusor-striated sphincter dyssynergia is present. As previously discussed, patients with this syndrome exhibit contraction instead of relaxation of the striated pelvic floor musculature at the time of detrusor contraction. Functional obstruction to urine flow in the area of the membranous urethra may occur. This diagnosis should be considered in all patients with reflex neurogenic bladder disease who carry high residual urine volumes. A combined cystometrogram–striated muscle electromyogram will show a dyssynergic pattern, and a voiding cystourethrogram will show the level of obstruction to be in the area of the membranous urethra.

The majority of patients with reflex neurogenic bladder disease are traumatic paraplegics. Transverse myelitis, multiple sclerosis, spinal cord vascular disorders, abscesses, and tumors are also responsible for this disorder.

Uninhibited Neurogenic Bladder (Fig. 44-11)

When a lesion develops in the cortical regulatory pathways, the ability to suppress reflex bladder contractions (either pontine or sacral) is lost. During bladder filling, all is normal until the point of first sensation. At this point, a sudden desire to void occurs; the patient is unable to inhibit this desire, and normal coordinated micturition occurs. The bladder empties completely and the stream is uninterrupted. Patients with cortical lesions and uninhibited neurogenic bladder disease do not exhibit detrusor-striated sphincter dyssynergia.[6]

Patients with this type of neurogenic bladder disease usually have urgency and urgency incontinence. A cystometrogram will reveal a small residual urine volume, intact

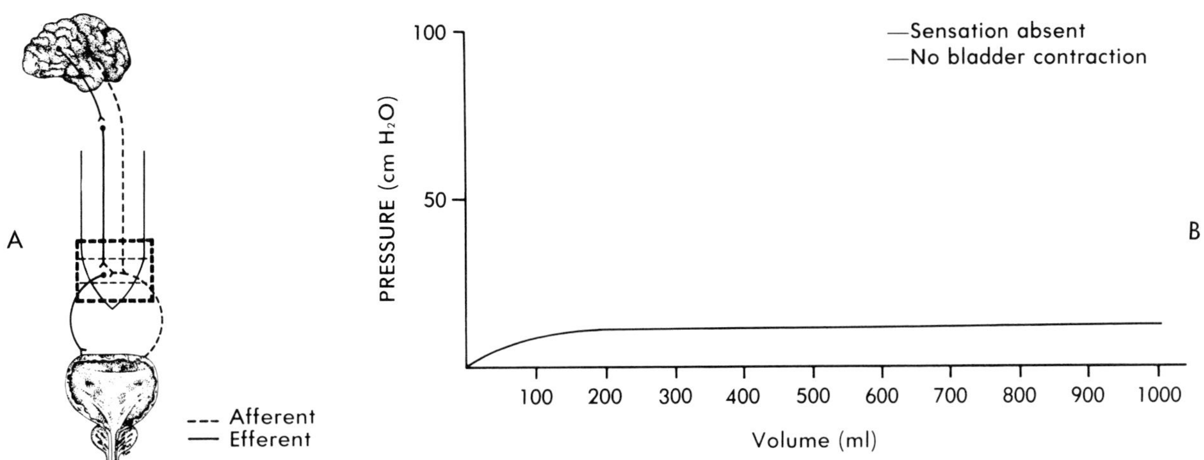

Fig. 44-9 Autonomous neurogenic bladder. **A,** Site of lesion indicated by box. **B,** Cystometrogram.

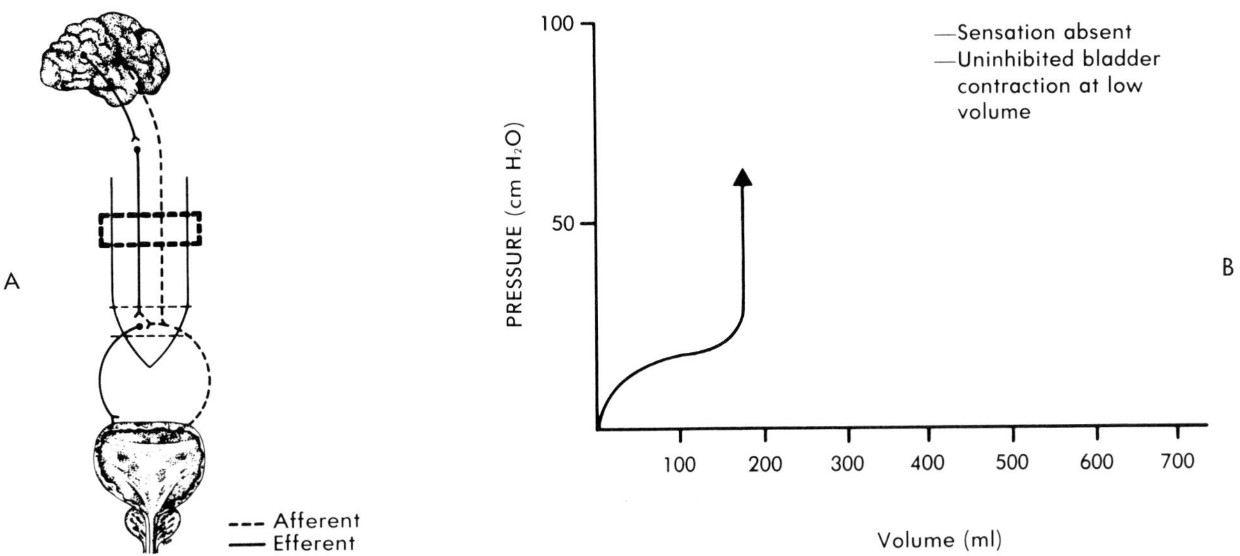

Fig. 44-10 Reflex neurogenic bladder. **A,** Site of lesion indicated by box. **B,** Cystometrogram.

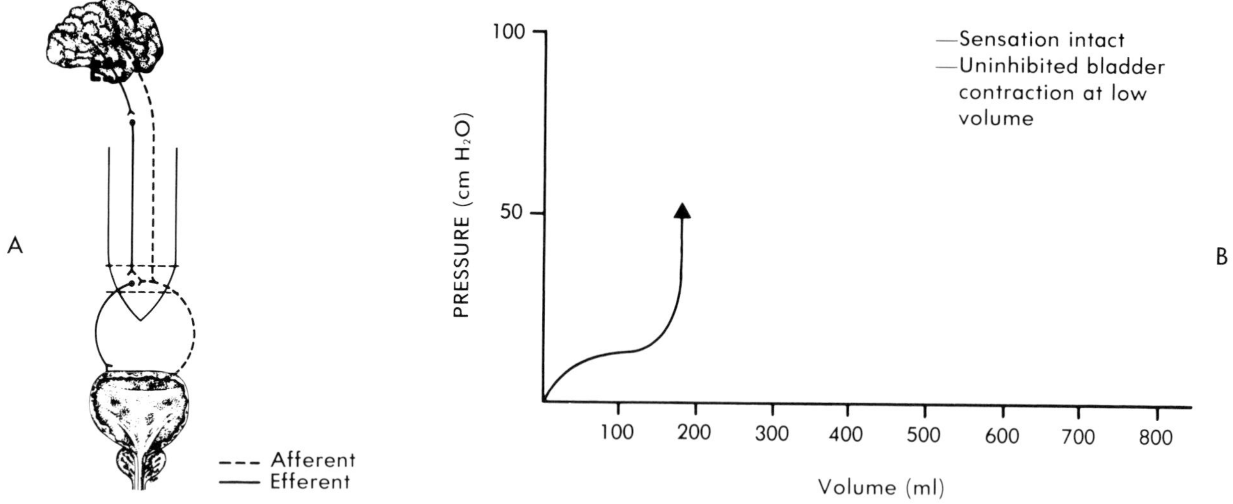

Fig. 44-11 Uninhibited neurogenic bladder. **A,** Site of lesion indicated by box. **B,** Cystometrogram.

sensation, and uninhibited bladder contractions. The cystometrogram findings are very similar to those seen with reflex neurogenic bladder disease. Bladder sensation, however, is absent in the presence of a reflex bladder and present in patients with an uninhibited neurogenic bladder.

Uninhibited neurogenic bladder disease is common in elderly patients. Cerebrovascular disease and Parkinson's disease are common causes. Multiple sclerosis may occur with any type of neurogenic bladder disease, and the patient with an uninhibited neurogenic bladder is no exception.

MANAGEMENT OF NEUROGENIC BLADDER DISEASE

A working knowledge of a classification scheme for neurogenic bladder disease, such as the Lapides classification previously discussed, is essential to an understanding of the pathophysiology involved. A simpler scheme, however, has been devised to assist in the therapy for these patients and is based on the premise that the urinary bladder has two functions: urine emptying and urine storage.[40] Despite the varied neurologic lesions that can lead to bladder dysfunction, patients with neurogenic bladder disease have either failure of urine emptying or failure of urine storage. If the patient's symptoms are the only factor taken into consideration, clinical mistakes regarding management are often made. For example, without a careful examination, which many times requires urodynamic assessment, the patient with overflow incontinence secondary to urinary retention may be viewed as having a failure of bladder storage rather than as having primarily a problem in bladder emptying.

In addition to control of the patient's bladder symptoms, the status of the patient's upper urinary tracts should always be kept in mind. Bladder dysfunction commonly results in renal deterioration because of hydronephrosis, vesicoureteral reflux, infection, or stone disease. The most common long-term cause of death in traumatic paraplegics, for example, is renal disease.[20]

Failure to Empty

Various methods are presently used to achieve bladder emptying; the method of choice will vary depending on the status and compliance of each individual patient.

Catheter Drainage

Although efficacious for short-term use, catheter drainage (either urethral or suprapubic) is usually not the best treatment for the long-term problem of bladder emptying. In males complication rates (urethral strictures and fistulas, infection, bladder stones) are particularly high with urethral catheter drainage. Long-term catheter drainage should be used only when other therapeutic options are not effective.

Clean Intermittent Self-Catheterization

Clean intermittent self-catheterization (CIC) is the therapy of choice in most patients with failure of bladder emptying secondary to neurogenic bladder disease. During the last decade, this form of therapy has gained widespread popularity because of patient acceptance and relatively low complication rates.[26] Many patients who formerly would have been treated with more radical therapeutic alternatives (urinary diversion) are presently being managed successfully with CIC (Fig. 44-12).

Patients are taught to catheterize themselves at approximately 4-hour intervals using a clean (not sterile) technique. Some degree of manual dexterity is required; the patient's neurologic disease cannot greatly limit use of the upper extremities. The use of CIC is applicable to children and adults and is particularly useful in those children with neurogenic bladder disease secondary to myelodysplasia.

Urinary tract infection is the most common complication in patients treated with CIC. These infections are usually easily treated, and the infection rate with CIC is far lower than that seen in patients with permanent indwelling catheters. Patients using CIC need periodic urine cultures and assessment of the upper urinary tracts by excretory urography or ultrasonography because renal deterioration has been reported in these patients.

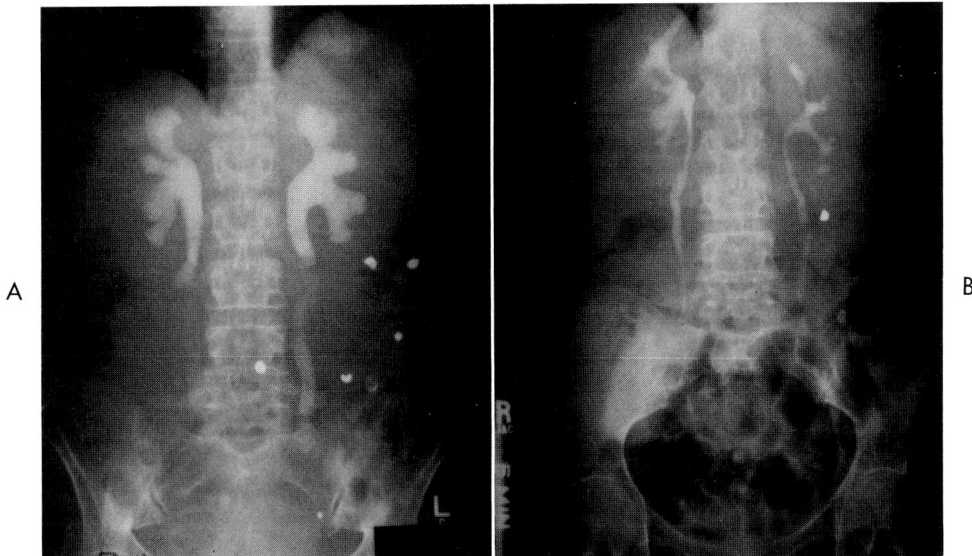

Fig. 44-12 Patient with sensory neurogenic bladder secondary to diabetes mellitus. Patient had 1000 ml of residual urine. **A,** Excretory urogram at time of diagnosis demonstrating bilateral hydroureteronephrosis. **B,** Excretory urogram after 6 months' treatment with clean intermittent self-catheterization demonstrating resolution of the hydroureteronephrosis.

Pharmacologic Therapy

Theoretically, any drug that causes the bladder to contract or causes the bladder outlet to relax should promote bladder emptying. Bethanechol chloride, a muscarinic cholinergic agonist, has been used for over 30 years for this purpose. This acetylcholinesterase-resistant drug is pharmacologically active and does cause bladder contraction. Recent studies, however, have questioned the clinical usefulness of this compound.[42] Specifically, patients treated with bethanechol have shown no improvement in objective measurements such as residual urine volumes or voiding flow rates. These results are not surprising when one considers that a coordinated bladder contraction is probably not produced by bethanechol and that stimulation of muscarinic receptors also results in urethral smooth muscle contraction, thereby increasing outlet resistance. Although the use of bethanechol to promote bladder emptying remains controversial, evidence favors the position that its use in most clinical situations is not efficacious.

An attempt has also been made to use drugs to promote bladder emptying by decreasing outlet resistance. As previously discussed, stimulation of alpha-adrenergic receptors in the bladder base and urethra causes contraction of smooth muscle in this area and thereby increases outlet resistance. Alpha-adrenergic blocking agents do decrease outlet resistance and have been used clinically.[9] However, the responses seen with such agents as phenoxybenzamine and prazosin are often not clinically significant, and troublesome side effects, notably postural hypotension, do occur.

External Sphincterotomy

Patients with spinal cord lesions above the sacral spinal cord may not achieve bladder emptying because of detrusor-striated sphincter dyssynergia. Patients with demyelinating diseases and occasionally neurologically intact children also manifest this syndrome. Many patients, particularly paraplegics with detrusor-sphincter dyssynergia, can be successfully managed with CIC. When CIC is not a viable therapeutic option (e.g., in patients with neurologic disease who have limited or no use of their upper extremities) or when persistent infections or upper tract deterioration occur while CIC is being perfomed, a surgical procedure designed to decrease urethral resistance in the area of the membranous urethra is usually warranted.

Although pudendal neurectomy has been used successfully in some patients, external sphincterotomy is the surgical treatment of choice at the present time. External sphincterotomy is performed endoscopically by resecting a portion of the urethra and periurethral striated musculature in the area of the membranous urethra with a resectoscope. Tissue is preferably removed from the 12 o'clock position. Incisions in the 3 o'clock and 9 o'clock positions have been reported to result in a high incidence of postsphincterotomy impotence.[21] Damage to the paired penile cavernosal nerves that course near the membranous urethra may be the cause of the impotence.

Cutaneous Vesicostomy

Cutaneous vesicostomy is an excellent method of treating young children with neurogenic bladder disease with failure to empty. In children the dome of the bladder can be easily mobilized and brought to the skin; the bladder wall is sutured to the anterior rectus fascia, and a stoma flush with the skin is created in the midline of the lower abdominal wall. This simplified Blocksom technique results in few complications (primarily stomal stenosis and bladder herniation) and is now preferred over previously used types of vesicostomy in which skin flaps were mobilized and brought down to the bladder wall.[14]

Urine exiting the stoma can be collected in diapers. When the child reaches an age when other therapy such as CIC can be instituted, the vesicostomy can be closed. This form of urinary diversion is generally not suitable for adults, primarily because of problems with collecting devices.

Failure to Store

In general, patients whose primary problem is one of urine storage (incontinence) are more difficult to treat than those whose primary problem is failure to empty. Patients with neurogenic bladder disease who fail to store urine and are therefore incontinent will have either uninhibited bladder contractions or decreased bladder neck and urethral resistance.

Pharmacologic Therapy

Although evidence does exist that demonstrates that the urinary bladder in in vivo models is relatively atropine-resistant, uninhibited bladder contractions associated with reflex or uninhibited-type neurogenic bladder disease can be treated with anticholinergic agents. Many patients, particularly those with uninhibited-type neurogenic bladders, obtain significant relief from their symptoms of urgency and urgency incontinence when so treated. A variety of drugs with anticholinergic activity, including propantheline, methantheline, and oxybutynin, have been used.

Drugs are also occasionally effective in increasing bladder outlet resistance. α-adrenergic receptor agonists (phenylpropanolamine, ephedrine, and pseudoephedrine) have been used with some success. Imipramine, a tricyclic antidepressant, is a clinically efficacious drug that promotes urine storage. The mechanism by which this drug acts on the lower urinary tract is not entirely understood. Imipramine does possess anticholinergic and direct smooth muscle depressant activity. In the central nervous system, imipramine has been demonstrated to have a cocainelike effect in that it blocks the reuptake of norepinephrine into nerve terminals. The net effect of this action is to enhance adrenergic activity. Peripherally, this sympathomimetic effect would increase outlet resistance (α-adrenergic receptor stimulation) and relax the bladder body (β-adrenergic receptor stimulation) and thus, at least theoretically, promote continence.[3]

In some clinical situations, drugs are intentionally used to convert a bladder that fails to store into a bladder that does not empty. For example, a patient with a spinal cord injury and incontinence secondary to uninhibited bladder contractions can be treated with anticholinergic agents with the hope of causing urinary retention. The urinary retention then can be managed by CIC.

Clean Intermittent Self-Cathetrization

Occasionally, patients with incontinence secondary to uninhibited bladder contractions can be treated by CIC alone. Patients who are successfully treated with this technique usually not only have uninhibited bladder contractions, but also carry high postvoiding residual volumes. If the bladder can be periodically drained and never reaches a volume high enough to initiate a reflex detrusor contraction, continence may be achieved.

Long-Term Catheter Drainage

For these previously discussed reasons, long-term catheter drainage is not the preferred method to achieve continence in most patients. However, in some patients, particularly elderly females, catheter drainage may be a reasonable choice of therapy.

Artificial Urinary Sphincter

In the past, numerous mechanical devices have been used in an attempt to achieve continence secondary to low outlet resistance. Many of the initial devices were implanted perineally, compressed the urethra, and increased urethral resistance essentially by creating an artificial stricture. The artificial sphincter, the most widely used device at present, consists of an inflatable cuff inserted around either the bladder neck or the bulbous urethra.[34] Patients can deflate the cuff to void and inflate the cuff to achieve continence by transferring fluid to and from a reservoir by a pump mechanism implanted into the scrotum or labia.

SUPRAVESICAL URINARY DIVERSON

When all other forms of therapy fail in patients with either failure to empty or failure to store, a supravesical urinary diversion can be performed as a last resort. Tube diversions (i.e., nephrostomy) are generally not suited for long-term urinary diversion for multiple reasons (infection, stone formation, and the necessity for frequent tube changes). In most patients, supravesical urinary diversion is best achieved by either an ileal or colon conduit or, in rare situations, by a ureterosigmoidostomy. Before the development of many of the treatment modalities discussed previously (particularly CIC, drug therapy, and the artificial urinary sphincter), many patients, particularly children with neurogenic bladder disease, underwent supravesical urinary diversion. Because of the success of other forms of treatment, many of these patients have undergone "undiversion."[1]

Ureters brought directly to the skin usually undergo stomal stenosis. For this reason, most operations designed to divert urine supravesically have either (1) used a segment of bowel, which is interposed between the ureters and skin (ileal or colon conduit), or (2) anastomosed the ureters directly into the intact bowel (ureterosigmoidostomy) (Fig. 44-13). Most patients with neurogenic bladder disease have undergone urinary diversion with either an ileal or colon conduit. An absolute contraindication to ureterosigmoidostomy is an incompetent anal sphincter, and many patients with neurogenic bladder disease also have significant problems with fecal, as well as urinary, control.

Although descriptions of surgical technique vary greatly, the performance of each of these procedures uses several basic principles. The ureters are divided well into the pelvis to ensure adequate ureteral length. One ureter is tunneled behind the colon mesentery to reach the opposite side. In performing an ileal or colon conduit, an appropri-

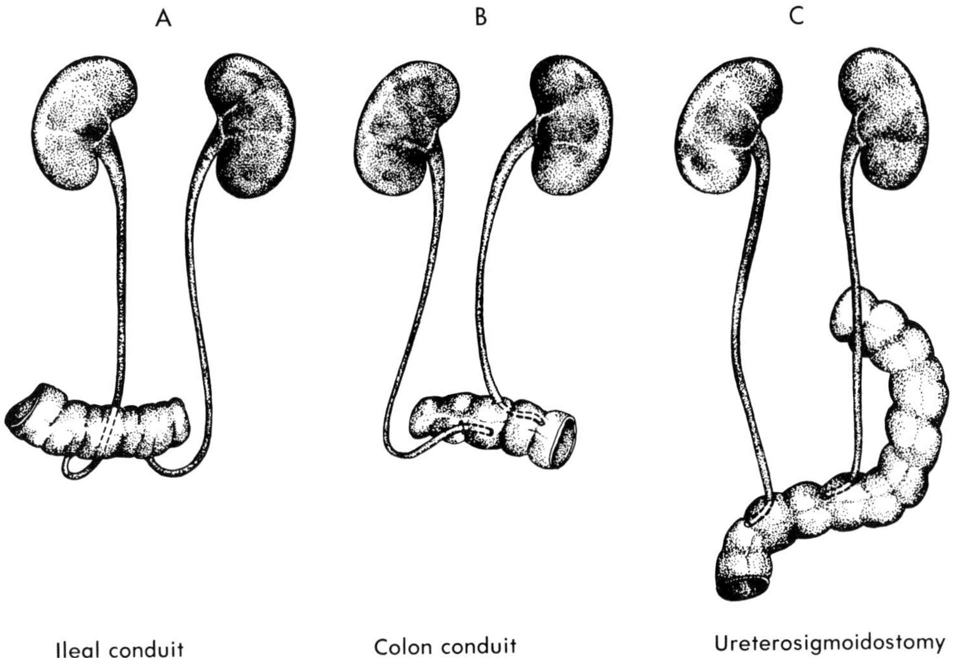

Fig. 44-13 Types of supravesical urinary diversion. **A,** Ileal conduit. **B,** Colon conduit. **C,** Ureterosigmoidostomy.

ate length of bowel is isolated for use as the conduit and then a bowel anastomosis is performed to reestablish bowel continuity. One end of the conduit is closed. Both ureters are attached to the ileum or colon by using a ureteral mucosa–to–bowel mucosa anastomosis. The open end of the conduit is then anastomosed to the skin. Some surgeons prefer colon conduits over ileal conduits because the thicker colon wall allows the ureters to be "tunneled," thereby creating an antirefluxing anastomosis. In a ureterosigmoidostomy, the colon is left in continuity and the ureters are usually anastomosed to the sigmoid by means of a "tunneled" antirefluxing technique.[17]

Early surgical complications seen with ileal and colon conduits include ureteral leak at the site of anastomosis, intestinal obstruction or fistula, ureteral obstruction, and rarely, necrosis of the conduit. Late surgical complications include pyocystis (secondary to the bladder being defunctionalized), stomal stenosis, intestinal obstruction, ureteral obstruction, calculi, and parastomal hernia. Long-term follow-up of patients (particularly children) who have undergone ureteroileal diversion has shown a high rate of upper tract deterioration (increasing hydroureteronephrosis, calculi, and pyelonephritis).[35] This realization has led to increasing reluctance to perform urinary diversion into ileal conduits on children with neurogenic bladder disease.

Surgical complications from uretersigmoidostomy include pyelonephritis, ureterocolonic anastomosis stricture, and calculi. In addition, a late complication of ureterosigmoidostomy is adenocarcinoma of the colon, which usually occurs at the site of the ureteral anastomosis.[32] The incidence of colon cancer associated with ureterosigmoidostomy has been calculated to be 500 times greater than the incidence in the normal population. Studies in rats have indicated that the presence of a fecal stream is necessary for the development of carcinoma. Whether carcinogenic factors are present in urine or feces or both is unclear. Only one case report exists of a carcinoma in a colon conduit urinary diversion where the fecal and urinary streams have been divided.[10] Most surgeons agree that patients with ureterosigmoidostomy should be followed up with stool examinations for blood and routine sigmoidoscopy or colonoscopy.

In addition to local surgical complications, systemic effects relating primarily to fluid and electrolyte disorders occur in patients whose urine has been diverted into bowel segments. In 1950 Ferris and Odel[15] reported that 80% of patients who had undergone a ureterosigmoidostomy had an elevated serum chloride level and 77% had at least some degree of metabolic acidosis. The primary event leading to this syndrome appears to be colonic absorption of chloride.[37] Hyperchloremia and acidosis may also occur in patients with ileal and colon conduits. The incidence and severity of this syndrome in conduits, however, is much less than with ureterosigmoidostomy. This difference is most likely related to both the amount of time urine is in contact with the bowel mucosa and the smaller mucosal surface area of conduits. In addition, patients with ureterosigmoidostomies tend to have slightly decreased serum potassium levels but markedly reduced total body potassium. The mechanism for potassium loss is probably potassium secretion by the colon. Patients with ileal or colon conduits uncommonly demonstrate clinical manifestations of electrolyte imbalance and rarely need treatment. Patients with ureterosigmoidostomies, however commonly need therapy to correct their acidosis and hypokalemia.

Patients undergoing ureteral diversion into a jejunal conduit develop a syndrome that differs from that described for other types of diversions.[16] Specifically, these patients

Table 44-1 **ELECTROLYTE CHANGES WITH URETERAL DIVERSION**

	Ureterosigmoidostomy	Ileal or Colon Conduit	Jejunal Conduit
Serum chloride	↑ ↑	↑	↓
Serum sodium	Normal	Normal	↓
Serum potassium	Normal to reduced	Normal	↑
Acidosis	Present (50%-80%)	Present (2%-15%)	Present (35%)

exhibit hypochloremia, hyponatremia, hyperkalemia, and acidosis (Table 44-1). Sodium and chloride are lost and potassium is absorbed from the conduit. Hypovolemia and hyponatremia decrease the glomerular filtration rate, which further aggravates the acidosis and hyperkalemia. Treatment of these patients is the administration of salt.

Diversion of urine into the bowel is occasionally complicated by encephalopathy associated with hyperammonemia.[28] This syndrome is usually seen when coexistent hepatic disease interferes with urea synthesis. Increased blood ammonia levels are thought to be secondary to absorption of urinary ammonia by the bowel coupled with the action of bacterial urease, which increases urinary ammonia levels.

SUMMARY

Although knowledge of the anatomy, neurophysiology, and neuropharmacology of the lower urinary tract is far from complete, clinically useful classification systems exist that allow accurate diagnosis and effective therapy for most patients with neurogenic bladder disease. In addition, the widespread use of increasingly sophisticated urodynamic studies has made possible more accurate diagnoses and for objective values to evaluate therapeutic modalities. Relatively new forms of therapy (including pharmacologic manipulation, self-intermittent catheterization, and the artificial sphincter) have obviated the need for supravesical urinary diversion in most patients.

REFERENCES

1. Allen, T.D.: Undiverting the ileal conduit, J. Urol. **124:**519, 1980.
2. Barrett, D.M.: Evaluation of psychogenic urinary retention, J. Urol **120:**191, 1978.
3. Benson, G.S., et al: Adrenergic and cholinergic stimulation and blockade of the human bladder base, J. Urol. **116:**174, 1976.
4. Benson, G.S., et al.: Bladder muscle contractility: comparative effects and mechanisms of action of atropine, propantheline, flavoxate, and imipramine, Urology **9:**31, 1977.
5. Bissada, N.K., and Finkbeiner, A.E.: Lower urinary tract function and dysfunction, New York, 1978, Appleton-Century-Crofts.
6. Blaivas, J.G.: The neurophysiology of micturition: a clinical study of 550 patients, J. Urol. **127:**958, 1982.
7. Blaivas, J.G., et al.: Detrusor-external sphincter dyssynergia, J. Urol. **125:**542, 1981.
8. Bradley, W.E., Timm, G.W., and Scott, F.B.: Innervation of the detrusor muscle and urethra, Urol. Clin. North Am. **1:**3, 1974.
9. Caine, M., Perlberg, S., and Meretyk, S.: A placebo-controlled double-blind study of the effect of phenoxybenzamine in benign prostatic obstruction, Br. J. Urol. **50:**551, 1978.
10. Chiang, M.S., et al.: Carcinoma in a colon conduit urinary diversion, J. Urol. **127:**1185, 1982.
11. Clark, S.L.: Some remarks on the anatomy and physiology of the urinary bladder and sphincter of the rectum. J. Anat. Physiol. **17:**442, 1883.
12. DeGroat, W.C., and Saum, W.R.: Adrenergic inhibition in mammalian parasympathetic ganglia, Nature **321:**188, 1971.
13. Donker, P.J., Droes, J.T.P.M., and Van Ulden, B.M.: Anatomy of the musculature and innervation of the bladder and urethra. In Williams, D.I., and Chisholm, G.D., editors: Scientific foundations of urology, vol. 2, Chicago, 1976, Year Book Medical Publishers.
14. Duckett, J.W., Jr.: Cutaneous vesicostomy in childhood: the Blocksom technique, Urol. Clin. North Am. **1:**485, 1974.
15. Ferris, D.O., and Odel, H.M.: Electrolyte pattern of the blood after bilateral ureterosigmoidostomy, JAMA **142:**634, 1950.
16. Golimbu, M., and Morales, P.: Electrolyte disturbances in jejunal urinary diversion, Urology **1:**432, 1973.
17. Goodwin, W.R., and Scardino, P.T.: Ureterosigmoidostomy, J. Urol. **118:**169, 1977.
18. Gosling, J.: The structure of the bladder and urethra in relation to function, Urol. Clin. North Am. **6:**31, 1979.
19. Gosling, J.A., et al: A comparative study of the human external sphincter and periurethral levator ani muscles, Br. J. Urol. **53:**35, 1981.
20. Hackler, R.H.: A 25-year prospective mortality study in the spinal cord injured patient: comparison with the long-term living paraplegic, J. Urol. **117:**486, 1977.
21. Hackler, R.H.: Surgical treatment of the adult neurogenic bladder dysfunction. In Krane, R.J., and Siroky, M.B., editors: Clinical neuro-urology, Boston, 1979, Little, Brown & Co.
22. Harris, J.D., and Benson, G.S.: Positive bethanechol chloride supersensitivity test in hereditary sensory neuropathy, J. Urol. **124:**923, 1980.
23. Hinman, F., Jr.: Urodynamic testing: alternatives to electronics, J. Urol. **121:**643, 1979.
24. Lapides, J.: Cystometry, JAMA **201:**618, 1967.
25. Lapides, J., et al.: Denervation supersensitivity as a test for neurogenic bladder, Surg. Gynecol. Obstet. **114:**241, 1962.
26. Lapides, J., et al.: Further observations on self-catheterization, J. Urol. **116:**169-171, 1976.
27. Levin, R.M., and Wein, A.J.: Quantitative analysis of alpha and beta adrenergic receptor densities in the lower urinary tract of the dog and rabbit, Invest. Urol. **17:**75, 1979.
28. McDermott, W.V.: Diversion of urine to the intestines as a factor in ammoniagenic coma, N. Engl. J. Med. **256:**460, 1957.
29. McGuire, E.J., and Woodside, J.R.: Diagnostic advantages of fluoroscopic monitoring during urodynamic evaluation, J. Urol. **125:**830, 1981.
30. Merrill, D.C., and Rotta, J.: A clinical evaluation of detrusor denervation supersensitivity using air cytometry, J. Urol. **111:**27, 1974.
31. Michaelson, R.G., Benson, G.S., and Friedman, H.M.: Urinary retention as the presenting symptom of acquired cytomegalovirus infection, Am. J. Med. **74:**526, 1983.
32. Parsons, C.D., Thomas, M.H., and Garrett, R.A.: Colonic adenocarcinoma: a delayed complication of ureterosigmoidostomy, J. Urol. **118:**31, 1977.
33. Raezer, D.M., et al.: Autonomic innervation of canine urinary bladder: cholinergic and adrenergic contributions and interaction of sympathetic and parasympathetic systems in bladder function, Urology **2:**211, 1973.
34. Scott, F.B.: The artificial sphincter in the management of incontinence in the male, Urol. Clin. North Am. **5:**375, 1978.
35. Shapiro, S.R., Lebowitz, R., and Colodny, A.H.: Fate of 90 children with ileal conduit urinary diversion a decade later: analysis of complications, pyelography, renal function, and bacteriology, J. Urol. **114:**289, 1975.
36. Siroky, M.B., Olsson, C.A., and Krane, R.J.: The flow rate nomogram. II. Clinical correlation, J. Urol. **123:**208, 1980.

37. Stamey, T.A.: The pathogenesis and implications of the electrolyte imbalance in ureterosigmoidostomy, Surg. Gynecol. Obstet. **103:**736, 1956.
38. Tanagho, E.A., and Smith, D.R.: The anatomy and function of the bladder neck, Br. J. Urol. **38:**54, 1966.
39. Turner-Warwick, R., et al: A urodynamic view of prostatic obstruction and the results of prostatectomy, Br. J. Urol. **45:**631, 1973.
40. Wein, A.J.: Classification of neurogenic voiding dysfunction, J. Urol. **125:**605, 1981.
41. Wein, A.J., and Raezer, D.M.: Physiology of micturition. In Krane, R.J., and Siroky, M.D., editors: Clinical neuro-urology, Boston, 1979, Little, Brown & Co.
42. Wein, A.J., et al.: The effects of bethanechol chloride on urodynamic parameters in normal women and in women with significant residual urine volumes, J. Urol. **124:**397, 1980.
43. Woodburne, R.T.: Anatomy of the bladder and bladder outlet, J. Urol. **100:**474, 1968.

45

James C. Stanley, Linda M. Graham, and Walter M. Whitehouse, Jr.

Renovascular Hypertension

Renovascular hypertension secondary to renal artery occlusive disease is the most common form of surgically correctable hypertension. High blood pressure in patients with this disease follows critical reductions in renal perfusion with activation of the renin-angiotensin system. This physiologic response results in restoration of renal blood flow toward normal, but it does so at the expense of producing systemic hypertension. This chapter will discuss the functional basis for increased blood pressure associated with renal artery stenoses, the histologic and morphologic character of the most common renal artery diseases, the clinical manifestations and means of diagnosing renovascular hypertension, and the therapeutic options in treating this disease entity.

PHYSIOLOGIC SEQUELAE OF RENAL ARTERY STENOSES

Physiologic derangements causing renovascular hypertension are complex. The most important elements contributing to blood pressure elevations in this disease include (1) renin, produced in the kidney; (2) renin substrate, produced in the liver; (3) converting enzyme, which is most active in the lung; (4) angiotensin II, produced from angiotensin I by converting enzyme; and (5) aldosterone, produced in the adrenal gland (Fig. 45-1).

The importance of renal contributions to this form of hypertension was firmly established by the classic canine experiments of Goldblatt and associates[29] first published in 1934. In these and subsequent studies sustained hypertension was produced by gradual reductions in renal artery blood flow using an intricate vascular clamp (Fig. 45-2).[28] Although Goldblatt's investigations suggested that renovascular hypertension was simply a consequence of renal ischemia, subsequent studies have disproven the importance of ischemia per se. Other hemodynamic signals appear more essential in the control of renin release, the most obvious being decreased mean perfusion pressure. In this regard stenoses causing at least a 70% to 80% reduction in the renal artery's cross-sectional area are necessary to induce a pressure gradient. Although this represents advanced stenotic disease, it may be difficult to recognize clinically. For example, the severity of stenoses caused by posterior atherosclerotic plaques may not be obvious on standard anterioposterior arteriograms, and the extent of fibrodysplastic lesions with their irregular webs may be difficult to document unless multiple arteriographic projections are obtained. Nevertheless, critical renal artery stenoses are a cause of renin release from the kidney.

Renin is produced by the juxtaglomerular apparatus of the kidney (Fig. 45-3). Major components of this anatomic region include (1) myoepitheloid cells or granular cells, located on the wall of the afferent arterioles; (2) the macula densa, which is a specialized region of tubular epithelial cells, located in the glomerular hilus at the transition of Henle's loop to the distal convoluted tubule; and (3) lacis cells, located in the region of the efferent glomerular arteriole and the macula densa. The lacis cells are intimately associated with the glomerulus and are anatomically similar to mesangial cells. An interrelationship clearly exists between the macula densa, glomerular arteriole vasomotion, and renal tubular function.[31]

Control of renin production and its release from the kidney is very complex.[12,44,63,98] Renal baroreceptors may be responsible for release of renin from juxtaglomerular cells, with these cells specifically acting as stretch receptors.[97] The cellular basis for activation of these receptors is speculative but may involve the calcium ion.[22] Increasing evidence indicates that renin release and intracellular levels of calcium are inversely related. Alternatively, the stimulus for renin release may be related to pressure change at the afferent renal arteriole level, as well as to renal interstitial volume and pressure changes.

The importance of the tubular fluid milieu and the macula densa has been well established, with changes in sodium and chloride content of tubular fluid altering renin release. An inverse relation may exist between renin release and the intratubular sodium load at the macula densa.[99] However, the relative importance of macula densa receptors in activation of the renin-angiotensin system in renovascular hypertension is uncertain.

Stimulation of postganglionic sympathetic neurons to renal arterioles, many of which end in the region of the juxtaglomerular apparatus, also causes increased renin release. This may be related to afferent arteriolar constriction with decreased stretch of intrarenal vascular receptors and decreased sodium load to the macula densa, but it is more likely a direct result of catecholamine action on beta-adrenergic receptors of the juxtaglomerular cells.[24,25] Although the importance of these receptors in the pathogenesis of renovascular hypertension is poorly defined, the efficacy of beta-blockers in reducing pressure in this disease entity is well recognized.

Renin is a proteolytic enzyme, synthesized and stored as granules within the juxtaglomerular cells, and in some instances as granules within the arteriolar wall. It has a molecular weight ranging from 35,000 to 43,000 daltons, probably reflecting that human renin exists in many forms. Renin has a half-life of approximately 20 to 30 minutes. Peripheral levels of circulating renin appear to be in a steady state; the sum of renin activity from both renal

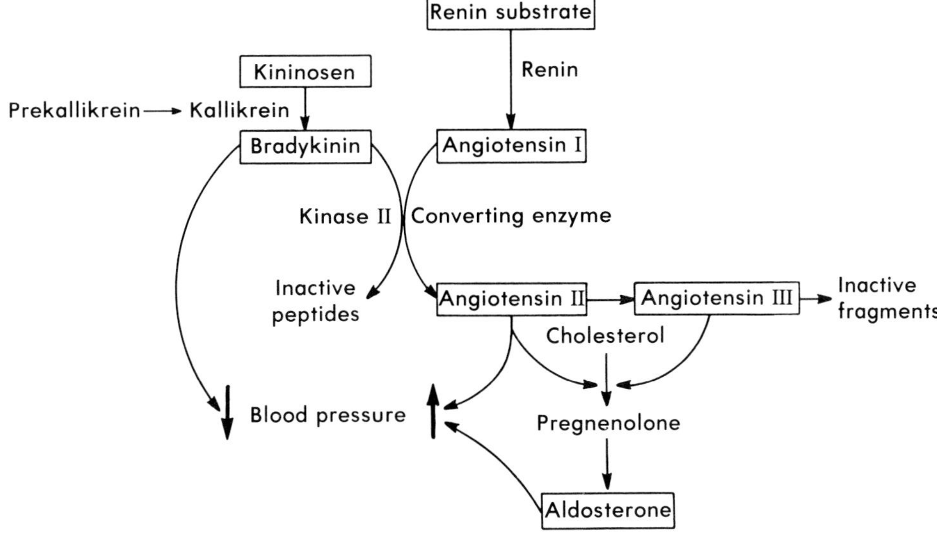

Fig. 45-1 Renin-angiotensin system interrelation with aldosterone and bradykinin in regulation of blood pressure.

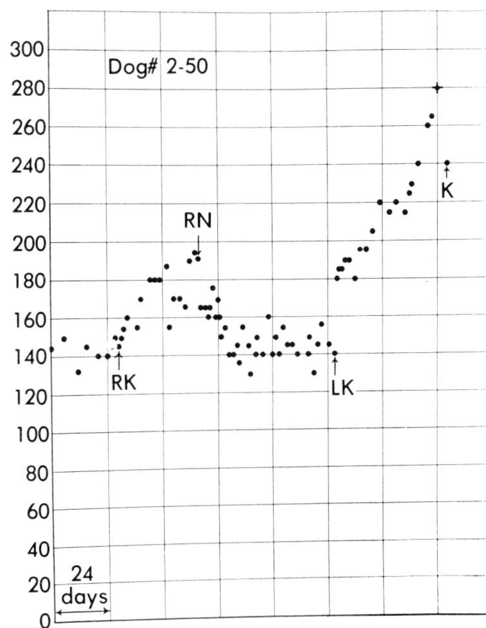

Fig. 45-2 Graph of mean blood pressure of the dog in Goldblatt's experiment. *RK,* Right main renal artery moderately constricted; *RN,* right nephrectomy; *LK,* severe constriction of left main renal artery; *K,* animal sacrificed. (Reproduced with permission from Goldblatt, H.: Ann. Intern. Med. **11**:69, 1937.)

veins is approximately 48% greater than that in the infrarenal vena cava or arterial circulation.[67] The major site for removal and clearance of renin is the liver.[37,66]

Extrarenal renin or reninlike enzymes *(isorenins)* have been found in the submaxillary salivary gland, uterus, placenta, and brain. No clear documentation has shown that these substances are functionally important in elevating blood pressure. *Prorenins* are another substance that has been extracted from the kidneys, with molecular weights higher than renin. Controversy exists as to whether these relatively inactive substances are precursors of renin or are altered postsynthetic forms of the enzyme.

Biochemical events related to the renin-angiotensin system have been relatively well defined (Fig. 45-4). The primary and perhaps only function of renin is the hydrolysis of the circulating peptide, *renin substrate* (also known as *hypertensinogen* or *angiotensinogen*) to form angiotensin I. Renin substrate is an alpha$_2$-globulin produced in the liver, has a molecular weight of approximately 110,000 daltons, and exists in several different forms. This substrate is itself not vasoactive.

Angiotensin I, the decapeptide produced by the renin substrate–renin reaction, is relatively inactive. It does exert some effect on the adrenal medulla, the sympathetic and central nervous systems, and the renal arterioles. Quantitation of this intermediary is the basis for many assays of renin activity.

Angiotensin II is produced when two C-terminal peptides are cleaved from angiotensin I by a carboxypeptidase known as converting enzyme. This octapeptide is the major contributor to the vasoactive element of renovascular hypertension. Angiotensin II stimulates liver production of renin substrate, but in normal individuals it provides a continuous negative feedback on the renal release of renin.[65] Angiotensin II has a half-life of approximately 4 minutes.[68]

Angiotensin III is derived by aminopeptidase cleavage of angiotensin II to I-desaspartyl-angiotensin II. Angiotensin III is a heptapeptide fragment that does have biologic activity, although its levels are so low that its physiologic importance is questioned. Angiotensin III inhibits angiotensin II. Perhaps its most relevant effect is stimulation of aldosterone synthesis.[30]

Aldosterone, a mineralocorticoid, is secreted from the zona glomerulosa of the adrenal cortex. The biosynthesis of this substance initially involves cleavage of the side chain of cholesterol to form pregnenolone. This step is facilitated by both angiotensin II and III. Aldosterone increases renal conservation of sodium and water, with a

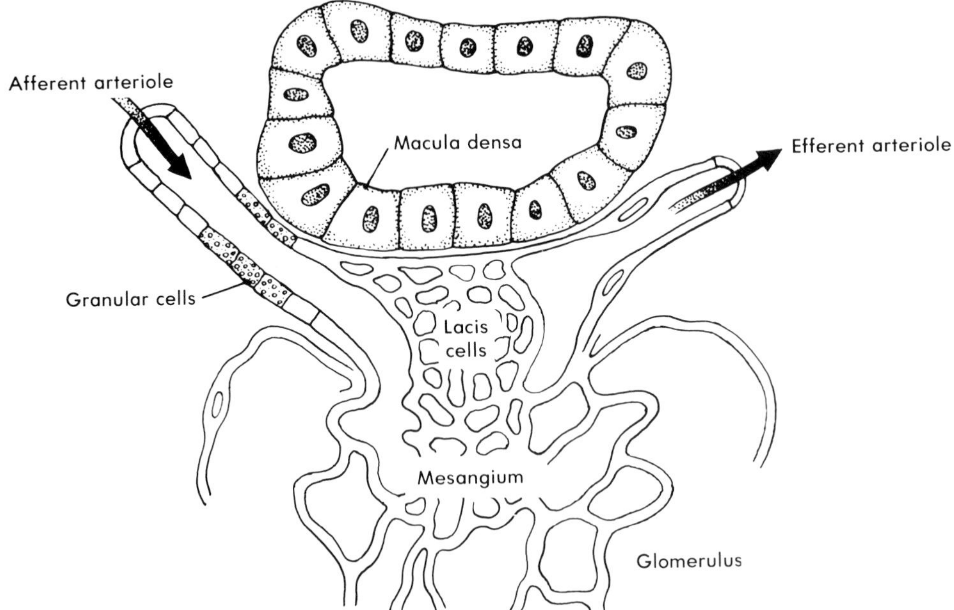

Fig. 45-3 Anatomic components of the juxtaglomerular apparatus.

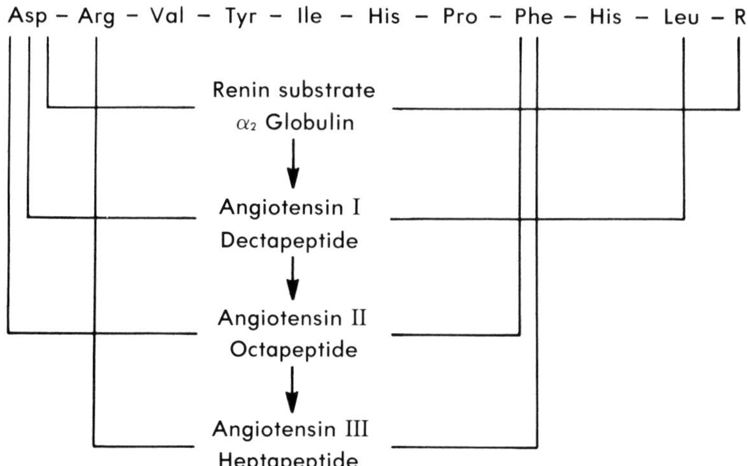

Fig. 45-4 Biochemical composition of renin substrate and the angiotensins.

resultant expansion of the extracellular fluid volume and an eventual increase in blood pressure.

Converting enzyme is a dipeptidylcarboxypeptidase responsible for the generation of angiotensin II from angiotensin I by removing C-terminal peptides. This enzyme has its highest concentration in the lung on the surface of endothelial cells. It also can be found at lower levels in the blood and kidney, as well as in other vascular beds.[1] Conversion of angiotensin I, at physiologic concentrations, has been shown to occur in a single passage thorugh the lungs.[59]

Converting enzyme also plays an important role in the metabolism of the vasodepressor *bradykinin*. At least two enzymes appear responsible for the inactivation of bradykinin.[106] The first is kinase I, which cleaves the carboxyl terminal arginine of bradykinin. The second enzyme, kinase II, cleaves the carboxyl terminal dipeptide group, Phe-Arg. Kinase II and angiotensin converting enzyme are considered the same in that they have nearly identical substrate specificities, cofactor requirements, and antigenic specificities.[60]

The most common technique for determination of plasma renin activity involves measurement of angiotensin I generation using a modified radioimmunoassay.[36] Plasma renin activity is expressed as the hourly rate of angiotensin I generation per unit of volume assayed. The assay involves two phases: (1) incubation of plasma to generate angiotensin I and (2) measurement of generated angioten-

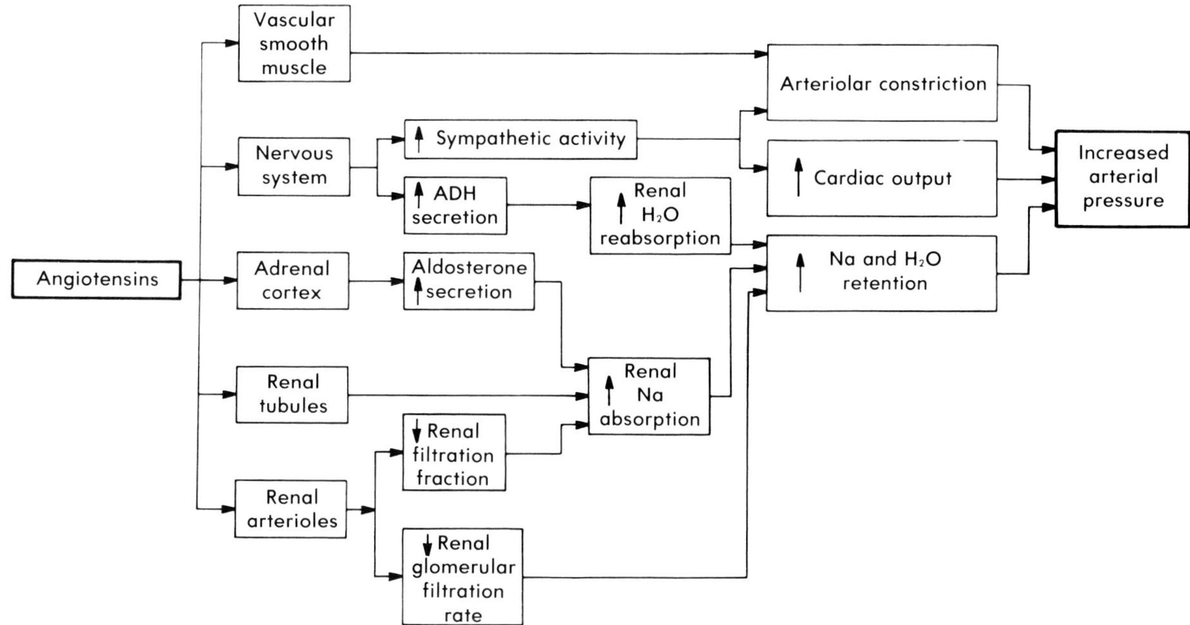

Fig. 45-5 Effects of angiotensins contributing to increased arterial pressure.

sin I by the radioimmunoassay. Assay methods vary among laboratories, often making interlaboratory comparisons difficult. Actual renin secretion is calculated as the renal arteriovenous difference in renin activity multiplied by renal plasma flow, and it is usually expressed as nanograms per milliliter per hour.

The physiologic role of the renin-angiotensin system in cardiovascular homeostasis was first proposed by Tigerstedt and Bergman,[96] who in 1898 demonstrated that intravenous injection of saline extracts of rabbit kidney caused immediate elevations in blood pressure of up to 20 minutes. They introduced the term *renin* as the substance responsible for this phenomena.

The humoral basis of renovascular hypertension was advanced further nearly a half century ago when investigators noted that renal venous blood in hypertensive animals exhibited greater vasoconstrictor activity than that from normal dogs.[18] Braun-Menendez and colleagues[7] called the vasopressor substance responsible for this activity "hypertensin," whereas Page, and Helmer[61,62] named this nonrenin vasoactive substance "angiotonin." These two groups subsequently agreed to call this substance "angiotensin." Skeggs and associates[70] later documented that angiotensin existed in two forms, known as angiotensins I and II.

Angiotensins have actions on the cardiovascular system, central nervous system, adrenal gland, and kidneys (Fig. 45-5). The effects on cardiac activity, vascular smooth muscle reactivity, and salt and water metabolism are profound, and all contribute to increased arterial pressure. The most important consequence of renal artery occlusive disease is the production of angiotensin II, which by weight is the most powerful pressor substance known. Angiotensin II acts directly on the arteriolar smooth muscle of nearly all vascular beds, with perhaps the exception of pulmonary vessels. The splanchnic, renal, and cutaneous circulations are most sensitive to its effects. Despite an acceptance of the central importance of angiotensin in the generation of renovascular hypertension, the relevance of absolute plasma levels remains unknown. The end-organ sensitivity to these vasoactive substances is often impossible to predict because it is different in various physiologic and pathologic settings. In addition, the exact role of cellular or locally secreted renin and generated angiotensin is undetermined in renovascular hypertension.

Hemodynamic responses to activation of the renin-angiotensin system depend on the rate at which renal blood flow is decreased, as well as whether one or both kidneys are at risk. Acute reductions in renal blood flow result in prompt blood pressure increases and increased plasma renin levels.[27,35,103] Experimental models are defined as one kidney–one clip (1K-1C), two kidney–one clip (2K-1C), or two kidney-two clip (2K-2C) Goldblatt's hypertension, depending on whether one or both kidneys are present and whether one or both renal arteries are constricted. Pioneering studies nearly half a century ago documented the importance of renin in both initiating and maintaining the hypertensive state in the 2K-1C form of renovascular hypertension. Recent confirmation of these findings has been possible with 2K-1C experiments employing renin antiserum, angiotensin II antibodies, angiotensin antagonists, and converting enzyme inhibitors.*

In instances of 2K-1C renovascular hypertension, where the total renal mass is not at risk, the hypertension is characterized by renin hypersecretion from the affected kidney and contralateral suppression of kidney renin production.[80,100] Sodium avidity within the affected kidney is counterbalanced by continuous sodium excretion from the

*References 3, 11, 17, 54, 55, and 64.

contralateral kidney, resulting in relative intravascular volume depletion.[93,94] This form of hypertension is angiotensin II dependent and responds to angiotensin antagonists and converting-enzyme inhibitors.[2,90]

Pathophysiologic alterations when the entire renal mass is at risk with 2K-2C or 1K-1C models are quite different and undoubtedly relate to changes other than vasoconstriction. Angiotensin II is known to be involved with sodium retention, decreases in glomerular filtration, stimulation of aldosterone production, and stimulation of norepinephrine release from the adrenergic nervous system. These effects may occur acutely, but in chronic 2K-2C or 1K-1C renovascular hypertension it appears that sodium retention accounts for late reductions in renin secretion, although the absolute renin activity may be abnormal with regard to the existing state of sodium balance. Studies have been unable to demonstrate that blood pressure elevations depend on the renin-angiotensin system in the sodium-replete condition of chronic renovascular hypertension. In fact, angiotensin antagonists or converting-enzyme inhibitors are effective in reducing elevated blood pressures only when the subjects are depeleted of sodium.[26]

PATHOLOGY OF RENAL ARTERY STENOTIC AND OCCLUSIVE DISEASE

Various types of occlusive disease affect the renal arterial circulation, ranging from unusual microvascular disease associated with connective tissue arteriopathies to common macrovascular diseases. Although relatively uncommon, renal artery emboli, spontaneous dissections, and traumatic occlusions are occasionally associated with acute forms of renin-mediated hypertension. The most often encountered causes of hypertension secondary to renal artery occlusive disease are those associated with atherosclerosis and arterial fibrodysplasia.[73,74]

Atherosclerosis

Atherosclerosis is the most common renal artery occlusive disease, accounting for approximately 70% of reported cases of renovascular hypertension. The frequency of this type of renovascular hypertension may be even higher because most reported series are surgical cases, which excludes many elderly patients who are not operative candidates. Atherosclerotic renovascular disease is usually recognized in the sixth decade of life. It is important to note that some degree of atherosclerotic renal artery stenotic disease affects nearly half the elderly population and that this is not always associated with elevated blood pressures.

Atherosclerotic renal artery occlusive disease typically involves the proximal third of the vessel with eccentric or concentric stenoses (Fig. 45-6). In nearly 75% of patients these lesions represent a "spill-over" stenosis associated with aortic atherosclerosis. Such lesions are bilateral in more than half the patients. When unilateral, they seemingly affect the right and left sides with equal frequency, although the left renal artery often appears more severely diseased. Subendothelial and medial accumulation of cholesterol-laden foam cells and fibrosis invariably are identified in these lesions. Necrosis, hemorrhage, and calcification are characteristic of more complicated atherosclerotic plaques associated with advanced stenoses.

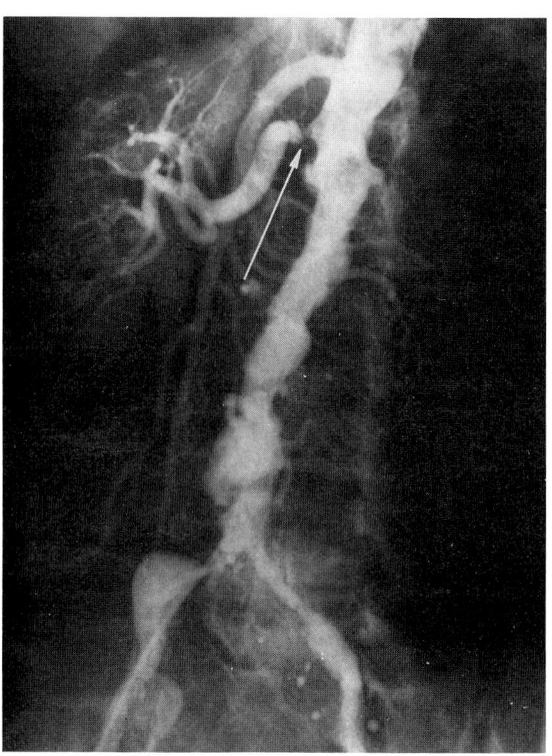

Fig. 45-6 Characteristic proximal disease in atherosclerotic renal artery stenosis.

Arterial Fibrodysplasia

Arterial fibrodysplasia is the second most common type of renal artery disease, affecting approximately 20% to 25% of renovascular hypertensive patients. Renal artery stenoses caused by dysplastic disease are a heterogenous group of lesions classified by the specific pathologic process and region of the vessel wall most affected. These lesions include intimal fibroplasia, medial hyperplasia, medial fibroplasia, and perimedial dysplasia.[81] The latter two entities appear to be a continuum of the same disease process. Each category has certain characteristic features that deserve mention.

Intimal Fibroplasia

Intimal fibroplasia accounts for approximately 5% of all dysplastic renal artery lesions. It affects infants and young adults more often than the elderly and occurs with equal frequency in female and male patients. The cause of primary intimal fibroplasia is unknown. Secondary intimal fibroplasia has been attributed to trauma, as well as to the sequela of earlier arteritis. Progression of intimal fibroplasia may cause an accelerated deposition of fibrous tissue and rapid compromise of the arterial lumen.

Intimal fibroplasia usually appears as long, tubular stenoses of the main renal artery in young patients or as smooth, focal stenoses in adults. Proximal ostial lesions are most often associated with aortic hypoplasia and coarctations or with neurofibromatosis.[83] Subendothelial accu-

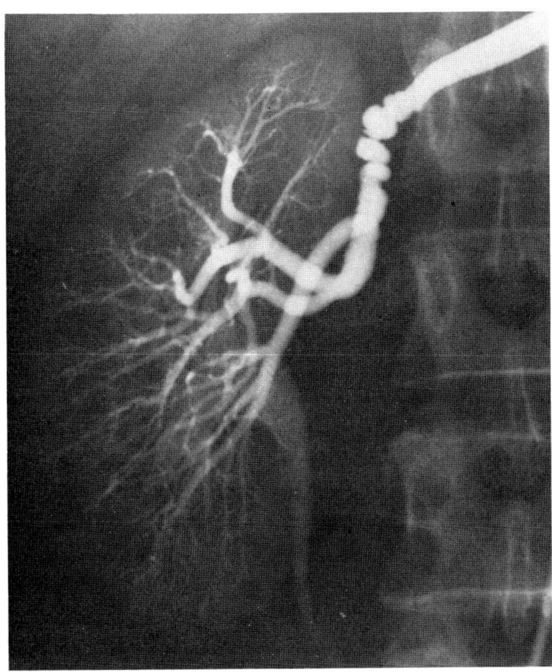

Fig. 45-7 Arterial fibrodysplasia. Serial stenoses and intervening macroaneurysmal outpouchings are characteristic of medial fibroplasia.

mulations of irregularly arranged mesenchymal cells surrounded by loose fibrous connective tissue are typical of these intimal lesions. The internal elastic lamina is usually intact, but partial fragmentation may occur.

Medial Hyperplasia

Medial hyperplasia is rare, accounting for less than 1% of dysplastic renal artery stenoses. Most patients affected with this entity are women in the 30- to 50-year-old age-group. Medial hyperplasia occurs most often as a focal stenosis in the midportion of the main renal artery and is characterized by excess numbers of minimally disorganized medial smooth muscle cells. Fibroproliferative changes are not present in these lesions.

Medial Fibroplasia

Medial fibroplasia is the most common dysplastic renal artery disease, accounting for 85% of such stenoses. Females are affected nine times more often than males, with clinical presentation occurring most often between 25 and 45 years of age. Medial fibroplasia appears to be a systemic arteriopathy, with the internal carotid, superior mesenteric, and external iliac arteries the extrarenal vessels most often affected. The etiology of medial fibroplasia remains poorly defined but appears associated with estrogenic stimuli on smooth muscle in females during their reproductive years, unusual stretch forces on affected vessels, and mural ischemia from impairment of vasa vasorum blood flow.[81]

Morphologic changes of medial dysplasia range from solitary stenoses in the middle and distal main renal artery to multiple constrictions with intervening mural dilations. The latter produce this lesion's classic string-of-beads appearance (Fig. 45-7). Actual macrovascular aneurysms, usually occurring at branchings, affect nearly 13% of patients with arterial fibrodysplasia[75] but are a very unusual cause of the hypertensive state.[82] Extension of stenotic disease into segmental branches occurs in approximately 20% of cases. Bilateral disease affects nearly 70% of patients and is usually most severe on the right. Unilateral lesions affecting the left renal artery occur in less than 10% of patients. Progression has been recognized in approximately 20% of patients, occurring more frequently in premenopausal women.

A spectrum of changes in medial fibroplasia occurs, including a diffuse and peripheral form of the disease. Gradations of these two lesions may be encountered in the same vessel. Diffuse medial fibroplasia is typified by severe disorganization of smooth muscle and the predominance of myofibroblasts, which appear responsible for excessive accumulations of ground substance encroaching on the vessel lumen.[72,81] These stenoses occur adjacent to areas of smooth muscle necrosis and medial thinning, resulting in mural dilations. Peripheral medial fibroplasia is characterized by fibroproliferative changes and loss of normal smooth muscle in the outer portion of the media. The latter findings are usually associated with less severe stenoses than occur with diffuse disease.

Perimedial Dysplasia

Perimedial dysplasia accounts for nearly 10% of dysplastic renal artery disease. It invariably affects women between the ages of 30 and 50 years. This particular dysplastic lesion appears to be more progressive than medial fibrodysplasia. Certain histologic and ultrastructural features are common to both perimedial dysplasia and medial fibroplasia, and although perimedial dysplasia is classified as a separate pathologic entity, this may not be an appropriate distinction. Angiographically, perimedial disease appears as solitary or multiple constrictions without intervening dilations. These stenoses involve distal portions of the main renal artery without branch involvement. Excessive accumulation of elastic tissue in inner adventitial regions is characteristic of perimedial dysplasia. Abnormal increases in medial ground substances may also accompany this type of renal artery dysplasia.

CLINICAL MANIFESTATIONS

The exact prevalence of renovascular hypertension among all patients with elevated diastolic blood pressures is unknown but is probably close to 1%. It clearly occurs much more often in individuals with moderate or severe diastolic blood pressure elevations; as many as 5% of such patients will have an underlying renovascular cause for their hypertension.

The Cooperative Study on Renovascular Hypertension documented the clinical manifestations of essential hypertension as well as of atherosclerotic and fibrodysplastic forms of renovascular hypertension.[69] Patients with atherosclerotic disease were older than patients with fibrodysplastic disease. Those with atherosclerotic disease were more likely to be males, and those with the fibrodysplastic form were more often women. In general, essential hypertensive patients had longer-standing disease and were more apt to have a family history of elevated blood pressure. Cooperative Study patients with atherosclerotic renovascular hypertension were more likely to exhibit accelerated hypertension and Grade III or IV retinopathy. Renovascular hypertensive patients had abdominal or flank bruits more often than patients with essential hypertension. Regardless of these findings, renovascular hypertension can affect either sex at any age, and its severity may range from mild to severe when first discovered.

Evidence suggestive of renovascular hypertension includes (1) systolic-diastolic upper abdominal bruits, (2) initial diastolic blood pressures greater than 115 mm Hg or sudden worsening of mild preexisting essential hypertension, (3) development of hypertension during childhood, or (4) development of high blood pressure after age 50. Drug-resistant hypertension and malignant hypertension are also more likely to be associated with this secondary form of hypertension. Patients who demonstrate deterioration of renal function while receiving multiple antihypertensive drugs, especially angiotensin-converting-enzyme inhibitors, must be suspect for underlying renal artery stenotic disease and renovascular hypertension. Clinical screening of patients is necessary before undertaking diagnostic studies for suspected renovascular hypertension. The costs of indiscriminate evaluations for this form of hypertension would otherwise be prohibitive.[53]

DIAGNOSIS OF RENAL ARTERY STENOSIS AND SECONDARY HYPERTENSION

Many diagnostic and prognostic tests for renovascular hypertension represent methods of assessing pathophysiologic derangements of renal function. The more important tests are discussed in this section.

Conventional Arteriography

Conventional arteriography is essential in the evaluation of all patients with suspected renovascular hypertension. Oblique aortography and multiple-plane selective renal arteriography have improved the accuracy of radiographic diagnosis of this disease entity. Arteriographic studies precisely define the morphologic character and extent of renal artery stenoses.

Collateral vessels circumventing a stenosis are evidence of the lesion's hemodynamic importance. Pressure gradients of approximately 10 mm Hg are necessary for development of collateral circulation, and the same degree of pressure change is associated with activation of the renin system. Accordingly, collateral vessels circumventing a renal artery stenosis are invariably associated with increased renin release. Thus the importance of an otherwise benign-appearing stenosis may be established when collateral vessels are present (Fig. 45-8) or when dilution defects representing noncontrast-containing blood from collaterals entering the poststenotic portion of the vessel are identified with selective renal arteriography.

Pharmacoangiographic vasodilatory and vasoconstrictive manipulations have been advocated as a means to demonstrate collateral vessels.[6] Selective renal artery infusions of acetylcholine or epinephrine may be used to reverse flow in nonparenchymal renal artery vessels originating beyond a critical stenosis. If reversed flow is identified, these vessels are assumed to be functioning as collateral channels.

Arteriographic evidence of arterial nephrosclerosis should not be considered an indication that renal revascularization or angioplasty will not have a beneficial effect on blood pressure. This is in keeping with previous reports that biopsy evidence of nephrosclerosis is of limited prognostic value.[102]

Digital Subtraction Arteriography

Digital subtraction arteriography following intravenous administration of contrast agents and computed enhancement of arterial images has been proposed to be an excellent diagnostic study for renovascular hypertension.[38,39] Although some have advocated this as an approproate first-step screening procedure, certain limitations must be addressed. For example, segmental renal artery disease such as that occurring in medial fibroplasia is difficult to demonstrate by digital subtraction arteriography. The sensitivity of this type of arteriography in identifying renal artery disease approaches 85%, and its specificity is in the range of 90%. An important application of this technology is its use following intra-arterial contrast injection. This allows the use of smaller amounts of contrast agents as compared to conventional arteriography, lessening potential nephrotoxicity. This is especially relevant in patients with preexisting impairment of renal function.

Renin Activity of Peripheral and Renal Venous Blood

Renin activity of peripheral and renal venous blood is an important method for determining the functional importance of renal artery disease. The renin-angiotensin system should be stimulated before sampling to reduce interpretive

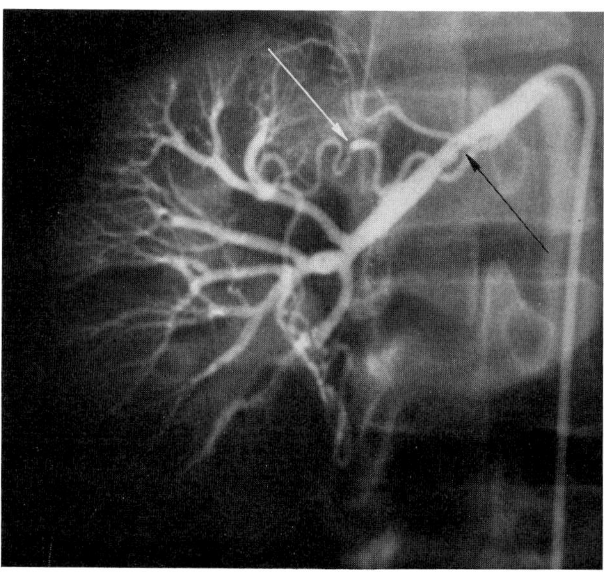

Fig. 45-8 Arteriogram of a benign-appearing stenosis *(black arrow)* associated with a large collateral vessel *(white arrow)* circumventing the lesion, defining hemodynamic significance of the stenosis and implicating its functional importance. (From Stanley, J.C., Graham, L.M., and Whitehouse, W.M., Jr.: Renovascular hypertension: limitations and errors of diagnostic and prognostic investigations. In Bernhard, V.M., and Towne, J.M., editors: Complications in vascular surgery, Orlando, 1985, (Grune & Stratton, Inc.)

errors of assay data evolving from minor fluctuations in basal renin activity. In general, sodium intake is limited to 20 mEq/day, and a diuretic is administered for 3 days before testing. Renin-suppressing drugs are discontinued whenever possible. Blood pressure in such circumstances may be controlled with renin-stimulating agents such as hydralazine. The effect of converting-enzyme inhibitors in stimulating renin release and altering test results remains to be defined in patients with renovascular hypertension. Blood samples for renin assay should be obtained simultaneously, or nearly simultaneously, with the patient tilted to an upright position.

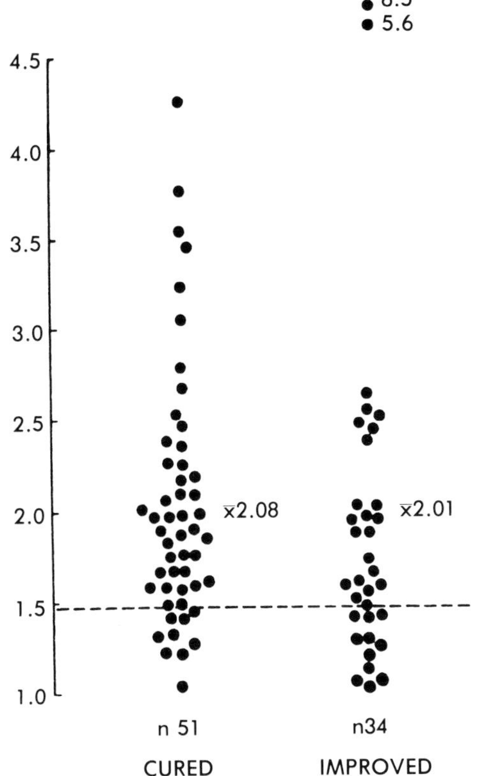

Fig. 45-9 Renal vein renin ratios, reflecting their limited diagnostic and prognostic value. (Modified from Stanley, J.C., Gewertz, B.L., and Fry, W.J.: J. Surg. Res. **20:**149, 1976.)

Renal Vein Renin Ratios

Renal vein renin ratios (RVRR) are calculated by dividing the renin activity in venous blood from the affected kidney by that from the contralateral kidney. A RVRR greater than 1.48 indicates functionally important renovascular disease.[80,100] Because this test compares one kidney to another, it may not be helpful in the presence of bilateral disease when both kidneys exhibit equal elevations of renin secretion. Approximately 15% of patients benefiting from surgery have a RVRR less than 1.48 (Fig. 45-9). Renovascular hypertension in such patients would not be identified if RVRR were the only criterion for diagnosis. An additional disadvantage of applying RVRR to clinical decision making is that this test cannot differentiate those patients most likely to be cured from those who will improve following technically successful surgical intervention.[76,80]

Renal/Systemic Renin Index

Renal/systemic renin index (RSRI) is an expression of an individual kidney's renin secretion. It is calculated by subtracting systemic renin activity from the individual renal venous renin activity and dividing the remainder by systemic renin activity.[80] In nonrenovascular hypertensive patients renal venous activity from each kidney is usually 24% higher than systemic activity.[67] Thus the total of both kidneys' activity is usually 48% higher than systemic levels, balancing hepatic degradation and establishing a steady state.

In renovascular hypertension the RSRI of the affected kidney becomes greater than 0.24 as renal blood flow de-

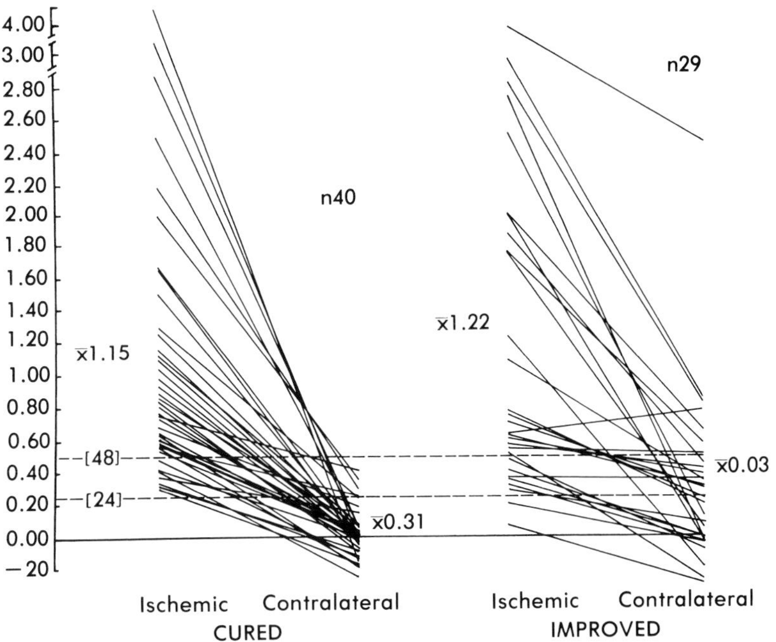

Fig. 45-10 Renal/systemic renin indices, depicting their prognostic usefulness. (From Stanley, J.C., and Fry, W.J.: Arch. Surg. **112:**1291, 1977. Copyright 1977, American Medical Association.)

creases. This is normally balanced by suppression of the contralateral kidney renin production with a drop in its RSRI below 0.24. With bilateral renal artery disease this servomechanism may be lost, and autonomous release of renin from both kidneys may cause the sum of the individual RSRI's to be greater than 0.48. Renin production then exceeds the capacity of normal hepatic degradation, and a hyperreninemic state evolves.

RSRI documentation of renin hypersecretion and suppression allows identification of patients most likely to be cured or improved following unilateral treatment (Fig. 45-10). Renin secretion from the kidney opposite the one being treated surgically must be suppressed if a cure is to be expected. The validity of ischemic renin hypersecretion (RSRI $>$ 0.48) and contralateral renin suppression (RSRI $<$ 0.24, approaching 0.0) in discriminating between cured and improved surgical outcomes has been well documented.[76,80,100] However, the prognostic usefulness of RSRI may be limited in that approximately 8% of patients who are cured do not exhibit contralateral renin suppression.[76] Although the RSRI represents an important refinement in interpretation of renin activity in renovascular hypertensive patients, one must be cautious in rigidly applying these data to clinical decision making.

Angiotensin II Antagonists

Angiotensin II antagonists, such as saralasin acetate (P113, 1-Sar, 8-Ala angiotensin II), may be used to document renin-dependent hypertension in patients with renal artery stenotic disease.[4,23,51,91] This antagonist competitively blocks angiotensin II receptor sites, causing decreased vascular smooth muscle contractility and subsequent diminutions in blood pressure.[91] A positive saralasin test, revealing angiotensinogenic hypertension, is usually associated with a decrease in blood pressure ranging from 5 to 15 mm Hg. Saralasin invariably causes a depressor effect in patients with high renin activity. In this regard blood pressure reductions are more obvious when patients are prepared with agents such as furosemide before testing. A potential problem in using saralasin without stimulation is a pressor effect that may occur in patients with low or normal renin activity. Earlier reports noted a depressor response in most patients with surgically correctable renovascular hypertension. Recent studies have shown that the sensitivity of saralasin testing is much less.[32,46] Some investigators have correlated blood pressure changes to renin activity as a means of improving the test's accuracy.[50] In general, the sensitivity of saralasin studies appears to be approximately 75%, and the specificity approaches 85%.

Angiotensin-Converting Enzyme Inhibitors

Angiotensin-converting enzyme inhibitors may reveal the angiotensinogenic character of renovascular hypertension by inhibiting angiotensin II generation.[10,11,90] Use of converting-enzyme inhibitors offers a more sensitive means than saralasin for detecting angiotensin II–dependent blood pressure elevations. However, the specificity of such studies is very low, perhaps because converting enzyme is the same as kinase II, and its inhibition causes accumulations of bradykinin with its subsequent depressor effect in nonrenin-mediated forms of hypertension.

Hypertensive Urography

Hypertensive urography is a poor diagnostic test for renovascular hypertension because of its limited sensitivity.[95] Bilateral or segmental disease often precludes recognition of gross differences in contrast excretion between the two kidneys. However, rapid-sequence urography may contribute to the diagnosis of renovascular hypertension when: (1) at least a 1-minute delay in contrast appearance occurs within the collecting system of the affected kidney compared to that of the contralateral kidney; (2) a length discrepancy is found, with the right kidney 2 cm shorter than the left or the left 1.5 cm shorter than the right; and (3) hyperconcentration of contrast in the collecting system of the affected kidney is observed on late x-ray films. Ureteral or pelvic irregularities caused by large collateral vessels may also accompany these urographic features. In a large series of patients with proven renovascular hypertension, urograms were abnormal in 27% of pediatric patients, 48% of patients with arterial fibrodysplastic disease, and approximately 72% of patients with atherosclerotic lesions.[84] These generally accepted findings do not support continued use of hypertensive urography as a diagnostic or prognostic test for renovascular hypertension.

Isotopic Renography

Isotopic renography has been used with both imaging and analysis of the washout curve of several tracers, the most common being radioactive iodine-131 (^{131}I) orthoiodohippurate. This compound provides an assessment of both renal blood flow and excretory function. Unfortunately, different states of hydration and intrarenal vascular resistance often result in flow abnormalities and false-positive studies in nonrenovascular hypertensive patients. The specificity and sensitivity of current studies are both approximately 75%.

Renal perfusion-excretion ratios and more sophisticated computer programs offer a potential means of increasing the predictive value of radionuclide screening for renovascular hypertension.[45,49] Use of technetium-99m (^{99m}Tc) DMSA and ^{99m}Tc DPTA in these instances may improve the ability to measure differential excretory function. Measurement of transit times by this methodology is another important advance in the diagnostic use of renography for the study of renovascular hypertension.

Split Renal Function Studies

Split renal function studies that assess altered individual renal function were among the first tests used in evaluating patients with suspected renovascular hypertension.[14] These studies require ureteral catheters for sampling of urine from each kidney. Two specific tests have been used most widely: (1) the Howard test, designed to document reduced urine volume, as well as increased sodium and creatinine concentration from the affected kidney; and (2) the Stamey test, performed after a urea-induced osmotic diuresis and an infusion of *p*-aminohippurate (PAH), with the affected kidney usually producing a smaller volume of urine and greater concentration of PAH than the normal kidney.

Vanderbilt University investigators have proposed a liberalization of diagnostic criteria for split renal function studies.[14] In their experience using classic criteria, few patients with essential hypertension had abnormal split renal function studies, but only half those with proven renovascular hypertension had diagnostic studies performed. A positive test, according to these researchers' modified criteria, was defined as constant lateralization on the affected kidney with 25% less urine volume and a 15% increase in creatinine concentration from this kidney. A greater sensitivity was obtained using such a definition, but appreciable numbers of studies in patients without renovascular hypertension became positive.

TREATMENT

Therapeutic results in renovascular hypertension relate to an accurate diagnosis and proper execution of an appropriate intervention, whether this is a vascular reconstructive procedure, ablative surgery or transcatheter renal infarction, percutaneous transluminal angioplasty, or institution of drug therapy. The specific type of renovascular hypertension being treated also plays a major role in determining the outcome of therapy.

Data from a prospective Mayo Clinic series suggest increased patient survival among individuals with both fibrodysplastic and atherosclerotic renovascular disease treated surgically compared to those treated medically.[41] Unfortunately, a prospective *randomized* study comparing medical and surgical therapy has yet to be published. Nevertheless, long-term drug therapy has not been favored by most practicing physicians responsible for the care of these patients, although recent pharmacologic advances may change this pattern.

Drug Therapy

New antihypertensive drugs have resulted in major improvements in the medical management of patients with renovascular hypertension.[101,107] The principles involved in drug therapy of renovascular hypertension are unlikely to change since they are based on an understanding of the underlying pathophysiologic sequelae of renal artery stenotic disease. Vasoconstriction assumes greatest importance with unilateral disease in patients having a normal contralateral kidney. Excessive sodium retention and hypervolemia become the dominant factors in patients with bilateral renal artery stenoses, as well as in those with unilateral stenoses associated with contralateral parenchymal disease or renal absence.

Blood pressure elevations in most if not all patients with renovascular hypertension may be controlled by appropriate drug interventions. However, issues that must be considered regarding drug treatment include (1) the side effects of treatment, (2) the degree of patient compliance in carefully structured programs, and (3) whether blood pressure control will result in decreased renal function, either as a direct effect of the drug or by insidious progression of renal artery occlusive disease. These issues are often controversial.

In instances of known renovascular hypertension, beta-blocking agents should probably be the first drug administered. Reduction in renin release with these agents is probably the primary factor in causing a lowering of blood pressure.[9] Propranolol and atenolol are the drugs most frequently used, although metoprolol, nadolol, timolol, and pindolol are similar agents producing antihypertensive effects in renovascular patients. High doses of these drugs may be required to control the blood pressure, although in most cases the primary effect of suppressing renin release may be accomplished with very small doses. In instances of more refractory hypertension, especially that caused by bilateral renal artery stenoses or unilateral lesions with contralateral parenchymal disease, addition of a standard diuretic is advised. The thiazide drugs, a hydrogenated thiazide, or substituted compound is recommended for such patients. In those with impaired renal function secondary to decreased blood flow, a loop diuretic such as furosemide will provide a more effective diuretic action.

Converting-enzyme inhibitors are among the newer agents for treating hypertension in general and renovascular hypertension in particular. Clinically useful inhibitors are related to various snake venom substances and their synthetic congeners. Antihypertensive effects other than decreased angiotensin II generation, such as those involving bradykinin and prostaglandins, probably occur with the use of these agents. Captopril, currently the most frequently used converting enzyme inhibitor, may be supplemented with beta-blockers or diuretics in resistant hypertension. In more severe hypertension, vasodilators such as minoxidil may be required.

It is important to recognize the effects of captopril on renal function, which result from either decreasing systemic blood pressure or altering intrarenal autoregulation. This becomes especially relevant in patients with bilateral renal artery stenoses, in cases of unilateral stenosis together with contralateral parenchymal disease, or when stenosis occurs in a solitary kidney.[40] In these instances severe deterioration of glomerular filtration may occur, and use of captopril is contraindicated. Other angiotensin-converting inhibitors, such as enalapril maleate and teprotide, may have less profound effects when the entire renal mass appears affected by renovascular disease, but this remains to be documented.

Percutaneous Transluminal Renal Angioplasty

In 1978 Gruntzig and associates[34] were the first to report the use of percutaneous transluminal angioplasty in the management of renovascular hypertension. This method of treatment has important patient safety and cost benefits. However, certain issues remain poorly defined, including (1) differences in treating various types of renal artery disease, (2) the frequency of being unable to catheterize or dilate a given type of stenosis, (3) the long-term effects of angioplasty on the vessel wall, (4) the incidence of renal and extrarenal complications, and (5) the durability of a successfully performed dilation.

Percutaneous transluminal angioplasty is usually undertaken after selective renal arteriography has defined the extent of the stenotic disease. A heavy guide wire is passed beyond the catheter used for the arteriography; a balloon

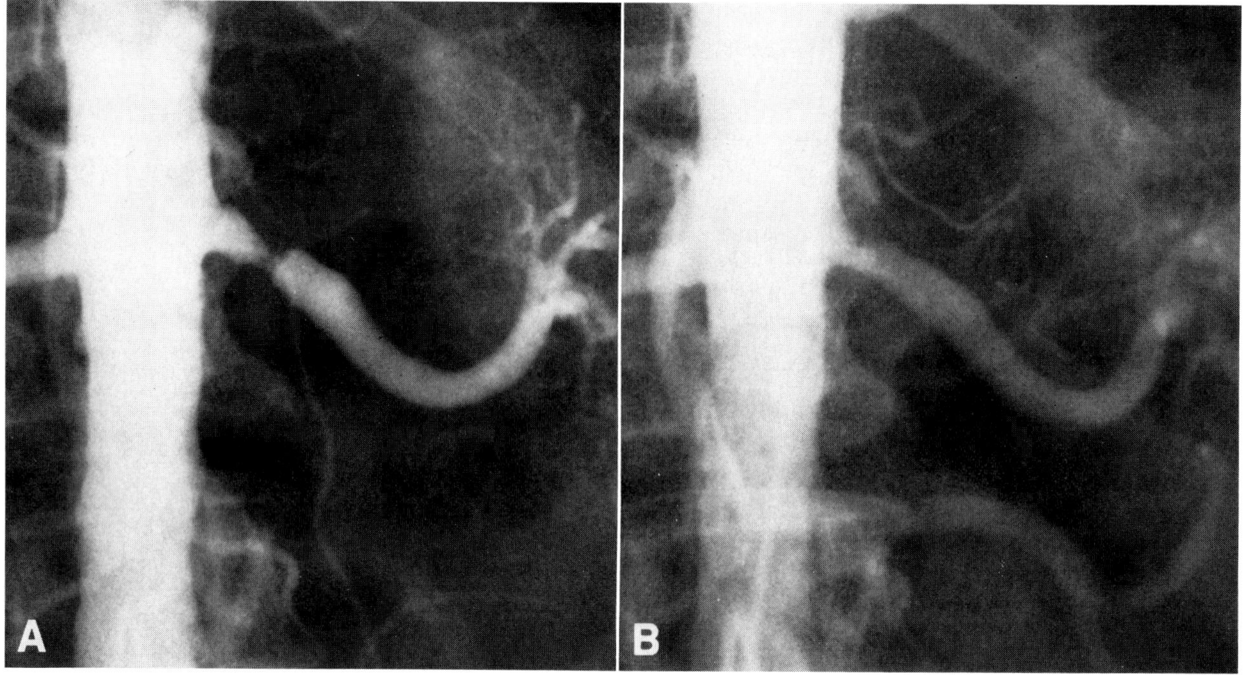

Fig. 45-11 Percutaneous transluminal angioplasty. Renal artery stenosis. **A**, Before dilation; **B**, after dilation.

catheter made of polyvinyl chloride or polyethylene is then exchanged for the angiographic catheter; and the balloon catheter is positioned within the stenosis. It is usually inflated two or three times at pressures ranging from 4 to 8 atmospheres, although newer balloons may be inflated at much greater pressures. Arteriographic confirmation of the adequacy of the procedure is obtained immediately after dilation (Fig. 45-11).

Intimal and medial dysplastic stenoses appear most amenable to percutaneous angioplasty. Ostial lesions associated with developmental aortic anomalies or neurofibromatosis represent hypoplastic vessels with considerable elasticity that are less likely to be successfully dilated.[52] Medial fibroplasia with multiple stenoses in series can often be easily dilated, but difficulties may occur in traversing extensive disease with the guide wire. Percutaneous transluminal angioplasty of atherosclerotic stenoses may be limited by an inability to dilate "spill-over plaque" from extensive aortic disease. These aortic-associated lesions appear most responsible for the high recurrence rate of atherosclerotic occlusive stenoses.[33]

Percutaneous transluminal angioplasty causes predictable disruption of the vessel wall. Intimal disruption probably results more often with dilation of the proximal renal artery, where elasticity of the vessel is greater and medial disruption is less likely. Medial tears are more likely with distal renal artery dilation, where vascular elasticity is less. Complications following dilation of both atherosclerotic and dysplastic lesions are uncommon, with renal complications probably not occurring in more than a few percent of cases. Extrarenal complications most often relate to hemorrhage at the site of arterial catheterization, which rarely threatens the patient's limb or life. The potential benefit following successful percutaneous transluminal angioplasty in carefully selected patients with renovascular hypertension approaches 90%.[71,92] Percutaneous transluminal renal angioplasty must be considered as an alternative to other therapies for renovascular hypertension, but carefully documented long-term clinical studies are needed before it becomes a routine therapeutic intervention.

Surgical Options

A variety of operative interventions for the treatment of renovascular hypertension has evolved over the past few decades. The most common procedures are discussed in this section.

Bypass Procedures

Bypass procedures are the most frequently used means of renal revascularization for both atherosclerotic and fibrodysplastic stenoses (Fig. 45-12). Autogenous saphenous vein is the graft material employed most often. Autogenous internal iliac arteries are preferred when undertaking reconstructions of pediatric renal arteries[88] since vein grafts placed in younger patients are often associated with late aneurysmal changes.[77,78] Prosthetic grafts are used when autogenous conduits are not available. Knitted Dacron or expanded Teflon conduits are the most frequently used synthetic grafts. Limitations of prosthetic grafts relate to their potential for infection and technical difficulties in anastomosing them to small segmental arteries.

Ex Vivo Renal Artery Reconstruction

Ex vivo renal artery reconstruction is an alternative to in situ repair for treating select cases of renovascular hypertension.[5,87] This technique allows temporary removal of the kidney with precise microsurgical repair of the dis-

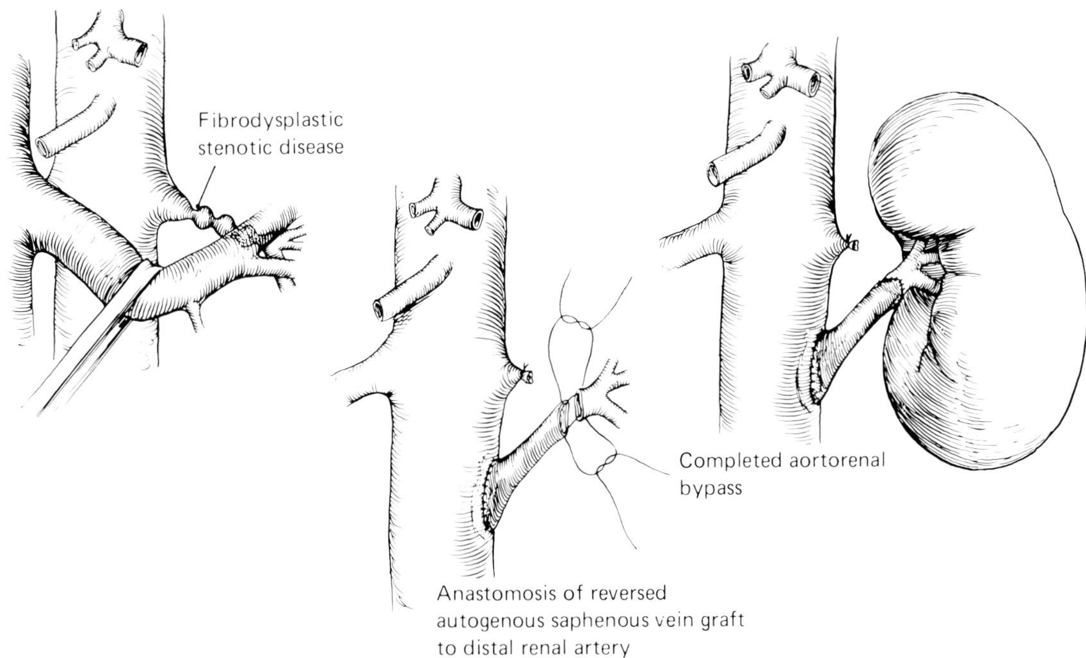

Fig. 45-12 Renal revascularization. Bypass procedure with autogenous saphenous vein.

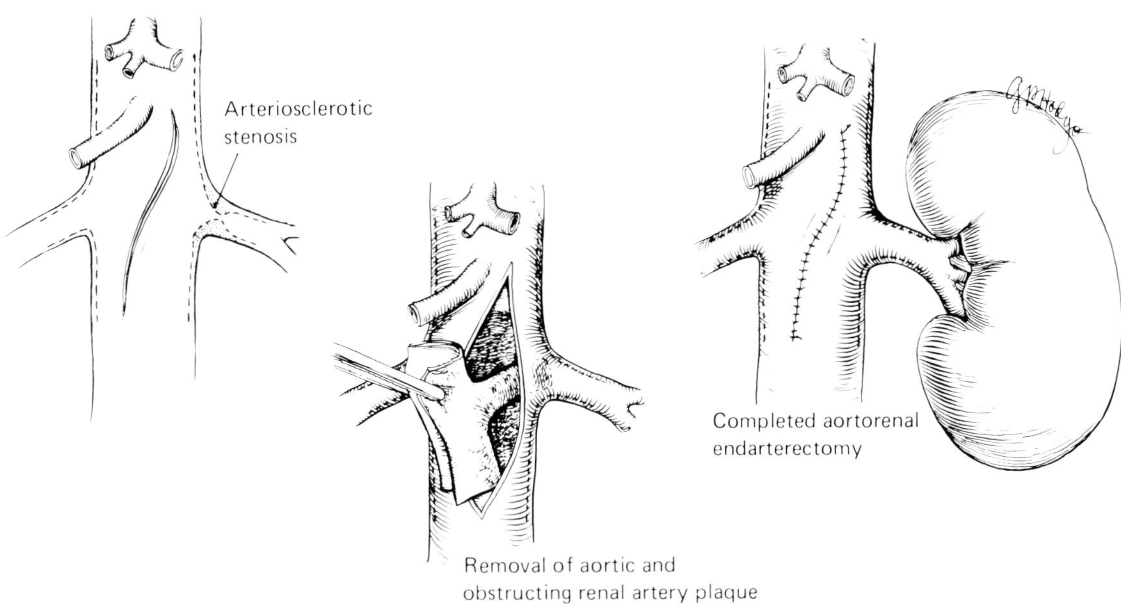

Fig. 45-13 Renal revascularization by performance of an endarterectomy.

eased vessel. Disruption of preexisting collateral channels and the longer duration of such procedures are disadvantages of ex vivo reconstructions. This form of reconstruction is most applicable when treating intraparenchymal stenoses and aneurysms or dissections of segmental vessels.

Endarterectomy

Endarterectomy has been advocated in the treatment of many atherosclerotic renal artery stenoses.[86] A transaortic approach with an aortotomy extending along the lateral aorta from the level of the superior mesenteric artery to below the renal orifices anteriorly may be preferable to a direct longitudinal renal arteriotomy and local endarterectomy (Fig. 45-13). The latter represents an acceptable alternative but usually requires patch graft closure of the artery.

Results of Surgical Therapy

The benefits of surgical therapy for renovascular hypertension were evaluated nearly 2 decades ago at 15 centers in the United States as the Cooperative Study of Renovascular Hypertension.[20,21] Included in this study were a total of 577 surgical procedures, of which only 315 were vas-

Table 45-1 **SURGICAL TREATMENT OF RENOVASCULAR HYPERTENSION—COMPARATIVE OVERALL RESULTS**

Institution	Time Period	Number of Patients	Ratio of Atherosclerotic/ Nonatherosclerotic Disease	Surgical Outcome*			Surgical Mortality (%)
				Cured (%)	Improved (%)	Failure (%)	
University of California, Los Angeles†[43]	1958-1977	503	1:2	64	23	13	2.1
Baylor College of Medicine[47]	1959-1979	489	3.2:1	36	29	35	1.8
University of Michigan[84]	1961-1980	313	1:1.5	47	42	11	1.9
Cleveland Clinic‡,[56-58,89]	1962-1978	225	1.5:1	50	34	16	3.1
University of California, San Francisco‡,[48,86]	1958-1977	128	2:1	39	34	27	1.6
Vanderbilt University[19]	1961-1972	122	1.8:1	59	31	10	5.4§
Columbia University‖,[8]	1962-1976	116	1.3:1	66	19	15	1

*Criteria for blood pressure response defined in cited publications.
†Series includes 230 primary, secondary, or partial nephrectomies; stated mortality is that from 1972-1977 experience with 142 patients.
‡Data from overlapping publications, not inclusive of entire experience.
§Mortality from more recent experience was 0.5% among 200 reconstructions, excluding those associated with aortic surgery.[13]
‖Series includes 42 nephrectomies.

cular reconstructions. Primary nephrectomy was undertaken in 168 patients, partial nephrectomy in 10, and contralateral nephrectomy with ipsilateral revascularization in nine. Thus 32% of the study's surgical interventions led to loss of renal mass. This would be unacceptable in contemporary practice.

Overall results of the Cooperative Study regarding hypertension were categorized as 51% patients cured, 15% improved, and 34% failures. Surgical mortality among all study patients was an unusually high 5.9%, with a 3.4% mortality in patients having fibrodysplastic lesions and a 9.3% mortality among those with atherosclerotic disease. Loss of life during renovascular surgery occurs infrequently today, with overall operative mortality in most large series usually less than 0.5% in patients undergoing renal artery reconstructive surgery alone.

Many current surgical experiences have great differences in nephrectomy rates. Renal preservation and maintenance of renal function is clearly very important in assessing clinical experiences. Cumulative primary and secondary nephrectomy rates should probably not exceed 10%. Nephrectomy may provide good early results but obviously leaves the patient at considerable risk if contralateral disease evolves later. The incidence of nephrectomy during second surgery for failed primary procedures approaches 43% and emphasizes the importance of an appropriately performed primary revascularization.[85]

Contemporary surgical treatment of renovascular hypertension has resulted in much better results than those reported by the Cooperative Study (Table 45-1). Differences among more recent series usually reflect the most prevalent disease entity causing the secondary hypertension at a given institution since results vary with different disease categories.[79] Pediatric patients with renovascular hypertension are the most likely to be cured after restoration of renal blood flow. A beneficial response following surgery may be expected in approximately 95% of such cases, and operative mortality is very unusual. Adults with arterial fibrodysplasia benefit from surgery more often than those with atherosclerotic disease, which reflects less coexisting essential hypertension or nephrosclerosis in these younger patients.

Atherosclerotic renovascular hypertension has often been considered a homogenous disease entity. Overall outcomes in contemporary surgical experiences are similar to those of the Cooperative Study, although higher nephrectomy and mortality rates were associated with the latter. Apparently at least two subgroups of patients with atherosclerotic lesions exist: (1) those having focal renal artery disease, with the only clinical manifestation of their atherosclerosis being secondary hypertension; and (2) those with clinically overt extrarenal atherosclerosis. Although the severity and duration of hypertension, age, and sex distribution in these two subgroups are similar, the surgical outcomes are very different. Although not addressed in most large series, improved renal function following revascularization is a well-recognized event, most likely occurring among patients with atherosclerotic disease and profound preoperative impairment in renal function.[15,16,42,104]

Surgical treatment of renovascular hypertension may be best assessed by reviewing results within four specific subgroups from the University of Michigan (Table 45-2). Patients were categorized as (1) pediatric patients up to 17 years in age, (2) adults with fibrodysplastic disease, or (3) adults having atherosclerotic renal artery lesions *without* or (4) *with* overt extrarenal atherosclerotic cardiovascular disease.[84] Patients in the fourth subgroup included those with extracranial cerebrovascular disease (cerebrovascular accident or transient ischemic attacks); coronary artery disease (angina pectoris or myocardial infarction), aneurysmal disease of the abdominal aorta or its branches, and symptomatic peripheral arterial occlusive disease. All patients subjected to surgical intervention in the Michigan experience were failures of previous medical management. However, none was receiving angiotensin-converting enzyme inhibitors, which clearly might have rendered some of them normotensive.

Surgical therapy was most beneficial in the pediatric and adult fibrodysplastic categories; 97% and 94% of patients,

Table 45-2 SURGICAL TREATMENT OF RENOVASCULAR HYPERTENSION—RESULTS IN SPECIFIC PATIENT SUBGROUPS, UNIVERSITY OF MICHIGAN EXPERIENCE, 1961-1980*

		Primary Surgical Procedures		Surgical Outcome‡			
Subgroup†	**Number of Patients**	**Arterial Reconstruction**	**Nephrectomy**	**Cured (%)**	**Improved (%)**	**Failure (%)**	**Surgical Mortality§ (%)**
Fibrodysplasia, pediatric	34	39	2	85	12	3	0
Fibrodysplasia, adult	144	160	6	55	39	6	0
Atherosclerosis, focal renal artery disease	64	63	3	33	58	9	0
Atherosclerosis overt generalized disease	71	70	6	25	47	28	8.5‖

*Represents results of 405 procedures (346 primary, 59 secondary).[84]

†See text for subgroup definition.

‡Effect of surgery on blood pressure. *Cured* indicates that blood pressures were 150/90 mm Hg or less for a minimum of 6 months, during which no antihypertensive medications were administered (lower pressure levels were used in evaluating pediatric patients). *Improved* indicates that patient was normotensive while receiving drug therapy, or that diastolic blood pressures ranged between 90 and 100 mm Hg but were at least 15% lower than preoperative levels. None of the improved patients was receiving converting-enzyme inhibitors. Failure indicates that diastolic blood pressures were greater than 90 mm Hg but less than 15% lower than preoperative levels, or that levels were greater than 110 mm Hg. Appropriate lower pressures, considering age and sex, were used in assessing outcome in pediatric cases.

§Surgical mortality includes all deaths within 30 days of surgery.

‖Four of the six deaths in this subgroup were associated with concomitant aortic reconstructive surgery.

respectively, were cured or improved. Outcomes were also satisfactory in adults with focal atherosclerotic disease; 91% were cured or improved. Adults exhibiting clinically overt generalized atherosclerosis had a 72% positive response to surgery, but only 25% were cured. It was among this subgroup of patients with widespread atherosclerosis that this series' only surgical mortality existed. Operative deaths did not occur in the other three renovascular hypertension subgroups.

SUMMARY

Renovascular hypertension, the most common cause of surgically correctable high blood pressure, results from altered renal circulatory hemodynamics causing the release of renin. Renin is produced in the juxtaglomerular apparatus of the kidney and released into the systemic circulation. Renin acts on renin substrate, an alpha$_2$-globulin produced in the liver, to form the decapeptide, angiotensin I. This latter substance is cleaved of two amino acids by angiotensin-converting enzyme to produce angiotensin II. Angiotensin II, an octapeptide, is a potent vasopressor responsible for contraction of vascular smooth muscle and the vasoconstrictive component of renovascular hypertension. Indirectly, angiotensin II acts to increase production of aldosterone with subsequent retention of sodium, the latter representing the volume component of renovascular hypertension. This renin-mediated form of hypertension can be altered by several drug interventions, including those (1) diminishing release of renin, (2) blocking the conversion of angiotensin I to angiotensin II, and (3) causing direct relaxation of vascular smooth muscle. Derangements of renovascular hypertension are best reversed by correction of the altered renal hemodynamics that usually result from renal artery stenosis. Surgical intervention with renal revascularization and percutaneous transluminal angioplasty are presently the most appropriate means available to this end.

REFERENCES

1. Aiken, J.W., and Vane, J.R.: The renin-angiotensin system: inhibition of converting enzyme in isolated tissues, Nature **228:**30, 1970.
2. Atkinson AB, et al.: Hyponatremic hypertensive syndrome with renal artery occlusion corrected by captopril, Lancet **2:**606, 1979.
3. Atkinson, A.B., et al.: Captopril in the management of hypertension with renal artery stenosis: its long-term effect as a predictor of surgical outcome, Am. J. Cardiol. **49:**1460, 1982.
4. Baer, L., et al.: Detection of renovascular hypertension with angiotensin II blockade, Ann. Intern. Med. **86:**257, 1977.
5. Belzer, F.O., and Raczkowski, A.: Ex vivo renal artery reconstruction with autotransplantation, Surgery **92:**642, 1982.
6. Bookstein, J.J., et al.: Pharmacoangiographic manipulation of renal collateral blood flow, Circulation **54:**328, 1976.
7. Braun-Menendez, E., et al.: La substancia hipertensora de la sangre del rinon isquemiado, Rev. Soc. Argent. Biol. **15:**420, 1939.
8. Buda, J.A., et al.: Predictability of surgical response in renovascular hypertension, Arch. Surg. **111:**1243, 1976.
9. Buhler, F.R., et al.: Propanolol inhibition of renin secretion, N. Engl. J. Med. **287:**1209, 1972.
10. Case, D.B., and Laragh, J.H.: Reactive hyperreninemia in renovascular hypertension after angiotensin blockade with saralasin or converting enzyme inhibitor, Ann. Intern. Med. **91:**153, 1979.
11. Case, D.B., et al.: Estimating renin participation in hypertension: superiority of converting enzyme inhibitor over saralasin, Am. J. Med. **61:**790, 1978.
12. Davis, J.O., and Freeman, R.H.: Mechanisms regulating renin release, Physiol. Rev. **56:**1, 1976.
13. Dean, R.H.: Indications for operative management of renovascular hypertension, J.S.C. Med. Assoc. **73:**523, 1977.
14. Dean, R.H., and Rhamy, R.K.: Split renal function studies in renovascular hypertension. In Stanley, J.C., Ernst, C.B., and Fry, W.J., editors: Renovascular hypertension, Philadelphia, 1984, W.B. Saunders Co.
15. Dean, R.H., Lawson, J.D., and Hollifield, J.W.: Revascularization of the poorly functioning kidney, Surgery **85:**44, 1979.
16. Dean, R.H., et al.: The effect of renal vascularization on kidney function, J. Surg. Res. **22:**443, 1977.
17. Dzau, V.J., et al.: Renin-specific antibody for study of cardiovascular homeostasis, Science **207:**1091, 1980.
18. Fasciolo, J.C., Houssay, B.A., and Taquini, A.C.: Blood-pressure raising secretion of the ischemic kidney, J. Physiol. (Lond.) **94:**281, 1938.
19. Foster, J.H., et al.: Ten years experience with surgical management of renovascular hypertension, Ann. Surg. **177:**755, 1973.

20. Foster, J.H., et al.: Renovascular occlusive disease: results of operative treatment, JAMA **231**:1043, 1975.
21. Franklin S.S., et al.: Operative morbidity and mortality in renovascular disease, JAMA **231**:1148, 1975.
22. Fray, J.C.S.: Stimulus-secretion coupling of renin: role of hemodynamic and other factors, Circ. Res. **47**:485, 1980.
23. Frohlich, E., and Maxwell, M.H.: Use of saralasin as a diagnostic test in hypertension: report of a consensus committee, Arch. Intern. Med. **142**:1437, 1982.
24. Ganong, W.F.: Biogenic amines, sympathetic nerves, and renin secretion, Fed. Proc. **32**:1782, 1973.
25. Ganong, W.F.: The renin-angiotensin system and the central nervous system, Fed. Proc. **36**:1771, 1977.
26. Gavras, H., et al.: Angiotensin-sodium interaction in blood pressure maintenance of renal hypertensive and normotensive rats, Science **180**:1369, 1973.
27. Gavras, H., et al.: Reciprocation of renin dependency with sodium volume dependency in renal hypertension, Science **188**:1316, 1317, 1975.
28. Goldblatt, H.: Studies on experimental hypertension. V. The pathogenesis of experimental hypertension due to renal ischemia, Ann. Intern. Med. **11**:69, 1937.
29. Goldblatt, H., et al.: Studies on experimental hypertension. I. The production of persistent elevation of systolic blood pressure by means of renal ischemia, J. Exp. Med. **59**:347, 1934.
30. Goodfriend, T.L., and Peach, M.J.: Angiotensin III: (des-aspartic acid)-angiotensin II—evidence and speculation of its role as an important agonist in the renin-angiotensin system, Circ. Res. **36-37**(suppl. I):38, 1975.
31. Goormaghtigh, N.: Facts in favour of an endocrine function of the renal arterioles (abstract), J. Pathol. Bacteriol. **57**:392, 1945.
32. Grim, C.E., et al.: Sensitivity and specificity of screening tests for renal vascular hypertension, Ann. Intern. Med. **91**:617, 1979.
33. Grim, C.E., et al.: Percutaneous transluminal dilatation in the treatment of renovascular hypertension, Ann. Intern. Med. **95**:439, 1981.
34. Gruntzig, A., et al.: Treatment of renovascular hypertension with percutaneous transluminal dilatation of a renal-artery stenosis, Lancet **1**:801, 1978.
35. Gutmann, F.D., et al.: Renal arterial pressure, renin secretion, and blood pressure control in trained dogs, Am. J. Physiol. **224**:66, 1973.
36. Haber, E., et al.: Application of a radioimmunoassay for angiotensin I to the physiologic measurements of plasma renin activity in normal human subjects, J. Clin. Endocrinol. **29**:1349, 1969.
37. Heacox, R., Harvey, A.M., and Vander, A.J.: Hepatic inactivation of renin, Circ. Res. **21**:149, 1967.
38. Hillman, B.J.: Digital imaging of the kidney, Radiol. Clin. North Am. **22**:341, 1984.
39. Hillman, B.J., et al.: The potential impact of digital subtraction angiography on screening for renovascular hypertension, Radiology **142**:577, 1982.
40. Hricik, D.E., et al.: Captopril-induced renal insufficiency in patients with bilateral renal-artery stenosis or renal-artery stenosis in a solitary kidney, N. Engl. J. Med. **308**:373, 1983.
41. Hunt, J.C., and Strong, C.G.: Renovascular hypertension: mechanisms, natural history and treatment. In Laragh, J.H., editor: Hypertension manual, New York, 1975, Dun-Donnelly.
42. Jamieson, G.G., et al.: Reconstructive renal vascular surgery for chronic renal failure, Br. J. Surg. **71**:338, 1984.
43. Kaufman, J.J.: Renovascular hypertension: the UCLA experience, J. Urol. **112**:139, 1979.
44. Keeton, T.K., and Campbell, W.B.: The pharmacologic alteration of renin release, Pharmacol. Rev. **31**:81, 1981.
45. Keim, H.J., et al.: Computer-assisted static/dynamic renal imaging: a screening test for renovascular hypertension? J. Nucl. Med. **20**:11, 1979.
46. Krakoff, L.R., et al.: Saralasin infusion in screening patients for renovascular hypertension, Am. J. Cardiol. **46**:609, 1980.
47. Lawrie, G.M., et al.: Late results of reconstructive surgery for renovascular disease, Ann. Surg. **191**:528, 1980.
48. Lye, C.R., et al.: Aortorenal arterial autografts: late observations, Arch. Surg. **110**:1321, 1975.
49. Machay, A., et al.: Assessment of total and divided renal plasma flow by ^{123}I-hippuran renography, Kidney Int. **19**:49, 1981.
50. Marks, L.S., Maxwell, M.H., and Kaufman, J.J.: Renin, sodium, and vasodepressor response to saralasin in renovascular and essential hypertension, Ann. Intern. Med. **87**:176, 1977.
51. Marks, L.S., et al.: Renovascular hypertension: does the renal vein renin ratio predict operative results? J. Urol. **115**:365, 1976.
52. Martin, E.C., Diamond, N.G., and Casarella, W.J.: Percutaneous transluminal angioplasty in nonatherosclerotic disease, Radiology **135**:27, 1980.
53. McNeil, B.J., et al.: Measures of clinical efficacy: cost-effectiveness calculations in the diagnosis and treatment of hypertensive renovascular disease, N. Engl. J. Med. **293**:216, 1975.
54. Miller, E.D., Jr., et al.: Inhibition of angiotensin conversion in experimental renovascular hypertension, Science **177**:1108, 1972.
55. Miller, E.D., Jr., et al.: Inhibition of angiotensin conversion and prevention of renal hypertension, Am. J. Physiol. **228**:448, 1975.
56. Novick, A.C., et al.: Splenorenal bypass in the treatment of renal artery stenosis, Trans. Am. Assoc. Genitour. Surg. **69**:139, 1978.
57. Novick, A.C., et al.: Diminished operative morbidity and mortality in renal revascularization, JAMA **246**:749, 1981.
58. Novick, A.C., et al.: Surgical treatment of renovascular hypertension in the pediatric patient, J. Urol. **119**:794, 1982.
59. Oparil, S., et al.: Mechanism of pulmonary conversion of angiotensin I to II in the dog, Circ. Res. **29**:682, 1971.
60. Oshima, G., Gecse, A., and Erdos, E.G.: Angiotensin I-converting enzyme of the kidney cortex, Biochim. Biophys. Acta **350**:26, 1974.
61. Page, I.H.: On the nature of the pressor action of renin, J. Exp. Med. **70**:521, 1939.
62. Page, I.H., and Helmer, O.M.: A crystalline pressor substance (angiotonin) resulting from the reaction between renin and renin-activator, J. Exp. Med. **71**:29, 1940.
63. Peach, M.J.: Renin-angiotensin system: biochemistry and mechanisms of action, Physiol. Rev. **57**:313, 1977.
64. Re, R., et al.: Inhibition of angiotensin-converting enzyme for diagnosis of renal artery stenosis, N. Engl. J. Med. **298**:582, 1978.
65. Samuels, A.I., et al.: Renin-angiotensin antagonists and the regulation of blood pressure, Fed. Proc. **35**:2512, 1976.
66. Schneider, E.G., et al.: The hepatic metabolism of renin and aldosterone: a review with new observations on the hepatic clearance of renin, Circ. Res. **26-27** (suppl. I):175, 1970.
67. Sealey, J.E., et al.: The physiology of renin secretion in essential hypertension: estimation of renin secretion rate and renal plasma flow from peripheral and renal vein renin levels, Am. J. Med. **55**:391, 1973.
68. Semple, P.F., et al.: Angiotensin II and its heptapeptide (2-8), hexapeptide (3-8), and pentapeptide (4-8) metabolites in arterial and venous blood of man, Circ. Res. **39**:671, 1976.
69. Simon, N., et al.: Clinical characteristics of renovascular hypertension, JAMA **220**:1209, 1972.
70. Skeggs, L.T., Jr., et al.: Existence of 2 forms of hypertension, J. Exp. Med. **99**:275, 1954.
71. Sos, T.A., et al.: Percutaneous transluminal renal angioplasty in renovascular hypertension due to atheroma or fibromuscular dysplasia, N. Engl. J. Med. **309**:274, 1983.
72. Sottiurai, V., Fry, W.J., and Stanley, J.C.: Ultrastructure of smooth muscle, myofibroblasts and fibroblasts in human arterial dysplasia, Arch. Surg. **113**:1280, 1978.
73. Stanley, J.C.: Morphologic, histologic and clinical characteristics of renovascular fibrodysplasia and arteriosclerosis. In Bergan, J.J., and Yao, J.S.T., editors: Surgery of the aorta and its body branches, New York, 1979, Grune & Stratton, Inc.
74. Stanley, J.C.: Pathologic basis of macrovascular renal artery disease. In Stanley, J.C., Ernst, C.B., and Fry, W.J., editors: Renovascular hypertension, Philadelphia, 1984, W.B. Saunders Co.
75. Stanley, J.C., and Fry, W.J.: Renovascular hypertension secondary to arterial fibrodysplasia in adults, Arch. Surg. **110**:992, 1975.
76. Stanley, J.C., and Fry, W.J.: Surgical treatment of renovascular hypertension, Arch. Surg. **112**:1291, 1977.
77. Stanley, J.C., and Fry, W.J.: Pediatric renal artery occlusive disease and renovascular hypertension: etiology, diagnosis, and operative treatment, Arch. Surg. **116**:669, 1981.

78. Stanley, J.C., Ernst, C.B., and Fry, W.J.: Fate of 100 aortorenal vein grafts: characteristics of late graft expansion, aneurysmal dilatation, and stenosis, Surgery **74**:931, 1973.
79. Stanley, J.C., Ernst, C.B., and Fry, W.J.: Surgical treatment of renovascular hypertension: results in specific patient subgroups. In Stanley, J.C., Ernst, C.B., and Fry, W.J., editors: Renovascular hypertension, Philadelphia, 1984, W.B. Saunders Co.
80. Stanley, J.C., Gewertz, B.L., and Fry, W.J.: Renal:systemic renin indices and renal vein renin ratios as prognostic indicators in remedial renovascular hypertension, J. Surg. Res. **20**:149, 1976.
81. Stanley, J.C., et al.: Arterial fibrodysplasia: histopathologic character and current etiologic concepts, Arch. Surg. **110**:551, 1975.
82. Stanley, J.C., et al.: Renal artery aneurysms: significance of macroaneurysms exclusive of dissections and fibrodysplastic mural dilations, Arch. Surg. **110**:1327, 1975.
83. Stanley, J.C., et al.: Developmental occlusive disease of the abdominal aorta and the splanchnic and renal arteries, Am. J. Surg. **142**:190, 1981.
84. Stanley, J.C., et al.: Operative therapy of renovascular hypertension, Br. J. Surg. **63**(suppl.):S63, 1982.
85. Stanley, J.C., et al.: Reoperation for complications of renal artery reconstructive surgery undertaken for treatment of renovascular hypertension, J. Vasc. Surg. **2**:133, 1985.
86. Stoney, R.J.: Transaortic renal endarterectomy. In Rutherford, R.B., editor: Vascular surgery, Philadelphia, 1984, W.B. Saunders Co.
87. Stoney, R.J., Silane, M., and Salvatierra, O., Jr.: Ex vivo renal artery reconstruction, Arch. Surg. **113**:1271, 1978.
88. Stoney, R.J., et al.: Aortorenal arterial autografts: long-term assessment, Arch. Surg. **116**:1416, 1981.
89. Straffon, R., and Siegel, D.F.: Saphenous vein bypass graft in the treatment of renovascular hypertension, Urol. Clin. North Am. **2**:337, 1975.
90. Streeten, D.H.P., and Anderson, G.H., Jr.: Angiotensin antagonists and angiotensin-converting enzyme inhibitors in renovascular hypertension. In Stanley, J.C., Ernst, C.B., and Fry, W.J., editors: Renovascular hypertension, Philadelphia, 1984, W.B. Saunders Co.
91. Streeten, D.H.P., et al.: Use of an angiotensin II, antagonist (saralasin) in the recognition of angiotensinogenic hypertension, N. Engl. J. Med. **292**:657, 1975.
92. Tegtmeyer, C.J., Kellum, C.D., and Ayers, C.: Percutaneous transluminal angioplasty of the renal artery: results and long-term follow-up, Radiology **153**:77, 1984.
93. Textor, S.C., et al.: Responses of the stenosed and contralateral kidneys to (sar-1-Thr-8) AII in human renovascular hypertension, Hypertension **5**:796, 1983.
94. Thompson, J.M.A., and Dickinson, C.J.: The relation between the excretion of sodium and water and the perfusion pressure in the isolated, blood-perfused rabbit kidney, with special reference to changes occurring in clip-hypertension, Clin. Sci. Mol. Med. **50**:223, 1976.
95. Thornbury, J.R., Stanley, J.C., and Fryback, D.G.: Hypertensive urogram: a nondiscriminatory test for renovascular hypertension, Am. J. Roentgenol. **138**:43, 1982.
96. Tigerstedt, R., and Bergman, P.G.: Niere und kreislauf, Scand. Arch. Physiol. **8**:223, 1898.
97. Tobian, L.: Interrelationship of electrolytes, juxtaglomerular cells and hypertension, Physiol. Rev. **40**:280, 1960.
98. Vander, A.J.: Renin angiotensin system. In Stanley, J.C., Ernst, C.B., and Fry, W.J., editors: Renovascular hypertension, Philadelphia, 1984, W.B. Saunders Co.
99. Vander, A.J., and Miller, R.: Control of renin secretion in the anesthetized dog, Am. J. Physiol. **207**:537, 1964.
100. Vaughan, E.D., Jr., et al.: Renovascular hypertension: renin measurements to indicate hypersecretion and contralateral suppression, estimate renal plasma flow, and score for surgical curability, Am. J. Med. **55**:402, 1973.
101. Vidt, D.G.: Advances in the medical management of renovascular hypertension, Urol. Clin. North Am. **11**:417, 1984.
102. Vidt, D.G., et al.: Surgical treatment of unilateral renal vascular disease: prognostic role of vascular changes in bilateral renal biopsies, Am. J. Cardiol. **30**:827, 1972.
103. Watkins, B.E., et al.: Incidence and pathophysiological changes in chronic two-kidney hypertension in the dog, Am. J. Physiol. **231**:954, 1976.
104. Whitehouse, W.M., Jr., et al.: Chronic total renal artery occlusions: effects of treatment on secondary hypertension and renal function, Surgery **89**:753, 1981.
105. Wylie, E.J., Perloff, D.L., and Stoney, R.J.: Autogenous tissue revascularization technics in surgery for renovascular hypertension, Ann. Surg. **170**:416, 1969.
106. Yang, H.Y., and Erdos, E.G.: Second kininase in human blood plasma, Nature **215**:1402, 1967.
107. Zweifler, A.J., and Julius, S.: Medical treatment of renovascular hypertension. In Stanley, J.C., Ernst, C.B., and Fry, W.J., editors: Renovascular hypertension, Philadelphia, 1984, W.B. Saunders Co.

46

Gage Van Horn and Alan H. Lockwood

Altered States of Consciousness

The relationships between mind and body have been a source of intense thought by philosophers and scientists throughout history. In early medical manuscripts, Platonic notions of consciousness and its localization in the head were supported by clinical descriptions of unconsciousness following head injuries. Descartes attributed consciousness to the pineal gland, but operated from a philosophic rather than an observational base. Franz Joseph Gall's concept that specific mental faculties were attributable to specific brain centers set the stage for the modern era of neurologic investigation that relates structure and function through careful experimentation and observation. The development of this structure-function approach was facilitated by the work of Cajal, who developed the neuronal theory of cerebral function, and by Brodmann, who identified and mapped anatomically distinct regions of the cerebral cortex that have been linked subsequently with specific neural functions.

Surgeons are frequently involved in the care of patients with impaired consciousness. Major surgical procedures are performed in patients rendered unconscious by the administration of general anesthetics. Drugs useful in alleviating postoperative pain and potentiating anesthetic agents also affect consciousness and may prolong postoperative lethargy. Surgeons are often the first physicians called on to provide care for unconscious patients, particularly in emergency rooms. Some must serve as the only treating physician for a comatose patient. Successful approaches to the diagnosis and management of patients with altered consciousness are highly dependent on an understanding of the pathophysiologic principles that relate neural structure and function. This chapter attempts to deal with those principles.

ANATOMIC AND PHYSIOLOGIC BASIS OF NORMAL CONSCIOUSNESS

In 1949 Moruzzi and Magoun[22] reported that stimuli applied to the reticular formation in the brainstem and the lower diencephalon interrupted high-voltage, slow synchronous electroencephalographic (EEG) activity and replaced it with low-voltage, fast activity. This activation was the same type observed after environmental stimuli such as eye opening and was interpreted as evidence for a reticular origin of EEG and behavioral activation. Additional studies led to the conclusion that the neural pathways involved in activation were multisynaptic and depended on the integrity of thalamic projection areas (Fig. 46-1). French and Magoun[13] placed lesions in the reticular formation of monkeys and induced coma that persisted until the animal died or was killed, confirming the importance of the reticular formation in the mediation of consciousness. Clinical and neuropathologic findings from five patients with persistent coma were reported by French[12] in 1952. Three patients had extensive destructive lesions in the reticular formation, one had lesions in the rostral projections of the reticular formation, and the fifth patient had nearly complete cortical ablation as a result of presumed tertiary syphilis. French concluded that destruction of the ascending reticular activating system, its rostrally projecting fibers, or the entire cerebral cortex would produce coma. These conclusions have withstood careful scrutiny by Plum and Posner[28] who reported similar conclusions.

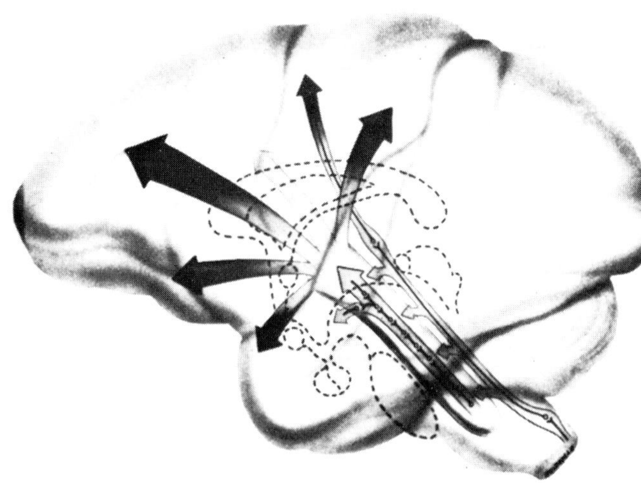

Fig. 46-1 Multisynaptic neural pathway activation *(arrows)* originating in the reticular formation. (From Magoun, H.W.: Brain mechanisms in consciousness, Oxford, 1954, Blackwell Scientific Publications, Ltd.)

Although the reticular formation has a homogeneous appearance grossly, even early microscopic studies by Cajal indicated that the region was anatomically heterogeneous. More recently, combined anatomic and physiologic studies have shown that the reticular formation is the site of origin of neurons that have very large projections and complex neurophysiologic interrelationships.

Neuropharmacologic studies of the reticular formation have shown additional heterogeneity. Neurons containing norepinephrine, serotonin, dopamine, and enkephalins have all been described and can be identified by using specific fluorescent techniques, autoradiographic ligand binding studies, or immunohistochemical stains directed at enzymes or metabolites related to specific neurotransmitters. Among the catecholaminergic nuclei in the reticular formation, the locus ceruleus has been the most completely described because of its characteristic appearance when viewed through the light microscope and because of the large amount of norepinephrine in the neurons. Lesions of the locus ceruleus increase the length of time that animals spend in a quiet but wakeful state.[2] This nuclear group appears to be important in coordinating neural inputs from the environment and viscera and relating them to the rest of the brain.[6]

Although no single homogeneous neuronal group has been identified in the reticular formation as the site of neural activity that determines wakefulness, the notion that this region of the brainstem does in fact control vigilance retains clinical usefulness. The complexities within the reticular formation, demonstrated by the types of studies mentioned previously, make it likely that the region identified by Moruzzi and Magoun[22] is the site where neural interactions determining consciousness have their highest density, either at a synaptic level or because of the physical proximity of neuronal elements. This region is the site where minimum lesions have maximum effects on consciousness.

In humans, a quantitative element and a qualitative element of consciousness are recognized. The quantitative aspect, or level of consciousness, is rated by an examiner on a continuum between complete alertness through lethargy and stupor to coma and is mediated by the reticular formation. Qualitative consciousness—including cognition, memory, language, and special sensory processing—is mediated by regions of the cerebral cortex and their interaction with subcortical, often thalamic, centers. In a clinical setting, an examiner describes the quantitative, on-off aspect of the level of consciousness on the basis of responses to alerting stimuli such as a spoken word or shout, or, in more extreme cases, to noxious stimuli. Qualitative aspects of consciousness can be evaluated only in individuals with a quantitative aspect of consciousness that is sufficient to permit interpersonal communication. The mental status examination—tests designed to measure orientation, memory, and cognition—evaluates this qualitative aspect of consciousness and the integrity of cerebral regions mediating the activity.

Although it is usually easy to determine whether or not patients are conscious, there are occasional patients in whom this is difficult. Certain patients with severe low-brainstem destructive lesions may be conscious but unable to interact with the environment because of quadriplegia and the inability to move the oral and pharyngeal muscles required for speech. Plum and Posner[28] describe these patients as being "locked in" by their neurologic lesions. Akinetic mutism or, more properly, the persistent vegetative state[15] is an increasingly common condition in which the patient gives the appearance of consciousness, possibly by visual tracking, but exhibits no evidence of cognition. This condition may be seen after head injury, cardiopulmonary arrest, or, less frequently, following other causes of nontraumatic coma.

MECHANISMS FOR ALTERED CONSCIOUSNESS

Lesions that affect consciousness do so by destroying, damaging, or interfering with the normal function of the reticular formation or the cerebral cortex. The mechanisms for altered consciousness can be divided broadly into structural vs. metabolic categories. In nearly 400 cases of coma of unknown origin, just over 30% of the patients had either supratentorial or infratentorial destructive lesions such as subdural hematomas, tumors, infarcts, and hemorrhages, and nearly 70% of the patients had metabolic abnormalities such as drug intoxication, infections, or anoxia.[28] In a surgical practice, trauma is a common cause of reduced consciousness and may coexist with a metabolic encephalopathy. The intoxicated alcoholic may have a subdural hematoma, or a metabolic abnormality may cause a driver to lose control of a car, resulting in an injury that may divert attention from an underlying medical problem.

Structural Lesions

Structural lesions alter consciousness by one or more mechanisms. Relatively small lesions confined to the rostral brainstem produce coma by destroying the reticular formation. Large lesions may produce a shift in brain structures, secondarily compressing the reticular formation. Altered consciousness also occurs if sufficiently large amounts of the cortex or underlying white matter are destroyed. The clinical diagnosis of structural lesions is made on the basis of neuroanatomic localizations that depend on the physician's ability to correlate observable neurologic deficits with a knowledge of functional neuroanatomy. For example, coma associated with bilateral complete oculomotor (third) nerve palsies indicates the presence of a lesion in the tegmentum of the midbrain where there is anatomic proximity between third-nerve nuclei and the reticular formation. A left hemiparesis associated with a dilated, fixed right pupil indicates the presence of a lesion affecting the corticospinal system in the right cerebral hemisphere, secondary compression of the reticular formation, and compression of the third nerve as it passes between the tentorium and the uncus of the temporal lobe.

Metabolic Disturbances

Metabolic disturbances affect most areas of the brain simultaneously, although specific regions vary in their sensitivity to metabolic abnormalities. The healthy brain has a very high metabolic rate. Representing only 2% of the total body weight, it accounts for nearly 20% of whole-body oxygen consumption and receives between 15% and 20% of the cardiac output. In spite of this high metabolic rate, the brain cannot store energy or energy substrates and is highly sensitive to interruptions in blood and metabolic supplies. This sensitivity is dramatized in Fig. 46-2.[20] Within seconds, adenosine triphosphate (ATP) stores show

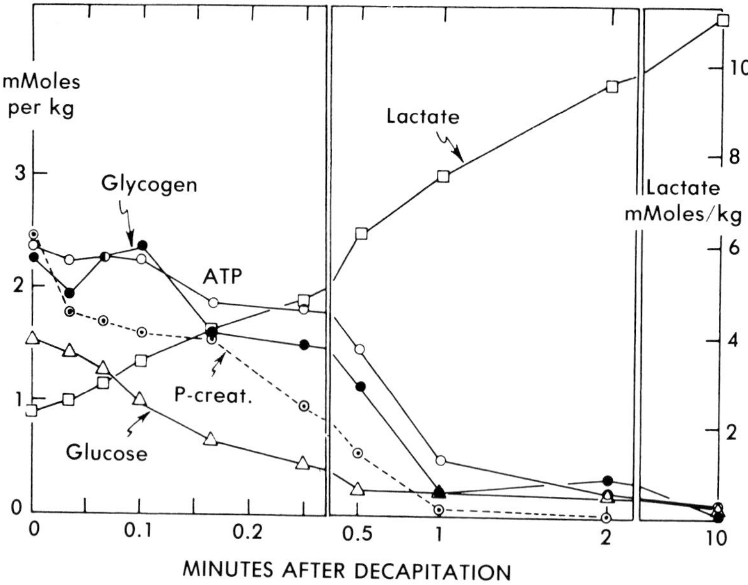

Fig. 46-2 Metabolic consequences of decapitation. (From Lowry, O.H., et al.: J. Biol. Chem. **239**:24, 1964.)

evidence of depletion. Within 1 minute, ATP and glucose are virtually absent as a result of their continued use with no replacement. Metabolic waste in the form of lactate, which is produced by anaerobic glycolysis, accumulates to high levels, produces acidosis, and contributes further to brain dysfunction. Clinically, loss-of-consciousness is observed within seconds of a cardiopulmonary arrest, and permanent brain damage follows within minutes if treatment is not successful.

Altered consciousness is the hallmark of metabolic encephalopathy, and early in its course, brainstem function is relatively preserved. Characteristically, the pupils are slightly smaller than normal and constrict in reaction to a bright light stimulus. As the patient's level of consciousness declines, the light reflex becomes sluggish and incomplete. In patients with profound metabolic coma such as occurs in severe barbiturate intoxication, the pupillary light response may be absent. Hypoxia and certain drugs such as glutethimide and the anticholinergics affect pupillary function out of proportion to the alteration in the level of consciousness. As the depth of coma increases, abnormalities of ocular motility emerge. In stuporous patients, eye movement is often dysconjugate and roving. Alerting stimuli such as deep pain may cause the eyes to become conjugate. As coma deepens, spontaneous eye movements cease. However, stimuli such as passive head movement or irrigation of the external ear with ice water usually elicit eye movements, providing evidence for the structural integrity of the brainstem.

Although metabolic causes for altered consciousness are common and have been the subject of intense experimentation, important questions regarding underlying mechanisms have not been answered. For example, turtle brain is much more resistant to hypoxia than mammalian brain, but the reason for this difference is unknown. Even though knowledge of mechanisms at the molecular level is absent, it is possible to classify metabolic encephalopathies into three clinically and pathophysiologically relevant categories: (1) encephalopathies attributable to deficient or absent metabolic substrate; (2) encephalopathies attributable to the presence of endogenous or exogenous toxin; or (3) encephalopathies attributable to an alteration of the normal internal cerebral milieu.

Substrate Deficiency

During the course of normal brain function, neurons are continually depolarized as potassium and sodium move through ion channels. The majority of brain work is exerted in pumping these ions back to where they belong. As progressive deficiency of required brain metabolites (usually glucose or oxygen) develops, cerebral blood flow and metabolite extraction increase in an effort to maintain fuel supplies and preserve brain function. These compensatory measures are not complete, and measurable decrements in brain performance begin to emerge (Fig. 46-3).[33] Experimental investigations have shown that ATP tends to remain at near-normal levels in comatose animals even during extreme hypoxia, suggesting that the brain has undescribed mechanisms that shut down brain function in an orderly fashion to preserve structural integrity during adverse conditions. At a critical threshold, near an arterial partial pressure of oxygen of 20 mm Hg, these mechanisms fail, cardiac arrhythmias develop, cerebral circulation fails, and the metabolic sequence depicted in Fig. 46-2 develops. Thus it is imperative to diagnose hypoxia promptly and to begin appropriate therapy immediately.

Although the brain depends on adequate glucose supplies (just as it requires oxygen), the body's resistance to the sudden development of hypoglycemia is greater than it is to the sudden development of hypoxia. Therefore the correct diagnosis and treatment of hypoglycemia, as com-

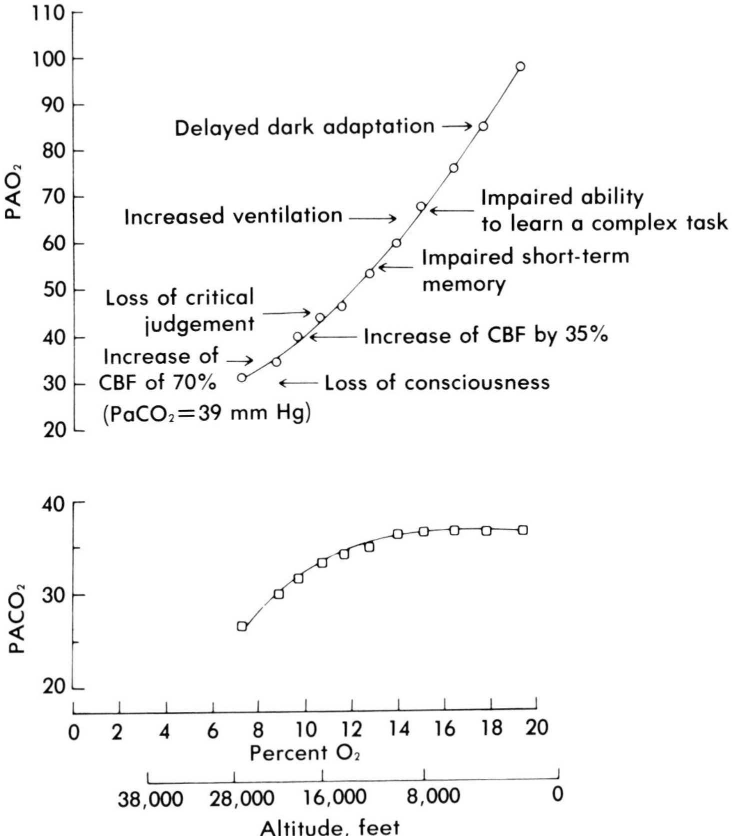

Fig. 46-3 Progression of neurologic abnormalities observed during increasing hypoxia. (From Siesjö, B.K.: Brain dysfunction and cerebral hypoxia and ischemia. In Plum, F.: Brain dysfunction and metabolic disorders, New York, 1974, Raven Press.)

pared with anoxia, is not as urgent. However, hypoglycemia cannot be diagnosed reliably on the basis of clinical criteria, and diagnostic delays, even using the most efficient laboratories, may lead to the development of irreversible brain injury. Therefore anyone with an altered level of consciousness, including a delirious patient, should be considered hypoglycemic until proven otherwise. The routine administration of glucose under these circumstances is warranted.

Toxins

Because of the complexity of normal cerebral function, there are innumerable opportunities for toxins, either endogenous or exogenous, to affect the way the brain works. Almost all toxins act by inhibiting normal brain function and reducing consciousness. Exceptions to this rule are seen in the cases of toxins that block neural inhibitory pathways, such as the bicuculine blockade of the inhibitory neurotransmitter gamma-aminobutyric acid, which produces epileptic seizures. Several principles of toxin action can be developed. These principles are illustrated by the actions of specific-function toxins including neurotransmitter blocking agents, pathophysiologic mechanisms that depend on the production of a common toxin such as ammonia, and production of common physical signs by seemingly unrelated toxins such as the hyperventilation seen in patients with salicylate intoxication, hyperammonemia, or acidosis.

Drugs affecting the brain often work by mechanisms related to their ability to influence a specific cerebral process. Thus antipsychotic agents that bind to dopaminergic postsynaptic sites in the brain produce clinical signs similar to those seen in dopamine-deficiency states or Parkinsonism, and organophosphates affect brain function by interfering with cholinergic neurotransmission. The majority of toxins act by means of unknown mechanisms. Hepatic encephalopathy caused by hyperammonemia in patients with cirrhosis of the liver is an excellent example of a toxin with an action that is not explained at the molecular level. However, cirrhosis of the liver is the second-ranked cause of death in adults in metropolitan areas, and hepatic encephalopathy after gastrointestinal hemorrhage is very common in these individuals, making ammonia intoxication an important clinical problem in a surgical practice.

Because ammonia is the final product in the catabolism of a variety of nitrogenous compounds, hyperammonemia is a feature of a wide variety of seemingly unrelated metabolic problems.[19] Valproic acid administration for the treatment of epilepsy is thought to produce symptomatic hyperammonemia in susceptible patients by depleting mitochondrial acetylcoenzyme A. Bacterial infections of ileal conduits may also produce symptomatic hyperammonemia through the action of urease, and hyperammonemia develops in association with hypercapnia.

Although most toxins are respiratory depressants, hyperventilation is characteristic of salicylate poisoning, hyperammonemia, and metabolic acidoses such as diabetic ketoacidosis. Hyperventilation is a physiologically normal response to acid stimulation of the medullary respiratory centers. Ammonia and salicylates act as irritant stimulators of the respiratory control systems.[28]

Altered Internal Milieu

In addition to constant supplies of oxygen and glucose, the brain depends on a normal internal environment for optimum function. Regulatory mechanisms in the brain maintain water, electrolyte, and acid-base balance within very narrow tolerance levels. Water metabolism is regulated by complex interactions between neurons located in the hypothalamus adjacent to the supraoptic nuclei, which mediate thirst, and antidiuretic hormone (ADH) production. Ordinarily, small deviations in osmolarity result in thirst, an increase in water consumption, and ADH release. Excess water causes production of dilute urine as ADH levels fall and thirst is abolished.

During uncontrolled water loss and dehydration or water intoxication, water molecules move freely across the blood-brain barrier toward the compartment with the highest solute concentration. During dehydration, water leaves and the brain shrinks. During water excess, water enters and the brain swells. Altered brain water content causes brain dysfunction that is probably the consequence of distortions of brain volume. A shrinking brain tears veins bridging the space between the cortex and the dural sinuses causing subdural hematomas; a swelling brain compresses the reticular formation. The brain is relatively defenseless against sudden dramatic changes in water content. However, large changes that develop over long periods of time are relatively well tolerated. The brain is able to produce osmotically active particles in the form of amino acids that help the brain retain its water and hence its volume during hyperosmolar states.[18] During conditions of water excess, the brain ejects potassium ions causing it to lose water and maintaining a more nearly normal volume.[31] It is quite possible for severe abnormalities in osmolarity to produce few symptoms if the abnormality develops slowly.

Just as the rapid development of hyperosmolarity or hypoosmolarity is dangerous to brain function, so too is rapid correction of a relatively asymptomatic, long-standing osmotic abnormality. Under these conditions, the replenishment to normal must be done with caution to avoid iatrogenic water intoxication or dehydration.

PATHOPHYSIOLOGIC BASIS UNDERLYING THE SIGNS AND SYMPTOMS IN PATIENTS WITH ALTERED CONSCIOUSNESS

A great deal of emphasis is placed on the bedside physical examination of the patient in determining the cause of diminished consciousness.[9] Such an examination is occasionally exceeded in importance by the acquisition of an accurate patient history, something not always available during the initial evaluation, but it can never be replaced

Table 46-1 **TYPICAL SYNDROMES OF ALTERED CONSCIOUSNESS**

Syndromes	Consciousness	Respirations	Pupils	Extraocular Muscle Function	Motor Function
Early metabolic or diffuse encephalopathy	Lethargy or delirium	Eupnea or posthyperventilation apnea	Equal, sluggishly light-reactive; pinpoint if opiates are cause of encephalopathy	Spontaneously roving; conjugate or disconjugate; extraocular movements full to reflex testing	Bilateral paratonia; ± bilateral upgoing toes; no asymmetry
Late metabolic or diffuse encephalopathy	Stupor to coma	Hypopnea to apnea; hyperventilation if acidotic	Small; may be unreactive	Directed straight ahead; fixed or very sluggish to extraocular reflexes	Flaccidity; no toe signs or bilateral upgoing toes
Large lateralized supratentorial lesion with early uncal herniation and early-to-late diencephalic dysfunction	Lethargy to stupor	Eupnea to Cheyne-Stokes respirations	Ipsilateral dilated and light-fixed pupil	Ipsilateral oculomotor palsy; eyes may be conjugately deviated to side of lesion but move past midline with extraocular reflexes	Contralateral hemiparesis or hemiplegia; contralateral decorticate or decerebrate posturing; ipsilateral decorticate posturing or purposeful movement; contra ± ipsilateral ↑ toes

by a screening battery of laboratory tests. The portions of the neurologic examination that should be stressed are:

Level of consciousness
Respirations
Pupils
Extraocular muscle function
Motor system function

A careful analysis of the abnormalities found in these systems can nearly always localize the anatomic lesions responsible for coma (Table 46-1). In some instances, the constellation of findings allows a precise diagnosis. In others, a narrowed list of differential diagnoses is produced. The systems listed are intimately related and are affected to some degree in every comatose patient. In addition the tests involving these systems do not require patient cooperation, i.e., they can easily be performed on the unconscious patient.

Level of Consciousness

The physiology and pathophysiology of consciousness have been discussed earlier in the chapter. Recording an initial accurate description of the patient's level of consciousness is very important to provide subsequent evaluators a basis for determining clinical improvement or deterioration. We have frequently been called into consultation about patients whose consciousness had been impaired for days but whose charts contained no physician's notes describing those levels of reduced consciousness.

In determining the patient's level of consciousness, observation should be the first step. What is the patient doing when unstimulated? If the patient is conscious, a few direct questions that require some cerebral function by the patient may be all that is needed to ascertain the level of consciousness. In other cases, a more detailed mental status examination is necessary to pinpoint minor abnormalities in content. If patients are asleep or unconscious, the examiner can first call the patient's name. If this action fails to alert the patient, the examiner can then try shaking the bed or the patient's shoulder in conjunction with repeating the patient's name more firmly. If the patient appears to be comatose, a painful stimulus must usually be delivered somewhere near the midline. Applying painful stimuli distally in the extremities, e.g., nailbed stimulus, is better suited for demonstrating spinal withdrawal reflexes but may be effective in arousing patients.

The words commonly used to describe various levels of consciousness are defined in the boxed material on p. 756. The definitions are imprecise, and some terms have multiple meanings.[9,10,28] In general, the level of consciousness is best described by indicating the patient's reaction to stimuli and his/her environment.

Some examples of good descriptions of states of consciousness follow:

- "This patient is fully conscious, alert, oriented, and cognizant."
- "This patient was found to be lethargic. When unstimulated for several minutes, she would lapse off to sleep from which she could be aroused by firmly calling her name. When awakened, she appeared dull, inattentive, inactive, and indifferent."

Table 46-1 **TYPICAL SYNDROMES OF ALTERED CONSCIOUSNESS—cont'd**

Syndromes	Consciousness	Respirations	Pupils	Extraocular Muscle Function	Motor Function
Large paramidline supratentorial lesion with early central transtentorial herniation and upper-brainstem dysfunction	Stupor to coma	Cheyne-Stokes respirations	Midposition, usually symmetric and light-fixed	Eyes may be deviated to side of lesion or downward; may be fixed to extraocular reflexes	Contralateral decerebrate and ipsilateral decorticate posturing or bilateral decerebrate or decorticate posturing
Supratentorial lesion with advanced transtentorial herniation and pontine dysfunction	Coma	Sustained tachypnea with hypocapnia	Midposition and light-fixed	Eyes are directed straight ahead and fixed to extraocular reflexes	Bilateral decerebrate posturing or flaccidity with bilateral ↑ toes
Large intrinsic brainstem lesion affecting pontine base and tegmentum	Coma	Sustained tachypnea with hypocapnia	Equal; near pinpoint but light-reactive with magnification	Eyes are directed straight ahead and fixed to extraocular reflexes	Flaccidity with bilateral ↑ or mute toes; no posturing
Extrinsic subtentorial lesion with pontine or medullary compression	Lethargy to stupor	Eupneic (early) to ataxic or apneustic (late)	Ipsilateral Horner's syndrome; light-reactive	Usually disconjugate with ipsilateral sixth nerve palsy	Contralateral ↑ toe or bilateral ↑ toes without posturing

- "This patient was deeply comatose. He could not be aroused by shouting his name. A midline painful stimulus produced bilateral decerebrate posturing but no arousal."

Patterns of Abnormal Respiration

Several distinct respiratory patterns can be seen in patients with reduced consciousness.[28] In many cases, these patterns can be produced only by structural lesions highly localized in the brainstem. However, altered respirations may be caused by both structural and metabolic abnormalities, sometimes acting in concert. In many cases information from arterial blood gas determinations must be integrated with bedside observations to pinpoint the cause of abnormal respiratory patterns. Before attempting to arouse the unconscious patient, examiners should note the rate, depth, and regularity of respirations. Any changes that occur with the application of stimulation should also be noted.

The brainstem respiratory centers reside in the reticular areas from the mid-pons to the caudal medulla. These centers receive input from higher cortical centers (forebrain), peripheral oxygen chemoreceptors in the great vessels, pH receptors near the ventral medullary surface, and stretch and irritant receptors in the upper- and lower-respiratory tracts. A comprehensive review of the neural regulation of respiration was published in 1977.[1] The influence of the neocortex over brainstem respiratory centers is maximum in the conscious patient but is present in lesser degree in the obtunded one.

Posthyperventilation apnea is a pattern seen in conscious patients with diffuse metabolic or structural hemispheric disease.[28] It may be induced by having the patient voluntarily hyperventilate for 30 seconds to 1 minute. In healthy patients, the rhythm of regular breathing is resumed with no more than a 12-second delay after hyperventilation. In impaired individuals, usually those individuals with diffuse or metabolic encephalopathies, there may be a prolonged period of apnea (up to 30 seconds) following the hyperventilation. The cause of posthyperventilation apnea is believed to be reduced forebrain input to the brainstem respiratory centers.

Cheyne-Stokes respiration (CSR) is a pattern of periodic breathing in which hyperpnea regularly alternates with apnea.[28] In most cases, there is a smooth crescendo and decrescendo with the hyperpneic period lasting longer than the apneic phase. In CSR, there is an exaggerated sensitivity to changes in partial pressure of carbon dioxide in arterial blood ($Paco_2$). When $Paco_2$ is elevated, there is an increased ventilatory response with a 30- to 40-second period of hyperpnea. The hyperpnea produces a lowered $Paco_2$ that leads to posthyperventilation apnea. During apnea, carbon dioxide reaccumulates, and the cycle begins again. The common denominator for most patients with CSR appears to be intact lower-brainstem respiratory centers that have been deprived of forebrain influences, analogous to the hyperactive tendon reflexes seen in patients with corticospinal tract disease. Structural lesions of both hemispheres or upper-brainstem and diffuse metabolic dysfunction can produce CSR.[4,5] In patients with a supratentorial mass lesion, the development of CSR suggests transtentorial herniation.

Structural lesions in the rostral brainstem tegmentum are frequently associated with sustained, rapid hyperpnea and hypocapnia, a condition that was formerly called central neurogenic hyperventilation.[28] Since lesions in the rostral brainstem often produce coma, this respiratory pattern is particularly common in comatose patients with head injury or transtentorial herniation. Hyperventilation of this sort, now called by some "central reflex hyperpnea," has also been observed in patients with meningitis, subarachnoid hemorrhage, and some metabolic abnormalities such as hepatic coma. The diagnosis of central neurogenic hyperventilation requires a normal to elevated partial pressure of oxygen in arterial blood (Pao_2), a reduced $Paco_2$, a nor-

---

LEVELS OF CONSCIOUSNESS

Consciousness
From Latin—literally means the ability to know. A normally conscious person is fully aware of self and environment, i.e., responds to stimuli with critical awareness.

Coma
From Greek—deep sleep; the opposite of consciousness; a state of profound unconsciousness from which the patient cannot be aroused. Patients with coma may respond reflexly to painful stimuli by posturing or withdrawing an extremity (brainstem or spinal reflexes), but there is no psychologic response that indicates cerebral cortical function.

Stupor
From Latin—to be benumbed, astonished, stupified; as used by neurologists, a state of deep unconsciousness from which the patient can be aroused only by continuous, vigorous stimulation. When the stimulus ceases, the patient lapses back into unconsciousness. In this context, stupor implies diffuse organic neurologic disease.

Confusion
From Latin—indicates a condition marked by disorder, disarray, uncertainty, and indecisiveness. Although this word conveys some meaning, it is not precise and cannot be used to denote a level of consciousness.

Delirium
From Latin—to be crazy; a transient mental disturbance that is characterized by confusion, disorientation, disordered speech, restlessness, excitement, and often delusions and hallucinations. It is seen in drug or alcohol withdrawal states, with high fever, and in many encephalopathies caused by trauma, seizures, and anoxia. Delirium always indicates organic disturbance.

Lethargy
From Greek—forgetfulness; a state marked by abnormal or morbid drowsiness. Neurologists use this term to denote a state of indifference, inactivity, inattentiveness, sluggishness, and apathy from which the patient may lapse into unconsciousness when there is infrequent stimulation. Obtundation implies a more profound degree of lethargy.

Sleep
A natural, regular suspension of consciousness from which the patient can be easily aroused. *Hypersomnia* is an excess of apparently normal sleep that is distinguishable from lethargy only by the increased level of cognition during arousal.

mal-to-basic cerebrospinal fluid pH, and no evidence of subarachnoid hemorrhage or central nervous system infection. In recent years, the central origin of this respiratory pattern has been questioned. Most comatose, brainstem-injured patients with tachypnea and hypocapnia do not meet all the criteria for central neurogenic hyperventilation since few have a normal-to-elevated PaO_2 and most have some lung congestion. Despite the unclear mechanism, sustained tachypneic hypocapnia in comatose patients with near-normal PaO_2s suggests structural upper-brainstem disease and a poor prognosis.

Apneustic breathing is characterized by a prolonged inspiratory phase with a pause at the end of respiration. This pattern is observed in patients with structural lesions affecting the rostral brainstem respiratory centers in the mid to lower pons. Apneusis is seen most commonly in patients with pontine infarction.

Ataxic and *cluster* breathing are observed in patients with structural lesions in or compressing the medulla. These respiratory patterns have localizing value but are not commonly associated with coma. Patients with ataxic, cluster, and apneustic respirations almost always use hypoxia as the stimulus to breathe and are insensitive to carbon dioxide. Administration of oxygen may therefore cause apnea.

Pupils

Examination of the pupils is critical to the neurologic examination of the comatose patient.[9] Sympathetic and parasympathetic pathways essential to pupillary function course through the upper-brainstem in juxtaposition to areas necessary for maintenance of consciousness. The examination is simple and should begin with observation for size, equality, and regularity in ambient light. Then a strong, concentrated light should be directed into first one eye and then the other, observing the response of both pupils simultaneously. If there is a question of light reactivity, magnification should be used.

The pupillary light reflex traverses a multisynaptic neuronal pathway from the retinas through the chiasm, optic tracts, pretectal nuclei, nuclei of the posterior commissure, Edinger-Westphal nuclei, and ciliary ganglia to the postganglionic fibers ending in the sphinctor pupillae.[3,26] This neuronal pathway crosses the midline in at least two places, the chiasm and posterior commissure, so that unilateral interruption of the pathway abolishes the pupillary light reflex unilaterally only when that interruption is distal to the Edinger-Westphal nuclei. More proximal interruption, unless it occurs bilaterally, will not abolish the light reflex. Parasympathetic pupillary fibers traveling in the peripheral oculomotor nerve are eccentric and are particularly vulnerable to compression (e.g., by a large aneurysm or by a herniating uncus). If third-nerve fibers are unilaterally interrupted in the presence of an intact brainstem, i.e., there is a relatively intact pupillary sympathetic system, the pupil becomes widely dilated and light fixed.

Sympathetic fibers mediating pupillary dilation originate primarily in the hypothalamous.[26] These fibers descend laterally in the brainstem tegmentum and cervical spinal cord to synapse with preganglionic neurons in the intermediolateral column of the upper three thoracic cord segments. The preganglionic fibers exit the cord, ascend in the sympathetic chain, and synapse with postganglionic neurons in the superior cervical ganglion. Postganglionic fibers travel along with the internal carotid artery, the ophthalmic branch of the trigeminal (V) nerve, and the nasociliary nerve to reach the pupillodilator muscle. The pathway is largely uncrossed so that unilateral interruption, presuming intact parasympathetic fibers are present, causes ipsilateral pupillary constriction (Horner's syndrome).[32] The intactness of this lateralized pathway can be tested by pinching one side of the patient's face or neck, which should produce ipsilateral pupillary dilation (ciliospinal reflex).[30] In this reflex, afferent pain fibers synapse with the descending sympathetic pathway at the cervical cord, medullary, and pontine levels.

Pupillary abnormalities have reliable localizing value in evaluating the comatose patient. Examples include the following.

1. In *diffuse or metabolic encephalopathies,* the pupils are usually equal and light-reactive, although that reaction may be sluggish. Because narcotics excite preganglionic parasympathetic pathways, coma produced by narcotic overdose is accompanied by very small (pinpoint) but light-reactive, pupils.
2. *Hypothalamic damage* produces ipsilateral pupillary constriction, narrowing of the palpebral fissure, and anhidrosis involving the entire body (not just the face as would be the case if the Horner's syndrome were caused by a more peripheral lesion).[32]
3. *Midbrain lesions* provide precise localization because both sympathetic and parasympathetic fibers are often involved and cause midposition (4 to 5 mm), light-fixed pupils.[28]
4. *Large pontine lesions* involving descending sympathetic fibers yield small-to-pinpoint, light-reactive pupils.
5. *Uncal herniation,* which may be produced by large subdural, epidural, or parenchymatous hematomas, frequently entraps the ipsilateral oculomotor nerve producing a widely dilated, light-fixed pupil.

Extraocular Movements

The neural pathways necessary for extraocular muscle function also lie adjacent to areas important for consciousness.[3,26] Therefore patients with altered consciousness frequently have abnormalities in extraocular muscle function. The pathways described in the following discussion are complex and incompletely understood but can be simplified for use in diagnosis.

Examination of the patient's extraocular function includes both observation and determination of reflex movements (extraocular reflexes). The eyelids and then the eye position with the eyelids lifted should be noted. Are the eyes conjugate? Do they move spontaneously? What is their position? Horizontal and vertical eye movements can be induced by either passive head turning (oculocephalic reflexes, or doll's eye movements) or caloric stimulation (oculovestibular reflexes). In the unconscious patient with intact brainstem function, passive head rotation induces conjugate eye deviation opposite the direction of the head rotation. Flexing and extending the head produces conjugate vertical movements opposite the direction of head movement. Cold-water stimulation of the unconscious, supine patient whose head is elevated approximately 30 degrees above the horizontal level and whose brainstem function is intact induces conjugate horizontal deviation of the eyes toward the stimulated side. Bilateral cold-water stimulation produces conjugate downward movement, and bilateral warm-water stimulation produces conjugate upward deviation.[28]

Voluntary or saccadic extraocular movements begin in the "frontal-gaze" or "frontal-eye" centers (Brodmann's Area 8). Parietooccipital areas subserve pursuit, but these areas are not as important as the frontal centers when considering the unconscious patient. Information moving from the frontal centers travels in axons through the internal capsule and upper-brainstem with other corticobulbar fibers. These fibers cross the midline in the upper-pons and synapse with neurons in the contralateral pontine paramedian reticular formation. From there, axons are sent to the adjacent abducens nucleus or through that nucleus, across the midline, and up the medial longitudinal fasciculus to the contralateral oculomotor nucleus. These pathways can be sorted by remembering that the stimulation of one frontal gaze center, such as might occur during focal seizures, drives the eyes to the opposite side or away from the gaze center that is being stimulated.

The supranuclear pathways for vertical gaze are less well understood. Those fibers controlling vertical eye movements from the frontal gaze fields presumably descend with the fibers controlling horizontal gaze. Important centers for vertical gaze are located in the pretectal region near the posterior commissure because vertical eye movements can be abolished by selective lesions in this region.[25] From the pretectal area, fibers descend through the medial longitudinal fasciculus to the oculomotor and trochlear nuclei.

The oculocephalic (passive head turning) and oculovestibular (caloric) reflexes are mediated through the vestibular nuclei and are connected to the extraocular muscle nuclei and the pontine paramedian reticular formation by the medial longitudinal fasciculus. In the oculocephalic reflex, afferent information comes from the peripheral vestibular apparatus (primarily the horizontal semicircular canals) and proprioceptive fibers in cervical muscles. Afferent stimulation in the oculovestibular reflex originates in the horizontal semicircular canals. The importance of these reflexes is primarily in demonstrating the intactness of all the brainstem structures involved. If the extraocular movements are full in response to passive head turning or to caloric stimulation, then it can safely be concluded that the comatose patient is not unconscious because of a structural brainstem lesion.

The following guidelines are helpful in localizing lesions within the brain based on determination of extraocular muscle function:

1. Unconscious patients with *diffuse or metabolic encephalopathies* and structurally intact brainstems have random eye movements that are usually conjugate.[28] Random eye movements must be observed for several seconds to be certain of their presence and to be sure that the mean direction is straight ahead. Patients with diffuse encephalopathies initially have intact extraocular (oculocephalic and oculovestibular) reflexes. As coma deepens, the random movements decrease or stop, and the extraocular reflexes disappear.
2. *Large, acute, destructive lesions in one hemisphere* affecting the frontal gaze center or fibers projecting from this center produce conjugate deviation of the eyes toward the side of the lesion and away from the associated hemiparesis. This deviation is most marked in the first few hours after insult and then diminishes rapidly. Within 3 to 4 days, the patient's eyes are usually midline, even though associated neurologic signs may be unchanged. In the acute stages of a large hemispheric lesion, moving the patient's eyes past the midline should be possible using the extraocular reflexes. After 1 to 2 days, the eyes can be moved fully to the "paretic" side with reflex stimulation. Large, destructive hemispheric lesions are the most common cause of tonic, conjugate eye deviation in unconscious patients. Irritative lesions, through the production of partial epilepsy, may stimulate the frontal gaze centers and drive the eyes away from the side of the lesion. In most cases, however, epilepsy producing coma is obvious because of associated clonic or tonic movements.
3. *Acute unilateral lesions in the pontine tegmentum* affecting the pontine paramedian reticular formation also produce tonic deviation of the eyes. In this relatively uncommon situation, the eyes deviate away from the side of the lesion and cannot be moved to the midline by using vigorous oculocephalic or oculovestibular stimulation.
4. *Large bilateral pontine tegmental lesions* affecting the pontine paramedian reticular formation symmetrically produce eyes that are directed straight ahead and that are fixed to extraocular reflexes.
5. *Lesions compressing the brainstem tectum* usually affect the midline center for upward conjugate gaze and produce tonic downward deviation of both eyes. Slight deviation may occur with extraocular reflexes.

Motor Function

An examination of the motor system provides valuable localizing information even though motor tracts are not necessarily adjacent to centers regulating consciousness. The signs and symptoms of motor dysfunction can be divided into two separate groups: (1) loss of function; and (2) release phenomena. Hemiparesis is an example of the former, and decerebrate rigidity is an example of the latter. Since this chapter concerns unconscious patients, the release phenomena are relatively more important. The previously considered neural systems occupy little volume in the central nervous system. By comparison, the motor system, which includes the precentral frontal cortex, motor-association areas, basal ganglia, cerebellum, cortical spinal tracts, and all of the interconnecting pathways, is enormous. Our knowledge of motor system physiology and pathophysiology comes from carefully observed clinicopathologic correlations, ablation experiments in animals and man, and stimulation experiments.[16]

Voluntary movement originates in the precentral frontal cortex. The most direct pathway to the anterior horn cell is through the cortical spinal tract, which courses through the internal capsule, the cerebral peduncles, the pontine base, the pyramid, and the anterior and lateral columns of the spinal cord. Numerous feedback loops modify this system at all levels. Anterior horn cells are constantly bombarded by input from a variety of sources, including muscle spindle and cutaneous afferent fibers. The cerebellar, basal ganglia, brainstem reticular, vestibular, and proprioceptive systems modify either the cortical spinal activity or the motoneurons directly. Through selective destruction of these subsystems or, more properly, the release of some systems to act unchecked, the various motor syndromes are produced.

When the motor system of a patient with impaired consciousness is examined, emphasis is placed on observation, resistance to passive motion, and reflex phenomena. Attention should be given to spontaneous movements or the lack thereof. Many observations about motor responses are made when the physician stimulates the patient to assess the level of consciousness. Those phenomena that are commonly observed in patients with impaired consciousness include purposeful movements toward the stimulus, decorticate posturing, decerebrate posturing, asymmetrical signs such as unilateral flaccidity, and no response at all. One or two joints of each limb should be moved through a full range of motion to assess tone. The tendon reflexes should be checked and plantar responses should be elicited.

Those signs that have localizing value include the following findings.

Paratonia

Paratonia or gegenhalten, is defined as a relatively constant increase in tone in both flexion and extension as if the patient were voluntarily resisting all movements.[28] This is an abnormality seen frequently in elderly, demented patients. Paratonia is differentiated from the rigidity seen in patients with Parkinsonism in whom rigidity is usually associated with "cogwheeling." The presence of paratonia usually indicates diffuse cerebral dysfunction such as might be seen in patients with atrophy or a metabolic encephalopathy.

Decorticate Rigidity

Decorticate rigidity, which may be seen spontaneously or as a response to stimuli, is defined as flexion at the wrist, fingers, thumb, and elbow with adduction at the shoulder and extension at the hip and knee.[16] This posturing mimics that of the chronic hemiplegic, is seen with lesions rostral to the midbrain, and implies a relatively intact brainstem. Decorticate posturing is frequently unilateral and may be opposed by purposeful movements or decerebrate posturing.

Decerebrate Posturing

Decerebrate posturing may also occur spontaneously but is more frequently observed following administration of a noxious stimulus.[28] In the fullest expression, decerebrate posturing includes internal rotation and adduction at the shoulders, opisthotonus (extreme extension of the spine), and contraction of all antigravity muscles in the extremities. Decerebrate posturing differs from decorticate posturing mainly in the upper-extremities where extension replaces flexion. Incomplete responses are common, even with administration of intensely noxious stimuli, and include extension of the spine, internal rotation of the arm, or extension at the wrist. In experimental animals, decerebrate rigidity is produced by transecting the midbrain at the midcollicular level and leaving intact the reticulospinal, vestibulospinal, and cerebellospinal influences on the spinal cord motoneurons. In humans, the level of dysfunction producing decerebration is at least localized to the rostral brainstem.[8] The common causes of decerebrate posturing are: (1) massive hemispheric lesions such as head trauma or large hematoma; (2) transtentorial herniation; (3) superior posterior fossa lesions with upward herniation; and (4) severe metabolic disturbances such as hepatic coma. Decerebrate posturing is an important clinical sign in patients with expanding supratentorial lesions such as subdural hematoma and implies transtentorial herniation.

Flaccidity

Flaccidity (absence of tone) indicates dysfunction at the ponto-medullary levels. Lesions such as pontine hematomas or large ponto-medullary infarcts frequently cause this response. Flaccidity may also be seen in patients with acute spinal cord transections ("spinal shock"), with diffuse motor-unit dysfunction (muscle relaxants such as curare), and with severe metabolic disturbances such as profound barbiturate intoxication.

LABORATORY EVALUATION

The laboratory evaluation of patients with reduced consciousness is important in confirming or establishing an etiology. The laboratory evaluations that are generally useful are as follows:

1. Blood—complete blood count, blood urea nitrogen, glucose, sodium, potassium, calcium, magnesium, liver function, arterial blood gases, and toxicology screen
2. Urine/gastric contents—toxicology screen
3. Computed tomography of brain
4. Electroencephalogram
5. Lumbar puncture
6. Cerebral angiography

Each test should be ordered for a specific indication. None of the tests, alone or in combination, is intended to replace the bedside evaluation.

Blood Tests

A battery of blood tests (including evaluation of complete blood count, blood urea nitrogen, glucose, serum electrolytes, liver function, and arterial blood gases) is usually performed for all comatose patients and is a screen for determining the cause of metabolic encephalopathies. Since many of these blood tests are repeated throughout the course of management of critical care patients, this initial set also serves as a baseline. Most physicians use a toxicology screen of blood, urine, and gastric contents, particularly in patients with apparent diffuse or metabolic encephalopathies. More specific determinations such as serum barbiturate levels are indicated, depending on the degree they are suspected. It would not be cost effective, for example, to order expensive toxicology determinations in patients with obvious structural brain disease.

Computed Tomography

Computed tomography (CT) of the brain is also judged by many neurologists to be a screening test for patients who have experienced a recent onset of reduced consciousness. CT, which images the distribution of tissue radiodensity, has revolutionized the practice of neurology.[24] Small differrences in x-ray absorption exist between cerebrospinal fluid, white matter, gray matter, and most central nervous system structural lesions such as tumor or infarct. Much larger differences exist between brain, air, blood, and calcified material. In most institutions, scans of the head are done before and after the intravenous administration of an iodinated contrast agent. Such administration results in a substantial iodine level in the extracellular space of lesions that have an impaired blood-brain barrier. Thus contrast enhancement causes many focal lesions to "light up." Almost all supratentorial and infratentorial lesions large enough to cause coma can be visualized by the late-generation scanners. CT is particularly useful in visualizing intracerebral hematomas, subdural hematomas or infections, cerebral tumors, and cerebral edema. Cerebral infarcts may be more difficult to visualize in the first 2 to 3 days, but the diagnosis of an infarct can usually be made on clinical grounds, particularly if a hematoma is excluded by CT. In most cases, CT obviates the need for more invasive brain examinations such as angiography. CT, therefore, is probably the most important laboratory investigation to use for patients with coma and should be performed early in the course of the patient's illness.

Electroencephalography

An electroencephalogram (EEG) is a voltage vs. time graph composed of from 8 to 16 parallel, complex lines. Each line represents the activity in one channel, i.e., from one amplifier. At a single point in time, the activity in any one channel is simply the potential difference between two scalp electrodes. Waves that are recorded from the scalp represent summated synaptic potentials from cells near the cortical surface.[23] When electrode pairs are systematically arranged in groups (montages), a topographic array of cortical surface electrical activity is produced. EEG is most useful in correlation with and in confirmation of the clinical diagnosis of seizure disorders. However, the examination has some usefulness in patients with reduced consciousness. EEG provides an indirect measure of cerebral function and response to stimulation and as such provides proof of an organic encephalopathy. The only way to establish the diagnosis of status epilepticus when convulsions are absent is through the use of EEG. EEG is an aid in the definition of cerebral death and may provide prognostic information in patients with a severe encephalopathy.[14,29] Patients with little or no EEG response to noxious stimuli have a very poor prognosis no matter what the cause of the encephalopathy. Generalized triphasic waves are seen in EEGs of patients with hepatic and other metabolic encephalopathies. Periodic sharp-wave discharges may also be observed in patients with encephalitides such as Creutzfeldt-Jakob disease. In summary, EEG may have some usefulness in the diagnosis of patients with coma, particularly in those who have diffuse encephalopathies, but it is not a routine test to be ordered without forethought. In many cases, a competent electroencephalographer can aid the clinician in deciding whether the EEG will be useful in any particular patient.

Lumbar Puncture

A lumbar puncture (LP) provides the clinician with the cellular and chemical composition of the cerebrospinal fluid (CSF) and a crude measure of the CSF but not necessarily intracranial pressure.[7,27] The two diagnoses that can be confirmed with confidence using LP are meningitis and subarachnoid hemorrhage. Therefore the two major indications for an LP in patients with clouding of consciousness are evidence of meningeal inflammation and an elevated temperature. However, most patients with coma of unknown etiology will eventually need an LP. It is important to realize that the lumbar puncture is invasive and can be deleterious or fatal to patients with intracranial herniation syndromes. An LP is contraindicated when there is evidence of uncal herniation (ipsilateral oculomotor palsy and contralateral hemiparesis), tonsillar herniation (rigid head tilt or neck retraction), or central transtentorial herniation (midposition light-fixed pupils, Cheyne-Stokes respiration, and decerebrate posturing). In patients with coagulation defects, papilledema, or suspected mass lesions, the risk of an LP must be carefully compared with the possible information to be gained.[27] Most clinicians avoid performing LPs in patients with focal neurologic signs and obtain a CT scan before performing an LP in any unconscious patient. It is inexcusable to miss a treatable purulent meningitis. Comfort is derived from the fact that, other than the elderly or immunosuppressed, most adult patients with purulent meningitis have meningeal signs.

Cerebral Angiography

Cerebral angiography provides an image of the blood space (vasculature) in the intracranial and extracranial areas.[24] However, neurologic specialists are very restrictive in their use of angiography as a diagnostic tool. In most instances, angiography is limited to those patients who are being considered for carotid surgery or neurosurgery. A good indication for its use would be to delineate the blood supply of a meningioma before its removal. There is limited usefulness for angiography in almost all patients with coma or clouding of consciousness. For instance, angiography is not ordinarily performed in comatose patients with suspected subarachnoid hemorrhage. A CT scan gives the clinician all the information needed for the patient's initial management. Cerebral arteritis is one of the few diagnoses that can be made exclusively with angiography. Almost all other structural lesions that cause clouding of consciousness can be seen better with CT.

Radionuclide Studies

Radionuclide studies such as the older static brain scan are included in this section for historic interest only. The radionuclide brain scan provided an indistinct image of large cerebral venous channels and areas of blood-brain barrier breakdown.[24] Both of these conditions can be much better appreciated on a CT scan after an intravenous contrast injection. Rapid head scanning after bolus intravenous injection of a radionuclide provides a crude image of blood flow in major cerebral vessels and is used in some centers as an aid in the diagnosis of cerebral death.[29]

THE TREATMENT OF PATIENTS WITH DISTURBED CONSCIOUSNESS

The treatment of specific conditions that cause coma or reduced consciousness is beyond the scope of this chapter. However, recognition of the etiology of coma carries a pointed objective—treat and remove the cause. The rationale of some of the modes of therapy are discussed in the following sections.

Supratentorial Mass Lesions

Patients with supratentorial mass lesions secondarily causing coma through transtentorial herniation must be treated early in the course of their reduced consciousness. If not, they will eventually develop secondary brainstem (Duret) hemorrhages, which are usually fatal.[28] The exact treatment of these lesions depends on their specific cause, but some generalities can be made. In most emergency situations, i.e., when a patient is brought to the emergency room, it must be assumed that the supratentorial lesion is acute and treatable. After first stabilizing the patient's vital signs, most physicians empirically treat the patient for cerebral edema. The patient will be intubated, controlled hyperventilation will be instituted, mannitol will be administered, and high doses of intravenous glucosteroids will be administered.[11,21] These remedies frequently "buy time" until the exact diagnosis can be made by using CT and more specific therapy can begin. It is important to recognize which patients are potentially salvageable and which ones will succumb no matter how much treatment is administered. Patients who are still posturing are salvageable and should be treated vigorously until it is proved that the offending lesion, such as a large central hematoma, is untreatable. Patients with treatable lesions, particularly subdural or epidural hematomas, should be taken to surgery as soon as possible after the diagnosis is made. The patient who has developed pontine signs (generalized flaccidity, pinpoint pupils, extraocular movements that are fixed to ocular reflexes, and sustained hyperventilation) from transtentorial herniation is not salvageable and will usually die even when given vigorous support.[17]

Supratentorial Lesions

Subtentorial lesions cause coma by direct involvement or compression of the reticular activating areas in the rostral brainstem. No interventional therapy is possible for large intrinsic lesions such as a brainstem infarct or hematoma. However, similar symptoms may be produced by lesions "extrinsic" to the brainstem such as a cerebellar hematoma. Surgical drainage of such a hematoma is life saving and may result in the patient's full recovery. The emergency treatment of coma secondary to a structural lesion in the posterior fossa is similar to that used in patients with supratentorial lesions. Intubation is perhaps even more imperative since many patients with supratentorial lesions have irregular, ineffective respirations. Controlled hyperventilation and administration of hyperosmolar agents and intravenous steroids are indicated and are usually administered at the same time the patient is being transported for CT to determine a definitive diagnosis. If a surgically treatable lesion is found and if the patient does not exhibit flaccidity and unresponsiveness, immediate decompression is indicated. If the lesion is intrinsic to the brainstem, such as infarct or hematoma, only supportive care is indicated. Patients who exhibit unresponsive flaccidity from a subtentorial lesion have the same poor prognosis as do similar patients with supratentorial lesions.

Metabolic or Diffuse Encephalopathies

The treatment of patients with metabolic or diffuse encephalopathies is important because this category constitutes the largest group of comatose patients and many of them have a potentially reversible condition. In addition, patients with diffuse encephalopathies are likely to be seen originally by nonneurologic specialists whose job it is to preserve the brain from permanent damage. If available, the patient's history frequently indicates the cause of the encephalopathy. Patients with metabolic encephalopathies often have asterixis, multifocal myoclonus (nonstereotyped, arrhythmic, asynchronous, twitching movements that occur multifocally in many muscle groups—particularly the facial and proximal extremity muscles), tremor, and seizures. Many patients hypoventilate or hyperventilate, but the irregular or periodic respirations of patients with structural lesions are usually not present. In general, patients with metabolic encephalopathies have no focal signs.

After a rapid initial appraisal of the patient and stabilization of vital signs, blood and urine for the metabolic studies listed in the section "Laboratory Evaluation," p. 759, should be obtained. Then 50 ml of 50% glucose is usually immediately administered in the event that hypoglycemia is the cause of the coma. If the patient is febrile or immunosuppressed, a lumbar puncture is indicated after the vital signs are stabilized. If acid/base imbalances are present, particularly acute metabolic acidosis, treatment must be begun early to prevent cardiac arrhythmias. Alcohol or sedative drug abuse is the most common cause of stupor and coma in emergency room patients, so the toxicology screen will probably be diagnostic. If the patient is comatose and a sedative drug overdose is the probable cause, gastric lavage is indicated after the administration of cuffed endotracheal intubation. In most patients with metabolic encephalopathies, the diagnosis is obvious after the initial screening laboratory evaluation. If not, the most likely diagnoses are postanoxic encephalopathies or postictal (seizure) depression. When no diagnosis can be reached, patients are usually supported maximally.

FUTURE DIRECTIONS

Two recent technologic developments—positron emission tomography (PET) and magnetic resonance imaging or spectroscopy—promise to provide new, previously unobtainable information about brain function during altered consciousness. PET is based on the detection of the products of positron emission from atoms that label a molecule, the behavior of which is to be investigated. The images are similar to those of CT but depict tracer content rather than tissue density. With the aid of appropriate data collection, strategies, and mathematic models of physiologic processes such as blood flow or glucose metabolism, the PET image of isotope concentration can be transformed into an image of flow or metabolism. This technique has provided valuable information about brain metabolism during stroke or in epileptic foci but is too expensive, cumbersome, and complex for routine clinical use.

Magnetic resonance imaging is based on the detection of electromagnetic energy released by the nuclei of atoms after perturbations in very strong, controlled magnetic fields. Clinically useful images related to the behavior of protons are now available in many centers and can be used to detect plaques in multiple sclerosis and to measure intraluminal blood flow in moderate-sized blood vessels. Additional applications will be forthcoming. Magnetic resonance spectra from nuclei other than protons have been recorded in experimental laboratories and may ultimately provide bedside information about the brain metabolism and physiology. At the present time, most magnetic resonance and PET investigations in research laboratories are likely to produce information that will lead to better treatment for patients in clinical settings without requiring every hospital to have these complex technologies.

SUMMARY

This chapter presents an approach to the examination of unconscious patients that is based on neuroanatomic, physiologic, and biochemical principles. Consciousness is mediated by the reticular activating system and the sum of the activity of the cerebral hemispheres. Consciousness may be altered by a variety of medical and surgical problems such as infarction and trauma that destroy brain tissue directly or by biochemical abnormalities that remove required metabolites, introduce toxins, or alter the internal cerebral environment, thus impairing brain metabolism and producing abnormalities of brain function. Typically, structural abnormalities of the brain produce focal neurologic signs that permit localization of the abnormality to a specific brain region. On the other hand, metabolic abnormalities are characterized by nonfocal signs of brain dysfunction. Pupillary light reactivity and ocular motility are the most useful clinical signs for making this differential diagnosis—absent function implies a structural lesion, but even minimum function usually presists with severe metabolic disturbances. Obtaining a prompt, accurate diagnosis for patients with altered consciousness is essential before the physician initiates the appropriate medical or surgical therapy to arrest or reverse the pathophysiologic process causing coma and to avoid or minimize irreversible neurologic deficits.

REFERENCES

1. Berger, A.J,, Mitchell, R.A., and Severinghaus, J.W.: Regulation of respiration, N. Engl. J. Med. **297:**92, 1977.
2. Braun, C.M., and Pivik, R.T.: Effects of brainstem lesions on tonic immobility in the rabbit (Oryctolagus cuniculus), Brain Res. Bull. **10:**127, 1983.
3. Brodal, A.: Neurological anatomy, New York, 1981, Oxford University Press.
4. Brown, H.W., and Plum, F.: The neurologic basis of Cheyne-Stokes respiration, Am. J. Med. **30:**849, 1961.
5. Cherniack, N.S., et al.: Experimentally induced Cheyne-Stokes breathing, Respir. Physiol. **37:**185, 1979.
6. Cooper, J.R., Bloom, F.E., and Roth, R.H.: The biochemical basis of neuropharmacology, ed. 4, New York, 1982, Oxford University Press.
7. Cutler, R.W., and Spertell, R.B.: Cerebrospinal fluid: a selective review, Ann. Neurol. **11:**1, 1982.
8. Davis, R.H., and Davis, L.: Decerebrate rigidity in humans, Neurosurgery **10:**635, 1982.
9. De Jong, R.N.: The neurological examination, ed. 4, Hagerstown, 1979, Harper and Row Publishers, Inc.
10. Fisher, C.M.: The neurological examination of the comatose patient, Acta Neurol. Scand. **45**(suppl 36):1, 1969.
11. Fishman, R.: Steroids in the treatment of brain edema, N. Engl. J. Med. 306:359, 1982.
12. French, J.D.: Brain lesions with prolonged unconsciousness, Arch. Neurol. Psychiatry **68:**727, 1952.
13. French, J.D., and Magoun, H.W.: Effects of chronic lesions in central cephalic brainstem of monkeys, Arch. Neurol. Psychiatry **68:**591, 1952.
14. Gloor, P., Kalabay, O., and Giard, N.: The electroencephalogram in diffuse encephalopathies: EEG correlates of grey and white matter lesions. Brain **91:**779, 1968.
15. Jennett, W.B., and Plum, F.: The persistent vegetative state: a syndrome in search of a name, Lancet **1:**734, 1972.
16. Lance, J.W.: The control of muscle tone, reflexes and movement: Robert Wartenberg lecture, Neurology **30:**1303, 1980.
17. Levy, D.E., et al.: Prognosis in nontraumatic coma, Ann. Intern. Med. **94:**293, 1981.
18. Lockwood, A.H.: Acute and chronic hyperosmolality: effects on cerebral amino acids and energy metabolism, Arch. Neurol. **32:**62, 1975.
19. Lockwood, A.H.: Ammonia-induced encephalopathy. In McCandless, D., editor: Cerebral energy metabolism and metabolic encephalopathy, New York, 1985, Plenum Publishing Corp.
20. Lowry, O.H., et al.: Effect of ischemia on known substrates and cofactors of the glycolytic pathway in the brain, J. Biol. Chem. **239:**18, 1964.
21. McGraw, C.P., and Howard, G.: Effect of mannitol on increased intracranial pressure, Neurosurgery **13:**269, 1983.
22. Moruzzi, G., and Magoun, H.W.: Brainstem reticular formation and activation of EEG, Electroencephalogr. Clin. Electrophysiol. **1:**445, 1949.
23. Niedermeyer, E., and deSilva, F.L.: Electroencephalography, Baltimore, 1982, Urban & Schwarzenberg, Inc.
24. Oldendorf, W.H.: The quest for an image of brain: a brief historical and technical review of brain imaging techniques, Neurology **28:**517, 1978.
25. Pasik, P., Pasik, T., and Bender, M.B.: The pretectal syndrome in monkeys, Brain **92:**521, 871, 1969.
26. Peele, T.L.: The neuroanatomic basis for clinical neurology, ed. 3, New York, 1977, McGraw-Hill Book Co.
27. Petito, F., and Plum, F.: The lumbar puncture, N. Engl. J. Med. **290:**225, 1974.
28. Plum, F., and Posner, J.B.: The diagnosis of stupor and coma, ed. 3, Philadelphia, 1980, F.A. Davis Co.
29. President's commission for the study of ethical problems in medicine and biomedical and behavioral research: guidelines for the determination of death, JAMA **246:**2184, 1981.
30. Reeves, A.G., and Posner, J.B.: The ciliospinal response in man, Neurology **19:**1145, 1969.
31. Rymer, M., and Fishman, R.A.: Protective adaptation of brain to water intoxication, Arch. Neurol. **28:**49, 1973.
32. Shafar, J.: The syndromes of the third neurone of the cervical sympathetic system, Am. J. Med. **40:**97, 1966.
33. Siesjo, B.K., et al.: Brain dysfunction in cerebral hypoxia and ischemia, Res. Publ. Assoc. Res. Nerv. Ment. Dis. **53:**75, 1974.

47

Donald P. Becker, Larry W. Jenkins, and Lennart Rabow

Pathophysiology of Head Trauma

Traumatic injury to the brain creates a complex interaction of primary and secondary processes that may require days to evolve. The secondary processes and related to the magnitude and the type of traumatic injury and the resulting systemic and neural complications. Thus the ultimate brain injury that is incurred may result not only from direct mechanical injury but from other complications imposed by additional factors or insults (e.g., apnea, arterial hypotension or hypertension, intracranial hypertension, and subarachnoid, subdural, and/or epidural hemorrhage), which may result in secondary brain hypoxia, ischemia, and/or edema. Thus the causes of traumatic brain injury represent a multitude of factors that may vary in their temporal and spatial relationships.

Because of the frequency of occurrence of secondary ischemia and hypoxia in human head trauma, the pathophysiology of trauma and of ischemia is sometimes considered as one. There are important distinctions to be made, however, and it is useful to make a comparison of the injury mechanisms between these two situations alone and in combination. It is also useful to distinguish between mechamisms of injury that result in cell dysfunction but are compatible with cell viability vs. those mechanisms that interfere with cell function but also have lethal consequences for the cell. This distinction is important because, even if the point is reached where effective strategies can be designed that increase cellular survival after neural trauma, such cells must also be able to resume function if they are to contribute to an improvement in the recovery of brain function and if their survival is to have significance.

Several major mechanisms of tissue injury have been identified in the pathologic processes such as ischemia, hypoxia, status epilepticus, and hypoglycemia. These mechanisms have been emphasized in several recent reviews, which should be consulted for more details.[5,76-78]

BASIC MECHANISMS OF BRAIN INJURY

The brain injury represents the most serious problem in head trauma. Brain injuries from head trauma range from mild, in which a person is momentarily stunned and sees "stars," to severe, in which extensive brainstem damage rapidly leads to death. Brain injuries produce various degrees of pathologic damage, ranging from cellular and subcellular reversible injury to shearing and tearing of brain cells and even disruption of brain tissue by contusion, brain hemorrhage, or laceration. The lesions vary in location and degree from patient to patient. Following the initial brain damage, the brain may be further damaged by secondary hypoxemia resulting from respiratory distress, cerebral ischemia from elevated intracranial pressure, or brain shift caused by accumulation of an intracranial hematoma or brain swelling. Definition of the locations, extent, and nature of the brain damage must be sought, treatment must be planned accordingly.

The most common mechanisms of brain injury are brain movement and deformation within the skull—the "acceleration-deceleration" injury. In deceleration injury, the rapidly moving head is suddenly stopped, such as occurs in an auto-tree collision. The skull movement is immediately arrested, but the gelatinous and viscoelastic brain continues to move during a 20-msec time period. The brain may also rotate in the skull around the axis of the brainstem. Different loci of the brain substance are deformed to different degrees, and internal shearing and stress forces can traumatize and disrupt cells and their process in the depths of the brain. If blood vessels are not disrupted, there may be no intracerebral hemorrhage, even in patients with severe injury that leads to early death. The immediate loss of consciousness results from the deformation affecting the brainstem and its reticular activating system.

In acceleration injury, the head is suddenly accelerated, such as occurs during a boxing injury when the head jolts backward and inertial forces strike the still unmoving brain against the accelerating skull. If the brainstem cells have been severely traumatized, the victim may remain unconscious for days or longer. If the brainstem trauma was mild, he may be unconscious for just a few seconds or less than a minute. In this case most of the traumatized brain cells are presumed to recover.

The other major mechanism of brain damage is direct tissue injury under the site of impact. Extensive local brain injury can occur even among patients who remain alert. For example, a crushing injury to a fixed head can drive a large plate of skull inward and destroy a large area of the hemispheres, yet the patient need not lose consciousness despite focal neurologic signs of injury (i.e., weakness or visual loss). With the head fixed, only the directly traumatized cerebrum is damaged; the brainstem is not deformed, and there is no loss of consciousness.

Varieties of Brain Injury

"Conclusion" describes head trauma associated with brief unconsciousness but with no physical signs in the sensorimotor systems or observed through radiographic tests to indicate residual structural brain damage. Brief vegetative paralysis may occur at the moment of impact. The physiologic basis for the loss of consciousness and the rapid recovery is not well understood, but sudden diffuse neurotransmitter release has been postulated.

Gunshot wounds cause brain damage along the tract of

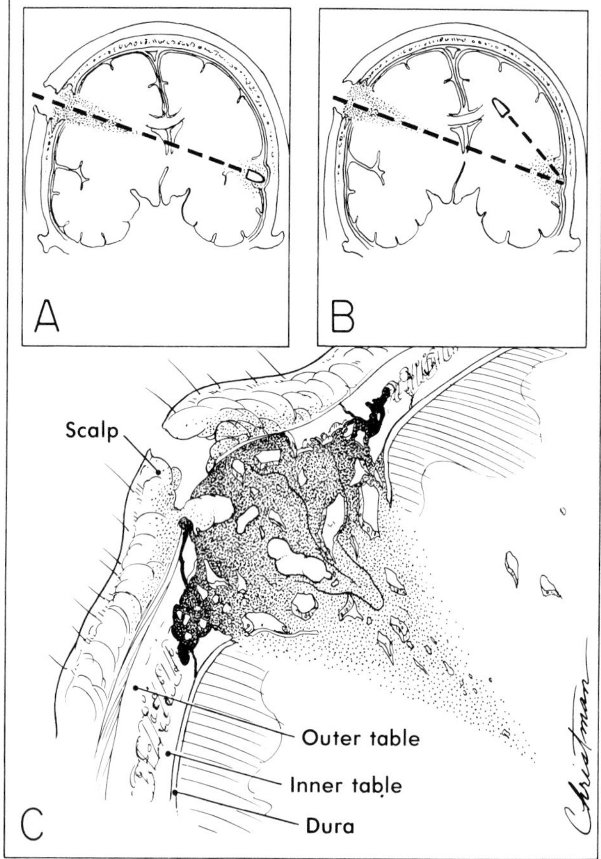

Fig. 47-1 Gunshot wound. **A,** The usual kind of path that a missile follows when traversing the brain. **B,** The capability of a missile, once traversing the brain substance, to bounce off the bony skull and cause further damage. **C,** The energy forces extending radially from the missile path and the extensive diffuse damage that can result therefrom.

the missile and extending radially outward from the path in proportion to the size and velocity of the missile. The shock wave will cause loss of consciousness if it reaches the brainstem with sufficient force (Fig. 47-1).

Most mild brain injuries are caused by acceleration or deceleration brain movement. The mildest form is represented by a sensation of being dazed or stunned that lasts seconds to several minutes. The next degree is immediate unconsciousness. With a clean knockout blow, there is prompt flaccidity in the patient accompanied by apnea, bradycardia, and widely dilated pupils that are unresponsive to light. Rarely a generalized seizure follows the blow. Oculovestibular reflexes may be lost transiently. In experimental animals given this "mild" injury, simultaneous transient arterial hypertension and slowing of the electroencephalograph occur. The signs and symptoms usually resolve within 30 to 60 seconds, and the individual progressively becomes oriented.

The duration of postconcussion signs and symptoms is variable and is related to the intensity of the blow and the degree of brain deformity. Recovery from mild injury takes place within 3 to 5 minutes. With stronger blows the physiologic response can be prolonged, and apneic periods lasting 8 to 12 minutes following the blow have been recorded in humans with subsequent excellent recovery. Nevertheless, a major cause of death from acute head injury is prolonged apnea that progresses successively to hypoxemia, arterial hypertension, hypotension, and cardiac arrest. Early artificial respiration administered by a well-trained rescue worker undoubtedly saves some lives.

Most persons who lose consciousness probably suffer at least some irreversible injury to brain cells. Although most of the traumatized cells rapidly regain normal function, some recover only over a protracted period of time, and others never do. The "punchdrunk" boxer shows evidence of the cumulative effect of recurrent brain damage. Affected persons are dysarthric, absentminded, and argumentative. They have difficulty concentrating, have a poor memory for recent events, and walk on a wide base with a stiff, spastic gait.

Within minutes after the injury, patients with mild brain trauma are characteristically alert and oriented. They can usually describe what they were doing up to the moments before the injury and have little or no retrograde amnesia. They rarely remember the blow itself and often cannot remember events that occurred for up to 10 minutes after the accident. This period of memory loss following the injury is called the time of antegrade amnesia or posttraumatic amnesia.

Patients with moderate brain injury characteristically remain lethargic or stuporous after emerging from periods of unconsciousness lasting 5 to 10 minutes or more. They are often intermittently restless and sometimes combative but return to sleep if undisturbed. They may speak in short sentences or phrases or repeatedly say the same word. Most are sufficiently in contact to follow at least a simple single-stage command. Some have symptoms of a mild-to-moderate delirious reaction. Although a mild focal neurologic deficit such as a hemiparesis may exist, these patients do not show signs of motor posturing such as decorticate or decerebrate positioning of the limbs spontaneously or in response to noxious stimuli.

Patients with moderate brain injury usually make a reasonably satisfactory recovery even when they have suffered subarachnoid hemorrhage, cerebral contusions, or a small intracerebral hematoma. A few have reduced mental performance, which reflects the presence of permanent brain damage. Over a period of several days to 1 to 2 weeks, these patients gradually recover orientation and alertness. Mild focal neurologic deficits usually disappear. However, during the acute stages these patients are vulnerable to secondary brain insults from respiratory insufficiency and hypoxemia, the growth of an intracranial blood clot, or development of brain edema, and they require close observation and carefully applied medical care.

With severe brain injury, patients do not regain consciousness for at least 20 minutes and often much longer after injury. When seen at the hospital, they do not speak understandable words or follow simple commands. This state remains after cardiopulmonary resuscitation. Other serious neurologic signs are common, and prognosis is related largely to evidence of brainstem injury. Motor posturing (decorticate and decerebrate responses) indicating extensive deep cerebral injury occurs in 30% of these patients. Decerebrate (extensor) posturing denotes a poorer prognosis than decorticate posturing. Impaired eye movements in response to the doll's eye maneuver (oculocephalic test) or to ice water irrigation of the ear canal (oculovestibular test) are seen in 40% of patients in this group and represents brainstem damage or, less often, inner ear or cranial nerve III, IV, VI, or VIII injury. Bilateral pupillary unresponsiveness to light also signifies brainstem damage. Bilateral decerebrate (extensor) posturing with impaired or absent oculocephalic responses implies a very extensive brain injury involving both the hemispheres and the brainstem. Most such severely damaged patients (80%) die, and the survivors can be expected to remain severely disabled or vegetative, even in the absence of an intracranial hematoma or elevated intracranial pressure.

Patients with decerebrate motor posturing but with normal eye movements have a less extensive brain injury and sometimes recover well. Likewise, patients with normal motor responses to noxious stimuli but who have impaired eye movements or fixed pupils occasionally recover well because of the more limited extent of the brain damage. Patients with severe head injury who have normal withdrawal or normal flexor response of their limbs to noxious stimuli can be expected to recover well unless they harbor an intracranial mass lesion that causes a major brain shift or elevates intracranial pressure to levels over 40 mm Hg for a prolonged period or unless they develop systemic complications such as septic shock or pulmonary edema. The presence of flaccidity or paralysis of all four limbs in response to noxious stimuli may be caused by a concomitant spinal cord injury, but even if related to the brain injury, flaccidity is an ominous sign.

Approximately 40% of patients with severe brain injury harbor an intracranial hematoma that causes brain compression and displacement as well as a high intracranial pressure. These patients almost always require prompt surgery to evacuate the mass lesion. If the physician waits for signs of neurologic deterioration, further permanent brain damage will usually occur. Patients who are initially seen with bilateral decerebrate posturing, impaired eye movements, and pupils fixed in response to light can, on rare occasions, recover if they are harboring a subdural or epidural hematoma and the clot is quickly evacuated. Unless checked by prompt treatment, such expanding masses threaten to produce potentially fatal uncal or central transtentorial herniation. It is imperative that the signs of impending transtentorial herniation be recognized because rapid appropriate treatment with osmotic diuretics and surgical evacuation of a mass can save life and, perhaps more important, brain function.

Sublethal Functional and Metabolic Derangements Following Traumatic Brain Injury

Frequently the injuries produced in head-injury models are so severe that it is not possible to sort out the primary effects of mechanical injury from those of secondary insults such as ischemia and hypoxia. Consequently, with severe traumatic injury it is extremely difficult to determine cause and effect because so many factors become involved that the isolation of individual variables for scientific study is severely compromised. Examining the historic difficulty of the study of human head injury quickly convinces the researcher of the complex pathophysiology involved. Experimental models that mimic this complexity are certainly relevant to the human situation and serve as more appropriate vehicles for examining the full spectrum of events involved in clinical head injury and for testing preclinical therapeutic regimens. However, such models are usually too complex for the study of isolated molecular mechanisms of injury. Thus head-injury models that allow for graded injury and in which secondary insults can be either minimized or prevented offer a better chance to isolate cause-and-effect relationships.

The study of mild-to-moderate injury in these models additionally affords the opportunity to identify those mechanisms producing the initial metabolic and functional derangements that may prove causative in the generation of irreversible traumatic brain injury but that may be obscured at higher injury levels. The fluid percussion head-injury model, in which cerebral trauma is produced by the release of a weighted pendulum that pounds a saline-filled plexiglas column, is particularly well suited for the study of mild-to-moderate trauma without extensive secondary complications. Results from fluid percussion injury will be emphasized, not only because of our familiarity with this model, but because there is substantial documentation that at mild-to-moderate injury levels ischemia and hypoxia are not involved. Thus we can be relatively confident that the pnenomenon to be discussed is the result of trauma uncomplicated by ischemia and hypoxia.

The measurement of both regional and total cerebral blood flow in the fluid percussion head-injury model has demonstrated that ischemia does not occur acutely following injury.[14,44,45] Furthermore, acute studies of the redox state of cytochrome oxidase (the last cytochrome in the electron transport chain) following injury have also confirmed that there is no limitation of oxygen that would impair or limit mitochondrial function.[15,69] Finally, acute metabolite studies of various substrates and products of the energy production pathway do not demonstrate cerebral ischemia or hypoxia.[90] Thus there is significant documentation that ischemia or hypoxia do not consitute a part of the mild-to-moderate traumatic insult acutely.[30] Although changes in autoregulation and vascular responsiveness to carbon dioxide and oxygen are altered acutely,[39,44,45] preliminary studies have demonstrated no secondary reductions in cerebral blood flow during the first 24 hours following trauma. In chronic studies with survival periods of a few days to 6 weeks, no morphologic changes that are indicative of hypoxia or ischemia have been observed in any brain region.

The fluid percussion model at mild and moderate injury levels produces primarily a concussive injury. There is a transient period of unconsciousness followed by periods of faulty locomotion and escape responses, nonresponsiveness to visual stimuli and a general decrease in resting muscle tone, altered righting and placing reactions, and increased reflex thresholds that last up to 12 hours after injury. Following 48 hours of posttraumatic survival, the animals had completely recovered from such behavioral deficits.[23]

Thus, on the basis of conventional neurologic criteria, mild-to-moderate fluid percussion injury appears to result in a concussion in which overt neurologic changes are transient. However, in contrast to the more classical concept of concussion in which transient unconsciousness is produced without any persistent cellular damage, there is some persistent structural damage observed even with mild fluid percussion injury within the brainstem that consists of axonal injury with occasional neuronal-somal changes.[66] Subtle axonal changes are observed within the first hour following trauma at the ultrastructural level, but longer periods of survival (12 to 24 hours) were required before reactive axonal swellings and the formation of classical retraction balls were seen. However, most injury of this type in the fluid percussion model has been confined to the brainstem with apparent sparing of the supratentorial compartment. This finding is consistent with the predilection of brainstem structural injury in this model when uncomplicated by secondary ischemia but does not necessarily hold true for metabolic dysfunction. Morphologic examination of various regions of the neocortex not directly under the injury site, of the caudate nucleus, and of the hippocampal cortices after survival from hours to 21 days following mild-to-moderate fluid percussion has not revealed any evidence of neuronal cell death or even obvious structural change at the light microscopic level in high-resolution, 2-micron plastic sections. As previously discussed, no evidence of morphologic changes indicative of cerebral ischemia and hypoxia have been seen in any brain region including areas traditionally vulnerable to ischemia or in brainstem regions. Quantitative studies are presently underway to confirm that there is no undetected progressive or delayed neuronal cell loss in these supratentorial structures. Structural changes, which result from the production of prostaglandins and the generation of free radicals, have also been found in the cerebral vasculature.[66]

Jane and associates[29] have that, even reported following mild head injury in patients who overtly recover neurologically, a substantial number may display persistent functional deficits (including information-processing abnormalities) at 3-month posttrauma evaluations. A number of impairments of mental function have been reported following concussive head injury and have been referred collectively as the ''postconcussional syndrome.'' Symptoms include memory deficits, headaches, dizziness, mental fatigue, and irritability as well as depression. These symptoms were originally thought to involve psychologic processes since concussion was considered not to result in structural damage.[33]

Based on the findings that axonal injury is consistently present even after mild injury in both the cat and the primate, such functional deficits have been attributed to axonal damage that occurs after even minor head injury.[29,66] This conclusion is also consistent with the suggestions of Gennarelli and associates[20] that link the extent of diffuse axonal injury with the duration of traumatic coma and the degree of functional damage in head injury. Substantial evidence has now accumulated from studies by these investigators that the extent of axonal injury correlates with the magnitude of the neurologic deficits following trauma. However, temporal and spatial correlation of two variables does not necessarily confirm cause and effect. Obviously, a decrease in information flow through axonal interruption has important functional consequences in an organ whose primary function is the flow, storage, and processing of information, and the importance of axonal injury cannot be denied. However, as pointed out by Povlishock,[66] functional failure may also occur in axons that remain intact, and the possibility of functional changes in other neuronal sites, such as at the synapse in both the presynaptic and the dendritic and somal postsynaptic membrane domains, exists. Additionally, functional changes may exist where no obvious structural change occurs, and to view even mild traumatic injury only as a diffuse axonal injury is probably an oversimplification.

Recent studies of mild fluid percussion trauma in which the activation of certain cholinergic pontine nuclei have been linked with postconcussive unconsciousness support this latter contention. Following concussive injury, an increase in glucose uptake and presumably in functional activity was observed in certain pontine nuclei when glucose uptake and functional activity were depressed in other brain regions. If these same nuclei were microinjected with the acetylcholine agonist carbachol in healthy cats, behavioral suppression and unconsciousness similar to that seen following concussion were observed. The effects of carbachol microinjections could be antagonized with atropine.[23] Such studies demonstrate the potential for changes in neurotransmitter functions following trauma to produce marked functional changes. Although the anatomic projections of these pontine nuclei are unknown, changes that produce a postsynaptic spatial or temporal input imbalance of neurotransmitters and/or neuromodulators can result in pronounced functional consequences following trauma even in the absence of obvious structural damage. However, one of the major questions to be answered is—can irreversible long-term changes in function be mediated without structural damage, by changes in the existing mechanisms for information flow and signal transduction between and within neurons?

Memory and Learning

The processes of memory and learning remain poorly understood. Several mechanisms for these processes have been proposed including the growth and formation of new synapses, reverberating circuitry, the swelling of both presynaptic and postsynaptic processes, and the modification of existing circuits by increased usage. Existing evidence suggests that the hippocampus is involved in the formation and retrieval of memory and that the cerebral cortex is associated with the storage of information.[47] Three types of processes appear to mediate and interact in the encoding and storage of memory: (1) recall of immediate events; (2) short-term memory of events that occurred within hours or seconds in the past; and (3) long-term memory of the remote past. The memory of recent events is frequently impaired in patients with some neurologic diseases and traumatic concussion, but remote memory can persist even in patients with severe brain damage. Retrograde amnesia of immediate events preceding neural trauma is common, and it lasts longer in humans than animals. Such memory loss may persist from days to years with long-term memory remaining intact. Lesion studies and the association of short-term memory loss with the hippocampus have provided considerable evidence that the encoding of memory occurs in the hippocampus and associated structures. The process responsible for the stable long-term memory mechanism is unknown, but it has been speculated that its resistance to injury and disease may be mediated by biochemical storage involving protein synthesis. There is evidence that protein synthesis inhibitors do interfere with the encoding of memory, and it has been proposed that the synthesis of new proteins in response to memory-induced biochemical changes may alter aspects of synaptic function such as transmitter synthesis, receptor sites, or ion channels.[19]

Mitochondrial Function Following Fluid Percussion Injury

Rosenthal and colleagues[69] have demonstrated that immediately after fluid percussion injury, there is increased oxidation of cytochrome oxidase (cyt aa_3) which persists for up to 15 minutes. This response is also seen in a number of conditions that result in an increased energy demand and an enhanced glycolytic and respiratory chain flux such as occurs during increased electrical stimulation, spreading cortical depression, and seizure activity.[69] Although there are a number of possible mechanisms for increased oxidation of cyt aa_3 during this acute posttraumatic period, we suggest the most likely candidates are increased metabolic carbon dioxide production (through increased citric acid cycle turnover), a decrease in mitochondrial matrix pH, and increases in oxygen availability secondary to increased cerebral blood flow.

There is evidence that the reduction of oxygen by the respiratory chain is more complex than depicted in this equation since the univalent reduction of oxygen by some other members of the respiratory chain occurs. This is especially true for coenzyme Q (a constituent of mitochondrial lipids and a member of the respiratory chain), which exists in several transitory states (quinone, semiquinone, and hydroquinine forms), one of which is a free radical depending on redox status. The univalent reduction of oxygen results in the production of various toxic products such as the superoxide and hydroxyl radicals and hydrogen peroxide. It has been proposed that under certain pathologic conditions the increased formation of such oxygen-dependent radicals may result in mitochondrial membrane damage that may challenge cell viability.[77]

As can be seen from the previous equation, the transfer of reducing equivalents from cyt aa_3 to molecular oxygen increases cyt aa_3 oxidation. Any increase in the concentration of matrix oxygen or hydrogen ions would increase the rate of the reaction toward the right. This reaction occurs more quickly than the passage of reducing equivalents down the respiratory chain and would thus increase the state of cyt aa_3 oxidation. Likewise, a reduction in the flow of reducing equivalents would also increase the oxidation state of cyt aa_3 in the absence of any change in matrix oxygen and hydrogen ion content because of the quicker reaction rate of the water-forming reaction compared to the passage of reducing equivalents between members of the respiratory chain.[35]

Intracellular Acidosis and Lactate Accumulation

Decreases in intracellular pH and increases in intracellular lactate occur acutely following fluid percussion trauma and last as long as 8 hours.[31,74,90] The cause of this persistent acidosis is probably a result of mitochondrial dysfunction that may be related to changes in the phosphorylation state of pyruvate dehydrogenase as documented in other situations.[4,8,47,73] A decrease in the activity of this key regulatory enzyme complex would limit the ability of brain mitochondria to use pyruvate as a generator of reducing equivalents for oxidative phosphorylation and mitochondrial ion transport. It would also decrease the ability of the mitochondria to oxidize lactic acid that may accumulate because of an enhanced glycolytic flux that exceeds pyruvate dehydrogenase activity. Such changes may limit the ability of the neuronal mitochondria to respond to increases in energy demand and Ca^{++} uptake and may also make the traumatized brain more likely to develop lactic acidosis.

If the lactate dehydrogenase (LDH) reaction is rearranged so that the reaction products can be viewed from how changes in their concentrations may affect lactate levels, the following equation is obtained.[11] Based on the LDH equilibrium, three major factors may result in increased lactate production:

$$\text{Lactate} = K_{LDH}\,(Mg^{++})\,\text{Pyruvate} \times \text{NADH/NAP}^{+} \times H^{+}$$

As can be seen, increases in pyruvate and the NADH/NAD^+ ratio or decreases in intracellular pH would increase the formation of lactate. Furthermore, the LDH equilibrium is affected by the concentration of intracellular Mg^{++}, and changes in Mg^{++} can shift the reaction to the right or the left. In addition, numerous factors affect these variables. In general, changes in the intracellular hydrogen ion concentration involve changes in the production of various organic acids such as lactic acid, citric acid or other critic acid cycle intermediates, and phosphoric acid as the result of adenine nucleotide dephosporylation and changes in tissue carbon dioxide content. All of these changes are mediated or affected greatly by changes in mitochondrial metabolism. Additionally, changes in pyruvate concentration are also dependent on the balance between glycolytic activity as mediated through hexokinase and phosphofructokinase and mitochondrial activity as controlled through pyruvate dehydrogenase activity. Finally, the cytoplasmic redox state ($NADH/NAD^+$) is determined by the balance between glycolytic flux, which produces NADH, and the speed of reducing equivalent flow within the mitochondria, which reoxidizes NADH to NAD^+ Thus all the factors of this reaction that contribute to increased lactic acid and intracellular acidosis reflect the balance between changes in glycolytic flux and mitochondrial function.

The cause of lactic acidosis is frequently very difficult

to determine without careful analysis. If attempts are made to identify cause and effect relationships only from the LDH reaction, it is quite difficult to determine, for example, if lactic acid production causes intracellular acidosis or intracellular acidosis causes lactic acid formation. Other sources of metabolic acids also have to be considered as the temporal genesis of various factors, requiring a global approach. The examination of the entire energy metabolism pathway is frequently necessary to determine cause-and-effect relationships in intracelluar acidosis. The most logical approach in evaluating changes in the flux and the reaction products involved in the energy production pathway is first to examine the major rate-controlling reactions of the pathway and the enzymes and regulatory factors that control these reactions.

Arachidonic Acid Metabolism and Free Radical Damage Following Trauma

There is direct evidence that a surge in prostaglandin synthesis[16] and in free radical damage occurs following even mild-to-moderate fluid percussion trauma that involves changes in cerebrovascular function and structure.[38-41,66] Previous studies have demonstrated a number of morphologic and functional abnormalities of the pial vasculature following traumatic injury that have been linked to free radical production as a result of trauma-induced increases in prostaglandin synthesis.[38-41] Subsequent topical administration of various radical scavengers blocks or significantly reduces the vascular abnormalities that result from traumatic injury.[39,40] Some specifics from these studies warrant discussion so that this evidence may be placed in perspective as it relates to the importance of radical formation as a mechanism of cellular injury to trauma.

First, functional and structural changes that have been documented to occur as the result of radical formation in traumatic injury are limited to the cerebral circulation. This does not mean that radical pathology does not occur in neurons and glia but only that evidence of such processes has not yet been documented directly. Obviously, some of the previously discussed metabolic consequences of traumatic injury within the parenchyma may be related to free fatty acid cascades involving prostaglandin and free radical surges. The surge in prostaglandin synthesis and the associated cerebrovascular changes following fluid percussion injury occur in response to the increase in arterial blood pressure that constitutes a hypertensive insult just after impact in this model. If the increase in arterial blood pressure is prevented, no cerebrovascular changes occur. The dependence of these changes on an acute rise in arterial blood pressure has been further documented in a model of acute hypertension.[38] The vascular abnormalities seen after both traumatic and hypertensive insults include sustained dilation of pial arterioles for hours, impaired or abolished vascular responsiveness of the pial circulation to changes in arterial blood pressure or carbon dioxide, and reduced oxygen consumption by pial arterioles and endothelial lesions in both pial and intraparenchymal blood vessels.[38-41,66] Additionally, despite the fact that no platelet aggregates were observed following trauma, platelet aggregation in response to additional stimuli was increased following fluid percussion injury. These adverse effects are either prevented or inhibited by pretreatment with cyclooxygenase inhibitors or a number of free radical scavengers. Furthermore, the topical application of agents that produce various free radicals produces similar functional and structural changes of the pial circulation.[40] The evidence to date indicates that the hydroxyl radical and superoxide anion radical are involved in the production of functional and structural changes of the pial vasculature in response to trauma and hypertension. However, the mechanisms by which an increase in intravascular pressure may stimulate prostaglandin synthesis and subsequent free radical formation are not known.

It is not presently known if all cells or just specific cell types of the brain parenchyma or cerebrovasculature participate in the prostaglandin surge[39]; however, based on the ratio of prostaglandin production, apparently parenchymal production predominates following trauma.[16,39] Measurements of free fatty acids have not been performed directly in this model, but an increase in the activity of phospholipase C activity has been demonstrated;[88] however, the mechanism by which hypertension activates phospholipase C remains obscure. A number of hypotheses about the mechanism have been suggested such as the entry of blood constituents into the blood vessel wall because of permeability changes as the result of vessel wall distention.[39] If the distention of the vessel wall allows for membrane depolarization both in the cellular elements of the vasculature and brain parenchyma, Ca^{++} influx, phospholipase activation, and an increase in free fatty acids and prostaglandin synthesis may occur.

Secondary Insults

Secondary insults such as ischemia, hypoxia, or epilepsy represent significant causes of additional brain damage following head trauma. It is well documented that the normal cerebrovascular responses to physiologic stress (e.g., hypoxia, hypercapnia, systemic hypotension, and intracranial hypertension) are impaired or absent following traumatic injury, and secondary ischemia and/or hypoxia is also more likely to occur in the traumatized brain than in the uninjured brain with normal cerebrovascular status.[33,42,44,45,58] Such protective changes in cerebral blood flow to ensure adequate substrate delivery and metabolite removal are an important defense system of the brain against injury. These effects have been stressed elsewhere[33] and are not the primary concern of our discussion since it is recognized that secondary insults are more likely following central nervous system trauma caused by the impairment of such protective vascular mechanisms. Instead, the concept of increased brain sensitivity to obvious and not so obvious secondary insults will be examined.

Flow-Metabolism Coupling

The concept of flow-metabolism coupling has become a popular window from which to view and evaluate primary and secondary vascular insults to the brain. Experimental evidence has confirmed that in both experimental animals and man, cerebral blood flow (CBF) is coupled to the metabolic demand or metabolism of the brain in such a way that a nearly linear relationship exists. Brain regions with low metabolic rates have corresponding low flows, and brain regions with high metabolic rates have proportionally high flows. Likewise, physiologic and metabolic stimuli that increase or decrease the metabolic rate in the healthy brain result in predictable compensatory changes in CBF unless the stimulus alters the flow-metabolism relationship (uncouples CBF and metabolism). When CBF and metabolism are coupled in the healthy brain, changes in CBF are produced by changes in metabolism, and it is widely believed that certain metabolites representative of the metabolic status of the tissue are the major regulators of this type of vascular reactivity (metabolic regulation). There is considerable disagreement over the role various metabolites (e.g., H^+, K^+, adenosine, and the prostaglandins, prostacyclin and thromboxane A_2) play, but there is a growing body of evidence that such metabolites may mediate their effects on vascular smooth muscle through changes in Ca^{++} flux.[77] For example, it has been proposed that increasing hydrogen ion production affects the tone of the vascular smooth muscle through a decrease in Ca^{++} permeability by producing conformational changes in Ca^{++} channels, by direct competition with Ca^{++} for passage across Ca^{++} channels, or by changing the activity of Na^+-K^+ ATPase, which indirectly affects intracellular Ca^{++} levels through the Na^+-Ca^{++} exchange system. Regardless of the mechanism, the effect of pH on vascular smooth muscle can be reversed by increasing extracellular Ca^{++}.

Under pathologic conditions the uncoupling of CBF and metabolism may occur in two directions. CBF may be inadequate for metabolic demand, a condition that is known to be harmful, or CBF may be increased in excess of metabolic demand, a condition that may be potentially harmful, although this possibility remains undocumented. In addition, various flow thresholds for general metabolic and physiologic events such as energy failure, ion redistribution, and edema development have been proposed for the healthy brain that has been subjected to cerebral ischemia.[77] However, to our knowledge there is no corresponding documentation that such thresholds are altered in the "injured" brain following various type of primary insults. Changes in such thresholds in response to secondary ischemia or hypoxia may indicate that the sensitivity of the injured brain to reductions in CBF is increased. In fact, even with minor brain injury in which the metabolic changes appear minimum and compatible with survival, the true significance of such changes may not become apparent until the brain is subjected to some secondary stress in which the inadequacy of compensatory vascular or metabolic mechanisms may become life threatening.

Primary and secondary vascular insults may occur whenever substrate and oxygen availability is inadequate to meet the metabolic demands of the tissue. Thus ischemia, hypoxia, or hypoglycemia is relative to the metabolic rate of the tissue. A CBF that is adequate for the maintenance of metabolism under hypometabolic conditions may represent relative ischemia when metabolism increases. The assessment of metabolic-flow relationships in both experimental animals and humans traditionally involves the use of CBF measurements and glucose and/or oxygen extraction from the circulation by the brain. Thus the cerebral metabolic rate of oxygen use ($CMRO_2$) and glucose use (CMRglu) is used to determine the metabolic requirements of the brain. It has been suggested that during normal physiologic activity as much as 50% of the oxygen and 10% of the glucose is extracted from the blood by the brain.[26] Thus the physiologic buffer range for increases in glucose or substrate demand is much more robust than that for oxygen.

Traditionally, changes in flow-metabolism uncoupling are viewed as significant secondary insults following head trauma only if it becomes obvious that the metabolic demands of the brain exceed the delivery of oxygen and substrate as determined by changes in the cerebral extraction of oxygen and/or glucose from blood. However, long-term reduction in the activity of pyruvate dehydrogenase reduces the ability of neuronal mitochondria to increase the reducing-equivalent flow through pyruvate, which affects ATP production as well as Ca^{++} accumulation. This limits the ability of the cell to respond to increases in metabolic demand even though substrate and oxygen delivery may be adequate to meet increased energy demand; however, the neuron could not use this increased availability of glucose and oxygen. This situation could occur because of the decreased ability of pyruvate dehydrogenase activity to convert glucose into reducing equivalents that could be used by the respiratory chain to restore the decreased transmitochondrial hydrogen ion potential that would result from increased ATP use and ADP formation. Such a situation can exist when blood flow is adequate, but there is less extraction of oxygen and glucose than should occur with a normal response to a similar increase in energy demand. Another disruption of the traditional flow-metabolism concept would occur if the process of ATP production became uncoupled from reducing equivalent flow and oxygen consumption either through competition of ATP formation with Ca^{++} uptake for the transmembrane hydrogen ion potential (such as has been proposed during the recirculation period following cerebral ischemia) or through altered inner-membrane permeability that would uncouple both ATP production and Ca^{++} uptake from reducing equivalent flow. In the latter event, increased $CMRO_2$ and CMRglu would be associated with increased reducing-equivalent flow to restore the decreased transmitochondrial hydrogen ion potential, but this increased metabolic consumption of substrates and oxygen would not be associated with any increase in ATP production or ion transport work. In this case the neuron could suffer from lack of adequate ATP despite increases in CBF, $CMRO_2$ and/or CMRglu that in healthy cells would be adequate to restore ATP production and meet increased energy demands. Furthermore, the conventional assessment of flow and metabolism using only CBF and $CMRO_2$ and/or CMRglu measurements may not be sensitive to this type of intracellular metabolic uncoupling, which makes additional evaluations of mitochondrial function by direct biochemical assessment in animals or by in vivo measurements of phosphates with magnetic imaging in patients an important adjunct. Thus the metabolic derangements after concussive traumatic injury may have very significant influences on the capability of neurons to respond to secondary stresses that involve the mitochondrial functions of increased ATP production and Ca^{++} accumulation.

Increased Sensitivity of the Traumatized Brain to Cerebral Ischemia

In addition to increasing the metabolic and functional damage already incurred, the inability of neurons to increase mitochondrial function in response to increased demand may potentially have lethal effects. To test this possibility we evaluated the effect of secondary insults on the mildly traumatized brain.

The major approach taken in these studies was to compare the morphologic response of the brain following mild fluid percussion trauma to the morphologic response of the healthy brain after each has experienced comparable insults of cerebral ischemia. If the sensitivity of the traumatized brain to cerebral ischemia was increased compared to that of the healthy brain, the morphologic consequences would be expected to become more severe and extensive. To maximize the detection of an increased sensitivity phenomenon to ischemic injury following trauma, we used the maximum ischemic insult that results in minimum and reversible morphologic changes even in the selectively vulnerable regions of the healthy brain. An insult of diffuse incomplete cerebral ischemia (95% reduction in CBF) of 7 minutes duration was used—a period of time that, in our laboratories, has demonstrated structural preservation in all brain regions after 24 hours of postischemic survival when inflicted on the healthy uninjured brain.[30]

There was no evidence of prolonged morphologic damage in the forebrain except directly at the impact site following mild-to-moderate fluid percussion injury even after survival of several weeks. Thus with either trauma or ischemia alone, the insult appeared reversible as determined by morphologic criteria in the supratentorial compartment. Axonal injury has been documented in the brainstem as have scattered somal changes in some brainstem nuclei following fluid percussion injury. The patterns of injury that occurred when either insult was produced alone were very important in clarifying the results observed when both insults were combined. When mild-to-moderate fluid percussion injury was followed by a 7-minute insult of incomplete ischemia 1 hour after trauma and allowed to survive for 1 to 12 hours after the secondary ischemia, progressive neuronal changes consisting of dark and shrunken neurons and swollen astrocytes typical of some types of ischemic neuronal changes were observed. With 1-hour survival after the combined insults of trauma and ischemia, such morphologic changes were seen only in neocortical regions; however, with 12-hour survival dark and shrunken neurons were observed in layers 3, 5, and 6 of the neocortex, all sectors of the hippocampus, the basal ganglia, and the cerebellar cortices. No progression of neuronal changes were seen in the brainstem proper after the combined insults. Cerebral blood flow was measured before, during, and after each insult, and the level and duration of ischemia that was inflicted on the traumatized brain was comparable to that used with the healthy brain. Thus an enhancement of the phenomenon of selectively vulnerable neuronal ischemic damage was produced when secondary ischemia was administered to the traumatized brain. This finding is quite important because it suggests that trauma has increased the sensitivity of the brain to ischemic injury and that the increased injury is not just the cumulative effects of both insults in which the morphologic damage produces by each insult was additive. This is further evidenced by the fact that no neuronal changes were seen when this same level and duration of cerebral ischemia was inflicted on the healthy brain. In addition, ischemic neuronal damage was increased with survival time following the combined insults, suggesting a maturation process.[30]

Systemic Factors that May Increase Ischemic Vulnerability Following Concussive Trauma

A number of possible mechanisms for the increased sensitivity of traumatized brain to cerebral ischemia should be considered. It is well known that both trauma and ischemia result in a sympathoadrenal surge that produces systemic changes in circulating catecholamines stored in sympathetically innervated target tissues.[37,70,72] The production and release of catecholamines by the adrenal medulla has been reported to be species specific[19] despite reports that at least the cardiovascular effects of concussion appeared to be very similar in a number of species.[72] Some species primarily release norepinephrine, and other species such as humans mainly release epinephrine. Much of the norepinephrine released from nerve endings contributes to the circulating levels with the half-life of circulating catecholamines approximately 2 minutes. An additional complication is that the adrenal medulla appears to produce and release different ratios of norepinephrine and epinephrine depending on the type of stress involved. In conditions of asphyxia and hypoxia, the ratio of norepinephrine to epinephrine is increased, and during hemorrhage epinephrine release is proportionally increased. Changes in the ratio of catecholamine release by the adrenal medulla do not always appear advantageous in minimizing the particular stress that evokes adrenal activation; consequently, such changes are not always part of purposeful evolutionary defense mechanisms.[19]

Regardless of the species, the quantity and relative ratio of norepinephrine to epinephrine released determines the exact nature of the sympathoadrenal response since most of the systemic effects of circulating catecholamines involve catabolic processes with norepinephrine and epinephrine participating to different degrees in various responses. The most important effects relevant to the present discussion are the changes in cardiopulmonary function, glycogenolysis in the liver and skeletal muscle, and general metabolic effects such as increases in basal temperature and the mobilization of free fatty acids.

The cardiopulmonary effects of the sympathoadrenal surge in fluid percussion trauma appear to vary with the intensity of the injury. Three major types of cardiovascular responses were observed following fluid percussion injury.[72] The first type consisted of minor changes in circulating catecholamines, slight bradycardia, and decreases in mean arterial blood pressure. These changes result from vagal stimulation and are found following very mild impacts. The second response was characterized by massive increases of catecholamines, mean arterial blood pressure, and cardiac arrhythmias that resulted from a sympathoadrenal response that was proportional to the injury level. This type of response was observed at the level of trauma used in our study described previously of the effects of concussive trauma on ischemic vulnerability. The third type of response was characterized by various types of cardiac arrhythmias and by progressive systemic hypotension that led to cardiovascular collapse, which was evident at severe levels of trauma that, in the fluid percussion model, are associated with severe structural damage to the brainstem.[72] Such variability is probably caused by differences in the amount and the relative ratio of norepinephrine and epinephrine released from the adrenal medulla and the noradrenergic nerve endings and by the level of the pathologic brainstem dysfunction and the structural damage produced by fluid percussion injury.

Although norepinephrine increases arterial pressure through $alpha_1$ receptor stimulation and vasoconstriction in most target organs, epinephrine produces vasodilation in the liver and skeletal muscles through $beta_2$ receptors, which exceeds the vasoconstriction produced by epinephrine in other target organs and usually results in a net decrease in total peripheral vascular resistance.[19] Thus the net effect of isolated intravascular norepinephrine infusion is general vasoconstriction and increases in mean arterial blood pressure, and the net effect of isolated intravascular epinephrine infusion is relative vasodilation and decreased mean arterial blood pressure.

Since the net response observed during the sympathoadrenal surge in the fluid percussion model at the injury levels used in our study of secondary ischemia is acute systemic hypertension, the norepinephrine response predominates despite massive increases in plasma epinephrine as well. In other trauma models that produce posttraumatic hypertension, alpha blockade impairs and beta blockade potentiates the hypertension response.[72] It is well documented that such systemic increases in mean arterial blood pressure following trauma frequently impair cerebral autoregulation[14,42,44,45] and possibly alter the transport status of the blood-brain barrier[66]; however, other organ systems may also be affected. A number of other organs (e.g., the kidneys, myocardium, liver, skeletal muscle, and mesentery) also demonstrate autoregulation and may also be affected by this sudden surge in arterial blood pressure. Since most of these other organ systems do not have an effective barrier to circulating catecholamines such as that in the vascular endothelium of the brain, a direct effect on vascular smooth muscle could be expected. Preliminary measurements of cardiac and renal blood flow with microspheres indicate that the myocardium and the kidneys also demonstrate significant hyperemia during trauma-induced systemic hypertension but subsequently show decreases in blood flow of a much greater percentage than has been reported for the brain. Such data indicate that the systemic hypertension overcomes the direct vasoconstrictor effects of catecholamines on renal and cardiac blood flow. Thus the possibility of hypertension-induced vascular damage to other organ systems in addition to the brain must be considered as results of massive sympathoadrenal discharges following traumatic injury.

Both norepinephrine and epinephrine increase heart rate and myocardial contractility in the isolated heart through $beta_1$ receptors. In addition, they increase myocardial excitability and result in cardiac arrhythmias. In the intact animal the hypertension produced by intravascular norepinephrine infusion results in reflex bradycardia through the stimulation of carotid and aortic baroreceptors that overcome the direct excitatory effects of norepinephrine on the cardiac conduction system with a resultant decrease in cardiac output. In contrast, although epinephrine results in a widened pulse pressure, the direct cardiac effects result in an increased heart rate, contractility, and cardiac output.[19]

From the results observed in studies of mild-to-moderate fluid percussion injury, a number of cardiac abnormalities developed as a consequence of the sympathoadrenal response. Tachycardia and bradycardia were observed almost equally in animals with injury levels in the mild-to-moderate range.[71] This indicates that the predominant net effect of norepinephrine or epinephrine on heart rate in the cat was observed equally during the period of the acute sympathoadrenal response. Cardiac output has not been measured in this model, but there is evidence from others that changes in cardiac output do occur in other models. In general, decreases in cardiac output have been observed following closed head injury, but this decrease usually occurs after the initial surge in catecholamines.[72] A significant long-term cardiac effect that may be mediated by catecholamines is that of cardiac necrosis, which has been reported both in experimental animal models and in humans.[10,72] However, if such events occur with mild fluid percussion injury, they are minimal since these animals demonstrate good long-term survival.[66] In addition, the release of opioid peptides by the adrenal medulla as part of the sympathoadrenal response following trauma has also been implicated as a possible cause of posttraumatic hypotension following the initial effects mediated by the surge in circulating catecholamines.[72] In our experience, the usual cause of death in animals subjected to fluid percussion injury and receiving constant respiratory support is cardiovascular collapse that may be analogous to cardiogenic shock (heart failure with resulting decreased cardiac output) or low-resistance shock (vasodilation despite adequate cardiac output and blood volume). However, the exact mechanisms involved await further confirmation. It is likely that this phenomenon is a result of brainstem injury with damage to vasomotor control centers produced in this model from higher impacts and systemic factors that impair myocardial and systemic vasomotor function involving the release of catecholamines and various opioid peptides as suggested by Rosner and associates.[72]

The pulmonary effects mediated by the sympathoadrenal surge following fluid percussion injury are more indirect and less clear. Various degrees of initial apnea accompany most traumatic injuries in experimental animals and may lead to respiratory arrest or varying degrees of hypoventilation or hyperventilation.[20,81] However, these respiratory changes are not relevant in ventilated animals with controlled respiration as performed in our studies with the fluid percussion model. However, other features of pulmonary dysfunction have been reported following fluid percussion injury such as pulmonary edema, which was considered neurogenic in origin and could be prevented with alpha adrenergic blockade.[72] High left ventricular end diastolic pressure occurred in animals that developed pulmonary edema, suggesting that systemic hypertension may have contributed to pulmonary hypertension that in turn may have resulted in pulmonary edema. We have also observed significant increases in left atrial pressure during the acute period of systemic hypertension following concussive trauma. The pulmonary circulation is a low-pressure, highly distensible system with the lowest arterial pressure (15 mm Hg) of any vascular bed during normal conditions and with pulmonary venous pressure normally ranging from 0 to 5 mm Hg, depending on left-sided heart function, pleural pressure, and pulmonary blood volume. Thus pulmonary capillary pressure is normally approximately 10 mm Hg with an oncotic pressure of approximately 25 mm Hg resulting in an inward driving force of approximately 15 mm Hg. In ventilated animals subjected to the concussive injury levels used in our studies, the increases in left atrial pressure have not consistently been high enough to overcome this net 15 mm Hg of inward pressure, and it is unlikely that such a mechanism may be involved in the production of pulmonary edema during the systemic hypertension period. In addition, there is no evidence that diffusion of oxygen and carbon dioxide between arterial blood and alveolar air is impaired acutely during the catecholamine surge; thus the relevance of pulmonary edema at the injury levels examined in our studies appears minimal.

Increased circulating catecholamines, transient systemic and pulmonary hypertension, and cardiac arrhythmias also occur at injury levels that are associated with long-term survival. Structural preservation of the forebrain of these unsupported animals, which require only transient ventilatory assistance at impact to prevent posttraumatic apnea, has already been documented. Since the type of ischemia used in our studies of secondary ischemia following trauma also results in a massive sympathoadrenal response, an additional catecholamine surge would again produce such systemic effects with the exception of arterial hypertension, which is prevented by exsanguination during the ischemia. However, since ischemia was confined to the brain, no direct ischemic effect on other organ systems occurred. However, even more pronounced short- and long-term effects in systemic organs may be mediated by this second catecholamine surge that may be modified even further by changes in adrenergic receptor sensitivity to agonist stimulation. Such systemic factors cannot be ruled out as contributing to the increased vulnerability of the brain to secondary ischemia as seen in our preliminary studies. However, the secondary ischemia was not followed by any additional decrease in cerebral blood flow or by arterial hypoxia, which would result in additional insults that may be mediated by adverse changes in cardiopulmonary function. For this reason, it appears unlikely that additional cardiopulmonary dysfunction resulted in any direct effect on the traumatized brain's vulnerability to a secondary ischemic insult.

Following trauma, the major systemic metabolic effects that most likely alters the vulnerability of the brain to cerebral ischemia is the production of serum hyperglycemia. Serum hyperglycemia decreases the tolerance of the healthy brain to cerebral ischemia, and there is considerable evidence that this decreased tolerance is the result of an increased level of lactic acidosis that develops during the insult.* However, with this fact in mind it should be emphasized that the hyperglycemia that develops during the insult is the most critical effect because, next to the duration and the level of ischemia, it is what determines the degree of acidosis that develops during the insult. Thus even if traumatized animals demonstrate hyperglycemia before the ischemic insult, the level of hyperglycemia during the secondary ischemic insult in our combined insult model is only slightly greater than that seen in healthy animals subjected to cerebral ischemia. For this reason preischemic hyperglycemia in the animals subjected to trauma should not render the brain more vulnerable to secondary ischemia since serum glucose levels during the ischemic insult are comparable. A more plausible mechanism may involve intrinsic changes in brain metabolism that result from trauma that renders the nervous system more vulnerable to ischemic acidosis.

Since lactic acidosis increases ischemic injury, the decreased ability of the dysfunctional mitochondria to regulate intracellular pH by having less latitude to change flux in pyruvate dehydrogenase to accelerate lactate metabolism may result in a more marked acid-base disequilibrium following trauma-plus-ischemia than is seen in ischemia alone. This may lead to more marked decreases in intracellular pH during the ischemic insult and to more impaired pH compensation during the postischemic recovery period. Although intracellular acidosis has been targeted as a major threat to cell viability if pH decreases below 6.5 and lactate levels exceed 20 μm, a recent theory has claimed that acidosis is harmful only when coupled with energy failure and that it may mediate its harmful effects through changes in the pathologic Ca^{++} signal by altering inner-mitochondrial membrane permeability and reducing the transmitochondrial hydrogen ion potential, resulting in decreased mitochondrial Ca^{++} buffering and ATP production. This effect of intracellular acidosis may be mediated through the activation of inner-mitochondrial membrane phospholipase A_2 with generalized increases in inner-membrane permeability.[36] Thus one hypothesis regarding the increased vulnerability of the brain to secondary ischemia concerns whether or not the traumatized brain develops greater levels of intracellular lactic acidosis during the ischemic insult when compared to the healthy brain despite comparable levels of serum hyperglycemia.

The impairment of pH-regulating mechanisms at the mitochondrial level following even mild fluid percussion injury is reflected by the persistent, although mild, lactic acidosis that is still present 8 hours after trauma. This lactic acidosis is in contrast to cerebral ischemia of up to 15-minutes duration,[49] spreading cortical depression,[62] and even that following sustained seizure activity[79] in which intracellular acidosis recovers acutely. All these pathologic situations also produce acute acidosis and pathologic intracellular Ca^{++} surges yet can still metabolize accumulated lactate following severe increases in energy demand. This finding may indicate that the derangements in the ability of mitochondria to oxidize lactate after even mild trauma are specific to some aspect of traumatic injury.

*References 24, 30, 49, 67, and 75-79.

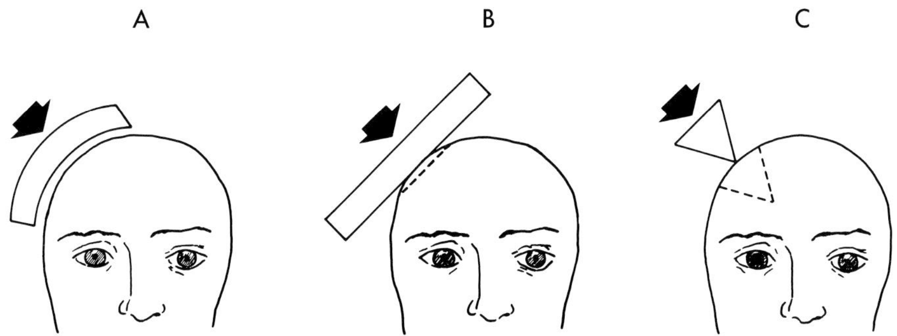

Fig. 47-2 Variable degree of injury related to the form of an object hitting the head with the same force (mass and velocity are constant). In **A** there may be no or only minimum injury. **B** will probably cause a depressed fracture and perhaps a small brain contusion, and **C** may create a severe brain laceration.

DEFINITION AND DIFFERENTIATION OF BRAIN INJURIES

The important thing in connection with a head injury is not so much what has happened to the exterior (i.e., the scalp and the skull) but what has occurred within the brain and its coverings. Although a cranial fracture occasionally needs special treatment, its presence is mainly proof that there has, in fact, been a head injury of a certain magnitude. Whether the trauma will give rise to a fracture is dependent not only on the forces involved but also on their direction (angle against the skull bone), the deceleration distance, the quality of the object hitting the head (whether it is hard or soft), its form (blunt or sharp) (Fig. 47-2), and also on the density and thickness of the skull bone where it is hit. The bone thickness varies from 3 to 11 mm within an area of 3 cm^2 in the temporal region.

The forces exerted on the brain in a head injury are proportional to the product of mass and acceleration (deceleration),[1] meaning that velocity is the major factor. Consequently, an object with a small mass and a high speed, such as a bullet, will cause considerably more brain damage than a larger object with a lower velocity, such as a basketball thrown from a human hand. Another essential factor is, however, that the latter blow may very well cause a concussion, while the former may not. A vise will not cause a concussion either, although it is certainly capable of compressing the brain to death. Thus it is evident that the essential feature of a concussive force is that it be sufficient to jar or shake the head. The word concussion is even derived from a Latin word, *concutere,* meaning to shake. Thus from a biomechanical point of view there are two types of phenomena involved in direct trauma to the head—contact phenomena and inertial loading. Contact phenomena include skull bending, compression, and penetration, which may be trivial or significant, but which are principally focal.

Inertial loading involves the forces causing concussion and has two components—translation and rotation. The two are usually associated; however, the rotational forces are probably those that produce the diffuse injuries since the brain is relatively resistant to pure compression (translation) but is easily deformed by shear forces or tension (rotation). Biomechanically it can be postulated that the effect of trauma to the mobile head would be greater on the surface than in the center, i.e., greater in the cerebral hemispheres than in the brainstem. This effect has also been shown by neuropathologists who, in a study of a large series of patients who died after head trauma, could find brainstem injuries only in those patients who also had extensive damage in the hemispheres.[1,2] The old clinical concept that patients initially seen in very poor condition but without any hematoma when arriving at the hospital have only brainstem injuries is thus probably wrong.[59] This does not mean, however, that the clinical picture of deep coma, motor posturing, and dilated and unresponsive pupils is not a sign of brainstem injury but only that this brainstem damage may also be associated with extensive cerebral hemisphere injury.

Fractures

Closed

A fracture, apart from being just a sign telling that head trauma has occurred, may also give hints to the risk of complications. Closed fractures in the temporal region are more often associated with epidural hematomas than are other fractures. Fractures transversing major dural sinuses have a greater chance of causing life-threatening hemorrhage. Fractures in the occipital region may be associated with infratentorial hematomas. A depressed fracture, similar to intracranial mass lesion, may diminish the volume of the intracranial cavity, but this is seldom of practical importance. The clinical implication of depressed fractures is that they may exert local pressure on the cerebral cortex thus causing focal neurologic deficits and constituting a focus for posttraumatic epilepsy. Most neurosurgeons recommend surgery when the fracture is depressed more than 5 mm, although many believe that the injury that will later become the epileptic focus is sustained at the moment of impact when the bone is fractured and hits the cortex.[32] Decompartmentalization of iron and heme compounds is associated with an increased incidence of epilepsy.[89]

A fracture that involves and changes the outer aspect of the skull is sometimes of more than cosmetic interest. It may affect the fixation points of the orbital muscles and cause double vision, or it may compromise the upper airways.

Open

A fracture can be open into the intracranial cavity, either directly through the scalp, which is obvious or at least suspected in most cases, or indirectly through the nasopharynx, the paranasal sinuses, or the middle ear, which is often not so obvious and, therefore, easily overlooked, especially in the unconscious patient.

The risk of meningitis makes it vital to detect this complication. Meningitis can change a comparatively trivial injury into a life-threatening one and is, in fact, responsible for almost 10% of those patients who "talk and die," i.e., patients who have been able to utter some words following head trauma but who will later die.[68] Thus open fractures must be closed as soon as possible. The dura should be sutured, or when this is not possible, a biologic dural substitute should be used, even though a wound revision often cannot be performed.

Cerebrospinal fluid (CSF) fistulas are the most common causes of posttraumatic meningitis since they may constitute a permanent entry to the subarachnoid space. The CSF leak must be stopped before an epithelialized pathway has been established, which usually takes a few days. Within this time period almost every CSF fistula through the ear will stop spontaneously. Many openings through the paranasal sinuses, if not too large, will respond similarly, probably at least in part because of compression of the subarachnoid space from brain swelling. If there is still a leak after 3 or 4 days (or earlier in the absence of clinical and radiologic signs of hematoma or increased intracranial pressure [ICP]), the subarachnoid pressure (equal to the ICP) must be lowered to zero to ascertain that there will be no spontaneous leak of CSF. This reduction can be accomplished through repeated lumbar punctures or, better, through an indwelling lumbar catheter (lumbar drainage). However, a lumbar puncture in a head-injured patient is risky and is *only* to be performed after thorough clinical and radiologic investigation. Such caution is necessary because the subarachnoid pathways may be blocked with a pressure gradient between the supratentorial space and the infratentorial space or between the intracranial cavity and the spinal canal. In both cases the pressure gradient will increase after a spinal tap, and the patient may deteriorate. This deterioration does not necessarily follow immediately but can often be seen a few hours after the lumbar puncture, probably as a result of CSF leakage through the punctured dura.

A CSF fistula, spontaneous or iatrogenic, will cause a headache as a result of the subnormal ICP, but it will usually disappear after a few days when the patient becomes accustomed to his new, low ICP level. Headache from low ICP is, in fact, often worse than the type resulting from high ICP, with the latter troublesome but, as a rule, not so intense.

Skull fractures may also damage the dural venous sinuses. An open fracture that lacerates the superior sagittal sinus or, more seldom, the transverse sinus may cause considerable bleeding and lead to profound shock and even death before the patients at the hospital. With closed fractures the symptoms are more vague, but the bleeding may again become profuse when the surgeon tries to elevate the depressed bone fragment. In such cases bleeding can generally be controlled simply by elevating the patient's head since this will decrease venous pressure. However, this procedure carries the risk of air embolism.

Traumatic thrombosis of the dural venous sinuses is a rather rare, but important, event associated with a high mortality. Those patients who survive fairly often develop chronically increased ICP, supposedly as a result of impaired venous outflow.

Brain Injury

The effects on the brain from head trauma are classically defined in the following terms: (1) brain concussion; (2) traumatic brain edema; (3) brain contusion/laceration; and (4-6) intracranial hematoma (epidural, subdural, and intracerebral). Our present understanding of its pathophysiology and neuropathology reveals that the damage to the brain is probably graded, and what is clinically designated as brain edema is a fairly complicated and dynamic event; however, this classification may still have clinical as well as didactic merit.

Brain Concussion

Brain concussion can be defined clinically as a transient (lasting not more than 10 minutes) loss of consciousness followed by immediate and complete recovery and accompanied by a period of retrograde and, as a rule, posttraumatic (anterograde) amnesia without morphologic changes visible through gross examination or light microscopy. According to this definition, a patient who has not been unconscious cannot be said to have sustained a concussion, and a patient who is not lucid after half an hour or who has some neurologic signs may certainly have had a concussion but most probably has a more advanced brain injury as well. In the latter circumstances the final diagnosis should not be that of a "simple" cerebral concussion. Many authors prefer to use the term "mild concussion" for cases in which the person is capable of continuing his activities after the head injury but does not remember what happened afterward, as is frequently seen in conjunction with sports-related injuries. Accepting the idea of a continuous scale of injury to the brain after trauma, it seems appropriate to recognize mild concussion as the first step on that scale.[64] The punch-drunk syndrome in boxers, who may develop serious signs of brain injury without suffering anything worse than multiple mild head injuries, indicates that these injuries may not be as harmless as previously believed.

Although there is a consensus that coma is caused by a sudden loss of neuronal function with disruption of connections between cortical and subcortical and/or brainstem structures, the exact mechanism of this process and the so-called concussive response (systemic hypertension, pulse changes, apnea, and pupillary dilation)[56] is not yet known.

Traumatic Brain Edema

The term traumatic brain edema is often used by clinicians to denote a state in which no major brain injuries are seen on an x-ray or during surgery, but nevertheless, the patient deteriorates with clinical signs of increased intracranial pressure (ICP). This course may be especially dramatic in children whose status can change from full alertness to deep unconsciousness accompanied by posturing and dilated, nonreactive pupils within a few hours.

It is true that an edematous reaction, focal and/or generalized, follows most cases of parenchymal brain damage, but it probably is very unusual for significant edema to develop in the absence of such a damage, i.e., after a concussion as defined previously. Modern x-ray techniques (computed tomography [CT] scan) often reveal that these patients have some contusions or a small intracerebral hematoma and a local or general low attenuation as viewed on an x-ray as a sign of increased water content in the brain tissue. Brain edema can be either vasogenic, caused primarily by a blood-brain barrier disturbance accompanied by protein leakage and an increased interstitial water content, or cytotoxic, caused by toxic or metabolic damage of brain cells and giving rise to an increase of intracellular water. The edema usually will not manifest clinically until 24 to 48 hours after injury, in contrast to hematomas, which usually give rise to symptoms within the first 24 hours.

In many patients with raised ICP there will not, however, be any proof of actual edema, although the CT scan may show signs of increased intracranial content (e.g., very small ventricles and obliteration of the cisterns normally surrounding the brainstem). In these cases, the increased ICP is probably caused by increased cerebral blood flow (CBF) and congestion. In some of the patients seen with the clinical symptoms supposedly caused by brain edema, the reason for neurologic deterioration may be the opposite, i.e., decreased CBF caused by cerebral vasospasm as a reaction to subarachnoid blood. Increased, as well as decreased, CBF may sooner or later lead to cerebral edema. However, the relationships between CBF, ICP, and brain edema are so complex and interrelated that all these parameters must be considered when defining the pathology and mechanisms causing the abnormalities.

Brain Contusion/Laceration

A macroscopic traumatic injury of the brain parenchyma is called a contusion, and if the integrity of the pia mater is broken, such as occurs in a gunshot injury, it is called a laceration of the brain. Because of the anatomy of the skull, almost 90% of all contusions are located in the frontal and/or temporal lobes, although a so-called contrecoup lesion is commonly seen on the opposite side of the brain, i.e., in the occipital or contralateral temporal lobe.[55] Sometimes a frontal contrecoup contusion will be the only lesion resulting from an occipital blow. The cerebellum is fairly well covered by strong musculature and bone, and although occipital fractures are relatively common, traumatic injury to the cerebellum is not (Fig. 47-3).

A contusion localized in the frontal or temporal lobe of the nondominant hemisphere does not necessarily give rise to any impressive neurologic symptoms, at least not in the first day before any complicating edema has developed. A patient with a contusion in such a ''silent zone'' may well regain consciousness after the initial concussion and thus show a ''free interval'' (see section on Epidural Hematoma), although, if examined carefully, he will probably not be entirely alert.

An open brain injury looks terrifying but is not necessarily associated with a bad prognosis. In many cases it appears that this type of injury has resulted from an elongated deceleration distance, thereby decreasing the forces exerted on the brain. Thus the outcome may be quite good if the injury is in a silent zone and if no infection follows. Because of the viscosity changes of an injured brain, it may certainly look as though a considerable amount of brain tissue is extruding through the wound, but during surgery the actual parenchymal defect is often found to be quite small.

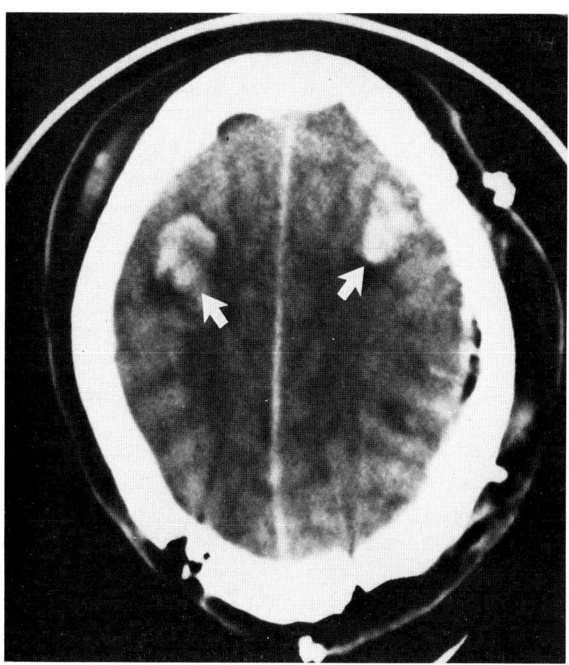

Fig. 47-3 Bilateral anterior contusions *(arrows)* seen in brain parenchyma during computerized tomographic scanning (edema is seen around the lesion).

Gunshot injuries, on the other hand, often do not appear too serious but may still have a very poor prognosis. While traversing the head, the shock waves from high-velocity missiles frequently cause considerable damage far afield from the bullet canal, in which case the patient seldom survives. In fact, even high-velocity shots to other parts of the body may cause severe brain injury from this shock wave. Most civilian-type missiles (i.e., smaller caliber with less velocity) do not traverse the opposite side of the skull (apart from large-caliber bullets); instead, they ricochet so that the line between the entry and the bullet may not represent the canal. Rapid increases in ICP from the shock wave may also result in a sudden downward displacement of the cerebellum causing contusion of the cerebellar hemispheres or tonsils.

The types of contusions described previously are the most obvious, representing one aspect of injury; the other type is the so-called diffuse axonal injury.[2] This term refers to the destruction of axons in the white matter of the hemispheres, a process that becomes more centrally distributed in the brain with increasing degrees of acceleration (retardation) force and that eventually includes the brainstem according to the biomechanical principles mentioned previously. An exclusive brainstem contusion probably does not exist as a separate entity but only in connection with very severe hemispheric injury. Since the axonal injury occurs at the same moment as the trauma, these patients will be in very poor state from the beginning. They are not able to talk after the trauma; they arrive at the hospital deeply unconscious, posturing, and with dilated, nonreactive pupils, reflecting a bad prognosis.

Epidural Hematoma

The most dramatic and feared complication associated with head injury is the extradural hematoma. Since a patient with this type of hematoma need not have any primary brain damage and thus should have a good prognosis, it is of utmost importance not to overlook this complication. It has been postulated that the percentage of head trauma patients dying from epidural hematoma within a geographic region is a measure of the quality of the organization of the head injury care, including the transportation facilities in that area.

The classic picture is that of a patient who is initially seen totally alert after a cerebral concussion, with a temporal fracture traversing the fissure of the middle meningeal artery. After a free interval of one to several hours, the patient becomes drowsy and restless, perhaps with a headache, and experiencing bradycardia and some arterial hypertension. His responsiveness continues to drop, and he soon becomes unconscious and develops a unilateral dilated pupil. Hemiparesis sometimes develops contralateral to the dilated pupil. If decompression is not performed immediately, both pupils will become dilated and fixed, and respiratory arrest and death will follow.

Unfortunately, all patients with epidural hematoma do not demonstrate this classic picture. Some have never been unconscious, and others, with concomitant brain damage, may not have any free interval. In many patients, especially children, in whom sutures can split apart for a moment, x-ray films will not reveal any demonstrable fracture line. The basic pathophysiologic events are, however, the same—the fracture, or just the shock wave itself, may shear the middle meningeal artery, or there will be massive

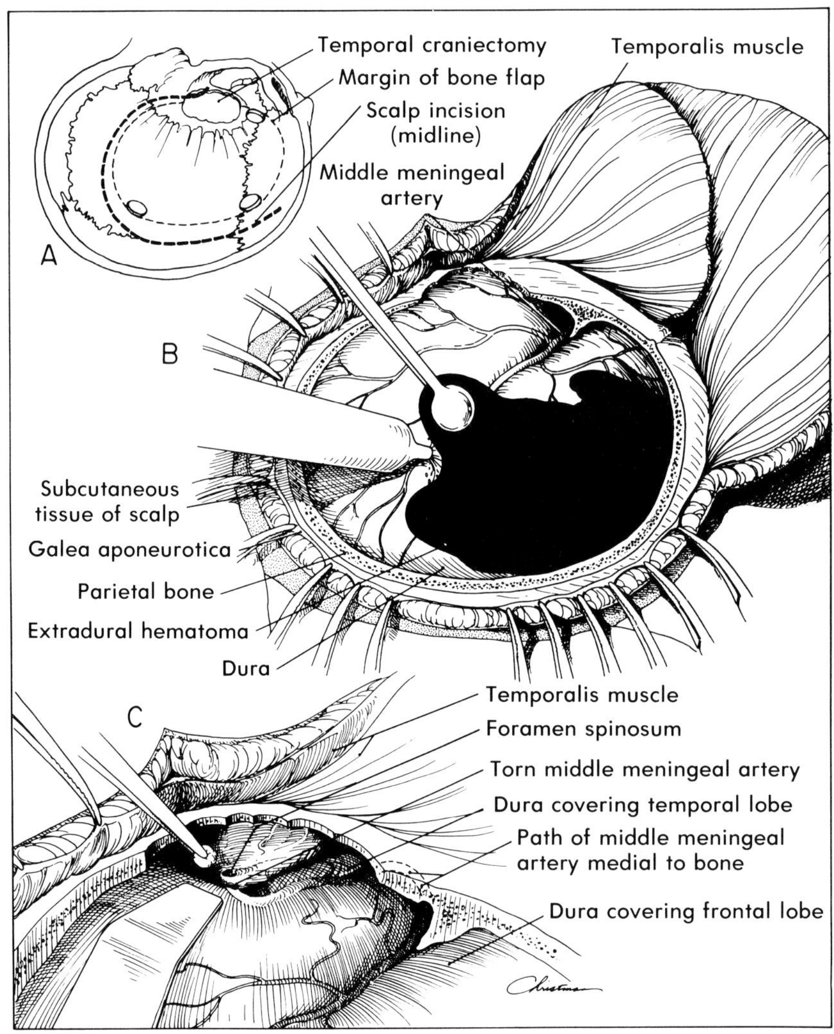

Fig. 47-4 Large epidural hematoma is removed through a craniotomy. The clot originated from the laceration of the middle meningeal artery at the foramen spinosum. **A,** The scalp incision site and the margins of the bone flap. **B,** The skull has been removed, and the blood clot is being evacuated. **C,** The anatomic relationships of the base of the skull, dura, brain, and middle meningeal artery.

bleeding from a dural venous sinus or from a large emissary vein in the fracture line. The bleeding will grow and will partly strip the dura off the inner table of the bone. Even if the blood is capable, to some extent, of reentering the circulation through ruptured veins or through vessels in the bone, an expanding mass will develop in most cases. If the bleeding is of arterial origin, it will not stop until it exerts a considerable compression on the brain. If the hematoma develops from a ruptured venous sinus, its pressure is lower; these hematomas sometimes tend to grow very large before causing coma.

Because of its origin near the foramen spinosum, middle meningeal arterial hemorrhage is usually located basally in the middle fossa, and compression of the ipsilateral oculomotor nerve will be a relatively early event. For the same reason contralateral hemiparesis is not a regular symptom and may, in fact, often be ipsilateral because of compression of the contralateral peduncle toward the tentorium. The bradycardia and arterial hypertension mentioned previously constitute the so-called Cushing response to increased ICP (Fig. 47-4).

Subdural Hematoma

Acute Subdural Hematoma. The brain parenchyma has a dense vasculature, and any damage to it will cause bleeding. A traumatic injury to the brain surface will injure the arachnoid, and a contusion will always be associated with a subdural hematoma, although this hematoma may not be of any significant size. An acute, symptomatic subdural hematoma without concomitant parenchymatous brain damage is, on the other hand, relatively rare because bleeding from surface arteries without brain injury is uncommon. Bleeding from veins bridging from the brain to the sagittal sinus, although probably fairly common, will in most cases be tamponaded by the brain before it causes serious problems. Alcoholics and other people with a history of multiple head trauma may have secondary adhesions between the dura and the cortex and are sometimes observed during surgery to have bled from a "bridging artery," i.e., they have developed a "true" acute subdural hematoma without a parenchymal brain injury (Figs. 47-5 to 47-7).

Many cases of acute subdural hematoma are combined not only with a focal contusion but with widespread contusions and hematomas within the lobe, usually the temporal lobe. The expression "burst lobe" has been suggested for this state and is a good description of the picture as it is seen during surgery.[33]

The syndrome associated with an acute subdural hematoma is seldom a clear-cut entity; in most cases, it is associated with severe parenchymatous brain damage. If this damage is limited and occurs in a silent zone, the symptoms, including the free interval, may not differ much from those of an epidural hematoma.

Subacute Subdural Hematoma. When the subdural hematoma is fairly small, i.e., when it has been tamponaded by the brain, it may not be suspected or detected for a few days, at which point the combined volume of the hematoma and the cerebral edema will give rise to symptoms. This is called a subacute subdural hematoma, although the hematoma has been there all the time. It may be said that the brain compresses the hematoma, rather than vice versa. With the frequent use of the CT scan, these hematomas are often revealed before they become "subacute." CT scans also reveal that many of them disappear spontaneously, although a few will become chronic.

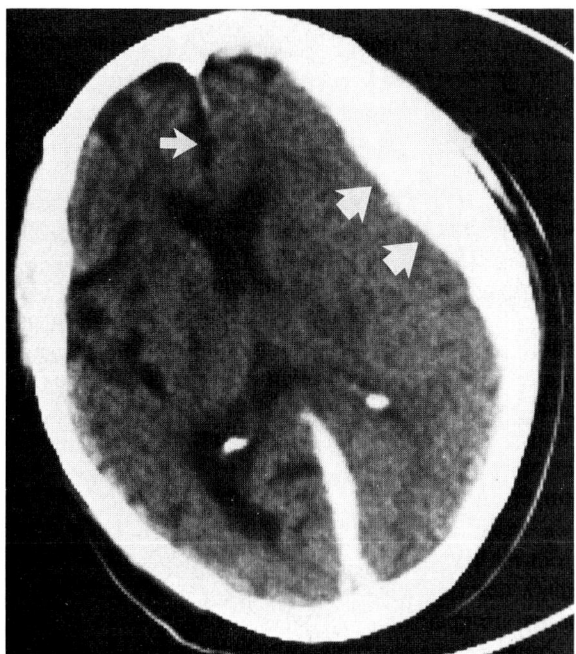

Fig. 47-5 Acute subdural hematoma *(double arrows)* seen on CT scan. The midline is markedly shifted *(single arrow)*.

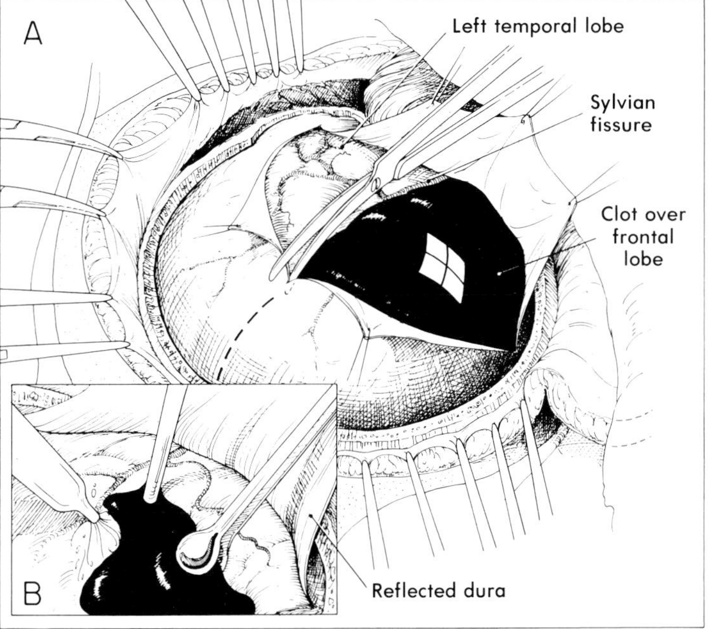

Fig. 47-6 Subdural hematoma is evacuated through a large craniotomy flap. **A,** Removal of the bone, opening of the dura, and identification of the hematoma (clot). **B,** The clot being removed.

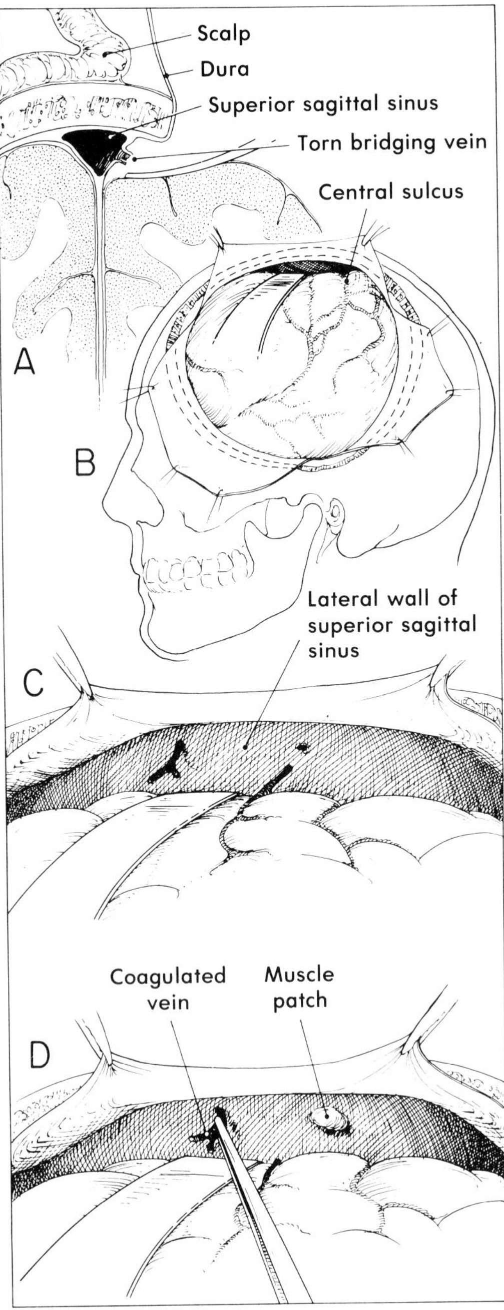

Fig. 47-7 Bridging veins, torn by the brain movement, are often responsible for the subdural hematoma. **A,** A coronal cut through the skull demonstrating anatomic relationships. **B,** The skull removed, dura opened, and lateral view of **A. C,** Corticol veins approaching the superior sagittal sinus. **D,** Two methods used to control venous bleeding—coagulation and placement of a muscle patch.

CHRONIC SUBDURAL HEMATOMA. Chronic subdural hematoma is a complication that appears after mild and moderate, but seldom severe, head injury. These hematomas emanate, as a rule, from a small vein bridging from the cortex to the superior sagittal sinus. In patients with severe head trauma, other brain injuries dominate the picture, and surgical procedures are used to evacuate the hematoma and secure its source, thus preventing it from becoming chronic. The common type of causative injury is a blow to the head in the sagittal direction, such as occurs when a person enters a car or passes through a low door jam. People with elongated and therefore tense bridging veins, i.e., thse with brain atrophy such as is seen in elderly patients and in alcoholics, are more apt to develop a chronic subdural hematoma.

The pathophysiologic events in this condition are not clear, but it has been suggested that the primary venous bleeding is tamponaded by the brain but because of the large subdural space in these patients, not until a fairly large clot is there. This clot is then dissolved, starting from the center, and it ends as a fibrinous capsule filled with clear fluid. The capsule, being semipermeable, grows slowly as the osmotic gradients draw water into it from the surrounding subarachnoid space. The hematoma thus acts as a slowly expanding mass, very much like a brain tumor. According to the site of its origin, the localization will be high up on one or both cerebral hemispheres. Paresis, on one or both sides, serves as an early sign, followed by general signs of elevated ICP. Because of variations in ICP, the symptoms, including the paresis, may vary from day to day, although steady deterioration will be seen over a longer period of time. Pupillary symptoms are a late sign, seen first when there is a substantial brain shift and an imminent temporal lobe herniation. If not decompressed, the process will continue, leading to brain compression, herniation, and death. Since chronic subdural hematomas may be bilateral in many cases, there may not always be any midline shift.

Intracerebral Hematoma

Apart from being associated with a brain contusion or a burst lobe, traumatic intracerebral hematomas are most commonly seen in patients with penetrating injuries. In some cases of closed injury, however, small intracerebral hematomas can be visualized on the CT scan. They are often located in the internal capsule or the basal ganglia and may cause severe neurologic focal deficits.

It is not uncommon to find that an intracerebral hematoma has developed within a contusion after one or a few days. Usually in a CT scan performed within a few hours after the trauma, discrete injury is evident in these patients. It is true that the primary event is the contusion, but it is the hematoma that is responsible for the patient's deterioration and that must be evacuated.

Apart from intracranial expansive lesions, there are a few other rather unusual complications of severe head injury. They are secondary to injury of the intracranial arteries. Trauma to the carotid artery in the neck may cause thrombosis with the patient initially seen with serious neurologic symptoms. After trauma a carotid-cavernous fistula can sometimes be seen engaging the skull base in the region of the carotid canal. Otherwise, posttraumatic arteriovenous fistulas in the brain are very rare. Posttraumatic arterial aneurysms, probably originally false aneurysms that develop within a small hematoma where the vessel was injured, are sometimes seen. Since many aneurysms do not have any real arterial wall, they bleed easily, most often within 3 weeks. They differ from congenital aneurysms in that they are usually located near the surface of the brain and not at a major arterial bifurcation.

PATHOPHYSIOLOGIC CORRELATES UNDERLYING THE SIGNS AND SYMPTOMS OF BRAIN INJURY

Even in today's computer age, the clinical examination is still the basis for diagnosis, therapy, and prognosis after a head injury. Changes in consciousness or, better perhaps, responsiveness are the most evident and the most valuable signs in evaluating a brain-injured patient. Such changes reveal that there has been some interruption between the reticular system in the brainstem and the cerebral cortex but do not disclose exactly where, to what extent, or whether this dysfunction is reversible or not, i.e., whether there is permanent anatomic damage.

There have been many attempts to correlate coma depth with the severity of brain injury, but problems arise because severity itself must first be defined. Should severity be determined by the volume of brain parenchyma that is primarily damaged, by some physiologic parameter such as ICP, CBF, or $CMRO_2$, or just by neurologic outcome? Or might some neurophysiologic parameter give the answer?

The Glasgow Coma Scale[83] (Table 47-I), the clinical scale that is most often used today, is still basically an empirical scale, originally using the patients' outcome as a yardstick.[84] One of its advantages is that nurses and general surgeons can be as consistent as neurosurgeons when using the scale. Its most important drawback, which it shares with other scales of the same type, is that it cannot be used in patients who are undergoing modern intensive care treatment with endotracheal intubation and pharmacologic paralyzation; in addition, the Glasgow Coma Score is not appropriate when the patient is aphasic. Comparing grades of responsiveness with severity of the injury to determine outcome is furthermore complicated by the well-known fact that the most important factor determining outcome after a brain injury is the patient's age since children (at least after the first few years) and young adults may recover from injuries that would invariably lead to severe disability in an older person.

The word coma needs a definition. The Head Injury Committee of the World Federation of Neurosurgical Societies has defined coma as "an unrousable, unresponsive state, regardless of duration; eyes continuously closed." Using this definition, patients who react to painful stimuli would not be in coma since they are not unresponsive. Plum and Posner[65] discussed several physiologic functions (i.e., state of consciousness, pupillary reaction, eye movements, ocular reflexes, motor responses, and breathing patterns) to be taken into consideration when evaluating the degree of coma. The Glasgow Coma Scale does not, in spite of its name, exactly determine if the patient is in coma or not, although a patient with a coma score of less than 7 to 8 will certainly be in coma.[84] The duration of the coma state is also important. Coma immediately following trauma does not indicate per se any permanent injury, although the patient who is still in coma 6 hours later probably has sustained severe damage and diffuse axonal injury. Patients who have been able to speak some understandable words after the trauma, on the other hand, are not too badly injured, and any decreased responsiveness later must be caused by what might be called a second insult, such as hematoma, brain swelling, and hypoxia.[56]

Table 47-1 **GLASGOW COMA SCALE**

Response	Points
Eye Opening	
Spontaneous	4
To sound	3
To pain	2
None	1
Motor Response	
Obeys commands	6
Localizes pain	5
Normal flexion (withdrawal)	4
Abnormal flexion (decortication)	3
Extension (decerebration)	2
None	1
Verbal Response	
Oriented	5
Confused conversation	4
Inappropriate words	3
Incomprehensive sounds	2
None	1

From Teasdale, G., and Jennett, B.: Lancet **2:**81, 1974.

It is important to administer repeated neurologic examinations to detect the small changes that warn that something is changing intracranially. The essential neurologic tests to perform are (apart from evaluation of responsiveness) checking pupil size and reaction, eye movements, and movements of face and extremities and, if the patient is not in coma, determining if he is able to talk and understand speech and to see and hear on both sides. Any epileptic seizures should be carefully noted with special emphasis on whether they are generalized or focal.

The purpose of the neurologic examination is to judge if the positive findings are results of generalized brain injury (such as occurs in coma) or a local injury (such as occurs with aphasia or a monoparesis). This judgment is often far from easy since most signs may represent both local and general disturbances of brain function. Epilepsy, for example, may be elicited by a focal cortical injury but may also be a sign of increased ICP. As already implied, it is the dynamic process rather than the actual state that has to be evaluated. A discussion follows of the various pathophysiologic events that may follow a severe head injury and their clinical consequences.

The most important "secondary insult" associated with head trauma is the development of an expanding intracranial mass—a hematoma, abscess, or localized edema. The mass usually is unilateral or at least predominantly on one side and is located frontally or temporally. As the mass grows, it compresses the brain and usually raises ICP. Headache, restlessness, and, sometimes, focal signs such as expressive dysphasia, depending on the site of the mass, often result. Then the medial part of the temporal lobe, the uncus gyri, is displaced over the free edge of the tentorium and later becomes herniated through the tentorial hiatus. Compression of the brainstem causes a deterioration of responsiveness and, especially if the ICP is raised, bradycardia and arterial hypertension. The oculomotor nerve will then be compressed between the posterior cerebral and superior cerebellar arteries, causing an ipsilateral dilated and fixed pupil. Further compression on the brainstem causes deep coma, abnormal motor response (decerebrate rigidity), and abnormal eye movements. Finally, the vasomotor centers in the medulla are affected with an increase in arterial pressure and a decrease in heart rate (symptoms that most often follow, rather than preceded, coma) and respiratory arrest.

When the expanding mass is mainly frontal, the entire brain is compressed downward with an axial displacement of the brainstem toward the foramen magnum, causing stretching of the brainstem branches of the basilar artery, with ischemia and hemorrhage into the brainstem, in which case bilateral symptoms are more apt to occur from the beginning. A paresis may become visible at any stage of this series of events. Also, a hemiparesis can be contralateral as well as ipsilateral to the growing mass, a result of either direct compression on the pyramidal tract or compression of the contralateral peduncle toward the tentorial edge. This is in contrast to the early pupillary symptoms, which are always ipsilateral to the expansive mass. When the mass is infratentorially located, the cerebellar tonsils will prolapse through the foramen magnum, and apnea and heart arrest from compression of the medulla oblongata may appear almost without warning.[55]

Some patients with chronic intracranial hypertension, e.g., those with pseudotumor cerebri, can tolerate very high ICP without much disturbance of brain function, and many of the symptoms traditionally attributed to raised ICP are probably a result of brain displacement, as discussed previously, or of the effect of the increased ICP on cerebral blood flow.[55] The healthy brain is capable of autoregulating its blood flow within very large limits of arterial blood pressure, as well as of ICP, but this ability is usually impaired after severe head injury.[17] A prolonged period of increased ICP may also further disturb the autoregulative mechanisms. In head injury patients, an ICP of 60 mm Hg or higher, even for a short period, is a very serious sign with a bad prognosis.[57] There are some patients who, in the absence of any significant mass, develop a generalized edema that is visualized on a CT scan as low attenuation of the brain parenchyma associated with very small ventricles and nonvisible brainstem cisterns. If monitored, elevated ICP will be found.[86] But even in these cases it is hard to say if it is the pressure per se or the compression on vital structures from the swollen brain that is responsible for any deterioration. When angiography was the method of choice for diagnosis after head injury, these patients often had very slow intracerebral circulation or had a spasm in one or more of their main cerebral arteries. During surgery these patients would have a very tense dura, a sign of high ICP. This high ICP is generally unaffected by mannitol, urea, and hyperventilation because of impaired autoregulation. It is difficult to say if the decreased CBF and/or the vasospasm is caused by the raised ICP or by the direct effect of blood in the CSF causing vasospasm in the pial vessels, in which case the high ICP is secondary to the hypoxic brain edema.

Rationale Underlying Diagnostic Tests

To accurately plan for treatment and to determine the prognosis after a severe head injury, obtaining exact information regarding the extent of primary brain damage and the potential influence of any secondary insult is fundamental. It is often difficult and sometimes impossible to evaluate individually the influence of raised ICP, compression of the brain, increased or decreased cerebral blood flow, hypoxia, arterial hypotension and hypertension, and metabolic disturbances. The clinical examination alone, although necessary as a basis for further analysis, cannot satisfactorily answer many of these questions and must be supplemented by objective information on anatomic and physiologic data whenever possible.

CT Scan

The CT scan[27] makes possible the good visualization of any intracranial mass, learning its extent, localization, and in most cases, its nature. Since the examination is quick and noninvasive when using the new generation of scanners, it can be performed in patients who are restless and in poor condition and in children. Since a hematoma may well be present long before it gives rise to any symptoms and since it should be evacuated, a CT scan should be performed on every head-injured patient who is not totally alert and free of neurologic symptoms on arrival at the hospital. Apart from revealing a possible hematoma, the CT scan also can reveal signs of edema and of raised ICP. If the water content of the brain is increased, the attenuation seen on x-ray film will diminish, resulting in a darkening on the films when compared with the surrounding nonedematous parenchyma or when compared with normal in cases of generalized brain edema. This finding is not necessarily indicative of raised ICP except when seen with small ventricles (in adults). Another sign, commonly related to raised ICP, is compression of the subarachnoid space so that the cisterns surrounding the brainstem are not visualized.[86] Although cerebral contusions are visible as areas of mixed density, diffuse anoxal injury can usually not be visualized on the CT picture.

Blood in the subarachnoid space is sometimes the only pathologic finding seen on a CT scan after a head injury. If the history of an accident is not clear, the presence of subarachnoid blood sometimes leads to the suspicion of a primary subarachnoid hemorrhage as the cause of the accident, especially if no fracture is seen. Fractures are easily seen on a CT scan, and depressed fractures are usually better visualized through a CT scan than routine x-ray films. Consequently, there is no need to perform a skull x-ray on patients for whom a CT scan is indicated.

Magnetic Resonance

Magnetic resonance[80] represents a totally new modality for visualization of the skull's interior, eliminating the use of ionizing radiation. It is based on the principle of the nucleus' rotation or ''spin'' around its axis and the magnetic field it generates. By measuring the distribution of hydrogen, predominantly in water and fat, the organs of the body can be displayed ''biochemically.'' Magnetic resonance clearly defines white and gray matter because the latter contains 14% more water. Magnetic resonance also identifies the structures of the posterior fossa better than CT because of the absence of artifacts from bone in the skull base. It is also easier than when using CT to get images in more than one dimension, but it is an expensive technique that probably will not be commonly available for some time, and many carefully controlled studies remain to be performed, especially regarding its long-term safety.

Angiography

Angiography can give more information about the brain's blood circulation than the CT scan, but its capacity to show the anatomic details and, especially, the nature of a pathologic change is so much inferior that it no longer has any role in examining acute head injuries when a CT scanner is available. Four-vessel angiography is, however, still the best way to certify brain death and is used routinely for this purpose in many countries whenever the question of taking organs for transplantation arises. If contrast injection in the aortic arch visualizes the peripheral branches of the external carotids and the internal carotids are distal at the base of the skull but with no contrast entering the brain and if the same results are obtained after a second injection 20 minutes later, the brain is dead.

When carotid angiography was the method of choice to diagnose posttraumatic intracranial pathology, a prolonged cerebral circulation time (the time from complete contrast filling of the arterial tree until the contrast has left the capillaries and the intracerebral venous circulation is visualized)[22] and/or a segmental or generalized spasm of a major intracranial artery could often be observed in patients with severe head injuries. Patients with a cerebral circulation time of 10 seconds or more were usually in a very poor state, and, during surgery, they often had a very high ICP caused by "malignant brain swelling" that did not react to hyperventilation, mannitol, or urea. The pulsations of the brain were weak or almost absent, and the outcome was poor. These patients were in the state that just precedes brain death. On the other hand, patients with segmental vasospasm but with a fairly normal overall circulation time often survive with focal neurologic signs only, such as aphasia or hemiplegia, and the recovery rate is not too poor.

Positron Emission Tomography

Positron emission tomography (PET) is a noninvasive scanning method that produces a cross-section picture of brain radioactivity following intravenous injection of a labeled indicator.[28] It was first applied to measurements of the local cerebral metabolic rate using methods similar to quantitative autoradiography. When fluorine-18–labeled deoxyglucose is used as a glucose-equivalent (i.e., the molecule is metabolized through the same pathways as glucose but only to a certain point where it will remain fixed without further metabolism), the density of locations on the films will be related to the regional metabolic rate of glucose. Other tracers include oxygen-15–labeled carbon dioxide and molecular oxygen used to quantitate regional CBF and carbon-11– or oxygen-15–labeled carbon monoxide used to quantitate cerebral blood volume. The PET technique relies on the fate of positrons emitted by certain radionuclides, the annihilation of which releases energy in the form of gamma rays. Measuring the attenuation on a calibrated scanner makes it possible to determine the regional concentration of a radioisotope within the brain in μCi/ml. Thus the PET picture is effected from internal radiation rather than from conventional external radiation as in a CT scan. PET can also show other aspects of metabolism such as the state of the blood-brain barrier, but it will probably continue to be available only in highly specialized centers.

Brain Scintigraphy

Brain scintigraphy, or brain scan, using intravenous radioactive isotopes (usually ^{99}Tc) is of no value in evaluating head injury except in diagnosing certain subchronic and chronic hematomas. When the components of a blood clot are disintegrated during the formation of a chronic subdural hematoma, the attenuation changes from high in fresh blood to very low in chronic hematoma effusion. Somewhere during this process, the hematoma attains the same attenuation as the surrounding brain tissue at which stage the hematoma, especially if bilateral, may be hard to detect on the CT scan, although it is easy to see on the scintigram. A brain scan is a very good screening test when a chronic subdural hematoma is suspected and a CT scan is not available, especially when used with the elderly, nonambulatory patient.

Echoencephalography

A mass, which is in most cases unilateral, is the most important complication in head injury, and since this mass is supposed to cause a midline shift of the brain, any diagnostic examination that can rapidly and easily detect such a shift is of value as a screening test. A frontal x-ray of the skull will, in approximately 25% of the adult population, reveal a calcified pineal body, which should normally not deviate more than 3 mm from the midline.[34] When the pineal gland cannot be visualized on an x-ray and in children, echoencephalography makes it possible to get an accurate determination of the midline. It works with ultrasound impulses that are transmitted through the bone from the temporal region. Since the velocity of the wave is known, the distance to the midline can be calculated from the time the impulse takes to travel a round trip, which is visualized on an oscilloscope directly as a distance.[34] The examination is quick and very accurate when performed by an experienced investigator but has lost importance since introduction of the CT scan.

Intracranial Pressure Monitoring

Since the introduction of long-term continuous registration of intracranial pressure (ICP) by Lundberg in 1960,[46] monitoring of ICP has become a standard procedure in many head injury centers. A rise in ICP is often the first warning of a hematoma before the patient's vital signs start to change.[82] With treatment in a modern intensive care unit of patients who are often paralyzed by muscle relaxants and depressants, ICP may be the only objective parameter available. The importance of ICP monitoring has been confirmed by the findings that ICP levels above 60 mm Hg, even for very short periods of time, are associated with a poor prognosis and must be avoided (Table 47-2).

If the numeric levels of ICP are important, even more vital information can be obtained from measurements of the brain's compliance or its reciprocal, elastance, i.e., the

Table 47-2 **TECHNIQUES FOR MONITORING INTRACRANIAL PRESSURE**

Method	Insertion	Accuracy	Infection	VPR and CSF drainage*
Ventricular catheter	Problem with small ventricles	Excellent	3%-5%	Yes
Subarachnoid screw	Little difficulty	Good	Less	No
Epidural transducer	Little difficulty	Variable	Negligible	No

*VPR, volume pressure ratio; CSF, cerebrospinal fluid.

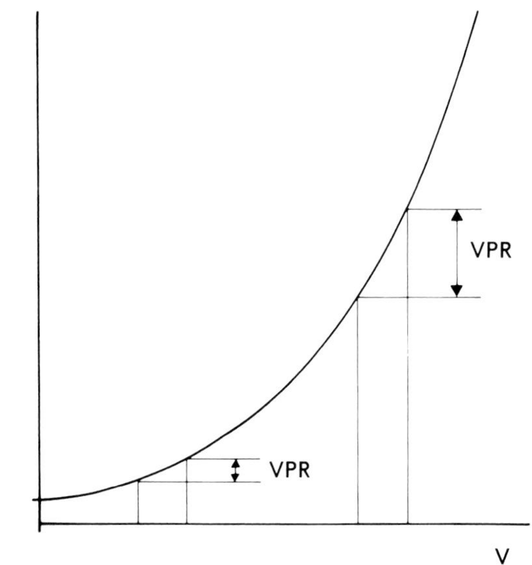

Fig. 47-8 Volume-pressure response *(VPR)*. A small addition of volume causes only an insignificant increase in intracranial pressure (ICP) when ICP is low; the same amount of volume increase may cause a considerable rise of ICP when the pressure is already high. *P*, pressure; *V*, volume.

relation between volume changes and pressure changes.[50] In an ''ideal'' container, pressure varies linearly with volume. The CSF compartment is not ideal, but the CSF volume pressure curve plotted on a linear axis has been found to be exponential. Plotted on a semilogarithmic axis, the curve can be approximated by a straight line, and the slope of that line is the pressure volume index, which is the amount of volume necessary to raise pressure by a factor of 10.[51] This theory has been adapted practically by Miller[54] who introduced the volume pressure ratio, which is the increase of ICP when 1 ml saline is introduced into the CSF (Fig. 47-8). A high-pressure response indicates that the margins for further intracranial expansion are small and that the patient is in great danger.

Cerebral Blood Flow Measurements

At the cellular level, metabolic activity determines the function and survival capacity of the neurons. Oxygen and glucose are the most important molecules involved, without which the whole mechanism stops working.[75] There are no direct methods to measure oxygen tension in brain tissue, but the metabolic consumption of oxygen ($CMRO_2$) can be calculated by measuring the difference in oxygen between arterial and venous (jugular bulb) blood ($AVDO_2$) and the cerebral blood flow (CBF). $CMRO_2$ is the product of $AVDO_2$ and CBF. This is, unfortunately, still a rough estimation since it does not take into account any regional differences.[9]

CBF is usually estimated from the velocity by which a radioactive molecule is ''washed out'' from the brain. Practically, the isotope, normally ^{133}Xe, is injected intravenously (or into the carotid artery), and the peak and the subsequent decrease of radioactivity are registered above the head with one or several detectors on each side of it. Since xenon is eliminated from the blood almost totally during its first passage through the lungs, the decrease of radioactivity will be proportional to the blood flow in the area covered by the detector. The radioactivity is decreased along a logarithmic curve with a fast component and a slow component that represent the gray and white matter respectively. Severe head injury may be associated with a low or a high CBF, and there may be marked regional differences. CBF studies can also determine if autoregulation is impaired.

When the CBF is too low to meet metabolic demands, brain cells will suffer from substrate and oxygen deficiency. Normal aerobic metabolism cannot continue but must switch to anaerobic pathways, a less effective method of energy production. Pyruvate cannot be metabolized through the Krebs cycle and may be converted to lactate, which will be reflected in the CSF as lactic acidosis; this condition is associated with a bad prognosis, although it is not certain if lactic acid is the cause or just an epiphenomenon. The fact that neutralization of the CSF through treatment with tromethamine (ThAM) has a favorable effect on outcome[70] favors the former alternative, as do results obtained by Rehncrona and associates.[67] CSF lactic acid is not, on the other hand, significantly correlated with CSF creatine phosphokinase BB (see section on Biochemical Tests), which may be a better indicator of the actual parenchymal brain damage.

Neurophysiologic Examinations

It is possible to get information concerning the condition of the brain by means of neurophysiologic studies, mainly an electroencephalogram (EEG) and evoked potentials. The normal alpha rhythm switches over to a pattern dominated by slow waves (delta rhythm) in patients with severe head injuries (and in many other types of injury). However, the enormous quantity of data accumulated when using a routine EEG for monitoring ICP makes the raw EEG impractical for head injury studies. For these reasons techniques have been developed to condense the EEG into a more compact form, of which the compressed

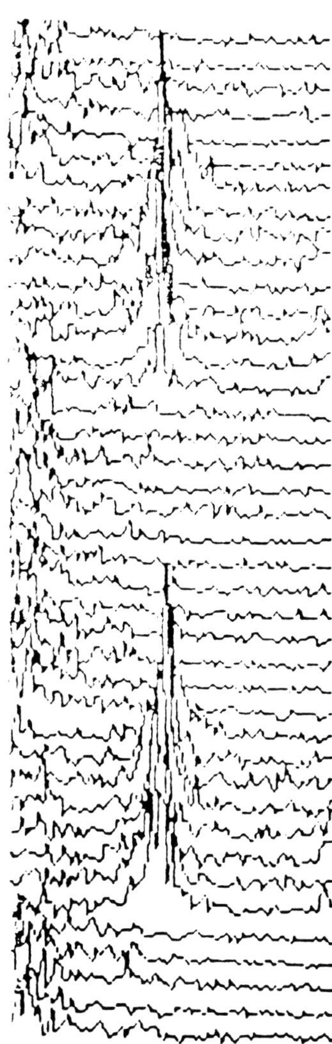

Fig. 47-9 Normal compressed spectral array of the electroencephalogram with a dominance of alpha rhythms (8 to 12 Hz).

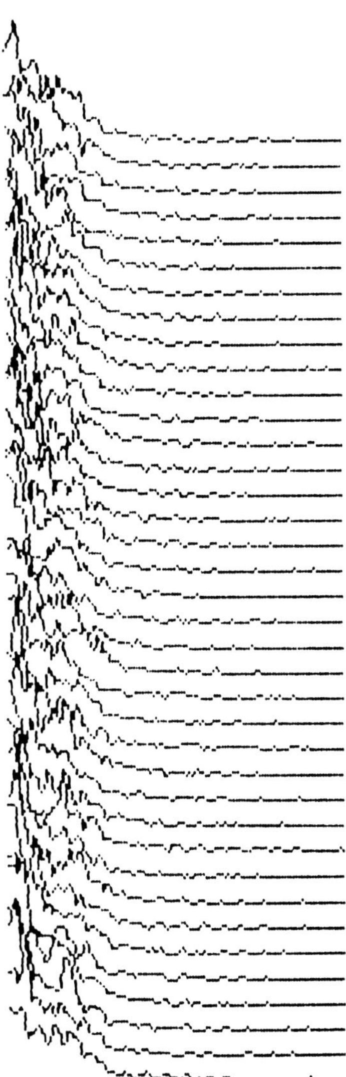

Fig. 47-10 Compressed spectral array showing excessive delta activity in a patient with severe brain injury.

spectral array seems the most promising. Compressed spectral array is a three-dimensional graphic display that demonstrates the amount of power within each frequency band (delta, theta, alpha, and beta) (Fig. 47-9). The compressed spectral array is generated by a digital computer that records the raw EEG for a given short epoch. It is possible with this method to obtain the percentage of power for each frequency band and to study the variations over a period of time. There seems to be some indications that the amount of power in the beta frequency band and, although perhaps to a lower degree, in the delta band and the variability of the frequency spectrum are related to the severity of the traumatic brain injury.

The sensory evoked potential is brain electrical activity that is recorded from the scalp, overlying the cerebral cortex, in response to a sensory stimulus. Visual, auditory, and somatosensory responses are the ones commonly used. Abnormalities in the evoked response pattern are related to outcome and, hence, are related to the severity of brain injury (Fig. 47-10).[63] In contrast to EEG results, the evoked potentials are not as affected by deep coma, drugs such as central nervous system depressants, or epileptic seizures, which makes them very useful in the study of head injury patients.

Biochemical Tests

The determination of certain biochemical markers of brain injury in blood or CSF is based on the concept that the markers reflect either a metabolic change (lactic acid) or mechanical damage to the cell membrane accompanied by the release of intracellular structural proteins or enzymes (myelin basic protein,[85] lactic dehydrogenase isoenzymes, or creatine phosphokinase BB).[48] All of these changes correlate with outcome and, therefore, with the severity of damage after head injuries.

Rationale Underlying Medical and Surgical Treatment of Head-Injured Patients

There are two basic principles underlying the management of patients with head trauma: (1) to anticipate and to prevent any additional brain insult from an abnormal physiologic event; and (2) to provide an ideal healing milieu for those brain cells that are partially injured but that can potentially recover.

It is well known that severely brain-injured patients can make an astonishingly good recovery weeks and even months after the trauma. Whether recovery is a result of central nervous system plasticity with uninjured cells taking over the functions of those that were destroyed or if it represents a true recovery of traumatized, but only partially injured, neurons is not totally clear; however, it seems both mechanisms are in operation.

Immediate Care

A study from three large neurosurgical institutes has shown that almost a third of head-injury patients who later die were able to utter at least a few understandable words at some stage after the trauma before they developed persistent coma.[33] This could mean that the primary insult to the brain was not incompatible with reasonable brain function and that it was a secondary insult that was responsible for the deterioration and death of these patients. This second insult was a hematoma in a majority of cases but was also fairly often of extracranial origin, such as hypoxia, anemia (from bleeding), or arterial hypotension (shock). These types of secondary insults cause severe generalized or focal disturbances that result in irreversible neuropathologic changes when the metabolic demands of the brain tissue cannot be adequately satisfied. The best measure to prevent these insults is to organize competent care beginning at the scene of the accident, through emergency care, to the specialized neurosurgical intensive care unit. The purpose of immediate care is to secure the brain's need for oxygen and blood, i.e., to ensure that the airway is free from obstruction, that respiration is satisfactory, and, if not, that artificial respiration is instituted. If there are no signs of dangerous bleeding or shock, the patient should be transported directly to a hospital where the essential neurosurgical expertise and resources are available, even if the choice of a hospital would mean a somewhat longer transportation time since a hematoma usually takes at least an hour to develop before it becomes critical. Often in treating patients with severe multiple injuries the neurosurgeon should be present from the beginning to help plan management so that valuable time is not lost before diagnosis of a hematoma and to ensure that drugs or anesthetics that may increase intracranial pressure are not used.[3,18]

If, on the other hand, a patient is found in shock after trauma, it must be remembered that shock is never caused by intracranial bleeding (since the patient would be dead long before the bleeding had become great enough to cause shock) and that the cause has to be found elsewhere. Patients with open fractures to the venous dural sinuses may bleed profusely, but a simple elevation of the patient's head well above the level of the heart is often enough to stop this bleeding.

Every head injury patient who is in coma must be treated as if he also has a cervical spine injury until the contrary has been proven.

Surgical Treatment

The most obvious and the most dramatic of the secondary insults in a head-injury patient is the intracranial hematoma that, within a couple of minutes, is capable of changing the patient's status from full alertness to deep coma. Although theoretically a hematoma is evacuated rather than prevented, if surgery is performed early, a second insult to the brain may, in fact, be prevented. Consequently, we believe that any expansive mass should be evacuated before deterioration and other signs indicating tentorial herniation appear.[7] Any patient with a severe head injury, i.e., a patient who is unable to follow a simple command and who has a lateral mass that causes a midline shift, should have this mass evacuated. If the mass is intra-axial, if no localized mass is demonstrable, or if there are multiple intracerebral lesions, surgery is indicated if there is a midline shift of 5 mm or more. If a small mass is found in a patient with clinical signs of a moderate head injury (has impaired responsiveness but still able to follow commands) or a mild head injury (has had a transient loss of consciousness but is alert, oriented, and without neurologic deficits), this patient should be monitored very carefully, and the CT scan should be repeated to confirm that the mass is not expanding. All severe head injuries, whether they undergo surgery or not, should have intracranial pressure monitoring with repeated measurements of volume-pressure response and, if possible, repeated studies also of CBF and $CMRO_2$. Using these aggressive indices for surgical treatment of intracranial masses, the mortality and mobidity rates decrease when compared to results using more conventional indications for operative treatment.[6,33]

An acute subdural hematoma is, in almost every case, only one element of the injury; the other and often more important element is the brain contusion, and a surgical approach planned only to allow evacuation of a clot may be doomed to fail. A bone flap that is large enough to provide for inspection of the underlying frontal and temporal lobes should always be turned.[7]

Open brain injuries constitute a special problem. Potentially infected material has to be extracted but not if to do so would further impair brain function. To avoid adhesions between the brain and the skin that may potentially cause posttraumatic epilepsy and also to prevent brain herniation, the dura should always be closed (if necessary, with a fascia transplant). Contaminated bone should not be replaced because of the risk of osteitis, but every effort must be made to get safe skin covering.

Although the symptoms caused by a hematoma are mainly ascribable to the direct compression and shift of the brain, raised intracranial pressure (ICP) is always an important feature in patients with intracranial hematomas. However, most patients with increased ICP after a head injury do not have a hematoma, and in these cases the increased ICP is usually associated with brain edema or brain swelling. The nomenclature regarding this state of increased volume of the intracranial contents is not yet defined in terms that are generally accepted, a fact that causes some confusion. But a consensus seems to be developing regarding the use of "brain edema" to represent a condition in which there is increased water content of the brain, intracellularly or extracellularly, and the use of "brain swelling" to indicate vascular engorgement (which certainly may also lead to some edema). A special type of extra-cellular edema is hydrocephalus, i.e., an increased volume of intracranial CSF causing ventricular enlargement. After head trauma, hydrocephalus may be caused very rapidly by an infratentorial hematoma compressing the CSF pathways or, somewhat later, by subarachnoid blood interfering with CSF circulation and/or resorption. The acute ventricular dilation observed in connection with infratentorial hematomas is associated with a very high ICP and is a life-threatening condition that demands immediate decompression by means of a ventricular puncture. Late posttraumatic hydrocephalus is usually less dramatic and is best treated with a permanent shunting device, which drains the CSF to the peritoneal cavity or directly to the blood.

Although use of a ventricular catheter or a shunt may sometimes be of value in patients with generalized edema, the ventricles are compressed in most of these patients and therefore will be difficult to puncture and, if punctured and drained, will produce a limited volume decrease that is often quickly refilled by the progressive edema. Even the evacuation of a hematoma does not always restore ICP to normal levels if the processes responsible for edema production have already started.

Hyperventilation

When the head-injured patient has no localized intracranial mass and no ventricular dilation, there will be no way to affect the raised ICP surgically. However, knowledge of normal and pathologic brain physiology, as described earlier in this chapter, enables the physician to tackle this problem etiologically, i.e., to influence the mechanisms responsible for the development of brain edema/swelling or at least to prevent its harmful effects on the nervous structures.

Since an essential part of the intracranial (brain) volume consists of blood vessels that are susceptible to volume changes from variations in extracellular pH[43] and since this extracellular pH is dependent on the partial pressure of carbon dioxide (P_{CO_2} within the cerebral capillaries, it seems rational and is effective to decrease intracranial volume and thereby ICP by decreasing arterial P_{CO_2}. Although responsiveness to P_{CO_2} changes (chemical regulation) is reduced after severe head injury, it still persists in most patients, and reduction of arterial P_{CO_2} from normal (40 mm Hg) down to 25 to 30 mm Hg by means of artificial hyperventilation is now a well-established treatment.[21]

Many severe head-injury patients hyperventilate spontaneously, but since this hyperventilation is associated with strenuous muscular work, it leads to systemic lactic acidosis and has to be counteracted. For this reason and to make it easier for the patients to adjust to the ventilator, they should receive muscle relaxants. There is still some controversy about the exact indications for instituting hyperventilation. British neurosurgeons and anesthesiologists especially advocate normoventilation, meaning that the main goal is that the patient is not underventilated. But most experts agree to hyperventilate every patient whose Glasgow Coma Scale score remains 8 or less 1 to a few hours after injury. Hyperventilation is also indicated if the partial pressure of oxygen (P_{O_2}) is less than 70 mm Hg or if it is expected that the patient will develop respiratory problems. If the patient undergoes surgery, hyperventilation should be continued at least until the following morning. The P_{CO_2} level must be checked, preferably by continuous monitoring, because hypocarbia around 20 mm Hg may cause ischemia and because hypercarbia, even for a very short period, such as when the patient's airways are suctioned, causes the ICP to rise to dangerous levels.

Hypertonic Solutions

Hypertonic solutions have long been used to counteract brain edema. Intravenously administered mannitol (20% in water) is most widely used at present, although some physicians are still using urea (carbamide) and/or glycerol, which can also be given orally. Mannitol cannot cross the blood-brain barrier. It establishes an osmotic gradient between the brain and the blood so that water is drawn out of the extracellular space into the vascular system. Mannitol reduces brain water content from 80% to 87%. It remains unclear, however, whether it acts differentially on the healthy brain or on regions with cerebral edema. Therefore the total reduction in brain volume is estimated as 5 to 20 ml with the use of mannitol. Recently an additional or alternative explanation has been given for the effects of hypertonic solutions.[60,61] Mannitol reduces blood viscosity. According to Poiseuille's law, the decreased viscosity should lead to an increase in cerebral blood flow (CBF). If autoregulation is intact, the brain does not need this extra CBF, and it will react with vasoconstriction, analogous to increased blood pressure.[38] In the presence of intact autoregulation, it has been estimated that the arteriolar vasoconstriction, after the administration of a bolus of 1 g mannitol/per kilogram of body weight, decreases cerebral blood volume by at least 5 to 20 ml, which is equal to the volume decrease resulting from the dehydrating effects of mannitol. This mechanism also explains why mannitol administration leads to an increase in CBF without much change in ICP when autoregulation is not intact. Therefore the use of hypertonic solutions may (temporarily) be beneficial even in the absence of ICP changes.[60]

Fluid Restriction

Fluid restriction for head-injury patients (still commonly prescribed) does not have a sound rationale. Brain edema may well exist in spite of a relative deficit of total body water. Water reduction may even be harmful because the increased viscosity of the blood may lead to cerebral vasodilation, i.e., a brain swelling, to keep CBF constant. There may also be negative systemic effects of dehydration. Thus even if liberal water intake should be avoided, indications for subnormal water intake do not seem to exist.

Glucocorticoids

Glucocorticoids have a positive effect on the edema surrounding malignant brain tumors and have been used in patients with many varieties of brain lesions, including traumatic head injury. Their effect on the electrolyte balance of central nervous tissues is well established, particularly in the reversal of pathologic water and ionic imbalances associated with edema. Animal studies have demonstrated that steroids ameliorate histopathologic changes created by a variety of insults to the brain. There are many hypothetical mechanisms—membrane stabilization preventing release of lysosomes and excessive Ca^{++}-influx into cells, alteration of ionic-clearing mechanisms, and improvement of CBF.[89] Antioxidant properties of steroids may play a role in inhibiting free radical reactions.[13] Randomized trials have not, however, demonstrated an improved outcome in head-injury patients who received these drugs in what is supposed to be adequate doses.[12] The only result is a tendency toward more pulmonary complications in patients in whom glucocorticoids had been administered. The chance that glucocorticoids would activate a peptic ulcer is, on the other hand, probably very much overemphasized. In a few patients, however, a diabetic tendency may grow into manifest diabetes with the very large doses of glucocorticoids used.

Hypothermia

Based on experience gained from performing intracranial aneurysm surgery where it was demonstrated that it is safe to clip a major cerebral artery for 10 to 12 minutes at a body temperature of 27° to 29° C, as opposed to 3 minutes at normal body temperature, hypothermia was introduced in the treatment of severe head injuries as a means of lowering the cerebral metabolism so that "demand could correspond to supply." However, the clinical results were not encouraging since all the usual complications of brain injury nevertheless appeared. Deep hypothermia might possibly afford some advantages, but its use would require a heart-lung machine, and this machine has not been tried clinically.

Hyperthermia must be avoided in brain-injured patients since even a limited rise of body temperature increases the metabolism and thereby increases the oxygen demand of the brain substantially. Fever can be counteracted by various means, such as administering antipyretic drugs (salicylates must be used with care since they may decrease coagulability of blood), maintaining a low room temperature, or cooling the body with a fan or by washing it with alcohol.

Barbiturates

Barbiturates were originally introduced to decrease metabolism, thereby protecting the brain from the effects of ischemia and hypoxia.[53] Barbiturates also controlled ICP in severely brain-injured patients.[52] Thus the use of barbiturates, specifically pentobarbital, in continuous coma-causing doses or as bolus injections has become widely used in the treatment of these patients. Barbiturates were primarily thought not to exert any direct actions on CBF and the tone of cerebral vascular smooth muscle, but there are now some indications that they may have a relaxant effect on cerebral blood vessels.[3] There is evidence that barbiturates penetrate into membrane lipid and alter its physical state. Resultant changes in ion channels and membrane-bound enzymes have been hypothesized as a mechanism of action of barbiturates.[25]

The most important and undesirable side effect of pentobarbital is arterial hypotension that is thought to be caused by peripheral vasodilation and, to some extent, by pentobarbital's depressive effect on cardiac contractility. Therefore, even if pentobarbital-caused coma can lower ICP, there is still no evidence that pentobarbital improves the outcome when used prophylactically in severely head-injured patients.[87]

RECOVERY FROM HEAD INJURY

Most recovery from traumatic brain injury occurs in the first 6 months, but some neurologic improvement can continue for 12 to 18 months. Improvement thereafter is usually a result of retraining or learning of special skills. Few patients with severe brain injury fully recover their neurologic and psychologic faculties. Even patients with mild brain injury frequently have annoying subjective symptoms that last 1 to 2 years or longer.

The location and extent of the initial and secondary brain injuries determine the quality of the ultimate outcome. Focal residual neurologic deficits such as hemiparesis or hemianopsia are relatively uncommon. Unfortunately, deficits and alterations in intellectual function, memory, and behavior are frequent and reflect injury to the frontal and temporal lobes and limbic structures. Most patients who survive severe brain injury recover independence; 80% are able to function without assistance in daily living. Of the remainder, 15% end up severely disabled, and a further 5% are severely demented or vegetative.

Rehabilitation after head injury should include neuropsychologic testing and therapy tailored to specific handicaps in the motor, emotional, behavioral, and mental spheres. Endogenous depression is common and may be related to a reduced level of brain biogenic amines. Drug treatment with antidepressants is often effective. Family counseling is critical.

Postconcussion Syndrome

Many patients who suffer brain injury experience annoying symptoms that may last for months and, rarely, years. Those patients who had a mild or moderate injury are thus expecting an early, complete recovery complain the most. Often there are no obvious abnormal neurologic signs, and the physician is at a loss to explain the complaints. The symptoms usually include headache, irritability, and a feeling of lightheadedness or dizziness but not true vertigo. Other complaints include difficulty with concentration, worry and apprehension, a preoccupation with self, a lack of interest in others' affairs, mild difficulty with memory, intolerance to loud noises and alcohol, insomnia, and loss of sexual interest. Quick movements or turning the head up or side-ways may bring on lightheadedness or a dazed, weak feeling. Perhaps as many as half of these patients show mild, subtle neurologic signs such as abnormal electronystagmography.

The anatomic basis for the postconcussive syndrome is not known. Presumably many patients have had an injury to the vestibular apparatus. Associated neck injuries (whiplash) are often a part of the complex. Neural connections between damaged neck muscles and the brainstem may be a contributing cause. Minimum brainstem injury could conceivably be responsible for some of the symptoms. The syndrome is so frequent and the complaints so consistent that it must have a consistent biologic substrate, out whether it is structural, neuropharmacologic, or psychologic remains a mystery. The symptoms are not merely a reflection of compensation claims or pending litigation, although such concerns undoubtedly influence the length and degree of the complaints. The most important aspect of treatment is firm and immediate reassurance that the symptoms are not unusual, have no serious implications, and will eventually disappear. Patients who are told there are no reasons for complaints become even more preoccupied with the symptoms. Recovery is the rule but may take as long as several years in some cases.

SUMMARY

The significance of head trauma relates not so much to what has happended to its exterior (i.e., the scalp and the skull) but to what has occurred within the brain and its coverings. Depending on the mass of the object striking the head and its accompanying velocity, the resulting brain injury may be mild, in which the patient is momentarily stunned and sees "stars," to severe, in which extensive brainstem damage rapidly leads to death. In addition to the direct mechanical injury giving rise to brain damage, the ultimate course and outcome in a given patient is also influenced by a number of additional factors including changes in the cerebral circulation with concomitant hypoxia and/or ischemia, the development of brain edema, accompanying mass lesions such as subarachnoid, subdural, or epidural hemorrhage, and various metabolic aberrations including both hypoglycemia and hyperglycemia. An understanding of this complex interplay of both primary and secondary processes and their influence on traumatic injury to the brain have greatly influenced the way that head-injury patients are currently managed. Although no specific therapeutic breakthrough has occurred in the treatment of head injuries, despite extensive research, newer diagnostic equipment and a better understanding of the pathologic physiology underlying brain damage have, however, substantially improved the prognosis for severe head-injury patients over what it was a decade ago.

REFERENCES

1. Adams, J.H., Graham, D.I., and Dyk, D.: Ischemic brain damage in fatal non-missile head injuries, J. Neurol. Sci. **39:**213, 1978.
2. Adams, J.H., et al.: Diffuse brain damage of immediate impact type, Brain **100:**489, 1977.
3. Altura, B.T., and Altura, B.M.: Effects of barbiturates, phencyclidine, ketamine and analogs on cerebral circulation and cerebrovascular muscle, Microcirc. Endothel. Lymph **1:**169, 1984.
4. Baudry, M., et al.: Entorhinal cortex lesions induce a decreased calcium transport in hippocampal mitochondria, Science **216:**411, 1982.
5. Becker, D.P., and Povlishock, J.T., editors: Central nervous system trauma status report—1985, Richmond, 1985, William Byrd Press.
6. Becker, D.P., et al.: The outcome from severe head injury with early diagnosis and intensive management, J. Neurosurg. **47:**491, 1977.
7. Becker, D.P., et al.: Diagnosis and treatment of head injuries in adults. In Youmans, J., editor: Neurological surgery IV, Philadelphia, 1982, W.B. Saunders Co.
8. Browning, M., Baudry, M., and Lynch, G.: Evidence that high frequency stimulation influences the phosphorylation of pyruvate dehydrogenase and that the activity of this enzyme is linked to mitochondrial calcium sequestration. In Gispen, W.I., and Routtenberg, A., editors: Brain phosphoproteins: characterization and function, progress in brain research, vol. 56, Amsterdam, 1982, Elsevier/North Holland Biomedical Press.
9. Bruce, D.A., et al.: Regional cerebral blood flow, intracranial pressure and brain metabolism in comatose patients, J. Neurosurg. **38:**131, 1973.
10. Clifton, G.L., Ziegler, M.G., and Grossman, R.G.: Circulating catecholamines and sympathetic activity after head injury, Neurosurgery **8:**10, 1980.
11. Cohen J.J., et al.: Acid/base, Boston, 1982, Little, Brown and Co., Inc.
12. Cooper, P.R., et al.: Dexamethasone in severe head injury, J. Neurosurg. **51:**307, 1979.
13. Demopolos, H.B., et al.: The free radical pathology and the microcirculation in the major central nervous system disorders, Acta Physiol. Scand. (Suppl.) **492:**91, 1980.
14. DeWitt, D.S., et al.: Effects of fluid percussion brain injury on regional cerebral blood flow and pial vessel diameter, J. Neurosurg. **64:**787, 1986.
15. Duckrow, R.B., et al.: Oxidative metabolic activity of cerebral cortex after fluid-percussion head injury in the cat, J. Neurosurg. **54:**607, 1981.
16. Ellis, E.F., et al.: Cyclooxygenase products of arachidonic acid metabolism in cat cerebral cortex after experimental concussive brain injury, J. Neurochem. **37:**(4):892, 1981.
17. Enevoldsen, E.M., and Jensen, F.T.: Autoregulation and CO_2 responses of cerebral blood flow in patients with acute severe head injury, J. Neurosurg. **48:**689, 1978.
18. Fitch, W., and McDowall, D.G.: Effect of halothane on intracranial pressure gradients in the presence of intracranial space occupying lesions, Br. J. Anaesth. **43:**904, 1971.
19. Ganong, W.F.: Review of medical physiology, ed. 11, Los Altos, 1983, Lange Medical Publications.
20. Gennarelli, T.A., et al.: Physiological response to angular acceleration of the head. In Grossman, R.G., et al., editors: Head injury: basic and clinical aspects, New York, 1982, Raven Press.
21. Gordon, E.: Controlled respiration in the management of patients with traumatic brain injuries, Acta Anaesthesiol. Scand. **15:**193, 1971.
22. Greitz, T.: A radiologic study of the brain circulation by rapid serial angiography of the carotid artery, Acta Radiol. (Suppl.) **140:**1, 1956.
23. Hayes, R.L., et al.: Activation of pontine cholinergic sites implicated in unconsciousness following cerebral concussion in the cat, Science **223:**301, 1984.
24. Hillered, L.: Mechanisms of mitochondrial damage in brain ischemia. In Fiskum, G., editor: Mitochondrial physiology and pathology, New York, 1985, Van Nostrand Reinhold Co.
25. Ho, I.K., and Harris, R.A.: Mechanisms of action of barbiturates, Annu. Rev. Pharmacol. Toxicol. **21:**83, 1981.
26. Hossmann, K.A.: Treatment of experimental cerebral ischemia, J. Cereb. Blood Flow Metab. **2:**275, 1982.
27. Hounsfield, G.N.: Computerized transverse axial scanning (tomography), Br. J. Radiol. **46:**1016, 1973.
28. Huang, S.C., et al.: Quantitative measurement of local cerebral blood flow in humans by positron computed tomography and $_{15}$O-water, J. Cereb. Blood Flow Metab. **3:**141, 1983.
29. Jane, J.A., et al.: Outcome and pathology of head injury. In Grossman, R.G., et al., editors: Head injury: basic and clinical aspects, New York, 1982, Raven Press.
30. Jenkins, L.W., et al.: Increased vulnerability of the traumatized brain to early ischemia. In Baethmann, A., Go, G.K., and Unterberg, A., editors: Mechanisms of secondary brain damage: NATO—Advanced research workshop, Italy, Mauls Sterzing, 1986, Plenum Publishing Corp.
31. Jenkins, L.W., et al.: Brain acidosis in mechanical injury. II. Metabolic changes. (In preparation.)
32. Jennett, B.: Epilepsy after Nonmissile head injuries, ed. 2, London, 1975, William Heinemann Medical Books, Inc.
33. Jennett, B., and Teasdale, G.: Management of head injuries, Philadelphia, 1982, F.A. Davis Co.
34. Jeppsson, S.T.: Echo-encephalography IV. The midline echo, Acta Chir. Scand. (Suppl.) **121:**1, 1961.
35. Jobsis, F.F.: Oxidative metabolism effects of cerebral hypoxia. In Fahn, S., Davis, J.N., and Rowland, L.P., editors: Advances in neurology, vol. 26, New York, 1979, Raven Press.

36. Jurkowitz, M.S., and Brierley, G.P.: H^+-dependent efflux of Ca^{2+} from heart mitochondria, J. Bioenerg. Biomembr. **14:**435, 1982.
37. Kapuscinski, A., et al.: Is acute failure of adrenals an important factor limiting recovery from cerebral ischemia? In Cervo-Narvarro, J., et al., editors: Cerebral microcirculation and metabolism, New York, 1981, Raven Press.
38. Kontos, H.A., et al.: Responses of cerebral arteries and arterioles to acute hypotension and hypertension, Am. J. Physiol. **234:**371, 1978.
39. Kontos, H.A., et al.: Prostaglandins in physiological and certain pathological responses of the cerebral circulation, Fed. Proc. **40:**2326, 1981.
40. Kontos, H.A., et al.: Free oxygen radicals in cerebral vascular responses, Physiologist **26:**165, 1983.
41. Kontos, H.A.: Appearance of superoxide anion radical in cerebral extracellular space during increased prostaglandin synthesis in cats, Cir. Res. **57:**142, 1985.
42. Langfitt, T.W., and Obrist, W.D.: Cerebral blood flow and metabolism after intracranial trauma, Prog. Neurol. Surg. **10:**14, 1981.
43. Lassen, N.H.: Brain extracellular pH: main factor controlling cerebral blood flow, Scand. J. Clin. Lab. Invest. **22:**247, 1968.
44. Lewelt, W., Jenkins, L.W., and Miller, J.D.: Autoregulation of cerebral blood flow after experimental fluid-percussion injury of the brain, J. Neurosurg. **53:**500, 1980.
45. Lewelt, W., Jenkins, L.W., and Miller, J.D.: Effects of experimental fluid-percussion injury of the brain on cerebrovascular reactivity to hypoxia and to hypercapnia, J. Neurosurg. **56:**332, 1982.
46. Lundberg, N.: Continuous recording and control of ventricular fluid pressure in neurosurgical practice, Acta Psychiat. Scand. (Suppl.) **149:**1, 1960.
47. Lynch, G., and Baudry, M.: The biochemistry of memory: a new and specific hypothesis, Science **224:**1057, 1984.
48. Maas, A.I.R.: Cerebrospinal fluid enzymes in acute brain injury, J. Neurol. Neurosurg. Psychiatry **40:**655, 1977.
49. Mabe, H., Blomqvist, P., and Siesjo, B.K.: Intracellular pH in the brain following transient ischemia, J. Cereb. Blood Flow Metab. **3:**109, 1983.
50. Marmarou, A., and Tabaddor, K.: Intracranial pressure: physiology and pathophysiology. In Cooper, P.R., editor: Head injury, Baltimore, 1982, The Williams & Wilkins Co.
51. Marmarou, A., Schulman, K., and Rosende, R.M.: A nonlinear analysis of the cerebrospinal fluid system and intracranial pressure dynamics, J. Neurosurg. **48:**332, 1978.
52. Marshall, L.F., Smith, R.W., and Shapiro, H.M.: Outcome with aggressive treatment in severe head injuries. II. Acute and chronic barbiturate administration in the management of head injury, J. Neurosurg. **50:**26, 1979.
53. Michenfelder, J.D., Milde, J.H., and Sundt, T.M., Jr.: Cerebral protection by barbiturate anaesthesia, Arch. Neurol. **33:**345, 1976.
54. Miller, J.D.: Clinical aspects of intracranial pressure-volume relationships. In McLaurin, R.L., editor: Head injuries, New York, 1976, Grune & Stratton, Inc.
55. Miller, J.D.: Physiology of trauma, Clin. Neurosurg. **29:**103, 1982.
56. Miller, J.D., and Becker, D.P.: Pathophysiology of head injury. In Youmans, J., editor: Neurological surgery IV, Philadelphia, 1982, W.B. Saunders Co.
57. Miller, J.D., et al.: Significance of intracerebral hypertension in severe head injury, J. Neurosurg. **47:**503, 1977.
58. Miller, J.D., et al.: Early insults to the injured brain, JAMA **240:**439, 1978.
59. Mitchell, D.E., and Adams, J.H.: Primary focal impact damage to the brainstem in blunt head injuries: does it exist? Lancet **2:**215, 1973.
60. Muizelaar, J.P., Lutz, H.D., and Becker, D.P.: Effect of mannitol on ICP and correlation with pressure autoregulation in severely head-injured patients, J. Neurosurg. **61:**700, 1984.
61. Muizelaar, J.P., et al.: Mannitol causes compensatory cerebral vasoconstriction and vasodilation in response to blood viscosity changes, J. Neurosurg. **59:**822, 1983.
62. Mutch, W.A.C., and Hansen, A.J.: Extracellular pH changes during spreading depression and cerebral ischemia: mechanisms of brain pH regulation, J. Cereb. Blood Flow Metab. **4:**17, 1984.
63. Newlon, P.G., and Greenberg, R.P.: Evoked potentials in severe head injury, J. Trauma **24:**61, 1984.
64. Ommaya, A.K., and Gennarelli, T.A.: Cerebral concussion and traumatic unconsciousness, Brain **97:**633, 1974.
65. Plum, F., and Posner, J.B.: Diagnosis of stupor and coma, ed. 3, Philadelphia, 1980, F.A. Davis Co.
66. Povlishock, J.T.: The morphopathologic responses to head injuries of varying severity. In Becker, D.P., and Povlishock, J.T., editors: Central nervous system trauma status report—1985, Richmond, 1985, William Byrd Press.
67. Rehncrona, S., Rosen, I., and Siesjo, B.K.: Brain lactic acidosis and ischemia cell damage. I. Biochemistry and neurophysiology, J. Cereb. Blood Flow Metab. **1:**297, 1981.
68. Rose, J., Valtonen, S., and Jennett, B.: Avoidable factors contributing to death after head injury, Br. Med. J. **2:**615, 1977.
69. Rosenthal, M., et al.: Consequences of cerebral injury on oxidative energy metabolism measured in situ. In Grossman, R.G., et al., editors: Head injury: basic and clinical aspects, New York, 1982, Raven Press.
70. Rosner, M.J., and Becker, D.P.: Experimental brain injury. Successful therapy with the weak base thromethamine with an overview of CNS acidosis, J. Neurosurg. **60:**961, 1984.
71. Rosner, M.J., Bennett, M.D., and Becker, D.P.: The clinical relevance of laboratory head injury models: prerequisites of therapeutic testing. In Grossman, R.G., et al., editors: Head injury: basic and clinical aspects, New York, 1982, Raven Press.
72. Rosner, M.J., Newsome, H.H., and Becker, D.P.: Mechanical brain injury: the sympathoadrenal response, J. Neurosurg. **61:**76, 1984.
73. Routtenberg, A.: Identification and back-titration of brain pyruvate dehydrogenase: functional significance for behavior. In Gispen, W.I., and Routtenberg, A., editors: Brain phosphoproteins: characterization and function, progress in brain research, vol. 56, Amsterdam, 1982, Elsevier/North Holland Biomedical Press.
74. Sakamoto, H., et al.: Brain acidosis in mechanical injury. I. Dynamic changes in pH. (In preparation.)
75. Siesjö, B.K.: Brain energy metabolism, New York, 1978, John Wiley & Sons, Inc.
76. Siesjö, B.K.: Cell damage in the brain: a speculative synthesis, J. Cereb. Blood Flow Metab. **1:**155, 1981.
77. Siesjö, B.K.: Cerebral circulation and metabolism, J. Neurosurg. **60:**883, 1984.
78. Siesjö, B.K., and Wielock, T.: Brain injury: neurochemical aspects. in Becker, D.P., and Povlishock, J.T., editors: Central nervous system trauma status report—1985, Richmond, 1985, William Byrd Press.
79. Siesjö, B.K., et al.: Extra- and intracellular pH in the brain during seizures and in the recovery period following the arrest of seizure activity, J. Cereb. Blood Flow Metab. **5:**47, 1985.
80. Smith, F.W.: Nuclear magnetic resonance in the investigation of cerebral disorder, J. Cereb. Blood Flow Metab. **3:**263, 1983.
81. Sullivan, H.G., et al.: Fluid percussion model of mechanical brain injury in the cat, J. Neurosurg. **45:**520, 1976.
82. Sullivan, H.G., et al.: The physiological basis of intracranial pressure change with progressive epidural brain compression, J. Neurosurg. **47:**532, 1977.
83. Teasdale, G., and Jennett, B.: Assessment of coma and impaired consciousness, Lancet **2:**81, 1974.
84. Teasdale, G., and Jennett, B.: Aspects of coma after severe head injury, Lancet **1:**878, 1977.
85. Thomas, D.G.T., Rabow, L., and Teasdale, G.: Serum myelin basic protein, clinical responsiveness and outcome of severe head injury, Acta Neurochir. (Suppl.)**28:**93, 1979.
86. vanDongen, K.J., Braakman, R., and Gelpke, G.J.: The prognostic value of computerized tomography in comatose head injured patients, J. Neurosurg. **59:**951, 1983.
87. Ward, J.D., et al.: Failure of prophylactic barbiturate coma in the treatment of severe head injury, J. Neurosurg. **62:**383, 1985.
88. Wei, E.P., Lamb, R.H., and Kontos, H.A.: Increased phospholipase C activity after experimental brain injury, J. Neurosurg. **56:**695, 1982.
89. Wilmore, L.J., and Triggs, W.J.: Effect of phenytoin and corticosteroids on seizures and lipid peroxidation in experimental post-traumatic epilepsy, J. Neurosurg. **60:**467, 1984.
90. Yang, M.S., et al.: Regional brain metabolite levels following low levels of experimental head injury in the cat, J. Neurochem. **63:**617, 1985.

48 Dennis R. Kopaniky

Pathophysiology of Spinal Cord Disruption and Injury

Severe spinal cord injury is a low-incidence but catastrophic disability. In the population of the United States the frequency of severe spinal cord injury resulting in paraplegia or quadriplegia has been estimated to be 30 to 35 injuries per million per year. Thus approximately 8000 spinal cord injuries occur every year in the United States. Of note is the youthful population most commonly involved in spinal cord injuries, with the most likely age for spinal cord injury being nineteen.[95] Furthermore, approximately 80% of all victims are under the age of 40, and it is estimated that about 50% are in the 14- to 24-year age range. The combination of generally youthful victims and severe permanent neurologic disabilities makes spinal cord injury a major health care problem.

Vehicular or pedestrian-related accidents account for the majority of traumatic spinal cord injuries (48%). Other causes include sports injuries (15%), falls (15%), and penetrating wounds (14%). Most vertebral fractures occur in the regions of greatest mobility, involving the cervicothoracic junction or the thoracolumbar junction. These include the spinal levels C5 to T1 and T11 to L2.

Remarkably, only within recent decades has the medical profession looked on spinal cord injury as a disability that can effectively be treated with the expectation that the patient will have a life of reasonable fulfillment. Nevertheless, rehabilitation for the patient with this type of injury is a lengthy undertaking at great expense. For paraplegic patients rehabilitation most often requires 100 to 160 days, whereas that of the quadriplegic patient requires 180 to 300 days.[71] The total national medical cost for treatment of spinal cord injuries in the United States has been estimated to be approximately $1.5 billion annually.[94] A large portion of this expense covers the cost of treating the many unique complications that form a continuum of threats to the patient with spinal cord injury. This chapter will discuss the pathophysiology of spinal cord injuries and provide a rational basis for its management and the prevention of its many complications.

CLINICAL ASSESSMENT OF SPINAL CORD INJURY

The association of spinal cord injury with other bodily injuries is common and can lead to diagnostic and treatment difficulties if a high index of suspicion is not maintained in the treatment of the patient with polytrauma. Results of spinal cord injury admissions to one acute care facility have recently been reviewed[85] and revealed some enlightening observations. Especially noteworthy was the incidence of associated injuries. Over 12% of patients with cervical cord injuries had other associated serious injuries. Equally impressive were the injuries to other body systems in 46% of patients with thoracic cord injuries and in 22% of patients with cauda equina injuries. Problems commonly associated with spinal cord injury included injury to the head, thoracic contents, abdominal cavity, and the extremities. In patients with cervical spinal cord injury, 67% had associated limb fractures with approximately equal involvement of the upper and lower extremities, 53% had intrathoracic injuries, and 33% had associated head injury. Not unexpectedly approximately 70% of patients with thoracic spinal cord injury had hemothorax, pneumothorax, or other associated intrathoracic injuries.

Medical personnel who deal frequently with patients who are unconscious such as victims of motor vehicle accidents all too frequently become aware of spinal cord injury late during the resuscitation of the patient. Thus all unconscious trauma victims must be *assumed* to have a spinal cord injury until proven otherwise by appropriate x-ray film studies and clinical examination. This simple rule can often save patients from needless spinal movement and consequent additional spinal cord injury.

As with all trauma victims, the initial assessment of a patient with possible spinal cord injury must include an evaluation of the respiratory and circulatory status. During the initial resuscitation, to save life it may be necessary to manipulate the spine to support ventilation or circulation. Once the threat to life is removed, all precautions for immobilizing the potentially injured spine must be resumed. Every effort must be made to adequately immobilize patients for transportation and medical assessment. Ideally the patient can best be transported strapped to a hard board, with the head immobilized by sandbags placed on either side of the head and neck and adhesive tape across the forehead. Patients with obvious traumatic spinal deformities may best be moved in the same position as they are found. This will prevent any unnecessary movement of the spine and spinal structures and further injury to a potentially damaged cord.

It may be possible to make a more accurate initial assessment of neurologic deficit if the patient is awake. Complete or partial loss of motor or sensory function at or below the level of the neck is likely to be the result of a spinal cord injury. A high index of suspicion must be maintained when pain is encountered anywhere along the spine, *even in the absence of neurologic deficit*. Such patients should be regarded as having potential spine or spinal cord injury until proven otherwise.

X-ray film examination of the spine is most accurately completed following the clinical neurologic examination,

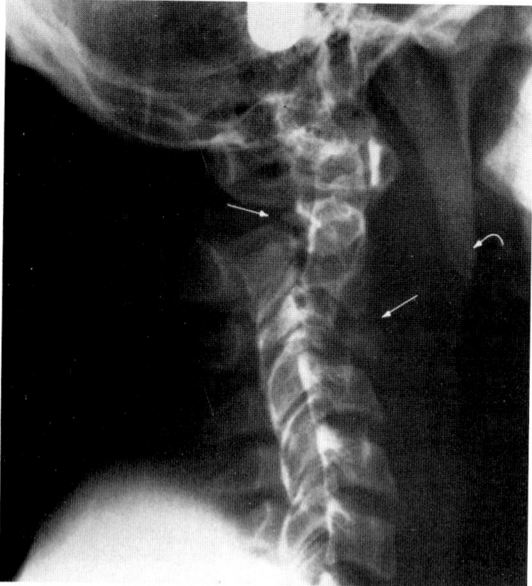

Fig. 48-1 Lateral cervical spine x-ray film showing a flexion crush fracture of the C3 vertebral body *(anterior straight arrow)* and a pedicle fracture *(posterior right arrow)*. Hemorrhagic swelling of the soft tissue anterior to the vertebral bodies *(curved arrow)* is an indirect indication of spinal injury.

which establishes the appropriate injury level. The thorough radiologic examination of the cervical spine includes an odontoid view and anteroposterior and lateral projection with complete visualization of the C7 vertebral body and the C7-T1 interspace. Although the majority of spinal injuries are readily visualized on standard x-ray film views, patients with signs and symptoms suspicious for spinal injury may require an intensive search for direct or indirect evidence of injury (Fig. 48-1). A "swimmer's" view or computed tomography scan of the cervical spine may be useful if heavy body build does not permit proper visualization of the C7 vertebral body (Fig. 48-2). If necessary, oblique views of the cervical spine without turning the patient may be necessary to fully visualize the facet joints. As standard procedure the routine x-ray film views of the spine should be obtained in areas of sensory loss to rule out hidden spine fractures.

Although the majority of cervical spine fractures will be treated by cervical traction in tongs, effective initial immobilization may be obtained by continued taping and sandbagging the head (Fig. 48-3). The thoracolumbar spine can be effectively immobilized by keeping the patient strapped to the examining surface, with bedrolls placed on either side of the body to minimize movement. These methods of temporary immobilization are effective in maintaining spinal sta-

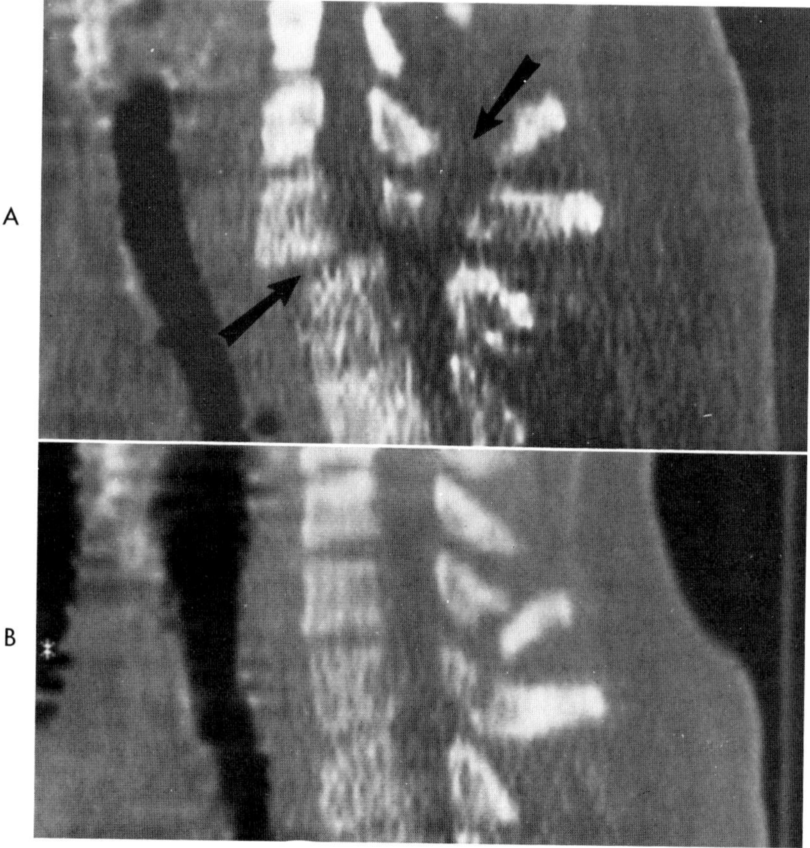

Fig. 48-2 **A,** On standard cervical spine x-ray film, low cervical spine in this patient with massive shoulder girth was not visualized, but on a sagittal CT scan of the low cervical and high thoracic spine a severe subluxation of the C7 and T1 vertebral bodies *(left arrow)* and fracture of the posterior spinous processes *(right arrow)* were visualized. **B,** After appropriate cervical traction was applied for spinal realignment, this subsequent CT scan showed improved alignment of the vertebral bodies.

bility until a definitive treatment plan can be determined after diagnostic testing. This should be done in consultation with a neurosurgeon or orthopedic surgeon experienced in the treatment of spinal cord injury.

Injury to the spinal cord is clinically defined both by the extent of the lesion (i.e., complete or incomplete) and the spinal level of the lesion. A complete injury is defined as a total loss of neurologic function below the level of cord injury, whereas an incomplete lesion denotes partial preservation of neurologic function below the injury site. The spinal level of lesion is designated as the most distal uninvolved segment of the spinal cord. Thus a patient with a spinal cord lesion involving the C7 segment of the spinal cord and neurologic dysfunction at C7 and below would be designated a C6 spinal level.

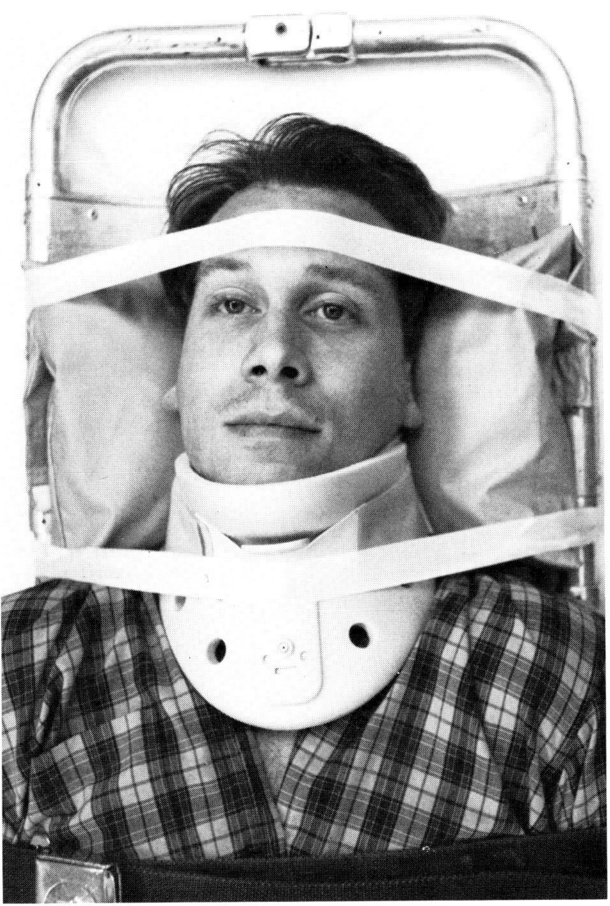

Fig. 48-3 Good immobilization of the cervical spine is achieved with the patient strapped to a hard board or scoop stretcher. Head and neck are further immobilized by sandbags placed on both sides of the head and by adhesive tape over the forehead and over the hard collar.

The neurologic deficit produced after spinal cord trauma may involve not only motor and sensory dysfunction but autonomic and inhibitory dysfunctions as well. Incomplete spinal cord injuries can often be characterized by specific syndromes, each having a particular clinical pattern of neurologic deficit. Frequently observed syndromes include the central cord syndrome, anterior spinal cord syndrome, and Brown-Séquard's syndrome (Fig. 48-4).

The *central cord syndrome* arises as a consequence of hemorrhagic necrosis in the central portion of the spinal cord. The extent of involvement of the spinal cord depends on the degree of injury, with mild injuries initiating small central lesions and increasingly severe injuries giving rise to centripetal extension of injured tissue toward the periphery of the spinal cord (see Fig. 48-4). Because of the anatomic arrangement of motor and sensory tracts, the outcome is *relative sparing* of motor and sensory function in the body areas distal to the injury. Classically, a central cord syndrome in the cervical spinal cord region produces neurologic impairment affecting the upper extremities more than the lower extremities, with greater neurologic loss in the proximal portions rather than distal.

The *anterior spinal cord syndrome* is a consequence of trauma directed toward the anterior portion of the spine and spinal cord. Although some of the destruction is mechanical, a large portion of neurologic disruption is a consequence of trauma to the anterior spinal artery and loss of vascularization to the anterior volume of the cord. There is loss of motor function and pain and temperature sensation below the injured segment. Since there is relative preservation of the dorsal columns, position sense remains intact.

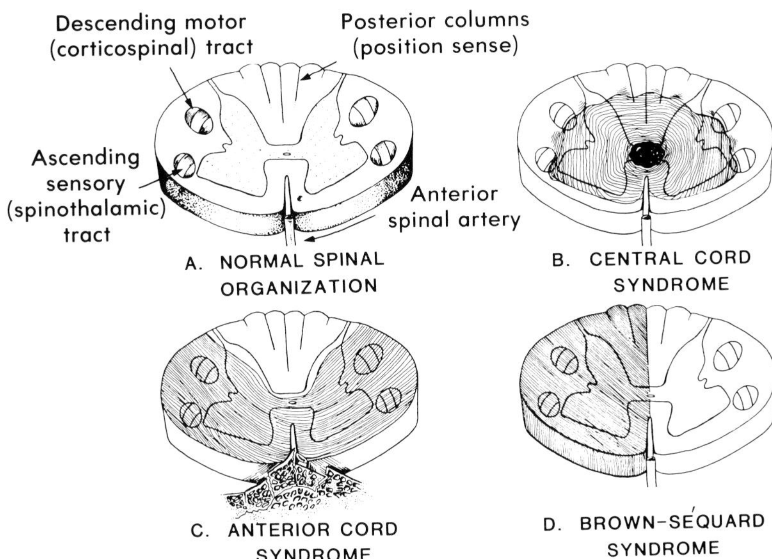

Fig. 48-4 Neurologic deficit following an incomplete spinal cord injury reflects the neurologic function subserved by those spinal cord fractures involved in the injury. **A,** Normal spinal organization. **B,** Central cord syndrome. Motor deficit affects the upper limbs more than the lower limbs. Note that the volume of the central necrotic region will determine the neurologic dysfunction since various neural structures such as the corticospinal tracts are progressively involved in the region. **C,** Anterior cord syndrome. Motor function and pain sensation are lost below the level of spinal cord injury. Position sense in the posterior columns is relatively preserved. **D,** Brown-Séquard syndrome. This syndrome reflects loss of motor function on the side ipsilateral to the spinal cord legion and loss of pain and temperature sensation on the contralateral side.

Classically, *Brown-Séquard's syndrome* is the result of injury to one half of the spinal cord. There is interruption of motor function ipsilateral to the injury site and interruption of pain and temperature on the contralateral side.

INDICATIONS FOR SURGICAL TREATMENT

A large number of treatment modalities for acute spinal cord injury have been used with varying degrees of success. These range from aggressive operative programs involving emergent decompressive surgery of the spinal cord[78,87] to totally nonoperative approaches.[8,38] The role of early surgery in the management of acute traumatic spinal cord injury remains highly controversial.[91] Despite this continued controversy, controlled studies comparing surgical and nonsurgical treatments have not been completed. The arguments for and against early surgery have been summarized elsewhere.[19] Arguments supporting early surgical intervention in spinal cord injury include: (1) restoration of anatomic bone alignment, (2) decompression of neural tissue, (3) stabilization of the spine by fusion or instrumentation, and (4) early mobilization of the patient. Counterarguments include the following: (1) alignment can be obtained by skeletal traction and closed manipulation; (2) removal of bone fragments and disk from the spinal canal might not assist in the recovery of neurologic function; and (3) adequate mobilization of patients confined to a bed may be obtained by a program of active physiotherapy.

Whether routine early surgery for acute spinal cord injury has specific advantages remains controversial,* and a decision to decompress the spinal cord should be made only after weighing the possible advantages against the inherit risks in a given patient with such an injury. Reasonable indications for early or emergent surgery may include: (1) progressively worsening neurologic deficit, (2) contaminated penetrating spinal wounds, and (3) failure to achieve reduction or restore spinal alignment by closed methods. Late surgical intervention for stabilization of the spine is far less controversial, and the decision for late surgery is made particularly on the basis of continued stability of the spine.

INTRAOPERATIVE MANAGEMENT AND CONSIDERATIONS FOR INTENSIVE CARE OF SPINAL CORD INJURY

Actual mechanical transsection of the spinal cord is rare, but it is common for the injured spinal cord to electrophysiologically mimic actual transsection. The severely injured cord will not allow neural action potentials to cross the area of the lesion, resulting in interruption of cerebral interaction with voluntary motor, sensory, and inhibitory activities in areas innervated by the cord distal to the site of the lesion. Spinal cord pathways that interact with the sacral component of the parasympathetic system and the descending sympathetic pathways are also interrupted. Disruption of these neural pathways results in isolation of the distal segment of the spinal cord, with inherent changes in the homeostatic physiology involving multiple body systems.

*References 9, 21, 41, 42, 62, 66, 88.

It is apparent that the secondary problems may have more of an effect on morbidity and mortality of patients with spinal cord injury than does injury to the spinal cord itself. As an indirect result of spinal cord pathophysiology, the management of patients with acute spinal cord injury requires primary attention to dysfunction of other organ systems.

Cardiovascular Dysfunction

Spinal cord trauma at the cervical or high thoracic level results in loss of sympathetic vasomotor tone. The major sympathetic tracts descend in the spinal cord to the peripheral sympathetic outflow areas between T1 and L2. Loss of the sympathetic vasomotor tone results directly in hypotension. A systolic blood pressure of 90 to 100 mm Hg is common during the acute period following spinal cord injury. In most patients this degree of hypotension does not severely intervere with tissue perfusion, but the ability to compensate may be lacking, and careful fluid administration and possibly use of agents such as dopamine may be required if the blood pressure continues to fall or the patient becomes symptomatic. The traumatologist must ensure that the hypotension is strictly the result of spinal cord injury and not a result of other bodily trauma such as injury to thorax, abdomen, or the extremities. In most cases judicious fluid administration will maintain an adequate blood pressure, and attempts need not be made to elevate blood pressure above 100 mm Hg in an otherwise asymptomatic patient. Attempts to elevate the blood pressure back to "normal" values are unnecessary and may even be detrimental to the patient. On the other hand, systolic blood pressure below 80 mm Hg indicates little margin for compensation, and blood pressures in patients with this problem should be controlled by sympathomimetic medications in a prophylactic manner. The goal is to maintain adequate blood pressure to provide good tissue perfusion.

Sinus bradycardia following spinal cord injury generally will not require treatment in previously healthy individuals. The bradycardia is initiated by loss of sympathetic input to the heart, with unopposed parasympathetic input through the intact vagus nerve. Following spinal cord injury the combination of hypotension and bradycardia is commonly observed and is referred to as neurogenic shock. Excessive parasympathetic stimulation of the heart, as may be produced by intense tracheal suctioning at the carina, may exacerbate bradycardia and even cause asystole. Although it is uncommon to encounter a patient so very sensitive to parasympathetic stimulation, intermittent use of anticholinergic drugs such as atropine (0.4 mg) may be necessary in this clinical setting. In rare cases a pacemaker may be required to adequately protect a patient.

Changes in the electrocardiogram have been observed following spinal cord injury. These changes are consistent with subendocardial ischemia and have been described both clinically and experimentally following severe cord injury in the cervical region.[33,34] This tissue damage and the loss of sympathetically mediated compensatory cardiovascular reflexes result in a myocardium that may be only marginally competent. Other observed changes in the electrocardiogram have included sinus pauses, shifting sinus pacemaker, nodal escape beats, runs of atrial fibrillation, multifocal premature ventricular contractions, ventricular tachycardia, and ST- and T-wave changes. A failing myocardium, often coupled with the necessity for controlled ventilation during resuscitation or anesthesia, may compromise venous return, cardiac output, systemic blood pressure, and tissue perfusion in the spinal cord injury patient. This patient lacks the ability to increase venous return when intrathoracic pressure is raised during controlled ventilation. Thus an expiratory pause may be required to allow adequate venous return,[5] and a high intrathoracic pressure during inspiration may be better tolerated when expiration is at least twice as long as inspiration.[68]

In the patient with acute spinal cord injury, fluid and electrolyte balance may be disturbed by both pathophysiologic or iatrogenically induced respiratory and metabolic changes in the acid/base balance. Examples include respiratory acidosis as a result of alveolar hypoventilation, metabolic alkalosis from emesis or gastric suction, and hypokalemia caused by loss from or into dilated gut. In patients with an intact renal system fluid and electrolyte balance will generally be achieved by judicious administration of appropriately balanced fluids. Over a longer period of time following spinal cord injury, fluid and electrolyte alterations may be encountered as a result of changes in the renin/aldosterone system.

Patients with either complete or nearly complete spinal cord injury in the high thoracic or the cervical region may experience syncopal episodes when first assuming an upright position. This complication is also the result of loss of sympathetic vascular tone. If such patients are to be brought into an upright position, this should be done by slowly advancing levels of incline, with close monitoring of blood pressure. From a physiologic standpoint, syncopal episodes may be minimized in the patient with spinal cord injury by use of elasticized stockings and an abdominal binder, both of which aid venous return to the heart.

Because of immobilization and direct trauma to the venous endothelium, patients with spinal cord injury are at risk for developing thromboembolic disease. The use of low-dose heparin to minimize these complications has been advocated by some, whereas other clinicians have found more value in instituting a routine of leg elevation while the patient is confined to bed, thigh-high elastic hose, and frequent passive range-of-motion exercises to the extremities. These treatment techniques appear to reduce the incidence of thrombembolism in the patient with spinal cord injury and offer excellent extremity mobilization in a patient who is otherwise confined to bed.

Immediately following trauma to the spinal cord, there ensues a period of "spinal cord shock," during which no neurologic function exists below the level of the spinal cord lesion. This state may exist for a period of several days to 8 weeks following the injury. After the period of shock the spinal reflexes return to the isolated distal segment of the spinal cord. A unique set of signs and symptoms referred to as autonomic hyperreflexia[22,59] may then be seen in patients with high thoracic or cervical spinal cord injuries. Autonomic hyperreflexia results when a strong sensory stimulus enters the isolated segment of the spinal cord below the injury level, initiating a mass reflex of sympathetic and somatic activity. Common stimuli initiating this response include an overdistended bladder or gut, irritation of cutaneous pressure sores, and sudden decreases in arterial blood pressure during the induction of anesthesia.[89] The sympathetic mass reflex produces strong vasoconstriction *below* the level of the spinal cord lesion, resulting in severe hypertension with consequent headaches, complex seizures, or even intracerebral hemorrhage. The hypertension triggers a compensatory parasympathetic reaction with vasodilation confined to body parts *above* the level of the spinal cord lesion. The dichotomy of vasodilated, flushed, warm skin above the lesion level and vasoconstricted, mottled skin below the lesion level is perhaps unique in clinical physiology. The parasympathetic effects also produce marked bradycardia despite the presence of severe hypotension. Autonomic hyperreflexia may be severely detrimental to the patient, and proper measures of control must be taken immediately. Fortunately the majority of these patients will simply respond to removal of the initiating stimulus such as evacuating a full bladder or bowel. On the other hand, if a clear response is not noted rapidly, alpha-adrenergic blocking agents may be used to interrupt the sympathetic portion of the syndrome.

Pulmonary Dysfunction

In the patient with spinal cord injury, respiration is impaired secondary to partial or total loss of intercostal muscle or diaphragmatic function.[29] Intercostal muscle function accounts for approximately 60% of the tidal volume[10,18] by expanding the thoracic cage. The combination of intercostal and diaphragmatic functional loss results in a significant decrease in vital capacity from approximately 5L/min in the normal adult to 1 or fewer L/min in the patient with spinal cord injury. The forced vital capacity is a good indicator of "respiratory reserve," and sequential measurements revealing a rapid decline in vital capacity may assist in determining a need for intubation or continued ventilatory assistance. In addition, there is impaired cough effectiveness with consequent pulmonary fluid accumulation and increased physiologic arteriovenous shunting or ventilation/perfusion mismatching. Patients with spinal cord injury require intensive *prophylactic* respiratory therapy, including intermittent positive-pressure breathing, chest percussion, postural drainage, and assisted cough. These measures must be used prophylactically because patients with spinal cord injury are at continued high risk for catastrophic pulmonary complications.

The high cervical spinal cord injuries may be the most difficult to manage because of involvement of phrenic nerve rootlets in the lesion. Phrenic nerve rootlets originate at spinal levels C3, C4, and C5 and innervate the diaphragms. However, even in patients with spinal injury below C5, the initial neurologic levels may ascend in the spinal cord because hemorrhage and edema in the central portion of the cord tend to relieve pressure by moving along the path of least resistance within the cord substance. Thus patients with injuries to the low cervical area must be monitored carefully for acute *delayed* changes in respiratory ability attributable to an "ascending lesion." Injuries to cervical cord segments C3 through C5 are unusual but potentially catastrophic; they may be associated with sleep apnea, sometimes referred to as "Ondine's curse," and patients thus affected may ventilate adequately while awake but lose their central respiratory drive while asleep. This syndrome may be enhanced by any pharmacologic agent that depresses the central nervous system[74]; thus use of such agents should be allowed only in appropriately monitored patients.

The initial loss of sympathetic vasomotor tone in the patient with spinal cord injury is associated with a significant increase in total vascular volume. Although this loss in tone might require administration of additional fluids to maintain adequate blood pressure in the early stages following spinal cord injury, a portion of the vascular tone may return autonomously during the initial 5 days following injury. During the compensatory phase, the vascular volume partially contracts, and the consequent fluid shifts may result in pulmonary edema. This can be a catastrophic complication for the patient with spinal cord injury and most often is related to iatrogenic causes. Difficulty maintaining adequate blood pressure or fluid balance suggests a need for placement of a Swan-Ganz catheter to provide direct measurement of pulmonary artery diastolic pressure and wedge pressure to detect changes that may be early indications of developing pulmonary edema.[86] Physiologic information obtained from the Swan-Ganz catheter has a distinct advantage over central venous pressure changes, which generally become apparent only *after* cardiopulmonary decompensation has occurred. If early surgery for any reason is to be contemplated for a patient with spinal cord injury, the preoperative placement of a Swan-Ganz catheter is advisable for intraoperative and postoperative management.

Intubation of patients with cervical spine trauma requires that the neck be maintained in a neutral position with the assistance of traction by skull tongs or immobilization with sandbags or collars for stabilization of the neck. Nasotracheal intubation may be attempted in the awake patient using "blind" technique, or a fiberoptic bronchoscope may be used for assisting insertion of the endotracheal tube. These methods are appropriate even in patients immobilized in a halo-vest apparatus (Fig. 48-5). A tracheostomy might be necessary in patients requiring long-term respiratory assistance.

Although sedation is indicated before intubation, muscle relaxant drugs must be used with caution since the stability of a spinal lesion may depend in part on muscle spasm in the area and this mechanical support will be lost secondary to the action of these drugs. If muscle relaxants are to be used, appropriate external immobilization must be ensured. Furthermore, muscle relaxants, especially the depolarizing agents, should be avoided in severerly traumatized patients. Depolarizing agents such as succinylcholine may cause a rise in serum potassium sufficient to initiate cardiac arrest. Thus use of this agent is contraindicated in spinal cord injury.[12]

Gastrointestinal and Nutritional Complications

Peristalsis of the gut stops within 24 hours following spinal cord injury. This ileus is a consequence of spinal cord shock. In uncomplicated cases of spinal cord injury peristalsis generally resumes within 3 to 5 days. However,

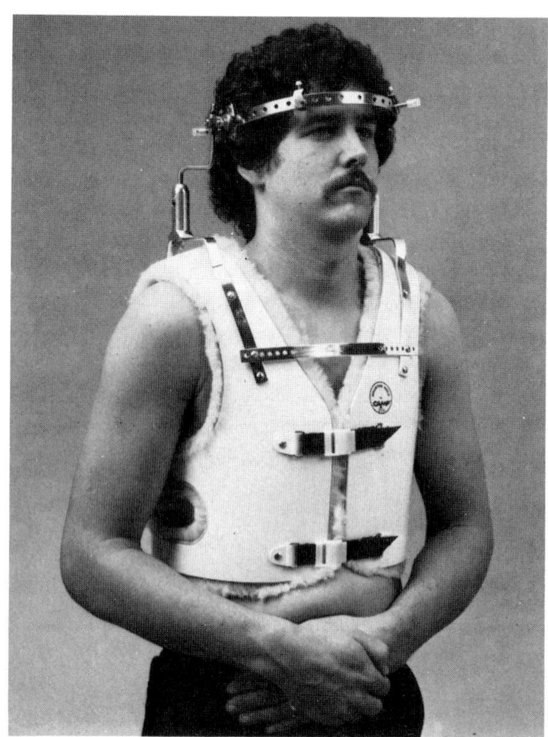

Fig. 48-5 Halo vest apparatus minimizes movement of the head and neck with respect to the body. Halo ring is applied to the skull by four-point fixation and is in turn attached to the vest apparatus by sturdy upright bars. (From Camp International, Inc., Jackson, Mich.)

associated injuries to the abdomen, chest, and retroperitoneum may delay resolution of the ileus. It is imperative that, in patients with either complete or incomplete spinal cord injury, a nasogastric tube be inserted and connected to suction. Because the ileus may be delayed for as long as 24 hours, prophylactic nasogastric suction should begin immediately.

In the patient with spinal cord injury, dilated viscera not only interfere with an already compromised respiratory mechanism but may actually result in viscous perforation. Since the patient with spinal cord injury has lost activity of the sympathetic nervous system, the unopposed parasympathetic system can exert unchecked influence and thus increase gastric secretions, thereby contributing to the development of gastric ulcers. The incidence of ulcer disease and gastrointestinal bleeding is elevated in the patient with spinal cord injury. The use of steroids directed toward the cord injury itself may act to enhance the risk of gastrointestinal bleeding and ulcer disease. Presently the use of steroids in treating spinal cord injury is under debate. The theoretic benefits of steroids are clear in animal experimental models[40]; however, the benefits are not so clear in the clinical situation in humans.[26]

Disastrous nutritional complications may be encountered in the patient with spinal cord injury.[72,81] These patients enter an obligatory phase of negative nitrogen balance almost immediately after their injury. This is the result of a combination of inactivity, severely increased metabolic demands secondary to trauma, and essential muscle "denervation" secondary to spinal cord shock. The skeletal muscle mass and the visceral mass of the body enter a catabolic phase. The muscular diaphragm, upon which many of these patients depend for respiratory effort, is also weakened by protein catabolism, and this may be a mechanism for progressive loss of respiratory reserve during the early stages of spinal cord injury.

Multiple pathophysiologic processes in the spinal cord–injured patient are associated with a poor nutritional state. For example, poor nutrition encourages development of skin pressure sores and is associated with development of an incompetent immunologic state[67,69,70] and compromise of cardiac and respiratory functions.[44]

To deliver adequate caloric requirements, parenteral nutrition[15,20] may be required when the patient has sustained polytrauma in addition to spinal cord injury. Although it may be preferable to use the gut for feeding purposes,[43] it is important to deliver adequate calories throughout the acute period of spinal cord injury. Thus it is often most beneficial to administer nutrition by way of intravenous hyperalimentation during the period of loss of gut peristalsis and progress to a system of nasogastric or oral feedings when peristalsis returns.

Since most patients with spinal cord injury lose both the urge to defecate and voluntary control of the anal sphincter, a bowel program is necessary to train the bowel to empty regularly as soon as the patient is receiving oral or nasogastric feedings. A simple but effective routine bowel program might include a daily stool softener and suppository to stimulate peristalsis at appropriate intervals.

Genitourinary Complications

The neural innervation of the bladder is derived from the autonomic and somatic nervous systems. The sympathetic component is derived from T11 to L2 and the parasympathetic innervation from S2 to S4. During the period of spinal shock the contractile ability of the bladder is lost (areflexic bladder). Following resolution of spinal shock, reflex activity returns (automatic bladder) since the spinal micturitional reflex arc is intact in the segment of cord isolated by the lesion.

The acute management of the patient with spinal cord injury requires catheterization of the bladder by either indwelling or intermittent methods. An indwelling catheter is most helpful during the phase immediately following injury when accurate fluid input and output are necessary. This may later be changed to intermittent catheterization, thus decreasing the risk of urinary tract infection, the frequency of which is high in both quadriplegic and paraplegic patients. Infection is of concern in patients with spinal cord injury because of the close association of urinary tract infections with renal disease and renal failure, which continue to be major causes of morbidity and mortality among patients with spinal cord injury.[39] Related to relative inactivity, these patients experience increased excretion of calcium in the urine with a high incidence of urinary tract calculi and polynephritis, which is related to relative inactivity. Calculi and long-standing indwelling bladder catheters may also result in formation of urinary tract fistulae and diverticulae with their own variety of complications.

During the stage of spinal shock all sexual functions cease in the male. When spinal shock resides and reflex activity returns, erections may occur in response to local stimuli. The ability to ejaculate will depend on the degree of completeness of the cord injury. Because of inability to ejaculate and generally decreased motility of sperm,[53] it is rare for males with spinal cord injury to sire children. On the other hand, spinal cord injury in females generally produces only transient interruption of the menstrual cycle, and these individuals can become pregnant and bear normal children.[39]

Musculoskeletal Complications

The importance of immediate immobilization of the spine has been addressed. While diagnostic tests are being performed and during periods of anesthesia, continued appropriate immobilization of the spine must be stressed. The simplest and perhaps the most effective method of immobilization of the cervical spine may be the application of sandbags to both sides of the head and neck, with adhesive tape applied across the forehead for strict immobilization. Cervical collars of a hard quality such as the "Philadelphia collar" will provide similar immobilization when adhesive tape is applied across the collar and across the forehead to secure the position of the head. However, the various cervical collars have a disadvantage in that the neck structures are hidden from view of the attending medical personnel. Although the majority of cervical spine injuries are managed with tongs and cervical traction, injuries resulting from distraction-type forces may at times be managed more appropriately in a halo-vest apparatus (see Fig. 48-5) that "impacts" rather than distracts the spine. Such decisions must be made by medical personnel experienced in managing spinal injury.

Many patients with spinal injury, particularly those with complete spinal cord injuries, may be managed in a nonsurgical fashion such that the area of spinal injury is allowed to autofuse. In these selected cases, patients are generally confined to bed for a period of as long as 6 weeks, during which time the area of injury begins to heal and form new bone or callus. In patients with highly unstable fractures or partial spinal cord injuries in whom chances for neurologic recovery are high, operative spinal fusion techniques may be used to ensure stability.

Classification of acute injuries to the spine assumes that each type of injury is the result of a pure force (flexion, extension, vertical compression, rotation, distraction) or a combination of pure forces (e.g., flexion-rotation).[46,92] This type of classification is important for determining the degree of stability and thus the specific treatment for a spinal injury.

From a practical standpoint, recognition of unstable spinal injuries is of primary importance in determining which diagnostic studies and which course of therapy might best be instituted. A stable spinal injury refers to maintenance of the integrity of the ligamentous and skeletal components of the spine following trauma such that further controlled motion has a low risk of producing spinal cord or nerve root damage.[2] Conversely, the unstable spinal injury allows actual or potential abnormal excursion of one vertebral segment on another, implying potential or actual compromise of neural elements.[27] Some clinicians[2,6,46] relate stability of a spinal injury to the integrity of the posterior ligamentous complex. These authors suggest that an intact posterior ligamentous complex maintains a stable fracture. Conversely, others[7] contend that additional damage must involve portions of the anterior ligamentous structures before spinal injury can be considered unstable. The degree of stability cannot be predicted in every instance of acute spinal injury. However, as informed an estimation of stability as possible must be made to render the most appropriate treatment.

Patients with spinal cord injury who are to undergo anesthesia and surgery will have many of the unique problems discussed in this chapter. Of special note during induction and maintenance of anesthesia is the use of muscle relaxants. In patients with unstable fracture dislocations of the spine, there may be further instability imposed on the injured site by relaxation of paraspinal muscles that, while in spasm, may splint the injury site. Thus appropriate precautions such as traction, halo-vest, or hard collar, must be used during a period of anesthesia and surgery to ensure continued stability during the procedure.

The use of intraoperative sensory-evoked potentials may aid in immediate surgical decision-making concerning the degree of decompression, continued spinal stability during turning or positioning, and surgical manipulation of neural or vascular structures.[36,73,93] These techniques are feasible only in cases of *incomplete* spinal cord injury so that intraspinal sensory-evoked potentials may propagate through the lesion in the cord. During spinal surgery, sensory-evoked potentials have been recorded from scalp,[37] spinous processes,[13] posterior spinous ligaments,[63] or from the epidural space[65] following stimulation of peripheral nerves below the area of surgery. Although these recordings reflect primarily dorsal column sensory functions, motor and other sensory functional changes appear to correspond reasonably well.[83] Variations on these techniques have been reported.[64,93] It is important to recognize that a steady pharmacologic and physiologic state must be ensured by the anesthesiologist so that the changes in evoked potentials may be accurately attributed to the surgical manipulation of interest. The possible pitfalls of anesthetic management during electrophysiologic monitoring have been reviewed.[93]

There are several problems peculiar to the more chronic phase of spinal cord injury that may be minimized with simple but appropriate care during the acute phase of management. These problems include heterotopic ossification, joint contractures, and spasticity. Heterotopic ossification (myositis ossificans) is an inflammation of the voluntary muscles around a joint and is characterized by calcium deposits within the muscle tissue, with a resultant loss of range of motion and consequent inability to attain functional goals. This occurs in areas below the level of the spinal cord lesion, most commonly in the hips, knees, and elbows. Although the joints are not affected per se, the ossification can become massive enough to cause an extra-articular ankylosis. Closely allied is contracture of the joints resulting from a loss of the elastic properties and shortening of the ligaments surrounding the bony articulations. Heterotopic ossification and joint contractures may be minimized by correct positioning and appropriate physical and occupational therapeutic intervention during the acute phase following spinal cord injury.

Similarly, early therapeutic intervention may minimize the degree to which spasticity will interfere with later rehabilitation of the patient with spinal cord injury. Spasticity, i.e., a combination of hyperactive reflexes and increased muscle tone below the level of spinal cord injury, occurs after the period of spinal cord shock has ended. The inhibitory influences from the cerebrum have been lost as a consequence of spinal cord injury, and the monosynaptic stretch reflex arc in the area of the isolated spinal cord below the lesion level reacts in an unrestrained manner. Spasticity can become severe enough to cause pain and interfere with nursing care such as turning or sitting the patient.

Skin Complications

Of all the complications of spinal cord injury, the complications of the integument may by far be the most costly in terms of dollar amount. Pressure ulcers developing over bony prominences are the single most frequent cause of extension of hospitalization and increased medical cost to the patient with spinal cord injury. Ulcerations of the skin are produced by ischemic conditions, and both degree and time of ischemia are important factors in their development. Prevention of pressure sores must begin at the time the patient is admitted to the hospital since ulcerations result within as short a period of time as one-half hour of occurrence of ischemia. The consequent risks of infection, difficulty of nursing care, and additional nutritional requirements imposed by the presence of ischemic ulcers are self-evident.

Ischemic ulcers are prevented by minimizing points of high pressure against any body surface and frequent redistribution pressure over the body such as by "log-rolling" the patient side-back-side every 2 hours. The pressure of traction devices need not interfere with good skin care. A standard hospital bed equipped with appropriate traction devices and an astute nursing care team to frequently turn patients and attend to their unique requirements may outperform the variety of mechanical beds that are presently available. The mechanical beds, providing motorized continuous side-to-side motion, may give better results in selected patients with multiple trauma such as grossly unstable spinal fractures with associated extremity or pelvic fractures.

PATHOPHYSIOLOGY OF SPINAL CORD INJURY

In humans and in multiple animal models, histologic studies of traumatized spinal cord tissue have been described.[4,5,49,50] A general pattern of structural changes has been noted following impact injury to the spinal cord. Almost immediately there is disruption of vascular structures,[77] followed next by development of punctate areas of hemorrhagic necrosis initially in the central grey matter of the cord.[4] Within minutes, small volumes of hemorrhagic necrosis tend to coalesce into much larger volumes; and in centripetal fashion the lesion extends outward toward the peripheral white matter of the cord. The degree to which the cross-sectional area of the spinal cord is damaged by hemorrhagic necrosis appears to be related directly to the severity of the initial injury. In areas of the spinal cord immediately surrounding the hemorrhagic necrosis, significant edema forms within the first several hours following injury.[51] Axons are seen to swell and later rupture, spilling their contents of lysosomal enzymes into the extracellular space,[48] forming larger cavities in the medullary substance of the cord, and producing gross focal metabolic changes.[52,90] The necrotic lesion is primarily an effect of vascular injury and is evident immediately following the trauma.[4] Histologically there is also capillary obstruction by fibrin, platelets, and red blood cells, suggesting compromise of the microcirculation by microthrombi. However, the effect of microthrombi is generally seen after a 30-minute delay following injury and may be secondary to the disruption of larger vessels or tissue necrosis rather than a primary effect of the trauma itself. Spinal cord blood flow at the area of spinal cord trauma has been shown to decrease dramatically within minutes following injury,[80] with the grey matter affected more than white matter.[76]

The precise mechanisms that block electrical conduction in the injured spinal cord are unclear. Three mechanisms already implicated are (1) compression-related structural changes or mechanical disruption in axons and other neural elements at the cellular or subcellular levels, (2) spinal cord edema, and (3) ischemia of the spinal cord with resultant metabolic deficiencies. Mechanical trauma to spinal cord structures with either disruption or deformation of axons and other neural elements clearly results in interruption of neural conduction across the area of injury.[30] Spinal cord ischemia[32] and edema, however, may have more subtle but no less important interruptive effects on electrical conduction. The controversy surrounding this issue is unresolved. The major problem appears to be an inability to separate the mechanical, ischemic, and edematous conditions. For example, extracellular potassium released from mechanically injured cells may result in a sudden increase in membrane permeability with (1) subsequent metabolic changes that interfere with neural conduction, and (2) tissue edema resulting in compressive changes in spinal cord blood flow and, consequently, further changes in metabolism.

The role of *continued* neural tissue distortion or compression following an injury to the spinal cord has not been clarified. It is for this reason that the advisability of early decompressive surgery following spinal cord injury is under debate. The surgical and nonsurgical approaches to management of spinal cord injury have already been discussed, and these clearly are significant areas for further laboratory and clinical research.

Spinal Cord Blood Flow

Anoxia or compression applied along any local segment of a peripheral nerve will halt electrical conduction across that segment, but conduction along the remainder of the axon remains intact. This indicates that the ability to conduct action potentials is a local phenomenon. Conduction of action potentials along axons in the spinal cord, as well as along peripheral nerves, is a local phenomenon. In peripheral nerves it has been shown that complete anoxia resulted in loss of ability to conduct action potentials within 10 to 20 minutes.[60] Similarly, by manipulating systemic blood pressure in a spinal cord compression model, a time delay of 10 to 20 minutes was observed before loss of conduction.[11] A similar time delay has been described in a nontraumatized ischemic,[57] anoxic, and compressed[5] spinal cord, which would suggest a common mechanism for loss of conduction in all of these models. Conduction in spinal cord axons or peripheral nerves appears to depend on oxidative phosphorylation through the energy-requiring sodium pump, which reasonably may be considered the common pathway.

That maintenance of spinal cord blood flow might be necessary for neural conduction to continue in the compressed spinal cord has been shown indirectly in an acute compression model in cats.[11] Brodkey and associates[11] recorded somatosensory-evoked potentials during submaximal cord compression or hypotension. In either case the somatosensory-evoked potential was unchanged. On the other hand, if both submaximal stimuli were applied simultaneously, the influence of each appeared to be additive, and the somatosensory-evoked potential was blocked. Furthermore, if sufficient compression was applied to the spinal cord so that the somatosensory-evoked potential was blocked, elevation of the systemic blood pressure resulted in return of somatosensory-evoked potential recordings, despite continued spinal cord compression. In these experiments spinal cord compression and blood pressure were used to manipulate spinal cord perfusion pressure and thus spinal cord blood flow. With the use of a radiolabeled microsphere technique to measure spinal cord blood flow, it has been demonstrated that spinal cord compression severe enough to block electrical conduction is associated with a significantly reduced spinal cord blood flow and that elevation of systemic blood pressure sufficient to cause return of electrical conduction is associated with return of spinal cord blood flow to at least control levels, despite continued compression.[58]

In an ischemic, nontraumatized spinal cord model, conduction remained intact at ischemic levels as high as 20% of normal spinal cord blood flow.[57] On the other hand, further levels of ischemia for periods of at least 10 minutes completely blocked conduction. This model would suggest an "on-off" concept of neural conduction, even though other investigators have found a gradual decline in the amplitude of spinal-evoked potentials as spinal cord compression was increased and spinal cord blood flow maintained.[35] On the other hand, after the lower limit of autoregulation was passed, there was a closely correlated decline in both evoked potential amplitude and spinal cord blood flow. In still another model[79] the amplitude of the spinal-evoked potential was maintained until a high degree of compression was attained, when the evoked potential was abruptly blocked. The results recorded in these various models are inconsistent, perhaps as a consequence of the use of different animal models and different methods of compression. However, these findings are good indirect evidence that continued spinal cord perfusion is required for the injured spinal cord to continue electrical conduction.

Autoregulation and carbon dioxide responsiveness are two vascular physiologic responses observed in both cerebral tissue and spinal cord.[54,82] Vascular autoregulation is mediated by the autonomic nervous system and ensures that tissue blood flow remains relatively constant over a wide range of systemic blood pressure. Thus the metabolic requirement of that tissue is maintained despite changes in blood pressure. Carbon dioxide responsiveness ensures that decreasing P_{CO_2} results in vasoconstriction and thus decreased tissue blood flow. Contusion injury to the spinal cord destroys both autoregulation and carbon dioxide responsiveness,[82] but whether a sustained compression injury to the spinal cord would also result in loss of autoregulation and carbon dioxide responsiveness remains unclear. The sympathetic nervous system appears to play a major role in the response to contusion injury to the spinal cord.[96] Loss of autoregulation in normal spinal cord has been observed following paravertebral thoracic sympathectomy. Furthermore, sympathectomy appears to be associated with maintenance of spinal cord blood flow to the injured segment of the spinal cord and to a return of neural conduction. Autoregulation of spinal cord blood flow has been studied with the use of alpha- and beta-adrenergic blockade.[55,56] It appears that the alpha-adrenergic component of the sympathetic system mediates autoregulation at low systemic blood pressures through progressive vascular constriction in response to blood pressure elevation. On the other hand, the beta-adrenergic component appears to be involved with "breakthrough" of autoregulation by initiating vasodilation and consequent increase in spinal cord blood flow. Whether attempts at maintenance of this blood flow following spinal cord injury will assist in preserving neurologic function and the precise degree to which the sympathetic nervous system controls autoregulation and spinal cord blood flow are matters for further laboratory and clinical investigation.

Multiple promising pharmacologic agents that assist in maintaining spinal cord blood flow are being investigated in the acute phase of spinal cord injury. On the other hand, in the subacute or chronic phases of spinal cord injury during which mechanisms of *regeneration* might be operational, it is clear from animal experimentation that vascular perfusion at the injury site may be suboptimal or entirely absent. In these later phases of spinal cord injury, revascularization procedures such as placement of a vascularized pedicle of omentum in the area of spinal cord injury have been investigated in experimental models[31] and may show reasonable promise for future clinical therapy of spinal cord injury in humans.

Spinal Cord Edema

Swelling of spinal cord tissue in the area of injury and in nearby tissue tends to occur rapidly following spinal cord injury.[51] Water content in injured tissue rises significantly, and initially this appears to be a vasogenic phenomenon, with intravascular fluids readily escaping into the extracellular space. Immediately following spinal cord trauma there is increased capillary permeability at the injury site secondary to direct vascular tissue damage, as well as to the indirect effects of vasoactive substances released by damage to surrounding neural matter. Furthermore, there is a significantly decreased spinal cord blood flow for reasons already discussed, and this results in hypoxic injury to the neural tissue with further increases in capillary permeability. This is a positive feedback mechanism that tends to perpetuate itself after initiation of the process. During the first 48 hours following injury, the fluid shifts continue but become cytotoxic in nature. The cellular membranes break down, allowing fluid in the extracellular space to shift into the intracellular space, with intracellular swelling and concomitant shrinkage of the extracellular space.

The process of edema formation has the effect of deforming neural elements and occluding vascular flow. In either case the outcome may be loss of electrical conduction in the local area by either direct or indirect mechanisms.

INNOVATIVE TREATMENTS FOR SPINAL CORD INJURY (SCI)

Naloxone

If it is accepted that the neurologic deficit following spinal cord trauma may in part be the result of spinal cord ischemia, it can be argued that maintaining spinal cord blood flow may potentially reverse these deficits, particularly if treatment is applied early. Multiple vasoactive pharmaceutic agents have been tried experimentally or clinically in an attempt to minimize the vascular changes in the focal areas of spinal cord injury. The opiate antagonist naloxone appears to be most promising from a clinical standpoint. Various plasma endorphins (endogenous opioids) abound in the mammalian organism and are active in regulation of the autonomic nervous system. Some of the endorphins are known to increase significantly following spinal cord injury, and these substances are further associated with diminution of arterial blood pressure and spinal cord blood flow. By blocking endorphin receptors in the spinal cord, naloxone may directly help maintain a more physiologic spinal cord blood flow following spinal cord injury.[25,28] Furthermore, naloxone may act indirectly through its ability to block the fall in systemic arterial blood pressure routinely seen immediately following spinal cord injury.

Naloxone may also act through nonopiate mechanisms such as stabilization of lysosomal membranes[14] or inhibition of free-radical reactions.[17] Free-radical particles are presumably formed in the respiratory chain in mitochondria during hypoxic or ischemic episodes. With any available oxygen, these highly reactive substances peroxidize unsaturated fatty acids in cellular membranes and cause damage to the membrane. Thus, acting as a free-radical "scavenger," naloxone may prevent damage to cellular membranes.

In a feline model of spinal cord injury, animals treated with naloxone regained neurologic function substantially faster than those untreated.[24] Other opiate antagonists and thyrotrophin-releasing hormone have also been used in various models of spinal cord injury and experimental shock models of various causes.[23,45]

Dimethyl Sulfoxide

The physiologic mechanism of action of dimethyl sulfoxide (DMSO) in trauma to the central nervous system is not clear. In an animal model of spinal cord injury, administration of DMSO appeared to accelerate return of motor function.[47] Electron microscopic studies have revealed that rapid administration of DMSO following spinal cord injury resulted in protection of axons and the myelin sheath and reduced associated tissue swelling. DMSO may act by inhibiting platelet aggregation and preventing vascular occlusion to the neural tisssue.[84] DMSO interacts with cyclic adenosine monophosphate, prostaglandins, and thromboxane A_2, a powerful platelet aggregator. Thus the effect of DMSO on spinal cord blood flow may relate to its effect on the platelet-aggregating mechanism[16] and on the various mechanisms that relate to vasospasm or vasoconstriction.[75] In addition, DMSO appears to have a stabilizing or protective effect on cellular and subcellular membranes.[61]

Spinal Cord Cooling

Local cooling as a treatment for spinal cord injury has had waxing and waning enthusiasm since its inception in 1967.[1] There appear to be multiple good reasons for using local cooling, and the procedure is relatively simple to implement. Although spinal cord cooling through percutaneously placed subarachnoid needles may provide an easily accessible route for continuous perfusion, most authors have preferred an open surgical technique such as a laminectomy (Fig. 48-6). The posterior bony covering of the spinal cord, the lamina, must be removed to expose the dural sac. The dura is then opened widely to allow constant irrigation of the injured tissue. If it is begun within 4 hours of the initial injury, spinal cord cooling of 50° F (10° C) has been noted to reduce the volume of neural tissue by approximately 10%.[3] At the same time neuronal metabolism and oxygen requirement are decreased. While the cord is cooling, electrolyte balance in the local area of

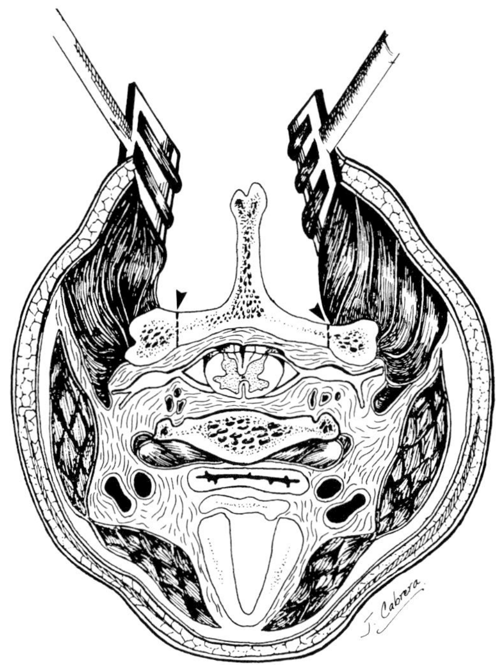

Fig. 48-6 Laminectomy involves removal of the posterior portion of the bony covering of the spinal cord. In this schematic drawing the bony portion between the arrows is surgically removed to expose the spinal dura.

spinal cord injury is controlled by manipulation of these substances in the irrigation fluid. A marked washout of biochemical breakdown products, catecholamines, and histamine-like substances can also be achieved. These are substances that have been shown to have a detrimental effect on injured spinal cord. Although spinal cord cooling may produce vasoconstriction in the irrigated area with potentially disastrous decreases in spinal cord blood flow, this detrimental effect of cooling may be reversed by judicious use of vasodilatory substances in the irrigation fluid.

Thus, from the standpoint of experimental spinal cord injury in laboratory animals, spinal cord cooling has been an effective adjunct to the total treatment of spinal cord injury. On the other hand, in the clinical situation in humans the effects of this treatment modality are yet to be tested. The reluctance of many surgeons to do a laminectomy following spinal cord injury is perhaps one reason why this method of treatment has not been used routinely. The several advantages of spinal cord cooling must be weighed carefully.

Spinal Cord Regeneration

Although the peripheral nervous system has the capacity to regenerate its own damaged axons, the process of regeneration does not appear to be applicable to spinal cord or brain injury. On the other hand, it is important to note that transected spinal cord axons can *initiate* a "sprouting" process but that this process appears to abort within 10 days. That axonal sprouting is initiated but aborted in the injured spinal cord may indicate a lack of specific nerve growth factors, which may be in ready supply in the peripheral nervous system. The identity of specific nerve growth factors is particularly unclear. The term "growth factor" may refer to neurotrophic substances, neurotransmitters, hormones, or other neurosecretory material. On the other hand, growth factor may refer, not to pharmacologic agents, but rather to morphologic components that produce a favorable tissue environment for regeneration as opposed to conditions that might form a barrier to such a process such as tissue necrosis, glial scar, and cavitation.[4,5,50,51,77] Clearly, the entire process cannot proceed without adequate vascular perfusion and delivery of oxygen and obligatory nutrients required for the regenerative process. This is an area requiring substantial research efforts before becoming available for clinical treatment in humans.

SUMMARY

Since spinal cord injury is being assessed as a major medical problem, an increasing number of patients are surviving the initial resuscitation and transportation to a major medical center. Furthermore, the proportion of patients with incomplete spinal cord injury, which carries a better overall prognosis than does complete injury, has increased significantly in recent years. These changes may be attributed to the increased sophistication of emergency medical services across the nation. Given increasing numbers of surviving patients with this injury, it is critical to note that the quality of life for these patients is significantly improved when their management is optimized by preventing common complications that comprise the greatest threat of morbidity and mortality to them. Prevention of complications common to the spinal-cord–injured patients has significantly lengthened their life spans and is a compelling reason for the development of regional spinal cord injury centers where knowledgeable medical management may be provided to these patients.

REFERENCES

1. Albin, M.S., et al.: Localized spinal cord hypothermia: anesthetic effects in application to traumatic injury, Anesth. Analg. **46**:8, 1967.
2. Apley, A.G.: Fracture of the spine, Ann. R. Coll. Surg. Engl. **46**:210, 1970.
3. Austin, G.M., Cushman, A., and Horn, N.M.: Spinal cord edema. In George M. Austin, editor: Spinal cord, New York, 1983, IGAKU-SHOIN, Ltd Publishers.
4. Balentine, J.D.: Pathology of experimental spinal cord trauma. I. The necrotic lesion as a function of vascular injury, Lab. Invest. **39**:236, 1978.
5. Balentine, J.D.: Pathology of experimental spinal cord trauma. II. Ultrastructure of axons and myelin, Lab. Invest. **39**:254, 1978.
6. Beatson, T.R.: Fractures and dislocations of the cervical spine, J. Bone Joint Surg. (Br) **45**:21, 1963.
7. Bedbrook, G.M.: Stability of spinal fractures and fracture-dislocations, Paraplegia **9**:23, 1971.
8. Bedbrook, G.M.: The care and management of spinal cord injuries, New York, 1981, Springer-Verlag.
9. Bedbrook, G., and Clark, W.B.: Thoracic spine injuries with spinal cord damage, J. R. Coll. Surg. Edinb. **26**:264, 1981.
10. Bergofsky, E.H.: Mechanism for respiratory insufficiency after cervical cord injury, Ann. Intern. Med. **61**:435, 1964.
11. Brodkey, J.S., et al.: Reversible spinal cord trauma in cats: additive effects of direct pressure and ischemia, J. Neurosurg. **37**:591, 1972.
12. Brooke, M.M., and Donovan, W.H., and Stolov, W.C.: Paraplegia: succinylcholine-induced hyperkalemia and cardiac arrest, Arch. Phys. Med. Rehabil. **59**:306, 1978.
13. Brown, R.H., and Nash, C.L., Jr.: Current status of spinal cord monitoring, Spine **4**:466, 1979.
14. Curtis, M.T., and Lefer, A.M.: Protective actions of naloxone in hemorrhagic shock, Am. J. Physiol. **239**:H416, 1980.
15. Deitel, M., and Kaminsky, V.: Total nutrition by periphral vein—the lipid system, Can. Med. Assoc. J. **111**:152, 1974.
16. de la Torre, J.C., et al.: Pharmacologic treatment and evaluation of permanent experimental spinal cord trauma, Neurology **24**:508, 1975.
17. Demopoulos, H.B., et al.: The free radical pathology and the microcirculation in the major central nervous system disorders, Acta Physiol. Scand. (suppl.) **492**:91, 1980.
18. DeTroyer, A., and Heilporn, A.: Respiratory mechanics in quadriplegia: the respiratory function of the intercostal muscles, Am. Rev. Respir. Dis. **122**:591, 1980.
19. Donovan, W.H., and Bedbrook, G.: Comprehensive management of spinal cord injury, Clin. Symp. **34**(2):2, 1982.
20. Dudrick, S.J., et al.: Parenteral hyperalimentation—metabolic problems and solutions, Ann. Surg. **176**:259, 1972.
21. Durward, Q.J., Schweigel, J.F., and Harrison, P.: Management of fractures of the thoracolumbar and lumbar spine, Neurosurgery **8**:555, 1981.
22. Erickson, R.P.: Autonomic hyperreflexia: pathophysiology and medical management, Arch. Phys. Med. Rehabil. **61**:431, 1980.
23. Faden, A.I., and Holaday, J.W.: Opiate antagonist: a role in the treatment of hypovolemic shock, Science **205**:317, 1979.
24. Faden, A.I., Jacobs, T.P., and Holaday, J.W.: Opiate antagonist improves neurologic recovery after spinal injury, Science **211**:493, 1981.
25. Faden, A.I., et al.: Endorphins in experimental spinal injury: therapeutic effect of naloxone, Ann. Neurol. **10**:326, 1981.
26. Faden, A.I., et al.: Megadose corticosteroids therapy following experimental traumatic spinal injury, J. Neurosurg. **60**:712, 1984.
27. Fielding, J.W., and Hawkins, R.J.: Roentgenographic diagnosis of the injured neck. In AAOS Instructional course lectures, vol. 25, St. Louis, 1976, The C.V. Mosby Co.
28. Flamm, E.S., et al.: Experimental spinal cord injury: treatment with naloxone, Neurosurgery **10**:227, 1982.
29. Frost, E.A.M.: The physiopathology of respiration in neurosurgical patients, J. Neurosurg. **50**:699, 1979.
30. Gelfan, S., and Tarlov, I.M.: Physiology of spinal cord, nerve root and peripheral nerve compression, Am. J. Physiol. **185**:217, 1956.
31. Goldsmith, H.S., et al.: Application of intact omentum to the normal and traumatized spinal cord. In Kao, C.C., Bunge, R.P., and Reier, P.J., editors: Spinal cord reconstruction. Proceedings of the First International Symposium on Spinal Cord Reconstruction, New York, 1983, Raven Press.
32. Goodging, M.R., Wilson, C.B., and Hoff, J.T.: Experimental cervical myelopathy: effects of ischemia and compression of the canine cervical spinal cord, J. Neurosurg. **43**:9, 1975.
33. Greenhoot, J.H., and Reichembach, D.: Cardiac injury and subarachnoid hemorrhage: a clinical pathological correlation, J. Neurosurg. **30**:521, 1969.
34. Greenhoot, J.H., Shiel, F.O., and Mauck, H.P., Jr.: Experimental spinal cord injury: electrocardiographic abnormalities and fuchsinophilic myocardial degeneration, Arch. Neurol. **26**:524, 1972.
35. Griffiths, I.R., Trench, J.G., and Crawford, R.A.: Spinal cord blood flow and conduction during experimental cord compression in normotensive and hypotensive dogs, J. Neurosurg. **50**:353, 1979.
36. Grundy, B.L.: Monitoring of sensory evoked potentials during neurosurgical operations: methods and applications, Neurosurgery **11**:556, 1982.
37. Grundy, B.L., Nash, C.L., Jr., and Brown, R.H.: Arterial pressure manipulation alters spinal cord function during correction of scoliosis, Anesthesiology **54**:249, 1981.
38. Guttman, L.: Initial treatment of traumatic paraplegia, Proc. R. Soc. Med. **47**:1103, 1954.
39. Guttmann, L.: Spinal cord injuries: comprehensive management and research, ed. 2, London, 1976, Blackwell Scientific Publications.
40. Hall, E.D., Baker, T., and Riker, W.F. Jr.: Glucocorticoid effects on spinal cord function, J. Pharmacol. Exp. Ther. **206**:361, 1978.
41. Harris, P., et al.: The prognosis of patients sustaining severe cervical spine injury (C2-C7 inclusive), Paraplegia **18**:324, 1980.
42. Heiden, J.S., et al.: Management of cervical spinal cord trauma in Southern California, J. Neurosurg. **43**:732, 1975.
43. Heymsfield, S.B., et al.: Enteral hyperalimentation: an alternative to central venous hyperalimentation, Ann. Intern. Med. **90**:63, 1979.
44. Hodges, R.E.: Nutrition in medical practice, Philadelphia, 1980, W.B. Saunders Co.
45. Holaday, J.W., and Faden, A.I.: Naloxone reversal of endotoxin hypotension suggest role of endorphins in shock, Nature **275**:450, 1978.
46. Holdsworth, F.W.: Fractures, dislocations, and fracture-dislocations of the spine, J. Bone Joint Surg. (Am.) **52**:1534, 1970.
47. Kajihara, K., et al.: Dimethyl sulfoxide in the treatment of experimental acute spinal cord injury, Surg. Neurol. **1**:16, 1973.
48. Kakari, S., et al.: Distribution of biogenic amine in contused feline spinal cord, J. Histochem. Cytochem. **21**:403, 1973.
49. Kakulas, B.A., and Bedbrook, G.M.: A correlative clinico-pathologic study of spinal cord injury, Proc. Aust. Assoc. Neurol. **6**:123, 1969.
50. Kakulas, B.A., and Bedbrook, G.M.: Pathology of injuries of the vertebral column. In Vinken, P.J., and Bruyn, G.W. editors: Handbook of clinical neurology, vol. 25, New York, 1976, John Wiley & Sons.
51. Kao, C.C., Chang, L.W., and Bloodworth, J.M.B., Jr.: The mechanism of spinal cord cavitation following spinal cord transection: electron microscopic observation, J. Neurosurg. **6**:745, 1977.
52. Kelly, D.L., Jr., et al.: Effects of hyperbaric oxygenation and tissue oxygen studies in experimental paraplegia, J. Neurosurg. **36**:425, 1972.
53. King, R.B., and Dudas, S.: Rehabilitation of the patient with a spinal cord injury, Nurs. Clin. North Am. **15**:225, 1980.
54. Kobrine, A.I., Doyle, T.F., and Rizzoli, H.V.: Spinal cord blood flow as affected by changes in systemic arterial blood pressure, J. Neurosurg. **44**:12, 1976.

55. Kobrine, A.I., Evans, D.E., and Rizzoli, H.V.: The effects of alpha adrenergic blockade on spinal cord autoregulation in the monkey, J. Neurosurg. **46:**336, 1977.
56. Kobrine, A.I., Evans, D.E., and Rizzoli, H.V.: The effects of beta adrenergic blockade on spinal autoregulation in the monkey, J. Neurosurg. **47:**57, 1977.
57. Kobrine, A.I., Evans, D.E., and Rizzoli, H.V.: The effects of ischemia on long tract neural conduction in the spinal cord, J. Neurosurg. **50:**639, 1979.
58. Kopaniky, D.R., and Brodkey, J.S.: Unpublished data, 1984.
59. Lambert, D.H., Deane, R.S., and Mazuzan, J.E.: Anesthesia and the control of blood pressure in patients with spinal cord injury, Anesth. Analg. **61:**344, 1982.
60. Leone, J., and Ochs, S.: Axonic block and recovery of axoplasmic transport and electrical excitability of nerve, J. Neurobiol. **9:**229, 1978.
61. Lim, R., and Mullan, S.: Enhancement of resistance of glial cells by dimethyl sulfoxide against sonic disruption, Ann. N.Y. Acad. Sci. **243:**358, 1975.
62. L'Laoire, S.A., and Thomas, D.G.T.: Surgery in incomplete spinal cord injury, Surg. Neurol. **17:**12, 1982.
63. Lueders, H., et al.: A new technique for intraoperative monitoring of spinal cord function: multichannel recording of spinal cord and subcortical evoked potentials, Spine **7:**110, 1982.
64. Lueders, H., et al.: Surgical monitoring of spinal cord function: cauda equina stimulation technique, Neurosurgery **11:**482, 1982.
65. Macon, J.B., et al.: Spinal conduction velocity measurement during laminectomy, Surg. Forum **31:**453, 1980.
66. Maynard, F.M., et al.: Neurological prognosis after traumatic quadriplegia: three-year experience of California Regional Spinal Cord Injury Care System, J. Neurosurg. **50:**611, 1979.
67. Miller, S.E., Miller, C.L., and Trunkey, D.D.: The immune consequences of trauma, Surg. Clin. North Am. **62:**167, 1982.
68. Morgan, B.C., et al.: Hemodynamic effects of intermittent positive pressure respiration, Anesthesiology **27:**584, 1966.
69. Mullin, T.J., and Kirkpatrick, J.R.: The effect of nutritional support on immune competency in patients suffering from trauma, sepsis, or malignant disease, Surgery **90:**610, 1981.
70. Nair, K.S., and Garrow, J.S.: Depression of cellular immunity as an index of malnutrition in surgical patients, Br. Med. J. **282:**698, 1981.
71. Panchal, P.D.: Rehabilitation of the patient with spinal cord, Curr. Probl. Surg. **17:**254, 1980.
72. Peiffer, S.C., Blust, P., and Leyson, J.F.J.: Nutritional assessment of the spinal cord injured patient, J. Am. Diet. Assoc. **78:**501, 1981.
73. Power, S.K., Bolger, C.A., and Edwards, M.S.B.: Spinal cord pathways mediating somatosensory evoked potentials, J. Neurosurg. **57:**472, 1982.
74. Quimby, C.W., Jr., Williams, R.N., and Griefenstein, F.E.: Anesthetic problems of the acute quadriplegic patient, Anesth. Analg. **52:**333, 1973.
75. Rao, C.V.: Differential effects of detergents and dimethyl sulfoxide on membrane prostaglandin E_1 and F_2 receptors, Life Sci. **20:**2013, 1977.
76. Sandler, A.N., and Tator, C.H.: Effect of acute spinal cord compression injury on regional spinal cord blood flow in primates, J. Neurosurg. **45:**660, 1976.
77. Sasaki, S.: Vascular change in the spinal cord after impact injury in the rat, Neurosurgery **10:**360, 1982.
78. Schneider, R.C., et al.: Traumatic spinal cord syndromes and their management, Clin. Neurosurg. **20:**424, 1973.
79. Schramm, J, et al.: Experimental spinal cord injury produced by slow graded compression: alterations of cortical and spinal evoked potentials, J. Neurosurg. **50:**48, 1979.
80. Senter, J.H., and Venes, J.L.: Altered blood flow and secondary injury in experimental spinal cord trauma, J. Neurosurg. **50:**198, 1979.
81. Silberman, H., et al.: Nutrition-related factors in acutely injured patients, J. Trauma **22:**907, 1982.
82. Smith, A.J.K., et al.: Hyperemia, CO_2 responsiveness, and autoregulation in the white matter following experimental spinal cord injury, J. Neurosurg. **48:**239, 1978.
83. Spielholz, N.I., et al.: Somatosensory evoked potentials and clinical outcome in spinal cord injury. In Popp, A.J., et al. editors: Neural trauma, New York, 1979, Raven Press.
84. Tateson, J.E., Moncada, S., and Vane, J.R.: Effects of prostacyclin (PGX) on cyclic AMP concentrations in human platelets, Prostaglandins **13:**389, 1977.
85. Tator, C.H., editor: Early management of acute spinal cord injury, New York, 1982, Raven Press.
86. Troll, G.F., and Dohrmann, G.J.: Anesthesia of the spinal cord injured patient: cardiovascular problems and their management, Paraplegia **13:**162, 1975.
87. Verbiest, H.: Anterolateral operations for fractures or dislocations of the cervical spine due to injuries or previous surgical interventions, Clin. Neurosurg. **20:**334, 1972.
88. Wagner, F.C., and Chehrazi, B.: Early decompression and neurological outcome in acute cervical spinal cord injuries, J. Neurosurg. **56:**699, 1982.
89. Walters, F.J.M., and Nott, M.R.: The hazards of anesthesia in the injured patient, Br. J. Anaesth. **49:**707, 1977.
90. White, A., Handler, P., and Smith, E.L.: Principles of biochemistry, New York, 1968, McGraw-Hill Book Co.
91. White, R.J.: Advances in the treatment of cervical cord injuries, Clin. Neurosurg. **26:**556, 1979.
92. Whitesides, T.E., and Ali Shah, S.G.: On the management of unstable fractures of the thoracolumbar spine: rationale for use of anterior decompression and fusion and posterior stabilization, Spine **1:**99, 1976.
93. Yates, B.J., Thompson, F.J., and Mickle, J.P.: Origin and properties of spinal cord field potentials, Neurosurgery **11:**439, 1982.
94. Young, J.S., Burns, P.E., and Wilt, G.A.: Medical charges incurred by the spinal cord injured the first six years following injury, Model Systems SCI Digest **4**(2):19, 1982.
95. Young, J.S., et al.: Spinal cord injury statistics: experience of the Regional Spinal Cord Injury Systems, Phoenix, 1982, Good Samaritan Medical Center.
96. Young, W., et al.: The role of the sympathetic nervous system in pressor responses induced by spinal injury, J. Neurosurg. **52:**473, 1980.

49

Irvine G. McQuarrie and Christine Idzikowski

Injuries to Peripheral Nerves

The management of nerve injuries poses special difficulties for the surgeon. Although the majority of nerve lesions will heal satisfactorily without surgical intervention, a year may pass before it is evident that a particular injured nerve will not heal of its own accord. By then it is too late to do a nerve repair *(neurorrhaphy)* and expect satisfactory motor recovery. To obtain a good result from neurorrhaphy, it must be performed within 3 to 6 months of injury. On the other hand, the result from neurorrhaphy is not as good as the result from spontaneous recovery. Thus neurorrhaphy is to be avoided unless clearly indicated, and this decision usually must be reached before spontaneous recovery could be manifested by changes in the neurologic examination or electromyogram. This chapter will address the pathophysiology of nerve injury and the physiologic basis of nerve repair and provide a strategy for the timely identification of nerve lesions that require operative care. To accomplish these goals, only mechanical trauma to large mixed (motor and sensory) nerves will be considered.

ANATOMY AND PHYSIOLOGY OF MIXED NERVES

Fascicular Anatomy

Although physicians agree that the effective and safe treatment of injuries to tissues and organs is based on a sound knowledge of the anatomy and physiology of the relevant structures, this is especially true for nerve injuries. In these, the most important consideration is the intraneural anatomy. This relates to the fact that each mixed nerve contains 4 to 20 bundles *(fascicles)* of nerve fibers (axons within myelin sheaths) that combine, divide, and rotate within the nerve as they travel distally (Fig. 49-1). This continuous plexuslike interaction delivers motor and sensory axons to nerve branches in a manner that connects end organs with their appropriate spinal cord segments and cell columns. As shown in Fig. 49-1, an unbranched 3-cm length of a relatively simple mixed nerve, e.g., the musculocutaneous nerve, contains 5 to 10 fascicles that interconnect to such an extent that most axons come to lie in a different quadrant and have different neighbors after traveling for that short distance.[62]

Because of this anatomic circumstance, it is impossible for the surgeon performing a neurorrhaphy to perfectly match fascicles in a proximal nerve stump to those in a distal nerve stump—even after a segment of nerve no longer than 1 cm has been removed. Thus the surgeon may want to carry out an electrophysiologic investigation at the operating table before deciding whether or not to resect an incomplete nerve lesion *(neuroma-in-continuity)*. These fusiform enlargements usually occur within weeks following a nontransecting nerve injury. Although a variable fraction of axons were broken at the time of injury *(axonotmesis),* the mass effect is less a result of the proliferation of axonal sprouts than of the proliferation of Schwann cells, fibroblasts, and collagen caused by the force of injury (Fig. 49-2). If the *perineurium* enclosing any of the fascicles has been breached, misdirected axonal sprouts grow for short distances in the *epineurium* (connective tissue that separates fascicles) before rounding up into small neuromas. Had the perineurium remained intact, sprouts would remain within the fascicle; then there would be a better than 90% chance that a good recovery would occur spontaneously.[30] However, there is less than a 60% chance of a good result from excising a neuroma-in-continuity and performing a neurorrhaphy[30] because regenerating axons have a reduced chance of entering the correct fascicle in the distal nerve stump.[6,33,66]

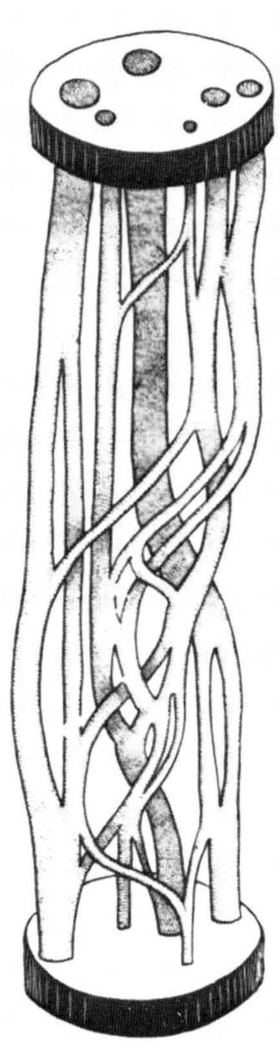

Fig. 49-1 Intraneural fascicular anatomy of a 3-cm segment from the musculocutaneous nerve of a human cadaver. (From Sunderland, S.: Nerves and nerve injuries. Edinburgh, 1978, Churchill Livingstone Inc.)

If the neuroma-in-continuity contains broken fascicles (perineurial rupture in addition to axonotmesis—a pathology now termed *neurotmesis*),[58] most of the resulting axon

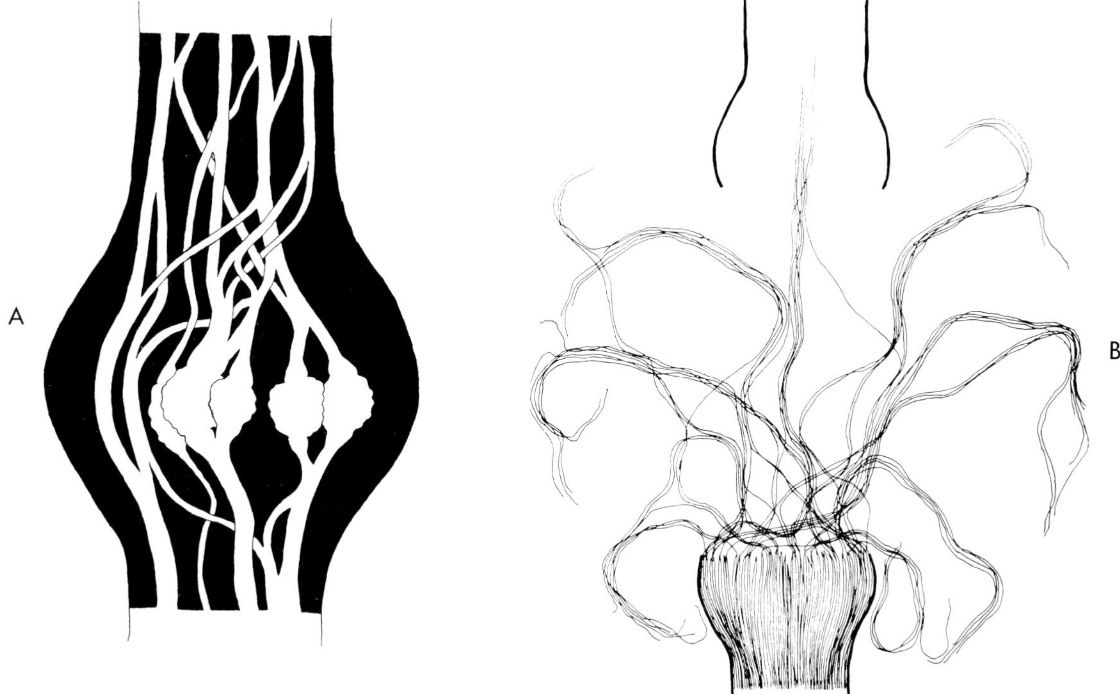

Fig. 49-2 Schematic representation of a neuroma-in-continuity. **A,** Intraneural fascicular anatomy is depicted in contrast with a dark background representing the proliferation of Schwann cells, fibroblasts, and collagen that occurs at any site of nerve contusion; five of the fascicles have sustained perineurial rupture, producing a neurotmesis-type lesion.[53] **B,** Intrafascicular axonal anatomy is depicted at a site of perineurial rupture (distal fascicle stump is at top of figure); a number of "minifascicles" have formed in response to a complete axotomizing lesion, and one of these has found its way to the distal fascicle stump.

sprouts would not be able to traverse the lesion. In that event the only possibility for recovery lies in neurorrhaphy. Since the majority of civilian nerve injuries result in a neuroma-in-continuity that is initially associated with a complete loss of nerve function, it is obvious that the decisions of whether and when to operate are of paramount importance.[30]

Homeostasis and Microvasculature

The special environment of central nervous system tissues is maintained by the blood-brain barrier, which is physically enforced by tight junctions between capillary endothelial cells. Active transport mechanisms within the endothelial cells permit the transfer of specific substances into the extracellular fluid of the brain. Similar mechanisms remove metabolic waste products and toxic substances from the extracellular fluid since the central nervous system has no lymphatic vessels. In mixed nerves the fibers in each fascicle are located within the endoneurium—a protected extension of the central nervous system environment. Thus there are no lymphatics, and the endoneurial capillaries are nonfenestrated and mostly have tight junctions;[1] the perineurial cells that enclose the endoneurial space also are joined by tight junctions. A breakdown of the perineurial barrier causes a total loss of function in the nerve fibers of the affected fascicle. This pathophysiologic event is not associated with any change in the ultrastructure of the fibers, and function is restored upon restitution of the perineurium.[28]

The intraneural blood supply is from longitudinally directed arterioles and venules located in both the epineurium and endoneurium and from capillaries within fascicles (Fig. 49-3). These capillaries lie between nerve fibers in the endoneurial space; the mean distance between capillaries is only 0.15 mm.[62] Although the largest nerves (median, sciatic) have nutrient vessels that are larger than arterioles, more than 90% of the intraneural vessels are less than 10 μm in diameter. These run for such great distances in the axial direction that considerable lengths of nerve have no nutrient vessels, e.g., the median and ulnar nerves between the shoulder and elbow joints.

Because of the long axial arterioles and venules and the extensive collateralization of the intraneural vascular network, blood flow rates are not affected by mobilization of the nerve or nerve transection. Experimental studies in cats show that flow returns to the normal range of 40 to 50 ml/100 g/min in both stumps by 1 hour after transection.[61] Thus the surgeon can safely mobilize 20- to 30-cm lengths of nerve without being concerned about the blood supply,[62] a maneuver that makes it possible to bridge a 5-cm gap if the extremity is splinted in a position of functional flexion.

Impulse Conduction

Nerve impulses are conducted over the axon surface to the axon terminal by a propagated reversal of charge that maintains the movement of the impulse at a constant amplitude and velocity. Although the rate of conduction in

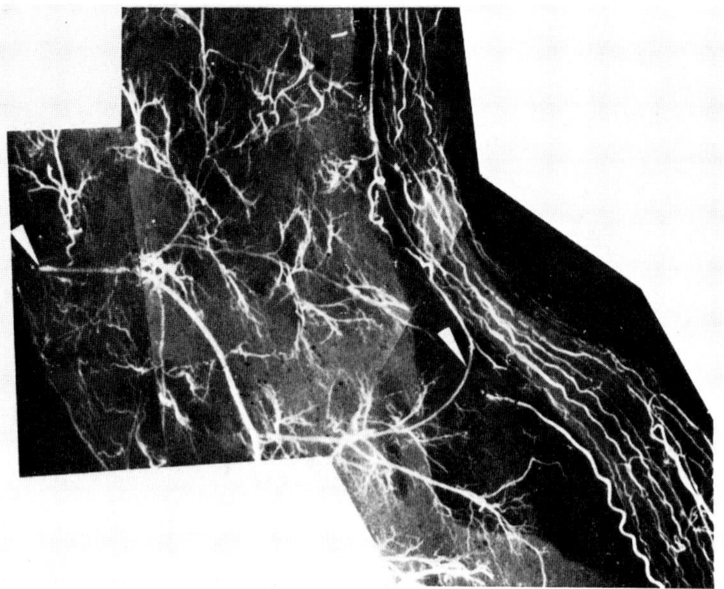

Fig. 49-3 Microradiograph of the rat sciatic nerve *(right)* and the caudofemoralis muscle *(left)* after intraarterial injection of 25% micropaque. The two arrowheads mark the course of the anastamotic artery as it arises in the muscle, emerges from the anterior muscle border, and joins the arteria comitans along the posterior surface of the nerve (×9.) (From Bell, M.A., and Weddell, A.G.M.: A descriptive study of the blood vessels of the sciatic nerve in the rat, man, and other mammals, Brain **107:**871, 1985.)

some fibers exceeds 100 m/sec, that rate is much slower than electrical conduction over a copper wire. Axons are actually poor electrical conductors: a 30-V stimulus could not produce a potential of 1 V at the end of an axon 1 m long without the energy-requiring process that mediates the reversal of charge at the axon surface.

If a nerve is interrupted by injury, the nerve action potential cannot be propagated across the point of injury. However, the axons of the distal nerve stump retain the ability to propagate for as many as 4 days after injury. Thereafter the axon surface loses its functional integrity as a result of segmentation of the axon into myelin-bounded "ovoids" or "digestion chambers" where the axon is phagocytosed—a process termed *Wallerian degeneration.*[12,58]

Pathology of Nerve Injury

With acute nerve compression of mild degree and short duration, the local pathology is limited to *paranodal demyelination* (a retraction and thinning of myelin at the nodes of Ranvier)[18]; greater compression results in a loss of myelin between two adjacent nodes of Ranvier *(segmental demyelination).* These forms of demyelination block the transmission of action potentials without interrupting the axon, producing a Class 1 injury or *neurapraxia* (Fig. 49-4, *A*).[58,67] Greater degrees of compression cause a break in the axon without disrupting the basement membrane of the Schwann cell (endoneurial tube) or the perineurium. This is termed a Class 2 injury or *axonotmesis* (Fig. 49-4, *B*).[58] Finally, cutting objects, shearing forces, and percussive forces produce varying degrees of connective tissue disruption, the most significant being a breach of the perineurium. These are termed Class 3 injuries or *neurotmesis.*[58] This literally means "a break in the nerve" and was originally used only to describe that event. Now that the perineurium is known to be the basis for the anatomic and physiologic integrity of the fascicles, the term is used to denote a break of either a nerve or a fascicle.

Myelin is readily displaced and thinned by pressure, especially at the paranodal regions. When this occurs, impulse transmission is interrupted even though the axon remains intact. Thus the susceptibility of axons to pressure increases with the degree of myelination, and nonmyelinated axons are more resistant to pressure than myelinated axons. This is best illustrated in a pure neurapraxia such as "Saturday night palsy," wherein a person intoxicated by ethanol develops paralysis and loss of sensation in an extremity because of sleeping for prolonged periods in a position that either stretches major mixed nerves or compresses them against a hard surface. The examination often shows total paralysis associated with an absence of proprioception and touch sensation in the distribution of one or more nerves to an extremity. However, the extremity withdraws in response to pinprick and a normal density of sweat droplets can be discerned by examining the skin with an ophthalmoscope set at +20 diopters. In other words, the functions served by large myelinated axons have been lost, but those served by unmyelinated axons have been retained. These patients typically begin to recover within 2 weeks and fully recover by 3 months.

When the force of compression is greater, there is a break in the axon *(axotomy).* Axonal transport is interrupted at the point of breakage; the axon distal to that point undergoes segmentation followed by phagocytosis (Wallerian degeneration). This process occurs simultaneously at all levels, and all axons show degeneration by the fifth day after injury.[12,58]

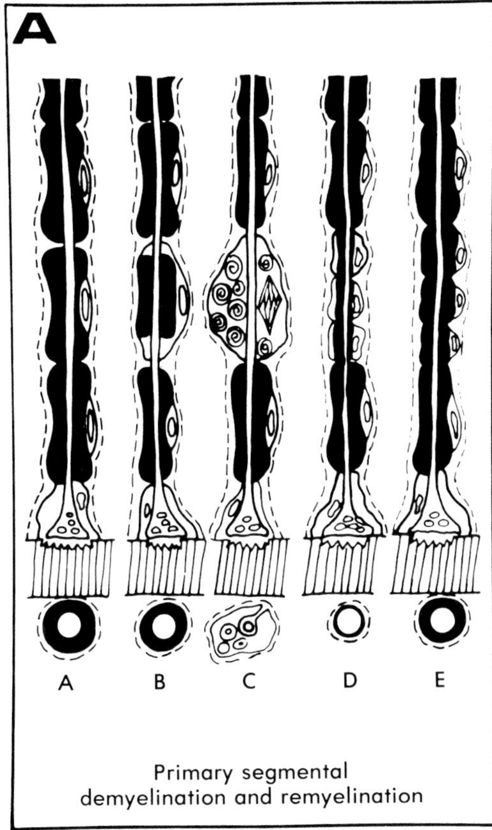

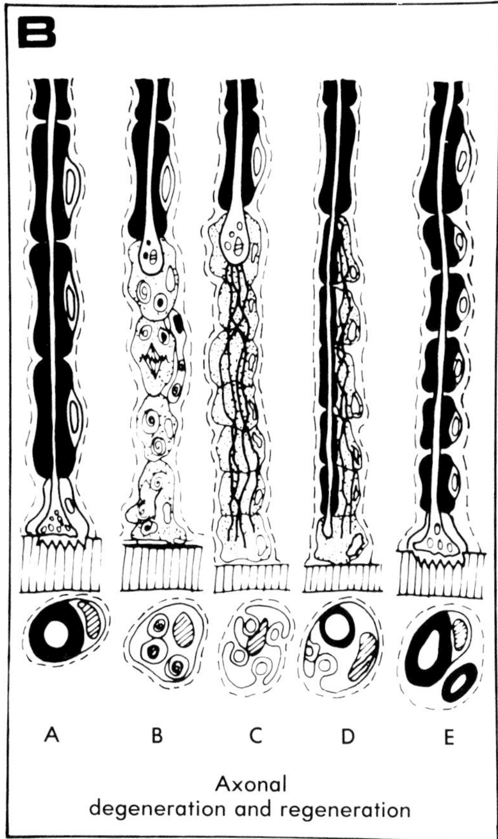

Fig. 49-4 Sequence of changes in a myelinated fiber sustaining a neurapraxia-type injury (**A**) vs. an axonotmesis-type injury (**B**) as a result of nerve compression. **A,** Neurapraxia-type injuries produce segmental demyelination and remyelination. *A,* Normal fiber; *B,* retraction of paranodal myelin with widening of nodal gap; *C,* destruction of myelin sheath and Schwann cell mitoses; *D* and *E,* remyelination through the intercalation of short internodes. **B,** Axonotmesis-type injuries produce axonal degeneration and regeneration. *A,* Normal fiber; *B,* by 1 week after axotomy, Schwann cells containing axon and myelin debris have divided to form *bands of Bungner; C,* during the second week, axon sprouts extend from the enlarged terminus of the proximal axon stump; *D,* one of the newly formed sprouts becomes myelinated; *E,* end-organ reconnection occurs. (From Weller, R.O., and Cervos-Navarro, J.: Pathology of peripheral nerves, London, 1977, Butterworth Publishers, Inc.)

Nerve Cell Body Reaction

The possibility of axonal regeneration depends on the survival of the injured neuron. Since 95% to 99% of the cytoplasm in peripherally projecting neurons is located in the axon[13] and a large fraction of the axonal volume is in the terminal arborization,[38] any axotomizing injury to a large mixed nerve amputates a majority of the cell mass. Because of this severe degree of neuronal trauma, most nerve lesions cause the death of at least a small percentage of neurons. The reason why most neurons survive is unknown but probably relates to the fact that none of the protein synthesis machinery is located in the axon.[13,23,40]

In response to axotomy, the nerve cell body undergoes a series of biochemical, physiologic, and anatomic changes that have traditionally been termed *chromatolysis* because of the commonly seen reduction in cytoplasmic basophilia. This tinctorial change is attributable to the diffusion of polyribosomes within the perikaryon—secondary to a disruption of the rough endoplasmic reticulum (where polyribosomes are normally concentrated) and an increase in cell volume.[23] The biochemical changes include an early and sharp reduction in the synthesis of proteins that are used for neurotransmitter production. This decrease is roughly balanced by an increase in the synthesis of proteins that are essential for rebuilding an axon: tubulin, actin, and other "growth-associated proteins."[2,23,40,60] Physiologic changes include a prompt internalization and degradation of cell surface receptors, a marked reduction in the amplitude of excitatory postsynaptic potentials, and a reduction in the velocity of impulse conduction in the surviving or *parent* axon.[19,23] Anatomic changes vary with the type of neuron but commonly include a withdrawal of axon terminals from the soma and dendrites of the injured neuron, a reduction in dendritic volume and length, enlargement of the nucleolus, eccentric positioning of the nucleus, an increase in perikaryal volume, disruption of the Nissl bodies (stacks of rough endoplasmic reticulum), an increase in free polyribosomes, and a thinning of the parent axon.[23,27]

There is abundant evidence that the nerve cell body reaction plays a prominent role in axonal regeneration.[23] However, there is increasing evidence suggesting that changes in the "terrain" that the *daughter axon* traverses are more critical to the success of regeneration.[5,40] Two recent developments support the primacy of neuronal events. First, studies over the past decade have shown that axonal outgrowth can be accelerated by the use of a conditioning lesion: this axotomizing lesion initiates the first crop of regenerating axons and is then removed by a second (testing) lesion. The second crop begins to sprout earlier and advances more rapidly than the first crop.[36,37,39-42] This acceleration appears to be based on the increased synthesis of tubulin, actin, and other growth-associated proteins, coupled with an increased anterograde transport of these materials through the axon.[40,42] Several lines of evidence indicate that the environment faced by the second crop of axons, an environment of degenerating nerve, is not the primary cause for accelerated outgrowth,[37,39,40,41] even though it is clear that this environment can facilitate outgrowth.[40,50] Second, the nerve cell body is able to promptly gain information concerning the status of the outgrowing axon tip and respond accordingly. Regardless of whether the growth cone meets with an obstruction or makes a successful synapse, the nerve cell body receives that information quickly by means of *retrograde axonal transport* and changes its protein synthesis program accordingly.[2,16] It is by this process, for example, that the nerve cell body knows within a few hours that it has sustained an axotomy.[59]

Axonal Transport

The motive force for axonal outgrowth appears to be the axonal transport system, which is responsible for supplying all the protein needs of the axon.[38,40,42,68] The axon contains no ribosomes, and exogenous proteins cannot cross the axon surface *(axolemma)* without the intervention of specific receptors. Thus protein requirements are met by the axonal transport of newly synthesized proteins from the neuronal perikaryon, with each protein carried by one of the five anterograde rate-components of axonal transport.[22] Nonmitochondrial proteins are mainly carried by *fast transport* and two subcomponents of *slow transport*.[22] The proteins that are used for synaptic transmission and renewal of the axolemma are conveyed in tubulovesicular form by fast transport at approximately 400 mm/day. During regeneration fast transport provides the glycoproteins and other membrane constituents that form the new axolemma.[13] In experimental studies of regeneration, fast transport is labeled with radioactive proteins to measure the axonal outgrowth distance.[13,36]

The principal cytoskeletal proteins are tubulin, actin, and the neurofilament triplet. These are conveyed through the axon by slow transport, mainly as polymers (microtubules, actin microfilaments, and neurofilaments). The 30 to 40 proteins that are associated with actin microfilaments move at 2 to 6 mm/day to form a group that is called slow component *b* (SC*b*). The protein triplet that forms the intermediate filaments of the axon, termed neurofilaments, is transported more slowly (1 to 2 mm/day) in association with most of the microtubules. This is the slowest of the five rate-components and is termed slow component *a* (SC*a*). During regeneration there are changes in the relative amounts of several proteins moving with each rate-component, but no proteins are added or deleted from the mix, and the rates of transport do not appear to change.[13,38,68] The most consistent change in slow transport within newly formed axons appears to be an increase in the amounts of actin and tubulin being carried by SC*b*.[38,40] This correlates with several lines of evidence, suggesting that the rate of axonal outgrowth cannot exceed the rate at which the SC*b* proteins advance.[38,40,42,68] The governing role of SC*b* may relate to the dependence of growth cone function on the polymerization of actin into microfilaments and the dependence of axonal elongation on the assembly of tubulin into microtubules.[38,40]

Axonal Regeneration

There are four stages of axonal regeneration that precede the onset of voluntary motor activity: (1) the *initial delay*, consisting of sprout formation and the advance of sprouts to the lesion site; (2) the *scar delay*, during which sprouts cross the lesion site; (3) the *outgrowth period*, during which axons elongate within the endoneurial tubes that they chance to enter, and (4) the *maturation delay*, during which the axons that contact an appropriate end organ initiate a series of recovery events. Maturation events include the reversal of end-organ atrophy, radial growth of the axon, and myelination.

If the time of onset of voluntary movement in a proximal-to-distal series of muscles served by an injured nerve and the distance from the lesion site to the point at which each muscle is innervated are noted,[62] the regression function of distance on time can be plotted. When this curve is extrapolated to zero distance, the number of days indicated on the x-axis is the *latent period* (Fig. 49-5). This delay represents a combination of the initial delay, the scar delay, and the maturation delay. In a classic study that used this procedure in a number of patients following neurorrhaphy, the latent period was estimated to be about 13 weeks.[3] For closed crush injuries (axonotmesis), which have a negligible scar delay, the latent period was about 9 weeks. Thus the average scar delay was 4 weeks. Since most of the nerve repairs in this study of World War II injuries were carried out after more than 6 months, the maturation delay would not have been the optimal 4 weeks; it can be assumed that it was 6 to 8 weeks.[32,54] This leaves an initial delay of 1 to 3 weeks. Thus there was a 5- to 7-week delay before axons began to elongate within the distal nerve stumps following neurorrhaphy. Experience with testing the nerve action potential across the lesion site during surgery has validated this estimate. Thus an operation for the purpose of recording the nerve action potential through a neuroma-in-continuity must be delayed until 8 to 10 weeks after injury.[30]

In experimental studies on rat sciatic nerves, sprouts begin to form within a few hours of injury, and many have stabilized (acquired a cytoskeleton) by 27 hours.[41] The zone of *traumatic degeneration* (involving the same pathology as Wallerian degeneration but located proximal to the injury site) must be traversed before these sprouts can attempt to bridge the neurorrhaphy.[37] The average initial delay in rats is approximately 36 hours, and the scar delay at a neurorrhaphy site is approximately 48 hours.[14] In monkeys the combined initial and scar delay after neuro-

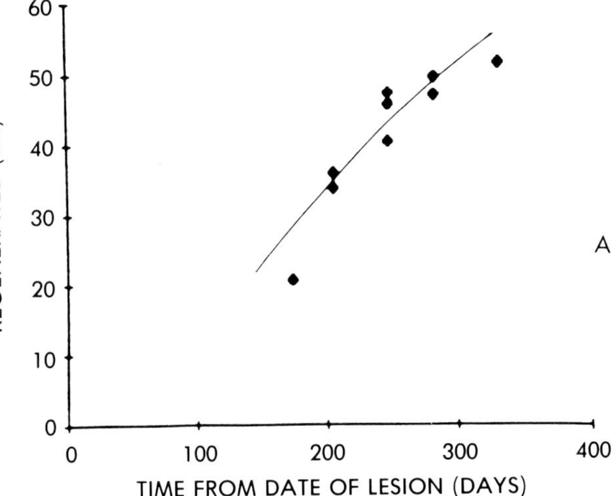

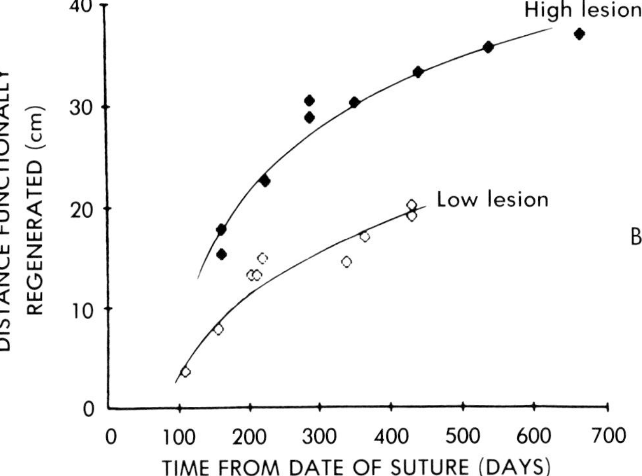

Fig. 49-5 Functional motor recovery in patients sustaining radial nerve injuries, illustrating the progress seen after an axonotmesis-type injury within a neuroma-in-continuity, **A**, vs. a neurotmesis-type injury repaired by nerve suture, **B.** Distances from the lesion site to the muscle nerve entry point are plotted on the ordinate, and the time from injury (or nerve suture) to the onset of recovery (voluntary contractions) is plotted on the abscissa. *Latent period* is estimated by extrapolating the regression function of distance on time to zero distance. **A,** Radial nerve axonotmesis: high lesion; the regression function indicates that the motor axon outgrowth rate is approximately 3 mm/day. **B,** Radial nerve sutures: low vs. high lesion; regression functions indicate that the axon outgrowth rate is approximately 1 mm/day. (From Bowden, R.E.M., and Sholl, D.A.: The advance of functional recovery after radial nerve lesions in man, Brain **73:**17, 1950.)

rrhaphy is 1 to 3 weeks.[7,31,32] This is much shorter than the 5 to 7 weeks required by chimpanzees[31] and humans, suggesting that the evolutionary step from monkeys to anthropoid apes involves a quantitative change in neuronal growth potential.[31]

The outgrowth period terminates with the arrival of axons at an end organ. If an incompatible end organ is encountered, as in the case of a sensory axon reaching a motor end plate, the maturation phase is not initiated, and the axon remains small in caliber.[56] If the contact is appropriate, the fiber undergoes radial growth—through the laying-down of neurofilaments within the axon and the induction of myelin formation by the Schwann cells.[27,51] The axon initiates myelin formation through both a chemical influence on the Schwann cell and the physical influence of its radial growth on the Schwann cell.[15,51] After the nerve fiber has matured and end-organ atrophy has been reversed through the resumption of neurotrophic activity, function is recovered. The mismatches between motor axons and muscle fibers (e.g., when a motor axon that had originally projected to a flexor muscle regenerates into an extensor muscle) are partially compensated by adaptive changes in connections along central nervous system sensory pathways[33,66] and by the neurotrophic induction of changes in muscle fiber type.[21]

CHARACTERIZATION OF THE LESION: TYPE AND LOCATION

Influence of Cause on Pathophysiology

The most straightforward classification of acute nerve injuries is to separate them first into open and closed categories, depending on whether there is a break in the skin. If closed, the lesion is either an *acute compression injury* (closed crush) or a *traction injury*. Acute compression injuries are usually secondary to fractures, with the radial nerve being involved most often.[52] The pathology is paranodal demyelination,[58] apparently secondary to increased endoneurial fluid pressure.[34] A traction component is often present because of angulation of the nerve over a bone fragment. Pure traction injuries are commonly seen in emergency rooms because of motorcycle accidents. The nerve injury occurs because the rider tries to maintain a grip on the handlebars in an attempt to stay with the motorcycle during an accident. The upper brachial plexus is involved if the motorcycle stops suddenly, throwing the rider over the handle bars; the lower plexus is involved if the rider is thrown off while the motorcycle keeps moving. Acute compression injuries are rarely severe enough to rupture a nerve fascicle, whereas traction injuries commonly do so.

Of the open injuries there are two types—those caused by bullet wounds and those caused by cutting objects such as glass. A bullet often causes a loss of nerve function without directly striking the nerve. This is because a *percussion injury* occurs as the bullet makes its transit: the kinetic energy of the bullet creates a temporary but large cavity in the tissues. The pathology is usually a combination of segmental demyelination and Wallerian degeneration, to give a mixed neurapraxia/axonotmesis injury.[18,53] The extent of nerve damage depends on the proximity of the bullet to the nerve and its kinetic energy. With a high-velocity bullet that is moving at more than 2500 f/sec when it enters the body, nerve fascicles can be ruptured even though the bullet misses the nerve. This is because the kinetic energy is proportional to the weight of the bullet and the *square* of its velocity. Obviously, a small bullet moving at several thousand feet per second is going to cause much more damage than a large bullet moving at several hundred feet per second. A military assault rifle such as the M-16 used by U.S. Forces discharges the former type of bullet, whereas a pistol such as the 0.38 Special used by detectives discharges the latter type. Both types cause a neuroma-in-continuity when they pass near a nerve, but the high-velocity bullet more often causes neurotmesis. Both types cause a prolonged initial delay because the zone of traumatic degeneration is longer than it would be with a simple laceration; the length of the initial delay is proportional to the kinetic energy of the bullet.[62] Thus after a low-velocity bullet wound it is appropriate to wait 8 to 10 weeks before exploring the nerve to test whether the nerve action potential is transmitted across the lesion, but 12 to 16 weeks is required in the case of a high-velocity bullet wound.[62]

When there are skin lacerations over a nerve that has lost all function, it can be assumed that neurotmesis is the diagnosis. Unless there are specific contraindications, immediate neurorrhaphy is the appropriate treatment.

Localization of Lesion and Assessment of Deficit

After an acute nerve injury, the sensory disturbances that occur in the autonomous cutaneous zone of a nerve are important for assessing the deficit. Loss of sensation (anesthesia) in these areas cannot be reversed by collateral sprouting from intact nerves, so such anesthesia denotes a complete nerve lesion (axonotmesis or neurotmesis). The autonomous cutaneous zones for specific mixed nerves are listed in the following section. With incomplete nerve lesions, sensation is retained in the autonomous zones, and there can be abnormal spontaneous sensations (paresthesias) or abnormal responses to stimuli (dysesthesias) in the skin regions innervated by the damaged nerve. Dysesthesias can include decreased or increased sensitivity of a normal type (hypesthesia, hyperesthesia). All of these symptoms, including anesthesia, can have a painful component.

The pathophysiology of pain after nerve injury has been studied in great detail in recent years, and an excellent review has been published by Wall.[65] The most important pain syndrome caused by nerve injury is *causalgia*. This occurs after approximately 2% of incomplete transections[55] and is rarely seen after complete transections that are promptly repaired. It is diagnosed when there are constant burning paresthesias in the skin area served by the injured nerve, in association with hyperesthesias and autonomic changes (skin that is excessively cold, moist, and cyanotic). With the passage of time, trophic changes develop. These consist of (1) glossy, smooth skin; (2) tapered digits of the denervated hand or foot; and (3) long and thickened nails. The pathophysiology of causalgia apparently involves an excess of activity in sympathetic motor axons and the transmission of this activity to somatic sensory axons my means of synapse-like connections in the proximal stump neuroma.[11]

Autonomic function is lost in the areas of cutaneous anesthesia, and loss in the autonomous zones similarly denotes a complete nerve lesion (axonotmesis or neurotmesis). Sweat secretion is undetectable when the skin is examined with the +20 D lens of an ophthalmoscope. The ninhydrin sweat test can be used to document both the absence of sweat formation and any recovery caused by collateral sprouting or axonal regeneration. The *erectores pillae* muscles at the base of each hair follicle will not erect the hairs in response to cooling, and the skin will be warm because of the absence of innervation to arterial smooth muscle. Later, as the adrenergic receptors on these muscle cells become supersensitive to congeners of the missing neurotransmitter norepinephrine, there is an overresponse to the circulating epinephrine that is released from the adrenal medulla during environmental or emotional stress. The affected part may become chronically underperfused, resulting in atrophy of subcutaneous tissues, poor healing from skin lesions, and lower growth of hair and nails.

Assessment of the response of muscles to voluntary effort is achieved through manual testing techniques that are specific to the nerve injury in question. For these to be diagnostic, the examiner must be aware of trick movements or substitution patterns. The distribution and extent of wasting (atrophy) is recorded as mild to severe, and is quantified by measuring the circumference of extremities at fixed distances from bony landmarks. Deformities of posture must be described and interpreted. For example, a *claw hand* deformity denotes an ulnar nerve lesion. The extent of muscle contractures in the hand is determined by applying standard tests for intrinsic and extrinsic tightness.[29] Joint contractures are measured in degrees by passive goniometric measurements and are judged to be either reducible or fixed.[46]

For motor disturbances the principal problem is muscle atrophy. Both disuse and the lack of neurotrophic influences contribute to this problem. If the muscle is not reinnervated within 2 to 3 years, all of the muscle cells will be replaced by connective tissue. If the muscle is not maintained in dynamic activity (by range-of-motion exercises) while it is denervated, much of the rehabilitative potential will be lost because of muscle fiber atrophy occurring in concert with endomysial fibrosis. Immobilization and paralysis also cause venous and lymphatic stasis, which further reduce blood flow and cause edema. Finally, joint changes occur because of decreased muscular support, edema, contractures, and the unopposed action of normally innervated muscles; joint stiffness and ankylosis are the result.

Examination of Specific Mixed Nerves

For the *median nerve* the autonomous zone of skin innervation includes the digital pads of the thumb and index finger and the dorsum of the terminal phalanx of the index finger. An absence of pin sensation and sweat formation in these areas indicates a total nerve lesion. The equivalent loss in terms of motor function is the lack of voluntary contractions in the abductor pollicus brevis muscle; without this muscle it is impossible to rotate the thumb to a position of grasp. If the median nerve injury is near the elbow, other movements will be impossible after a total nerve lesion. These include flexion of the distal thumb and index finger joints and pronation of the forearm.

For the *radial nerve* there is no autonomous sensory zone. In most individuals, however, a total nerve lesion causes loss of sensation over the radiodorsal forearm and the dorsum of the thumb. On the motor side the fingers cannot be extended at the metacarpophalangeal joints, the thumb cannot be extended at any joint, and the hand cannot be extended at the wrist.

For the *ulnar nerve,* the autonomous zone is over the terminal phalanx of the fifth finger. None of the fingers can be adducted or abducted, and the metacarpophalangeal joints cannot be flexed without flexing the interphalangeal joints. A claw hand deformity is common. This involves hyperextension of the metacarpophalangeal joints and flexion of the interphalangeal joints.

In the lower extremity the *common peroneal nerve* does not have a definite autonomous zone of skin sensation, but a total nerve lesion commonly causes a loss of sensation over part of the middorsum of the foot and the web space between the great and second toes. On the motor side there is an inability to evert the foot, dorsiflex the ankle, or extend the toes. For the *tibial nerve* the autonomous zone is the entire sole of the foot. The motor deficit is a loss of plantar flexion at the ankle and metatarsophalangeal joints. Axotomizing lesions of the *sciatic nerve* produce combinations of the tibial and common peroneal nerve patterns of loss.

Neurophysiologic Tests

Hoffmann's sign indicating sensory axon regeneration was described by military surgeons during World War I. It is elicited by light percussion of the distal nerve stump, beginning distally and proceeding proximally. When the leading sensory axons are percussed, the patient feels a tingling sensation in the cutaneous distribution of the injured nerve. Percussion of the nerve within 10 cm of the lesion may produce a false-positive result by producing traction on the lesion. This stimulates regenerating sensory axons that have not yet entered the distal nerve stump. Thus the sign must be elicited at progressively more distal points along the nerve before it can be interpreted as evidence of sensory axon regeneration, and the rate of progression must be appropriate, e.g., 1.5 to 5 mm/day at points proximal to the wrist or ankle.[35,62] Following neurorrhaphy the sign should be elicited at 10 cm below the repair site after 9 to 12 weeks, assuming an initial delay of 2 weeks and a scar delay of 4 weeks (Fig. 49-6).[35,62] Before surgery the presence of a propagated Hoffmann's sign suggests a diagnosis of axonotmesis. However, neurotmesis is also a possibility because a few sensory axons can bridge a nerve gap as wide as 1 to 2 cm and produce a propagated Hoffmann's sign in the distal nerve stump.[45] In the setting of such a gap, there is no possibility of functional recovery. Thus Hoffmann's sign is only useful if a neurorrhaphy has been done or a nerve action potential has been demonstrated across a neuroma-in-continuity.

Another simple neurophysiologic test is to block transmission in undamaged nerves that can contribute branches to a damaged nerve. This is especially worthwhile if the damaged nerve appears to retain some function. For example, function can be retained in median-innervated intrinsic hand muscles following a complete transection of the median nerve at the wrist in 15% of patients because of the anatomic Martin-Gruber anastomosis between the median and ulnar nerves in the forearm.[62] A *procaine block* of the ulnar nerve at the wrist would demonstrate this by eliminating all remaining intrinsic muscle activity.

Electromyography is of great value in evaluating nerve injuries that do not require immediate repair; i.e., whenever there is a total loss of nerve function as a result of acute compression, traction, or percussion injuries.[20] The most useful information is obtained if the test is carried out 3 weeks after nerve injury. By this time Wallerian degeneration has eliminated the neurotrophic influence on the denervated muscle, and sufficient time has passed to allow the muscle fiber to develop a supersensitivity to its neurotransmitter, acetylcholine, by producing extrajunctional receptors.

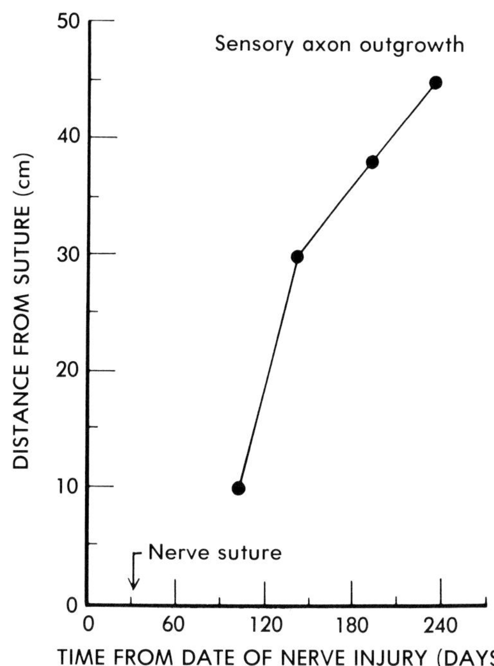

Fig. 49-6 Progress of Hoffmann's sign of sensory axon outgrowth in a patient sustaining a neurotmesis injury of the ulnar nerve at the elbow. By extrapolating the regression function to zero distance, the *latent period* can be estimated to be 7 to 8 weeks after nerve suture. With this test of nerve function there is no maturation delay; the axon terminal is continuously and exquisitely sensitive to mechanical stimuli.[35,39,45,62] Thus the latent period simply represents the sum of the initial delay and the scar delay. (From McQuarrie, I.G.: J. Neurol. Sci. **26:**499, 1975.)

As applied to the evaluation of nerve lesions, the electromyogram uses a concentric needle electrode to record from the nonfunctioning muscles in the distribution of the lesioned nerve. The object is to determine whether any of these are innervated by intact fibers. After the needle is placed in a muscle, the patient is asked to attempt a movement that uses that muscle. If no motor unit action potential is recorded, the nerve is stimulated at a point distal to the lesion by inserting a needle electrode.[20] When the nerve lesion is a severe neurapraxia (local demyelination), motor unit action potentials will be elicited without difficulty, even though none can be elicited by voluntary effort and the muscle is electrically silent when the nerve is not being stimulated. After an axotomizing nerve lesion (axonotmesis or neurotmesis), motor unit action potentials cannot be elicited by stimulation of the distal nerve. The muscle is electrically active at rest, and nerve stimulation does not alter that activity. The spontaneous activity mainly consists of fibrillation potentials (Fig. 49-7, *A*). These are never seen in normally innervated muscles but almost invariably appear within 3 weeks after an axotom-

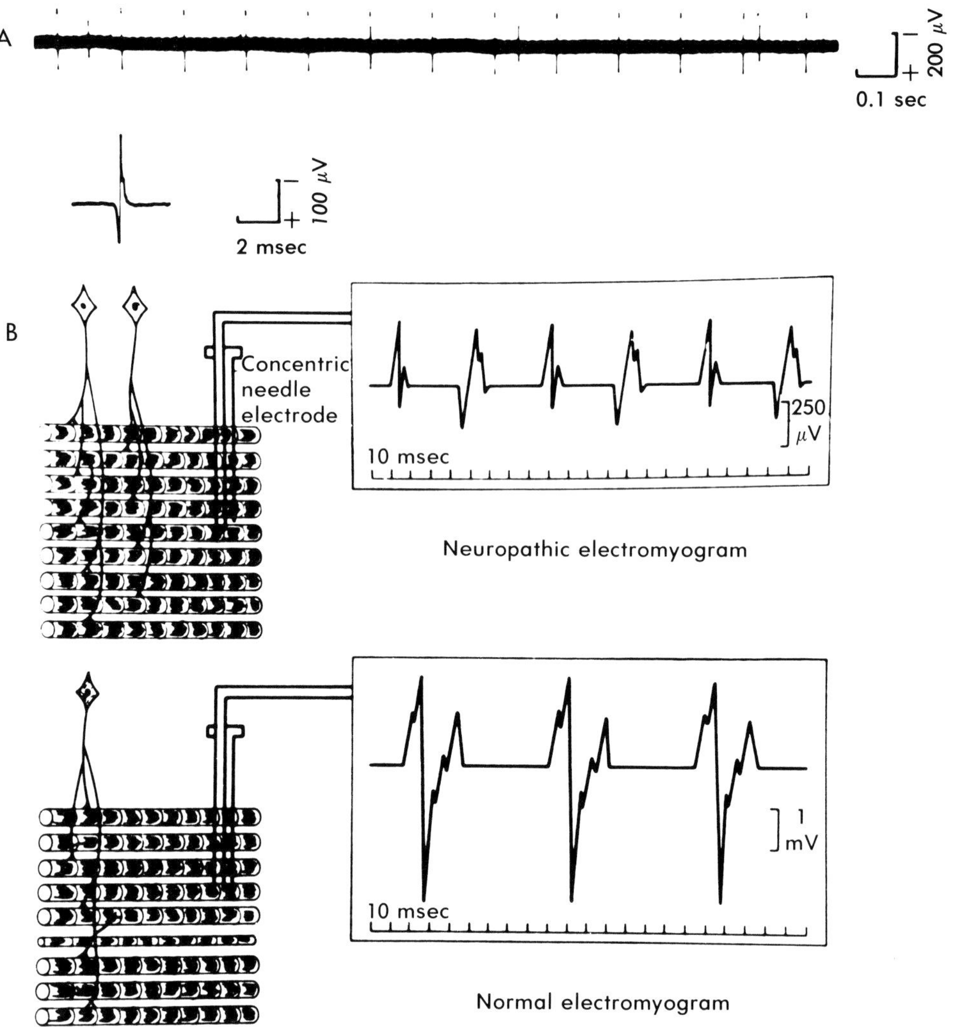

Fig. 49-7 **A,** Fibrillation potentials recorded at slow and fast sweep speeds. **B,** Electromyogram (EMG) responses during weak voluntary contractions: normal EMG contrasted with neuropathic EMG seen following axonal regeneration. (**A,** From Goodgold, J., and Eberstein, A.: Electrodiagnosis of neuromuscular diseases, Baltimore, 1978, The Williams & Wilkins Co. **B,** From Bradley, W.G.: Disorders of peripheral nerves, Oxford, 1974, Blackwell Scientific Publications.)

izing injury to the motor nerve. However, they can also occur infrequently with primary myopathic disease, polymyositis, botulism, and hyperkalemic familial periodic paralysis. (In any of these conditions, muscles outside the distribution of the injured nerve would be affected.) Fibrillations differ from motor unit action potentials by being shorter in duration, having a lower amplitude, and starting with a positive (rather than a negative) deflection.[4,20] Fibrillations occur at a frequency of 5 to 15 per second and apparently arise from single muscle fibers. The cause of fibrillations is unknown, but they are thought to be the result of supersensitivity of the muscle fiber membrane to acetylcholine-like molecules carried by the bloodstream to the extracellular fluid. Positive sharp waves, which are longer in duration than fibrillations, may also be seen with denervation. They appear to come from denervated fibers that are damaged by needle insertion, since they usually disappear a few seconds following insertion. The electromyogram is very helpful for detecting axonal reconnection at motor end plates: fibrillations disappear and are replaced by nascent motor unit action potentials that mature into the large polyphasic potentials characteristically seen with axonal regeneration (Fig. 49-7, *B*).

From the previous paragraph it is evident that motor nerve conduction studies are carried out concomitantly with the electromyography. *Sensory conduction* can also be examined, usually by stimulaing distally with digital cuff electrodes and recording proximally with needle or skin electrodes.[20] If the nerve action potential is not of sufficient amplitude, the effect of nonspecific fluctuations in the baseline can be subtracted from the nerve action potential with the use of a small computer and a signal-averaging program. By 5 to 7 days after injury, the sensory axons distal to an axotomizing lesion will no longer be able to conduct nerve action potentials because of Wallerian degeneration.[12,20] It is important to place the recording electrodes slightly distal to the lesion site since a neurapraxia would block conduction across the lesion even though the axons are intact. Thus motor and sensory conduction studies can be used to differentiate a neurapraxia from an axotomizing injury by 7 days after injury. The use of these tests for differentiating axonotmesis from neurotmesis is taken up in the following section.

RATIONALE FOR NERVE EXPLORATION AND REPAIR

Indications and Timing

The main goals of treatment are to preserve fascicular anatomy[57,62] and ensure that end organs become reinnervated within 8 months after nerve injury.[54,62] To achieve the first goal, axonotmesis must be differentiated from neurotmesis with certainty. This is not difficult if there is a skin laceration directly over the course of a nerve that has lost all function below the level of the laceration. The wound should be explored immediately, and, if the nerve has been transected, neurorrhaphy should be carried out. Any delay results in scar information that will necessitate trimming 1 to 2 cm off each nerve stump when the delayed neurorrhaphy is performed. However, if the soft tissues show evidence of extensive contusion (petechial hemorrhages and discoloration) or a bacterial infection is likely because the wound was not closed within 12 to 24 hours of injury, delayed neurorrhaphy (2-3 weeks) is preferable.

When there is a high-velocity bullet wound and the initial debridement does not reveal a nerve lesion, any loss of nerve function must be attributed to the percussive force of the bullet. During the Vietnam war, 69% of the casualties of this type recovered spontaneously after 3 to 9 months.[49] If spontaneous recovery is going to occur, axons will have crossed the lesion site within 10 to 16 weeks after injury. Most patients who are going to recover spontaneously have electromyographic evidence of recovery in the most proximal denervated muscles by 3 months.[39] This evidence includes the disappearance of fibrillation potentials and the appearance of nascent motor unit action potentials, changes that occur 1 to 2 months before voluntary contractions can be elicited.[30] Those patients who do not show electromyographic evidence of recovery by 3 to 4 months should be explored to demonstrate that the nerve action potential can be transmitted across the lesion. Techniques for carrying out these tests were originated by Kline and Hackett[30] and by Kline, Hackett, and May[32] and were further developed by Terzis, Dykes, and Hakstian.[63] For nerves that travel near the surface of the extremity, these tests can sometimes be carried out with needle electrodes.[70]

Nerve injuries caused by acute compression from a fracture, traction on an extremity, or mild percussion from a low-velocity bullet often recover spontaneously.[52] An element of neurapraxia is usually present, so that nerve conduction studies can identify patients with a favorable prognosis, occasionally as early as 7 days after injury. However, the nerve should be explored for nerve action potential testing if these studies remain negative and electromyographic evidence of recovery is not seen within 10 weeks for compression and percussion injuries[30,32,63] or 16 weeks for traction injuries (because of the longer zone of traumatic degeneration).[62]

Treatment of Neuroma-in-Continuity

From the point of view of pathology, this fusiform enlargement of the nerve involves a proliferation of connective tissue elements that may, if a fascicle has been ruptured, include thin axons that lack linear organization. Ruptured fascicles must be identified and repaired within 4 months if the patient is to have a reasonable chance for satisfactory motor recovery.[30,54,63] Ruptured fascicles are identified by intraoperative nerve action potential testing[63] at a time when regeneration can be detected in the intact fascicles: 8 to 10 weeks after injuries caused by acute compression or low-velocity missiles; 12 to 16 weeks after injuries caused by traction or high-velocity missiles.

It is not reasonable to carry out nerve exploration earlier than 2 months after injury unless there is reason to think that the diagnosis is neurotmesis. Even if all fascicles are intact, one cannot expect to demonstrate nerve action potentials across the lesion site if testing is carried out before 7 to 8 weeks.[30] For high-velocity missile wounds and traction injuries, there should be at least a 12-week wait because of the greater extent of traumatic degeneration in the proximal stump. However, to delay definitive diagnosis and treatment any longer than 4 months only serves to increase the likelihood of a poor result should neurorrhaphy prove necessary. This is because axonal regeneration proceeds slowly, at an overall rate of 1 mm/day,[39] and distances of over 300 mm often must be overcome before end-organ atrophy can be reversed by the arrival of regenerating axons. After 8 to 12 months, the effects of atrophy and endomysial fibrosis on striated muscle fibers reach a stage that is not compatible with good motor recovery.[54,62] This means that muscles more than 250 mm distal to a nerve lesion are likely to show a good recovery only if neurorrhaphy is carried out on the day of injury.

When nerve lesions caused by a bullet or fracture are explored, a great amount of scarring is encountered in the region where the bullet had passed through the tissues or the fracture fragments had lacerated the tissues. In these cases the nerve lesion is best approached by first finding the nerve in normal tissues that are well above or below the site of injury. These operations can be facilitated by consulting a useful guide that has been written by Henry.[26]

Treatment of Nerve Gap

When neurotmesis is diagnosed and the nerve stumps have been trimmed back to the point at which normal endoneurial tissue can be seen through the operating microscope, the gap between stumps can be measured. (Endoneurial tissue normally has a gel-like consistency and bulges beyond the cut edge of the nerve.) When the extremity is flexed to a position of function and the residual gap is more than 3 to 5 cm, it is unreasonable to expect that a tension-free neurorrhaphy can be achieved with extensive mobilization of the nerve. In this situation it is preferable to reconnect the fascicles with several free autogenous nerve grafts of small caliber taken from a long cutaneous nerve serving a small skin area.[24,44] The sural nerve is most commonly used for this purpose. To restore fascicular anatomy most effectively, it is important to make a map of the location and size of fascicles in the proximal and distal stumps and to use the position of blood vessels on the surface of the nerve as a guide for reconnecting appropriate quadrants of the nerve and matching major fascicles.[44]

RATIONALE FOR REHABILITATION METHODS

Modern rehabilitation methods can successfully address most of the sensory, autonomic, and motor disturbances that result from denervation.[69] Although in this discussion we recognize that most nerve lesions consist of a neuroma-in-continuity and that many of these have a neurapraxic element that does not involve denervation, the discussion focuses on the rehabilitation of patients with transsection of a major mixed nerve. Accordingly, three phases of rehabilitation can be recognized: the *denervation phase* that precedes end-organ reconnection, the *recovery phase* during which end-organ atrophy is reversed, and the *adaptation phase* during which the central nervous system and the new peripheral connections are reorganized in response to the changed pattern of connection. In each of these phases, rehabilitation methods are aimed at preventing unnecessary disability. This is accomplished by using the existing motor and sensory functions and by taking measures to enhance the rate of recovery in denervated structures.

Throughout the rehabilitation program the outlook of the injured person is an important element in recovery. Beginning with that first moment of despair, patients see their skills destroyed, their careers ruined, and their family life jeopardized. Self-worth and identity invariably suffer. During the slow and tedious recovery process the personality of the patient is truly tested. Some patients will devote considerable time and effort to assist in the recovery process, whereas others will remain indifferent and apathetic. To some the injured part will remain useless despite reinnervation; to others even a permanently disabled part will be able to serve in a useful capacity. Still other patients will exploit their injury for monetary and secondary gains.

The rehabilitation program must respect the importance of the human interactions between the patient and the health professional. These play a vital role in rebuilding the patient's feelings of confidence and trust—feelings that are indispensable to the success of the rehabilitation program. Even the most optimal professional attention can be rendered ineffectual if the patient does not receive the interest and support of friends and family members. At every stage both the patient and these key people need to be advised together about the problems and expectations of the rehabilitation effort. To a large extent the rehabilitation program depends on the faith, courage, and determination of the patient.[29]

The performance of the activities of daily living is promoted throughout the rehabilitation program, regardless of the extent of motor and sensory recovery or the degree to which the patient has made a psychologic adjustment to the injury. Focus is placed on the patient's existing strengths, with the use of adaptive techniques and devices to allow the patient to achieve the highest level of performance possible. In this process the activities that are important for self-care, homemaking, recreation, school, and work are stressed.

Denervation Phase

The denervation phase begins at the onset of injury and continues until there is evidence of neural function. Before the onset of recovery, the emphasis of rehabilitation is on keeping denervated tissues in optimal condition pending reinnervation. Patients must be educated to appreciate the degree and extent of their sensory deficit, learn to compensate for it, and adopt appropriate safety precautions. They must learn to rely more heavily on their vision while performing activities and to avoid applying excessive pressure to denervated skin by looking for signs of trauma—redness, edema, and warmth.[29] Skin that is dry and smooth because of the absence of sweating should be treated to prevent cracking. Daily soaks and the application of oils will help to retain moisture. Decreased circulation should be attended to by applying retrograde massage, elevating involved parts, and protecting these from extremes of temperature. Passive range-of-motion exercises and active exercises that use uninvolved muscles are useful for improving circulation and maintaining muscle and joint flexibility.[29] This program can minimize the trophic changes in denervated skin areas by improving blood flow and reducing the frequency and severity of minor trauma.

Denervated muscles must be maintained in dynamic activity to slow the process of fibrillar atrophy and endomysial fibrosis. Immobilization beyond that which is needed to prevent tension on the neurorrhaphy must be avoided since it promotes tissue edema and reduces blood flow in addition to encouraging the development of muscle contractures. Splinting can be used for several purposes: (1) to prevent overstretching of paralyzed muscles, (2) to support joints, (3) to provide for a balancing of forces on joints and tendons, and (4) to facilitate the active contraction of noninvolved muscles in a manner that substitutes for paralyzed muscles. The type and design of these splints must be individualized to the patient's needs, and relief from the splint must be provided several times daily to combat the adverse effects of immobilization.

The application of heat in the form of warm water or oil increases circlation without harming sensitive, denervated tissues. Blood flow through denervated muscles can also be improved by actively contracting nonparalyzed muscles, thereby exerting a pull on paralyzed muscles through interconnecting fascial sheaths. Retrograde massage and passive range-of-motion exercises are also helpful in this regard.

Joint stiffness and ankylosis can occur as a result of decreased muscular support, edema, contractures, and the unopposed action of normally innervated muscles. Joint mobility and the ranges of tendon excursion are preserved by daily passive exercises. Edema, which is caused largely by the inactivity of muscle masses, is combated by elevation, active contraction of noninvolved muscles, massage, use of the Jobst intermittent pressure pump, and the application of Ace wraps.

The use of electrical stimulation to prevent denervation atrophy of affected muscles remains controversial because there are no controlled studies in human subjects.[58,69] Although end-organ stimulation cannot prevent denervation atrophy, there is considerable experimental evidence that its use reduces the rate and degree of atrophy and that the electrical properties of the muscle more closely resemble those of normal muscle.[47] However, there is no benefit in terms of final twitch tension or tetanic tension. To reduce the degree of atrophy, treatment must begin soon after injury. The stimulus strength must be sufficient to cause long contractions without pain or discomfort; 15 to 20 contractions per session with low-frequency stimulation in the range of 10 to 12 Hz is used three to four times per day. Treatment is abandoned in favor of active contraction after reinnervation has been documented.[62]

Recovery Phase

The recovery phase begins with axonal reconnection at an appropriate end-organ. Early signs of sensory recovery include feelings that "something is happening," tenderness to pressure exerted on muscles, and an advancing Hoffmann's sign.[69] The reinnervation of sensory receptors results in altered sensations. Normal tactile stimuli may be perceived as noxious, leading patients to complain of pain, paresthesias, or hyperesthesias. The desensitization modalities that are used to control hyperesthesias include exposing the sensitive skin to graded textures (cotton progressing to sandpaper), increasingly strong vibratory stimuli, and a variety of solid particles (popcorn progressing to plastic). Finally, normal stimuli are applied to the skin until they are readily tolerated.[29]

The principles of pain treatment following nerve injury include measures directed at the pain itself and use of the involved part. The latter is of value because the pain is largely a result of the combined effects of vasomotor dysfunction, scar tissue near the proximal nerve stump, and traction on this scar from movement of the limb. One of the most valuable methods for addressing the pain directly is transcutaneous electrical nerve stimulation. This uses an electrical device that emits a pulsed current in the form of a biphasic asymmetric wave to skin electrodes. Peripheral nerve stimulation is so effective in treating pain from peripheral nerve injuries that mild transcutaneous stimulation using needle electrodes or surface electrodes is considered to be sufficient even for the treatment of causalgia.[8,43] Different forms of stimulation are achieved by adjusting the amplitude, frequency, and duration of the pulse. Constant stimulation of large-diameter, myelinated, afferent fibers reduces the perception of pain, which occurs by means of the slowly conducting nonmyelinated fibers. Transcutaneous electrical nerve stimulation is not a cure for pain but rather an adjunct to treatment. Its purpose is to decrease pain to a degree that allows patients to participate in the rehabilitation program and perform functional activities.

With nerve regeneration, a pattern of sensory recovery has been recognized; pain and temperature appreciation return first, followed by awareness of vibration of 30 c/s, moving touch stimuli, and vibration at 256 c/s. The accurate localization of tactile stimuli and two-point discrimination are the last to recover.[10] Modality tests include pinprick, temperature discrimination, vibration, moving touch/pressure, and constant touch/pressure. The return of function is assessed from tests of moving and static two-point discrimination, the response to a ridge-shaped sensitometer, and tactile gnosis (the ability to feel the shape, weight, and texture of objects well enough to identify them).[29] The Moberg pickup test is particularly useful since the ability to pick up a series of 10 to 12 small objects of various sizes and place them into a small container is readily timed and compared to results for the normal hand.[29] An effort must be made to standardize the conditions for these tests at follow-up examination since there are many uncontrollable factors affecting sensory impulses between the periphery and the cortex.

Muscle atrophy is reversed by reinnervation of the motor end plate, provided that endomysial fibrosis is not advanced. Rehabilitative efforts are aimed at maximizing voluntary motion, motor control, and strength. The therapist needs to be familiar with the expected order of reinnervation following repair of the particular nerve lesion being treated, information that is readily obtained from standard texts.[62] Treatment methods during the recovery phase include muscle reeducation, biofeedback, resistive exercises (initially resisting gravity alone), proprioceptive facilitation techniques (to maximize the stimulation of muscle afferents), and the use of patterns of movement wherein the maximal number of muscle fibers are recruited.[46]

Adaptive Phase

Once end-organ function has been restored, higher nervous centers receiving information from these end organs undergo changes that reflect adaptation to a new pattern of connectivity. An important part of this phase that can be influenced by the rehabilitation program is the reeducation of integrative mechanisms in the central nervous system so that new patterns for acquiring sensory information and distributing commands to muscle groups can be learned as quickly as possible.

Sensory recovery may slowly progress for more than 3 years before it is complete. Improvement occurs as a result of the maturation of reunited axon-receptor systems and the subliminal reeducation of integrative mechanisms in the central neurvous system. Since the central nervous system acquires sensory information differently after neurorrhaphy as a result of the nonspecificity of end-organ reinnervation, the sensations that occur early in the recovery phase may be foreign to the part of the cerebral cortex in which they are perceived.[25,66] Sensory reeducation involves a graded series of specific sensory exercises instituted at appropriate times in the recovery process. Central reorganization is facilitated so that patients are able to learn to reinterpret the altered profile of neural impulses reaching their conscious level. In the early stages of recovery patients are reeducated to modality-specific perceptions such as moving vs. constant touch and pressure. In the later stages patients are educated to regain tactile gnosis (name recognition of objects in the hand; two-point discrimination). This program is continued until the patient resumes self-education functions and returns to working, avocations, and self-care. With sensory reeducation the maximum stage of recovery can be achieved within 2 years,[10] thereby shortening the adaptive phase by a year or more.

Surgical procedures for the relief of pain caused by peripheral nerve injuries include the excision of any neuromas and sympathectomy. However, the former is rarely effective[48]; and the latter has largely been replaced by transcutaneous electrical nerve stimulation, ganglion blocks, and phenoxybenzamine.[17,43] Muscle mass is regained through repeated exercises and use of the injured part in activities of daily living.

Permanent Denervation

Specific adaptive techniques, support personnel, or appliances may be required if the functional impairment is substantial and permanent.[64] Sufficient time should elapse before evaluating the extent and significance of recovery with a view to offering delayed reconstructive procedures. Although these are effective and need to be performed in a timely manner, they do signal the patient that the hoped-for recovery will never occur. These procedures include arthrodesis, tendon transfers, tendon translocation, tenodesis, nerve transfers,[9] microsurgical free muscle transplants, muscle transfers using an intact neurovascular island pedicle, and amputation with prosthetic fitting. After these procedures, specific rehabilitation methods and goals are required.

SUMMARY

Peripheral nerve injuries are rarely followed by a full recovery of function and often leave the patient significantly disabled. Most of the injuries involve an upper extremity and often leave the patient with impaired hand function. To minimize the extent and incidence of permanent disability, it is important to preserve as much of the microanatomy of the injured nerve as possible. Often this means "leaving well enough alone." To know when to intervene surgically and, more importantly, when not to intervene, is the theme of this chapter. It is necessarily important to have an in-depth understanding of the anatomy and physiology of normal nerve trunks before the complex events that follow nerve injury can be appreciated to provide an opportunity for recovery. Similarly, the importance of using active rehabilitation measures cannot be overemphasized. Therapy should begin soon after injury, continue during the phases of recovery, and ultimately maximize the patient's independence in the performance of daily activities.

REFERENCES

1. Bell, M.A., and Weddell, A.G.M.: A descriptive study of the blood vessels of the sciatic nerve in the rat, man, and other mammals, Brain **107:**871, 1985.
2. Benowitz, L.I., Yoon, M.G., and Lewis, E.R.: Transported proteins in the regenerating optic nerve: regulation by interactions with the optic tectum, Science **222:**185, 1983.
3. Bowden, R.E.M., and Sholl, D.A.: The advance of funtional recovery after radial nerve lesions in man, Brain **73:**17, 1950.
4. Bradley W.G.: Disorders of peripheral nerves, Oxford, 1974, Blackwell Scientific Publications.
5. Bray, G.M., Rasminsky, M., and Aguayo, A.J.: Interactions between axons and their sheath cells, Annu. Rev. Neurosci. **4:**127, 1981.
6. Brushart, T.M., and Mesulam, M. M.: Alteration in connections between muscle and anterior horn motoneurons after peripheral nerve repair, Science **208:**603, 1980.
7. Cabaud, H.E., Rodkey, W.G., and Nemeth, T.J.: Progressive ultrastructual changes after peripheral nerve transection and repair, J. Hand Surg. **7:**353, 1982.
8. Campbell, J.N., and Long, D.M.: Peripheral nerve stimulation in the treatment of intractable pain. J. Neurosurg. **45:**692, 1976.
9. Chacha P.B., Krishnamurti, A., and Soin, K.: Experimental sensory reinnervation of the median nerve by nerve transfer in monkeys, J. Bone Joint Surg. **59A:**386, 1977.
10. Dellon A.L.: Evaluation of sensibility and reeducation of sensation in the hand, Baltimore, 1981, The William & Wilkins Co.
11. Devor, M., and Janig, W.: Activation of myelinated afferents ending in a neuroma by stimulation of the sympathetic supply in the rat, Neurosci. Lett. **24:**43, 1981.
12. Donat, J.R., and Wisniewski. H.M.: The spatio-temporal pattern of Wallerian degeneration in mammalian peripheral nerves, Brain Res. **53:**41, 1973.
13. Forman, D.S.: Axonal transport and nerve regeneration. In Kao, C.C., Bunge, R.P., and Reier, P.J., editors: Spinal cord reconstruction, New York, 1983, Raven Press.
14. Forman, D.S., Wood, D.K., and DeSilva, S.: Rate of regeneration of sensory axons in transected rat sciatic nerve repaired with epineurial sutures. J. Neurol. Sci. **44:**55, 1979.
15. Friede, R.L.: Control of myelin formation by axon caliber (with a model of the control mechanism), J. Comp. Neurol. **144:**233, 1972.
16. Frizell, M.: The effect of ligation combined with section on anterograde axonal transport in rabbit hypoglossal nerve, Brain Res. **250:**65, 1982.
17. Ghostine, S.Y., et al.: Phenoxybenzamine in the treatment of causalgia: report of 40 cases, J. Neurosurg. **60:**1263, 1984.
18. Gilliatt, R.W.: Physical injury to peripheral nerves. Physiologic and electrodiagnostic aspects, Mayo Clin. Proc. **56:**361, 1981.
19. Goldring, J.M., et al.: Reaction of synapses on motoneurones to section and restoration of peripheral sensory connexions in the cat, J. Physiol. (Lond.) **309:**185, 1980.
20. Goodgold, J., and Eberstein, A.: Electrodiagnosis of neuromuscular diseases, ed. 2, Baltimore, 1978, The Williams & Wilkins Co.
21. Gordon, T., and Stein, R.B.: Reorganization of motor-unit properties in reinnervated muscles of the cat, J. Neurophysiol. **48:**1175, 1982.
22. Grafstein, B., and McQuarrie, I.G.: Role of the nerve cell body in axonal regeneration. In Cotman, C.W., editor: Neuronal plasticity, New York, 1978, Raven Press.
23. Grafstein, B., and Forman, D.S.: Intracellular transport in neurons, Physiol. Rev. **60:**1167, 980.
24. Haase, J., Bjerre, P., and Simensen, K.: Median and ulnar nerve transections treated with microsurgical interfascicular cable grafting with autogenous sural nerve. J. Neurosurg. **53:**73, 1980.
25. Hallin, R.G., Wiesenfeld, Z., and Lindblom, U.: Neurophysiological studies on patients with sutured median nerves: faulty sensory localization after nerve regeneration and its physiological correlates, Exp. Neurol. **73:**90, 1981.
26. Henry, A.K.: Extensile exposure, ed. 2, Edinburgh, 1973, Churchill Livingstone.
27. Hoffman, P.N., et al.: Changes in neurofilament transport coincide temporally with alterations in the caliber of axons in regenerating motor fibers, caliber by neurofilament transport, J. Cell Biol. **101:**1332, 1985.
28. Hudson, A., and Kline, D.: Progression of partial experimental injury to peripheral nerve. II. Light and electron microscopic studies. J. Neurosurg. **42:**15, 1975.
29. Hunter, J.M., et al.: Rehabilitation of the hand, ed. 3, St. Louis, 1987, The C.V. Mosby Co.
30. Kline, D.G., and Hackett, E.R.: Reappraisal of timing for exploration of civilian peripheral nerve injuries, Surgery **78:**545, 1975.
31. Kline, D.G., Hayes, G.J., and Morse, A.S.: A comparative study of response to species to peripheral nerve injury, J. Neurosurg. **21:**980, 1964.
32. Kline, D.G., Hackett, E.R., and May, P.R.: Evaluation of nerve injuries by evoked potentials and electromyography, J. Neurosurg. **31:**128, 1969.
33. Lisney, S.J.W.: Changes in the somatotopic organization of the cat lumbar spinal cord following peripheral nerve transection and regeneration, Brain Res. **259:**31, 1983.
34. Lundborg, G., Myers, R., and Powell, H.: Nerve compression injury and increased endoneurial fluid pressure: a "miniature compartment syndrome," J. Neurol. Neursurg. Psychiatry **46:**1119, 1983.
35. McQuarrie, I.G.: Nerve regeneration and thyroid hormone treatment, J. Neurol. Sci. **26:**499, 1975.

36. McQuarrie, I.G.: The effect of a conditioning lesion on the regeneration of motor axons, Brain Res. **152**:597, 1978.
37. McQuarrie, I.G.: Accelerated axonal sprouting after nerve transection, Brain Res. **167**:185, 1979.
38. McQuarrie, I.G.: Role of the axonal cytoskeleton in the regenerating nervous system. In Seil, F.J., editor: Nerve, organ, and tissue regeneration: research perspectives, New York, 1983, Academic Press, Inc.
39. McQuarrie, I.G.: Clinical signs of peripheral nerve regeneration. In Wilkins, R.H., and Rengacharay, S.S., editors: Neurosurgery, Baltimore, 1984, The Williams and Wilkins Co.
40. McQuarrie, I.G.: Effect of a conditioning lesion on axonal transport during regeneration: the role of slow transport. In Elam, J., and Cancalon, P., editors: Advances in Neurochemistry vol. 6, New York, 1984, Plenum Press.
41. McQuarrie, I.G.: Effect of a conditioning lesion on axonal sprout formation at nodes of Ranvier, J. Comp. Neurol. **231**:239, 1985.
42. McQuarrie, I.G., and Grafstein, B.: Protein synthesis and axonal transport in goldfish retinal ganglion cells during regeneration accelerated by a conditioning lesion, Brain Res. **251**:25, 1982.
43. Meyer, G.A., and Fields, H.L.: Causalgia treated by selective large fibre stimulation of peripheral nerve. Brain **95**:163, 1972.
44. Millesi, H.: Interfascicular grafts for repair of peripheral nerves of the upper extremity, Orthop. Clin. North Am. **8**:387, 1977.
45. Napier, J.R.: The significance of Tinel's sign in peripheral nerve injuries, Brain **72**:63, 1949.
46. Nickel, V.L.: Orthopedic Rehabilitation, Edinburgh, 1982, Churchill Livingstone.
47. Nix, W.A.: The effect of low-frequency electrical stimulation on the denervated extensor digitorum longus muscle of the rabbit, Acta Neurol. Scand. **66**:521, 1982.
48. Noordenbos, W., and Wall, P.D.: Implications of the failure of nerve resection and graft to cure chronic pain produced by nerve lesions, J. Neurol. Neurosurg. Psychiatry **44**:1068, 1981.
49. Omer, G.E.: Injuries of nerves of the upper extremity, J. Bone Joint Surg. **56A**:1615, 1974.
50. Politis, M.J., Ederle, K., and Spencer, P.S.: Tropism in nerve regeneration in vivo: attraction of regenerating axons by diffusible factors derived from cells in distal nerve stumps of transected peripheral nerves, Brain Res. **253**:1, 1982.
51. Politis, M.J., et al: Studies on the control of myelinogenesis. IV. Neuronal induction of Schwann cell myelin-specific protein synthesis during nerve fiber regeneration, J. Neurosci. **2**:1252, 1982.
52. Pollock, F.H., et al: Treatment of radial neuropathy associated with fractures of the humerus, J. Bone Joint Surg. **63A**:239, 1981.
53. Richardson, P.M., and Thomas, P.K.: Percussive injury to peripheral nerve in rats, J. Neurosurg. **51**:178, 1979.
54. Richter, H-P.: Impairment of motor recovery after late nerve suture: experimental study in the rabbit. Part 1: Functional and electromyographic findings, Neurosurgery **10**:70, 1982.
55. Rothberg, J.M., Tahmoush, A.J., and Oldakowski, R.: The epidemiology of causalgia among soldiers wounded in Vietnam, Milit. Med. **148**:347, 1983.
56. Sanders, F.K., and Young, J.Z.: The influence of peripheral connexion on the diameter of regenerating nerve fibers, J. Exp. Biol. **22**:203, 1946.
57. Schady, W., et al.: Peripheral projection of fascicles in the human median nerve, Brain **106**:745, 1983.
58. Schaumberg, H.H., Spencer, P.S., and Thomas, P.K.: Disorders of peripheral nerves, Philadelphia, 1983, F.A. Davis Co.
59. Singer, P.A., Mehler, S., and Fernandez, H.L.: Blockade of retrograde axonal transport delays the onset of metabolic and morphologic changes induced by axotomy, J. Neurosci. **2**:1299, 1982.
60. Skene, H.H.P., and Willard, M.: Axonally transported proteins associated with axon growth in rabbit central and peripheral nervous systems, J. Cell Biol. **89**:96, 1981.
61. Smith, D.R., Kobrine, A.I., and Rizzoli, H.V.: Blood flow in peripheral nerves: normal and post severance rates, J. Neurol. Sci. **33**:341, 1977.
62. Sunderland, S.: Nerves and nerve injuries, Edinburgh, 1978, Churchill Livingstone.
63. Terzis, J.K., Dykes, R.W., and Hakstian, R.W.: Electrophysiological recordings in peripheral nerve surgery: a review, J. Hand Surg. **1**:52, 1976.
64. Trombly, C.A., and Scott, A.D.: Occupational therapy for physical dysfunction, Baltimore, 1977, The Williams and Wilkins Co.
65. Wall, P.D.: The painful consequences of peripheral injury, J. Hand Surg. **9B**:37, 1984.
66. Wall, J.T., Felleman D.J., and Kaas, J.H.: Recovery of normal topography in the somatosensory cortex of monkeys after nerve crush and regeneration, Science **221**:771, 1983.
67. Weller, R.O., and Cervos-Navarro, J.: Pathology of Peripheral Nerves, London-Boston, 1977, Butterworth Publishers, Inc.
68. Wujek, J.R., and Lasek, R.J.: Correlation of axonal regeneration and slow component *B* in two branches of a single axon, J. Neurosci. **3**:243, 1983.
69. Wynn Parry, C.B.: Rehabilitation of the hand, ed. 3, London, 1978, Butterworth Publishers, Inc.
70. Zalis, A.W., et al.: Evaluation of nerve regeneration by means of nerve evoked potentials, J. Bone Joint Surg. **54A**:1246, 1972.

50

Brian L. Thiele and Dennis F. Bandyk

Physiology of Arterial, Venous, and Lymphatic Flow

Accurate evaluation of patients with diseases of the circulatory system requires a thorough understanding of the anatomy and flow dynamics of the arterial, venous, and lymphatic circulations. The development of noninvasive techniques that accurately measure and monitor arterial system function has resulted in improved understanding of the pathophysiology of arterial disease, more accurate diagnostic methods, and the ability to estimate the physiologic significance of anatomic disease. Similarly, new knowledge over the past decade concerning the dynamics of venous and lymphatic flow has directly impacted on our ability to more effectively treat diseases affecting these circulatory systems. In this chapter the functional anatomy of the various components of the circulatory system will be discussed, and the essentials of arterial, venous, and lymphatic flow will be reviewed. Special emphasis will be placed on how certain biophysical properties of the circulation (e.g., pressure, flow velocity, turbulence) can be measured in man and how such measurements can be used as an essential part of the evaluation of patients with vascular disease. Although this discussion will focus primarily on the principles of arterial, venous, and lymphatic flow in the lower extremity, they are equally germane and applicable to flow in these various circulations in the upper extremity.

PERIPHERAL ARTERIAL SYSTEM

The purpose of the arterial system is to deliver blood to the tissue capillaries in amounts sufficient to maintain normal cellular function. Metabolic demands of different tissues vary widely, both in normal and diseased states. The ability of the arterial circulation to respond to these various demands is related to the anatomic and physical properties of the system and is mediated through two main regulatory mechanisms: local control of blood flow through the tissue according to its metabolic state (autoregulation) and neural control of peripheral vascular resistance. These factors, acting in concert, control tissue blood flow and consequently regulate the output of the heart. Control of blood flow is also strongly influenced by other factors such as those regulating extracellular fluid volume and urinary output.

The functional elements of the arterial system include the heart, which generates the energy necessary to maintain arterial pressure and blood flow at the appropriate level; arteries, which transport blood to the periphery; arterioles, which regulate the flow of blood into the microcirculation; and capillaries, which are the site of nutrient and metabolite exchange to the tissues. Depending on their position in the arterial system, arteries can act as storers of the pressure energy produced by the heart, cushioning vessels that convert the pulsatile flow of blood into smooth flow, and/or resistance vessels connected to the microcirculation. Arterial wall structure and neural innervation accordingly reflect the specialized function of the various arterial system elements.

As blood proceeds through the arterial system, the network of conducting vessels undergoes repeated branching and decreases in caliber with many parallel distributing vessels, finally terminating in the capillary bed. In the arterial system of the lower extremity, branching produces potential collateral networks that can bypass blood around a hemodynamically significant obstruction in a conduit artery (Fig. 50-1). The total cross-sectional area progressively increases each time branching occurs, with a concomitant decrease in mean flow velocity (Table 50-1). At the capillary level the cross-sectional area is approximately 1000 times that of the aorta. Each red blood cell remains in the microcirculation only 1 to 3 seconds, an exceedingly short time during which all diffusion and fluid exchange must occur.

Approximately 20% of the entire blood volume of the body is in the arterial system in contrast to the 64% in the venous system. The heart contains 7% of the blood, and the pulmonary vessels 9%. Surprisingly, only 5% of the total blood volume resides in the capillaries. Although total capillary volume is small, surface and cross-sectional areas are immense to facilitate the transfer of oxygen, carbon dioxide, water, nutrients, and electrolytes through the capillary walls.

The heart, through cyclic muscle wall contraction, generates a complex pressure pulse and provides the energy for blood flow. The ability of the heart to vary its output is based on its three fundamental properties: the capacity to vary the rate of contraction (chronotropism); the rate of isometric tension development, which is a function of car-

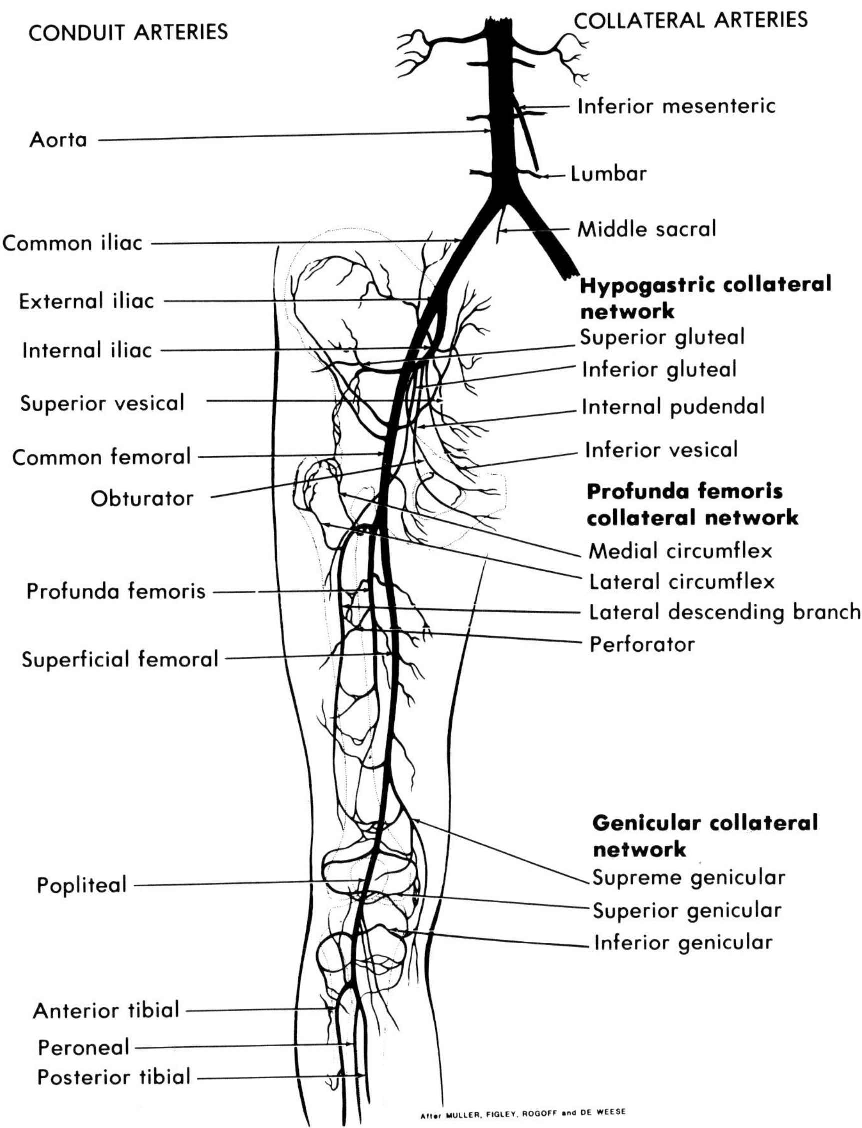

Fig. 50-1 Diagram of the arterial circulation to the lower extremity, indicating the main conduit arteries and corresponding potential collateral arteries.

Table 50-1 **PHYSICAL AND HEMODYNAMIC CHARACTERISTICS OF THE ARTERIAL SYSTEM IN HUMANS**

	Total Blood Volume (%)	Cross-Sectional Area (cm^2)	Mean Flow Velocity (cm/sec)	Pressure (mm Hg)	Resistance (%)
Aorta	8	2.5	14-18	100	4
Branching arteries	5	20	12	90	21
Arterioles	2	40		55	41
Capillaries	5	2500	0.07	25	27

diac muscle fiber length (Frank-Starling mechanism); and the ability to alter the velocity of muscle fiber shortening (inotropism). From these properties four factors that are independent determinants of cardiac output can be defined. These are commonly referred to as ventricular preload, ventricular contractility, ventricular afterload, and heart rate. The output of the heart reflects the demands of the peripheral circulation. The frequency of contraction is determined by the interplay of neural and humeral adrenergic and neural cholinergic activity on the sinoatrial node. The velocity and force of ventricular muscular contraction are influenced by both circulating and neurally released catecholamines acting on the muscle fibers themselves. The work output of the heart is the amount of energy that the heart transfers to the blood. This energy is in the form of potential energy of pressure and kinetic energy of blood flow used to accelerate blood to its velocity of ejection through the aortic valve. In the distribution of blood to the various capillary beds, the viscoelastic properties of the artery walls and the tapered, converging vessel caliber are important physical characteristics maintaining blood pressure and minimizing fluid energy losses.

Arterial Wall: Structural Features

The composition and structure of the arterial wall in the different segments of the arterial system reflect the local wall mechanics and its functional role. With the exception of the capillaries, the walls of arteries consist of three concentric layers: tunica intima, tunica media, and tunica adventitia. The tunica intima is the innermost layer and consists of a monolayer of endothelium lining the vessel wall, a thin basal lamina, and a subendothelial layer (present in the large elastic arteries of the thorax and abdomen) composed of collagenous bundles, elastic fibrils, and smooth muscle cells. The tunica media is the middle layer and is made up of predominantly smooth muscle cells in a varied number of elastic sheets (laminae), bundles of collagenous fibrils, and a network of elastic fibrils. The tunica adventitia consists of dense fibroelastic tissue without smooth muscle cells. The adventitia also contains the nutrient vessels of the arterial wall (vasa vasorum) and both vasomotor and sensory nerves for the vascular wall itself.

Arteries can be classified by the respective amounts of elastin, smooth muscle, and collagen in their walls. The distensibility of an artery generally correlates with the elastin content in the vessel wall. The large arteries of the thorax and abdomen such as the aorta, innominate, iliac, subclavian, and common iliacs are referred to as elastic or "pressure storer" arteries since their walls contain a predominance of elastin and few smooth muscle cells. The large elastic arteries instantaneously accommodate each stroke volume of the heart, storing a portion during systole and draining this volume during diastole (windkessel effect). This helps to propel the blood toward the periphery during diastole and promotes continuous flow to the capillaries. The internal pressure in the large arteries is normally about 120 to 180 mm Hg.

Proceeding distally from the conducting arteries, the muscular or branching arteries such as the brachial, radial, femoral, and popliteal have a media with primarily smooth muscle and collagen and little elastic tissue. The varying viscoelastic wall properties distant from the heart are related to the proportions of collagen and elastin in the media, the linkage between these two elements, the insertions of elastin and muscle on collagen fibers, and the contractile state of the vascular smooth muscle. Proceeding from the thoracic aorta distally there is a gradual decline in the elastin-collagen ratio. This results in a low vascular impedance for the initial segment of the arterial tree, thereby reducing the oscillatory component of work required distally to maintain cardiac output. The increased relative stiffness of the distal muscular arteries may be important to ensure that undampened transmission of the pressure pulse to baroreceptors occurs, for example, at the carotid bifurcation. At the level of the arterioles the arterial wall is composed almost entirely of smooth muscle. The smooth muscle of the media is well innervated by sympathetic nerves. These vessels provide the major site of resistance in the arterial system and provide for the regulation of blood flow to the microcirculation (see Table 50-1). Internal pressure in the arterioles ranges from 40 to 60 mm Hg.

The collagen content of the arterial wall is correlated with its tensile strength, with the adventitial collagen accounting for the majority of wall stability. This is evident from the maintenance of vessel integrity by the adventitia following surgical endarterectomy, which removes the intima and a large portion of the media. In naturally occurring aneurysms the collagen content of the adventitia is decreased, and failure of wall integrity occurs. Only degradation of collagen results in arterial wall rupture. The circumferential tension (T) in the arterial wall is calculated as the product of the transmural pressure, P_t (inside pressure minus outside pressure), and the radius (R). This relationship can be expanded to include the factor of wall thickness (μm):

$$T = \frac{P_t R}{\mu m} \text{ (dynes/cm)}$$

In arteries with a radius and wall thickness of equal proportions, wall tension varies with transmural pressure. For example, the small radius and low pressure of a capillary requires only a thin wall to support the wall tension, whereas the aorta with its greater pressure and radius requires a thicker wall to prevent rupture.

The elastic properties of any blood vessel can be described by Young's modulus (E), which is stress divided by strain. Because arteries are subject to pulsatile pressure, measurements of elasticity are determined from the strain that accompanies a period of time in which stress is varied, producing what is called a dynamic modulus (Edyn). The most important component of stress in arteries is the first harmonic of the pressure pulse, i.e., heart rate. The dynamic elastic modulus of an artery is also a determinant of pulse wave velocity. In vivo arterial wall motion occurs predominantly in the circumferential direction. The variation of diameter oscillations closely resembles the waveform of the pressure pulse. Intrathoracic arteries vary 8% to 18% in diameter with each cardiac cycle, whereas peripheral arteries change 8% to 10% in diameter. The distensibility characteristic of arteries also depends on the extent of stretch (transmural pressure). At low pressure and small diameters, arteries are very distensible, whereas they become gradually stiffer with increasing pressure and diameter.

The viscoelastic properties of arteries are altered not only in diseased states but also change with age. In the aging artery the arterial diameter dilates, and the wall thickness and collagen-to-elastin ratios increase. These changes result in increased arterial stiffness, an increase in the pulse wave velocity, and an increase in vascular impedance. Although an increase in the thickness of the intima, which initially occurs in atherosclerosis, has little effect on the elastic properties of the artery, the accompanying changes within the media and adventitia, particularly if the wall nutrition through vasa vasorum is involved, may have marked effects of hemodynamic characteristics and further disease progression.

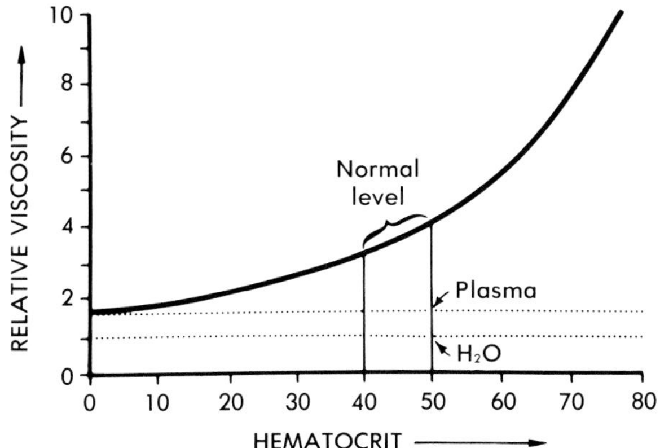

Fig. 50-2 Effect of hematocrit on relative viscosity of blood. Note that, as hematocrit increases, the relative viscosity increases disproportionately. (From Smith, J.J., and Kampine, J.P.: Circulatory physiology, ed. 2, Baltimore, 1984, The Williams & Wilkins Co.)

Essentials of Arterial System Hemodynamics

Hemodynamics is a discipline concerned with the interrelationships of the physical characteristics of blood and the pulsatile flow conditions in the viscoelastic arterial and venous circulations. As a first step toward understanding the complexity of arterial flow, it is useful to discuss the viscous properties of blood itself and the interrelationships between pressure, flow, and resistance under steady flow conditions.

Viscous Properties of Blood

Blood is a viscous fluid composed of cells and plasma. When blood flows, frictional forces develop primarily between the cellular components of blood, causing it to exhibit the property of viscosity. Since the red blood cells comprise the majority of the cellular component, the hematocrit is a major determinant of blood viscosity, as illustrated in Fig. 50-2. If measured with reference to water, the relative viscosity of blood at a hematocrit of 40 is about 3.6 compared to water. This means that three to four times as much pressure is required to force blood through a tube than to force water through the same tube. Blood viscosity is not constant in the arterial system but exhibits a non-Newtonian fluid property: the faster it flows, the lower is its viscosity. The chief determinants of this property are the red cell concentrations and plasma concentration of fibrinogen and globulins. The viscosity of blood decreases in small caliber tubes (less than 200 μm) that include arterioles, capillaries, and venules. This phenomenon is known as the Fahraeus-Lindqvist effect and is related to red cell orientation and lower hematocrit in small vessels. The rheology of blood in the capillary circulation is poorly understood, although the deformability of the red cell membrane and erythrocyte velocity are important factors.

The viscosity of blood is important not only from its effect on the resistance to blood flow but in producing impairment of tissue perfusion in pathologic states such as severe polycythemia, gross elevations of plasma concentrations of fibrinogen or globulins, and the other hyperviscosity syndromes that occur following severe tissue trauma, e.g., thermal burns. These low flow states promote erythrocytes to aggregate into stocks or "rouleaux" with resultant tissue ischemia.

Resistance to Flow

The relations between flow and pressure in cylindric tubes were first accurately described by the French physician, Poiseuille, in 1846. Under the conditions of his experiments, the volume flow (Q) through a vessel is determined by:

$$Q = \frac{P\pi r^4}{8\, l\mu}$$

where P is perfusion pressure, or the pressure gradient between the ends of the vessel; r is vessel radius; l is length of the vessel; and μ is viscosity of the fluid. Poiseuille's law describes the viscous energy losses that occur in a steady-flow, idealized fluid model. The theoretic derivation rests on the assumptions that each particle of fluid moves at a constant velocity parallel to the vessel wall, that the force opposing this motion is proportional to fluid viscosity, and that the velocity gradient is perpendicular to the direction of flow. This means that in a cylindrical tube fluid moves in a series of concentric lamina and flow is laminar. Steady laminar flow results in a parabolic velocity profile in the tube. As predicted by this law, the resistance to flow is most dependent on vessel radius. Resistance is proportional to vessel length and viscosity but inversely proportional to the fourth power of the radius. Assuming a constant blood viscosity, doubling the length of a conduit will double the resistance, whereas halving the radius increases the resistance 16 times. In the human peripheral arterial system, flow is primarily determined by active changes in the diameters of arteries less than 200 μm in diameter and the resistance in the arteriole and capillary. Artery caliber varies according to the state of contraction of the vascular smooth muscle, which depends on perfusion pressure, activity of the sympathetic nervous system, and local mechanisms involving metabolic, humeral, and physiologic factors.

In the flow model governed by Poiseuille's law, the physical properties of the system (tube dimensions and fluid viscosity) determine how large a pressure gradient is required to produce a given flow. The ratio of mean pressure gradient to mean flow is thus a measure of the opposition to flow, commonly termed *vascular resistance*. When Poiseuille's law is simplified to an expression of pressure = flow times resistance, it is exactly analogous to Ohm's law of electric circuits, V = I × Re, when Poiseuille's equation is rearranged to:

$$P = Q\,\frac{8\, l\mu}{\pi r^4}$$

where the term $8\, l\mu/\pi r^4$ expresses electrical resistance (Re), P is voltage (V), and Q is flow of current (I). Vascular and electrical resistance both express the dissipation of energy per unit flow within a system. In the arterial system, resistance is expressed as peripheral resistance units (PRU) where 1 PRU equals the resistance to flow

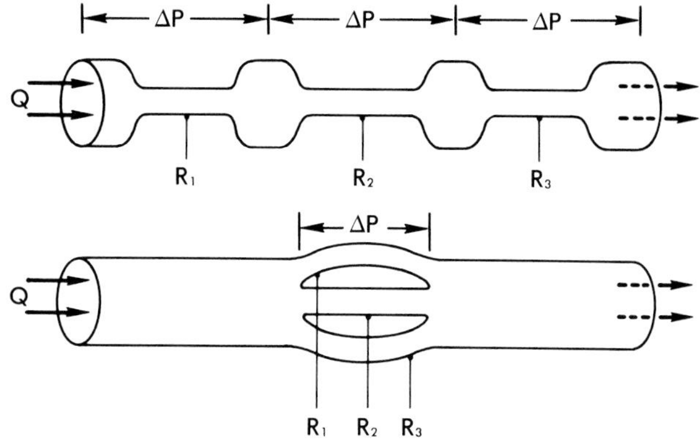

Fig. 50-3 Vascular resistance in series and parallel. *Top,* total resistance (Rt) of a conducting system with individual resistances in series is the sum of the resistances: Rt = $(R_1+R_2+R_3)$. *Bottom,* if the resistance vessels are in parallel, the total resistance is the sum of the reciprocals of the individual resistance: Rt = $1/(R_1+R_2+R_3)$. Note that in a parallel conducting system total resistance is less than any individual resistance level. Q, blood flow.

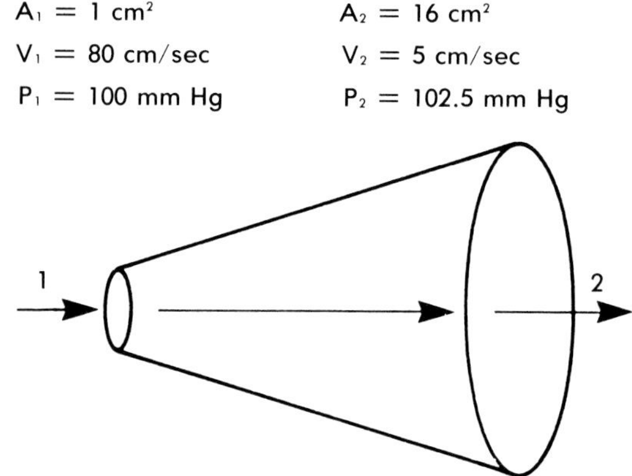

Fig. 50-4 Effect of increasing cross-sectional area on pressure in frictionless fluid system. Although pressure increases, total fluid energy remains constant because of a decrease in velocity. *A,* area; *V,* velocity; *P,* pressure. (From Zierler, R.E., and Strandness, D.E.: In Moore, W.S.: Vascular surgery—a comprehensive review, New York, 1983, Grune & Stratton, Inc. Modified from Sumner, D.S. In Rutherford, R.B.: Vascular Surgery, Philadelphia, 1984, W.B. Saunders Co.)

when there is a pressure difference between two points of 1 mm Hg and flow is 1 ml/sec. The resistance of the entire systemic circulation is approximately 1 PRU, calculated using a 100–mm Hg pressure gradient between the left ventricle and the right atrium and an average blood flow of 100 ml/sec.

The total resistance of a conducting system depends on whether the vessels are in series or in parallel (Fig. 50-3). When vessels are in series, total resistance is equal to the sum of the individual resistances. On the other hand, if the conducting vessels are in parallel, total resistance is the reciprocal of the total conductance. This means that in a parallel conducting system total resistance is less than any of the individual resistance vessels.

Fluid Energy

Although in general blood flows from a point of high pressure to one of lower pressure, the differential in total fluid energy is the true driving force. Total fluid energy associated with blood flow is of three types: intravascular pressure, gravitational, and kinetic. The intravascular pressure (P) has three components: (1) the dynamic pressure produced by the contraction of the heart; (2) the hydrostatic pressure; and (3) the static filling pressure. Both the gravitational energy and the hydrostatic pressure are determined by the product of the specific gravity of blood (p), the acceleration of gravity (g), and the distance (h) above the right atrium. Gravitational energy (+pgh) is the ability of the blood to do work on the basis of its height and is of the opposite value of the hydrostatic pressure (−pgh). The static filling pressure is the residual pressure that exists in the absence of arterial flow. This pressure is determined by the volume of blood and the compliance of the arterial system and is usually in the range of 5 to 10 mm Hg. Since the hydrostatic pressure and the gravitational potential energy cancel each other out and static filling pressure is relatively low, the dynamic pressure produced by the heart is the major source of potential energy used in moving blood.

Kinetic energy (Ek) is the ability of blood to do work on the basis of its motion. It is proportional to the specific gravity of blood (p) and the square of the blood velocity (v):

$$Ek = \tfrac{1}{2}\, pv^2$$

Omitting the term for gravitational energy (i.e., +pgh), the total fluid energy per volume of blood (E) can be expressed as:

$$E = P + \tfrac{1}{2}\, pv^2$$

where P is intravascular pressure. In an idealized fluid system of steady flow and/or frictional energy losses, total fluid energy along a streamline remains constant with the relationship between the different energy forms described by Bernoulli's principle of the conservation of energy:

$$P_1 + \tfrac{1}{2}\, pv_1^2 = P_2 + \tfrac{1}{2}\, pv_2^2$$

In the horizontal diverging tube shown in Fig. 50-4, steady flow between two points is accompanied by an increase in cross-sectional area and a decrease in flow velocity. Although fluid energy moves against a pressure gradient of 2.5 mm Hg (p_2-p_1, Fig. 50-4) and there gains potential energy, total fluid energy remains constant because of a lower velocity and a proportional loss of kinetic energy. In the normal arterial system in which ideal flow conditions are absent and vessels change diameter only gradually, the pressure gradients caused by viscous losses as predicted by Poiseuille's law far outweigh the extremely small interconversions to kinetic energy and pressure. In certain disease states, however, such as sudden vessel widening into an aneurysm or narrowing as a result of an atherosclerotic plaque, the Bernouilli effect and the production of turbulence with the associated changes in kinetic energy explain the pressure and flow change under such conditions.

It is important to emphasize that the pressure-flow relationship described in Poiseuille's law is based on assumptions involving idealized fluid mechanics that significantly underestimate the energy losses present in the viscoelastic, pulsatile flow conditions of the human circulation. Poiseuille's law represents the minimum pressure gradient produced by viscous losses that may be expected in arterial flow. In addition to energy loss caused by friction, inertial energy losses related to changes in the velocity and the direction of flow occur. In the arterial system, particularly in the presence of disease, energy losses caused by inertial effects usually exceed viscous energy loss.

Energy losses related to inertia are proportional to the specific gravity of blood and the square of the blood velocity. Since the density of blood is a constant, inertial losses result when blood accelerates, decelerates, or changes direction. Inertial energy losses therefore occur at bifurcations and points of curvature and from variations in lumen diameter, all of which are normally present in the arterial system. The acceleration and deceleration of blood in pulsatile flow adds inertial forces to the constant kinetic energy of steady flow.

Arterial Flow Patterns

The combination of viscous (frictional) and inertial forces acting on the blood determines whether flow is *laminar* or *turbulent*. The transition to turbulent flow is physiologically important because a greater pressure gradient is needed to maintain flow. Frictional interactions at the inner wall of an artery can also produce flow pattern variations referred to as boundary layer separation. The clinical importance of local flow patterns in arteries resides in their role in the pathogenesis of atherosclerosis and the ability of current instrumentation to detect disease by identifying the abnormal flow patterns produced.

Laminar and Turbulent Flow

As previously discussed, the flow pattern is streamlined or laminar in the steady flow conditions specified by Poiseuille's law. The velocity profile is parabolic in shape (Fig. 50-5). In contrast to the concentric laminae of laminar flow, turbulence is a condition in which the flow velocity vectors are moving in a random fashion with respect to space and time. The point at which flow changes from laminar to turbulent, termed the critical velocity, depends on the ratio of inertial forces to viscous forces and is best defined in terms of a dimensionless entity known as Reynold's number:

$$Re = pdv/\mu$$

where p is the blood density, d is the vessel diameter, v is the mean velocity, and μ is the viscosity. Below a Reynold's number of 2000, flow is laminar because viscous forces predominate and damping of random inertial forces on the flow stream occur. At a Reynold's number above 2000, the inertial forces may disrupt the laminar flow pattern, the result being increased energy dissipation as sound and heat. Energy dissipation in laminar flow is proportional to flow velocity, whereas losses in turbulent flow occur with the velocity squared. Flow conditions that predispose to the development of turbulence include an increased flow velocity, a decreased vessel diameter, or a reduced blood viscosity. An important clinical sign of turbulence is the presence of a *bruit*. Streamlined (laminar) flow is silent, but turbulence produces wall vibrations that

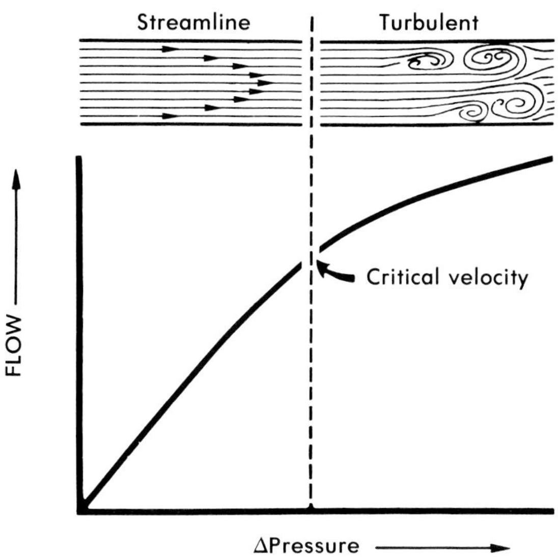

Fig. 50-5 Relationship between velocity of flow and turbulence. (From Ruch, T.C., and Patton, H.D.: Physiology and biophysics, Philadelphia, 1974, W.B. Saunders Co.)

can often be heard with a stethoscope. Sounds used in the conventional auscultatory method of arterial pressure measurement are audible because of turbulence in the flow stream. Bruits produced by stenoses are loudest over the stenotic segment and are transmitted in a distal direction.

Projections or obstacles in the flow stream and roughness of the luminal surface also influence flow patterns. For example, whether turbulence develops downstream to an atherosclerotic plaque depends not only on the Reynold's number but also on the size and shape of the projection. For a sharp-edged plaque, laminar flow is preserved if:

$$\frac{h}{r} < \frac{4}{\sqrt{RE}}$$

where h is the height of the plaque, r is the radius of the vessel, and $\sqrt{RE}$ is the square root of Reynold's number. In reviewing this equation, it can readily be seen that the adverse effects that the shape of a plaque has on vessel radius are of more importance than the relative height of the obstruction resulting therefrom.

Under conditions of turbulent flow, the velocity profile changes from the parabolic shape of laminar flow to a blunt shape. Although turbulent flow is uncommon in arteries, a condition of disturbed flow commonly occurs. Disturbed flow is a transient perturbation in the laminar streamlines that disappears with time or as flow proceeds downstream. Flow disturbances have been identified in the thoracic aorta during the flow deceleration of each heart cycle, in regions of branching and bifurcations, and as a result of atherosclerotic lesions that narrow the lumen. The recognition of the kinetic energy losses of disturbed flow further helps to explain the gross underestimation of energy loss when Poiseuille's law is used to evaluate arterial flow.

The magnitude of disturbed flow can be divided into three categories on the basis of the velocity waveform pattern: highly disturbed, disturbed, and undisturbed. As

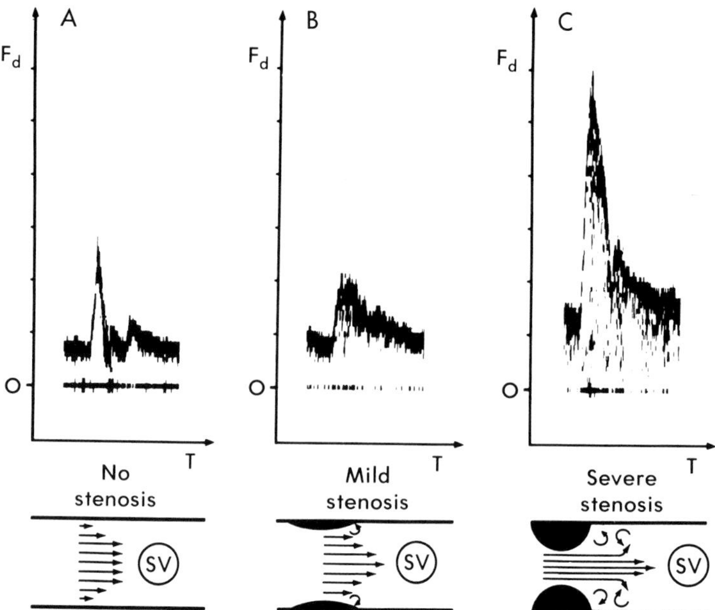

Fig. 50-6 Centerstream flow from a normal artery is laminar and is demonstrated on the spectrum **(A)** as a narrow band of frequencies during systole, with a clear window beneath the frequency envelope. Disturbed flow caused by mild stenosis appears as spectral broadening on the frequency spectrum **(B)** without producing changes in the peak systolic velocity. Highly disturbed flow (turbulence) is characterized by high peak velocities and spectral broadening throughout the cardiac cycle. Also note the increase in end-diastolic velocity associated with severe stenosis **(C)**. *SV*, systolic velocity; *T*, time. (From Roederer, G.O., et al.: Comprehensive noninvasive evaluation of extracranial cerebrovascular disease. In Noninvasive diagnosis of vascular disease, Pasadena, 1984, Appleton Davies.)

shown in Fig. 50-6, Doppler spectrum analysis of flow through a stenosis demonstrates the localized disruption of laminar flow in the arterial segment. Highly disturbed velocity waveforms are those with high-frequency disturbances that persist all the way through systole, including the deceleration phase. Disturbed velocity waveforms are those with high-frequency components only at peak systole and probably represent a transitional flow condition. Undisturbed velocity waveforms exhibit negligible high-frequency content and are representative of laminar flow.

Boundary Layer Separation

The outer layer of fluid in a flow stream adjacent to the vessel wall is referred to as the *boundary layer*. Radially directed velocity gradients exist as a result of the frictional interactions of fluid with the vessel wall and the more rapidly moving fluid in the center of the vessel. When vessel geometry changes suddenly such as at points of curvature and bifurcations, small pressure gradients are created that cause the boundary layer to stop or reverse direction. This results in a complex, localized flow pattern known as an area of flow separation. Areas of flow separation have been observed in models of arterial anastomoses and bifurcations. The endothelial cells adjacent to separation zones are subject to relatively low shear stresses. In the carotid bifurcation depicted in Fig. 50-7, an area of flow separation has formed along the outer wall as a result of the converging diameter of the carotid bulb. A complex flow pattern has been identified in normal human carotid bifurcations and includes vortices and regions of flow reversal.

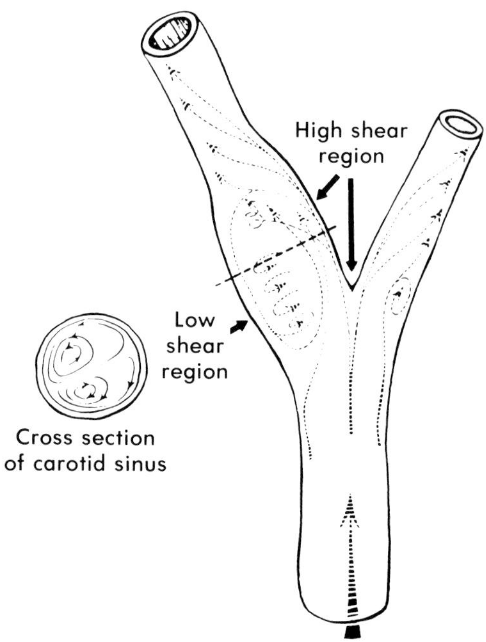

Fig. 50-7 Flow patterns at model carotid bifurcation. Adjacent to the outer wall of the bulb, flow is stagnant (a region of flow separation), may reverse, or may be diverted across the vessel lumen. Rapid flow is associated with high shear stress, whereas the slow flow in the separation zone produces a region of low shear. (From Sumner, D.S.: Pitfalls on noninvasive cerebrovascular testing and angiography. In Bernhard, V.M., and Towne, J.B., editors: Complications in vascular surgery, ed. 2, New York, 1985, Grune & Stratton, Inc.)

The local flow disturbances and low shear stress in regions of boundary layer separation may contribute to the formation of atherosclerotic plaques. Examination of carotid and iliac bifurcations, both at autopsy and during surgery, indicates that intimal thickening and plaque formation tend to occur in these regions of flow separation. The influence of localized flow disturbances on the initiation or progression of atherosclerotic disease awaits further investigation.

Principles of Pulsatile Flow

In the pulsatile arterial system, pressure and flow vary continuously with time, and the velocity profile changes throughout the cardiac cycle. The pressure-flow relationships defined under steady flow conditions do not take into consideration the inertia foces of acceleration and decelerating blood, the compliant nature of the arterial wall, and the influence of vessel tapering and bifurcations on the shape and size of the pulsatile pressure and flow wave. The addition of a pulsatile component on steady flow increases fluid energy expenditure. As much as 30% of the energy in cardiac output is dissipated as a result of pulsatile flow. With increasing heart rate, energy losses caused by pulsatile flow decrease exponentially up to a heart rate of approximately 150 beats per minute. The remainder of the energy of cardiac output is used for tissue perfusion; it is primarily lost in the arteriolar and capillary bed. Although the true nature of pulsatile energy loss remains poorly defined, contributing factors include the inertia energy loss with acceleration; the skewing of the velocity profile related to geometric tapering, curvature, and bifurcation; the production of disturbed flow; and the non-Newtonian character of blood.

Of importance to the surgeon is that in pulsatile flow the energy losses produced by arterial reconstructions, which commonly have anatomic and physical characteristics much different from the normal arterial system, are likely to be much greater than predicted by the equations governing steady flow. Although pulsatile flow appears less efficient than steady laminar flow, studies indicate that individual organs require pulsatile flow for optimum function. Perfusion of a kidney with steady flow instead of pulsatile flow results in a reduction of urine volume and sodium excretion. Pulsatile flow and pressure probably exert their effect at the microvascular level. Although the exact mechanism is unknown, transcapillary exchange, arteriolar and venular tone, and lymphatic flow are all responsive to pulsatile pressure.

With each stroke volume of the heart, blood is pumped into the distensible arterial tree, which acts as an elastic reservoir or windkessel absorbing the cardiac energy that is later released during ventricular diastole. The physiologic effect is to damp the flow/no-flow effect of the heart so that pressure and flow are maintained during diastole. As blood is forced into the aorta, the instantaneous increase in volume is transmitted along the artery as a pressure and flow wave. As shown in Fig. 50-8, the increase in flow starts almost synchronously with the rise in pressure, but the peak flow velocity precedes peak pressure. The instantaneous flow rate is not determined by the magnitude of the pressure pulse but by the pressure-gradient developed along the artery. The pressure-gradient can be determined by recording the pressure at two points a short distance apart and subtracting the downstream pressure from that of the upstream pressure during the cardiac cycle. The effect of the traveling pressure wave is to produce an oscillatory pressure-gradient. The magnitude of the pressure-gradient determines both instantaneous flow velocity and the direction of flow. Unless there is a marked decrease in the mean pressure along the artery, there will always be a period during the pulse cycle when the pressure gradient is reversed. This reversal of gradient causes a rapid deceleration of the flow; and, if it continues after the forward flow has been brought to a halt, flow reversal can occur. Indeed, flow reversal during diastole is a normal pattern of blood flow in peripheral limb arteries.

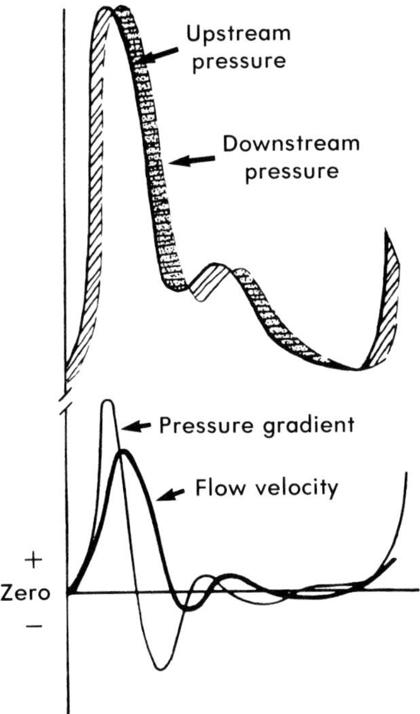

Fig. 50-8 Generation of flow velocity waveform by traveling pulse rate. Simultaneous pressure pulse and flow velocity pulse recordings from an arterial segment. Although similar in configuration when drawn in comparable scale, the fact that peak flow occurs before the pressure peak shows there is no simple relationship between these hemodynamic parameters. Flow is determined by the pressure gradient that develops along the arterial segment.

As the pressure pulse wave travels from the aorta to the periphery, its rates of travel, magnitude, and configuration are altered. The pressure wave is produced by the sudden ejection of blood into the aorta. The pressure wave velocity increases from 4 to 6 cm/sec to approximately 13 cm/sec in the muscular arteries of the lower limb. The velocity of the pressure wave is 20 times greater than the mean velocity imparted to the blood in the aorta (20 to 40 cm/sec), illustrating that the pressure wave has no direct relationship to flow and can occur when there is no flow at all. The acceleration of the pressure wave in the peripheral arteries is caused primarily by increasing wall stiffness. Because of this relationship, the transmission velocity of the pressure wave has been used as an index of arterial distensibility.

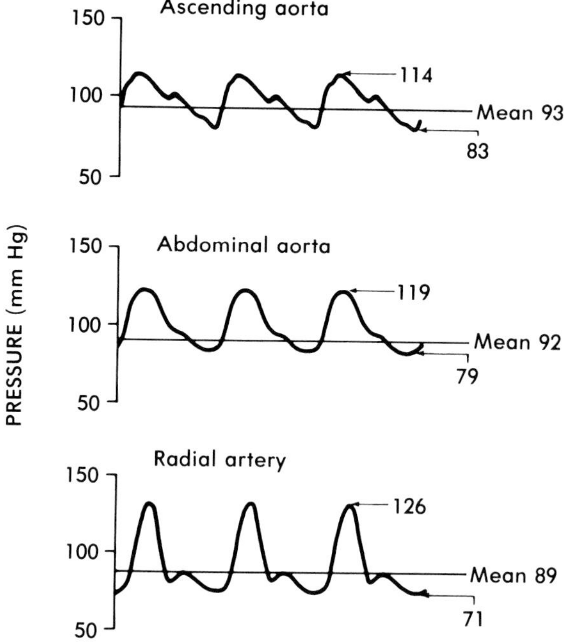

Fig. 50-9 Pressure waves at different sites in the arterial tree. With pressure wave transmission into the distal aorta and large arteries, the systolic pressure increases and the diastolic pressure decreases, with a resultant increase in pulse pressure. Note that mean arterial pressure declines steadily.

Table 50-2 **MAIN DETERMINANTS OF AORTIC SYSTOLIC AND DIASTOLIC PRESSURES**

Systolic Pressure	Diastolic Pressure
Stroke volume	Systolic pressure
Aortic distensibility	Aortic distensibility
Ejection velocity	Heart rate
	Peripheral resistance

The amplitude of the pressure wave, otherwise known as the *pulse pressure,* increases, and wave configuration changes during transmission through the arterial system (Fig. 50-9). With increasing distance from the heart, the rate of systolic pressure rise increases, the sharp inflection of the downslope known as the *dicrotic notch* becomes rounded and disappears in the abdominal aorta, and dicrotic waves appear. In the arteries of the lower limb systolic pressure is higher, and diastolic pressure lower than in the aorta. This is the result of the viscoelastic characteristics of the arterial conduits, the effect of pressure waves being reflected from sites of increased peripheral resistance (i.e., from sites of tapering and branching), and the abrupt increase in resistance at the level of the arterioles. It is important to note that the mean pressure decreases with the distance from the heart but the pressure loss in the large arteries of the thorax and abdomen is small because of their large radius. As shown in Table 50-2, systolic and diastolic pressures recorded from large arteries are influenced by various hemodynamic factors. Careful analysis of the pressure wave configuration and its transmission can provide useful clues to important cardiac and peripheral arterial physiology.

The pulsatile characteristics of the pressure wave are dampened considerably at the level of arterioles at which mean pressure reaches values of 40 to 60 mm Hg. In general, perfusion pressure in the capillaries is nonpulsatile, and pressure waves in the venous system are caused primarily by pressure changes in the right heart and not the left.

Measurement of Arterial Pressure

A major advance in the understanding and approach to patients with arterial occlusive disease came with the recognition that the physiologic disturbance responsible for symptoms is predominantly related to development of a pressure gradient in the proximal arterial segment. Pressure measurement is a more sensitive index of an occlusive process than is the measurement of flow because in the presence of moderate arterial disease blood flow is essentially normal, owing to the reduction of resting arteriolar resistance compensating for the increased resistance of the proximal arterial system. Although flow measurement techniques (i.e., indicator dilution methods, impedance flowmeter) have clinical value in the determination of cardiac output, flow volume measurement in the limbs are of limited value as a clinical or diagnostic tool. For these reasons a variety of techniques are available for the measurement of arterial pressure both directly and indirectly using noninvasive instrumentation.

Direct pressure measurement involves the placement of a needle or catheter into the artery and recording the pressure waveform with the aid of manometer or strain-gauge transducers. The hydraulic system that couples the transducer to the arterial lumen should be maximum bore and minimum length to avoid damping of the pressure wave. From a continuous recording of the pressure waveform, *systolic pressure* is the peak pressure during the pulse cycle, and *diastolic pressure* is the lowest pressure. The difference between these two pressures is the *pulse pressure. Mean pressure,* the force responsible for the mean flow of blood to an organ, can be determined electronically by calculating the area of the pulsatile waveform or estimated from systolic and diastolic pressure measurements (mean pressure = diastolic pressure + ⅓ pulse pressure). Although direct pressure measurements provide the most accurate data, their routine clinical use is not warranted since the technique is invasive and requires sterile conditions, and pressure data obtained indirectly are sufficiently accurate for diagnostic purposes.

Indirect pressure measurements depend on (1) the production of Korotkoff sounds, which are the result of turbulence in the flow stream, (2) the appearance and disappearance of the pressure pulse, or (3) the reappearance of flow when a proximally located pneumatic cuff has been inflated and slowly deflated above the regional perfusion pressure (Figs. 50-10 and 50-11). Auscultatory (Riva-Ricci method) and palpatory techniques to measure upper limb arterial pressure are the most common hemodynamic assessments of the arterial circulation. To avoid measurement errors, the occluding cuff should be 20% wider than

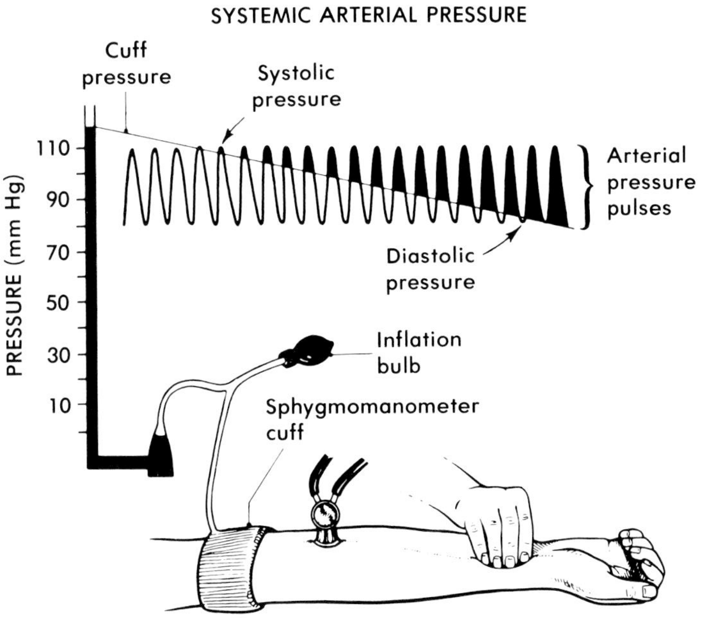

Fig. 50-10 Illustration of the auscultatory and palpatory techniques for the indirect method of measuring arterial blood pressure. Appearance and disappearance of the auscultatory sounds are illustrated.

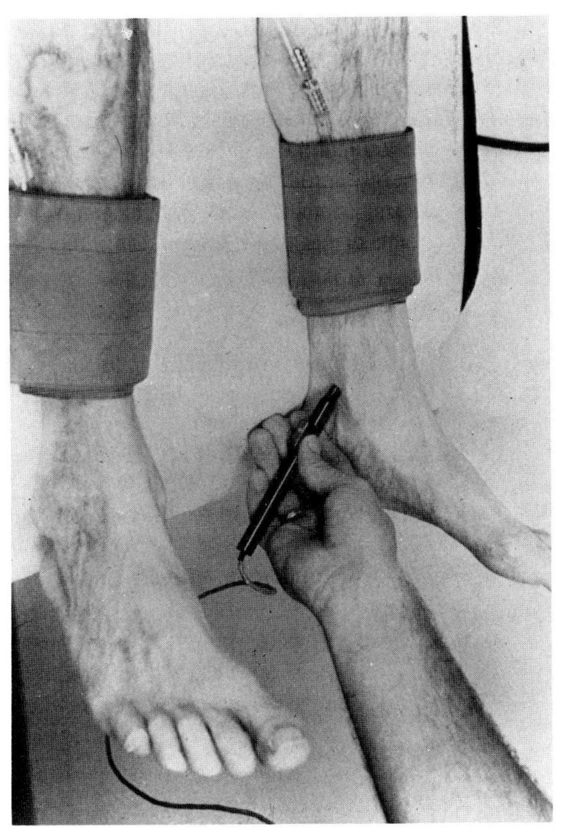

Fig. 50-11 Measurement of ankle systolic pressure. Doppler probe is positioned over the posterior tibial artery.

the limb diameter. If it is too narrow, the pressure will be erroneously high; if it is too wide, the reading may be erroneously low.

A variety of techniques developed to measure systolic pressure in the limbs include the mercury strain gauge and air plethysmograph, the photoplethysmograph, and the ultrasonic velocity detector. All of these instruments are used as sensors to indicate return of flow with cuff deflation. Plethysmography operates on the principle that changes in the circulation of the blood to a body part (e.g., leg) will result in corresponding changes in the size of that part that are measurable. Such changes in size can be measured by displacement of air or mercury in a strain gauge or emission of light in a photoelectric cell as is done in photoplethysmography. In general, devices with ultrasound are most commonly used because these instruments are inexpensive and simple to use and the Doppler-derived pressure measurements have been thoroughly evaluated and have been noted to be as accurate as plethysmographic measurements.

The assessment of arterial flow with ultrasound is made on the basis of the Doppler effect, which refers to the shift in frequency that occurs when sound is reflected from a moving object. Moving red blood cells reflect the ultrasound beam and shift the frequency proportional to the flow velocity. The Doppler signal can be (1) amplified to provide an audible sound with pitch directly proportional to blood velocity, (2) converted into an analog waveform using a zero-crossing frequency meter, or (3) analyzed for its frequency-amplitude content. Failure to obtain a Doppler signal from an artery usually indicates occlusion; however, an extremely low flow rate (under 2 cm/sec) may not produce detectable Doppler frequency shift.

The systolic pressure at any level of an extremity can be

measured by applying a pneumatic cuff and positioning the Doppler probe over a patent artery distal to the cuff (Fig. 50-11). The arterial signal is distinguished from the adjacent venous signal by its characteristic high pitch sound that corresponds to the cardiac cycle. When the cuff is inflated above systolic pressure, the arterial flow signal disappears. As cuff pressure is gradually lowered, the point at which flow resumes is recorded as the systolic pressure. In the lower limb, the use of multiple cuffs placed at the high-thigh, above- and below-knee, ankle, and digital levels permits the measurement of segmental pressures. The level of pressure measurement is determined by cuff placement and not the site of Doppler flow detection. The difference in systolic pressure between any two adjacent cuffs or between corresponding segments in the opposite limb is less than 20 mm Hg in normal individuals. Because of cuff artifact, proximal thigh systolic pressure normally exceeds brachial pressure by 30 to 40 mm Hg.

Because of amplification of the pressure wave with distance from the heart, the systolic pressure measured at the ankle is normally higher than that in the brachial artery, which in the absence of disease is nearly equal to central aortic pressure. To compensate for variation in central perfusion pressure and to permit comparisons of serial measurements, the ankle systolic pressure is expressed as a ratio of brachial pressure, termed the *ankle-brachial pressure index*. The normal ankle-brachial pressure index is always greater than 1 (mean value 1.11 × ± 0.1). The ankle-brachial pressure index also correlates with the degree of arterial insufficiency. In limbs with intermittent claudication, the ankle-brachial pressure index (mean ± S.D.) is 0.58 × ± 0.15; in limbs with ischemic rest pain, 0.26 × ± 0.13; and in limbs with gangrene, 0.05 × ± 0.08.

The measurement of toe pressures can be used to identify obstructive disease distal to the ankle and to measure pressure in diabetic patients in whom ankle pressure measurement by the cuff method is artifactually high because of the incompressibility of calcified arteries. Normal systolic toe pressure is approximately 80% of the brachial systolic pressure. Photoplethysmographic techniques are better suited than the ultrasonic methods of flow determination at the digital level because of the smaller size and lower-flow velocity in the digital arteries.

Real-Time Ultrasound Arterial Imaging and Flow Analysis

In the last decade ultrasonic techniques have been developed to both image the peripheral arteries and analyze the flow patterns within the lumen. The technique referred to as echo-Doppler (duplex) ultrasonic scanning combines real-time pulse-echo imaging units (B-mode) with pulsed Doppler flow detectors. B-mode ultrasound provides a two-dimensional image of the vascular anatomy and the spatial relationships with surrounding tissues (Fig. 50-12, *A*). Echos from a pulse of ultrasound are reflected from tissue boundaries and displayed as dots on a screen. The intensity of the echos is indicated by dot brightness (B-mode). Image quality depends on the transmitting frequency and the vessel depth. Vessel walls are easily distinguished from surrounding tissues, and characterization of the wall morphology or vessel lumen anatomy depends on its echogenicity. Spatial resolution is sufficient to permit accurate measurement of vessel diameter and wall thickness.

Velocity of blood within the visualized vessels is characterized with the use of a Doppler velocity detector. Accurate characterization of blood flow patterns requires the use of a pulsed Doppler whose sample volume (the point in space from which blood flow is detected) is small in relation to the vessel diameter. The Doppler signal is processed by a real-time spectrum analyzer to determine the velocity of blood, the direction of flow, and the velocity distribution of the red blood cells. When the sample volume of a pulsed Doppler flow detector is placed in the midstream of nondisturbed (laminar) arterial flow, the Doppler signal will contain a narrow range of frequencies (spectral width) of similar amplitude corresponding to uniform movement of red blood cells at this site during the pulse cycle. This produces a "clear window" in the spectra beneath the frequency envelope that is characteristic of normal arterial flow (Fig. 50-12, *B*).

Calculation of flow velocity requires measurement of the angle between the incident Doppler beam and the blood velocity vector. An operator-controlled line on the B-mode image indicates the direction of the sound beam from the pulsed Doppler probe. In general the Doppler beam is adjusted to intersect the flow stream at an angle of approximately 60 degrees. A "dot" on the Doppler beam cursor indicates the location of the sample volume. The sample volume is placed in the center of the vessel lumen, and the Doppler angle is calculated electronically by the operator positioning a cursor parallel to the longitudinal axis of the vessel. Blood flow velocity is calculated from the frequency spectra waveform measurements using the Doppler equation:

$$\text{Flow velocity} = \frac{\text{C Fs}}{2\ \text{Fo}} \cos\theta \qquad \text{(cm/sec)}$$

where C is the average speed of sound in tissue (1.54×10^6 mm/sec), Fs is the shift in frequency between the transmitted and reflected Doppler beam, Fo is the frequency of the transmitted Doppler beam, and θ is the Doppler beam angle.

If the mean frequency shift can be electronically extracted from the Doppler spectrum, the spatial average velocity (Vsa) as a function of time can be calculated. Volumetric blood flow (Q) can then be determined from a measurement of lumen diameter (D) by the equation:

$$Q = \frac{\text{Vsa}\ \pi\ D^2}{4}$$

Although the determination of volumetric flow is attractive, the accurate calculation of Vsa can be quite difficult, since it requires complete insonation of the flow stream across the vessel lumen, knowledge of the velocity profile configuration, and a correction for both the forward and reverse components of pulsatile flow.

Duplex scanning provides both anatomic and physiologic information regarding arterial flow. This method has been applied clinically to the evaluation and classification

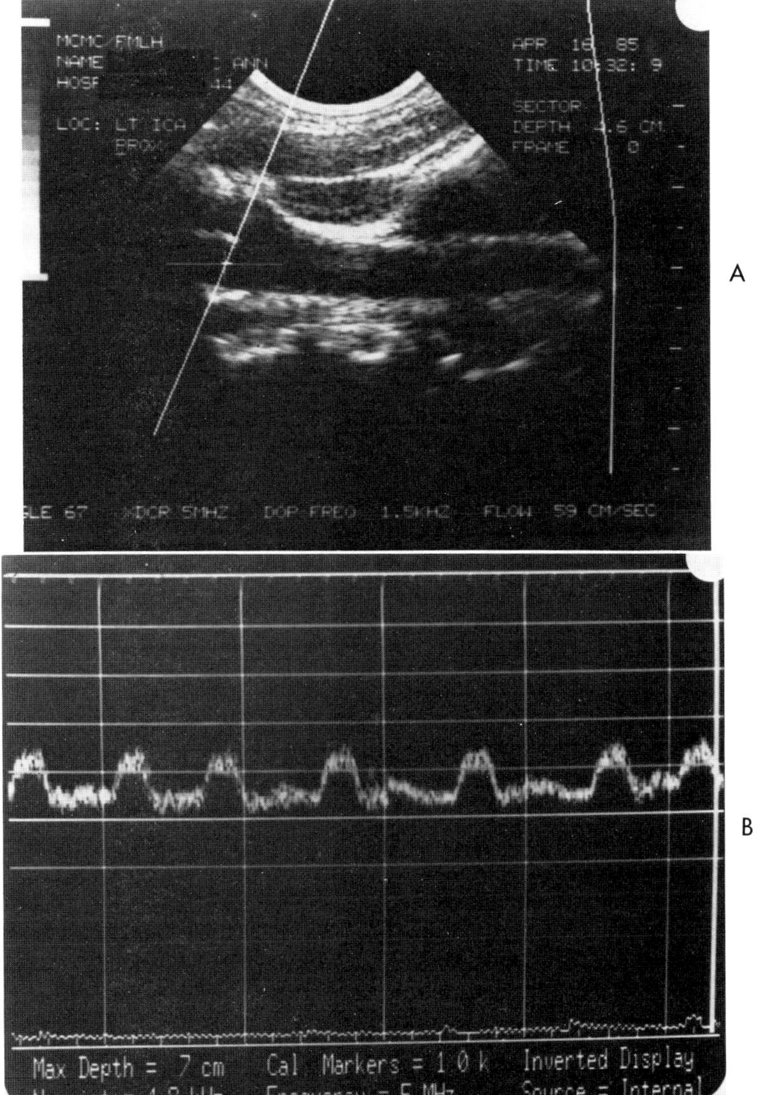

Fig. 50-12 Ultrasound imaging of the carotid artery. **A,** B-mode image of the carotid artery bifurcation. Sample volume of the pulsed Doppler probe is positioned in the proximal internal carotid artery. **B,** Narrow band of frequencies during the pulse cycle and the clear area beneath the waveform are characteristics of laminar flow in a normal carotid artery.

of atherosclerotic occlusive disease involving the carotid bifurcation, visceral arteries (renal, celiac, and superior mesenteric), the abdominal aorta, and the arteries of the lower limb. Under normal conditions flow in peripheral arteries is nondisturbed (Figs. 50-12 and 50-13). As discussed previously, turbulence is responsible for most of the fluid energy loss associated with arterial disease. Because turbulence occurs at lesser degrees of stenosis than detectable changes in mean flow and pressure, assessment of arterial flow by duplex scanning permits a more accurate diagnosis of altered hemodynamics than is available using techniques that monitor pressure and flow. Distal to a site of stenosis, turbulence is evident in the Doppler signal by an increase in peak systolic velocity, an alteration in the velocity waveform, and the presence of spectral broadening corresponding to the disordered, random movement of red blood cells in the flow stream. Accurate characterization of vessel anatomy and flow in both normal and diseased states is possible by duplex mapping of the peripheral arterial system. Long-term studies with this technique may clarify the natural history of arterial disease, including important hemodynamic factors involved in the initiation and progression of vascular disease.

THE PERIPHERAL VENOUS SYSTEM

The primary function of the venous system is to return blood to the right heart for reoxygenation by the lungs. As such it serves a conduit function similar to the arterial system. In the latter, however, this is accomplished by left ventricular contraction at high pressure with high velocity. Venous return is accomplished at low pressure and low velocity without cardiac contraction. The mechanisms responsible are best addressed by considering first the anatomic configuration and unique structure of the venous

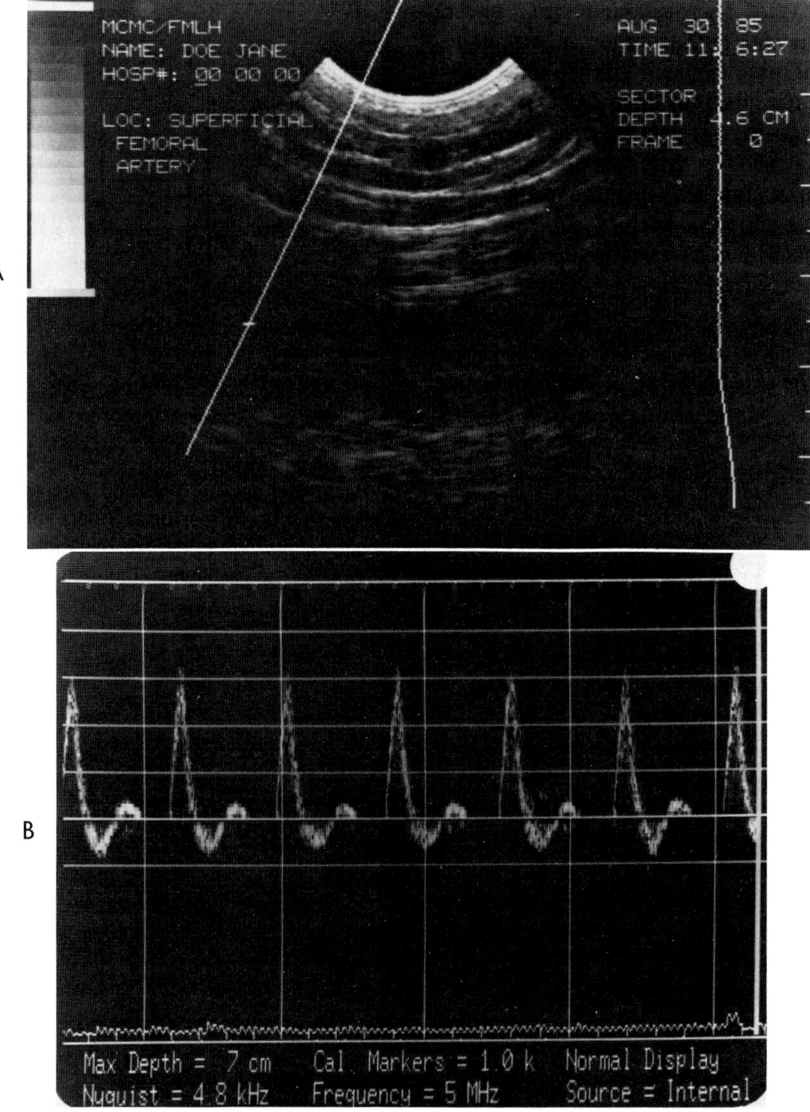

Fig. 50-13 Duplex examination of normal superficial femoral artery flow. Velocity spectra **(A)** and waveform configuration, **(B)** are typical of normal flow in a limb artery.

channels and then the interaction of the structural characteristics with the forces responsible for normal venous return.

Venous Anatomy

For descriptive purposes the venous system of the lower extremity is divided into a superficial and deep component. The superficial system consists of the greater and less saphenous veins that are located in the subcutaneous tissue superficial to the deep fascia (Fig. 50-14). These channels are responsible for collection of venous blood from the skin and subcutaneous tissues and terminate by penetrating the deep fascia at the groin and popliteal fossa, respectively, to enter the deep venous channels. The superficial veins are subjected to a very large hydrostatic pressure and are therefore relatively thick walled. These superficial veins contain numerous bicuspid valves that facilitate flow from the periphery of the limb to the central portion of the limb and prevent flow in a retrograde direction.

The deep system of veins consists of the venous channels accompanying the major muscular arteries and are similarly named. In the periphery of the limb these channels are frequently present in duplicate and, because they are protected from the force of gravity by the muscles in the lower extremity, are relatively thin walled. Bicuspid valves are also present in these veins, with the greatest density occurring peripherally and relatively few valves being located in the more central larger channels. For example, the inferior vena cava, and the common iliac veins are devoid of valves, whereas the external iliac vein infrequently has a single bicuspid valve present.

A second major component of the deep venous system is the soleal sinuses, a group of endothelial-lined venous reservoirs located within the substance of the gastrocnemius and soleus muscles that communicate with the deep veins (Fig. 50-15). It is these structures that the calf muscles compress and empty during contraction, facilitating venous emptying of the lower limb.

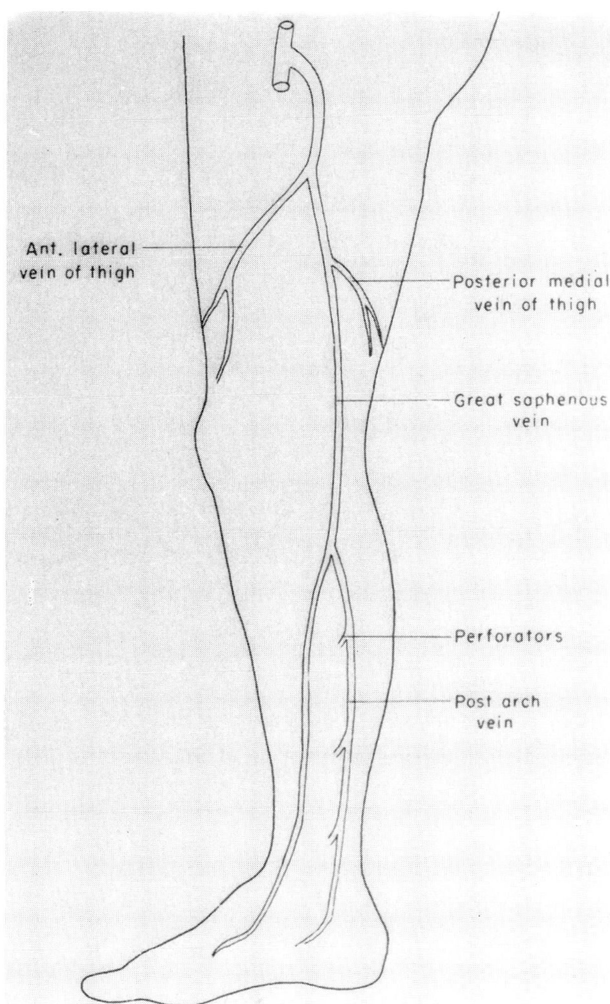

Fig. 50-14 Diagrammatic representation of the major anatomic features of the great and lesser saphenous veins and their tributaries.

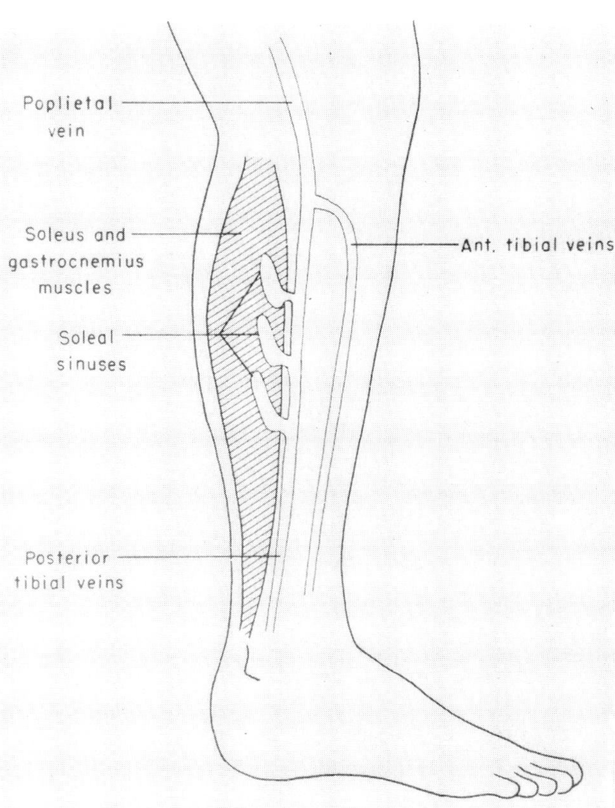

Fig. 50-15 Schematic representation of the soleal sinuses and their relationship to the calf muscles and deep venous system. It should be noted that these empty directly into the deep venous system and also on occasion receive communications from the superficial system.

The superficial and deep venous systems of the lower extremity are united by a series of perforating veins that pass from the superficial venous system through the deep fascia to the deep venous channels. These venous conduits range in number from 100 to 200 and are also most frequently located below the level of the knee. Bicuspid valves are also located in these channels so that under normal circumstances flow occurs only from the superficial to the deep venous system (Fig. 50-16). Venous flow in the lower extremity therefore always travels in centripetal direction from peripheral to central channels. The presence of valves prevents reflux in the superficial, deep, and connecting systems. The necessity for these valves is greatest at the most peripheral locations where the gravitational force is greatest and is least important in the central venous channels where the pressure changes generated by respiration are sufficient to overcome the effects of gravity.

In addition to blood traveling from the peripheral to central regions, it also moves preferentially from the superficial to the deep system with only 10% of the venous outflow being conducted by the superficial veins and 90% by the deep veins.

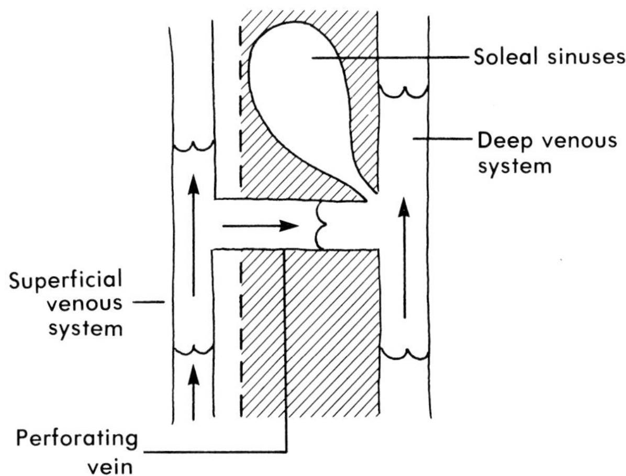

Fig. 50-16 Schematic representation of the valvular relationships in the superficial veins, the connecting veins or perforators, and the deep venous system. It can be seen that under normal circumstances flow only occurs from the superficial to deep channels.

Structural Features

The vein varies from one third to one tenth of the thickness of the systemic arteries. It contains considerably less elastin than the arterial wall but, like arteries, also contains a variable amount of smooth muscle. The major factor influencing the smooth muscle content is not the necessity

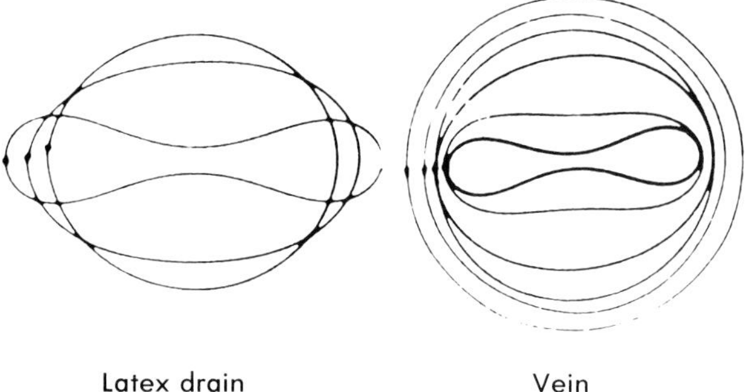

Fig. 50-17 Capacitance of collapsible tubes. Effect of volume change on the cross-sectional area of veins showing the small cross-sectional area in the collapsed ellipsoid state and the significant increase in cross-sectional area associated with filling. This change occurs without a change in circumference and, because the wall is not stretched, can occur with the application of relatively minor force.

for control of regional blood flow as in arteries but the gravitational force the wall is required to withstand. The great saphenous vein has the highest percentage of smooth muscle because it is located subcutaneously in the lower extremity where it is exposed to the maximum gravitational force. At the foot and ankle smooth muscle may account for as much as 80% of the total wall thickness, whereas in the central axillary vein it composes only 5% of the vein wall.

The smooth muscle fibers are arranged in helical bundles united by strands of connective tissue with a tough outer layer of predominately collagen fibers constituting the adventitia. Deep to the smooth muscle layer is the intima, the most important component of which is the single layer of endothelial cells responsible for the blood/vessel wall interface integrity. Perhaps because of the relatively low velocity in the venous system, these cells contain abundant quantities of fibrinolytic agents, with the veins in the lower extremity having higher concentrations than the intimal cells of the upper extremity. The lowest concentration of fibrinolytic active substances is found in the deep veins of the calf region and may in part explain the predisposition for thrombi to form in this location.

The deep veins are surrounded by skeletal muscle that protects them from the adverse effects of gravity. Thus they contain relatively small amounts of smooth muscle and large amounts of collagen. This structural feature is the major factor responsible for the relative nonstretchability of veins as compared to arteries. In the large central veins contained within the body cavities such as the vena cava, this property is of major importance in determining the shape changes induced by alterations in pressure-volume characteristics. Reductions in the volume of blood in these vessels result in collapse of the wall and assumption of an elliptical shape (Fig. 50-17). Restoration of volume to normal is associated with a resumption of the normal resting circular cross section. This shape change can also occur with the application of minimal external force, and, although the pressure generated by respiration may produce similar changes, it is primarily a response of the major central veins to the volume of blood in the system.

These changes in venous volume are accomplished with minimal changes in pressure. The importance of this is appreciated when it is realized that 40% of the total blood volume may be found in these large central veins at a pressure of 5 mm Hg, whereas a reduction to 5% is accompanied by a fall in pressure of only a few millimeters of mercury. Thus the central venous system may be classified as a high-compliance, high-capicitance system compared to the low-compliance, low-capacitance arterial system. In the clinical state of hypovolemic shock the central veins collapse and autotransfuse their volume to the arterial system to maintain nutritional blood flow. Of practical clinical importance is the fact that the pressure measured in the central veins may be used as an index of the moment-to-moment blood volume; i.e., high pressures represent an expanded blood volume, and low pressures a volume deficiency. These pressure changes have a major effect on cardiac performance and are discussed elsewhere in this book.

Pressure-Flow Relationships

In contrast to the arterial system, blood flow throughout the venous system is not mediated by a central pumping mechanism. The forces affecting pressure and therefore flow in the venous system are generated by respiration and exercise. The relative importance and interaction of these forces is best understood by considering the independent effects of each one and how they impact on the gravitational forces that must be overcome in the erect posture.

Gravitational Effects

Gravitational forces have a negative effect on venous flow from the lower extremity and are best appreciated by considering the pressure relationships first in the supine position where gravity is not a factor. In the venular end of the capillaries the pressure is normally approximately 15 mm Hg, and the pressure in the right atrium 5 mm Hg. There is a point in the venous system located in the inferior vena cava close to the diaphragm termed the hydrostatic indifference point where the pressure is always zero, regardless of attitude (Fig. 50-18). These pressure gradients are adequate to sustain normal venous return in the supine position but are augmented, as will be detailed later, by respiratory-induced pressure changes.

Assumption of the erect position results in profound changes in these pressure relationships. The system can then be likened to a vertical column of fluid approximately 180 cm in height in a hypothetic six-foot "dead man," although certain modifications of this model are required to parallel the real circumstances (see Fig. 50-18). As noted earlier, the pressure at the hydrostatic indifference point is unchanged by the erect position, and right atrial pressure is normally 0 mm Hg. The veins above this point will either fill or collapse, depending on the degree of filling in the system and the effects of respiration. This is best seen in the external jugular vein clinically where intermittent filling and decompression are readily apparent. The skull acts as a protective barrier against these collapsing forces and maintains the intracerebral venous channels distended even in the erect position. Below the hydrostatic indifference point the pressure gradually increases so that at the foot level a hydrostatic pressure of 80 mm Hg is

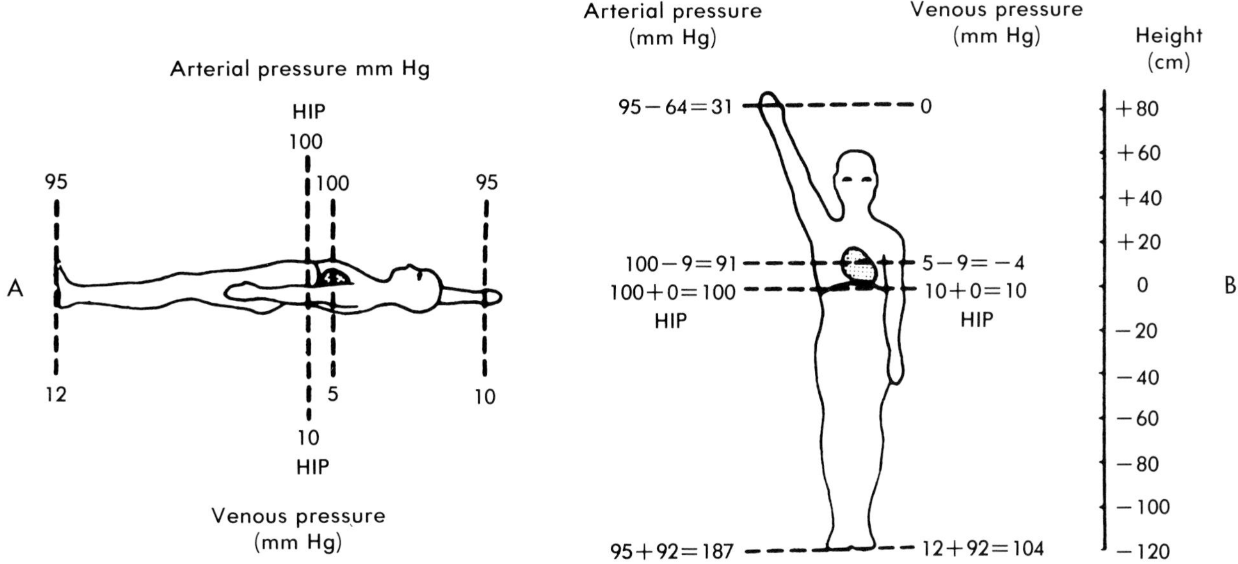

Fig. 50-18 Pressure relationships in the various levels of the arterial and venous system shown in the supine, **A,** and the erect positions, **B.** Hydrostatic indifference point *(HIP)* is located just below the diaphragm.

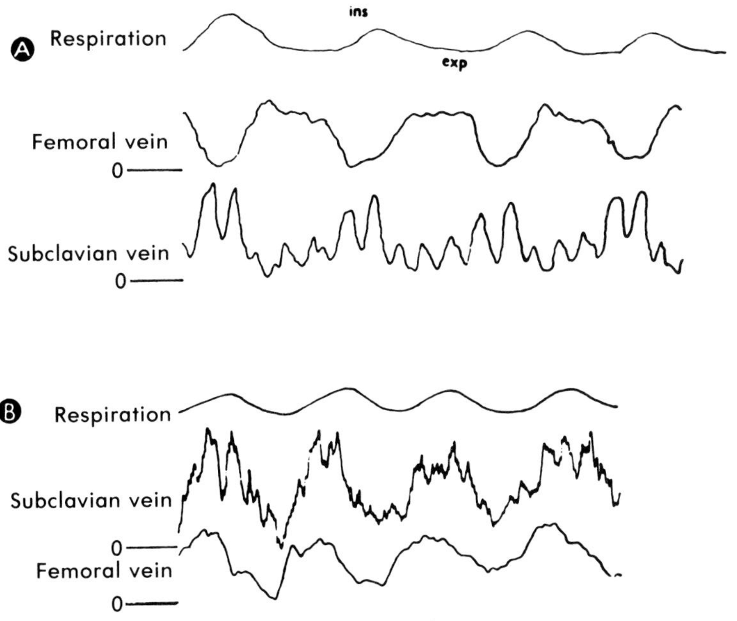

Fig. 50-19 Relationship between respiration and flow in the femoral and subclavian veins in the supine **(A),** and in the erect position, **(B)**. *ins,* inspiration; *exp,* expiration.

produced. This has two profound effects, the first of which is cessation of flow from the lower extremities and progressive pooling in the leg veins. This associated reduction in venous return secondarily produces a major decrease in cardiac output and, if the stimulus is long enough, may activate the syncope reflex. This pressure is also apparent in a change of the fluid dynamics at the tissue level; and, again, if it persists for any prolonged period, massive extravascular fluid extravasation may occur, further depleting venous return.

This negative effect on venous circulation by gravity is overcome by the combined effects of respiration and exercise.

Effects of Respiration

The effects of respiration on venous flow are, again, most easily understood by first considering the pressure characteristics and changes that occur with the subject in the supine position.

During inspiration negative pressure is generated in the thoracic cavity, which facilitates flow into the superior mediastinum from the venous channels in the head, neck, and upper extremity. Descent of the diaphragm produces an increase in intraabdominal pressure that compresses the inferior vena cava and is associated with a marked reduction in flow from the lower extremities. The pressure changes produced by respiration are insufficient to overcome the gradient that exists between the peripheral venules and the right atrium, and therefore even during inspiration there is some venous outflow from the lower extremities. Cessation of flow may be relatively easily produced, however, by increasing the pressure a few millimeters of mercury, as occurs with a Valsalva maneuver. Conversely, during expiration venous return from the upper extremities and head and neck is interrupted, and flow from the lower extremities augmented (Fig. 50-19).

Assumption of the erect position, however, introduces the force of gravity that drastically alters the pressure-flow relationships. Without the pulsatile pump of the arterial system, the venous circulation does not contain an intrinsic mechanism capable of overcoming this effect. Clearly the relatively small changes induced by respiration are inadequate for normal venous return, and additional forces must be activated. Prolonged assumption of the erect position without activation of other mechanisms results in a serious disturbance of the hydrostatic forces at the tissue level, with the development of both peripheral edema and venous pooling in the lower extremities.

The major force responsible for maintenance of normal venous return in the erect position is contraction of the calf muscles of the lower extremities.

Pressure Changes with Exercise

The calf muscle pump is to the venous system what the left ventricle is to the arterial system. The changes produced by calf muscle contraction are best considered by reviewing (1) the overall net effect after multiple muscle contractions and (2) the step-by-step pressure relationships. Calf muscle contraction exerts a force in excess of 80 mm Hg on the walls of the veins in the calf, thus exceeding that exerted by gravity and resulting in a net efflux of blood out of the limb. With each contraction the venous pressure is progressively lowered until after 10 contractions the mean pressure at the ankle level falls to approximately 15 mm Hg, similar to that in the quiet resting supine state (Fig. 50-20). This is responsible for an overall reduction in the resistance of the peripheral vascular system and an associated increase in arterial inflow to the extremity necessary for normal exercise requirements. Although this is the mean effect of exercise, the moment-to-moment pressure changes are more complex.

During the phase of calf muscle relaxation or diastole, the large venous channels are distended, and the pressure in the deep veins falls below that in the superficial veins. During calf muscle contraction, however, the pressure in the deep veins increases dramatically to exceed the pressure in the superficial veins, with a pumping effect being generated and forcing venous blood out of the extremities in an antegrade direction. During calf mucle relaxation, therefore, flow occurs from the superficial venous system to the deep venous system through the perforating veins; this flow is facilitated by the unidirectional valves contained in the perforating veins. During calf muscle contraction the unidirectional valves in the deep venous system result in blood being forced to flow in a centripetal direction, with the valves in the perforating veins preventing blood from entering into the superficial system from the deep. At the completion of calf muscle contraction, the cycle is again repeated (Fig. 50-21). The increase in frequency and depth of respiration associated with exercise acts to facilitate overall venous return.

Changes Induced by Disease

Acute Venous Thrombosis

The development of occlusive thrombi in the major axial veins of the venous system will obviously have the effect of preventing normal venous outflow from the extremities (Fig. 50-22). This effect can be used as a diagnostic test with plethysmographic methods to identify this condition. Physiologically the presence of a major axial vein obstruction will result in a gradual rise in the pressure at the venular end of the capillaries, with the subsequent development of edema. This effect, however, is quite variable and

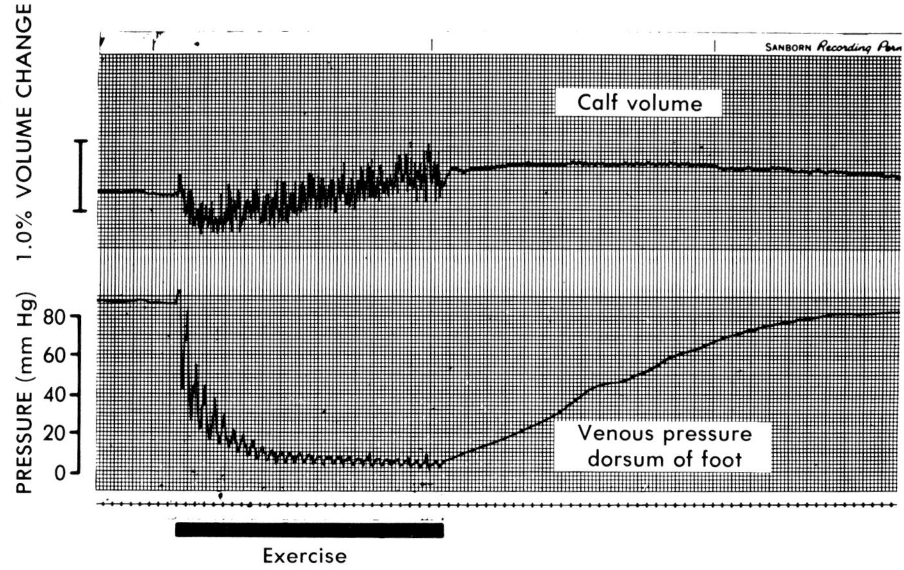

Fig. 50-20 Effect of exercise on venous pressure. With each contraction of the calf muscle, there is a rapid fall in venous pressure reaching a plateau after approximately 10 contractions.

depends not only on the location and extent of the venous thrombosis but also on the availability of collateral venous channels to compensate for the obstruction. It is therefore not infrequent to observe that venous thrombosis may not be associated with significant edema because of the presence of a well-functioning collateral network.

A secondary effect of an occlusive thrombus and the development of peripheral venous hypertension is that the minor pressure changes produced by respiration are not transmitted beyond the area of obstruction. Therefore flow distal to the obstruction loses its normal phasic relationship to respiration and becomes continuous. This effect can be detected with simple Doppler devices that evaluate velocity in the venous system and can easily detect increases

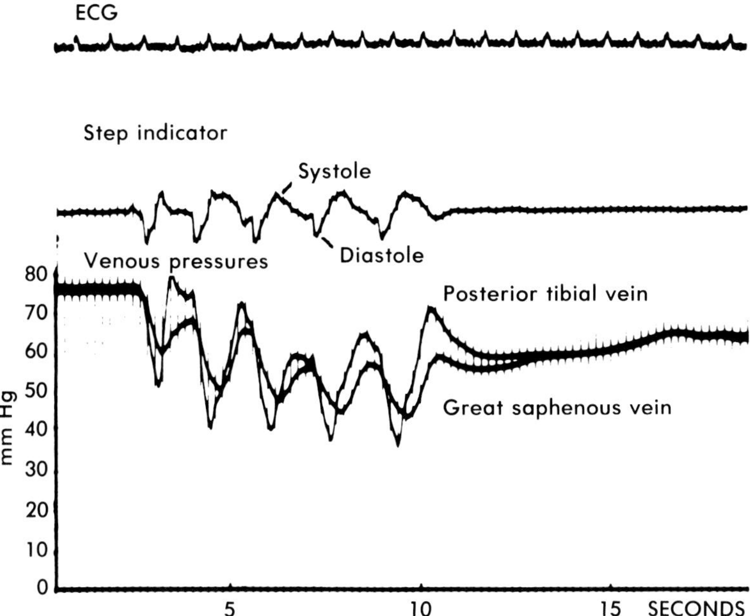

Fig. 50-21 Pressure relationships between the superficial and deep venous system during walking. It should be noted that, during calf muscle contraction or systole, the pressure in the deep system exceeds that in the superficial; whereas during calf muscle relaxation pressure in the deep system is less than that in the superficial. Filling of the calf muscle pump therefore occurs as with the heart during diastole. *Posterior tibial vein,* deep vein; *great saphenous vein,* superficial vein.

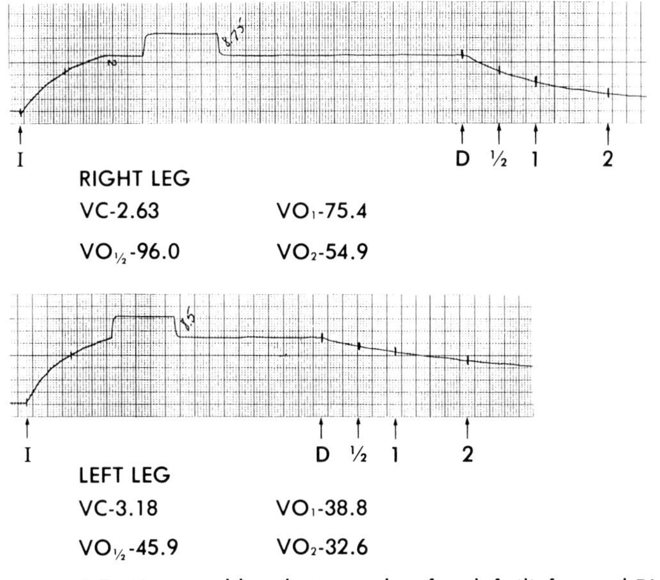

Fig. 50-22 Plethysmographic recordings from 60-year-old male 4 months after left iliofemoral deep vein thrombosis. Recordings were obtained from right leg with no deep vein thrombosis and left leg with superficial femoral vein thrombosis. Recordings are obtained by inflating a pressure cuff above venous pressure followed by instantaneous release of the pressure. Rate of emptying is significantly less in right leg compared to left leg, a fact that can be used in a diagnostic investigation.

and decreases in velocity in the normal system produced by respiration and, conversely, the uniform velocity present in cases of venous obstruction (Fig. 50-23).

Postthrombotic Venous Insufficiency

The adverse long-term sequelae of venous thrombosis are produced by residual venous obstruction and the destruction of valves in both the deep axial veins and the perforating veins. This latter effect in particular produces profound changes in the dynamics of the venous circulation during exercise, which at least in part are responsible for the clinical changes of edema, hyperpigmentation, and ulceration.

The most significant changes are seen during exercise. Valve destruction adversely affects the flow patterns produced by the pressure changes seen with exercise, and, instead of flowing in a centripetal direction and from superficial to deep, blood may be forced under high pressure from the deep system during calf muscle contraction through incompetent perforating veins into the superficial system producing severe superficial hypertension. In the deep system the normal antegrade flow pattern is completely interrupted, and venous return from the leg is significantly reduced.

Instead of a gradual reduction in venous pressure in the lower extremity produced by exercise, in severe cases exercise may actually be associated with an increase in the venous pressure in both the deep and superficial systems as depicted in Fig. 50-24. The likelihood of developing severe complications such as venous ulceration is closely related to the degree of ambulatory venous hypertension that occurs in such patients as shown in Table 50-3.

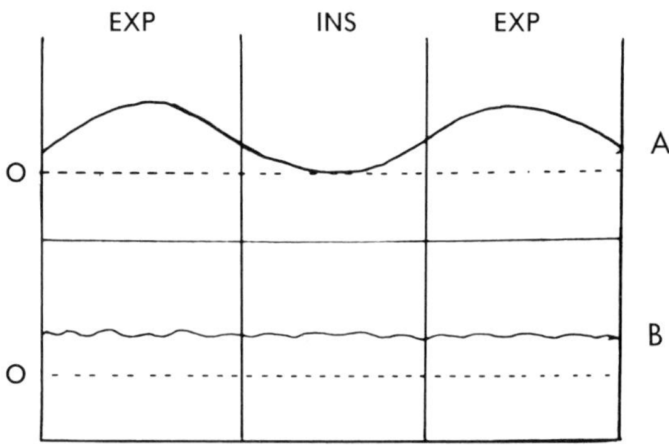

Fig. 50-23 Venous flow patterns in the normal state, **A,** and in the presence of venous obstruction, **B.** It should be noted that in the latter there is a loss of the oscillatory pattern produced by respiration. *EXP*, expiration; *INS*, inspiration.

LYMPHATIC SYSTEM

Just as the venous system is primarily responsible for the return of fluid and blood constituents from the extremity to the heart, the lymphatic system provides a conduit for the return of other molecular constituents (e.g., protein) in the interstitial space, in large part independent of the fluid exchanges occurring at the capillary level. Al-

Table 50-3 **RELATION OF AMBULATORY VENOUS HYPERTENSION TO INCIDENCE OF ULCERATION**

Ambulatory Venous Pressure (mm Hg)	Incidence of Ulceration (%)
45	0
45-50	5
50-59	15
60-69	50
70-79	75
80	80

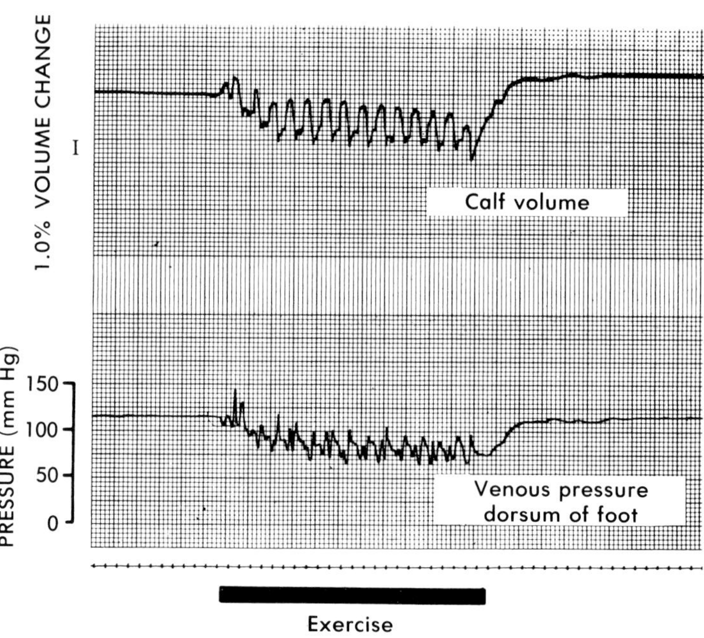

Fig. 50-24 Effect of calf muscle exercise on ankle pressure in patients with the postthrombotic syndrome. There is no significant decrease in venous pressure associated with exercise as is seen in the normal state. Compare with Fig. 50-20.

though the lymphatics also provide a medium for lymphocyte transport, that function will not be considered in this section. As with the arterial and venous systems, knowledge of the lymphatic anatomy is essential to a further understanding of the physiologic characteristics of this system.

Lymphatic Anatomy

As with the venous system, the lymphatics in the lower extremity may be divided into superficial and deep. The majority of the lymphatic effluent from the lower extremity travels through the superficial lymphatics. These channels commence as minute blind sacs in the soft tissues that coalesce to form a plexus of small vessels subjacent to the skin termed the subpapillary dermal plexus. They progressively unite to form the definitive lymph channels located in the subcutaneous tissues.

Similar to the venous system, the major channels of the lower limb begin in the dorsum of the foot on the medial side and course predominately along the medial side of the leg intimately related to the great saphenous vein and through the thigh to the superficial group of inguinal lymph nodes adjacent to the termination of this vein. These channels empty their lymphatics into the superficial nodes and subsequently into the deep inguinal lymph nodes around the common femoral vein. The lymphatic vessels are approximately 1 to 2 mm in diameter throughout the extremity with unidirectional valves located every few millimeters. In the thigh region there are usually five of these trunks, and on occasion as many as seven or eight are visualized with x-ray film techniques.

The deep lymphatic channels in the lower extremity are less numerous than the superficial channels and, like their deep venous counterparts, course in close proximity to the deep muscular arteries. In the calf region these channels are relatively small but progressively enlarge in the thigh and terminate in the deep inguinal group of lymph nodes. Efferents from the deep inguinal lymph nodes course along the brim of the pelvis, usually in three different groups of channels intimately related to the major vessels in these locations. In the region of the lumbosacral joint these channels coalesce on each side to form the para-aortic lymph channels that are, again, numerous. Throughout the course from the groin to the region of the abdominal aorta, there are numerous large pelvic lymph nodes interspersed along these channels. Lymph from the lower extremity is eventually joined by chyle from the intestinal lymphatics in the cisterna chyle and transported through the thorax by way of the thoracic duct, terminating in the posterior triangle on the left side at the junction of the internal jugular and subclavian veins.

Lymphatic Structure

The actual structure of the lymphatics provides important clues to the functional characteristics of the lower extremity lymphatic system. The structural features of most functional import are the presence of bicuspid valves throughout the lymphatics and smooth muscle located uniformly in the wall of the lymphatic channel. The bicuspid valves are located every few millimeters along the course of the lymphatic channels and enable lymph flow to occur from the periphery to the central regions. The smooth muscle in the lymphatics is innervated by the sympathetic nervous system, although the exact anatomic details of this interaction are relatively poorly understood. However, it is clear that lymphatic channels are capable of independent contraction, exerting pressures in the vicinity of 50 mm Hg during these contractions, which may occur up to 4 to 5 times per minute.

Characteristics of Lymph Flow

The primary function of the lymph vessels is to transport large molecules such as protein from the tissues back to the central venous system. A small amount of water also passes through the lymph channels from the tissues, but this is negligible compared to other constituents of the lymph circulation and serves primarily as a vehicle for these constituents.

An understanding of the lymph circulation is integrally related to the exchanges that occur at the capillary level, of which two main processes can be implicated; i.e., filtration and diffusion. Filtration is primarily responsible for the movement of fluid across the capillary membranes and is governed by the forces expounded by Starling in 1896. At the arterial end of the capillary there is a net efflux of fluid into the tissues, whereas at the venous end there is a net return of fluid from the tissues back into the venular end of the capillary. Under normal circumstances there is a slight excess of fluid filtered over that reabsorbed, and it is this fluid that is removed from the tissues by the lymphatics. It should be emphasized, however, that fluid exchange at the capillary level is primarily a function of the capillaries and not the lymphatics. It is now apparent that diffusion plays a major role in the exchange of molecules across the capillary membrane and may occur independently of the fluid fluxes present. The only factor influencing the diffusion process is the semipermeable nature of the capillary membrane and the size of the pores in this membrane. However, molecules of protein that diffuse into the tissues can easily enter the highly permeable lymphatics by which they are subsequently transported out of the tissues.

Once this fluid and large molecular complex enters the lymphatic circulation, the dynamics of the return of the lymph fluid to the major central channels must be considered. As in the venous system, flow of lymph depends on the presence of the bicuspid valves, contraction of smooth muscle in the walls of the lymphatic vessels, and compression of the vessels by extrinsic forces. Factors such as respiration are also likely to influence lymphatic flow, although the contribution of this mechanism is not well understood.

As noted earlier, the unidirectional valves encourage flow to occur from the periphery of the limb to the central locations, although valves are absent in the minute lymphatic capillaries of the dermal plexus where flow may occur in any direction. Although spontaneous rhythmic contractions have been observed in virtually all lymphatics of the body, as indicated above, the major factors responsible for lymph efflux from the lower extremity are probably those produced by extrinsic compression of skeletal muscle contraction and also by the regular pumping action of the arterial channels intimately related to the lymphatic vessels.

In addition to these forces acting as a means of propelling lymph fluid along the lymph channels, they also probably provide an explanation of the way in which the terminal lymphatics may function as a suction pump facilitating the entry of interstitial fluid into the lymphatics in both normal and pathologic states. Contraction of the lymphatic wall may result in the generation of a positive pressure proximal to the area of contraction and a negative pressure at the bulbous terminal portion of the lymphatic that facilitates entry of interstitial fluid. A mechanism such as this is essential for the movement of fluid into the lymphatic system because recent evidence suggests that interstitial fluid pressure is, in fact, negative.

Lymphatics in Disease

Although a detailed pathologic description of the various disease states affecting the lymphatics is beyond the scope of this chapter, each has a final common denominator in that lymphatic outflow from the extremity is impaired. The changes with lymphatic obstruction or inefficient lymphatic outflow are very different from those seen with vascular obstruction and are best understood by comparing the changes that occur at the tissue level in each. If flow in the arteriolar and venular side of the capillary ceases, the supply of essential nutritional requirements to tissues is impaired, resulting eventually in tissue necrosis. With lymphatic obstruction, however, there is merely a gradual accumulation of large protein molecules in the tissue, increasing the oncotic pressure, with a net accumulation of fluid and the development of the condition known as lymphedema. The diffusion of essential nutritional elements may still proceed unimpeded, and thus tissue necrosis will not occur even in the presence of quite severe edema. Eventually a steady state will be reached at which the hydrostatic pressure exerted by the fluid in the tissues will balance the oncotic pressure, and essentially normal fluid exchange will then continue. Despite a new balance in fluid dynamics, however, the presence of this interstitial edema will remain unless altered by external pressures. The practical importance of this knowledge is that it is possible to forcefully expel this edematous fluid from the extremity with the application of external pumps that exceed the hydrostatic interstitial fluid pressure, resulting in a reduction in the extremity edema.

SUMMARY

The circulatory system as a whole serves to maintain normal tissue nutrition under conditions of rest and peak exercise, with both the arterial and venous systems, like many others in the body, having a major functional reserve capacity. The arterial and venous systems are primarily involved in the maintenance of a favorable tissue milieu for normal metabolism, with the lymphatics functioning as a scavenger system to remove macromolecules and any excess of fluid that is extravasated from the capillary mechanism. Whereas the arterial system is dynamic with the energy being provided intrinsically by contraction of the left ventricle, both the venous and lymphatic systems are uniquely designed to facilitate movment of fluid under relatively low pressures and to rely predominately on extrinsic forces such as respiration and skeletal muscle contraction to offset the negative effects of gravity.

SUGGESTED READINGS

1. Arnoldi, C.C.: Venous pressure in the leg of healthy human subjects at rest and during muscular exercise in the nearly erect position, Acta Chir. Scand. **130:**520, 1965.
2. Basmajian, J.V.: Distribution of valves in femoral, internal iliac and common iliac veins and their relationship to varicose veins, Surg. Gynecol. Obstet. **95:**537, 1952.
3. Burton, A.C.: Physiology and biophysics of the circulation, Chicago, 1972, Year Book Medical Publishers, Inc.
4. Cockett, F.B., and Dodd, H., editors: The pathology and surgery of the veins of the lower limb, Edinburgh, 1976, Churchill Livingstone.
5. Folkow, B., and Neil, E.: Circulation, Oxford, 1971, Oxford University Press.
6. Geddes, L.A., and Baker, L.E.: Principles of applied biomedical instrumentation, ed. 2, New York, 1975, John Wiley & Sons.
7. Guyton, A.C.: Human physiology and mechanisms of disease, ed. 2, Philadelphia, 1982, W.B. Saunders Co.
8. Ludbrook, J.: Functional aspects of the veins of the leg, Am. Heart J. **64:**796, 1962.
9. McDonald, D.A.: Blood flow in arteries, London, 1974, Edward Arnold.
10. Milnor, W.R.: Hemodynamics, Baltimore, 1982, The Williams & Wilkins Co.
11. Moreno, A.H., et al.: Mechanics of distension of dog veins and other thin-walled tubular structures, Circ. Res. **27:**1069, 1970.
12. Rhodin, J.A.: Architecture of the vessel wall. In Handbook of physiology: the cardiovascular system, Baltimore, 1982, The Williams & Wilkins Co.
13. Smith, J.J., and Kampine, J.P.: Circulatory physiology — the essentials, ed. 2, Baltimore, 1984, The Williams & Wilkins Co.
14. Stegall, H.F.: Muscle pumping in the dependent leg, Circ. Res. **19:**180, 1966.
15. Strandness, D.E., and Sumner, D.S.: Hemodynamics for surgeons, New York, 1975, Grune & Stratton, Inc.
16. Todd, A.S., and Nunn, A.: The histological localization of fibrinolysin activator, J. Pathol. Bacteriol. **78:**281, 1959.
17. Yoffey, J.M., and Courtice, F.C.: Lymphatics, lymph and lymphoid tissue, Baltimore, 1967, The Williams & Wilkins Co.

51

Christopher K. Zarins and Alan M. Graham

Aorta and Arterial Disease of the Lower Extremity

Atherosclerosis is the major disease process affecting the aorta and arteries of the lower extremity. It is a degenerative disease characterized by the formation of intimal plaques that may obstruct the lumen and reduce blood flow through the vessel. Plaques may ulcerate, with embolization of atherosclerotic debris or thrombotic material to the distal arterial bed, or they may cause thrombosis of the lumen. In addition, the artery wall may degenerate, resulting in thinning and weakening of the wall and aneurysm formation. Each of these processes may result in a spectrum of clinical presentations and may require different diagnostic and therapeutic approaches. In this chapter we will consider some of the general features of atherosclerosis, along with its pathologic and clinical manifestations in the lower extremities, and discuss diagnostic modalities and treatment alternatives.

ATHEROSCLEROSIS

Risk Factors of Atherogenesis

Although atherosclerotic plaques develop in most people, epidemiologic studies have identified a number of risk factors that are important in the development of complications of atherosclerotic lesions. These include the following:

- Hypercholesterolemia
- Hypertension
- Cigarette smoking
- Diabetes mellitus
- Physical inactivity
- Obesity
- Type A behavior
- Heredity

Certain factors may be more closely associated with manifestations of atherosclerosis in some arterial beds than in others. For example, serum cholesterol and low-density lipoprotein levels are strongly and directly related to coronary heart disease, whereas hypertension is more closely associated with complications of cerebrovascular disease. Cigarette smoking and diabetes appear to have a greater impact on peripheral vascular disease than on coronary and cerebrovascular disease.[13] In addition, each factor appears to have an additive effect on the cardiovascular risk. For example, smoking has been shown to dramatically increase the rate of progression of atherosclerosis in the hypercholesterolemic patient. Another example of additive risk factors is apparent in the marked development of peripheral occlusive disease in women with hypertension and diabetes who smoke. These women develop atherosclerosis at the same rate as men.

An understanding of risk factors is important, and efforts should be made to control them since there is evidence that this may have a beneficial effect on the expression of the disease. For example, it has been shown that control of serum cholesterol and low-density lipoprotein levels is beneficial in preventing coronary atherosclerosis.[18] Control of hypertension has a beneficial effect on both coronary and cerebrovascular disease. Cessation of smoking has a beneficial effect on the manifestations of peripheral occlusive disease, and limb loss rates are much lower in these patients than in those who continue to smoke.[15] Physical exercise, weight reduction, and diminution of stress all are felt to have a beneficial effect on disease manifestations.[24] However, it is not clear that control of hyperglycemia will prevent vascular complications in patients with diabetes mellitus.[29] In addition to a great body of knowledge with regard to general risk factors, local hemodynamic or metabolic conditions may be equally important in plaque formation since plaques deposit in certain focal areas of the vascular tree, whereas other areas are spared. The aorta and arteries of the lower extremity are among the particularly susceptible sites for the development of atherosclerotic lesions.

Localizing Factors in Development of Atherosclerotic Lesions

The areas of the vascular tree such as the carotid bifurcation, the coronary arteries, the abdominal aorta, and vessels of the lower extremity that are particularly prone to the development of atherosclerotic lesions are areas of branching and are characterized by alterations in local hemodynamic conditions. A number of hemodynamic theories to explain plaque localization have been proposed, including high shear stress, low shear stress, turbulence, and flow separation. Elevated shear stress has been thought to contribute to plaque formation by causing endothelial injury or denudation of the lumen surface with exposure of subendothelial connective tissue that results in platelet deposition. Subsequent release of platelet growth factor would stimulate smooth cell proliferation and intimal thickening.[25] However, there is little or no evidence that high shear stress and endothelial injury are major initiating or sustaining mechanisms in human or experimental plaque formation. Clinical observations on plaque localization suggest, rather, that lesions localize in areas of low shear stress and flow separation such as the upstream rim of aortic ostia and the outer wall of the internal carotid sinus.[39]

Relatively slow flow and low wall shear stress may also be predisposing factors in abdominal aortic and peripheral atherosclerosis. The renal arteries alone carry 25% of the entire cardiac output at rest. The renal arteries together with the celiac and superior mesenteric arteries ensure a constant high volume flow in the thoracic and suprarenal aortas, which are rarely involved with significant atherosclerosis. However, the volume of flow in the aorta below the renal arteries depends greatly on the muscular activity of the lower extremities. Although a physically active bipedal existence ensures intermittent high volume flow, a sedentary life-style and a dependence on motorized vehicles may expose the human abdominal aorta to relatively slower flow velocites than a vessel of its caliber should carry and slower than the rest of the suprarenal aorta. This may predispose the aorta to plaque deposition over a long period of time such as is necessary for plaque formation. The relative slow flow in the abdominal aorta may be further accentuated by the tendency of all arteries, including the aorta, to dilate as a function of age.

Configuration and Composition of Atherosclerotic Lesions

Atherosclerotic lesions are focal intimal accumulations of cells, lipids, connective tissue, fibrous tissue, calcium, and necrotic debris. A lesion typically has a fibrous cap, which is a densely compact structure containing smooth muscle cells and fibrous connective tissue. Beneath this fibrous cap is a region known as the necrotic center that contains lipid-laden cells, cell debris, amorphous cholesterol and cholesterol crystals, and calcium. The fibrous cap serves to sequester or wall off the necrotic center from the lumen. Thus plaques are well tolerated in the circulation for many years and produce clinical manifestations only if the fibrous cap breaks down to produce a complicated plaque. These complicated lesions can lead to thrombosis, ulceration, calcification, or aneurysm formation.

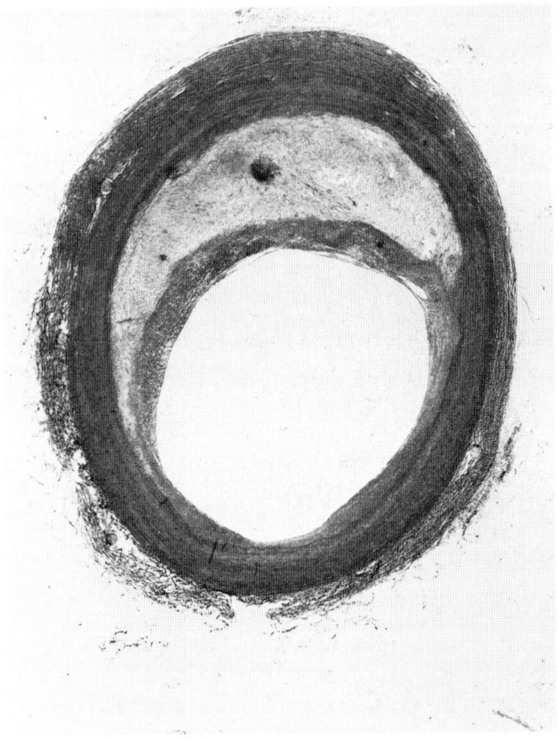

Fig. 51-1 Atherosclerotic plaque demonstrating the fibrous cap over a necrotic center. Note the oval external contour with the round lumen typical of these plaques.

As plaques enlarge, there is a compensatory dilation of the artery wall to counteract the tendency of the enlarging plaques to produce stenoses. Plaques viewed on cross section usually are eccentric, resulting in an oval external vessel contour with a rounded lumen contour (Fig. 51-1). The commonly held belief that plaques bulge or protrude into the lumen to produce obstruction to flow arises from the fact that most plaques are observed in opened, collapsed arteries either at operation or at postmortem. With loss of distending pressure, plaques do indeed appear to bulge into the lumen, but this is not the case in vivo. The angiographic impression of plaques bulging into the lumen arises because the vessels are viewed in a longitudinal plane rather than on cross section. Irregular cross-sectional lumen contours in vivo usually arise from lesion ulceration or thrombosis. Ulcerations probably occur at least as commonly in the aortoiliac and femoral vessels as they do in the carotid bifurcation. However, a small ulcer and embolization in the carotid bifurcation become immediately apparent to the patient and physician because of neurologic symptoms, whereas embolization to the lower extremity may proceed without any symptoms for many years, with progressive obstruction of the distal outflow vessels and the development of gangrene only as a late manifestation.

PATHOPHYSIOLOGIC PROCESSES AFFECTING THE AORTA AND LOWER EXTREMITY ARTERIES

The processes affecting the arteries to the lower extremity include plaque formation with obstruction of the lumen and subsequent limitation of flow, thrombosis resulting in acute ischemia, ulceration of the plaque with distal embolization, and weakening of the arterial wall with aneurysmal formation resulting in rupture or thrombosis.

Stenosis

Progressive intimal plaque deposition may result in narrowing of the lumen, or stenosis. Mild degrees of stenosis producing less than 50% reduction in lumen diameter usually do not obstruct blood flow. It is not until lumen diameter falls below a critical point that resistance to blood flow increases. This is referred to as *critical arterial stenosis,* or the percentage by which the lumen diameter must be reduced in order to produce a measurable drop in blood flow. Under experimental conditions there is no significant pressure drop and no reduction in flow until there is more than 80% reduction in lumen cross-sectional area (equivalent to 55% diameter reduction).[20] However, pressure drops across stenoses are critically dependent on flow, and noncritical stenoses at rest may develop significant pressure gradients when flow is increased with exercise. This can account for the clinical observation of disappearing pedal pulses after exercise and symptoms of claudication in patients with palpable pedal pulses.

The extent of disability from an obstruction is related to the location of the lesion, the degree of obstruction, length and number of obstructions, the metabolic needs of the tissues distal to the obstruction, and the ability of collateral vessels to provide the necessary flow. *Collateral blood flow* may be quite extensive in occlusive disease. Collateral vessels are naturally existing branches of large and medium-sized arteries that enlarge to carry blood flow around an obstruction. They do not represent neovascularization but adaptation of existing vessels to an increased demand of blood flow. The collateral blood flow that develops in the face of a developing, progressive obstruction usually can supply the demands of resting tissue. However, it often is unable to supply the flow necessary for an exercising muscle group.

There are a number of well-recognized collateral beds that develop in the presence of atherosclerosis of the aorta and distal tree:

1. Intercostal and lumbar arteries
2. Superior and inferior mesenteric arteries
3. Hypogastric artery
4. Profunda - geniculate arteries
5. Peroneal - tibial arteries

Patients may have a totally occluded abdominal aorta for several years with relatively mild symptoms of hip and buttock claudication. Under these circumstances the intercostal arteries, superior epigastric arteries, and visceral arteries become important sources of collateral flow to the lower extremity (Fig. 51-2). For example, blood supply to the distal aorta may be through the inferior mesenteric artery, which derives collateral supply from the superior mesenteric artery. In addition, the inferior mesenteric artery can be an important source of collateral flow to the lower extremities through the superior hemorrhoidal network.

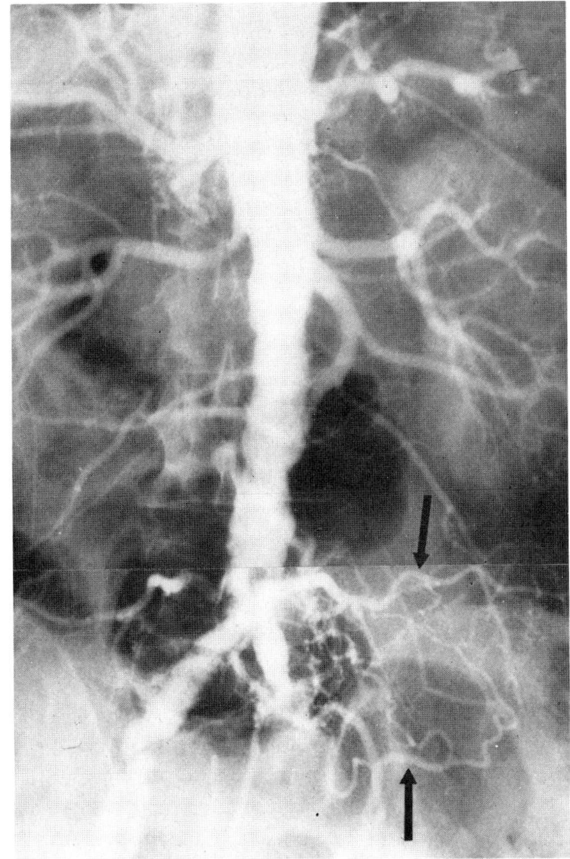

Fig. 51-2 Angiogram revealing severe aortoiliac disease. Note the large collaterals *(arrows)* that have developed in response to occlusion of the left iliac artery.

Thrombosis

The causes of *acute arterial obstruction* can be divided into two categories: embolism and thrombosis (see boxed material below). Emboli arise from a proximal source, most commonly the heart, and obstruct the tapering arterial tree at a branch point or at the point where the embolus is larger than the lumen diameter. Mural thrombus that forms in a fibrillating atrium is the most common source of arterial emboli,[31] but emobli can also arise from areas of recent transmural infarction, ventricular aneurysms, and diseased valves. Spontaneous thrombosis usually occurs in arteriosclerotic arteries as a result of slow flow caused by severe stenotic lesions or as a result of sudden dissection of hemorrhage under a previously nonstenotic plaque.

Acute thrombosis usually results in very sudden and severe symptoms of arterial ischemia. The severity of clinical symptoms is related to the site of the obstruction, the size and extent of the thrombus, and the adequacy of collateral vessels. In severe ischemia, one or more of the often described five P's may be present; pulselessness, pallor, paresthesia, pain, and paralysis. The loss of motor power and sensation in the toes and foot indicate very severe ischemia and limb loss unless the ischemia is relieved promptly. Acute thrombosis of a previously stenosed artery that has excellent collateral vessels about it may occur with only mild symptoms and little risk of limb loss.

Ulceration

Ulceration occurs when breakdown of the fibrous cap over a lesion exposes the necrotic core of the plaque to the circulation. This may be the site for platelet deposition and thrombus formation or may result in embolization of the plaque contents itself producing cholesterol emboli in the distal arterial tree.

The most common clinical syndrome in the peripheral circulation associated with distal embolization from a proximal ulcerated plaque is the *blue toe syndrome*. Patients may have normal pedal pulses but suddenly develop one or more cold, blue, painful toes, a condition that resolves in 3 to 4 days. These symptoms may be caused by

CAUSES OF EMBOLISM AND THROMBOSIS

Embolism
Atrial fibrillation
Valvular disease
Mural thrombus
Cardiac prosthesis
Aortic aneurysm
Atherosclerotic vessels

Thrombosis
Atherosclerotic vessels
Aneurysm (proximal vessel)
Aortic dissection
Degenerative arteriopathies
Hematologic
Malignancy

cholesterol emboli in the digital arteries of the feet. The source of the emboli usually is a proximal ulcerated lesion in the aorta, iliac, or femoral vessels. Unrecognized and untreated repeated embolization to the foot results in obstruction of the small arteries of the foot, gangrene, and limb loss.

Aneurysm Formation

An aneurysm is a localized arterial dilation. A *true aneurysm* is one in which there is thinning or atrophy of all layers of the artery wall with enlargement of the lumen. This should be distinguished from a *false aneurysm,* which results from a rupture of the artery wall, usually caused by trauma, with containment of the bloodstream by fibrous tissue surrounding the vessel. Thus in a true aneurysm there is an inadequate artery wall, whereas in a false aneurysm there is absence of the artery wall.

As the lumen radius of an aneurysm enlarges, there is an increase in *tension* on the vessel wall (T) according to the Law of LaPlace (T = Pr) where P is pressure and r is radius. The larger the radius, the greater the tension and the greater the tendency for further enlargement of the lumen. This explains why larger aneurysms have a greater tendency to rupture than smaller aneurysms. Blood flow in the dilated aneurysms have a greater tendency to rupture than smaller aneurysms. Blood flow in the dilated aneurysmal sac is slower than normal, producing an increased tendency to thrombosis. Most large abdominal aortic aneurysms are lined by laminated mural thrombus. Mural thrombus may be so thick that lumen caliber on angiography does not appear enlarged. However, mural thrombus provides little, if any, support for the artery wall and no protection from aneurysm rupture.

ARTERIAL OCCLUSIVE DISEASE OF THE AORTA AND PERIPHERAL ARTERIES

The manifestations of atherosclerosis in the aorta and peripheral arteries are either occlusive disease or aneurysm formation. The general risk factors are the same for both conditions, but aneurysmal disease tends to occur approximately one decade later than occlusive disease. The arteries of importance in the circulation to the lower extremities are diagrammed on Fig. 51-3. Obstructive plaques may occur in each of the vessels shown but are most common in the infrarenal abdominal aorta, iliac arteries, and superficial femoral arteries. The profunda femoris artery is relatively spared, and diabetics are more prone to develop lesions in the tibial arteries.

Clinical Manifestations of Peripheral Occlusive Disease

The clinical manifestations and physical findings of peripheral occlusive disease are as follows:

Symptoms	Physical Findings
Claudication	Absent or diminished pulses
Rest pain	Bruits
Skin ulceration	Skin pallor
Gangrene	Dependent rubor
Impotence	Hair loss
	Skin and muscle atrophy
	Trophic changes of the nails
	Decreased temperature

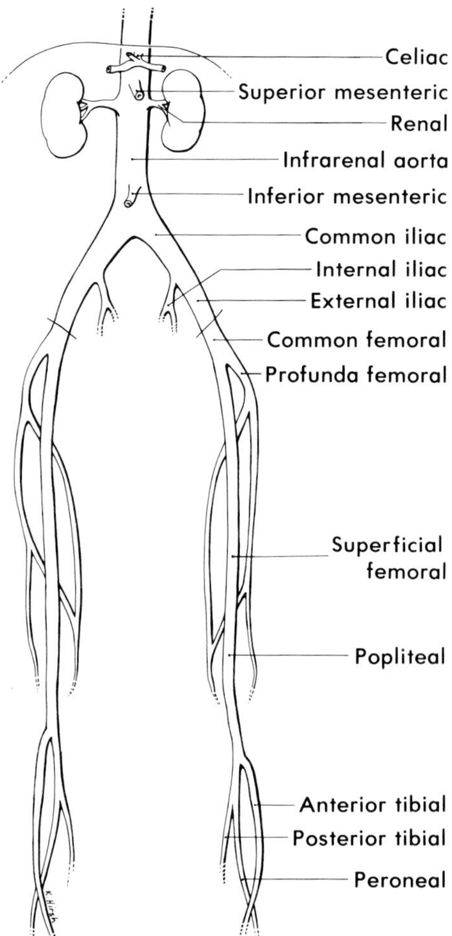

Fig. 51-3 Arterial supply to the viscera and lower extremities. Obstructive or aneurysmal changes can occur in each of these vessels. The clinical signs and symptoms will vary depending on the location and blood supply distribution of a given artery. Full angiographic evaluation of the aorta and lower extremity vessels should demonstrate each of these arteries.

Claudication

Claudication arises from the term *"claudicatio,"* which means to limp. It is a clinical syndrome of pain on exercise that is relieved by rest and results from a fixed obstruction or stenosis in arteries to the lower extremity. Although circulation may be adequate at rest, with exercise there is an increasing demand for flow. When such flow is obstructed by a stenosis, the muscle served by that vessel becomes ischemic and begins to function with anaerobic metabolism. This results in pain and symptoms of fatigue, causing the patient to stop and rest. Typically the patient rests for 1 to 2 minutes, allowing the circulation to again restore aerobic conditions, after which the patient can again exercise. Patients with aortoiliac occlusive disease have symptoms of claudication in the hips and buttocks, whereas patients with superficial femoral artery obstruction have symptoms of claudication in the calf. The level of claudication is always below the level of the arterial obstruction.

Most patients with claudication, though symptomatic, are at low risk for developing gangrene. In the Framingham study,[22] only 5% of patients with claudication required major amputation for gangrene within 5 years of diagnosis if treated conservatively. On the other hand, 20% of these patients died during that period, with the majority of deaths resulting from coronary artery disease. Thus patients with stable, nonlimiting claudication may be safely followed, and revascularization should be reserved for those with disabling symptoms.

Rest Pain

Patients with worsening ischemia develop a clinical syndrome called rest pain. The condition of rest pain indicates a much more severe degree of ischemia than claudication and, unlike claudication, indicates that the patient is at high risk for developing gangrene and limb loss. Typically the patient experiences pain in the toes and forefoot during the night that causes him to awaken from sleep. The patient usually sits up in bed, dangles his legs over the side of the bed, and frequently relieves his symptoms by getting up and walking. After a short period to time, the patient's symptoms have disappeared and he can return to sleep. The symptoms of rest pain occur because of severe ischemia in the forefoot and toes brought about by two conditions: (1) the patient is recumbent and thereby eliminates the hydrostatic pressure gradient that assists the arteriolar perfusion pressure when erect; and (2) during sleep there is a diminution of cardiac ouput that correspondingly diminishes the volume of peripheral blood flow. When the patient dangles his feet, he restores the hydrostatic gradient; and, when he gets up to walk, he increases his cardiac output and thereby improves the perfusion of his lower extremities. Patients frequently complain of nocturnal cramps in the calf muscles. This should not be confused with nocturnal rest pain, which typically is in the toes and forefoot rather than in the calf.

Ulceration

Cutaneous ulcers may be the first evidence of peripheral vascular disease. These ulcers are caused by severe ischemia from proximal arterial occlusions and are often associated with minor skin trauma. However, there are many causes of skin ulceration that must be differentiated from ischemic ulcers:

- Vascular insufficiency (ischemic)
- Venous stasis
- Hypertension
- Infection
- Neoplasm
- Neurotrophism
- Hematology

Each type of ulcer has certain clinical and physical characteristics. The ischemic ulcer is most commonly found on the toes, heel, dorsum of the foot, or lower third of the leg. The pain is usually severe, persistent, and worsens at night. The ulcer itself is generally irregular with a pale or necrotic base.

At times patients have ulcerations that are attributed to venous disease that may in fact be the result of a combination of arterial ischemia and venous stasis. Ulcerations not in the classic position for venous disease (at the medial malleolus) should be considered as potentially being of an arterial origin. Even if a component of venous disease is present, the arterial component must be evaluated if effective therapy is to be instituted.

Gangrene

Progressive ischemia caused by atherosclerosis can result in gangrenous changes of the tissues. Most commonly the digits are affected initially, but progression to the forefoot is not unusual. Small amounts of infection superimposed on a severe chronic ischemic state can progress very rapidly to gangrene. Clinically, dry and wet gangrene should be differentiated. *Dry gangrene* represents mummification of tissue, and active purulent tissue and cellulitis are absent. *Wet gangrene* is characterized by active infection with cellulitis and purulent tissue planes and is an indication for urgent amputation to prevent ascending infection.

Impotence

Penile erection requires a threefold increase in blood flow through the penile arteries that is shunted into the vascular spaces of the corpora cavernosa. Arterial obstruction that prevents this increase in blood flow can result in erectile impotence in much the same way that symptoms of claudication are brought about by exercise when there is an unmet demand for increased blood flow. Rene Leriche in 1923 first noted the association among atherosclerotic occlusion of the aorta, hip claudication, buttock atrophy, and erectile impotence. This is now known as the *Leriche syndrome*. Obstruction can occur at any level from the abdominal aorta, the common iliac arteries, the internal iliac arteries, internal pudendal arteries, or penile arteries, resulting in erectile impotence. Although the majority of cases of impotence have psychogenic or urologic causes or are the result of the side effects of medication, the importance of an adequate vascular supply is becoming increasingly recognized and can be objectively assessed, as is discussed below.

EVALUATION OF PERIPHERAL VASCULAR OCCLUSIVE DISEASE

Peripheral vascular occlusive disease is evaluated on the basis of a thorough clinical examination, noninvasive vascular testing, and, finally, angiography.

Clinical Examination

Peripheral vascular occlusive disease will often be accurately diagnosed with a careful history and thorough physical examination of the patient. In addition to the important determination of symptoms of claudication or rest pain, the patient's level of activity and walking distance should be noted. Often patients with very severe disease do not walk enough to develop symptoms. A careful evaluation of all pulses should be made, although the presence of a palpable pulse does not rule out the possibility of significant arterial occlusive disease. The presence or absence of *bruits* should also be determined. Bruits are produced by the turbulence of blood just distal to a stenosis but may also be produced by angulations and bends in arteries. Bruits may be audible with a stethoscope over and distal to an area of stenosis. A high-pitched bruit is particularly indicative of a severe stenosis. Finally, the temperature, quality, and color of the skin, hair, and nails should be noted, including the presence of skin ulcerations or gangrenous changes (see list on p. 840).

Noninvasive tests are used after the clinical examination to confirm the presence of occlusive disease, identify the level and severity of the disease, and assess whether angiography will be required to further evaluate these patients.

Objective Assessment with Vascular Laboratory Techniques

Doppler Ankle Pressure

The ready availability of the handheld Doppler ultrasound has made measurement of lower extremity blood pressure simple and convenient and has permitted the development of objective means of assessing lower extremity perfusion. The Doppler ultrasound probe emits high-frequency sound waves in the range of 2 to 10 MHz. The sound is reflected by the movement of red blood cells in the vessel that produces a frequency shift that is picked up by the receiving crystal of the Doppler probe. This frequency shift is proportional to the blood flow velocity. This *Doppler shift* can be expressed by the following formula:

$$\Delta f = \frac{2f \; V \cos \theta}{C}$$

where V is velocity, f is frequency of the incident sound beam; C is velocity of sound in tissue, and Θ is the angle of the incident sound beam to the vessel examined. Because V, C, and Θ can be constant, the shift in frequency is proportional to the velocity of the blood flow.

To measure the blood pressure in the legs, a blood pressure cuff is placed at the ankle just above the malleoli and inflated while a handheld Doppler is used to listen to flow in the dorsalis pedis and posterior tibial artery. Inflation of the cuff above systolic pressure causes obliteration of the Doppler signal, and systolic blood pressure can be recorded as the cuff is deflated and flow resumes in the measured vessel. Since a patient's blood pressure may fluctuate, more precision can be gained by comparing the ankle pressure to the brachial pressure. Usually the ankle systolic pressure is divided by the brachial systolic pressure to produce an *ankle/brachial index*. Such an index is quite useful in assessing the severity of peripheral occlusive disease. Patients without occlusive disease have an ankle pressure index of 1, whereas patients with claudication have an ankle presssure index of 0.5 to 0.6. Patients with rest pain, gangrene, and ulceration have an ankle pressure index of 0.4 and less. This measurement is useful for differentiating patients with lower extremity pain caused by spinal stenosis, arthritis, or other nonvascular conditions. Patients with diabetes frequently have calcified vessels that cannot be compressed by the blood pressure cuff. This may lead to a false elevation of the ankle/brachial index.

It is important to note that the pressure measured is determined by the location of the cuff rather than the location of the listening probe. Thus an ankle pressure can be recorded by placing a cuff at the level of the malleoli, and a below-knee or above-knee pressure by appropriate blood pressure cuff placement. Patients with superficial femoral artery occlusion will have a normal pressure in the upper thigh but will have an abnormal pressure below the knee and at the level of the ankle. The resting ankle index is the most accurate of the noninvasive techniques of objectively assessing the presence or absence of occlusive disease. It is reproducible, and hence the index can be followed to identify the progression of disease.

It should also be recognized that listening and hearing flow in the dorsalis pedis and posterior tibial artery does not represent a pulse. A pulse is palpated with the fingers. Flow can be heard at very low levels of circulation in the dorsalis pedis and the posterior tibial artery, and patients may have frank gangrene of their foot even though audible Doppler signals are heard. One should not be lulled into a false sense of security of good perfusion of the foot if Doppler flow signals in the foot are heard but pulses cannot be palpated.

Stress Testing

Since patients with claudication develop their symptoms only with exercise, stress testing is a useful means for documenting the degree of walking impairment. Treadmill exercise can be performed at a standard pace of 1.5 miles per hour at a 7-degree grade. Normally one has no diminution of the ankle blood pressure following exercise. On walking to the point of claudication, there is a substantial drop in ankle pressure index because blood flow is shunted to the proximal thigh muscle and cannot pass through the obstruction to the distal vascular bed. There is return of ankle pressure to normal with rest. The symptom of reduction in ankle pressure is similar to the finding of disappearing pulses with exercise seen on clinical examination.

Doppler Waveform Analysis

Doppler detectors can provide an analog signal that is porportional to the velocity of the blood in vessels studied. The shape of the waveform reflects the status of the vessel. Normally a *triphasic* waveform is seen, indicative of reversal of flow in early diastole. Stenosis proximal to the vessel examined first eliminates this reversed flow. As the stenosis becomes more severe, the peak of the waveform is blunted, and the wave form widens (Fig. 51-4). Quantitative analysis of these waveforms at different levels of the extremity can identify the level and severity of occlusive lesions.

Analysis of the Doppler waveforms in conjunction with systolic pressures at several levels in the leg can allow the clinician to make an accurate diagnosis of the location and extent of peripheral vascular occlusive disease. For example, Fig. 51-5 illustrates the decrease in the waveform and systolic pressures across an obstructed superficial femoral artery. A decrease in systolic blood pressure of 30 mm Hg or more between any two levels in the leg usually indicates total occlusion of the intervening artery.

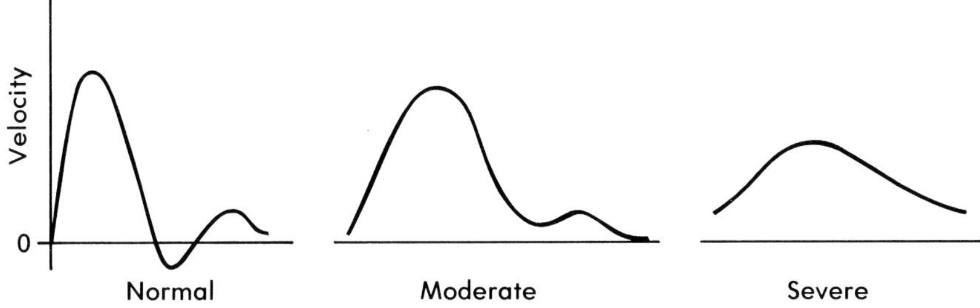

Fig. 51-4 Doppler ultrasound velocity waveforms indicating the normal triphasic waveform, the loss of the reverse flow component seen in moderately stenotic vessels, and the blunted waveform of a severely stenotic vessel.

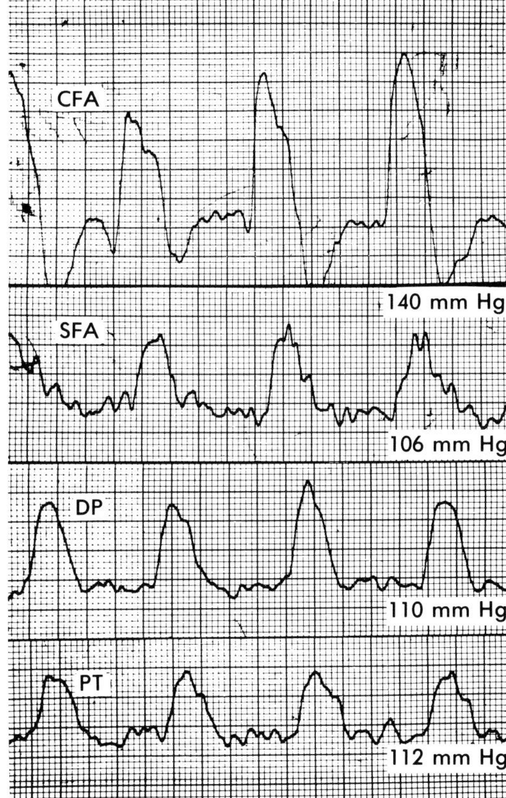

Fig. 51-5 Doppler flow velocity waveforms recorded at four places in an extremity with superficial femoral artery occlusion demonstrated by angiography. Recordings were made at the common femoral artery *(CFA)*, superficial femoral artery *(SFA)*, dorsalis pedis *(DP)*, and posterior tibial *(PT)* arteries. Associated systolic blood pressures were measured to be 140 mm Hg in the thigh and 106 mm Hg below the knee. This 34–mm Hg drop in pressure indicates occlusion of the intervening artery (in this case, the superficial femoral artery). Distal arteries fill through collateral vessels. Note change in Doppler velocity waveforms.

Doppler Ultrasound Imaging and Duplex Scanning

B-mode ultrasound imaging of arteries and plaques combined with pulsed Doppler ultrasound flow determination and sound spectral analysis is becoming available in the common femoral, superficial femoral, and popliteal artery. This technique provides the ability to noninvasively image arteries and to assess flow and is particularly useful for evaluating anastomoses in grafts following surgery. Its use can also be expanded to the evaluation of aneurysms and ulcerated lesions as a source of distal embolization in these vessels.

Penile Brachial Pressure Index

The simplest and most reliable assessment of the adequacy of penile perfusion is the measurement of arterial pressure in the corpora cavernosa supplied by the penile arteries. A Doppler velocity probe is positioned directly over one of the six penile arteries, and a small pneumatic cuff is placed around the penis proximal to the probe. The cuff is inflated until arterial flow is abolished and is then allowed to slowly deflate until flow returns, which indicates the systolic blood pressure. The penile systolic pressure is divided by the brachial systolic pressure to provide a penile:brachial index (PBI). A PBI greater than 0.9 is normal. A PBI less than 0.7 is consistent with a vascular occlusive cause of the impotence.

Angiography

Angiography provides the most definitive assessment of obstructing vascular lesions and is performed before vascular reconstruction. Since atherosclerosis is a diffuse disease, careful assessment of the arteries, both proximal and distal to the lesion, is required. This includes visualization of the abdominal and infrarenal aorta, the iliac arteries, and the femoral, popliteal, and tibial vessels throughout their length (see Fig. 51-3). Angiography is usually performed through a transfemoral approach, which has the advantage of allowing selective catheterization and the study of individual arteries as needed. Transaxillary and translumbar aortography can also be used successfully. Newer techniques of digital subtraction and computer enhancement of images permit the use of smaller volumes of iodinated contrast materials. Patients should be well hydrated before and after angiography to minimize the possibility of renal failure caused by the osmotic diuresis produced by the hypertonic contrast medium.[27]

TREATMENT OF PERIPHERAL VASCULAR OCCLUSIVE DISEASE

The treatment of peripheral vascular occlusive disease is determined by the severity of the patient's symptoms and the anatomic location and extent of obstructing lesions.

Treatment options include nonoperative measures, minimally invasive procedures such as transluminal angioplasty, and operative revascularization.

Nonoperative Measures

Patients with peripheral occlusive disease usually have one or several risk factors for the development of vascular disease, including cigarette smoking, hyperlipidemia, hypertension, and diabetes mellitus. Every effort should be made to control these factors to prevent progression of obstructive disease. Patients with symptoms of claudication that are not physically limiting have a low risk of limb loss[22] and usually respond well to a program of cessation of smoking and walking exercise to stimulate enlargement of collateral circulation and to condition the muscles to function at a higher level with the available blood supply. Exercise programs are effective in improving walking distance but must be maintained. Cessation of the exercise program will usually return the patient to the same level of claudication as present originally. Patients often adjust their levels of activity and coexist with occlusive disease well for many years. Those who continue to smoke have the poorest outlook.

Medical therapy for peripheral vascular disease has in general been ineffective. A number of vasodilating drugs have been used in an attempt to diminish vasospasm, improve perfusion of ischemic limbs, and help the development of collateral vessels. These agents as a group have been ineffective, and most have been removed from the market.

In recent years four new classes of drugs have been described that may potentially benefit the patient with vascular disease: (1) calcium channel blockers (nifedipine); (2) prostaglandins (PGE_1 and PGI_2); (3) pentoxifylline; and (4) thromboxane synthetase inhibitors.

Nifedipine has been found useful in the treatment of vasospasm as seen in Raynaud's syndrome,[28] and many currently consider it the drug of choice for this disease. The complex biologic activity of the prostaglandins has only recently evolved. PGE_1 is a vasodilator and a strong inhibitor of platelet aggregation. No single trial has yet to demonstrate the benefits of PGE_1 in the improvement of rest pain or healing of ischemic ulcers.

Pentoxifylline is a xanthine derivative that has been used in the medical treatment of peripheral vascular occlusive disease. It has been suggested that it exerts its effect by decreasing the rigidity of erythrocytes so that they can more readily deform and pass through the small capillary beds, thereby increasing tissue perfusion. A recently completed trial of patients with claudication has shown a slight increase in walking distance in patients treated with pentoxifylline as compared to placebo.[23] This drug has been recently classified as effective in the treatment of intermittent claudication by the Food and Drug Administration, but long-term benefits have not been established. There is no evidence that pentoxifylline is effective in patients with ulceration, rest pain, or gangrene.

Thromboxane synthetase inhibitors exert their effects by blocking the function of thromboxane, which produces vasoconstriction and platelet aggregation. Prevention of these events in the microcirculation might improve distal circulation. However, no clinical benefits have yet to be realized with these agents.

Transluminal Angioplasty

Transluminal balloon angioplasty is a percutaneous method of dilating arterial stenoses or recanalizing occluded vessels. The procedure is usually performed in the angiography suite after completion of diagnostic angiography. Proper patient selection is important, and clinical criteria similar to those used to select patients for surgery should be used. Dilation of lesions that appear significant on angiography but that produce minimal or no symptoms must be avoided. The best candidate for transluminal angioplasty is one with severe claudication caused by an isolated hemodynamically significant iliac artery lesion or a proximal superficial femoral artery stenosis. Other clinical situations include patients with a short-segment, superficial femoral artery occlusion or a short stenosis of a previously placed bypass graft.

In transluminal angioplasty a catheter with a balloon that has a predetermined maximum diameter at its tip is used. The catheter with balloon deflated is passed over a guidewire under x-ray control through an obstructing lesion. Inflation of the balloon disrupts the plaque and stretches the arterial wall, resulting in enlargement of the lumen. This enlargement of the lumen cross-sectional area occurs by separating the plaque from the underlying tunica media and stretching the artery wall (Fig. 51-6). At times the media is stretched and thinned to the point of media rupture, in which case vessel integrity is maintained by the adventitia.[38] There is no plaque compression on removal of the lesion, and long-term patency depends on the vessel wall remaining in the overstretched state. When the vessel contracts to its predilated state, restenosis occurs. This occurs in a substantial number of patients and is a limitation of the procedure.

Results from transluminal angioplasty depend on the site dilated, the length of the stenosis, whether a complete obstruction is being dilated, and the degree of calcification in the plaque. In the iliac region, 90% to 95% of the lesions can be successfully dilated, whereas 70% to 85% will have a 2-year patency.[16,17] Angioplasty of the superficial femoral artery has less impressive results. Initial success rates of 76% to 84% fall to 57% and 75%, respectively, at 2 years.[19,34]

Transluminal angioplasty can also be a useful adjunct in the treatment of end-stage atherosclerosis when no surgical bypass option is available. Initial limb salvage in these patients has been reported at 76%.[26]

Endarterectomy

Endarterectomy is a surgical procedure in which the diseased intimal plaque is removed from an artery to enlarge the lumen. The cleavage plane for endarterectomy is usually just below the internal elastic lamina, although the media below extensive plaque is often degenerated and is removed along with the intimal plaque. In these circumstances the cleavage plane is at the external elastic lamina and thus only the adventitial layer contains the blood-

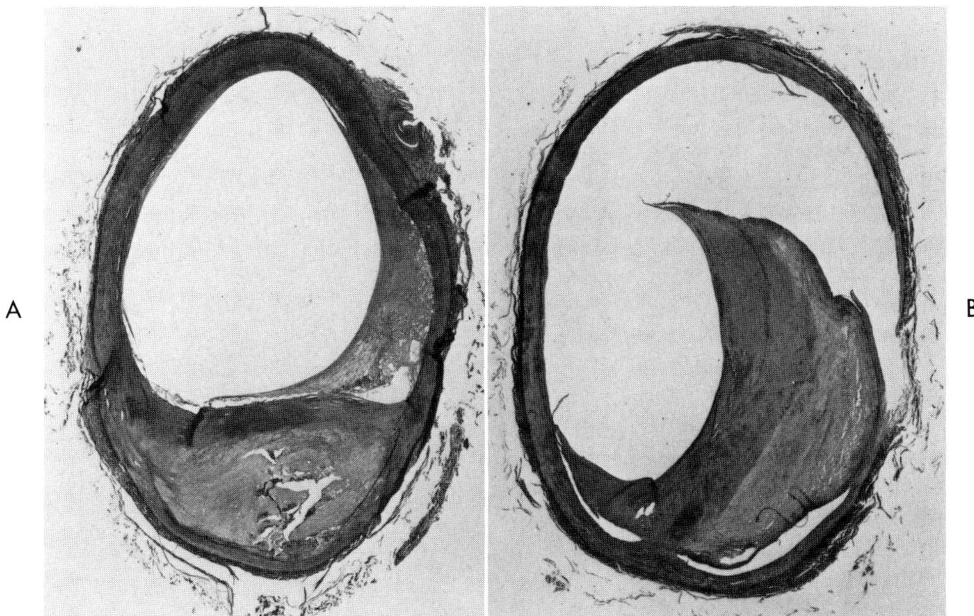

Fig. 51-6 Mechanism of balloon dilation of arteries. **A,** Human superficial femoral artery that has been fixed with an intraluminal pressure of 100 mm Hg and cut in cross-section. Note the eccentric plaque and round lumen. **B,** Segment of the same artery after balloon dilation. Note the separation of plaque from the media and protrusion of the plaque into the lumen. The media is thinner and has ruptured, and lumen integrity is maintained by the adventitia. Disruption and stretching of the artery wall results in a larger lumen area. There is no plaque compression. (From Zarins, C.K., et al.: Arterial disruption and remodeling following balloon dilatation, Surgery **92:**1086, 1982.)

stream. The adventitial layer alone provides sufficient structural support, and aneurysmal dilation of endarterectomized arterial segments does not occur.

Although endarterectomy is the standard mode of treatment for carotid bifurcation atherosclerosis, it has a more limited usefulness in the treatment of peripheral vascular occlusive disease. This is because carotid plaques are very localized in the carotid bifurcation, whereas lower-extremity atherosclerosis usually is extensive with no discrete starting or end points. Some patients with localized aortoiliac disease and no distal occlusive disease are candidates for local aortoiliac endarterectomy, but bypass procedures are more commonly performed. If a local endarterectomy is to be considered, these patients must not have aneurysmal disease or fibrotic small-caliber vessels. Results of *local* aortoiliac endarterectomy compare favorably to aortobifemoral bypass grafts.

Most surgeons occasionally use local endarterectomy as an adjunctive procedure to aortobifemoral bypass grafting. Such local endarterectomies are frequently performed in the common and profunda femoral arteries at the time of anastomosis of bypass grafts, but primary endarterectomies have limited usefulness in the peripheral circulation.

Bypass Procedures

Procedures to bypass occlusive lesions are the standard surgical methods for treatment of lower-extremity peripheral occlusive disease. Procedures are usually considered as inflow or outflow procedures, depending on the level of obstruction. Inflow procedure refer to those used for aortoiliac obstructions, and outflow procedures are those used for superficial femoral and popliteal artery obstructions, with the level of the groin usually being the dividing line. Angiographic, vascular, laboratory, and clinical criteria are used to determine the primary level of obstruction. If a patient has both inflow and outflow disease, the proximal, or inflow, obstruction is treated first and usually is sufficient to relieve symptoms.

Aortofemoral Bypass

The indications for surgical intervention in patients with aortoiliac occlusive lesions are severe claudication and limb-threatening ischemia as defined by rest pain, ulcerations, and gangrene. The standard surgical treatment for bypass of aortoiliac obstructions is the aortofemoral bypass graft. In this procedure a knitted or woven Dacron bifurcation graft is sutured from the infrarenal aorta, which is usually free of disease, to the common femoral arteries. This graft bypasses the entire aortoiliac segment, which includes the inferior mesenteric artery and internal iliac arteries. The proximal anastomosis is placed just below the level of the renal arteries and may be performed in either an end-to-end or an end-to-side fashion (Fig. 51-7). When an *end-to-end anastomosis* is used, the distal aorta is ligated, and the entire aortic outflow passes through the graft. Blood is supplied to the distal aorta, and the inferior mesenteric and internal iliac arteries by retrograde flow from the common femoral artery through the external iliac artery. With an *end-to-side proximal anastomosis,* blood flows in parallel in the bypass graft and in the distal aorta.

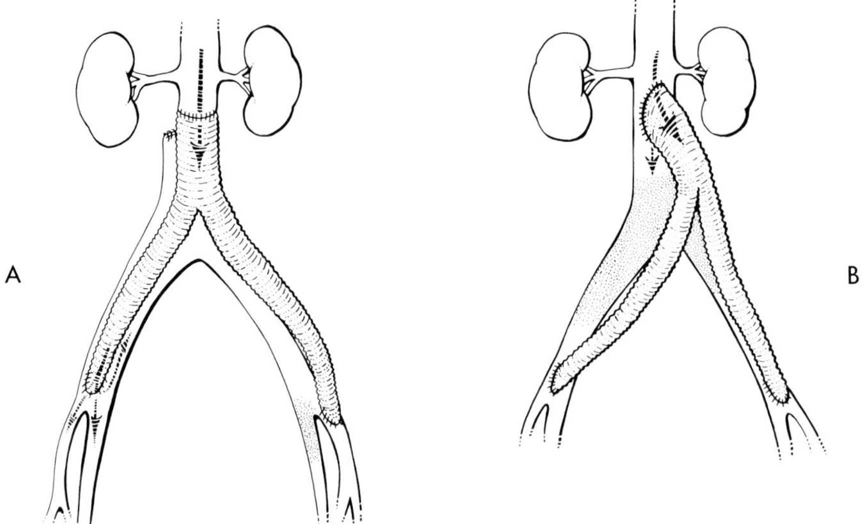

Fig. 51-7 Aortofemoral bypass for aortoiliac obstruction. Proximal anastomosis may be performed end-to-end **(A)** or end-to-side of the aorta **(B)**. With an end-to-end anastomosis, perfusion of the internal iliac arteries and distal aorta is retrograde from the common femoral artery in the groin.

This anastomosis is preferred when the external iliac arteries are occluded and would prevent retrograde fill of the aorta from the groin. The distal anastomosis is usually placed on the common femoral artery with outflow through the superficial femoral and profunda femoris vessels. If there is associated superficial femoral artery occlusion, the profunda artery alone can serve as the outflow bed with relief of symptoms. Concomitant endarterectomy of the orifices of the superficial femoral and profunda can be undertaken to improve the distal anastomosis. *Profundaplasty* is performed by extending the opening of the common femoral artery onto the profunda femoris artery and suturing the Dacron graft onto the profunda artery. This results in enlargement of the lumen of the proximal profunda artery and is useful when there is a stenosis at that site.

Aortofemoral bypass graft is a stable and durable operation that effectively eliminates the inflow obstruction. Surgical mortality rate is less than 2%, and the 5-year graft patency rate is greater than 90%.[4] Should these operations fail, they generally do so because of progression of disease in the arteries at or distal to the groin anastomosis rather than because of failure of the Dacron graft itself.

Early complications of aortobifemoral grafts are caused mainly by technical misadventures. These include postoperative hemorrhage, early graft thrombosis, distal embolization, groin hematomas, and lymph leaks. Long-term complications include graft infection, pseudoaneurysm formation, and aorta duodenal fistula. Details of these problems will be expanded on below.

Extraanatomic Bypass

Patients who require bypass of aortoiliac lesions but are too ill to withstand an intra abdominal operation for placement of an aortobifemoral graft may be revascularized with an *axillofemoral* or *femorofemoral* bypass graft (Fig.

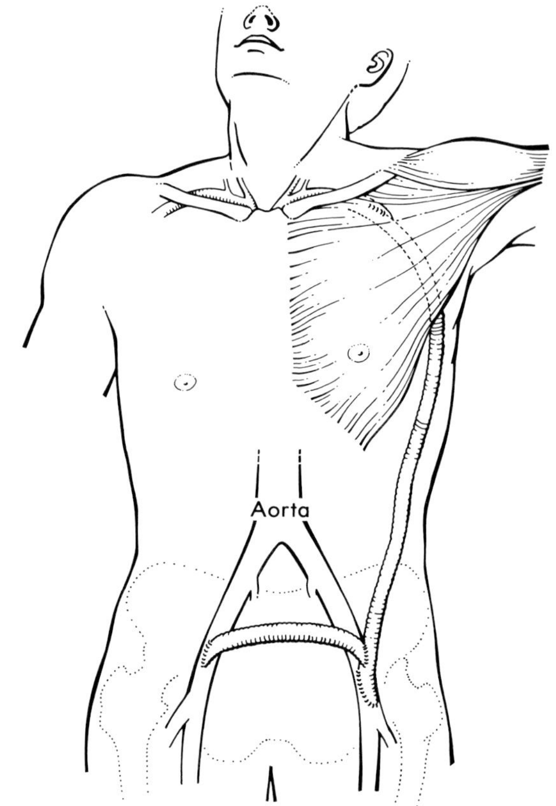

Fig. 51-8 Illustration of extraanatomical bypasses for aortoiliac obstruction. Axillofemoral bypass courses in the subcutaneous space in the midaxillary line and brings blood from the subclavian artery to the femoral artery to bypass an aortic obstruction. Femorofemoral bypass brings blood from one femoral artery across to the other. ''Steal'' phenomena does not occur if there is no obstruction to the inflow of the donor artery.

51-8). These operations are effective in relieving aortoiliac, or inflow, obstruction but do not require that the abdominal cavity be entered. The bypass is tunneled in the subcutaneous space, and incisions to expose the axillary and femoral vessels can be performed under local anesthesia. Thus they are safer and more amenable to use in high-risk patients. *Axillofemoral bypasses* are also useful to bypass the aorta in situations of infection within the abdominal cavity. There is no steal of blood from the upper extremity when an axillofemoral bypass is placed because there is an increase in flow in the feeding subclavian artery. This increase is sufficient to supply the arm and both legs. However, the great length of the axillofemoral graft makes it prone to thrombosis.

A *femorofemoral* graft can be used to bypass an iliac artery occlusion if the opposite patent iliac artery is disease free. In this situation one iliac artery is able to deliver enough flow to supply both legs. Five-year patency rates for femorofemoral grafts vary from 44% to 74%.[9,11] Axillofemoral bypass grafts have a poorer patency rate than aortofemoral grafts, with 5-year patency rates reported near 75%. These grafts fail more commonly than an aortobifemoral graft because of their longer course and the risk of external compression in the subcutaneous tunnel. Thus extraanatomic grafts should be considered only when aortobifemoral grafts or local aortoiliac endarterectomies are not feasible.

Femoropopliteal and Femoral Distal Bypass Grafts

Claudication or severe ischemia of the legs despite a good aortoiliac segment is usually the result of obstruction of the superficial femoral or popliteal artery and its branches. A preoperative angiogram will identify the level of arterial obstruction and demonstrate which distal vessels are patent and of adequate caliber to accept a bypass graft. If the popliteal artery is patent with runoff through at least one of the tibial vessels, a *femoropopliteal bypass* is the procedure of choice. If the popliteal artery is occluded, bypass should be performed to the tibial artery that best fills the plantar arch.

The saphenous vein is the most suitable conduit for bypasses below the inguinal ligament. It may be used as a reversed or in situ vein bypass (Fig. 51-9). In a *reversed saphenous vein femoropopliteal bypass,* the saphenous vein is excised, and all branches are ligated and divided. The vein position is reversed so that the distal end of the vein is sewn to the common femoral artery, whereas the proximal portion of the vein is sewn to the popliteal artery. This permits arterial flow to course in the vein in the direction of the valves. An *in situ vein bypass* is left in its normal position.[5] The proximal vein is sewn to the common femoral artery, and the distal portion sewn to the popliteal (or tibial) artery. To permit blood to flow in the vein against the direction of the valves, the valve leaflets must be cut to render them incompetent. The in situ graft avoids extensive dissection of the vein and disruption of the vasa vasorum, provides a better size match between the smaller distal artery and vein, and allows the use of smaller veins that might not be suitable for reversed vein bypass.

If the saphenous vein has been previously excised or is varicose, thrombosed, or otherwise not suitable for a bypass, prosthetic materials such as *polytetrafluoroethylene* or gluteraldehyde-tanned *umbilical vein* can be used. These prosthetic materials have lower long-term patency rates than saphenous vein bypasses but provide good results in the femoropopliteal position. For bypasses to the anterior tibial, posterior tibial, and peroneal arteries, saphenous vein is far superior, and every effort should be made to use vein.

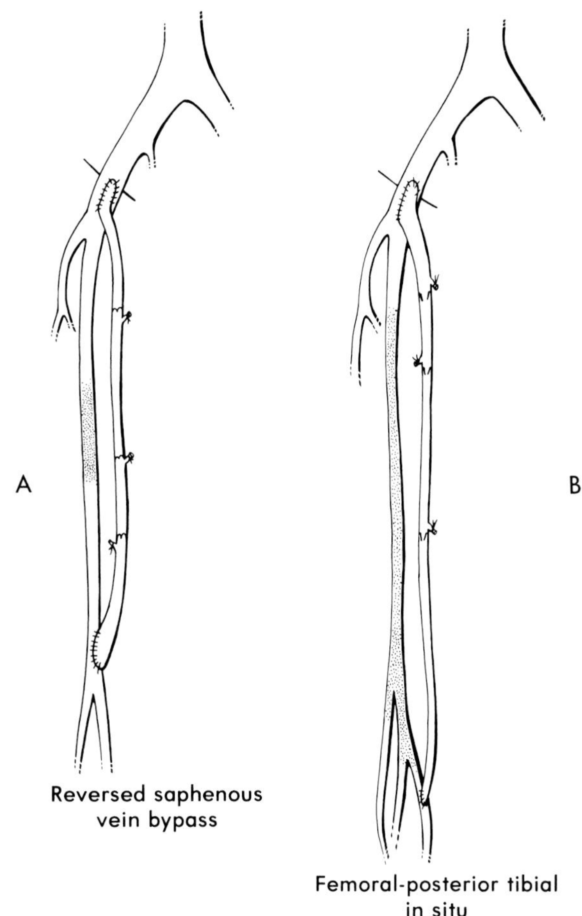

Fig. 51-9 Saphenous vein bypasses in the lower extremity for treatment of femoropopliteal occlusions. These may be performed as a reversed saphenous vein bypass (**A**) or an in situ saphenous vein bypass (**B**). In the in situ bypass, the saphenous vein valves must be cut to render them incompetent. Selection of the site of distal anastomosis depends on angiographic demonstration of the patency of distal arteries.

Limb salvage rate for patients undergoing femoropopliteal bypass grafting is 73% at 5 years; for femoral distal bypass grafts limb salvage is 51% at five years.[33] The limb salvage rates are usually 15% higher than the actual graft patency rates. The patency of each individual graft depends on the adequacy of inflow, the type of graft material used, the quality of the outflow vessels, and the technical aspects of the procedure.

The complications of femoropopliteal and femoral distal bypass grafts are similar to an aortobifemoral procedure. Early thrombosis is the most serious early problem and

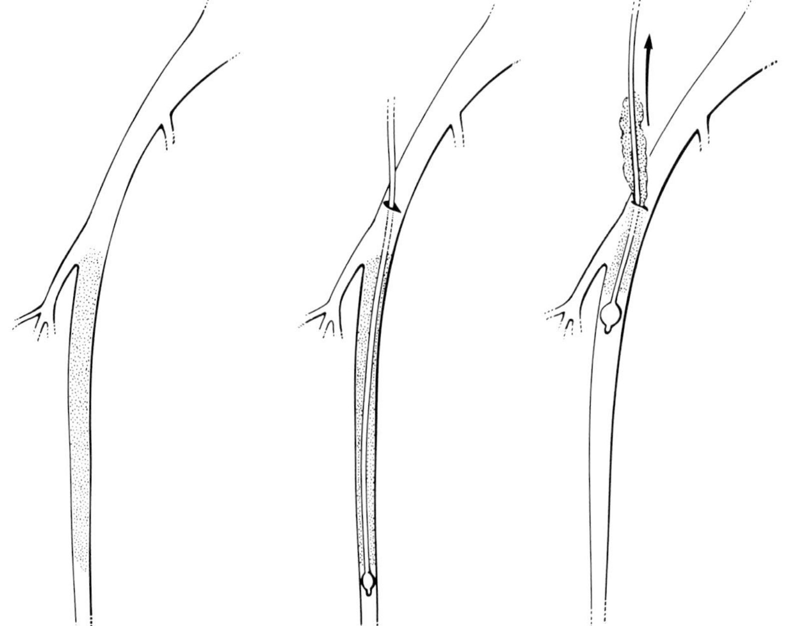

Fig. 51-10 Fogarty catheter balloon embolectomy. Deflated balloon is passed through the thromboembolus. Balloon is inflated and withdrawn, and the embolus is extracted from the artery.

usually represents technical error or inadequate runoff vessels. Prompt thrombectomy and recognition of the technical problem will return function to the graft but usually results in reduction of long-term patency.[6]

Sympathectomy

Lumbar sympathectomy produces vasomotor paralysis, which increases blood flow by decreasing peripheral resistance. Before the advent of direct arterial surgery, sympathectomy was the chief surgical therapeutical approach for peripheral occlusive disease. With progressive improvement in the ability to directly revascularize ischemic tissue, lumbar sympathectomy has fallen into disfavor. It has no beneficial effect in the treatment of claudication but has been reported to improve rest pain in approximately 50% of patients. It has been shown to increase cutaneous, but not muscle, blood flow and thus has been recommended for the treatment of ischemic ulcers. Some surgeons use sympathectomy as an adjunct to arterial reconstruction, believing that sympathectomy adds to the total improvement of blood flow to the extremity by causing vasodilation in the small vessels of the foot. However, there is little evidence that there is improved flow over and above the benefit derived from arterial reconstruction alone. In addition, there are potential complications of lumbar sympathectomy, including postsympathectomy neuralgia and failure of ejaculation. Although sympathectomy has limited usefulness in arteriosclerosis obliterans, it is effective in the treatment of causalgia, Raynaud's disease, and hyperhidrosis.

Embolectomy/Thrombectomy

Acute arterial occlusion with severe ischemia may be caused by emboli, which usually arise from the heart, or by thrombosis of a diseased artery. In addition to the ischemia caused by the embolus, the limb is threatened by propagation of thrombus in the arteries distal to the embolus where blood flow is slow. Therefore patients with acute arterial occlusion should be immediately anticoagulated with heparin. In addition to preventing clot propagation, anticoagulation will help prevent recurrent embolization from the heart.

Removal of the obstructing embolus is readily accomplished using the Fogarty *balloon catheter* (Fig. 51-10). An incision is made in the femoral artery, and the catheter with balloon deflated is passed through the thrombus. The balloon is then inflated, and the clot extracted. This procedure is very effective in removing fresh thrombus and restoring blood flow in patients with embolism. However, bypass may be required to restore flow in patients who have thrombosis induced by severe stenotic plaques.

In some instances thrombi and emboli may be lysed with *thrombolytic* agents such as urokinase or streptokinase administered intravenously or intraarterially directly into the thrombus. These thrombolytic agents are very effective in lysing the thrombus but carry a significant risk of inducing hemorrhage.

ANEURYSMAL DISEASE OF AORTA

The abdominal aorta is particularly vulnerable to aneurysm formation and contains 90% of all aneurysms. Aneurysms are usually located in the infrarenal abdominal aortic segment with sparing of the first 1 to 2 cm below the level of the renal arteries. Aneurysms are usually clinically silent but may enlarge, cause symptoms, and rupture.

Cause of Aortic Aneurysms

Special anatomic features of the infrarenal abdominal aorta may make it vulnerable to the development of aneurysms. The aortic media is composed of groups of smooth muscle cells surrounded by layers of elastin in a network of collagen fibers. The elastin layers serve to allow distensibility of the aortic wall in pulse propagation, whereas the collagen fibers provide tensile strength and prevent overdistention and rupture. The number of medial lamellar units increases proportionally with the aortic diameter to support the tensile stress. The aortic media is nourished by diffusion from the lumen to a depth of approximately 29 medial lamellar units.[35] However, if the aorta is thicker than 29 layers, adventitial vasa vasorum penetrate the media to supply nutrition. The relationship between the number of medial layers and the depth of penetration of vasa in the aortic media applies to both the thoracic aorta and abdominal aortic segment in most mammals. However, the human abdominal aorta is a noticeable exception in that it contains fewer lamellar units than would be expected for its diameter and the media is devoid of vasa vasorum.[36] Thus each layer is thicker than expected and sustains an increased tension per lamellar unit. This may make the aorta vulnerable to relative ischemic injury of the medial smooth muscle cells, leading to medial atrophy in aneurysm formation.[37]

Atherosclerotic plaques are also prone to develop in the infrarenal abdominal aorta and may be a factor in aneurysm formation. Intimal plaques may obstruct diffusion of nutrients from the lumen to the media. Usually there is ingrowth of new medial vasa to supply the media and plaque under these circumstances. When this does not occur, aneurysmal degeneration may take place because of inadequate medial nutrition. Vasa vasorum usually arise from the renal arteries, and the immediate infrarenal aortic segment may have a better vasa vasorum supply than the rest of the aorta. This may explain the relative protection from aneurysm formation in this area.

Other etiologic factors in aneurysm formation have been proposed, including increased elastase or collagenase activity, hemodynamic factors in the infrarenal aorta, copper deficiency, and genetic predisposition.

Aneurysms are also found in the femoral and popliteal arteries, although much less commonly. Patients with peripheral aneurysms usually have coexistent abdominal aortic aneurysms, suggesting a more general aneurysmal diathesis.

Clinical Manifestations

The biologic fate of an aneurysm of the abdominal aorta is to increase in size with eventual rupture. When first detected in a patient, aneurysms may be asymptomatic, symptomatic, or ruptured. In addition, slow flow within the dilated aneurysm may result in thrombus formation along the wall that occasionally may totally occlude the lumen, causing acute ischemia, or may embolize to the distal arterial tree.

Asymptomatic Aneurysms

Aneurysms are remarkable by their clinical silence in the majority of cases. Asymptomatic aneurysms are frequently discovered by palpating a pulsatile mass during physical examination of the abdomen. Since the aortic bifurcation is located at the level of the umbilicus, the pulsatile mass is usually in the epigastrium. Such pulsatile masses must be distinguished from normal aortic pulsations transmitted through a solid organ or tumor that pulsates mainly in a sagittal plane, whereas an aneurysm also pulsates laterally. This is best appreciated by palpation with both hands deep along the lateral margins of the mass. However, aneurysms less than 5 cm in diameter are difficult to palpate, especially in corpulent people; and these aneurysms are usually discovered incidental to x-ray film examination for gastrointestinal, genitourinary, orthopedic, or other lesions.

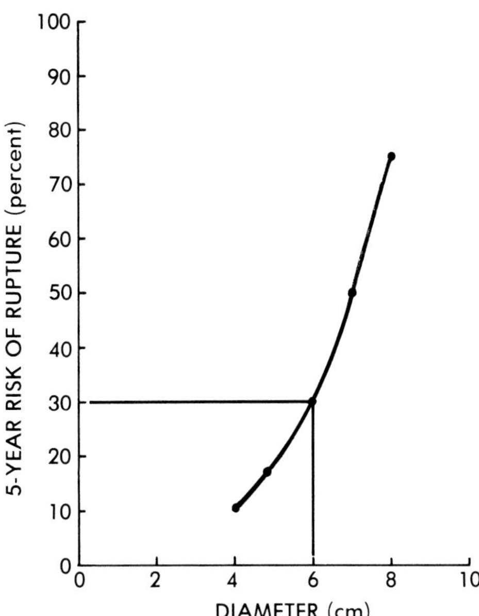

Fig. 51-11 Relationship between the 5-year risk of rupture and the diameter of infrarenal abdominal aortic aneurysms. A 6-cm abdominal aneurysm has a 30% risk of rupturing within 5 years.

The single most important prognostic feature of asymptomatic abdominal aortic aneurysms is the size, or transverse diameter. Small abdominal aortic aneurysms less than 4 cm in diameter have a risk of rupture of less than 15% in 5 years, whereas aneurysms greater than 8 cm in diameter have a 75% risk of rupture over 5 years (Fig. 51-11).

Enlarging and Symptomatic Aneurysms

Aneurysms tend to progressively enlarge because of the increased tension on the artery wall and thinning of artery wall. If this process is slow, symptoms do not appear or are very late in appearing. If, however, enlargement is relatively rapid, symptoms of pain may arise as a result of pressure on the somatic sensory nerve elements of the retroperitoneal soft tissue in the vicinity of the aneurysmal sac. The pain is usually severe, constant, unrelated to posture, and boring in character; it is most commonly located in the lumbar spine region, in the midabdomen, or in the pelvis. Such symptoms indicate impending rupture of the aneurysm and require immediate clinical attention.

Serial follow-up examinations using clinical and radiologic methods will identify the patient with an aneurysm that is expanding and yet asymptomatic. The rate of enlargement can be very variable and unpredictable. The mean rate of expansion of infrarenal abdominal aortic aneurysms is 0.4 cm/year[3]; but some do not change at all, whereas others enlarge at twice that rate.

Ruptured Aneurysms

Aneurysms that rupture usually do so into the retroperitoneal space with the development of severe back pain and sudden hypotension. If the rupture occurs anteriorly, free intraperitoneal hemorrhage results with rapid exsanguination. Rupture can also occur into the inferior vena cava, resulting in the development of an *aortocaval fistula* with hypotension and an elevated central venous pressure. The overall survival of patients with ruptured abdominal aortic aneurysms who survive to reach the hospital averages approximately 50% if treated surgically. The mortality rate of patients with minor contained leaks is not much greater than for elective repair, but if free intraperitoneal bleeding and shock are present, survival is less than 20%. On physical examination ruptured aneurysms, even large ones, may be difficult to palpate because of hypotension and because the aortic aneurysm is often diffuse and ill defined as a result of obliteration of the margins of the aneurysm by retroperitoneal hematoma.

Diagnosis

The diagnosis of abdominal aortic aneurysm may be made on physical examination. However, physical examination commonly overestimates the true size of the aneurysm by 1 to 2 cm when compared to ultrasound or (CT) computed tomography examination. *A cross table lateral x-ray* may demonstrate a rim of clacium outlining the anterior wall of the abdominal aorta and indicate the presence of an aneurysm. This x-ray film is taken with the patient lying supine with the x-ray beam running horizontally allowing intestinal gas to rise superiorly and the retroperitoneum to be visualized. Physical examination and a lateral x-ray film were in the past the predominant methods of evaluation for an abdominal aortic aneurysm. However, in view of the new development of ultrasound, the lateral abdominal x-ray film is currently used infrequently.

B-mode ultrasound is the most commonly used method of diagnosing an abdominal aortic aneurysm. It is simple, safe, noninvasive and accurate and can be readily repeated for serial evaluation of aneurysms. It provides information on the presence or absence of an aneurysm and on the transverse diameter, length, and presence or absence of mural thrombus. It is the procedure of choice for routine evaluation for aneurysm.

CT scan provides better resolution and imaging of aneurysms than ultrasound, especially when intravenous contrast enhancement is used. It provides the most detailed evaluation of the aortic wall and mural thrombus, and the most accurate assessment of aneurysm size. It also allows the evaluation of retroperitoneal extravasation and rupture. However, the procedure is more expensive than ultrasound and usually is not essential for most abdominal aneurysms. The CT scan offers significant advantages over ultrasound in assessing the thoracoabdominal aorta since ultrasound will not pass through the air in the lung and cannot visualize the thoracic aorta. Thus it is particularly helpful in assessing thoracoabdominal aneurysms. In addition, CT is very useful in evaluating the pelvis for the presence of internal iliac aneurysms.

Angiography is useful in the evaluation of abdominal aortic aneurysms but provides little information on aneurysm size since only the aortic lumen is visualized. Aneurysms frequently contain mural thrombus, which may result in a normal or relatively normal lumen contour and diameter. This mural thrombus provides no structural strength to the aortic wall, and such aneurysms are just as likely to rupture as those without extensive mural thrombosis. Despite the fact that aortic angiography may not accurately represent aneurysm size, other important information can be obtained, including (1) accurate assessment of the proximal extent of the aneurysm in relation to the renal arteries, (2) the status of the renal arteries and the presence of accessory renal arteries arising from the aneurysm itself, (3) the inferior mesenteric artery and its collateral blood supply to the left colon, (4) coexistent occlusive disease of the iliac and femoral vessels, and (5) identification of congenital abnormalities of the kidneys such as horseshoe kidney.

Treatment

Indications for Surgery

Indications for surgical repair of abdominal aortic aneurysms depend on the presence or absence of symptoms, the size of the aneurysm, and the general medical condition of the patient. If a patient has a ruptured aortic aneurysm, immediate surgical treatment is imperative. No diagnostic tests should be performed, and resuscitation should be carried out in the operating room. External compression of the legs and abdomen with a G-suit and fluid resuscitation may be useful during transport.

Patients with symptoms attributable to an aneurysm but without hypotension or signs of rupture should undergo confirmatory ultrasound or CT examination and urgent operative repair of the aneurysm. Similarly, if there is evidence of rapid enlargement of the aneurysm on routine physical examination or x-ray film follow-up such as B-mode ultrasound, urgent repair of the aneurysm is advised.

The absolute size of the aneurysm also determines whether repair should be undertaken. Studies of the natural history of aneurysms reveal that the risk of rupture of untreated aneurysms is directly proportional to their size.[2,30] Aneurysms greater than 5 cm in transverse diameter as measured by ultrasound or CT scan or aneurysms that have more than twice the diameter of the adjacent, nonaneurysmal aorta should be surgically repaired if the patient has no medical contraindications to surgery such as severe cardiac, pulmonary, renal, or neoplastic disease. However, it must be realized that aneurysms smaller than 5 cm can also rupture and must be carefully observed.

Surgical Repair

The surgical treatment of an abdominal aortic aneurysm consists of excluding the aneurysm from the circulation and replacing it with a Dacron prosthetic bypass graft. The aorta is clamped proximal to the aneurysm, below the level of the renal arteries, and distal to the aneurysm. The aneurysm sac is opened, and the graft sutured to the normal,

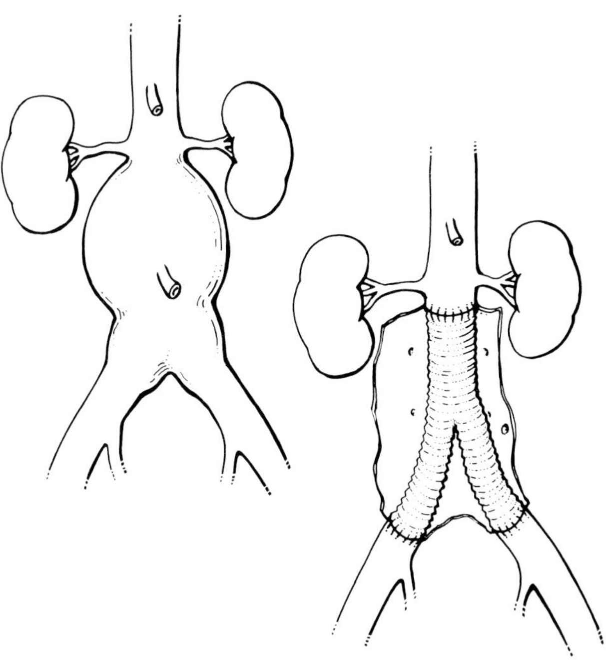

Fig. 51-12 Repair of abdominal aortic aneurysm. Aneurysm sac is opened, and a Dacron graft is sutured to the normal, nonaneurysmal artery. Aneurysm is not excised, but it is excluded from the circulation.

nonaneurysmal aorta from within the aneurysm. The graft may be a straight "tube" graft confined to the abdominal aorta or a bifurcation graft to the iliac arteries if the aortic bifurcation and iliac arteries are involved (Fig. 51-12). The aneurysm sac is not excised but closed over the graft after it is in place in order to isolate the graft from the bowel. This prevents possible erosion of the bowel, aortoduodenal fistula formation, and graft infection. The inferior mesenteric artery, which always arises from the aneurysm, is usually ligated. Collateral circulation from the celiac and superior mesenteric arteries and internal iliac arteries maintains flow to the sigmoid colon. Occasionally, when collateral flow is insufficient, the inferior mesenteric artery must be reimplanted into the bypass graft in order to avoid colonic ischemia.

Results and Long-Term Outlook

The results of abdominal aortic aneurysm repair differ depending on whether the procedure is performed electively for an asymptomatic aneurysm, urgently for a symptomatic aneurysm, or emergently for a ruptured aneurysm. Elective aneurysm repair and urgent repair of nonruptured aneurysms have a mortality rate of less than 3%.[8,32] Operations for ruptured abdominal aortic aneurysms have a mortality rate of 50% to 80% or higher.[12] Thus every effort should be made to repair abdominal aortic aneurysms before rupture. Improved operative techniques with better preoperative and perioperative care, including central hemodynamic monitoring, earlier diagnosis, improvements in fluid management, and refinements in anesthesia techniques, have allowed elective aneurysm repair to be carried out with a similar low mortality rate even in octogenarians.[21] Thus age alone is not a contraindication to aneurysm repair.

The long-term survival of patients who have undergone abdominal aortic aneurysm repair is approximately 50% at 5 years. Associated coronary artery disease is responsible for the majority of deaths in the long-term follow-up of these patients. In a matched group, the expected 5-year survival is 80%.[32] It is possible that with more aggressive treatment of coexistent coronary disease that this mortality rate can be decreased. The overall survival and long-term outlook with elective repair of abdominal aortic aneurysms is significantly better than nonsurgical treatment, which is associated with a 50% 1-year mortality.

PERIPHERAL ARTERY ANEURYSMS

Although it is not common, aneurysms can form in arteries other than the aorta. The most commonly involved peripheral arteries are the common femoral and popliteal arteries that together account for 90% of all peripheral aneurysms. The popliteal artery accounts for 70% of these aneurysms. *Popliteal aneurysms* are unique in that they are found almost exclusively in males and the vast majority are atherosclerotic in origin. Approximately two thirds of the patients have bilateral aneurysms, with one half of these patients having associated abdominal aortic aneurysms.

Popliteal aneurysms are usually symptomatic when discovered, and over 50% present with complications.[10] The most common complication is thrombosis of the aneurysm, which is associated with a 33% amputation rate. Embolization of mural thrombus from within the aneurysm to the distal arterial tree also occurs and is associated with a high amputation rate. Rupture of popliteal aneurysms is unusual but can occur. Compression of the popliteal vein with lower extremity edema and neurologic pain syndromes from nerve compression are also possible.

Treatment of popliteal aneurysms consists of ligation of the aneurysm to exclude it from the circulation, followed by bypass grafting from the femoral artery to either the popliteal or tibial vessels. Results of surgery are influenced by the status of the leg at the time of presentation and the extent of coexistent occlusive disease in the tibial vessels and vessels of the foot. If these are obstructed because of prior and repeated embolization from the aneurysm, prospects for revascularization are poor. There is minimal limb loss in patients with asymptomatic aneurysms, but 34% of limbs are lost if the patient presents with symptoms.[10] Therefore popliteal aneurysms should be repaired electively when found, before symptoms of embolization or thrombosis occur.

Femoral artery aneurysms are similarly found in elderly males and are caused by atherosclerosis. Associated hypertension is extremely common. Associated abdominal aortic aneurysms are present in 51% to 85% of patients[7,14] and in the popliteal artery segment in 17% to 44% of patients,[1,14] suggesting an aneurysmal diathesis. As in the popliteal artery, symptoms may be caused by local pressure from the expanding aneurysm on the adjacent femoral vein or nerve, distal embolization, acute or chronic thrombosis, or rupture of the aneurysm. Because of the risk of limb loss from acute thrombosis and distal embolization, surgical management of these aneurysms is advised in all patients who are reasonable medical risks. Surgical techniques include replacement of the aneurysm with an interposition graft.

COMPLICATIONS OF VASCULAR PROCEDURES

Complications following vascular procedures fall into two categories: those involving the generalized disease process of atherosclerosis and those involving local factors related to the vascular procedure or bypass graft.

The generalized process of atherosclerosis involves not only the peripheral arteries but also the carotid and coronary arteries. The risk factors of hypertension, hyperlipidemia, diabetes mellitus, and cigarette smoking are important in whether there is disease progression, stabilization or regression; and control of these factors is important. The major cause of morbidity and mortality in the vascular surgical patient is disease progression in the coronary arteries, with myocardial infarctions accounting for the majority of deaths in these patients despite successful peripheral vascular procedures. Stroke from progression of cerebrovascular disease is also a major problem. These same risk factors play a major role in the progression of distal disease following bypass grafts and are a common reason for restenosis and subsequent graft occlusion and its related morbidity.

Local factors related to vascular procedures may produce a number of complications following vascular procedures. Graft thrombosis in the early postoperative period may be the result of a technical error in the graft-to-artery anastomosis or caused by an obstructed outflow bed with slow flow in the graft. Late graft occlusion is usually caused by progression of atherosclerotic occlusive disease in the inflow or outflow vessels or by a hypertrophic proliferative response of intima at the anastomosis and can usually be corrected by reoperation.

Pseudoaneurysms may form at the sites of vascular anastomoses and must be distinguished from true aneurysms that involved dilation of all layers of the artery wall. In a pseudoaneurysm there is separation of the vascular graft from the artery wall, and the bloodstream is contained by surrounding fibrous tissue. The integrity of an anastomosis of prosthetic graft to artery is forever dependent on the integrity of the suture line. Failure of the suture or excess tension on the suture line can result in the disruption of the anastomosis with pseudoaneurysm formation. In addition, anastomotic breakdown with pseudoaneurysm formation may be a harbinger or sign that infection of the prosthetic bypass graft has occurred. Treatment of a pseudoaneurysm mandates replacement of that segment with a prosthetic graft if it is not infected. However, infected grafts must be totally removed because prosthetic grafts are foreign bodies and infection cannot be eradicated until all foreign material is excised.

Revascularization under these circumstances is complex and usually involves the use of an "extraanatomic" bypass in a clean, noninfected area. An example of such a bypass is an axillofemoral bypass to bypass an infected intra-abdominal aortoiliac bypass graft.

SUMMARY

Atherosclerosis is a degenerative disease process that affects the aorta and peripheral arteries, as well as coronary and carotid arteries. It can result in occlusive disease, obstructing the lumen or aneurysmal disease with dilation of the lumen. Occlusive disease can result in stenosis and diminished blood flow or embolization with occlusion of distal arteries. Obstruction of blood flow can result in ischemia of the lower extremities, producing symptoms of claudication, rest pain, ulceration or gangrene. Obstructions can be detected with the use of clinical, noninvasive, and angiographic diagnostic techniques. Revascularization of the lower extremities with a bypass or with transluminal balloon angioplasty can restore circulation and avoid limb loss.

Aneurysmal disease results in progressive arterial enlargement and weakening of the aortic wall, with eventual rupture unless the patient dies of intercurrent disease. The larger the aneurysm, the higher the risk of rupture. Most aneurysms are asymptomatic and are detectable by noninvasive techniques. Operative replacement of aneurysmal segments of artery with a Dacron graft will prevent further degeneration and aneurysm rupture.

REFERENCES

1. Baird, R.J., et al.: Arteriosclerotic femoral artery aneurysms, Can. Med. Assoc. J. **117:**1306, 1977.
2. Bernstein, E.F.: The natural history of abdominal aortic aneurysms. In Najarian, J.S., and Delaney, J.P., editors: Vascular surgery, Miami, 1978, Symposia Specialists.
3. Bernstein, E.F., et al.: Growth rates of small abdominal arotic aneurysms, Surgery **80:**765, 1976.
4. Brewster, D.C., and Darling, R.C.: Optimal methods of aortoiliac reconstruction, Surgery **84:**739, 1978.
5. Corson, J.D., et al.: In situ vein bypasses to distal tibial and limited outflow tracts for limb salvage, Surgery **96:**756, 1984.
6. Craver, J.M., et al.: Hemorrhage and thrombosis as early complications of femoropopliteal bypass grafts: causes, treament, and prognostic implications, Surgery **74:**839, 1971.
7. Cutler, B.S., and Darling, R.C.: Surgical management of arteriosclerotic femoral aneurysms, Surgery **74:**764, 1973.
8. DeBakey, M.D., et al.: Aneurysms of abdominal aorta: analysis of results of graft replacement therapy one to eleven years after operation, Ann. Surg. **160:**622, 1964.
9. Eugene, J., Goldstone, J., and Moore, W.S.: Fifteen-year experience with subcutaneous bypass grafts for lower extremity ischemia, Ann. Surg. **186:**177, 1976.
10. Evans, W.E., Conley, J.E., and Bernhard, V.: Popliteal aneurysms, Surgery **70:**762, 1971.
11. Flanigan, P., et al.: Hemodynamic and angiographic guidelines in selection of patients for femorofemoral bypass, Arch. Surg. **113:**1257, 1978.
12. Garrett, H.E., and Ilabaca, P.A.: The ruptured abdominal aortic aneurysm. In Bergan, J.J., and Yao, J.S.T., editors: Aneurysms: diagnosis and treatment, New York, 1982, Grune & Stratton, Inc.
13. Gordon, T., and Kannel, W.B.: Predisposition to atherosclerosis in the head, heart, and legs: the Framingham study, JAMA **221:**661, 1972.
14. Graham, L., et al.: Clinical significance of arteriosclerotic femoral artery aneurysms, Arch. Surg. **115:**502, 1980.
15. Jeurgens, J.L., Barker, N.W., and Hines, E.A.: Arteriosclerosis obliterans: review of 520 cases with special reference to pathogenic and prognostic factors, Circulation **21:**188, 1960.
16. Johnston, K.W., and Colapinto, R.F.: Transluminal dilatation—a surgeon's viewpoint, Vasc. Diagn. Ther. **2:**15, 1981.
17. Kumpe, D.A., and Jones, D.N.: Percutaneous transluminal angioplasty radiological viewpoint, Vasc. Diagn. Ther. **3:**19, 1982.

18. Lipid Research Clinics Program: The lipid research clinic coronary primary prevention trial results, Parts I and II, JAMA **251**:351, 1984.
19. Martin, E.C., et al.: Angioplasty for femoral artery occlusions: comparison with surgery. Am. J. Roentgenol. **137**:915, 1981.
20. May, A.G., DeWeese, J.A., and Rob, C.G.: Hemodynamic effects of arterial stenosis, Surgery **53**:513, 1963.
21. O'Donnell, T.F., Jr., Darling, R.C., and Linton, R.R.: Is 80 years too old for aneurysmectomy? Arch. Surg. **111**:1250, 1976.
22. Peabody, C.N., Kannel, W.B., and McNamara, P.M.: Intermittent claudication: surgical significance, Arch. Surg. **109**:693, 1974.
23. Porter, J.M., et al.: Pentoxifylline efficacy in the treatment of intermittent claudication, Am. Heart J. **104**:66, 1982.
24. The Pooling Project Research Group: Relationship of blood pressure, serum cholesterol, smoking habit, relative weight, and EEG abnormalities to incidence of major coronary events: final report of the Pooling Project, J. Chronic Dis. **31**:201, 1978.
25. Ross, R., and Harker, L.: Hyperlipidemia and atherosclerosis, Science **193**:1094, 1976.
26. Rush, D.S., et al.: Limb salvage in poor-risk patients using transluminal angioplasty, Arch. Surg. **118**:1209, 1983.
27. Shehadi, W.H., and Tonielo, G.: Adverse reactions to contrast media, Radiology **137**:299, 1980.
28. Smith, C.D., and McKendry, R.J.: Controlled trial of nifedipine in the treatment of Raynaud's phenomenon, Lancet **2**:1299, 1982.
29. Stemmer, E.A.: Vascular complications of diabetes mellitus. In Moore, W.S., editor: Vascular surgery: a comprehensive review, Orlando, 1984, Grune & Stratton, Inc.
30. Szilagyi, D.E., Elliott, J.P., and Smith, R.F.: Clinical fate of patients with asymptomatic abdominal aortic aneurysm and unfit for special treatment, Arch. Surg. **104**:600, 1972.
31. Thompson, J.E., et al.: Arterial embolectomy: a 20-year experience with 163 cases, Surgery **67**:212, 1970.
32. Thompson, J.E., et al.: Surgical management of abdominal aortic aneurysms: factors influencing mortality and morbidity—a 20-year experience, Ann. Surg. **188**:654, 1975.
33. Veith, F.J., et al.: Progress in limb salvage by reconstructive arterial surgery combined with new or improved adjunctive procedures, Am. Surg. **194**:386, 1981.
34. Waltman, A.C., et al.: Transluminal angioplasty of the iliac and femoropopliteal arteries: current status, Arch. Surg. **117**:1218, 1981.
35. Wolinsky, H., and Glagov, S.: Nature of species differences in the medial distribution of aortic vasa vasorum in mammals, Circ. Res. **20**:409, 1967.
36. Wolinsky, H., and Glagov, S.: Comparison of abdominal and thoracic aortic medial structure in mammals: deviation of man from the usual pattern, Circ. Res. **25**:677, 1969.
37. Zarins, C.K., and Glagov, S.: Aneurysms and obstructive plaques: differing local responses to atherosclerosis. In Bergan, J.J., and Yao, J.S.T., editors: Aneurysms: diagnosis and treatment, New York, 1982, Grune & Stratton, Inc.
38. Zarins, C.K., et al.: Arterial disruption and remodeling following ballon dilatation, Surgery **92**:1086, 1982.
39. Zarins, C.K., et al.: Carotid bifurcation atherosclerosis: quantitative correlation of plaque localization with flow velocity profiles and wall shear stress, Circ. Res. **53**:502, 1983.

52 Bruce L. Gewertz

Cerebrovascular Disease and Upper Extremity Vascular Disease

In each calendar year nearly 500,000 Americans suffer cerebral infarctions; 175,000 strokes are fatal, whereas the remaining patients experience variable disability. The emotional and economic consequences of advanced cerebrovascular disease are staggering; the cost of care and loss of earnings secondary to permanent disability or death have been estimated at more than $10 billion annually.

In contrast to these depressing statistics, there has been a persistent 10-year decline in the death rate from stroke that has exceeded the general decline in cardiovascular mortality observed over the same time period.[36] It is difficult to explain this phenomenon. Although surgery for extracranial occlusive disease has become much more common in the last 15 years, improved medical and surgical care can account for only a small fraction of the change in death rate. It is most likely that the decline in cardiovascular mortality reflects better control of arterial hypertension, changes in life-style, and the general reduction in cigarette smoking.

Although the natural history of stroke in the United States was defined in an earlier era, studies performed from 1950 to 1975 provide useful information regarding the indications and timing of cerebrovascular surgery.[32,53] The following are now accepted facts.

1. Patients who have survived one cerebral infarction have a high incidence of *recurrent strokes* (approximately 25%). More than half of these recurrent strokes are fatal.
2. Prodromal symptoms of stroke such as *transient cerebral ischemic attacks* identify patients at greatest risk of suffering later completed strokes. The cumulative stroke rate approaches 50% at 5 years and is highest in the first year after the transient ischemic episode.[52]

In this chapter the anatomy and physiology of cerebral blood flow will be reviewed, the variable clinical presentations of cerebral ischemia characterized, and the diagnostic and therapeutic options considered. It has become clear that only through better understanding of cerebrovascular physiology can the care of patients with advanced vascular disease be improved.

CEREBRAL BLOOD FLOW

Anatomy

The brain is perfused by paired carotid and vertebral arteries that communicate with each other through the circle of Willis at the base of the skull. Although there is substantial variation in the effectiveness of this collateral network (less than 20% of patients have "complete" circles), occlusion of one vessel is frequently compensated for without neurologic deficit. In general terms a carotid artery supplies only the ipsilateral cerebral hemisphere through the middle, anterior, and posterior cerebral vessels. The vertebral arteries join to form a single basilar artery that supplies the brainstem and cerebellum with additional contributions to the posterior aspect of the circle of Willis (Fig. 52-1).

Boundary zones or "watershed" areas between the primary perfusion territories of the middle, anterior, and posterior cerebral arteries can be demonstrated by anatomic studies. These areas are most at risk for ischemia and infarction during hypotension or vascular occlusion. Perhaps because of the lower basal vascular tone of these vessels, boundary zones are frequently the site of intracerebral hemorrhages associated with acute hypertension.

The subclavian origin of both vertebral arteries makes possible the unique subclavian steal syndrome that will be discussed in greater detail later in this chapter (Fig. 52-2). This syndrome occurs when an occlusive lesion proximal to the origin of the vertebral vessels decreases perfusion pressure in the distal subclavian artery. The vertebral artery then functions as a collateral pathway for the arm, and reversal of flow (away from the cranium) can be demonstrated angiographically. This flow pattern "steals" blood from the basilar system and may result in cerebellar ischemia or infarction.

Characteristics of Flow

The cerebral circulation is supplied with nearly 15% of cardiac output. Resting total blood flows range from 50 to 60 ml/min/100 g of tissue, with higher values in the cellular grey matter (100 ml/min/100 g) and lower flows in the cell poor white matter (20 ml/min/100 g).[17,37] Cerebral blood flow is regulated by both metabolic and myogenic mechanisms that tend to maintain or "autoregulate" perfusion to avoid cerebral infarction during hypotension and cerebral hemorrhage during hypertension.[26] Cerebral infarcts may result when regional blood flows decline below 15 ml/min/100 g, although the metabolic state of the brain strongly influences the likelihood of cell death.[34] Barbiturate coma has been shown to decrease the ischemic limit to as low as 5 ml/min/100 g.[50]

The cerebral circulation is further distinguished by a *blood-brain barrier* that effectively isolates brain tissue from serum ionic changes and humoral factors.[1] The barrier is both a physical and biochemical impediment to the transport of protein and polar substances into cerebral extracellular fluid. Anatomic features include very tight junctions between endothelial cells, with only a few scattered pores and minimal transport by pinocytotic vesicles. A membrane-bound enzyme system, primarily composed of monoamine oxidase, effectively degrades circulating catecholamines and limits cerebral extraction to less than 5%. It is noteworthy that the areas of the brain responsible for hormone regulation such as the hypothalamus, pituitary gland, and pineal gland, do *not* demonstrate the anatomic or functional characteristics of the blood-brain barrier.

The blood-brain barrier is disrupted in areas of tissue infarction and during periods of severe hypertension.[30] These observations are clinically important since breakdown of the blood-brain barrier (1) facilitates the diagnosis of cerebral infarcts by radionuclide scanning, and (2) explains the occurrence of late hemorrhage in previously "bland" infarcts when patients become severely hypertensive.

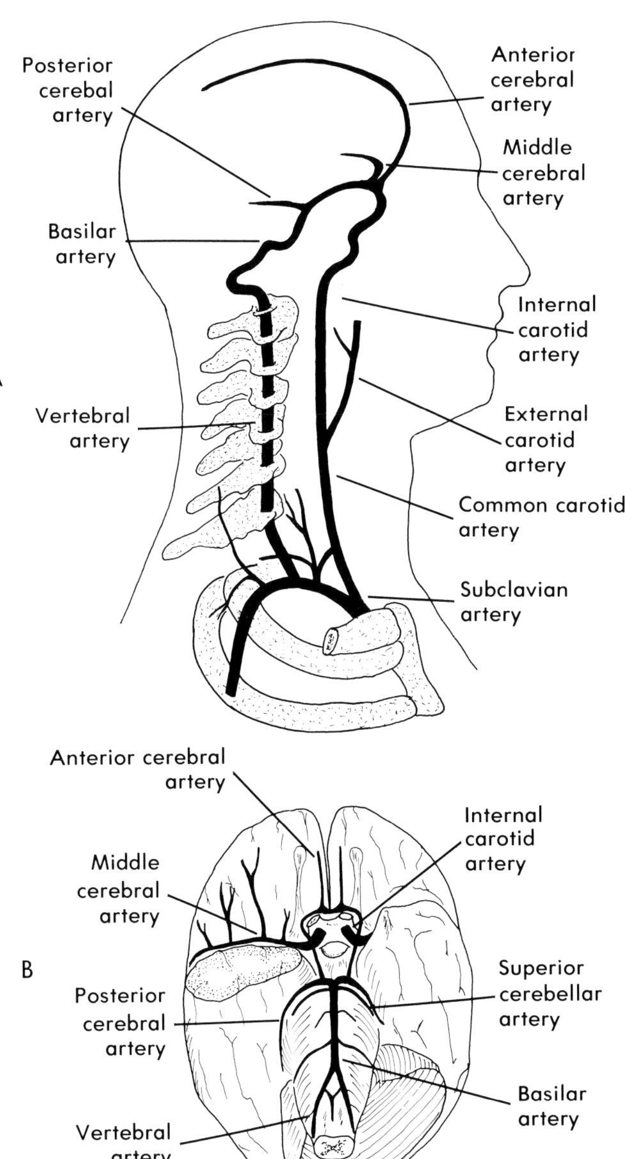

Fig. 52-1 **A,** Carotid artery supplies middle cerebral and anterior cerebral arteries predominantly with major contributions to posterior cerebral artery. **B,** Vertebral arteries form the basilar artery that supplies cerebellar vessels and posterior cerebral arteries.

Measurement Techniques

Diverse methods have been used to measure cerebral blood flow in experimental settings, including venous outflow collections, radioactive microspheres, autoradiography, and heat or hydrogen clearance.[6] In clinical practice most measurements of total and regional cerebral blood flow are made on the basis of the clearance of inhaled inert gases including xenon-133. Using the modified Kety-Schmit technique, xenon-133 washout is monitored by external gamma scintillation counters and subjected to "curve stripping" to remove any component of extracranial blood flow. This technique is most accurate in the middle cerebral distribution and least helpful in evaluating the posterior cerebral or cerebellar circulations.

The recent introductions of positive emission tomography allows repeated imaging of radionuclide concentration in any transverse section of the brain.[43] Depending on the labeled element, regional blood flow ($H_{2O}{}^{15}$), or substrate use (C^{11}-glucose) can be measured. Although this technology is still regarded as a research tool, it provides the most precise metabolic and flow data available.

Flow Regulatory Mechanisms

Pressure-flow autoregulation is the ability of an organ to maintain normal blood flow despite variations in blood pressure. This protective mechanism is well documented in the cerebral circulation. Most physiologists agree that the process is an intrinsic property of blood vessels involving a continuous readjustment of the myogenic activity of vascular smooth muscle that depends on changes in transmural pressure and the local (extracellular) chemical environment. Increased intravascular pressure (hypertension) predictably results in compensatory vasoconstriction,

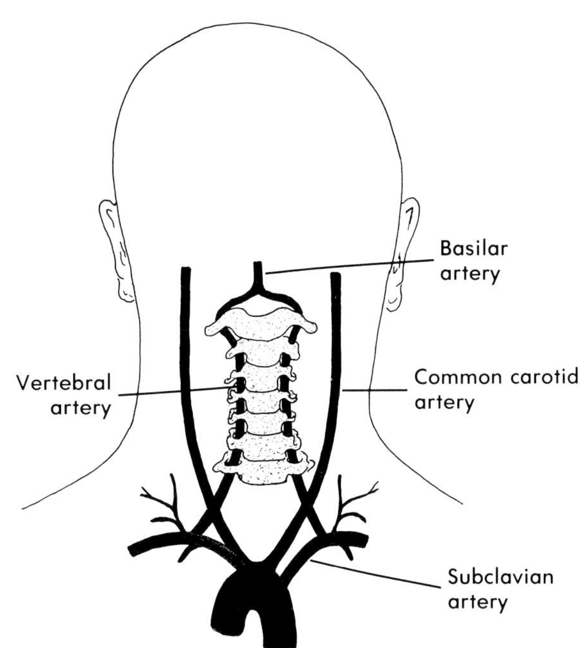

Fig. 52-2 Subclavian origin of vertebral arteries allows these vessels to function as collateral pathways for upper extremity. Cerebellar ischemia may result from the "steal" of blood flow.

whereas decreased pressure (hypotension) elicits vasocilation.[19] Although early experiments suggested that Pco_2 was the primary chemical regulator of vascular tone, it has become well accepted that the hydrogen ion concentration in the extracellular space provides the vasodilatory influence.[3,25]

Decreasing Pco_2 results in lower hydrogen ion concentration, and vasoconstriction is observed. An elevated Pco_2 leads to higher hydrogen ion concentration and vasodilation. This relationship is applied clinically in the management of severe head injuries; hyperventilation with resultant hypocarbia and decreased hydrogen ion concentration decreases cerebral blood flow and attenuates posttraumatic cerebral edema. Responses to changes in Po_2 are less vigorous, although hypoxia does result in moderate cerebral vasodilation.

Sympathetic stimulation and other neural stimuli have only a small influence on cerebrovascular resistance and blood flow autoregulation.[14] In fact, there is minimal histologic evidence of adrenergic vasoconstrictive fibers on cortical vessels.[42] Neurally mediated vasoconstriction is limited to large vessels outside the brain proper and as such does not represent a primary regulatory mechanism.[27]

CLINICAL PRESENTATION OF CEREBROVASCULAR DISEASE

Definitions

For purposes of discussion, clinicians have grouped neurologic deficits into four categories. *Transient ischemic attacks* are classically defined as short-lived, often repetitive alterations of mentation, vision, motor, or sensory function that are completely reversed within 24 hours. Although transient ischemic attacks often involve the middle cerebral artery distribution and present with contralateral arm, leg, and facial weakness, perhaps the most well-recognized episodes involve transient monocular blindness (*amaurosis fugax* or "fleeting blindness"). Transient ischemic attacks that last only a few minutes may be prognostically different from those deficits that persist for longer than 2 hours. For this reason, longer lasting episodes (2 to 72 hours) that still result in no permanent neurologic deficit or radiologic evidence of brain infarction are usually designated *reversible ischemic neurologic deficits*.

A documented cerebral infarction *(stroke* or *cerebrovascular accident)* implies a permanent neurologic deficit that is usually associated with computed tomography scan evidence. Neurologic recovery is quite variable and may be complete, but the time course of recovery (weeks or months) cleary distinguishes infarcts from transient ischemic attacks or reversible ischemic neurologic deficits. A "stuttering stroke" in which the neurologic deficit "waxes and wanes" has been termed *stroke-in-evolution*. This type of presentation is not as common but has received much recent attention because of the potential that therapeutic maneuvers could improve the eventual outcome.[28,38]

Although the above definitions have aided communication, they can be criticized for arbitrarily grouping diverse mechanisms with quite variable prognoses. For example, transient ischemic attacks can be caused by migraines, seizure disorders, and intracranial aneurysms, as well as carotid artery lesions. This "lumping" phenomena is most confusing when large multicenter studies attempt to characterize the natural history of a clinical presentation without rigorous preselection on the basis of cause.

Mechanisms

Symptoms of cerebrovascular disease reflect both the mechanism of ischemia and the specific areas affected. In general, ischemia and infarction result from either *low flow* in large or medium-sized vessels associated with obstructive lesions or hypotension or *emboli* to smaller vessels from proximal ulcerative lesions or turbulent flow. Hemodynamic derangements predisposing to the low flow are manifest clinically by neurologic deficits corresponding to the "watershed areas" between main cerebral artery perfusion territories. Symptoms of embolic occlusion depend on the site of distal impaction. Predictably the size of the embolus determines the vessel it will occlude. Both mechanisms can result in permanent and reversible deficits.[40] In particular, repetitive short-lived neurologic deficits (i.e., transient ischemic attacks) are compatible with either (1) recurrent ischemia of watershed areas or (2) impaction and lysis of intermittent platelet emboli following a consistent route mandated by hemodynamics and anatomy.

The most common disease process involving the cerebral and extracranial vessels is atherosclerosis.[46] Although the disease is most prevalent in patients over the age of 50, presentations of younger patients are not rare. In roughly half of the cases the atheroma is localized to the extracranial bifurcation of the common carotid into the internal and external carotid arteries. Such atherosclerotic plaques may slowly encroach on the arterial lumen or suddenly occlude following intraplaque hemorrhage.[29]

Other pathologic processes are less common and may more frequently involve younger patients. These include spontaneous subintimal dissections of the internal carotid and fibromuscular dysplasia.

Although it is generally accepted that the majority of emboli arise from ulcerated atherosclerotic lesions in the common or internal carotid artery, the intracranial carotid siphon near the origin of the ophthalmic artery can also harbor symptomatic ulcerative lesions. Stenoses and occlusions can involve either the extracranial or intracranial carotid arteries, both areas simultaneously (tandem lesions), or any portion of a specific cerebral artery.[12,18]

TYPES OF CEREBROVASCULAR DISEASE

Extracranial Carotid Artery Disease

Clinical presentation

The symptoms of extracranial carotid disease can be described by the timing of impairment (permanent, transient, relapsing) and the type of neurologic deficit (motor, sensory, cognitive, or communicative). As discussed earlier in this chapter, both decreases in cerebral blood flow and embolic occlusions can produce the entire clinical spectrum. The persistence of any neurologic deficit is synonymous with death of brain tissue. Transient and relapsing episodes unassociated with infarctions are distinguished by the return of the neurologic examination to normal.

The exact nature of a deficit can be directly correlated with the area of brain rendered ischemic. The most commonly involved area is the perfusion territory of the middle cerebral artery (the parietal lobe) that is the main outflow vessel of the carotid artery. The patient with middle cerebral ischemia presents with contralateral hemiparesis or hemiplegia, usually more severe in the arm, and paralysis of the contralateral lower part of the face ("central seventh nerve paralysis"). Associated findings including some degree of hypesthesia (decreased sensation) on the paralyzed side and a contralateral homonymous hemianopsia (visual field deficit). Aphasia (difficulty with speech) is noted if the dominant hemisphere is involved. The left hemisphere is dominant in nearly all right-handed people and roughly 50% of left-handed people. Such defects can be expressive (Broca's aphasia), receptive (Wernicke's aphasia), or complete. If the nondominant hemisphere is affected, a curious "neglect response" is noted in which the paralyzed extremity is essentially ignored by the patient.

Ischemia of the anterior cerebral artery most commonly presents with contralateral monoplegia involving only the lower extremity; visual-spatial problems and cortical sensory loss are also common.

Posterior cerebral artery ischemia may result from carotid occlusive disease but is also closely related to vertebral-basilar lesions. Presentations often include visual field defects and may overlap with symptoms of ischemia of the posterior portion of the middle cerebral distribution such as language disturbances and contralateral hemiparesis. Other neurologic signs consistent with posterior cerebral artery ischemia include ipsilateral third cranial nerve palsy and contralateral complete sensory loss (thalamic syndrome).

Diagnosis

Symptomatic carotid artery disease is commonly associated with the above neurologic presentations. However, it is essential to exclude other causes for such syndromes, including migraines, brain tumors, intracranial hemorrhage, and vascular malformations.

The physical finding most consistent with extracranial carotid disease is a demonstration of a *bruit* on auscultation of the upper cervical region reflecting turbulent blood flow at a stenosis. Classic carotid bruits have the following characteristics: they are (1) high pitched and fade into diastole, (2) localized to the angle of the jaw, and (3) best heard with the bell rather than the diaphragm of the stethoscope. Unfortunately, even experienced examiners frequently cannot distinguish internal or common carotid bruits from clinically irrelevant turbulence in the distal external carotid artery or other cervical blood vessels. As many as 50% of symptomatic ulcerations may be unassociated with stenoses and hence may not present with bruits. Finally, when a stenosis exceeds 90% of vascular cross-sectional area, the intensity of the bruit often decreases because of lower volume flow. This lack of specificity of cervical bruits is most disturbing in asymptomatic patients with bruits since physical examination alone does not allow assessment of the degree or even the presence of carotid disease.

Many noninvasive tests have been developed to better characterize extracranial carotid disease without the risk of angiographic procedures. They are most widely used in asymptomatic patients with cervical bruits and in the long-term follow-up of patients already treated with carotid endarterectomy.

Indirect noninvasive tests

Indirect noninvasive tests use hemodynamic criteria to assess the patency of the extracranial carotid system. These include oculoplethysmography (OPG) and directional supraorbital doppler examination. OPG measures volume changes in the eye with each heartbeat. Since the ophthalmic artery is the first intracranial branch of the internal carotid artery, a hemodynamically significant stenosis in the carotid artery would be expected to delay or damp the ipsilateral pulse volume recording. With a modification of this principle (OPG-Gee), the actual perfusion pressure in the ophthalmic artery (and by extension the internal carotid artery) can be quantitated. Supraorbital doppler examination is made on the basis of the observation of reversed flow in the supraorbital vessels with severe internal carotid artery occlusive disease. The decrease in distal internal carotid artery pressure changes blood flow in the branches of the external carotid artery from the normal pattern (outward to extracranial tissue) to retrograde perfusion (inward providing collateral flow to the middle cerebral through the ophthalmic artery). It is important to note that these indirect tests cannot detect nonstenotic ulcerative lesions; in addition, the OPG is potentially inaccurate in bilateral disease and/or intrinsic obstruction of the ophthalmic artery.

Direct tests

Direct tests use ultrasound techniques (especially B-mode) to image the extracranial vessels. When combined with sophisticated range-gated pulsed doppler instruments (duplex scanning), the velocity and volume flow can be determined.[35] The resolution of duplex scanning has improved recently such that ulcerative nonstenotic lesions can be detected in most patients.

Arteriography remains the definitive study of the extracranial carotid system. Recent advances in digital processing have improved resolution, allowing use of both intravenous and arterial contrast injection. Arterial studies are advantageous in that they allow selective injections, superior definition, and lower contrast volumes with less renal and cardiac risk (Figs. 52-3 and 52-4). Complications of arterial catheterization include embolization of atherosclerotic debris and puncture site hemorrhage.[20] Intravenous digital angiograms avoid some of the local complications of arterial studies but require larger dye loads and provide less resolution for complex problems suchas intracranial lesions and ulcerations.

Operative indications

Most surgeons agree that carotid endarterectomy is indicated in patients with classic transient ischemic attacks associated with ulcerations or stenoses of the ipsilateral carotid artery.[48,51] This approach is based on clinical studies that indicate that transient ischemic attacks are reliable indicators of future strokes. The incidence of stroke after transient ischemic attack approaches 10% per year.[15,24] It remains more controversial whether patients with com-

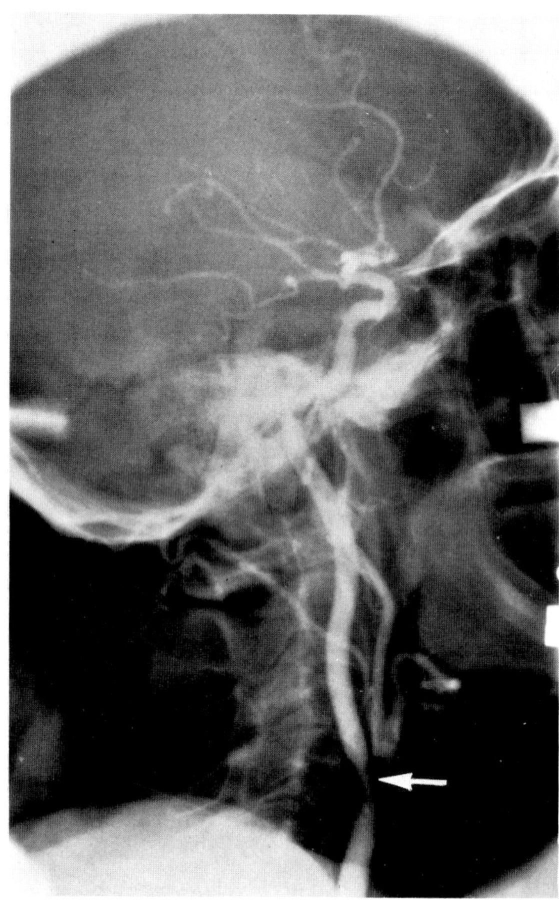

Fig. 52-3 Preoperative angiogram of patient presenting with repeated episodes of contralateral hemiparesis demonstrates severe stenosis of both internal *(arrow)* and external carotid arteries.

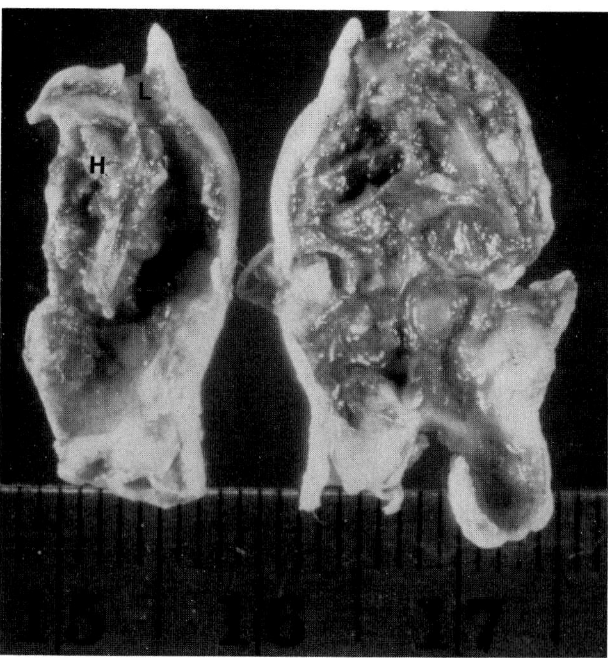

Fig. 52-4 Operative specimen (bivalved) reveals narrow lumen *(L)* with fresh hemorrhage *(H)* within atherosclerotic plaque. Extensive ulcerations are noted.

pleted strokes and appropriate carotid disease should undergo endarterectomy following recovery or at least 4 weeks after the neurologic event. The high incidence of recurrent strokes in these patients (15% to 35%) supports an aggressive surgical approach. Nonetheless, many surgeons will not operate if severe intracranial disease or cardiac risk factors would decrease the effectiveness or increase the morbidity of the procedure.

The prognosis of asymptomatic patients with highly stenotic carotid lesions remains difficult to characterize.[7,28] Long-term follow-up of patients with persistent disease of the contralateral carotid artery following unilateral carotid endarterectomy documents a 20% incidence of cerebrovascular symptoms; the incidence of stroke without antecedent transient ischemic attacks is approximately 3% to 5%.[41] Since experienced surgeons document a perioperative stroke rate of less than 2%, operative intervention may be appropriate in asymptomatic patients with limited anesthetic risk factors and those undergoing major surgical procedures that may predispose to hypotension.

Nonoperative treatment

The most significant risk factor for stroke is hypertension. Hence the control of hypertension is most important in the medical management of patients with cerebrovascular disease. Evaluation of serum lipoproteins will likely assume a greater role in the prevention and retardation of atherosclerosis as dietary and drug therapies for specific abnormalities become more clear.

Direct medical therapy for cerebrovascular disease has focused on anticoagulation (heparin and warfarin) and antiplatelet drugs (aspirin, dipyridamole, and sulfinpyrazone).[5,39] Mechanisms of action differ considerably, but the common rationale includes prevention of sudden thrombosis of stenotic lesions and inhibition of platelet activation on ulcerative lesions. Although many studies have suggested a benefit of long-term anticoagulation, the methodologies of these investigations have been seriously questioned, especially regarding their lack of randomization and precise patient selection. Furthermore, the statistically significant reduction in stroke rate (from 19% to 12% in one series) does not compare to the better results achieved by carotid endarterectomy.[8,21]

Many clinicians believe antiplatelet agents are most appropriate in patients with minimal ulcerative nonstenotic lesions and only one episode or one closely spaced series of transient ischemic attacks. If symptoms recur in such patients, endarterectomy remains an option. Other candidates for anticoagulation include patients with very high operative risk or those with severe associated intracranial disease.

Operative techniques, results, and complications

Carotid endarterectomy is the procedure of choice for disease of the common carotid artery or the extracranial portion of the internal carotid artery. The procedure can be performed under general or local anesthesia. Patients at greatest risk for a perioperative ischemic stroke include patients with previous infarcts, those with contralateral carotid occlusions, and those with unstable neurologic deficits. Some surgeons routinely use an indwelling vascular shunt to maintain carotid cerebral perfusion during endarterectomy, whereas others use shunts selectively or not at all. Intraoperative monitoring of electroencephalograms or retrograde carotid perfusion pressure ("stump pressure") have been used to assess the need for shunt placement. Since it is likely that embolic events account for the majority of perioperative strokes, precise dissection technique is crucial in patients with thrombotic or ulcerative plaques.[47]

The incidence of perioperative stroke varies with operative indication. Most large series report stroke rates of 1% to 2% in patients with transient ischemic attack and 3% to 5% in patients with previous strokes or contralateral carotid occlusion. Other postoperative complications include cranial nerve injury (especially the hypoglossal and recurrent laryngeal nerves) and myocardial infarction. Because the carotid sinus regulates blood pressure homeostasis, postoperative hypotension or hypertension is noted in many patients during the 24 hours required for baroreceptor reacclimation.[4]

Recurrent stenoses occur in approximately 8% to 10% of patients if followed closely, although the incidence of symptomatic recurrence is much lower (3%). Restenosis within 24 months usually represents exuberant intimal regeneration, whereas later presentations reflect recurrent atherosclerosis.[13]

Vertebrobasilar Disease

Clinical presentation

As noted earlier, the paired vertebral vessels join to form the basilar artery. For this reason, proximal occlusion or ligation of only one vertebral vessel will not cause symptoms unless the contralateral vessel is diseased or hypoplastic. More distal disease of one vertebral vessel with occlusion of the small branches supplying the lateral medulla can result in neurologic deficits.

The most frequent symptoms of basilar insufficiency include nausea, vertigo, ipsilateral facial numbness, ipsilateral Horner's syndrome, and limb ataxia. Although ischemic symptoms are generally mild, true posterior fossa infarction can be progressive and lethal as a result of extensive edema and midbrain compression. Emboli can contribute to posterior cerebral and cerebellar ischemia, but occlusive disease of the vertebral arteries or the basilar artery is the most common mechanism. The thrombotic process may involve the basilar artery proper or the basilar branch vessels that penetrate into the brain stem.[8]

A classic syndrome of vertebrobasilar insufficiency (subclavian steal syndrome) is associated with subclavian or innominate arterial occlusive disease.[22] The subclavian origins of the vertebral arteries allow the vessels to function as collaterals for the upper extremity. During arm exercise, flow is reversed in the vertebral artery, and basilar arterial blood flow and perfusion pressure are decreased. Symptoms of posterior cerebral and cerebellar ischemia can result, especially if any flow-limiting carotid lesions are present. The anatomic relationship favors left-sided involvement approximately 4:1.

The diagnosis of subclavian steal syndrome is supported by complaints of intermittent vertigo, light-headedness,

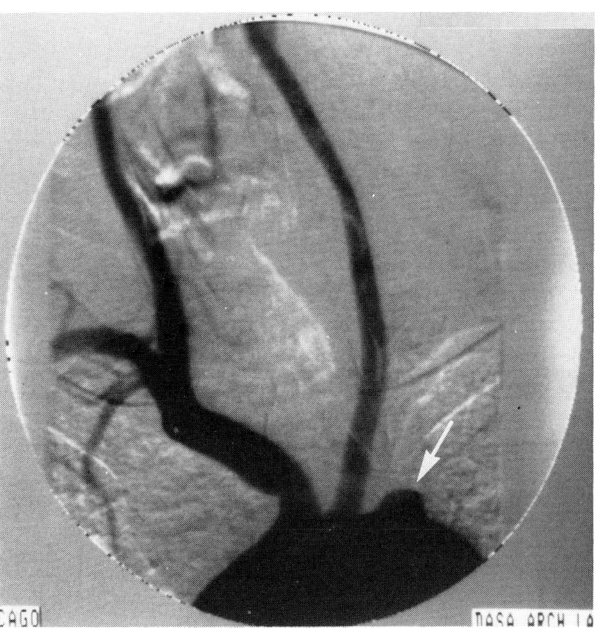

Fig. 52-5 Preoperative angiogram in patient presenting with stroke in basilar distribution (superior cerebellar) demonstrates complete occlusion of left subclavian artery *(arrow)*.

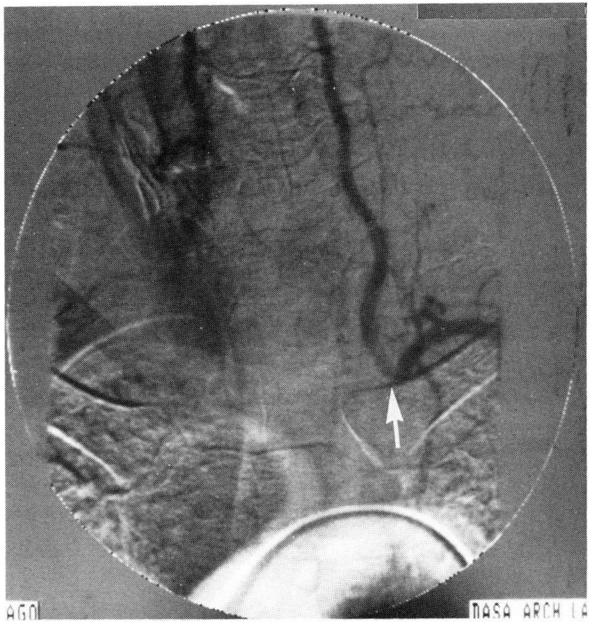

Fig. 52-6 Delayed films document reversed flow in large left vertebral artery *(arrow)* with reconstitution of distal subclavian artery (subclavian steal syndrome).

and nausea and vomiting intensified by arm exercise. Physical findings include supraclavicular bruits and 40- to 60-mm Hg blood pressure discrepancies between the arms.

Diagnosis

Measuring blood pressure in both upper extremities is essential in any patient with cerebral symptoms. More sophisticated tests include B-mode imaging of the subclavian and vertebral vessels and the use of directional dopplers to document reversal of vertebral artery blood flow.

The primary diagnostic test remains arteriography.[10] It is important to obtain delayed films to adequately demonstrate retrograde flow through the vertebral into the distal subclavian (Figs. 52-5 and 52-6). The origin of the contralateral vertebral artery and the status of the basilar artery should also be evaluated with oblique films if necessary. The incidental demonstration of subclavian steal during arteriography for some other reasons is, in itself, not cause for concern or surgical therapy.

Operative indications and techniques

Symptomatic patients with multiple vertebral occlusive lesions or subclavian steal syndrome should be considered for elective surgery. Procedures include endarterectomy of the proximal vertebral artery or carotid subclavian bypass to restore antegrade vertebral flow.[11] The latter can be accomplished by bypass graft or division of the cervical subclavian artery with reimplantation into the common carotid artery. These procedures can be performed through a cervical incision (Fig. 52-7). Subclavian or innominate artery endarterectomies usually require thoracotomy or sternotomy and are less frequently applied.

In patients with associated carotid artery disease, carotid endarterectomy alone may relieve symptoms of vertebral-basilar insufficieny by increasing collateral flow to the posterior cerebral artery and cerebellum.[46] This is most appropriate in symptomatic patients with severe carotid stenoses and those with more distal vertebral or basilar occlusion.

Results and complications

Patency of vertebral endarterectomies and carotid subclavian bypass grafts exceeds 90%. In most cases, symptoms are completely relieved by successful bypass. Failure to achieve symptomatic improvement may be caused by continued carotid disease or intracranial lesions.[2]

Perioperative complications include injuries to the phrenic nerve, cervical sympathetic ganglia (with Horner's syndrome), or the thoracic duct. Basilar territory infarction after carotid subclavian bypass is very rare; even early graft failure should not further compromise vertebral flow.

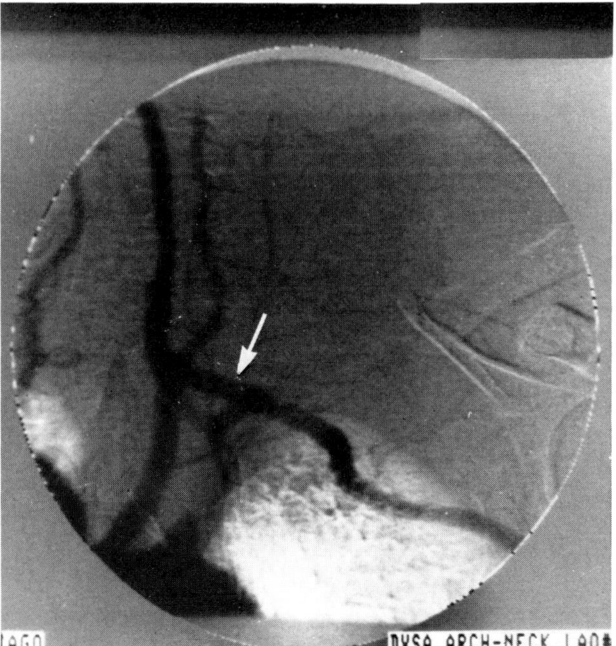

Fig. 52-7 Postoperative intravenous digital angiogram demonstrates patent carotid-subclavian bypass *(arrow)* with return of cephalad flow in left vertebral artery.

THORACIC OUTLET SYNDROME

Clinical Presentation

Thoracic outlet syndrome is best described as an intermittent but reproducible compression irritation of the brachial plexus caused by congenital fibromuscular bands, cervical ribs, or the anterior scalene muscle (Fig. 52-8).[33,44] Classic symptoms include shoulder pain with radiation to the occiput and down the arm along the C8 to T1 distribution. Numbness and tingling frequently accompany the pain. In advanced cases, weakness of the hands and forearm may be noted. Although the subclavian artery may also be compressed by the same anatomic configuration, most symptoms of thoracic outlet syndrome relate directly to neurologic rather than vascular compromise.

A history of neck or shoulder trauma can be elicited in many patients, suggesting to some clinicians that scalene muscle spasm is an initiating event. Whiplash injuries are frequently implicated, but documentation of a cause-and-effect relationship is nearly impossible. The differential diagnosis includes carpal tunnel syndrome, cervical disk compression, arthritis, tendinitis, and angina pectoris.

Diagnosis

The chronicity and lack of specificity of the clinical presentation is paralleled by a lack of definitive diagnostic tests other than chest x-ray film demonstration of an abnormal cervical rib. The Adson maneuver is a positional test long associated with thoracic outlet syndrome. The test is considered positive if the radial pulse disappears during abduction and external rotation of the arm. Unfortunately, the Adson maneuver is frequently positive in asymptomatic patients and negative in patients with classic symptoms of thoracic outlet syndrome, again emphasizing the neurologic as opposed to vascular origin of the pain syndrome. Angiographic demonstration of subclavian artery compression also does not contribute significantly to the diagnosis unless there is evidence of a persistent blood pressure gradient in the involved arm.[31]

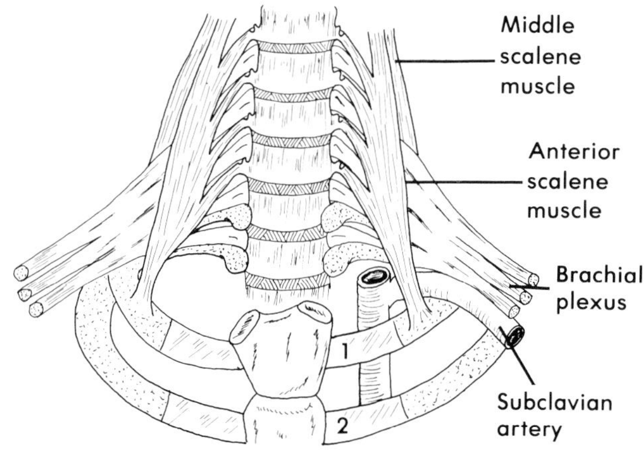

Fig. 52-8 Brachial plexus compression occurs at triangular outlet between scalene muscles and first rib.

Electromyograms and nerve conduction velocities have been suggested as objective measures of thoracic outlet nerve compression. Unfortunately, enthusiasm for these studies has decreased recently because of the difficulty of electrically stimulating nerves proximal to the presumed sight of compression and the intermittent nature of the syndrome. Furthermore, clinical correlations between positive nerve conduction studies and symptomatic relief following surgery have not been very convincing.

Operative Indications and Techniques

Initial therapy should include shoulder girdle exercises and avoidance of extreme posturing. If pain remains and symptoms are fully consistent and reproducible, surgical therapy is appropriate. Unfortunately, even experienced surgeons report complete relief in only 80% to 85% of patients.

The most common operation is transaxillary resection of the first rib or the cervical rib if present. In some patients merely transecting the insertion of the anterior scalene muscle onto the first rib may suffice.[45] Although there has been some enthusiasm for concurrent cervical sympathectomy, this is usually unnecessary unless symptoms of post-traumatic sympathetic dystrophy (causalgia) are evident.

Complications

The failure rate from all procedures remains relatively high in thoracic outlet syndrome.[49] Complications of surgery include Horner's syndrome, direct injury to the brachial plexus, and pneumothorax.

SUMMARY

Although cerebrovascular disease remains a major cause of morbidity and mortality in our population, improved understanding of the mechanisms and pathologic processes involved has allowed a wider application of preventive medical and surgical therapies. Appropriate selection of noninvasive tests to evaluate asymptomatic patients with signs of extracranial cerebrovascular disease have further characterized the natural history of these disorders. Although specific recommendations for medical or surgical therapy will continually be modified, it is generally accepted that patients with repetitive neurologic deficits (transient ischemic attacks) associated with extracranial atherosclerotic disease benefit significantly from surgical intervention.

REFERENCES

1. Abboud, F.M.: Special characteristics of the cerebral circulation, Fed. Proc. **40:**2296, 1981.
2. Allen, G.S., Cohen, R.J., and Preziosi, T.J.: Microsurgical endarterectomy of the intracranial vertebral artery for vertebrobasilar transient ischemic attacks, Neurosurgery **8:**56, 1981.
3. Borgstrom, L., Johannson, H., and Siesjo, B.K.: The relationship between arterial PO_2 and cerebral blood flow in hypoxic hypoxia, Acta Physiol. Scand. **93:**423, 1975.
4. Bove, E.L., et al.: Hypotension and hypertension consequences of baroreceptor dysfunction following carotid endarterectomy, Surgery **85:**633, 1979.
5. Brust, J.C.M.: Transient ischemic attacks: natural history of anticoagulation, Neurology **27:**701, 1977.
6. Brusija, D.W., Heistad, D.D., and Marcus, M.L.: Continuous measurement of cerebral bloodflow in anesthetized cats and dogs, Am. J. Physiol. **241:**H228-H234, 1981.
7. Busuttil R.W., et al.: Carotid artery stenosis—hemodynamic significance and clinical course, JAMA Assoc **245**(14):1438, 1981.
8. Canadian Cooperative Study Group: A andomized trial of aspirin and sulfinpyrosane in threatened stroke, N. Engl. J. Med. **229:**53, 1978.
9. Caplan, L.R.: Vertebrobasilar disease: time for a new strategy, Stroke **12:**111, 1981.
10. Caplan, L.R., and Rosenbaum, A.E.: Role of cerebral angiography and vertebrobasilar occlusive disease, J. Neurol. Neurosurg. Psychiatry **38:**601, 1975.
11. Clark, K., and Perry, M.O.: Carotid vertebral anastomsis: an alternate for repair of the subclavian steal syndrome, Ann Surg. **163:**414, 1966.
12. Craig, D.R., et al.: Intracranial internal carotid artery stenosis, Stroke **13:**825, 1982.
13. Crossman, D., et al.: Early restenosis after carotid endarterectomy, Arch. Surg. **113:**275, 1978.
14. D'Alecy, L.G., and Feigl, E.O.: Sympathetic control of cerebral blood flow in dogs, Circ. Res. **31:**267, 1972.
15. DeWeese, J.A., et al.: Results of carotid endarterectomies for transient ischemic attacks—five years later, Ann. Surg. **178:**258, 1973.
16. Diaz, F.G., et al.: Combined reconstruction of the vertebral and carotid artery in one single procedure, Neurosurgery **12:**629, 1983.
17. Dinsdale, H.B., Robertson, D.M., and Haas, R.A.: Cerebral blood flow in acute hypertension, Arch. Neurol. **31:**80, 1974.
18. Eisenberg, R.L., et al.: Relationship of transient ischemic attacks and angiographically demonstrable lesions of the carotid artery, Stroke **8:**483, 1977.
19. Ekstrom-Jodal, B.: Effect of increased venous pressure on cerebral blood flow in dogs, Acta Physiol. Scand. (suppl) **350:**51, 1970.
20. Faught, E., Trader, S.D., and Hanna, G.R.: Cerebral complications of angiography for transient ischemia and stroke: prediction of risk, Neurology (Minneap) **29:**4, 1979.
21. Fields, W.S., et al.: Controlled trial of aspirin in cerebral ischemia, Stroke **8:**301, 1977.
22. Fisher, C.M.: A new vascular syndrome: "the subclavian steal." N. Engl. J. Med. **265:**912, 1961.
23. Goldner, J.C., Whisnant, J.P., Taylor, W.F.: Long-term prognosis of transient cerebral ischemic attacks, Stroke **2:**160, 1971.
24. Goldstone, J., and Moore, W.S.: A new look at emergency carotid artery operations for the treatment of cerebrovascular insufficiency, Stroke **9:**599, 1978.
25. Greenberg, J.H., et al.: Local cerebral blood volume response to carbon dioxide in man, Circ. Res. **43:**324, 1978.
26. Gregory, P.C., et al.: Effects of hemorrhagic hypotension on the cerebral circulation, Stroke **10:**719, 1979.
27. Heistad, D.D., and Marcus, M.L.: Evidence that neural mechanisms do not have important effects on cerebral blood flow, Circ. Res. **42:**295, 1978.
28. Humphries, A.W., et al.: Unoperated, asymptomatic significant internal carotid artery stenosis: a review of 182 instances, Surgery **80:**695, 1976.
29. Javid, H., et al.: Natural history of carotid bifurcation atheroma, Surgery **67:**80, 1970.
30. Johansson, B., et al.: The effect of acute arterial hypertension on the blood-brain barrier to protein tracers, Acta Neuropathol. **16:**117, 1970.
31. Judy, K.L.,and Heymann, R.L.: Vascular complications of thoracic outlet syndrome, Am. J. Surg. **123:**521, 1972.
32. Kannel, W.B., et al.: Components of blood pressure and risk of atherothrombotic brain infarction: the Framingham Study, Stroke **7:**327, 1976.
33. Kirgis, H.D., and Reed, A.F.: Significant anatomic relations in the syndrome of the scalene muscles, Ann. Surg. **127:**1182, 1948.
34. Lassen, N.A., Henriksen, L., and Paulson, O.: Regional cerebral blood flow in stroke by ^{133}xenon inhalation and emission tomography, Stroke **12:**284, 1981.
35. Lees, R.S., Kistler, J.P., and Sanders, D.: Duplex Doppler scanning and spectral bruit analysis for diagnosing carotid stenosis, Circulation **66:**(suppl:1) 102, 1982.
36. Levy, R.I.: Stroke decline: implications and prospects, N. Engl. J. Med. **300:**490, 1979.
37. Marcus, M.L., Bischof, C.J., and Heistad, D.D.: Comparison of microsphere and xenon-133 clearance method in measuring skeletal muscle and cerebral blood flow, Circ. Res. **48:**748, 1981.

38. Mentzer, R.M., et al.: Emergency carotid endarterectomy for fluctuating neurologic deficits, Surgery **89:**60, 1981.
39. Olsson, J-E., et al.: Anticoagulant vs. antiplatelet therapy as prophylactic against cerebral infarction in transient ischemic attacks, Stroke **11:**4, 1980.
40. Pessin, M.S., et al.; Mechanisms of acute carotid stroke, Ann. Neurol. **6:**245, 1979.
41. Podore, P.C., et al.: Asympatomatic contralateral artery stenosis: a five year follow-up study following carotid endarterectomy, Surgery **88:**748, 1980.
42. Raichle, M.E., et al.: Central noradrenergic regulation of cerebral blood flow and vascular permeability, Proc. Natl. Acad. Sci. USA **72:**3726, 1975.
43. Raichle, M.E., et al.: Measurement of regional substrate utilization rates by emission tomography, Science **199:**986, 1978.
44. Roos, D.B.: Congenital anomalies associated with thoracic outlet syndrome: anatomy, symptoms, diagnosis, and treatment, Am. J. Surg. **132:**771, 1976.
45. Sanders, R.J.: Scalenectomy versus first rib resection for treatment of the thoracic outlet syndrome, Surgery **85:**109, 1979.
46. Solberg, L.A., and Eggen, D.A.: Localization and sequence of development of atherosclerotic lesions in the carotid and vertebral arteries, Circulation **43:**711, 1971.
47. Steed, D.L.,et al.: Causes of stroke in carotid endarterectomy, Surgery **92:**634, 1982.
48. Thompson, J.E., and Talkington, C.M.: Carotid surgery for cerebral ischemia, Surg. Clin. North Am. **59:**539, 1979.
49. Urschel, H.D., Jr., et al.: Reoperation for recurrent thoracic outlet syndrome, Ann. Thorac. Surg. **21:**19, 1976.
50. Wechsler, R.L., Drips, P.O., and Kety, S.S.: Blood flow and oxygen consumption of the human brain during anesthesia produced by thiopental, Anesthesiology **12:**308, 1951.
51. West, H., et al.: Comprative risk of operation and expectant management for carotid artery disease, Stroke **10:**117, 1979.
52. Whisnant, J.P.: Epidemiology of stroke: emphasis on transient cerebral ischemic attacks and hypertension, Stroke **5:**68, 1974.
53. Wolf, P.A., et al.: Asymptomatic carotid bruit and risk of stroke, JAMA **245:**1442, 1981.

53 Kenneth G. Swan and Joyce M. Rocko

Venous and Lymphatic Abnormalities of the Limbs

In 1628 Harvey's epic work awakened man's interest in extremity veins by demonstrating the valvular function that enables the circulation of blood. His treatise, *De Motu Cordis on the Motion of the Heart and Blood in Animals,* published in Latin in the German city of Frankfurt, is universally regarded as a classic because it is the magic window through which the inquirer into the nature of science can discern its most hidden meanings and mode of advancement.[29] Since Harvey's classic contribution, knowledge of the pathophysiology of the various venous and lymphatic abnormalities of the limbs has evolved greatly. This chapter will discuss our current understanding of these abnormalities and their management. Particular attention will be directed to venous thrombotic disease and lymphedema.

VENOUS DISORDERS OF THE LOWER EXTREMITIES

Varicose Veins

The term varicose vein refers to the tortuous and dilated superficial veins that commonly involve the greater and lesser saphenous venous systems of the lower extremities. The common physiologic derangement associated with such varicosities is regurgitant blood flow in which blood normally being propelled toward the heart is now reversed and flows toward the feet. This occurs because of the loss of elasticity within the venous walls and the accompanying incompetency of the venous valves. As the loss in elasticity becomes pronounced and the affected vein undergoes dilation, the delicate bicuspid valve cusps tend to pull apart from each other, allowing retrograde flow toward the feet and stagnation of blood. Once the disease affects a given vein, it becomes a self-perpetuating process in that the retrograde flow of blood dilates the vein distally, producing incompetence of the next valve downstream. As retrograde flow continues to increase venous pressure, further varicosities develop so that ultimately the vein involved is affected from the site of origin to the level of the foot.

Two types of varicosities have been recognized. *Primary* varicose veins develop de novo without any prior problems with deep venous thrombosis. The exact cause in this circumstance has not been clearly defined. Although the upright position of the human being is probably a contributing factor, it is clearly not the only one, since many people whose jobs and life-styles require them to spend large portions of their time standing do not develop varicosities. That congenital factors probably play a role is supported by the finding that 30% to 40% of patients with varicosities have a family history of this disease.[30] Further, females are clearly at a greater risk for its development (three-to-one female-to-male incidence), possibly related to the effects of female sex hormones, which have a smooth muscle-relaxing effect that is often manifested by a dilation of veins during each menstrual cycle.[30] In females with this propensity, pregnancy will often initiate the onset of varicosities or aggravate them further if they already exist. Other etiologic factors that appear to be important in the development of primary varicosities include obesity, advancing age, and an increase in intraabdominal pressure.

Secondary varicosities arise either in patients who have previously developed thrombosis of the deep veins of the lower extremities in which the valves in this system have been destroyed, leading to a reflux of blood pedally, or when a state of venous obstruction exists.[30,68] In either event, the increased venous pressure within the deep system produces dilation of the communicating veins and a resultant incompetency of their valves, allowing reversal of blood flow from the deep veins to the superficial venous system. Thus the superficial veins behave as a collateral system to drain blood from the deep compartment of the leg and thereby become dilated and tortuous.

Clinical Presentation

Depending on the extent to which varicosities exist, symptoms may be absent entirely or characterized as a dull, nagging ache or discomfort that is most pronounced in the calves and ankles and is usually aggravated with prolonged standing. Not uncommonly a sensation of fullness with an associated ankle edema may be noted at the end of the day. Most patients who have these symptoms usually have obvious dilation, tortuosity, and elongation of the superficial veins and unsightly bluish discoloration of the affected leg. It is usually such cosmetic findings that bring a patient, particularly a woman, to the attention of a physician. If varicosities have been long-standing or have been affected by an episode of thrombophlebitis, edema, eczematoid dermatitis, hyperpigmentation, and superficial skin ulcerations may exist, particularly in the region of the medial malleolus of the ankle, although this problem is more commonly seen in patients with deep venous disease. Such varicose ulcers may be secondarily infected. On rare occasions a varix may actually rupture when locally traumatized.

In the evaluation of a patient with varicose veins, it is important to define the extent of the varicosities and whether one or both of the greater and lesser saphenous venous systems are involved. It is also important to determine whether the varicosities are primary or secondary, since the treatment of these two conditions is different. If the varicosities are secondary to deep venous disease, it is generally inappropriate to excise or ligate the superficial

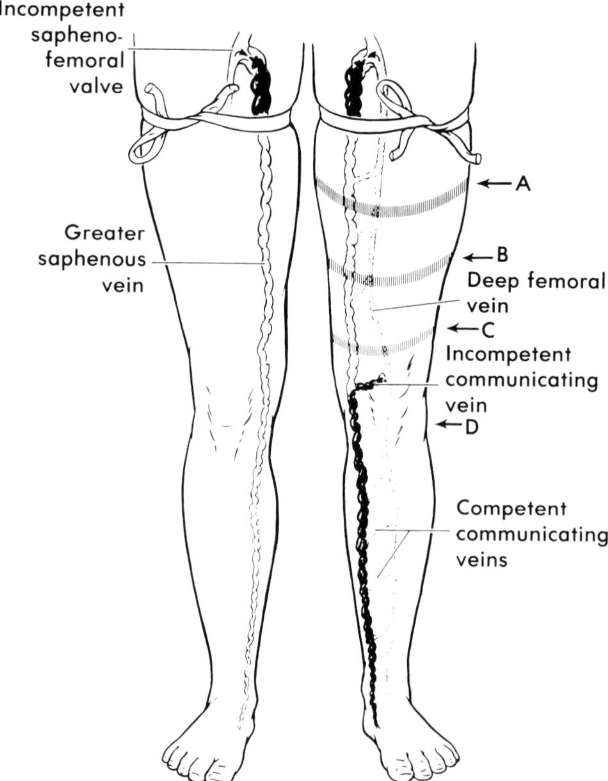

Fig. 53-1 Modified Trendelenburg (tourniquet) test for varicose veins. The tourniquet on the patient's *right* leg prevents filling of the varicosed greater saphenous vein distally, proving competency of all the communicating valves and incompetency of the saphenofemoral valve. On the patient's *left* leg, an incompetent communicating vein valve at the knee allows filling of the greater saphenous vein distal to this point, but the tourniquet prevents filling of the vein above the knee. A second tourniquet at points A, B, or C would not alter the findings. However, had a second tourniquet been placed at point D, the greater saphenous vein would have filled only from the knee down to this level. (From Soper, R.T., and Furnas, D.W.: Peripheral veins. In Liechty, R.D., and Soper, R.T., editors: Synopsis of surgery, St. Louis, 1976, The C.V. Mosby Co.)

veins, since such veins are now serving as important collateral channels to empty blood from the extremity.

To distinguish between primary and secondary varicosities, two clinical tests are generally used. The first is the *Perthes test,* which is performed by placing a tourniquet around the groin of sufficient snugness to occlude normal flow in the superficial venous system. When this has been accomplished, the patient is then asked to walk briskly. If pain and edema develop, obstruction of the deep venous system is assumed. The other maneuver is the *Trendelenburg test*. With this procedure the leg is elevated to empty the veins, and a tourniquet is placed over the saphenofemoral junction. The leg is then quickly placed in the dependent position. If no filling of the varicosities is seen during such dependency but rapidly occurs on release of the tourniquet to allow retrograde filling of the superficial venous systems, the communicating or perforating veins are competent, and the varicosities are of the primary type. If rapid filling of the varicosities occurs during such dependency when the tourniquet is in place, it can be assumed that incompetent perforating veins exist secondary to deep venous disease. This test is of further value in demonstrating the extent to which previous deep venous disease is present by placing the tourniquet at different positions on the thigh as shown in Fig. 53-1.

Treatment

Treatment of varicosities is generally conservative and depends on the extent to which symptoms may be present. Any constricting garments (garters or girdles) should be avoided, and prolonged periods of leg inactivity when the legs may be dependent should be minimized. Most patients feel better wearing some type of elastic hose. If excessive weight is a contributing factor, attempts at reduction should be encouraged. The cosmetic appearance of varicosities bothers some patients, even though symptoms may be minimal. If cosmesis is a concern, ligation and stripping of the varicosities can be performed and generally give excellent results both cosmetically and functionally.

Vein stripping is accomplished by passing a semimalleable instrument, known as a stripper, down the length of the involved vein, tying the divided vein to be removed to the instrument, and pulling out the entire vein on removal of the instrument[39,75] (Fig. 53-2). This approach avulses the main venous channel from its associated perforating veins. On completion, the stripped portion of the leg is wrapped in a cephalad direction, starting with the toes; this wrapping allows the exposed perforators to thrombose. Such wrappings are generally continued for several weeks, after which normal leg function is resumed. Ligation and stripping are generally reserved for primary varicosities, since those developing from previous deep venous disease represent an important collateral pathway to drain blood from the leg. If varicosities are small, sclerotherapy may be used by injecting a sclerosing agent (e.g., sodium tetradecyl sulfate) directly into the involved vein.[70] This procedure results in obliteration and permanent fibrosis of the injected veins.

In the circumstance in which varicose ulcers have developed secondary to long-standing varicosities, excision of the ulcer bed and the surrounding skin to the level of the muscle fascia is generally performed, following which epithelialization is achieved with the use of a split thickness skin graft.

Venous Thrombosis

Venous thrombosis can occur in any vein involving the superficial and deep venous systems of the leg. Usually one or the other system is involved, but thrombosis involving both systems does occasionally occur. In this latter setting it usually begins in the deep veins, with extension to the superficial system as a later event.

In understanding venous thrombosis, two terms need to be distinguished. *Thrombophlebitis* represents the formation of a clot within a vein in which there are associated signs of inflammation, typically erythema, pain, and tenderness. Because of the acute inflammatory response in this condition, the developing clot is usually firmly adherent to the intima of the vessel wall so that embolization to a distant site such as the lungs is distinctly uncommon. *Phlebothrombosis* also indicates clot formation within a

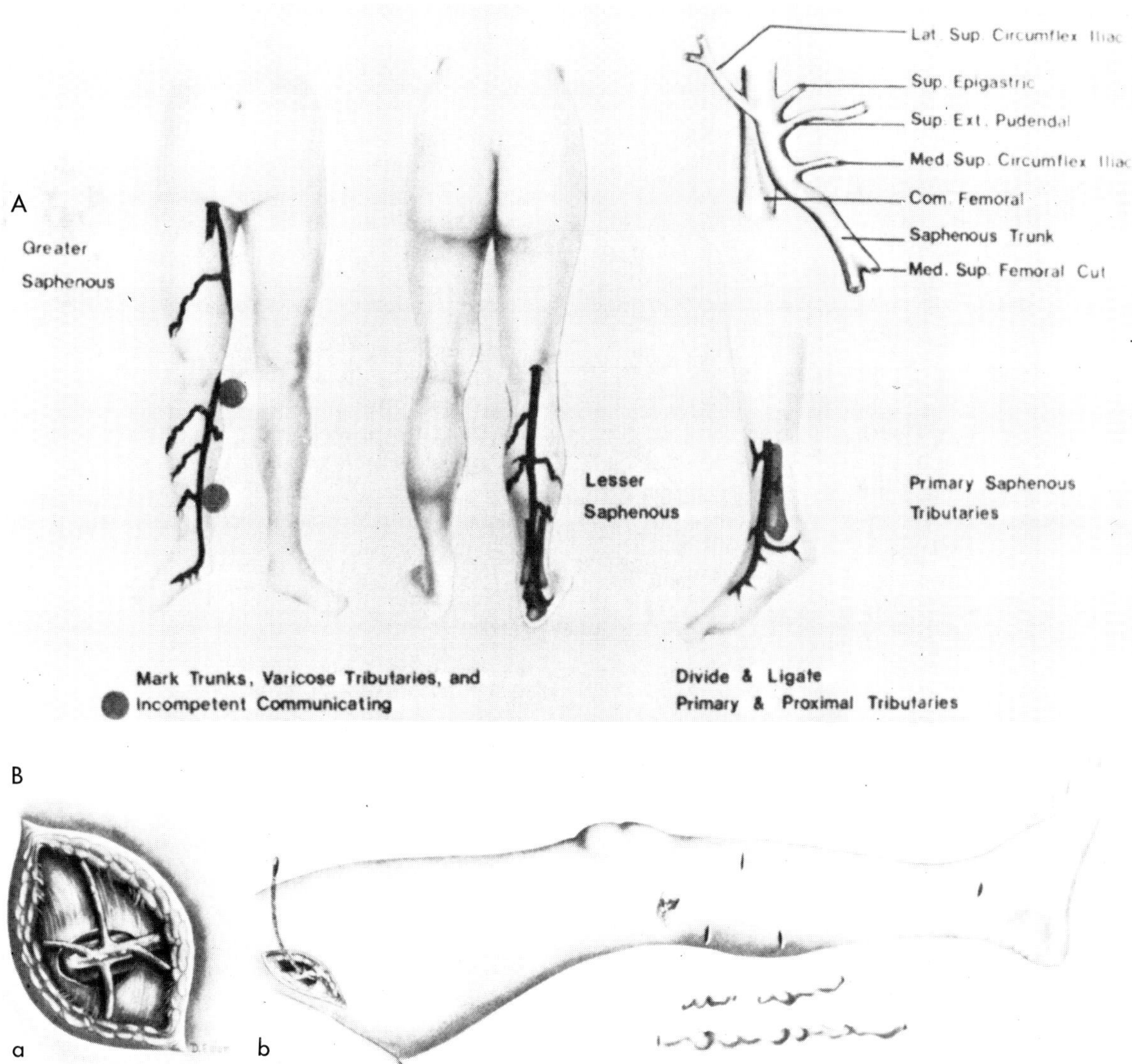

Fig. 53-2 **A,** Sketched proximal tributaries of the involved greater saphenous vein and the distal primary tributaries of the trunks to be stripped are divided and ligated. The varicose trunks and tributaries are completely stripped. The dots indicate the most common locations of incompetent communicating veins that are divided and ligated. (From Keith, L.M., and Turnipseed, W.D.: Am J. Surg. **128:**612, 1974.) **B,** Ligation and stripping of saphenous vein. *a,* Groin incision, showing junction of greater saphenous and femoral veins. Note four major branches of saphenous vein that required ligation and division. *b,* Counterincision at knee or ankle to permit stripping of saphenous vein. Additional incisions to permit removal of branch varicose veins. (From DeWeese, J.A.: Venous and lymphatic disease. In Schwartz, S.I., editor: Principles of surgery, ed. 2, New York, 1974, McGraw-Hill Book Co.)

vein, but without the associated signs of acute inflammation. Clot formation typically develops in an asymptomatic fashion, and, because of its loose attachment to the venous intima, embolization is a more likely possibility. Although these two forms of venous thrombosis can be distinguished clinically, some degree of overlap of the two is commonly present and thus should be considered as a continuum of a common underlying process generally requiring similar approaches to prevention and treatment.

A variety of etiologic factors may be responsible for the development of venous thrombosis, but stagnation of blood flow is usually a common antecedent. Thus conditions that result in such stagnation are commonly associated with the development of venous thrombosis. These include varicosities, direct trauma to veins, prolonged bed rest, stasis during an operation or illness, any factor that may result in diminished arterial blood flow such as cardiac disease or shock, and various states of blood hypercoagulability.[55,64,81] Collagen vascular diseases and a number of malignant processes are also associated with a higher than normal incidence of venous thrombosis.[49]

Superficial Thrombophlebitis

Thrombophlebitis usually involves the superficial veins in the lower extremities, in contrast to phlebothrombosis, which is more typically seen in deep veins. Varicose veins are usually a preexisting condition of superficial thrombophlebitis involving the lower extremities, although not an absolute prerequisite.[34,47] Additional causes of this condition include occult malignant neoplasia, local trauma, and parenteral drug abuse. In a substantial number of cases the condition may be idiopathic. The common clinical presentation is localized pain, erythema, and induration (often tender) of the thrombosed vein. A low-grade fever may also be present.

When thrombophlebitis exists below the level of the knee, therapy is usually performed on an outpatient basis and consists primarily of symptomatic relief of the signs and symptoms. Such treatment consists of bed rest, leg elevation, and local heat (usually in the form of hot packs) to the affected vein. The disease is usually self-limiting and results in obliteration of the involved segment of the superficial venous system, thus precluding subsequent attacks. Anticoagulant therapy is almost never indicated because the bleeding complications resulting therefrom far outweigh the risks of thromboembolism, which is distinctly rare.

When the disease process extends above the knee, the condition has the potential of becoming considerably more serious because the possibility of embolization exists. Such patients should be hospitalized. In-hospital therapy consists of the same treatment indicated for infragenicular disease, but closer attention is given to the possibility of the progression of the disease and the accompanying thrombus formation more cephalad. The administration of anticoagulants (see discussion under deep venous thrombosis for agents and dosage) depends on the response to conservative management. It must be emphasized that anticoagulant therapy is used solely for the prevention of thromboembolism and not as an effort to erradicate the underlying condition. Should the disease progress proximally despite these treatment measures, emergency surgery may be indicated, consisting of ligation of the saphenous vein at the saphenofemoral junction as in standard surgical procedures for phlebectomy for varicose veins (see Fig. 53-2).

Deep Venous Thrombosis

Deep venous thrombosis is a much more serious threat to life than phlebitis involving the superficial veins. This relates to the fact that the inflammatory response commonly associated with involvement of the superficial veins is generally absent and the clot, at least initially after formation, is much more loosely adherent to the intima and consequently more likely to embolize to the lungs. In addition, symptoms are often lacking in patients with deep venous thrombosis so that the risk of embolization is not appreciated and the appropriate prophylactic measures to prevent this complication are consequently delayed. In fact, as many as 40% to 50% of patients who develop pulmonary emboli have no antecedent symptoms of deep venous disease.[15,49]

Virtually any patient may develop deep venous thrombosis, but certain patient populations are clearly at risk. These include those who are immobilized for long periods of time such as those with long bone fractures, paraplegia, or quadriplegia[23]; patients who have sustained trauma to the chest and/or abdomen, elderly and obese patients, those with central nervous system disease, and those with malignancies. Other risk factors adversely influencing the incidence of deep vein thrombosis include oral contraceptive use, a group A blood type, a history of previous venous thromboses, congestive heart failure, pregnancy,[66,73] and any condition requiring prolonged bed rest (medically indicated or otherwise). Finally, surgical procedures themselves are associated with an increased risk for the development of venous thromboses. This is not only related to the immobilized state but may be a reflection of the type of anesthetic used, since epidural anesthesia appears to be associated with a lower incidence of deep venous thrombosis than other types of anesthetic approaches.[50]

CLINICAL PRESENTATION. In those patients who develop symptomatology, mild ankle edema and superficial vein dilation are usually the earliest findings. Pain is also usually present in the calf, especially on walking, although this is not an invariable symptom. However, the inflammatory picture so characteristic of superficial thrombophlebitis is usually lacking in deep vein thrombosis. Physical examination usually reveals tenderness on palpation of the calf; occasionally the thrombosed vein may actually be felt. This can be demonstrated anywhere from the plantar aspect of the foot to the femoral triangle in the groin, depending on the extent of the thrombosis, but usually is best appreciated on palpation in the popliteal space. Active or passive dorsiflexion of the foot with the leg extended often reveals tenderness and tightness in the back of the calf (termed Homan's sign), providing further evidence of the presence of thrombosis. This sign, however, may be present with any type of calf muscle irritation so that it is not pathopneumonic for thrombotic disease.

Although most forms of deep venous thrombosis involve the popliteal vein and its tributaries, occasionally the thrombus will extend proximally to involve the femoral vein and at times even the iliac vein. If femoral vein involvement is present, swelling is much more prominent and may extend to the level of the knee. In addition, considerable pain is also usually present in the distal thigh. If iliofemoral involvement exists, the affected extremity may demonstrate massive swelling extending from the toes to the inguinal ligament. This condition, known as *phlegmasia cerulea dolens,* is also characterized by severe pain and tenderness involving the entire extremity with obvious cyanosis.[9] A variant of this disorder, known as *phlegmasia alba dolens,* has, in addition, an associated arterial spasm so that the leg is pale and cool with diminished pulses.

Although the more severe forms of deep venous thrombosis are clinically obvious, particularly when involving the iliofemoral system, thrombotic disease confined to the popliteal vein and its tributaries may be confused with other conditions. Rupture of the plantaris muscle or various disorders involving the knee, particularly a ruptured Baker's cyst, may present with many of the symptoms suggestive of deep venous thrombosis. Since the treatment of these conditions obviously differs, it is important to confirm the presence of venous thrombosis in such patients.

TESTS TO CONFIRM DIAGNOSIS. The most specific way of confirming the diagnosis is with the use of *ascending phlebography* (venography).[32,35,57] This technique is the gold standard for establishing the diagnosis of venous thrombosis and involves the injection of a radiopaque contrast medium into a vein on the dorsum of the foot, and the use of fluoroscopy and serial x-ray films to follow the opacification of its drainage through the popliteal, femoral, and iliac veins. If thrombotic disease is present, abrupt termination of the dye column, filling defects, or inadequate filling of various portions of the venous system will be demonstrated. This technique is highly accurate, and the negative phlebogram virtually excludes the presence of a venous thrombosis. Nonetheless, it is not a practical means of screening most patients, and a small but definite risk of developing venous thrombosis from the test itself is known to occur.[45,80] In addition, extravasation of the contrast media at the site of injection may produce a severe perivasculitis, cellulitis, and even skin ulceration.[78] For these reasons, most patients are screened with one of the available, less invasive techniques and not subjected to phlebography unless the diagnosis is still in doubt. Another venographic approach involves the use of radioisotopes instead of contrast medium. Early results with this technique suggest that it may be as reliable as the contrast method.[60]

Of the noninvasive techniques, *Doppler ultrasound* is clearly the most practical diagnostic modality available.[5,8,32,60] This technique can evaluate the flow characteristics across veins (whether normal or static), can indicate whether a vein is patent or occluded, and can assess all of the major deep veins of the lower limb. It cannot, however, exclude the presence of thrombi in small veins and is less accurate in diagnosing thrombotic disease in the calf than with more proximal disease. In experienced hands, though, it has an accuracy approaching 90%. In addition, it is inexpensive and can be repeated many times in patients that may need to be reassessed frequently.

Plethysmography is a technique that measures volume changes in the extremity. It is useful in the diagnosis of deep venous thrombosis because of the associated edematous changes that occur with this disorder. It is generally performed by placing a blood pressure cuff around the proximal thigh and inflating it to a level between normal arterial and venous pressures. When this is done, a previously positioned calf plethysmograph will record a volume increase. On deflation of the blood pressure cuff, a reduction in calf volume will occur. The rate at which this volume change occurs reflects the efficiency of venous outflow. As with ultrasound, plethysmography is more helpful in diagnosing proximal thrombotic disease than that occurring in the calf; but, when a positive result is obtained, the accuracy rate approaches 90%.[5,8,10,60]

Intravenously injected *radioactive fibrinogen* is yet another technique to diagnose deep venous thrombosis, but is not especially practical because 12 or more hours may elapse between the time of injection and the availability of results.[5,8] This technique involves the intravenous injection of ^{125}I-labeled fibrinogen, following which the legs are scanned hours and sometimes days later. The principle underlying this technique is that an active ongoing thrombosis incorporates fibrinogen; thus any increase in radioactivity indicates that a thrombus is forming. This test is especially accurate for thromboses in the calf, but because of the high background radiation from bones and bladder, it is not particularly useful diagnostically in assessing veins of the upper thigh.

Treatment. The mainstay of treatment of deep venous thrombosis is anticoagulation.* The purpose of such therapy is to limit propagation of the original thrombus and prevent new thrombi from developing and to ensure adequate provision against pulmonary embolization. To accomplish these goals, heparin is the best initial anticoagulant because it acts rapidly and can be reversed with protamine sulphate, should excessive dosage be given, and thereby can decrease the possibility of bleeding complications. The initial dose of heparin is usually 10,000 U given as an intravenous bolus followed by 1000 to 2000 U hourly as a continuous intravenous infusion. Although subcutaneous and intramuscular approaches have been used for heparin administration in other situations, adequate levels of anticoagulation and the potential for bleeding complications (when administered intramuscularly) cannot be ensured with these approaches. Consequently, the intravenous route is preferred.

To monitor the adequacy of anticoagulation, one of the coagulation tests should be followed because heparin inhibits thrombin formation and platelet release and blocks the formation of thromboplastin. The partial thromboplastin time (PTT) is quite satisfactory for this purpose and should generally be maintained around 80 seconds. The activated partial thromboplastin time (APTT) or the activated coagulation time (ACT) can also be used for monitoring if preferred. During anticoagulation, the patient should be maintained at bed rest until symptoms abate. Gradual ambulation is then permitted as tolerated with elastic support of the involved extremity.

Generally after the patient has been on heparin therapy for a week or more, oral anticoagulation should be commenced[15,21] by overlapping the oral therapy with the heparin treatment. The drug usually used for this purpose is warfarin (coumadin). Such oral therapy is continued for 3 to 6 months to prevent a late pulmonary embolus and to ensure adequate lysis of the thrombus with recanalization and collateralization of the affected vein or veins. Since coumadin blocks prothrombin production, the adequacy of anticoagulation is monitored with a prothrombin time. The dosage of coumadin is monitored in such a fashion that the prothrombin time is maintained at about two to two and one-half times the control value. When warfarin treatment is first being started, heparin therapy is continued until the prothrombin time has reached this level.

Although the foregoing anticoagulant approach is the current standard of managing most patients with deep vein thrombosis, fibrinolytic agents have also been used to treat this problem.† The two that have been evaluated clinically are urokinase and streptokinase. Both of these fibrinolytic agents can lyse fresh intravascular clots and in that regard are superior to the other two conventional anticoagulants (i.e., coumading and heparin). Unfortunately, the bleeding complications associated with they has made their routine use prohibitive. In addition, once a thrombus has been present for more than 72 hours, their anticoagulant capabilities greatly decrease. Further, they have no decided ad-

*References 11, 14, 16, 31, 49, and 59.

†References 3, 13, 19, 37, 40, 61, 67, and 76.

vantages over heparin for the prevention of recurrent venous thrombosis. Thus their role in managing deep venous disease is limited and will require further study and definition. It may be that their greatest use will be in patients with extensive thrombotic disease such as those involving the iliofemoral system.

Although various types of surgical approaches have been used over the years to extract venous thrombi with varying degrees of enthusiasm, success with such approaches has been greatly limited.[7,33] Rethrombosis is high following these procedures and, when compared with heparin therapy, has no decided advantages in terms of morbidity and mortality. The only specific circumstance in which venous thrombectomy may play an important role is in the individual with extensive ileofemoral disease in which limb loss is threatened. Even in this situation, however, heparin therapy is generally more efficacious.

Complications of Venous Thrombosis

Pulmonary Embolism. The most feared complication of venous thrombosis is that which results when a portion of the clot separates from its in situ position and is transported to the lungs, a condition known as pulmonary embolism. This disorder can occur in almost any clinical thrombotic setting, but is especially common in patients with thromboses involving the deep veins of the legs. In fact, 90% to 95% of pulmonary emboli are thought to arise from venous thromboses of the legs; the other major source is thrombotic disease of the pelvic veins.[6,71] Pulmonary embolism is probably responsible for as many as 250,000 deaths annually in the United States. As pointed out by Sir Reginald Murley in his Bradshaw lecture of 1981, this condition has been recognized as a distinct entity since 1882, and as many as 5% of hospitalized patients are afflicted by this condition at any given time.[52] Although the majority of pulmonary emboli result in nonfatal attacks, the fact that many patients succumb to this disease who otherwise are suffering from a nonlethal condition emphasizes the importance of recognizing its pathogenesis, instituting appropriate prophylactic measures to prevent its development, and ensuring the optimum in treatment should it occur. The patient populations at particular risk for the development of pulmonary embolus have already been discussed in the section on deep venous thrombosis. It cannot be stressed too strongly, however, that a significant number of patients in whom pulmonary emboli occur have no history of previous venous disease or evidence of thrombophlebitis or venous thrombosis on careful examination. Thus the possibility that a pulmonary embolus may develop in any patient cannot be overemphasized.[6,44,71]

Pathophysiology and clinical presentation. The majority of pulmonary emboli of clinical significance arise from thromboses originating in large veins such as the iliac and femoral veins. Although thromboses may also develop in smaller veins such as those in the calf, it is only when such thromboses extend to the level of the iliac and femoral veins that major clinical sequelae may ensue. When embolization occurs, the lobar arteries in the lungs are usually affected. The hemodynamic consequences are related to this mechanical occlusion and include increases in pulmonary arterial resistance, pulmonary arterial pressure, and right ventricular work.[6] Usually there is some degree of bronchospasm that probably occurs from the release of vasoactive substances (possibly prostaglandins) that arises from the embolus itself. If preexisting cardiopulmonary disease is present, these pathophysiologic aberrations may be pronounced even further. Usually, though, the extent of such derangements correlates quite closely with the extent of pulmonary arterial obstruction.

Clinically the most frequent findings in a patient with pulmonary embolus are dyspnea and tachypnea.[6,44,71] Other findings commonly seen include a pleuritic type pain, coughing, a sensation of precordial pressure, tachycardia, an altered mental state, and hemoptysis. In some patients, symptoms may be absent entirely except for a low-grade fever. If the embolus has been massive, a state of cardiovascular collapse may ensue, including shock, cyanosis, extreme dyspnea, restlessness, and massive chest pain. Unless such patients have a previous history of venous thrombosis, this constellation of symptoms is often misdiagnosed as a massive myocardial infarction.

Confirmation of the diagnosis. In addition to the clinical presentation just described, a number of other findings provide further support for the diagnosis.[6,44,71] These include an exaggerated second heart sound with electrocardiographic evidence of right ventricular strain or bundle branch block. Likewise, the sudden onset of atrial fibrillation in a patient without a prior history of cardiac disease suggests the presence of a pulmonary embolus. Similarly, arterial blood-gas analysis may also prove helpful, since the absence of hypoxemia makes the diagnosis of a pulmonary embolus quite unlikely. If a major embolus is present, the carbon dioxide tension may be higher than expected because the increased hypercarbia from the poorly perfused lung offsets any hypocarbic effect from the tachypnea. Finally, the triad of an elevated lactic dehydrogenase (LDH) and bilirubin in combination with a normal serum glutamic-oxaloacetic transaminase (SGOT) suggests the presence of a pulmonary embolus. Unfortunately, this combination of findings is rarely seen, except when the embolus is massive and more urgent diagnostic maneuvers are needed. Similarly, although a chest x-ray film may provide supportive evidence of a pulmonary embolus, there are no pathopneumonic radiologic signs of this disease. Findings suggestive, but certainly not diagnostic, of a pulmonary embolus include a prominent pulmonary artery shadow, blanched peripheral lung fields because of diminished blood flow secondary to the embolus, and the occasional demonstration of a wedge-shaped peripheral infiltrate.

To confirm the presence of an embolus, pulmonary scanning or arteriography will almost always be needed before justification and commencement of therapy with anticoagulation (see p. 869). Because the scanning technique is less invasive, this is the initial diagnostic procedure of choice. With this technique, the lungs are scanned after the intravenous infusion of human serum albumin labeled with ^{99m}Tc or ^{131}I. In areas of the lung perfused by vessels plugged with emboli, poor uptake of these macromolecules is seen. Unfortunately, this technique may yield a false positive result, since diseases such as pneumonia, atelectasis, and even asthma may demonstrate a defect on scan-

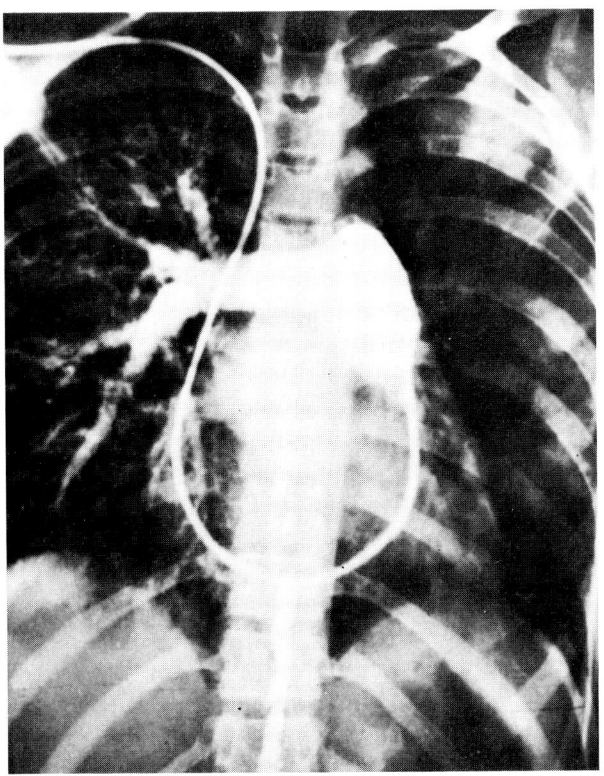

Fig. 53-3 Pulmonary angiogram demonstrating absence of filling of left pulmonary arterial branches indicative of large embolus obstructing left main pulmonary artery. (From DeWeese, J.A.: Venous and lymphatic disease. In Schwartz, S.I., editor: Principles of surgery, ed. 2, New York, 1974, McGraw-Hill Book Co.)

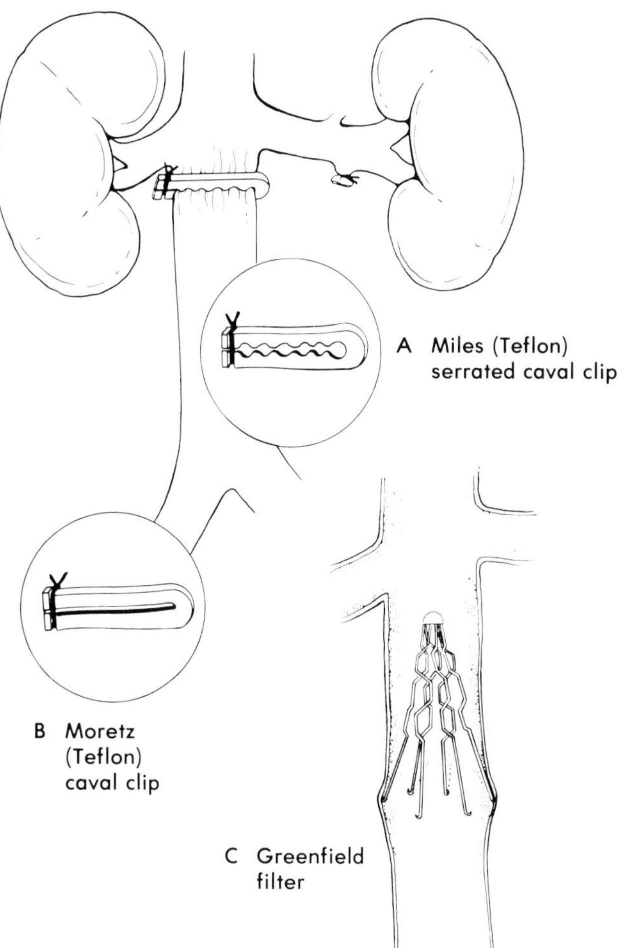

Fig. 53-4 Surgical prevention of pulmonary embolism. Large emboli can be trapped by partial interruption of the inferior vena cava. **A,** Serrated Teflon (Miles) clip. **B,** Smooth Teflon (Moretz) clip. These should be placed just distal to the renal veins, and the gonadal veins should be ligated. **C,** Greenfield filter, which is inserted transvenously through a jugular cutdown. Some surgeons prefer to simply ligate the cava. (From Goldstone, J.: Veins and lymphatics. In Way, L.W., editor: Current surgical diagnosis and treatment, ed. 7, Los Altos, Calif. 1985, Lange Medical Publications.)

ning. By combining this technique with a radioactive ^{131}I xenon ventilation scan (which demonstrates the distribution of this inhaled gas throughout the lung), a correct interpretation of the perfusion scan becomes more likely. In a patient with pulmonary embolus, a defect on the perfusion scan in an area of normal xenon ventilation is typically seen.[44,71]

The only definitive means of establishing the diagnosis of a pulmonary embolus is with the use of a pulmonary arteriogram that selectively evaluates the pulmonary arteries for evidence of embolization.[44,71] This technique allows radiographic visualization of the pulmonary arterial tree and a careful outline of those branches that may be occluded by a clot (Fig. 53-3). Unfortunately, this technique as conventionally performed is associated with significant risks and thus is usually carried out only when results with ventilation-perfusion pulmonary scanning are sufficiently confusing that more precise information is needed. An intravenous angiographic approach (that is less risky than the conventional approach), using a digital video subtraction technique, is currently being evaluated as an alternative approach to diagnosing pulmonary embolus. Early results are quite encouraging and have demonstrated excellent images of the pulmonary arterial tree.

Treatment. Once the diagnosis of pulmonary embolus has been established, intravenous heparin is the treatment of choice.[7,44,52,71] The dosage and approach to monitoring are the same as those already considered in the section on deep venous thrombosis. As with this latter entity, intravenous anticoagulation should be substituted with oral therapy (using warfarin) following the recommendations previously outlined. Patients with pulmonary embolus should be maintained on anticoagulation for at least 3 months. Many authorities believe that this should be lengthened to 6 months.

Occasionally a patient will develop a recurrent embolus while receiving anticoagulation or not be a suitable candidate for anticoagulation because of some bleeding diaphysis or recent bleeding problem such as gastrointestinal or intracranial hemorrhage. In such situations interruption of the inferior vena cava should be performed. Vena caval interruption should also be carried out in patients with known deep venous thromboses (but in whom no emboli have occurred) when anticoagulation is contraindicated to prevent embolic disease.

Several approaches have been used[4,26,28] (Fig. 53-4).

The first involves surgical placement of a caval clip that is positioned around the inferior vena cava just below the renal veins. Both retroperitoneal and transperitoneal approaches have been used to position such clips. The transperitoneal approach allows the concomitant ligation of the left ovarian vein in female patients that usually drains into the renal vein and may be an additional source of pulmonary emboli from the pelvic veins. In another approach to interrupting the vena cava, a balloon or filter is inserted into the inferior vena cava under fluoroscopic control. To accomplish this, an incision is usually made in the skin overlying the jugular vein, and the occluding balloon or filter is inserted transvenously through a jugular cutdown. A variety of trapping devices have been developed over the years, but the most popular one currently is the Greenfield filter.[37a] The advantages of the Greenfield filter over balloon techniques are that the vena cava is not totally occluded and the venous stasis complications in the lower extremity commonly associated with the balloon approach are less a problem. The transvenous approach of inserting a caval filter is especially attractive in the critically ill patient in whom direct surgical interruption of the vena cava is associated with considerable risk.

Occasionally a patient will be a victim of a massive pulmonary embolus with refractory hypotension. In this rare circumstance an emergency pulmonary embolectomy may be a life-saving procedure.[48] This operation, first performed by Trendelenburg nearly a century ago (and referred to by his name), involves the direct surgical removal of the embolus through a thoracotomy. In another approach devised by Greenfield and associates, a large suction catheter is inserted through the femoral vein for the removal of a pulmonary embolus.[27,28] Early results with this technique have been quite promising and may ultimately replace surgical embolectomy as the procedure of choice. Finally, thrombolytic therapy (i.e., urokinase and streptokinase) has also been used as an alternative to pulmonary embolectomy but has been fraught with a number of problems, including allergic reactions from these macromolecules and significant bleeding complications.[67]

Prophylaxis. Since as many as 95% of patients developing pulmonary embolism have as the source of emboli thromboses that arise in the deep veins of the legs, any prophylactic measures that can be used to reduce the incidence of postoperative deep venous thrombosis will also have direct bearing on the likelihood of pulmonary embolic disease occurring.[15,44,65,71] Thus measures to improve venous return and prevent venous stagnation are especially helpful and should include early ambulation after surgery, active leg exercises, and the avoidance of prolonged sitting and standing. Although their clinical value is still a debatable issue, most clinicians believe that elastic stockings are an important adjunctive prophylactic measure because they increase femoral venous blood flow. Intermittent compression devices that clearly enhance venous blood flow may also be applied during and/or after surgery; but, because of the cumbersome nature of these approaches, they have not gained widespread acceptance among most clinicians. Nonetheless, in patients at particularly high risk for the development of venous thrombosis, such maneuvers appear to decrease the development of venous thromboses. They are particularly suitable in patients requiring prolonged bed rest, as are passive exercises and the elevation of the foot of the bed at 15 to 25 degrees to increase venous return.

When to use prophylactic anticoagulation remains an unsettled issue. A number of studies have clearly shown that prophylactic heparinization can clearly prevent deep venous thrombosis.* The usual dosage scheme is to administer 5000 U of heparin subcutaneously 2 hours before surgery and every 8 to 12 hours after surgery until the patient has resumed ambulation. Although this dosage does not alter the normal coagulation time, it does activate antithrombin III, and through this effect low-dose heparin therapy mediates its beneficial action. Proponents of prophylactic heparinization emphasize the importance of instituting this treatment in patients who are at high risk for the development of deep venous thrombosis and stress that bleeding complications and transfusion requirements are only minimally increased when this approach is used. Other anticoagulant approaches that have been used in high-risk patients include the use of prothrombin depressants such as warfarin and platelet function suppressants such as aspirin and dipyridamole. Whereas low-dose heparin therapy has generally been ineffective in patients undergoing hip surgery, these other anticoagulant strategies have clearly decreased the incidence of postoperative deep venous thrombosis in this patient setting. It must be stressed, however, that any type of anticoagulant prophylaxis is contraindicated where even small amounts of bleeding could elicit disastrous complications. Examples would include operations on the brain and the eye.

Postphlebitic Syndrome. The postphlebitic syndrome (also called the chronic venous stasis syndrome) represents a state of chronic venous insufficiency with severe stasis dermatitis resulting from extensive thrombotic disease of the deep venous system of the leg.[36] Clinically the disease is characterized by varying degrees of edema (usually brawny and nonpitting), hyperpigmentation, and superficial ulceration (usually in the region of the medial malleolus) and dilated superficial veins. This constellation of findings occurs because the valves in the deep veins are destroyed and recanalization of previously thrombosed main veins is inadequate to sufficiently drain blood from the leg. Consequently, blood is diverted through the communicating veins into the superficial system, resulting in obvious secondary varicosities. This circumstance and the resulting venous hypertension is responsible for the findings just enumerated.

Treatment of the postphlebitic syndrome is both taxing and frustrating, both for the patient and physician. Therefore every effort should be made to prevent the development of this problem. In the patient who has been unfortuante enough to develop this disorder, effective external compression to increase venous return is the mainstay of therapy. Thus, as soon as the patient arises in the morning, a carefully wrapped elastic bandage or fitted stocking should be applied. Although pain may discourage any vigorous activity, the patient should be encouraged to exercise the leg when in the standing position. Prolonged standing

*References 2, 15, 38, 44, 51, 58, 65, 71, and 77.

or sitting is contraindicated and, when the affected leg is not active, the involved extremity should be elevated at a 45-degree angle. During sleep at night, the stocking or dressing may be removed, but the foot of the bed should be elevated so that the legs are higher than the heart to encourage venous return. Since the skin, particularly in the medial part of the ankle, is extremely fragile in these patients, care must be taken to resist even minor episodes of trauma. Even though itching is commonly encountered, scratching must be resisted, since this may also traumatize such skin and result in breakdown.

If skin ulcerations are present, effort should be made to encourage their healing with the application of saline dressings or with Unna's paste boot. This latter technique is especially helpful in that it maintains constant pressure over the leg and thereby enhances venous return, prevents irritation from external sources, and reduces the likelihood of bacterial infection. As healing is a slow process with these ulcers, it is not uncommon that a patient may need to be managed with such a boot for many months. If these conservative measures fail to heal the ulcer, formal surgical excision may be necessary, and a skin graft applied.[7,63] When this occurs, the incompetent venous perforators in the area of the ulcer are ligated and removed. Although grafting of this nature will generally heal the ulcer, a prolonged period of hospitalization to ensure proper wound care, leg elevation, and the appropriate application of compressive dressings is usually required.

VENOUS DISORDERS OF THE UPPER EXTREMITIES

With the more common use of synthetic intravenous cannulae for fluid and antibiotic administration and the increasing incidence of drug abuse in this country, thrombophlebitis involving superficial veins in the upper extremity has clearly become a more important problem in recent years. When intravenous access is required and the upper extremity is the preferred choice, care must be directed toward prevention of the infiltration of the infusing solution into the surrounding soft tissues. This is best accomplished by the routine use of metallic needles for short-term therapy and Teflon cannulae for longer courses of intravenous therapy.[79] The myriad of drugs used for care of the hospitalized patient and the potential for extravasation of such drugs into the perivascular tissues compound the likelihood of thrombophlebitis. Should superficial thrombophlebitis develop, treatment is similar to phlebitis of lower-extremity veins following removal of the access device. If a question of infection exists, antibiotics should also be instituted. If the involved vein is a true focus of infection (i.e., septic thrombophlebitis), the diseased vein should be surgically excised, since such a vein can be a source of major sepsis and even death.[54] Anticoagulant therapy is usually not necessary for upper-extremity superficial thrombophlebitis, since the incidence of a pulmonary embolus arising from this lesion is distinctly uncommon.

In addition to superficial thrombophlebitis of the upper extremity, thrombosis of the axillary and/or subclavian veins occasionally occurs. In contrast to deep venous thrombosis of the lower extremity, such thromboses are quite uncommon and account for only about 3% of all deep venous thromboses.[18] This low incidence is probably related to the continual movement of the upper extremity, virtually eliminating problems with venous stasis.

Thrombosis of the axillary vein is occasionally seen when the upper extremity is subjected to vigorous exercise, either related to sports or occupational activities, in which the arm is vigorously abducted on the shoulder. This type of thrombosis is frequently referred to as "effort thrombosis" and probably occurs in response to progressive trauma to the vein initiating thrombus formation. Obstruction most frequently occurs where the vein crosses the first rib and presumably results from compression of the vein between the clavicle and first rib. If the vein is totally occluded, an insidious swelling quickly develops that usually involves the entire arm and is nonpitting. Associated with these findings is a cyanotic mottling of the skin and a feeling of tightness, often pronounced in the axilla, with clear evidence of distention of the superficial veins. Other conditions that occasionally give rise to axillary vein thrombosis include congestive heart failure, indwelling venous catheters, any type of external trauma, and neoplastic disease (usually metastatic) in the region of the axilla. Diagnosis is usually obvious on clinical grounds alone and is supported by the demonstration of an elevated venous pressure in the anticubital veins that rises with muscular exercise in contrast to the usual fall in the nonoccluded state. In doubtful cases the diagnosis can be confirmed with venography. Treatment consists of arm rest and elevation in combination with anticoagulation (i.e., heparin) to prevent progression of the thrombus and potential embolization to the lungs. The dosage scheme is the same as that used for deep venous thrombotic disease in the legs. This approach generally results in rapid recovery. In occasional circumstances venous thrombectomy is performed to remove the occluding thrombus with the goal of preserving valvular integrity. Since rethrombosis following this procedure is commonly encountered, it is seldom used at present.

Occlusion of the subclavian vein may result as an extension of axillary vein thrombosis or as a separate entity. A particularly common cause is intimal injury from an indwelling venous catheter that is more frequently seen today with the increasing use of total parenteral nutrition than it was a decade ago.[22] Management considerations are similar to those discussed for axillary vein thrombosis.

Although the superior vena cava is not technically an upper extremity vein, because treatment of occlusive disease of this vein is so similar to that of axillary (subclavian) vein thrombosis, it is appropriate to consider discussion of this problem in this section. Occlusion of the superior vena cava usually occurs from extrinsic compression by some neoplastic process or enlarged lymph nodes.[46,69] Rarely direct trauma and/or infection from insertion of a foreign body such as a central venous catheter may also lead to thrombosis. The *superior vena caval syndrome* that may result from any of these circumstances is usually dramatic clinically and consists of cyanosis of the skin involving the head and neck with edema of the upper chest and extremities and varying degrees of venous distention. Such findings may also be associated with varying degrees of vertigo, headache, epistaxis, and occasionally fainting. As with acute axillary vein thrombosis, an elevated upper-extremity venous pressure can be demonstrated in this condition, but venography will be necessary to definitely confirm and define the level and extent of obstruction. Treatment is generally directed to the underlying source of disease. Occasionally this will require surgical resection of the underlying neoplastic process; at other times radiation therapy has been successful in relieving the compression if the underlying disease is neoplastic (particularly that arising from bronchogenic carcinoma). Whatever the underlying cause, anticoagulation is clearly indicated.

LYMPHEDEMA

Just as the primary function of veins is to return blood to the heart, the major function of the lymphatic system is resorption of macromolecules (particularly albumin) from the interstitial space and their delivery to the subclavian veins through the lymphatic and thoracic ducts.[42] The magnitude of this feat becomes apparent when it is realized that in a given 24-hour period greater than 50% of the circulating albumin is lost into the interstitial space. Over a similar time period, as much as 4 L of lymph flow are returned to the large veins containing as much as 100 to 200 g of protein. Failure of the lymphatics to accomplish this function in the extremities will result in the accumulation of excess amounts of protein in the interstitial space, a condition known as lymphedema. This may be the result of a developmental abnormality of the lymphatics or arise secondarily from lymphatic obstruction.

The primary form of lymphedema is a developmental defect of the lymphatics.[1,43] It may involve any extremity, but more frequently is observed in the legs, and often the left lower extremity alone. Several subtypes have been recognized. When present at birth, it is called *congenital lymphedema* (10%). The hereditary form of congenital lymphedema has been termed Milroy's disease and apparently follows a sex-linked dominant pattern; it is permanent, progresses in severity over time, and has no associated constitutional symptoms. *Lymphedema praecox* (80%) is similar to congenital lymphedema, except that it becomes clinically obvious sometime between the adolescent years and the age of 35. The third form of primary lymphedema is known as *lymphedema tarta* (10%) and is seen in patients over the age of 35 years. In all three forms, a variety of patterns can be identified microscopically, including aplasia, hypoplasia, and dilation and tortuosity of the lymphatics.

Primary lymphedema clearly affects women more often than men by a ratio of 3:1 and initially usually involves one lower extremity, generally the left leg. As many as 50% of these patients will ultimately have involvement of both legs. Because of the high incidence of this disease in adolescent females, a hormonal cause has been suggested.[1,43] Of further potential etiologic importance is the lower subcutaneous hydrostatic pressure that has been identified in women in contrast to men, a circumstance that would favor edema formation.[20] Why the left leg is more commonly involved than the right remains uncertain, but may be related to the known compression of the left common iliac vein by the right common iliac artery that has been identified in patients with lymphedema.[12]

The acquired (secondary) form of lymphedema typically occurs in later life (over 40 years) and may have a number of different causes.[42] Worldwide, the most common cause is lymph node blockage by the parasite *Filaria bancrofti*. Other causes include recurrent lymphangitis or chronic bacterial infections, changes in the circulation following thrombophlebitis (such as the postphlebitic syndrome), scarring and fibrosis from radiation burns or other types of trauma, neoplastic invasion of the lymphatics, tuberculosis, sarcoidosis, lymphogranuloma venereum, and allergic reactions. In the United States, removal of inguinal or axillary regional nodes by surgical excision or ablative radiation in the management of malignant disease is a common cause. Lymphatic obstruction from prostate carcinoma in men and lymphoma or intrapelvic carcinoma in women is also a frequent cause. In patients undergoing radical mastectomy for breast cancer, lymphedema may affect the ipsilateral upper extremity in as many as 15% to 20% of patients secondary to the number of lymph nodes removed or the concomitant radiation therapy used for treatment.

Pathophysiology and Clinical Presentation

Whether primary or secondary, the pathology underlying lymphedema is basically the same, i.e., obstruction of normal lymphatic drainage.[42] This results in inadequate transport of lymph from the interstitial space, giving rise to an increased protein concentration within this tissue compartment. Accompanying this increase in protein concentration is an increase in fluid accumulation by the osmotic attraction of the protein, eventuating in tissue distention and stretching of the fibrous supportive tissue, skin, and lymphatics. The net effect of all of these changes as the protein concentration increases in the edema fluid (from a normal of 0.1 to 0.5 g/100 ml to a concentration of 1 to 5 g/100 ml) is the stimulation of tissue fibrosis involving the connective tissue components within the subcutaneous fat. Such aberrations eventually lead to skin thickening and hyperkeratosis that ultimately give the appearance of elephantiasis (Fig. 53-5).

Early in the development of lymphedema, the edema is soft, pitting, and often limited to the ankle. As the process worsens, the lymphedema becomes firm, rubbery, and nonpitting and ultimately involves most of the leg. In contrast to the edema associated with chronic venous insufficiency, lymphedema is rarely associated with hyperpigmentation or ulceration and does not decrease with overnight leg elevation. In addition, recurrent episodes of cellulitis and lymphangitis are common complications of lymphedema and may develop even following minor injuries to the involved extremity. When these problems occur, erythema, pain, and systemic signs of infection are usually present. The infection is often visible as red streaks in the skin of the involved extremity and not infrequently spreads from the foot to the groin. The causative organism is most commonly beta hemolytic streptococcus.

A less frequent, but more devastating, complication of lymphedema is lymphangiosarcoma.[72] This lesion is virtually always associated with lymphedema and usually occurs in the upper extremity following mastectomy for breast carcinoma. It arises from the lymphatic endothelium and presents clinically as blue, red, or purple macular or

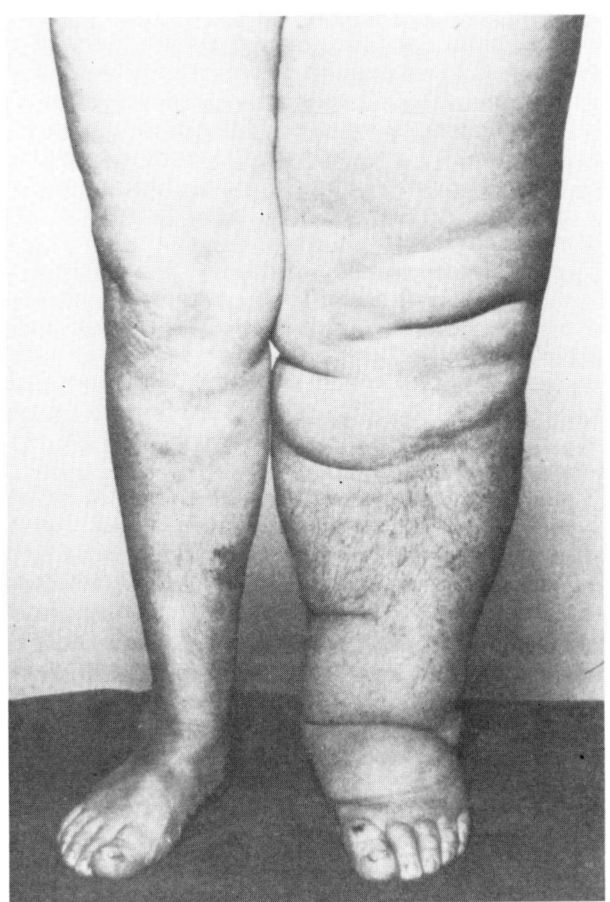

Fig. 53-5 Massive unilateral lymphedema of the leg. (From Mansfield, A.O.: Vein and lymphatic surgery. In Cuschieri, A., Giles, G.R., and Moossa, A.R., editors: Essential surgical practice, Bristol, England, 1982, John Wright & Sons, Ltd.)

papular lesions in the skin or subcutaneous tissue. Occasionally it may present as a large ulcerating mass. The prognosis for this lesion is dismal, and most patients succumb to this disease within 2 years of diagnosis.

Treatment

Although there is no known cure for lymphedema (whether primary or secondary) at the present time, most patients can be managed effectively without surgery.[41,42] The major objectives are to control the edema as much as possible and prevent infectious complications. To reduce lymph formation, a variety of measures can be used. These include avoiding prolonged periods of standing and frequently elevating the foot and ankles throughout the day. During sleep the foot of the bed should be elevated on blocks at least 6 to 8 inches. External compression is particularly important, and heavy duty elastic stockings (preferably of the leotard type) should be worn at all times when the patient is awake. Although knee-length stockings may be more practical, they usually are not as effective as the longer hose. In patients in whom the disease has not progressed to the stage of severe fibrosis, externally applied air compression devices are often of value in milking edema fluid from the extremity. In all patients dietary sodium should be restricted, and in many patients intermittent diuretic therapy is of value in controlling the swelling, particularly if the fibrotic stage has not developed. Great care should be taken to protect areas of vulnerable skin from injury to prevent cellulitis and lymphangitis. When infection develops, intravenous antibiotics should be initiated. In patients with repeated episodes of cellulitis and lymphangitis, long-term prophylactic antibiotic treatment may be necessary.

In those patients in whom the lymphedema is not satisfactorily controlled by the measures just outlined (20% or less), some type of surgical management scheme will be required.[24,41,42,62] Unfortunately, no single surgical procedure will work in all patients, and the large number of procedures that have been developed attest to the difficulty in managing this problem. Generally, two broad types of surgical approaches have been used to treat lymphedema. These include excisional procedures in which varying amounts of the involved subcutaneous compartment are removed and those in which some physiologically designed approach is fashioned to reconstruct lymphatic drainage.

An excisional procedure is the operation of choice when moderate lymphedema is present, and the degree of skin fibrosis is not extensive. With this surgical approach the affected skin and the underlying lymphedematous subcutaneous tissue are totally excised, and split-thickness skin grafts are placed on the investing fascia or bared muscle. To be effective, total excision of the involved lymphedematous tissue must be removed; lesser procedures are usually associated with recurrent swelling.

Of the physiologic approaches available to improve lymphatic drainage, the Thompson procedure has been particularly successful and has enjoyed considerable popularity among surgeons who deal with lymphedema problems.[74] This procedure involves the use of a shaved dermal flap that is positioned beneath the muscles along the medial and lateral aspects of the involved extremity and thereby enables drainage of the involved subcutaneous compartment into the deep lymphatics, presumably through connections that have developed between the normal muscle and abnormal subcutaneous lymphatic systems. Whether such connections do indeed develop remains to be documented, but clinical results have generally been good with this surgical approach. Another physiologic approach to lymphedema management involves the construction of an omental pedicle that is tunneled subcutaneously from the abdominal cavity to the affected limb, thereby allowing lymph to return from the limb to the abdomen.[25] This approach has been fraught with a number of complications and has generally not been as successful as the Thompson procedure. Finally, using various microvascular techniques, direct anastomoses have been created between major veins and various lymphatic vessels and between lymphatic vessels themselves.[17,53] It remains to be seen whether such surgical maneuvers will provide significant long-term improvement in lymphatic flow.

SUMMARY

Although a variety of venous disorders may affect the arms and legs, the most important abnormality in terms of morbidity and potential mortality is that of deep venous thrombosis of the lower extremity. Not only may this condition give rise to the postphlebitic syndrome, management of which can be taxing and frustrating both for the patient and the physician, but more importantly deep venous thrombosis is responsible for the majority of the more than 250,000 deaths that occur annually in the United States from pulmonary embolism. As the pathogenesis of deep venous disease has become more clearly defined, knowledge concerning those patients at particular risk for the development of this disorder has also become clarified so that appropriate prophylactic measures can be instituted. Of these, prophylactic heparinization has been clearly shown to prevent deep venous thrombosis when administered subcutaneously before surgery and every 8 to 12 hours following surgery until normal ambulation has been resumed. In those patients in whom anticoagulation is contraindicated, either because the patient has a concomitant bleeding disorder or has suffered a pulmonary embolus in spite of presumed adequate anticoagulation, interruption of the vena cava has also proven to be a worthwhile approach in preventing pulmonary embolization, even though it does not alter the thrombotic process within the legs. Such interruption can be accomplished directly surgically by placing a clip across the vena cava just below the renal veins or indirectly by passing a filter transvenously through a cut down in the jugular vein to trap emboli.

Of the lymphatic diseases that may affect the extremities, lymphedema is clearly the most important. This disorder may result from a primary developmental abnormality in which the lymphatic vessels are either absent entirely or malformed or may occur secondarily from lymphatic blockage as a result of a condition such as scarring and fibrosis from ablative radiation or neoplastic invasion of the lymphatics. Whatever the cause, there is no known cure for lymphedema; but most patients can be managed effectively without surgery with the use of a variety of conservative measures such as external compression of the affected limb to enhance lymphatic drainage. In the event that conservative measures are not effective, a number of surgical procedures have been used, the most common being excision of the affected skin and the underlying lymphedematous subcutaneous tissue in the involved limb.

REFERENCES

1. Allen, E.V.: Lymphedema of the extremities: classification, etiology, and differential diagnosis—a study of 300 cases, Arch. Intern. Med. **54:**606, 1934.
2. Andersson, G., et al.: Subcutaneous administration of heparin: a randomized comparison with intravenous administration of heparin to patients with deep vein thrombosis, Thromb. Res. **27:**631, 1982.
3. Arnesen, H., Hoiseth, A., and Ly, B.: Streptokinase or heparin in the treatment of deep vein thrombosis, Acta Med. Scand. **211:**65, 1982.
4. Barker, W.F.: Milestones in the use of interruption in venous thromboembolism: David M. Hume Memorial Lecture, Am. J. Surg. **138:**192, 1979.
5. Barnes, R.W.: Current status of noninvasive tests in the diagnosis of venous disease, Surg. Clin. North Am. **62:**489, 1982.
6. Bell, W.R., and Simon, T.L.: Current status of pulmonary thromboembolic disease: pathophysiology, diagnosis, prevention, and treatment, Am. Heart J. **103:**239, 1982.
7. Bergan, J.J., Flinn, W.R., and Yao, J.S.T.: Venous reconstructive surgery, Surg. Clin. North Am. **62:**399, 1982.
8. Bernstein, E.F., editor: Noninvasive diagnostic techniques in vascular disease, St. Louis, 1978, The C.V. Mosby Co.
9. Bertelsen, S., and Anker, W.: Phlegmasia coerulea dolens: pathophysiology, clinical features, treatment, and prognosis, Acta Chir. Scand. **134:**107, 1968.
10. Brakkee, A.J., and Kuiper, J.P.: Plethysmographic measurement of venous flow resistance in man, VASA **11:**166, 1982.
11. Buckler, P., and Douglas, A.S.: Antithrombotic treatment, Br. Med. J. **287:**196, 1983.
12. Calran, J.: Lymphoedema: the case for doubt, Br. J. Plast. Surg. **21:**32, 1968.
13. Consensus Development Center Summaries: Thrombolytic therapy in thrombosis, **3:**13, 1980.
14. Conti, S., Daschbach, M., and Blaisdell, W.: A comparison of high-dose versus conventional-dose heparin therapy for deep vein thrombosis, Surgery **92:**972, 1982.
15. Coon, W.W.: Venous thromboembolism: prevalence, risk factors, and prevention, Clin. Chest Med. **5:**391, 1984.
16. Copplestone, A., and Roath, S.: Assessment of therapeutic control of anticoagulation, Acta Haematol. **71:**376, 1984.
17. Degni, M.: New technique of lymphatic-venous anastomosis for the treatment of lymphedema. VASA **3:**479, 1974.
18. Demeter, S.L., et al.: Upper extremity thrombosis: etiology and prognosis, Angiology **33:**743, 1982.
19. Duckert, F.: Thrombolytic therapy, Semin. Thromb. Hemostas. **10:**87, 1984.
20. Emmett, A.J., Barron, J.N., and Veall, N.: The use of I^{131} albumin tissue clearance measurements and other physiological tests for the clinical assessment of patients with lymphoedema, Br. J. Plast. Surg. **20:**1, 1967.
21. Errichetti, L.J.: Management of oral anticoagulant therapy: Experience with an anticoagulation clinic, Arch. Intern. Med. **144:**1966, 1984.
22. Freund, H.R.: Chemical phlebothrombosis of large veins: a not uncommon complication of total parenteral nutrition, Arch. Surg. **116:**1220, 1981.
23. Frisbie, J.H., et al.: Venous thrombosis and pulmonary embolism occurring at close intervals in spinal cord injury patients, Paraplegia **21:**270, 1983.
24. Glenn, W.W.: The lymphatic system: some surgical considerations, Arch. Surg. **116:**989, 1981.
25. Goldsmith, H.S.: Long-term evaluation of omental transposition for chronic lymphedema, Ann. Surg. **180:**847, 1974.
26. Gomez, G.A., Cutler, B.S., and Wheeler, H.B.: Transvenous interruption of the inferior vena cava, Surgery **93:**612, 1983.
27. Greenfield, L.J.: Pulmonary embolism: diagnosis and management. In Current Problems in Surgery, Chicago, 1976, Year Book Medical Publishers, Inc.
28. Greenfield, L.J., and Langhan, M.R.: Surgical approaches to thromboembolism, Br. J. Surg. **71:**968, 1984.
29. Harvey, W.: On the motion of the heart and blood of animals, Chicago, Ill., 1962, Henry Regnery Co.
30. Hobbs, J.J., editor: The treatment of venous disorders, Philadelphia, 1977, J.B. Lippincott Co.
31. Holm, H.A., et al: Heparin treatment of deep venous thrombosis in 280 patients: Symptoms related to dosage, Acta Med. Scand. **326:**57, 1984.
32. Hull, R.D., et al.: Cost-effectiveness of clinical diagnosis, venography, and noninvasive testing in patients with symptomatic deep-vein thrombosis, N. Engl. J. Med. **304:**1561, 1981.
33. Husni, E.A.: Reconstruction of veins: the need for objectivity, J. Cardiovasc. Surg. **24:**525, 1983.
34. Husni, E.A., and Williams, W.A.: Superficial thrombophlebitis of lower limbs, Surgery **91:**70, 1982.
35. Husted, S.E., et al.: Deep vein thrombosis detection by ^{99m}Tc-plasmin test and phlebography, Br. J. Surg. **71:**65, 1984.
36. Jacobs, P.: Pathogenesis of the postphlebitic syndrome, Ann. Rev. Med. **34:**91, 1983.
37. Johansson, L., et al.: Comparison of streptokinase with heparin: late results in the treatment of deep venous thrombosis, Acta Med. Scand. **206:**93, 1979.

37a. Jones, D.K., Barnes, R.W., and Greenfield, L.J.: Greenfield vena caval filter: rationale and current indications, Ann. Thorac. Surg. (suppl.): **42:**S48-S55, 1986.

38. Kakkar, V.V.: Low-dose heparin—present status and future trends, Scand. J. Haematol. (suppl.) **36:**158, 1980.
39. Keith, L.M., Jr., and Smead, W.L.: Saphenous vein stripping and its complications, Surg. Clin. North Am. **63:**1303, 1983.
40. Kiil, J., et al.: Urokinase or heparin in the management of patients with deep vein thrombosis? Acta Chir. Scand. **147:**529, 1981.
41. Kinmonth, J.B.: Lymphoedema and its treatment, Br. J. Plast. Surg. **7:**193, 1954.
42. Kinmonth, J.B.: The lymphatics: surgery, lymphography, and diseases of the chyle and lymph systems, ed. 2, Arnold, 1983.
43. Kinmonth, J.B., Tracey, G.D., and Marsh, J.D.: Primary lymphedema: clinical and lymphangiographic studies of a series of 107 patients in which the lower limbs were affected, Br. J. Surg. **45:**1, 1957.
44. Knight, B., and Zaini, M.R.: Pulmonary embolism and venous thrombosis, Am. J. Forensic Med. Pathol. **1:**227, 1980.
45. Kristiansen, P., et al.: Thrombosis after elective phlebography as demonstrated with the ^{125}I-fibrinogen test, Acta Radiologica Diag. **22:**577, 1981.
46. Lochridge, S.K., Knibbe, W.P., and Doty, D.B.: Obstruction of the superior vena cava, Surgery **85:**14, 1979.
47. Lofgren, E.P., and Lofgren, K.A.: The surgical treatment of superficial thrombophlebitis, Surgery **90:**49, 1981.
48. Mattox, K.L., et al.: Pulmonary embolectomy for acute massive pulmonary embolism, Ann. Surg. **195:**726, 1982.
49. Menzolan, J.O., et al.: Therapeutic and clinical course of deep venous thrombosis, Am. J. Surg. **146:**581, 1983.
50. Modig, J., et al.: Comparative influences of epidural and general anesthesia on deep venous thrombosis and pulmonary embolism after total hip replacement, Acta Chir. Scand. **147:**125, 1981.
51. Multicenter Trial Committee: Prophylactic efficacy of low-dose dihydroergotamine and heparin in postoperative deep venous thrombosis following intra-abdominal operations, J. Vasc. Surg. **1:**608, 1984.
52. Murley, R.: Venous thromboembolism: challenge and fulfillment? Ann. R. College of Surgeons of England **64:**151, 1982.
53. O'Brien, B.M., and Shafiroff, B.B.: Microlymphaticovenous and resectional surgery in obstructive lymphedema, World J. Surg. **3:**3, 1979.
54. O'Neill, J.A., Jr., et al.: Suppurative thrombophlebitis—a lethal complication of intravenous therapy, J. Trauma **8:**256, 1968.
55. Penner, J.: Hypercoagulation and thrombosis, Med. Clin, North Am. **64:**743, 1980.
56. Plate, G., et al.: Thrombectomy with temporary arteriovenous fistula: the treatment of choice in acute iliofemoral venous thrombosis, J. Vasc. Surg. **1:**867, 1984.
57. Ruckley, C.V., and Buist, T.A.: Venography in the diagnosis and management of deep vein thrombosis, Letter to the Editor. Br. Med. J. **286:**1512, 1983.
58. Salzman, E.W.: Progress in preventing venous thromboembolism, N. Engl. J. Med. **309:**980, 1983.
59. Salzman, E.W., et al.: Management of heparin therapy, N. Engl. J. Med. **292:**1046, 1975.
60. Sandler, D.A., et al.: Diagnosis of deep vein thrombosis: comparison of clinical evaluation, ultrasound, plethysmography, and venoscan with x-ray venogram, Lancet **2:**716, 1984.
61. Sasahara, A.A., Sharma, G.V., and Tow, D.E.: Clinical use of thrombolytic agents in venous thromboembolism, Arch. Intern. Med. **142:**684, 1982.
62. Savage, R.C.: The surgical management of lymphedema, Surg. Gynecol. Obstet. **160:**283, 1985.
63. Schanzer, H., and Pierce, E.C.: A rational approach to surgery of the chronic venous stasis syndrome, Ann. Surg. **195:**25, 1982.
64. Schaub, R.B., et al.: Early events in the formation of a venous thrombus following local trauma and stasis, Lab Invest. **51:**218, 1984.
65. Scholz, P.M., Jones, R.H., and Sabiston, D.C.: Prophylaxis of thromboembolism, Adv. Surg. **13:**115, 1979.
66. Secker-Walker, R.H.: On purple emperors, pulmonary embolism and venous thrombosis, Letter to the Editor, Ann. Intern. Med. **98:**1006, 1983.
67. Sharma, G.V., et al.: Thrombolytic therapy. N. Engl. J. Med. **306:**1268, 1982.
68. Shepard, T.J., and Vanhoutte, P.M.: Role of the venous system in circulatory control, Mayo Clin. Proc. **53:**246, 1978.
69. Skinner, D.B., and Salzman, E.W.: The challenge of superior vena caval obstruction, J. Thorac. Cardiovasc. Surg. **49:**824, 1965.
70. Sladen, J.G.: Compression sclerotherapy: preparation, technique, complications, and results. Am. J. Surg. **146:**228, 1983.
71. Stein, P.D., and Willis, P.W., III: Diagnosis, prophylaxis, and treatment of acute pulmonary embolism, Arch. Intern. Med. **143:**1983, 1983.
72. Stewart, F.S., and Treves, N.: Lymphangiosarcoma in postmastectomy lymphedema: report of 6 cases in elephantiasis chirurgica, Cancer **1:**64, 1948.
73. Tawes, R.L., Kennedy, P.A., and Harris, E.J.: Management of deep venous thrombosis and pulmonary embolism during pregnancy, Am. J. Surg. **144:**141, 1982.
74. Thompson, N.: The surgical treatment of chronic lymphoedema of the extremities, Surg. Clin. North Am. **47:**445, 1967.
75. Tolins, S.H.: Treatment of varicose veins: an update, Am. J. Surg. **145:**248, 1983.
76. van de Loo, J.C., et al.: Controlled multicenter pilot study of urokinase—heparin and streptokinase in deep vein thrombosis, Thromb. Haemostas. **50:**660, 1983.
77. Wessler, S., and Gitel, S.N.: Low-dose heparin: is the risk worth the benefit? Am. Heart J. **98:**94, 1979.
78. Wheeler, H.B., Patwardhan, N.A., and Anderson, F.A.: The place of occlusive impedance plethysmography in the diagnosis of venous thrombosis. In Bergan, J.J., and Yao, J.S.T., editors: Venous problems, Chicago, 1978, Year Book Medical Publishers, Inc.
79. Williams, D.N., et al.: Infusion thrombophlebitis and infiltration associated with intravenous cannulae, National Intravenous Therapy Assoc. Inc. **5:**379, 1982.
80. Winter, J.H., et al.: Case report: thrombosis after venography in familial antithrombin III deficiency. Br. Med. J. **283:**1436, 1981.
81. Winter, J.H., et al.: Preoperative antithrombin III activities and lipoprotein concentrations as predictors of venous thrombosis in patients with fracture of neck and femur, J. Clin. Pathol. **36:**570, 1983.

54

O. Howard Frazier and Rolando Colon

Disorders of the Thoracic Aorta

Surgically significant lesions of the thoracic aorta include aneurysms, dissections, and traumatic ruptures. The surgical cure of intrathoracic aortic lesions represents an important achievement in modern surgery. With the advent of cardiopulmonary bypass, the introduction of safer anesthetic techniques, and the development of synthetic grafts, these complex lesions are now amenable to operative therapy with excellent results.

In the past syphilitic aneurysms were common, but now most thoracic aortic disease results from degenerative processes. Early recognition and diagnosis, along with timely surgical intervention and improved preoperative and postoperative care, have resulted in long-term survival for this group of patients. This chapter will discuss the pathophysiologic aberrations responsible for the development of thoracic aneurysms and aortic dissections and the physiologic principles underlying their management.

INTRINSIC THORACIC AORTIC DISEASE

Thoracic Aneurysms

Classification

Aneurysms of the thoracic aorta can be classified according to type, shape, and location. An organized categorization allows the surgeon to use a systematic approach to the treatment of these complex vascular lesions. Aneurysms in the thoracic aorta involving the three layers of the arterial wall are called "true aneurysms," whereas those involving only the adventitia are called "false aneurysms" or "pulsating hematomas." False aneurysms usually result from trraumatic rupture, most commonly seen in decelerating blunt chest trauma.

Fusiform aneurysms, in which the vessel assumes a spindle shape, result in circumferential dilation of all layers of the aorta. They can affect a localized portion or an extensive segment of the aorta, and they are usually secondary to degenerative diseases, such as arteriosclerosis and cystic medial necrosis.[50] Saccular aneurysms are localized spherical dilations that affect one segment of the vessel wall and are connected to the lumen by a mouth. The aneurysmal sac is usually filled by thrombus. These lesions are usually secondary to syphilis or other bacterial infections following an episode of bacterial endocarditis.

Aneurysms involving the aortic arch are classified into four categories according to location.[12] Type A lesions are localized and saccular, involving only the transverse arch. Type B lesions are fusiform and involve the ascending aorta and arch. Type C lesions extend into the proximal descending aorta, and Type D lesions are more extensive, involving the entire descending aorta (Fig. 54-1). Although Type D lesions are the least common, they are the most challenging in terms of surgical therapy.

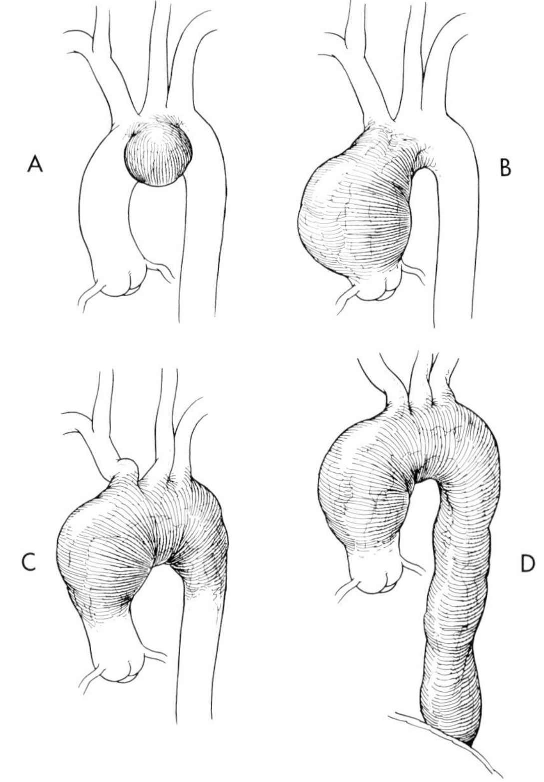

Fig. 54-1 Cooley classification of aortic arch aneurysms. **A,** Type A lesions are saccular lesions, confined to the arch. **B,** Type B lesions are fusiform, involving the ascending aorta and proximal arch. **C,** Type C lesions extend into the proximal descending aorta; and **D,** Type D lesions involve the entire descending aorta. (From Cooley, D.A.: Surgical treatment of aortic aneurysms, Philadelphia, 1986, W.B. Saunders Co.)

Aneurysmal disease of the aorta is often a multifocal disease. In a review of 1510 patients with aortic aneurysms, Crawford and Cohen[15] identified 191 patients (12.6%) with multifocal disease. Abdominal aortic aneurysms are the most common lesions accompanying thoracic aneurysms. For this reason the entire aorta should be evaluated when a patient is being considered for surgical treatment of an aortic aneurysm because better results are obtained when both lesions are corrected at the same time.

Traumatic rupture of the aorta produces a false aneurysm, usually located distal to the left subclavian artery at the level of the ligamentum arteriosum. This type of lesion is usually saccular and constitutes a surgical emergency most commonly seen in major trauma centers. It is discussed in a separate section later in this chapter.

Pathophysiology

Saccular and fusiform aneurysms of the aorta result from loss of structural integrity of the aortic wall and its individual components.[52] Alterations in the adventitia[21] and loss of lamellar units in the tunica media[45] have been cited as the major causes of aneurysmal dilation of the aorta. Unusual hemodynamic stresses and impaired blood flow can cause these pathologic changes as a result of deficient delivery of nutrients and ischemia of the vessel wall secondary to involvement of vasa vasorum by various degenerative, inflammatory, and infectious disease states. This assumption is supported by the fact that aneurysms are more common in the abdominal than in the thoracic aorta, and the observation that the thoracic aorta has more vasa vasorum originating from a system of paired intercostal arteries compared with the abdominal aorta, which has single lumbar vessels.[5]

In the case of syphilitic aortitis, active inflammatory destruction of all elements of the arterial wall occurs at a faster rate than that at which the damage can be repaired by fibrous tissue proliferation, and it is aggravated by severe endoarteritis of the vasa vasorum with subsequent ischemia of the vessel wall.[21] Most syphilitic aneurysms are saccular, and they are usually located in the ascending aorta and arch.[31,48] Fortunately, the early diagnosis and treatment of syphilis and the use of penicillin have made this complication a rare cause of aortic aneurysms today.

Most aneurysms of the ascending aorta presently encountered exhibit the histologic characteristics of cystic medial necrosis,[33] which were originally described by Gsell and Erdheim. This type of pathologic lesion is found in patients suffering from Marfan's syndrome[3,4] and usually affects the aortic root, an area of high stress caused by the velocity and turbulence of blood flow in this region. The histologic pattern reveals necrosis and disappearance of muscle cells in the middle third of the media with disintegration of elastic laminae and collagen. A mucoid material fills the cystic spaces. The primary lesion is accompanied by secondary tears caused by the underlying focal weakness.[4,53] Annuloaortic ectasia represents a severe form of cystic medial necrosis with electron microscopic changes similar to those found in patients both with and without Marfan's syndrome.[54] This ectatic condition affects the entire ascending aorta, extending from the aortic annulus to the innominate artery. When present, it can cause severe congestive heart failure secondary to aortic insufficiency, with a high risk of aortic rupture or dissection.[9]

The concept of cystic medial necrosis (CMN) as an intrinsic disease of the media that caused aneurysms of the aorta has been challenged by Schlatmann and Becker.[55] They studied histologic changes in the media of the normal aortas of 100 patients at different ages and found that the changes atrributed to CMN were present in these subjects, the frequency of which increased with age. They proposed that these changes are the result of hemodynamic stress on the vessel wall and represent a process of injury and repair in the normal aging aorta. Therefore the ascending aorta, which is subjected to higher hemodynamic stress, is the most common site for histologic changes caused by CMN.

With the steady increase in the number of older persons in the population and with the control of the late complications of syphilis, arteriosclerosis has emerged as a more common cause of aortic aneurysmal disease today. Arteriosclerotic aneurysms are confined mainly to the descending and distal thoracic aorta and are fusiform. Once the media and adventitia have been weakened by arteriosclerosis, the disease progresses steadily, and it is aggravated by the presence of hypertension, progression of the dilation, and further ischemia of the aneurysmal wall. The primary factors contributing to the formation of arteriosclerotic aneurysms are alterations in blood flow to the vasa vasorum of the vessel wall and disturbances in intraluminal flow patterns.[21] It is also known that flow across stenotic plaques creates high lateral pressures and that turbulent reversed flow likewise impacts against the wall. This results in structural fatigue and subsequent dilation,[29] suggesting another factor of etiologic importance.

Infections of the vessel wall, by suppurative or granulomatous processes, result in formation of mycotic aneurysms.[34] These aneurysms are usually saccular and can develop in any part of the aorta. Previously damaged vessels are more likely to be affected, with the resultant symptoms depending on the size and location of the lesion. Aortitis of unknown cause or that arising in association with different autoimmune disorders is also characterized by aortic dilation and the formation of aneurysms. The exception is Takayasu's arteritis, which is primarily an inflammatory disease associated with severe stenotic lesions of the aorta and other large and medium-sized vessels.[34] Nonspecific aortitis can also result in multiple saccular aneurysms of the aorta, with death attributed to rupture.[28]

Inflammatory aneurysms of the aorta are usually located in the terminal aorta, accompanied by a severe inflammatory process in the retroperitoneal space, encasing the ureters and sometimes the vena cava. Histologic analysis reveals destruction and replacement of both the media and adventitia with a thick, fibrotic wall. Both layers are infiltrated with lymphocytes, plasma cells, lymphoid follicles, and multinucleated giant cells.[18] However, the occurrence of these aneurysms in the thoracic aorta usually will not involve the surrounding mediastinum and the pleura.

Diagnosis

Clinical Presentation. The clinical presentation and symptomatology of thoracic aneurysms are related to the location of the lesion and the compression of adjacent structures. The erosion of large masses through ribs and sternum is a late finding, and fortunately this type of aneurysm now occurs rarely. Symptoms include pain, stridor, and coughing produced by the aneurysm's compressing the vagus nerves, trachea, and bronchi. Congestive heart failure is common in aneurysms of the ascending aorta involving the aortic annulus as a result of aortic insufficiency. Free rupture into the pericardial sac or pleura is catastrophic and is diagnosed post mortem.

Occasionally, the diagnosis is suspected in an asymptomatic patient who is found to have an upper mediastinal mass contiguous with the aortic shadow in routine chest x-ray film. Further studies are then indicated to confirm the diagnosis.

Special Diagnostic Techniques. The patient with thoracic aortic aneurysmal disease requires a thorough multidisci-

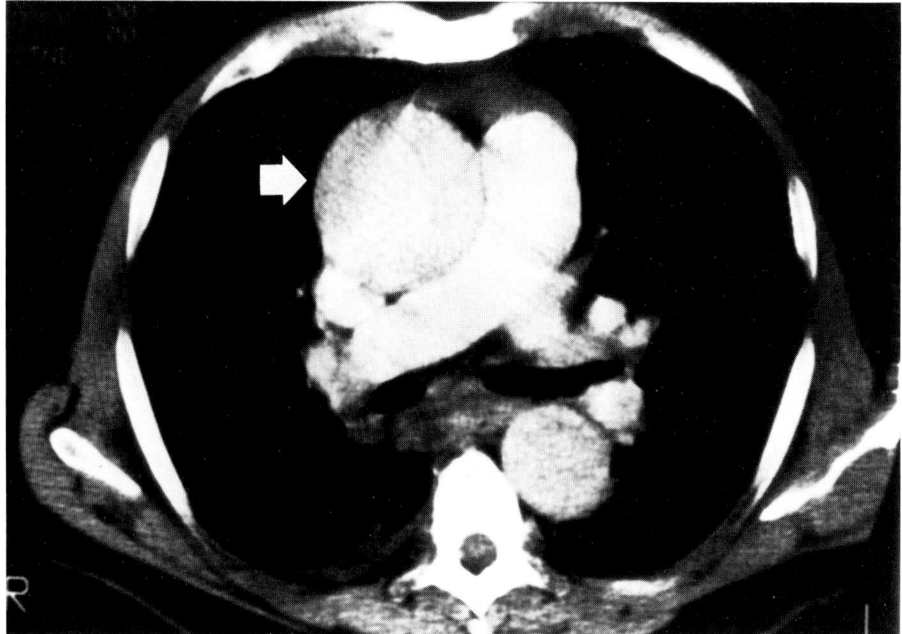

Fig. 54-2 Computerized axial tomography showing aneurysm of the ascending aorta *(arrow)*.

plinary evaluation so that the surgeon will have all information necessary to plan the surgical procedure. Routine chest x-ray films and arteriography remain the standards to which newer techniques are compared. However, arteriography is an invasive technique with specific risks for critically ill patients. Thus a trend toward using noninvasive techniques for diagnosis is developing with promising results. Of these, computerized axial tomography is useful in describing certain characteristics of thoracic aneurysms, including their configuration and location, the extension of the disease process, and tissue modifications (Fig. 54-2).

Another new technique for evaluating aortic disease is that of magnetic resonance imaging (MRI). MRI produces images of mediastinal vessels along their axes and creates sagittal and coronal views without degradation of spatial resolution.[40] It has been especially helpful in the identification of aortoannular ectasia and serial evaluation of postoperative results and disease progression. Unlike conventional angiography, however, MRI cannot determine the presence and degree of aortic valve insufficiency or the condition of the coronary arteries, which is important information for planning the surgical approach.[2]

Although such noninvasive techniques are attractive, aortography is preferred for preoperative evaluation of patients with aneurysmal diseases of the thoracic aorta because it provides a detailed image of the lesion, the coronary arteries, and the branches of the aortic arch.[24] However, the noninvasive techniques provide important information that, when used in combination with aortographic studies, gives the surgeon a better anatomic picture of the diseased aorta and its branches.

Treatment

With the introduction of cardiopulmonary bypass, the development of safer hypothermic circulatory arrest techniques, and the use of better synthetic vascular grafts, surgical treatment of aortic aneurysms has become the standard approach to these complex vascular lesions.

Most patients who do not undergo surgery for treatment of aneurysms die of rupture. Furthermore, overall survival following emergency surgery is also dismal, with elective intervention being clearly associated with less mortality and morbidity.[47] For these reasons, elective surgical repair is recommended when the patient suffers from symptoms related to the aneurysm, the diameter of the lesion is over 10 cm, or enlargement of a smaller lesion has been documented.[41] It is also recommended for patients with Marfan's syndrome whose ascending aorta is over 5.5 to 6 cm in diameter.[41] Early and late mortality are related to advanced age, the urgency of surgery, and the presence of congestive heart failure and arterial hypertension.

The surgical approach to these aneurysms varies according to their location and their specific anatomic characteristics. Therefore unique surgical techniques and complications associated with aneurysms of the different segments of the thoracic aorta will be discussed.

Ascending Aorta. The treatment of choice for most ascending aortic aneurysms is surgical resection and graft replacement. Cardiopulmonary bypass using right atrial and femoral artery cannulation is instituted for perfusion of the brain and other vital organs during cross-clamping of the distal ascending aorta. A modified technique is used when there is associated aortic valve insufficiency and coronary ostia involvement. When the sinuses of Valsalva are not grossly dilated, supracoronary grafting and conventional aortic valve replacement is the procedure of choice, and care must be taken to prevent damage to the coronary ostia, hemorrhage, or formation of pseudoaneurysms. If the sinuses of Valsalva are involved in the aneurysmal dilation and the coronary ostia are displaced cephalad 2 cm or more, a valved conduit with reimplantation of the coronary ostia to the graft is indicated (Fig. 54-3).[10]

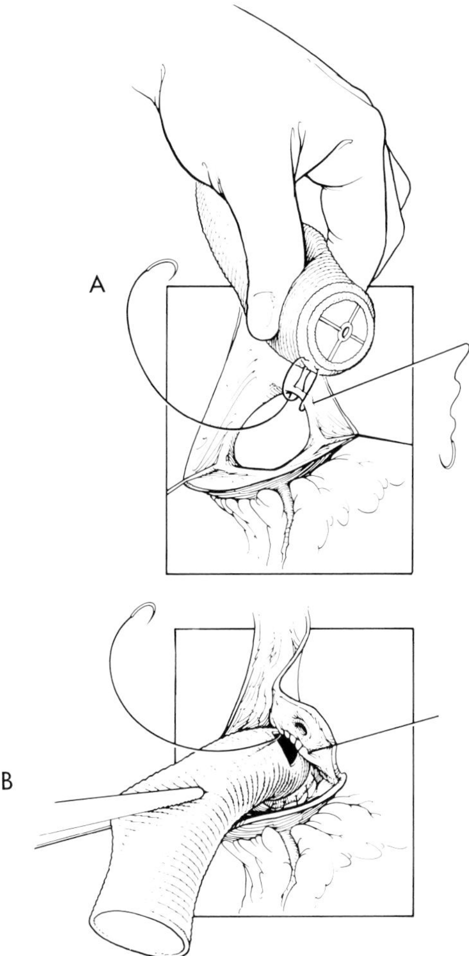

Fig. 54-3 **A,** Graft replacement of ascending aorta using valve conduit. **B,** Reimplantation of coronary ostia to conduit. (From Cooley, D.A.: Surgical treatment of aortic aneurysms, Philadelphia, 1986, W.B. Saunders Co.)

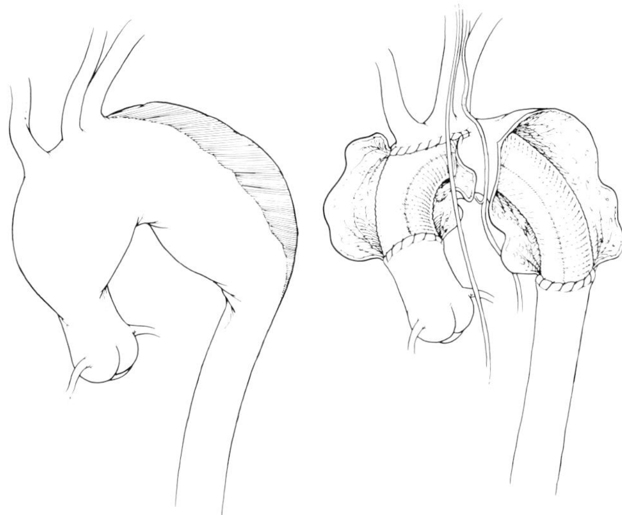

Fig. 54-4 Graft replacement of Type C aortic arch aneurysm with reimplantation of great vessels into graft. (From Cooley, D.A.: Surgical treatment of aortic aneurysms, Philadelphia, 1986, W.B. Saunders Co.)

Transverse Arch. The surgical treatment of transverse aortic arch aneurysms presents a special challenge to the cardiovascular surgeon. The most serious surgical complications are cerebral damage resulting from cerebral ischemia and the occurrence of air or particulate emboli during graft replacement. For this reason, indications for surgery should be evaluated on an individual basis, and elective surgical intervention reserved for those lesions approaching 6 to 8 cm in diameter and causing symptoms related to compression of vital structures.

Several techniques have been used to approach these lesions, including temporary tube bypass, temporary and permanent bypass grafts, cardiopulmonary bypass with separate perfusion of the brachiocephalic vessels, and cardiopulmonary bypass with profound hypothermia and circulatory arrest.[10,16,32] Bypass techniques and separate perfusion to brachiocephalic vessels are complicated, and the results are inconsistent.

Surgeons at the Texas Heart Institute in Houston have used hypothermic circulatory arrest, which provides adequate cerebral protection during arch replacement, as well as a simplified operative field because the need for perfusion cannulas and excessive clamps is eliminated.[37] The patient's core temperature is lowered to between 22° and 26° C using a pump oxygenator and heat exchanger. The aneurysm is then repaired using a low-porosity woven Dacron graft that has been preclotted with autologous plasma and autoclaving.[13] Proximal and distal anastomoses are performed with a running, nonabsorbable, monofilament suture (Fig. 54-4). The patient is gradually rewarmed at the rate of 1° C every 3 minutes to avoid production of gaseous microemboli.

This simplified technique of moderate hypothermia satisfactorily protects the cerebrum and myocardium for periods of 20 to 30 minutes during circulatory arrest. Furthermore, preclotting the graft with autologous plasma has prevented the excessive bleeding associated with the use of deep hypothermia (14° to 18° C). Most of the neurologic deficits resulting from this technique are transient; however, most fixed deficits appear to be caused by emboli, so special precautions should be taken to avoid particulate embolization from atherosclerotic aneurysms during graft replacement.

Descending Aorta. Although most cardiovascular surgeons consider graft replacement the best surgical treatment for descending aortic aneurysms, they disagree about which approach should be used to avoid the complications related to this procedure.

Since the early days of Carrel,[8] who identified it in experimental animals, postoperative paraplegia is the most dreaded complication associated with operations on the descending thoracic aorta. The mechanism that causes spinal cord injury following cross-clamping of the proximal descending thoracic aorta is not well understood. Several factors are probably responsible, but the primary ones appear to be interruption of blood flow and distal ischemia to the spinal cord, in addition to elevation of the cerebrospinal fluid pressure secondary to proximal hypertension.[6,43] Accordingly, special attention has been given to understanding how blood is supplied to the distal spinal cord.[60,61] The arteria radicularis magna anterior, also known as the artery of Adamkiewicz, originates somewhere between T9 and T12, and it is responsible for supplying most of the blood to this segment of the spinal cord. Isolated ligature of this vessel in experimental animals without proximal cross-clamping or other hemodynamic alterations results in a paraplegia rate of 72%,[61] which establishes its importance.

During the early days of aortic surgery, Cooley and associates,[10] DeBakey, Cooley, and Creech,[20] and Pontius and co-workers[46] demonstrated experimentally and clinically the value of systemic hypothermia as an adjunct to prevent ischemic spinal cord injury. However, the risk of developing cardiac arrhythmias and coagulopathies resulting from systemic hypothermia remained a problem.[12] Other researchers recommend the use of various shunts and partial bypass techniques,[22,35,36,62] but the results are inconsistent; furthermore, the techniques are more complicated, which unnecessarily prolongs the operation.

After reviewing their experience with these complex lesions, two major vascular surgical centers advocate simple cross-clamping technique without the use of adjuncts to avoid ischemia.[14,17,32,38] They also recommend the prevention of hypotension, expeditious removal of the aneurysm and restoration of distal flow, and the avoidance of cross-clamping over 30 minutes, which is associated with a higher risk of postoperative paraplegia.

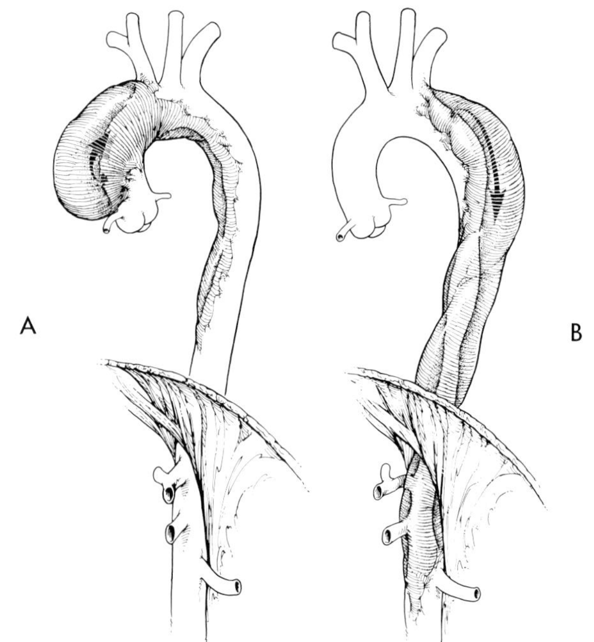

Fig. 54-5 Classification of aortic dissections. **A,** Type A lesions comprise the ascending aorta and may extend into the aortic arch. **B,** Type B lesions originate in the proximal descending aorta, extending distally. (From Cooley, D.A.: Surgical treatment of aortic aneurysms, Philadelphia, 1986, W.B. Saunders Co.)

Aortic Dissection

Pathophysiology

Aortic dissection is a unique entity involving the thoracic aorta that is characterized by a spontaneous tear of the intima and part of the media of the aortic wall, which allows blood to escape under pressure into the aortic laminae and results in a pathologic separation of the media along the longitudinal axis of the aorta, parallel to the flow of blood. This "false" channel of dissection in the middle of the aortic wall spreads downstream for a variable distance. It usually starts 2 cm distal to the aortic valve cusps.[10,51] In most cases, a transverse intimal tear marks the beginning of the dissection, but this can vary. A tear in the ascending aorta is usually located in the right lateral aortic wall, and the dissection progresses along the greater curvature of the aorta. The occurrence of a reentry tear is much less frequent and difficult to identify. Dissections can also begin in the transverse arch or the proximal descending thoracic aorta, usually at the level of the isthmus, distal to the origin of the left subclavian artery. Once the dissecting process has begun, it progresses rapidly, depending mainly on the systemic blood pressure and the velocity of blood flow. The extent of the dissection appears to be influenced by intrinsic characteristics of the vessel wall itself, but medial scarring secondary to atherosclerotic plaquing seems to be the most common cause of interruption of progression of the dissection.[51]

A working classification of aortic dissection based on the site of origin and extension provides a practical approach to these lesions and aids in the plan of management.[19] Type A dissections originate from a tear in the ascending aorta and may extend distally into the descending aorta. These dissections have the greatest risk of rupture and are associated with acute aortic regurgitation and myocardial infarction secondary to dissection and obstruction of the coronary arteries. Type B dissections originate in the descending aorta, distal to the arch (Fig. 54-5). The dissecting process usually extends distally, but proximal dissection is also possible.

The cause of aortic dissection is still a subject of debate. This lesion was previously called a "dissecting aneurysm," but the term "acute aortic dissection" is more appropriate because its pathologic process is different from that of a true aneurysm, and aneurysmal expansion is usually not a particularly prominent feature of the process. Although dissection was attributed to cystic medial necrosis in the past, the studies of Schlatmann and Becker[55] revealed that the morphologic changes of aortic dissection might result from a process of injury and repair within the aortic wall. Such changes give rise to alterations in the structural properties of the vessel wall, leading to dilation. The local hemodynamic circumstances determine whether further dilation, dissection, or rupture will occur. Patients with Marfan's syndrome who most frequently suffer from aortic dissections have an underlying connective tissue disorder that makes them more susceptible to developing aortic complications at an earlier age.[56] Arterial hypertension is present in approximately 70% of patients with aortic dissection, and it is the most common predisposing factor for this condition. Other associated factors include the presence of a bicuspid aortic valve, aortic isthmic coarctation, trauma, and the iatrogenic situation where an aortic incision has been made for cannulation in cardiopulmonary bypass.

Diagnosis

CLINICAL PRESENTATION. The presenting symptoms of aortic dissection vary according to the location of the tear and the associated complications and ischemia to vital organs with a blood supply that has been compromised by the dissecting process. The most common symptom is the acute onset of severe chest pain that radiates to the back and abdomen. The patient may also complain of numbness or pain in the right arm when the dissection extends into the innominate artery, compromising the right subclavian artery. Proximal dissections may result in aortic valve insufficiency, in which case a diastolic murmur can be heard. In severe cases, signs and symptoms compatible with congestive heart failure may be the clinical presentation.

Complications of acute aortic dissection are varied. Rupture of the aorta is the most devastating complication, leading to immediate exsanguination. Rupture can occur anywhere from the pericardial sac to the abdominal cavity. Obstruction of blood flow to vital organs by a medial hematoma of the vessel wall supplying that particular organ can result in ischemia, producing a myriad of symptoms depending on which organ or organs are involved. Myocardial infarction, cerebral insufficiency, renal failure, mesenteric ischemia, and even paraplegia can be the presenting manifestation of aortic dissection. As described earlier, proximal dissection can result in dilation of the aortic annulus with acute aortic regurgitation and congestive heart failure.

SPECIAL DIAGNOSTIC TECHNIQUES. As in the diagnosis of thoracic aneurysmal disease, aortography remains the technique of choice in establishing the diagnosis of aortic dissection. The most common angiographic findings of aortic dissections are opacification of the false lumen, visualization of the intimal flap, and deformity of the true lumen (Fig. 54-6).

Other less invasive techniques are being used with increasing frequency, but their role in the diagnosis of aortic dissection remains to be defined. Two-dimensional echocardiography is especially useful in the diagnosis of aortic dissection involving the ascending aorta. The technique has the advantage of being a bedside procedure, and it provides other useful information regarding the differential diagnosis. The criteria for aortic dissection are: (1) an aortic root measuring at least 42 mm, (2) an intraluminal structure within the proximal aorta consistent with an intimal flap, and (3) a high frequency of intimal flap operations, which is the most specific sign.[26] Other physicians have reported adequate visualization of the descending thoracic aorta using transesophageal echocardiography, adding further means of bedside evaluation in suspected cases of aortic dissection.[7] Computerized arterial tomography may also be useful in describing various features of aortic dissection, but when compared to two-dimensional echocardiography, the latter has better resolution because it makes identifying the intimal flap in cases of dissection easier.[30]

Ultimately MRI may prove to be the most useful of the noninvasive techniques and when further refined could conceivably supplant the need for aortography to diagnose aortic dissection. For example, the absence of an intraluminal signal from blood flowing at normal velocities eliminates the need for administering contrast material, and MRI readily identifies intimal flaps and the origin of aortic branches from true and false lumens in cases of aortic dissection.[1]

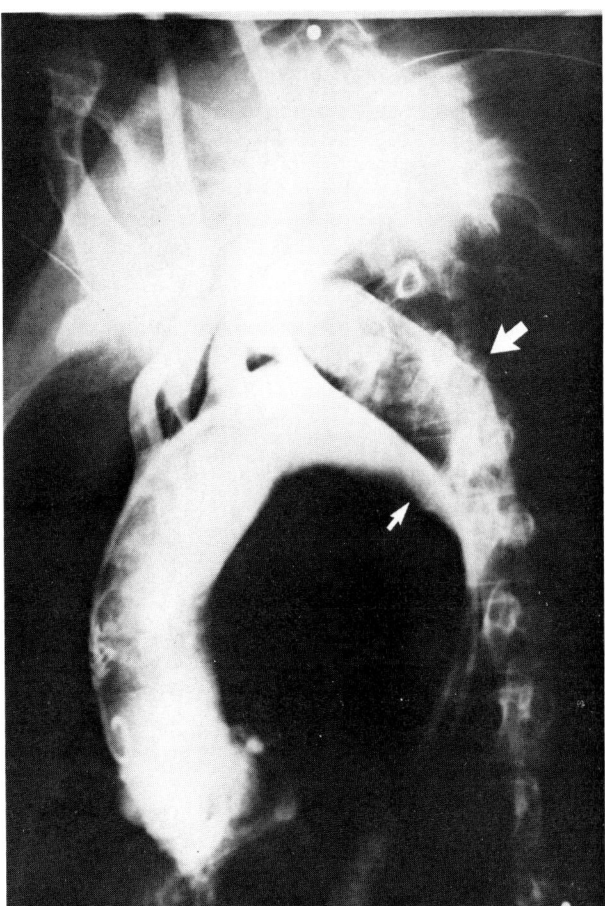

Fig. 54-6 Arteriography of a Type B aortic dissection. Notice opacification of false lumen *(large arrow)* and compression of true lumen *(small arrow)*.

Treatment

Treatment of aortic dissection depends on its location and associated complications. The treatment for Type A dissections is immediate surgical intervention and repair.

Uncomplicated Type B lesions can be managed medically by close observation, administration of intravenous peripheral vasodilators to lower the systemic blood pressure, and beta-adrenergic blockers to reduce the ejection velocity of the heart.[23] However, such patients must be followed carefully to avoid associated complications, and not all authorities agree that medical management is the best approach. After analyzing their results with surgical treatment of Type B lesions, Reul and colleagues[49] recommended early surgical repair as definitive treatment of acute and chronic descending aortic dissection before extension, rupture, or massive enlargement occurs.

Prophylactic surgery for aortic dissection is indicated in those patients with Marfan's syndrome in whom the ascending aorta reaches a diameter of 6 cm as measured by echocardiography. These patients are candidates for com-

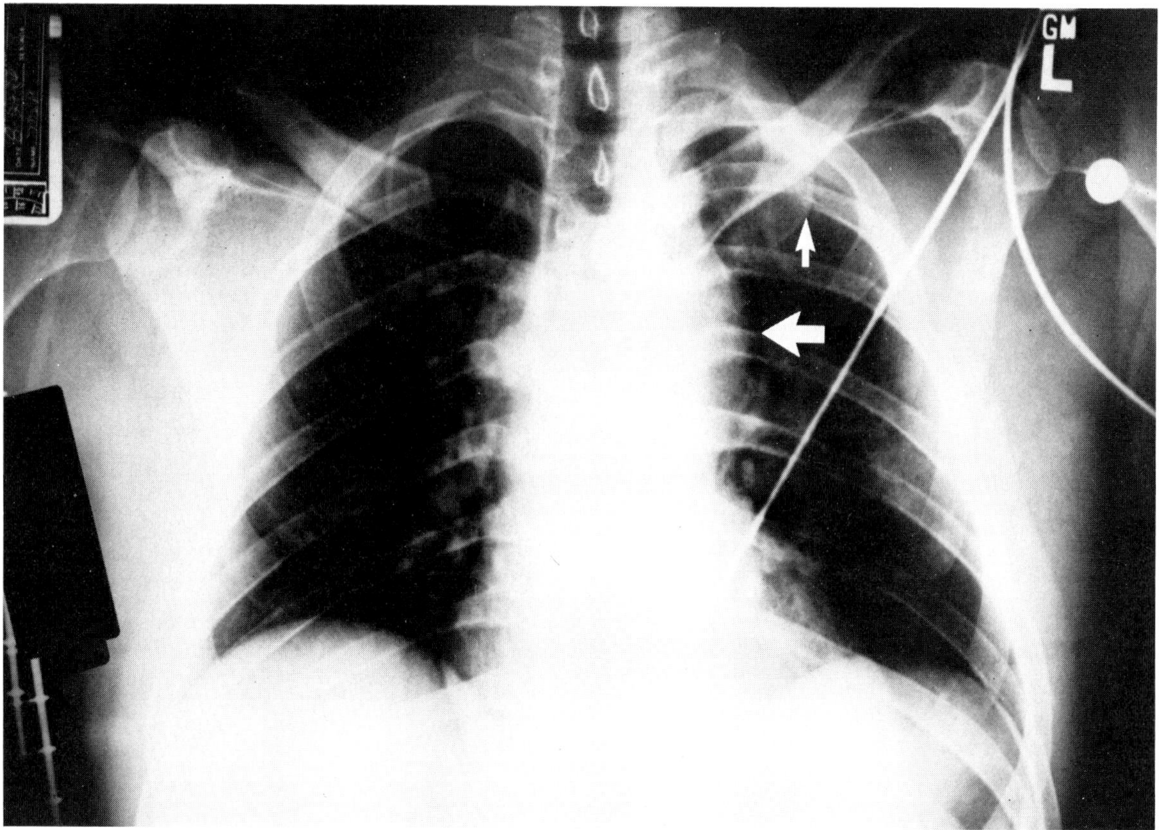

Fig. 54-7 Chest x-ray film of a patient with aortic transection. Notice presence of a widened mediastinum *(large arrow),* evidence of a mediastinal hematoma. Loss of aortic knob contour, a left apical cap, and fracture of left second and third rib is present *(small arrow).*

posite graft repair, and early intervention has proven to be highly beneficial.[25]

TRAUMATIC ANEURYSMS

Modern methods of ground transportation have resulted in a steady increase in the incidence of blunt decelerating injuries to the chest. Traumatic rupture of the thoracic aorta occurs in approximately 10% to 17% of fatal motor vehicle accidents.[27] Only 20% of patients survive the initial injury when traumatic aortic transection occurs. For this small group of patients, mortality increases with time, 49% of them dying within the first 49 hours, and only 2% surviving for more than 4 months if left untreated.[44] Death results from rupture and immediate exsanguination.

Disruption is a result of shearing stresses at the junction of the fixed and mobile parts of the aorta,[42] usually distal to the left subclavian artery, at the ligamentum arteriosum. If the tear is complete, exsanguination is immediate, resulting in death at the scene. In patients whose adventitia remains intact with disruption of the intima and media, a false aneurysm forms. The adventitia containing the pulsating hematoma cannot withstand the bursting pressure that the intact aorta can and is more susceptible to rupture at the time of aggressive fluid resuscitation in the emergency room or at induction of anesthesia, when measures to counteract hypotension are taken.[58] For this reason, if aortic rupture is suspected, careful monitoring of the systemic blood pressure is mandatory to avoid the extremes of pressure and rapid changes.

The diagnosis of aortic transection should be suspected in any patient who has sustained blunt chest trauma. The chest x-ray film is the initial study that is used to make the diagnosis in these patients. Loss of the aortic knob contour appears to be the most consistent and reliable sign of aortic tear. Other findings include: (1) a mediastinal width to chest width ratio of greater than 0.25 in a supine chest film, (2) a left apical cap, (3) displacement of the nasogastric tube and/or trachea to the right, (4) displacement of the right paraspinous interface, and (5) depression of the left mainstem bronchus[57] (Fig. 54-7). Once the chest x-ray film is considered suspicious, immediate aortography is indicated to confirm the diagnosis and localize the tear, allowing the surgeon to plan a surgical approach (Fig. 54-8).

Treatment of acute aortic transection and the formation of a false aneurysm is immediate surgical repair through a left thoracotomy. Most of these lesions can be repaired primarily or with the use of an interposition graft. Whether adjunctive measures are necessary and even useful to avoid spinal cord ischemia and renal failure remains controversial. As a rule, during operation for aortic transsection, special attention is given to avoid excessive stress on the left ventricle as a result of proximal cross-clamping and to keep the total distal ischemic time to a minimum. Numer-

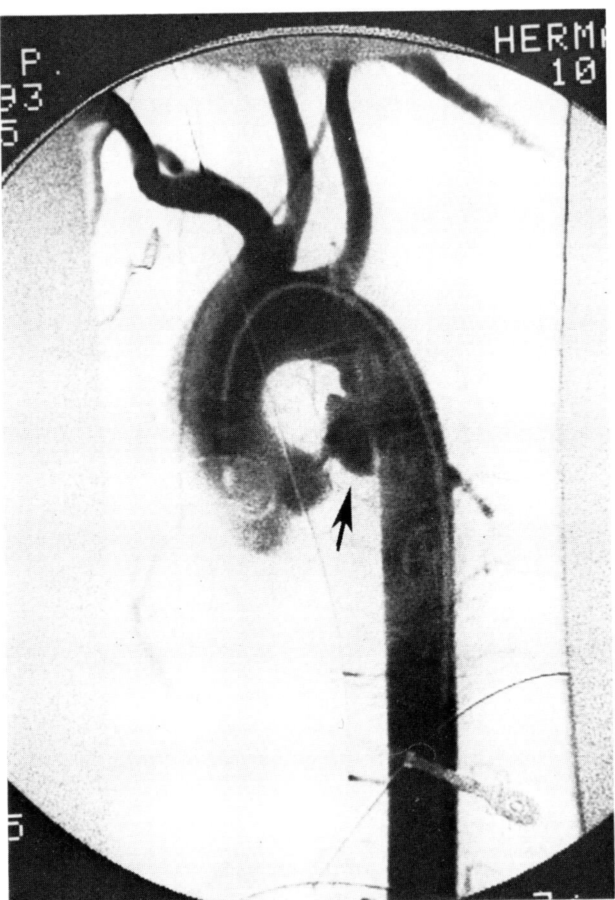

Fig. 54-8 Digital subtraction angiography of the thoracic aorta in a patient with traumatic aortic transection and development of a false aneurysm distal to the left subclavian artery at the level of the ligamentum arteriosum *(arrow)*.

ous adjuncts have been used to accomplish these goals, including the use of partial bypass techniques and different types of shunts. The use of bypass techniques carries a higher mortality than shunting and simple cross-clamping,[39] probably because of the need to use heparin with its attendant complications in patients suffering from multiple body trauma when bypass procedures are used. The experience of various groups indicates that simple aortic cross-clamping with an expeditious surgical technique to keep ischemic time to less than 30 minutes is the procedure of choice for repair of acute traumatic rupture of the aorta.[39,59]

SUMMARY

Because of the increase in the number of elderly people, most aneurysmal disease of the thoracic aorta is now most commonly secondary to chronic degenerative processes involving the different layers of the vessel wall. The concept of cystic medial necrosis as a primary disease of the ascending aorta has been challenged. Aneurysms are now believed to be a response to local hemodynamic factors inflicting stress on the aortic wall. Distal to the ascending aorta, arteriosclerosis is most commonly responsible for aneurysmal dilation of the aorta. The cause of arteriosclerosis is still uncertain, and preventive measures controversial.

The clinical presentation of thoracic aneurysms and dissections has been well described, and aortography has generally been the procedure of choice in confirming the diagnosis. But the need to develop better techniques still exists. Some of the new, noninvasive techniques have partially addressed this need. Magnetic resonance imaging is among the most promising developments in the noninvasive field, and early results with this diagnostic tool have been encouraging. Whether this technique will ultimately supplant the need for conventional angiography remains to be determined.

The treatment of thoracic aneurysms and dissections is surgical repair. The development of cardiopulmonary bypass, safer anesthesia, newer hypothermic techniques, and better prosthetic grafts have resulted in improved survival of these complex lesions.

REFERENCES

1. Amparo, E., et al.: Magnetic resonance imaging of aortic disease: preliminary results, Am. J. Radiol. **143**(6):1203, 1984.
2. Amparo, E., et al.: Aortic dissection: magnetic resonance imaging, Radiology **155**(2):399, 1985.
3. Baer, R.W., Taussig, H.B., and Oppenheimer, E.H.: Congenital aneurysmal dilatation of the aorta associated with arachnodactyly, Bull. Johns Hopkins Hosp. **72:**309, 1943.
4. Bahnson, H.T., and Nelson, A.R.: Cystic medial necrosis as a cause of localized aortic aneurysms amenable to surgical therapy, Ann. Surg. **144**(4):519, 1956.
5. Benjamin, H.B., and Becker, A.B.: Etiologic incidence of thoracic and abdominal aneurysms, Surg. Gynecol. Obstet. **125**(6):1306, 1967.
6. Blaiswell, F.W., and Cooley, D.A.: The mechanism of paraplegia after temporary thoracic aortic occlusion and its relationship to spinal fluid pressure, Surgery **51:**351, 1962.
7. Borner, N., et al.: Diagnosis of aortic dissection by transesophageal echocardiography, Am. J. Cardiol. **54**(8):1157, 1984.
8. Carrel, A.: On the experimental surgery of the aorta and heart, Ann. Surg. **52:**83, 1910.
9. Chapman, D.W., and Cooley, D.A.: Annulo-aortic ectasia with cystic medial necrosis, Am. J. Card. **16**(5):679, 1965.
10. Cooley, D.A.: Surgical treatment of aortic aneurysms, Philadelphia, 1986, W.B. Saunders Co.
11. Cooley, D.A., and DeBakey, M.E.: Hypothermia in the surgical treatment of aortic aneurysms, Bull. De La Societe Int. de Chirurgie **15:**206, 1956.
12. Cooley, D.A., et al.: Surgical treatment of aneurysms of the transverse aortic arch: experience with 25 patients using hypothermic techniques, Ann. Thorac. Surg. **32**(3):260, 1981.
13. Cooley, D.A., Romagnoli, A., and Milam, J.D.: A method of preparing dacron grafts to prevent interstitial hemorrhage, Cardiovascular Disease (Bull. Texas Heart Instit.) **8:**48, 1981.
14. Crawford, E.S., and Rubio, P.A.: Reappraisal of adjuncts to avoid ischemia in the treatment of aneurysms of descending thoracic aorta, J. Thorac. Cardiovasc. Surg. **66:**693, 1973.
15. Crawford, E.S., and Cohen, E.S.: Aortic aneurysm: a multifocal disease, Arch. Surg. **117**(1):1393, 1982.
16. Crawford, E.S., Saleh, S.A., and Schuessler, J.S.: Treatment of aneurysms of transverse aortic arch, J. Thorac. Cardiovasc. Surg. **78**(3):383, 1979.
17. Crawford, E.S., et al.: Graft replacement of aneurysms in descending thoracic aorta: Results without bypass of shunting, Surgery **89:**73, 1981.
18. Crawford, J.L., et al.: Inflammatory aneurysms of the aorta, J. Vasc. Surg. **2**(1):113, 1986.
19. Daily, P.O., et al.: Management of acute aortic dissections, Ann. Thorac. Surg. **10**(3):237, 1970.

20. DeBakey, M.E., Cooley, D.A., and Creech, O.: Resection of the aorta for aneurysms and occlusive disease with particular reference to the use of hypothermia: analysis of 240 cases, Surgery **5**:153, 1955.
21. de Takats, G., and Pirani, C.L.: Aneurysms: general considerations, Angiology **5**:173, 1954.
22. Donahoo, J.S., Brawley, R.K., and Gott, V.L.: The heparin-coated vascular shunt for thoracic aortic and great vessel procedure: a ten-year experience, Ann. Thorac. Surg. **23**:507, 1977.
23. Doroghazi, R.M., Slater, E.E., and DeSanctis, R.W.: Medical therapy for aortic dissections, J. Cardiovasc. Med. **6**:187, 1981.
24. Earnest, F., Muhm, J.R., and Sheedy, P.F.: Roentgenographic findings in thoracic aortic dissection, Mayo Clin. Proc. **54**(1):43, 1979.
25. Gott, V.L., et al.: Surgical treatment of aneurysms of the ascending aorta in the Marfan's syndrome, N. Engl. J. Med. **314**(7):1070, 1986.
26. Granato, J.E., Dee, P., and Gibson, R.S.: Utility of two-dimensional echocardiography in suspected ascending aortic dissection, Am. J. Cardiol. **56**(1):123, 1985.
27. Greendyke, R.M.: Traumatic rupture of the aorta: special reference to automobile accidents, JAMA **195**:527, 1966.
28. Henochowicz, S.I., et al.: Multiple saccular aortic aneurysms in nonspecific aortitis, Am. J. Cardiol. **57**(4):377, 1986.
29. Holman, E., and Peniston, W.: Hydrodynamic factors in the production of aneurysms, Am. J. Surg. **90**(2):200, 1955.
30. Iliceto, S., et al.: Diagnosis of aneurysm of the thoracic aorta: comparison between two noninvasive techniques—two-dimensional echocardiography and computed tomography, Eur. Heart J. **5**(7):545, 1984.
31. Kampmeier, R.H.: Saccular aneurysms of the thoracic aorta: a clinical study of 633 cases, Ann. Intern Med. **12**(5):624, 1938.
32. Kay, G.L., et al.: Surgical repair of aneurysms involving the distal aortic arch, J. Thorac. Cardiovasc. Surg. **91**(3):397, 1986.
33. Klima, T., et al.: The morphology of ascending aneurysms, Human Pathol. **14**(9):810, 1983.
34. Lande, A., and Berkmen, Y.M.: Aortitis: pathologic, clinical, and arteriographic review, Radiol. Clin. North Am. **14**(2):219, 1976.
35. Laschinger, J.C., et al.: Experimental and clinical assessment of the adequacy of partial bypass in maintenance of spinal cord blood flow during operations on the thoracic aorta, Ann. Thorac. Surg. **36**:417, 1983.
36. Lawrence, G.H., et al.: Results of the use of the TDMAC-heparin shunt in the surgery of aneurysms of the descending thoracic aorta, J. Thorac. Cardiovasc. Surg. **73**:393, 1977.
37. Livesay, J.J., et al.: Resection of aortic arch aneurysms: comparison of hypothermic techniques in 60 patients, Ann. Thorac. Surg. **36**(1):19, 1983.
38. Livesay, J.J., et al.: Surgical experience in descending thoracic aneurysmectomy with and without adjuncts to avoid ischemia. Ann. Thorac. Surg. **39**(1):37, 1985.
39. Mattox, K.L., et al.: Clamp/repair: a safe technique for treatment of blunt injury to the descending thoracic aorta, Ann. Thorac. Surg. **40**(5):456, 1985.
40. Moore, E.H., et al.: Magnetic resonance imaging of chronic post-traumatic false aneurysms of the thoracic aorta, Am. J. Radiol. **143**(6):1195, 1984.
41. Moreno-Cabral, C.E., et al.: Degenerative and atherosclerotic aneurysms of the thoracic aorta: determinants of early and late surgical outcome, J. Thorac. Cardiovasc. Surg. **88**(6):1020, 1984.
42. Newman, R.J., and Rastoji, S.: Rupture of the thoracic aorta and its relationship to road traffic accident characteristics, Injury **15**(5):296, 1984.
43. Oka, Y., and Miyamoto, T.: Prevention of spinal cord injury after cross-clamping of the thoracic aorta, JPN J. Surg. **14**:159, 1982.
44. Parmley, L.F., et al.: Nonpenetrating traumatic injury of the aorta, Circulation **17**:1086, 1958.
45. Pomerance, A., Yacoub, M.H., and Gula, G.: The surgical pathology of thoracic aortic aneurysms, Histopathology **1**(3):257, 1977.
46. Pontius, R.G., et al.: The use of hypothermia in the prevention of paraplegia following temporary aortic occlusion: experimental observations, Surgery **36**:33, 1954.
47. Pressler, V., and McNamara, J.J.: Aneurysms of the thoracic aorta: review of 260 cases. J. Thorac. Cardiovasc. Surg. **89**(1):50, 1985.
48. Reich, N.E.: Syphilis of the aorta. In Diseases of the aorta: diagnosis and treatment, New York, 1949, MacMillan Co.
49. Reul, G.J., et al.: Dissecting aneurysm of the descending aorta: improved surgical results in 91 patients, Arch. Surg. **110**(5):632, 1975.
50. Richards, M.A.: Medionecrosis aortae idiopathica cystica, Am. J. Pathol. **8**(6):717, 1932.
51. Roberts, W.C.: Aortic Dissection: anatomy, consequences, and causes, Am. Heart J. **101**(2):195, 1981.
52. Robicsek, F., et al.: The applicability of Bernoulli's Law in the process of enlargement and rupture of aortic aneurysms, J. Thorac. Cardiovasc. Surg. **61**(3):472, 1971.
53. Rotino, A.: Medial degeneration, cystic variety in unruptured aortas, Am. Heart J. **19**(3):330, 1940.
54. Savunen, T., and Aho, H.J.: Annuloaortic ectasia: light and electron microscopic changes in the aortic media, Virchows Arch. Path. Anat. **407**(3):279, 1985.
55. Schlatmann, T.J.M., and Becker, A.E.: Histologic changes in the normal aging aorta: implications for dissecting aortic aneurysm, Am. J. Cardiol. **39**(1):13, 1977.
56. Schlatmann, T.J.M., and Becker, A.E.: Pathogenesis of dissecting aneurysm of the aorta, Am. J. Cardiol. **39**(1):21, 1977.
57. Sefczek, D.M., Sefczek, R.J., and Deeb, Z.L.: Radiographic signs of acute traumatic rupture of the thoracic aorta, AJR **141**(6):1259, 1983.
58. Stiles, Q.R., et al.: Management of injuries to the thoracic and abdominal aorta, Am. J. Surg. **150**(1):132, 1985.
59. Svensson, L.G., Antunes, M.D.J., and Kinsley, R.H.: Traumatic rupture of the thoracic aorta, S. Afr. Med. J. **67**(21):853, 1985.
60. Svensson, L.G., et al.: Relationship of spinal cord blood flow to vascular anatomy during thoracic aortic cross clamping and shunting, J. Thorac. Cardiovasc. Surg. **91**:71, 1986.
61. Wadouh, F., et al.: The arteria radicularis magna anterior as a decisive factor influencing spinal cord damage during aortic occlusion, J. Thorac. Cardiovasc. Surg. **88**:1, 1984.
62. Zacharopoulos, L., and Symbas, P.N.: Internal temporary aortic shunts for managing lesions of the descending thoracic aorta, Ann. Thorac. Surg. **35**:240, 1983.

55

Glenn W. Geelhoed

Calcium and Phosphorus Metabolism and the Parathyroid Gland

Tucked behind the thyroid gland or in close proximity to it are a group of endocrine structures (usually four in number) known as the parathyroid glands. Despite their small size, they play an extremely important role in the maintenance of normal calcium and phosphorus balance, both ions being critical components of a number of metabolic systems. The function of the parathyroid glands is vital to such crucial processes as neuromuscular excitability, membrane permeability, blood coagulation, and muscular contraction through maintenance of calcium homeostasis. When these glands fail to perform their normal activities, a state of hypocalcemia or hypercalcemia may ensue, resulting in a variety of potentially serious and possibly lethal pathophysiologic aberrations. This chapter will review the intricate control systems that exist in the body to maintain calcium and phosphorus balance and how this is effected through normal parathyroid function.

CALCIUM COMPARTMENTS

Calcium, a mineral required in structural support in bone, also functions in muscle action and membrane repolarization. Calcium is the body's principal divalent cation, with over 1 kg of this element locked in storage form where it functions principally in structure. Approximately 1% of this total is available in extracellular fluids and in intracellular position in such tissues as muscle where it is available for metabolic function. The small fraction of metabolically accessible total body calcium is critical in physiology, and this compartment is in dynamic equilibrium with the large reservoir of inactive calcium forms through interaction with one or more other cations, several anions, and multiple hormones. A competing divalent cation is magnesium; counterbalancing anions are chloride, phosphate, and bicarbonate; hormones principally involved in calcium metabolism include parathyroid hormone (parathormone), calcitonin, and vitamin D and its metabolites. Through intricate interaction of these competing and regulating biochemical systems, a relative constancy is maintained in the active form of ionic calcium in circulation. The body senses and regulates a disturbance in this critical ionic calcium level through compensatory metabolic and endocrine reactions, with disease resulting when the limits of these compensatory mechanisms are exceeded and hypocalcemia or hypercalcemia results.

Intracellular Calcium Functions

Calcium is required in both the electrical and mechanical activation of cardiac muscle, vascular smooth muscle, and skeletal muscle. Muscle cell membranes are semipermeable to calcium by means of specific "channels" through which calcium flux occurs at different rates. The rate of calcium passage is voltage dependent or phosphorylation dependent. The voltage-dependent calcium channels are open to intracellular influx of calcium when the membrane is depolarized, and drugs called "calcium channel blockers" may moderate arrhythmias by dampening this calcium current. Beta-adrenergic receptor stimulation may trigger phosphorylation through cyclic AMP (cAMP) kinase. Through the voltage-dependent and phosphorylation-dependent gates, membrane excitation occurs.[35]

Electrical excitation (i.e., transmembrane calcium influx in muscle cells) is necessary but not sufficient for muscular contraction. The increase in intracellular calcium from the influx and from the calcium release by sarcoplasmic reticulum that it triggers causes binding to an intracellular regulatory protein. This protein is troponin in myocardial cells and calmodulin in vascular smooth muscle cells. The complex between calcium ion and the intracellular proteins causes tertiary structural changes in myosin, and contraction results from a force generation between myosin and actin.

Relaxation occurs with the efflux of calcium as troponin and calmodulin dissociate from the complex and calcium is bound again within the sarcoplasmic reticulum. The degree of muscle tension depends on intracellular calcium concentration, and the rate of these contractions depends on the rapidity of calcium fluxes in and out of the myofilaments (Fig. 55-1).

Thus calcium and its transmembrane movement have a pivotal role in both excitation and contraction of cardiac, vascular, and skeletal muscle through these channels and under regulatory control of kinases sensitive to catecholamine. This role suggests the physiologic principles behind normal and stress metabolism, tetany, and susceptibility to hormones and drugs such as epinephrine and calcium-channel blocking agents. In contrast to this normal physiology, pathophysiology frequently is caused by an excess or deficit in the metabolically active calcium made available to the cells through the circulating plasma.

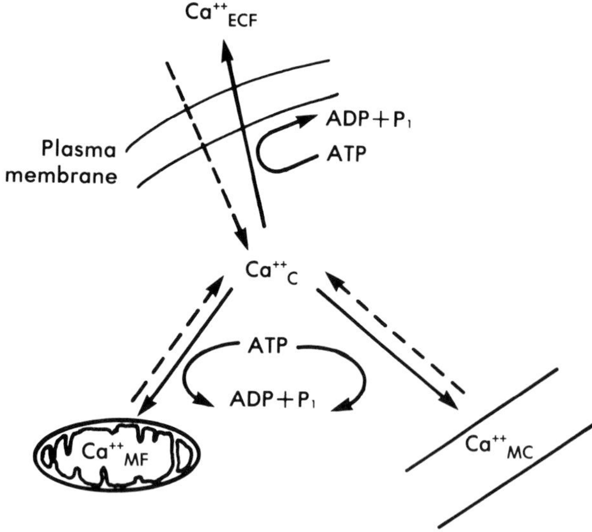

Fig. 55-1 Intracellular calcium ($Ca^{++}{}_c$) comes from extracellular calcium ($Ca^{++}{}_{ECF}$) through the plasma membrane by voltage-dependent and phosphorylation-dependent calcium channels. The $Ca^{++}{}_c$ is complexed by protein (troponin in myocardium and calmodulin in vascular muscle) from which it can be taken up by myofilaments *(MF)* or sarcoplasmic reticulum *(MC)*; each Ca^{++} transition involves ATP energy.

Extracellular Calcium Compartments

One half of the measurable plasma calcium is in the metabolically active ionized form. This active calcium compartment is in equilibrium with a protein-bound moiety and with a third fraction that is chelated. Homeostatic regulation involves the ionized half of the total serum calcium, and shifts from the numerator to denominator in this fraction are sensitive to a number of influences exerted in the plasma. The first of these factors is the quantity of serum albumin available to bind calcium. Because the bound calcium is not counted in the metabolic effects of the total plasma calcium, with a very low serum protein a patient can quite possibly have hypercalcemia and its metabolic consequences with readings in the low-normal range by blood chemistry report. Under normal conditions of physiologic pH, 1 g/100 ml in serum albumin binds 0.8 mg/100 ml in total serum calcium.

A second dynamic factor interactive with the first is the pH of the blood. Plasma protein is a principle component of the buffer capacity in the bloodstream, and acute changes in hydrogen ion concentration affect both protein binding and the chelation of calcium by the physical chemistry rules reflected in the Henderson-Hasselbach equation. Acidosis is buffered in blood proteins, which have less capacity for binding calcium when these binding sites competitively occupy hydrogen ions displacing more of the calcium into the ionized fraction in plasma. A change in pH in the alkaline direction causes greater calcium binding to protein and a subsequent decrease in the ionized plasma calcium. A patient bordering on hypocalcemia may induce an acute decrease in ionized calcium by hyperventilation. The resulting alkalosis may be sufficient to reduce ionized calcium to the point of clinical manifestation by the patient in hypocalcemic tetany, even though the total plasma calcium remains the same.

Technique used in drawing blood for calcium determination and the methods used in assay are important in judging truly normal or abnormal values. A prolonged tourniquet application may cause hemoconcentration and elevate the total serum calcium; at the same time, a tourniquet inflated to arterial pressure may cause ischemia and consequent acidosis, which would shift blood calcium toward the measured ionized fraction. If blood is not drawn anaerobically (as into a vacuum container), carbon dioxide leaves, raising the pH. The same may happen with the "alkaline tide" after a meal or, as previously noted, with the patient's breathing pattern. Ionized calcium may be measured directly through the specialized use of an ion-selective electrode. This specialized measurement of the metabolically active calcium compartment is useful if the test is done correctly. However, ion-selective electrodes are sensitive to the multiple factors in blood that have calcium consequences, e.g., body temperature, presence or absence of calcium-chelating anticoagulants, and loss of CO_2 at the blood-air interface with a consequent rise in pH. Most of the measurement errors tend to sum in the direction of underestimating the ionized calcium, which is a value protected at considerable metabolic expense even in critically ill patients.

PHOSPHORUS

Phosphate, the principal intracellular divalent anion, is abundant in metabolically active cells. In the adult human body nearly 1 kg of phosphate exists. It is so directly involved in energy-transfer processes that the "phosphorus gate" is taken as an indicator of metabolic activity in nuclear magnetic resonance. Phosphate compounds of adenosine (e.g., adenosine triphosphate) are the "common currency" in cellular energy exchanges.

The average daily adult dietary intake of calcium and phosphate approximates 1 g each, and active and passive transfer mechanisms sensitive to intimately interrelated endocrine control for each regulate absorption and secretion. Phosphate is generally abundant in metabolic systems. The principal control mechanisms are by renal excretion of phosphate excess. Typical serum concentrations measure 3.5 mg/100 ml ± 1 mg/100 ml in adults, 1.5 mg/100 ml higher in children.[8] This serum phosphate is under constant surveillance by the renal tubule because almost all of the plasma phosphate that passes into the glomerular filtrate is reabsorbed in the proximal tubule. Reabsorption of phosphate in the renal tubule is a process that requires energy; it is sensitive to many influences, including pH (and competitive bicarbonate concentration) and parathormone, which has a phosphaturic effect. Consequently, major changes in serum phosphate occur as a result of renal failure, and phosphate retention may be the principal driving force in disturbances in calcium level and parathormone secretion in the patient with renal insufficiency.

Hyperphosphatemia

Since active reabsorption in the proximal tubule is necessary for maintenance of the generally abundant serum phosphorus, hyperphosphatemia occurs from a decrease in renal filtration or stimulation of lower thresholds in its reabsorption. Vitamin D may increase both phosphate and calcium in the blood, and an acute deficit in parathormone may cause hyperphosphatemia and hypocalcemia. Over the long term, metastatic calcification in soft tissues may be seen with chronic hyperphosphatemia, but the symptoms of hyperphosphatemia are usually related to the induced hypocalcemia. For that reason, phosphate is regulated by both a normal diet and by control of blood calcium, with which it is inextricably related.

Hypophosphatemia

Hypophosphatemia may be present in critical illness and have consequences with impairment in the role that phosphate plays in energy transfer, membrane phospholipids, or oxyhemoglobin dissociation through its presence in 2,3-diphosphoglycerate. Over the long term, hypophosphatemia may result in demineralization of bone, and this osteomalacia may lead to pathologic fractures.

Starvation may be a cause of hypophosphatemia, but a more specific cause in the critically ill patient is diabetic ketoacidosis.[20] The acidosis itself may induce shifts of calcium and phosphorus from storage depots, and the osmotic diuresis may result in a total body deficit of phosphate. Hypophosphatemia is also regularly encountered in management of the chronic alcoholic suffering from malnutrition. In carbohydrate loading of the patient with chronic malnutrition, phosphate is shifted intracellularly, and both hypophosphatemia and hypomagnesemia can be seen in the alcoholic under treatment.[31] In severe illnesses superimposed on chronic malnutrition, parenteral administration of phosphate may be necessary because intestinal absorption may be unreliable. A major manageable cause of hypophosphatemia is primary hyperparathyroidism. Therapy may be directed principally at reducing the hypercalcemia, but a consequence of a reduction in parathormone is an elevation in the depressed serum phosphate.

PARATHORMONE

Parathyroid hormone (i.e., parathormone) is the principle homeostatic regulator of calcium and phosphate at the sites of bone, kidney, and gut. In turn, the ionized fraction of blood calcium controls parathormone's secretion from the parathyroid gland. This biofeedback loop is rapid and sensitive and may be disordered in primary pathology of the parathyroid gland(s), kidney, bone, or gut.

The Molecule

Parathormone is a single-chain polypeptide of 84 amino acids in sequence, with a 34-amino acid peptide comprising the N-terminal portion. This N-terminal fragment has biologic activity nearly the equal of the intact parathormone, but a further reduction in the size of this peptide inactivates it. A prohormone somewhat larger than parathormone is synthesized and secreted by the parathyroid gland, but the principal storage form within the gland is the 84–amino acid polypeptide parathormone (PTH).[26] The hormone activates receptors in kidney and bone, but it is also subject to cleavage in the circulation, with components of that cleavage detectable by radioimmunoassay in the circulation (Fig. 55-2). Excretion or disposal of these fragments is not as rapid a process as the PTH cleavage, nor is the clearance rate the same for each portion. Both the intact PTH and the biologically active N-terminal have short serum half-lives, and each represents approximately 10% of the circulating PTH immunoreactivity. The remaining 80% of the circulating hormone detected by radioimmunoassay is the two thirds of the molecule represented by the carboxy terminal fragment, which has a long serum half-life and is principally excreted through the kidneys. In renal failure the C-terminal fragments accumulate; however, for screening patients thought to have hyperparathyroidism, C-terminal assay may be superior to N-terminal assay because of the greater proportion of this species in the circulation and its longer circulating half-life.

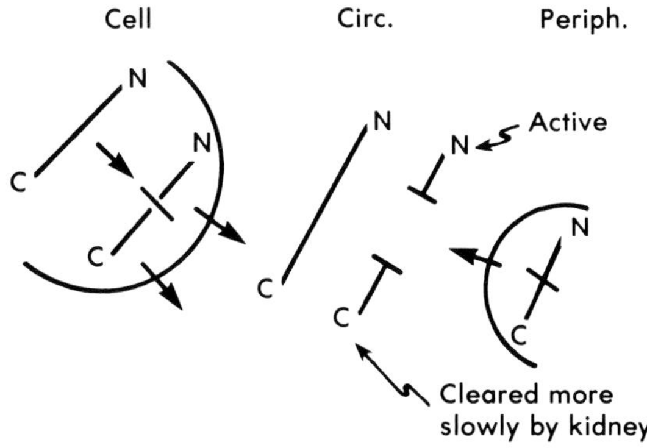

Fig. 55-2 Parathyroid hormone is an 84–amino acid single-chain polypeptide existing in the circulation as PTH and as a biologically active 34–amino acid N-terminal portion with a short half-life, and an inert C-terminal residue with a long half-life is serum dependent on renal excretion.

Action of Parathormone

The parathyroid gland's role is especially critical in sensing and responding to hypocalcemia. At each point in the circulation reached by PTH and its active N-terminal metabolite, the net result is an increase in blood calcium. The gut effect is to facilitate vitamin D in improving the efficiency of intestinal calcium absorption. PTH is the principal hormone in control of phosphate excretion at the kidney. If calcium absorption in the gut and phosphate excretion from the kidney are the principal parathormone actions for a net increase in calcium and decrease in circulating phosphate, the action of parathormone on bone is to release both calcium and phosphate from bone storage into circulation (Fig. 55-3). In each of the three sites of parathormone action, there is interaction with vitamin D with synergy in their combined activities.

Control of PTH Secretion

The parathyroid gland is principally sensitive to the circulating ionized calcium concentration. The parathyroid cells sense an increment or decrement in ionized calcium

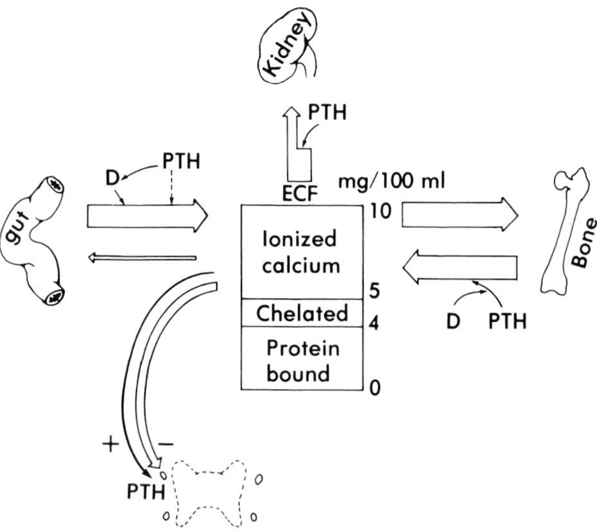

Fig. 55-3 Parathormone and vitamin D are interactive at gut, bone, and kidney for the synergistic result of an increase in blood calcium.

or magnesium but are apparently insensitive to serum phosphate concentrations. Conversely, parathormone degradation is sensitive to high serum ionized calcium and inhibited by hypocalcemia.[17]

Parathyroid hormone release may be sensitive to other hormones, the receptors of which (e.g., beta-adrenergic and H_2-receptors) have been found in parathyroid glands. Catecholamines in stress levels increase PTH secretion by elevating cAMP activity.

Conversely hypercalcemia inhibits PTH synthesis in the parathyroid gland and further inhibits response to PTH, at least at the renal receptors.[30] The total effect of hypocalcemia is to elevate parathormone synthesis, secretion, and activity, raising blood calcium. The net effect of an increase in blood calcium is to diminish synthesis, release, and activity of parathormone at its receptor sites. This stimulation and inhibition is rapid and delicately attuned for stability in the ionized calcium homeostasis.

VITAMIN D

Vitamin D, and especially one of its metabolites—vitamin D_3—are hormones in the body with high biologic activity in calcium metabolism. The precursors for the active hormone are calciferol produced by skin exposed to ultraviolet irradiation or absorbed in the gut from foods or vitamin supplementation. The kidney is the principle endocrine organ to create an active hormone of these calciferol precursors. An important distinction from parathormone production is that synthesis does not depend on calcium or phosphate concentrations in the blood.

As seen in Fig. 55-3, the sites of vitamin D and its principal actions are primarily on the gut and on bone as an adjunct to facilitate parathormone action. Because of its primary role in calcium absorption, vitamin D was first identified as a "vital amine," or vitamin, because its deficiency state results in hypocalcemia and demineralized bones or rickets. Vitamin D deficiency and the resultant hypocalcemia and hypophosphatemia from absorption failure lead to secondary hyperparathyroidism. Because vitamin D plays only an ancillary role in mobilization of calcium from bones, the osteomalacia occurs even with deficient vitamin D activity at the site of bone resorption and especially because of deficient vitamin D at the site of gut calcium absorption. In addition to the dietary deficit of the precursor or lack of sunlight exposure, failure of the specific secretory organ, the kidney, may also produce a deficiency in the active form of vitamin D. A hydroxylase found in the kidney is necessary for the activation of vitamin D, and a deficiency in this renal hydroxylase can produce renal osteodystrophy or renal rickets.

Normal calcium and phosphate metabolism requires normal function in kidney, gut, bone, and parathyroid gland. Ionized calcium within a rather restricted and protected range for membrane excitation, muscular contraction, and relaxation is the end result, which is also the biofeedback most specifically sensed by the parathyroid glands. A number of other hormones and substances are involved in some physiologic capacity, and others in pathologic imbalance in this homeostatic servosystem.

OTHER HORMONES

Calcitonin

When first discovered, calcitonin was named thyrocalcitonin from its origin in the parafollicular C cells of the thyroid. These cells are of neuroectodermal origin, and they are part of the amine precursor uptake and decarboxylation system, the capability of which is the common biochemical denominator. Any of the cells of this amine precursor uptake and decarboxylation origin can secrete calcitonin. This peptide has been isolated from several species; salmon calcitonin has been synthesized and, when given in pharmacologic doses, is more active in man than is human calcitonin in lowering blood calcium from pathologically elevated levels to normal. However, in spite of its original calcium-lowering effect and notwithstanding the therapeutic application of large quantities of the synthetic hormone, no direct inference can be drawn as to calcitonin's physiologic role. No evidence to date demonstrates that calcitonin plays a physiologic role in calcium or phosphate metabolism. It may have physiologic functions quite apart from its demonstrated pharmacologic action on extracellular calcium in metabolic systems quite different from those initially investigated; recent evidence suggests that it may be a pulmonary hormone.[1]

On the basis of evidence seen in patients dying of widespread medullary thyroid cancer with very elevated serum calcitonin levels and normal calcium and phosphate metabolism, calcitonin's role in calcium and phosphate metabolism seems negligible or is unknown. A subtype of a hereditary syndrome called multiple endocrine adenopathy (MEA) III (or MEA IIb) exists in which patients have early aggressive medullary thyroid cancer and correspondingly high blood calcitonin levels, but no abnormalities in the parathyroid glands and normal calcium and phosphate metabolism. The pharmacologic role of calcitonin may be through inhibition of bone resorption, an effect independent of parathyroid hormone.

Thyroxine

The iodinated thyronines, and specifically thyroxine, may have a pathologic effect that leads to hypercalcemia, but they do not have an apparent role in the normal calcium and phosphate physiology. In hyperthyroidism, one of the results of the generally increased metabolism is a direct increase in bone resorption mediated by thyroxine.[23] Phosphate metabolism is generally affected in the hypermetabolism that follows excess thyroxine circulation. However, thyroid hormone has no clearly proven role in normal physiology.

Cortisol and Other Steroids

The adrenal and gonadal steroids influence mineral homeostasis and skeletal remodeling. Again, these putative roles are remarkable in pathologic conditions but are rarely clear in normal calcium homeostasis. Cortisol can block calcium resorption from bone, but in high-dose corticosteroid treatment, demineralization of bone is seen as a rule. Paradoxically, in Addisonian crises hypercalcemia may also occur, stemming from vitamin D effect on bone resorption unopposed by cortisol or decreased renal calcium clearance. Estrogen failure is widely known in association with osteoporosis, yet patients treated with estrogens, progesterone, or androgens (e.g., for therapy of metastatic breast cancer) may develop rapid hypercalcemia. Much controversy surrounds the primary or ancillary role of steroids of either adrenal or gonadal origin in the postmenopausal osteoporosis syndrome; but, except for pathologic deficits or therapeutic excesses of these hormones, the role of such steroids in normal calcium homeostasis is unknown.

Insulin and Catecholamines

As previously noted, diabetic ketoacidosis may result in total body depletion of phosphate, even though serum phosphate is not affected until insulin therapy is begun. However, insulin administration with sugar causes a rapid shift of phosphate, potassium, and glucose into cells, and an immediate hypophosphatemia occurs. The hypoglycemia that follows insulin administration may also be a strong stimulus to catecholamine release. As previously noted, beta-adrenergic receptors are found present on parathyroid cells and may cause increased release of the parathormone. However, catecholamines also affect the phophokinase systems, and phophorylation-dependent calcium channels may change in their sensitivity to unchanged levels of ionized calcium in serum.[7]

Malignancy-Associated Factors

Among patients found to have hypercalcemia, the single most common association is a malignant disease. The majority of this malignancy-associated hypercalcemia is easily understood from osteolytic metastases and bone absorption. However, some parathormone-like substances or other humoral agents have been postulated, and some have been identified in patients with cancers notorious for producing hypercalcemia.[22] Some of these factors have been characterized as activating osteoclasts, which may be the principle mechanism in the hypercalcemia of myeloma.[22] Prostaglandins are implicated, since prostaglandin blockade seems to inhibit the severity of hypercalcemia in some malignancies, and glucocorticoids may have a similar therapeutic effect through perhaps related mechanisms. Some malignancies, particularly those of APUD origin, such as small-cell carcinoma of the lung, may produce multiple peptides; not all of these peptides are characterized, but some may be parathyroid hormone–like in their activity. In the majority of patients with cancer who have severe hypercalcemia, the origin of their hypercalcemia is most often obvious by the extent of the skeletal metastases.

The evidence is scant that each of the other hormones described, aside from those principally active in calcium and phosphate metabolism, have a humoral effect on normal physiologic mineral homeostasis, at least with respect to ionized calcium. These other factors come into play in pathologic states in which one tries to explain the extent of the deviation from normal calcium balance or because these agents or their congeners have been used with suggestive therapeutic response. The control of normal calcium physiology appears to reside in the interplay of parathormone and vitamin D and their responses through cAMP activation.

CLINICAL CONDITIONS OF DISORDERED CALCIUM METABOLISM

With respect to the critical constancy of ionized calcium in the blood, the fundamental disorders in calcium balance that disturb function are hypocalcemia and hypercalcemia. The "buffer capacity" of the compensatory systems is amazingly effective in protecting this infinitesimal fraction of the total body calcium pool, and these compensations blunt major shifts before disease is evident. When we see the clinical result, we are measuring the disease process with the failed best efforts of these compensatory mechanisms before the decompensation has occurred. The causes, consequences, and care of hypocalcemia will be examined first.

Hypocalcemia

Hypocalcemia results from a failure of the effect of parathormone or vitamin D secretion or the sequestration of calcium in compartments not susceptible to mobilization by this humoral control. The compensatory response is an increase in parathormone and vitamin D synthesis and release, thus increasing calcium absorption from gut, liberation from bone, and resorption by the kidney. These compensatory mechanisms may be adequate to protect the serum ionized calcium for a period of time, and the disease is principally reflected in the target organs that have been affected in the compensatory stress. Or the clinical result is tetany if one of the critical components is missing or if over time the reserves are exhausted and an actual decrease in ionized serum calcium occurs.

Causes of Hypocalcemia

Common causes of hypocalcemia are listed in Table 55-1. Deficiency in the action of vitamin D may be the result of dietary deprivation, lack of sunlight on exposed skin, or hereditary or acquired resistance to the hormone. The first and most direct deficit is that calcium absorption decreases and total blood calcium declines. Parathyroid hormone increase chiefly mediates immediate compensatory mecha-

Table 55-1 **HYPOCALCEMIA**

Cause	Mechanism	Compensatory Condition
Vitamin D deficiency	See Fig. 55-4	Compensatory PTH ↑ ↑ with Ca^{++} ↓ sparing at expense of $PO^{=}_4$ ↓ ↓
Hypoparathyroidism	Surgical absence of PTH or defect in PTH synthesis or release	Ca^{++} ↓, $PO^{=}_{4}$↑, PTH absent
Pseudohypoparathyroidism	End-organ failure of PTH *effect*	Ca^{++} ↓, $PO_4^{=}$ ↑, PTH ↑, but no urinary cAMP response to PTH administration
Hypomagnesemia	↓ Mg ↛ PTH release and peripheral response	Ca^{++} ↓ $PO_4^{=}$ ↑ ↓ PTH absent MG <1 mEq/L
Malabsorption	↓ Absorption vitamin D and Ca^{++}	Same as 1
Pancreatitis	Unknown	Ca chelation (saponification ?)
Hypoalbuminemia	Normal ionized Ca^{++} Total blood Ca^{++} ↓ ↓	Hypoalbuminemia
vs.	vs.	vs.
Hyperventilation	Normal total blood Ca^{++} but ionized Ca^{++} ↓ ↓	Alkalosis
Chelation	Calcium-binding	Citrate anticoagulants in blood transfusion

nisms. Parathormone excess decreases urinary calcium loss but does not considerably increase intestinal calcium absorption—the most important role of the action of vitamin D. Thus ionized serum calcium may be protected by parathormone compensation; but, with mobilization from bone and continuing absorption deficit, the (even diminished) renal losses mean that total body calcium *balance* becomes negative. Further increases in parathormone may maintain the hypocalcemia in mild form at the expense of increasing phosphate loss through the kidney. Because both the calcium and phosphate are mobilized from bone, osteomalacia, pathologic fractures, and the deformities of rickets begin to be apparent. As calcium is protected, severe hypophosphatemia results. Late in rickets, as seen through the compartment shifts in Fig. 55-4, phosphate wasting may be the principal disorder in the presence of parathormone excess. The parathyroid gland still receives the hypocalcemic signal, and increased synthesis and release of parathyroid hormone may be able to maintain the diminished serum ionized calcium pool, but maintenance is accomplished at the considerable expense of further phosphate wasting.

Hypoparathyroidism. Lack of parathyroid hormone may stem from a failure in synthesis or release of the hormone, but most frequently it results from intentional surgical excision or incidental damage to the blood supply of the parathyroid glands. Because parathyroid hormone is deficient or absent, it cannot block renal excretion, stimulate bone resorption of calcium, or facilitate vitamin D in enhanced gut calcium absorption.

To make compensation effective, a high dose of vitamin D could be given in the range of 100,000 units or more per day. When vitamin D is administered in very high therapeutic doses to the patient with hypoparathyroidism, calcium absorption from the gut is increased, but bone resorption is activated as well. This absorption may raise serum calcium, but parathyroid hormone is the principal agent of reclamation of calcium from urine, and in its absence calciuria continues unopposed. In this form of compensated hypocalcemia, ionized serum calcium may thus be protected at the cost of a negative calcium balance.

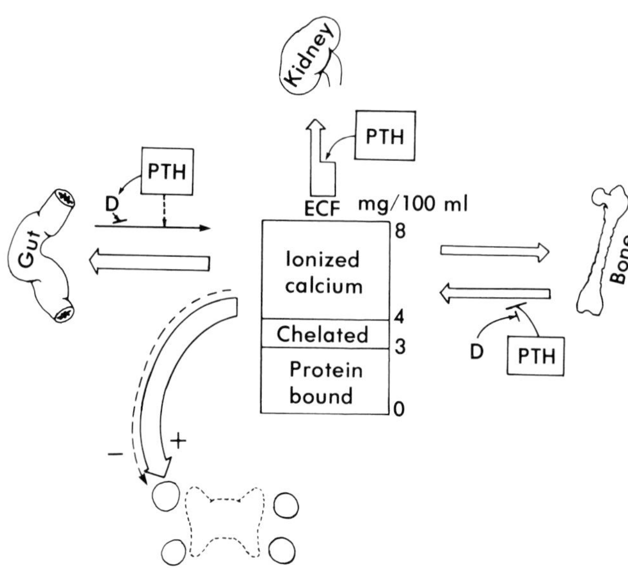

Fig. 55-4 In vitamin D deficiency parathormone excess barely compensates for the hypocalcemia caused by loss of absorption from the gut, but this is accomplished by severe phosphate wasting through the kidney, which has been mobilized out of bone—hence the skeletal deformities of rickets.

Hypoparathyroidism may be transient following cervical parathyroid exploration or thyroidectomy. However, the hypocalcemia stimulates the residual parathyroid tissue, and return to function is likely if some blood supply persists. Idiopathic hypoparathyroidism may exist as a component of a polyglandular failure thought to be based in an autoimmune process. It is rare and, like postoperative hypoarathyroidism, is treated with vitamin D in high doses. Improved treatment of the long-term aparathyroid state might be ideally managed by parathyroid transplantation, which has been carried out in patients already immunosuppressed for reasons of a concomitant kidney transplant. At present, administration of parathyroid hormone extracts from animal organs is not practical, analogous to commercial insulin production, and the quantities of parathyroid hormone that have been synthesized are inconsequential for therapeutic use. So presently hypoparathyroidism is managed by a superabundant calcium diet and vitamin D in therapeutic doses in anticipation of some return of endogenous parathyroid function.

PSEUDOHYPOPARATHYROIDISM. Neither parathyroid transplantation nor administration of parathormone extract benefits pseudohypoparathyroidism (see Table 55-1). This condition is usually familial and exhibits hypocalcemia with increased phosphorus but normal parathyroid hormone response to the hypocalcemia. In this case the hypocalcemia is caused not by a failure of the parathyroid gland to respond by increasing its hormone secretion but by the failure of the end organ to respond to this appropriately increased parathormone. When exogenous parathyroid hormone is administered to such patients, the cAMP response is lacking. This disease is familial and associated with a characteristic phenotype. The treatment is similar to that for hypoparathyroidism following neck exploration, i.e., large doses of vitamin D to compensate for the lack of parathormone response at the end organ.

HYPOMAGNESEMIA. Hypomagnesemia blocks both peripheral response to parathormone at the end organ and release of parathormone from the parathyroid gland. A number of nephrotoxic drugs may result in magnesium urinary losses and hypomagnesemia. Restoration to normal of serum magnesium levels that were low because of drug toxicity or nutritional deficits, as can be seen in the chronic alcoholic, restores normal parathormone release and end-organ response. Paradoxically, hypermagnesemia may suppress parathyroid hormone release, a response similar to that seen with hypercalcemia.

MALABSORPTION. Some gastrointestinal tract disorders may result directly in deficient absorption of vitamin D and/or calcium. For example, in some instances such as short gut syndrome or extensive intestinal bypass, vitamin D may be given parenterally. However, if the surface for calcium absorption is inadequate to be facilitated by vitamin D's action, calcium absorption may remain impaired despite optimum vitamin D and parathormone activity. However, if vitamin D is absorbed and not activated, the result is a deficit in the active form of vitamin D because of intestinal, hepatic, or renal disease. With some drug administrations such as diphenylhydantoin, vitamin D is not activated in the liver but is metabolized more quickly.

PANCREATITIS. With soft tissue destruction and digestion, calcium may be trapped or taken out of solution in the retroperitineum and other sites. Hypocalcemia results, but not from fundamental failure in calcium homeostasis as much as from sequestration by mass action. Rapid saponification of calcium has been implicated in pancreatitis and also in some syndromes in which sepsis is prominent such as in septic abortion.

HYPOPROTEINEMIA. As we know, calcium exists in circulation bound and inactive for as much as 50% of the total plasma calcium. Deficit of total plasma calcium must always be measured next to the albumin level and, if a severe hypoalbuminemia is present, the calculated ionized calcium may be normal. Only the metabolically active ionized calcium will be counted in the judgment of true hypocalcemia. However, malabsorption, hypoalbuminemia, and liver failure may all combine in some patients who have real hypocalcemia from common proximate causes for the deficits in circulation of each of these complexed pairs.

Table 55-2 **CLINICAL SIGNS OF HYPOCALCEMIA**

Neural	Muscle	General
Chvostek's sign	Tetany	Hypotension
Trousseau's sign	Cramps	Bradycardia
Seizures	Weakness	Cataracts
Irritability	Fatigue	Osteomalacia
Laryngeal spasm	Cardiac arrhythmia	Depression
Tingling paresthesias	Carpopedal spasms	Urinary frequency
Lightheadedness	Involuntary twitching	Anticoagulation

Similarly, as discussed above, hypoventilation would not change total serum calcium but would result in hypocalcemia by a shift from the ionized active fraction to the protein-bound portion. In hypoalbuminemia, these mirror image situations reflect an absolute decrease in serum calcium without a decrease in the ionized active fraction. In hyperventilation they reflect identical readings in total serum calcium but a decrease in ionized calcium with the change in pH.

CHELATION. Other circulating substances or administered drugs can complex calcium, and the complex that results may be bound with high affinity or may not be susceptible to the action of parathormone, vitamin D, or hydrogen ion in dissociation. Examples of such agents are the anticoagulants such as citrate used to bind calcium in transfused blood. Some drugs such as mithramycin have as a major side effect a reduction in blood calcium. Consequently, their indication has been shifted to use in hypercalcemic crises.

From all of these causes, the common result is a decrease in the biologically active ionized calcium compartment in blood. This decrease is experienced through the compensatory mechanisms that dampen this effect. However, when hypocalcemia is seen, calcium-dependent functions begin to change, and clinical consequences occur.

Consequences of Hypocalcemia

The clinical consequences of hypocalcemia are increased excitability in cellular membranes of nerves and muscles with tetany, spasms, and seizures. Clinical signs of this irritability are listed in Table 55-2.

NEURAL MANIFESTATIONS. Tetany, the principal feature of hypocalcemia may be latent or evident in intractable seizures. Latent tetany may be demonstrated by inducing the facial twitching or carpal spasm. Chvostek's sign is contraction of facial musculature induced by light tapping over the facial nerve just ahead of the tragus. Trousseau's sign is the carpal spasm produced by inflation of a blood pressure cuff above systolic pressure.

The initial symptoms the patient experiences usually are tingling paresthesias around the lips or in the fingertips.

Later these early neural symptoms can be uncovered in motor signs such as the Chvostek. However, more dangerous progression to laryngeal spasm or contraction of other smooth muscle because of hyperirritability may develop, and cardiac arrythmia may result. Muscle cramps may proceed to carpopedal spasm. This is usually quite frightening to the patient. The anxiety that follows is compounded further by the hyperventilation exhibited in response to this bizarre behavior, which the patient may never have previously experienced. Seizures may ultimately result.

CONTROL OF CLINICAL SYMPTOMS OF HYPOCALCEMIA. Some immediate help in symptom control may come from having the patient rebreathe or slowing down the patient's anxiety response with sedation. Hydantoin drugs may relieve the annoying paresthesias and tingling prodrome the patient may have in latent tetany. However, the obvious solution to the symptoms of hypocalcemia is immediately to raise the serum calcium and address the underlying cause of the hypocalcemia. The immediate effect of increased ionized calcium in the blood can be achieved with administration of a calcium salt solution. Some available calcium compounds are complexed to molecules that require metabolism before the calcium is available to replenish the ionized calcium. For immediate treatment, one must be aware of the type of calcium compound and the dose of elemental calcium it contains.

TREATMENT OF HYPOCALCEMIA. Calcium is an ion that comes readily out of solution in intravenous admixtures. Patients who are being resuscitated are often given sodium bicarbonate, which will precipitate any calcium salt administered through the same intravenous line. Moreover, calcium salts irritate the vein through which they are administered and should be diluted, but they are likewise a source of irritation to cardiac and other neuromuscular membrane surfaces. Large, rapid doses of calcium chloride contain a very high quantity of elemental calcium in readily available ionized form, so the dosage should be diminished, and the rate slowed. Calcium gluceptate or gluconate can be prepared in 10% solution and slowly infused over 10 minutes until tetany or paresthesias has stopped.

For longer-term treatment of hypocalcemia, treating symptoms rather than numbers is generally safer. If the patient requires continuing calcium support to prevent symptomatic hypocalcemia, oral treatment is initiated using a calcium wafer preparation. If a 4-g daily oral calcium supplementation does not result in freedom from symptoms or if the hypocalcemia persists at levels at which symptoms are anticipated with a high degree of likelihood, a vitamin D analog is added. The fastest-acting vitamin D preparation is 1,25-dihydroxycholecalciferol (Rocaltrol), which may be administered as 0.5 μg in daily dosage. When the patient is on both vitamin D and calcium supplementation, monitoring the blood calcium is important because hypercalcemia may develop insidiously. With a rise in the serum calcium toward normal, the vitamin D analog is discontinued first; the patient can be tapered off the calcium supplementation over the period of time that he remains asymptomatic. Special considerations are due those patients with renal insufficiency or liver failure because of the enzyme systems required for activating the furnished vitamin D precursors.

For long-term treatment of hypoparathyroidism in those patients requiring sustained calcium and vitamin D therapy, parathyroid hormone administration might be considered, but at present the quantities of parathormone congener are available only for diagnostic testing of the pseudohypoparathyroidism syndrome (see boxed material below). A reasonable alternative to freeing parathyroprival patients from dependence on calcium supplementation and vitamin D therapy is parathyroid transplantation. Parathyroid allografting[33] has been carried out in patients who have already been immunosuppressed and are recipients of renal allografts, having had previous total parathyroidectomy for secondary hyperparathyroidism. Such a parathyroid gland transplant can function, but an interesting speculation is that the renal allograft itself constitutes the transplantation of an endocrine gland with respect to activation of vitamin D precursors to the hormonally active vitamin D_3. As a consequence, the patients are more easily managed on calcium and vitamin D supplementation, and, as noted the boxed material below, even the patients with renal failure or anephric patients can benefit from some species of the vitamin D that will not require renal activation. As will be pointed out later, the majority of patients with hypoparathyroidism either recover some parathyroid function or are more easily managed by the newer forms of vitamin D therapy, which have fewer risks than parathyroid allografting. In some hypoparathyroid patients following reoperation with excision of pathologic parathyroid glands, parathyroid autotransplantation has been attempted.[3] However, the risk involved with grafting possibly autonomous pathologic parathyroid is that recurrence of hyperparathyroidism can occur, with

MANAGEMENT OF HYPOCALCEMIA[35]

A. Determination of cause
   Measure Ca^{++}, $PO_4^{=}$, albumin, mg^{++}, pH, PTH
B. For hypomagnesemia (< 0.8 mEq/L serum)
   mg Cl_2 IV 1-2 mEq/kg/24 hrs
C. For symptomatic latent tetany
   Diphenylhydantoin
D. Calcium supplementation
   1. IV
      10 ml 10% Ca gluconate in 50 ml D_5/W over 10 minutes
   2. PO
      1 g Ca gluconate wafers p.o. q.6h.
E. Vitamin D
   1. Normal liver and kidneys
      1.2 mg calciferol p.o. q.d.
   2. Liver disease
      50 μg calderol p.o. q.d.
   3. Renal disease
      0.5 μg rocaltrol p.o. q.d.
F. Parathormone
   1. Synthetic PTH—only as test for pseudohypoparathyroidism syndrome
   2. Parathyroid grafting—only in parathyroid patients already immunosuppressed with renal allograft

From Zaloga, G.P., and Chernow, B.: Calcium metabolism. In Geelhoed, G.W., and Chernow, B., editors: Endocrine aspects of acute illness, Clinics in critical care medicine, New York, 1985, Churchill-Livingstone.

the new source of the disease being the heterotopic site of the grafted gland. At present, treatment of persistent hypoparathyroidism is chronic support with calcium and vitamin D, which can successfully maintain serum calcium at a level at which the patient does not experience hypocalcemic symptoms.

Hypercalcemia

In hypercalcemia the body makes physiologic compensatory responses to lower ionized serum calcium by decreasing absorption, decreasing bone calcium resorption, and allowing unimpeded calciuresis. Hypercalcemia induces these changes by an inhibition of parathormone synthesis and release and a decrease in synthesis and activation of vitamin D. The dynamic pool of calcium in the blood expands either when absorption or resorption increases or when excretion decreases (i.e., when the capacity of these compensatory mechanisms to maintain a constant ionized serum calcium is exceeded).

Hypercalcemia is found in a number of pathologic conditions and has many clinical consequences. It is a finding generated by multiphasic biochemical screening of even asymptomatic patients. The finding of hypercalcemia always deserves investigation because it is a principle harbinger of disease. The hypercalcemia also usually indicates a significant disease for which further information should be gathered for diagnosis or prognosis. Hypercalcemia may be "an incidental finding," but rarely is the only abnormal laboratory value and is of little clinical significance to the patient. Most causes of hypercalcemia are serious diseases; a very significant few are caused by disease treatable for cure. Cancer causes hypercalcemia in the single biggest fraction of these patients, and often the cancer has spread beyond surgically curative treatment. However, the second most common cause of hypercalcemia, and the fraction that is increasing in frequency, is based in hyperparathyroidism, for which curative surgical treatment is a high probability.

Given the significance of hypercalcemia as a finding, its determination must be made with precision, on repeated observations, with investigations of the interrelated ions and hormones. Attention to the details of blood-drawing technique will reduce artifacts in repeated observation of hypercalcemia, proving it to be a true finding compelling a differential diagnosis as to its cause.

Causes

Primary Hyperparathyroidism. In many ways the most satisfying differential diagnosis of hypercalcemia's causes may be primary hyperparathyroidism because of its hopeful prognosis (Table 55-3). Currently, hyperparathyroidism accounts for nearly one third of the patients with hypercalcemia in large population surveys.

Since initial professional awareness of this diagnosis, the character of the population found to have hyperparathyroidism has changed. The initial patients were symptomatic with advanced disease. In current practice, patients are rarely encountered with end-stage target organ consequences such as Brown tumors, pathologic fractures, staghorn calculi with renal destruction, and metastatic calcification in soft tissue. The presentation of primary hyperparathyroidism today is much more subtle. As a rule, today's index case is an asymptomatic patient discovered through the exercise of differential diagnosis on the finding of hypercalcemia. Hypercalcemia resulting from primary hyperparathyroidism is most often mild, prolonged, asymptomatic, with subtle findings even in retrospect. Parathyroid poisoning is a very notable exception to this rule.

Table 55-3 **HYPERCALCEMIA**

Cause	Mechanism	Features
BENIGN		
Primary hyperparathyroidism	see Fig. 55-5	PTH ↑ ↑, Ca^{++} ↑, PO_4 ↓, Cl^- ↑
Vitamin D toxicity	↑ Ca absorption ↑ Ca bone resorption	Ca^{++} ↑, $PO_4^=$ ↑ ↓, PTH O
Sarcoidosis	Vitamin D hypersensitivity	Ca^{++} ↑, $PO_4^=$ ↑ ↓, PTH O, Chest x-ray$^+$
Thyrotoxicosis	Hypermetabolic bone breakdown	Ca^{++} ↑, $PO_4^=$ ↓ ↑, PTH O, T_3 ↑, T_4 ↑
Drug (e.g., thiazides)	Renal tubular Ca^{++} reabsorption, hemoconcentration	Ca^{++} ↑, K^+ ↓, PTH O
High bone turnover (e.g., immobilization, Paget's disease)	Outward flux of bone Ca stores	Ca^{++} ↑ $PO_4^=$ ↑, PTH O
Familial (e.g. familial hypocalciuric hypercalcemia)	Increased renal sensitivity to PTH	Ca^{++} ↑, PTH Nl ↓ urine Ca^{++}
Doubtful (e.g. milk-alkali syndrome)	Increased availability of Ca^{++} for absorption	Ca^{++} ↑ PO_4 ↓ ↑, pH ↑, PTH ↓ ↓, urinary $CO_3^=$
MALIGNANT		
Metastatic cancer (e.g, breast, prostate)	Osteolytic release of Ca^{++}, $PO_4^=$	Ca^{++} ↑, $PO_4^=$ ↑, alk p'tase ↑, PTH ↓
Parendocrine (PTH-like or OAF)	APUD cells or nonendocrine tumors, multiple myeloma	Ca^{++} ↑, PO_4 ↑ ↓, direct assay of osteoclast activity

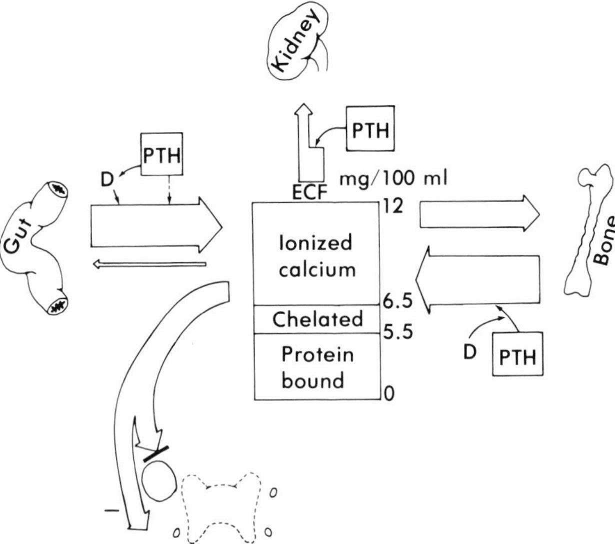

Fig. 55-5 In primary hyperparathyroidism, autonomous parathyroid tissue (in this case, a parathyroid adenoma) secretes parathormone in excess with increased calcium absorption from gut, resorption from bone, and urinary calcium reclamation, leading to hypercalcemia.

Table 55-4 **INCIDENCE OF HYPERPARATHYROIDISM**

Age	Men	Women
<39	4.5/100,000	8/100,000
40-59	26/100,000	1/1000
>60	1/1000	2/1000

From Heath, H.S., et al.: Reprinted by permission of N. Engl. J. Med. **302:**189, 1980.

Autonomous parathyroid tissue (often an adenoma) secretes parathormone in an excess that the hypercalcemia does not inhibit. This hyperparathyroidism increases calcium absorption from the gut, resorption from the bone, and reclamation of urinary calcium (Fig. 55-5).

The incidence of primary hyperparathyroidism is higher in females than in males and varies with the age, increasing in frequency in both genders with advancing age (Table 55-4). The most dramatic prevalance of primary hyperparathyroidism occurs in the elderly female,[24] and its discovery and treatment in this group is often gratifying. In all age groups, however, primary hyperparathyroidism as a cause of hypercalcemia is among the leading endocrinologic reasons a patient undergoes operations.[12]

Hyperparathyroidism is classified as primary, secondary or tertiary, depending on whether the hypersecretion of parathyroid hormone is primary or appropriately reactive to some other stimulus. However, primary hyperparathyroidism is the principle concern in the differential causes of hypercalcemia, and it is the most frequent type of hyperparathyroidism seen in the human populations submitted to health screening tests.

The clinical manifestations of primary hyperparathyroidism range from asymptomatic without evidence of disease apart from the biochemical findings, which is most frequently seen, to an acute life-threatening crisis, fortunately rare, called "parathyroid poisoning."[34] Patients may progress through the clinical scale from those who are asymptomatic to those who experience hyperparathyroid complications.[29] However, it is not proven that treatment of asymptomatic patients with isolated biochemical findings of primary hyperparathyroidism influences longevity in the absence of the development of hyperparathyroid complications. Longitudinal studies have been undertaken to follow the natural history of the untreated disease with intervention occurring immediately on disease complication or progression, defined by a rise in serum calcium above some arbitrary level set prospectively. This "bail out" is built into protocols for the study of primary hyperparathyroidism's natural history because of the increased incidence of complications seen in patients with higher calcium values. Also an approximate linear correlation exists between the mass of autonomous parathyroid tissue and the degree of symptoms, rate of complication, and absolute increment in the serum calcium.

Although diagnosing primary hyperparathyroidism as a cause of hypercalcemia is a very valuable contribution to the patient's care, it is not the only, or even the leading, cause (see Table 55-3). It must be differentiated from the other diagnoses that also cause hypercalcemia.

Vitamin D Toxicity. Excessive vitamin D activity is an easily treatable cause of hypercalcemia. If excessive exogenous vitamin D is given, calcium resorption from bone increases, and intestinal absorption of calcium increases greatly. The fundamental mechanisms of hypercalcemia based in vitamin D toxicity are the reverse of the pathophysiology of hypocalcemia caused by vitamin D deficiency. Reading Fig. 55-5 in reverse illustrates this mechanism. Though calcium is up, phosphate may be unchanged, and parathormone is near zero. These features distinguish this cause from primary hyperparathyroidism in which phosphate is depressed and parathormone reading is high.

Drug manufacturers of vitamin supplements now restrict the supply of vitamin D in multivitamin tablets to prevent the toxicity of overfeeding vitamin D. Factitious hypervitaminosis D may still occur if patients take excessive vitamin pills without regard to the package labeling restrictions. This was a particular risk with flavored children's vitamin supplements; and the higher serum calciums generally seen in children with high bone turnover, remodeling, and growth complicated the differential diagnosis.

Sarcoidosis. Sarcoidosis can cause hypercalcemia because the sarcoidosis granulomas are involved directly in accelerating vitamin D activation. As in vitamin D toxicity, serum phosphate levels are variably affected, and parathormone values should reflect the hypercalcemic inhibition of parathormone with assays showing near zero circulating parathormone. Chest x-ray film study may further substantiate the sarcoidosis diagnosis. Corticosteroids frequently are used in the management of this form of hypercalcemia on the basis of counteracting the accelerated vitamin D activation.

Thyrotoxicosis. Hyperthyroidism may accelerate bone breakdown and thereby cause hypercalcemia. As seen in vitamin D intoxication, parathormone levels reflect parathyroid suppression, an appropriate response to the hypercalcemia. Other features of hyperthyroidism should give clinical indication for measuring T_3 and T_4 to detect their elevation. Antithyroid drugs that slow down the hypermetabolism of thyrotoxicosis by blocking synthesis or release of thyroid hormones effect a gradual return toward normal calcium values.

Thiazides and Other Drugs. Thiazide diuretics act principally on renal tubular function and at this site enhance calcium reclamation from urine. To the extent that they accomplish an effective diuresis, an elevated serum calcium may reflect hemoconcentration in much the same way as inappropriate tourniquet technique elevates serum calcium reading. Potassium and phosphate are often depressed; thus they are often supplemented in the patient taking diuretics to maintain normal plasma values. The appropriate response of the parathyroid glands to hypercalcemia is depressed parathormone.

Active Bone Turnover. Some patients may exhibit hypercalcemia during periods of high bone turnover activity; for example, children whose blood normally contains higher calcium measurements; previously active adults who are abruptly immobilized such as might occur with an accidental spinal cord injury and paralysis, or older patients with Paget's disease. Both calcium and phosphate may be elevated, and parathormone is low.

Familial Hypocalciuric Hypercalcemia. A familial syndrome that has tricked surgeons into operating on patients with hypercalcemia despite normal or variable parathormone is characterized by low urinary calcium excretion and serum calcium retention through apparent increased renal sensitivity to parathormone. This familial hypocalciuric hypocalcemia (FHH)[21] can be distinguished from primary hyperparathyroidism, which may also have a familial occurrence, by specialized studies of urine calcium clearance and a careful examination of the relationship of parathormone and simultaneous ionized serum calcium. These studies are often occasioned by a repeat operation in a patient or family member with no findings based in the parathyroid gland that would explain the hypercalcemia and with postoperative results that indicate a surgical procedure has failed to control hypercalcemia. In this population of patients, urinary calcium clearance studies should exclude FHH before a repeat operation, particularly if a positive family history of hypercalcemia exists.

Milk-Alkali Syndrome. Patients with peptic disease may be taking large volumes of calcium salts and acid neutralizers. Hypercalcemia may result, probably less from the increased calcium made available for intestinal absorption than from acid/base imbalance because vitamin D_3 suppression should increase the fecal calcium loss in the presence of the resulting hypercalcemia. However, the ingestion of alkali changes acid/base balance at the kidney, the ultimate regulator of acid/base balance, and urinary bicarbonate secretion may be decreased. Under most circumstances of dietary calcium intake, the finely tuned vitamin D parathormone regulators are able to adjust absorption and excretion to maintain a constant ionized serum calcium, and this alleged syndrome is a doubtful exception to this rule. The caution the surgeon should apply before presuming this diagnosis in someone with peptic ulcer disease is that hyperparathyroidism may coexist with peptic ulcer disease, particularly in familial syndromes. Even with this caveat, some investigators question whether the milk-alkali syndrome exists at all,[5] and the putative mechanisms of milk-alkali intake should not dissuade the clinician from further differential diagnosis of hypercalcemia.

Metastatic Cancer. Unfortunately, the group that constitutes the largest number of patients differentiated from those with hypercalcemia are patients who first come to medical attention with cancer that is metastatic, usually to bone. Five principal primary tumors in sites other than bone have a proclivity to spread to osseous sites of metastases: breast cancer, lung cancer, prostate cancer, thyroid cancer, and hypernephroma. Because of its very high prevalence in Western populations, breast cancer leads the list of tumors responsible for hypercalcemia. In the osteolytic action of metastatic cancer, calcium and phosphorus are both released; this heavy load of these metabolites in the catabolic patient may overwhelm the renal clearance capacity. In some cancers the hypercalcemia seems out of proportion to the evident bone destruction, and for these tumors additional humoral factors are postulated and in some cases proven. Alkaline phosphatase may rise in parallel with the hypercalcemia; in the case of prostate cancer acid phosphatase may be elevated. These metabolic consequences are usually accompanied by skeletal pain, often at the specific site where the disease is most active.

Paraendocrine Tumors. It would not be surprising if metastatic parathyroid carcinoma produced hypercalcemia because presumably this parathormone excess would have mechanisms identical to the primary hyperparathyroidism seen with benign hyperfunctioning parathyroid tissue. However, primary malignancies in nonparathyroid tissues can also give rise to parathyroid-like hormones or their effect. Epithelial carcinomas arising from multiple organs have been recorded with parathormone-like activity. In addition, other paraendocrine products may also contribute to the hypercalcemia of special groups of cancers.

Hematologic malignancies with proliferation in bone marrow are known for hypercalcemia. In particular, multiple myeloma has been well recognized for hypercalcemia production, not only on the basis of its intraosseous location, but also from its production of a paraendocrine substance identified as osteoclast-activating factor. Multiple peptides and prostaglandins have also been implicated in the paraendocrine consequences of these nonendocrine tumors; among the consequences associated with release of these humoral factors is hypercalcemia. Parathormone of ectopic origin in malignant cells may occasionally cross-react with some antibodies used in radioimmunoassay of parathyroid hormone. However, parathyroid hormone of parathyroid gland origin has a much greater and more immediate response by cAMP measured in urine than does ectopic parathormone. This response may be useful in distinguishing those infrequent cases in which other clinical data do not make this difference apparent.

Consequences of Hypercalcemia

The signs and symptoms of hypercalcemia are protean, may range from subtle to lethal, and are not often associated with the specific cause that gave rise to the hypercalcemia. The absolute elevation in serum calcium is important, but the rate at which the hypercalcemia has progressed is nearly as important. Acute hypercalcemia from calcium infusion in a normal patient with an abrupt rise in total serum calcium of several milligrams per 100 ml may be lethal; the same patient might accommodate a gradual elevation in serum calcium of twice the same increment over a year and not show any disability. Because of this insidious progression, the hypercalcemia of primary hyperparathyroidism is more often clinically silent than is the rapidly progressive hypercalcemia of metastatic malignancy, which is often a principal cause of death.

Clinical Presentation. Clinical discrimination of patients' complaints has passed well beyond the "stones, bones, and abdominal groans" of the mnemonic first used to describe the features of hypercalcemia. Much more subtlety is now demanded of the astute clinician, who often sensitively screens new patients by retrospective questioning after they have been treated for hyperparathyroidism. Often patients recall symptoms after they have subsided following successful reduction of serum calcium; the patients may not even recognize the symptoms as present preoperatively because of the insidious progression that led the patient to accept these minor aberrations as accompaniments of advancing age or to attribute them to other known illness. Patients may express some or none of the principal features listed in the boxed material below, or they may have symptoms not listed; and the only direct evidence that they are part of the hypercalcemia complex is their improvement with treatment or recurrence with the return of hypercalcemia. Few of these listed symptoms fulfill "Koch's postulates" as invariably associated with the disease. The one invariable finding, i.e., an elevation in ionized serum calcium, is not a clinical symptom.

Of the symptoms and signs in the boxed material at left, many are of degree rather than qualitative presence or absence. For example, specific responses regarding mentation in the "review of systems" include a complaint by one middle-aged gentleman that he could no longer complete the book of crossword puzzles that he had started successfully some time before. A patient in a nursing home had incontinence attributed to senility until it was cured following treatment for hyperparathyroidism. Arthritis frequently turns out to be myalgia or bone pain on closer questioning. Headache is a prime presenting sign of hypercalcemia, and a screening blood chemistry analysis has a much higher yield than CT scanning of such patients and is far more cost effective in its application.

CLINICAL CONSEQUENCES OF HYPERCALCEMIA

Eye, Ear, Nose, Throat
Band keratopathy
Cataracts
Conjunctivitis
Change in vision
Change in ocular prescription
Pruritis

Gastrointestinal
Weight loss
Polydipsia
Weakness
Pancreatitis
Peptic ulcer
Calcific stippling
Anorexia
Thirst
Malaise
Nausea/Vomiting
Abdominal pain
Constipation

Genitourinary
Urinary calculi
Polyuria
Uremia
Ureteral colic
Nocturia
Hematuria

Musculoskeletal
Osteoporosis
Resorption of clavicle ends
Decreased reflexes
Decreased tone
Backache
Bone pain
Ataxia
Myalgia

Cardiovascular
ECG changes
Hypertension

Central Nervous System
Confusion
Incontinence
Disorientation
Lethargy
Coma
Headache
Memory loss ("can't do crossword puzzles")
Depression
Hearing loss
Stupor

Testing Patients with Hypercalcemia

A simple screen of the patient found to have confirmed hypercalcemia (Fig. 55-6) is based on the chloride/phosphate ratio that is suggestive, but not diagnostic, of hyperparathyroidism if this ratio is greater than 30. With some degree of confidence, one can diagnose primary hyperparathyroidism without a parathormone assay, if the chloride to phosphate ratio is greater than 30, with a distinctly elevated calcium and a serum albumin that also allows a calculated ionized calcium value estimated to be elevated.

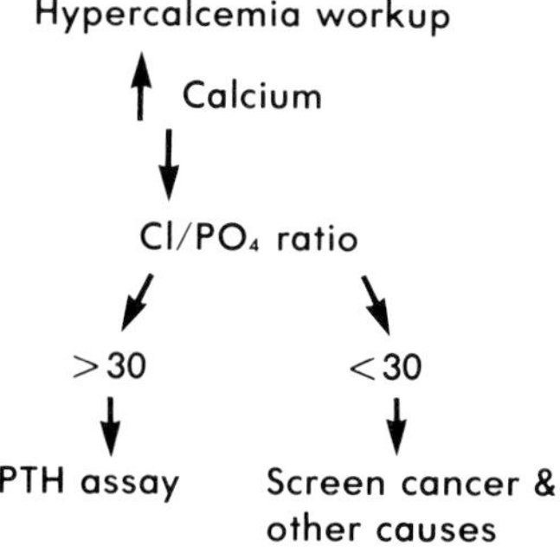

Fig. 55-6 A simple screen of the hypercalcemic patient makes use of the ratio of chloride to phosphate for an initial approximation of whether hyperparathyroidism or oncogenic hypercalcemia is likely.

Disease	Blood			Urine		
	Ca	P_i	^{125}(OH)D	NcAMP	$^{F}Ca_{E}$	TRP/GFR
1° HPTH	↑	↓	↑	↑	↑↔	↓
Malignancy	↑	↑↔	↓↔	↑	↑↑	↓
Osteolytic Metastases	↑	↔	↓↔	↓	↑↑	↔

Fig. 55-7 Further differentiation in blood and urine tests can be carried out deliberately for a reliable diagnosis before confident recommendations for treatment, particularly in the asymptomatic patient.

Parathormone assays have improved considerably with the further speciation of antibodies recognizing different portions of the intact molecule of parathormone or different fragments in the circulation. Consequently, surgeons with some knowledge of the type of assay available can have confidence in the parathormone assay if it confirms the biochemical impression obtained from the quicker analysis of calcium, phosphate, chloride, and albumin. If the chloride/phosphate ratio is less than 30, typically further work is needed to differentiate among the causes seen in Table 55-4.

Further differentiating tests on blood and urine are exhibited in Fig. 55-7. In most instances the diagnosis of primary hyperparathyroidism can be made with all the leisure required to approach clinical certainty. If applied, the treatment of this disorder is elective and is not described until tests have eliminated any lingering doubt about the correct diagnosis. Cervical operation has no role in the *diagnosis* of primary hyperparathyroidism. Some urgency may be associated with diagnosis and management of certain malignant disorders that can lead to hypercalcemia, particularly if compromise in organ function is a risk. A rare indication for a truncated laboratory workup and accelerated treatment plan is the patient in hypercalcemic crisis because of acute hyperparathyroidism. Treatment should immediately be directed at reducing the serum calcium. A biochemical pattern that suggests primary hyperparathyroidism and hand x-ray films that show subperiosteal resorption along the radial aspect of the phalanges in the patient who is dangerously hypercalcemic constitute sufficient diagnostic information to indicate urgent parathyroidectomy.[9] This presentation is rare, however, and all other hypercalcemic cases, particularly the asymptomatic patients, deserve deliberate workup with a high reliability assigned to the final diagnosis.

The majority of patients will have had at least the primary laboratory evaluation outlined in the boxed material below. The serum calcium determination is the most important because a second, later confirmation of hypercalcemia with the patient off medication and under circumstances of normal diet and activity patterns is required. For practical purposes the ionized calcium, which is strictly controlled within the body, can be calculated under conditions of known pH by the simultaneous measurement of protein in the blood. The calculated ionized calcium value is typically higher than the ionized calcium levels measured by an ion-sensitive electrode, but the number of patients with low calculated ionized calcium is fewer than the number of the patients found to have absolute decrease in total serum calcium. Under normal circumstances the calculated ionized calcium value is sufficient; in the dynamic state of critical illness an ionized serum calcium might be measured directly by a selective electrode. The phosphate determination, already used in the screening test of chloride/phosphate ratio, is typically depressed in the patient with hyperparathyroidism and may be elevated in those patients with renal failure or metastatic cancer. Parathyroid hormone excess causes a lowered serum phosphate through a decrease in renal tubular resorption of phosphate. This urinary test can be used to confirm directly the hyperparathyroidism through a measurement of tubular resorption of phosphate (TRP). The TRP is the ratio expressed in percentage of urinary phosphate times serum creatinine/urinary creatinine times serum phosphate.

Of hyperparathyroid patients on a normal diet and without renal failure, 81% have a TRP less than 78%.[9]

Although the N-terminal fragment of parathormone is biologically active, its half-life in serum is short. Consequently, the C-terminal parathormone assay is more helpful in testing patients for hyperparathyroidism. However, the clearance of C-terminal parathyroid fragments is through the kidney, and in renal failure an elevation in circulating parathormone will be measured on a basis of this excretion failure, with or without an increase in secretion. Highly specialized radioimmunoassay antibodies against other components of parathyroid hormone or parathyroid-like hormones have been developed to detect the atypical hyperparathyroidism from ectopic sources in the paraendocrine malignancies.[2]

The repeated measurements of elevated serum calcium, depressed phosphate, and elevated serum parathormone may be the only laboratory diagnostic tests required following the screening studies mentioned in the discussion of the patient with classic primary hyperparathyroidism. Thereafter further ancillary studies are necessary to differentiate patients with other causes for their hypercalcemia or to make the difficult diagnosis of primary hyperparathyroidism in the early appearance of the syndrome or in the patient with only marginally elevated hypercalcemia. Many ancillary studies focus on establishing the normalcy of other laboratory values such as magnesium and creatinine before looking further to see if an abnormality in the patient's bones or kidneys accounts for the hypercalcemia. Alkaline phosphatase levels may be elevated in the metastatic malignancy and slightly elevated in hyperparathyroidism. Uric acid is mildly elevated in most patients with primary hyperparathyroidism. The elevation may also be a function of impaired renal clearance of uric acid and can be checked against the creatinine and blood urea nitrogen.

One of the helpful urine tests is a stone analysis for those patients who have passed renal calculi. Calcium calculi are more suggestive of primary hyperparathyroidism than are urate stones. Urinary calcium assay is helpful because a quantitative hypercalciuria suggests primary hyper-

LABORATORY EVALUATION OF CALCIUM AND PHOSPHATE DISORDERS

Primary	**Ancillary**
Serum calcium	Alkaline phosphatase
(Ionized calcium)	Magnesium
Phosphate	Creatinine
Chloride	BUN
Albumin	Uric Acid
Parathormone	pH
1,25 $(OH)_2$ D	$HCO_3^=$
Urine	**X-ray Films**
Stone analysis	Hands
Calcium	Skull
TRP	Chest
cAMP	

parathyroidism and helps to distinguish this diagnosis from familial hypocalciuric hypercalcemia (FHH).[21] Urinary cAMP is a very sensitive test of a very rapid change in the urine reflecting the presence or excess of parathormone. Well over 90% of patients with primary hyperparathyroidism have elevated levels of nephrogenous cAMP, and mild renal failure does not dampen the measurement of cAMP in the urine. Because cAMP in the urine is a very sensitive and rapid indicator of the presence of parathyroid hormone, the urinary measurement of cAMP can confirm the ablation of excess parathyroid activity and serve as a useful indicator during operation that the offending pathology has been resected.

Radiographic examinations may be helpful in some instances, but not for the majority of those patients who have asymptomatic hypercalcemia. The rare patient who has had long-standing hyperparathyroidism and may be symptomatic or even toxic may have radiographically identifiable bone lesions (Fig. 55-8). Bone cysts and subperiosteal resorption of bone in phalanges or distal clavicles (see Fig 55-8, *C*) or diffuse "ground-glass" demineralization of the skull (see Fig. 55-8, *B*) may still be seen in patients with hypercalcemia. However, "Brown tumors" of von Recklinghausen's disease are rare enough to be of historic significance, except in cases of very neglected hyperparathyroidism. Fig. 55-8, *A* shows long bone cystic changes in a patient with such a long and neglected course of primary hyperparathyroidism, but a more useful study may be the chest x-ray film, routinely performed in patients admitted to the hospital for evaluation or treatment of hypercalcemia. The chest x-ray film can exclude either primary lung cancer or metastatic cancer as one possible cause of

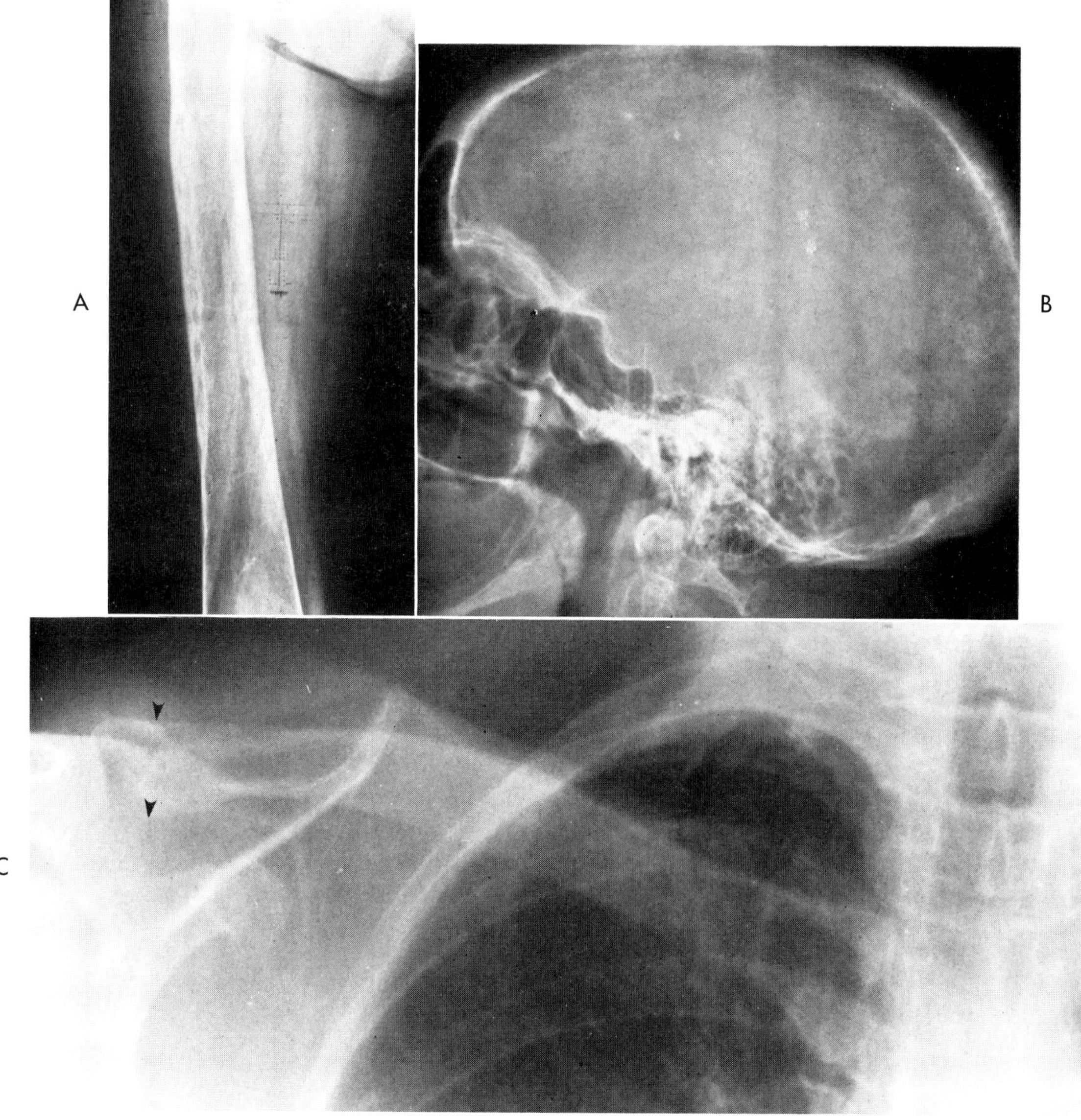

Fig. 55-8 Radiographic findings in hyperparathyroidism include the bone cysts **(A)** or ground-glass demineralization seen on skull film **(B)** that is increasingly rare except in neglected cases of prolonged hypercalcemia; an earlier and nearly pathognomonic sign seen in another patient's chest film is the resorption of the distal clavicles **(C),** or so-called "Higginbotham's sign."

the hypercalcemia, but a nearly pathognomonic sign in hyperparathyroidism may be noted in absorption of the distal clavicles, the so-called "Higginbotham's sign" (see Fig. 55-8, *C*). Occasionally, nuclear medicine scans are used to determine bone density as an estimate of demineralization, occurring in hyperparathyroidism and other disorders such as osteoporosis. An improved test of demineralization is dual photon absorptiometry (DPA). The preoperative appearance of demineralization on such scans can often be associated with a postoperative problem of remineralization termed the "hungry bone syndrome." As postoperative hypoparathyroidism and a return to normal calcium dynamics occur, the heavy shift of calcium back into the bones from which it was mobilized during the hyperparathyroidism may cause changes in blood phosphate, magnesium, and calcium as these minerals return to the "bone sink" from which they had been released. A late postoperative bone density scan reveals the restoration of this mineral density in successfully treated hyperparathyroidism. A number of other radiographic tests have been used in hyperparathyroidism for localization of the source of the excess parathyroid hormone, and these will be considered in the section on parathyroid localization studies.

Treatment of Hypercalcemia

Asymptomatic hypercalcemia requires no urgent treatment if indicated solely by the determination of elevated numbers on laboratory tests. In fact, if severely elevated calcium levels are reported in an asymptomatic patient, one should first suspect the numbers to represent laboratory error and repeat the tests, along with determination of the ancillary studies listed in the boxed material below. Treatment attempts to prevent the long-term consequences of hypercalcemia in the asymptomatic patient typically is through a deliberate diagnostic process and an elective surgical treatment. For such patients the suggestions about general management recommendations listed below may be adequate. Particularly if troubled by intercurrent complications of chronic hypercalcemia such as urinary tract calculi, some patients may have added to their general management oral neutral phosphates and a low calcium diet. The general management recommendations are typically for the outpatient who is found to have hypercalcemia and is undergoing the deliberate diagnostic testing before recommendations of treatment or continued observation. The urgent treatment of hypercalcemia by means of intravenous agents to prevent hypercalcemic crisis is limited to inpatients.

General Hypercalcemic Management Recommendations. For the patient with hypercalcemia detected by outpatient blood testing, rational recommendations include a decrease in dietary calcium intake. This reduction is particularly valuable if the patient is taking calcium supplements or is experiencing high calcium intake as an indirect consequence of treatment directed toward some other end such as antacid treatment for peptic ulcer disease. Generally, a decrease in milk and other dairy products, discontinuation or suspension of antacid tablets or a shift to magnesium and aluminum salts for antacid therapy, and discontinuation of thiazide diuretics or antihypertensives are effective. Quite clearly patients should suspend use of any vitamin D preparations they might be taking, including the use of most multiple vitamin supplements.

Increased mobilization should be encouraged. Stress along long bones and exercise through the activities of normal daily living prevent an increase in the rate of bone demineralization. Neutral phosphate may be administered through the gastrointestinal tract for long-term calcium-lowering action. However, its effect is mild, and its side effect is diarrhea because the same agents are given as phospha-soda as for cathartics. One of the consequences of repeated Fleet's enema administration is an increase in phosphate in the serum and a corresponding decrease in blood calcium. For patients who are undergoing long-term observation and treatment for prevention of recurrent renal calculi, sodium brushite may be useful for binding calcium in the gastrointestinal tract to lower its rate of absorption.

Inpatient Treatment of Hypercalcemic Crisis. For the symptomatic patient with dangerously elevated serum calcium, hospitalization and intravenous therapy are indicated. As seen in the boxed material below, a sequence of steps may be taken to lower serum calcium gradually to safe levels while simultaneously determining its cause. Rarely are these hypercalcemic treatment steps indicated

TREATMENT OF HYPERCALCEMIC CRISIS

General: D/C dietary Ca^{++}, Thiazides, Vitamin D ↑ Mobilization Oral Neutral Phosphates, Brushite

Hydration and Diuresis, Calciuresis

1. Saline infusion	2 L/3 hours
2. Furosemide	100 mg IV/4 hours
Complexing Ca^{++} in serum	
3. Phosphate	1.5 g IV/8 hours
4. Citrate or EDTA (dangerous)	1 g IV/4 hours
Drugs decreasing Ca^{++} from bone and gut	
5. Hydrocortisone	100 mg IV q.8h.
6. Salmon Calcitonin	5 Medical Research Council (MRC) U/kg/hour IV
7. Mithramycin	25 mg/kg/24 hours IV
Dialysis	Acute hemodialysis/4 hours
Urgent parathyroidectomy	As indicated by x-ray film bone resorption

for a total serum calcium less than 12 mg/100 ml or ionized calcium less than 5.5 mg/100 ml, but the absolute number measured in the blood is less significant than the severity of the patient's symptoms attributed to the hypercalcemia.

The first treatment indicated, and the mainstay of hypercalcemic management, is intravenous hydration and diuresis. The symptomatic, hypercalcemic patient may be dehydrated because the symptoms most often include nausea and vomiting. However, hypertension and cardiac arrythmias may also be reflections of hypercalcemia. They may limit the rate of rehydration, unless simultaneous diuretic treatment is administered. Saline solutions are preferred over dextrose in water, but Ringer's lactate is contraindicated because of the presence of small quantities of calcium in the infusion. Saline diuresis should be induced rapidly by administration of 2 L of saline over 3 hours, usually accompanied by intravenous furosemide given in high doses with frequency dependent on its effect. With vigorous saline hydration and diuretic treatment, as much as 1 g of elemental calcium may be cleared through the urine in 24 hours, and serum calcium may drop from 2 to 3 mg/100 ml. Cardiac and renal function and chest x-ray film should be carefully observed and serum potassium and magnesium monitored during this treatment. The end point in this treatment is not to achieve an arbitrary level for blood calcium but to reduce patient symptoms, particularly to effect a return to consciousness from stuporous obtundation. The kind of symptomatic hypercalcemia seen with hyperparathyroidism or vitamin D toxicity is usually managed successfully with hydration and diuresis therapy alone and the initiation of brisk calciuresis. For hypercalcemia based in malignancy, very severe symptoms associated with extremely high calcium levels require further treatment beyond these initial steps. In addition, some rare forms of primary hyperparathyroidism, i.e., parathyroid

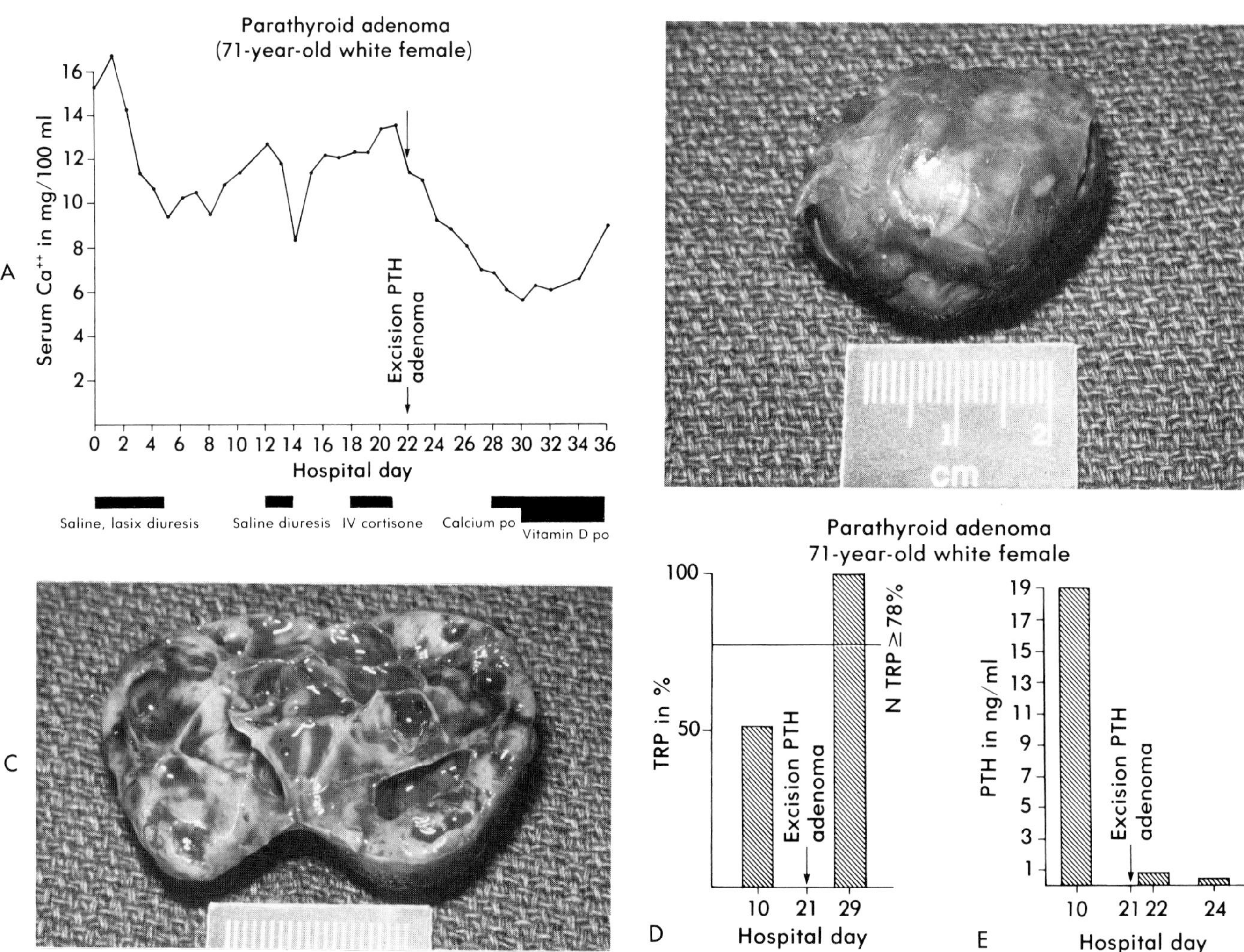

Fig. 55-9 Measurements and management in "parathyroid poisoning." A stuporous 71-year-old woman was admitted in hypercalcemic crisis and begun on saline diuresis while diagnostic studies to prove hyperparathyroidism were being performed. **A**, Serum calcium (16.5 mg/100 ml on admission) was moderated to still-symptomatic levels of 12 mg/100 ml by saline, furosemide, and cortisone, until parathyroidectomy of an adenoma (inset **B**) that had undergone cystic degenerative changes (inset **C**). Changes in preoperative and postoperative tubular resorption of phosphate **(D)** and parathormone **(E)** reflect the hypocalcemia postoperatively supported with transient vitamin D and calcium supplements.

poisoning (Fig. 55-9), may also require further treatment measures to return serum calcium toward normal.

The next steps in a rapid decrease in ionized serum calcium include complexing the calcium in the serum or shifting it to the un-ionized form by acid/base manipulation. Intravenous phosphate may be administered up to 1.5 g intravenously over 8 hours. Citrate or ethylene diamine tetraacetic acid (EDTA) may be given to complex the calcium in circulation, but these agents are dangerous and unpredictable in their effects, particularly on the kidneys. They should be used only in extreme circumstances because safer drugs may be used to decrease calcium absorption from bone and gut if calciuresis has not returned the patient from dangerously elevated hypercalcemic levels.

Hydrocortisone administration (100 mg intravenously) may be helpful in decreasing calcium absorption and encouraging calcium renal excretion. However, the use of hydrocortisone is nearly specific for hypercalcemia based in sarcoidosis, some malignant neoplasms, or vitamin D toxicity because rarely do patients with hyperparathyroidism respond to steroid treatment. In fact, because only about 5% of patients whose hypercalcemia is based in hyperparathyroidism respond, the use of hydrocortisone to reduce serum calcium has been standardized as a "hydrocortisone suppression test" to rule out hyperparathyroidism. Newer agents used in hypercalcemia management are H_2-receptor blocking agents such as cimetidine or ranitidine.

The introduction of calcitonin therapy has introduced a significant treatment agent with less toxicity than others that are used in serious hypercalcemia. Salmon calcitonin is currently the largest therapeutic molecule commercially, biochemically synthesized. In hypercalcemia, it has been used in pharmacologic levels at which it inhibits bone resorption and increases renal clearance of calcium. Salmon calcitonin is the species of this peptide used because it is more potent than mammalian calcitonin. This hormone may be used in levels of 5 MRC U/kg/hour with fewer side effects than the other somewhat more potent but considerably more dangerous intravenous agents.

Mithramycin's side effect of lowering serum calcium has been known for some time. Now this cytotoxic agent chemotherapeutic may be used therapeutically for hypercalcemia. It is especially useful in patients with hypercalcemia based in malignancy, although other agents such as streptozocin have also been used for hypercalcemia based in specific malignancy such as islet cell carcinoma. Mithramycin has a cumulative toxicity but an immediate calcium-lowering effect. Therefore it may be administered when diuresis fails to bring serum calcium under control, and its prolonged hypocalcemic effect may continue for several days after this initial administration. If only one or two doses are needed, the nephrotoxicity and other side effects are limited. Often administration of this agent in those intervals brings the hypercalcemia under control.

At times intravenous hydration, diuresis, and hypocalcemic agents successfully lower serum calcium from crisis levels, but the cause persists and drives the calcium back up again. In other cases the presence of organ failures such as renal failure contraindicate further use of toxic agents or diuresis. In such instances urgent hemodialysis may be considered for maintaining the blood calcium at reduced levels. Hemodialysis is indicated in any event if renal failure is part of the patient's problem. By regulating the bath against which dialysis occurs, a net calcium loss can be achieved in each dialysis. However, the small dynamic serum pool of calcium is backed up by an enormous reserve in calcium stores, and the hemodialysis must be frequently repeated to keep serum calcium under control as it equilibrates again with the released bone stores. In one specific hypercalcemic crisis, the unusual case of acute hyperparathyroidism, a rapid diagnostic determination can be made, and an urgent parathyroidectomy is indicated.

The application of diagnostic measures and management of parathyroid poisoning may be shown in a clinical example of a patient in hypercalcemic crisis (see Fig. 55-9). A 71-year-old woman was admitted in coma found to be based in hypercalcemia with levels of 16.5 mg/100 ml despite a low serum albumin. Immediate saline diuresis with furosemide treatment was begun (see Fig. 55-9, *A*) with reduction of the serum calcium to levels of 12 mg/100 ml at which the patient remained symptomatic. During the management of the hypercalcemic crisis, tubular reabsorption of phosphate (see Fig. 55-9, *D*) and serum parathormone (see Fig. 55-9, *E*) suggested primary hyperparathyroidism, which was further supported by x-ray film examination of the hands showing subperiosteal phalangeal bone resorption on fine grain industrial film. She was taken to the operating room for urgent parathyroidectomy when these results were known, and a parathyroid adenoma was encountered and excised (Fig. 55-9, *B*). The pathophysiology of this acute hyperparathyroidism is probably based in the findings of acute cystic degeneration (Fig. 55-9, *C*) which the pathologist suggested was a recent change in this adenoma. Postoperatively the patient experienced symptomatic hypocalcemia and was supported by transient oral calcium and vitamin D administration. Vitamin D therapy was discontinued 2 weeks following discharge from the hospital; in 1 month calcium supplementation was stopped; at 6 weeks the patient was asymptomatic and found to have normal calcium, phosphate, chloride, and parathormone values when studied as an outpatient. This patient reflects the problems seen with both hypercalcemic and hypocalcemic crises, the measurements needed for management of each, and medical and surgical control of hypercalcemia with transient medical support of hypocalcemia until endogenous hormone autoregulation restores the patient's normal calcium homeostasis.

HYPERPARATHYROIDISM

Primary, Secondary, and Tertiary Hyperparathyroidism

Hyperparathyroidism is classified as primary, secondary, or tertiary. In *primary* hyperparathyroidism (PHPT), an idiopathic disorder in biofeedback of calcium control, secretion of parathyroid hormone is inappropriate considering the elevation in serum calcium. *Secondary* hyperparathyroidism is an increased activity in the parathyroid glands stimulated by low serum calcium or elevated serum phosphate. The appropriate hyperfunction of the parathyroid gland under this chronic stimulation may evolve into autonomous parathyroid hyperfunction. If this condition continues unabated in the absence of appropriate stimulation, it is called *tertiary* hyperparathyroidism. In all three forms parathyroid gland activity is increased, and parathormone secretion is elevated. In secondary hyperparathyroidism this elevated activity is an appropriate sensing of and responding to the hypocalcemic signal (see Fig. 55-4). It serves a physiologically useful role in compensatory release and retention of calcium by protecting against the impaired cellular function that would develop if the hypocalcemia were unopposed. In primary and tertiary hyperparathyroidism this overactivity is autonomous and continues despite the signals of hypercalcemia and hypophosphatemia that should inhibit parathyroid action and parathormone effect. What signal is ignored or what sensors misfire in autonomous primary and tertiary hyperparathyroidism? The cause appears to be based in a loss of calcium-sensitivity or a change in the ionized serum calcium "set-point" by the offending parathyroid tissues. This change may take place in one or more glands and be triggered by congenital or acquired defects in this autoregulatory mechanism. Brown and associates[4] studied the response of normal and abnormal parathyroid glands to calcium stimulation or inhibition of parathormone in the gland's native position in the neck, in tissue transplanted in the forearm, or in tissue culture. The exact point at which parathyroid cells undergo transformation and lose sensitivity to the calcium signal is not known in the sporadic cases of primary or tertiary hyperparathyroidism, but it appears to be genetically predetermined in some hereditary cases of primary HPT.

Cause

Hyperparathyroidism is familial in some pedigrees with or without association to other synchronous endocrine abnormalities. This genetic predisposition in families with isolated primary hyperparathyroidism may result from an altered "set point" in at least some parathyroid cells. A genetically co-determined hyperparathyroidism is present in two major types of hereditary multiple endocrine adenopathy (MEA). The malfunctioning parathyroid gland, the one common abnormality shared by MEA-I and MEA-II, is often one of the earliest manifestations, occurring frequently in children in such families. However, it is not uniformly part of all multiple endocrine adenopathies; one subtype of MEA-II is distinctive in part because of the normalcy of parathyroids and their calcium response.[12]

In MEA-I (Wermer's syndrome) the primary hyperparathyroidism is associated with abnormalities in pancreatic islets and pituitary gland form and function. In MEA-II (Sipple's syndrome) the parathyroid problem is associated with medullary thyroid cancer and chromaffin system abnormalities such as pheochromocytoma. In these familial syndromes the relationship of the parathyroid hormone and calcium metabolism changes to the involved other hormones is interesting. However, to suggest that the parathyroids were reacting to stimuli mediated by calcium from these other abnormalities would be facile. For example, in Wermer's syndrome an intimate relationship exists among calcium, gastrin release, and peptic ulceration from hyperacidity, the ulcer is often treated with calcium-containing antacids and associated with the multiple endocrine products of pancreatic islets and pituitary. Similarly, gastrin and calcium stimulate calcitonin release from medullary carcinoma as may be found in Sipple's syndrome. Furthermore, multiple connections exist within the MEA-II of APUD hormone synthesis and release. For example, it might be postulated that calcitonin decreases calcium; the parathyroids react appropriately to this hypocalcemia; and, much as in tertiary hyperparathyroidism, the parathyroids may become autonomous in their function, thereby accounting for the linkages in MEA-II of the other endocrine abnormalities with hyperparathyroidism. However, as already noted, in one subtype of MEA-II the parathyroids and the serum calcium are normal, despite early, widespread, and frequently lethal medullary thyroid cancer with abundant calcitonin secretion. Patients dying of sporadic medullary thyroid carcinoma with very high levels of calcitonin also have no detectable abnormality in their serum calcium, so even pathologically elevated levels of calcitonin may produce little effect in extracellular calcium. The current conclusion is that hyperparathyroidism is genetically co-determined with the other defects in these hereditary syndromes.[16]

Chronic stimulation of the parathyroid glands occurs in patients with renal failure, phosphate retention, and calcium wasting. This appropriate stimulus-response may continue, even after successful renal allografting has returned calcium and phosphate to normal on the basis of normalized renal function. However, one might speculate that the parathyroid glands have been unalterably switched on during this period of chronic stimulation, thus accounting for tertiary hyperparathyroidism. A similar prolongation of diet or drug-induced hyperphosphatemia and hypocalcemia in animal experiments can produce hyperparathyroidism.[25] Further, as seen in Table 55-4, hyperparathyroidism is most common in humans in postmenopausal women, coincidentally the group with the highest rate of osteoporosis and shifts in calcium and phosphate metabolism. These clinical coincidences and the forced circumstances in laboratory experiments suggest that some primary hyperparathyroidism may be induced by environmental circumstances such as diet, drugs, or metabolic changes associated with aging and that this parathyroid stimulation may switch parathyroid hyperfunction into autonomy. However, these suggestions are not conclusive because the majority of patients with secondary hyperparathyroidism treated by successful transplantation or carefully regulated dialysis do not develop tertiary hyperparathyroidism, the majority of postmenopausal women do not develop parathyroid neoplasms, and solitary gland involvement is the rule among most patients with primary hyperparathyroidism, except in the familial kindreds in which hyperplasia is predominant. At the present time the mechanism of neoplastic transformation of parathyroid glands is unknown.

One further bit of evidence comes from studies of patients who have developed thyroid abnormalities secondary to radiation. Studying population cohorts in each direction, i.e., groups of patients with proven hyperparathyroidism for history of cervical radiation[27] and larger populations of patients who have had cervical radiation for hyperparathyroidism,[32] investigators have shown an association between radiation to the head and neck and hyperparathyroidism. Multiple investigators have found an increased incidence of parathyroid pathology in patients being operated on for thyroid abnormalities, and the reverse. Radiation may change the rate at which the fundamental neoplastic transformation occurs, but this explanation is not satisfactory as the only one because the vast majority of patients with primary hyperparathyroidism have had no proven exposure to ionizing radiation, at least of a therapeutically significant level.

Morphology

The most important distinction in the morphologic basis of hyperparathyroidism is between single and multiple gland disease. If the parathyroid tissue is responding appropriately to stimulation (as with secondary hyperparathyroidism) or if the hyperparathyroidism is based in a genetic defect carried uniformly with each parathyroid cell (as, presumably, would be the case in the familial primary hyperparathyroidism in MEA, all the parathyroid cells present would be expected to be the seat of pathology. Thus correction of hypersecretion should involve a systemic change in the stimulus or identification and ablation of all parathyroid tissue. If neoplastic transformation was a "single hit" or a monoclonal proliferation of a single line of hyperfunctioning cells, the location of the hypersecretory locus should be a point source susceptible to ablation without disturbing the other parathyroid tissues that retain autoregulatory control. Surgically important for management, the distinction between single and multiple gland disease is also pathologically significant because the morphologic diagnosis is indistinguishable from a single specimen of overactive parathyroid tissue and indications for further therapy or prognosis cannot be drawn from a histologic observation of one specimen.

Further morphologic distinction in patients in whom all parathyroid glands are involved with hypercellularity and presumed hyperfunction may take the form of chief cell or clear cell hyperplasia. The early predominance of clear cell hyperplasia appears to be decreasing[6] and that of chief cell hyperplasia appears to be increasing.[10] Although oxyphil cells are also present, they appear to be functionally insignificant at least when encountered as adenomas, as individual cells when stained with parathyroid hormone-specific stains, and by electron microscopy, which shows absence of secretory granules. Oxyphil cells increase in number with aging and do not appear to be a pathologic part of the process of hyperparathyroidism.

In addition to the histologic characterization of cell types, the pathologist often is called on to distinguish benign from malignant parathyroid neoplasms. As with most endocrine tissues, in parathyroid tissue this distinction is difficult to make on cytologic grounds; and sometimes even with histologic evidence it is not easy. The surgeon's observations and the pathologist's determinations are subservient to the patient's clinical course, which can contradict the impressions of either professional or both. Before a gross adenoma is viable to the surgeon, microadenomata may be present within an externally undeformed gland that may still give rise to chemical and even clinical hyperparathyroidism.[28] Adenomas may become surgically detectable

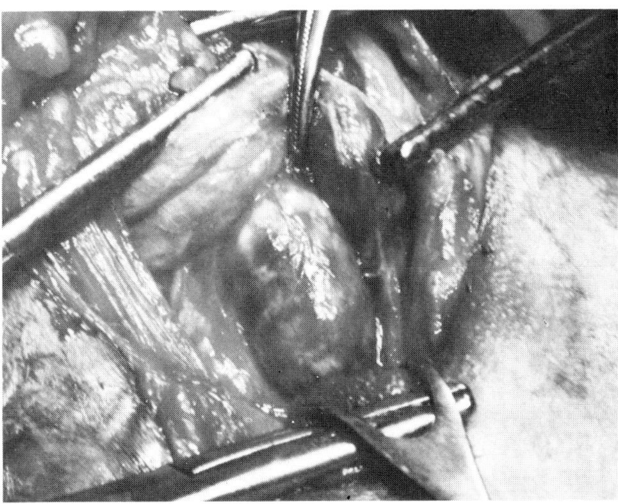

Fig. 55-10 A parathyroid adenoma may have a characteristic appearance as seen here, but no conclusion is drawn about single-gland or multiple-gland origin of the patient's primary hyperparathyroidism unless this gland is compared surgically and pathologically to the other parathyroid glands in the same patient.

and pathologically characteristic when they reach an arbitrary size that causes them to have a characteristic appearance surgically and histologically distinctive from the normal glands in the same patient (Fig. 55-10).

In sporadic, most often asymptomatic cases, primary hyperparathyroidism is most often based in parathyroid adenoma involving a singular gland. This is true for 90% of patients with primary hyperparathyroidism in many large series reported, with an additional 9% based in primary hyperplasia of either chief or clear cell type involving multiple glands. Normally, four parathyroid glands are present in distributions determined by the embryologic origin from the pharyngeal arches, the inferior parathyroid glands derived from the third arch, and the superior glands derived from the fourth. However, more than four glands are present in some patients, and typically all are involved in the parathyroid hyperplasia of secondary hyperparathyroidism or in familial parathyroid disorders. Whether multiple adenomas occur is a moot point because we will retain our fundamental distinction between single and multiple gland disease. Therefore more than one gland involvement will be classified as multiple gland disease, whether that glandular pattern appears to be multiple adenomas or hyperplasia in multiple glands. An earlier histologic distinction that does not appear to be useful is the presence of a compressed rim of apparently normal parathyroid tissue by the expansion of the adenoma, yet this same finding can also be present in hyperplastic glands. In my experience and in other studies, parathyroid adenocarcinoma is the cause of primary hyperparathyroidism in 0.5% of cases when the carcinoma is defined by its metastasizing rather than by histologic criteria of parathyroid carcinoma.[19] This group may include an equal number of additional patients in whom the clinical behavior of the tumor appears similar to that of the benign adenoma or suggests its complete excision by simple removal of the enlarged gland.

Goal of Surgical Treatment in Hyperparathyroidism

Within half a century surgical therapy for hyperparathyroidism has expanded from its first deliberate undertaking in the United States to its widespread application to asymptomatic disease. Because of this relatively rapid development, the natural history of the untreated disease has not been followed throughout a lifetime; the indications for operation are still based in presumption of probable complications from the untreated disorder. At some serum calcium levels, these predictions can be made with a high degree of confidence, particularly if the hypercalcemia is already symptomatic. That the disease requires treatment at marginal levels of hypercalcemia in the asymptomatic patient is less apparent. However, in the United States the majority of patients who have a confidently established diagnosis of primary hyperparathyroidism are typically operated on at their elective convenience. The single criterion that remains as sine qua non before operation is that a diagnosis of primary hyperparathyroidism be made with confidence. Particularly in marginal diagnostic calls, the operating surgeon and the patient commit to the undertaking of a meticulous operation to find the site of the pathology and correct it so as to restore normal calcium balance. Operation is the most precise localizing technique, but it is *not* a diagnostic procedure for primary hyperparathyroidism.

The goal of the surgical procedure is to reduce parathyroid hypersecretion to normal and restore autoregulatory calcium balance. In the event of single gland disease, this procedure entails identifying and removing the solitary focus of the pathology in distinction to the patient's normal or suppressed parathyroid glands with which the pathology is compared. For the patient with multiple gland disease, subtotal resection is the rule, with a residual mass of parathyroid tissue capable of producing approximately 150 mg total, usually in multiple identified sites. Normal parathyroid glands should be identified and preserved with intact blood supply. Their removal will not effect hyperparathyroidism, but it may cause an increased likelihood of hypoparathyroidism following this or subsequent operation. Primary surgical exploration is 95% successful in accomplishing the goals of reduced parathormone and restored calcium autoregulation. In approximately 3% of cases the primary exploration will not find or fix the pathologic problem in the thyroid, and in the remainder the disease may return after initial success in managing the hypercalcemia surgically. Using the arbitrary duration of 6 months, the distinction is made between *persistence* of hypercalcemia following a failed primary cervical exploration and *recurrence*, which means hyperparathyroidism reappears following 6 months of low or normal calcium levels after surgical treatment.

Special techniques are considered for the peculiar problems of persistence, recurrence, ectopic or supernumerary glands, sequence of treatment in other endocrinopathy associated with PHPT, parathyroid transplantation, and nonsurgical techniques of both localization and control of persistent hyperparathyroidism. The goals of each of these special management techniques remain the same, reduction of parathormone toward normal and autoregulatory calcium homeostasis.

Primary Cervical Exploration for Primary Hyperparathyroidism

In the first attempt at treatment, a cervical exploration by an experienced surgeon is the most precise localizing technique for pathologic parathyroids. Preoperative physical examination is performed in all such patients, but rarely would one expect positive findings related to the parathyroid gland, except in patients with toxic parathyroid single gland disease such as cystic degeneration of a large adenoma or a parathyroid carcinoma. The most likely palpable abnormality in a patient undergoing exploration for asymptomatic hypercalcemia is a thyroid nodule or lymph node because rarely can a parathyroid adenoma of the size and texture usually associated with this form of hyperparathyroidism be clinically palpable. The name of the operation is "parathyroid exploration"—not excision of parathyroid adenoma—because adenoma is a presumptive diagnosis in a patient who might have multiple gland disease as the cause for the syndrome even though the majority have single gland disease. The name suggests the procedure: i.e., careful dissection for and identification of all visible parathyroid tissue in its normal, likely, or abnormal locations. If the referring physician or patient requests a preoperative study, it should be limited to a noninvasive simple procedure such as sonography. The sonography for parathyroid adenoma requires specialized small parts equipment, and it is operator dependent. However, at present sonography is more reliable than the radioisotopic method with which promising experience has been gathered at the date of this writing. However, neither of these methods is required preoperatively because *no* nonoperative method currently available identifies visually and confirms pathologically all visible parathyroid tissue. Because the localization studies do not identify the normal or suppressed glands, the early identification of a solitary large gland may be misleading and at least makes the dissection of the remaining glands somewhat tedious after the encounter with the presumptive site of pathology. However, failure to complete this tedious dissection to identify the remaining glands increases the chance of persistence or recurrence of hyperparathyroidism.

Anatomic variants make parathyroid exploration interesting; exciting as a skilled application of anatomic, embryologic and pathologic information to intricate technique in a vital dissection field; and sometimes frustrating. The surgeon must have a thorough knowledge of cervical anatomy. He must know not only where parathyroid glands are normally found, but also where they might be found because often the abnormal parathyroid gland is found in ectopic locations. The landmarks useful in locating normally situated parathyroid glands include the recurrent laryngeal nerve, the inferior cornu of the thyroid cartilage, and the inferior thyroid artery. If the parathyroid glands are successfully located on one side of the trachea, the mirror image position on the opposite side is the most likely site of the comparable glands. The enlargement of a single gland in an adenoma may distort or displace the structures around it, making the normal parathyroid adjacent to it somewhat more difficult to identify (Fig. 55-11). Besides serving as a landmark, enlargement of the inferior thyroid artery can suggest lateralization of a single gland abnor-

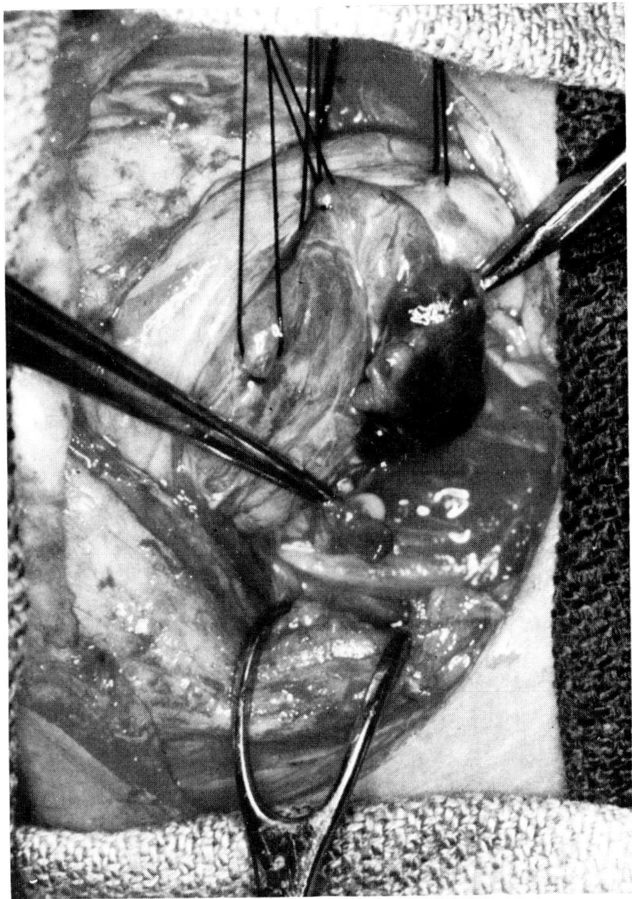

Fig. 55-11 A parathyroid adenoma is seen in situ in this primary parathyroid exploration and is compared with the normal parathyroid gland at the end of the forceps.

mality. If the enlarged parathyroid gland does not lie in its normal anatomic location, searching the inferior thyroid artery for principle branches may indicate hidden adenomas, e.g., adenomas located in lateral clefts in the thyroid gland and, rarely, a wholly intrathyroidal adenoma. By following any thyroid artery branches that go down in the submanubrial space, careful dissection of the superior mediastinum can be accomplished through a cervical approach.

Following preliminary parathyroid dissection, the surgeon may know the locations of three glands, but not the fourth. This situation tests the mettle of the surgical team because the normal locations have been searched and the fourth gland, particularly if a pathologic gland was not seen in the first three, must be identified during this first cervical exploration or be excluded by careful dissection as not within reach of the extended cervical exploration. The areas of this extension include the tracheoesophogeal groove, the retroesophageal space, the carotid sheath, the thyroid gland, and especially the substernal superior mediastinum (see boxed material below). Teasing up the tongue of thymus suspended from the thyrothymic ligament along the inferior thyroid artery is a part of any cervical exploration that has not identified four glands or any that has identified four glands without a clear pathologic diagnosis. Although some surgeons recommend the use of a vital staining as an intraoperative adjunct, I suggest this as a technique only in reoperation. Other ancillary tests may suggest that the pathologic parathyroid tissue has been removed, even if this is not confirmed by the pathologist. The cAMP measurement in urine is a sensitive indicator of parathyroid hormone; if the parathyroid source of hyperparathyroidism has been ablated, the urine content of

PROCEDURE FOR SEARCH FOR FOURTH GLAND

A. Intraoperatively; pathologist's report confirms three glands; parathyroid "map" indicates position of missing gland; search posterior thyroid capsule in this position; examine "mirror image" position opposite confirmed gland
   1. If superior gland:
      a. Search above superior thyroid pole, taking down superior thyroid artery
      b. Palpate tracheoesophageal groove
      c. Explore retroesophageal area
      d. Dissect carotid sheath on suspected side
      e. Perform thyroidotomy
   2. If inferior gland:
      a. Trace any branches of inferior thyroid artery
      b. Palpate submanubrial space
      c. Tease up thymic fat pad
      d. Perform limited thyroidectomy in area where gland is missing
   3. cAMP urinary excretion monitoring
   4. If convinced that there is no evidence of additional parathyroid tissue in neck, close!
      No indication for sternotomy at a primary exploration

B. Postoperatively
   1. Test for persistent hypercalcemia
   2. CT and ultrasonic scanning
   3. Venous sampling and venography
   4. Arteriography
      a. If adenoma encountered in neck—cervical reexploration
      b. If mediastinal adenoma with inferior thyroid arterial blood supply—cervical reexploration
      c. If mediastinal adenoma with internal mammary arterial blood supply—contrast staining

cAMP dramatically decreases, even during the course of the parathyroid exploration. A special case will be made for the mediastinal glands that may be present and their selective management in initial cervical operation, in subsequent localization studies, and in sternotomy for mediastinal excision. Finally, sternal-splitting chest exploration during the primary operation is almost never indicated because that operation is not an exploration but an excision of known or strongly suspected pathology based on the application of localizing techniques before reoperation, if indicated.

An example of a surgical procedure that will require persistence based on the confident preoperative diagnosis of primary hyperparathyroidism is a parathyroid exploration that encounters four apparently normal glands, possibly even in their normal anatomic locations. If the surgical certainty indicating this operation is that the patient had primary hyperparathyroidism, the dissection continues for the identification of the fifth gland that might be the locus of disease, more especially because it is not seen in the normal anatomic locations. In the example illustrated in Fig. 55-19, the suspected parathyroid pathology was not identified despite verified presence of four parathyroid glands in the normal locations. No apparent fifth gland was within the reach of cervical dissection. At this point the surgeon was satisfied that he had exhausted cervical exploration as the primary localizing technique; thus he used angiography to assist in localizing the fifth gland.

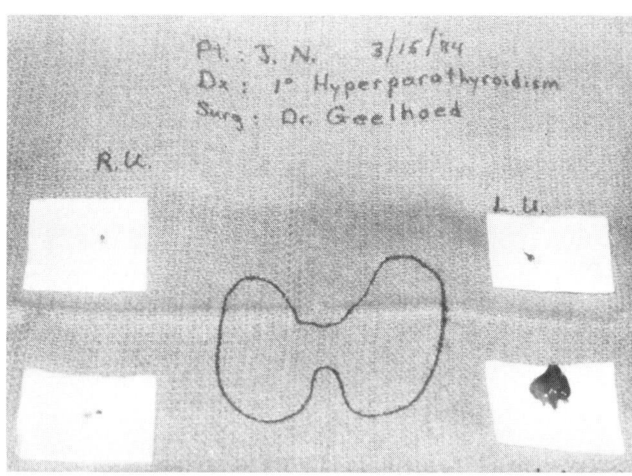

Fig. 55-12 After identification of all visible parathyroids by the surgeon, surgical pathology consultation is requested, and biopsies of the normal-appearing parathyroid glands and excision of the enlarged gland are carried out with specimens placed on a "parathyroid map" for identification of their location.

Pathology Consultation and Confirmation of Successful Parathyroid Exploration

In addition to the urinary cAMP, which is especially helpful in confirming excision of the offending parathyroid tissue after reoperation, pathology consultation is involved in every parathyroid exploration. As a courtesy to the surgical pathologist, the surgeon avoids requiring the pathologist to be on a continuous standby to receive serial frozen section specimens to determine the presence or absence of parathyroid tissue or to satisfy surgical curiosity as to the nature of abnormal tissues present. Courtesy, efficiency, and accuracy are best served by first directly visualizing all accessible parathyroid tissues. After identifying the four glands, the surgeon can perform biopsy of the normal-appearing glands and excision of the abnormal ones in total (adenoma, carcinoma) or subtotal (hyperplasia). The surgeon then passes the specimens to the pathologist who, after viewing the multiple glands passed to him on a "parathyroid map" identifying their locations in situ (Fig. 55-12), gives an opinion of the parathyroid pathology. The pathologist's options include cytologic identification of the presence or absence of parathyroid tissue or histologic determination of the same tissue with an additional attempt made at specifically diagnosing the source of parathyroid pathology. The more important determination is the identification of tissue as parathyroid or nonparathyroid because multiple or single gland disease is grossly apparent to both the surgeon and the pathologist. Consequently histologic diagnosis of an adenoma or suppressed normal parathyroid gland can be reserved for permanent pathology sections or can be suggested on frozen section determination on those specimens already proven to be parathyroid tissue by touch preparation.

A new technique for determining the presence or absence of parathyroid tissue is the use of intraoperative imprints for cytologic identification of parathyroid tissue.[16] The rapid imprint technique is very useful in screening the specimens handed over for pathologic consultation at the conclusion of the surgical exploration while the patient remains anesthetized.

Extent of Parathyroid Excision

Any decision regarding the extent of parathyroid resection is made on the basis of the gross and microscopic determination of the parathyroid disease during the operation. Removal of single gland disease is curative in nearly all patients who undergo this excision; biopsies of the other parathyroid glands substantiate the belief that the disease is of a single gland. However, if the other glands are enlarged or hypercellular on biopsy, the suspicion that hyperparathyroidism may be based in multiple gland disease might indicate more extensive parathyroid reduction. Typically this involves total excision of two parathyroid glands and subtotal excision of the remaining two glands with a marker left with them to identify their sites[14] and parathyroid remnants of approximately 75 mg in each location.

The ultimate confirmation of successful parathyroid exploration comes from the patient's clinical and biochemical course after surgical therapy. Excision of a large adenoma or a major reduction in parathyroid tissue in hyperplasia usually results in postoperative hypoparathyroidism reflected in a fall in serum calcium to hypocalcemic levels; thus the hypoplastic glands adjacent to what had been the adenoma may return to normal function. Following operation the patient may require calcium supplementation and/or vitamin D support. If this calcium and vitamin D therapy is required for a prolonged period of time, hypoparathyroidism is suspected. If the vitamin D and calcium are decreased and the patient is maintained in asymptomatic biochemical hypocalcemia, this stimulus should be adequate to return to function any residual parathyroid tissue. However, if 1 year after parathyroidectomy the patient still requires these treatments to avoid symptoms, permanent hypoparathyroidism is suggested. If within 6 months from successful parathyroid operation the patient has recurrent hypercalcemia, the burden of parathyroid tissue is once again excessive. Possible causes of this excess are: (1) stimulation of the transient hypocalcemia that developed and acted on glands with a predetermined genetic propensity for hyperfunction, and (2) disturbance of the blood supply to hyperfunctioning tissue so that the blood supply was effectively isolated from the circulation or infarcted. Any viable cells around the periphery may have resumed function over the interval; if they retained their tendency toward autonomous hyperfunction, they may be the source of recurrence. The retention of any incompletely excised, autonomous parathyroid cells is the predictable source of recurrent hyperparathyroidism some time later. A distressing sequel of parathyroid exploration is the patient with persistent hypercalcemia. This condition indicates a failed primary cervical exploration, and the patient now has indication for localization studies to assist in reoperative correction of the hyperparathyroidism not resolved at the primary cervical exploration. Such patients are screened carefully to rule out some nonparathyroid cause for their hypercalcemia such as FHH or for some ectopic source of hyperparathyroidism not based in the parathyroid glands themselves.

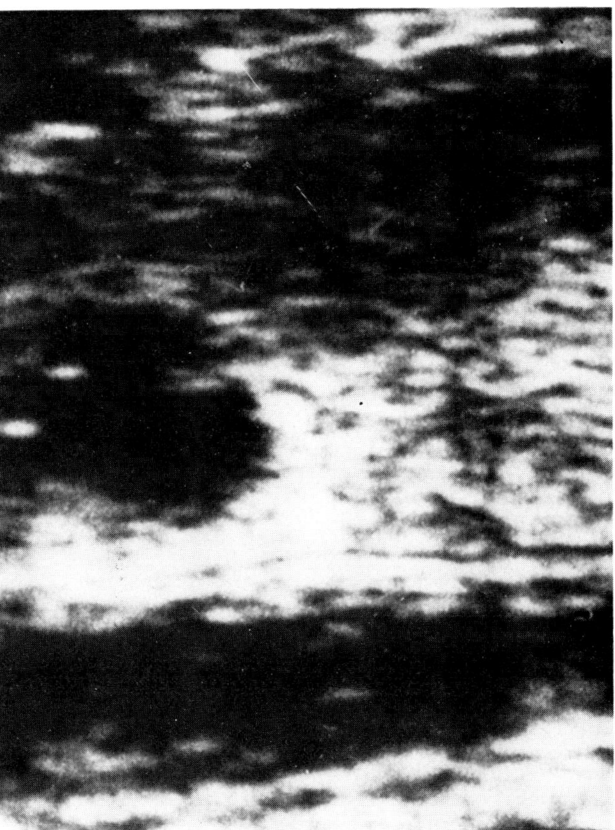

Fig. 55-13 Sonography demonstrated this large parathyroid adenoma, which would be unlikely to be overlooked in this position in surgical exploration.

Parathyroid Localization Studies

Preoperative localization studies are not required before primary cervical exploration, but they are advisable preceding a second surgical attempt at control of hyperparathyroidism or, in some instances, as a substitute for it.

Sonogram

Sonography may be helpful, and it is sometimes used in primary cases. Like most radiographic or isotopic tests, the ultrasound study is a "shadow-producing procedure" and may tell of the presence and location of a mass, but does not confirm the nature of that mass. In the neck multiple masses are possible, including those that are normal structures such as thyroid or lymph nodes or abnormalities within those structures.

Fig. 55-13 shows a sonogram of a large parathyroid adenoma that was present in a symptomatic patient with very elevated serum calcium. Its size is such that it would be readily encountered in cervical exploration, and it is in a position where this exploration would take place. The ultrasound scan is less helpful in the ectopic locations that the surgeon has not reached in primary exploration such as the mediastinum. Furthermore, the specific type of sonogram requires a 10-mHz small parts, real-time dedicated machine and an interested and experienced operator. Both the expertise and the machinery are not readily available at all centers, whereas CT scanning with high resolution is available in most United States referral centers.

Isotopic Scanning

Previous scanning techniques have been disappointing when applied to the parathyroid area, and selenium-methionine and technetium scan alone are probably of historic interest only. However, a newer technique combining thallium/technetium is an advance in subtraction scanning. This method can identify enlarged parathyroid glands, including those in ectopic locations,[11] but it does not identify normal parathyroid glands and has been associated with a higher than acceptable rate of false-positive readings in early series. Though its reliability is variable, it is a less invasive method of positive identification of solitary enlarged parathyroids in ectopic locations (Fig. 55-14).

Computed Tomography

Computed tomography (CT) scanning is a very helpful noninvasive localization study, particularly if coupled with contrast augmentation in examining the areas less accessible to sonography. As seen in Fig. 55-15, on the basis of a CT scan in one patient a preoperative diagnosis of parathyroid carcinoma, suggested on the CT scan because the irregular borders of the mass appeared to invade tissues adjacent to it and a calcific rim, was confirmed on exploration. The best application of CT is in the area of the mediastinum not accessible to submanubrial inspection and

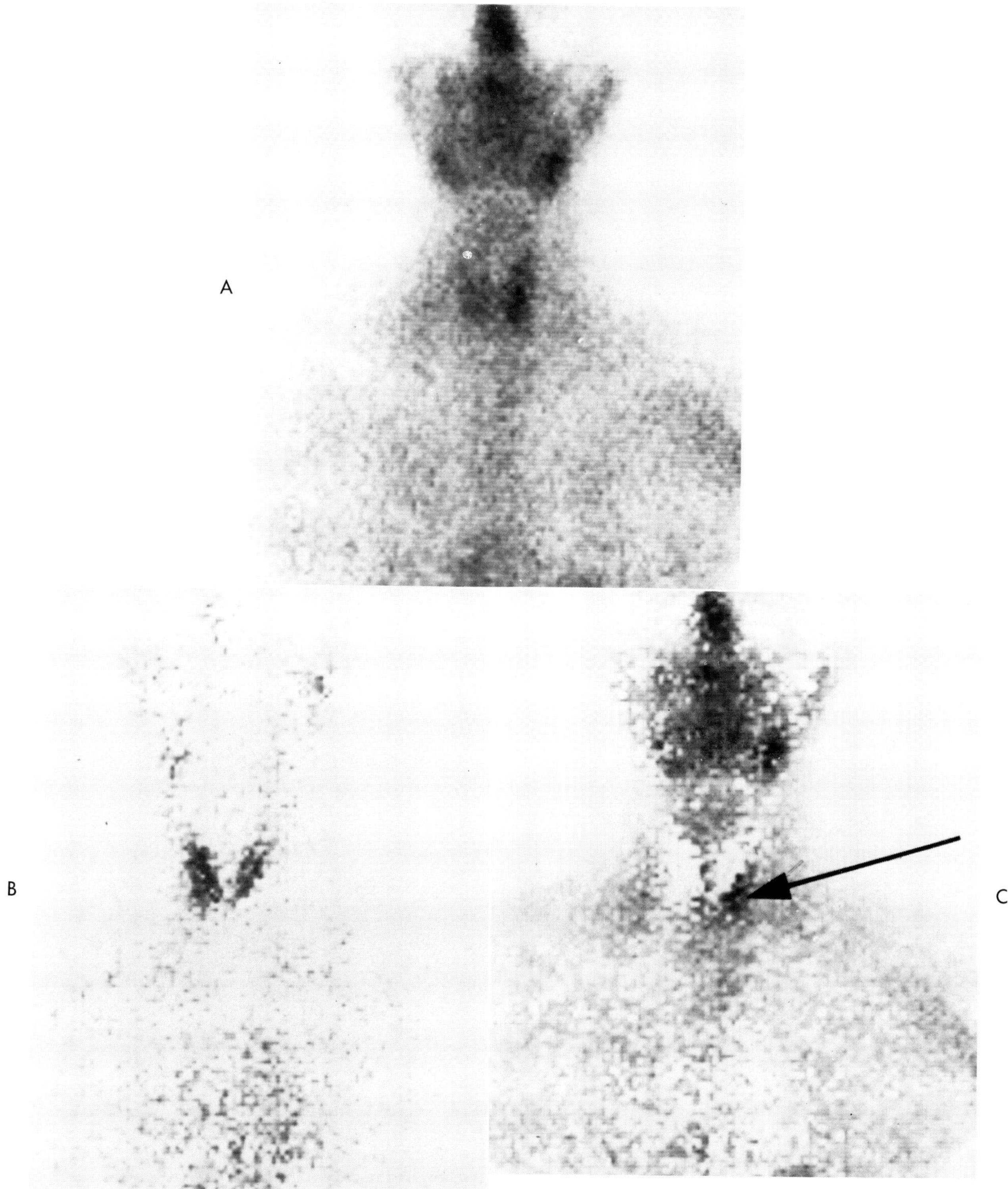

Fig. 55-14 Thallium/technetium subtraction isotopic scan shows promise for localization of enlarged parathyroids, but no noninvasive study yet devised demonstrates normal parathyroid glands—a requirement of primary cervical exploration. **A,** Thallium scan of neck; **B,** technetium scan of thyroid; **C,** thallium/technetium subtraction film showing left lower pole parathyroid adenoma.

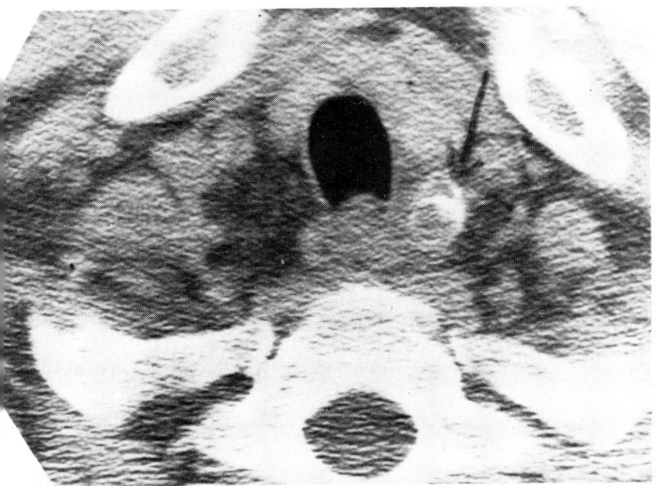

Fig. 55-15 Computed tomography not only demonstrated this large and unusual parathyroid lesion, but preoperatively suggested that it might be a parathyroid carcinoma, which it proved to be after surgical excision.

palpation from the cervical approach at the time of the primary cervical exploration.

Fine-Needle Aspiration

A rarely used, recent development in parathyroid localization has been the sonography-directed or CT-directed fine-needle aspirate. Aspiration cytology can give evidence of the presence of parathyroid cells in the mass within range of the needle. Like the touch preparation intraoperatively, this sample is studied by cytologic technique to identify presence or absence of parathyroid tissue. With the use of immunoperoxidase-specific parathormone staining, this identification can be very specific even if rapid. Several patients have already been diagnosed by percutaneous fine-needle aspiration with a subsequent suggestion that ablation might be possible by alcohol injection through the same needle that identifies the parathyroid cells.[15]

Venous Sampling

Selective venous catheterization and sampling for parathyroid hormone assay is the most specific radiologic localization test that can correlate form and function. Since the hormone that is biologically active is best measured by the N-terminal–recognizing antibody, this radioimmunoassay should be used with specimens obtained by selective venous catheterization. Fig. 55-16 illustrates a patient problem managed successfully with the help of venous catheterization data. A patient who had undergone a pri-

A

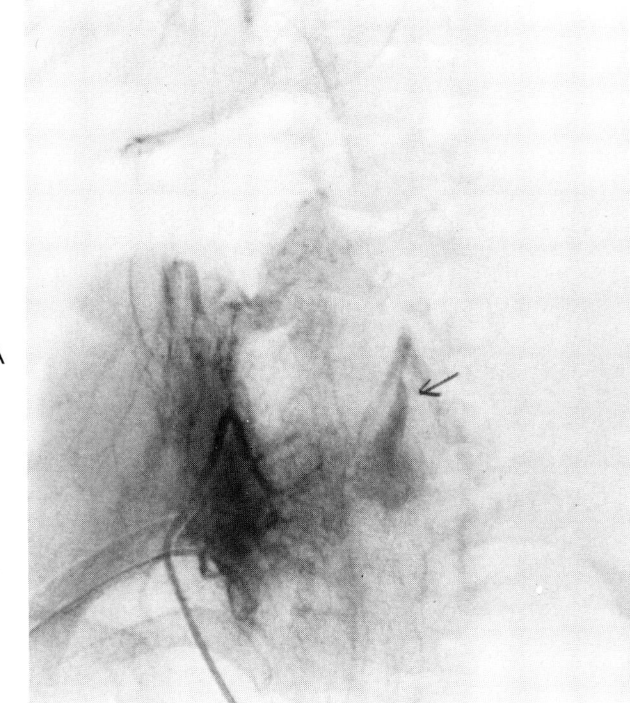

B

4. Right common jugular
5. Inferior thyroid
3. Left superior thyroid
1. Vertebral
2. Internal and external jugular

1. 42 pg/ml (11-24 pg/ml)
2. 45
3. 45
4. 48
5. 63
6. >35 (peripheral)

Fig. 55-16 Following initial failure to locate an adenoma, arteriography demonstrated a tumor blush not well distinguished from thyroid **(A)**, but venous sampling of parathormone added other hypersecretion information shown on this localizing map **(B)**, with the adenoma identified and excised upon reoperation **(C)**.

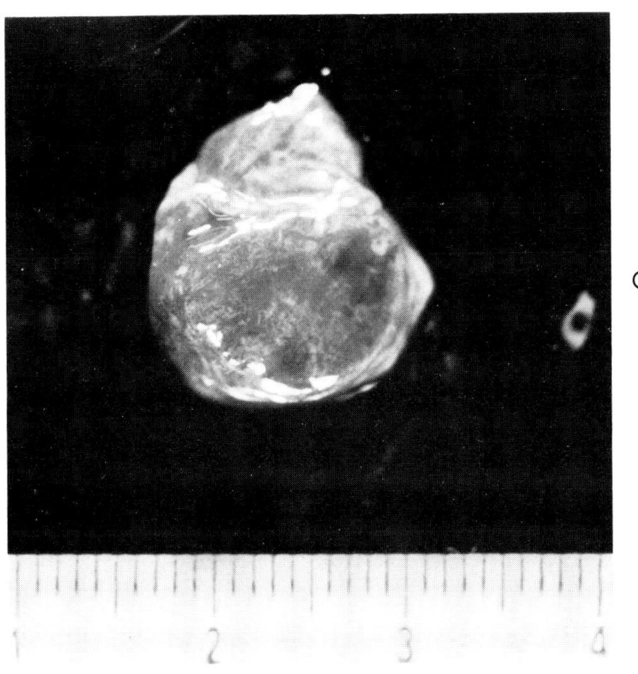

C

mary failed cervical exploration had arteriography (see Fig. 55-16, *A*), which suggested an abnormality that could not be clearly distinguished from the thyroid blush seen on arteriography. The venous blood sampling pattern of N-terminal parathormone suggested a high parathyroid hormone reading in the inferior thyroid sample draining the same site suggested on arteriography, giving functional significance to the morphologic abnormality confirmed in the excision of the adenoma at that site (see Fig. 55-16, *C*). Despite these advantages, parathyroid localization by venous assay depends on the expertise of the radiologist. Furthermore, a disruption based on previous thyroid or parathyroid surgery may have ligated many of the venous drainage patterns normally seen, and neovascularity may result after the passage of some time since the first cervical operation.

Digital Subtraction Angiography

Use of digital subtraction angiography is quite limited because the technique does not have the high resolution of selective arteriography, although it is not as operator dependent. The major use of digital subtraction angiography is in combination with venous catheterization sampling to identify major vessels or their anomalies that might be otherwise confusing in data interpretation. The resolution of this technique does not exceed that of CT scanning, which is more applicable in checking mediastinal or other ectopic sites.

Selective Arteriography

In skilled hands selective arteriography is the "gold standard" of radiographic localization of morphologic abnormality. This very invasive technique requires nearly as much time and concentrated effort as surgical reexploration. Further, its high yield in information may be attended with corresponding toxicity. Excess contrast material may lead to renal failure, and injection of cervical arteries has raised concern regarding the anterior spinal artery and any transient paresis risk.

However, the advantage of arteriography is that the localization and treatment of an ectopic parathyroid adenoma not accessible to cervical reexploration might be accomplished by the same arteriographic catheter. In addition, if the arteriogram suggests the presence of an adenoma in a cervical location where it had been overlooked in previous operation (Fig. 55-17, *A*), the adenoma can be retrieved through reoperation (Fig. 55-17, *B*). If the arteriogram suggests that the adenoma is located in the mediastinum and is supplied by an internal mammary artery branch that might make it less amenable to cervical reoperation retrieval, the same arteriographic catheter can be advanced into this feeding vessel and wedged. Hypertensive injection of concentrated contrast material then creates an osmotic shock to the parathyroid tissue, and a prolonged angiographic stain is seen persisting for even days following this procedure. This modification of the original technique of embolization[14] has been used in a number of patients who have been cured of their persistent hyperparathyroidism for as long as 14 years following angiography.[15] Arteriography can localize adenoma by the pattern of neovascularity and "tumor blush" for surgical retrieval in the good-risk patient or may serve as an alternative to sternotomy in the patient who has an internal mammary arterial supply to a mediastinal adenoma causing persistent symptomatic hypercalcemia. A series of patients with mediastinal adenoma is presented in Figs. 55-18 to 55-20, illustrating the appropriate application of cervical retrieval, mediastinotomy, and transcatheter ablation using arteriographic indications for treatment.

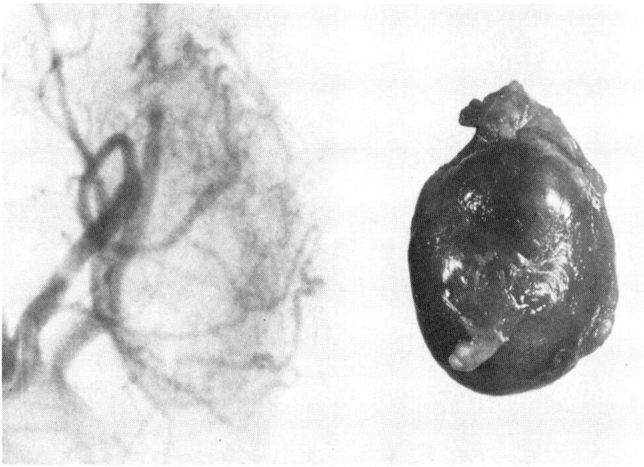

Fig. 55-17 A patient referred for persistent hypercalcemia was studied arteriographically with demonstration of a large tumor blush; the adenoma thus shown was excised by reoperation.

Additional Localization Studies

Additional localization studies include primary studies such as thyroid scan to test for intrathyroidal filling defects. The same information might be obtained from sonography or CT scan or by the thalium/technetium subtraction study, but any one of those tests might be indicated

PARATHYROID LOCALIZATION STUDIES

Before operation:	Physical examination of neck (±, low yield)
	Sonography (not required before operation, special equipment and expertise required)
Primary:	*Surgical exploration* of all glands by experienced surgeon (intraoperative staining)
	Surgical pathology consultation: touch prep cytology, frozen section histology
Reoperation:	Thyroid-scan—filling defects
	1. Sonogram (small parts, real-time, 10 mHz, operator-dependent)
	2. Thallium/technetium scan (reliability variable)
	3. CT with contrast study
	4. (FNA—aspiration cytology, immunoperoxidase PTH staining)
	5. Venous sampling—PTH lateralizing—form/function correlation
	6. (Digital subtraction angiography)
	7. Selective arteriography

by the suspicion based in preliminary findings on thyroid scan conclusions.

No patient should have all of the localization studies listed in the boxed material on p. 910; each should have only those with highest yield used in series until a positive test is achieved in a patient in whom the diagnosis of primary hyperparathyroidism remains undisputed. Before the application of these localization studies and certainly before the reoperation they indicate the patient should have the biochemical testing to differentiate FHH or other nonparathyroid sources of hypercalcemia. One would probably not use multiple localization studies if reoperation were not anticipated or acceptable to the patient. The one exception to this rule might be the parathyroid selective arteriography, which can serve an additional role besides localization technique and may be used as a percutaneous treatment for persistent hyperparathyroidism based in a selected group of ectopic parathyroid adenomas.[15]

Special Considerations in the Treatment of Unusual Hyperparathyroidism

Reoperation or Extension of Primary Cervical Operation Techniques

For a persistent hyperparathyroidism based in a cervical adenoma, arteriography as seen in Fig. 55-17 demonstrates the lesion, and reoperation was directed at the excision of this demonstrated mass. The reoperation differs from a primary cervical "parathyroid exploration." In this instance exploration is not intended to identify all sites of parathyroid tissue in virgin tissue planes but rather to provide a primary excision of a demonstrated mass through the preoperative application of these radiologic localization techniques. Often reoperation may be at risk for removing the last functioning parathyroid tissue—albeit hyperfunctioning. The risk of postoperative hypoparathyroidism is consequently increased, and preserving some of the excised parathyroid tissue may have some purpose should the patient require it for later transplantation (considered below).

Mediastinal Adenoma. Ectopic parathyroid adenomas may be managed differently, as suggested above, by the origin of their arterial blood supply. Examples of three different methods of managing mediastinal adenomas can be seen in the three patients illustrated in Figs. 55-18 to 55-20.

In the first patient (see Fig. 55-18) careful primary cervical exploration revealed three glands in the normal parathyroid locations. When the left inferior parathyroid gland was not found in the usual cervical areas searched, a suspicious branch of the inferior thyroid artery was traced down into the superior mediastinum. With careful blunt dissection, a digital plane was developed past the manubrium down to the level of the gladiolus. At the level of the third intercostal space a small mass was palpable at the tip of the thymic remnant. After passing a metallic ligating clip down this retrosternal space by a right angle clip applier, the surgeon teased this thymic remnant into the neck and excised it. This thymic remnant contained the missing fourth gland (see Fig 55-18, *A*), and the histologic examination confirmed the fourth gland as the adenoma. After operation the patient had a transient hypocalcemia not requiring treatment; he has remained normocalcemic for the subsequent 12 years since operation. The mediastinal location of this adenoma retrieved through the cervical approach is proven by the postoperative chest x-ray film (see Fig. 55-18, *B*), which reveals the location of the metallic clip placed just below the adenoma when it was in situ.

Cervical exploration was carried out in another patient who had urinary calculi and unquestioned primary hyperparathyroidism on repeated biochemical analysis (see Fig. 55-19). The cervical exploration was performed carefully, with the identification of four parathyroid glands in the usual locations; however, nothing was unusual about the four glands on histologic examination except for some degree of hypocellularity. A careful but limited submanubrial exploration was unrevealing. When the patient's hypercalcemia persisted postoperatively, selective arteriography demonstrated a fifth parathyroid gland in the mediastinum that was enlarged in the arteriographic blush (see Fig. 55-19, *A*). On the patient's request, sternotomy to excise the demonstrated adenoma was carried out (see Fig. 55-19, *B*)

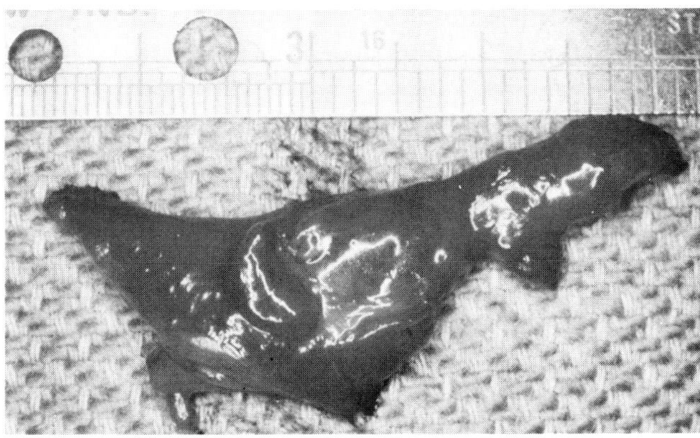

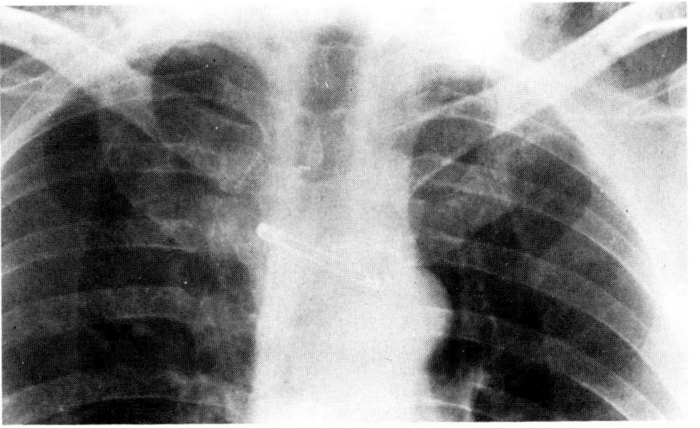

B

Fig. 55-18 Three glands were found in the normal parathyroid positions, but the fourth was found by diligent search at the time of primary operation and delivered from the anterior mediastinum. Found within the substance of the thymus **(A)**, the location of this adenoma is suggested postoperatively on the chest x-ray film **(B)** by the metallic clip that had been placed before teasing it up through the cervical incision. (Patient previously demonstrated in Geelhoed, G.W., and Doppman, J.L.: Am. Surg. **114:**71, 1978.)

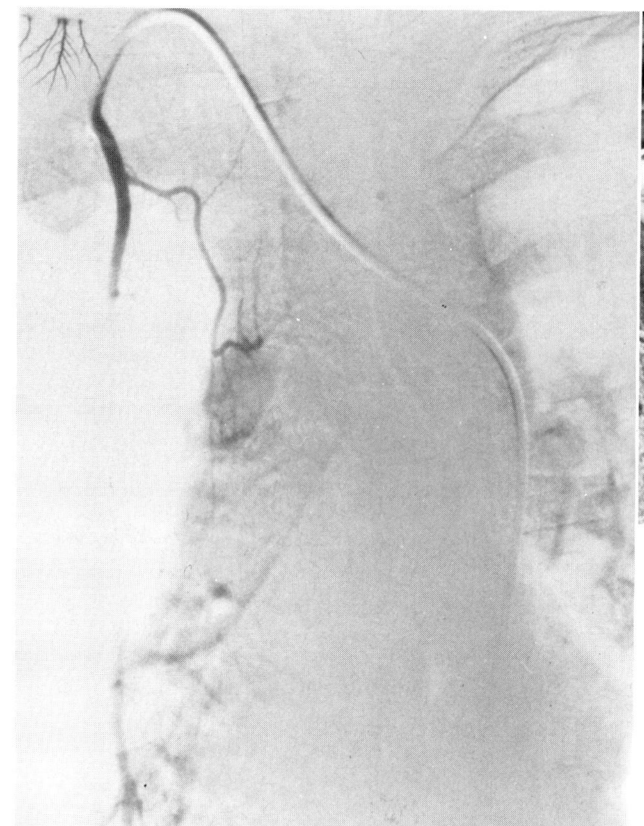

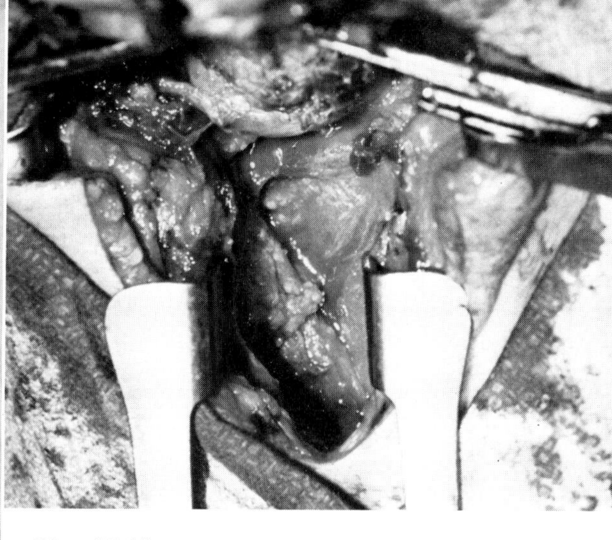

Fig. 55-19 Another patient had persistent hyperparathyroidism despite four-gland identification at primary cervical exploration; an adenoma in a fifth gland was demonstrated angiographically **(A),** and the patient underwent successful excision of this adenoma by sternotomy **(B).**

with a successful long-term cure of the hyperparathyroidism based in this fifth-gland ectopic parathyroid adenoma.

In another patient with hyperparathyroidism initial cervical exploration revealed three normal parathyroid glands (see Fig 55-20). When hyperparathyroidism persisted, she had selective arteriography that showed no abnormalities demonstrable in the neck. However, by injection of internal mammary arterial supply, a tumor blush was seen deep in the mediastinum (see Fig. 55-20, *A*). This patient's request for an attempt at percutaneous ablation through transcatheter contrast staining was carried out with the intense staining noted immediately after injection (see Fig. 55-20, *B*). This adenoma staining was persistent for a period of several hours after the arteriogram (see Fig. 55-20, *C*), and the patient had immediate hypocalcemia as occurs after successful ablation of a parathyroid adenoma. Her calcium balance returned to normal, and she has been followed 14 years since this percutaneous treatment with normal parathyroid hormone and calcium values.

Transplantation of the Parathyroid Glands. In some instances of thyroid or parathyroid operation, a normal parathyroid gland may become dislodged, or its arterial blood supply interrupted. A normal parathyroid gland should not be discarded, even though the remaining parathyroid tissues should have reserves sufficient to sustain a normal calcium balance. The parathyroid gland may be minced and implanted in the strap muscles at the site of the primary incision. However, one would not wish to implant presumably autonomous parathyroid tissue, but rather to excise this completely so as not to have recurrent hyperparathyroidism at a later date.

In secondary hyperparathyroidism, the glands are hyperplastic but responsive to the stimuli that gave rise to the secondary hyperparathyroidism in the first place. If that hypocalcemic and hyperphosphatemic stimulus should be resolved such as through successful kidney transplantation, such hyperplastic parathyroid tissue would regress to normal function in autoregulatory control. If, during the course of the patient's renal failure, operation for secondary hyperparathyroidism were carried out, total parathyroidectomy might be followed by hypoparathyroidism when kidney function is restored. As a consequence, the tissue excised might be preserved and retain cell viability by the same techniques of cryopreservation as are used in blood-banking of frozen blood cells by means of slow-freeze techniques. Small portions of these glands may be transplanted in the forearm of the patient at a later date, should the patient require this form of support for persistent hypocalcemia on vitamin D and calcium supplementation later. It should be noted that autonomous tissue may hyperfunction in whatever site it is implanted.[3] Routine parathyroid excision and autotransplantation should be discouraged because occasionally patients are seen who have an "unnatural disease," i.e., hyperparathyroidism originating from the neck and arm. Parathyroid tissue transplanted into the forearm is more easily measured by parathormone arteriovenous differences across the implantation site and can also be retrieved by a simple procedure under local anesthesia. However, implantation of autonomous hyperfunctioning parathyroid tissue is better prevented than treated, and the determination of autonomy can be made by in vitro study.

If the tissue culture of the excised hyperplastic parathyroid tissue produces parathormone in calcium-poor milieu, but no parathormone is produced in calcium-rich culture medium, the parathyroid tissue seems to be normally responsive in sensing the ionized calcium at the appropriate

A

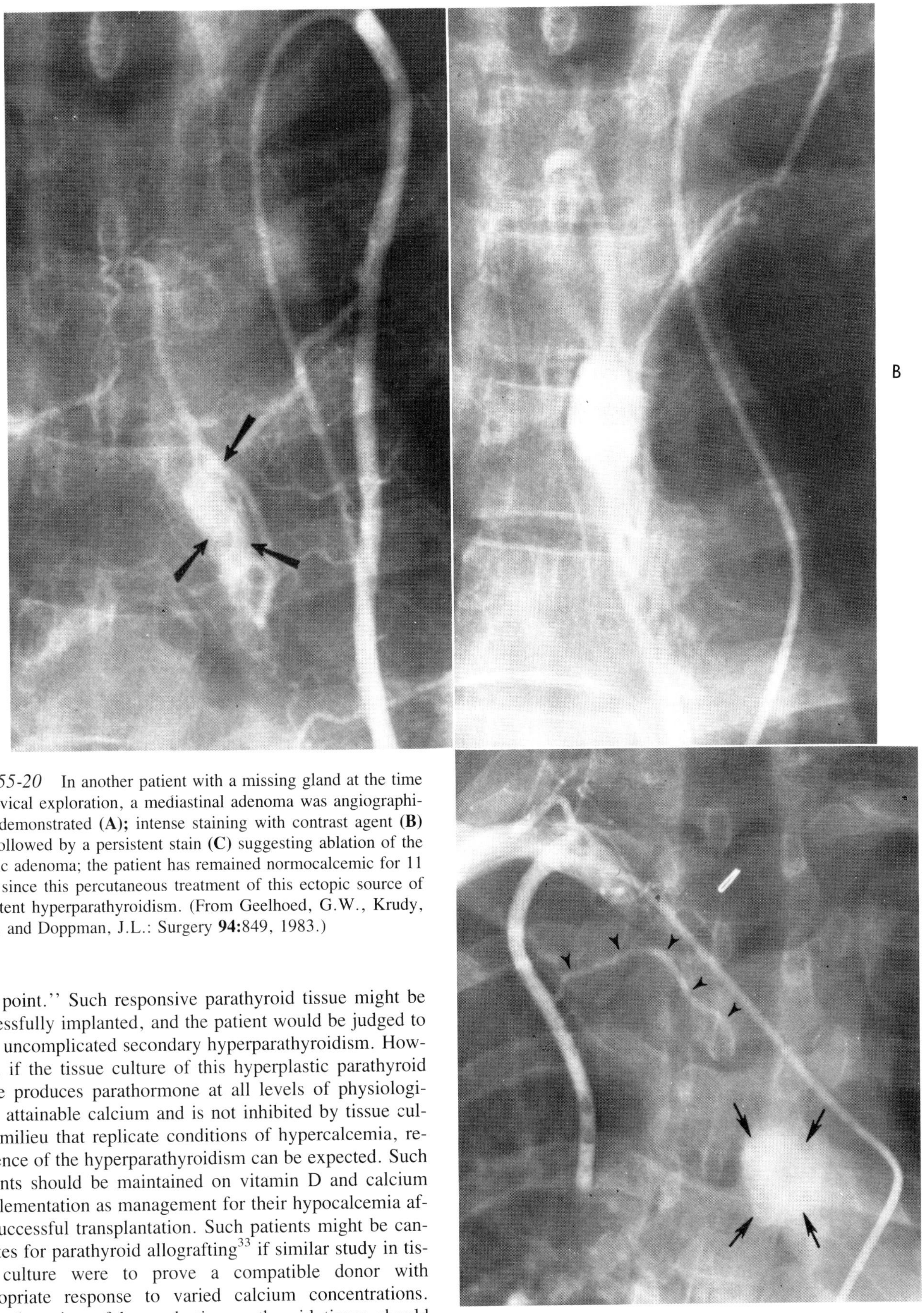

B

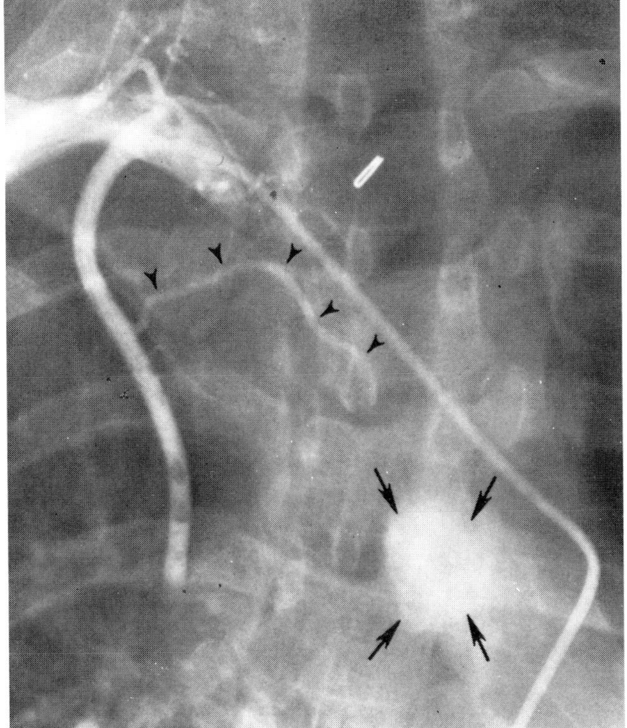

C

Fig. 55-20 In another patient with a missing gland at the time of cervical exploration, a mediastinal adenoma was angiographically demonstrated **(A)**; intense staining with contrast agent **(B)** was followed by a persistent stain **(C)** suggesting ablation of the ectopic adenoma; the patient has remained normocalcemic for 11 years since this percutaneous treatment of this ectopic source of persistent hyperparathyroidism. (From Geelhoed, G.W., Krudy, A.G., and Doppman, J.L.: Surgery **94:**849, 1983.)

"set point." Such responsive parathyroid tissue might be successfully implanted, and the patient would be judged to have uncomplicated secondary hyperparathyroidism. However, if the tissue culture of this hyperplastic parathyroid tissue produces parathormone at all levels of physiologically attainable calcium and is not inhibited by tissue culture milieu that replicate conditions of hypercalcemia, recurrence of the hyperparathyroidism can be expected. Such patients should be maintained on vitamin D and calcium supplementation as management for their hypocalcemia after successful transplantation. Such patients might be candidates for parathyroid allografting[33] if similar study in tissue culture were to prove a compatible donor with appropriate response to varied calcium concentrations. Transplantation of hyperplastic parathyroid tissue should not be undertaken in patients with familial hyperparathyroidism, since the genetic defect that changed the "set point" of their calcium-sensors would presumably be abnormal in all parathyroid cells. The same caveat should be followed with any presumably autonomous adenoma, with the additional risk that parathyroid carcinoma might be transplanted because it is poorly distinguished from adenoma by histologic criteria.

Hyperparathyroidism in MEA

As a rule, hyperparathyroidism as part of MEA is based in multiple gland disease. The genetic defect carried in all parathyroid cells makes identification of all parathyroid glands and their subtotal excision a requirement of parathyroid operation. Generally the patients are more likely to have symptomatic hypocalcemia after the operation than is the case with the excision of a sporadic parathyroid adenoma. Hyperparathyroidism is more likely to recur in these patients as well, when compared with the primary hyperparathyroidism based in parathyroid hyperplasia in sporadic cases.

In MEA-I hyperparathyroidism is often the earliest feature of the endocrinopathy and is frequently symptomatic. Moreover, hypercalcemia is a strong stimulus to gastrin release and the hyperacidity that may follow. For that reason, the first attack on the endocrine abnormalities in MEA-I is cervical, first correcting hyperparathyroidism. In some instances patients with MEA-I have a decrease in their serum gastrin and even regression of the pancreatic islet abnormalities, at least transient, following successful treatment of the hyperparathyroidism.[12]

In MEA-II the life-threatening abnormality is the pheochromocytoma that may be present. Under no circumstances should the coincidental hyperparathyroidism be approached first until the much more significant threat of catecholamine excess is controlled. Whereas the cervical surgical approach to correct primary hyperparathyroidism is the first priority in MEA-I, the hyperparathyroidism is the last priority in MEA-II. The physiologic threat of pheochromocytoma takes priority over the oncologic importance of medullary thyroid carcinoma, the primary reason for the cervical exploration. At the time of the total thyroidectomy for medullary thyroid carcinoma, the parathyroid glands can be inspected and reduced as appropriate to the hyperparathyroidism the patient may exhibit.

Hyperparathyroidism in Pregnancy

Normal pregnancy is a time of very large changes in calcium metabolism in the pregnant woman, when over 30 g of calcium must be transferred across the placenta into the fetal skeleton. Parathormone, however, does not cross the placenta. Fetal calcium requirements are met, regardless of calcium intake or demineralization in the maternal skeleton, particularly if hyperparathyroidism is associated with pregnancy. Maternal hyperparathyroidism, however, is associated with a high rate of fetal wastage.[13] If hyperparathyroidism is symptomatic, surgical treatment should be carried out during pregnancy. In the pregnant patient with asymptomatic hypercalcemia, parathyroid exploration can be postponed until after delivery if there is careful monitoring to prevent the loss of the pregnancy. Management of hypercalcemia in the pregnant patient can include hydration and diuretics, but administration of cytoxic drugs such as mithramycin are precluded.

The effect on the fetus of maternal hyperparathyroidism is not apparent in utero. However, when the fetus is separated from the maternal circulation, the resulting hypoparathyroidism may be exhibited as irritability or tetany. Vitamin D and calcium are required for treatment of an infant born of a hypercalcemic mother. The vitamin D and calcium must be carefully tapered so as to avoid prolonging the suppression of the infant's parathyroid glands. Hypoparathyroidism should be anticipated in the fetus born of a hyperparathyroid mother. On rare occasions, neonatal tetany has been the presenting sign of previously undiagnosed maternal hyperparathyroidism.

Results of Treatment of Hyperparathyroidism

After excision of single gland disease in primary hyperparathyroidism when primary cervical operation reveals the normal or suppressed parathyroid glands, less than 1% of patients experience late recurrence of hyperparathyroidism. However, persistent hyperparathyroidism occurs in approximately 5% of treated patients, usually on the basis of multiple gland disease not appreciated or inadequately reduced at the time of the primary cervical procedure.

The success rate of control of hyperparathyroidism treated by reoperation is much lower than the success rate of the initial operation, depending on the nature of the disease that gave rise to the persistence of hypercalcemia. In multiple gland involvement both persistence and recurrence of hypercalcemia is higher following both primary operation and reoperation than for the sporadic incidence of single-gland disease.

The recurrence rate is highest in those patients who have a familial occurrence of multiple-gland disease or in those patients who still have parathyroid stimulation, as from the persistence of azotemia managed by dialysis but with persistent hyperphosphatemia.

For most patients with persistent hypercalcemia, if this disorder is not based in some nonparathyroid problem such as FHH, the source is probably a single-gland, diseased parathyroid, most often overlooked in some ectopic location in the neck. For satisfactory treatment of persistent hypercalcemia, preoperative localization studies that precede reoperation can aid in the often difficult dissection that occurs in areas of the scarring of previous operation.

Hypercalcemia should always be investigated. If the hypercalcemia is based in primary hyperparathyroidism, treatment is very satisfying with the usual identification of a solitary adenoma, the excision of which is curative. The vast majority of patients so treated remain normal in their calcium homeostasis in long term follow-up.

SUMMARY

Calcium and phosphorous are critical components of metabolic systems. Intricate control systems exist in the body, especially to maintain serum ionized calcium within a narrow range upon which neuromuscular excitation, contraction, and relaxation depend. Sites of calcium regulation include absorption from the gut, resorption from large reservoirs in bone, and excretion via the kidney.

The parathyroid glands are both ionized calcium sensors and the effectors of normal calcium homeostasis through the role of parathormone in controlling bone resorption and renal excretion of calcium. Other factors involved in calcium balance include ions (phosphate, chloride, hydrogen and magnesium), buffers (albumin and chelators), and other hormones (vitamin D, thyroxine, calcitonin, corticosteroids, catecholamines and malignancy—associated paraendocrine products).

Hypocalcemia is the result of inadequate intake of calcium, vitamin D precursors, magnesium or protein, or failure of absorption from the gut or unopposed excretion from lack of vitamin D or parathormone secretion. Consequences of hypocalcemia include irritability and tetany, and careful replacement of the inadequate hormone or mineral substrates is used in acute and chronic treatment.

Hypercalcemia arises from a number of causes, including excess calcium, vitamin or drug ingestion, mobilization of calcium from bones or blocked renal excretion, or primary hypersecretion of parathormone.

Primary hyperparathyroidism may be differentiated from these other causes of hypercalcemia by study of the mineral metabolites and hormone assay. Most patients with primary hyperparathyroidism are asymptomatic when first discovered now by multiphasic biochemical screening tests; but hypercalcemia may give a variety of symptoms from loss of organ reserves, obtundation, seizures, coma, and death. Acutely elevated serum calcium may be safely lowered by a series of medical means, whereas its cause is determined and differentiated for further recommendations on fixing the underlying source. Cervical exploration is a usually successful method of locating and correcting primary hyperparathyroidism, often by excision of an autonomously hyperfunctioning single gland source.

Special consideration is given persistent or recurrent hyperparathyroidism and that associated with hereditary syndromes or pregnancy. Reconfirmation of the primary hyperparathyroidism diagnosis is often followed by radiologic localization techniques before reoperation for persistent parathyroid problems, often stemming from hyperfunctioning multiple, supernumerary, or ectopic glands.

Hypercalcemia as a finding in patient screening always warrants investigation, since it represents an abnormality in view of the sensitive control systems for calcium homeostasis. If based in malignancy, this discovery is valuable in prognosis. If based in primary hyperparathyroidism, successful parathyroid correction is achieved in most patients who undergo operation, which restores calcium metabolism to delicate intrinsic autoregulatory balance.

REFERENCES

1. Becker, K.L., et al.: The pathophysiology of pulmonary calcitonin. In Becker, K.L., and Gazdar, A.F., editors: The endocrine lung in health and disease, Philadelphia, 1984, W.B. Saunders Co.
2. Benson, R.C. Jr., et al.: Immunoreactive forms of circulating parathyroid hormone in primary and ectopic hyperparathyroidism, J. Clin. Invest. **59:**175, 1974.
3. Brennan, M.F., et al.: Recurrent hyperparathyroidism from an autotransplanted parathyroid adenoma, N. Engl. J. Med. **299:**1057, 1978.
4. Brown, E.M., et al.: Calcium regulated parathyroid hormone release in primary hyperparathyroidism, Am. J. Med. **66:**923, 1979.
5. Carroll, P.R., and Clark, O.H.: The milk-alkali syndrome: does it exist and can it be differentiated from primary hyperparathyroidism? Ann. Surg. **197:**427, 1983.
6. Castleman, B., Schantz, A., Roth, S.I.: Parathyroid hyperplasia in primary hyperparathyroidism, Cancer **38:**1668, 1976.
7. Chernow, B., and Zaloga, G.P.: Ions for society members, SCCM. In Schoemaker, W.C., editor: Critical care state of the art, Vol. 5, Fullerton, California, 1984, Society of Critical Care Medicine.
8. Chester, W.L., Zaloga, G.P., and Chernow, B.: Phosphate problems in the critically ill patient. In Geelhoed, G.W., and Chernow, B., editors: Endocrine aspects of acute illness, clinics in critical care medicine, New York, 1985, Churchill Livingstone.
9. Clark, O.H., and Way, L.W.: The hypercalcemic syndrome: hyperparathyroidism. In Faissen, S.R., editor: Surgical endocrinology: clinical syndromes, Philadelphia, 1978, J.B. Lippincott Co.
10. Cope, O., et al.: Primary chief cell hyperplasia of the parathyroid gland: a new entity in the surgery of hyperparathyroidism, Ann. Surg. **148:**375, 1958.
11. Ferlin, C., et al.: New perspectives in localizing enlarged parathyroids by technetium—thallium subtraction scan, J. Nuclear Med. **24:**438, 1983.
12. Geelhoed, G.W.: Problem management in endocrine surgery, Chicago, 1983, Yearbook Medical Publishers, Inc.
13. Geelhoed, G.W.: Surgery of the endocrine glands in pregnancy, Clin. Obstet. Gynecol. **26:**865, 1983.
14. Geelhoed, G.W., and Doppman, J.L.: Embolization of ectopic parathyroid adenomas: a percutaneous treatment of hyperparathyroidism, Am. Surg. **44:**71, 1978.
15. Geelhoed, G.W., Krudy, A.G., and Doppman, J.L.: Long-term follow-up of patients with hyperparathyroidism treated by transcatheter staining with contrast agent, Surgery **94:**849, 1983.
16. Geelhoed, G.W., and Silverberg, S.A.: Intraoperative imprints for the identification of parathyroid tissue, Surgery **96:**1124, 1984.
17. Habener, J.F., and Potts, J.T.: Biosynthesis of parathyroid hormone, N. Engl. J. Med. **299:**580, 635, 1978.
18. Heath, H., Hodgson, S.F., and Kennedy, M.A.: Primary hyperparathyroidism: incidence, morbidity and potential economic impact in a community, N. Engl. J. Med. **302:**189, 1980.
19. Kay, S., and Hume, D.M.: Carcinoma of the parathyroid glands, Arch. Pathol. **96:**316, 1973.
20. Keller, V., and Berger, W.: Prevention of hypophosphatemia by phosphate infusion and during treatment of diabetic ketoacidosis and hyperosmolar coma, Diabetes **29:**87, 1980.
21. Marx, S.J., et al.: The hypocalciuric or benign variant of familial hypercalcemia: clinical and biochemical features in fifteen kindreds, Medicine **60:**397, 1981.
22. Mundy, G.R., et al.: Evidence for the secretion of an osteoclast stimulating factor in myeloma, N. Engl. J. Med. **291:**1041, 1974.
23. Mundy, G.R., et al.: Direct stimulation of bone resorption by thyroid hormones, J. Clin. Invest. **58:**529, 1976.
24. Peskin, G.W., Greenburg, A.G., and Saik, R.P.: Expanding indications for early parathyroidectomy in the elderly female, Am. J. Surg. **136:**45, 1978.
25. Pickleman, J.R., et al.: Thiazide-induced parathyroid stimulation, Metabolism **18:**867, 1969.
26. Potts, J.T.: Mineral ion homeostasis and its control. Part II, Harvard Medical School Pathophysiology Course Outline Musculoskeletal Section, 1982.
27. Prinz, R.A. et al.: Radiation—associated hyperparathyroidism: a new syndrome? Surgery **82:**296, 1977.
28. Rasbach, D.A., et al.: Solitary parathyroid microadenoma, Surgery **96:**1092, 1984.
29. Scholz, D.A., and Purnell, D.C.: Asymptomatic primary hyperparathyroidism—10 year prospective study, Mayo Clinic Proc. **56:**473, 1981.
30. Spiegel, A.M., and Marx, S.J.: Parathyroid hormone and vitamin D receptors, Clin. Endocrinol. Metabol. **12:**221, 1983.
31. Stern, J.N., Smith, W.D., and Ginn, H.E.: Hypophosphatemia in acute alcoholism, Am. J. Med. Sci. **252:**78, 1968.
32. Tisell, L.E., et al.: Hyperparathyroidism in persons treated with x-rays for tuberculous cervical adenitis, Cancer **40:**846, 1977.
33. Wells, S.A., et al.: Transplantation of the parathyroid glands: current status, Surg. Clin. North Am. **591:**167, 1979.
34. Yeager, R.M., and Krementz, E.T.: Acute hyperparathyroidism, South. Med. J. **69:**797, 1971.
35. Zaloga, G.P., and Chernow, B.: Calcium metabolism. In Geelhoed, G.W., and Chernow, B., editors: Endocrine aspects of acute illness, clinics in critical care medicine, New York, 1985, Churchill-Livingstone.

56

Michael E. Miner and Juan A. Cabrera

Pituitary Dysfunction

The skeleton of Hunter's giant, O'Bryan, is now over 200 years old, but it still provides one of the first clear evidences of the clinicopathologic correlation between pituitary pathology and systemic hormonal effects.[90] Dr. Hunter believed that giantism was caused by a tumor of the pituitary and, despite O'Bryan's strenuous objections, the enlarged sella turcica and skeleton of the giant can still be found in the museum of the Royal College of Surgeons.[66] Although this is not the first recognition of the potential role of pituitary gland dysfunction as a cause of human disease, it remains one of the most dramatic early observations.

The history of the notions concerning pituitary dysfunction have enticed some of the leading minds in medicine for the past century.[35] Marie's detailed observations and naming of the syndrome of acromegaly in 1886,[42] Babinski's report in 1900 of what was to become Frohlich's hypopituitarism syndrome,[2] and Cushing's description in 1933 of the syndrome that bears his name[18] all witness to the rapid explosion of knowledge concerning the pathologic manifestations of pituitary tumors that occurred during the early part of this century. Throughout the same time period, other conditions affecting pituitary function were also being described. Simmond's patient with polyuria secondary to metastatic breast cancer to the pituitary[18] and Frank's patient who developed diabetes insipidus and other signs of hypopituitarism after a gunshot wound to the sella[16] were early evidence that pituitary function could be influenced by conditions other than tumors.

No sooner were the diagnoses being made of pituitary and parasellar tumors than surgeons were devising approaches to treat them.[90] Sir Victor Horsley exposed the pituitary gland to excise a tumor as early as 1889.[42] By 1907 Schloffer had recorded the first transsphenoidal approach to the pituitary gland followed 2 years later by Gramengas' report of a prompt but brief remission of acromegalic symptoms following x-ray treatment.[42,90] However, it was Cushing who brought together the clinically relevant data and demonstrated that sellar and parasellar tumors could be routinely approached with safety. His monumental work on both the treatment and physiology of pituitary disorders still stands as classic medical literature.[17,18] The past 20 years have witnessed another information explosion, extending knowledge of hormone control systems, interaction, and medical regimens to treat pituitary dysfunction.

ANATOMY OF PITUITARY GLAND

The pituitary gland weighs approximately 525 mg. It is significantly larger in females than males and grows even larger during pregnancy. It is approximately 5 mm in height, 10 to 14 mm in width, and 10 mm in depth. It is confined on its anterior, posterior, and inferior surfaces by the sella turcica, a bony depression in the sphenoid bone. Immediately below the sella is the sphenoidal air sinus, and lying lateral to it are the cavernous venous sinuses. Within each trabeculated cavernous sinus are the carotid artery (Fig. 56-1); the ocular motor, trochlea, abducens; and the first two major divisions of the trigeminal nerve. The dura mater that lines the sella forms an incomplete diaphragm above the pituitary gland through which traverses the pituitary stalk from the median eminence of the hypothalamus, the portal veins, and the superior hypophyseal artery (Fig. 56-2). The arterial supply to the pituitary gland and infundibulum is through branches of the superior and inferior hypophyseal arteries that are direct tributaries of the carotid artery. Venous drainage is through a series of veins that directly connect to the dural venous sinuses. The optic chiasm is immediately anterior to the stalk of the pituitary, and the tip of the basilar artery lies in close proximity posteriorly to the sellar diaphragm. The arachnoid membrane does not normally enter through the diaphragm but lies immediately above it. A pouch of arachnoid may herniate into the sella and compress the pituitary gland, resulting in an "empty sella."[56,61,69]

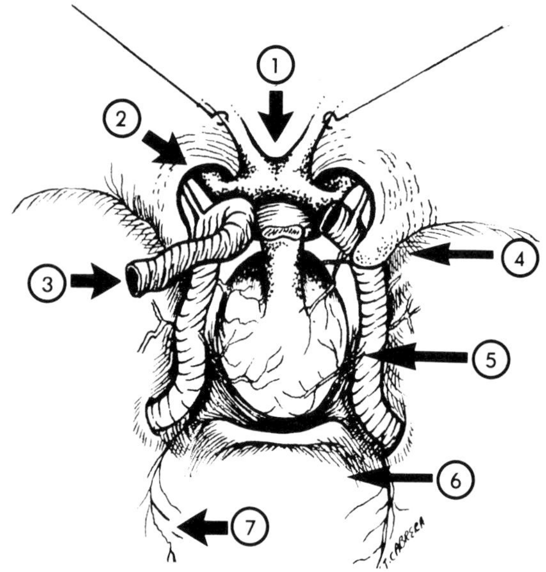

Fig. 56-1 Anatomy of the sellar region. Optic tracts are retracted anteriorly to demonstrate the relationship between the optic chiasm and foramen, pituitary gland and stalk, carotid arteries, and bony confines of the pituitary gland. *1,* Optic tracts; *2,* optic foramen; *3,* internal carotid arteries; *4,* anterior clinoid processes; *5,* meningeal-hypophyseal vessels; *6,* dorsum sellae; and *7,* tentorial vessels.

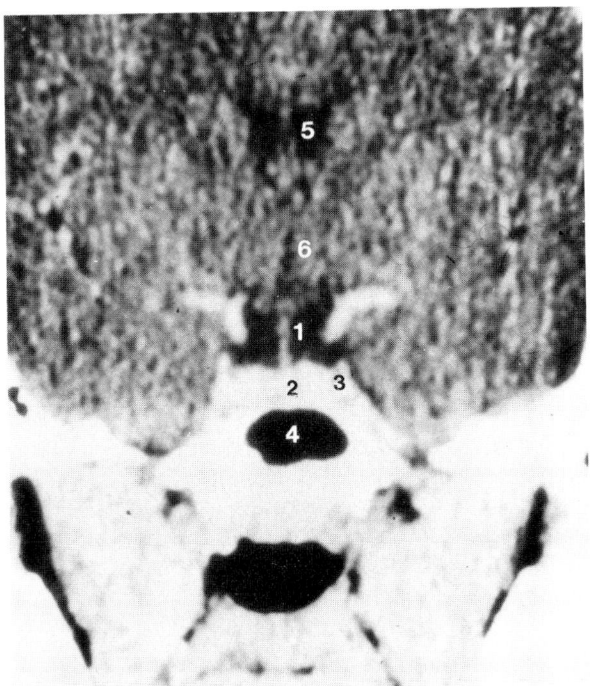

Fig. 56-2 Coronal computed tomogram demonstrating the normal relationship between the pituitary stalk *(1)*, pituitary gland *(2)*, both internal carotid arteries *(3)*, and the sphenoidal air sinuses *(4)*. Note the lateral *(5)* and third *(6)* ventricles superior to the pituitary gland.

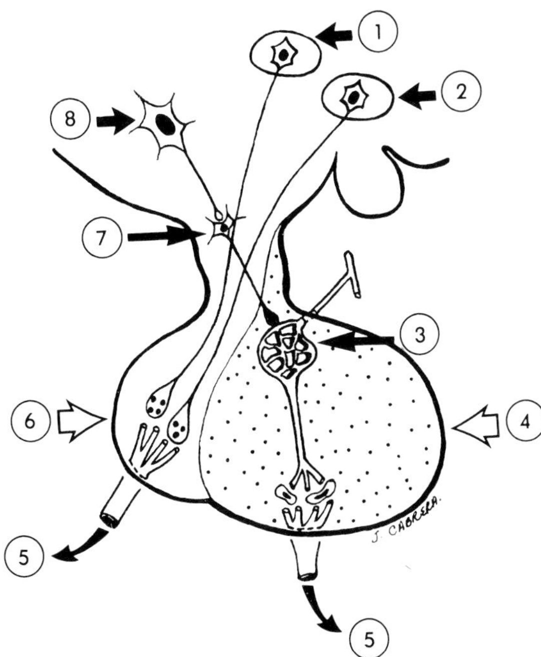

Fig. 56-3 Schematic representation of hypothalamohypophyseal vascular and neuronal relationships. Hormones manufactured in neurons of the paraventricular and supraoptic hypothalamic nuclei are released in the posterior lobe of the pituitary gland (neurohypophysis). Monoaminergic neurons produce releasing and inhibiting hormones to be released into the portal veins to control the secretion of anterior pituitary (adenohypophysis) hormones. *1*, Paraventricular nuclei; *2*, supraoptic nuclei of the hypothalamus; *3*, portal venous system; *4*, adenohypophysis; *5*, efferent vein to dural sinuses; *6*, neurohypophysis; *7*, tuberal infundibular neuron; and *8*, monoaminergic neuron.

Within 1 cm of the pituitary gland lies a portion of half of the cranial nerves, the entire blood supply to the cerebral hemispheres, the cavernous sinuses, the hypothalamus, the brainstem, the cerebrospinal fluid (CSF), a paranasal air sinus, and the nasopharynx. Thus it should not be surprising that abnormalities of the pituitary gland might well affect these structures or that a wide variety of lesions involving those structures should secondarily affect pituitary function.

EMBRYOLOGY OF THE PITUITARY GLAND

Two separate ectodermal sources combine embryologically to form the pituitary gland. A hollow invagination of oral pharyngeal epithelium extends dorsally to form Rathke's pouch, which then separates from the tissue of origin to form the adenohypophysis. In contrast, the neurohypophysis is a downward extension from the diencephalon of the brain. Therefore the neurohypophysis should be considered a direct extension of the central nervous system, which is directly linked to two sets of hypothalamic nuclei, i.e., the supraoptic and paraventricular nuclei. On the other hand, the adenohypophysis is not in anatomic connection with the central nervous system but maintains communication with the hypothalamus by means of the portal venous system through which blood flows from the hypothalamus along the pituitary stalk toward the adenohypophysis. This portal blood carries regulatory hormones from the hypothalamus to the adenohypophysis. Thus both the adenohypophysis and neurohypophysis are in close communication with the hypothalamus. An ever-growing literature on hypothalamic pituitary "cross-talk" is developing that indicates that physiologically the system should

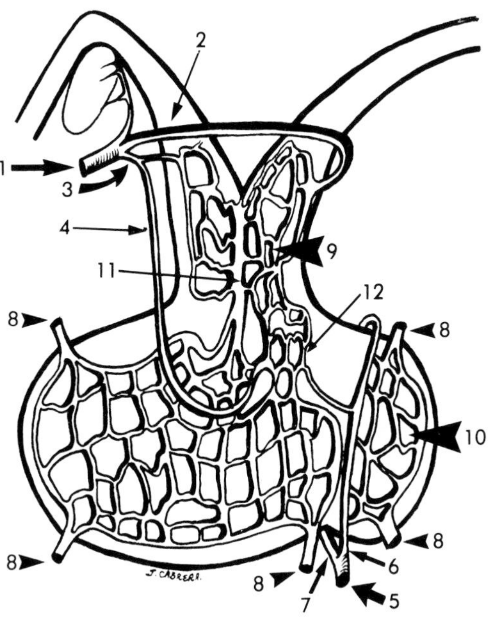

Fig. 56-4 Detailed schematic representation of the vascular supply to the pituitary gland. *1*, Superior hypophyseal artery; *2*, posterior branch; *3*, anterior branch; *4*, artery of trabecula; *5*, inferior hypophyseal artery; *6*, lateral branch; *7*, medial branch; *8*, efferent vein to dural sinus; *9*, primary portal system; *10*, secondary portal system; *11*, long hypophyseal portal vein; and *12*, short hypophyseal portal vein.

be thought of as a highly dependent one with multiple feedback loops, i.e., the hypothalamohypophyseal system (Figs. 56-3 and 56-4).

PITUITARY FUNCTION

The function of the hypothalamohypophyseal system is to manufacture, store, and control the release of the eight known pituitary hormones. Even though the pituitary can be viewed as a single endocrine organ, for purposes of understanding its function it is more fruitful to consider it as two independent organs that have subtle, but important interactions (see Fig. 56-3).

The site of production of the pituitary hormones of the posterior pituitary gland is in the hypothalamic nuclei. The supraoptic and paraventricular nuclei appear to manufacture these polypeptide hormones, which are then released in the neurohypophysis.[56,61,69] The anterior pituitary hormones, on the other hand, are manufactured in the adenohypophysis, but their release into the bloodstream is under the influence of releasing and inhibiting hormones that arrive by means of the hypophyseal portal venous system. Thus the release of hormones from both the adenohypophysis and neurohypophysis is controlled by the hypothalamus, but the mechanisms underlying this control are quite different. Furthermore, the structure of the hormones of the adenohypophysis and the neurohypophysis are strikingly different (see Fig. 56-4). The interactions between the pituitary hormones and their releasing and inhibiting substances are the subject of exciting, ongoing investigation. Current evidence indicates that each of the eight pituitary hormones is associated with a well-described clinical syndrome resulting either from its overproduction or absence.

Hormones of Neurohypophysis

Antidiuretic hormone (ADH) and oxytocin are the two nonapeptide hormones of the neurohypophysis.[28] ADH is produced primarily in the supraoptic nuclei of the hypothalamus, whereas oxytocin is formed in the paraventricular nuclei. However, although these hormones are produced in the hypothalamus, they are not simply transported down the axons to the neurohypophysis. Polypeptides that facilitate the transport of ADH and oxytocin are also produced in the hypothalamus. These polypeptides, called neurophysines, are released into the bloodstream along with the active hormones at the level of the neurohypophysis with minimal storage in the neurohypophysis. Thus the neurohypophysis serves as little more than an immediate site for the release of ADH and oxytocin. The neurophysines appear to be taken back up by the nerve terminals for another trip down the axon with new hormones. There are no known physiologic activities of the neurophysines other than to facilitate intracellular hormone transport.

Oxytocin primarily stimulates the uterus during labor and appears to play an integral part in normal delivery. In addition, it has a role in causing the alveolar cells of the mammary glands to constrict and thus aids with milk ejection. Although it has some antidiuretic activity, the effect appears to be quite minimal when compared to that of ADH.

ADH plays a major role in water metabolism.[29] Normally the kidneys form approximately 180 L of glomerular filtrate every day. Under the influence of ADH, more than 99% of this is resorbed in the nephrons, thus serving to conserve water. ADH appears to affect the renal tubular cells by interacting with receptors on the peritubular surface rather than by entering the cell per se. On the surface membrane ADH activates adenylate cyclase, which catalyzes the formation of cyclic AMP (cAMP) from adenosine triphosphate (ATP). cAMP activates protein kinases, which then phosphorylate specific membrane proteins that control the pore size of the luminal membrane in the nephron. When the size of the pores is changed, the flow characteristics of the membrane are altered, and the rate at which water flows from the tubular lumen into the cells of the tubular walls is controlled. ADH closely regulates water conservation, but it is certainly not the only mechanism important in renal water resorption. Interposed on this system are other influences such as the effect of renal prostaglandins E_1 and E_2. These prostaglandins appear to decrease the concentration of cAMP on the luminal membrane and thereby aid in fine tuning the effect of ADH on water resorption.[27]

The release of ADH from the neurohypophysis is primarily directed by plasma osmoreceptors thought to be located in the supraoptic nuclei. As osmolality increases the secretion of ADH also increases, and more water is reabsorbed from the renal ultrafiltrate back into the plasma, thereby decreasing osmolality. Accordingly, a decrease in plasma osmolality reduces or halts further release of ADH, which promotes excretion of water by the kidney. This negative feedback control system is physiologically well defined, even though the structure of the osmoreceptors has not been well demonstrated.

It has been observed that altering plasma volume also affects the release of ADH, independent of its effect on osmolality. A decrease in plasma volume results in the release of ADH and a subsequent increase in plasma volume secondary to increased water reabsorption by the kidney. Although it has been postulated that volume receptors initiating these ADH effects are located in the right atrium of the heart and that the afferent neural impulses are transmitted through the vagus nerve, such receptors have not been clearly identified.

Many well-known factors common to everyday experience influence ADH secretion.[63] Affect, mood, and anxiety clearly stimulate ADH secretion. Cholinergic and beta-adrenergic stimulation increase ADH secretion, whereas alpha-adrenergic stimulation is inhibitory. Multiple pharmacologic agents, including nicotine, morphine, barbiturates, vincristine, and some tricyclic antidepressants stimulate ADH secretion; whereas hydantoin, ethanol, and reserpine inhibit it. Although the final common pathway for ADH secretion is from the hypothalamus, there are clearly many other influences, both endogenous and exogenous, that modulate the secretion of this hormone.

Hormones of Adenohypophysis

Three polypeptide hormones (i.e., growth hormone, prolactin, and adrenocorticotropin [ACTH]) and three glycoprotein hormones (i.e., thyroid-stimulating hormone [TSH], follicle-stimulating hormone [FSH] and luteinizing hormone [LH]) are secreted by the adenohypophysis. In contrast to the neurohypophysis, hormones of the adenohypophysis are produced and stored in the gland before secretion, and the influence of the hypothalamus is purely one of regulating their release.

Two subunits of the glycoprotein hormones have been identified: alpha and beta. Although neither of the subunits has been completely characterized, the alpha subunit appears to be exactly the same for TSH, FSH, and LH. However, the beta subunits are unique for each hormone and therefore confer the specificity to the hormone for a particular receptor site. The beta subunit does not possess biologic activity by itself and only becomes biologically active when coupled with the alpha subunit. Thus these hormones function as though the receptor required both a general and a specific key to cause effect. In both males and females the glycoprotein TSH stimulates the production and secretion of thyroid hormone. In females FSH stimulates the maturation of ovarian follicles and the secretion of estrogens by those follicles. In males it stimulates development of testicular tubules and spermatogenesis. LH in the female induces ovulation and causes luteinization to develop in the mature ovarian follicle, with the subsequent production and secretion of progesterone. In males it stimulates the development of Leydig cells in the testes and the production and secretion of testosterone.

Of the polypeptide hormones, prolactin is the largest, consisting of 198 amino acid residues. In females it stimulates the growth of breast tissue and induces production and secretion of breast milk. In males the function of prolactin is less obvious, but it appears to be essential to normal spermatogenesis.[59] ACTH is a single-chain polypeptide composed of 39 amino acids. The primary function of ACTH is to cause the cortex of the adrenal gland to produce and secrete cortisol and other adrenal steroids. However, the adrenal cortical hormone, aldosterone, is a clear exception to this principle because it is primarily under the influence of renin and angiotensinogen.

Human growth hormone (hGH) is a polypeptide consisting of 191 amino acids, which, unlike the other pituitary hormones, has no specific target organ but has an effect on virtually all tissue. The growth resulting from hGH stimulation is not a direct effect but rather is induced by a group of substances known as somatomedins. These growth hormone–dependent polypeptides are thought to be produced in the liver and not in the pituitary gland.[26] Five different somatomedins have been identified, all of which stimulate growth in responsive tissues.

Hypothalamic Control of Adenohypophyseal Hormone Secretion

For many years it was thought that hormone secretion by the anterior pituitary resulted in stimulation of a specific target organ. This target organ then released a second hormone. Thus the pituitary was thought to orchestrate the entire hormonal system by a straightforward series of independent negative feedback systems. For example, TSH stimulates the thyroid to release the hormones of the thyroid. The level of the secondary hormones (i.e., the thyroid hormones) is increased in the blood; this is detected by the pituitary, and TSH secretion is turned off by means of a simple negative feedback loop. However, the elegant work of Schally and Arimura[74] and Schally and associates[75] has clearly shown that the pituitary hormone control system is much more complex.[74,75] On the basis of their work, it is currently accepted that there are a series of releasing and inhibiting substances that are secreted by the hypothalamus into the hypophyseal portal venous system. It is these substances that cause specific cells of the adenohypophysis to selectively secrete their distinctive hormones. There appears to be good evidence for a hypothalamic-releasing hormone for all of the anterior pituitary hormones and an inhibiting substance for at least hGH and prolactin. This complex system is interactive in that (1) the releasing hormones may effect the release of further releasing hormone and (2) although the releasing and inhibiting hormones are specific for the adenohypophyseal hormones, they may not be totally selective. Stated another way, there appears to be some crossover of function between the various releasing hormones. All of the releasing and inhibiting hormones characterized at this point consist of three or more amino acids.

A few of these releasing and inhibiting hormones have also been found in other areas of the brain and in sites outside of the central nervous system. This implies that, in addition to being influenced by the pituitary hormones themselves and the target gland hormones, the stimulatory and inhibitory hormones of the hypothalamus are influenced by stimuli from many portions of the body and higher cortical centers. The pituitary gland may well be the grand orchestrator of all of the hormones, but the physiologic control of the pituitary hormones is a complex system, the nature of which is still unfolding.

Growth hormones

Both an hGH-releasing factor (GHRF) and an inhibiting hormone (somatostatin) have been demonstrated in hypothalamic extracts. However, somatostatin has other activities in addition to inhibiting the release of hGH. It also has activities that inhibit the release of thyrotropin from the pituitary and insulin and glucagon from the pancreas. This broad range of actions points to a more integrated and complex system of hormonal control than previously appreciated.

The control of hGH release ultimately occurs at the level of the hypothalamus. In addition to the normal negative feedback mechanisms involved in the other hormone control systems, the blood concentrations of glucose, fatty acids, estrogens, and most interestingly, sleep, also affect the release of hGH. The increase in hGH identified during sleep perhaps validates the notion that children need their sleep to grow properly. Although norepinephrine, dopamine, and serotonin stimulate the release of hGH in the normal person, in those people with hGH-secreting tumors, metergoline, an antiserotonin drug, and bromocriptine, an agent that binds to dopamine receptors, suppress hGH levels; indeed, both have been used successfully to treat acromegaly.[23,86]

Prolactin

The hypothalamus primarily inhibits rather than stimulates the release of prolactin from the adenohypophysis. It follows that in the absence of hypothalamic control there is excessive secretion of prolactin with an associated galactorrhea. A prolactin-releasing factor that stimulates prolactin release has been identified, but its role under normal circumstances is not clear. Thyrotropin-releasing hormone (TRH) also stimulates prolactin release from the adenohypophysis. The control of prolactin secretion is, like growth hormone, complex, and the feedback systems are not clearly characterized. Other hormones, particularly estrogens, also affect the secretion of prolactin.

Thyroid-stimulating hormone

TSH was the first pituitary hormone to be characterized. However, the thyroid hormones thyroxin and triiodothyronine act directly on the pituitary gland to decrease the production of TSH. Exactly how TRH modulates this response is unclear. A thyrotropin-inhibiting hormone has not been demonstrated. See Chapter 58 for a further discussion of these considerations.

Follicle-stimulating hormone and luteinizing hormone

A decapeptide-releasing hormone that functions to increase both FSH and LH has been characterized. With this single gonadtropin-releasing hormone, FSH and LH are released sequentially rather than simultaneously during the normal menstrual cycle. This control system is not well characterized but may be related to the positive and negative feedback control of the gonadal steroids on the pituitary gland itself.

Adrenocorticotropin

The hypothalamic control of ACTH is poorly understood. A corticotropin-releasing factor has been demonstrated in the hypothalamus but hypothalamic-inhibiting factor has not.[74,75]

PITUITARY DYSFUNCTION

Since the pituitary gland is an endocrine organ, dysfunction is expressed as the result of overproduction or underproduction of one or more hormones. Tumors secreting each of the anterior pituitary hormones have been described. In most reported series of pituitary tumors there are also a large proportion of "nonfunctioning" tumors. However, with the advent of more sophisticated diagnostic techniques the proportion of nonfunctional pituitary adenomas seems to be diminishing. Whether these are tumors that have minimal secretion or are truly nonfunctional hyperplasia is the subject of debate. The controversy centers around the histologic appearance of many of these nonsecreting "tumors" that have characteristics that would predict hormone secretion. One hypothesis is that they do, in fact, secrete hormones, but at very low concentrations. This low concentration is so near normal that the target organ sees this as normal pituitary hormone secretion and responds appropriately. This in turn results in a decrease in the hypothalamic-stimulating hormone, and thus the normal secreting cells of the adenohypophysis are functionally inhibited. However, it should be assumed that, in patients who have the signs and symptoms of an overproduction of adenohypophyseal hormone, a tumor is present. There are exceptions to this assumption, but they are few.

It is important to recognize that pituitary adenomas can be induced, at least in animals, by large dosages of estrogens, the classic example being the inducement of prolactin-secreting tumors by exogenous administration of high dosages of estrogen.[36] The point at which such lesions become independent of hypothalamic control is critical. Those subclinical tumors that remain dependent on hypothalamic control may be very common and may either require minimal or no treatment. On the other hand, when they escape from hypothalamic control and become independent of the normal regulatory mechanisms, they become enlarging pituitary adenomas and are clearly detrimental to the patient. Certainly not every microadenoma will become an autonomous tumor, but the distinction is frequently difficult to ascertain.

Adenohypophyseal hyposecretion is also well described. Although panhypopituitarism literally means total pituitary failure, in the common use of the term it denotes loss of function of only the adenohypophyseal hormones. Primary causes of pituitary failure are becoming increasingly more uncommon as more and more secondary causes are identified. Simmond's disease is the term applied to pituitary failure from any cause, whereas Sheehan's syndrome refers to pituitary necrosis secondary to shock, hemorrhage, or sepsis associated with child birth.[78,79] Pituitary apoplexy, on the other hand, is similar to Simmond's disease in that pituitary insufficiency develops; but pituitary apoplexy is generally reserved for cases in which there was a preexisting tumor that suffered acute hemorrhage or necrosis. The absence of any adenohypophyseal hormones except prolactin may result in a specific syndrome. Nonetheless, absence of a single anterior pituitary hormone is comparatively less common than panhypopituitarism and may be idiopathic or familial. This absence of a single hormone is commonly the result of abnormalities in the hypothalamus, but most cases are associated with subclinical hyposecretion of other hormones as well.

Diabetes insipidus is the result of a deficiency of ADH secondary to an impairment in the hypothalamoneurohypophyseal system. Although diabetes insipidus can be familial and idiopathic, it is much more commonly secondary to either primary neoplasms, vascular insufficiency of the pituitary, infections within the pituitary gland, or mass lesions in the parasellar region such as aneurysms or tumors. Diabetes insipidus may be quite transient as occurs in a resolving head injury or permanent as is seen after destruction of the hypothalamoneurohypophyseal system.

The syndrome of inappropriate ADH secretion is associated with a wide variety of other conditions ranging from malignant tumors of the lung and pancreas that secrete ADH to prolonged positive pressure ventilation. Although this syndrome is well documented following prolonged ventilation, the cause underlying this condition has remained elusive. The neurohypophysis may also be invaded by an astrocytoma or ependymoma from the surrounding tissues and for unknown reasons may result in ADH secretion. Primary tumors of the neurohypophysis are exceedingly rare. Such tumors, designated choristomas, have only been described in approximately 20 patients (Fig. 56-5).[48]

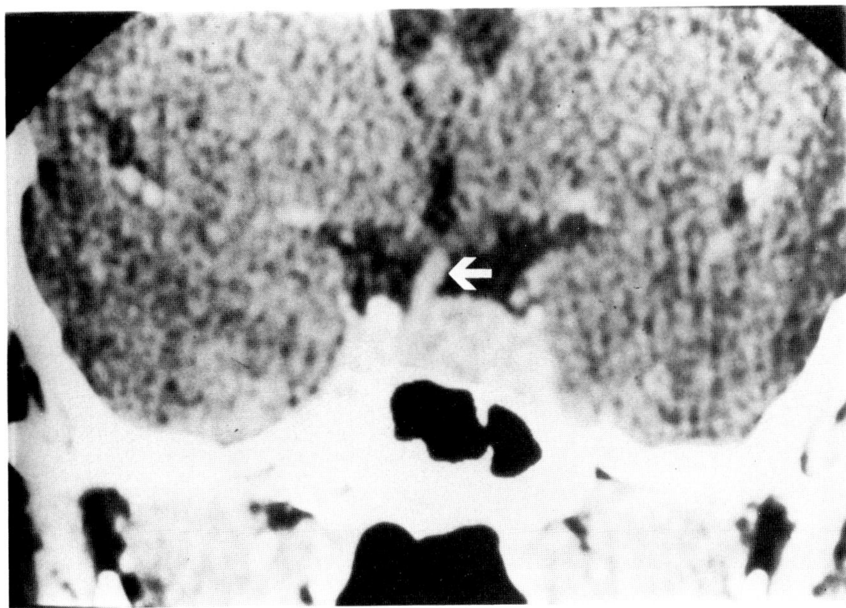

Fig. 56-5 Coronal computed tomogram demonstrating deviation of the stalk *(arrow)* of the pituitary gland to the right as result of a tumor.

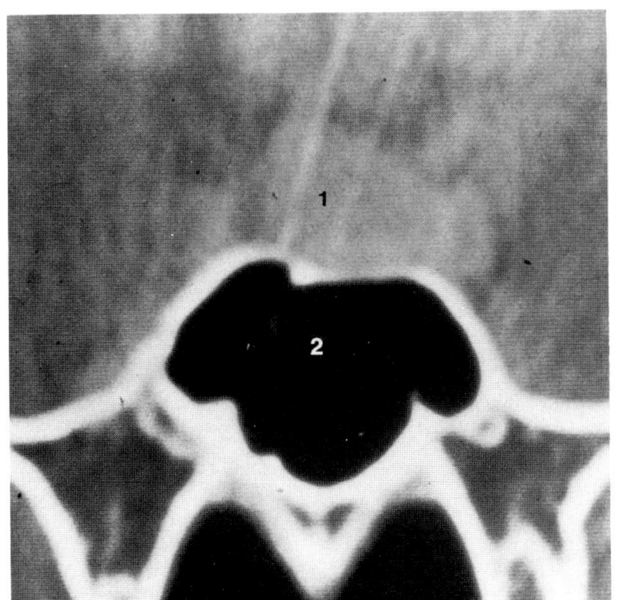

Fig. 56-6 Coronal computed tomogram demonstrating the relationship between an eccentrically placed pituitary tumor *(1)* and the sphenoidal air sinus *(2)*. This view is particularly helpful in planning transsphenoidal surgery.

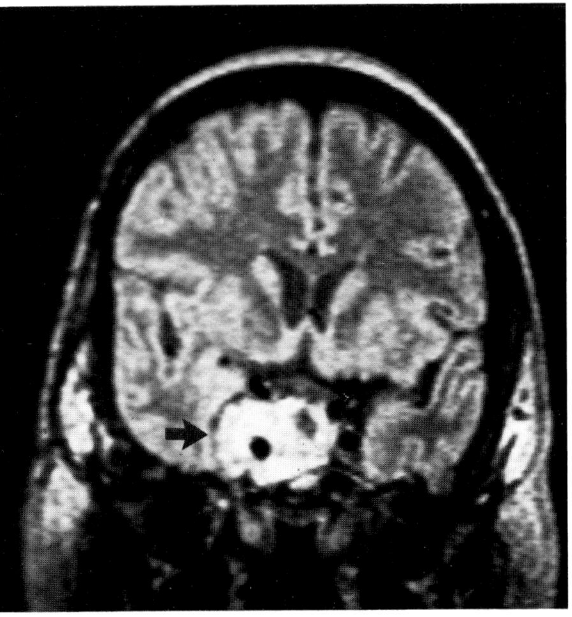

Fig. 56-7 Nuclear magnetic resonance study (coronal view) demonstrating a large adenoma with suprasellar extension and invasion of cavernous sinus *(arrow)*.

Pituitary Tumors

Adenomas of the pituitary are almost always histologically benign.[50] The ability to visualize the pituitary gland by noninvasive computerized tomography (CT) has opened new vistas for diagnosing these tumors[30] (Fig. 56-6). The use of magnetic resonance imaging to visualize the sellar region (Fig. 56-7) provides another potentially exciting diagnostic modality, but its precise role in visualizing pituitary tumors is undetermined and is currently undergoing active evaluation. Sophisticated endocrinologic investigations have also improved the ability to diagnose these tumors while they are small. Careful sectioning of the pituitary gland at autopsy has shown that between 10% and 25% of the normal population have abnormal tissue within the pituitary gland that may represent subclinical adenomas or hyperplasia.[14,15] Such observations make the question of who should be treated and how aggressive this treament should be of utmost relevance.

New medical treatment regimens are being tried, and even more effective regimens are on the horizon for man-

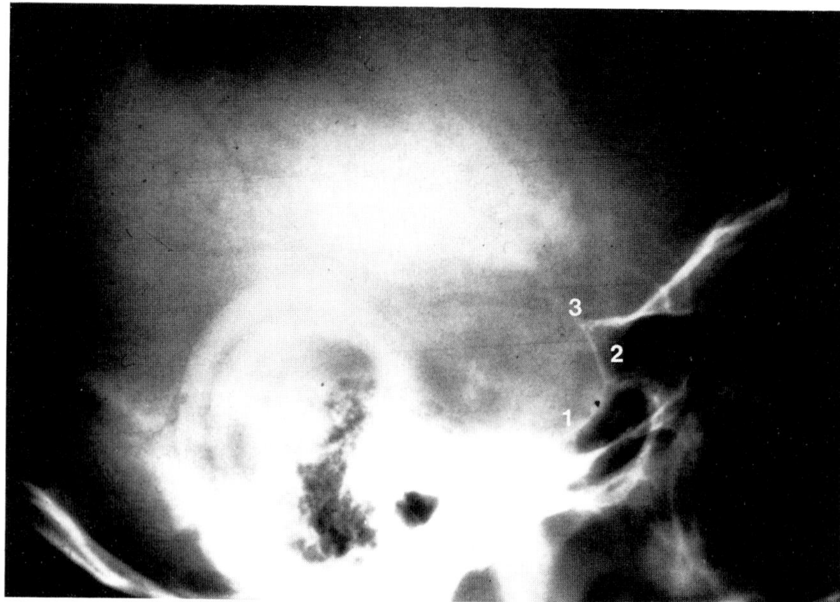

Fig. 56-8 Lateral skull x-ray film demonstrating extreme erosion of the sella turcica *(1)*. Note the double floor of the sella *(2)* and absence of the dorsum sella and erosion of the anterior clinoid processes *(3)*.

aging small hormone-secreting tumors without surgery.[68] The surgical treatment for pituitary tumors has also improved because ever smaller tumors are being identified and resected earlier and because of significantly improved postoperative management and intraoperative anesthetic care. The relative value of surgical therapy compared to medical management for small, hormonally active tumors is still evolving.

Clinical Presentation of Pituitary Tumors

Signs and symptoms of pituitary tumors occur because of the hormones they secrete and the mass effect of the tumor on adjacent structures. Such tumors may encroach on any of the surrounding anatomic structures, but frequently a characteristic clinical picture develops.[44] The resulting syndrome points to the location of the lesion, but other studies are required to elucidate the nature of the underlying pathology.

Visual field defects are commonly encountered in patients with pituitary tumors but often go unnoticed until they are relatively severe. The characteristic visual field deficit caused by an intrasellar mass is a bitemporal hemianopsia.[17] This condition is usually asymmetric and may result in a variety of patterns, depending on the rapidity of tumor growth, the precise location of the optic chiasm with regard to the tumor, and the age and general health of the patient. The fundi are usually benign but may show signs of optic atrophy. Papilledema may occur but is generally a late sign that strongly suggests the presence of hydrocephalus secondary to the tumor extending posteriorly and superiorly into the third ventricle.

Although hormone overproduction may cause the patient to seek medical attention, in certain cases the lack of the effect of specific hormones may be the presenting symptom. The tumor may so compromise the remainder of the gland that panhypopituitarism develops. Similar phenomenona may occur with other mass lesions in the vicinity of the pituitary, including intracavernous carotid artery aneurysms, metastatic tumors, or infectious processes within the sella turcica.

The radiologic sine qua non of pituitary tumors is ballooning of the walls and thinning of the floor of the sella. If thinning of the floor is asymmetric, a double floor will be seen on lateral skull x-ray films, which virtually requires an intrasellar mass lesion to be present (Fig. 56-8). Generally sellar enlargement caused by mass lesions can easily be differentiated from the sellar enlargement associated with increased intracranial pressure. However, since pituitary tumors can cause increased intracranial pressure by obstructing the normal flow of CSF, the cause of sellar changes as seen on x-ray films may occasionally be quite difficult. Furthermore, as pituitary tumors increase in size, the sella may become so distorted that it is virtually impossible to differentiate the underlying cause of the lesion. Skull x-ray films may give other hints as to cause of the sellar mass lesion. The typical calcifications of carotid artery aneurysms, tumors such as meningiomas and craniopharyngiomas, or the destructive lesions associated with infections or malignancies are well described. Nonetheless, histologic differentiation of pituitary tumors is generally not apparent from viewing the sella turcica.

CT scanning has revolutionized intracranial imaging (see Figs. 56-6 and 56-7) (Fig. 56-9). With 1-mm sectioning of the sellar and parasellar regions, the stalk of the pituitary and basilar artery can be seen routinely. Using this technology, microtumors can often be visualized, and their location within the gland can be predicted. Although CT investigation is clearly valuable in diagnosing certain tumor types, its major benefit to the surgeon is in planning surgical strategies. Thus, before surgical intervention in the patient with a pituitary lesion, CT of the sella, sphenoid sinuses, and suprasellar tissues is required since other

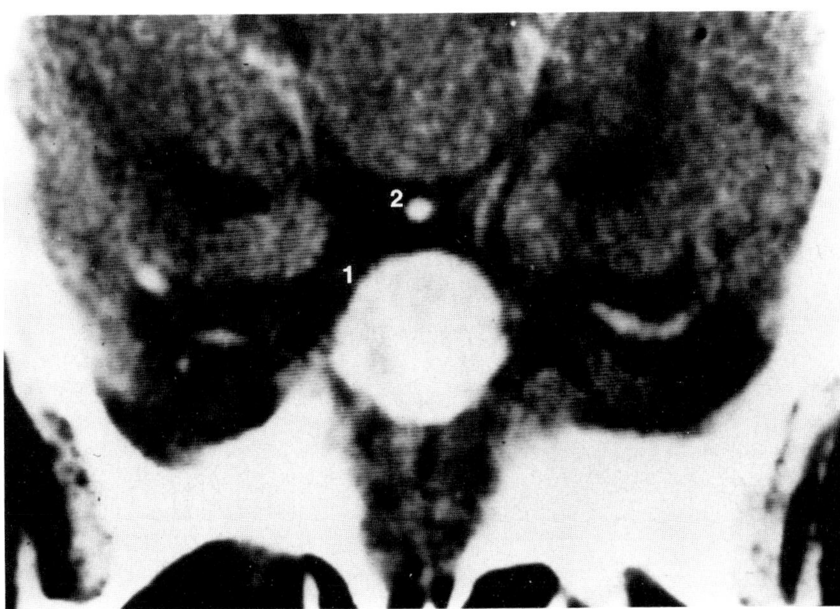

Fig. 56-9 Contrast enhanced computed tomogram demonstrating a large pituitary tumor *(1)* and its relationship to the basilar artery *(2)*.

parasellar structures can be invaded by pituitary tumors. Lateral extension into the sphenoid sinuses with thrombosis of the sinuses or pressure on the cranial nerves can occur, even though this is rare. Posterior and superior extension affects the optic chiasm and can push the brainstem backward and involve the basilar artery. More commonly, suprasellar extension occurs with invagination into the third ventricle, compression of the hypothalamus and, ultimately, blockage of the cerebral aqueduct with subsequent hydrocephalus.

Growth Hormone–Secreting Tumors. A pituitary tumor producing excessive amounts of growth hormone results in gigantism in prepubertal patients and in acromegaly if secretion continues after the epiphyses of the long bones are closed. There have also been reports of patients with acromegaly associated with extrapituitary tumors, particularly carcinoids of the lung, with regression of the acromegalic features upon removal of the tumor.[19,80] Evidence suggests that these extremely rare, nonpituitary tumors do not actually release growth hormone itself, but rather a growth hormone–releasing factor. Whether growth hormone–secreting tumors of the pituitary arise de novo or as a response to an imbalance between growth hormone–releasing and inhibiting factors from the hypothalamus is still speculative. However, increasing knowledge concerning the interplay physiologically between the hypothalamus and the pituitary strongly suggests that a primary hypothalamic disorder may in fact induce the development of growth hormone–secreting tumors.

The syndromes of gigantism and acromegaly are not difficult to distinguish clinically and have virtually no differential diagnosis in their full-blown expression. Before closure of the epiphyses of the long bones, gigantism ensues; other than stature, gigantism has many of the features of acromegaly. Gigantism secondary to excessive growth hormone production can be mistaken for cerebral gigantism, but in the latter situation there is no enlargement of the pituitary gland, the height is generally not as extreme, and it does not, of course, progress to acromegaly. In rare instances acromegaly could be mistaken for pachydermoperiostosis, a rare form of inherited hypertropic osteoarthropathy.

The term acromegaly originally was used to denote the striking changes in the acral portions of the body. In this condition there is certainly a "tufting" of the terminal phalanges that is quite characteristic on x-ray films. However, the hands and feet are also large and have a particular doughy feel to them. Often a handshake with the patient will call into suspicion the diagnosis of acromegaly. On x-ray film examination there is clear prognathism of the mandible, and the paranasal air sinuses are markedly enlarged (Fig. 56-10). Marked overgrowth of the supraorbital rim creating disfigurement to the face is frequently present. The excessive growth of the jaw, nose, and orbital ridge, with relative sparing of the remainder of the facial bones, results in a very characteristic facies. It is this grotesque appearance that often brings the patient to the physician; however, because these facial changes slowly evolve over many years, they may be quite extreme before the patient realizes the marked alterations that have occurred. These changes are often noticed by someone who has not seen the patient in many years or on reviewing an old photograph. It is striking how significant the facial appearance can become before the patient is truly aware of it.

In approximately 50% of patients with acromegaly there is also a myopathy that is most marked in the proximal musculature. Serum enzymes characteristic of muscle dysfunction are usually normal as are muscle biopsies, except for a general hypertrophy of individual muscle fibers. The carpal tunnel syndrome is commonly associated with acromegaly and has the expected characteristics of numbness and weakness in the distribution of the median nerve. This syndrome may be secondary to encroachment of the carpal

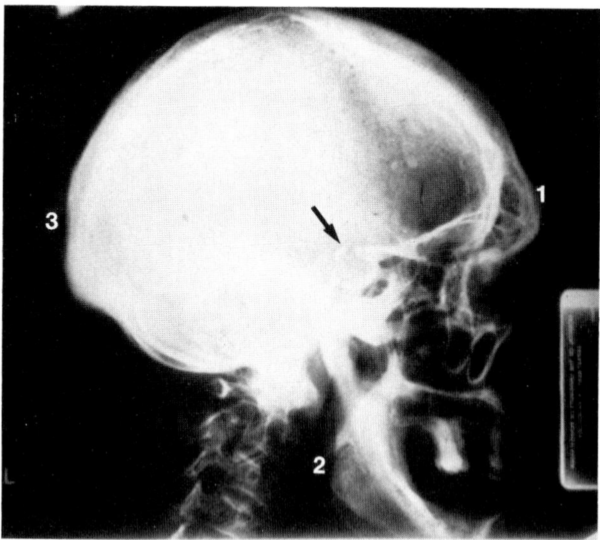

Fig. 56-10 Lateral skull x-ray film of a patient with acromegaly. Note the large frontal sinuses *(1)*, enlarged sella turcica with erosion of the dorsum sella *(arrow)*, prominent mandible *(2)*, and generalized thickening of the calvarium *(3)*.

bones and soft tissues on the median nerve and involvement of the nerve by a hypertrophic neuropathy or by primary changes in nerve metabolism. Quite possibly all of these factors play a role in its development. It is striking how rapidly this problem improves with appropriate therapy to reduce the growth hormone levels.

A generalized thickening of the subcutaneous tissues characteristically occurs in patients with acromegaly. A heel pad thickness of greater than 25 mm is characteristic. Of patients with acromegaly, 80% or more complain of hyperhidrosis and a distinctive oiliness of the skin. Many patients with acromegaly also complain of a dull throbbing headache that apparently is secondary to distortion of the diaphragm of the sella turcica or stretching of the nearby large blood vessels.

The spine on x-ray film examination has a striking demineralization, osteophytic formation, and loss of disk space height in acromegalic patients. Whether this is true osteoporosis is a subject of debate since the incidence of compression fractures in these patients does not appear to be strikingly increased over the normal population. The abdominal viscera are also diffusely enlarged in these patients. Kidney, liver, and spleen enlargement are the rule.

The most serious clinical abnormality in acromegaly is that frank diabetes mellitus develops in approximately 25% of patients and another 50% have prediabetic glucose intolerance. Their diabetes is frequently resistant to insulin, presumably because of an alteration in insulin receptors by growth hormone. Associated with the diabetes mellitus is a striking incidence of hypertension, atherosclerosis, and congestive heart failure, in addition to a high incidence of primary cardiomegaly. Indeed, the most common cause of death in patients with acromegaly is myocardial infarction. This high incidence of myocardial infarction necessitates aggressive care in acromegaly and emphasizes the life-threatening potential of this disease.

Patients with acromegaly may be quite large and appear very strong, but in fact they are generally easily fatigued and frequently have decreased thyroid, adrenocortical, and gonadotropic hormonal levels because of the adverse mass effects of the growth hormone tumor on other portions of the pituitary responsible for the secretion of these hormones. The thyroid is enlarged in as many as 25% of these patients, presumably because of the decreased blood levels of TSH. Gonadotropic hormones are commonly reduced in concentration with resultant impotence in males and menstrual irregularities in females. Serum and organic phosphate levels may be increased secondary to defective growth hormone effects on renal tubular secretion.

The syndrome of multiple endocrine neoplasia is associated with growth hormone–secreting adenomas, prolactin and nonfunctioning adenomas of the pituitary, parathyroid adenomas, and islet cell tumors of the pancreas, including insulinomas and gastrinomas. Thus the usual clinical abnormalities in acromegalic patients can be compounded by the hypersecretion of parathyroid hormone, insulin, and gastrin.

Prolactin-Secreting Tumors. Prolactinoma is the most common type of pituitary tumor that comes to medical attention. This is in contrast to what existed two decades ago because of the better diagnostic capabilities of the endocrinologist and radiologist that presently exist. Approximately one third of all pituitary tumors secrete increased amounts of prolactin; however, a serum prolactin level above 260 ng/ml is required for a diagnosis of prolactinoma to be made.[1,95]

Of patients with prolactin-secreting tumors, only a third will actually have galactorrhea.[38] To add to the confusion, galactorrhea is not necessarily related to the magnitude of the serum prolactin concentration. Furthermore, patients with galactorrhea and increased prolactin serum levels may not have a prolactin-secreting tumor. Rather, a tumor that is impinging on the hypothalamus and inhibiting the release of prolactin-inhibiting factor may mimic the clinical syndrome caused by a prolactin-secreting tumor. Thus the Forbes-Albright syndrome, originally describing galactorrhea, specifically refers only to women with amenorrhea and galactorrhea secondary to a pituitary tumor.[11]

Although hyperprolactinemia is classically associated with galactorrhea, irregular menses, and anovulation, it should be clear that the syndrome is truly a spectrum ranging from normal menstruation to total amenorrhea, no ovulatory cycle, and galactorrhea. In men the spectrum ranges from no clinical manifestations at all through galactorrhea with changes in libido, oligospermia, and occasionally gynecomastia. Fortunately the successful treatment of hyperprolactinemia commonly restores fertility and cures the galactorrhea. The normal prolactin level is approximately 20 ng/ml. When patients with galactorrhea or infertility have increased prolactin levels, they should be evaluated for a prolactin-secreting pituitary tumor.

Cushing's Disease. There are several causes of Cushing's syndrome, but Cushing's disease refers to that spectrum of the syndrome in which signs and symptoms result from an ACTH-dependent hyperplasia of the adrenal cortex.[96] It is currently felt that Cushing's disease is a primary hypothalamic disorder rather than one that arises in the pituitary itself.[37] However, the adenomas resulting from the excessive production of the ACTH-releasing factor may over time become independent of hypothalamic control. The clinical manifestations of Cushing's syndrome are secondary to hypercortisolism, but hypercortisolism may be caused by a primary disorder of the adrenal cortex; a lesion of the hypothalamus or pituitary may not be necessary for hypercortisolism. Thus, since the clinical findings in patients with Cushing's syndrome, whether caused by an abnormality in the pituitary gland, hypothalamus, or adrenal cortex, are the same. However, defining the specific cause of hypercortisolism is especially important because treatment is strikingly different.

Perhaps the most common complaint of patients with Cushing's syndrome is weakness and fatigue. Patients with this disease are generally obese with significant loss of muscle mass. Their obesity is particularly pronounced in the trunk and minimal in the extremities. They have a characteristic moon-shaped appearance to their face and a dorsal kyphosis with a "buffalo hump" comprised of subcutaneous fatty tissue over the upper thoracic spine. Their hirsutism, ruddy complexion, ease of bruising, purple stria, and centripetal fat distribution make the diagnosis classic. At least three fourths of these patients have hypertension and diabetes mellitus. Further, they have calcium wasting that results from demineralization of their bones and an associated increased incidence of long bone and spine fractures.

The diagnosis of Cushing's syndrome can frequently be made on first evaluation of the patient. However, the underlying cause may be significantly more difficult to define. In addition to pituitary hyperplasia and adenomas, multiple other causes must be considered. Adrenocortical adenomas, adrenocortical carcinoma, and ectopic ACTH secretion by nonpituitary tumors, especially carcinoma of the lung, must be included in the differential diagnosis. Other tumors such as carcinoma of the thymus, pancreas, and bronchial carcinoids may also secrete ACTH and cause Cushing's syndrome. Thus a thorough investigation of these patients is required. Differentiation of Cushing's disease from other causes of Cushing's syndrome can generally be accomplished by endocrinologic investigation. For a comprehensive discussion of the pathophysiology of Cushing's syndrome and its differential diagnosis, see Chapter 57.

Nelson's Syndrome. Nelson's syndrome is characterized by excessive production of ACTH in combination with beta-melanocyte–stimulating hormone.[47,49,65] This disease may occur because of an ACTH-secreting pituitary tumor developing after bilateral adrenalectomy. However, it is more likely that Nelson's syndrome is a continuum of an untreated Cushing's disease. The striking feature in these patients is the dark skin pigmentation that may occur over relatively short periods of time. Unfortunately the pituitary tumors in these patients are often quite large and are particularly difficult to surgically remove.[45,62]

TSH, FSH, and LH-Secreting Tumors. TSH- and FSH-secreting tumors are rare neoplasms that produce the characteristic radiologic changes in the sella turcica similar to other pituitary tumors and the expected secondary hormonal effects on the respective target organs. Approximately 20 patients have been identified with either a primary gonadotropin-secreting or thyrotropin-secreting pituitary tumor. Their manifestations and treatment are similar to those that would be expected from an overproduction of TSH or FSH. A tumor that secretes only LH has not been identified.

Treatment of Pituitary Tumors. The treatment of pituitary tumors historically quickly followed the recognition of the clinical syndromes associated with such lesions and the characterization of these lesions on plain skull x-ray films. The successful removal of pituitary tumors is one of the earlier neurosurgical procedures that found acceptance. Currently, however, the appropriate treatment of pituitary tumors is a much more individualized decision. With a clearer understanding of the clinical correlates of pituitary dysfunction and the advent of more sophisticated neuroradiologic and endocrinologic evaluation techniques, extremely small tumors are being recognized. Coincident with these advances in diagnosis have been similar advances in medical and surgical management of these tumors. We now have the ability to decrease hormonal hypersecretion by the pituitary in various disease states and to perform safer, more effective surgical therapy. Furthermore, the capability of detecting "subclinical" tumors has necessitated the continued reassessment of which patients need any treatment at all. At the other end of the spectrum are tumors that behave invasively and therefore make complete surgical extirpation necessary but potentially hazardous. The role of radiotherapy is still controversial even after 75 years of experience with this treatment modality. Clearly there is real justification for the controversy regarding the optimal treatment of pituitary tumors because in some cases there are two or more safe, effective treatment possibilities.[53] Although it could therefore be argued that medical and surgical therapy are each reasonable options in some cases, few patients would believe that decisions concerning the "risks" of surgery vs. the need to remain on indefinite medications were equivalent, but rather that such decisions require more than statistic judgment.

Medical Therapy

Medical therapy is directed at decreasing the hormonal hypersecretion of the tumor. Generally its usefulness has only been clearly demonstrated in the treatment of prolactinomas and growth hormone–secreting tumors. There is evidence with both of these tumors that dopamine agonists cause morphologic regression of the tumor while on treatment. L-DOPA inhibits growth hormone secretion in most acromegalic patients, but the effect is short-lived.[6] In contrast, bromocryptine (2-bromo-alpha-ergocryptine), an agent that binds to dopamine receptors, has been demonstrated to suppress growth hormone levels for 6 to 12 hours after a single dose. Although the response to prolonged administration is rapid, growth hormone levels continue to fall for several weeks with a maximum response evident at approximately 8 to 12 weeks.[12] The overall response is clearly dose dependent. The site of action of bromocriptine appears to be at the level of the pituitary gland rather than the hypothalamus. Long-term studies have shown bromocryptine to be effective in 70% to 80% of acromegalic patients in lowering the growth hormone levels to a normal range.[13] Improvement in glucose tolerance and cardiac function, reduction in soft tissue volume, improvement in facial appearance, amelioration of the symptoms of the carpal tunnel syndrome,[58] and a decrease in sweating have all been observed in conjunction with the decrease in growth hormone levels.[32,39,55] In fact, there have been a few reports of pituitary apoplexy (see below) occurring in patients taking bromocriptine.

Lergotrile mesylate has demonstrated effectiveness in reducing growth hormone levels in acromegaly; however, it is currently unavailable for clinical use because of the occurrence of genital tumors in animal studies in which the drug has been used.[23] Cyproheptadine and methysergide partially inhibit the normal growth hormone elevation observed with hypoglycemia, intravenous arginine infusion, and exercise. However, long-term data on their use to treat hormonally active growth hormone tumors are lacking. Somatostatin (hGH-inhibiting factor) has been used in experimental situations, and it does suppress hGH secretion in essentially all acromegalic patients. The question of toxicity (suppression of insulin and glucagon secretions and platelet dysfunction) also needs to be resolved before somatostatin can be considered for routine clinical use.

Prolactin secretion is principally controlled by inhibitory factors, of which dopamine is one of the more effective. As with growth hormone–secreting tumors, dopaminergic drugs would be expected to decrease prolactin secretion. Indeed, bromocryptine has been successful in controlling hyperprolactinemia in 80% to 90% of cases with a variety of causes, including prolactin-secreting tumors.[87,88] Such treatment results in cessation of galactorrhea in approximately 90% of patients and restores normal menstration in 80% to 90%.[34,77,81,82] The drug has the side effects of nausea, dyspepsia, headaches, postural hypotension, and occasionally depression or anxiety. Nausea and headaches are the most common patient complaints. Unfortunately, when the drug is withdrawn, the tumor once again expresses itself.

If medical therapy is to be used, bromocriptine is the current drug of choice for acromegalic patients, but 10% to 20% will not respond.[85,91] It is also the drug of choice for patients with prolactin-secreting tumors. The advantages of medical therapy in these conditions primarily center around not subjecting the patient to the risks of surgery, especially the risk of injury to the normal tissue in the pituitary when microtumors are present. An additional benefit may be that a period of treatment with bromocriptine makes surgical planes better defined and surgery therefore easier to perform. The major disadvantages to medical therapy are patient compliance, uncertain long-term untoward effects, possible untoward effects on the fetus (one of the common reasons patients with prolactinomas seek medical attention is infertility), and the concern that the tumor is perhaps not being followed closely.

Surgical Therapy

Two general surgical approaches to the sella turcica have been devised. These include an approach by means of craniotomy from above the optic chiasma[54] and an approach from below the sella turcica through the sphenoidal sinus.* The approach from above the pituitary entails either a frontal or temporal craniotomy and removal of the tumor through the diaphragm.[67] The safety of this approach depends primarily on the size of the tumor and the position of the chiasma. There is always some manipulation of the brain tissue, but the craniotomy approach does allow visualization of the third ventricle and a clear exposure of the structures surrounding the sella. However, it is frequently difficult to remove a tumor without removing the pituitary gland entirely. Further visualization within the sella turcica may be difficult.

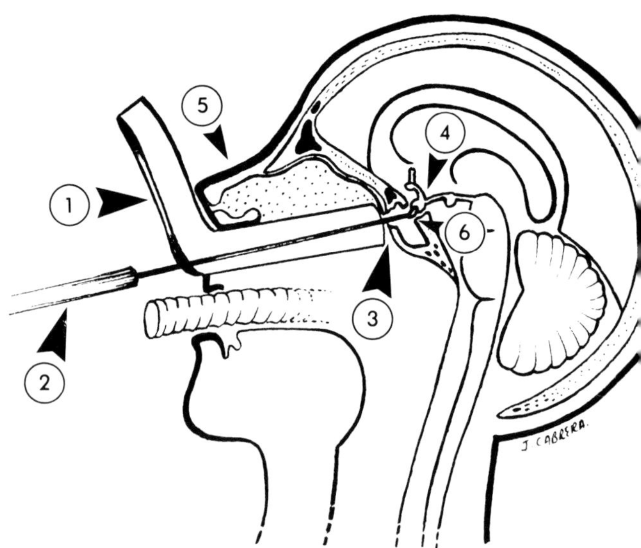

Fig. 56-11 Schematic representation of the transnasal, transseptal, transsphenoidal approach to the pituitary gland. *1,* Bivalve speculum in place; *2,* ring curette in the sella; *3,* open sphenoidal sinus; *4,* pituitary gland; *5,* resected nasal cartilage; and *6,* open sellar floor.

The transseptal, transsphenoid approach (Fig. 56-11) as originally devised was a very formidable surgical procedure.[46] However, with the use of the surgical microscope and detailed fluoroscopy, the technique has become part of the armamentarium of many neurosurgeons. The procedure has many advantages over the craniotomy approach. Obviously cerebral retraction and manipulation and potential damage to the olfactory nerves are eliminated. The need for blood transfusions is virtually eliminated, and patients generally feel better after surgery. However, the major advantage is that small tumors can be totally removed with preservation of the remaining pituitary gland, and the contents of the sella turcica can generally be well visualized. This technique is especially well suited for small tumors in the anterior lobe of the pituitary. Because the neurohypophysis can frequently be left intact, the incidence of diabetes insipidus following this procedure is quite small, and the need for long-term hormonal replacement is significantly reduced. With the advent of sophisticated CT of the sellar region, many tumors can be visualized within the gland, and decisions made before surgery as to precisely where to incise it to remove the tumor. The major disadvantage to the transsphenoidal approach lies in the inability to view the other side of the tumor. Specifically the optic chiasm cannot be visualized until the tumor is removed. Thus torrential bleeding could occur from injury to the ca-

*References 1, 3-5, 31, 40, 41, 52, 71, 84, 95, and 97.

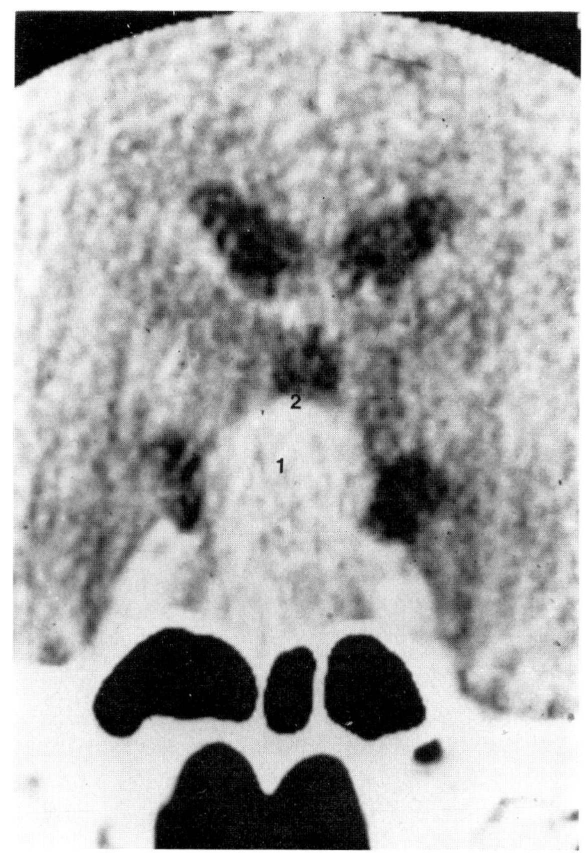

Fig. 56-12 Contrast-enhanced computed tomogram demonstrating suprasellar extension of a tumor *(1)*. Compression of the optic chiasm was present. Note encroachment of the tumor on the third ventricle *(2)* and presence of hydrocephalus.

rotid arteries, which may well be fatal. With the use of contrast enhancement of the carotid arteries on preoperative CT of the sphenoid sinus, the details of arterial anatomy can be defined and thereby greatly minimize the incidence of this complication.

Current experience with microsurgical procedures indicates that surgical excision of small tumors of the pituitary is a safe, effective treatment modality with a low complication rate.[25] Radiation therapy is also effective in these patients, and the choice between radiation therapy and surgery depends on the characteristics of the tumor, the expectation of the patient, and the experience of the physician. Radiation therapy is appropriate for small or medium-sized tumors with minimal suprasellar extension (Fig. 56-12), patients in whom surgery is refused or contraindicated, and as postoperative adjunctive therapy in patients with invasive or incompletely excised tumors. Radiotherapy may also be of benefit in treating some patients with a craniopharyngioma. This latter tumor is a benign, congenital neoplasm, usually suprasellar in position, and represents a secretory vestige of Rathke's pouch. It affects pituitary function by invading the gland and causing hypopituitarism.

As a sole therapy, radiation treatment is contraindicated in large tumors with suprasellar extension, patients with major visual field defects, acromegalics with serum hGH levels greater than 50 ng/ml before treatment, and in patients with prolactinomas who wish fertility restored. Approximately 5% of patients treated with radiotherapy can be expected to develop pituitary apoplexy, with the acute onset of severe headache, loss of vision, extraocular nerve palsies, and loss of consciousness. The long-term effects of radiation to the sellar region are not insignificant, especially with regard to vision. Radiotherapy is contraindicated in small children with pituitary and extrapituitary lesions because of the risk of small vessel occlusion resulting in visual disturbances and stroke.

In addition to the primary role of medical therapy in the treatment of acromegaly and prolactinomas, as discussed above, it may also be efficacious in these patients following surgery or radiotherapy.[51] Ten percent to 40% of patients with hGH-secreting tumors will continue to have persistent hGH elevations (more than 10 ng/ml) after surgery and/or radiation and continue to exhibit progression of their disease. In this circumstance, bromocriptine therapy has proven useful in decreasing growth hormone levels in the blood. Similarly in patients with persistent hyperprolactinemia following ablative surgery, bromocriptine has effectively suppressed serum prolactin and restored normal gonadal function in the majority of these individuals. Dosages of 2.5 to 10 mg daily by mouth are usually adequate for both acromegaly and prolactin-secreting tumors. Of note, bromocriptine may also produce tumor regression in some of these patients.

Pituitary Apoplexy

A sudden, unexpected, life-threatening hemorrhage can occur in pituitary tumors. This complication does not appear to be associated with a particular tumor type, and an obvious triggering event is not required. In autopsy studies, between 4.6% and 10% of patients with pituitary tumors have areas of hemorrhagic necrosis.[57,94] Wakai and associates[89] noted that, in over 9% of 560 patients with documented pituitary tumors, the initial presentation was a major or minor hemorrhage into the tumor. However, even though pituitary apoplexy has been associated with head trauma, mechanical ventilators, bromocriptine therapy, hypertension, and a variety of other conditions, it frequently occurs without a precipitating event.[9,21,22,89] In our present state of knowledge, the precise cause of this condition remains unclear.

The most common presenting signs and symptoms are sudden severe headache, loss of vision, nausea and vomiting, ocular disorders, fever, stiff neck, and almost invariably, an alteration in the state of consciousness. Obviously such a syndrome can easily be confused with fulminating meningitis or subarachnoid hemorrhage from other causes; however, in patients with known pituitary tumors, the diagnosis should always be suspected. Plain skull x-ray films or CT should increase the suspicion to virtual certainty in nearly all cases.

Pituitary apoplexy is such a life-threatening event that, once the diagnosis is made, treatment with high dosages of intravenous steroids should be immediately instituted. Plans to excise the tumor, preferably by means of the transseptal, transsphenoidal approach, need to be formulated on an emergent basis. Following surgery, specific hormone replacement therapy is initially given as though the pituitary were totally destroyed. However, with time and recovery of residual pituitary function, replacement therapy can be individualized to meet the precise needs of the patient.

Nontumorous Causes of Enlarged Sella Turcica

Although it is common to equate enlargement of the sella turcica with an expanding neoplasm, it can enlarge from several nontumorous causes:

1. Empty sella syndrome
   a. Primary
   b. Secondary
2. Carotid artery aneurysms
3. Arachnoid cyst
4. Granuloma
5. Increased intracranial pressure
6. Pseudotumor cerebri
7. Hydrocephalus

An empty sella is an abnormal extension of the subarachnoid space into the pituitary fossa. Although this is generally an incidental pathologic observation on radiologic evaluation, an empty sella may cause signs and symptoms if it leads to enlargement of the sella turcica and compression of the normal intrasellar contents. The primary type of empty sella results from a development defect of the diaphragm of the sella, allowing the arachnoid to herniate into the sella turcica. Secondary empty sella syndromes result from a similar process that occurs after the intrasellar contents have been destroyed by surgery, irradiation, or infarction.[7,33,43,60,70]

The typical patient with the primary empty sella syndrome is a middle-aged, multiparous, obese, hypertensive woman. The common presenting symptoms are frequently nonspecific and vague, but headache and fatigue are virtually ubiquitous. Although they are rare, suspicious findings are visual field disturbances suggesting herniation of the optic chiasm into the sella and CSF rhinorrhea.[8-10, 92] In the vast majority of cases no endocrine syndromes develop, but on occasion exceptions to this general rule have been reported.[64,72] Except in the rare situations noted above, the neurologic examination is entirely normal. No treatment is required for the patient with uncomplicated primary empty sella syndrome. Surgical treatment is needed, however, for CSF rhinorrhea and visual field defects. Usually the transphenoidal approach is sufficient, but on occasion craniotomy is required for "chiasmapexy" to relieve traction on the optic nerves.[55,93]

Secondary empty sella syndrome must always be considered when evaluating patients for recurrence of pituitary tumors after surgery or irradiation.[94] Impairment of vision may occur within a few months or several years after ablation of the intrasellar contents because of herniation of the optic chiasm into the sella. Exquisite CT of the sella or pneumoencephalography may be required to distinguish the diagnosis of an empty sella from tumor recurrence. Treatment may be needed for relief of chiasmal signs or CSF rhinorrhea as noted in the preceding paragraph.

Panhypopituitarism

Panhypopituitarism is characterized by decreased or absent function of the target organs stimulated by the pituitary hormones. It is expressed as insufficiency of the target organs rather than the pituitary gland. Signs and symptoms of the primary pituitary lesion such as bitemporal hemanopsia may be present, but more commonly it is the generalized endocrinopathy that brings patients to medical attention. Panhypopituitarism in its strictest sense refers to failure of all of the pituitary hormones, but, in fact, only adenohypophyseal failure usually occurs. Clearly panhypopituitarism should be viewed as a spectrum of disease with total pituitary failure at one end and multiple endocrinopathies at the other. Patients with "isolated" hormone deficits should be under suspicion for subclinical disorders, in the production of other hormones. The location of lesions that cause panhypopituitarism can also be viewed as a spectrum ranging from small isolated lesions of the hypothalamus to large destructive lesions of the hypothalamopituitary system. The boxed material above lists the various lesions frequently associated with panhypopituitarism.

The clinical findings of panhypopituitarism will naturally vary with the degree of pituitary dysfunction and are related to the diminished function of the target organs. Patients complain of generalized fatigue and weakness and have a particular lack of resistance to cold weather and fasting, reflecting abnormalities in thyroid and adrenal gland function. They are frequently small in stature with reduced bone age compared to their chronologic age. Their skin is remarkably pale and dry. They tend to have a low blood pressure and are commonly troubled by orthostatic hypotension. Amenorrhea and galactorrhea in women and impotence in men are reflections of diminished gonadotrophic hormone function. A lack, or even regression, of secondary sexual characteristics is common. Mental retardation is associated with pituitary failure occurring early in life. In addition to the effects of the primary lesion,

CAUSES OF PANHYPOPITUITARISM

Hypothalamic-Pituitary Disorders

Organic
- Congenital: hypophyseal infantilism
- Traumatic: basilar skull fractures
- Inflammatory: granulomas
- Degenerative: irradiation
- Vascular: Sheehan's syndrome
  - Pituitary necrosis secondary to systemic hypotension in postpartum period
- Simmond's disease: hypophyseal cachexia
- Neoplastic: large pituitary adenomas
- Surgical hypophysectomy

Functional
- Medications: hormonal replacement
- Systemic disease
- Endocrinopathies: primary thyroditis, adrenal dysfunction, and diabetes mellitus
- Extreme malnutrition

Extrasellar Structural Disorders

Neoplastic: craniopharyngioma, meningiomas and metastatic lung malignancies
Vascular: carotid aneurysms invading the sella
Trauma: severe intracranial pressure

REPLACEMENT THERAPY FOR PITUITARY INSUFFICIENCY

CHRONIC PITUITARY INSUFFICIENCY	
ACTH	25 mg cortisone acetate or 5 mg prednisone daily in two divided doses
	Additional steroids as required for physiologic stress such as injury, surgery, or infection
Thyroid	100 to 200 μg L-thryroxine daily as a single dose
Gonadotropin	Males: Testosterone 12 to 15 mg intramuscularly every 2 weeks
	Females: Ethinyl estradiol 10 to 15 μg/day, or standard estrogen-progesterone regimen as for birth control
Growth hormone	Only considered in pediatric age group
Prolactin	No replacement required
REPLACEMENT THERAPY AFTER PITUITARY SURGERY	
Steroids	Cortisone acetate 50 mg every 6 hours
	Tapering dosage after 5 days except in patients with Cushing's disease
	May require chronic replacement
Thyroid	If normal thyroid function before surgery, no replacement
	If abnormal before surgery, Synthroid (thyroxine) 0.1-0.15 μg daily
Persistent prolactinemia	Reoperation or bromocriptine
REPLACEMENT FOR LIFE-THREATENING PITUITARY FAILURE	
Hydrocortisone or cortisone 100 to 300 mg/day intravenously thryroxine 200 μg/day	

patients with panhypopituitarism are physiologically fragile and may develop overwhelming fever, cardiovascular shock, coma, and death as a result of relatively minor stressful situations.

The evaluation of panhypopituitarism is made primarily on the basis of clinical suspicion, assessment of endocrinologic function, and determination of the specific cause of the pituitary failure. Because hypopituitarism generally develops insidiously and may escape detection for years, its diagnosis will depend on a high index of suspicion. Thus patients who are unusually fatigued, appear to be aging more rapidly than is suggested by their chronologic age, have unexplained imbalances in body temperature regulation, and are unable to respond to infection or stress in an appropriate manner should be considered possible candidates for hypopituitarism and endocrinologically evaluated for this disorder.

The demonstration of a low level of hormone secreted by a pituitary target organ in the presence of a low level of pituitary trophic hormone is strongly suggestive of hypothalamic or pituitary dysfunction. Patients with panhypopituitarism have the expected limited ACTH reserve on Metopirone (metyrapone) testing; radioactive iodine uptake is depressed in the thyroid gland but increases following exogenous thyrotrophic hormone administration; urinary 17-ketosteroids and hydroxycorticosteroids, as well as cortisol, are low but slowly rise after ACTH administration; and growth hormone assay yields low levels with little response to stimulation with insulin, hypoglycemia, arginine infusion, or L-DOPA administration. Of course, the pituitary trophic hormone levels are also depressed. As a single test, the most useful aid in diagnosing panhypopituitarism is measurement of serum thyroxine. Virtually all patients with pituitary deficiency will be found to have low values of this hormone. If serum thyroxine is normal, it is highly unlikely that hypopituitarism exists.

The diagnosis of the specific cause of panhypopituitarism rests primarily on the results of x-ray film evaluation of the sella turcica and the measurement of serum levels of the various pituitary hormones both under basal conditions and after administration of the specific hypothalamic releasing factors or stimulation of the endogenous hypothalamic hormone. Treatment is aimed at the primary cause if possible. However, endocrine substitution must be used as soon as the diagnosis of panhypopituitarism is made and continued through the treatment period or, in some cases, permanently. With the exception of corticotropin, there is no available effective pituitary replacement preparation, and therapy must therefore aim at correction of the end-organ deficiencies. Virtually complete hormone replacement can be obtained for the corticosteroids, thyroid hormones, and sex steroids. Growth hormone replacement is generally not practical. The boxed material above outlines replacement needs for acute pituitary failure that may occur after pituitary surgery or immediately after pituitary apoplexy, chronic replacement required for patients with chronic panhypopituitarism, and emergency treatment of acute life-threatening hypopituitarism.

The prognosis for patients with panhypopituitarism depends on the specific cause of the disorder, the duration of the disorder, the age of the patient at onset, and the secondary effects that have occurred before the initiation of treatment. For example, patients suffering pituitary apoplexy may recover spontaneously and only require short-term therapy. In contrast, patients having more chronic forms of hypopituitarism will often require prolonged treatment with replacement hormones normally secreted by target organs that have been adversely affected by the pituitary dysfunction. If pituitary function never recovers, this therapy will of necessity be lifelong. These individuals will need to be under the constant care of a physician skilled in the management of panhypopituitarism, and both patient and doctor alike will need to be prepared to manage the potentially disasterous consequences that may occur from the common stresses of life such as relatively minor episodes of starvation, infection, or trauma.

ADH Abnormalities

Diabetes Insipidus

Diabetes insipidus results from either a decrease in secretion of ADH or a decreased responsiveness to ADH by the renal tubular apparatus of the nephron of the kidney. The diagnosis should be suspected in an individual who excretes unusually large volumes of urine of low osmolality. Nocturia and nighttime thirst are often the first manifestations. The serum osmolality may be only slightly elevated, particularly if the patient drinks enough water in response to thirst. However, in those patients whose thirst mechanism is either deficient or who cannot satisfy their thirst, diabetes insipidus can quickly lead to its full-blown effects: severe dehydration, hypovolemia, serum hyperosmolality, fever, hyperpnea, stupor, coma, and even death. These changes can take place in a remarkably short period of time.

To distinguish primary diabetes insipidus from that arising from a lack of responsiveness of the nephron to ADH, proof that the kidney can conserve water is obtained.[73] This is accomplished by injecting ADH (i.e., 5 pressor units) either subcutaneously or intravenously, and measuring effects on urinary output. The expected response in an intact kidney is a decrease in the urine volume and an increase in urine osmolality and specific gravity within 30 to 60 minutes. In less severe situations the ability to conserve water can be determined by water deprivation for 6 to 8 hours. In normal individuals the urine osmolality will increase to greater than the serum osmolality, and the urine specific gravity to greater than 1.015, without a significant change in serum osmolality. Radioimmunoassays are available for ADH but are not usually necessary to establish the diagnosis, except in those cases in which it appears to be the renal tubules that are not responding properly to adequate concentrations of ADH in the serum. The normal ADH level is 2.7 + 1.4 pg/ml.

Familial or congenital diabetes insipidus is a rare disorder that comes to medical attention in infancy or early childhood. Both sexes are affected. It appears to be the result of a failure of development of the supraoptic nucleus of the hypothalamus. This circumstance results in a reduction in the size of the posterior pituitary gland. This condition must be distinguished from congenital nephrogenic diabetes insipidus, which is a consequence of an inherited defect in renal tubular responsiveness to ADH.

Posttraumatic diabetes insipidus (i.e., from head trauma) may be a part of panhypopituitarism or an "isolated" abnormality of pituitary function. Fortunately many cases are transient and incomplete but require treatment for short periods of time. Tumors may infiltrate the stalk of the pituitary from above as in the case of astrocytomas of the third ventricle or from below as in the case of lymphomas or leukemic infiltrates. Small circumscribed granulomas and pyogenic meningitides may similarly result in diabetes insipidus. Sarcoidosis is the most common type of granulomatous disease that results in diabetes insipidus. Virtually any metastatic tumor or infectious agent can lodge in the infundibulum or upper pituitary stalk; however, carcinoma of the lung is particularly notorious in this regard.

Vascular lesions, either carotid aneurysms within the cavernous sinus or pituitary necrosis secondary to hypotension (Sheehan's postpartum necrosis), may cause diabetes insipidus presumably because of vascular insufficiency to the upper pituitary stalk. Obviously surgical interventions in the region of the pituitary or hypophysectomy for tumor or pain relief can result in diabetes insipidus that may be permanent or transient. The frequency of diabetes insipidus following pituitary surgery depends in great measure on the level of the stalk section; (i.e., the higher the level of section the greater the chances of diabetes insipidus).[20] Idiopathic causes of diabetes insipidus continue to account for approximately half of all cases of this syndrome. If the cause for diabetes insipidus is not readily apparent after diagnosis, it is unusual to ultimately identify one precisely.

The management of patients with diabetes insipidus must, of course, be individualized. The person most responsible for the patient's long-term management is the patient himself. Each patient should be aware of the symptoms of diabetes insipidus, especially the potential for electrolyte imbalance and dehydration. He needs to establish a method of recording urine output and measuring urine specific gravity. Diabetes insipidus is not an all-or-none phenomenon but rather varies in severity from one individual to another. Many patients can be directed to be especially conscious of their own thirst and can be managed with minimum or no medications. Chlorpropamide in oral dosages of 100 to 200 mg/day or hydrochlorthiazide in dosages of 50 to 100 mg/day are effective regimens to control polyuria in the milder forms of the disorder. These oral agents paradoxically control diabetes insipidus by stimulating renal medullary adenylate cyclase and inhibiting renal prostaglandin synthetase and renal phosphodiesterase. Each of these effects augments the response to ADH in the renal collecting duct and overshadows the expected diuretic effect of these agents. Frequently encouraging intermittent medication with these drugs and allowing the patient to control the dosage are the most successful methods of treatment.

If the oral drugs are not sufficient, one of the forms of ADH becomes necessary. ADH can be administered in a variety of ways, but unfortunately it is not available in an oral preparation. Aqueous ADH (vasopressin) (20 IU/ml) is a partially purified extract of neurohypophysis. Since its effect after subcutaneous injection is short-lived (i.e., approximately 2 hours), it is used in crisis situations or acute onset diabetes insipidus such as is encountered after surgical procedures on the pituitary gland. It is also an excellent medication in those situations in which there may be vacillation in the production of endogenous ADH and diabetes insipidus is thought to be a transient situation (e.g., the patient with mild head injury).

In the situation in which diabetes insipidus will be permanent, a longer-acting ADH preparation is needed. Vasopressin tannate in oil (5 IU/ml) is such a preparation. This substance is a tannic acid salt of partially purified vasopressin suspended in oil for delayed absorption and thus provides a longer effect. Patients generally require intramuscular injections every 3 to 4 days with this preparation. This regimen is not the favorite among patients needing long-term treatment because of the pain of intramuscular injection. Lysine 8-vasopressin nasal spray contains 50 IU/ml and provides good control of symptoms in most patients but only lasts for 3 to 4 hours. Therefore it is usually used in conjunction with some other regimen for "fine tuning." D,D, arginine vasopressin is a synthetic analog of arginine vasopressin that can be taken by nasal insufflation. The dosage can be controlled by the patient, and it is frequently sufficient as a sole medication. However, the most important variable in treating chronic diabetes mellitus is the patient himself. In most situations undertreatment with medications and reliance on matching of urine output with intravenous fluids in the acute situation and volume replacement on the basis of the patient's thirst in the chronic situation is superior to the control of diabetes insipidus of solely with ADH administration.[83]

Inappropriate Secretion of ADH

The syndrome of inappropriate ADH secretion (SIADH), the Schwartz-Bartter syndrome, is a relatively common disorder associated with a wide variety of clinical situations.[24,76] Symptoms occur because of the dilutional hyponatremia that results from inappropriate and excessive retention of water.[69] It derives its name because the signs, symptoms, and results from laboratory experiments are similar to those produced experimentally by chronic ADH administration.

The pathophysiology of SIADH is complex and seemingly paradoxic because of the excessive water retention and dilutional hyponatremia in the face of high sodium excretion in the urine. Because renal clearance is not depressed, nitrogenous waste products are adequately cleared, and blood urea and creatinine remain at normal levels. The patients have the same signs and symptoms as would be expected from extreme hyponatremia or water intoxication. In patients with previous neurologic disorders, the clinical abnormalities may appear at moderate levels of hyponatremia. On the other hand, in patients in whom the disorder is slowly evolving, extreme levels of hyponatremia may develop before the onset of symptoms. In general, symptoms do not develop until the serum sodium falls to 120 to 125 mEq/L. Early symptoms are anorexia, nausea, vomiting, lethargy, and irritability. Subtle personality changes, inattentiveness, and forgetfulness may progress to paranoia and delusions. As the disorder progresses and the serum sodium levels fall to 100 to 110 mEq/L, the neurologic manifestations become more severe and include stupor, coma, and intractable generalized seizures.

The list of disorders associated with SIADH is quite long but they can be categorized as follows: excessive secretion of ADH from hypothalamic disorders, excessive secretion of ADH secondary to other diseases, excessive production of ADH from nonhypothalamic sites (ectopic ADH production), and SIADH associated with a variety of medications. It stands to reason that hypothalamic disorders such as tumors, trauma, or infarcts might result in SIADH. However, acute intermittent porphyria, myxedema, subarachnoid hemorrhage and many metabolic encephalopathies are associated with SIADH as well. Cerebral hemispheric infarcts and subdural hematomas along the convexities of the brain are also associated with a high incidence of SIADH. Simply lying in the recumbent position appears to be a cause of SIADH, but in general SIADH should be thought of as a disorder secondary to some other abnormality. SIADH is associated with a variety of pulmonary lesions, especially tumors and tuberculosis. Many drugs including vincristine, chlorpropamide, chlorpromazine, and carbamazepine are also associated with SIADH. Thus the possible causes of SIADH are great, and all patients with low serum sodium should have SIADH in their differential diagnosis.

Treatment is primarily by strict water restriction (e.g., 400 to 600 ml/day). This regimen is generally all that is needed in patients in whom the disorder is mild or moderate. After the serum sodium has recovered to normal, in most patients fluid intake can be liberalized without SIADH relapsing. However, serious brain disturbances demand urgent treatment with hypertonic saline and fluid restriction. Corticosteroids and anticonvulsants may be indicated in extreme cases. A major diuretic such as furosemide may also be needed. In extreme cases the outlook may be very grave, but incredible neurologic recoveries have been reported with prompt, aggressive care.

SUMMARY

Although the pituitary gland has long been recognized as an important endocrine organ, its role as the grand orchestrator in mediating or modulating virtually every major metabolic process in the body has only become appreciated in the last 20 years as information concerning the mechanisms underlying the synthesis and release of its eight hormones has unfolded. The ability to safely and conveniently totally replace these hormones or those secreted by their target organs has allowed physicians to increase the possibilities of treating a wide variety of pituitary dysfunctions. The future for the further understanding of pituitary disorders, both on a fundamental and therapeutic level, is exciting. New noninvasive imaging techniques such as magnetic resonance are being explored and may offer a different way to evaluate the sella and parasellar anatomy. In addition, safer and more effective medical regimens for treatment may allow further definition concerning the precise indications for surgery. With this explosion in knowledge relating to the physiology of the pituitary, the patient with dysfunction of this gland has many possible treatment alternatives that were not heretofore available. The challenge in management is for each patient to be seen as a unique opportunity for individualized care and to enlist the cooperative skills of endocrinologists, surgeons, and radiation therapists to provide the most rational and optimal therapy.

REFERENCES

1. Aubourg, P.R., et al.: Endocrine outcome after transsphenoidal adenomectomy for prolactinoma: prolactin levels and tumor size as predicting factors, Surg. Neurol. **14:**141, 1980.
2. Babinski, J.: Tumeur du corps pituitaire sans acromegalie et avec arret de development des organes genitaux, Rev. Neurol. **8:**531, 1900.
3. Balagura, S., Derome, P., and Guiot, G.: Acromegaly: analysis of 132 cases treated surgically, Neurosurgery **8:**413, 1981.
4. Baskin, D.S., Boggan, J.E., and Wilson, C.B.: Transspenoidal microsurgical removal of growth hormone-secreting pituitary tumors: a review of 137 cases, J. Neurosurg. **56:**634, 1982.

5. Belopavlovic, M.: Transfrontal pituitary surgery: clinical results, intraoperative management and postoperative monitoring, Acta Neurochir. **64**:9, 1982.
6. Boyd, A.E., Lebovitz, H.E., and Pfeizzer, J.B.: Stimulation of human-growth-hormone secretion by L-DOPA, N. Engl. J. Med. **283**:1425, 1970.
7. Brisman, R., et al.: The empty sella syndrome-intrasellar cisternal herniation-in "normal" patients and in patients with communicating hydrocephalus and intracranial tumors, Neuroradiology **17**:35, 1978.
8. Brisman, R., Hughes, J.E.O., and Mount, L.A.: Cerebrospinal fluid rhinorrhea and the empty sella, J. Neurosurg. **31**:538, 1969.
9. Broughan, M., Heusner, A.P., and Adams, R.D.: Acute degenerative changes in adenomas of the pituitary body with special reference to pituitary apoplexy, J. Neurosurg. **7**:421, 1950.
10. Buckman, M.T., et al.: Primary empty sella syndrome with visual field defects, Am. J. Med. **61**:124, 1976.
11. Chang, R.J., et al.: Detection, evaluation, and treatment of pituitary microadenomas in patients with galactorrhea and amenorrhea, Am. J. Obstet. Gynecol. **128**:356, 1977.
12. Chiodini, P.G., et al.: Stable reduction of plasma growth hormone (hGH) during chronic administration of 2-Br-α-ergocriyptine (CB-154) in acromegalic patients, J. Clin. Endocrinol. Metab. **40**:795, 1975.
13. Corenblum, B.: Bromocryptine in pituitary tumors, Lancet **2**:786, 1978.
14. Costello, R.T.: Subclinical adenoma of the pituitary gland, Am. J. Pathol. **12**:205, 1936.
15. Cuse, S.A., and Kernohan, J.W.: Squamous cell nests of the pituitary gland, Cancer **8**:623, 1955.
16. Cushing, H.: Surgical experiences with pituitary disorders, JAMA **63**:1515, 1914.
17. Cushing, H.: Pituitary Body, Hypothalamus and Parasympathetic Nervous System, Springfield, Ill., 1932, Charles C Thomas, Publisher.
18. Cushing, H.: "Dyspituitarism": twenty years later. Arch. Intern. Med. **51**:487, 1933.
19. Dabek, J.T.: Bronchial carcinoid tumor with acromegaly in two patients, J. Clin. Endocrinol. **38**:329, 1974.
20. Daniel, P.M., and Prichard, M.M.L.: Human hypothalamus and pituitary stalk after hypophysectomy or pituitary stalk section, Brain **95**:813, 1972.
21. Daniel, P.M., Spicer, E.J.F., and Triep, C.S.: Pituitary necrosis in patients maintained on mechanical respirators, J. Pathol. **111**:135, 1973.
22. Dawson, B.H., and Kothandaram, P.: Acute massive infarction of pituitary adenomas: a study of five patients, J. Neurosurg. **37**:275, 1972.
23. Delitala, G., et al.: Growth hormone and prolactin release in acromegalic patients following metergoline administration, J. Clin. Endocrinol. **43**:1382, 1976.
24. Dila, C.J., and Pappius, H.M.: Cerebral water and electrolytes, Arch. Neurol. **26**:85, 1972.
25. Domingue, J.N., Richmond, I.L., and Wilson, C.B.: Results of surgery in 114 patients with prolactin-secreting pituitary adenomas, Am. J. Obstet. Gynecol. **137**:102, 1980.
26. Doughaday, W.H.: Hormonal regulation of growth by somatomedin and other tissue growth factors, Clin. Endocrinol. Metab. **6**:117, 1977.
27. Dousa, T.P.: Cellular action of antidiuretic hormone in nephrogenic diabetes insipidus, Mayo Clin. Proc. **49**:188, 1974.
28. du Vigneaud, V.: Hormones of the posterior pituitary gland: oxytocin and vasopressin. In The Harvey lectures 1954-55, New York, 1956, Academic Press, Inc.
29. Edwards, C.R.W.: Vasopressin and oxytocin in health and disease, Clin. Endocrinol. Metab. **6**:223, 1977.
30. Endocrinology 1980: "Proceedings of the VI International Congress of Endocrinology", Melbourne, Australia, Feb. 10-6, 1980, Elsevier, 1980, North Holland Biomedical Press.
31. Faria, M.A., and Tindall, G.A.: Transsphenoidal microsurgery for prolactin-secreting pituitary adenomas: results in 100 women with the amenorrhea-galactorrhea syndrome, J. Neurosurg. **56**:33, 1982.
32. Feldman, J.M., Plonk, J.W., and Bivens, C.H.: Inhibitory effects of serotonin antagonists on growth hormone release in acromegalic patients, Clin. Endocrinol. **5**:71, 1976.
33. Foley, K.M., and Posner, J.B.: Does pseudotumor cerebri cause the empty sella syndrome? Neurology **25**:565, 1975.
34. Friesen, H.G., and Tolis, G.: The use of bromocryptine in the galactorrhea-amenorrhea syndrome: Canadian Cooperative Study, Endocrinology (suppl. 6): 91, 1977.
35. Frohlich, A.: Ein Fal von Tumor der Hypophysis cerebri ohne Akromegalie, Wien. Klin. Rundschau. **15**:883, 1901.
36. Furth, J., Ueda, G., and Clifton, K.H.: The pathophysiology of pituitaries in their tumors: methodological advances. In Husch, H., editor: Methods in cancer research, vol. 10, New York, 1973, Academic Press, Inc.
37. Gold, E.M.: The Cushing syndromes: changing views of diagnosis and treatment, Ann. Intern. Med. **90**:829, 1979.
38. Gomes, F., Reyes, F.I., and Farman, C.: Non-peripheral galactorrhea and hyperprolactinemia, Am. J. Med. **62**:648, 1977.
39. Gonzales, E.: Update on pituitary tumor regression with bromocriptine therapy, JAMA **244**:1535, 1980.
40. Hardy, J.: Transsphenoidal microsurgery of the normal and pathological pituitary, Clin. Neurosurg. **16**:185, 1969.
41. Hardy, J.: Trans-sphenoidal hypophysectomy, J. Neurosurg. **34**:581, 1971.
42. Haymaker, W., and Schiller, F.: The Founders of Neurology, Springfield, Ill., 1953, Charles C Thomas Publisher.
43. Hodgson, S.F., et al.: Empty sella syndrome: report of 10 cases, Med. Clin. North Am. **56**:897, 1972.
44. Jenkins, J.S.: Pituitary tumors, London, 1973, Butterworth Publishing Co.
45. Kleinberg, D.L., Noel, G.L., and Frantz, A.G.: Galactorrhea: a study of 235 cases including 48 with pituitary tumors, N. Engl. J. Med. **296**:589, 1977.
46. Knappe, G., et al.: 10 year follow-up of transphenoidal pituitary surgery in acromegaly, Endokrinologue **79**:423, 1982.
47. Krieger, D.T.: Pharmacological therapy of Cushing's disease and Nelson's syndrome. In Linfoot, J.A. editor: Recent advances in the diagnosis and treatment of pituitary tumors. New York, 1979, Raven Press.
48. Krieger, D.T., Amorosa, L., and Linick, F.: Cyproheptadine induced remission of Cushing's disease, N. Engl. J. Med. **293**:893, 1975.
49. Kriezer, D.T., and Luria, M.: Effectiveness of cyproheptadine in decreasing plasma ACTH concentrations in Nelson's syndrome, J. Clin. Endocrinol. Metab. **43**:1179, 1976.
50. Landolt, A.M., and Wilson, C.B.: Tumors of the sella and parasellar area in adults. In Youmans, J.R., editor: Neurological surgery, Philadelphia, 1982, W.B. Saunders Co.
51. Lawrence, A.M., Pinsky, S.M., and Goldfine, I.D.: Conventional radiation therapy in acromegaly, Arch. Intern. Med. **128**:369, 1971.
52. Laws, E.R., and Kern, E.B.: Pituitary tumors treated by transnasal microsurgery: 7 years of clinical experience with 539 patients. In Sano, K., Takakura, K., and Fukushima, T. editors: Functioning pituitary adenoma: proceedings of the first workshop on pituitary adenomas, New York, 1980, Excerpta Medica.
53. Laws, E.R., and Randall, R.: Management of pituitary adenomas and related lesions, New York, 1982, Appleton-Century-Crofts.
54. Laws, E.R., Randall, R., and Abboud, C.F.: Surgical treatment of acromegaly: results in 140 patients. In Givens, J., editor: Hormone-secreting pituitary tumors, Chicago, 1982, Year Book Medical Publishers, Inc.
55. Laws, E.R., Trautmann, J.C., and Hollenhorst, R.W.: Transsphenoidal decompression of the optic nerve and chiasma: visual results in 62 patients, J. Neurosurg. **46**:717, 1977.
56. Locke, W., and Schally, A.V.: The hypothalamus and pituitary in health and disease, Springfield, Ill., 1972, Charles C Thomas, Publisher.
57. Lopez, J.A.: Pituitary apoplexy, J. Oslo City Hosp. **20**:17, 1970.
58. Luboshitzky, R., and Barzilac, D.: Bromocriptine for an acromegalic patient, improvement in cardiac function, and carpal tunnel syndrome, JAMA **244**:1825, 1980.
59. Magrini, G., et al.: Study on the relationship between plasma prolactin levels and androgen metabolism in man, J. Clin. Endocrinol. **43**:944, 1955.
60. Malarkey, W.B., Goodenow, T.J., and Lanese, R.R.: Diurinal variation of prolactin secretion differentiates pituitary tumors from the primary empty sella syndrome, Am. J. Med. **69**:886, 1980.

61. Martin, J.B., Reichlin, S., and Brown, G.: Clinical neuroendocrinology, Philadelphia, 1978, F.A. Davis Co.
62. McGregor, A.M., et al.: Reduction in size of a pituitary tumor by bromocryptine therapy, N. Engl. J. Med. **300**:291, 1979.
63. Moses, A.M., Miller, M., and Streeten, D.H.P.: Pathophysiologic and pharmacologic alterations in the release and action of ADH, Metabolism **25**:697, 1976.
64. Neelon, F.A., Goree, J.A., and Lebovitz, H.E.: The primary empty sella: clinical and radiographic characteristics and endocrine function, Medicine **52**:73, 1973.
65. Nelson, D.H., et al.: ACTH-producing tumor of the pituitary gland, N. Engl. J. Med. **259**:161, 1958.
66. Paget, S.: John Hunter, man of science and surgeon (1728-1793), London, 1897, Longmans, Green and Co.
67. Patterson, R.H., Jr., and Danylevich, A.: Surgical removal of craniopharyngiomas by a transcranial approach through the lamina terminalis and sphenoidal sinus, Neurosurgery **7**:111, 1980.
68. Post, K.D., and Jackson, I.M.D.: The pituitary adenoma, New York, 1980, Plenum Publishing Corp.
69. Randall, R.V.: Neuroendocrinology. In Youmans, J.R., editor: Neurological surgery, Philadelphia, 1982, W.B. Saunders Co.
70. Raskind, R., Brown, H.A., and Mathis, J.: Recurrent cyst of the pituitary: 26-year follow-up from first decompression: case report, J. Neurosurg. **28**:595, 1968.
71. Ray, B.S., Intracranial hypophyesectomy, J. Neurosurg. **28**:180, 1968.
72. Ridgway, E.C., et al.: Thyrotroin and prolactin pituitary reserve in the "empty sella syndrome," J. Clin. Endocrinol. **41**:968, 1975.
73. Robinson, A.G.: DdAVP in the treatment of central diabetes insipides, N. Engl. J. Med. **294**:177, 1976.
74. Schally, A.V., and Arimura, A.: Physiology and nature of hypothalamic regulatory hormones. In Martini, L. and Besser, G.M., editors: Clinical neuroendocrinology, New York, 1977, Academic Press, Inc.
75. Schally, A.V., et al.: Purification of corticotropin releasing factor from porcine hypothalamus, Endocrinology **100**:95, 1977.
76. Schwartz, W.B., Bartler, F.C.: The syndrome of inappropriate secretion of antidiuretic hormone, Am. J. Med. **42**:790, 1967.
77. Seki, K., Seki, M., and Okamura, T.: Effect of CB-154 (2-BR-a-ergocryptine) on serum follicle stimulating hormone, lutenizing hormone and prolactin in women with amennorrhea-galactorrhea syndrome, Acta Endocrinol. **79**:25, 1975.
78. Sheehan, H.L., and Davis, J.C.: Pituitary necrosis, Br. Med. Bull. **24**:59, 1968.
79. Simmonds, M.: Uber embolische prozesse in der hypophysis, Virchows Arch. **217**:226, 1914.
80. Sonksen, P.H., et al.: Acromegally caused by pulmonary carcinoid tumors, Clin. Endocrinol. **5**:503, 1976.
81. Sorbrinko L.G., et al.: Effect of treatment with bromocriptine on the size and activity of prolactin producing pituitary tumors, Acta Endocrinol. **96**:24, 1981.
82. Sorbrinko, L.G., et al.: Radiologic evidence for regression of prolactinoma after treatment with bromocryptine, Lancet **2**:257, 1978.
83. Sridhar, C.B., Calvert, G.D., and Ibbertson, H.K.: A new interpretation in diabetes insipidus, J. Clin. Endocrinol. Metab. **38**:890, 1974.
84. Stern, W.E., and Batzdorf, V.: Intracranial removal of pituitary adenomas, J. Neurosurg. **33**:564, 1970.
85. Summers, V.K., et al.: Treatment of acromegaly with bromocriptine, J. Clin. Enodcrinol. Metab. **40**:904, 1975.
86. Thorner, M.O., et al.: Bromocriptine treatment of acromegaly, Br. Med. J. **1**:299, 1975.
87. Thorner, M.O., et al.: Rapid regression of pituitary prolactinomas during bromocriptine treatment, J. Clin. Endocrinol. Metab. **51**:438, 1980.
88. Velentzas, C., et al.: Regression of pituitary prolactinoma with bromocriptine administration, JAMA **245**:1149, 1981.
89. Wakai, S., et al.: Pituitary apoplexy: its incidence and clinical significance, J. Neurosurg. **55**:187, 1981.
90. Walker, E.A.: A history of neurological surgery, Baltimore, 1982, The Williams & Wilkins Co.
91. Wass, J.A.H., et al.: Long term treatment of acromegaly with bromocryptine, Br. J. Med. **1**:875, 1977.
92. Weiss, M.H., Kaufmann, B., and Richards, D.E.: Cerebrospinal fluid rhinorrhea from an empty sella: transsphenoidal obliteration of the fistula; technical note, J. Neurosurg. **39**:674, 1973.
93. Welch, K., and Stears, J.C.: Chiasmapexy for the correction of traction on the optic nerves and chiasm associated with their descent into an empty sell turcica: case report, J. Neurosurg. **35**:291, 1971.
94. Wersberg, L.A.: Clinical study of pituitary apoplexy with emphasis on five cases precipitated by radiotherapy, Neurology **26**:353, 1976.
95. Wilson, C.B., and Dempsey, L.C.: Transphenoidal microsurgical removal of 250 pituitary adenomas, J. Neurosurg. **48**:13, 1978.
96. Wilson, C.B., et al.: Cushing's disease and Nelsons's syndrome, Clin. Neurosurg. **27**:19, 1980.
97. Zervas, N.T., and Martin, J.B.: Management of hormone secreting pituitary adenomas, N. Engl. J. Med. **302**:210, 1980.

57 Adrenal Glands

Heber H. Newsome, Jr.

The adrenal glands are physiologically complex structures. As with other endocrine glands, they participate in hyperfunctioning and hypofunctioning states, both under physiologic conditions and during many disease processes. Anatomically and physiologically they possess two distinctly different components, a cortex and medulla. The hormonal output of the two components differs in control and in effect, but the complexity is compounded by the cortex's ability to secrete several types of steroids and the medulla's ability to produce two catecholamines, as well as other recently appreciated substances. This chapter focuses on the mechanisms of secretion and the effects of these hormones. More emphasis is placed on the less familiar areas, in terms of clinical relevancy; with the more familiar areas, such as adrenal tumors, for example, one can easily relate the basic observations to the clinical features.

ADRENAL GLAND ANATOMY

The adrenal glands are paired structures located cephalad of each kidney.[44] Their shape approximates that of an elongated triangle with somewhat rounded points. Whereas the left adrenal gland is slightly folded into a shallow saucerlike configuration, the right adrenal tends to be relatively flat. The dimensions are approximately 4 to 5 cm in length, 3 to 4 cm in width, and only 0.3 to 0.8 cm in thickness. The normal adult adrenal gland weighs approximately 4 to 5 g. The rubbery consistency and the bright-yellow color serve to delineate the structure from the typical surrounding fat. On the cut section it is apparent that the gland has two distinct portions. The thin (1 to 2 mm), bright-yellow *cortex* envelops an even thinner layer of dark, reddish gray tissue that is the adrenal *medulla*. The adrenal medulla is soft and comprises approximately 20% of the total adrenal gland weight.

Histologically the adrenal cortex is divided into three distinct zones. Just under the capsule is a thin layer designated as the *zona glomerulosa*. It is composed of small, round, compact cells with a high nuclear/cystoplasmic ratio. They are arranged in small clusters to give them a glomerular appearance. Aldosterone is produced exclusively in this zone. Just under the zona glomerulosa is the *zona fasciculata,* composed of clear cells loosely arranged in strands oriented from the capsule toward the medulla. The *zona reticularis* is deep to the zona fasciculata and adjacent to the adrenal medulla. This zone is composed of small, compact cells arranged homogeneously in sheets. Although cortisol production is evenly divided between the zona fasciculata and the zona reticularis, the former is more responsive to short-term adrenocorticotropic hormone exposure and produces more of the 17-hydroxycorticosteroids compared to the inner zone. The zona reticularis is primarily responsible for sulfoconjugation of steroids and produces the preponderance of adrenal androgens and deoxycorticosterone. The cells of the adrenal medulla are typical ganglion cells interspersed with nerve fibers. The central vein runs through the medulla.

The blood supply to the adrenal glands is composed primarily of many small arteries arising from the diaphragm, phrenic artery, aorta, and renal artery. These form a capsular arterial plexus that enters the cortex to form capillaries coursing through the cortical cells. The capillaries form a venous portal system that drains into the adrenal medulla, where they reach confluence with the central adrenal vein. This corticomedullary venous portal system provides a high concentration of adrenal steroids in the medullary tissue. The adrenal medulla is also supplied by *arteriae medullae* directly into the substance of the adrenal medulla. Although some small veins drain from the surface of the adrenal cortex, most arterial blood flows from the capsule to the medulla and out the central venous vein. The adrenal vein on the right drains into the vena cava, approximately 5 to 7.5 cm above the right renal vein; on the left, the adrenal vein drains into the superior aspect of the renal vein, approximately 1 to 3 cm from the vena cava.

Innervation of the adrenal gland arises from the greater splanchnic nerve and the abdominal sympathetic plexus and from contributions of the vagus nerve. The neural fibers are primarily associated with the arteriae medullae, which go directly to the adrenal medulla, and with connective tissue trabeculae entering through the capsule of the gland. Most of the nerves terminate in the adrenal medulla and on major arteriolar walls. Nonmyelinated fibers have been described as passing close to the adrenocortical cells, but the functional significance of these is not clear. The cells of the adrenal medulla function essentially as sympathetic ganglionic neurons, with the secretion products, norepinephrine and epinephrine, passing into the systemic circulation by way of the central adrenal vein. The lymphatics of the adrenal gland are found primarily in the capsule and drain medially into the thoracic duct or cisterna chyli (chylecistern).

ADRENOCORTICAL PHYSIOLOGY

Cortisol

Physiology of Cortisol Secretion

The control of cortisol secretion by the zona fasciculata of the adrenal cortex begins in the central nervous system (CNS). Neural projections originating from almost every part of the brain impinge on the hypothalamus and modulate both internal and external influences to regulate the release of a 41-amino-acid peptide, *corticotropin-releasing*

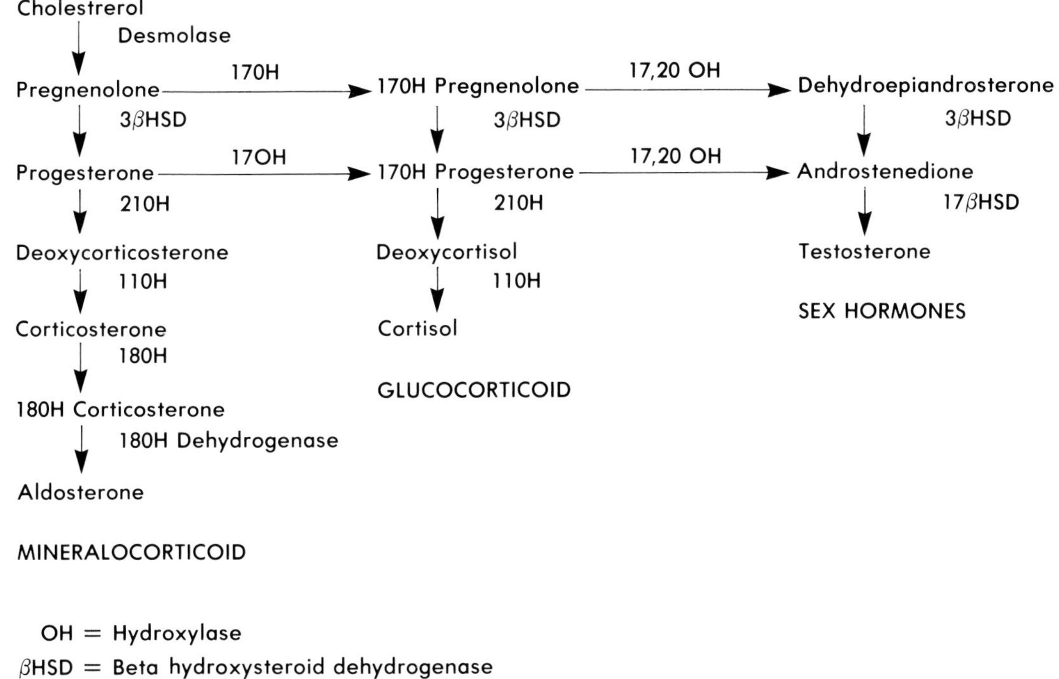

Fig. 57-1 Metabolic pathways in the adrenal cortex.

factor (CRF), from the hypothalamus. After its release, CRF reaches the anterior pituitary by way of a direct portal venous system, where CRF in turn stimulates synthesis and release of *adrenocorticotropic hormone (ACTH),* a 39-amino-acid peptide. Interestingly, ACTH is a portion of a large precursor molecule from which is also derived beta-lipotropin. Beta-lipotropin can be cleaved to produce beta-endorphin and beta-melanocyte-stimulating hormone (beta-MSH). The ACTH molecule contains the amino acid sequence for alpha-MSH. The release of ACTH by CRF occurs very rapidly, perhaps within 1 minute. ACTH is released into the general circulation, where it reaches the adrenal cortex to stimulate synthesis and release of cortisol. An increase in adrenal secretion of cortisol is seen almost immediately with stimulation by ACTH. Both the magnitude and the duration of increased cortisol secretion are directly proportional to the concentration of ACTH in the adrenal arterial blood.

With the advent of relatively simple, precise, and sensitive assay techniques, frequent sampling of plasma has revealed interesting details of ACTH-cortisol secretion in the basal state. ACTH is secreted intermittently in bursts throughout the day. With a plasma and biologic half-life measured in minutes, ACTH intermittently stimulates the adrenal cortex to produce cortisol. However, cortisol has a plasma half-life of approximately 70 minutes, and although the plasma cortisol pattern fluctuates somewhat, a less irregular pattern to cortisol exists compared to ACTH concentrations in the plasma. Under basal conditions the CNS, CRF, ACTH, and adrenocortical cascade results in a circadian rhythm of fluctuating mean plasma cortisol concentration. A peak in plasma cortisol concentrations normally occurs in the early morning hours, with a nadir in the late afternoon.

Stimulation of cortisol secretion by ACTH proceeds along a steroidogenic pathway, shown in Fig. 57-1. The primary focus of action of ACTH is at the conversion of cholesterol to delta-5-pregnenolone. The adrenal cortex is also capable of producing androgens, which has implications that are discussed later in this chapter. Of further interest is the production of the major mineralocorticoid, aldosterone, by enzymes found in the zona glomerulosa. Control of aldosterone secretion is also covered in a later section.

Under basal conditions plasma cortisol concentrations are maintained within fairly narrow limits by an interplay between the concentrations of circulating cortisol and CRF-ACTH secretion. Basal plasma ACTH concentrations range between 20 to 200 pg/ml, whereas cortisol remains approximately within the range of 5 to 15 μg/100 ml of plasma. As cortisol increases above this physiologic limit, ACTH secretion is suppressed. Such suppression of ACTH secretion by cortisol is exerted through at least three mechanisms, as shown in Fig. 57-2. Cortisol acts directly on the pituitary to inhibit synthesis of ACTH. Cortisol also suppresses the release of ACTH by CRF. Finally, cortisol inhibits the synthesis of CRF itself. Through these mechanisms the negative feedback effect of cortisol on the ACTH release obviously serves to maintain circulating plasma cortisol below a certain concentration.

The negative feedback suppression of ACTH by acute administration of cortisol exogenously apparently has at least two aspects.[28] One is a *rate-sensitive feedback inhibition,* which is a rapid suppression of ACTH release related to the rate at which plasma cortisol concentration is being increased. Another aspect is the *delayed negative feedback phase,* which is apparently related to the maximum concentration of cortisol achieved. It is speculated

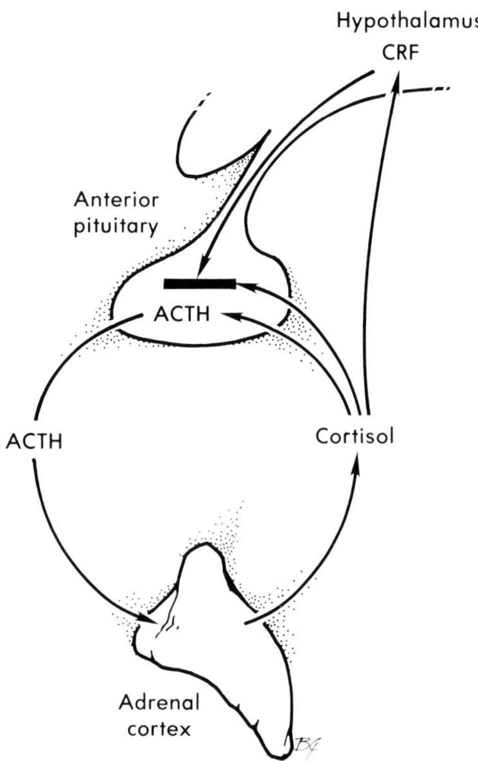

Fig. 57-2 Interactions between the hypothalamus, pituitary gland, and the adrenal cortex in the regulation of plasma cortisol levels.

that the rate-sensitive feedback effect is caused by a membrane phenomenon preventing release of ACTH, whereas the concentration-sensitive feedback mechanism is an effect on ACTH synthesis. On the other hand, when cortisol drops below a certain level, about 5 μg/100 ml plasma in human beings, ACTH release is stimulated, and this in turn restores plasma cortisol to the normal range.

In general, the increased secretion of ACTH and cortisol, brought about by acute stress, fever, pain, and hemorrhage, overrides the negative feedback effect of acute endogenous or exogenous hypercortisolemia. ACTH secretion increases in proportion to the magnitude of stress, and the response of the adrenal secretion of cortisol is linearly related to the concentration of ACTH up to a range of 400 to 500 pg/ml. The maximum plasma concentration of cortisol produced by stress is in the range of 50 to 70 μg/100 ml. Concentrations above 70 to 80 μg/100 ml are distinctly unusual, even in situations of longstanding adrenal hyperplasia caused by ectopic ACTH production.

In contrast to the acute cortisol feedback on the CRF-ACTH mechanism, longstanding cortisol (or synthetic steroid) excess has a lasting suppressive effect on ACTH secretion. Prolonged cortisol excess prevents the ACTH response to stress and other factors. The length of time that excess cortisol or cortisol-like steroids must be administered before achieving chronic suppression of ACTH release has not been precisely determined in human beings. After approximately 2 to 3 weeks of chronic daily steroid therapy, the pituitary-adrenal axis may not respond to stress. At least in the case of exogenously administered steroids, the suppressive effect is clearly dose dependent. Using prednisone as an example, approximately 10 mg/day is the minimum required dose for chronic pituitary suppression. If the administration of a given steroid is spaced out so that its half-life permits an intermittent resurgence of ACTH, the hypothalamic-pituitary suppression may be avoided. This phenomenon is exploited clinically by the alternate-day dose regimen of steroid therapy. Once the cortisol excess is abolished, either from removal of an endogenous source or by cessation of administered steroids, return of pituitary-adrenal function follows a fairly predictable pattern. ACTH secretion returns within 3 to 4 months, followed in a few months by return of adrenocortical responsiveness and consequent cortisol secretion. The return of adrenal responsiveness can be hastened by exogenous administration of ACTH during the first period of pituitary-adrenal unresponsiveness.

Molecular Mechanisms of Steroid Action

Whether secreted by the adrenal cortex, testis, or ovary, steroids circulate in the plasma in a form in which they are primarily bound to particular globulins synthesized by the liver. A free, unbound portion of the steroid is always present in plasma equilibrium with the larger bound fraction. The process of plasma protein binding is partly responsible for the particular half-life of any given steroid species. The greater the plasma binding, the longer is the half-life. Chemical structural features that affect degradation are perhaps more important in determining half-life, such as degree of saturation of the steroid nucleus.

The circulating unbound form of the steroid passes freely through the membrane of the target cell and is attached to a protein in the cytosolic portion of the cell. The protein, a linear peptide with a molecular weight of approximately 87,000 g, is termed the *steroid receptor*. Steroid receptors are found in almost every type of cell in the body. The receptor conformational requirements are such that steroids may be received or excluded by the receptor based on steroid structure. The various types of steroids are thus separated into functional classifications depending on the functions of the receptive cell. For example, cortisol, prednisone, and dexamethasone are structurally correct to fit into the receptors of cells that lead to "glucocorticoid" activity. Other cytosolic receptors of steroids are activated only by testosterone, estrogens, or mineralocorticoids. The distribution of these latter receptors is more limited in the body so that actions of these steroids are not so widespread as compared to those of the glucocorticoids.

Steroids within a group share similar actions. As a rule, the activity of one type of glucocorticoid for a given action or cell type is produced by the other glucocorticoids, whether they are synthetic or endogenous. For any given steroid, the strength of the response is related to the concentration of the steroid available to the cells. In comparing potency among various steroids, the relative potency is related to several factors, such as the plasma half-life, the degree of binding by the circulating globulins, and the affinity coefficient for the cytosolic receptor. In contrast to the glucocorticoid receptors, which exclude nonglucocorticoid steroids, the mineralocorticoid receptors in the kidney are subtyped into groups that have various affinities for the glucocorticoids, as discussed later in relation to aldosterone.

The activation of the cytosol receptor by the steroid to effect a conformational change in the receptor-steroid complex is central to the action of steroids. The activated complex is translocated into the nucleus of the cell. There it is attached to the chromatin, and the replication of specific deoxyribonucleic acid (DNA) occurs. This transcriptional effect produces messenger ribonucleic acid (mRNA), which in turn produces new protein synthesis in the cell. Although the precise nature of this newly produced protein has been characterized in only a few steroid-responsive systems, most known actions of steroids in all cell systems are consistent with this view.[6]

A promising future possibility for manipulating steroid effects should be mentioned.[10] An interesting type of steroid-receptor interaction exists in which certain types of specifically structured steroids may bind to, but not activate, the receptor. The steroid receptor is thus prevented from translocating to the cell nucleus. These inactive steroids have the effect of occupying the cytosolic receptor to the exclusion of effective steroid agonists. These steroids are antagonists and therefore represent the possibility for blockage of steroid action at the cellular level. To date, antagonists have been demonstrated only in vitro.

At this point a simplified overview of the pituitary-adrenal effects can be outlined. Primarily through the neurogenic pathways, CRF is released to stimulate the synthesis and release of ACTH. ACTH in turn stimulates the secretion of cortisol from the adrenal cortex, and cortisol is presented to all cells by way of the arterial circulation. The particular effects of cortisol depend on the presence of steroid receptors that have specific conformational parity and bind the cortisol in such a way that the steroid-receptor complex is translocated into the cell nucleus and institutes new protein synthesis. The particular effect of cortisol on these cells depends on the cells' particular RNA-directed response.

Effects of Glucocorticoids

Almost every tissue in the body is affected by the glucocorticoids. Consideration of these effects here is limited to those actions relevant to the surgical patient. These actions and effects are listed in Table 57-1. Some of the indirect effects of the glucocorticoids on specific tissues are mediated through their direct effects on fuel substrates.[43]

Fuel Substrates. Glucocorticoid-related changes in carbohydrate metabolism have the net effect of producing hyperglycemia. The two primary events responsible for the hyperglycemia are (1) a decreased peripheral utilization of glucose and (2) an increased gluconeogenesis. A separate action of glucocorticoids is an increased hepatic glycogen synthesis, which is thought to be insulin dependent.

Decreased utilization of glucose by peripheral tissues is promoted by the glucocorticoids through two general actions. The first is an inhibition of glucose transport and metabolism, especially in fat cells, by a direct cellular effect of the glucocorticoids. The effect can be demonstrated in vitro in the absence of insulin. A second mechanism is glucocorticoids' production of resistance to the action of insulin. Decreased binding of insulin by insulin-sensitive tissues clearly occurs, probably because of a decrease in affinity of the insulin receptor for insulin. An insulin-dependent effect of glucocorticoids beyond the insulin-binding step also occurs. The resultant insulin resistance seen during glucocorticoid excess obviously blunts the hypoglycemic effect of insulin. Conversely, with low or absent glucocorticoid concentrations, the actions of insulin are accentuated. Consequently patients with adrenocortical insufficiency are exquisitely sensitive to the hypoglycemic effect of insulin.

Increased gluconeogenesis is caused by several mechanisms that probably involve both peripheral and hepatic actions of the glucocorticoids. By both direct and indirect effects, glucocorticoids increase the gluconeogenic precursors used for producing glucose. Glucocorticoids act on muscle to release branch-chain and other glucogenic amino acids for conversion in the liver to glucose. The mechanism for such a release is currently unclear but probably involves proteolysis. Although this action is consistent with an anti-insulin effect on muscle, it is demonstrable even in diabetic animals and therefore does not require the presence of insulin. A second mechanism for provision of gluconeogenic precursors is the permissive effect of glucocorticoids on epinephrine. Both the lipolytic effect of epinephrine to release glycerol from fat cells and the glycogenolytic effect of epinephrine on muscle to release lactate appear to depend partly on the presence of glucocorticoids. Thus glucocorticoids provide increased glucogenic amino acids, glycerol, and lactate from the periphery for glucose production in the liver through the process of gluconeogenesis. Third, the permissive effect of glucocorticoids accounts for the dependence of epinephrine and glucagon on these steroids for their gluconeogenic action. Fourth, glucocorticoids have a direct effect on gluconeogenesis, apparently by induction of several gluconeogenic hepatic enzymes. An indirect effect of the hyperglycemia seen in glucocorticoid excess is the stimulation of insulin secretion and the consequent relative hyperinsulinemia seen under these conditions.

The other effects of glucocorticoids on fuel substrates relate primarily to their action on adipocytes. Glucocorticoids apparently stimulate lypolysis, with a resulting increase in both circulating triglycerides and free fatty acids. The effect is probably a direct one, although the general anti-insulin properties of these steroids may be partly responsible. The interesting body fat distribution seen in clinical states of glucocorticoid excess may be related to a differential sensitivity of various adipose tissues to the two hormones. In body areas with a paucity of fat, such as the extremities, the fat cells are thought to be more sensitive to the lipolytic effect of glucocorticoids than to the lipogenic effect of insulin. Conversely, the fat cells distributed in the upper trunk and back are more sensitive to the lipogenic effect of insulin.

The glucocorticoids' mechanism of action on protein synthesis and metabolism is not clear. Although the proteolytic effect of excessive amounts of glucocorticoids has

Table 57-1 **ACTIONS AND EFFECTS OF GLUCOCORTICOIDS ON VARIOUS TISSUES AND PROCESSES**

Areas	Actions	Effects
Fuel substrates		
Glucose	Decreased peripheral utilization: Has direct effect on uptake; Causes insulin resistance Increased gluconeogenesis: Causes release of muscle amino acids as substrate; Allows epinephrine to work; Has direct effect	Hyperglycemia
Adipocytes	Lipolysis	Fat distribution
Muscle	Proteolysis	Muscle wasting
Immune functions	Eosinopenia Leukocytosis Lymphopenia (T-helper cells) Decreased antigenic and mitogenic lymphocyte stimulation Decreased interleukin I production	Immunosuppression
Inflammatory response	Decreased number of cells (monocytes) in wounds Decreased chemotaxis, phagocytosis, and bacterial activity Decreased production of soluble mediators ? Lysozomal stabilization	Increased susceptibility to infection
Wound healing	Decreased tensile strength Suppressed scar contraction Delayed epithelialization	Poor wound healing, abdominal striae
Bones	Decreased bone formation: Poor protein matrix; Delayed osteoblastic maturation Increased bone resorption: probable secondary hyperparathyroidism	Osteoporosis, delayed growth
Cardiovascular system	Inotropic and chronotropic cardiac effect Increased peripheral vascular resistance	Hypertension Sodium retention
Renal system	Increased renal tubular sodium resorption Increased free water clearance	
Gastrointestinal tract	Decreased mucosal cell turnover Decreased mucosal and pancreatic prostaglandin synthesis	? Increase in peptic ulcers, pancreatitis, and bowel perforation

been well documented and accounts for the pronounced muscle wasting seen in this condition, it has only recently been demonstrated that even physiologic concentrations of glucocorticoids probably exert a proteolytic effect with an increase in, for example, circulating leucine and alanine concentrations. The proteolytic effect with increased availability of glucogenic amino acids is probably one of the several indirect means by which glucocorticoids increase gluconeogenesis, as already mentioned.*

Regulation of Immune Functions. The effects of glucocorticoids on immune function are complex and numerous. In considering both in vivo and in vitro effects, as well as those seen with both low-dose or high-dose steroid administration, it is evident that almost every aspect of the immune response can be modified by steroid administration.

In general terms, the effects of the glucocorticoids are to suppress immune function. Investigation into the mechanism of this suppression has emphasized inhibition of cellular glucose transport and/or a decrease in protein synthesis as likely means by which steroids exert their suppressive action. Most research has focused on the various cellular components of the immune response. For convenience, these effects can be separated into (1) those related to the circulating populations of cellular components and (2) those having direct functional effects on these cells. In general, the effects on circulating populations can be achieved by relatively low-dose steroid administration, whereas those related to functional effects are usually obtained by high doses.

The effect of steroid administration on circulating populations of cells can be characterized by a polymorphonuclear leukocytosis, a lymphopenia, and an eosinopenia. In both steroid-sensitive species (rat, mouse) and steroid-resistant species (human being, monkey, guinea pig), the

*References 19, 25, 33, 56, and 57.

neutrophilia is thought to result from a release of these formed elements from the bone marrow. In the steroid-sensitive species the lymphopenia is caused by lympholysis. In resistant species normal nonactivated lymphocytes are believed to be sequestered in bone marrow in response to steroid administration. Although this has not been demonstrated directly in human beings, radioisotope studies in other steroid-resistant species have directly demonstrated the bone marrow sequestration. Human lymphopenia results from a redistribution primarily of thymic-derived lymphocytes (T cells). The bone marrow–derived lymphocytes (B cells) redistribute to a lesser degree than T cells. Furthermore, circulating T-helper cells, rather than T-suppressor cells, are apparently preferentially sequestered out of the circulation. Evidence in human beings suggests that activated lymphocytes are susceptible to lympholysis by steroids and are lysed by high-dose steroids. The summation of the steroid effects on circulating cells is obviously to suppress the immune response.

The effects of steroids on the function of particular lymphocytes are usually caused by high-dose steroid administration and have been shown mainly by in vitro experiments. Two notable exceptions are the in vivo demonstration in human beings of (1) a suppression of the late cutaneous hypersensitivity reactions and (2) a suppression of immunoglobulin synthesis. Many in vitro effects of steroids have been found. The stimulation of lymphocyte proliferation following exposure to mitogens is suppressed by glucocorticoids. Suppression of antigenic stimulation such as in the mixed lymphocyte reaction is obtained by addition of steroids to the culture media. Several components of the cell-mediated cytotoxicity reactions are suppressed by glucocorticoids in vitro. Although many of these in vitro effects are undoubtedly related to direct effects on the lymphocyte, some effects on blastogenesis (e.g., the suppression of interleukin I production by monocytes) may result from actions on precursor cells. Lack of this soluble mediator may then inhibit the complex cascade of events leading to lymphocyte proliferation.[12]

Modulation of Inflammatory Response. In addition to the steroidal effects on the immune system, the effects on the inflammatory response may be important in the increased susceptibility to infection in patients with excess glucocorticoid activity, either endogenous or exogenous. Both the incidence of infection and the resistance of the infection to treatment increase in those patients who have steroid excess.

The decreased response to tissue injury from any cause is apparent in the steroid-treated patient. A decreased number of inflammatory cells of all types are found in the wound. Two reasons for this have been suggested:

1. A well-documented decreased adherence of leukocytes to endothelial surfaces occurs in states of steroid excess, possibly from a direct effect of the steroids on the membranes of the circulating cells.
2. Effects on the capillary membrane may occur in the area of injury to prevent migration of the inflammatory cells into the injured tissue.

The second theory may also be consistent with the lack of edema seen in many such wounds.

Of the various inflammatory cellular components of the wound, the monocytes appear most sensitive to the steroidal effects. It has been well demonstrated that the chemotactic, phagocytic, and bactericidal functions of the monocytes are suppressed by the steroids. Steroids also inhibit production of many soluble factors elaborated by the inflammatory cells. Examples of these are plasminogen activator, interleukin I, and the prostaglandins and leukotrienes. Stabilization of lysosomal membranes has been well demonstrated in vitro. Although inhibition of the release of the lysozymes would be a ready explanation for the depression of the inflammatory response by steroids, the concentrations of steroids required in vitro to achieve this stabilization are far greater than those levels obtainable in tissues during in vivo steroid administration. It is not certain that stabilization of lysosomal membranes is an actual in vivo effect of high-dose steroids.[13]

Wound Healing. Excess glucocorticoids decrease the tensile strength of wounds, suppress contraction of the scar, and delay epithelialization. These effects have been demonstrated in several species, including human beings. In vivo studies have amply demonstrated the decrease in collagen synthesis. The decrease in protein synthesis usually seen with glucocorticoids is consistent with the decrease in collagen production.

Recent wound healing studies have focused on the early migration of inflammatory cells into the wound and on the importance of these cells for stimulating the subsequent events in wound healing, including migration of fibroblasts and the production of collagen. Steroids have a marked effect on the early migration of inflammatory cells into the wound, with consequent decreased collagen production and tensile strength of the wound. Data relating to the dose and timing of steroid administration on wound healing in human beings are scant. Animal studies, however, have clearly shown that a certain minimum steroid dose is required to affect wound healing. Regular, frequent steroid administration is needed. Alternate-day administration, for example, has a less deleterious effect on healing. The timing of steroid administration is also important. Although previous regular steroid treatment evidently will suppress wound healing, a particular time occurs after wounding beyond which steroids do not delay the healing process. Probably by 24 hours following wounding, steroid administration will have little, if any, effect on healing.[23]

Bones. The main effects of corticosteroids on bones are focused on the trabecular type of bone, such as the ribs and vertebral bodies. In patients with steroid-induced osteopenia, compression fractures of the vertebra and stressed rib fractures typically occur. Steroids decrease bone formation and increase bone resorption. As in wound healing, the steroids depress collagen synthesis, in this case by the osteoblast, and bone protein matrix is defective. Also, development of the osteoblastic cells from the precursor to the mature forms is delayed. Although a direct stimulatory effect of steroids on the osteoclastic function of bone resorption possibly exists, a more indirect effect has been postulated. A decrease occurs in intestinal calcium resorption through the action of steroids on the gut mucosa. The decreased gut absorption of calcium results in a secondary increase in parathyroid hormone secretion. This increased parathyroid secretion stimulates osteoclastic activity and consequent bone resorption. Delayed growth noted in children receiving steroid therapy is probably caused by the decreased maturation of precursor cells. The effect on bone formation or growth is seen with as low as 8 mg of prednisone per day.[47]

CARDIOVASCULAR SYSTEM. Administering glucocorticoid, either acutely to the patient with adrenal insufficiency or chronically in excess to produce a cushingoid state, increases the blood pressure. Glucocorticoid administration has an inotropic and chronotropic effect on the heart. An increase in peripheral vascular resistance also occurs. These central and peripheral effects increase the systemic blood pressure. The most plausible explanation for the glucocorticoid effects is a potentiation of the actions of circulating catecholamines.[54] Studies on heart muscle exposed to glucocorticoids have demonstrated an increase in the concentration of low-affinity calcium-binding sites on plasma membranes. The increased calcium influx produced in response to catecholamines, for example, is accentuated by the increase in low-affinity binding sites. The same mechanism of glucocorticoid action may explain the potentiation of catecholamine vasoconstriction after glucocorticoid administration.

RENAL SYSTEM. The endogenous glucocorticoids exert a mineralocorticoid action on the kidney. This action manifests as an increase in renal sodium retention. In addition to the classic mineralocorticoid receptor (Type I) found in the kidney, which has high affinity for aldosterone and low affinity for the glucocorticoids, two other receptors have been described.[38] Type II has a high affinity for corticosterone and dexamethasone, has a low affinity for aldosterone, and is designated as a glucocorticoid receptor. A third type, with a high affinity for corticosterone but a low affinity for dexamethasone and aldosterone, has also been described. Although no definite proof can show that the glucocorticoid receptors are responsible for the mineralocorticoid effect of these steroids, the presence of receptors would be consistent with this possibility. Administration of glucocorticoids also results in an increase in free water clearance and a suppression of circulating antidiuretic hormone (ADH). A proposed mechanism is a restoration of normal plasma volume with a consequent decrease in ADH and an increase in free water clearance.

GASTROINTESTINAL TRACT. The demonstration of an increase in both gastric acidity and frequency of peptic ulceration in response to glucocorticoid administration is controversial. Several actions of glucocorticoids have the potential to increase gastric ulcer formation. The decreases in cell turnover, in general wound healing, and in cytoprotective prostaglandin synthesis may point to at least a permissive role of glucocorticoid administration in peptic ulcer formation.

The precise relationship between pancreatitis and glucocorticoids is also unclear. A slightly increased incidence of pancreatitis may occur in patients, especially children, receiving steroid therapy compared to those who are not. In autopsy series 30% to 40% of these patients have either microscopic or grossly focal pancreatitis associated with steroid therapy. Steroid administration may impair cytoprotective mechanisms in the pancreas such as prostaglandin synthesis. As with gastric ulcer disease, the possible accentuation in ulcer formation and perforation of the small bowel and in diverticular perforation of the colon are controversial issues. No clear-cut evidence shows that the incidence of either increases with excess steroid. It is well demonstrated that glucocorticoid administration increases sodium and water reabsorption in the colon, as does mineralocorticoid administration.[53]

Glucocorticoid Excess

ACUTE PHYSIOLOGIC RESPONSE. The adrenal gland clearly is necessary for life. In several documented instances, adrenalectomized patients without maintenance steroids died after 6 to 8 days under basal conditions following cessation of replacement therapy. On the other hand, stressed patients with an inadequate hypothalamic-pituitary-adrenal (HPA) response have been known to die within hours from irreversible shock. In view of these reports, the well-documented increase in circulating cortisol concentrations during stress strongly implies that the physiologic response of hypercortisolemia is an essential component of the so-called stress response.

Studies in dogs focusing on the regulation of glucose have shown that steroids, along with glucagon and epinephrine, apparently are important mediators of the metabolic response to stress. An extension of these studies to human beings that includes other parameters, such as oxygen consumption, carbon dioxide production, glucose production and utilization, and nitrogen balance, points to the important effect of corticosteroids and the response of these parameters to stress. Although the low amplitude of the response to these hormones shows that other mediators are involved in the metabolic changes during significant stress, earlier studies have also shown that corticosteroids are essential for maintenance of the organism during these periods of stress.

As outlined in the previous section on actions of the glucocorticoids, steroids promote increased blood glucose, thus presumably providing increased availability of the substrate to glucose-dependent tissues, such as CNS. Ample evidence suggests that the circulating blood volume may depend on the integrity of the adrenal cortex and that normalization of blood volume is critically important in situations involving blood loss in trauma. Because of the permissive action of steroids on the cardiovascular effects of catecholamines, the sympathetic nervous system response to stress obviously would not reach its full extent in the absence of adrenal steroids.[4]

CHRONIC STATES OF GLUCOCORTICOID EXCESS. Although the previous section emphasized the crucial nature of the exaggerated steroid response to stress, on a chronic basis the circulating cortisol concentrations apparently must be kept below the supraphysiologic level. The reasons for the upper-limit requirements are readily seen. Excess steroids can produce problems with wound healing, the immune response, the inflammatory response, resistance to infection, and other processes. Fortunately the HPA system with its negative feedback control ordinarily keeps the circulating steroid concentrations within the physiologic range. However, both exogenous and endogenous sources of chronic steroid excess exceed the upper limit of the normal range and produce disease states. The clinical state of

CAUSES OF EXCESS CORTICOSTEROIDS

Exogenous administration
Excessive production of ACTH
  Pituitary origin
  Nonpituitary tumors (e.g., bronchial carcinomas)
Adrenocortical tumors
  Adenomas
  Carcinomas
Macronodular adrenal hyperplasia

chronic glucocorticoid excess was described by Harvey Cushing, and the syndrome now bears his name.[2,16,34,37]

Causes of excess corticosteroids. The most common cause of steroid excess is exogenous administration for treatment of diseases such as arthritis or for immunosuppression, particularly in organ transplantation (see boxed material above). The exogenous steroids are usually the synthetic glucocorticoids such as prednisone or methylprednisolone. Doses above a certain level per day are associated with the stigmata of steroid excess in a high percentage of cases. The daily doses for various steroids required to produce glucocorticoid excess range from 50 to 75 mg for cortisone, 10 to 15 mg for prednisone, 8 to 12 mg for methylprednisolone, and 0.75 to 1 mg for dexamethasone. The endogenous causes of glucocorticoid excess naturally relate to the HPA axis.

Excessive production of ACTH, accounting for 75% to 80% of patients with Cushing's syndrome, is termed *Cushing's disease*. Cushing's disease can arise either from adenomas of the pituitary or rarely from the ectopic production of ACTH by tumors such as bronchial carcinomas. The consequent elevation of circulating ACTH produces adrenal hyperplasia of varying degrees. About 20% to 25% of cases of endogenous excessive glucocorticoid secretion result from primary adrenal causes. Adrenal adenoma is slightly more common than adrenal carcinoma. Another condition known as macronodular adrenal hyperplasia, in which ACTH levels are variably elevated, occurs infrequently.

Diagnosis of endogenous glucocorticoid excess. Many of the following clinical features of steroid excess (Cushing's syndrome) can be anticipated from an understanding of the actions of glucocorticoids:

- Weakness
- Easy tiring
- Headaches
- Amenorrhea
- Poor wound healing
- Hypertension
- Abdominal striae
- Central obesity
- Muscle wasting
- Osteoporosis
- Hyperglycemia

For example, the abdominal striae and poor wound healing in these patients can be explained by the decrease in collagen synthesis. The characteristic hyperglycemia stems from decreased glucose tolerance. Osteoporosis and muscle wasting are the results of steroids' effect on protein metabolism. The peculiar central obesity is probably caused by the differential sensitivity of tissues to insulin and steroids, as mentioned previously.

Several diagnostic maneuvers are available for establishing the diagnosis of Cushing's syndrome and determining the specific cause. Some of the tests and their interpretations are listed in Table 57-2. Diagnosis of excessive glucocorticoid production can be made by demonstrating either increased plasma cortisol concentrations or increased urinary excretion of free cortisol or metabolic products that can be measured as 17-hydroxycorticosteroids. Loss of diurnal variation in plasma cortisol concentrations is typical of the endogenous causes of glucocorticoid excess. Diagnostic details of assay techniques, normal values, and various manipulative tests can be found in standard clinical texts.

Table 57-2 **DIAGNOSTIC CONSIDERATIONS IN CUSHING'S SYNDROME**

Test Findings	Interpretation
Increased plasma or urinary cortisol	Excessive cortisol production
Loss of diurnal variation of plasma cortisol	Endogenous source of cortisol
Dexamethasone (Dex):	
Suppressible cortisol production	Excessive pituitary ACTH production
Nonsuppressible cortisol production	Adrenal tumor or ectopic ACTH production
Elevated plasma ACTH:	
Dex suppressible	Excessive pituitary ACTH
Non–dex suppressible	Ectopic ACTH production
Suppressed plasma ACTH	Adrenal tumor

An understanding of the physiology of the HPA axis plus the recent availability of reliable ACTH assays and sensitive adrenal scanning techniques has greatly simplified the diagnosis of Cushing's syndrome. For example, an elevated ACTH concentration together with an elevated cortisol concentration would imply a pituitary source for the hypercortisolemia. In contrast, an adrenal tumor would produce an elevated serum cortisol with undetectable plasma ACTH concentrations because of the negative feedback suppression of ACTH synthesis and release. The infrequent entity of macronodular adrenal hyperplasia can be associated with both elevated cortisol and detectable plasma ACTH, but characteristically nodular, enlarged, bilateral adrenal glands on computed tomography (CT) scan confirm the diagnosis.

Therapeutic considerations. The mainstay of therapy for chronic steroid excess originating in the adrenals is surgical adrenalectomy. For the patient with Cushing's syndrome and resistant infection, however, the physician should consider the use of metyrapone before surgery. Metyrapone blocks the 11-beta-hydroxylase enzymes responsible for converting deoxycortisol to cortisol (see Fig 57-1). Metyrapone is successful in lowering cortisol in the patient with adrenal tumors because the normal rise in ACTH and the consequent overriding of the enzymatic block is not present in these patients because of chronic suppression of ACTH by hypercortisolemia. The consequent normalization or suppression of cortisol by metyrapone leads to the reversal of the hyperglucocorticoid state and usually renders the infection amenable to antibiotic and surgical therapy. Aminoglutethimide has also been used for this purpose (see following section on sex steroids). Disadvantages of this strategy include the 2 to 3 months' delay in removing the adrenal pathology, occasional reactions to the drugs, and noncompliance by the patient. Attention must also be given to possible drug-induced adrenal insufficiency, and dexamethasone is usually the replacement steroid of choice used with these steroidogenic blocking agents.

In considering adrenalectomy for glucocorticoid excess, the surgeon must remember several basic points. Since glucocorticoid effects last hours, or even months in the case of chronic excess, exogenous steroid replacement can be initiated in the operating room in the form of intravenous hydrocortisone. This schedule is in contrast to the appropriate lead time of 6 to 12 hours when, for example, patients are undergoing adrenalectomy for breast cancer palliation. The operative approach may be altered by the threat of wound infection and wound dehiscence. Many surgeons prefer a flank or paravertebral approach instead of a transabdominal incision. The thickened panniculus in these patients is an added incentive toward choosing the posterior, retroperitoneal approach. The incidence of pancreatitis is lower after left adrenalectomy through a posterior approach than through the transabdominal route; the latter approach necessitates disturbing the pancreas to locate and surgically remove the left adrenal gland. The posterior approach through the eleventh or twelfth rib bed does not allow removal of large tumors, and the choice of approach must be based on more than pathophysiologic aspects.

In the postoperative period infection in the wound may be difficult to detect because of the suppressed inflammatory response. In some instances only a high index of suspicion will lead to detection by needle aspiration or sterile wound probe of an early infection. The compromised rate of wound healing dictates that skin sutures or clips be left in place two to three times longer in these patients than in those with sutures or clips in a comparable location. Although adrenalectomy can be done for Cushing's disease, transsphenoidal hypophysectomy is currently the treatment of choice. Microsurgical techniques allow removal of the pituitary adenomas and leave behind normally functioning pituitary tissue. The increasing availability and success rate of this procedure have also led to the less frequent use of palliative measures such as pituitary suppression by cyproheptadine. Weaning the patient to maintenance doses of steroids after total adrenalectomy, or postoperative elimination of the steroids in the case of unilateral adrenalectomy, is discussed in the following section.

Hypoadrenocorticism

Recognition and Diagnosis. Many of the effects of inadequate or absent circulating concentrations of cortisol suggesting hypoadrenocorticism can be predicted from knowledge of the actions of the glucocorticoids. In most cases the diagnosis can be established by the measurement of plasma cortisol or the excretion of cortisol in the urine, which demonstrates low or absent amounts. However, this may not be true following an acute decrease in steroid administration to a normal level in those patients exposed to chronic, excessive amounts of cortisol. Also, the physician should not wait for confirmatory laboratory evidence before increasing therapy. The clinical presentation of the steroid deficit and the laboratory findings largely depend on the clinical context. The development of *chronic adrenocortical insufficiency (Addison's disease)* may be insidious. The major etiologies include the following:

- Surgical adrenalectomy
- Metastatic cancer to the adrenal cortex
- Tuberculosis of the adrenal cortex
- Adrenal hemorrhage
- Withdrawal of chronic steroid therapy
- Pharmacologic agents, e.g., aminoglutethimide, ortho,para-dichloro-diphenyl-dichloroethane
- Congenital steroidogenic enzyme defects
- Idiopathic causes

Surgical adrenalectomy may have been performed many years before, and now the patient may be inadequately replaced by maintenance steroids during stressful periods or for various reasons may have chosen not to take the steroids appropriately.

Patients with Addison's disease usually experience weight loss, dehydration, and perhaps diarrhea. In extreme cases they may develop fever, hypotension, and cardiovascular collapse. Hyperpigmentation of the skin may result from the compensatory increase in ACTH and the accompanying melanotropic hormone. Hyponatremia, hyperkalemia, and eosinophilia are characteristic. On the other hand, the clinical picture of acute adrenal insufficiency is usually different from that of the chronic form. Acute insufficiency is typically seen in the patient inadequately replaced during a stressful period such as surgical procedures. Significant weight loss and hyperpigmentation obviously will not develop during this short time. Hyponatremia and hyperkalemia are usually not prominent features. The patient may experience malaise, and hyperpyrexia and hypotension may ensue.

Other clinical syndromes that appear after withdrawal or tapering of steroids following a previous state of steroid excess are sometimes confusing. The plasma cortisol concentration may even be within the normal range; however, the patient may still experience anorexia, nausea, lethargy, headaches, arthralgias, and weight loss. The mechanisms for these symptoms are poorly understood, but presumably cortisol insufficiency is present relative to the preexisting level of available steroids on which the various physiologic functions had become dependent.

Treatment. In considering prevention of adrenal insufficiency, *timing* of treatment is the initial question. In patients with known adrenal ablation or destruction who have not received steroid treatment for several days, it is imperative to restart replacement therapy immediately. The patient who is facing surgery or is under other forms of stress and is taking only maintenance replacement doses of cortisone should have supplemental steroid therapy.

A more difficult question arises when the patient has been chronically placed on high-dose therapeutic steroids and is facing surgery. Should the patient receive increased steroid supplementation during a period of stress? The answer will depend on the dose of the particular steroid taken, the frequency of administration, and the duration of therapy. Suppression of the HPA axis can be expected if the patient has been receiving more than 50 to 75 mg of cortisone, 10 to 15 mg of prednisone, or 1 mg of dexamethasone daily. The HPA axis will probably not be suppressed if the patient has been taking steroids every other day rather than every day. Even alternate-day administration of a long-acting steroid, such as dexamethasone, may suppress the HPA axis, especially if the dose is high. Although anecdotal reports of an unresponsive HPA axis following only 1 to 2 weeks of steroid therapy exist, after more than 2 to 3 weeks of daily steroid therapy patients should be assumed to have a suppressed HPA system and should be covered accordingly by increased steroid administration during periods of stress.

Once the question of indications for steroid coverage is settled, the *dosage* of increased steroids must be decided. In the patient previously receiving maintenance steroid dosage, periods of stress can be safely covered by giving two to three times the normal steroid replacement, for example, 50 mg of cortisone acetate every 8 hours. Because of its short half-life, intravenous hydrocortisone should be given every 6 hours in 50- to 100-mg doses. For patients previously exposed to excessive glucocorticoid activity, whether exogenous during treatment of a disease process or endogenous from the pituitary and/or adrenal gland, the exact steroid dosage is more difficult to prescribe. Because of the relative adrenal insufficiency that may be present in patients who previously took high doses of steroids, a more liberal use of steroid replacement may be indicated. Following removal of an adrenal adenoma that produced Cushing's syndrome, for example, the patient may be treated with 100 mg of cortisone acetate every 8 hours for the first 24 to 48 hours. Although the inactive cortisone is rapidly converted to the active cortisol in vivo, some clinicians prefer the use of intravenous hydrocortisone administered every 6 hours in 100-mg doses.

The short-term tapering of steroid doses to maintenance levels is usually simple in those patients who previously received maintenance steroids. However, the physician often observes patients with previous chronic hypercortisolemia who experience withdrawal syndromes and have the symptoms described earlier. In such instances the acute tapering of the steroids must be done gradually over days or weeks to avoid these symptoms. When steroids must only be tapered to their preexisting therapeutic levels or when the adrenals were previously absent or nonfunctioning and tapering is at basal maintenance levels, patients usually experience no problems with symptoms. The more difficult situation is gauging dose schedules in patients following a unilateral adrenalectomy for Cushing's syndrome or in those taking high doses of therapeutic steroids who need to be weaned from these medications. Sudden cessation of steroid administration would lead to hypocortisolemia because of the chronically suppressed HPA axis.

The HPA axis recovers from steroid suppression in two stages. Within the first 3 months ACTH is secreted in normal amounts. In the ensuing several months the adrenal cortex regains its responsiveness to ACTH. After the initial 2 to 3 months, it is then possible to hasten the reappearance of adrenocorticoid responsiveness by infusing ACTH. Responsiveness can be tested by measuring pre- and post-ACTH serum cortisol concentrations. An alternative method is to switch after 2 or 3 months from daily to alternate-day steroid administration in order to accentuate stimulation of the adrenal cortex with endogenous ACTH. In most instances with either method, a certain trial-and-error element exists, the patient must be monitored by serum cortisol concentrations, and the clinical condition must be observed.

The question of mineralocorticoid replacement also often arises. In many patients with HPA axis suppression, mineralocorticoid replacement is unnecessary. Aldosterone secretion is largely regulated by the renin-angiotensin system, and ACTH is not necessary for stimulation of its secretion. Even in patients with adrenal ablation, administration of a mineralocorticoid may not be necessary since some activity resides in cortisone acetate, the oral maintenance form of cortisol typically used. In a substantial number of patients, however, cortisone is not sufficient to replace mineralocorticoid needs, and a mineralocorticoid such as 1 mg of fluorohydrocortisone daily is required. The need for such supplementation can be judged by a tendency toward hypotension, hyponatremia, and hyperkalemia. Additional precision may be added by measuring plasma renin activity, which will be elevated in the presence of sodium loss and a negative sodium balance.[30,61]

Sex Steroids

Although the surgeon does not often encounter problems arising from the adrenal gland relating directly to the secretion of androgens or estrogens, several relevant concerns in this area of adrenal physiology must be emphasized. The general surgeon will encounter adrenal tumors that secrete androgens and estrogens, either alone or in combination with the glucocorticoids or mineralocorticoids. The urologist may also encounter these tumors and may frequently deal with sexual ambiguity in children. In addition, both the urologist and the oncologist will be concerned with the derivation of estrogens from the adrenal cortex when choosing hormonal therapy for prostatic and breast cancer.

Physiologic Steroid Secretion

Normal secretion of androgens by the adrenal cortex has clinical implications mainly for steroid-sensitive cancer. To understand the role of the adrenal cortex in this regard, it is helpful to outline the secretion of adrenal androgens and the subsequent conversion of these androgens to estrogens in peripheral tissue.

Androgenic Secretion. As can be seen from Fig. 57-1, the three androgenic steroids arising from the adrenal cortex are dehydroepiandrosterone (DHEA), androstenedione, and testosterone. Quantitatively, DHEA is the most prominent androgenic product of the adrenal cortex. However, androstenedione is important for conversion to estrogen, whereas testosterone is the most potent of the three in terms of androgenic activity. The adrenal cortex clearly has the potential to produce virilization, either through secretion of androgens by tumors or as a consequence of enzyme defects that shunt steroidogenesis toward androgen formation.

Breast and Prostate Cancer. In terms of estrogen-sensitive cancer, the peripheral conversion of androstenedione to estrone and estradiol is the most important facet of adrenal androgen secretion. Androstenedione is converted to estrone by a series of hydroxylations that depend on the cytochrome P-450 system. This process of aromatization is the sole source of estrogens in men and postmenopausal women. Studies have now demonstrated that cancers of the breast and prostate having estrogen receptors respond favorably to adrenal ablation, either medical or surgical. An especially interesting agent, aminoglutethimide, illustrates the importance of both adrenal androgen secretion and the peripheral aromatization of the androgens to estrogens. This drug blocks the conversion of cholesterol to pregnenolone, with the consequent decreased production of adrenal androgens. Cortisol is also lowered, and a resultant outpouring of ACTH occurs unless inhibited by the use of such glucocorticoids as dexamethasone. However, even if dexamethasone is not employed and adrenal androgen secretion is significant, aminoglutethimide has a potent effect on blocking aromatization, as evidenced by extremely low peripheral estrogen concentrations.[51]

Excessive Secretion

In the surgical context excessive androgen secretion is related to (1) adrenal tumors in adults and children and (2) congenital adrenocortical enzymatic defects, which are seen primarily in newborns as sexual ambiguity.

Adrenal Tumors. Androgen secretion by adrenal tumors is associated with a predominance of cortisol secretion. Female patients with Cushing's syndrome have masculinizing features such as coarsening of facial hair and distribution of pubic hair into the male pattern. Although aspects of virilization may appear in patients with benign adrenocortical tumors, excessive adrenal androgen production, as evidenced by increased 17-ketosteroids in the urine, is almost always seen in adrenocortical carcinoma. The most striking clinical examples of virilizing adrenal tumors are those producing primarily androgens. These particular tumors may go undetected initially in the adult male, but the female patient undergoes a deepening of the voice, coarsening of the skin, thickening and darkening of the facial hairs, assumption of male hair distribution, clitoral hypertrophy, and menstrual cessation. These tumors also appear in childhood and result in precocious puberty in both males and females. Virilization is a prominent feature in female children, as in the female adult.

The converse situation is seen with the rare adrenal carcinoma that produces estrogens. These tumors are difficult to detect in the female patient, but menstrual irregularities may lead to definitive diagnosis by measurement of plasma or urinary estrogens. The male patient has loss of libido and onset of impotency, enlargement of breast tissue, and possible softening of facial hair with a regression of sexual hair from the male distribution.

Enzymatic Defects. An interesting syndrome, *congenital adrenal hyperplasia,* takes several forms depending on the exact enzymatic defect present. Placement of these enzymes in the steroidogenic pathway is represented in Fig. 57-1.

The two most common enzymatic defects, *21-hydroxylase deficiency* and *11-beta-hydroxylase deficiency,* both produce masculinization in the female infant that must be distinguished from female pseudohermaphroditism of chromosomal origin. Defects in the 11-beta-hydroxylase or 21-hydroxylase enzymes result in an overproduction of adrenal androgen by the fetus in utero. The circulating androgens, usually absent in the female, cause stimulation of the wolffian ducts, elongation of the genital tubercle with migration of the labioscrotal folds, and midline fusion of these folds and swellings to form the penis and scrotal sac. The urethral opening migrates to the tip of the phallus. In the normal fetus the ovary does not secrete testosterone, and the genital tubercle remains small, the labial folds unfused, and so on. Besides endogenous androgen producing masculinization, *exogenous* androgens from maternal ingestion of androgenic compounds during the first trimester of pregnancy or from an androgen-secreting tumor in the mother can produce virilization of the fetal external genitalia. Although the male infant may show no immediate effects of the enzymatic defect, subsequent masculinization and precocious puberty will become obvious.

The 11-beta-hydroxylase deficiency may be accompanied by hypertension because of excessive secretion of deoxycorticosterone. The 21-hydroxylase deficiency may be of the salt-wasting variety, with consequent dehydration and early fatality unless diagnosed promptly and treated adequately with glucocorticoids, mineralocorticoids, and sodium chloride. It is not clear why this particular deficiency occurs in two forms, but two hypotheses are most widely accepted: (1) the enzymatic defect is more complete in the salt-wasting than in the non-salt-wasting form, or (2) the zona glomerulosa 21-hydroxylase enzyme, distinct from that in the zona fasciculata, is deficient only in the salt-wasting variant.

Two other relatively rare disorders are *17-hydroxylase deficiency* and *3-hydroxysteroid dehydrogenase deficiency*. In the 17-hydroxylase deficiency hypertension is caused by the excessive secretion of deoxycorticosterone and corticosterone. Subnormal levels of plasma cortisol are also present. In males the testis fails to secrete androgens, and thus the normal male external genitalia may fail to develop. The ovary in females fails to secrete estrogen, and secondary sex characteristics fail to develop at the normal age of puberty. The 3-hydroxysteroid dehydrogenase deficiency results in decreased secretion of both mineralocorticoids and glucocorticoids but increased quantities of adrenal androgens. The cortisol and mineralocorticoid deficiency requires replacement of these steroids. Males fail to develop normal external genitalia because of the gonads' participation in this deficit. Partial masculinization in females results from the hypersecretion of the weak adrenal androgens.[45]

Aldosterone

Aldosterone is a steroid originating from the zona glomerulosa of the adrenal cortex. It is the end product of a steroidogenic pathway that includes corticosterone and deoxycorticosterone, as shown in Fig. 57-1. Aldosterone has a specific effect on sodium, potassium, and hydrogen ion transport. As with glucocorticoids, the specificity of the action of aldosterone is determined by its chemical configuration, by the conformational structure and location of steroid receptors, and by postreceptor intracellular events. In contrast to the glucocorticoids, the actions of aldosterone are comparatively circumscribed because of the limited distribution of the receptors. The receptors' location in the kidney tubule means that aldosterone plays a major role in the control of sodium, potassium, and extracellular fluid balance. Aldosterone receptors in the salivary glands and the colonic mucosa are less obviously important.

Control of Aldosterone Secretion

The primary control mechanism for aldosterone secretion is the renin-angiotensin system. Renin is released from the juxtaglomerular apparatus of the kidney in response to a decrease in vascular volume, such as occurs with hemorrhage, a negative sodium balance, or dehydration. Both a decrease in pressure in the afferent arteriole entering the glomerulus and a decrease in intratubular sodium concentration at the level of the macula densa (a sensing apparatus adjacent to the arterial juxtaglomerular apparatus) will stimulate renin secretion. Renin released into the bloodstream hydrolyzes a circulating protein substrate derived from the liver to produce a decapeptide designated *angiotensin I*. The peptide is then further cleaved by a converting enzyme in the lung to form an octapeptide, *angiotensin II*. As well as being a potent vasoconstrictor, angiotensin II is a trophic hormone to the adrenal zona glomerulosa and stimulates secretion of aldosterone. Thus hemorrhage, dehydration, and so on result in an increase in aldosterone secretion because of stimulation by angiotensin II. Conversely, conditions producing a replete blood volume, positive sodium balance, overhydration, and so forth lead to a suppression of angiotensin II formation and a decrease in aldosterone secretion.

Aldosterone secretion apparently is also controlled directly by the concentration of serum potassium. An increase in serum potassium results in the stimulation of aldosterone secretion, whereas a decrease results in a lowering of the aldosterone secretion rate. In the anephric patient, in the absence of the renin-angiotensin system, serum potassium appears to be the primary mechanism for control of aldosterone secretion.

ACTH is capable of stimulating aldosterone secretion. Such stimulation is obviously accompanied by an increase in cortisol secretion. In comparison, angiotensin II and serum potassium do not stimulate cortisol production. Although ACTH clearly can stimulate aldosterone, ACTH alone is not sufficient to restore the full secretory capacity of the zona glomerulosa.

Various other conditions modulate the sensitivity of the zona glomerulosa to stimuli. For example, increased potassium or decreased sodium intake enhances the sensitivity of the zona glomerulosa to angiotensin stimulation. An increased potassium intake enhances the responsiveness of the zona glomerulosa to increased potassium itself or to ACTH stimulation. Hypothyroidism decreases the response to angiotensin II, whether increased serum potassium or ACTH infusion. Recent studies have shown that dopamine directly inhibits the secretion of aldosterone. The physiologic significance of the dopamine observation is currently under investigation.[9,15,21]

The boxed material at top right lists the factors relevant to aldosterone secretion.

FACTORS IN CONTROL OF ALDOSTERONE SECRETION

Stimulators
Angiotensin
Serum K^+
ACTH

Inhibitor
Dopamine

Potentiators	**Stimuli**
Hyperkalemia	Angiotensin Hyperkalemia ACTH
Negative Na^+ balance	Angiotensin

Aldosterone Effects

Direct Mechanisms. Receptors for aldosterone have been found in such tissues as the parotid gland and colonic mucosa, but the primary site for physiologic control of electrolyte and fluid balance is in the kidney. Furthermore, those receptors responsible for the increased sodium reabsorption from the kidney appear to be located specifically in the cortical section of the collecting tubule. From work with the renal receptors and with those in the amphibian urinary bladder, the intracellular mechanism of receptor binding and so on, as described for the glucocorticoids, apparently applies to aldosterone. The 60- to 120-minute latent period seen in vivo between administration of aldosterone and its effects on the kidney can be related directly to the time during which binding to the cytosol receptor, activation of the receptor, translocation into the nucleus, and transcription to produce mRNA and new protein occur.

The primary effect of aldosterone on the kidney is a net sodium resorption in the proximal portion of the collecting tubule. Interestingly, no three types of mineralocorticoid receptors have been identified according to specificity and affinity for several classes of steroids. The Type I receptor, which is thought to be the specific receptor for aldosterone, also has a weak affinity for corticosterone and dysoxycorticosterone. Although the Type II receptor retains a strong affinity for aldosterone, it also has a strong affinity for the glucocorticoids; this particular type of receptor may be responsible for the effects of glucocorticoids on electrolyte and water excretion. Considering the effect of aldosterone on sodium resorption by the tubule, a deficit of aldosterone is associated with a negative sodium balance, whereas excess aldosterone together with continued sodium intake results in an overload in total body sodium. Under normal circumstances an upper limit is placed on the sodium and consequent fluid overload by an ill-defined renal mechanism sometimes referred to as the *escape phenomenon*. After an expansion by 2 to 3 L equivalent of normal saline in terms of total sodium balance, the kidney overrides excessive, inappropriate aldosterone effects, and natriuresis occurs. The responsible mediator for the escape may be a newly discovered substance in the myocardium named *auriculin*.

Another effect of aldosterone is increased potassium secretion. The exact mechanism for the kaliuresis is currently unclear. Initially it was thought to be a simple exchange of sodium for potassium across the tubular membrane, but recent evidence suggests that the secretion of potassium may not relate directly to the reabsorption of sodium. Several mechanisms for potassium secretion, such as changes in acid/base balance or changes in fluid flow through the renal tubule, could represent indirect means whereby aldosterone could influence potassium secretion. Regardless of the mechanism, a chronic aldosterone excess results in a depletion of body potassium through increased kaliuresis. Aldosterone also promotes a secretion of hydrogen ions into the renal tubule. This process may also not necessarily be associated directly with sodium reabsorption. The net result of chronic proton deficit is the development of a metabolic alkalosis.

The influence of aldosterone on water balance is best seen in the deficient state. In adrenal insufficiency both a defect in free water clearance, which may lead to water intoxication, and a decrease in maximum urinary concentration occur. Two mechanisms are probably responsible for the defect in free water clearance. The sodium depletion resulting from the deficit in aldosterone leads to a decreased extracellular fluid volume with a decreased delivery of filtrate to the ascending limb of Henle's loop. The resultant increase in the corticomedullary concentration gradient promotes increased reabsorption of water from the collecting duct. In addition, the contraction in extracellular fluid results in an increased secretion of ADH, which also inhibits the excretion of a water load. The decreased maximum urine concentration is not clearly explained, but it may relate to a demonstrated loss of sensitivity in the tubule to the action of ADH. Thus, although ADH secretion is above normal because of a contracted extracellular fluid, as already mentioned, the maximum concentration of urine is below normal because of the decreased renal tubular sensitivity to ADH. With normal aldosterone secretion, free water clearance is maintained and maximum urinary concentration is restored.[39,41]

Indirect Effects Of Excess Aldosterone. The most notable result of increased sodium reabsorption in response to excess aldosterone secretion is an increase in blood pressure. Two mechanisms have been proposed as being responsible. One invokes an increase in vascular intramural sodium concentration, with a subsequent fluid increase in the small precapillary arterioles that leads to increased vascular resistance and hypertension. The other possible mechanism relates to an increased extracellular volume resulting from the renal effects of sodium retention and consequent water retention. The expansion of extracellular fluid has another effect, important mainly in the diagnosis of primary aldosteronism. The positive sodium balance results in a chronic, sustained suppression of renin secretion from the kidney; thus hyporeninemia is a characteristic finding in primary hyperaldosteronism. Characteristically, no peripheral edema occurs in hyperaldosteronism because of the renal escape mechanism previously mentioned.

The loss of potassium from the kidney results in hypokalemia. The resulting hypokalemia has at least three systemic effects:

1. Hypokalemia can produce a change in renal tubular function, even progressing to nephropathy, which is manifested by an impairment of the kidney's ability to concentrate urine. The clinical features of polydipsia, polyuria, and nocturia result.
2. Hypokalemia can also result in muscle weakness, cramps, and even paralysis if it is severe.
3. Hypokalemia can influence the beta cells of the pancreas. The sensitivity of the beta cell for insulin release by glucose stimulation is lowered, and the resultant hypoinsulinemia accounts for a trend toward hyperglycemia in such patients.

In this setting a hypokalemic metabolic alkalosis can develop. As mentioned earlier, the loss of hydrogen ions in the urine produces systemic alkalosis. Both the reputed effect of aldosterone on chloride secretion by the kidney and the intrarenal mechanisms of chloride secretion related to systemic alkalosis lead to a characteristic hypochloremic alkalosis. The hypokalemia just mentioned is also characteristic of this alkalosis. Some of the actions of aldosterone and their effects are listed in Table 57-3.[32]

Hyperaldosteronism

Secondary Hyperaldosteronism. A variety of acute forms of secondary hyperaldosteronism may come to the attention of the surgeon. The acute HPA response to surgical stress is discussed in an earlier section. Even in the absence of blood loss, aldosterone may be stimulated to some degree by the effect of ACTH on the zona glomerulosa. The typical retention of sodium and excretion of potassium seen during acute surgical stress is partly caused by the renal effects of aldosterone. The increase in aldosterone secretion associated with significant blood loss is mediated primarily by the renin-angiotensin system. Similarly, dehydration or loss of extracellular fluid by any one of several mechanisms, such as diarrhea, vomiting, or major burns, will result in hyperaldosteronism. Under any of these circumstances the hyperaldosteronism has the effect of retaining sodium and thereby preventing a further decrease in extracellular volume through renal mechanisms.

Chronic secondary hyperaldosteronism may be seen in diseases affecting internal shifts in the extracellular fluid volume, such as congestive heart failure with peripheral edema or hepatic cirrhosis with the accumulation of fluid in the third space (i.e., ascites). A different mechanism provokes hyperaldosteronism in renal hypertension. The

Table 57-3 **RENAL ACTIONS OF ALDOSTERONE AND THEIR EFFECTS**

Actions	Effects
Increased renal tubular reabsorption of sodium	Positive sodium balance Hypertension Hyporeninemia
Decreased renal tubular reabsorption of potassium	Hypokalemia Polyuria, nocturia Muscle weakness, paralysis Hypoinsulinemia Hyperglycemia Metabolic alkalosis

sequential relationship of renal artery constriction or renal parenchymal damage, hyperreninemia, and angiotensinemia, as well as stimulation of the zona glomerulosa, explains the increased secretion of aldosterone. All these conditions leading to secondary hyperaldosteronism are associated with hyperreninemia, a finding in marked contrast to the hyporeninemia of primary aldosteronism.[14]

PRIMARY HYPERALDOSTERONISM

Etiology. Primary aldosteronism arises from an autonomous overproduction of aldosterone through intrinsic adrenal mechanisms. An adrenocortical adenoma arising from the zona glomerulosa is most often responsible for this condition. This diagnosis is particularly gratifying because surgical removal of such a lesion results in amelioration or cure of the hypertension in a high percentage of patients. On the other hand, primary aldosteronism may result from hyperplasia of the zona glomerulosa, and bilateral adrenalectomy may not eliminate the hypertension. The origin of hyperplasia of the zona glomerulosa is currently obscure. A rare, familial form of hyperplasia causing hyperaldosteronism is suppressible by dexamethasone administration.

Recognition and diagnosis. The typical clinical presentation of primary hyperaldosteronism is a normal-appearing patient with hypertension and hypokalemia. Both of these findings can be explained by the effect of aldosterone on the sodium and potassium balance. The patient may also have polyuria and polydipsia because of the hypokalemic effect on the kidney. Glucose intolerance may be present as a result of the hypokalemic effect on pancreatic beta-cell sensitivity. The diagnosis of aldosteronism is confirmed by either an elevated plasma aldosterone concentration or increased excretion of aldosterone in the urine. The condition can be identified as primary and distinguished from secondary hyperaldosteronism by the finding of suppressed plasma renin activity. As already stated, most causes of secondary hyperaldosteronism are associated with a contraction in effective blood volume and a consequent increase in plasma renin activity.

It is important from a therapeutic standpoint to distinguish between adenoma and hyperplasia, both of which can produce primary hyperaldosteronism. If available, adrenal vein catheterization and measurement of differential aldosterone concentrations in the adrenal effluent should be attempted. Monitored by plasma cortisol concentrations to validate the exact blood sampling location, adrenovenous aldosterone concentrations can distinguish hyperplasia from adenoma. With hyperplasia equal concentrations of aldosterone are found in each adrenal effluent, whereas with an adenoma aldosterone will be greatly increased in the adrenal effluent from the affected side. A promising imaging technique uses radioactive cholesterol to take advantage of cholesterol's incorporation into the steroidogenic pathway. The adrenal gland harboring a tumor will show up quite clearly on the scintillation scan, whereas the contralateral adrenal gland may not be visualized because of renin-angiotensin suppression and consequent unstimulated zona glomerulosa activity. In contrast, hyperplasia will result in highly visible adrenal glands bilaterally. Uptake of cholesterol by the glucocorticoid pathway must be suppressed, and dexamethasone is used for ACTH-cortisol inhibition. The effective use of a CT scan for diagnostic purposes is possible in some cases, but the gland in the zona glomerulosa hyperplasia usually does not increase to an appreciable size. Also, the occasional very small adenomas producing primary aldosteronism may be undectable by CT scan.

Since adrenal vein catheterization or radioactive imaging techniques may not be available, use of the *plasma aldosterone response* to an upright posture may be diagnostically beneficial. In patients with primary aldosteronism caused by an adenoma, the plasma aldosterone decreases in the morning following a 4-hour upright position. Such a decrease reflects two conditions: a decreasing plasma ACTH because of the circadian variation and the tumor's residual responsiveness to ACTH. The response of the tumor to angiotensin is slight. In contrast, hyperplasia of the zona glomerulosa is exquistitely sensitive to angiotensin, and the 4 hours of upright posture result in an increase in angiotensin and consequent elevation of serum aldosterone. Therefore, by measuring aldosterone after 4 hours of upright posture, the distinction between adenoma and hyperplasia can be made in a high percentage of patients.

Treatment. Preoperative preparation of the patient with primary aldosteronism takes advantage of aldosterone producing almost all its effects through renal mechanisms. Spironolactone is a specific aldosterone antagonist at the renal locus that blocks the action of aldosterone to promote sodium excretion and potassium retention. Thus spironolactone can be used in preoperative patients to lower the blood pressure and normalize the serum potassium. Because of a long-standing negative potassium balance, it may be prudent to supplement these patients' diet with oral potassium. Usually the serum potassium will return to normal in 7 to 10 days.

Postoperatively the only pathophysiologic aberration sometimes seen is selective mineralocorticoid deficiency. After removal of one adrenal gland, the zona glomerulosa of the contralateral gland remains inactive. The long-standing suppression of plasma renin lingers for days after removal of the tumor. In a process somewhat analogous to the ACTH-cortisol relationship following removal of a cortisol-producing tumor, circulating angiotensin normalizes after several weeks, and the responsiveness of the zona glomerulosa soon follows. During the interim, when the angiotensin-aldosterone system is unresponsive, it may be necessary to administer a mineralocorticoid; fluorohydrocortisone at 0.1 mg/day is usually sufficient. The tendency toward hypotension and hyperkalemia will be corrected by this regimen.[3,22,24]

ADRENOMEDULLARY PHYSIOLOGY

The medulla is the thin inner layer of the adrenal gland, sandwiched within the substance of the gland and surrounded by the cortex. In broad terms it functions similar to the adrenal cortex in that it discharges substances into the bloodstream that circulate to produce effects in distant tissues. On the other hand, the adrenal medulla is different from the adrenal cortex in several ways. The adrenal medulla is derived from the neural crest cells and may participate in conditions affecting other organs of this origin, such as the anterior pituitary, pancreatic islets, and C cells of the thyroid in multiple endocrine adenomatoses. Although circulating substances arising from a distance can modulate its secretion, the adrenal medulla is controlled mainly through direct apposition of sympathetic nerve fibers on its secreting cells. In general the stimuli that cause increased secretion of adrenomedullary products are also those that stimulate the sympathetic nervous system. Although many of these same stimuli also produce an increased secretion of steroids from the adrenal cortex, this increase from the cortex is mediated by a circulating substance, ACTH, rather than through direct neural stimulation by preganglionic sympathetic fibers.

The following sections outline anatomic and functional features of the adrenal medulla.

Adrenergic Nervous System and Adrenomedullary Secretion

Anatomic Arrangements

Since it lies within the adrenal gland, the adrenal medulla is situated above the kidney. Basically it is a suprarenal sympathetic ganglion and functions much as other sympathetic ganglia do. It is richly innervated by preganglionic sympathetic fibers arising in neurons in the spinal cord. These fibers arise predominantly at the level of T10 and T11. The ordinary sympathetic ganglia, such as the paravertebral ganglia of the "sympathetic chain," or the preaortic ganglia exemplified by the celiac, superior mesenteric, and inferior mesenteric locations, are also innervated by preganglionic fibers that employ cholinergic transmission of impulses to the ganglia. These ordinary sympathic ganglia contain neurons that send out fibers to various intraabdominal and lower extremity structures. The postganglionic neuronal terminals elaborate norepinephrine as the transjunctional neurotransmitter to these adjacent structures. With the adrenal medulla, however, the preganglionic cholinergic fibers transmit their signals to the chromaffin cells of the adrenal medulla, which in turn elaborate both epinephrine and norepinephrine into the surrounding vascular sinusoids. Thus the adrenal medulla communicates with distant target structures through hormones transported by the vascular system.

Adrenomedullary Secretion

Epinephrine and norepinephrine are the principal secretory products of the adrenal medulla. Dopamine is also a secretory product of undetermined functional significance. Enkephalins have recently been found in the adrenal medulla, but their significance is also unclear. In the human being, under basal conditions, approximately 80% of the catecholamine output is epinephrine.

Much of the information obtained concerning human adrenomedullary secretion depended on the development of sensitive and precise assays for circulating catecholamines. Two such general methods currently in use are radioenzymatic assays and those using high-pressure liquid chromatography. Interpretation of the peripheral concentrations of catecholamines as related to adrenomedullary secretion is somewhat difficult because norepinephrine spillover from peripheral sympathetic nerve terminals produces fluctuating plasma norepinephrine concentrations in response to a variety of stimuli. Therefore, in terms of circulating norepinephrine concentrations, it is not clear whether these changes represent increased adrenomedullary secretion specifically or increased general sympathetic neural discharge. The circulating concentrations of epinephrine have been used to indicate adrenomedullary secretion because the adrenal medulla is unique in being the only sympathetic tissue that elaborates epinephrine. The enzyme, phenylethanolamine-*N*-methyltransferase (PMNT), converts norepinephrine to epinephrine and is found only in the adrenal medulla. Thus, assuming disappearance rates are steady, a rise in peripheral epinephrine concentrations indicates an increase in adrenomedullary secretion. Stimuli that include anxiety, pain, upright posture, cold, isometric and other exercise, hypoglycemia, and hypotension clearly cause an increase in adrenomedullary secretion.

The mechanisms for adrenomedullary secretion involve the induction of certain enzymes in the synthetic pathway for catecholamines, as shown in the boxed material below. The precursor for the catecholamines is the amino acid, tyrosine. The conversion of tyrosine to dihydroxyphenylalanine (dopa) is accomplished by the action of tyrosine hydroxylase. Tyrosine hydroxylase is the rate-limiting enzyme of the entire synthetic pathway. Stimulation of the sympathetic nerves to the adrenal gland results in an increase in tyrosine hydroxylase content, as well as the subsequent increase in norepinephrine and epinephrine production. Next in the pathway, dopa is converted to dopamine by dopa decarboxylase, and the dopamine, now in catecholamine storage vesicles, is converted to norepinephrine by dopamine beta-hydroxylase. As mentioned, PNMT converts norepinephrine into epinephrine. Interestingly, PNMT depends on high concentrations of cortisol for its activity. Demonstrable vascular connections lead from the adrenal cortex through the adrenal medulla, presumably carrying high concentrations of cortisol to the enzyme.

During secretion the storage vesicles containing the catecholamines are brought to the surface of the chromaffin cells during adrenal stimulation and release their contents into the extracellular fluid. From there the catechol-

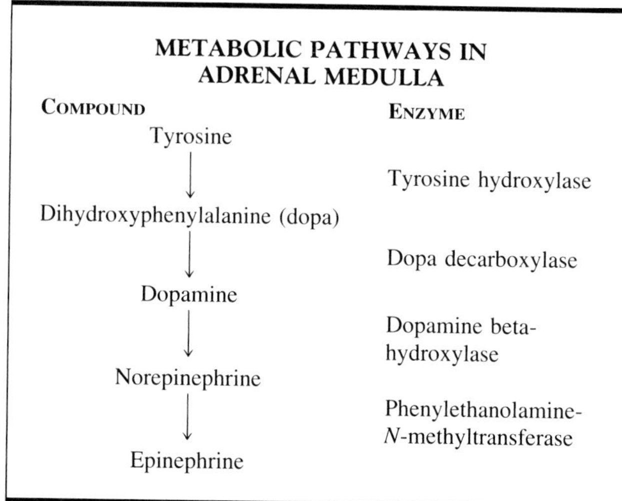

amines quickly enter the vascular circulation to be distributed throughout the body. Dopamine beta-hydroxylase is found exclusively in the secretory vesicles. Interest has focused on release of this enzyme as a separate indicator of adrenomedullary discharge. At present, difficulties with assay techniques and the wide range of its concentrations found in normal subjects limit the usefulness of dopamine beta-hydroxylase as a marker for adrenomedullary secretion.

Several mechanisms are capable of modulating adrenomedullary secretion. The adrenomedullary cells probably are under the same presynaptic control of secretion as exists for the peripheral sympathetic neurons. Receptors are known to exist in these latter structures and are called alpha$_2$-receptors; norepinephrine has an affinity for them. Through binding to the receptors, increased concentrations of norepinephrine serve to inhibit the discharge of neurotransmitters from the terminals. Another adrenomedullary mechanism is the high concentrations of norepinephrine, which result in suppression of tyrosine hydroxylase activity. Since this is the rate-limiting enzyme for catecholamine synthesis, the suppression of tyrosine hydroxylase by its eventual product represents a negative feedback mechanism. The relationship between catecholamine secretion and renin-angiotensin formation is a bidirectional control mechanism. Stimulation of the renal sympathetic nerves or infusion of catecholamines into the renal artery produces an increased renin release and subsequent angiotensin formation. Angiotensin in turn enhances the adrenomedullary response to the various stimuli already enumerated. Conversely, prostaglandins have been shown to suppress the adrenomedullary response to these stimuli.

Following release from either the adrenal medulla or peripheral sympathetic endings, the catecholamines are dissipated by several mechanisms. *Neuronal uptake* is a local phenomenon in which the catecholamines are returned to the storage vesicles, where they can be rereleased. A quantitatively more important mechanism is *enzymatic degradation*. Some catecholamines taken up by the neurons are metabolized by monoamine oxidase, eventually yielding vanillylmandelic acid (VMA). Extraneuronal inactivation occurs primarily through the enzyme carboxy-*O*-methyltransferase (COMT), which is located mainly in the liver and metabolizes catecholamines released into the circulation. The major metabolites of COMT are normetanephrine (in the case of norepinephrine) and metanephrine (in the case of epinephrine). A third means of catecholamine dissipation is the binding of epinephrine or norepinephrine with its receptor on the effector cell. A fourth and minor mechanism is the excretion of free circulating epinephrine and norepinephrine in the urine. A fifth and poorly defined pathway is conjugation to sulfur.*

Catecholamine Effects

Adrenergic Receptor Concept

Based on pharmacologic experiments, two types of responses to catecholamines have been described. In general terms the responses are (1) a contraction of smooth muscle and (2) a relaxation of smooth muscle; these responses are called alpha and beta, respectively. Furthermore, the potency of several specific catecholamines has been compared. The potency series for *alpha effects* is:

$$\text{Epinephrine} > \text{Norepinephrine} \geq \text{Isoproterenol}$$

On the other hand, the potency series for *beta effects* is:

$$\text{Isoproterenol} > \text{Epinephrine} \geq \text{Norepinephrine}$$

The beta-adrenergic agonists are further defined in their potency series by their relative lipolytic, cardiac, bronchodilatory, and vasodilatory effects. *Beta$_1$-receptors* are receptors found on cardiac muscle that result in inotropic and chronotropic responses. Beta-receptors on adipose tissues that mediate the lipolytic effect of epinephrine are also classified as beta$_1$-receptors. The term *beta$_2$-receptors* defines receptors on vascular and bronchial smooth muscle that mediate relaxation of these structures by isoproterenol. Although norepinephrine is almost equal in potency to epinephrine in terms of the beta$_1$-receptors, it is effective only in very high concentrations for beta$_2$ effects. The in vitro use of radioligands has further disclosed the complexities of the adrenergic receptor system.

The alpha receptors have been subdivided into alpha$_1$ and alpha$_2$. *Alpha$_1$-receptors* are found primarily on vascular and uterine smooth muscle to promote contraction. *Alpha$_2$-receptors* are found on platelets to produce aggregation and on presynaptic neuronal terminals to blunt the action potential–evoked release of norepinephrine or acetylcholine. Adrenergic antagonists have been recently developed that emphasize the difference in these two types of alpha-receptors. Prazosin has a greater potency than yohimbine for blockade of the alpha$_1$-norepinephrine effect of vascular smooth muscle contraction. On the other hand, yohimbine is more potent than prazosin in blocking the effects of the catecholamines on platelet aggregation as an alpha$_2$-receptor function. The boxed material below summarizes alpha and beta effects.

The myriad effects of epinephrine and norepinephrine can be explained by several features of the adrenergic re-

ADRENERGIC RECEPTOR–MEDIATED EFFECTS

Beta$_1$
Increased heart rate and force of cardiac contraction
Lipolysis
Decreased peripheral glucose utilization

Beta$_2$
Relaxation of smooth muscle

Alpha$_1$
Contraction of smooth muscle gluconeogenesis
Glycogenolysis
Stimulation of glucagon
Suppression of insulin secretion

Alpha$_2$
Contraction of smooth muscle
Increased platelet aggregation
Antilipolytic effect
Inhibition of noradrenaline release

*References 5, 7, 11, 17, 29, and 64.

ceptors. As mentioned, differential effects between the two catecholamines can be seen according to the amount of agonist present in the circulation. For example, the potency series shows that norepinephrine will have a beta$_2$-receptor effect only at extremely high concentrations that are seldom achieved in vivo, whereas epinephrine and certainly isoproterenol will have a bronchodilatory effect at lower concentrations. Another mechanism for a differential effect is the distribution of types of receptors among various tissues. Some tissues have an abundance of alpha-receptors while being totally devoid of beta-receptors; for example, circulating white blood cells have a predominance of beta-receptors.

One of the most important mechanisms for fine-tuning the catecholamine effects is the regulation of the number of receptors by the catecholamines themselves. The presence of agonists in the receptors has the effect of reducing receptor numbers. Of course, this "down-regulation" or reduction in receptor numbers has the effect of rendering a given tissue less sensitive to catecholamines. Conversely, the presence of antagonists or the lowering of agonist concentration, such as following sympathectomy, increases the number of adrenergic receptors and renders the affected tissue more sensitive to the catecholamines. These regulatory phenomena serve as feedback mechanisms in that the effects of catecholamines are blunted or increased, depending on catecholamine excess or deficit, respectively.

In addition to the regulation of receptor numbers, post-receptor events may be modulated as well. After the receptors are occupied by the catecholamine agonist, adenylate cyclase activity is increased, the cyclic adenosine monophosphate (cAMP) concentration is increased, and a physiologic effect is produced. This information has been derived from recent studies, such as investigations of the effect of hyper- and hypothyroidism on catecholamine sensitivity. Excessive or deficient thyroxine may produce an increase or decrease in adenylate cyclase activity or cAMP concentrations without necessarily producing a change in adrenergic receptor numbers. In some tissues where adrenergic receptors are regulated, the sensitivity to catecholamines may or may not be changed.

The adrenal medulla, fixed in place above the kidney and equipped with its simplistic hormonal output, can still achieve wide-ranging systemic effects through the complex mechanisms just outlined. Stimulatory input into the adrenal medulla can originate from almost all areas and systems of the body, be processed through the CNS, and arrive at the adrenal medulla by way of the afferent adrenal innervation. The resulting secretion of epinephrine and norepinephrine is carried by the bloodstream to all tissues of the body. By regulating the degree of secretion, the concentrations of catecholamines to which these tissues are exposed can be almost infintely varied. Furthermore, the conformation of adrenergic receptors is such that a selectivity of response for the various tissues is achieved according to the type of receptor present. The regulation of receptor number and activity serves as a buffer against the effects of wide fluctuation in the circulating concentrations of catecholamines. Against this background of information, it is useful to look at a few selected effects of adrenomedullary secretion.[35,42,58,59]

Effects of Catecholamines on Selected Systemic Functions

Perhaps because of the stimulation of both alpha- and some beta-receptors by peripheral neuronal norepinephrine, the absence of the adrenal medulla does not have obvious and widespread adverse effects on the body. Norepinephrine's spillover from peripheral nerve terminals along with the rich sympathetic innervation of most tissues and organs in the body, compensates for the absence of secretion from the adrenal medulla. A few exceptions can be cited, such as the slow recovery of blood glucose from insulin-induced hypoglycemia in the adrenalectomized patient. However, the adrenal medulla augments the generalized sympathetic discharge in response to the various stimuli already mentioned, and the effects of this discharge on several selected physiologic functions are outlined in this section.*

Metabolism. Adrenergic discharge has the effect of maintaining and/or raising the plasma glucose concentration.[1,63] This effect is mediated through several mechanisms. Through alpha-receptor stimulation, hepatic production of glucose is increased by the mechanisms of gluconeogenesis and glycogenolysis.

Gluconeogenesis is a result of both the direct effects of catecholamines on the liver and the indirect effects of alpha-receptor stimulation to increase pancreatic glucagon production, which promotes gluconeogenesis. Alpha stimulation of the pancreas concomitantly suppresses insulin secretion. Peripheral utilization of glucose is decreased both as a consequence of suppressed insulin secretion and as a direct effect on peripheral nonmuscular tissues, presumably through a beta-receptor mechanism. Interestingly, catecholamines produce increased glycolysis in the exercising heart and skeletal muscle. Presumably the glycolysis of vigorous exercise would tend to blunt the rise in plasma glucose that is produced by an accentuated adrenergic discharge.

Catecholamines also exert a *glycogenolytic effect* in muscle similar to that in the liver, but the glycogenolysis in muscle is thought to be mediated through a beta-receptor. The recovery from hypoglycemia produced by insulin infusion, for example, is mediated primarily by an increase in plasma glucagon. Also, in the adrenalectomized patient, glucagon is sufficient to promote a recovery from the hypoglycemia. In the absence of glucagon, however, the increased circulating epinephrine produced by hypoglycemia is sufficient to allow a prompt and full recovery of the blood glucose concentration.

Other metabolic effects of increased catecholamine stimulation are seen in fat and muscle. *Lipolysis* is stimulated through beta-receptors, and a resulting increase in serum glycerol and nonesterified fatty acids occurs. Adrenergic mechanisms stimulate hepatic *ketogenesis*. Catecholamines also suppress the release of amino acids, especially the branch-chain group, from muscle.

Catecholamines also promote *thermogenesis*. Increased

*References 1, 26, 49, 60, 63, and 66.

glucose ingestion in human beings and many other species, as well as fat ingestion in some lower animals, stimulates adrenergic discharge. Conversely, starvation suppresses sympathetic discharge. It is speculated that such an arrangement represents a feedback regulation for weight control in that increased food intake promotes adrenergically mediated thermogenesis, thereby increasing energy requirements and diverting calories from conversion to fat. Conversely, starvation and suppressed thermogenesis have the effect of more efficiently using scarce calories for tissue repair, locomotion, and so on rather than for heat production.

CARDIOVASCULAR EFFECTS OF ADRENERGIC STIMULATION. The most obvious and perhaps most important effect of adrenergic stimulation is an increase in systemic blood pressure. The maintenance of or increase in blood pressure is accomplished through various mechanisms. The adrenergic stimulation of the myocardium is predominantly carried out through sympathetic innervation and local release of norepinephrine from the nerve terminals. Circulating norepinephrine has an effect on the heart similar to that of local stimulation.

The effects of norepinephrine and epinephrine on the heart are mediated through beta$_1$-receptors. The two catecholamines share the common action of increasing the force of myocardial contraction. With norepinephrine the chronotropic effect of beta stimulation is masked by the peripheral alpha effect of norepinephrine to constrict blood vessels, increase blood pressure, and suppress heart rate through a feedback mechanism from baroreceptors. In contrast, epinephrine has a peripheral beta$_2$-receptor activity to promote peripheral vasodilation so that its cardiac action of increasing the force of contraction is counterbalanced by the peripheral vasodilatory effect; blood pressure tends to rise slightly, and little if any baroreceptor inhibition of heart rate occurs. Thus the beta stimulatory effect of epinephrine on heart rate is not reflexedly inhibited, in contrast to inhibition of tachycardia caused by the rise in blood pressure, as seen with norepinephrine. Whether accompanied by an increase in heart rate or not, adrenergic stimulation has the effect of increasing cardiac output.

The peripheral vasculature is richly endowed with alpha$_1$- and alpha$_2$-adrenergic receptors. Norepinephrine and epinephrine have a vasoconstrictive effect on these receptors. The vasoconstriction and consequent increase in resistance combines with the increased cardiac output to produce an elevated systemic blood pressure. It is postulated that the vascular alpha$_1$-receptor responds to the norepinephrine released from the adjacent sympathetic nerve terminal, whereas the alpha$_2$-receptors are primarily stimulated by circulating epinephrine and norepinephrine.

RENAL EFFECTS OF ADRENERGIC STIMULATION. As noted previously, renal adrenergic stimulation indirectly assists in blood pressure control through the stimulation of renin release and the increased formation of the potent pressor agent, angiotensin. Such an increase in renin and angiotensin has an indirect effect to reduce renal sodium excretion through angiotensin-stimulated aldosterone production. Beyond these indirect renal effects, direct sympathetic innervation of the renal tubule occurs. Stimulation of renal nerves results in decreased sodium excretion in the absence of a change in glomerular filtration rate, total renal blood flow, the distribution of intrarenal blood flow, or renin release. The decreased sodium excretion during hemorrhage is probably mediated through this mechanism because renal denervation or infusion of adrenergic antagonists can prevent the sodium retention of hypovolemia. The effects of adrenergic discharge under various conditions can also be blocked by alpha-adrenergic antagonists.

An important extrarenal mechanism for control of serum potassium has been ascribed to epinephrine. Mediated by a beta$_2$-adrenergic receptor, epinephrine activates a membrane-bound adenylate cyclase system that promotes stimulation of a sodium-potassium-ATPase system, with the result of pumping potassium into skeletal muscle. Such an effect can be blocked by beta-adrenergic inhibitors. In this regard, it is interesting that both the other immediate-acting mechanism for lowering serum potassium (i.e., insulin secretion) and the adrenergic discharge are activated by food ingestion.

ADRENERGIC EFFECTS ON WHITE BLOOD CELLS. The recent demonstration of beta-adrenergic receptors on human lymphocytes has focused attention on the possibility of adrenergic modulation of the immune response. The receptor numbers on lymphocytes can be modulated, both in vivo and in vitro, by changes in adrenergic activity such as epinephrine infusions or use of beta-antagonists. Other in vitro studies have shown, for example, that the formation of the second component of complement by monocytes can be enhanced by exposure to epinephrine or norepinephrine. The mitogen responsiveness of mononuclear cells from peripheral blood can be suppressed by epinephrine infusion in human subjects. Since earlier in vitro studies failed to demonstrate the catecholamines' effect in this regard, it is probably mediated by indirect mechanisms. Epinephrine-induced changes in distribution of lymphocyte subsets have even been demonstrated in the peripheral blood of human subjects. Specifically, epinephrine increases the percentage of natural killer cells in the lymphocyte population.

Other than augmentation of the general sympathetic response, ascribing an essential role to the adrenal medulla is difficult. As noted previously, recovery from hypoglycemia is retarded in the adrenalectomized patient. In the case of immune cells, studies have clearly demonstrated the adrenergic receptor to be the beta type. Furthermore, in vitro binding studies with leukocytes show that epinephrine is at least 10 times more effective in binding to these sites compared to norepinephrine. In view of these facts, a role for the adrenal medulla in regulating immune functions could be postulated. With so many other circulating substances and complex cell-cell interrelationships in the immune system, the importance of epinephrine in this regard may be slight.

Hypersecretion of Adrenal Medulla

Earlier discussion reviewed the physiologic stimuli to the adrenal medulla that result in increased secretion of the catecholamine products, epinephrine and norepinephrine. This section focuses on two causes of adrenomedullary hypersecretion that are most relevant for surgeons: pheochromocytoma tumors of the adrenal medulla and the response to stress.

Pheochromocytoma

Pheochromocytoma is a tumor arising from the cells of the adrenal medulla. It can be nonfunctioning, with a simple space-occupying character, or can be functioning and produce many signs and symptoms related to the excessive circulation of epinephrine and norepinephrine. Although the focus here is on the adrenal medulla, these tumors can occur anywhere in sympathetic ganglia, such as in the paravertebral area, the preaortic area, and even the urinary bladder.

Evidence suggests that tumors in either the adrenal or the extra-adrenal locations are not functionally innervated by the sympathetic nervous system. However, approximately one third of these tumors are associated with intermittent episodes of symptoms, suggesting bursts of increased release of catecholamines. One hypothesis speculates that catecholamines are released into the intramedullary blood pool, and that fluctuations in adrenomedullary blood flow serve to wash out these potent hormones into the general circulation.

Another variant of symptomatology seen with these tumors is a steady hypertension, unassociated with intermittent bursts of catecholamine activity. The reason for this lack of intermittence may be the well-known ability of these tumors to metabolize the bioactive products before they reach the general circulation. Both monoamine-oxidase and carboxy-*O*-methyltransferase enzymes that degrade the catecholamines into inactive products are present in the adrenal gland. Whether sustained or episodic, excess secretion of epinephrine and norepinephrine causes the characteristic signs and symptoms of the tumor.

Diagnosis. An increase in systemic blood pressure is a characteristic clinical finding with pheochromocytoma. Whether episodic, constantly sustained, or sustained with superimposed episodes, the occurrence of hypertension can be easily understood in light of the effects of the catecholamines on cardiac output and peripheral resistance, as outlined earlier. In addition to headaches, which are probably the result of the hypertension, patients with this disease may complain of palpitations, which may reflect the tachycardia resulting from the chronotropic effect of epinephrine or from the arrhythmias sometimes set off by the excess circulating catecholamines. Patients have described episodes of sweating, apprehension, and even feelings of impending doom. In general these CNS symptoms may be said to be related to a release of large amounts of catecholamines by the adrenal medulla. The actions of the catecholamines to raise blood glucose levels account for the hyperglycemia found during laboratory testing.

The laboratory diagnosis of pheochromocytoma is based on the demonstration of increased plasma catecholamines or increased excretion of urinary catecholamines or their metabolites, such as VMA and metanephrine. In patients with sustained hypertension or during episodes of hypertension, the plasma and urinary catecholamines and/or the urinary catecholamines and metabolites will be increased. In a few patients with mild hypertension or intervening episodes of normotension, the urinary metabolites may be substantially elevated with only a mild increase in the free catecholamines. Some pheochromocytomas, usually the larger ones, can degrade the catecholamines internally before their excretion into the general circulation. This phenomenon results in a marked increase in formation of metabolites but a relatively small output of the metabolically active catecholamines.

Localization of the tumor is a useful preoperative maneuver because of the possibility of their extra-adrenal location. One of the earliest means to detect tumors was intravenous pyelography, which demonstrated displacement of the kidney inferiorly by a large tumor. The arteriogram can be used to detect the smaller tumors, but the radiocontrast material injected into the adrenal gland sometimes causes a severe, dangerous increase in blood pressure. The more recent CT scan is noninvasive, safe, and relatively sensitive; it can detect most tumors greater than 1 cm in diameter. One of the more promising tests is the use of radiolabeled compounds structually similar to norepinephrine and guanidine. The most effective of these is iodine-131 metaiodobenzylguanidine (^{131}I MIBG). MIBG is taken up by the sympathetic ganglia cells and stored in the granules much as norepinephrine is stored. The advantages of this scan include the ability to detect adrenomedullary hyperplasia, to detect metastases from a malignant medullary tumor, and to distinguish adrenergic tumors from other tumors of the adrenal gland.

Therapeutic Considerations. Although no randomized studies have been reported, most experienced surgeons believe that the preoperative institution of adrenergic blockade has made surgery for pheochromocytomas safer than it was in the preblockade era. Two less obvious potential benefits of the preoperative preparation are (1) a normalization of the hypothesized contracted blood volume resulting from the lowered blood pressure and (2) the ability of the adrenergic receptor population to increase during blockade. Although untested by a randomized study, the hypotension following tumor removal may be averted by both these corrective mechanisms.

Hypertension produced by the pheochromocytoma is primarily caused by stimulation of the vascular alpha-adrenergic receptor. Blockade of this receptor would obviously lower the blood pressure. The most widely used alpha-blocker is phenoxybenzamine. This blocker is best administered in 10 mg daily doses and increased until orthostatic hypotension supervenes. The beta-receptor, chronotropic effect may also be present, as indicated by a resting pulse rate greater than 100/minute. Propranolol is the beta-blocker of choice for decreasing the tachycardia; 30 to 40 mg/day given orally may be necessary to control the heart rate. Because beta-adrenergic blockade may decrease the force of heart contraction, it is important to lower the blood pressure first by instituting alpha-adrenergic blockade.

Intraoperative management of the sudden bursts in catecholamine secretion, especially when the tumor is manipulated, requires the use of fast-acting hypotensive agents. Phenoxybenzamine has a slow onset of action measured over several days. Phentolamine is a ganglionic blocker with a rapid onset and disappearance of activity. Nitro-

> **PHARMACOLOGIC AGENTS FOR MANAGEMENT OF PATIENTS WITH PHEOCHROMOCYTOMA**
>
> **Preoperative**
> Phenoxybenzamine
> Propranolol
>
> **Intraoperative**
> Phentolamine
> Nitroprusside
> Lidocaine
> Propranolol
> Levophed
> Transfusions
>
> **Postoperative**
> Levophed
> Transfusions

prusside, which is thought to act directly on blood vessels, is also a popular antihypertensive agent used intraoperatively because of its more rapid onset and disappearance of activity. Intravenous propranolol is used for control of tachycardia, and lidocaine may be necessary to control the arrhythmic effect of the catecholamines.

A special problem, seen more often before the frequent use of properative adrenergic blockade, is hypotension after tumor removal. The hypotension is probably the result of down-regulation of adrenergic receptors caused by the preexisting, long-standing catecholamine excess. The residual baseline sympathetic tone coupled with the sparse receptor population is not sufficient to maintain the blood pressure. An alternate and perhaps complementary mechanism is the contracted blood volume that may result from long-standing hypertension. Although the use of norepinephrine infusion can normalize the blood pressure postoperatively, most clinicians believe that transfusion of blood lessens or eliminates the requirement for exogenous pressor administration. The various pharmacologic agents that may be required are listed in the boxed material above.*

Adrenergic Response to Stress

As enumerated previously, a prompt and marked sympathetic discharge occurs in response to a wide variety of noxious and potentially harmful events, such as traumatic injury, hemorrhage, and sepsis. The adrenal medulla's participation in the general sympathetic response to stress is evidenced by an increase in epinephrine, as well as norepinephrine, during these events. With hypovolemia, for example, the sympathetic nervous system plays a key role in the maintenance of blood pressure and consequent perfusion of vital organs such as the CNS and kidneys. During normovolemic traumatic injury, however, maintenance of blood pressure may not depend on excessive adrenergic responses. The question of the importance of the adrenergic response to stress may also be a consideration in the control of blood glucose. For example, although the catecholamines are one of the hormonal factors responsible for the hyperglycemia during stress, cortisol apparently is a more potent effector for the hyperglycemic response. Similarly, in the restoration of blood glucose following hypoglycemia, it appears that glucagon is the predominant hormone in this response, even though plasma catecholamines are clearly elevated during hypoglycemia.

The sympathetic nervous system may be the initiator of the stress response in that it is an extremely fast-acting system, and the increase in circulating catecholamines seems to precede that of other stress responders. The interaction of the sympathetic nervous system with other stress hormones may be one of the keys to its importance during stress. The catecholamines' modulation of the actions of angiotensin, thyroxine, and insulin on their target organs are examples of how the adrenergic system may function to enhance the response to stress. The catecholamines also have an effect on the secretion of other key stress hormones, such as ACTH, insulin, glucagon, and renin.

The particular role of the adrenal medulla is not clear. Does the adrenal medulla simply serve as a back-up system for the neurally organized sympathetic nervous system? One could argue that epinephrine has a more potent chronotropic effect on the heart and thus may produce a greater increase in cardiac output. In human beings almost all the circulating norepinephrine is simply a spillover from the neuronal sympathetic discharge. Furthermore, infusion studies have shown that norepinephrine is approximately 10 times less potent than circulating epinephrine in terms of its effect on the cardiovascular system and on hyperglycemia.

Epinephrine, and therefore the adrenal medulla, may be an important back-up system for the maintenance of blood glucose during glucagon or cortisol deficiency. Although the individual actions of the sympathetic nervous system have been clearly elucidated, the precise role of the sympathetic discharge and especially of the adrenal medulla in the survival of the organism during stress is far from clear.[18,50]

Hyposecretion of Adrenal Medulla

Hypoactivity of the sympathetic nervous system can be seen secondary to diseases such as diabetes mellitus and amyloidosis. A variant of the primary hypoadrenergic state is *familial dysautonomia,* in which orthostatic hypotension results from a failure to activate an intact sympathetic nervous system. The adrenomedullary response to hypoglycemia is intact in these patients.

Two other disorders of the sympathetic nervous system marked by orthostatic hypotension are *idiopathic orthostatic hypotension (IOH)* and orthostatic hypotension accompanying multiple neurologic deficits, known as *Shy-Drager syndrome*. Shy-Drager syndrome results from degenerative changes in several of the CNS structures responsible for the initiation of sympathetic discharges. The peripheral sympathetic nervous system is relatively intact. In contrast, IOH appears to be caused by the loss of peripheral sympathetic nerves, especially those to blood vessels. As predicted by the adrenergic receptor mechanism theory, patients with Shy-Drager syndrome have normal

*References 8, 20, 27, 36, 40, 46, 48, 52, 55, and 65.

pressor response to catecholamine infusions, whereas the patients with IOH are supersensitive to administered norepinephrine. Interestingly, some of these patients, both those with IOH and those with Shy-Drager syndrome, have no epinephrine response to insulin hypoglycemia. In such patients the initial rapid phase of recovery from insulin hypoglycemia is delayed. All other aspects of the hypoglycemic recovery are normal.

Treatment of sympathetic nervous system hyposecretion is difficult. Volume expansion with the synthetic mineralocorticoid fludrocortisone, along with increased salt intake, is the most frequently used regimen. Since hypertension and even congestive heart failure have been reported during recumbency with this regimen, waist-high fitted stockings or even an anti-G suit has been worn effectively by some patients. Other drugs such as propranolol or prostaglandin inhibitors have not been uniformly successful.[31,62,67]

SUMMARY

The adrenal glands are paired, flattened triangles, each situated on the superior aspect of a kidney. From this relatively inaccessible vantage point, they produce their diverse physiologic effects by release of hormones into the bloodstream. The thin, yellow cortex of the gland secretes steroids, whereas the even thinner, grayish inner medulla secretes catecholamines. The steroidogenic cortex is divided into three histologic layers: the zona glomerulosa, the zona fasciculata, and the zona reticularis. Aldosterone is produced by the zona glomerulosa, and cortisol and sex steroids are produced by the other two zones.

As the blood-borne steroids bathe the tissues of the body, specific receptors in the cytosol of the target cells bind the particular steroid stereochemically suitable for that receptor, and the chain of intracellular metabolic events is begun. Since the steroid-induced changes are mediated through nuclear receptors as new protein synthesis, steroidal effects are relatively slow in onset and slow to abate. The long list of steroid actions attest to the fact that many tissues contain these steroid receptors. Aldosterone effects are best seen in the kidney, salivary glands, and large bowel and are related to electrolyte transport. The sex steroids have many functions, centered primarily on the organs related to reproduction, such as the breast and prostate. The primary carbohydrate-active steroid, cortisol, has a myriad of effects, including modulation of fuel substrates (fats, carbohydrates, amino acids), immune functions, inflammatory response, wound healing, and bone metabolism and mineralization.

The importance of the adrenocortical function is obvious when one considers that death inevitably results in its absence. Adrenocortical function also becomes clinically apparent when it occurs in excess. Certain enzymatic defects in the steroidogenic pathway result in superabundant production of certain steroids, which leads to the clinical expressions of masculinization and precocious puberty. Other enzymatic defects produce steroid deficits that are incompatible with life unless corrected. The pituitary gland may develop microadenomas that produce excessive adrenocorticotropic hormone, which in turn stimulates the adrenal cortex to produce cortisol in excess. The adrenal can autonomously produce excess cortisol with development of a cortical adenoma, cortical carcinoma, or macronodular hyperplasia. A benign tumor arising from the zona glomerulosa produces a syndrome characteristic of an aldosterone excess. Finally, adrenocortical tumors can produce excessive androgens or estrogens to produce masculinization in the female or feminization in the male.

The thin, inner portion of the adrenal gland, the medulla, is an integral part of the sympathetic nervous system and represents a large cluster of ganglion cells. The two main secretory products of the adrenal medulla, norepinephrine and epinephrine, also reach peripheral tissues by means of the bloodstream. In contrast to steroids, the catecholamines have a very short plasma half-life, and their effects are mediated fairly rapidly through membrane receptors. These receptors are designed as alpha or beta, depending on the effects produced. For example, stimulation of beta-receptors results in an increased cardiac rate and force of contraction. Alpha-receptors mediate contractions of smooth muscle, glycogenolysis, or gluconeogenesis. Further subdivision of these receptors, such as relaxation of smooth muscle for $beta_2$- or increased platelet aggregation for $alpha_2$-receptors, has been useful in describing the widely divergent effects of the catecholamines.

In contrast to the adrenal cortex, the adrenal medulla does not appear to be essential for life. Other components of the sympathetic nervous system can compensate for absence of the medulla. Although the adrenal medulla participates in specific hypoadrenergic states, such as Shy-Drager syndrome, isolated adrenomedullary deficiency is seldom clinically detectable. On the other hand, a striking syndrome is produced by a tumorous overgrowth of the adrenal medulla known as pheochromocytoma. Hypertension, tachycardia, glucose intolerance, apprehension, sweating, and even sudden death are dramatic overstatements of the functional capabilities of the adrenal medulla.

The adrenal glands are interesting to the surgeon and vexing to the patient when abnormal function occurs. Considering their essential normal functions, however, such as fluid and electrolyte balance, fuel substrate utilization, and musculoskeletal integrity, the adrenal glands are fascinating structures worthy of respect and preservation, when possible.

REFERENCES

1. Altorfer, R.M., Ziegler, W.H., and Froesch, E.R.: Insulin hypoglycaemia in normal and adrenalectomized subjects: comparison of metabolic parameters and endocrine counter regulation, Acta Endocrinol. **98:**413, 1981.
2. Aron, D.C., et al.: Cushing's syndrome: problems in management, Endocr. Rev. **3:**229, 1982.
3. Auda, S.P., Brennan, M.F., and Gill, J.R.: Evolution of the surgical management of primary aldosteronism, Ann. Surg. **191:**1, 1980.
4. Axelrod, J., and Reisine, T.D.: Stress hormones: their interaction and regulation, Science **224:**452, 1984.
5. Badder, E.M., et al.: Adrenal medullary epinephrine secretion: effects of cortisol alone and combined with aminoglutethimide, J. Lab. Clin. Med. **96:**815, 1980.
6. Baxter, J.D., and Rousseau, G.G.: Glucocorticoid hormone action: an overview. In Baxter, J.D., and Rousseau, G.G., editors: Glucocorticoid hormone action, New York, 1979, Springer-Verlag New York, Inc.
7. Carballeira, A., and Fishman, L.M.: The adrenal functional unit: a hypothesis, Perspect. Biol. Med., Summer 1980, p. 573.

8. Causon, R.C., and Brown, M.J.: Catecholamine measurements in phaeochromocytoma: a review, Ann. Clin. Biochem. **19**:396, 1982.
9. Chan, J.C.M.: Control of aldosterone secretion, Nephron **23**:79, 1979.
10. Chrousos, G.P., et al.: Development of glucocorticoid antagonists, Pharmacol. Ther. **20**:263, 1983.
11. Cryer, P.E.: Physiology and pathophysiology of the human sympathoadrenal neuroendocrine system, N. Engl. J. Med. **303**:436, 1980.
12. Cupps, T.R., and Fauci, A.S.: Corticosteroid-mediated immunoregulation in man, Immunol. Rev. **65**:133, 1982.
13. Dannenberg, A.M.: The anti-inflammatory effects of glucocorticosteroids, Inflammation **3**:329, 1979.
14. Del Greco, F., et al.: The renin-angiotensin-aldosterone system in primary and secondary hypertension, Ann. Clin. Lab. Sci. **11**:497, 1981.
15. Dluhy, R.G.: Regulation of aldosterone secretion in normotensive and hypertensive man, Pathobiol. Annu. **10**:305, 1980.
16. Dluhy, R.G., and Williams, G.H.: Cushing's syndrome and the changing times, Ann. Intern. Med. **97**:131, 1982.
17. Eliasson, K.: Stress and catecholamines, Acta Med. Scand. **215**:197, 1984.
18. Engeland, W.C., et al.: The adrenal medullary response to graded hemorrhage in awake dogs, Endocrinology **109**:1539, 1981.
19. Fain, J.N.: Inhibition of glucose transport in fat cells and activation of lipolysis by glucocorticoids. In Baxter, J.D., and Rousseau, G.G., editors: Glucocorticoid hormone action, New York, 1979, Springer-Verlag New York, Inc.
20. Fedlman, J.M., et al.: Alterations in plasma norepinephrine concentration during surgical resection of pheochromocytoma, Ann. Surg. **188**:758, 1978.
21. Fraser, R., et al.: Control of aldosterone secretion, Clin. Sci. **56**:389, 1979.
22. Ganguly, A., and Donohue, J.P.: Primary aldosteronism: pathophysiology, diagnosis, and treatment, J. Urol. **129**:241, 1983.
23. Goforth, P., and Gudas, C.J.: Effects of steroids on wound healing: a review of the literature, J. Foot Surg. **19**:22, 1980.
24. Grant, C.S., Carpenter, P., and van Heerden, J.A.: Primary aldosteronism, Arch. Surg. **119**:585, 1984.
25. Grunfeld, C., et al.: Glucocorticoid-induced insulin resistance *in vitro:* evidence for both receptor and post-receptor defects, Endocrinology **109**:1723, 1981.
26. Güllner, H.G.: The role of the adrenergic nervous system in sodium and water excretion, Klin. Wochenschr. **61**:1063, 1983.
27. Juan, D.: Pharmacologic agents in the management of pheochromocytoma, South. Med. J. **75**:211, 1982.
28. Keller-Wood, M.E., and Dallman, M.E.: Corticosteroid inhibition of ACTH secretion, Endocr. Rev. **5**:1, 1984.
29. Kelly, R.B., et al.: Biochemistry of neurotransmitter release. In Cowan, W.M., editor: Annual review of neuroscience, Palo Alto, Calif., 1979, Annual Reviews, Inc.
30. Khalid, B.A.K., et al.: Steroid replacement in Addison's disease and in subjects adrenalectomized for Cushing's disease: comparison of various glucocorticoids, J. Clin. Endocrinol. Metab. **55**:551, 1982.
31. Kopin, I.J., et al.: Urinary catecholamine metabolites distinguish different types of sympathetic neuronal dysfunction in patients with orthostatic hypotension, J. Clin. Endocrinol. Metab. **57**:632, 1983.
32. Kotchen, T.A., and Guthrie, G.P., Jr.: Renin-angiotensin-aldosterone and hypertension, Endocr. Rev. **1**:78, 1980.
33. Kraus-Friedmann, N.: Hormonal regulation of hepatic gluconeogenesis, Physiol. Rev. **64**:170, 1984.
34. Krieger, D.T.: Physiology of Cushing's disease, Endocr. Rev. **4**:22, 1983.
35. Lefkowitz, R.J., Caron, M.G., and Stiles, G.L.: Mechanisms of membrane-receptor regulation, N. Engl. J. Med. **310**:1570, 1984.
36. Manger, W.R., and Gifford, R.W.: Pheochromocytoma, New York, 1978, Springer-Verlag New York, Inc.
37. Manolas, K.J., et al.: The pituitary before and after adrenalectomy for Cushing's syndrome, World J. Surg. **8**:374, 1984.
38. Marver, D.: Evidence of corticosteroid action along the nephron, Am. J. Physiol. **246**:F111, 1984.
39. Marver, D., and Kokko, J.P.: Renal target sites and the mechanism of action of aldosterone, Miner. Electrolyte Metab. **9**:1, 1983.
40. Modlin, I.M., et al.: Phaeochromocytomas in 72 patients: clinical and diagnostic features, treatment and long-term results, Br. J. Surg. **66**:456, 1979.
41. Morris, D.J.: The metabolism and mechanism of action of aldosterone, Endocr. Rev. **2**:234, 1981.
42. Motulsky, H.J., and Insel, P.A.: Adrenergic receptors in man, N. Engl. J. Med. **307**:18, 1982.
43. Munck, A., Guyre, P.M., and Holbrook, N.J.: Physiological functions of glucocorticoids in stress and their relation to pharmacological actions, Endocr. Rev. **5**:25, 1984.
44. Neville, A.M., and O'Hare, M.J.: The human adrenal cortex, New York, 1982, Springer-Verlag New York, Inc.
45. New, M.I., et al.: An update of congenital adrenal hyperplasia. In Greep, R.O., editor: Recent progress in hormone research, proceedings of the 1980 Laurentian Hormone Conference, vol. 37, New York, 1981, Academic Press, Inc.
46. Newsome, H.H.: The lack of catecholamine responses in patients with pheochromocytomas, Surgery **94**:932, 1984.
47. Peck, W., et al.: Corticosteroids and bone, Calcif. Tissue Int. **36**:4, 1984.
48. Ram, C.V.S., and Engleman, K.: Pheochromocytoma—recognition and management, Curr. Probl. Cardiol. **IV**:8, 1979.
49. Rosen, S.G., et al.: Epinephrine supports the post-absorptive plasma glucose concentration and prevents hypoglycemia when glucagon secretion is deficient in man, J. Clin. Invest. **73**:405, 1984.
50. Rosner, M.J., Newsome, H.H., and Becker, D.P.: Mechanical brain injury: the sympathoadrenal response, J. Neurosurg. **61**:76, 1984.
51. Santen, R.J., et al.: Aminoglutethimide as treatment of post-menopausal women with advanced breast carcinoma, Ann. Intern. Med. **96**:94, 1982.
52. Scott, H.W., et al.: Surgical management of pheochromocytoma, Am. Surg. **47**:8, 1981.
53. Scott, J.: Physiological, pharmacological and pathological actions of glucocorticoids on the digestive system, Clin. Gastroenterol. **10**:627, 1981.
54. Seleznev, I.M., and Martynow, A.V.: Permissive effect of glucocorticoids in catecholamine action in the heart: possible mechanism, J. Mol. Cell. Cardiol. **14**:49, 1982.
55. Shapiro, B., et al.: Malignant phaeochromocytoma: clinical, biochemical and scintigraphic characterization, Clin. Endocrinol. **20**:189, 1984.
56. Simmons, P.S., et al.: Increased proteolysis: an effect of increases in plasma cortisol within the physiologic range, J. Clin. Invest. **73**:412, 1984.
57. Stalmans W., and Laloux, M.: Glucocorticoids and hepatic glycogen metabolism. In Baxter, J.D., and Rousseau, G.G., editors: Glucocorticoid hormone action, New York, 1979, Springer-Verlag.
58. Starke K. Docherty JR: Alpha$_1$ and alpha$_2$-adrenoceptors: pharmacology and clinical implications, J. Cardiovasc. Pharmacol. **3**:S14, 1981.
59. Stiles, G.L., and Lefkowitz, R.J.: Cardiac adrenergic receptors, Ann. Rev. Med. **35**:149, 1984.
60. Struthers, A.D., and Reid, J.L.: The role of adrenal medullary catecholamines in potassium homeostasis, Clin. Sci. **66**:377, 1984.
61. Sullivan, J.N.: Saturday conference: steroid withdrawal syndromes, South. Med. J. **75**:726, 1982.
62. Thomas, J.E., et al.: Orthostatic hypotension, Mayo Clin. Proc. **56**:117, 1981.
63. Tse, T.P., et al.: Neuroendocrine responses to glucose in ingestion in man, J. Clin. Invest. **72**:270, 1983.
64. Ungar, A., and Phillips, J.H.: Regulation of the adrenal medullar, Physiol. Rev. **63**:787, 1983.
65. van Heerden, J.A., et al.: Pheochromocytoma: current status and changing trends, Surgery **91**:367, 1982.
66. Young, J.B., and Landsberg, L.: Catecholamines and the sympathoadrenal system: the regulation of metabolism. In Ingbar, S.H., editor: Contemporary endocrinology, vol. 1, New York, 1979, Plenum Medical Book Co.
67. Ziegler, M.G., Lake, C.R., and Kopin, I.J.: The sympathetic-nervous-system defect in primary orthostatic hypotension, N. Engl. J. Med. **296**:293, 1977.

58 Thyroid Disease and Pathophysiology

Philip R. Orlander and Alton L. Steiner

The thyroid gland, although small in size, is an important organ in modulating normal metabolic processes within the body. The thyroid gland is relevant to the surgeon because of the various neoplastic processes that may involve it and the need to remove all or substantial portions of it when the production of its normal hormones become excessive. A knowledge of the normal physiology of this organ is paramount if the dysfunctional states associated with it are to be successfully treated.

THYROID ANATOMY

The thyroid gland is a bilobed structure, covered by a thin fibrous capsule and attached to the thyroid cartilage of the trachea by connective tissue (Fig. 58-1). It normally weighs 20 to 25 g, with the right lobe being somewhat larger and more vascular than the left. Both lobes are connected by an isthmus, from which a fingerlike projection of varying lengths, known as the pyramidal lobe, protrudes to the left. The blood supply of the thyroid is derived from the external carotid and subclavian arteries that give rise to the superior and inferior thyroid arteries, respectively. A rich lymphatic network is also present. The cervical ganglia and vagus nerves bilaterally innervate the gland, thus giving it both adrenergic and cholinergic innervation. The infrahyoid muscles, carotid sheaths, and sternocleidomastoid muscles flank the gland, and the recurrent laryngeal nerves run between the lobes and the trachea. There are normally four parathyroid glands, two on each posterior surface of the thyroid lobes.

The thyroid has a large capacity for increased growth and vascularity in disease states. Being a particularly vascular structure, its blood flow may increase substantially in various pathologic states such as Graves' disease. Glandular function and growth are influenced by hormonal factors (e.g., thyroid-stimulating hormone [TSH]), blood flow, and direct adrenergic innervation. Goiters (enlargements of the thyroid gland) weighing in excess of 100 g are not rare.

THYROID FUNCTION AND NONTHYROIDAL DISEASE

The thyroid gland adapts to the metabolic needs of the body. Not only are the hormones it secretes intimately involved with the control of cellular metabolism, but they

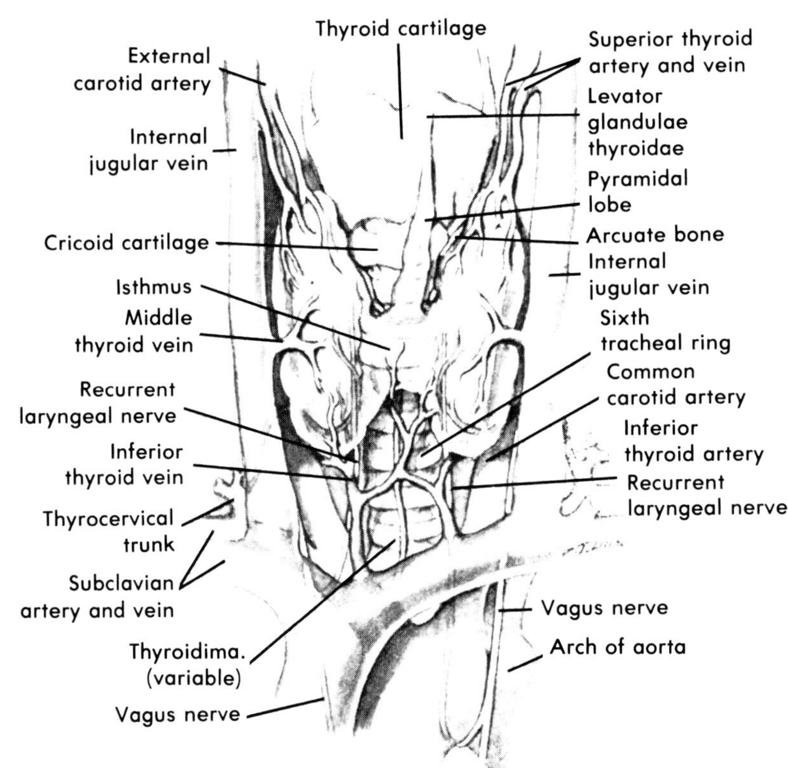

Fig. 58-1 Anatomy of the thyroid gland. (From Thorek, P., and Linden, C.T.: Anatomy in surgery, ed. 2, Philadelphia, 1962, J.B. Lippincott Co.)

also profoundly influence tissue growth and development, as well as tissue differentiation. Nonetheless, abnormal laboratory findings suggesting thyroid dysfunction may result from nonthyroidal disease. Thus an understanding of this adaptive mechanism is essential so as not to treat nonexistent thyroid disease and to appropriately treat disorders of this gland when present.

In the body's attempt to adapt to its environment, and stress in particular, higher brain centers transmit messages to the hypothalamus. The mechanisms underlying this transmission and the individual hormones responsible for it remain undefined but may include peptides such as somatostatin, adrenocorticotropic hormone (ACTH), endorphins, and possibly other as yet unidentified hormones. The importance of cerebral input on hypothalamic thyroid regulation remains unclear. Nonetheless, anecdotal reports of stress as a precipitating cause of hyperthyroidism are not uncommon.

Thyrotropin-releasing factor (TRF) is secreted by the hypothalamus into the hypophyseal portal system and stimulates pituitary secretion of (TSH). TSH in turn stimulates the thyroid gland to synthesize and release thyroxine

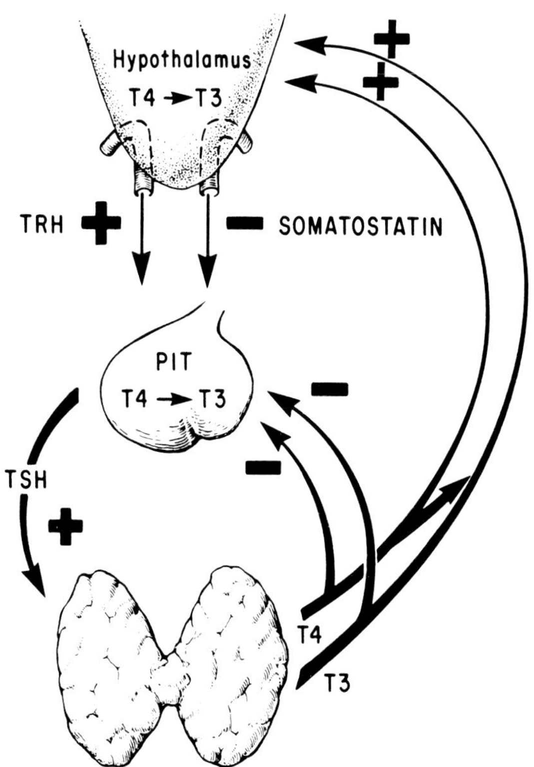

Fig. 58-2 Hypothalamic-pituitary-thyroid axis. Secretion of thyrotropin is regulated by the interaction of a releasing factor (thyrotropin-releasing factor [TRH]) and an inhibiting factor (somatostatin). Thyroid hormones, triiodothyronine and thyroxine (T_4 and T_3), act directly on the pituitary to inhibit thyrotropin secretion. Thyroid hormone also acts at the hypothalamic level to stimulate somatostatin release. The effect of thyroid hormone on secretion of TRH has not been established with certainty. Finally, T_4 is converted to T_3 in the periphery, the pituitary, and the hypothalamus; in all sites, T_3 is more potent than T_4. (From Martin, J., and Reichlin, S.: Clinical neuroendocrinology, ed. 2, Philadelphia, 1987, F.A. Davis Co).

(T_4) and triiodothyronine (T_3) into the bloodstream. Somatostatin is also secreted by the hypothalamus and has an inhibitory effect on TSH secretion. Although T_4 and T_3 have no known direct control of TRF, they do stimulate release of hypothalamic somatostatin secretion, which in turn inhibits TSH secretion. These considerations are summarized in Fig. 58-2.

Pituitary secretion of TSH depends on the prevailing levels of TRF, somatostatin, and thyroid hormone in the blood. Thus the pituitary plays a central role in thyroid hormone regulation, integrating messages from higher centers and feedback from the thyroid gland itself. The pituitary is able to convert T_4 to T_3, the latter hormone being 20 times more potent than T_4. This allows the pituitary to have exquisite control over the free thyroid hormone concentration in serum. TSH stimulates all steps in thyroid hormonogenesis, including iodine uptake, organification, coupling, and secretion of the hormone. In addition, TSH has a stimulating effect on growth and vascularity of the gland, possibly through a noncyclic adenosine monophosphate (cAMP)–mediated pathway. Thyrotoxic patients (in whom excessive quantities of T_4 and T_3 are made) classically have undetectable TSH levels as a result of the feedback inhibitory mechanisms of thyroid hormone on the pituitary.

Iodine plays a complex role in thyroid physiology. The thyroid avidly concentrates iodine, and small daily amounts of this substance are essential for normal gland function. Iodine deficiency is responsible for endemic goiters, hypothyroidism, and the mental retardation associated with it that continues to plague large segments of the developing world. When doses of iodine of 6 mg or greater are administered to patients, the iodine acutely but transiently blocks thyroid hormone secretion. This happens because, when intrathyroidal iodine concentration increases, iodine itself transiently inhibits further organification (Wolff-Chaikoff effect). In the absence of TSH, intrathyroidal organic iodine concentration has an inverse relationship on ^{131}I-uptake by the gland. Iodine appears to interfere with the coupling of TSH to adenylcyclase activation. This is one reason why large doses of iodine (called Lugol's solution) are effective therapeutically in thyroid storm and in preparing a patient with active Graves' disease for surgery (see discussion below).

In the normal gland, as TSH levels rise the Wolff-Chaikoff effect is overriden and will not last more than 2 weeks. In patients with compensated underlying thryoid disease (Hashimoto's thyroiditis, inherited biochemical defects, previously treated Graves' disease), the compensatory TSH rise may not be able to override the combined inhibitory force of the iodine and the underlying thyroid disease. Depending on the degree of organification block, the patient may develop a goiter with or without associated hypothyroidism. Discontinuation of iodine therapy will usually result in resolution of the goiter. The high incidence of compensated Hashimoto's thyroiditis in the United States and the common use of iodinated contrast substances in venous radiologic procedures increases the occurrence of iodine-associated thyroid disease.[34]

A compensated iodine-deficient goiter with autonomous or semiautonomous nodules may be able to absorb large amounts of iodine, rapidly synthesize thyroid hormone, and cause thyrotoxicosis (Jod-Basedow effect). Because of the increased iodine pool, the radioactive iodine (^{131}I) uptake of the gland is low. Thus neither ^{131}I therapy nor antithyroid medications are effective acutely in the treatment of iodine-induced thyrotoxicosis.[23] In this circumstance medications that decrease the adrenergic response (beta-blockers) should be administered until the iodine pool has decreased.

T_4 is the major secretory product of the thyroid gland. Only about 0.03% of total T_4 is free, the remainder being bound to various serum proteins, including thyroxin-binding globulin (TBG) (80%), thyroxine-binding prealbumin (15%), and albumin (see boxed material below). Approximately 80% of T_4 is converted peripherally to T_3, which is also bound to the above-noted proteins but with a relative affinity of only about 10%. Thus, T_3 is responsible for most, if not all, of the metabolic effects of thyroid hormone. Monodeiodination of T_4 occurs with varied activity in the liver, pituitary, kidney, and elsewhere, yielding T_3 and biologically inert reverse T_3 (Fig. 58-3). Actual direct thyroid secretion of T_3 is negligible. Administration of T_4 to athyreotic patients results in substantial elevation of total T_3 levels, confirming the efficacy and physiologic basis of replacement therapy for hypothyroidism with T_4 alone.[8]

The free thyroid hormone level determines the metabolic status of the patient. An accurate estimate of free hormone levels may be ascertained by directly measuring binding proteins in relation to total hormone values in serum, estimating binding sites on these proteins by using the T_3 resin uptake (RU) technique, or directly measuring free hormone levels by equilibrium dialysis. The latter assay is technically difficult and rarely adds information not obtained by the simpler and less expensive T_3 RU. To perform this latter test, isotopically label T_3 is added to the patient's serum and allowed to bind to available sites. A resin is then added that absorbs any unbound labeled T_3. Multiplying the T_3 RU by the total T_4 concentration yields an estimate of the free hormone concentration (free thyroid index).

Physiologic or pathologic states that increase binding proteins (e.g., pregnancy, estrogens, chronic liver disease, inherited abnormal proteins) result in a decreased T_3 RU but no change in the free hormone level, since the total T_4 level is increased in these conditions (see boxed material at left and below). Conversely, conditions that raise T_3 RU by decreasing thyroid-binding globulin (major systemic illness, hypoproteinemic states, glucocorticoid or anabolic steroid administration, nephrotic syndrome, and genetic causes) result in a lower total hormone level, but usually a normal free thyroid index. Unfortunately, this mathematic construction fails at the upper and lower limits of the nor-

COMMON CONDITIONS ASSOCIATED WITH TBG FLUCTUATION

INCREASED TBG CONCENTRATION (DECREASED T_3 RESIN UPTAKE)
1. Pregnancy
2. Estrogens
3. Oral contraceptives
4. Chronic active hepatitis
5. Inherited binding abnormalities
6. Hypothyrodism

DECREASED TBG CONCENTRATION (INCREASED T_3 RESIN UPTAKE)
1. Androgens
2. Glucocorticoids
3. Nephrotic syndrome
4. Severe acute or chronic illness
5. Inherited binding abnormalities
6. Hepatic failure
7. Hyperthyroidism

CONDITIONS THAT IMPAIR NORMAL PERIPHERAL THYROXINE METABOLISM (T_4 to T_3 CONVERSION)
1. Fasting (especially carbohydrate depletion)
2. Severe acute or chronic illness
3. Trauma, postoperative state
4. Hepatic failure
5. Radiologic contrast dyes
6. Glucocorticoids
7. Propranolol
8. Propylthiouracil
9. Amiodarone

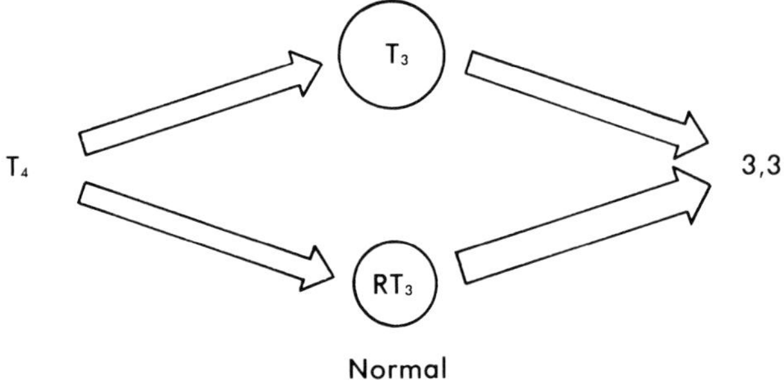

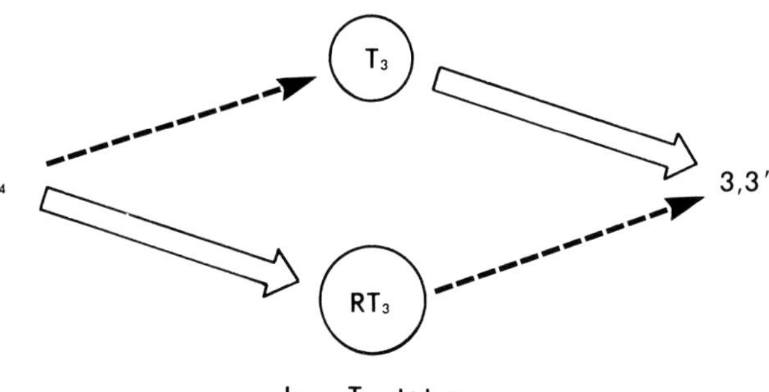

Fig. 58-3 Thyroxine deiodination. Pathways of T_4 deiodination in normals (upper) and in patients with low T_3 states (lower). The major abnormality is an impairment in 5′-deiodination both of T_4 and of reverse T_3 (RT_3). The size of each circle enclosing T_3 and RT_3 symbols depicts the relative change in serum concentration in the typical case. (From Cavalieri, R.R.: Peripheral metabolism of thyroid hormones, Deerfield, Ill., Thyroid today, vol. 3, 1980, Travenol Laboratories, Inc.)

mal range, and occasionally the free thyroid index will be outside of the normal range.

An interesting pathologic state that may affect thyroid function is the euthyroid sick syndrome. This occurs in patients who are sufficiently ill to impede normal metabolism of thyroid hormone.[13] In this condition normal deiodination of T_4 in the periphery is not accomplished, and a biologically inert metabolite (termed *reverse* T_3 because of its mirror image structure to T_3) accumulates (Fig. 58-3). Low values of T_3 may be an isolated abnormality; or, if the patient is severely ill with derangements of normal serum proteins (e.g., albumin, thyroid-binding globulin), a low T_4 and elevated T_3 RU may also be observed.[12] As distinct from patients with primary thyroid failure, patient with euthyroid sick syndrome are clinically euthyroid, have normal TSH levels, and do not improve with thyroid hormone replacement.[46] These patients are not truly hypothyroid but are attempting to conserve energy expenditure in the face of a severe insult. Extremely low values of T_3 by radioimmunoassay (RIA) correlate with an elevated morbidity and mortality, almost irrespective of the primary disease process.

In any patient suspected of having thyroid disease, laboratory evaluation of thyroid function should begin with a measurement of total T_4 by RIA and T_3 by RU (Table 58-1). A suspicion of hypothyroidism should be confirmed by an elevated TSH level. A total T_3 RIA is an unreliable screening test, since it may be normal in early hypothyroidism and low in euthyroid sick syndrome. An elevated T_3 by RIA confirms the suspicion of hyperthyroidism. Nonthyroidal disease should be suspected if there is a divergence between the T_4 and T_3 RU. An elevated T_4 and T_3 RU is seen in hyperthyroidism, and a decrease in both levels is seen in hypothyroidism. However, an elevated T_4 associated with a decreased T_3 RU or vice versa is indicative of protein-binding abnormalities and not thyroid pathology.

THYROTOXICOSIS

Thyrotoxicosis is a toxic-metabolic state resulting from abnormally elevated levels of circulating free thyroid hormone. The term hyperthyroidism is generally reserved for thyrotoxic states caused by increased hormone synthesis by the thyroid gland (e.g., Graves' disease, toxic multinodular goiter). Exogenous ingestion of thyroid hormone would be an example of thyrotoxicosis without hyperthyroidism.

Autoimmune Hyperthyroidism (Graves' Disease)

Autoimmune factors are generally thought to be responsible for a major portion of hyperthyroid disease, especially in the young. Autoimmune thyroid disease comprises a spectrum of clinical manifestations. The hypothyroidism secondary to Hashimoto's thyroiditis (see discussion under hypothyroidism) may result from a predominance of cytotoxic or inhibiting antibodies to the thyroid. In contrast, the hyperthyroidism secondary to Graves' disease appears to result from a predominance of thyroid-stimulating antibodies.

Graves' disease is a common cause of hyperthyroidism. There is a marked female predominance, especially during the reproductive years, although it may affect all ages. A positive family history for both Graves' disease and Hashimoto's thyroiditis is commonly seen. Twin studies show a high concordance rate and certain HLA types (e.g., DR3, DR4) are especially common in both diseases. These HLA types have also been associated with other disorders suspected of having an autoimmune cause, including Type I diabetes mellitus, Addison's disease, systemic lupus erythematosis, and pernicious anemia.

Although the precise cause of Graves' disease is un-

Table 58-1 **LABORATORY EVALUATION OF THYROID PATHOLOGY**

	T_4	T_3 Resin Uptake	Thyroid-Binding Globulin	T_3 by RIA	TSH	24-Hour ^{131}I Uptake
Normal	4.5-11.5 μg/100 ml	25%-35%	1-1.5 mg/100 ml	90-190 ng/100 ml	1-10 μU/ml	5%-30%
Mild hypothyroidism	↓	↓	N or ↑	N	↑	↓
Severe hypothyroidism	↓ ↓	↓ ↓	↑	↓	↑ ↑	↓ ↓
Graves' disease	↑ ↑	↑ ↑	↓	↑ ↑	Undetectable	↑ ↑ (>50%)
Nodular hyperthyroidism	↑ ↑	↑ ↑	↓	↑ ↑	Undetectable	↑ (>30%)
Factitious hyperthyroidism	↑ ↑	↑ ↑	↓	↑ or N	Undetectable	Undetectable
Thyroiditis with hyperthyroidism	↑	↑	↓	↑	N	↓ ↓
NONTHYROID DISORDERS						
Pregnancy or estrogen intake	↑	↓	↑	N	N	N*
Euthyroid sick syndrome	↓ or N	↑	↓	↓ ↓ ↓	N	Not known

*N, Within normal range.

Table 58-2 **MEASUREMENTS OF RECEPTOR ANTIBODIES**

Method	Species Used for Detection	Parameter Measured	Term Applied to Stimulator	Advantages	Disadvantages
Bioassays					
McKenzie	Mouse	Iodine release from thyroid	LATS*	Bioassay	Laborious, mouse assay
cytochemical bioassay	Guinea-pig	Alteration in lysosomal permeability	TSAb	Bioassay, very sensitive	Technically difficult, low throughput, guinea-pig assay
T_3 release	Pig	Release of T_3 by porcine thyroid slices	TSAb	Bioassay, very sensitive	Porcine assay, rather low throughput
cAMP	Man	Activation of adenylate cyclase in membranes, or increase in cAMP in slices, or human thyroid cells in tissue culture	TSAb	Bioassay, human	Laborious, needs normal human thyroid tissue
Receptor assays					
LATS-P	Man	Inhibition of binding of LATS	LATS-P†	Human	Laborious, not a bioassay
Receptor assay	Man	Inhibition of labeled TSH binding	Receptor antibodies or TBII‡	Simple, human	Not a bioassay

From Kaplan, E.L., editor: Surgery of the thyroid and parathyroid glands, New York, 1983, Churchill Livingstone.
*LATS, Long-acting thyroid stimulator.
†LATS-P, Long-acting thyroid stimulator-protector.
‡TBII, Thyroid-binding inhibiting immunoglobulins.

known, current evidence suggests that B lymphocytes produce a thyroid-stimulating antibody (TSab) that interacts with TSH receptors on the thyroid cells, resulting in enhanced T_4 production (Table 58-2). These or similar antibodies may interact with separate receptors, resulting in enhancement of growth and vascularity.[57] Such phenomena may be transient and/or recurring, resulting in remissions and exacerbations of the disease. As lymphocytic infiltration of the gland is common, one hypothesis is that the site of TSab production is the thyroid itself.[33]

Recent improvements in laboratory techniques with the use of human thyroid cells from patients with Graves' disease have shown TSabs in more than 80% of these individuals. Unfortunately, neither the presence, absence, or changes in the titers of these antibodies correlates well with the course of the disease. It is possible that several different antibodies may play a role in the pathogenesis of Graves' disease. This is based on the observation that several antithyroid antibodies (e.g., antithyroglobulin, antimicrosomal) are also frequently found in the serum of patients with Graves' disease, as well as in those with Hashimoto's thyroiditis. Although the titers of these antibodies are usually higher in Hashimoto's thyroiditis, it is generally not possible to distinquish between these disease states on the basis of the antibody titer. In fact, histologic examination of thyroid glands in patients with Graves' disease frequently reveals localized areas of Hashimoto's thyroiditis. It remains unclear whether these autoantibodies play a pathogenic role or are innocent bystanders.

Clinical Manifestations

The classic signs and symptoms of Graves' disease are well described. The diagnosis is made on the basis of clinical manifestations of a hypermetabolic state and include heat intolerance, weight loss, tremor, increased appetite, palpitations, rapid pulse, diarrhea, proximal muscle weakness, a diffusely enlarge goiter, exophthalmus, and rarely pretibial myxedema. Occasionally atypical presentations may obscure the diagnosis. Weight gain, for example, may be seen in younger patients whose increased appetite and calorie intake can exceed 9000 calories per day. Psychiatric manifestations, including frank psychosis, may predominate over the symptoms.

On physical examination the patient is usually fidgety, often is sweating, and possesses a warm, moist skin. Deep tendon reflexes are usually exaggerated, and the pulse pressure is increased. Lid lag and a widened palpebral fissure are common in all thyrotoxic states and thought to be secondary to adrenergic stimulation. Signs of Graves' ophthalmolopathy include periorbital infiltration, proptosis, extraocular muscle dysfunction and possible corneal ulceration. Chemosis and dysconjugate gaze may also be present. Diplopia on lateral superior gaze is a particularly early sign of extraocular muscle dysfunction.

The thyroid is almost always diffusely enlarged and nontender. Minor degrees of nodularity and asymmetry may be present, but a dominant nodule(s) is distinctly unusual. The pyramidal lobe is frequently enlarged. Rarely, especially in men, the goiter may be substernal and not easily visible.

Laboratory Findings

The diagnosis of Graves' disease is made on the basis of the clinical picture associated with laboratory evidence of ongoing excessive thyroid hormone production (see boxed material on p. 961, top left). An accurate assessment of the free thyroid hormone level may be obtained by comparing the total T_4 or T_3 level with the available protein-binding sites. Total T_4 or T_3 is easily measured by RIA. The T_3 RU is a commonly used test to determine free binding sites on various proteins in the blood (e.g., thyronine-binding globulin, thyronine-binding prealbumin,

COMMON CONDITIONS ASSOCIATED WITH RADIOACTIVE IODINE UPTAKE (RAIU OR ^{131}I UPTAKE)

Elevated

1. Graves' disease
2. Toxic nodular goiter
3. Iodine deficiency (may be associated with diuretics)
4. Hashimoto's thyroiditis (may be variable)

Decreased

1. Subacute thyroiditis
2. Exogenous thyroid hormone administration (may be surreptitious)
3. Recent iodine administration (dietary, radiologic contrast, or therapeutic)

and albumin). An elevation of the uptake on the resin (T_3 RU) suggests a decreased number of binding sites. An elevated T_4 level in the presence of an elevated T_3 RU suggests an increased free thyroid hormone level consistent with thyrotoxicosis. However, to confirm ongoing thyroid hormone production, it is necessary to show that the gland is actively concentrating iodine and replenishing its intrathyroidal iodine pool. This is easily accomplished with the radioactive iodine uptake test (RAIU) in which a small quantity (50 μ ci) of ^{131}I is administered intravenously and its uptake in the neck measured and compared to background uptake. The RAIU is markedly elevated in Graves' disease, whereas it is low in thyrotoxicosis because of exogenous intake of thyroid hormones or because of inflammatory states that interrupt the integrity of the gland (subacute thyroiditis). A technetium scan of the thyroid gland in Graves' disease should show an enlarged gland that intensely and diffusely traps the isotope.

Total T_3 levels (T_3 by RIA) are elevated in hyperthyroidism. The ratio of T_3/T_4 secreted from the gland is increased in hyperthyroidism, and on occasion the T_4 level may be normal in spite of an elevated T_3 level (i.e., T_3 toxicosis). This latter circumstance may occur as an early manifestation of Graves' disease or after medical (^{131}I therapy) or surgical (subtotal thyroidectomy) therapeutic intervention. It is occasionally seen in toxic nodular goiters. Thus a total T_3 by RIA should be obtained in a patient who is clinically hypermetabolic but with equivocal thyroid function studies.

Treatment

There is no available therapy that specifically attacks the autoimmune derangements thought to be the cause of the disease. Therapy is therefore aimed at decreasing thyroid hormone production, either by blocking organification of iodine with thionamide drugs (e.g., propylthiouracil [PTU], methimazole), destroying the gland with radioactive iodine, or surgically removing the hyperplastic gland.

Medical Therapy. Antithyroid medications (i.e., thionamide drugs) are an effective mode of therapy. PTU, in addition to blocking iodine organification, also blocks peripheral T_4-to-T_3 conversion. Recent in vitro studies suggest that PTU has an immunologic action on T lymphocytes.[59a] Further studies are necessary to determine if PTU therapy has any lasting effect on the suspected immune mechanisms of Graves' disease. Several studies have shown remission rates after 3 to 24 months of antithyroid therapy ranging from 15% to 50% (see boxed material above).[24a] There is no single marker that reliably predicts which patients will relapse. Larger goiters, thyroid glands with persistently high ^{131}I uptakes, high serum titers of thyroid-stimulating antibodies, and a DR3 HLA type are all associated with higher relapse rates.

FACTORS ASSOCIATED WITH SPONTANEOUS REMISSION OF GRAVES' DISEASE

1. Small goiter
2. Decrease in goiter size during therapy
3. Normalization of RAIU
4. Low levels or normalization of thyroid-stimulating antibody levels
5. ? DR3- or DR4-negative HLA types

A 6- to 9-month treatment course with antithyroid medications is a reasonable first step in the treatment of Graves' disease. Children may be treated for longer periods of time, whereas elderly patients usually receive other modes of therapy (i.e., radioactive iodine or surgical) as soon as they are eumetabolic. Disadvantages of this medical regimen include a 5% to 10% incidence of minor allergic reactions, a 0.01% incidence of agranulocytosis, and compliance problems associated with chronic therapy. The dose of medication may be titrated to make the patient euthyroid (average dose in an adult is 300 to 600 mg of PTU or 30 to 60 mg of methimazole daily), or a larger blocking dose can be used to make the patient hypothyroid, supplemented by replacement therapy with oral T_4. This latter regimen has the practical advantage of decreasing the frequency of clinic visits and the theoretic advantage of suppressing the immune system.

The amount of thionamide treatment necessary to control hyperthyroidism depends on the severity of the disease and the rapidity of hormone turnover. Increased doses of medication given at more frequent intervals (every 4 to 6 hours) will control even the most severely hyperthyroid patient. Since these medications do not affect already stored thyroid hormone, a treatment period of at least 4 to 6 weeks is necessary to attain a eumetabolic state. This period is related to the amount and half-life of T_4 already formed (7 to 10 days in normal man, shorter in hyperthyroidism).

Beta-adrenergic blocking agents such as propranolol will quickly relieve some of the symptoms of hyperthyroidism related to a hyperdynamic cardiovascular system. In addition, propranonol in large doses (160 to 320 mg/day) will decrease T_4 to T_3 conversion in the periphery. In symptomatic patients, beta blockade should be initiated in conjunction with antithyroid medication. Once a eumetabolic state is achieved, beta blockage may be tapered and discontinued.

Radiodine Therapy. Radioiodine is safe and effective therapy for adults with Graves' disease (Fig. 58-4). The theoretic concerns regarding the subsequent development of thyroid carcinoma, hematologic malignancies, and birth

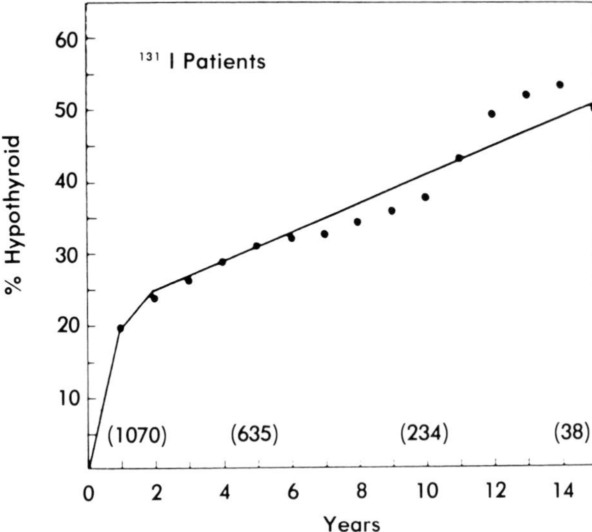

Fig. 58-4 Incidence of post-radioiodine hypothyroidism in relation to the duration of follow-up. Total number of patients followed for each of the indicated time periods is shown in parenthesis. (From Dunn, J.T., et al.: N. Engl. J. Med. **271:**1037, 1964.)

defects with such treatment have not been substantiated. Graves' disease is very sensitive to iodine, and usually small doses suffice. The radiation dose to the ovaries is approximately equivalent to that received during an intravenous pyelogram or barium enema. Nevertheless, radioiodine administration to women of reproductive age, adolescents, and children remains controversial.

It is not possible to accurately calculate a dose of radioiodine that will always result in euthyroidism. Small doses may result in an unacceptably high rate of recidivism. Although the incidence of hypothyroidism 1 to 2 years after radioiodine treatment is generally lower than after subtotal thyroidectomy (20% vs. 30% to 40%), the incidence of postradioiodine hypothyroidism increases by about 3% per year, reaching 50% to 70% after 10 years. Because of the unpredictability of radioiodine therapy and the necessity for life-long follow-up, many investigators argue that ablative radioiodine treatment followed by T_4 replacement therapy is the preferable plan.

As with surgery, radioiodine therapy administered to an uncontrolled hyperthyroid patient may precipitate a thyrotoxic crisis. Therefore in a severely hyperthyroid patient thionamides remain the first line of therapy. If radioiodine is chosen as definitive therapy, iodine administration (see discussion below) is avoided. Once the patient is eumetabolic, the thionamide is discontinued. A RAIU study and thyroid scan are performed approximately 4 days later, the dose of ^{131}I is calculated and administered, and the thionamide is restarted approximately 4 days after this. Beta blockade is usually given during this period to avoid any cardiovascular effects of a thyroid hormone surge. This sequence allows for accurate dosing and uptake of the radioiodine without placing the patient at substantial risk from thyrotoxicosis. Radiation thyroiditis, an inflammation of the thyroid resulting in a tender gland, and exacerbation of the thyrotoxic state may occur approximately 1 to 2 weeks after radioiodine therapy. Fortunately, this thyroiditis is not usually seen in Graves' disease, since the dose of ^{131}I is usually less than 20 mCi, much lower than is generally associated with this problem. Beta blockade is usually sufficient to control the transient and infrequent phenomenon of exacerbation of the thyrotoxic state.

The effect of radioiodine on thyroid function is slow and is usually not detected clinically for at least 6 weeks, and more frequently 3 to 6 months, after treatment. Medical therapy can be slowly tapered during this period. Uncontrolled hyperthyroidism after 9 to 12 months should warrant further evaluation and possibly a repeat dose of radioiodine.

Surgical Therapy. Thyroidectomy (i.e., generally subtotal) remains an important therapeutic option in the treatment of Graves' disease. As with radioiodine, it is not possible to reliably predict the size of the remnant that will render the patient euthyroid.[28,30,53] The relatively high percentage (30% to 40%) of patients that are cured by thyroidectomy suggests that somehow thyroid hemeostasis is reestablished by the procedure. Thyroidectomy not only removes the source of thyroid hormone production, it may decrease the population of antibody-producing lymphocytes.[33] Advantages of thyroidectomy include the speed of remission and the low rate of recurrence.

The argument over the extent of thyroidectomy (subtotal vs. total) mirrors the debate over the calculated dose of radioiodine.[10] A more complete thyroidectomy may be preferable in a child with Graves' disease, since the chances of regrowth of the remnant and recurrence of disease are fairly high. Depending on the published series examined, recurrent thyrotoxicosis occurs in 0.6% to 30% of cases following surgery.[30]

Evidence of coexisting Hashimoto's thyroiditis, as noted by antibody titers (antimicrosomal and antithyroglobulin antibodies), or lymphocytic infiltration microscopically is also associated with a higher incidence of postsurgical hypothyroidism. In this setting hypothyroidism may result from progressive fibrosis and inflammation of the thyroid remnant following surgery, since this situation can occur in the absence of definitive radioiodine or surgical therapy. Rather than being an adverse effect of therapy, hypothyroidism may be thought of as part of the natural history of the disease. Thus more agressive radioiodine or surgical approaches may only accelerate this natural course.

On the basis of these considerations, recurrence of thyrotoxicosis after thyroidectomy appears to be directly related to the size of the residual remnant, the severity of the hyperthyroidism, the age of the patient at the time of surgery, and the underlying immune aspects of the disease. One argument for total thyroidectomy is the removal of the source of autoimmune activity. However, it remains unclear if any mode of therapy, be it medical, radioiodine, subtotal, or total thyroidectomy, affects the ophthalmopathy presumed to be related to autoimmune mechanisms.

Although thyroidectomy can be performed on all patients with Graves' disease, certain individuals may benefit particularly from surgical treatment. These include: (1) children with unremitting Graves' disease where experience with radioiodine remains limited, (2) pregnant women with uncontrolled hyperthyroidism in the third trimester, (3) patients with suspicious "cold" nodules in an otherwise diffusely hyperplastic gland, and (4) patients who cannot tolerate antithyroid medications and require rapid resolution of the thyrotoxic state.

In spite of the benefits of surgery, it must be remembered that the unstable metabolic state associated with hyperthyroidism increases the risk of anesthesia and surgery. Thyroid storm may be precipitated by surgery in a poorly prepared patient. Thus thionamides should be given in large enough doses and at frequent enough intervals to achieve a euthyroid state in 4 to 6 weeks. Surgery may then be planned on an elective basis. In addition, iodine is very effective in decreasing the size and vascularity of the gland, in acutely blocking secretion of thyroid hormones by the gland, and in transiently interfering with organification (Wolff-Chaikoff effect). The mechanism by which iodine decreases the vascularity of the gland (involution) is unknown. Since the Wolff-Chaikoff effect is temporary, lasting only 10 to 14 days, it is important to administer iodine only in the presence of a thionamide. Iodine alone will supply a hyperplastic gland with unlimited substrate to synthesize thyroid hormone. Iodine is therefore administered only during the week before surgery, once the patient has been rendered euthyroid.

In patients unable to tolerate thionamide therapy, surgical preparation with propranolol and iodine is usually successful. A total thyroidectomy would be desirable in this circumstance to avoid either an exacerbation of hyperthyroidism or an eventual recurrence.

Toxic Nodular Goiter

Toxic nodular goiter is a form of hyperthyroidism that is more commonly encountered in patients over 40 years old and frequently occurs in the elderly. A marked female predominance is again noted. The patient may present with a long stable history of a multinodular goiter or with a predominant nodule in the neck. The addition of iodine, either in medications or contrast dye, may precipitate thyrotoxicosis is an iodine-deficient nodular goiter.

Cardiovascular effects of hyperthyroidism predominant in this condition and in the elderly may be the only clinical signs detected. Apathetic hyperthyroidism aptly describes a depressed, frequently constipated, elderly patient who presents to the physician with weight loss and cardiac arrhythmias. Eye signs are lacking, and, although a goiter is usually present, it may not be impressive. Therapy should be initiated with antithyroid medications and propranolol. Iodine should be avoided in these patients. The diagnosis should be confirmed with an elevated RAIU, T_4 level, and a thyroid scan revealing one or more hot nodules.

Large multinodular goiters do not concentrate iodine well compared to Graves' disease and generally require larger doses of radioiodine (i.e., 20 to 30 mCi for toxic multinodular goiter as opposed to 6 to 10 mCi for Graves' disease) for treatment. Recurrence or failure of initial radioiodine therapy is common, since destruction of one autonomous nodule may be replaced with another autonomously functioning nodule. Although thyroid carcinoma is unusual in this setting, an enlarging hypofunctioning nodule in a hyperthyroid gland may warrant biopsy or surgical exploration.

The size and vascularity of large, multinodular goiters makes surgical management more formidable. In contrast to the hyperplastic glands found in Graves' disease, the multinodular goiter may not shrink with iodine (Lugol's solution), and iodine may precipitate a thyrotoxic crisis. Therefore the preferred treatment of a toxic multinodular goiter is radioiodine. Hypothyroidism is unusual after such therapy in this setting.

Solitary hyperfunctioning adenomas occur in older patients, with a male predominance. These autonomous nodules may suppress the normal surrounding thyroid tissue and produce hyperthyroidism. More commonly the total thyroid hormone production remains in a normal range in spite of the autonomous nature of the nodule. The natural history of solitary "hot" nodules is that they remain small and stable or increase in size and produce thyrotoxicosis or degenerate after hemorrhage and become a "cold" nodule.

Solitary nodules that are greater than 3 cm in diameter, produce an increased T_3/T_4 ratio, or suppress all extranodular thyroid tissue on nuclear imaging are likely to produce thyrotoxicosis.[25] As with toxic multinodular goiters, the symptoms and signs of a toxic thyroid adenoma may be subtle, especially in the elderly. A solitary thyroid mass, usually greater than 3 cm, may be the only thyroid tissue palpable. RAIU may be only modestly elevated, but the thyroid scan will show intense uptake only in the area of the palpable abnormality. A T_3 by RIA should be obtained, especially if the total T_4 level is normal and in view of the high incidence of T_3 toxicosis in this circumstance.

Radioiodine therapy of toxic adenomas has the theoretic advantage of being taken up only by the hyperfunctioning tissue, destroying it, and rendering the patient euthyroid. The incidence of carcinoma in a hot nodule is extremely small, and there is no evidence that radioiodine is carcinogenic. However, recurrence of hyperthyroidism after radioiodine therapy is not uncommon, and repeated doses of radioiodine required to deliver 10 to 15 mCi ^{131}I to the nodule (30 mCi ^{131}I to the patient) may be undesirable in the younger patient. In a recent study of the long-term effects of ^{131}I on solitary autonomous nodules, 54% (12/23 patients) had no change in the size of the nodule, and 36% developed hypothyroidism.[24]

Surgery for toxic adenomas has the advantage of quickly resolving the thyrotoxic state and avoiding recurrences. A simple nodulectomy is usually sufficient because the remainder of the thyroid is normal and carcinoma is distinctly unusual in the nodule itself. If an image of the suppressed thyroid tissue is desirable before surgery, this may be accomplished by administering bovine TSH before a thyroid scan.

Thyroid Storm

Thyroid storm is an extreme form of hyperthyroidism. In addition to the recognized findings of hyperthroidism, the clinical diagnosis of thyroid storm is based on cardiovascular abnormalities (malignant arrhythmias resistant to medications), mental status changes (psychosis, confusion, obtundation, or coma), and pyrexia. Therapy is directed at acutely decreasing thyroid hormone secretion (iodine intravenously, glucocorticoids, PTU) and decreasing adrenergic tone (propranolol). Although rare, thyroid storm is associated with high morbidity and mortality. Severe stress may precipitate thyroid storm in a patient with unrecognized mild hyperthyroidism. Other common precipitating causes of thyroid storm include surgery, trauma, infection, and iodine administration. Iodine-containing radiographic contrast media are also common offending agents. Amiodarone, an effective antiarrhythmic, contains a large amount of iodine and has been associated with both hypothyroidism and hyperthyroidism. A medical regimen that allows the patient to be eumetabolic before surgery has essentially eliminated the danger of thyrotoxic crisis.

HYPOTHYROIDISM (MYXEDEMA)

Thyroid failure is the natural end point of several thyroid diseases, including thyroiditis and postirradiation atrophy of the thyroid gland following treatment of Graves' disease. Although iodine deficiency is the most common worldwide cause of hypothyroidism, Hashimoto's thyroiditis predominates in the United States. The absence of circulating thyroid hormones, so important to normal cellular metabolic function, also obviously occurs when the thyroid gland is totally removed surgically for whatever reason.

Thyroiditis and Hypothyroidism

Thyroiditis is the term given to various inflammatory processes involving the thyroid gland. Four types of thyroiditis have been recognized. These include Hashimoto's disease (the lymphocytic type), Riedel's thyroiditis, and both viral and acute suppurative types of thyroiditis. Of these, Hashimoto's thyroiditis is the most common and is thought to be caused by an autoimmune mechanism, resulting in an invasion of lymphocytes and fibrous tissue within the gland. Clinically the disease is characterized by a diffuse, rubbery, nontender goiter. All types of thyroid dysfunction have been associated with Hashimoto's thyroiditis, including transient hyperthyroidism, euthyroid goiter, hypothyroid goiter, and an atrophic thyroid gland with an associated hypothyroidism. In most patients some degree of hypothyroidism is present. Hashimoto's thyroiditis generally afflicts women between the ages of 20 and 50 years, but it also is commonly encountered in children. The diagnosis is usually confirmed by the finding of a firm goiter in the presence of a markedly elevated antithyroid antibody titer (i.e., antimicrosomal and antithyroglobulin). Thyroid imaging usually reveals a patchy uptake of isotope. Histologic examination of the thyroid gland reveals lymphocytic infiltration. If hypothyroidism is present in this disease, thyroid hormone replacement is the keynote of treatment.

The second most common form of thyroiditis is the viral type, also called subacute or de Quervain's thyroiditis (although 10 times less commonly encountered than Hashimoto's disease). Clinically the thyroid gland is tender and diffusely enlarged, and often the patient complains of a mild fever and generalized malaise, with an associated elevation in the sedimentation rate on laboratory evaluation. Treatment is usually supportive and includes bed rest, sedation, and the administration of antiinflammatory drugs such as aspirin. There are no permanent sequalae from this disease.

Both Riedel's thyroiditis and acute suppurative thyroiditis are extremely rare. Most authorities feel that the Riedel's type is the fibrous endstage of Hashimoto's disease. Pathologically the gland atrophies and is characterized clinically as being woody hard. Because of this firmness, cancer cannot be excluded on clinical grounds alone, and therefore biopsy is indicated to exclude that possibility. Since patients with Riedel's thyroiditis, similar to Hashimoto's disease, often have some form of hypothyroidism, replacement with thyroid hormones is usually indicated. Acute suppurative thyroiditis is usually bacterial in origin and generally results from abscessed lower teeth. Treatment therefore includes incision and drainage of the abscess, along with appropriate antibiotic coverage. In addition, appropriate dental care is indicated.

Clinical Presentation

The clinical presentation of hypothyroidism may be very subtle. The classic symptoms of weight gain, bradycardia, constipation, dry skin, cold intolerance, and somnolence are not always obvious. Children may present with a decreased attention span, difficulty at school, and short stature. An abnormal growth curve and delayed bone age should prompt a workup for hypothyroidism. Adolescents and young adults may come to the physician with difficulty in concentrating and depression. Elderly patients frequently have depression and signs of organic brain syndrome. In surveys of nursing home populations, approximately 10% of elderly females were found to have unsuspected primary hypothyroidism on thyroid screening tests.

Thyroid function studies in hypothyroid patients typically reveal a low total T_4 level, a low T_3 RU consistent with an increase in binding sites, and a low free thyroid index. Although RAIU is decreased in hypothyroidism, the quantity of iodine in the American diet impairs the use of this study diagnostically. The pituitary is exquisitely sensitive to a decreased T_4 level, and an elevated TSH level, especially greater than 20 mIU/ml, is diagnostic of thyroid failure. In an attempt to maintain metabolic homeostasis, a failing gland may secrete a higher ratio of T_3/T_4 in response to high values of TSH. This invalidates the measurement T_3 by RIA as a useful study in early hypothyroidism.

Two principal problems confront the surgeon in dealing with a patient with low T_4 levels:

1. Is the patient truly hypothyroid, or are the low values the result of a physiologic response to an acute or chronic illness?
2. If the patient is hypothyroid, what is the most appropriate replacement regimen in order to avoid anesthetic or surgical complications?

As previously noted, low thyroid function studies are common in severe acute or chronic illness. The finding of an extremely low T_3 by RIA has been observed to correlate with a high mortality. An elevated T_3 RU, a normal or low TSH, a normal free T_4 by dialysis, and a normal reverse T_3 are all consistent with the euthyroid sick syndrome. Thus thyroid replacement therapy is not indicated in this group of patients. The diagnosis of primary hypothyroidism must be confirmed by an elevated TSH level.

Pituitary or hypothalamic disease should be suspected in a patient with an inappropriately low or normal TSH value. Clinical suspicion and further evaluation can differentiate true hypothyroidism from the euthyroid sick syndrome.

Levothyroxine is the drug of choice to treat hypothyroidism. A euthyroid state is usually attained with a dose of approximately 2 μg/kg. In older patients or patients with cardiovascular disease, it is best to start with a low dose (0.025 to 0.05 mg daily) and slowly increase to a full dose.

It is not always possible to achieve a eumetabolic state before embarking on a major surgical procedure. A good example of this is the hypothyroid patient with severe coronary artery disease who experiences an exacerbation of his angina when the dose of levothyroxine is adjusted. Coronary bypass surgery may be performed on such a patient if there is close cooperation among the internist, surgeon, and anesthesiologist. Since the metabolism of most drugs will be slowed in the hypothyroid patient, adjustment of drug doses and avoidance of opiates and sedatives are necessary. Arterial blood gases and estimates of ventilatory effort should be monitored frequently. A recent retrospective study suggests a lower morbidity from coronary bypass surgery in hypothyroid patients than in patients having surgery after replacement with thyroid hormone.[46a]

Myxedema Coma

Severe myxedema should be suspected in a hypothermic, somnolent patient. Hypercapnia and hyponatremia are common metabolic findings. A puffy face; periorbital edema; evidence of previous neck surgery; doughy, dry, cool skin; and a delayed relaxation of deep tendon reflexes are usually present. Althouth absence of the lateral third of the eyebrows was previously thought to be a helpful clinical finding, it is only of significance in patients less than 40 years of age.

Myxedema coma may be precipitated in a patient with unrecognized hypothyroidism by infection, cold exposure (apartments for the elderly without heat in the winter), surgery, trauma, and drugs. The metabolism of most drugs, particularly sedatives and opiates, are slowed by hypothyroidism. Respiratory depression and hypercapnia caused by a sluggish respiratory center result in coma and respiratory failure. Anesthetics and postoperative opiates may precipitate a severely myxedematous state in an unrecognized hypothyroid patient. Thyroid hormone replacement therapy should be begun immediately after blood for thyroid studies are drawn (T_4, T_3 RU, TSH) in a patient suspected of myxedema coma.

Treatment of Myxedema Coma

Primary thyroid failure has an indolent course that frequently requires several years to develop into a myxedematous state. A large infusion of thyroid hormone may precipitate malignant cardiac arrhythmias. Levothyroxine administered intravenously is the preferred replacement regimen. Depending on the severity of the myxedema and the fragility of the patient's cardiovascular system, daily doses of 100 to 200 μg may be safer than the loading dose of 500 usually recommended. The patient should be carefully monitored in an intensive care unit for any potentially life-threatening arrhythmias.

Glucocorticoids are an important adjunctive therapy for patients with severe hypothyroidism because the sudden increase in the metabolic rate after the addition of T_4 may render the patient relatively adrenally insufficient. In addition, the autoimmune phenomena that result in Hashimoto's thyroiditis may be be more generalized, thus producing a syndrome of polyglandular endocrine failure. The most common manifestations of this syndrome are primary thyroid failure, primary adrenal insufficiency, and Type I diabetes mellitus. An evaluation of the pituitary-adrenal axis, including pretreatment cortisol levels, is therefore essential.

In patients with myxedema coma, treatment should result in prompt improvement in the pco_2, ventilatory status, and mentation. Glucocorticoids may be tapered and discontinued if the adrenal reserve is adequate. Replacement doses of T_4 in adults range from 0.1 to 0.2 mg daily, depending on body weight (2.25 μg/kg) and age. The TSH level should slowly decline toward the normal range if the replacement dose is adequate and the patient is compliant.

THYROID NODULES AND NEOPLASIA

Thyroid nodules are common. Approximately 5% of the population, with a 9:1 female predominance, have such nodules.[58] A small percentage of these nodules are malignant, and an even smaller percentage of such malignant nodules are life threatening. In the past the decision to proceed to surgical intervention after noting the presence of a thyroid nodule was based in large part on the anxiety of the patient and the physician. Improvements in our ability to obtain cytologic information have resulted in a decreased number of unnecessary surgical procedures and an increase in the percentage of actual malignant neoplasms found at surgery. Further, a better understanding of the biologic behavior of different thyroid tumors has permitted a more reasoned physiologic approach to their treatment.

Pathophysiology of Thyroid Nodules and Neoplasia

Clinical and pathologic study of thyroid disease is complicated by the fact that several different insults to the thyroid manifest themselves similarly. Any injury to the thyroid that impairs its ability to synthesize thyroid hormones will frequently result in the development of a goiter. The initial insult may be autoimmune thyroiditis, iodine deficiency, or inherited biochemical defects. Goiters of puberty and pregnancy are not nodular, and, although TSH is suspected as playing a role in their pathogenesis, the TSH levels by RIA are invariably normal as long as the patient is euthyroid. Thus the cause of these physiologic goiters remains unclear. They frequently resolve spontaneously, and therapy is rarely indicated. The presence of growth factors other than TSH is presumed but not proven to be responsible for their pathogenesis.

Increasing age is accompanied by an increased frequency of thyroid nodules (Fig. 58-5).[58] Radioautography of thyroid sections suggests the following natural history of thyroid nodules.[54] After a period of stimulation, presumably from TSH, a diffusely enlarged goiter with good

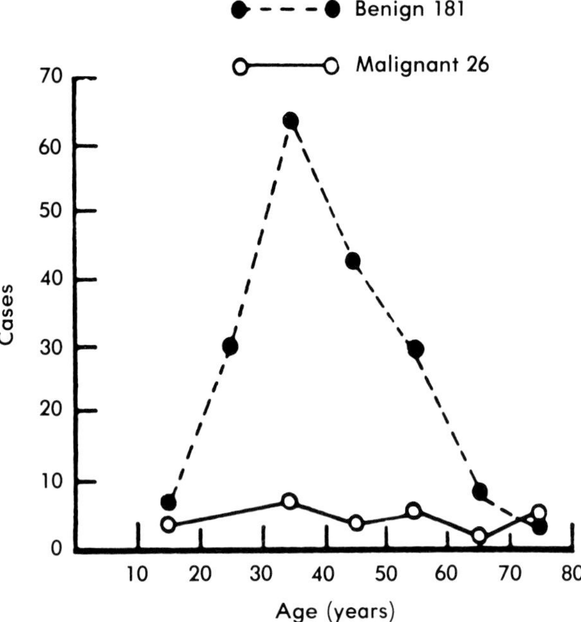

Fig. 58-5 Age distribution of 207 benign and malignant thyroid nodules. (From Werner, S., and Ingbar, S., editors: The thyroids, New York, 1978, Harper and Row, Publishers, Inc.)

vascularity and homogenous radioiodine uptake becomes a diffusely enlarged gland with patchy uptake of iodine. This difference in uptake slowly results in some area of the gland becoming relatively hypofunctioning and others becoming relatively hyperfunctioning; these latter areas of the gland slowly become nodular. Some of these nodules may spontaneously resolve, whereas others may enlarge secondary to hemorrhage in the nodule, and still others may become autonomously hyperfunctioning. This sequence of events will eventually result in a clinically multinodular goiter.

How can these events be explained on the basis of TSH stimulation, if in fact the TSH levels are invariably normal? The following hypotheses have been suggested:

1. A normal TSH level in the presence of iodine deficiency or dyshormonogenesis may be goitrogenic. The most common cause of multinodular goiters outside of the United States is iodine deficiency. Hashimoto's thyroiditis impairs hormonogenesis and is responsible for a major portion of sporadic nontoxic goiters. Further, inherited biochemical deficits in hormone synthesis are evident in selected populations.
2. Qualitative secretion of TSH may be abnormal when quantitative measurements are in a normal range. In other words, the RIA may not be sensitive enough to pick up small differences in TSH secretion.
3. Changes in the vascularity of the gland, including possibly arterial-venous shunts, may increase the TSH levels in certain parts of the gland, resulting in areas of hyperplasia.
4. Growth factors other than TSH are present.

Unfortunately, experimental evidence is lacking to verify or refute any of these hypotheses.

Table 58-3 **RADIATION-ASSOCIATED THYROID CARCINOMA**

	Thyroid Cancer Death Rates/100,000/Year		Occult Thyroid Cancer (Autopsy Studies, Similar Methods)(%)
	Males	**Females**	
Switzerland	1.51	1.56	1.2
America	0.4	0.8	5.7
Japan	0.21	0.46	17.9

(From Degroot, L.J., et al.: Radiation-associated thyroid carcinoma, New York, 1977, Grune & Stratton, Inc.)

The evaluation of thyroid nodules involves in a large part the evaluation of the benign sporadic nontoxic goiter. Stated another way, "solitary nodules" often are not solitary. In a study of 207 patients with presumed solitary nodules on clinical examination, only 60% were found to be solitary at surgery, and only 52% after histologic section.[54] In spite of the weak evidence for a role for TSH as a prime mover in the pathogenesis of thyroid nodules, it has been known for more than 100 years that the administration of suppressive doses of thyroid hormone will decrease the size of many nontoxic goiters and nodules. Failure of the gland to shrink when given thyroid hormone may be related to the presence of fibrosis, colloid lakes, hemorrhage in degenerating nodules, as well as the duration of the goiter. In addition, well-differentiated thyroid carcinomas are also frequently TSH dependent and may decrease in size with suppressive doses of thyroid hormone. It is unknown whether thyroid adenomas or carcinomas arise from TSH stimulation or de novo or whether there is a transition from adenoma to carcinoma.

Prevalence of Thyroid Nodules and Neoplasia

The major problem confronting the clinician in managing patients with thyroid nodules is differentiating the myriad benign thyroid lesions from the few malignant ones. It has been estimated that approximately 2% of nodules in a nontoxic nodular goiter are malignant. The malignancy rate increases to approximately 10% to 15% in solitary nodules. The incidence of benign thyroid nodules increases with age and appears to be maximum approximately at the age of 40, with a 7 to 9:1 predominance in women over men. The incidence of thyroid carcinoma may not change appreciably for different age groups; however, the decrease in benign nodules in childhood and in the elderly raises substantially the percentage of nodules that are malignant in these age groups. Deaths from thyroid carcinoma are rare and estimated to be approximately 1100 cases per year. Incidences of thyroid nodules and thyroid carcinoma may be on the increase and have been attributed to radiation-associated thyroid disease[40] (Table 58-3).

Occult thyroid carcinoma is a common autopsy finding. Estimates range from 2% to 28%, depending on the study quoted.[48] These tumors are nonpalpable and by definition are less than 1.5 cm in diameter. Suprisingly, when carcinoma death rates are compared to the prevalence of occult carcinoma, there appears to be either no relationship or possibly even an inverse relationship.[48] Survival curves for the general population and patients with occult thyroid carcinoma are virtually the same.[60] In Woolner's study from the Mayo Clinic in 1960, 140 cases of occult carcinoma were followed for as many as 30 years after surgery.[61] There were no deaths from thyroid carcinoma, in spite of the fact that 58 of the 140 cases were associated with metastases to the regional lymph nodes at the time of diagnosis. Six patients presented with nodal metastases thought to be lateral aberrant thyroid tissue with normal-appearing thyroid glands. Five of these patients have been followed for more than 20 years, and none have died of thyroid-related disease. Occult carcinoma has an excellent prognosis, possibly because of host resistance, and a limited thyroidectomy appears to be adequate for cure in many instances.

Classification of Benign Thyroid Nodules

The most common benign thyroid nodule is the follicular adenoma. It is a well-encapsulated tumor that may comprise as many as 70% of benign thyroid nodules. It may be particularly difficult to differentiate a benign follicular adenoma from a well-differentiated follicular carcinoma on the basis of either frozen section or needle biopsy.[45] Vascular invasion must be noted, and it is frequently necessary to take multiple sections of the tumor to verify the diagnosis of follicular carcinoma. The surgeon must therefore be wary of the diagnosis of follicular adenoma by needle biopsy or on frozen section.

Colloid adenomas are responsible for approximately 7% of benign, solitary, cold nodules and are usually not a diagnostic problem histologically. Cellular adenomas may include fetal, embryonal, and Hurthle cell types and may be responsible for as many as 20% of benign solitary nodules of the thyroid. Controversy exists over whether some of these cellular adenomas, in particular the Hurthle cell tumors, have malignant potential and should be included under the classification of malignant tumors. As in the case of follicular adenomas, it is important to perform multiple sections to be certain that there is no capsular or vascular invasion.

Thyroid cysts are frequently the result of degeneration of a benign adenoma. Occasionally a degenerating carcinoma can also present as either a mixed solid-cystic lesion or, rarely, a purely cystic lesion. In general, only cystic lesions greater than 4 cm in size have an appreciable incidence of carcinoma.[59] Although any cystic content can be associated with cancer, a bloody cystic aspirate is particularly worrisome for carcinoma.

Localized areas of Hashimoto's thyroiditis can present as benign thyroid nodules that may be hypofunctioning. In a diffusely abnormal thyroid gland, Hashimoto's thyroiditis may coexist with a malignant lymphoma.[27] A careful examination by the pathologist for lymphoma is therefore indicated. In addition, small-cell carcinoma is occasionally confused with thyroiditis on cytology.

Malignant Nodules of the Thyroid

Thyroid carcinomas have distinct differences in biologic behavior from benign nodules, and their malignant characteristics are greatly influenced by their histologic type. Papillary and follicular carcinomas comprise the differentiated carcinomas of the thyroid. Greater than 50% of thyroid carcinomas are of the papillary type. Approximately 20% are believed to be follicular, but, in fact, many of these have papillary characteristics microscopically within the tumors and behave as papillary carcinomas. Since their biologic activity is similar, papillary carcinomas and mixed follicular-papillary carcinomas are grouped together.

Types of Carcinomas (Figs. 58-6 and 58-7)

Papillary Carcinoma. Papillary carcinoma is the major thyroid cancer of childhood and young adults. Clinically it presents as a solitary nodule, but careful histologic examination of resected thyroid specimens reveals a 40% to 60% incidence of microscopic multicentric spread through intraglandular lymphatics to other parts of the gland and associated lymph nodes. Metastatic spread beyond the neck to lung and bone is uncommon. The rate of occult carcinoma may be as high as eight times the rate of clinical occurrence.[56] A microscopic tumor on occasion can present with cervical lymph node metastases as the predominant clinical finding, initially misdiagnosed as lateral aberrant thyroid tissue. Papillary carcinoma is more aggressive in patients older than 40 years of age, in whom death rates are substantially higher than in younger patients and are frequently due to recurrent local invasion.

The hallmarks of papillary carcinoma histologically are the papillary projections of epithelial cells, which are nonencapsulated and associated with psammoma bodies. This diagnosis can frequently be made by fine-needle aspiration biopsy. Because papillary carcinoma concentrates ^{131}I poorly, it appears hypofunctioning or nonfunctioning on radioisotope scans when compared with the remaining uninvolved gland. After thyroidectomy, the ability of the tumor to concentrate miniscule amounts of ^{131}I can be detected on scans. Thus ^{131}I can be used both diagnostically and therapeutically for follow-up purposes.

Follicular Carcinoma. Follicular carcinomas are encapsulated cellular tumors that spread hematogenously to the lung, bone, and liver. They occur more commonly in patients over 40 years of age, and the prognosis correlates with the invasiveness of the tumor. Clinically, follicular carcinoma may present as a solitary nodule, an enlarging nodule in a multinodular gland, or as a pathologic bone fracture from a metastasis. Lymph node involvement is uncommon. Histologically the cells may vary from being indistinguishable from normal thyroid tissue to grossly abnormal within the same lesion. For this reason the diagnosis of follicular carcinoma is made on the basis of careful examination of the capsule and blood vessels for invasion. Fine-needle aspiration and frozen section are often inaccurate, and reliance on these techniques may result in inadequate surgery or unnecessary multiple operations.

Follicular carcinoma can concentrate ^{131}I reasonably well and rarely may synthesize thyroid hormones. Thyro-

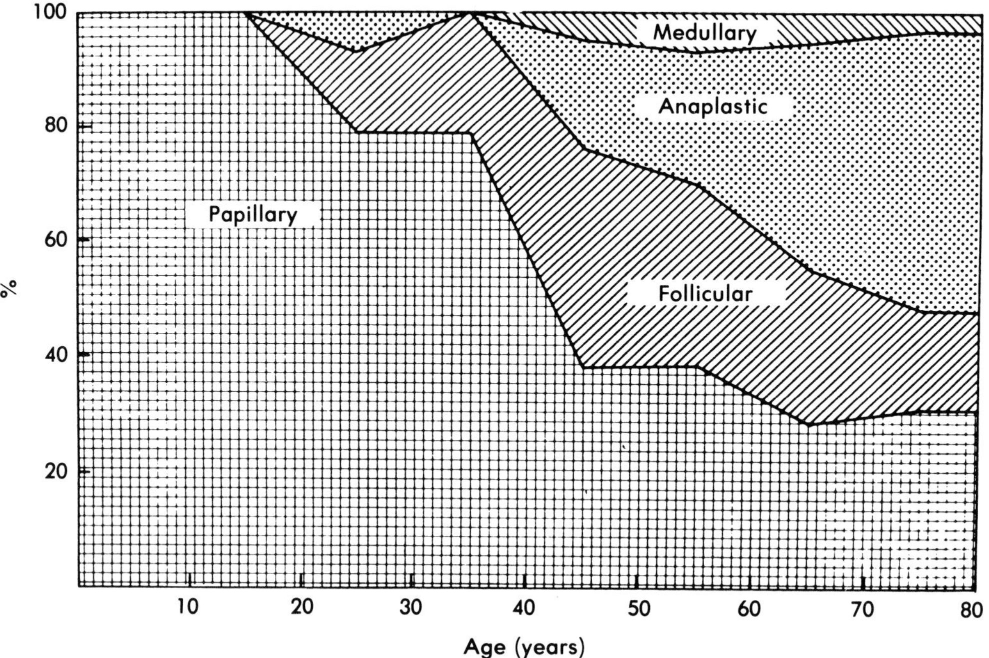

Fig. 58-6 Percentage distribution of 230 cases of thyroid carcinoma into histologic types, by age. (From Degroot, L.J., editor: Radiation-associated thyroid carcinoma, New York, 1977, Grune & Stratton, Inc.)

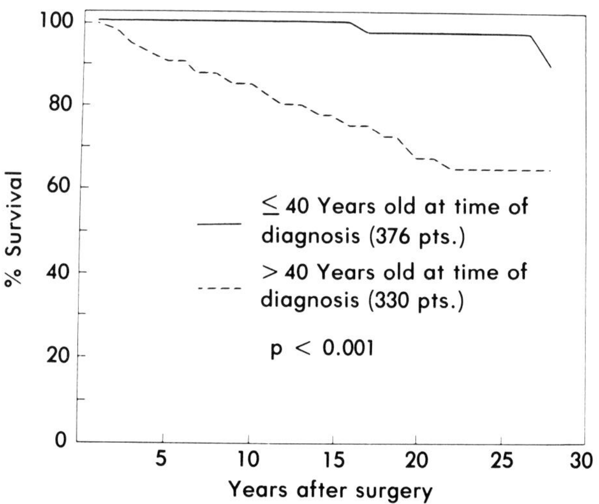

Fig. 58-7 Survival curves for patient diagnosed before (—) and after (----) the age of 40 years. (From Samaan, N.A.: J. Clin. Endocrinol. Metabol. **56:**1131, 1983.)

toxicosis, including T_3 toxicosis, can result from bulky functional metastases. In spite of a generally decreased capacity to concentrate ^{131}I vs. normal thyroid tissue, pulmonary metastases have been known to disappear on thyroid suppression alone, especially in younger patients who have more endocrinologically dependent tumors.[14]

Medullary Thyroid Carcinoma. Medullary thyroid carcinoma (MTC) is a rare neoplasm of the parafollicular cells (C-cells) that readily invades the intraglandular lymphatics and the bloodstream, spreading to the lungs, liver, and bone.[11] MTC may appear as part of the syndrome of multiple endocrine neoplasia, which is represented by a group of familial disorders of variable autosomal dominant penetrance. In these syndromes family members may have one or more of the following conditions: MTC, parathyroid hyperplasia, and pheochromocytomas, often bilateral. In addition, ganglioneuromas, mucosal neuromas, and a marfanoid habitus can be seen in the so-called ''bumpy-lips'' syndrome. For a more extensive discussion of these syndromes, the reader is referred to Chapter 60.

Calcitonin is secreted from the C-cells of the thyroid and is a sensitive marker for MTC.[31] Early detection and surgery of C-cell hyperplasia in affected children of family members with these syndromes can be curative.[31,49] Basal and stimulated calcitonin levels, after pentagastrin or calcium, should be performed yearly on suspected carriers, starting in childhood.[31,49] Total thyroidectomy with regional lymph node removal should be undertaken if the calcitonin levels are elevated. Hyperparathyroidism and pheochromocytoma should be ruled out biochemically before surgery. Because of the risk of hypertensive crises, pheochromocytomas should be removed first, if present.

More commonly, medullary thyroid carcinoma appears sporadically (greater than 60% of the time) in patients older than 50 years. It can appear simply as a nodule or nodules, with or without nodal or distant disease, and occasionally as Cushing's syndrome or carcinoid syndrome, depending on peptides that the tumor is able to secrete (i.e., ACTH, serotonin, vasoactive intestinal peptide, kinins, prostaglandins). Soft-tissue calcifications bilaterally of the neck, occasionally seen with this neoplasm, can sometimes be demonstrated on x-ray film.

Histologically the tumor is not encapsulated, and the cells may be somewhat undifferentiated with abundant stromal amyloid. MTC is more malignant than the differentiated thyroid tumors and carries a higher morbidity and mortality (50%), especially in the older patient with nodal or distant disease. With fine-needle aspiration biopsy, this condition can occasionally be diagnosed before surgery, with special stains for amyloid. Elevated calcitonin and carcinoembryonic antigen levels will confirm the diagnosis. These levels are excellent markers for recurrent disease after surgery. Since thyroid suppressive therapy does not affect growth of the tumor because it is not TSH dependent, surgical management is indicated.

Anaplastic Carcinoma. Anaplastic carcinoma is a particularly lethal and rapidly growing cancer that affects mostly the elderly. The tumor is usually well advanced at the time of diagnosis and is almost uniformly fatal within 2 years of diagnosis, in spite of aggressive therapy. Histologically one can see a variety of spindle-shaped and bizarre cells that can be confused with small cell carcinomas. These cells do not concentrate ^{131}I and are not responsive to TSH suppression. Anectodal reports suggest that patients with long-standing, well-differentiated thyroid cancer can develop anaplastic carcinoma. It is unknown if ^{131}I therapy contributes to this transformation. Anaplastic carcinoma frequently appears in patients with a history of long-standing nodular goiter. The relationship of goiter, papillary carcinoma, ^{131}I therapy, and anaplastic transformation requires further investigation. Fine-needle aspiration biopsy is frequently diagnostic. A multidisciplinary approach to therapy, including surgery, radiation, and chemotherapy has shown improved survival.

Rare Tumors of the Thyroid. Primary lymphoma of the thyroid is rare and frequently confused with other undifferentiated carcinomas. Hashimoto's thyroiditis frequently coexists with lymphoma. Improved experience with needle biopsies has increased the number of diagnoses being made preoperatively. The patient may present with a solitary nodule or, more commonly, with an enlarging diffusely abnormal gland. Radiation treatment and chemotherapy result in initial remission, but long-term survival is usually poor unless the tumor is still confined to the neck at the time of diagnosis.

Metastatic disease to the thyroid is not uncommon and may arise from primary tumors in the kidney, larynx, breast, esophagus, lung, and rectum. Fine-needle aspiration may be diagnostic and help avoid unnecessary surgery.

Prognostic Factors Related to Thyroid Cancer

The histologic type of tumor is the most important single prognostic factor in thyroid cancer.[9] Well-differentiated tumors have normal or near normal 10- and 20-year survival curves, especially in the young, even in the face of widespread metastases. Additional prognostic factors in order of decreasing importance include age, intraglandular invasion of the primary tumor, distant metastases, size of primary tumor, blood vessel invasion, multifocality, sex, and possibly lymph node metastases[9,43,47] (see boxed material at top right and Figs. 58-8 to 58-10).

Age is important both in evaluating a thyroid nodule and as a prognostic factor for a thyroid neoplasm. Benign nodules increase in number with age, especially in women, and therefore a solitary nodule in a young boy or an elderly man is more worrisome. The frequency of different types of thyroid carcinoma also is influenced by age. Pap-

PROGNOSTIC FACTORS IN THYROID CARCINOMA

1. Histologic type
2. Age
3. Extent of primary tumor
4. Distant metastases
5. Size
6. Blood vessel invasion
7. Multiple foci
8. Sex
9. Lymph node metastases (??)

From Degroot, L.J., et al.: Radiation-associated thyroid carcinoma, 1977, Grune & Stratton Inc.

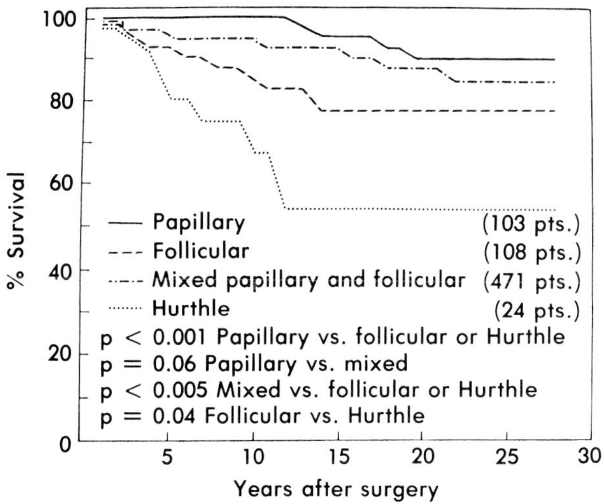

Fig. 58-8 Survival curves for patient with papillary (—), mixed papillary and follicular (-·-), follicular (----), and Hurthle cell (····) carcinomas. (From Samaan, N.A.: J. Clin. Endocrinol. Metabol. **56:**1131, 1983.)

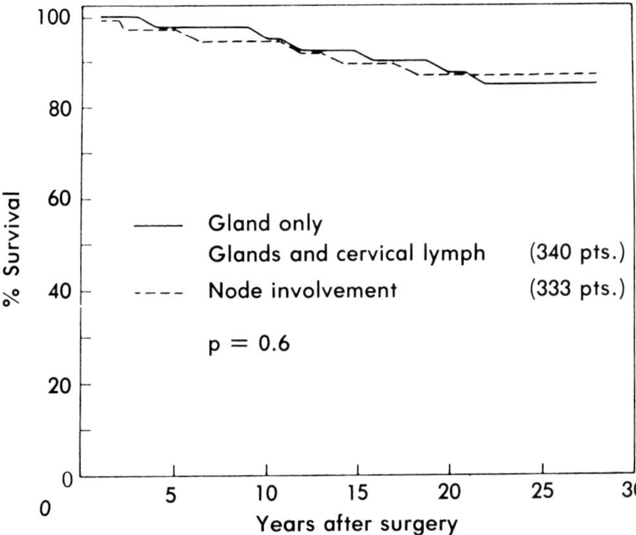

Fig. 58-9 Survival curves for patients with disease in the gland only (—) and those with disease in the gland and neck nodes (----). (From Samaan, N.A.: J. Clin. Endocrinol. Metabol. **56:**1131, 1983.)

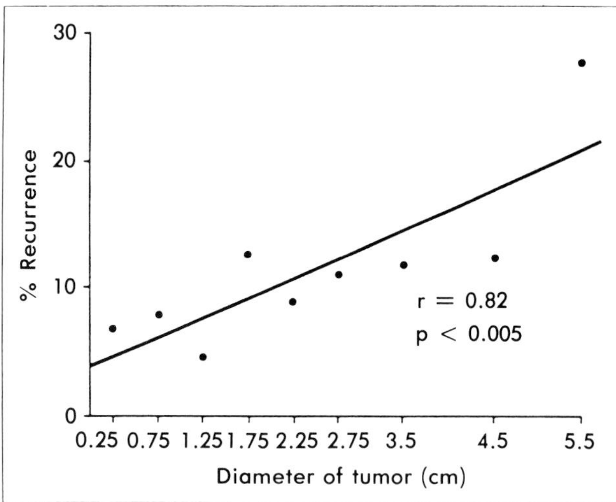

Fig. 58-10 The influence of primary tumor size on recurrence of papillary thyroid carcinoma, (From Mazzaferri, E.L., and Young, R.L.: Am. J. Med. **70:**511, 1981.)

illary carcinoma comprises the vast majority of thyroid carcinomas that occur under the age of 40. Follicular and anaplastic carcinomas become more common in the elderly. In addition, the prognosis is significantly worse for someone older than 40 years with differentiated thyroid carcinoma. In spite of a marked predominance of thyroid cancer in women, men appear to have a more somber prognosis.[47]

The size of the thyroid nodule plays a role both in its management and in the prognosis of the neoplasm. A cyst greater than 4 cm increases the risk of carcinoma. Mazzaferri[42,43] has shown an increase in mortality and recurrence for primary thyroid lesions greater than 2.5 cm, with negligible morbidity for lesions less than 1.5 cm. The significance of intraglandular and extraglandular invasion is even more important than the absolute size of the initial lesion. Minor intraglandular invasion is associated with a 9% mortality rate, whereas this quickly increases to 16% with major intraglandular disease.[9] With extraglandular disease, the mortality accelerates to 39%.[9]

One fascinating feature of differentiated thyroid carcinoma is the apparent lack of correlation between lymph node metastases and mortality. In Cady's study of 792 patients followed over a 40-year period, the mortality decreased with the increasing number of lymph nodes involved with metastatic disease.[9] No patient with 10 or more positive nodes died of thyroid carcinoma. Mazzaferri[43] has shown an inverse relationship between recurrence rates in papillary cancer and age of diagnosis, but a direct relationship between deaths and increasing age.[43] In addition, radical neck dissection has no effect on survival or recurrence.[43]

Approach To the Patient With a Thyroid Nodule

Several important historical points must be examined in order to arrive at an assessment of the patient's risk for thyroid carcinoma. A family history of medullary thyroid carcinoma necessitates a plan of action that would include a biochemical screening of the family, with basal and stimulated calcitonin levels, and a total thyroidectomy if the calcitonin levels were abnormal. Age and sex are also important factors to consider in the evaluation of a thyroid nodule. A solitary nodule in a male less than 20 years old has an increased frequency of carcinoma, approaching 50% in childhood. Mortality, however, is more directly associated with age over 40 years old.[9,43,47] A history of sudden pain in the nodule may result from a hemorrhage into a cyst and may be responsible for a sudden increase in the size of the nodule. Symptoms such as Horner's syndrome, hoarseness, or other signs of airway obstruction are worrisome, although objective signs of obstruction can frequently be caused by benign lesions. Evidence that the patient may have been iodine deficient would increase the incidence of both benign and malignant thyroid disease.

Controversy persists concerning the importance of radiation-associated thyroid carcinoma.[15] Radiation administration to animals increases the incidence of thyroid cancer, especially if there is a physiologic stimulus to TSH (i.e, iodine deficiency, thiourea administration, exogenous TSH administration). T_4 administration to animals before exposure to radiation results in a marked reduction of thyroid tumors. It remains unclear whether these data can be extrapolated to man.[15] Nonetheless, radiation appears to increase the incidence of both benign and malignant thyroid nodules in man. In an autopsy study[48] performed in Japan after the atomic bomb explosion, there was an increased incidence of occult thyroid carcinoma (28%) but no increase in mortality. In multiple studies of patients who received head and neck radiation during childhood, approximately 30% of the nodules were found to be carcinomatous vs. 15% to 20% of patients without a history of irradiation.[20] Latency from the time of irradiation to the development of carcinoma may be 5 to 35 years. Radiation greater than 2000 rad causes necrosis rather than carcinogenesis. The lowest amount of ^{131}I used to treat Graves' disease will deliver greater than 2000 rad to the thyroid and has not been associated with an increased incidence of thyroid carcinoma.

In spite of the laboratory and clinical evidence noted above for radiation-associated thyroid disease, it is important to point out the following:

1. A threshold for radiation-associated thyroid carcinoma has not been defined. Fifty rad may be sufficient to increase the risk.
2. More than 95% of the tumors that have been noted after radiation are well-differentiated papillary carcinomas that act biologically similar to nonirradiated papillary carcinomas. The vast majority of these tumors are less than 1 cm and would be considered occult carcinomas with no increase in mortality.

What action should be taken for a patient who presents with a normal thyroid examination and a history of irradiation as a child? The conservative approach of yearly thyroid palpations by an experienced physician has gained widespread acceptance. Routine radioisotope scans deliver small doses of radiation to the thyroid, and the results may be misleading. The administration of suppressive doses of T_4 would theoretically decrease the risk of benign or malignant thyroid nodules; however, several cases of radiation-associated thyroid carcinoma have been detected while on suppressive doses of T_4.[15] The thyroid nodule found in a gland that has been irradiated should be evaluated as any other thyroid nodule, in spite of the somewhat increased risk of carcinoma.

Evaluation of a Thyroid Nodule

Examination of the Thyroid Nodule. Inspection of the thyroid gland during swallowing allows the contour of the gland, its approximate size and the presence of one or more nodules to be seen. The patient should be positioned to take advantage of the light. Deep palpation of the gland both from a posterior and anterior direction allows assessment of the firmness and size of the nodule. Particular attention should be paid to examination of the lymph nodes, i.e., to their size, consistency, and mobility. Evidence of recurrent laryngeal nerve compression, Horner's syndrome, or growth in the nodule while on T_4 suppression raises the concern for a malignancy. Very few of the so-called classic signs of malignancy such as hardness of the nodule, its size, recent growth patterns, and associated airway obstructive symptoms have been shown to significantly increase the incidence of malignancy to warrant surgical intervention without further evaluation. Benign multinodular goiter may present with symptoms of obstruction, and calcification in benign adenomas is not rare.

After the thyroid nodule has been evaluated, the remainder of the examination should be directed toward the thyroid gland as a whole. A dominant nodule in an otherwise barely palpable or nonpalpable thyroid gland suggests a hyperfunctioning thyroid nodule and would greatly decrease the incidence of malignancy. A radioisotope scan would be helpful, and, if a hyperfunctioning nodule is found, an evaluation for hyperthyroidism should be initiated. The palpation of other smaller nodules in the gland with a dominant nodule would suggest the possibility of a multinodular goiter and also significantly decrease the incidence of malignancy. On the other hand, the palpation of a solitary nodule in an otherwise normal gland would raise the concern for malignancy.

A Biochemical Evaluation of Thyroid Nodules. A thyroid profile consisting of a blood T_4 level and an assessment of T_4 binding capacity, such as a T_3 RU, should be performed on all patients with nodules to assure that they are euthyroid. Laboratory values consistent with either hypothyroidism or hyperthyroidism would obviously require further evaluation. Massive infiltration by an undifferentiated carcinoma may cause enough destruction of the thyroid gland to precipitate hypothyroidism. Thyroid carcinoma coexisting with hyperthyroidism has been reported in the last few years. The thyroid carcinoma invariably is found in an area of hypofunction in an otherwise hyperfunctioning gland. Toxic adenomas may present with T_3 toxicosis in the face of normal T_4 levels.

Calcitonin is an exquisitely sensitive biochemical marker in the blood for medullary carcinoma of the thyroid.[11,51] Early diagnosis of MCT may be made by stimulating calcitonin secretion either with the use of pentagastrin or calcium.[31,49] These studies are routinely performed in children of families with a history of multiple endocrine neoplasia syndromes or medullary thyroid carcinoma. Calcitonin and CEA levels are also useful for early diagnosis of recurrence after surgery for MCT. The rarity of this histologic type of carcinoma makes routine screening of patients with thyroid nodules not cost effective.

Thyroglobulin is a large glycoprotein that is the principal iodoprotein of the thyroid gland. Sensitive RIAs have been able to detect elevated serum thyroglobulin levels in a variety of thyroid diseases. Unfortunately, the levels of this globulin are similarly elevated in benign and malignant diseases, making measurement of this protein not a useful diagnostic tool. Preliminary studies, however, suggest the measurement of thyroglobulin levels as a marker for recurrent thyroid carcinoma may be worthwhile.[3,6]

Thyroid Imaging. Multiple techniques for imaging the thyroid have been used in the past in an attempt to differentiate normal from abnormal thyroid tissue.[1] The limit of resolution of these techniques is approximately 1 to 1.5 cm. It is important to obtain lateral or oblique views, since small nonfunctioning nodules may be obscured by overlying functioning tissue. The most commonly used radioisotope is ^{99M}Tc-pertechnetate. This radioisotope is trapped in the thyroid gland, like iodine, but is not organified. The major advantages of technetium vs. other isotopes are a short half-life (6 hours) and a relatively low amount of radiation delivered to the thyroid. ^{131}I is no longer used in routine imaging of the thyroid because of its long half-life (8 days) and the relatively high degree of radiation exposure. On the other hand, ^{123}I has a particularly short half-life and delivers approximately 1% of the radiation dose that ^{131}I does. The disadvantages of ^{123}I are its expense and short shelf life.

The functional status of thyroid nodules judged by imaging techniques is only marginally helpful in making a clinical decision about the malignant potential of a given thyroid nodule. Of approximately 5300 patients included in 22 different studies, 85% of the nodules were nonfunctioning by radioiodine scan, and an additional 10% were "warm."[1,2] Sixteen percent of the cold nodules and 9% of the warm nodules were found to be malignant at operation, in contrast to hyperfunctioning nodules which were rarely malignant (Table 58-4). Therefore, on the basis of thyroid imaging alone, between 85 and 95% of patients with thyroid nodules would have been recommended for surgery.

Many other radioisotopes have been used in an attempt to improve the false-positive and false-negative results encountered with technetium. At this time, none has been shown to be superior to standard imaging techniques.

Ultrasound Examination of the Thyroid. Ultrasound examination of the thyroid is used to distinguish between solid and cystic lesions. The incidence of malignancy is believed to be markedly decreased in purely cystic lesions. In a total of 16 different studies, approximately 1200 patients had ultrasonographic examination before surgery.[1,2] Approximately 70% of patients had solid lesions on ultrasound, and an additional 12% had mixed solid-cystic lesions. Twenty-one percent of the solid lesions and 12% of the mixed lesions were found to be carcinomatous at operation. In contrast, only cystic lesions greater than 4 cm in diameter had a significant incidence of carcinoma.

Surgical evaluation on the basis of either thyroid imaging or ultrasound examination alone or in combination results in a high surgical rate, a low incidence of malignancy found at surgery, and a small number of thyroid carcinomas that would not have been removed on the basis of either technique.

Thyroid Suppression Therapy. In spite of the fact that thyroid suppressive therapy has been available for more than 100 years, its usefulness in differentiating benign from malignant nodules remains controversial. Benign thyroid adenomas and well-differentiated thyroid cancers have TSH receptors, and hypofunctioning nodules can be reduced in size by thyroid suppressive therapy (0.2-0.3 mg of levothyroxine per day). Unfortunately, many benign lesions continue to grow or do not decrease in size after administration of large doses of thyroid suppressive therapy.[7] Occasionally a low-grade thyroid carcinoma may decrease in size for a period of time following suppressive therapy. In spite of these drawbacks, thyroid suppressive therapy continues to be commonly used according to the following rationale: (1) A nodule that responds to thyroid suppressive medication by decreasing in size 50% or more is unlikely to be a carcinoma; (2) well-differentiated tumors are slow growing, and a 3- to 6-month period of observation is unlikely to be placing the patient at undue risk; (3) if the patient has an undifferentiated carcinoma, the morbidity and mortality of this disease is high, regardless of therapy. Although somewhat supplanted by fine-needle aspiration, thyroid suppressive therapy remains a valuable diagnostic and therapeutic adjunct.

Fine-Needle Aspiration of the Thyroid. Diagnostic thyroid gland puncture has been attempted since the early 1920s. Over the years several investigators have used 16- and 18-gauge needles in an attempt to make a diagnosis of thyroid disease from direct visualization of thyroid tissue. Because of complications, primarily bleeding, with such large needles, thyroid puncture as a standard technique failed to enjoy any substantial popularity. In 1952 the technique of fine-needle aspiration and cytologic evaluation was first described.[37] Although initially received with mixed favor, this technique is now commonly used in the United States (Figs. 58-11 to 58-13).

In experienced hands fine-needle aspiration is a simple technique without significant morbidity and with a high diagnostic yield.[26,44,45] An experienced aspirator and, more importantly, an experienced and interested cytopathologist are critical ingredients in obtaining diagnostic specimens. Experienced cytopathologists are now able to differentiate many benign and malignant lesions, and the number of false-negatives has decreased sharply in relation to the number of aspiration procedures being performed.

Needle biopsy of the thyroid has been divided into fine-needle aspiration using needle gauges between 20 and 25, large-needle biopsy using 16- and 18-gauge needles, and core needle biopsies using either a Vim-Silverman or a Trucut needle. The accuracy of the three techniques is virtually identical, and fine-needle aspiration is more avail-

Table 58-4 **RESULTS OF RADIOIODINE SCANS OF THYROID NODULES**

	Nonfunctioning		Hypofunctioning/Normal		Hyperfunctioning		Total	
	No. of cases (no. operated)	No. malignant	No. of cases (no. operated)	No. malignant	No. of cases (no. operated)	No. malignant	No. of cases (no. operated)	No. malignant
All Patients Sent to Surgery—Totals of 22 Separate Studies								
Subtotal	4457	708 (16%)	554	49 (9%)	283	10 (4%)	5294	767 (14%)

(From Ashcraft, M.W., and VanHerle, A.J.: Head Neck Surg. **3**:299, 1981.)

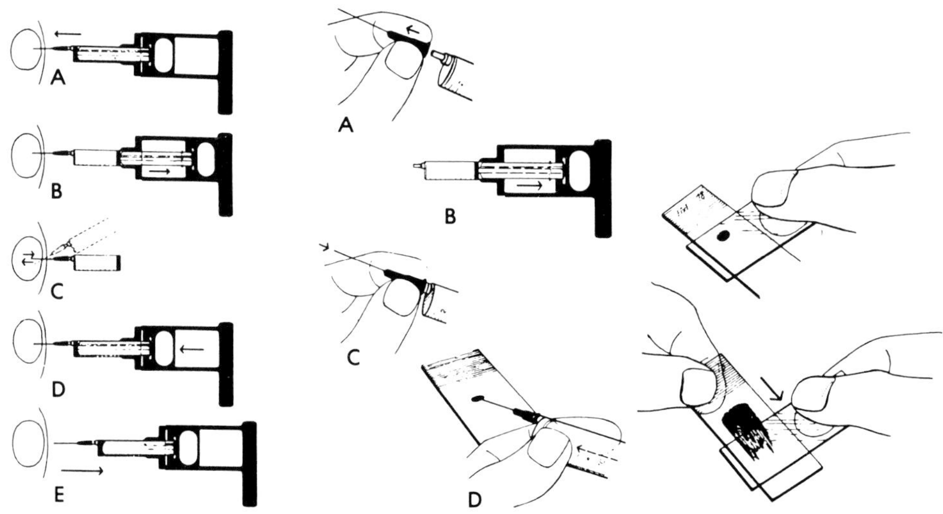

Fig. 58-11 Illustrations of technique for fine-needle aspiration biopsy of the thyroid. (From Lowhagen, T., et al.: Surg. Clin. North Am. **59**:1, 1979.)

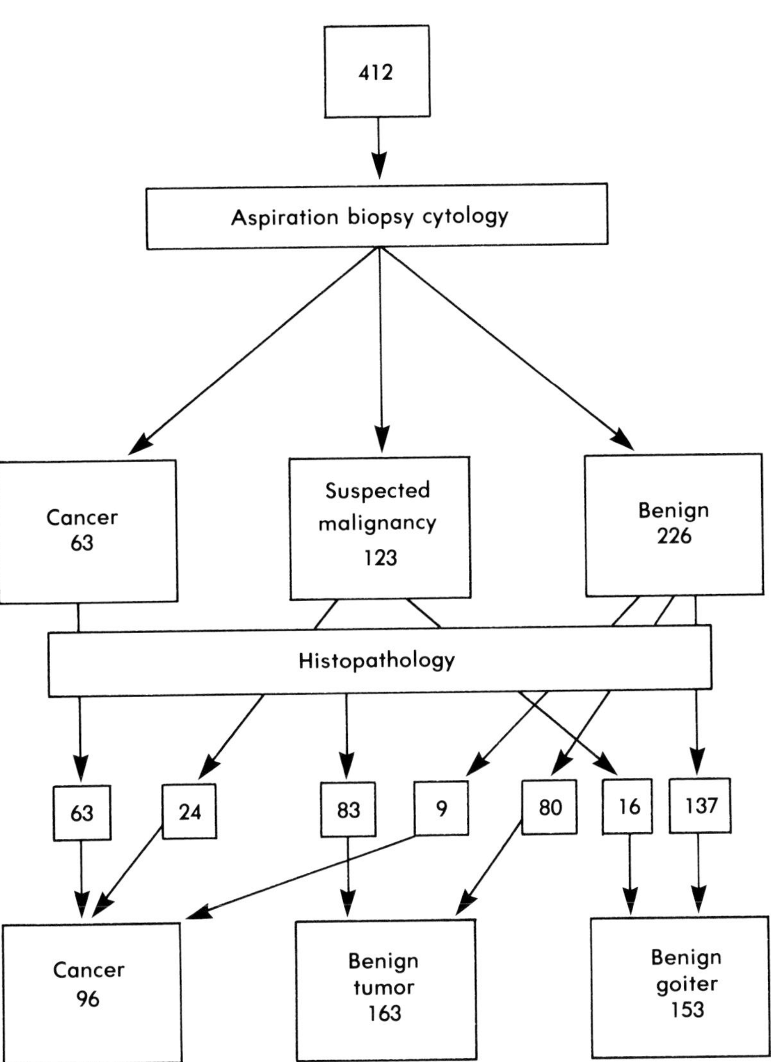

Fig. 58-12 Accuracy of diagnosis by fine-needle aspiration biopsy of the thyroid as compared with definitive histopathologic diagnosis. (From Lowhagen, T., et al.: Surg. Clin. North Am. **59:**8, 1979.)

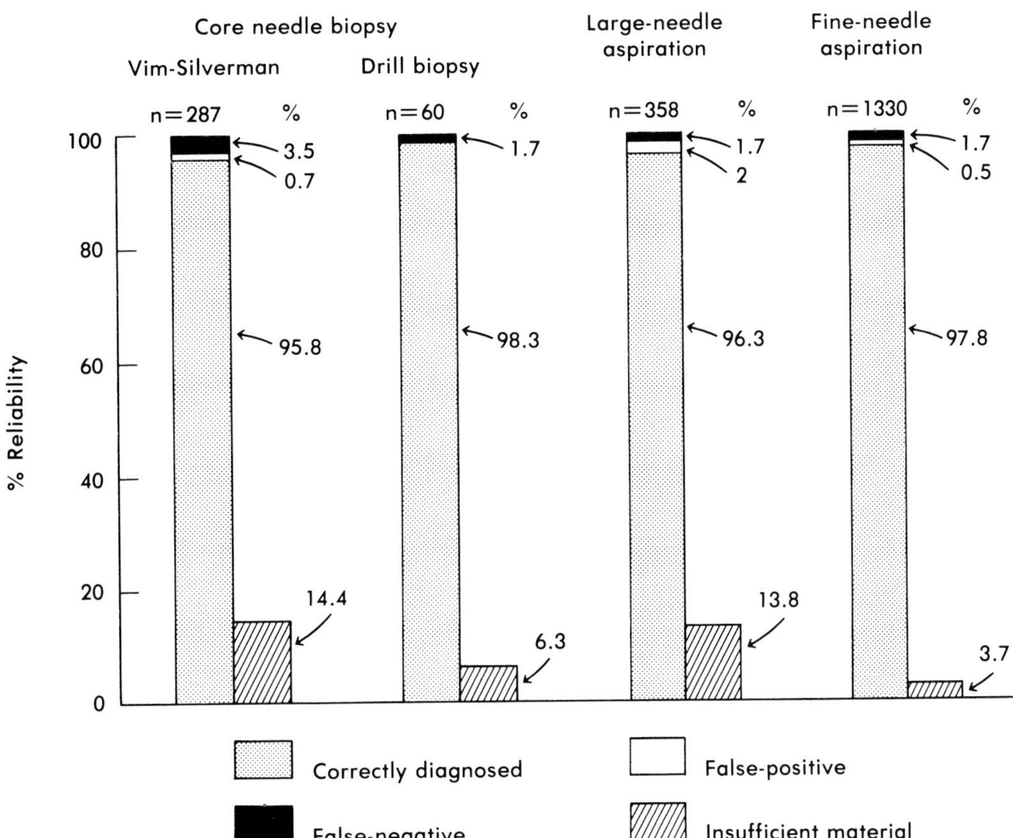

Fig. 58-13 Needle biopsy: reliability of various techniques. Fine-needle aspiration has a smaller number of insufficient sampling and is virtually without complications. (From Ashcraft, M.W., and VanHerle, A.J.: Head Neck Surg. **3:**297, 1981.)

able, easier, and has fewer complications than the other two techniques. Complementary information may be obtained from all three techniques.

Several recent monographs illustrate the technique of fine-needle aspiration in detail.[26,44,45] Complications are extremely rare and include minor hematomas and transient pain. Spread of tumor by needle biopsy is extremely unusual. If the nodule is fluid filled, it may be aspirated virtually completely and centrifuged for cytologic evaluation. A clear, watery fluid may be indicative of a parathyroid cyst and should be sent for parathormone levels. If the fluid is bloody, it should be discarded, since this is an uninterpretable specimen. Bloody aspirates may be indicative of degenerating thyroid carcinomas, and a biopsy on the advancing edge of the lesion may be more helpful in this circumstance. A fine-needle aspiration biopsy should be performed on the remnant after the cyst is evacuated. Attention must be paid to making the slide relatively thin and as bloodless as possible. If possible, a cytologist may help the aspirator make the slides and quickly review them in order to ensure a satisfactory specimen. If these details are followed, the patient may avoid having to return for a repeat aspiration, and a specific diagnosis at the time of aspiration will generally result.

Aspiration has proven very useful in diagnosing papillary carcinoma and Hashimoto's thyroiditis. Lymphoma may coexist with Hashimoto's thyroiditis and should be considered in a grossly abnormal gland. The technique of fine-needle aspiration has been particularly useful in the search for metastatic disease to the thyroid, making it possible to avoid unnecessary surgical procedures. It is not possible, however, to differentiate cellular adenomas (e.g., Hurthle cell, follicular cell) from carcinomas by cytologic examination.

Summary of Preoperative Approach to the Thyroid Nodule[1,2] (Fig. 58-14)

Physiologically a diseased portion of the thyroid will have disturbed function when compared to normal tissue. Radioisotope imaging techniques attempt to take advantage of this functional difference. Unfortunately, many benign disorders of the thyroid interfere with effective iodine uptake, and, conversely, well-differentiated follicular carcinoma may have near normal function. Thus the attempt to diagnose thyroid disease on the basis of functional status (e.g., technetium trapping, radioiodine organification) has not been successful. In spite of advances in ultrasonography, the impact of this modality on the management of thyroid nodules has not been substantive. Fine-needle aspiration biopsy of the thyroid is a technically simple, cost-effective procedure which, although not ideal, offers a higher sensitivity and specificity diagnostically than other available studies, short of surgical exploration.

On the basis of these considerations, after clinical evaluation of the patient a fine-needle aspiration should be the initial study. If an adequate sample showing benign cytology is obtained, the patient should be placed on thyroid suppressive therapy (levothyroxine 0.15 to 0.2 mg daily) unless there is overriding clinical concern of a malignancy. During suppressive therapy the patient should be followed for any change in the nodule. Shrinkage of the nodule by more than 50% is reassuring. No change or increase in nodule size on T_4 suppression should prompt a repeat biopsy or surgical intervention. Cellular aspirates (i.e., follicular adenoma, Hurthle cell adenoma) are frequently reported as suspicious, atypical, or indeterminant. Because of the inherent inability to differentiate cellular adenomas from carcinomas, such interpretations are not considered

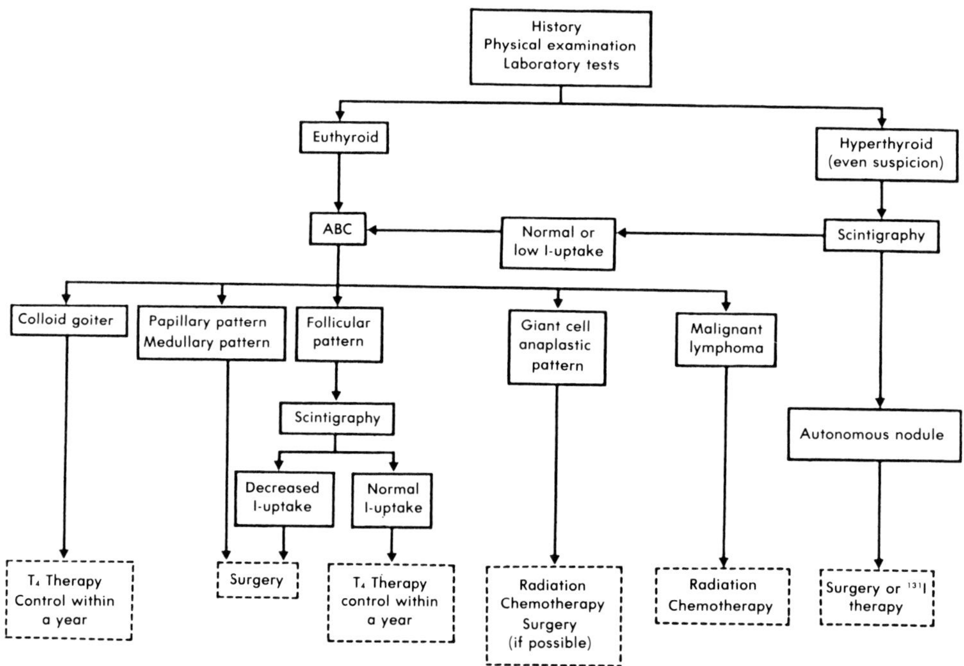

Fig. 58-14 Management of flowchart in the case of a solitary thyroid nodule. *ABC*, aspiration biopsy cytology. (From Kaplan, E.L., editor: Surgery of the thyroid and parathyroid glands, New York, 1983, Churchill Livingstone.)

false-positives. A radioiotope scan may help in differentiating the hyperfunctioning adenoma that has a negligible malignancy rate from the hypofunctioning cellular nodule. Surgery is indicated in a cold cellular nodule, especially if it does not respond to thyroid suppressive therapy.

In the case of thyroid cysts, the cyst should be drained as completely as possible with a larger needle (18 to 20-gauge). A fine-needle aspiration biopsy of the remaining remnant should then be sent for cytologic examination. Recurrent cysts may require surgery. Thyroid suppressive therapy should be given for benign cytology.

At the Mayo Clinic, the use of fine-needle aspiration has cut medical costs by 25%, decreased the percentage of patients referred for thyroid surgery, and increased the likelihood of diagnosing a malignancy at surgery from 14% to 29%. No adverse consequences of any possible missed malignancies have been reported.[24b]

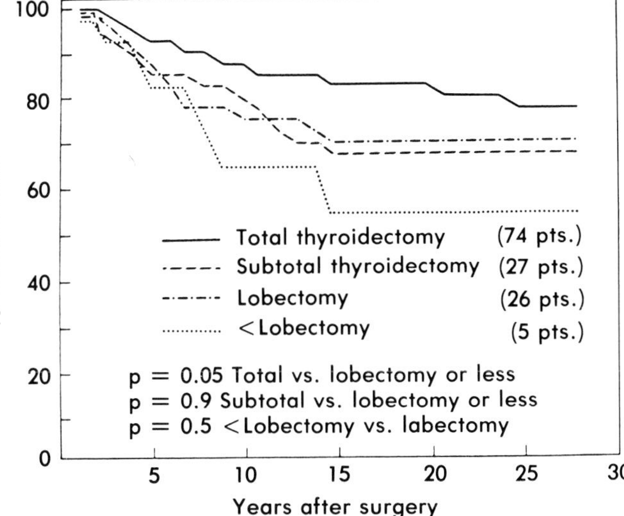

Fig. 58-15 Disease-free intervals of patients who had total thyroidectomy (—), subtotal thyroidectomy (----), lobectomy (-·-·-), and less than a lobectomy (····). (From Samaan, N.A.: J. Clin. Endocrinol. Metabol. **56:**1131, 1983.)

Surgical Treatment of Thyroid Nodules Suspected of Having Cancer (Figs. 58-15 and 58-16)

The extent of surgery required to cure thyroid cancer is unknown. Treatment should be based on knowledge of the biologic behavior of the tumor. All patients with suspicious nodules should be placed on lifelong thyroid hormone following surgery to suppress any new nodular growth. Therefore the surgical procedure is limited by the risks of hypoparathyroidism and laryngeal nerve damage, and not by a concern for hypothyroidism. For this reason a minimal operation would include a lobectomy, isthmusectomy, and possibly a partial contralateral lobectomy. Neither fine-needle aspiration nor frozen section can adequately differentiate follicular adenoma from follicular carcinoma. A more complete initial operation may avoid subsequent surgeries. Occult papillary carcinoma is occasionally found incidentally after a surgical procedure for a benign lesion. Given the low mortality of occult carcinoma, a subtotal thyroidectomy is usually adequate.

Head and neck irradiation in childhood increases the risk of multicentric tumors. A physiologic approach to this circumstance would include removal of all thyroid tissue to prevent recurrence. However, the vast majority of these tumors are occult papillary carcinomas of low malignant potential and should be treated with conservative surgery. Thus subtotal thyroidectomy (lobectomy, isthmusectomy, and possibly contralateral partial lobectomy) is adequate for a benign lesion in a previously irradiated thyroid.

Papillary thyroid carcinomas spread intraglandulary

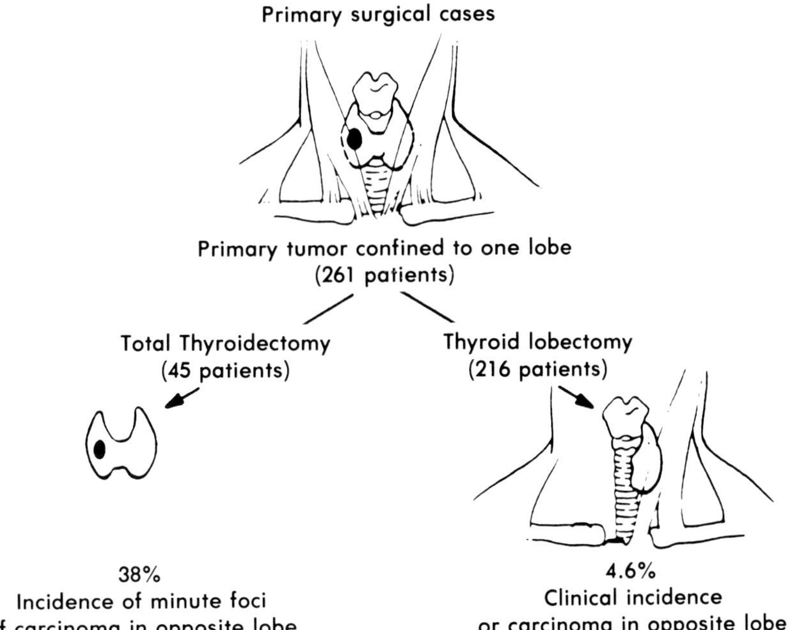

Fig. 58-16 Incidence of carcinoma in the opposite lobe in papillary carcinoma of the thyroid. (From Tollefson, H.R., et al.: Am. J. Surg. **124:**472, 1972.)

through the lymphatics. Therapy ideally should be directed at removing all involved and potentially involved thyroid tissue in order to prevent recurrences[55] and prepare the patient for radioiodine therapy if necessary. Total thyroidectomy, however, is a more technically difficult operation and associated with a complication rate that exceeds 10% in some series.[9,43] For this reason, near total thyroidectomy with the posterior capsule of the contralateral lobe left intact, associated with radioiodine ablation of the thyroid remnant, is recommended in patients believed to be at high risk for thyroid cancer. Several large retrospective studies[42,47] suggest that histologic type in decreasing order of aggressiveness—Hurthle cell carcinoma, follicular carcinoma, mixed papillary follicular, and pure papillary—age over 40 at diagnosis, male sex, extent of invasion, and size (greater than 2.5 cm), forebode a poorer prognosis. Total or near total thyroidectomy with radioiodine ablation is justified in this group and appears to prolong survival.[4,5,43,47,48] Lymph node metastases do not affect survival, and radical neck dissection is usually not indicated. Grossly involved nodal tissue can be removed. The current practice of autotransplantation of the parathyroid glands may dramatically decrease the incidence of permanent hypoparathyroidism. Papillary carcinomas 1.5 cm or less have a similar natural history as occult carcinoma, and subtotal thyroidectomy is justifiable.[42,43]

Follicular carcinoma spreads hematogenously to the lungs, bone, and liver; and the prognosis is proportional to the degree of invasion. Since follicular carcinoma is not multifocal, the rationale for complete thyroidectomy is predicted on preparing the patient for possible radioiodine therapy to treat metastases rather than a fear of local recurrence. A wide excision of thyroid tissue will decrease the necessary dose of radioiodine.

Medullary thyroid carcinoma is an aggressive multicentric tumor that spreads commonly to nodes. Early detection and an aggressive surgical approach, including total thyroidectomy and node dissection, improve the prognosis.

Anaplastic carcinoma is a rapidly lethal tumor of the elderly. It is hoped that aggressive therapy of well-differentiated cancers will decrease any tendency for anaplastic transformation. A multidisciplinary approach has been associated with remissions. Radical surgery increases morbidity without improving survival.

Radioiodine Therapy

Ablation of Thyroid Remnant

Routine radioiodine ablation of normal thyroid tissue following near-total thyroidectomy (Fig. 58-17) remains controversial.[5,50] Physiologically it seems appropriate to complete the surgical ablation of the thyroid with ^{131}I to prevent local recurrence and prepare the patient for diagnostic or therapeutic radioiodine studies. Thyroid remnant tissue will avidly concentrate ^{131}I as compared to thyroid carcinoma and thus prevent detection of nodal, pulmonary, or distant disease. However, in order to justify radioiodine ablation, the benefits must be balanced against the rare but present risks of leukemia (less than 1%) and possibly anaplastic transformation. Combined experience from several major centers suggest a decreased recurrence and an improved survival rate when near total thyroidectomy and

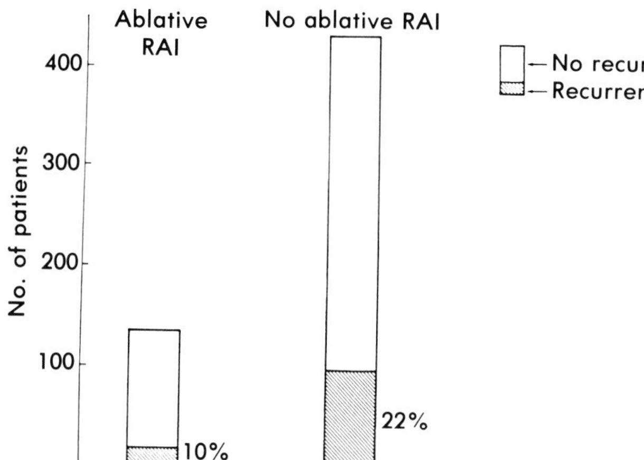

Fig. 58-17 Comparison of recurrence rates between ablative and nonablative ^{131}I therapy. Patients with no ablation had a higher recurrence rate. (From Samaan, N.A., et al.: J. Clin. Endocrinol. Metabol. **56:**131, 1983.)

^{131}I ablation are used adjunctively.[5,35,42,43,47] It is difficult to demonstrate a beneficial effect of ^{131}I on the extremely low mortality from papillary carcinomas in young patients, especially in tumors 1.5 cm or smaller. Radioiodine should not be given unless there is ^{131}I uptake present postoperatively in the thyroid bed, in the nodes, or distantly.

Treatment of Residual Disease (Fig. 58-18)

Radioiodine therapy is indicated for all patients with well-differentiated thyroid cancer suspected of haboring residual disease. Following surgery, thyroid hormone replacement is initially withheld; and 6 weeks after a total or near total thyroidectomy, an ^{131}I scan is performed with 10 mCi of ^{131}I. A TSH level is performed to confirm the hypothyroid state. ^{131}I is administered in an attempt to deliver at least 30,000 rad to the thyroid remnant and 8000 rad to the metastases.[41] Small remnants may be treated with a standard 30-50 mCi ^{131}I dose, but repeat treatment may be necessary.[16] Postradioiodine therapy, lifelong thyroid suppression therapy (0.2 to 0.4 mg of levothyroxine daily) should be administered to produce mild chemical hyperthyroidism with undetectable TSH levels. A lack of TSH response to TRF ensures complete suppression.

Follow-up of Established Thyroid Cancer

A follow-up ^{131}I scan is performed 1 year after therapy and, if negative, every 3 to 5 years (see boxed material on p. 977). Thyroxine is discontinued, and the patient is begun on T_3 50 to 100 μg daily for 2 weeks. All thyroid hormone is then discontinued, and the patient becomes acutely biochemically and clinically hypothyroid over the following 2 weeks. The clinical manifestations are significantly more severe than in spontaneous hypothyroidism. The switch from T_4 (half-life 7 to 10 days) to T_3 (half-life 24 hours) helps to shorten the patient's discomfort. A TSH level is performed to ensure a hypothyroid state before the ^{131}I scan. Any ^{131}I uptake is treated as previously described by dosimetry. T_4 is reinstituted after radioiodine treatment.

Radioiodine can successfully treat metastases to the

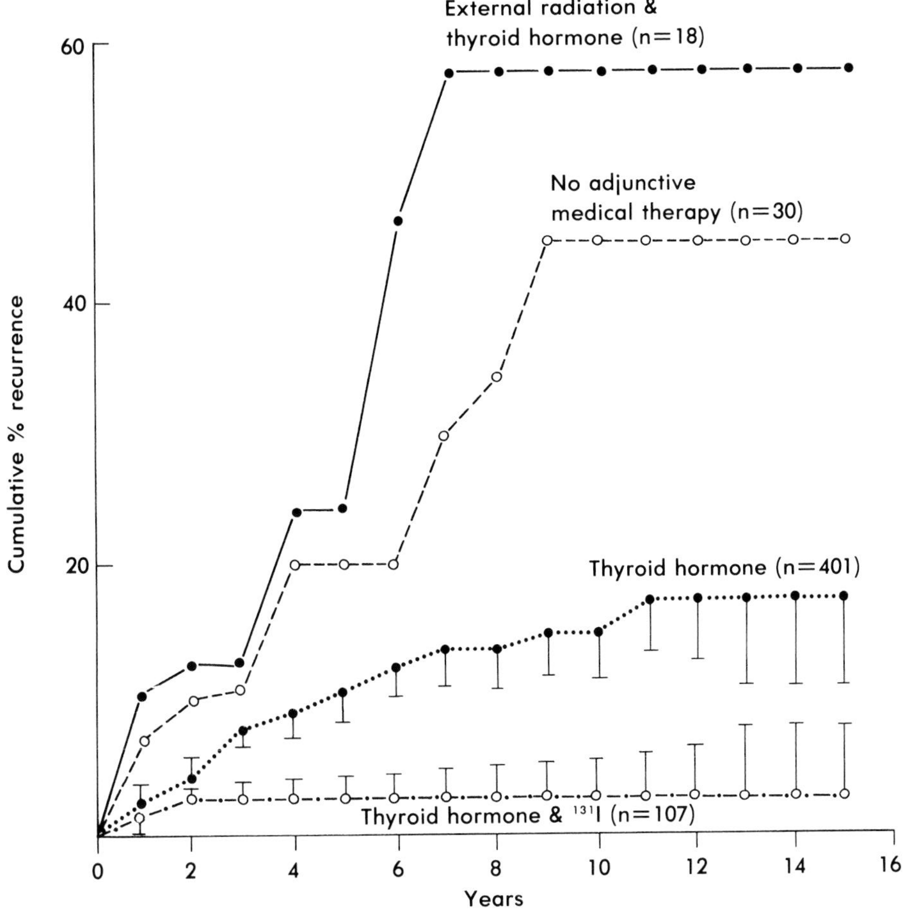

Fig. 58-18 The influence of mode of therapy on the rate of postoperative recurrence in patients with papillary thyroid carcinoma. (From Mazzaferri, E.L., et al.: Medicine **56:**171, 1977.)

"IDEAL" TREATMENT PROTOCOL OF UNIVERSITY OF MICHIGAN*

1. Thyroidectomy performed within 1 yr after a suspicious nodule has been detected.
2. Lobectomy with frozen section, and completion of total thyroidectomy within 6 months.
3. Withholding of thyroid hormones for 6 weeks before ^{131}I scan of the neck is performed.
4. Scintiscan performed within 3 months after the thyroidectomy.
5. Treatment with ^{131}I for residual ^{131}I uptake.
   a. Not less than 100 mCi for uptake in the thyroidal bed.
   b. Not less than 150 mCi for uptake in the cervical nodes.
   c. Not less than 175 mCi for distant metastases.
6. T_4 given between follow-up examinations.
7. Reexamination of the patient within 1 year after treatment with ^{131}I.
8. Reexamination of patient at 3 years if the 1-year scan is negative.

From Beierwaltes, W.H., et al.: J. Nucl. Med. **23:**562, 1982, The Society of Nuclear Medicine, Inc.

*Conformity with at least half of the above noted procedures correlated with improved survival.

nodes and lungs in almost all young patients with papillary carcinoma, in approximately 60% of young patients with follicular carcinoma, but in less than 50% of older patients with differentiated thyroid cancer.[35] Radioiodine significantly improves survival rates in patients with thyroid carcinoma outside of the neck.

Occasionally, a thyroid carcinoma that previously concentrated ^{131}I loses this capacity, and surgical removal of gross thyroid disease may be necessary. Inability to concentrate ^{131}I suggests a less differentiated tumor and forbodes a poor prognosis.

Medullary thyroid carcinoma is not TSH dependent and does not concentrate ^{131}I. However, ^{131}I has been given in an attempt to deliver a tumoricidal dose of radiation to the thyroid bed. Further evaluation of this therapy is necessary.

Complications from ^{131}I therapy are unusual if doses are appropriately spaced to allow for bone marrow recovery.[4,5] The incidence of leukemia is less than 1%, and pulmonary fibrosis is not seen when the recommended single-dose treatment is less than 200 mCi. There is a small but increased incidence of anaplastic transformation and second malignancies (especially breast) in patients with thyroid cancer, but there is no apparent influence of ^{131}I on these events. There is no increase in birth defects or infertility in young girls who have received ^{131}I therapy.

^{131}I scanning, although useful for follow-up, is uncomfortable to the patient and may be tumor promoting. Thyroglobulin levels have been known to correlate with thyroid cancer disease activity and is a possible adjunctive marker.[3,6] The test is limited by the fact that a fair percentage of patients have significant antibodies to thyroglobulin which interferes with the present assay. A biochemical marker that can be obtained while the patient is on T_4 therapy would greatly facilitate follow-up.

COMPLICATIONS ASSOCIATED WITH THYROID SURGERY

As indicated in the preceding sections of this chapter, operations on the thyroid gland are frequently necessary to manage the underlying pathophysiology. As is true with any operation, the benefits to be derived from a given surgical procedure must be balanced against the potential risks. For this reason, an understanding of the morbidity and mortality associated with thyroid surgery must be appreciated before recommending surgery to a patient. Although a wide variety of complications have been reported following thyroid surgery, the following discussion attests to the safety of operations on the thyroid gland when they are accomplished by an experienced surgeon.

Mortality

In 1917 Theodor Kocher reported a mortality of less than 0.5% after 5000 thyroidectomies and won the Nobel prize. Until that time, thyroid surgery was considered extremely hazardous with mortality rates in excess of 40%. Major advances in our understanding of thyroid pathophysiology, preoperative preparation of the hyperthyroid patients, and improvements in surgical and anesthetic techniques have made thyroid surgery one of the safest surgical procedures.[17,19,21] Published series of 1000 thyroidectomies without a mortality are not unusual. In Foster's extensive review [22] of 24,108 thyroidectomies (one third of all thyroidectomies performed in the United States in 1970), the overall mortality was 0.3%, with no deaths in patients less than 40 years of age with nontoxic goiters. Major factors affecting mortality were age, indication for thyroidectomy, and extent of surgery. The mortality for nontoxic goiters was 0.02% in patients less than 50 years of age, but rose to 0.66% in elderly patients (70 years or older). In spite of increased attention to preoperative preparation of patients with diffuse toxic goiters, mortality was five times greater than for nontoxic benign goiters. Total or near-total thyroidectomy comprised approximately 10% of the operations but carried a higher morbidity and mortality. Patients with malignant goiters had more extensive surgical procedures (one third treated by total thyroidectomy) and an increased morbidity and mortality (1.2%). However, in 766 patients less than 40 years old with malignant goiters, the in-hospital mortality rate was zero.[22]

Morbidity

Operations on the highly vascular, enlarged thyroid surrounded by vital structures may appear formidable to a surgical house officer, but careful attention to surgical technique has produced an exemplary tract record in terms of complications in many centers. Table 58-5 is a compilation of six recently published studies. Postoperative wound infections are distinctly unusual, and prophylactic antibiotics are generally considered unnecessary when operations on the thyroid gland are to be performed. The types of complications that may occur with thyroid surgery are discussed in the following paragraphs.

Hemorrhage

Postoperative hemorrhage and the danger of rapid asphyxiation are the most dramatic complications of thyroid surgery. Attention to hemostasis during surgery and close

Table 58-5 **SUMMARY OF SIX RECENTLY PUBLISHED STUDIES ON COMPLICATIONS OF THYROIDECTOMY***

Operation/Location (Year Published)	No. of Mortality (Operations)	Recurrent laryngeal Nerve Damage (%)	Permanent Hypoparathyroidism (%)	Hypothyroidism (%)	Recurrent Hyperthyroidism (%)
Subtotal thyroidectomy/ (Rochester, Minn., 1981)[18]	0 (100)	3	1	75	1
Subtotal thyroidectomy/ (Dublin, 1983)[52]	0 (306)	3.6	2.9	20.5	15.6
Subtotal thyroidectomy/ (Philadelphia, Penn., 1984)[38]	0 (83)	0	0	27%	6
Partial, subtotal, total thyroidectomy (Toronto 1983)[21]	0 (117)	3.2	0	NR†	NR
Subtotal, total thyroidectomy (Louisville, Ky., 1983)[39]	0.7% (407)	0.6	0.9	15.8%	NR
Total thyroidectomy (Nashville, Tenn., 1983)[32]	0 (234)	0.8	2.8	—	—

*Complications decreased to 0.8% after adoption of Thomson's technique of total thyroidectomy.
†NR, Not reported.

observation of a minimally dressed or undressed wound in the recovery room and the initial 8 postoperative hours are crucial to avoid this complication. Local warm compresses may be sufficient for a small hematoma or edema of the wound, but swelling of the neck, stridor, and hypoxia require prompt attention, with opening of the skin incision and strap muscles at the bedside, if necessary. Equipment for immediate endotracheal intubation and tracheostomy should be close by for all patients following thyroidectomy. An overly dressed neck wound, with or without drains, will not prevent postoperative hemorrhage and may delay its recognition, resulting in catastrophic hypoxic brain damage or death. Several authorities recommend placing the patient in a 30-degree head-down position coincident with tracheal stimulation before wound closure and extubation.[17,19] This maneuver will increase pressure and unmask any poorly sutured vessels.

Nerve Damage

Injury to the laryngeal nerves is closely related to the experience of the surgeon performing the operation and the extent of surgery. Injury to the recurrent laryngeal nerve is more common and more easily recognized than injury to the external branch of the superior laryngeal nerve. Indirect laryngoscopy before surgery, identification of the nerves throughout their course, and repeat indirect laryngoscopy after surgery results in a complication rate of less than 1% in surgery for benign disease. Mechanical disturbance of the nerve may result in transient, but rarely permanent, vocal cord paralysis. Delayed vocal cord dysfunction can occur up to 1 week following surgery but is usually transient. Aberrant left recurrent nerves are extremely rare, but 15% of the right recurrent nerves may be aberrant, again indicating the need for careful dissection. The superior laryngeal nerve may be injured during ligation of vessels of the upper pole of the thyroid.

Although unilateral paralysis of the recurrent laryngeal nerve can be easily detected by laryngoscopy and the patient's hoarseness, techniques to uncover postoperative superior laryngeal nerve damage are not routinely performed; and, except for patients who depend on their voice professionally, the symptoms may be quite subtle. On the other hand, bilateral recurrent nerve injury is a rare but life-threatening complication acutely evident after removal of the endotracheal tube and requiring emergency reintubation or tracheostomy.

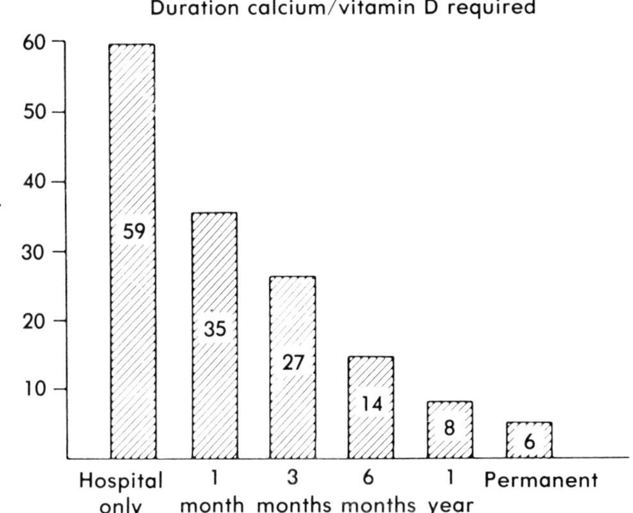

Fig. 58-19 Duration that calcium or vitamin D supplements were required to maintain normocalcemia after total thyroidectomy. (From Jacobs, J. K., et al.: Ann. Surg. **197**:542, 1983.)

Hypoparathyroidism

The parathyroid glands are particularly susceptible to ischemic or mechanical injury and inadvertent or unavoidable removal, depending on the extent of thyroid surgery performed. Transient or subclinical hypoparathyroidism may be substantially more common than the reported rate of permanent hypoparathyroidism (Fig. 58-19). A complication rate of 1% or less after subtotal thyroidectomy may rise quickly to more than 10% with near-total or total thyroidectomy. Meticulous dissection and identification of all four glands and their blood supply and preservation of the posterior capsule of the thyroid during total thyroidectomy should keep the complication rate to less than 5% even in the more extensive procedures. Preservation and autotransplantation of the parathyroids should reduce this complication rate further in patients requiring en bloc resection for advanced thyroid neoplasms.[36]

Symptoms of hypocalcemia may appear 1 to 7 days after surgery and include circumoral and acral parathesias, carpopedal spasm, laryngeal stridor, and, in extreme untreated cases, convulsions. Daily serum calcium determinations and frequent examination of the patient for the appearance of Chvostek's and Trousseau's signs are essential for early recognition of hypocalcemia. Since a small percentage of normal subjects will exhibit a positive Chvostek sign, it is important to verify a negative sign before surgery to accurately recognize a change after surgery.

Significant hypocalcemia resulting in the symptoms noted in the boxed material below should be treated promptly with intravenous calcium gluconate. Mild decreases in serum calcium (approximately 8 mg/100 ml) should be observed closely without therapy, in the hope that hypocalcemia will stimulate parathormone (PTH) secretion in the remaining glands. One ampule of calcium gluconate (10 ml of a 10% solution) can be given intravenously over several minutes for symptomatic hypocalcemia. A continuous intravenous infusion of calcium (20 to 40 ml of 10% calcium gluconate per liter) may be titrated to keep the serum calcium in the low normal range

INDICATIONS FOR CALCIUM OR VITAMIN D SUPPLEMENTATION AFTER THYROIDECTOMY

Severe circumoral or acral paresthesias
Carpopedal spasm
Electrocardiogram abnormalities
Calcium less than 7.5 mg/100 ml
Laryngeal stridor
Convulsions

and the patient comfortable until oral therapy can be started.

The symptoms of hypocalcemia are closely related to the level of ionized calcium. Serum protein abnormalities, particularly albumin, will affect the level of ionized calcium. A simple estimate of ionized calcium can be made by noting approximately a 1 mg/100 ml decrease in serum calcium for each 1 g/L decrease in serum albumin from normal (4 g/L).

Some degree of endogenous PTH secretion is frequent in surgical hypoparathyroidism, and the doses of calcium or vitamin D to maintain calcium homeostasis are smaller than in hypoparathyroidism from other causes. Frequently revascularization or hypertrophy of the remaining glands occur, and therapy may be discontinued after several months. If the patient has an adequate calcium intake, 1 to 2 g of elemental calcium with or without a vitamin D supplement may be sufficient. Vitamin D metabolites such as 25-hydroxycalciferol or the more potent 1,25-dihydroxycalciferol are extremely effective, fast-acting agents that may be used initially. The cast of these newer agents is a major disadvantage, and many patients can be adequately controlled on generic vitamin D 50,000 U twice a week or more frequently, depending on the severity of the hypoparathyroidism. However, vitamin D preparations will not be effective unless an adequate calcium intake is assured. The adjunctive use of a thiazide diuretic will decrease urinary calcium and thus decrease the need for oral supplementation.

The goal of therapy for hypoparathyroidism is to avoid symptomatic hypocalcemia and maintain the serum calcium in the low normal range. This will avoid renal complications caused by hypercalciuria. Insidious hypocalcemia may cause chronic malaise, cognitive dysfunction, and cataracts. Therefore serum calcium and phosphorus levels should be monitored in all patients after surgery, regardless of the lack of symptoms.

Hypothyroidism and Recurrent Hyperthyroidism

Hypothyroidism is common after surgical therapy and is somewhat, but not exclusively, related to the size of the remnant.[28-30] The presence of Hashimoto's thyroiditis (lymphocyte infiltration of the gland, antithyroid antibodies) increases the chances of hypothyroidism after therapy. Thyroid registries in England verify a bimodal pattern of hypothyroidism with a peak incidence in the first 18 months following surgery but a persistent 1% annual incidence for at least 5 to 10 years after surgery.[28] Late-onset hypothyroidism appears to be related to the natural history of the disease process and stresses the need for life-long follow-up. Large thyroid remnants may not protect against hypothyroidism and appear to increase the chance of recurrent hyperthyrodism, especially in those patients requiring surgery for the treatment of hyperthyroidism initially. Near-total or total thyroidectomy will by necessity cause myxedema, and the patient should be treated with levothyroxine replacement immediately following surgery.

Rare Complications

In radical surgery for malignant disease several rare neurologic complications have been reported. These include injury to the cervical sympathetic trunk during ligation of the inferior thyroid artery, causing Horner's syndrome; phrenic nerve damage with paralysis of the hemidiaphragm; and transection of the spinal accessory nerve with paralysis of the trapezius muscle. Rarely the right lymphatic duct or thoracic duct may be injured, requiring ligation. Tracheomalacia has been reported after removal of a large goiter but is a distinctly rare complication.

SUMMARY

In spite of its small size, the thyroid gland plays an important role in the maintenance of normal body cellular metabolism. This is exemplified by the pathologic aberrations that supervene in both hyperthyroid and hypothyroid states. The significance of this organ to the surgeon relates not only to the effect that thyroid dysfunction may have in ensuring the smooth performance of any operation and the resulting postoperative convalescence, but also to the important role that surgery plays in managing patients with various hyperthyroid states and in those individuals with thyroid lesions suspicious for malignancy. In this latter group of patients, the frequency of surgical intervention has diminshed greatly with the current availability of fine-needle aspiration. This technique provides the unique ability to aspirate cystic lesions previously requiring formal surgical exploration, as well as the ability to distinguish benign and malignant lesions from each other so that those individuals subjected to surgery will clearly benefit from such a procedure. Even when surgery is indicated, a good result can be expected, since current anesthetic management and surgical technique are associated with minimum morbidity and virtually no mortality.

REFERENCES

1. Ashcraft, M.W., and VanHerle, A.J.: Management of thyroid nodules, Part I, Head Neck Surg. **3:**216, 1981.
2. Ashcraft, M.W., and VanHerle, A.J.: Management of thyroid nodules, Part II, Head Neck Surg. **3:**297, 1981.
3. Barsano, C.P., et al.: Serum thyroglobulin in the management of patients with thyroid cancer, Arch. Intern. Med. **142:**763, 1982.
4. Beierwaltes, W.H.: The treatment of thyroid carcinoma with radioiodine, Semin. Nucl. Med. **8:**79, 1978.
5. Beierwaltes, W.H., et al.: Survival time and cure in papillary and follicular thyroid carcinoma with distant metastases: statistics following University of Michigan therapy, J. Nucl. Med. **23:**561, 1982.
6. Black, F.G., et al.: Serum thyroglobulin in thyroid cancer, Lancet **2:**443, 1981.
7. Blum, M., and Rothchild, M.: Improved nonoperative diagnosis of the solitary cold thyroid nodule, JAMA **243:**242, 1980.
8. Braverman, L.W., Ingbar, S.H., and Sterling, K.: Conversion of thyroxine to triiodothyronine in athyreotic human subjects, J. Clin. Invest. **49:**855, 864, 1970.
9. Cady, B., et al.: Changing clinical, pathologic, therapeutic, and survival patterns in differentiated thyroid carcinoma, Ann. Surg. **183:**541, 1976.
10. Catz, B., and Perzik, S.L.: Total thyroidectomy in Graves' disease, Am. J. Surg. **118:**434, 1969.
11. Chong, G.A., et al.: Medullary carcinoma of the thyroid glands, Cancer **45:**695, 1975.
12. Chopra, I.J., et al.: Misleading low free thyroxine level and usefulness of reverse triiodothyronine measurement in nonthyroidal illnesses, Ann. Intern. Med. **90:**905, 1979.
13. Chopra, I.J., et al.: Thyroid function in nonthyroidal illnesses, Ann. Intern. Med. **98:**946, 1983.

14. Crile, G., McNamara, J.M., and Hagard, T.B.: Results of treatment of papillary carcinoma of the thyroid, Surg. Gynecol. Obstet. **109**:315, 1959.
15. Degroot, L.J.: Clinical features and management of radiation-associated thyroid carcinoma. In Kaplan, E.L. editor: Surgery of the thyroid and parathyroid glands, London, 1983, Churchill Livingstone.
16. Degroot, L.J., and Reilly, M.: Comparison of 30 and 50 millicurie doses of iodine^{131} for thyroid ablation, Ann. Intern. Med. **96**:51, 1982.
17. Edis, A.J.: Prevention and management of complication associated with thyroid and parathyroid surgery, Surg. Clin. North Am. **59**:83, 1979.
18. Farnell, M.B., et al.: Hypothyroidism after thyroidectomy for Graves' disease, Am. J. Surg. **142**:535, 1981.
19. Farrar, W.B.: Complications of thyroidectomy, Surg. Clin. North Am. **63**:1353, 1981.
20. Favus, M.J., et al.: Thyroid cancer occurring as a late consequence of head and neck irradiation, N. Engl. J. Med. **294**:1019, 1983.
21. Fenton, R.S.: The surgical complications of thyroidectomy, J. Otolaryn. **12**:104, 1983.
22. Foster, R.S.: Morbidity and mortality after thyroidectomy, Surg. Gynecol. Obstet. **146**:423, 1978.
23. Fradkin, J.E., and Wolff, J.: Iodide-induced thyrotoxicosis, Medicine **62**:1, 1983.
24. Goldstein, R., and Hart, I.R.: Followup of solitary autonomous thyroid nodules treated with I^{131}, N. Engl. J. Med. **309**:1473, 1983.
24a. Greer, M.A., Kammer, H., and Bouma, D.J.: Short-term antithyroid drug therapy for the thyrotoxicosis of Graves' disease, N. Engl. J. Med. **297**:173, 1977.
24b. Hamberger, B., et al.: Fine needle aspiration biopsy of thyroid nodules, impact on thyroid practice and cost of care, Am. J. Med. **73**:381, 1982.
25. Hamburger, J.: The autonomously functioning thyroid adenoma: clinical considerations, N. Engl. J. Med. **309**:1512, 1983.
26. Hamburger, J.I., Miller, J.M., and Kini, S.R.: Clinical pathological evaluation of thyroid nodules: handbook and atlas (private publication), 1979.
27. Hamburger, J.I., Miller, J.M., and Kini, S.R.: Lymphoma of the thyroid, Ann. Intern. Med. **99**:685, 1983.
28. Hedley, A.J., et al.: Recurrent thyrotoxicosis after subtotal thyroidectomy, Br. Med. J. **4**:258, 1971.
29. Hedley, A.J., et al.: The effect of remnant size on the outcome of subtotal thyroidectomy for thyrotoxicosis, Br. J. Surg. **59**:559, 1972.
30. Hedley, A.J., et al.: Late onset hypothyroidism after subtotal thyroidectomy for hyperthyroidism: implication for long-term followup. Br. J. Surg. **80**:740, 1983.
31. Hennessy, J.F., et al.: A comparison of pentagastrin injection and calcium infusion as provocative agents for the detection of medullary carcinoma of the thyroid, J. Clin. Endocrinol. and Metabol. **39**:487, 1974.
32. Jacobs, J.K., Alaud, J.W., and Ballinger, W.F.: Total thyroidectomy: a review of 213 patients, Ann. Surg. **197**:542, 1983.
33. Kendall-Taylor, P., et al.: Evidence that thyroid stimulating antibody is produced in the thyroid gland, Lancet **1**:654, 1984.
34. Klein, I., and Levey, G.S.: Iodine excess and thyroid function, Ann. Intern. Med. **98**:406, 1983.
35. Leeper, R.D.: The effect of I^{131} therapy on survival of patients with metastatic papillary or follicular thyroid carcinoma, J. Clin. Endocrinol. and Metabol. **36**:1143, 1973.
36. Lore', J.M., and Pruet, C.W.: Retrieval of the parathyroid glands during thyroidectomy, Head Neck Surg. **5**:268, 1983.
37. Lowhagen, T., et al.: Aspiration biopsy cytology in nodules of the thyroid gland suspected to be malignant, Surg. Clin. North Am. **59**:3, 1979.
38. Maier, W.P., et al.: Long-term follow-up of Graves' disease after subtotal thyroidectomy, Am. J. Surg. **147**:266, 1984.
39. Max, M.H., Scheum, M., and Bland, K.I.: Early and late complications of thyroid operations, South Med. J. **76**:977, 1983.
40. Maxon, H.R., et al.: Ionizing Irradiation and the introduction of clinically significant disease in the human thyroid gland, Am. J. Med. **63**:967, 1977.
41. Maxon, H.R., et al.: Relation between effective radiation dose and outcome of radioiodine therapy for thyroid cancer, N. Engl. J. Med. **309**:937, 1983.
42. Mazzaferri, E.L., and Young, R.L.: Papillary thyroid carcinoma: a ten-year followup report of the impact of therapy in 576 patients, Am. J. Med. **70**:511-515, 1981.
43. Mazzaferri, E.L., et al.: Papillary thyroid carcinoma: the impact of therapy in 576 patients, Medicine **56**:171, 1977.
44. Miller, J.M., Hamburger, J.I., and Kini, S.: Diagnosis of thyroid nodules: use of fine needle aspiration and needle biopsy, JAMA **241**:481, 1979.
45. Miller, J.M., Kini, S.R., and Hamburger, J.L.: Needle biopsy of the thyroid, New York, 1983, Prager.
46. Milmed, S., et al.: A comparison of methods for assessing thyroid function in nonthyroidal illness, J. Clin. Endocrinol. Metabol. **54**:300, 1982.
46a. Paine, T.D., et al.: Coronary arterial surgery in patients with incapacitating angina pectoris and myxedema, Am. J. Cardiol. **40**:226, 1977.
47. Samaan, N.A., et al.: Impact of therapy for differentiated carcinoma of the thyroid: an analysis of 706 cases. J. Clin. Endocrinol. Metabol. **56**:1131, 1983.
48. Sampson, R.J.: Prevalence and signficance of occult thyroid cancer. In Degroot, L.J., editor: Radiation-associated thyroid carcinoma, New York, 1977, Grune and Stratton, Inc.
49. Sizemore, G.W., and Go, V.L.M.: Stimulation tests for diagnosis of medullary thyroid carcinoma, Mayo Clin. Proc. **50**:53, 1975.
50. Snyder, J., Gorman, C., and Scanlon, P.: Thyroid remnant ablation: questionable pursuit of an ill-defined goal, J. Nucl. Med. **24**:659, 1983.
51. Stepanas, A.V. et al.: Medullary thyroid carcinoma: importance of serial serum calcitonin measurement, Cancer **43**:825, 1979.
52. Sugrue, D.D., et al.: Long-term followup of hyperthyroid patients treated by subtotal thyroidectomy, Br. J. Surg. **70**:408, 1983.
53. Taylor, G.W., and Painter, N.S.: Size of remnant in partial thyroidectomy, Lancet, **1**:287, 1962.
54. Taylor, S.: Sporadic and nontoxic goiter: etiology and pathogenesis. In Werner, S., and Ingbar, S., editors: The thyroid, New York, 1978, Harper and Row.
55. Tollefson, H.R., and Decosse, J.J.: Papillary carcinoma of the thyroid gland after initial surgical treatment, Am. J. Surg. **106**:728, 1963.
56. Tollefson, H.R., and Shah, H.: Papillary carcinoma of the thyroid, Am. J. Surg. **124**:468, 1972.
57. Valente, W.A., et al.: Antibodies that promote thyroid growth, N. Engl. J. Med. **309**:1028, 1983.
58. Vander, J.B., Gaston, E.A., and Dawber, T.R.: The significance of nontoxic thyroid nodules, Ann. Intern. Med. **69**:537, 1968.
59. Walfish, P.G., et al.: Combined ultrasound and needle aspiration cytology in the assessment and management of hypofunctioning thyroid nodules, Ann. Intern. Med. **87**:270, 1977.
59a. Weiss, I., and Davies, T.F.: Inhibition of immunoglobulin secreting cells by antithyroid drugs, J. Clin. Endocrinol. Metabol. **53**:1223, 1981.
60. Woolner, L.V., Beahrs, O.H., and Black, B.M.: Thyroid carcinoma: general consideration and followup data on 1181 cases. In Young, S., Inman, D.R., editors: Thyroid neoplasia, New York, 1968, Academic Press, Inc.
61. Woolner, L.V., et al.: Occult papillary carcinoma of the thyroid gland: a study of 140 cases observed in a 30-year period, J. Clin. Endocrinol. Metabol. **20**:89, 1960.

59

Ronald C. Merrell, Giacomo Basadonna, and Kenji Kakizaki

Endocrine Pancreas

To coordinate the function of metazoan life forms for mutual, organismal benefit, the cells of the organism must communicate. In simple multicellular organisms, electrical coupling, cell contact events, and the local diffusion of metabolic and messenger molecules are sufficient. Neighboring cells are informed by mass action, allosteric enzyme interactions, or specific binding to receptors. In larger organisms with a circulatory system, coordinating messages in the form of small molecules may flow through the organism to arrive at tissues possessing specific receptors with complex postreceptor events. Also, neural fibers arborize over great distances to release communicating molecules to specialized receptors when triggered by propagated depolarization of the neuronal membrane.[36]

The pancreas demonstrates essentially all of the known mechanisms for cellular communication in a metazoan organism. In addition to cell-to-cell interaction among islet cells across gap junctions (Fig. 59-1), the simplest coordinate function, and complex adrenergic and cholinergic innervation, the pancreas engages in exocrine, paracrine, and endocrine interactions with the remainder of the body (Fig. 59-2). *Exocrine function* describes release of synthesized products into a nonvascular duct for delivery at another anatomic locus. *Paracrine function* requires release of a synthesized product into the extracellular space for delivery by diffusion to a target tissue no more than several microns away. *Endocrine interactions* call for release of a synthesized product that enters the circulation for transport to a distant target tissue. The intricacy and, indeed, redundancy of communication pathways for this islet cell mass underscore its crucial role in maintaining glucose homeostasis through the balance of glucose clearance mediated by insulin and glucose generation mediated by glucagon. The goal of this chapter is to describe the endocrine community of the islets of Langerhans; their origins and relationships, both internal and external; and their role in homeostasis and disease states.

In 1869 Paul Langerhans demonstrated the unique features of the islets that now bear his name. These structures, originally viewed as islands in the alien sea of the exocrine pancreas, are now more clearly seen as integral and not accidental features of the pancreas with extensive interaction with the exocrine portion of the gland. Von Mering and Minkowski[56] provided evidence for an endocrine function for the pancreas in 1889 when they found that total pancreatectomy led not only to the expected exocrine insufficiency but also to diabetes mellitus. Attribution of endocrine function to the islets followed and seemed to culminate with isolation of insulin and its clinical application for Type I diabetes mellitus by Banting and Best in 1922.[2] However, the full richness of islet interaction and regulation was only suggested by the recognition of insulin, and new data continue to enhance the importance of the islets in homeostasis.

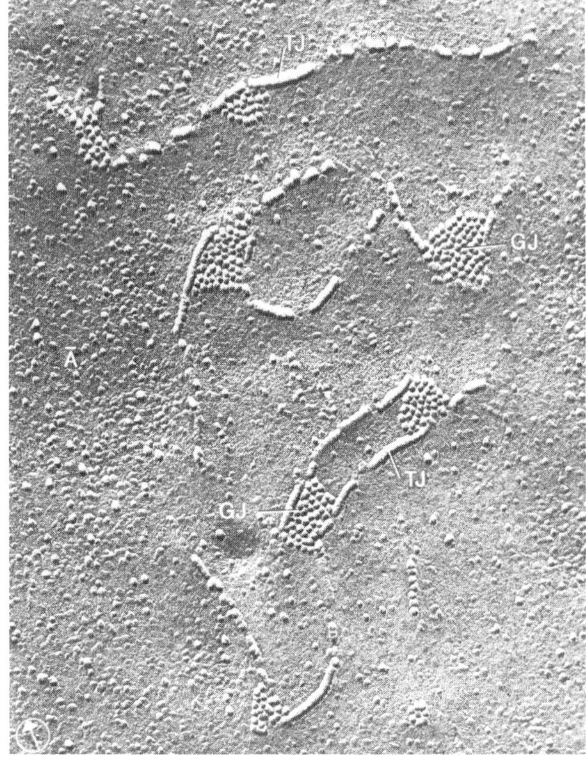

Fig. 59-1 Gap junctions *(GJ)* and tight junctions *(TJ)* between islet cells suggest the rich transcellular communication between component cells of islets of Langerhans. This freeze fracture electron micrograph shows extensive cellular contacts between islet cells. (Courtesy Lelio Orci, Geneva.)

ANATOMY AND EMBRYOLOGY OF THE ISLETS

The islets of Langerhans constitute individually an endocrine community engaged in active collaboration to secure glucose homeostasis. At least four distinct endocrine cells have been identified: (1) A cells, which secrete *glucagon,* a catabolic hormone that raises plasma glucose; (2) B cells, which produce *insulin,* an anabolic hormone that lowers plasma glucose; (3) D cells, which produce *somatostatin,* a regulatory hormone for A and B cells; and (4) F cells, which secrete *pancreatic polypeptide,* a hormone awaiting functional clarification. Each cell contains and secretes only one endocrine product. The lettering system for these cells stems from special chemical staining properties of the secretory granules. The letter C in the series was

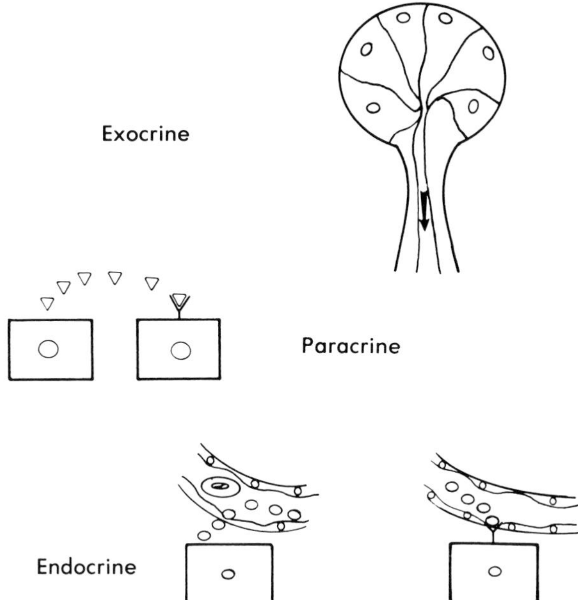

Fig. 59-2 *Exocrine* delivery of a secreted cellular product occurs along ducts that ultimately discharge into the gastrointestinal tract or outside the body. *Paracrine* secretions reach a target cell solely by diffusion over a short distance. (Schematic cell on the left is discharging a substance that is being received by the cell on the right). *Endocrine* secretions enter the circulation and arrive at a target tissue at some distance from the point of origin. (Schematic cell on the left is discharging a substance into the blood; the blood then transports this substance to a distant target cell, as shown on the right.)

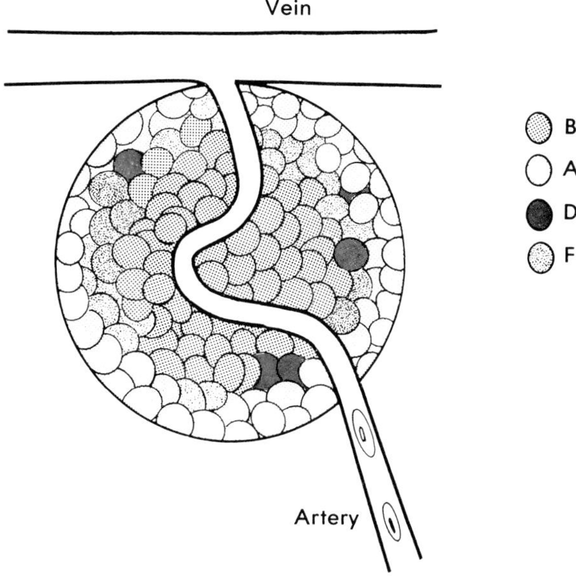

Fig. 59-3 B cells are centrally located in the islet in close approximation to incoming blood supply, whereas A cells are arrayed as a mantle at the periphery of the islet. D and F cells are interspersed. B cell secretions move through the islet toward the periphery before reentering the circulation. This flow determines the opportunity for paracrine interaction among the component cells. The modest suppression by insulin of A cells can be paracrine, whereas the more substantial stimulation of B cells by glucagon must be endocrine. D and F cells could interact with one another, with A cells or with B cells.

reserved for a cell in guinea pig islets that contained no granules. This cell may have been a degranulated B cell or a precursor cell but no longer has any valid stature among its lettered neighbors. Also, the E cell, described only in the opossum, must await further study before inclusion into this endocrine community. The cells were lettered in order of discovery, and the missing C and E cells in the islet serve to remind us of the enormous confusion that preceded our current meager understanding.[38] That understanding is based on staining islets with specific antibodies to the various secretory products and then using a variety of tactics to visualize that bound antibody over the secretory granules of the appropriate cell. This staining by immunocytochemistry forms the basis of our current understanding of islet anatomy.

The pancreas arises from foregut endoderm through a dorsal bud, first evident in the 3-mm embryo, and then by a ventral anlage, which is a branch of the liver bud. By clockwise rotation, the ventral structure ultimately fuses with the dorsal structure. The endocrine cells derive from precursors along the pancreatic ductal elements. By immunocytochemistry, A, B, and D cells can be recognized in organized islets by 8 weeks' gestation. By 10 to 11 weeks, islets can be identified. Islets are more numerous in the tail than in the head of the pancreas in adults, and this pattern is well established in fetal life. The islets organize away from ducts as discrete structures and then grow by cell division throughout fetal life and for the first few years after birth. Islets are not of uniform size in humans but average approximately 300 μm.[16] The A cells mature first, but by birth the distribution of the cells is the same as in adults: 60% to 70% B cells, 20% to 25% A cells, 10% to 15% D cells, and 5% to 10% F cells (Fig. 59-3). The distribution of the islets is not completely uniform throughout the pancreas with respect to constituent cells. For example, A and B cells are more numerous in tail islets, and F cells are much more numerous in the pancreatic head.

The origin of islet cells has been the subject of spirited debate for nearly 10 years. The islet cells have metabolic and morphologic features shared by all neuroendocrine cells, including amine precursor uptake and decarboxylase (APUD), and neuronal specific enolase. A common embryologic source for all these cells in the neuroectoderm of the neural crest has been proposed.[41] However, careful studies in developmental biology refute this origin for pancreatic islet cells and place them firmly in the same lineage as the exocrine cells. For example, elimination of the neural fold before the three-somite stage does not preclude B-cell development in rat embryo explants.[49] A great majority of the endocrine system derives from the gastrointestinal epithelium, including the pituitary (Rathke's pouch), the thyroid (second branchial arch and ultimobranchial body), and the parathyroid glands (branchial pouch III and IV). Nonetheless, the APUD concept has been of enormous value in predicting the properties of endocrine tissue in one site on the basis of knowledge of other endocrine systems. Also, the behavior of pathologic endocrine tissue

Table 59-1 **INSULOACINAR AXIS**

Hormone	Exocrine Effect
Insulin	↑ Uptake of amino acids ↑ Amylase synthesis ↑ Cell division Permits HCO_3^- release
Glucagon	↓ Enzyme synthesis ↓ Enzyme release ↑ HCO_3^- release
Somatostatin	↓ Pancreatic secretion
Pancreatic polypeptide	↓ Release of enzymes

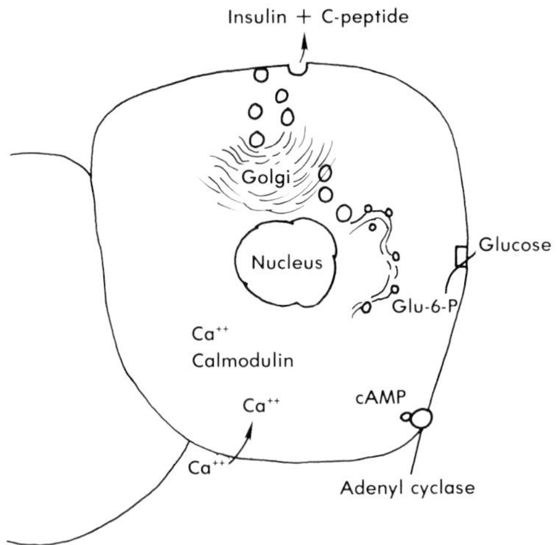

Fig. 59-4 The release of insulin from B cells is controlled at least by intracellular cAMP and Ca^{++}. Although glucose is the predominant secretagogue for insulin, many other metabolic or receptor-mediated events also modulate insulin secretion. Proinsulin is packaged from the endoplasmic reticulum after synthesis and moves through the Golgi. Proinsulin is cleaved in the secretory or storage vesicles to give C-peptide and insulin, which are released in equimolar quantities by exocytosis.

can be anticipated in less known tumors on the basis of knowledge of better characterized tumors. All cells in an organism have the same genome, and the differentiation of transcription during development can be convergent so that, after many different branch points in development, two cells serving similar (e.g., endocrine) functions are more alike than cells much closer in developmental lineage.

It is significant that the islets are in the pancreas and develop with the pancreas because this relationship suggests that islets function with the remainder of the pancreas. Indeed, there is an insuloacinar axis, which constitutes a portal system that delivers islet hormones in high concentration to much of the acinar pancreas (Table 59-1). Insulin increases amylase synthesis, permits bicarbonate secretion, and is permissive for the action of cholecystokinin. The pancreas of insulin-dependent diabetics is much smaller than normal as a result of atrophy, which may be caused by a relative lack of insulin locally or by the inhibitory effects of excess glucagon, which suppresses enzyme synthesis and release, although it stimulates bicarbonate secretion. The inhibitory effects of glucagon are so pronounced experimentally that this hormone was proposed for the treatment of acute pancreatitis; however, clinical results have not been impressive. Somatostatin and pancreatic polypeptide are also inhibitory to the exocrine pancreas and presumably are active in the insuloacinar axis.[19]

PHYSIOLOGY OF THE ISLETS

Insulin and the B Cell

The best studied of the islet cells is the B cell. The nucleus of this cell transcribes messenger ribonucleic acid (mRNA) for preproinsulin, which is synthetized in the rough endoplasmic reticulum. The amino terminal signal sequence is cleaved in the lumen of the endoplasmic reticulum, and the 9000-dalton product, proinsulin, passes through the Golgi apparatus where secretory vesicles are assembled. The vesicles are stored in the cytoplasm in the webbing of the cytoskeleton and, under secretory stimuli, move to the plasma membrane where the vesicle and plasma membranes fuse to release equimolar concentrations of insulin and C-peptide into the extracellular space. In the storage vesicles the single chain of proinsulin is doubly cleaved to give the A and B chains of insulin (molecular weight, 6000) bonded together by two disulfide bridges and the connecting chain, C-peptide. A third disulfide bond determines the shape of the A chain. In the vesicles insulin is a hexamer coordinated by two Zn^{++} ions. During release and dilution the hexamer dissociates to the active monomeric form.[12]

Stored insulin is abundant, and the number of B cells in the normal pancreas far exceeds the number required for insulin release. When insulin release is maximally stimulated, it is rare to release more than 5% of the total insulin available. As much as 95% of the normal pancreas can be resected without inducing insulin insufficiency or carbohydrate intolerance. The release of insulin is prompted by a movement of Ca^{++} into the B cell and by the accumulation of cyclic AMP (cAMP). There are many secretagogues that can accomplish one or both of these events, which are somewhat independent with respect to insulin release. It is convenient to view Ca^{++} and cAMP as the final events necessary for access to the insulin pool. Access to the Ca^{++} and the cAMP pools, in turn, can be achieved through a variety of routes, which are either receptor mediated or connected to the metabolism of the B cell (Fig. 59-4).[31] Pluralistic access to the insulin pool is important to explain even partially the wide range of secretagogues and inhibitors for the release of this crucial hormone. Glucose is the major secretagogue in humans (see boxed material on p. 985).

The B cells are generally concentrated at the center of an islet in close apposition to the arteriole that penetrates the islet to deliver blood first to its interior (see Fig. 59-3). These cells are coupled electrically to surrounding cells and have rich gap junction contacts transmitting sizable molecules among B cells and other adjacent endocrine cells.[35] The boxed material on p. 985 outlines the major secretagogues and inhibitors of insulin release. The insulin leaving the islets arrives like all islet hormones at the liver through the portal vein. Approximately 50% of insulin is

INSULIN RELEASE

Secretagogues	
Metabolic	***Receptor-mediated***
Glucose	Glucagon
Other hexoses (potentiate)	Gastric inhibitory peptide
Hexosamines (potentiate)	beta-Endorphin
Glycolytic products (potentiate)	beta-Adrenergic agonists
	Acetylcholine
Amino acids	Sulfonylurea
Fatty acids	Gastrin
Ca^{++} (Ionic)	Secretin
Calcium ionophores	Cholecystokinin
Islet activating protein	Cortisol
Suppressors	
Metabolic	***Receptor-mediated***
D-Manno-heptulose	Somatostatin
2-Deoxyglucose	alpha-Adrenergic agonists
Diazoxide	
Suppression of Electrical Activity	
Cytoskeleton blockade	
Diphanylhydantoin	
Colchicine	

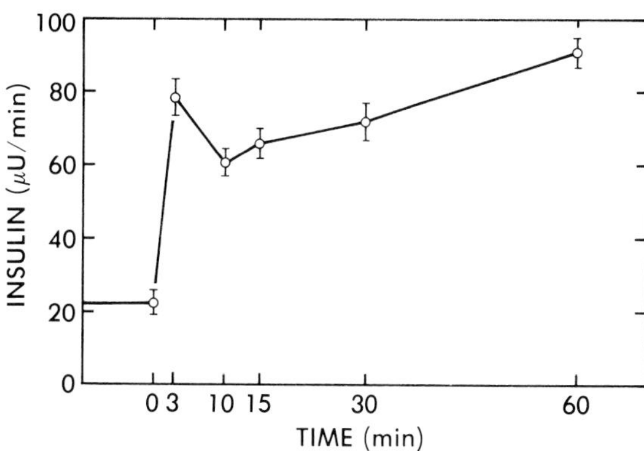

Fig. 59-5 Biphasic release of insulin after glucose stimulation is seen from either isolated islets of Langerhans, as in this figure, or from the in situ pancreas when pulsed with glucose. The initial sharp peak of insulin release at 3 minutes is followed by sustained insulin release, which peaks at 30 to 60 minutes. The significance of the biphasic nature of insulin secretion is probably great but poorly understood. Multiple insulin pools have been implicated to explain the discontinuity of insulin release.

removed on the first pass through the liver, which may be considered the major site of action for insulin.

The least understood of the mechanisms for insulin release are the metabolic pathways. Clearly flow of oxygen through the mitochondrial respiratory chain is critical, and lipoxygenase has been implicated.[37] It is possible that glucose has a membrane receptor that prompts release in addition to metabolic regulation. Although many hexoses and intermediates are secretagogues or facilitate glucose-mediated insulin release, galactose and 3-0-methylglucose participate in glycolysis but do not promote insulin secretion. Also, some agents that block glycolysis do not block glucose-stimulated insulin release. Therefore a glucose receptor is suggested.[33] However, the nature of a receptor that responds in a concentration range for glucose of 5×10^{-3} M to 15×10^{-3} M is obscure at best. The dissociation constant (K_D) K_D for hormone receptors favors regulatory interaction at 10^{-8} M to 10^{-9} M. The high molecular concentration of glucose that affects insulin regulation is more consistent with allosteric interaction with an enzyme rather than cell surface or cytosolic receptor kinetics. In general, three routes of stimulation may be distinguished: *metabolic,* typified by glucose and amino acids; *receptor-mediated,* typified by acetylcholine; and *ionic* as in Ca^{++} ionophores.

The interaction of insulin with secretagogues other than glucose and amino acids is important. The amount of insulin released after oral ingestion of glucose is two to three times that secreted after intravenous delivery of the same amount of this substance. This phenomenon has given us the term insuloenteric axis. The gastrointestinal hormones that cause this effect have not been specifically identified from among the rather long list of known secretagogue peptides in the gastrointestinal tract. Also, in apancreatic animals that have striking elevations in plasma glucose, the glucose returns to normal after hypophysectomy. Therefore counteracting or antagonistic hormones in metabolism can determine the need or superfluity of insulin.[20] Vagal stimulatory effects on insulin secretion are dramatic and can induce hypoglycemia with only the sight and smell of food. However, B cells can generally function in glucose homeostasis with or without this extraordinary amount of input. The checks and balances of insulin release are so numerous that failure of the B cell mass with glucose intolerance represents the collapse of a long series of protective endocrine and metabolic mechanisms.

There is a basal release of insulin that averages 4 mU/minute.[44] This level is biologically quite active. Therefore insulin is important in basal metabolism and not simply to reduce excursions in the glucose concentration. When an appropriate stimulus is given, the insulin is released in two phases. There is an initial or first-phase peak that reaches about five times basal insulin within 3 to 5 minutes. This phase deteriorates and a second, sustained phase of insulin release continues for 60 to 70 minutes. This second phase is quantitatively much more substantial.[47] The biphasic contour (Fig. 59-5) suggests that insulin is stored in at least two compartments under somewhat different control. Insulin release returns to basal after either a restoration of ambient glucose to normal or exhaustion of the B cell. Physiologic inhibitors do indeed modulate insulin release but are not important in a feedback loop. Insulin itself may not be directly involved in feedback in that infused insulin in vivo[26] can reduce insulin output but no such effect can be demonstrated with isolated islets in vitro.[32] All the modulators of insulin release are of modest importance compared to the primacy of glucose as the major regulator of B cell function.

Insulin lowers plasma glucose principally by facilitating the diffusion of glucose into tissues that have insulin receptors. After interaction with its receptors, a number of protein phosphorylations occur, and the entrance of glucose as glucose-6-phosphate is greatly accelerated.[54] The hormone promotes glycogen synthesis by reducing cAMP effects on glycogenolysis. Insulin also promotes amino acid uptake and protein synthesis and inhibits protein degradation. Fat synthesis is promoted by means of pyruvate dehydrogenase, and lipolysis is inhibited.[34] Insulin promotes the entry of K^+ and Mg^{++} into cells even in the absence of glucose (see boxed material below). The hormone generally supports cell growth and division by metabolic enhancement. Insulin is similar in primary structure to nerve growth factor, other growth factors, and relaxin. The wide array of insulin effects apparently does not have a common postreceptor second messenger. Rather, insulin has multiple intracellular actions after initial binding and internalization of the insulin-receptor complex. Insulin is also associated with a reduction in intracellular cAMP.

Insulin is so critical to the existence of life forms with a circulatory system, and therefore endocrine relationships, that its primary sequence is conserved with exquisite precision through speciation. Among mammals there is significant variation only at amino acid residue numbers 8, 9, and 10 of the A chain.[9] Human and porcine insulin differ by only one amino acid. Insulin from fishes has significant biologic activity in humans (Fig. 59-6).

INSULIN EFFECTS

Facilitates Entry into Cells of:
- Glucose
- Amino acids
- K^+
- Mg^{++}

Enhances	**Inhibits**
↑ Glycogen synthesis	↓ Glycogenolysis
↑ Lipogenesis	↓ Lipolysis
↑ Protein synthesis	↓ Protein degradation
	↓ Gluconeogenesis
	↓ cAMP

Although most tissues need insulin to modulate the metabolism of glucose, this hormone is not needed by the central nervous system. In fact, insulin does not readily pass the blood-brain barrier. Muscle tissue that has been physically conditioned by exercise has a great reduction in the need for insulin to transport glucose. Quantitatively the most important site for insulin activity in metabolism is the liver, and the most important site for rapid reduction of plasma glucose is the fat cell mass.

Glucagon and the A Cell

The complementary hormone to insulin is glucagon, which is secreted by A cells and acts to raise plasma glucose. Glucagon is a single peptide of 3485 daltons that has sequence homology with secretin, vasoactive intestinal peptide, gastric inhibitory peptide, growth hormone–releasing factor and placental lactogen.[40] A prohormone is synthesized that yields glucagon in the secretory granules after proteolytic cleavage. In health, glucagon is clearly as important as insulin, but, since it is not of primary importance in any common disease states, its discovery in 1923[24] received little notice. This crucial hormone has until recently been viewed as a probe to the primacy of insulin. However, glucagon in stress is so preponderant in driving catabolic metabolism that new knowledge concerning its actions and properties is received with great anticipation by those wishing to better understand stress physiology.

The principal stimulus for glucagon release is hypoglycemia. The mechanisms of release are probably similar to those of insulin but much less studied. Amino acids stimulate the release of both glucagon and insulin. The only gastrointestinal peptide known to stimulate glucagon secretion is cholecystokinin. Glucagon release is also prompted by epinephrine by means of alpha-adrenergic effects. Cortisol, growth hormone, and beta-endorphin all promote glucagon release. Glucagon release is suppressed by hyperglycemia, somatostatin, secretin, and insulin. It also exercises feedback inhibition on its own secretion.[22] After a glucose challenge the suppression of baseline glucagon

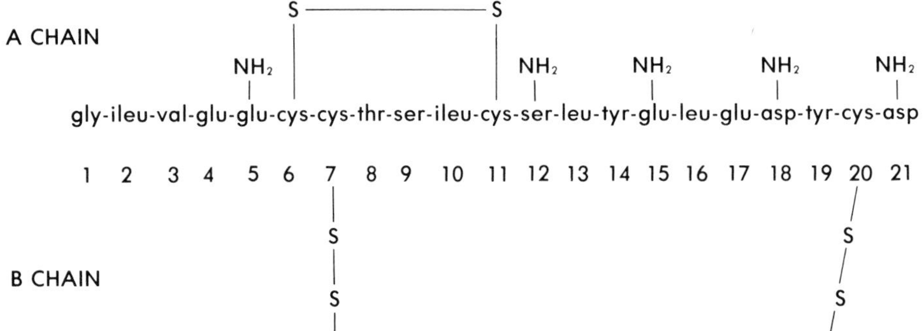

Fig. 59-6 The structure of insulin in all species is quite similar to that shown here for human insulin. Sequence variation among various species is most prominent at residues 8, 9, and 10 of the A chain. Both A and B chains are derived from the same proinsulin molecule by proteolytic removal of the C-peptide. The three sulfhydryl bridges coordinate the tertiary structure of the molecule.

release closely parallels insulin stimulation. The magnitude of the suppression is much greater after oral glucose intake than after intravenous delivery. The mirror image of insulin response is clear:

1. Secretagogues
   a. Hypoglycemia
   b. Amino acids
   c. Cholecystokinin
   d. alpha-Adrenergic agonists
   e. Cortisol
   f. Growth hormone
   g. beta-Endorphin
2. Suppressors
   a. Hyperglycemia
   b. Insulin
   c. Secretion
   d. Somatostatin

Basal glucagon is of great importance in countervening the effects of insulin. At steady-state glucose, basal insulin release describes an oscillation easily measured in portal venous blood. The period of the oscillation is about 10 minutes. Basal glucagon release follows a similar sine wave variation 180 degrees out of phase to that of insulin. The oscillatory delivery of insulin and glucagon to the liver cannot be explained on the basis of variable glucose delivery to the islets. Rather, an internal rhythm must be presumed in the islets themselves that does not require the circulatory system.[17] In spite of the extensive communication among the cells within an islet, there is no evidence for linkage between individual islets. However, rhythmic basal insulin release can be seen in cultured islets in vitro. The mechanism for this biologic clock is not known.

Approximately 25% of the portal venous glucagon remains in the liver after one pass. The liver is the most important target tissue for this hormone; in the liver specific receptors recognize portal venous glucagon and promote a rise in intracellular cAMP. Glycogenolysis follows by enzyme activation by means of protein kinases. On a molar basis glucagon is 20 to 30 times more potent than epinephrine in stimulating glycogenolysis. Gluconeogenesis is enhanced, whereas lipolysis in the liver and periphery is stimulated by this hormone. Glucagon is not as pervasive in its cell membrane effects as insulin. There are, for example, no important ion movements associated with glucagon, and it does not stimulate cell division. However, in addition to its metabolic effects, glucagon is a powerful suppressor of pancreatic exocrine activity and a powerful smooth muscle antagonist in the gastrointestinal tract (see boxed material below). This property is used mostly in endoscopy and radiology to temporarily paralyze the gut.

GLUCAGON EFFECTS

ENHANCES	INHIBITS
↑ Glycogenolysis	↓ Glycogen synthesis
↑ Lipolysis	↓ Lipogenesis
↑ Gluconeogenesis	
↑ cAMP	

Somatostatin and Pancreatic Polypeptide

Somatostatin is released by islet D cells that lie in juxtaposition to, and often between, A and B cells. It was first recognized in the brain as a suppressor of growth hormone release. Somatostatin modulates insulin and glucagon release by inhibiting both. Its regulatory action in the islets may be more paracrine than endocrine. One pathway to the inhibition of insulin release may be by means of somatostatin. The release of somatostatin is prompted by glucose, arginine, leucine, and glucagon.[11]

Pancreatic polypeptide is a hormone with a single peptide chain weighing 4240 daltons and is secreted by the F cells of the islets. Pancreatic polypeptide bears sequence homology to glucagon and secretin. Its potency to promote hepatic glycogenolysis rivals that of glucagon. It also causes gallbladder relaxation, decreases intestinal motility, and suppresses gastric acid secretion. This intriguing peptide, described first in 1968,[25] does not have a clear place in metabolic regulation and gastrointestinal physiology. Assignment of importance or consignment to obscurity must await further investigation.

ISLETS IN HEALTH AND DISEASE

As reviewed in the previous section, the islets of Langerhans regulate metabolism with the object of maintaining plasma glucose. The principal site for insulin and glucagon to accomplish this mission is the liver. At rest between meals, insulin and glucagon have a balanced, almost harmonic effect. After meals, the hormonal balance shifts according to the chemical nature of the meal to distribute the calorigenic nutrients for efficient use and storage. In prolonged fasting, glucagon is more important to support glucose synthesis from protein by gluconeogenesis and by hydrolysis of glycogen. Glucagon also permits use of the lipid stores. The glucose requirement in fasting is modest, and its provision generates little detriment to body protein. In times of severe stress or injury, glucagon is again important to provide the extra glucose needed for caloric consumption. Therefore the islet cell mass responds to disease states and metabolic derangements by ensuring a hormonal balance through insulin or glucagon release, which promotes the generation of endogenous fuel substrate.

The disease states of the endocrine pancreas are small in number, although they are great in terms of medical consequence. There are either states of deficiency or neoplasia. The only spontaneous deficiency involves the B cells. No natural deficiency diseases are recognized for glucagon, somatostatin, or pancreatic polypeptide. However, each cell of the islet may become neoplastic as a benign or malignant tumor secreting isotopic hormone (entopic), ectopic hormone, or no hormone.

Diabetes Mellitus

The B cells may be nearly eliminated, as occurs in Type I insulinopenic diabetes mellitus or may be functionally inadequate as occurs in Type II diabetes mellitus. In this latter condition, plasma insulin may be normal or high, but insulin insensitivity in target tissues hampers glucose clearance, and hyperglycemia develops.

Type I or insulinopenic diabetes mellitus results from the loss of B cells in childhood or early adult life. There is a strong familial tendency in the autosomal recessive mode with variable penetrance. Approximately 25% of diabetic patients have one or more first-order relatives with the disease. Children of diabetic fathers have a 6.1% likelihood of developing the disease; offspring of diabetic mothers have a diabetic incidence of only 1.3%. This disparity is not explained.[57] A close association with the antigens HLA-DR3 and HLA-DR4 has been noted. In families at risk for diabetes, the clinical disease is heralded for as long as a year by circulating autoantibodies to islet cells.[51] Although these antibodies are directed against all islet cells, the B cells are selectively destroyed by cell-mediated immunity in an insulitic process. The development of frank diabetes is also prefaced by a progressive decline in the first phase of insulin release. In a bold experiment, children recently diagnosed as diabetics were immunosuppressed with cyclosporine. After 1 year a startling one half of those children were in remission and required no insulin.[53] These newer data conflict with the previous picture of diabetes developing as an acute illness with perhaps a viral cause. There are, in fact, viruses that selectively destroy B cells in animals, and there are numerous B cell–specific toxins. However, the familial diabetes patients may not accurately represent the larger number (50% to 75%) of spontaneous diabetes cases. The final common pathway to the disease is loss of B cells, and a variety of approaches to this path can be imagined. However, among the diabetes-prone families, the recognition of prediabetes as an autoimmune event offers the prospect of immune suppression to delay or eliminate the emergence of overt diabetes.

Insulinopenic Type I diabetes is also called juvenile onset diabetes and accounts for about 10% of the 200,000 new diabetics diagnosed in the United States each year. Before the use of insulin, this acute illness was usually fatal, and the gene pool for diabetic propensity remained small. However, in the last 60 years the gene pool has enlarged considerably as treated diabetics have more consistently achieved reproductive maturity. What had been a devastating acute illness has now become a very important chronic illness. When all diabetics are grouped together, they represent 1% to 5% of the U.S. population. Diabetes is the leading cause of blindness in young Americans and is the most frequently reported diagnosis for patients beginning chronic dialysis for renal failure. The clinical ramifications of this disease are so extensive that it is appropriate to consider the condition as a syndrome rather than a single disease.

The most obvious effect of diabetes is hyperglycemia, which reflects the reduced capacity of glucose to enter cells that rely on insulin receptor occupation for facilitated glucose diffusion. Renal tubular capacity to reabsorb glucose is exceeded at 180 to 200 mg/100 ml (10 mM), and glycosuria follows. Glucose is osmotically important and causes an osmotic diuresis. Hemoconcentration and dehydration follow because of the diuresis. Hyperosmolar effects are significant when plasma glucose exceeds 540 mg/100 ml where the 30 mM glucose contributes 30 mOsm/L to the plasma osmolarity. Hyperosmolarity leads to coma, and the volume loss caused by osmotic diuresis leads to vascular collapse. Without treatment, hyperglycemia is fatal (see boxed material above).

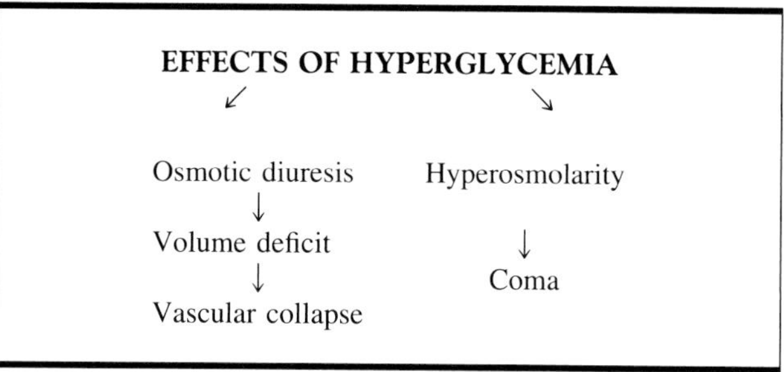

The metabolic response to reduced glucose movement into cells is prompt, damaging, and potentially fatal (Fig. 59-7). Intracellular metabolic compartments perceive the mass action message of insufficient glucose. Therefore protein catabolism is accelerated to support gluconeogenesis. Nitrogen loss is massive and is accompanied by substantial loss of potassium. The extra glucose leads further increases in plasma glucose. It is important to realize that the potentially fatal glucose in the plasma of uncontrolled diabetics does not represent ingested carbohydrate that arrives in the circulation directly from the jejunum. Rather, the source of the enormous glucose compartment in the plasma is endogenous, either glycogen or gluconeogenesis. The decrease in intracellular energy substrate also prompts lipolysis. The liberated glycerol participates in gluconeogenesis. Free fatty acids go to the liver where beta-oxidation in the mitochondria is associated with the release of acetoacetate and beta-hydroxybutyrate (ketogenic events). The generation of ketones involves acidic reactions sufficient to produce metabolic acidosis. There are no renal mechanisms to reabsorb these short carbon chains; therefore, ketonuria develops. Also, the ketones are volatile and may escape in expired air, lending a fruity odor to the breath. The released ketones are available for metabolism and energy generation. Beta-oxidation is the only event in the diabetic adaptation that helps to increase the generation of high-energy phosphate bonds. The respiratory response to the metabolic acidosis is hyperventilation in the form of air hunger called Kussmaul respiration. The clinical picture of diabetic ketoacidosis is now complete with hyperglycemia, dehydration, ketoacidosis, ketonuria, polyuria, and Kussmaul respiration. If this metabolic nightmare is not corrected by insulin, coma, vascular collapse, and death will follow.

Type II noninsulin-dependent diabetes mellitus is also called adult-onset diabetes mellitus or nonketogenic diabetes. This disease is quite distinct from Type I diabetes and only shares the common feature of derangement of carbohydrate metabolism tending toward hyperglycemia. The consequences of the hyperglycemia in terms of vascular complications are quite similar in the two diseases. Whereas Type I diabetes is marked by profound insulinopenia, Type II diabetes is a condition in which the circulating insulin levels may be normal or even greater than normal. However, the impact of circulating insulin in regulating total body carbohydrate metabolism is greatly di-

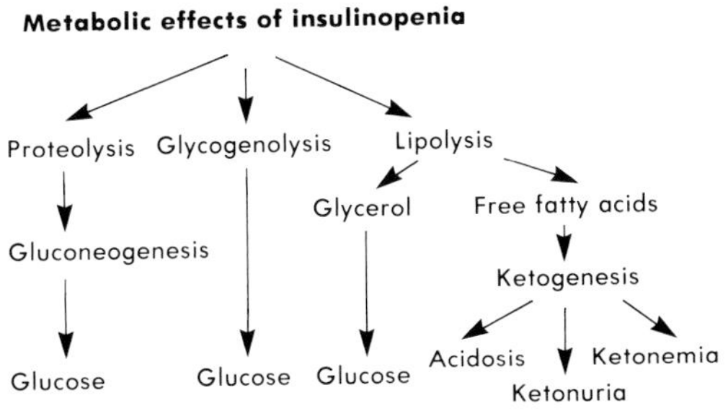

Metabolic effects of insulinopenia

Proteolysis → Gluconeogenesis → Glucose
Glycogenolysis → Glucose
Lipolysis → Glycerol → Glucose
Lipolysis → Free fatty acids → Ketogenesis → Acidosis, Ketonuria, Ketonemia

Fig. 59-7 When insulin levels are low, insulin mediation of glucose uptake in responsive tissues is greatly reduced, leading to a deficiency of intracellular glucose. The response to diminished intracellular carbohydrate is to increase the export of glucose from the liver by gluconeogenesis or glycogenolysis. In response to meager intracellular energy, substrate liposysis is encouraged, with export of ketone bodies, acetoacetate, and beta-hydroxybutyrate from the liver. Pathologically elevated plasma glucose, abundant plasma ketones with ketonuria, and the metabolic acidosis that attends ketogenesis define hyperglycemic ketoacidosis.

minished, and hyperglycemia develops. The sensitivity of peripheral tissue receptors for insulin seems greatly diminished, and there has been considerable confusion as to whether this disease arises because of any real pathology of the B cells of the islets of Langerhans or if, indeed, it represents a receptor problem at the periphery. Because insulin secretion and reception are so tightly linked, it is difficult to divorce the two events to obtain a better, if arbitrary, distinction between Types I and II diabetes. Type II diabetes, though, does occur in older patients with a striking propensity for obese patients. The hyperglycemia and hyperinsulinemia can be resolved in many obese patients by simply reducing the fat stores by dieting. There is a familial tendency in adult onset diabetes, but it more closely parallels the familial incidence of obesity. Control of hyperglycemia may require supplemental insulin in these patients with Type II diabetes mellitus, but the use of insulin still should not confuse the illness with the Type I variant. In Type II diabetes, the insulin is not required to sustain life but merely to better regulate plasma glucose. Therefore the term noninsulin-dependent diabetes mellitus is still applicable to the Type II diabetic.

The principal feature of Type II diabetes that causes clinical trouble is hyperglycemia. This can be associated with a striking and life-threatening syndrome of hyperosmolar coma when the blood sugar exceeds 800 mg/100 ml. The increase in blood glucose is osmotically quite important and can literally draw water out of the brain cells, resulting in a comatose state. However, ketosis is not associated with this drastic derangement in carbohydrate metabolism in which glucose clearance is so inadequate as to lead potentially to hyperosmolar death.

This lack of ketosis is not completely understood. The dehydration that is associated with the polyuria of hyperosmolar coma has been implicated. It is more likely that the hyperglycemic crisis in Type II diabetics is unique because insulin is, indeed, present in substantial quantities, unlike the situation in the hyperglycemic crisis of Type I diabetes. The impact of insulin in diminishing lipolysis is preserved in Type II diabetics in large measure. The adipocytes are 20 to 30 times more sensitive to the antilipolytic effects of insulin than to the facilitated entry of glucose under the influence of insulin. Therefore it is likely that, although a hyperglycemia crisis has followed because of poor insulin effect in Type II diabetics, lipolysis and, consequently, ketogenesis cannot occur. The treatment of nonketotic hyperosmolar coma in Type II diabetes is directed toward fluid resuscitation and sufficient insulin to clear the extracellular compartment of the extraordinary concentrations of free glucose.

Complications of Diabetes

Diabetes is a truly devastating disease in terms of curtailment of longevity and quality of life as a consequence of its complications and not as a consequence of its more dramatic metabolic manifestations such as ketoacidosis or nonketotic hyperosmolar coma. It is the leading cause of blindness in young Americans and may soon become the most common diagnosis for patients on chronic dialysis programs for end-stage renal disease. Although diabetes affects less than 10% of the population of the United States, it is the eighth leading cause of death. About one half of diabetics as a group die of coronary disease, whereas most juvenile onset diabetics die from ramifications of renal failure. The complications are not inherently different in Type I or II diabetes and may be considered to be neural, vascular, or infectious. These three categories are interrelated but are probably independent in their genesis. Nonetheless, they are all related to abnormal glucose metabolism.

Neuropathy is manifestated by autonomic motor and sensory problems. The autonomic problems include gastroparesis, impotence, orthostatic hypotension, and diarrhea. Sensory deficits include position sense and pin-prick. Radiculopathy is seen, and the pain can be disabling. The sensory deficit problems contribute to lower extremity injury, which cannot be healed because of poor blood supply. Such extremities tend to become infected because of poor response to bacteria with consequent limb loss.

The cause of the neuropathy is not well understood and tends to parallel the vascular complications in the course of the natural history of diabetes. However, recent work implicates abnormal metabolism of sugar alcohols through the enzyme aldose reductase. This enzyme is the rate-limiting step in the pathway to sugar alcohols, and that pathway is confined to Schwann cells, spinal roots, and lens epithelium. The enzyme is probably not abnormal in diabetics, but mass action events in hyperglycemia and intracellular glucoprevia activate this otherwise exotic pathway. The nature of the toxicity of sugar alcohols in these tissues has not been elucidated, but inhibition of aldose reductase has been clinically useful in improving autonomic function and in relieving the pain that can be a manifestation of sensory neuropathy.[23]

The vascular lesions of diabetes are numerous and perhaps distinct in their development. There is an acceleration of atherosclerosis in diabetics along lines that are indistinguishable from the peripheral vascular lesions seen in patients without carbohydrate intolerance. These lesions are associated with the hyperlidemia that accompanies diabetic metabolism. However, disease of small vessels develops along lines that are distinct to diabetics.[50] Capillary basement membranes thicken through the course of diabetes. Although this thickening may be something of an exaggeration of normal aging, the implications for the diabetic are important. If the capillary basal lamina is considered to be the framework for wound healing and the gate that must be passed in the diapedesis of inflammatory cells, the stiff, thickened layer can be seen as a significant part of other diabetic problems. The glycopeptides of basal lamina have not been extensively studied in diabetes, but the opportunity for abnormal glycosylation is certainly great in hyperglycemia and has been observed in patients with this disease. The convalent addition of glucose molecules to protein normally requires a glycosyl transferase. However, the enzymatic glycosylation, like all enzymatically catalyzed reactions, favors, through catalysis, a reaction that would normally occur without the enzyme, although at a much slower rate. In the presence of persistently high ambient glucose concentrations, glucose molecules apparently can be added to the amino acid backbone of many peptides to create new and potentially pathologic glycopeptides. The glycosolated hemoglobin, HbA1C, is easily measured, and the concentration of this substance in a diabetic's blood has a direct correlation with the degree of ambient hyperglycemia in recent weeks.[27] Therefore a high HbA1C level means that control of hyperglycemia has been poor, not just on the day of blood sampling, but within preceding weeks as well. Although HbA1C has not itself been associated with any malfunction of hemoglobin, the potential importance of glycosylation of other peptides in the evolution of diabetic pathology has been suggested. This glycosylated product can be measured readily and reflects the degree of hyperglycemia and therefore the degree of diabetic control in recent weeks. The ultimate significance of glycosylation in diabetic pathology remains to be determined.

The angiopathy in the retina takes the form of microaneurysms of capillaries. These lesions can rupture with escape of blood and opacification of the eye. Great progress has been made in controlling these lesions by photocoagulation with lasers to thrombose the aneurysms before they burst. Cataract formation is also prevalent in diabetics as a consequence of either derangement of carbohydrate metabolism or accelerated aging.

The renal vasculopathy seen in diabetics was first described by Kimmelstiel and Wilson in 1936. Accumulation of basement membrane material in the mesangium of the glomerulus may either be nodular or diffuse. This glomerulosclerosis leads to proteinuria and eventually to azotemia. All insulin-dependent diabetics who survive 20 years or more will manifest the microscopic lesion, and half of them will have significant renal impairment. The kidney may also be affected by hypertension, atherosclerosis, and infection in diabetes. End-stage renal disease in diabetics is treated by dialysis and renal transplantation.

Diagnosis and Treatment of Diabetes

The diagnosis of diabetes is precise and easily accomplished. Patients with polyuria, polydipsia, and weight loss and especially those with visual disturbances or frequent pyogenic infections should be evaluated for hyperglycemia. A fasting blood sugar ≥ 140 mg/100 ml on more than one occasion defines carbohydrate intolerance and demands for its evaluation oral glucose tolerance testing. After an overnight fast in a patient who has previously had unrestricted calories and unrestricted exercise, 75 g of glucose is given by mouth, and the blood glucose is measured periodically for the next 2 hours. A value of 200 mg/100 ml or greater at 2 hours and at one previous time point defines diabetes mellitus. The test is invalidated by stress from infection, surgery or trauma, prolonged fasting, prolonged physical inactivity, and glucocorticoid or thiazide administration. Therefore testing of hospitalized patients as a group is inappropriate. Furthermore, the benefit of diagnosing mild diabetes mellitus in truly asymptomatic patients is meager in that no treatment is indicated. Therefore oral glucose tolerance testing is not a routine screening test.[5]

The treatment of Type II adult-onset diabetes mellitus, in many, if not most, patients involves caloric restriction and weight loss to restore carbohydrate tolerance. If insulin is required, the goals and considerations for treatment become the same as for Type I. The use of oral hypoglycemic agents (i.e., tolbutamide) has been less important recently because the benefit to patients in the long term has been difficult to document and there has been more than a suggestion that vascular complications are made worse.[7] Perhaps oral agents were misused by patients as an apparently simple alternative to the rigors of dieting. Therefore patients on oral agents may have represented a rather noncompliant population. At any rate, when dietary measures fail to control diabetes Type II, the use of insulin to manage hyperglycemia is becoming more commonplace.

The goals of diabetic management are to keep blood glucose at normal levels, to recognize and treat complications promptly, and to enhance the life-style of patients with this disease. A significant advance has been realized in recent years by improved monitoring of plasma glucose. Traditionally diabetics estimated blood glucose control by monitoring the presence of glucose in the urine using test strips impregnated with glucose oxidase or tubules that tested for glucose as a reducing substance. When plasma glucose exceeded the maximum for renal tubular reabsorption (i.e., 180 mg/100 ml or 10mM), glucose spill in the urine occurred. The greater the plasma glucose, the greater the renal loss. Therefore the more intense the glucose reaction in urine, the greater the need for insulin administration. Despite the usefulness of glycosuria monitoring in most diabetics to determine insulin needs, it must be emphasized that its correlation with the status of glucose intolerance is generally unreliable in renal disease, pregnancy, and unstable or brittle diabetes.

Although urine glucose is preferred in monitoring patients who do not require insulin, blood glucose measurement at home is becoming the recommended parameter for insulin administration. Capillary blood obtained by fingerstick is made to react with glucose oxidase on paper strips and read by a color chart or in a reflectance meter. Plasma glucose is usually about 15% higher than these whole blood measurements. Home blood glucose monitoring offers precise monitoring for very close glucose control.

Another tactic to quantitate the precision of glucose control is the measurement of HbA1c. As previously indicated, this glycosylated hemoglobulin is generated by nonenzymatic means, has a relatively long half-life, and is directly proportional to average ambient glucose. Chromatographic analysis of HbA1c reflects the accumulation of the glycoprotein in recent weeks over the customary 4% of total hemoglobin. The accumulation of HbA1c is an excellent parameter of glucose control over time.

The use of home glucose monitoring and precise review of management by measuring HbA1c are only appropriate in highly trained diabetic patients. The training of diabetic patients to become actively involved in the management of their disease has been greatly promoted and advanced by the American Diabetes Association. The patient from a very early age is an active participant in therapy, recognition of complications, general health maintenance, and life goals. There are instructional peer group camps for children, instructional programs for all ages, mutual support groups, and active encouragement for patients to understand and question the scientific progress being made in the area of diabetes.

Dietary measures to limit disposable glucose have recently been greatly liberalized to permit the diabetic patient more freedom. The effect has been to generally improve adherence by better trained patients to a more acceptable dietary regimen. Carbohydrate constitutes 45% to 60% of daily calories, fat provides 30% to 35% and protein 12% to 20%. Total calories are carefully prescribed on the basis of physical activity.

Appropriate insulin therapy necessitates a familiarity with the various forms available. Insulin is purified from beef or pork pancreas and exists in several modifications. Regular, crystalline insulin, when given subcutaneously, has its onset of action at 30 to 60 minutes, peaks at 3 to 6 hours, and has a duration of action of 6 to 10 hours. Neutral protamine Hagedorn (NPH) insulin is complexed for slower absorption and has its onset of action at 1½ to 3 hours, peaks at 6 to 12 hours, and has a duration of action of 18 to 24 hours. Other forms are available for special purposes, but regular and NPH insulin form the basis for most diabetic management. Some patients develop allergies to the protein sequence of animal insulin. Porcine insulin only differs by one amino acid from human insulin, but standard preparations are contaminated with proinsulin, which is antigenically quite distinct in the C-peptide region. Porcine insulin can be highly purified for the allergic patients. Recombinant deoxyrubonucleic acid technology now offers human insulin for therapy in patients with significant allergy to animal insulins.

Maintenance insulin is administered to keep the plasma glucose below 150 mg/100 ml and above 80 mg/100 ml. Insulin is usually administered as a single morning dose subcutaneously with a supplemental evening dose as needed. The dosage in Type I diabetes varies from 15 to 90 NPH U/day. For apancreatic patients who lack the countervening effects of glucagon, 15 to 20 U/day is generally sufficient. The management of ketoacidosis is a very special case for insulin administration. The acidosis diminishes tissue sensitivity to insulin. Therefore very large amounts of insulin are required. The objectives in treating ketoacidosis are rehydration, restoration of normal plasma pH, reduction in plasma glucose, and replacement of glycolytic pathways for ketogenic pathways by moving glucose into cells. Rehydration is commenced with normal saline at 1 L/hour until heart rate, blood pressure, and urine output suggest improvement in volume status. In adults 2 to 3 L are commonly needed. Hypotonic saline (0.45%) is given at a rate of 1 L every 2 to 4 hours to resuscitate and reduce the hyperosmolarity that follows the osmotic diuresis and high glucose levels. When plasma glucose falls to 300 mg/100 ml, glucose should be added to the intravenous infusion. If the arterial pH is less than 7.1, buffering with intravenous bicarbonate is indicated. As the plasma glucose moves into cells under the influence of insulin, potassium is shifted also. Therefore vigorous potassium replacement is necessary.

The regimen for insulin administration in ketoacidosis is disputed among clinicians. Basically the glucose must be lowered in a patient with rapidly changing insulin sensitivity without inducing an overshoot and potentially fatal hypoglycemia. A safe approach calls for 20 U of regular insulin IV followed by an insulin drip (100 U in 500 ml of 0.45% saline) at 50 to 75 ml/hour. Blood glucose must be measured every 30 to 60 minutes initially until the insulin infusion rate stabilizes. The fatal components of ketoacidosis are dehydration and acidosis. There is no need to cause the glucose to plummet in a short period of time. In fact, rapid reduction can lead to fluid shifts with cerebral edema or fatal hypoglycemia.

Insulin administration in the diabetic patient undergoing surgery will vary depending on the complexity of the operation and the length of time it takes to perform. If the procedure is minor and the operation is performed early in the morning, the insulin dose is delayed until the procedure is completed. For major procedures involving a general anesthetic, a highly workable regimen calls for one half the usual morning dose given subcutaneously as NPH, continuous 5% dextrose infusion IV, and monitoring of the plasma glucose every 6 hours. Insulin is given to keep the glucose level between 150 and 250 mg/100 ml. After surgery insulin orders based on urine glucose are not as precise as orders based on plasma glucose. Continuous insulin infusion with 5% dextrose infusion is appropriate in monitored environments and may replace intermittent insulin administration in perioperative patients. Surgical patients undergoing prolonged operations or undue stress may require 25% to 50% more insulin.

In order to attain a constancy of plasma glucose impossible with bolus injection, continuous subcutaneous insulin infusion (CSII) has been developed in recent years. A programmable pump delivers short-acting regular insulin by means of a subcutaneous cannula. The baseline delivery rate can be increased to cover for the increased carbohydrate absorption after meals. CSII and home glucose monitoring offer the greatest precision in control of ambient glucose. The precision can be documented by following HbA1c levels. However, the impact of this precision on preventing or slowing the development of diabetic complications has not been particularly gratifying.[29]

An unstated belief has long prevailed in the management of diabetes that the complications associated with this disease are the consequence of inferior compliance by the patient and therefore inadequate control of blood glucose. By implication, perfect control of glucose with supplemental insulin should eliminate complications. Although there is some basis for this belief, it cannot be absolutely true. Vascular and retinal complications progress even in patients managed with infusion pumps. To explain the syndrome of diabetes mellitus, there is no reason to propose that the loss of beta cells leads to a deficiency of any hormone other than insulin. However, the exquisite balance between insulin and glucagon metabolism that occurs in the nondiabetic patient has not been achieved by exogenous insulin delivery. Plasma glucose is just a crude measure of the profound coordination that exists between insulin and glucagon release on the body's metabolic compartments and the movement of substrate through those compartments.

Until the interaction of A and B cells is more completely understood and mechanically reproducible, transplantation of islets of Langerhans may offer an option for normal glucose homeostasis in diabetic patients. In rodent models made diabetic with streptozocin, syngeneic islets purified from pancreas of healthy animals can be transplanted into the liver through the portal vein. These animals are permanently replenished and normoglycemic.[1,6] Apparently loss of innervation, acinar relationships, and the introduction of heterotopic relationships do not affect the capacity of the transplanted islets to serve the endocrine needs of these animals. However, the transplanted animals have a distinct advantage over diabetic rats treated with exogenous insulin. Streptozocin-induced diabetic rats maintained on insulin develop retinal and renal changes that resemble those seen in humans. Transplantation of islets of Langerhans can arrest and reverse these changes.[4,18] Therefore the prospect looms for controlling the diabetic syndrome in its entirety rather than controlling only the gross excursions of plasma glucose. The rodent experience with transplantation has been extended to autografts in dogs but not successfully to humans.

Allografting of islets has generally failed in all species in spite of the use of immunosuppression effective for renal or cardiac grafting. Mere immunogenicity of islets as an explanation for this failure seems extreme, but a more precise hypothesis has not been offered. Extensive work currently addresses the problem of islet immunogenicity, which can be reduced by tissue culture, carrier lymphocyte depletion, ultraviolet irradiation, and elimination of Class II antigen-bearing cells by immunotoxins.[28] Another problem in humans is more one of mechanics than species biology in that sufficient islet mass has not yet been retrievable from human pancreas. However, whole pancreas and segments of pancreas on a vascular pedicle have been transplanted in humans with about a 25% success rate. This method of providing an islet cell mass is surgically demanding, but the results have occasionally been spectacular. In addition to controlling hyperglycemia, mesangial changes in the kidneys transplanted to diabetic patients have been reversed by subsequent pancreas transplantation. Thus transplantation holds the promise of truly correcting the diabetic lesion. It remains to be seen whether the propensity for B cell loss will later affect the transplanted islets. However, studying the immune aspects of diabetes has been most revealing. Immune approaches might be useful in preventing the disease entirely.

ENDOCRINE TUMORS OF THE PANCREAS (Table 59-2)

The rich endocrine resources found within the pancreas can generate a wide variety of syndromes and clinical conundrums when one or more of the cell lines becomes neoplastic. The resulting tumors can secrete hormones that occur naturally or entopic to the endocrine pancreas. The tumors can also secrete hormones not normally released from the endocrine pancreas, in which case the secretions are ectopic. Although the endocrine tumors of the pancreas are rare, they have taught us a great deal about the nature of endocrinology in health and disease. For example, hypergastrinemia first described by Zollinger[59] in 1955 has, despite its rarity, greatly advanced our understanding of acid-peptic ulceration of the stomach. Proinsulin was first discovered in secretions of an insulinoma and introduced the concept of large-molecular-weight gene products that are subsequently tailored before secretion.[39]

Our understanding of the nature of endocrine tumors has been greatly advanced by the APUD concept of Pearse and Polak.[41] The capacity to diagnose these tumors has been profoundly enhanced by the availability of radioimmunoassays for the measurement of the endocrine products. Localization of the endocrine tumors has been tremendously aided by selective venous catheterization coupled with radioimmunoassay to identify the source of the abnormal concentrations of the hormones that are found in circulating blood. Localization and logistics for removal of endocrine tumors have been aided considerably by precise arteriography, ultrasound, and computerized tomographic images of the pancreas.[52] Unfortunately a significant number of pancreatic endocrine tumors are malignant with an early propensity to metastasis.

Types of Pancreatic Endocrine Tumors

Insulinoma

Insulinomas are the most common of the pancreatic endocrine tumors and arise from the B cells of the islets. Approximately 80% are solitary and benign; the incidence of malignancy is about 10%. The remainder are either multiple benign adenomas or hyperinsulinism caused by islet cell hyperplasia. In infants hyperinsulinism is usually a result of adenomatous hyperplasia of B cells, i.e., nesideoblastosis. The size of insulinomas is small; about 40% are 1 cm or less in diameter. Tumors are distributed in almost equal numbers throughout the head, body, and tail of the pancreas. Only 1% or less of all insulinomas are ectopic in location, but these are found close to the pancreas in most instances. The MEA-1 syndrome occurs in 4% of patients with insulinomas (see Chapter 60).

The major signs and symptoms of insulinoma are a result of the effects of hypoglycemia (from the hyperinsulinemia) on the central nervous system: these include apathy, sluggishness, irritability, excitement, changes in behavior, and occasionally convulsions and coma. Hypo-

Table 59-2 **PANCREATIC ENDOCRINE NEOPLASIA**

Cell of Origin	Pathology	Metabolic Change	Hormone	Symptoms
B	Adenoma Carcinoma (10%) Hyperplasia	Hypoglycemia Glycogenesis Gluconeogenesis Lipolysis Ketogenesis	Insulin Proinsulin	Those of hypoglycemia
A	Carcinoma (70%) Hyperplasia	Hyperglycemia Glycogenolysis Lipolysis Ketogenesis GI motor changes	Glucagon Enteroglucagon	Dermatitis Ileus Constipation
D	Carcinoma Adenoma	Mixed, mild glucose Biliary Pancreatic exocrine	Somatostatin Insulin Glucagon	Cholelithiasis Steatorrhea Dyspepsia
F	Adenoma	?	Pancreatic polypeptide	None
?	Carcinoma (80%)	H^+ secretion	Gastrin	Acid-peptic ulceration
(Zollinger-Ellison)	Adenoma Hyperplasia			Diarrhea
?	Carcinoma (50%)	Intestinal secretion	Vasoactive intestinal peptide	Diarrhea
(Verner-Morrison)	Adenoma	Gastric secretion Hypokalemia		Hypochlorhydria

glycemia also induces a release of epinephrine, which causes sweating, nervousness, tremor, palpitation, hunger, and pallor. The classic diagnostic criteria (Whipple's triad) are still valid. Whipple's triad includes central nervous system symptoms brought on by fasting, a fasting blood glucose of less than 50 mg/100 ml, and complete reversal of all symptoms by infusion of intravenous glucose.

Insulin levels are high relative to the blood glucose concentration. The insulin-to-glucose ratio is normally less than 0.4, but in patients with insulinoma the ratio is often close to 1 or even greater. The measurement of elevated plasma proinsulin is also helpful in the diagnosis of insulinoma. Furthermore, malignant tumors can be differentiated from benign islet cell lesions by documenting the greater percentage of proinsulin in the total insulin immunoreactivity in patients with malignant lesions.

The traditional diagnostic test for insulinoma is the demonstration of fasting hypoglycemia (less than 50 mg/100 ml). Fasting is continued for 72 hours or until hypoglycemic symptoms appear. Hypoglycemia occurs in two thirds of patients by 24 hours and in 95% by 48 hours. During fasting, insulin levels remain elevated in insulinoma patients because of the autonomous nature of insulin secretion. The provocation tests for insulin release (e.g., tolbutamide, glucagon, leucine, arginine) have been used to make the diagnosis of insulinoma but are thought to be of little value since serum insulin levels can be directly measured. The infusion of insulin secretagogues to normal patients should not result in pathologically low blood glucose levels. However, these secretagogues may provoke an insulinoma to release profoundly pathologic amounts of insulin with consequent hypoglycemia.

Selective angiography with subtraction and magnification techniques is the best way for preoperative localization of an insulinoma. The success rate of localizing these tumors approaches 90%. Selective pancreatic vein catheterization and venous sampling for insulin assay has also been used with considerable success to diagnose and localize the site of insulinomas. Ultrasound and computed tomography have been used to localize these lesions, but in comparison with the other diagnostic modalities available they are of limited usefulness.

Being predominantly benign, insulinomas are the only pancreatic endocrine tumors that can frequently be cured by surgery. Depending on their localization, enucleation or distal pancreatectomy are the treatments of choice. It is rarely necessary to perform a pancreaticoduodenectomy as the initial procedure for a small tumor of the head of the pancreas. The adjunctive therapeutic agent of choice in patients with metastases is streptozocin with a response rate approaching 50%. In patients in whom persistent hypoglycemia poses a problem following presumed successful removal of insulinoma or with metastases, diazoxide is frequently effective in suppressing insulin release.

Gastrinoma (Zollinger-Ellison Syndrome)

The first of the endocrine tumor syndromes identified in pancreatic islets was reported by Zollinger and Ellison in 1955. The tumors responsible for this syndrome, i.e., gastrinomas, not only occur in pancreatic islets but may also be found as isolated lesions within the proximal duodenum or in its vicinity. The cell that gives rise to gastrinoma has not been identified. Gastrin is not a normal product of the islet of Langerhans. The gastrinoma syndrome results from excessive quantities of gastrin released from these tumors and is usually manifested clinically by virulent acid-peptic ulceration of the upper gastrointestinal tract. Such ulceration may be found in the first portion or the duodenum where other forms of acid-peptic disease commonly occur; not infrequently, though, ulcers may occur in aberrant regions such as the distal duodenum and jejunum.[30] These ulcers usually are single, but on occasion they may also be multicentric. Generally the ulcer precedes identification of the tumor by 3 to 5 years; on occasion the ulcer itself is totally asymptomatic and is discovered accidentally. In approximately 20% of patients, diarrhea with steatorrhea is the only clinical symptom of the syndrome; this presumably occurs because of the excessive acid production of the stomach that inactivates pancreatic enzymes and thereby inhibits fat digestion and absorption by the duodenum and jejunum.

Approximately one third of patients with hypergastrinemia caused by gastrinoma have relatives with endocrinopathies. This condition is commonly suspected because of refractory or recurrent acid-peptic disease. Upper gastrointestinal x-ray films frequently show a suspicious multiplicity of ulcers throughout the duodenum and even the proximal jejunum. Hypertrophic mucosal folds are evident in the stomach secondary to the hypergastrinemia. Before the availability of radioimmunoassay enabling measurement of serum gastrin levels, the clinical diagnosis of gastrinoma was made on the basis of gastric analysis. The high volume of gastric secretion in gastrinoma patients displayed an acid output that approached the physiologic maximum elicited by histamine derivatives. Currently the diagnosis is made on the basis of the demonstration of hypergastrinemia under fasting conditions. A serum gastrin in excess of 200 pg/ml is suggestive of this syndrome. When the gastrin levels exceed 100,000 pg/ml, extensive tumor involvement, including hepatic metastasis, is highly probable. For equivocal levels of fasting gastrin, provocative testing with secretin has been useful. A rise of at least 100 pg/ml over a fasting baseline after 2 U/kg of secretin given as an intravenous bolus is diagnostic of the disease. Gastrin levels may also be elevated in some patients with hyperplasia of the G cells in the antrum. However, in this circumstance serum gastrin will not change during secretin provocation.[58]

The ulcerogenic gastrinoma may be localized in approximately one third of cases with angiography.[15] Computed tomography will often demonstrate pancreatic tumors if they are larger than 2 cm. Successful localization of pancreatic tumors by computed tomography approaches 32% overall for primary pancreatic tumors.[10] Preoperative ultrasound in the intact patient has not been as successful as desired; however, intraoperative ultrasound has been useful in identifying lesions not obvious. Percutaneous transhepatic portal and pancreatic venous sampling for gastrin can also localize the source of the systemic hypergastrinemia.[21]

Hypergastrinemia caused by gastrinoma is ideally treated by complete resection of the gastrinoma. Unfortunately this is possible in only approximately 20% of patients because the gastrinomas may be multiple or metastatic at the time of diagnosis. Until recently, total gastrectomy was uniformly accepted as the treatment of choice to control the acid-peptic disease in those patients for whom complete tumor excision was not possible. The concept of end-organ ablation by surgical removal has been challenged with the development of H_2 receptor antagonist therapy.[14] Parietal cell vagotomy can improve the effectiveness of cimetidine therapy,[48] but tumor plus end-organ ablation appears to be the only secure procedure to restore serum gastrin levels to normal. Of interest, an effect of the stomach on enhancing tumor growth has been proposed,[13] i.e., if the stomach is removed, tumor growth is slowed. Since 80% of gastrinomas are malignant, metastatic disease is not uncommon. In this circumstance palliation with streptozocin has produced a positive response in about half of patients with metastatic gastrinoma. For a more comprehensive discussion of gastrinoma, see Chapter 16.

Glucagonoma

Glucagonoma is a neoplastic condition of the A cells of the islets of Langerhans in which the entopic hormone glucagon is released. The tumor is malignant approximately two thirds of the time, with early metastases to regional lymph nodes or the liver. Distant metastases are uncommon. The tumors are more frequently found in the tail of the pancreas where there is the largest representation of A cells.

Glucagonoma causes a striking clinical syndrome manifested biochemically by hyperglycemia from the hyperglucagonemia. Patients with the syndrome sustain marked weight loss and demonstrate glossitis, frequent venous thrombosis, depression, and diarrhea. The most striking feature of this syndrome is called necrolytic migratory erythema.[42] This skin lesion consists of erythematous macules and pustules together with flaccid bullae. The necrolytic pattern is present on portions of the skin that are easily traumatized. Histologically there is superficial epidermal necrolysis and severe inflammation of the dermis with cellular infiltration. There is no explanation for this dermatologic phenomenon that resolves after resection of the glucagonoma. The patients also demonstrate a normochromic, normocytic anemia. The hyperglycemia is not usually particularly severe. The metabolic consequences of hyperglucagonemia include rapid movment of the plasma amino acids into gluconeogenic pathways in the hepatic cytosol. The consumption of amino acids for gluconeogenesis depletes the circulating pool of amino acids and results in a hypoaminoacidemia. This pool is not rapidly replenished by a complementary catabolism of muscle protein. The degree of hyperglucagonemia would be expected to cause a much sharper rise in blood glucose, but this is partially compensated for a slight hyperinsulinism because of the hyperglycemia and also because glucagon is a secretagogue for insulin. Although glucagon does not directly promote loss of muscle protein into the amino acid pool, the brisk gluconeogenesis deprives skeletal muscle of circulating amino acids that might be applied to muscle anabolism. Therefore muscle wasting and weakness are quite prominent. In many ways glucagonoma patients resemble chronically stressed patients who have received inadequate nutritional support.

When the disease is suspected, diagnosis is established by radioimmunoassay for glucagon.[3] In marginal elevations of glucagon, pathologic overresponse to arginine can be demonstrated. Intravenous tolbutamide similarly causes a spectacular rise in glucagon in patients with glucagonoma. Once glucagonoma has been diagnosed, anatomic localization of it by computed axial tomography has been useful because the tumors are frequently rather large in their position in the body and tail of the pancreas. Percutaneous transhepatic venous sampling has not been particularly helpful as a diagnostic aid because of the delicate nature of the glucagon assay and the large number of samples needed for adequate localization. Ultrasound can demonstrate the tumors only when large and bulky.

Radical surgical resection of the tumor is clearly the most satisfactory treatment for glucagonoma. Unfortunately, surgical resection is frequently palliative because of the presence of hepatic metastases. For unresectable or metastatic glucagonoma, streptozocin can be useful in reducing the size of the tumors, slowing the growth of metastases, and reducing the circulating levels of glucagon.[8] The clinical symptoms such as the skin lesion and anemia are ameliorated by streptozocin, but the carbohydrate intolerance does not undergo remission probably because of toxicity of the streptozocin to the B cells of the healthy islets of Langerhans.

Vipoma

Verner-Morrison syndrome was described in 1958 as the third islet-associated syndrome after insulinoma and the Zollinger-Ellison syndrome.[55] These islet cell tumors, called vipomas, secrete vasoactive intestinal polypeptide (VIP). It is not clear which cell in the normal islet gives rise to this tumor. The secreted product is clearly ectopic; and the 28-amino-acid peptide causes watery diarrhea, hypokalemia, hypochlorhydria, or achlorhydria. Only about 100 cases have been described, and in approximately 80% of these a single tumor of the endocrine pancreas has been held responsible for the syndrome. In the remaining 20%, hyperplasia of an uncertain member of the islet cell community has been implicated. Ductal proliferation and an increase in the number of cells in the islets has been described in patients with this syndrome. Approximately one half of the tumors are benign.

The VIP released by these tumors causes diarrhea, with volume losses in the range of 2 to 10 L/day. Associated potassium waste is observed, which leads to hypokalemia. Not infrequently the hypokalemia gives rise to flaccid paralysis and a nephropathy that can lead to renal failure. Hypomagnesemia and mild hypercalcemia have also been described in patients with this syndrome. The clinical effects of excessive VIP secretion are anticipated rather easily by its known biologic action. VIP has specific receptors on the small bowel mucosa, and binding of the peptide causes a sharp rise in AMP, causing the effect of VIP to be similar to that of cholera toxin. The fluid losses are quite similar to those expected in cholera, and therefore Verner-Morrison syndrome has been called pancreatic cholera. VIP has substantial sequent homology to other gastrointestinal hormones such as secretin, glucagon, and gastric inhibitory peptide. Therefore tumors secreting this peptide can (1) enhance the secretion of alkaline fluid by the pancreas, which suggests secretin overactivity; (2) induce hyperglycemia, which suggests a glucagon effect; and (3) strikingly suppress gastric acid secretion like an infusion of gastric inhibitory peptide. The release of VIP from these tumors can occur in paroxysms to give pictures of flushing caused by the vasodilatory reaction of VIP and can lead to some confusion with the carcinoid syndrome.

Diagnosis of the Verner-Morrison syndrome is not easily accomplished since radioimmunoassay for vasoactive intestinal polypeptide is not universally available. Further, a very similar syndrome is also caused by tumors that release prostaglandin E_2. Generally, when the clinical picture of the Verner-Morrison syndrome is encountered, the pancreas is studied by computed tomography, angiography, or ultrasonography for evidence of a pancreatic mass lesion. If a tumor is identified, preferred treatment is by surgical resection. In the presence of hepatic metastases, high-dose steroids and streptozocin have offered reasonable palliation.[43]

PP-oma

A few tumors of the endocrine pancreas have been described that apparently only secrete pancreatic polypeptide (PP). The importance of this is uncertain since there is no specific metabolic or clinical manifestation of these tumors, called PP-omas. Pancreatic polypeptide is released in abnormally large amounts by patients who harbor other kinds of non-B islet cell tumors. Therefore pancreatic polypeptide has been suggested as a marker for other pancreatic endocrine tumors, especially in families with a propensity to develop these lesions. Approximately half of patients with other pancreatic endocrine tumors have an elevation in pancreatic polypeptide. Furthermore, approximately 50% of patients with carcinoid tumors, regardless of site, will demonstrate an elevation in pancreatic polypeptide. When they are present, pancreatic polypeptide–secreting tumors are treated by surgical resection and are usually benign. Most commonly pancreatic polypeptide–secreting tumors present clinically because of the effect of the mass in the pancreas or because of metastases. Therefore the syndrome of pancreatic polypeptide–secreting tumors is not necessarily an endocrine syndrome but one more related to neoplasia. Pancreatic polypeptide is frequently secreted in high concentration in addition to the primary or symptoms-producing hormone in patients with islet cell tumors. Also, the hormone is quite often elevated in the plasma of patients with asymptomatic tumors. Therefore pancreatic polypeptide measurements can be used as a tumor marker to screen patients with multiple endocrine neoplasia—Type I syndrome (MEN-I) for the preclinical appearance of an islet cell tumor.

Somatostatinoma

The first reported case of a somatostatin-secreting tumor was published in 1977. Approximately 20 patients have now been described.[45] These tumors are usually malignant and accompanied by hepatic metastases. Somatostatinomas may be located in the pancreas or duodenum.

Metabolically, somatostatin inhibits numerous endocrine and exocrine secretory functions. Dyspepsia, mild diabetes, and cholelithiasis with steatorrhea constitute the expected pathophysiologic constellation for this endocrine condition. These effects are easily attributable to the inhibitory effects of somatostatin on a wide array of smooth muscle and endocrine secretory events. Somatostatin is inhibitory for essentially all gastrointestinal hormones, including insulin, pancreatic polypeptide, glucagon, gastrin, secretin, motilin, and gastric inhibitory peptide. The mild diabetes is directly attributable to inhibitory peptide. The mild diabetes is directly attributable to inhibition of insulin secretion, whereas diarrhea and steatorrhea are contributable to deficient secretion of pancreatic enzymes. The dyspepsia may be more a motor disturbance in smooth muscle function because, in fact, hypochlorhydria is observed when gastric acid studies are performed in somatostatinoma patients. The reduced muscular tone of the gallbladder presumably leads to gallbladder stasis with the formation of stones. Somatostatinoma patients also uniformly lose weight, which can be attibuted to neoplastic effects or malabsorption.

Somatostatinoma may be identified by elevated levels of somatostatin in the blood. Excessive secretion of somatostatin by these tumors can be induced in response to intravenous tolbutamide. These tumors are identified on computed tomography or angiography, and, if they have not metastasized, they are ideally treated by complete excision.

Other Islet Cell Tumors

A variety of non-B islet cell tumors apparently have no secretory product that can be identified. They generate no endocrine syndrome to lead to their diagnosis, even though they constitute approximately 20% of all islet cell tumors and are most commonly discovered by computed tomography or angiography as incidental structures or as the explanation for a large intraabdominal mass. These tumors can effect the biliary tree by obstruction, which leads to their discovery in approximately half the patients. A tumor marker for these lesions is plasma neuronal-specific enolase, a neural isomer of the glycolytic enzyme enolase. The glycolytic pathway in neural tissue could be very adversely affected by the lowered pH in neural cells, which is the consequence of intense metabolic activity. The enolase found in other tissues is an allosteric subunit enzyme that dissociates in the cytosolic pH found in neural cells. Neuronal-specific enolase is stable in its allosteric confirmation at the pH range associated with neural tissue. This enzyme is common to all APUD and neural cells. In fact, the enzyme is released into the plasma of patients with APUD tumors and can be used as a marker for all APUD tumors.[46]

In as many as 80% of patients with nonfunctioning islet cell tumors, the histology will reveal evidence of malignancy; however, these tumors grow slowly, and even patients with hepatic metastases can experience prolonged survival. Surgical removal is generally the preferred treatment; medical therapy with streptozocin has a good response in patients with metastases.

The endocrine tumors of the pancreas present a challenge to the endocrinologist and surgeon, with the prospect for occasional cure and frequently long-term palliation. Recently, substantial endocrine palliation has been achieved with almost all of the endocrine syndromes by administering long-acting somatostatin to suppress hormone release. This is not a chemotherapeutic agent, and no tumor remission has been seen. However, control of the endocrine syndrome in Zollinger-Ellison, insulinoma, Verner-Morrison, and glucagonoma represents a spectacular improvement in managing these unfortunate patients. A knowledge of the islet cell tumors of the pancreas is important to anyone treating pancreatic neoplasia. In fact, all masses in the pancreas are not evident for a hopeless adenocarcinoma of the pancreas. Indeed, pancreatic masses, even those that occlude the common bile duct, deserve careful attention. The identification of a resectable islet cell tumor can indeed be the very happy conclusion of a diagnostic work-up in which islet cell tumor was not the leading possibility at the outset of the investigation.

SUMMARY

The endocrine pancreas controls the movement of glucose through the extracellular fluid by regulating the generation of glucose and the facilitated diffusion of glucose into most cells. The islets of Langerhans that comprise the endocrine pancreas constitute a community of at least four cell types that are interactive in the islets for the purpose of regulating conflicting secretions that either raise or lower plasma glucose. The A (glucagon), B (insulin), D (somatostatin), and F (pancreatic polypeptide) cells respond to a vast number of secretagogues and antogonists to support a hormonal output compatible with an appropriate hormonal presentation, especially to the liver, to guarantee the movement of glucose in response to substrate demand. These cells join a large number of others strewn along the gastrointestinal tract to secrete the hormonally active gut peptides.

This chapter outlines the anatomy, embryology, and physiology of the islets. The only known spontaneous deficiency disease of the endocrine pancreas, diabetes mellitus, is discussed in some detail. The pathophysiology of the functioning neoplasms of these endocrine cells is also discussed. Although the endocrine neoplasms are quite rare, the metabolic and pathologic sequelae of excess states of these critical hormones serve to reinforce our understanding of metabolism and its hormonal regulation.

REFERENCES

1. Ballinger, W.F., and Lacy, P.E.: Transplantation of intact pancreatic islets in rats, Surgery **72:**175,1972.
2. Banting, F.G., and Best, C.H.L.: The internal secretion of the pancreas, J. Lab. Clin. Med. **7:**251, 1922.
3. Belchetz, P.E., et al.: ACTH, glucagon and gastrin production by a pancreatic islet cell carcinoma and its treatment, Clin. Endocrinol. **2:**307, 1973.
4. Bell, R.H., et al: Prevention by whole pancreas transplantation of glomerular basement membrane thickening in alloxan diabetes, Surgery **88:**31, 1980.
5. Clutter, W.E.: Diabetes mellitus and hyperlipidemia. In Campbell, J.W., and Frisse, M, editors: Manual of medical therapeutics, Boston, 1983, Little, Brown, & Co.
6. Cobb, L., and Merrell, R.: Intrasplenic islet autografts: insulin response to IV glucose challenge, Curr. Surg. **40:**36, 1983.
7. Cornfield, J.: The university group diabetes program: a further statistical analysis of the mortality findings, JAMA **217:**1676, 1971.
8. Danforth, D.N., et al.: Elevated plasma proglucagon-like component with a glucagon-secreting tumor: effect of streptozotocin, N. Engl. J. Med. **295:**242, 1976.

9. Dayhoff, M.O.: Atlas of Protein Sequence and Structure, Silver Spring, Maryland, 1969, National Biomedical Research Foundation Inc.
10. Dunnick, N.R., et al.: Computed tomographic detections of nonbeta pancreatic islet cell tumors, Radiology **135:**117, 1980.
11. Efendic, S., and Luft, R.: Somatostatin and its role in insulin and glucogen secretion. In Cooperstein, S.J., and Watkins, D., editors: The islets of Langerhans, New York, 1981, Academic Press, Inc.
12. Farnby, B., Schmid-Farmby, F., and Grodsky, G.M.: Relationship between insulin release and ^{65}Zinc efflux from rat pancreatic islets maintained in tissue culture, Diabetes **33:**229, 1984.
13. Friesen, S.R.: Treatment of the Zollinger-Ellison syndrome, Am. J. Surg. **143:**331, 1982.
14. Friesen, S.R., et al.: Cimetidine in the management of synchronous crises of MEAI, World J. Surg. **4:**123, 1980.
15. Giacobazzi, D., and Passaro, E.: Preoperative angiography in the Zollinger-Ellison syndrome, Am. J. Surg. **126:** 74, 1973.
16. Goldman, H., Wong, I., and Patel, Y.C.: A study of the structural and biochemical development of human fetal islets of Langerhans, Diabetes **31:**897, 1982.
17. Goodner, C.J., Hom, F.G., and Koerker, D.J.: Hepatic glucose production oscillates in synchrony with the islet secretory cycle in fasting Rhesus monkeys, Science **215:**1257, 1982.
18. Gray, B.N., and Watkins E.: Prevention of vascular complications of diabetes by pancreatic islet transplantation, Arch. Surg. **111:**254, 1976.
19. Henderson, J.R., Daniel, P.M., and Fraser, P.A.: The pancreas as a single organ: the influence of the endocrine upon the exocrine part of the gland, Gut **22:**158, 1981.
20. Houssay, B.A., and Penhos, J.L.: Diabetogenic action of pituitary hormones on adrenalectomized hypophysectomized dogs, Endocrinology **61:**774, 1957.
21. Ingemausson, S., et al.: Pancreatic vein catheterization with gastrin assay in normal patients and in patients with Zollinger-Ellison syndrome, Am. J. Surg. **134:**558, 1977.
22. Itoh, M., et al.: Secretion of glucagon. In Cooperstein, S.J., and Watkins, D., editors: The islets of Langerhans, New York, 1981, Academic Press, Inc.
23. Jaspan, J., et al.: Treatment of severely painful diabetic neuropathy with an aldose reductose inhibitor: relief of pain and improved somatic and autonomic nerve function, Lancet **2:**758, 1983.
24. Kimball, C.P., and Murlin, J.R.: Aqueous extracts of pancreas. III. Some precipitation reactions of insulin, J. Biol. Chem. **58:**337, 1923.
25. Kimmel, J.R., Pollack, H.G., and Hazelwood, R.L.: Isolation and characterization of chicken insulin, Endocrinology **83:**1323, 1968.
26. Klines, I., et al.: Normal insulin sensitivity of the islets of Langerhans in obese subjects with resistance to its glucoregulatory actions, Diabetes **33:**305, 1984.
27. Koenig, R.J., and Cerami, A.: Hemoglobin A, C, and diabetes mellitus, Annu. Rev. Med. **31:**29, 1980.
28. Lacy, P.E.: Experimental immuno-alteration, World J. Surg. **8:**198, 1984.
29. Lauritzen, T., et al.: Effect of one year of near-normal blood glucose levels on retinopathy in insulin-dependent diabetics, Lancet **1:**200, 1983.
30. Lomsky, R., Langr, F., and Vortel, V.: Demonstration of glucagon in islet cell adenomas of the pancreas by immunofluorescent technic, Am. J. Clin. Pathol. **51:**245, 1969.
31. Malaisse, W.J., Senor, A., and Malaisse-Lagae, F.: Insulin release: reconciliation of the receptor and metabolic hypothesis, Mol. Cell. Biochem. **37:**157, 1981.
32. Marincola, F., et al.: The independence of insulin release and ambient insulin in vitro, Diabetes **32:**1162, 1983.
33. Matschinksy, F.M., et al.: Glucoreceptor mechanisms in islets of Langerhans, Diabetes **21:**555, 1972.
34. McGarry, J.D., and Foster, D.W.: Regulation of hepatic fatty acid oxidation and ketone body production, Am. Rev. Biochem. **49:**395, 1980.
35. Meda, P., Perrelet, A., and Orci, L.: Increase of gap junctions between pancreatic B-cells during stimulation of insulin secretion, J. Cell Biol. **82:**441, 1979.
36. Merrell, R.C.: Cell-cell recognition in neuroembryology. In Bradshaw, R.A., and Schneider, D.M., editors: New York, 1980, Raven Press.
37. Metz, S.A., Fujimoto, W.Y., and Robertson, R.P.: Lipoxygenation of arichidoric acid: a pivotal step in stimulus secretion coupling in the pancreatic beta cell, Endocrinology **111:**2141, 1982.
38. Munger, B.L.: Morphological characteristics of islet cell diversity. In Cooperstein, S.J., and Watkins, D., editors: The islets of Langerhans, New York, 1981, Academic Press, Inc.
39. Oyer, P., et al.: Studies on human proinsulin, J. Biol. Chem. **246:**1375, 1971.
40. Pandol, S.J., et al.: Growth hormone-releasing factor stimulates pancreatic enzyme secretion, Science **225:**326, 1984.
41. Pearse, A.G.E., and Polak, J.M.: Endocrine tumours of neural crest origin: neurolophomas apudomas and the APUD concept, Med. Biol. **52:**3, 1974.
42. Pedersen, N.B., Jonsson, L., and Holst, J.J.: Necrolytic migratory erythema and glucagon cell tumour of the pancreas: the glucagonoma syndrome, Acta Derm. Venereol. (Stockh.) **56:**391, 1976.
43. Pignal, F., et al.: Streptozotocin treatment in pancreatic cholera (Verner-Morrison) syndrome, Digestion **24:**176, 1982.
44. Pilo, A., Ferranini, E., and Navalesi, R.: Measurement of glucose induced insulin delivery rate in man by deconvolution analysis, Am. J. Physiol. **233:**E500, 1977.
45. Pipeleers, D., et al.: Five cases of somatostatinoma clinical heterogenity and diagnostic usefulness of basal and tolbutamide induced hypersomatostatinemia, J. Clin. Endocrinol. Metab. **56:**1236, 1983.
46. Prinz, R.A., et al.: Serum markers for pancreatic islet cell and intestinal carcinoid tumors, Surgery **94:**1019, 1983.
47. Reaven, E., et. al.: Effect of age and environmental factors on insulin release from the perfused pancreas of the rat, J. Clin. Invest. **71:**345, 1983.
48. Richardson, C.T., et al.: Effect of vagotomy in Zollinger-Ellison syndrome, Gastroenterology **77:**682, 1979.
49. Rutter, W.J., et al.: An analysis of pancreatic development. In Papoconstautinou, J., and Rutter, W.J., editors: Molecules control of proliferation and differentiation, New York, 1978, Academic Press, Inc.
50. Siperstein, M.D., Unger R.H., and Madison, L.L.: Studies of muscle capillary basement membranes in normal subjects, diabetic and pre-diabetic patients, J. Clin. Invest. **47:**1973, 1968.
51. Srikanta, S., et al.: Pre-Type I diabetes: identical endocrinological course independent of HLA DR types or presence of cytoplasmic anti-islet antibodies, Diabetes **33:**10A, 1984.
52. Stark, D.D., et al.: Computed tomography and nuclear magnetic resonance imaging of pancreatic islet cell tumors, Surgery 94:1024, 1983.
53. Stiller, C.R., et al.: Effects of cyclosporine—Type I diabetes: clinical course and immune response, Diabetes **33:**13A, 1984.
54. Tepperman, J.: Metabolic and endocrine physiology, ed. 3, Chicago, 1973, Year Book Publishers, Inc.
55. Verner, J.V., and Morrison, A.B.: Islet cell tumor and a syndrome of refractory watery diarrhea and hypokalemia, Am. J. Med. **25:**374, 1958.
56. Von Mering, J., and Minkowski, O.: Diabetes mellitus nach pancreasextirpation, Arch. Exp. Pathol. Pharmakol. **26:**371, 1889.
57. Warren, J.H., et al.: Differences in risk of insulin-dependent diabetes in offspring of diabetic mothers and diabetic fathers, N. Engl. J. Med. 311:**149**, 1984.
58. Zollinger, R.M.: The ulcerogenic syndrome. In Fiesen, S.R., editor: Surgical endocrinology, Philadelphia, 1978, J.B. Lippincott, Co.
59. Zollinger, R.M., and Ellison, E.H.: Primary peptic ulcerations of the jejunum associated with islet cell tumors of the pancreas, Ann. Surg. **142:**709, 1955.

60 Clifford W. Deveney and Orlo H. Clark

Multiple Endocrine Neoplasia: Types 1 and 2

Although tumors of the endocrine system most often occur within a single gland and arise sporadically, the concurrence of neoplasms involving multiple endocrine tissues, developing familially in an autosomal dominant pattern, and giving rise to well-characterized clinical syndromes, is now solidly established. The familial association of tumors of the pituitary gland, the parathyroid glands, and the pancreatic islets has been referred to as multiple endocrine neoplasia Type 1 (MEN 1). The association of familial medullary thyroid carcinoma and pheochromocytoma has been termed multiple endocrine neoplasia Type 2 (MEN 2). MEN 2 is now known to occur in two variants. MEN 2a is characterized by medullary thyroid carcinoma, pheochromocytoma, and hyperparathyroidism, whereas the rarer but more lethal MEN 2b includes medullary thyroid carcinoma and pheochromocytoma in association with mucosal neuromas, intestinal and oropharyngeal ganglioneuromatosis, and a marfanoid habitus.

In both MEN 1 and 2 syndromes, most cells involved in tumors are cells of the *amine precursor uptake and decarboxylation (APUD)* series, a characteristic that all these cells share. The APUD cells are found in the central nervous system (CNS) (hypothalamus, pituitary axis, pineal gland), gut, thyroid, and placenta and possess common biochemical functions (i.e., the uptake of amine precursors and the production of peptides). The initial postulate that the APUD cells had a common origin from the neural crest has since been disputed, but they all do appear to originate from neural ectoderm. These cells also possess a common enzyme, *neuron-specific enolase*. The concept of a common origin for these cells in diverse locations is appealing because it might explain the secretion of common peptides by APUD cells in the gut, thyroid, and CNS. The APUD concept is also fascinating in relation to the MEN syndromes because these inherited syndromes involve hyperplasia and tumors of selected APUD cells.

MULTIPLE ENDOCRINE NEOPLASIA TYPE 1

MEN 1, or Wermer's syndrome, is an inherited disorder characterized by the development of endocrine tumors in the parathyroid gland, pancreatic islets, and pituitary gland. In 1954 Wermer[49] was the first to characterize the syndrome and postulate that it was inherited. Subsequent case studies of families with this syndrome have confirmed that the genetic trait is autosomal dominant with a high degree of penetrance. Thus approximately one half of the children of involved individuals will develop the syndrome.[50]

In patients with MEN 1 the pituitary, parathyroid glands, and pancreatic islet cells all contain multiple foci of hyperplasia or neoplasia[25]; however, discrete tumors or the clinical syndromes produced by these cells may not develop. When they become clinically demonstrable, these syndromes usually manifest themselves in a predictable sequence. Hyperparathyroidism appears first and by the end of the third decade of life is present in all affected kindreds. In more than 80% of these patients all parathyroid glands (usually four) are hyperplastic.[22] Multiple adenomas or even solitary parathyroid tumors have also been described but are less common.

Gastrin-secreting pancreatic islet tumors are the next most common entity, followed by insulinomas. Clinical manifestations resulting from islet cell tumors occur in only 50% to 60% of patients. Tumors secreting glucagon, vasoactive intestinal polypeptide (VIP), somatostatin, and pancreatic polypeptide (PP) have all been described, but their occurrence is unusual. Pancreatic islet cell tumors in patients with MEN 1 are multiple and involve the entire pancreas. Microscopically they may appear as multiple islet cell adenomas, islet cell hyperplasia, or nesidioblastosis.[38] A typical microscopic islet cell adenoma is seen in Fig. 60-1. One or several adenomas may enlarge and appear as a dominant tumor(s). These tumors may also be malignant, with the propensity to malignancy depending on the cell type and peptide hormone secreted. An islet cell tumor is demonstrated in Fig. 60-2.

In patients with MEN 1 islet cell tumors have a lower incidence of malignancy than in those patients who sporadically develop these tumors. The MEN 1 patient may eventually develop islet cell tumors secreting several different peptides. Thus a patient with a gastrinoma may subsequently or concomitantly have an insulinoma. Therefore these patients should be periodically screened for other peptide-secreting tumors. PP is usually elevated in MEN 1 patients when they have islet cell tumors or islet cell hyperplasia and thus appears to be a useful marker for the diagnosis of pancreatic tumors in this syndrome.[16] Overt pituitary tumors occur in only 10% to 30% of MEN 1 kindreds, but prolactin levels are elevated in a greater number of patients. Tumors secreting growth hormone (GH), prolactin, melanocyte-stimulating hormone (MSH), and adrenocorticotropic hormone (ACTH) have been described.[37,50]

In summary, the typical MEN 1 patient usually has hyperparathyroidism. If patients do not already have pancreatic islet cell tumors, they are likely to develop them subsequently (50% to 70% probability). The islet cell tumor will be a gastrinoma in 80% of cases, and more than one islet cell endocrinopathy will probably develop. Patients are likely to have or develop functioning pituitary adenomas (GH-, prolactin-, MSH-, ACTH-secreting tu-

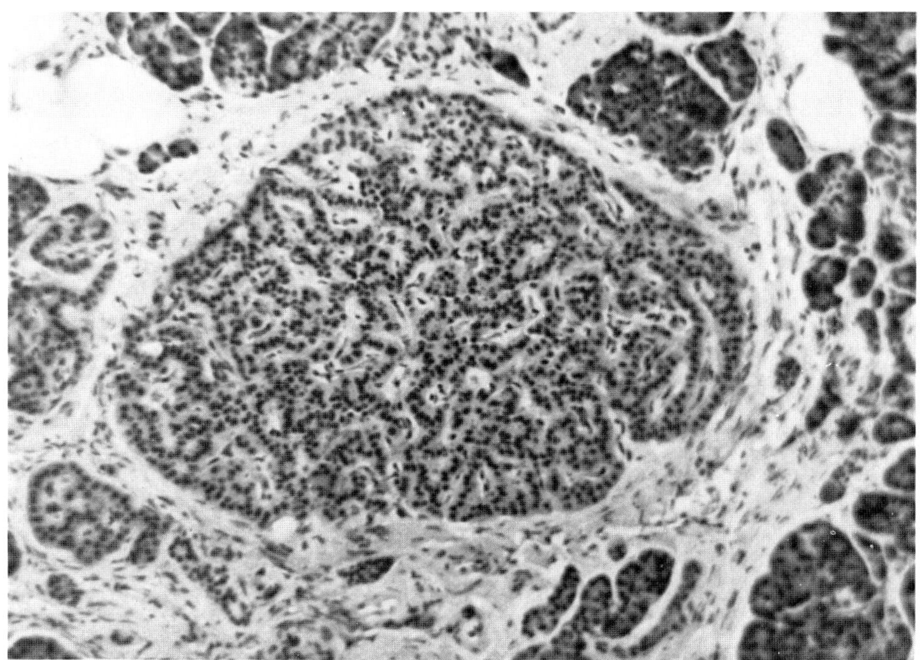

Fig. 60-1 Microscopic islet cell adenoma. Note that the islet has lost the normal architecture and has a uniform follicular pattern. The islet is well encapsulated. Many patients with multiple endocrine neoplasia Type 1 (MEN 1) have similar adenomas scattered throughout the pancreas.

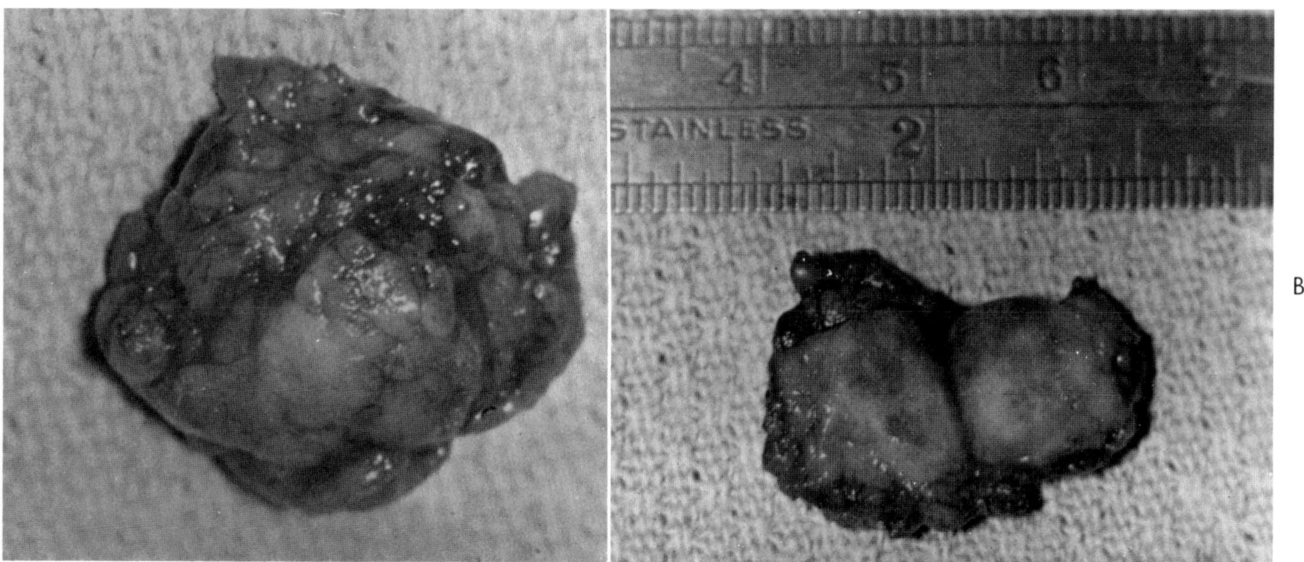

B

Fig. 60-2 Islet cell adenoma 1 cm in size. **A,** It is located within the pancreatic parenchyma and **B,** is more apparent on cut section.

mors) and the accompanying clinical syndromes associated with these hormones (10% to 30% probability).

The parathyroid, islet cell, and pituitary tumors in MEN 1 are multiple, usually involve the entire gland, and will probably continue to develop as long as these glands remain viable. This has therapeutic implications, which are discussed under each syndrome. It also means that these patients must be periodically screened for elevated hormone levels for their entire life. Radioimmunoassays are available for most of the peptides secreted by these tumors, and it is reasonable to screen these patients yearly with measurements of serum calcium, parathyroid hormone (PTH), prolactin, PP, and gastrin since these are the most common peptides secreted. If the patient has symptoms compatible with a syndrome caused by excess of another hormone, the workup for that hormone-secreting tumor should commence. Other tumors rarely occurring in patients with MEN 1 include lipomas and carcinoid tumors. The carcinoid tumors are usually of foregut (thymic, bronchial, or stomach) origin.

Hyperparathyroidism in MEN 1

As already stated, hyperparathyroidism is the most common endocrinopathy in MEN 1 and occurs in almost all patients with this endocrine disorder. It generally appears before the end of the third decade of life, which is earlier than the onset of sporadic hyperparathyroidism, but it rarely occurs before 10 years of age. Essentially all patients with MEN 1 will have parathyroid hyperplasia involving all glands. In contrast, 80% to 90% of patients with sporadic hyperparathyroidism will have a solitary parathyroid adenoma. As in sporadic hyperparathyroidism, elevated serum calcium and PTH levels confirm the diagnosis.

Because of the relatively constant association of parathyroid hyperplasia with MEN 1, any patient who has hyperparathyroidism secondary to parathyroid hyperplasia should be screened for MEN 1 with measurement of serum gastrin and prolactin. Conversely, any patient with a gastrinoma or insulinoma should have a calcium and PTH measurement. In patients with a solitary parathyroid adenoma, screening for MEN 1 is not justified unless symptoms suggest islet cell or pituitary tumors.

The symptoms of hyperparathyroidism are the same in MEN 1 as those in nonfamilial hyperparathyroidism. However, when hyperparathyroidism is detected because of a family history, the endocrinopathy is often diagnosed earlier, and symptoms such as lethargy, weakness, nervousness, constipation, anorexia, polyuria, polydipsia, and nocturia may be mild. These patients should be surgically treated for hyperparathyroidism because when left untreated, some will develop bony, renal, and neuropsychologic complications (see Chapter 55).

When gastrinoma and hyperparathyroidism are both concurrently present, the hyperparathyroidism should be treated first. Reduction of serum calcium to normal levels will facilitate control of gastric acid hypersecretion secondary to hypergastrinemia and will obviate the need for urgent surgery to control gastric acidity. In many patients with primary hyperparathyroidism and gastrinoma, the serum gastrin level will fall to normal for a prolonged period (1 to 5 years) following successful parathyroidectomy.

The surgical treatment of hyperparathyroidism in MEN 1 should consist of subtotal parathyroidectomy (removal of three and one-half glands), which is preferred, or total parathyroidectomy with transplantation of 50 g of parathyroid tissue into the forearm. The thymus should be removed at the time of parathyroidectomy. Thymectomy is performed because of the high frequency of an intrathymic fifth parathyroid gland or parathyroid rests (cell groups) within the thymus. The surgeon should assume that all patients with this syndrome have parathyroid hyperplasia. Hyperplastic glands vary considerably in size so that some glands may appear normal even though diffuse hyperplasia is present. Further, no reliable tests can be performed at surgery to differentiate an adenoma from hyperplasia. The distinction between hyperplasia and a normal gland can also be difficult at times. Thus neck exploration should be performed, with all glands identified and confirmed by biopsy and microscopic examination.

Before performing subtotal parathyroidectomy, one of the smaller parathyroid glands with a particularly good vascular pedicle and distant from the recurrent laryngeal nerve should be identified and partially resected, leaving 30 to 50 g of tissue (the size of a normal parathyroid gland). The gland should be marked with a clip to enable identification if hyperparathyroidism should recur at some point following surgery. Once it is confirmed that this remnant is viable, the other three glands and the thymus should be removed.

An alternate method of treatment is to perform a total parathyroidectomy with autografting of a portion (approximately fifteen pieces 1 mm in size) of one gland to individual pockets in the forearm muscle. The disadvantage of total parathyroidectomy is that at least a 5% chance exists of early or late graft failure and consequent hypoparathyroidism. An advantage of this method is that the autotransplanted parathyroid is easily accessible if hyperparathyroidism recurs. When total parathyroidectomy and autotransplantation are performed, approximately 500 mg of tissue should be cryopreserved to allow retransplantation if the initial transplant fails to function adequately.

In experienced hands the recurrence rate or persistence of hyperparathyroidism after subtotal or total parathyroidectomy is 20% to 30%.[28,40,47] In our experience hyperparathyroidism recurred in seven of 21 patients (33%) who underwent subtotal parathyroidectomy.[6] This high rate of recurrence is caused by the diffuse involvement of all glands.

Pancreatic Endocrinopathies in MEN 1

Fifty percent or more of patients with MEN 1 will develop islet cell tumors of the pancreas. Gastrinoma comprises 80% of these tumors. Insulinoma is the next most common tumor, occurring in about 20% of patients. Other tumors such as vipomas, glucagonomas, somatostatinomas, and PP-producing tumors develop but are rare.

Methods for localizing these tumors are the same as for sporadically occurring endocrine tumors of the pancreas. Computed tomography (CT) scanning will identify most tumors 1.5 cm in diameter or greater, but many tumors are smaller than this.[7,12] Our experience with CT scanning has been good in detecting lesions larger than 1 cm, but we have been unable to see smaller lesions.[35] Tumors larger than 1 cm are usually detectable at surgery. Selective arteriography is helpful in about 50% of patients but usually identifies tumors that are readily apparent to the surgeon. Intraoperative ultrasonography may also be helpful in localization.

Transhepatic portal venous sampling is probably the most sensitive test for diagnosis since it depends on function and not size of tumor. To perform this test, a catheter is placed percutaneously through the liver and into the portal vein. The catheter is then advanced through the portal vein and into the splenic, superior mesenteric, and gastroepiploic veins and their tributaries. Blood is sampled from different positions and assayed for hormones.[17,32,42] An elevation of the hormone production at a specific site suggests that hormone is coming from that area. When hormone levels are essentially the same from all sampling sites, the clinician must assume that hormone production is uniform throughout the pancreas. Selective venous catheterization requires several hours and an experienced radiologist.

Patients with MEN have multiple tumors diffusely scattered throughout the pancreas, and resection of individual tumors is unlikely to result in cure, especially in patients with gastrinomas.

Gastrinoma in MEN 1

The presence of hypergastrinemia and hypersecretion of gastric acid signifies the presence of gastrinoma. The symptoms produced by a gastrinoma are related to the hypersecretion of acid. These patients have intractable ulcer disease and diarrhea. The diarrhea appears to be related to the adverse effects of the excessive hypersecretion of acid on small bowel mucosa and the impairment of fat digestion. Because of the strong association of gastrinoma with MEN 1, every patient with gastrinoma should have a serum calcium level measured to screen for hyperparathyroidism. In most series of gastrinomas the incidence of MEN 1 is 20% to 30%.[43]

Diagnosis. A gastric acid secretion of greater than 15 mEq per H^+/hour accompanied by a serum gastrin concentration greater than 500 pg/ml is diagnostic for gastrinoma. Gastric acid secretion should always be measured when serum gastrin is elevated because gastrins can be elevated in patients with hyposecretion of acid when the gastric pH is 5 or greater.

One other cause of hypergastrinemia with hypersecretion of acid is antral G-cell hyperplasia. This entity can be differentiated from gastrinoma by the *gastrin response to a standard meal*. Patients with antral G-cell hyperplasia will respond to a meal by increasing serum gastrin 100% or more above basal levels, whereas those with hypergastrinemia secondary to pancreatic tumors will have a minimal response to a meal (Fig. 60-3, *A*). When gastrin values are elevated above the normal range (0 to 100 pg/ml) but not high enough to be diagnostic of a gastrinoma (100 to 500 pg/ml), the secretin test or calcium infusion test may be used to stimulate gastrin release from gastrinomas.[9,27]

The *secretin test* is performed by measuring serum gastrin concentration before and 2, 5, 10, and 15 minutes after the intravenous injection of 2 units of secretin/kg of body weight. Patients with gastrinoma will show a prompt increase in serum gastrin of 100 pg/ml or greater, the explanation for which has not been defined. The response is usually seen in the 2- or 5-minute sample. Those patients with hypergastrinemia from antral G-cell hyperplasia and normal individuals with peptic ulcer disease will respond slightly or not at all to secretin (Fig. 60-3, *B*).

The *calcium infusion test* is performed by infusing calcium either as gluconate or chloride at a rate of 5 mg Ca^{++}/kg/hour for 3 hours. Serum gastrin is measured before the infusion and at 30-minute intervals during the infusion. Patients with gastrinoma will demonstrate an absolute increase of 300 pg/ml or more, whereas those without gastrinoma will respond with a change of 100 pg/ml or less. The response in patients with antral G-cell hyperplasia is not as predictable, and some of these patients will have large increases in serum gastrin. Because the calcium infusion test takes much longer to perform than the secretin test and gives essentially the same results, the secretin test in combination with the gastrin response to a standard meal are the two tests most often used to confirm the diagnosis of gastrinoma. The gastrin responses to secretin, calcium, and a standard meal are summarized in Table 60-1.

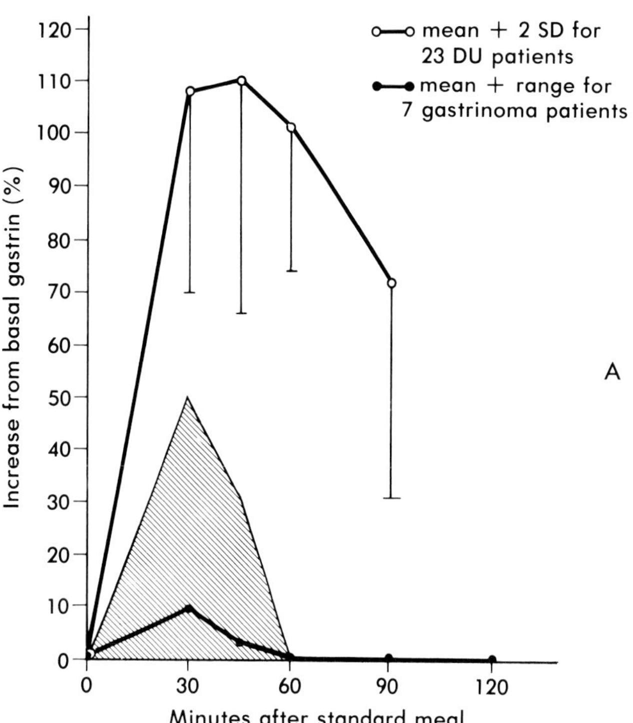

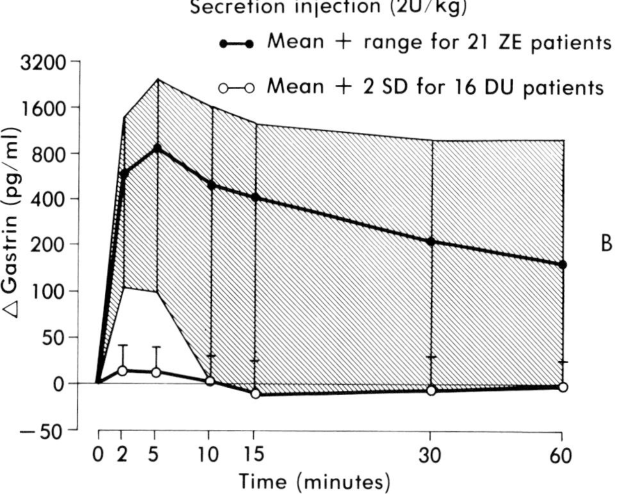

Fig. 60-3 **A,** Gastrin response to a standard meal. Note that the response is expressed as a percentage of the basal level. In patients without gastrinoma the gastrin response to a meal is 70% to 130% of the basal value. The highest increase in patients with gastrinoma is about 40% above the basal level. **B,** Increase in gastrin after secretin administration occurs within 5 minutes of injection.

Table 60-1 **GASTRIN RESPONSE TO PROVOCATIVE TESTS***

	Secretin	Standard Meal	Calcium
Duodenal ulcer	−	+	−
G-cell hyperplasia	−	+	±
Gastrinoma	+	−	−

*+, Positive response; ±, variable response; −, negative response.

TREATMENT. If left untreated, patients with gastrinoma will eventually succumb to the complications of peptic ulcer diathesis secondary to gastric hyperacidity. Therefore the primary objective of treatment is to control acid hypersecretion. The therapeutic options are (1) to treat with H_2-receptor antagonists, (2) to perform a total gastrectomy, and (3) to resect the gastrin-producing tumors.

The *H_2-receptor antagonists* effectively control acid secretion acutely in these individuals, although large doses are usually required (5 to 10 g/day of cimetidine or 0.9 to 1.5 g/day of ranitidine). When using H_2-receptor antagonists in patients with gastrinoma, it is important to measure the acid secretion and adjust the dose of the H_2-receptor antagonist so that the patient secretes less than 10 mEq H^+/hour in the hour preceding the next dose. With high doses of cimetidine, many male patients experience gynecomastia and impotence. For these reasons, ranitidine is the preferred drug.[3,9,10,19,30]

A newer, more potent, and longer-acting H_2-receptor antagonist, famotidine, is now available. In an initial trial, it appears to be superior to cimetidine and ranitidine.[18] Also, a new class of drugs (substituted benzimidazoles, i.e., omeprazole) that block acid secretion by inhibiting the hydrogen ion pump has been initially evaluated for treatment of gastrinoma and shows considerable promise therapeutically. Omeprazole lowers gastric acid 10-fold more than H_2-receptor antagonists and must be given only once daily.[26]

Total gastrectomy was the recommended treatment for gastrinomas before H_2-blockers were available. It effectively removes the acid-secreting organ and improves survival. The procedure can be performed with less than a 5% mortality by an experienced surgeon, and patients tolerate it with minimum dumping syndrome, diarrhea, or weight loss.[3,9,19] Before total gastrectomy is considered, the patient should have had a trial of management with H_2-receptor antagonists. If treatment with H_2-receptor antagonists is unsatisfactory, the patient should subsequently have a total gastrectomy.

Tumor resection conceivably is the ideal treatment. It attacks the problem at its source, that is, excess production of gastrin, and removes a tumor with malignant potential. Unfortunately, in MEN 1, gastrin-secreting tumors are most often multifocal, and tumor resection rarely produces a decrease in serum gastrin. Although curative resections have been reported in approximately 20% of patients with sporadic gastrinoma, the number of cures is considerably less for gastrinoma patients with MEN 1.[15] Even though it is unlikely that resection will result in cure in patients with MEN 1, it is reasonable to explore such patients surgically and resect large pancreatic neoplasms if technically possible. When malignant, these tumors are progressive and eventually lethal. Thus, if a tumor can be enucleated or removed by resecting the tail of the pancreas, this approach is the recommended treatment. The morbidity and mortality of more extensive surgery, such as the Whipple's procedure (pancreatoduodenectomy) or total pancreatectomy, cannot be justified for gastrinoma.

Because vagotomy potentiates the effect of H_2-receptor antagonists, some authorities recommend exploratory laparotomy, resection of the tumor when feasible, and parietal cell vagotomy. The laparotomy enables one to assess resectability of tumor. If resection is not possible, parietal cell vagotomy can be performed with minimum morbidity and will enhance reduction of acid secretion by H_2-receptor antagonists.[31]

Insulinoma in MEN 1

Insulinomas are the second most common pancreatic tumor in the MEN 1 syndrome. Symptoms in patients with insulinoma are secondary to the effect of hypoglycemia on the central and sympathetic nervous systems. Typical symptoms are confusion, hunger, dizziness, paresthesias, bizarre behavior, tachycardia, pallor, and sweating. Hypoglycemic episodes tend to occur in early morning before breakfast, late in the afternoon before dinner, or after exercise. Weight gain is common because the patient's symptoms are ameliorated by eating.

DIAGNOSIS. The diagnostic criteria for insulinoma are hyperinsulinism accompanied by hypoglycemia. Ninety percent of patients with insulinoma will become hypoglycemic after a 12-hour overnight fast. If the fasting period is continued for 72 hours and followed by a brief period of exercise, almost all patients with insulinoma will become hypoglycemic. The standard diagnostic method is to have the patient fast for 72 hours and measure blood sugar and insulin levels at frequent intervals and when the patient is symptomatic.[23] The insulin/glucose ratio is of key importance. In normal individuals this ratio is approximately 0.175 (14 μu/ml insulin at a time when the glucose is 80 mg%). In insulinoma patients this ratio will be increased and is 0.3 or greater.

Insulin is cleaved from a larger molecule called proinsulin. After cleavage, the remaining molecule is called *C peptide* (connecting peptide). Both insulin and C peptide are simultaneously released from the beta cell. The half-life of C peptide is longer than insulin (30 vs. 4 to 8 minutes), thus the molar concentration of C peptide is greater than insulin and is easier to measure in serum. Many investigators recommend measuring both C peptide and insulin in the diagnosis of insulinoma. The C-peptide concentration is especially helpful for distinguishing between patients with insulinoma and those with factitious hyperinsulinism caused by self-administered injections of insulin. Patients who have injected themselves with insulin will have low C-peptide and high insulin concentrations, whereas patients with insulinoma will have high C-peptide and high insulin-concentrations.

Another method for diagnosis of insulinoma is the *C-peptide test*. In this test an intramuscular injection of purified soluble insulin (0.1 u/kg body weight) is given to maintain blood glucose at approximately 40 mg%. This infusion will suppress insulin and C-peptide secretion in normal individuals but not in patients with insulinoma. Thus an elevated C peptide 30 minutes after the insulin injection is diagnostic for insulinoma. This test is recommended for patients in whom insulinoma is strongly suspected but cannot be diagnosed by a prolonged fast.

Proinsulin, which is insulin still connected to C peptide, is also elevated in insulinoma and can be measured by radioimmunoassay. Several provocative tests for insulin release have also been used in the past to diagnose insulinoma. Intravenous tolbutamide and glucagon release insulin. Both these tests have false-positive results and can produce severe hypoglycemia. They are therefore no longer recommended.

TREATMENT. The episodes of hypoglycemia resulting from insulinoma can be ameliorated by frequent small feedings high in carbohydrate. Diazoxide, a thiazide, strongly inhibits the release of insulin from the islet cells and is effective in preventing episodes of hypoglycemia. However, diazoxide can cause fluid retention in some patients, which may preclude its use. The initial dose of diazoxide is 50 mg orally three times daily. This may be increased to 600 mg/day, although most patients are controlled with 300 mg/day or less. The effectiveness of diazoxide is measured empirically by the reduction in the number of hypoglycemic episodes. It can be further quantified by measuring insulin/glucose ratios before and after diazoxide administration. In a patient with a good response, the number of hypoglycemic episodes will be abolished or significantly reduced, and the insulin/glucose ratio will fall to less than 0.3.

Before resection of insulinoma is attempted, all patients should receive a trial of diazoxide because when celiotomy does not reveal discrete tumor(s), the extent of pancreatic resection may be influenced by the response to treatment with diazoxide. In the patient with no obvious tumors who has diffuse microscopic islet cell adenomas, an 80% pancreatectomy is indicated in those who have a poor response to diazoxide, whereas a distal pancreatectomy of less than 80% should be performed in those with a good response to diazoxide.

In non-MEN 1 patients, 80% of insulinomas are benign and solitary, and enucleation of the tumor or resection of the portion of pancreas containing tumor will usually result in cure. In MEN 1, insulinomas are almost always multiple; if multiple insulinomas are present, one should suspect MEN 1. Multiple insulinomas can sometimes be enucleated or treated with distal pancreatectomy. However, because of the high likelihood of microscopic insulinomas or islet call hyperplasia in the remaining pancreas, recurrence of hyperinsulinism is high after local pancreatic resections in patients with MEN 1. For this reason, some have recommended 80% pancreatectomy as the treatment of choice for MEN 1 patients with insulinoma.[21,29]

Attempts should be made preoperatively to localize insulinomas using percutaneous transhepatic portal venous sampling. If a patient has been receiving diazoxide to control the hypoglycemia, this treatment must be discontinued before performing this procedure because it inhibits insulin release. If a localized insulin gradient exists in a certain area of the pancreas, that part should be included in the resection.

Other Islet Cell Tumors in MEN 1

Other islet cell peptide-producing tumors such as vipomas, glucagonomas, somatostatinomas, and PP-omas occur in MEN 1, but they are rare. The presence of these tumors should be suspected only if the patient displays characteristic symptoms.

VIPOMA. High circulating levels of VIP cause severe diarrhea secondary to jejunal secretion and not malabsorption. Gastric acid secretion in these patients is normal or low. Thus measurement of acid secretion can be used to differentiate the diarrhea in vipoma from that produced by gastrinoma, in which acid production is excessive.

Severe, watery diarrhea and hypokalemia, and sometimes hypercalcemia, with low or normal gastric acid secretion should lead one to suspect vipoma. Other causes of diarrhea, such as malabsorption, infection, and surreptitious laxative use, should be ruled out. A high serum or plasma VIP level in a symptomatic patient is diagnostic.

Resection of the tumor is the only means for cure and can be accomplished in about half the patients with vipoma. Half the tumors are also malignant. Streptozocin may produce a temporary remission of symptoms in patients with unresectable tumors. If no tumor is found, it is reasonable to remove the tail and body of the pancreas. In many patients the diarrhea will improve after subtotal pancreatectomy.

GLUCAGONOMA. Glucagonoma syndrome is characterized by a migratory necrolytic dermatitis (usually involving the legs and perineum), weight loss, stomatitis, hypoaminoacidemia, anemia, and mild diabetes mellitus. Visual scotomas and changes in visual acuity have been reported in some cases. The diagnosis may be suspected from the distinctive skin lesion; even the presence of a prominent rash in a patient with diabetes mellitus should be enough to raise suspicions. Elevated serum glucagon levels are diagnostic.

About 25% of glucagon-producing tumors are benign and confined to the pancreas. The remainder have metastasized by the time of diagnosis, most often to the liver, lymph nodes, adrenal glands, or vertebrae. Occasionally hyperglucagonemia is seen with islet cell hyperplasia. Although distinctly rare, glucagonomas have also been reported in the kidney, lung, and intestines.

Surgical removal of the glucagonoma and of resectable metastases is indicated if technically feasible. Even if it is not possible to remove all the tumor, considerable palliation may result from debulking the tumor. Oral zinc supplements may improve the dermatitis. Streptozocin and decarbazine are the most effective chemotherapeutic agents for unresectable lesions. Phenytoin (Dilantin) results in decreased serum glucagon levels. The clinical course generally parallels changes in serum levels of glucagon in response to therapy.

After appropriate preoperative localization studies (CT, angiography, transhepatic portal venous sampling), the patient should undergo laparotomy and attempted tumor resection.

SOMATOSTATINOMA. Somatostatinomas produce few symptoms. Diabetes mellitus (usually mild), diarrhea and malabsorption, and dilation of the gallbladder (usually with cholelithiasis) are common findings in patients with this disease. These tumors are most often malignant and are accompanied by hepatic metastases. The diagnosis may be made by recognizing the clinical syndrome and measuring increased concentrations of somatostatin in the serum. In most cases, however, the somatostatinoma syndrome has been unsuspected until discovered at surgery, and the diagnosis is confirmed by histologic evidence of metastatic islet cell carcinoma. If surgical treatment can only be palliative, chemotherapy with streptozocin, decarbazine, or doxorubicin hydrochloride is sometimes helpful.

PP-OMA AND "NONFUNCTIONAL" TUMORS. Pancreatic polypeptide (PP) is consistently elevated in the serum of MEN 1 patients with any pancreatic tumor and is considered a good tumor marker in the MEN 1 syndrome. PP-omas, or pure pancreatic polypeptide tumors, occur in MEN 1 but are extremely rare. Excess production of PP produces no symptoms so that these tumors are usually large, unresectable, and metastatic at the diagnosis. Islet cell tumors that are "nonfunctional," that is, producing no known peptides, have also been reported.

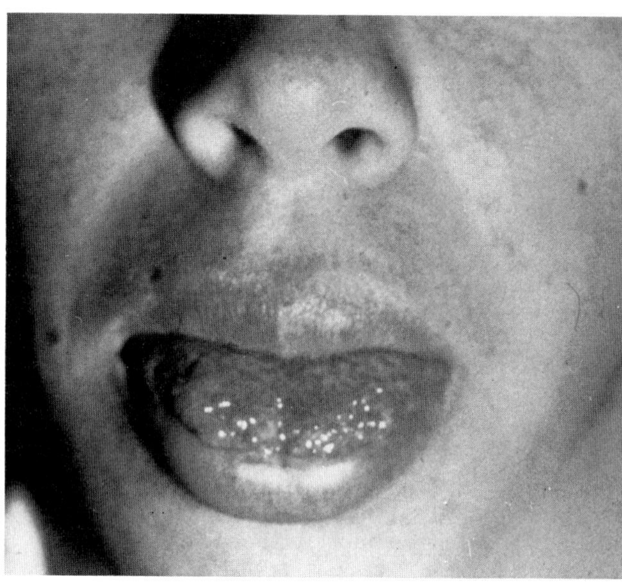

Fig. 60-4 Patient with MEN 2b. Note the small tumors on the tongue and the puffy lips.

Pituitary Lesions in MEN 1

Although all MEN 1 patients have microscopic pituitary lesions, only 30% are symptomatic. The symptoms may be caused by excess production of peptides by the tumors or may be secondary to neurologic impingement by tumor and decreased pituitary function.

Pituitary tumors may secrete a variety of hormones, including GH, ACTH, and MSH, but prolactin is the most common. Females with hyperprolactinemia usually are infertile and have irregular menses and galactorrhea. In males the symptoms are subtle and include loss of libido and impotence. Excess of the other hormones can produce typical syndromes, such as Cushing's disease (ACTH excess) and acromegaly (GH excess). If the tumor becomes large (i.e., greater than 5 mm), it can extend in the suprasellar space and impinge on the optic nerves and cause bitemporal visual field defects or headaches and cranial nerve deficits.

Transphenoidal hypophysectomy is the treatment of choice for small symptomatic tumors. Larger tumors may require treatment with surgery (transfrontal) and radiation therapy. Bromocryptine has been used successfully to treat symptoms in patients with functioning prolactinomas.

MULTIPLE ENDOCRINE NEOPLASIA TYPES 2A AND 2B

MEN Types 2a and 2b are inherited syndromes characterized by the development of medullary carcinoma of the thyroid (MCT) and pheochromocytoma. Patients with MEN 2a will also develop hyperparathyroidism, which is usually secondary to parathyroid hyperplasia. Patients with MEN 2b have a marfanoid habitus and hyperelastic joints and develop submucosal ganglioneuromas of the oropharynx at an early age. MEN 2b patients also have a characteristic facies with puffy lips and eyelids (Fig. 60-4). MEN 2b patients only rarely develop hyperparathyroidism, but medullary carcinomas appear at an earlier age, often in infancy, and are more virulent than in patients with MEN 2a.

Both MEN 2a and 2b are inherited through an autosomal dominant gene, which means that one-half the offspring of an affected individual will inherit the syndrome. MEN 2b also occurs as a spontaneous mutation, so many patients with MEN 2b will have no family history of this syndrome. Researchers initially believed that different genes were involved in the two syndromes, but recent evidence suggests that the defects producing MEN 2a and 2b are from different loci on the same gene.[1,8,36] The parafollicular or C cells of the thyroid, the tumor cell in MCT, and the adrenomedullary cell, the cell of the pheochromocytoma, are APUD cells and originate from the neural crest, as do the ganglioneuroma cells. Thus all the cells involved in these syndromes have a common neural origin. The parathyroid cells do not originate from the neural crest, but rather from neuroectodermal placodes.

All the tumors in MEN 2 are multifocal, diffuse, and bilateral. Neoplastic changes are usually preceded by hyperplasia. MCT will appear in 100% of patients with MEN 2a and 2b and is the most life-threatening lesion in this syndrome. Pheochromocytomas occur in about 40% to 50% of patients with MEN 2a and 2b.[48] The pheochromocytomas are almost always benign, although malignant forms with metastases have been reported.[5] Hyperparathyroidism occurs in about 60% of patients with MEN 2a and is most often secondary to parathyroid hyperplasia. A substantial number of these patients have normocalcemic hyperparathyroidism. The marfanoid habitus and oral submucosal ganglioneuromas occur in almost all patients with MEN 2b. Submucosal ganglioneuromas usually develop before MCT and may suggest the diagnosis of sporadic development of MEN 2b. These lesions are sometimes subtle and may go unnoticed for many years. Early rec-

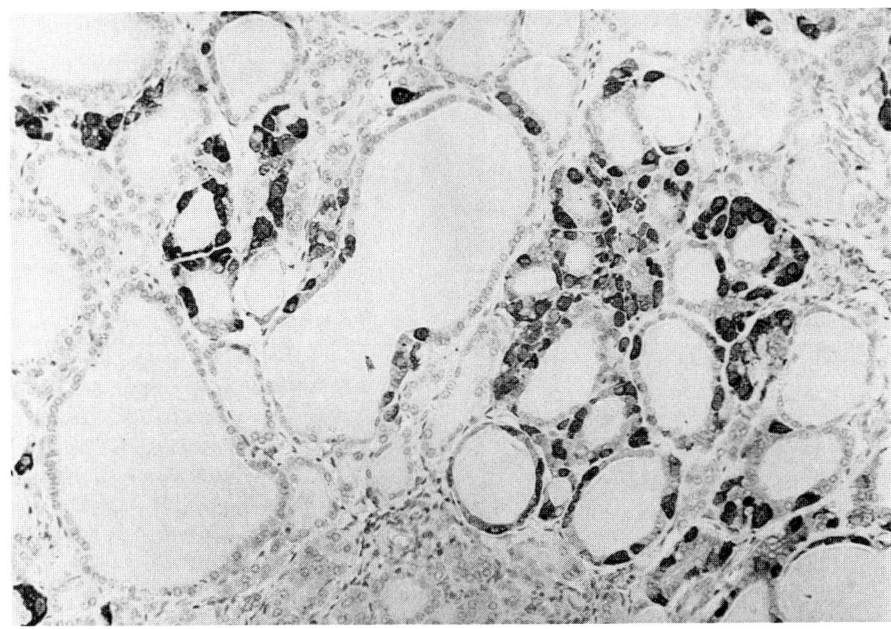

Fig. 60-5 C-cell hyperplasia. C cells are stained with an immunoperoxidase technique with antibodies directed to calcitonin. The parafollicular C cells are increased in number but have not formed discrete tumors.

ognition and diagnosis is important in MEN 2b because few patients can be cured of MCT when diagnosed after childhood.[20]

Medullary Carcinoma of Thyroid in MEN 2

MCT originates from the calcitonin or "C" cells that are located around the periphery of the thyroid follicles. These cells secrete calcitonin. The presence of elevated serum calcitonin basally or increased calcitonin levels in response to provocative stimuli can be used to diagnose patients with MEN 2 when they have C-cell hyperplasia that resembles MCT early in its evolution (Fig. 60-5).[41] About 80% of cases of MCT occur sporadically, and the remaining 20% occur with MEN 2a, MEN 2b, and in another inherited (familial) disorder without MEN. In sporadic MCT the tumor usually appears in the third to fourth decades of life and is usually confined to one lobe of the thyroid. In the MEN 2 syndromes MCT is always bilateral and generally appears before age 30 in MEN 2a and before age 5 in MEN 2b.

Diagnosis. Elevated serum calcitonin or increased calcitonin levels in response to provocative stimuli in patients suspected of having MEN 2 are diagnostic of MCT.[44,45] Since 100% of patients with MEN 2a and 2b will develop MCT, patients with known MEN 2a or 2b or those at risk to develop the syndrome should be screened with a serum calcitonin every 6 months. If the basal calcitonin level is normal, screening should also include levels in response to provocative stimulation (see following paragraphs). For those patients with MEN 2a, screening should begin early in the second decade of life; for those with MEN 2b, screening should begin in infancy since these tumors often develop at this time in this variant of MEN 2.

Calcitonin is often not measurable in individuals without MCT and is never greater than 200 pg/ml. Therefore a basal calcitonin level greater than 250 pg/ml is diagnostic for MCT. However, in patients with MEN 2a or 2b who have not yet developed elevated calcitonin levels, provocative tests for calcitonin release should be used to diagnose microscopic MCT or C-cell hyperplasia, which is a precursor of MCT.

Pentagastrin and *calcium* as calcium gluconate are both used as provocative agents for calcitonin release. As single agents, they are roughly equally effective, but the combination of the two increases the release of calcitonin significantly in patients with MCT, and the combination is the preferred method of testing. When combined, 5 μg/kg pentagastrin is given as an injection and calcium gluconate (2 mg Ca^{++}/kg) is infused over 1 minute. Blood for calcitonin measurement is collected before and at 1, 2, 3, 5, 10, and 15 minutes following injection. With a positive response, an abrupt increase in calcitonin occurs within 5 minutes of injection. Fig. 60-6 depicts a typical positive response after pentagastrin alone; the response to combined agents is similar but more pronounced. Normal subjects respond with an increase in calcitonin of less than 200 pg/ml, whereas patients with MCT respond with an increase of 300 pg/ml or greater.[44,46]

The calcium and pentagastrin test should routinely be performed in patients with MEN 2a and 2b who have normal serum calcitonin; when they become positive, they should have a total thyroidectomy. A basal calcitonin value of 250 pg/ml or greater or a stimulated increase of 300 pg/ml or more are both diagnostic for MCT. These values will vary somewhat in different radioimmunoassays. The routine use of these provocative tests in MEN 2a and 2b patients has enabled the physician to make an early diagnosis of MCT when patients still have C-cell hy-

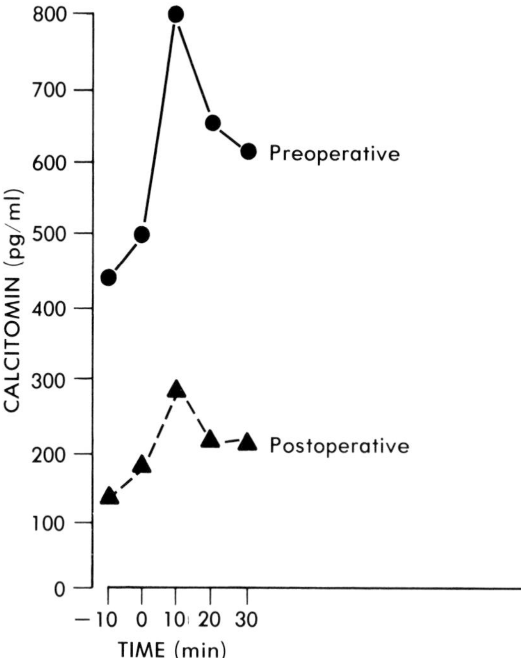

Fig. 60-6 Serum calcitonin response to pentagastrin pre- and postoperatively. Note the fall in serum calcitonin postoperatively. The reduction in calcitonin was not down to normal, and this patient probably has residual MCT. The time course of the response to pentagastrin is similar to the response seen with the combination of pentagastrin and calcium.

perplasia or small microscopic foci of tumor. The cure rate in these patients at this stage of disease is excellent. The importance of screening with calcitonin tests in MEN 2b patients in infancy cannot be overemphasized. To achieve cures in these patients, diagnosis and treatment must begin in infancy.

To increase the accuracy and sensitivity of screening, MEN 2 patients should be tested annually. If basal calcitonin exceeds 250 pg/ml or if the response to calcium and pentagastrin is greater than 300 pg/ml, total thyroidectomy is recommended. If basal and stimulated calcitonin levels are in an equivocal range (i.e., 200 to 250 pg/ml), one should attempt to localize calcitonin release to the thyroid gland. The inferior thyroid vein should be cannulated and blood collected for calcitonin. If calcitonin values are elevated basally or after provocative tests in the venous effluent of the inferior thyroid vein, the diagnosis of MCT or C-cell hyperplasia is made and total thyroidectomy is recommended. If serum calcitonin values are less than 300 pg/ml with provocative testing, the patient should be followed and tests repeated in 6 to 12 months.[44]

Serum calcitonin levels are also a good indicator of residual or metastatic tumor and have proved useful in following patients with MCT after thyroid resection. Patients with disease limited to the thyroid gland usually have calcitonin levels below 500 pg/ml, and those with metastatic disease have calcitonin levels greater than 1000 pg/ml. The calcitonin level does correlate with the number of metastases; that is, the larger the number, the higher is the level.

Calcitonin can also be secreted by other causes:

1. Malignant neoplasms: oat cell, breast, laryngeal, pancreatic, and prostatic cancer
2. Endocrine neoplasms: carcinoid tumors, pheochromocytoma, gastrinoma
3. Inflammatory bowel disease: regional enteritis
4. Organ failure: chronic pulmonary disease, renal failure, liver failure
5. Other: trauma, severe burns, pregnancy, breast-feeding

However, extraneous sources of calcitonin seldom present a problem in following MEN 2 patients after thyroidectomy or in making the diagnosis of MCT.

Patients with sporadic MCT usually have a thyroid nodule or a metastasis to a cervical lymph node. The physician should ask any patients with a thyroid nodule if they have hypertension, episodic headaches, sweating, or palpitations. One should also inquire about the family history of thyroid tumors or severe hypertension in relatives. If any of these factors is present, patients should be evaluated for pheochromocytoma and have the thyroid nodule aspirated with a fine needle for cytologic examination. If one fails to diagnose an associated pheochromocytoma in a patient with MCT, a hypertensive crisis and death may occur either with induction of anesthesia or during the surgical procedure to resect the thyroid.

About 40% of patients with MCT have calcification within the thyroid situated at the junction of the upper and middle one third of the thyroid gland (i.e., the site of the greatest concentration of C cells in the normal thyroid gland). Such a finding on a neck radiograph would suggest the presence of MCT. A needle aspiration of the nodule is helpful in determining the type of nodule. Screening tests for serum calcitonin levels or following provocation with pentagastrin and calcium are not recommended for routine evaluation of patients with thyroid nodules because of the low incidence (2% to 3%) of MCT in thyroid nodules.

Treatment. The minimum surgical treatment of MCT in MEN 2 is total thyroidectomy and removal of the lymph nodes in the central neck extending from the arch vessels in the superior mediastinum to the thyroid cartilage. This should include the thymus. If any of the cervical lymph nodes is involved, a modified radical or radical cervical lymph node dissection on the involved side should be performed. A careful examination of the parathyroid glands should also be performed because hyperparathyroidism secondary to hyperplasia or adenoma frequently accompanies MEN 2a.[33] The parathyroid glands in these patients should also be marked at surgery in the event that subsequent identification becomes necessary at a later date.

Several weeks after total thyroidectomy and node dissection the patient should have basal and stimulated calcitonin values measured. If the levels remain increased or are positive with provocative testing, the patient should have cervical and hepatic veins catheterized. If the elevated calcitonin levels localize on the side of the neck (i.e., the cervical levels are higher than the hepatic vein levels), the patient should have a modified neck dissection, if not already done, on the side of the most extensive tumor or where the serum calcitonin level was elevated. Most patients with persistent disease have tumor in the ipsilateral cervical nodes or in the superior mediastinal nodes. If the plasma calcitonin levels in the hepatic veins are equal to or higher than those in the cervical veins, distal metastases are present and a second procedure is not indicated. The most common sites for MCT to metastasize after the regional lymph nodes are lung, liver, adrenal glands, and bone.

Surgical resection is the only effective treatment for MCT. Anecdotal reports indicate that some of these tumors respond to iodine-131 (^{131}I); however, these reports are few, and no evidence suggests that C cells themselves take up iodine. MCT is also relatively insensitive to radiation therapy. Likewise, most chemotherapeutic agents such as cyclophosphamide (Cytoxan), methotrexate, and fluorouracil are ineffective, although several reports suggest that doxorubicin hydrochloride (Adriamycin) has produced palliation and partial remission in some patients.

The overall 5-year survival of patients with MCT varies from 25% to 75%. Survival can be predicted by the extent of tumor at the initial surgery. Patients with C-cell hyperplasia or microscopic MCT are almost always surgically cured, and 80% to 85% will be free of disease in 5 years. Patients with MEN 2b have a poorer prognosis than those with MEN 2a. Further, patients with a homogeneous distribution of C cells by immunoperoxidase staining of the tumor also have a better prognosis than those with a heterogeneous distribution.

Pheochromocytoma in MEN 2

Pheochromocytoma in MEN 2 usually becomes apparent after MCT. It is not known whether the actual tumor develops later or if the disease becomes clinically manifest later. Adrenomedullary hyperplasia probably occurs first and progresses to pheochromocytoma.[24] Unlike MCT, pheochromocytomas are almost always benign. These tumors are almost always bilateral, or a tumor may involve one adrenal gland and medullary hyperplasia may involve the other. The tumors are often multifocal within the gland. About half the patients with MEN 2a or 2b will develop pheochromocytoma.[48]

Diagnosis and Symptoms. The symptoms of pheochromocytoma are those of catecholamine excess, such as hypertension, palpitations, and headache. The primary risk in patients with pheochromocytoma is death from hypertensive crisis, which may be the first manifestation of the disease. Because pheochromocytoma is a part of MEN 2, all patients with this endocrinopathy or with MCT should be screened for pheochromocytoma before thyroid surgery.

Pheochromocytoma is diagnosed by measuring elevated catecholamines or their metabolites in plasma or urine. The substances measured are epinephrine, norepinephrine, and the metabolites metanephrine and vanillylmandelic acid (VMA). A urinary VMA greater than 11 mg/24 hours or urinary metanephrine greater than 1.8 mg/24 hours is diagnostic. Plasma catecholamines (epinephrine and norepinephrine) greater than 2000 pg/ml are also diagnostic for pheochromocytoma.

If these tests are equivocal, the diagnosis can be made by the *glucagon stimulation test* or the *clonidine suppression test*. Glucagon is given intravenously in a bolus of 1 to 2 mg and should produce a threefold increase in epinephrine and norepinephrine or an absolute increase greater than 2000 pg/ml 3 to 5 minutes after injection. The glucagon stimulation test will probably elevate the blood pressure and should not be used in patients with diastolic pressures of 110 mm Hg or greater. Clonidine is an alpha-adrenergic agonist and suppresses the release of catechols from neural tissue but not tumors. The clonidine suppression test is performed by giving 0.3 mg of clonidine and measuring plasma epinephrine and norepinephrine 2 to 3 hours later. In patients without tumor plasma, these catecholamines should be less than 500 pg/ml. Because clonidine has the potential to cause hypotension, marked volume depletion should be corrected, and concomitant use of antihypertensive agents, particularly beta-adrenergic blockers, should be avoided when performing this suppression test.[4] Patients in MEN 2 kindreds should be screened yearly or whenever symptoms suggesting pheochromocytoma appear.

When pheochromocytoma is diagnosed, one should attempt to localize the tumor. CT scanning is the least invasive method and will demonstrate tumors larger than 1 cm; however, the CT scan is not helpful for smaller tumors or for adrenomedullary hyperplasia. In adrenomedullary hyperplasia the adrenal medulla changes little in size, but the cortex thins out and the ratio of medulla to cortex increases.

Iodine-131 metaiodobenzylguanidine (MIBG), a radionuclide specific for catecholamine precursors in the adrenal medulla, demonstrates pheochromocytomas present in the adrenal, in ectopic positions, and in metastatic deposits.[2,13] This nuclide also reveals adrenomedullary hyperplasia. The test is relatively noninvasive and aids greatly in the localization of pheochromocytomas. It is especially helpful for localizing extra-adrenal pheochromocytomas. In a recent study MIBG had a 87.9% sensitivity and a 98.9% specificity.[34] MIBG has also been used to treat a few patients with unresectable pheochromocytomas in the same way that radioactive iodine is used to treat patients with metastatic, differentiated thyroid cancer. Its ultimate role as a therapeutic modality remains to be defined.

Arteriography is rarely necessary to identify the presence of a pheochromocytoma. Selective adrenal vein sampling of catechols is a very sensitive technique, but it is often difficult to perform because of problems catheterizing the right adrenal vein. Arteriography or selective venous sampling should only be done after the patient has been prepared with alpha-adrenergic blockers, as for surgery. (See also Chapter 57 and the following discussion.)

Treatment. After preoperative preparation the patient should undergo resection of the tumor. Preoperative preparation consists of blocking the potential effects of catechols released by the tumor. Phenoxybenzamine, a long-acting alpha-adrenergic blocker, is initially used at a dose of 10 mg orally three times daily. This dose is gradually increased along with vigorous hydration until the patient has mild orthostatic hypotension. This allows expansion of a contracted blood volume and may demonstrate an anemia. If anemic, the patient should receive blood transfusions as clinically indicated. If tachycardia or arrythmias persist after alpha-adrenergic blockade and rehydration, beta-blockade with propranolol should be instituted. One should initiate preoperative blockade at least 10 days before invasive localizing procedures or surgery. Intraoperative blood pressure should be monitored because even when preoperative blockade is adequate, hypertension can occur intraoperatively, particularly when the tumor is manipulated.

The incision for resecting pheochromocytoma in MEN 2 patients should allow access to both adrenal glands and the periaortic area because bilateral tumors, extra-adrenal tumors, or adrenomedullary hyperplasia may be present. If both adrenal glands contain tumors, bilateral adrenalectomy is recommended. When one gland appears normal following localizing studies and palpation, it is unclear whether the normal-appearing gland should be removed.[14,39,41] Some authorities recommend bilateral adrenalectomy for all MEN 2 patients with biochemical evidence for pheochromocytoma because the "grossly normal" gland is always involved with at least medullary hyperplasia or occult tumors. These investigators believe that the risk of recurrent pheochromocytoma and the attendant complications of hypertension and possible malignant degeneration warrant removal of the normal-appearing gland.

Control of the hypoadrenal state is usually easily managed by the daily administration of hydrocortisone (20 mg in the morning and 10 mg in the afternoon or evening). Others have elected to remove only the abnormal gland, stating that no evidence suggests that the remaining gland will eventually develop a functioning pheochromocytoma, even though hyperplasia is present. Several MEN 2 patients with unilateral adrenalectomies have been followed for 5 to 15 years without developing biochemical evidence of pheochromocytoma in the remaining adrenal gland. More experience and longer follow-up are needed to determine the natural history of these tumors and the role of unilateral or bilateral adrenalectomy when only one adrenal gland is clearly involved.

After resection, patients should be followed regularly with blood pressure measurements and yearly with determination of urinary catecholamines. About 30% of patients with pheochromocytomas will have some residual hypertension despite removal of both adrenal glands and reversal of catechol levels to normal.

Hyperparathyroidism in MEN 2

Hyperparathyroidism secondary to parathyroid hyperplasia occurs in 20% to 40% of patients with MEN 2a. Hyperparathyroidism rarely if ever occurs in MEN 2b. The parathyroid hyperplasia is probably genetically caused and is not secondary to the elevated calcitonin level (an antihypercalcemic hormone) that occurs in MCT.

DIAGNOSIS. Elevated serum calcium and PTH levels signify the presence of hyperparathyroidism in patients with MEN 2. The finding of one or more enlarged parathyroid glands by localization tests such as ultrasound or CT scanning or at surgery confirms the diagnosis. Some patients with MEN 2a and hyperparathyroidism will be normocalcemic, and the diagnosis is made by elevated PTH levels and the finding of enlarged parathyroid glands at the time of thyroidectomy for C-cell hyperplasia or MCT.

TREATMENT. Hyperparathyroidism is often diagnosed concurrently with MCT and can be treated during the thyroidectomy for MCT. All the parathyroid glands should be identified; if enlarged, three and one-half glands should be removed. The remaining parathyroid tissue may be left in the neck and marked with a suture clip, which we prefer, or transplanted to the forearm. One should also cryopreserve 500 mg of parathyroid for autotransplantation in case the patient has hypoparathyroidism after surgery. Hyperparathyroidism is more easily controlled in MEN 2a than in MEN 1. Also, hypoparathyroidism occurs more often after surgery in MEN 2 than persistent hyperparathyroidism, so great care must be taken to preserve a viable parathyroid remnant.

When performing thyroidectomy for MCT in a normocalcemic patient, one should inspect all four parathyroid glands. Most surgeons would recommend removing any parathyroid glands that are enlarged and carefully marking the remaining glands. It is also occasionally necessary to transplant biopsy-confirmed normal parathyroid glands because of the extensive surgery necessary to remove the thyroid gland and all the central neck nodes.

SUMMARY

Although the endocrine tumors associated with multiple endocrine neoplasia Types 1 and 2 are fascinating from the standpoint of their pathophysiology, they are potentially life threatening and require early diagnosis and treatment. The histologic distinction between hyperplasia and neoplasia and between benign and malignant tumors is often difficult. Many of these tumors can now be diagnosed early in the course of their symptomatic presentation before the lesion has progressed or transformed from its hyperplastic to its neoplastic form. By diagnosing these patients earlier, less extensive surgical procedures are effective in preventing these lethal tumors from developing.

REFERENCES

1. Babu, V.R., Van Dyke, D.L., and Jackson, C.E.: Chromosome 20 deletion in human multiple endocrine neoplasia types 2A and 2B: a double blind study, Proc. Natl. Acad. Sci. USA **81:**2525, 1984.
2. Beierwaltes, W.H: The localization and treatment of pheochromocytomas with ^{131}I MIBG. In Thompson, N.W., and Vinik, A.I., editors: Endocrine surgery update, New York, 1983, Grune & Stratton, Inc.
3. Bonfils, S., et al.: Results of surgical management in 92 consecutive patients with Zollinger-Ellison syndrome, Ann. Surg. **194:**692, 1981.
4. Bravo, B.L., and Gifford, R.W., Jr.: Pheochromocytoma: diagnosis, localization, and management, N. Engl. J. Med. **311:**1298, 1984.
5. Carney, J.A., Sizemore, G.W., and Sheps, S.G.: Adrenal medullary disease in multiple endocrine neoplasia type 2: pheochromocytoma and its precursors, Am. J. Clin. Pathol. **6:**279, 1976.
6. Clark, O.H., Way, L.W., and Hunt, T.K.: Recurrent hyperparathyroidism, Ann. Surg. **184:**391, 1976.
7. Damgaard-Peterson, K., and Stage, J.G.: CT screening in patients with Zollinger-Ellison syndrome and carcinoid syndrome, Scand. J. Gastroenterol. (Suppl.) **53:**117, 1979.

8. Deveney, C.W., and Way, L.W.: Regulatory peptides of the gut. In Greenspan, F.S., and Forsham, P.H., editors: Clinical endocrinology, Los Altos, Calif., 1983, Lange Medical Publications.
9. Deveney, C.W., Deveney, K., and Way, L.W.: The Zollinger-Ellison syndrome—23 years later, Ann. Surg. **188:**384, 1978.
10. Deveney, C.W., Stein, S., and Way, L.W.: Cimetidine as primary treatment for gastrinoma—long term follow up, Am. Surg. **146:**116, 1983.
11. Deveney, C.W., et al.: Resection of gastrinomas, Ann. Surg. **198:**546, 1983.
12. Dunnick, N.R., et al.: Computed tomography detection of nonbeta pancreatic islet cell tumors, Radiology **135:**117, 1980.
13. Farndon, J.R., Fagraeus, L., and Wells, S.A.: Recent developments in the management of pheochromocytoma, In Johnson, I.D.A., and Thompson, N.W., editors: Endocrine surgery, Boston, 1983, Butterworth Publishers.
14. Freier, D.T., et al.: Dilemmas in the early diagnosis and treatment of multiple endocrine adenomatosis, type II, Surgery **82:**407, 1977.
15. Friesen, S.R.: Treatment of the Zollinger-Ellison syndrome—a 25 year assessment, Am. J. Surg. **143:**331, 1982.
16. Friesen, S.R., Tomita, T., and Kimmel, J.R.: Pancreatic polypeptide update: its roles in detection of the trait for multiple endocrine adenopathy syndrome type I and pancreatic polypeptide-secreting tumors, Surgery **94:**1028, 1983.
17. Glowniak, J.V., et al.: Percutaneous transhepatic venous sampling of gastrin, N. Engl. J. Med. **307:**293, 1982.
18. Howard, J.M., et al.: Famotidine, a new, potent long-acting histamine H_2-receptor antagonist: comparison with cimetidine and ranitidine in the treatment of Zollinger-Ellison syndrome, Gastroenterology **88:**1026, 1985.
19. Jensen, R.T.: Basis for failure of cimetidine in patients with Zollinger-Ellison syndrome, Dig. Dis. Sci. **29:**363, 1984.
20. Jones, B.A., and Sisson, J.C.: Early diagnosis and thyroidectomy in multiple endocrine neoplasia type 2b, J. Pediatr. **102:**219, 1983.
21. Kaplan, E.L., and Fredland, A.: The diagnosis and treatment of insulinomas. In Thompson, N.W., and Vinik, A.I., editors: Endocrine surgery update, New York, 1983, Grune & Stratton, Inc.
22. Lamers, G.B.H.W., and Froeling, P.G.A.M.: Clinical significance of hyperparathyroidism in familial multiple endocrine adenomatosis type I (MEA I), Am. J. Med. **66:**422, 1979.
23. LeQuesne, L.P., and Daggett, P.R.: Insulin tumors of the pancreas. In Johnston, I.D.A., and Thompson, N.W., editors: Endocrine surgery, Boston, 1983, Butterworth Publishers.
24. Lips, K.M., et al.: Bilateral occurrence of pheochromocytoma in patients with the multiple endocrine neoplasia syndrome Type 2A (Sipple's syndrome), Am. J. Med. **70:**1051, 1981.
25. Majewski, J.T., and Wilson, S.D.: The MEA I syndrome: an all or none phenomenon? Surgery **86:**475, 1979.
26. McArthur, K.E., et al.: Omeprazole: effective, convenient therapy for Zollinger-Ellison syndrome, Gastroenterology **88:**939, 1985.
27. Modlin, I.M., et al.: The early diagnosis of gastrinoma, Ann. Surg. **196:**512, 1982.
28. Prinz, R.A., et al.: Subtotal parathyroidectomy for primary chief cell hyperplasia of the multiple endocrine neoplasia type I syndrome, Ann. Surg. **193:**26, 1981.
29. Rasbach, D., et al.: Surgical management of hyperinsulinism in the MEN 1 syndrome, Arch. Surg. **120:**584, 1985.
30. Raufman, J.P., et al.: Reliability of symptoms in assessing control of gastric acid secretion in patients with Zollinger-Ellison syndrome, Gastroenterology **84:**108, 1983.
31. Richardson, et al.: Treatment of Zollinger-Ellison syndrome with exploratory laparotomy, proximal gastric vagotomy, and H_2-receptor antagonists, Gastroenterology **89:**357, 1985.
32. Roche, A., Raisonnier, A., and Gillos-Savouret, M.D.: Pancreatic venous sampling and arteriography in localizing insulinomas and gastrinomas: procedure and results in 55 cases, Radiology **145:**621, 1982.
33. Russell, C.F., et al.: The surgical management of medullary thyroid carcinoma, Ann. Surg. **197:**42, 1983.
34. Shapiro, B., et al.: Iodine-121 metaiodobenzylguanidine for the locating of suspected pheochromocytoma: experience in 400 cases, Nucl. Med. **26:**576, 1985.
35. Stark, D.D., et al.: Computed tomography and nuclear magnetic resonance imaging of pancreatic islet cell tumors, Surgery **94:**1025, 1983.
36. Talpos, G.B., et al.: Phenotype mapping of multiple endocrine neoplasia II syndrome, Surgery **94:**650, 1983.
37. Thompson, N.W.: Surgical considerations in MEA I syndrome. In Johnston, I.D.A., and Thompson, N.W., editors: Endocrine surgery, Boston, 1983, Butterworth Publishers.
38. Thompson, N.W., et al.: MEN I pancreas: a histological and immunohistochemical study, World J. Surg. **8:**561, 1984.
39. Tibblin, S., et al.: Unilateral versus bilateral adrenalectomy in multiple endocrine neoplasia IIA, World J. Surg. **7:**201, 1983.
40. van Heerden, J.A., et al.: Primary hyperparathyroidism in patients with multiple endocrine neoplasia syndromes, Arch. Surg: **118:**533, 1983.
41. van Heerden, J.A., et al.: Surgical management of the adrenal glands in the multiple endocrine neoplasia Type II syndrome, World J. Surg. **8:**612, 1984.
42. Vinik, A.I., et al.: Localization of gastroenteropancreatic (GEP) tumors. In Johnson, I.D.A., and Thompson, N.W., editors: Endocrine surgery, Boston, 1983, Butterworth Publishers.
43. Welbourn, R.B., et al.: Tumors of the neuroendocrine system (APUD cell tumors—APUDomas), Curr. Probl. Surg. **21:**1, 1984.
44. Wells, S.A., et al.: The early diagnosis of medullary carcinoma of the thyroid gland in patients with multiple endocrine neoplasia Type II, Ann. Surg. **182:**362, 1975.
45. Wells, S.A., et al.: Medullary thyroid carcinoma: relationship of method of diagnosis to pathologic staging, Ann. Surg. **188:**377, 1978.
46. Wells, S.A., et al.: Provocative agents and the diagnosis of medullary carcinoma of the thyroid gland, Ann. Surg. **188**(2):139, 1978.
47. Wells, S.A., et al.: Long term evaluation of patients with primary parathyroid hyperplasia managed by total parathyroidectomy and heterotopic autotransplantation, Ann. Surg. **192:**451, 1980.
48. Wells, S.A., Jr., and Norton, J.A.: Medullary carcinoma of the thyroid and multiple endocrine neoplasia–II syndromes. In Friesen, S.R., editor: Surgical endocrinology: clinical syndromes, Philadelphia, 1978, J.B. Lippincott Co.
49. Wermer, P.: Genetic aspects of adenomatosis endocrine glands, Am. J. Med. **16:**363, 1954.
50. Wilson, S.D.: Wermer's syndrome: multiple endocrine adenopathy, Type 1. In Friesen, S.R., editor: Surgical endocrinology: clinical syndromes, Philadelphia, 1978, J.B. Lippincott Co.

61 Wound Healing

Thomas R. Stevenson and Stephen J. Mathes

Success of a surgical procedure depends on satisfactory wound healing. After any injury, the patient and his physician expect prompt healing and gradual restoration of wound strength. A basic understanding of the healing process helps the physician select the most appropriate wound management techniques among the many available options, anticipate the duration and extent of disability, recognize when a variation from the normal healing process is occurring, and intervene if necessary.

STAGES OF WOUND HEALING

A wound may be inflicted by physical trauma, heat, cold, electromagnetic radiation, chemical, injury, and infection.[1,2] Healing begins from the moment of injury, and in every wound, the stages of healing bear similarities. These stages overlap in time, each stage beginning before the completion of a previous one (Fig. 61-1). The example of a simple, clean laceration serves to illustrate the process of wound healing. A laceration that is closed promptly and heals primarily undergoes the stages of *inflammation*, *epithelialization*, *cellular phase*, and *maturation*. The healing of an open wound differs from that of a closed wound and is considered separately.

Inflammation

Inflammation is the result of trauma from any stimulus. Aurelius Cornelius Celsus in the first century AD characterized the signs of inflammation as heat, redness, swelling, and tenderness. They remain the cardinal signs of inflammation.

The inflammatory response involves both a vascular and a cellular reaction. Most wounds result in injury to blood vessels with a consequent hemorrhage. Vasoconstriction occurs almost immediately, followed 5 to 10 minutes later by vasodilation. Venules in the area become more permeable to fluid, and plasma escapes into the extravascular space.

Numerous substances participate in increasing the venule permeability to fluid. Histamine is both synthesized at the wound site and released from stores within mast cells. Histamine augments the permeability of arterioles, capillaries, and venules to albumin, globulin, and fibrinogen.[5] It increases permeability by causing the contraction of endothelial cells and by partially removing the diaphragms covering gaps in the endothelium.[5,24] Platelets and mast cells release-hydroxytryptamine (serotonin) that also enhances vascular permeability. Kinins are polypeptides produced at the site of inflammation from alpha globulin found in plasma. The kinins serve to increase venule permeability. Prostaglandins E_1 and E_2 are synthesized at the site of injury and participate in the acute inflammatory process including increasing in vascular permeability. Prostaglandins are also active in the later stages of wound healing.[12,22,23,25,37]

The inflammatory exudate includes fibrin and fibronectins. Fibrin is produced in the wound through the conversion of circulating plasma fibrinogen. It promotes hemostasis and provides a scaffolding for the ingrowth of cells. Fibronectins constitute a family of high-molecular-weight glycoproteins. They are present in an insoluble form in connective tissue and at cell surfaces and in a soluble form in plasma and other body fluids. Fibronectins play a role in the adherence of fibrin and collagen, as well as in the attachment of fibroblasts to fibrin.

Circulating plasma leukocytes adhere quickly to the vascular endothelium in the injured region. They traverse the vessel wall through a process of *diapedesis*. These cells migrate toward the injured area where they are stimulated to phagocytize particles and release substances that are in part responsible for inflammation.[43] Polymorphonuclear and mononuclear cells are present initially at the site of injury in proportions similar to those in the blood. Since polymorphonuclear cells are relatively short-lived, mononuclear cells are more abundant in an older inflammatory reaction. Polymorphonuclear leukocytes are essential in controlling any bacterial contamination that may occur at the time of wounding.

Within a few hours after injury, the wound fills with an exudate consisting of white cells, red cells, soluble plasma proteins, and fibrin. This acute inflammatory response usually decreases in intensity after a few days. In the presence of extensive injury or massive bacterial contamination, inflammation can be prolonged almost indefinitely.

Macrophages are as important as polymorphonuclear leukocytes in the inflammatory response.[20] The macrophage removes necrotic tissue and foreign bodies from the wound. More importantly, the macrophage may act as a *translator*, responding to the numerous stimuli of injury by translating these stimuli into chemical signals that initiate cell regeneration, fibroblast migration, collagen synthesis, and collagen degradation.[13,40]

Migratory fibroblasts develop from undifferentiated

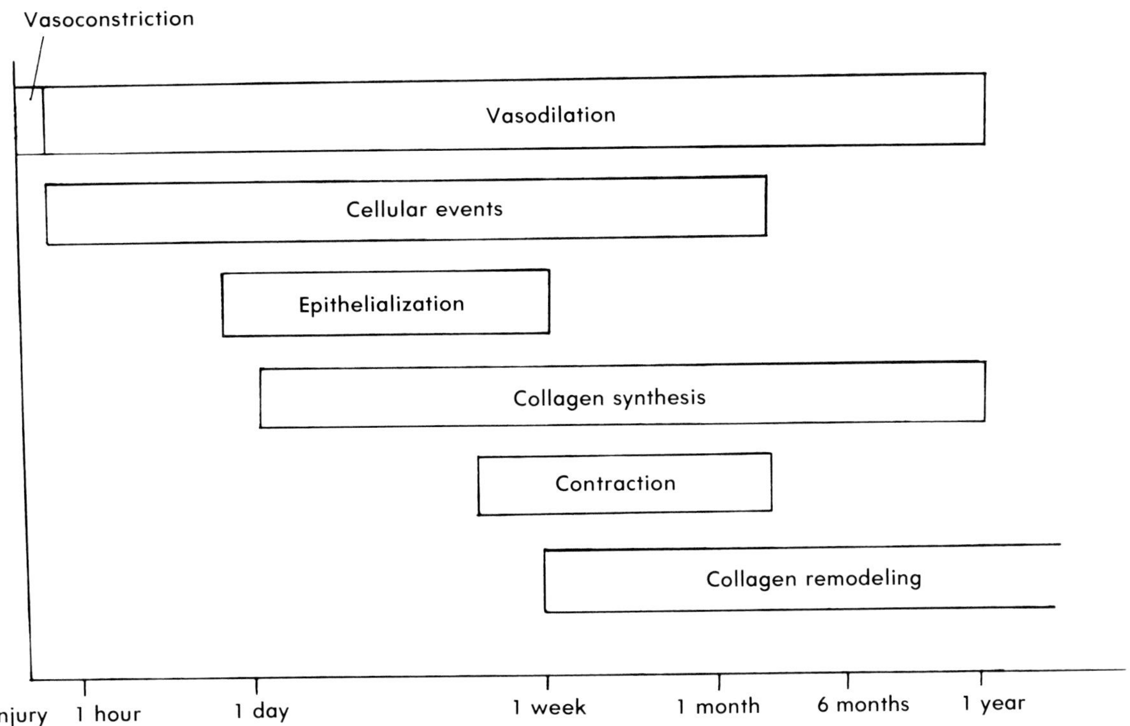

Fig. 61-1 Sequence of events in wound healing.

mesenchymal cells near the site of injury.[33,38] Chemotaxis refers to the attraction toward inflammatory cells exerted by various compounds; serotonin and other tissue hormones have chemotactic activity and draw the fibroblasts into the wound.[4] These fibroblasts become closely associated with the fibrin and fibronectin lattice laid down in the wound. Migration of fibroblasts into the traumatized area is followed closely by capillary formation and ingrowth. Endothelial cells secrete a powerful activator that converts plasminogen to plasmin. Fibrinolysis is mediated by plasmin, and dissolution of the fibrin network is accomplished quickly by the invading capillary mass.

In the wound, fibroblasts proliferate. They synthesize and secrete protein-polysaccharides and glycoproteins. Fibroplasia begins with the synthesis of collagen on the fourth or fifth day after injury. This phase lasts 2 to 4 weeks. At the end of that time, many of the new capillaries disappear. The number of active fibroblasts decreases, and the glycoprotein and mucopolysaccharide levels fall. The rate of collagen synthesis and degradation reaches equilibrium.

Epithelialization

Epithelialization of an incised and sutured wound occurs quickly. Within 24 hours after injury, basal cells along the wound margins lose their firm attachment to the dermis. A simultaneous increase in the mitotic rate of these basal cells is observed. The cells enlarge, flatten, and begin to move over the intervening defect. These cells cover any areas of exposed dermis and migrate across the base of the wound.[27] Two days after wounding, the defect is covered with epithelial cells. Mitosis also commences in those epithelial cells covering the gap. These cells go on to mature, differentiate, and keratinize.

Cellular Phase

The cellular phase is characterized by the deposition of collagen in the wound. Collagen is the most important component supporting the healed wound. It is a complex protein, unique in that it almost completely lacks the sulfur-containing amino acids cystine and tryptophan. Collagen incorporates hydroxyproline and hydroxylysine, two less common amino acids.

The structure of collagen is characterized by the presence of three peptide chains, each in a right-handed helical formation with the three chains aligned parallel to one another and twisted into a left-handed configuration. The resultant structure, termed tropocollagen, is initially held together by hydrogen bonds. As the molecule matures, stronger covalent bonds form among the three peptide chains. The tropocollagen molecule is very large, having a molecular weight of approximately 300,000 and dimensions of 15 Å in width and 2800 Å in length. Tropocollagen molecules aggregate to form collagen filaments, these collagen filaments join together as collagen fibrils, and collagen fibrils associate to form collagen fibers (Fig. 61-2).

There are at least five types of collagen, each differing in the amino-acid sequence or in the combination of the three basic polypeptide chains making up the tropocollagen.[19] The interstitial collagens, Types I, II, and III, are products of separate genes and have unique amino-acid sequences. Type I collagen is found in bone, skin, and tendon. It has two $alpha_1$(I) chains and one $alpha_2$(I) chain. Type I collagen is low in carbohydrate and hydroxylysine. Type II collagen is found primarily in cartilage and consists of three $alpha_1$(II) chains. It contains relatively more hydroxylysines per chain. Type III collagen is made up of three $alpha_1$(III) chains, contains cysteine, and is relatively low in hydroxylysine. It was originally believed to be *fetal* collagen. Type III collagen is commonly found in blood vessels, skin, and the parenchyma of internal organs. The collagen of adult skin is 80% Type I and 20% Type III. Type IV collagen appears to contain two chains distinct from the ones in other collagens: three alpha$_2$(IV) chains and three alpha$_2$(IV) chains. Type IV collagen is found primarily in basement membranes. Type V collagen consists of two alpha$_1$(V) chains and one alpha$_1$(V) chain. Type V collagen is present in skin, smooth muscle, bone, and placenta.

The synthesis of collagen occurs through a series of reactions that are begun within the cell, are continued on or near the cell-surface membrane, and are completed in the extracellular space (Fig. 61-3). Collagen is synthesized by fibroblasts, osteoblasts, smooth muscle cells, chondrocytes, epithelial cells, and endothelial cells. Amino acids in the intracellular space are synthesized into polypeptide chains at the ribosome. Nonhelical procollagen consists of three such chains aggregated together. Proline and lycine in the polypeptide chains are hydroxylated through the action of the enzymes prolyl hydroxylase and lysyl hydroxylase. Essential cofactors for these reactions are ferrous ions, alpha-ketoglutarate, oxygen, and ascorbic acid. After hydroxylation, the polypeptide chains fold into a helical formation. This helical procollagen consists of a collagen molecule with an attached nonhelical N-terminal and C-terminal polypeptide. Collagen appears to be excreted from a cell as a procollagen. On or near the cell surface, procollagen peptidase converts procollagen into tropocollagen.

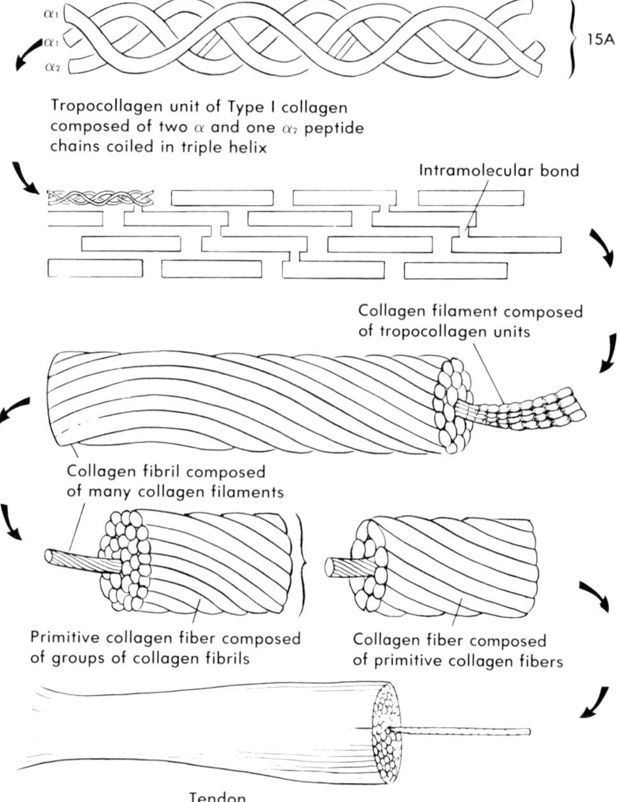

Fig. 61-2 Formation of collagen fiber.

The tropocollagen undergoes assembly into collagen filaments, and ultimately collagen fibers appear. As the collagen matures, the polypeptide chains comprising each tropocollagen unit form strong intramolecular bonds mediated by lysyl amine oxidase. Intermolecular cross-linking among the tropocollagen molecules also occurs and strengthens the collagen complex.

A complex of mucopolysaccharides, protein-polysaccharides, and glycoproteins is present in the wound within 24 hours of injury. These molecules compose the ground substance in conjunction with ions and water. Ground substance appears to participate in directing the aggregation of collagen.

The breakdown of collagen (collagenolysis) occurs in the maturing wound and in the stable scar. Collagenase is the most active collagenolytic enzyme. It is secreted by polymorphonuclear leukocytes, macrophages, and epithelial cells. The enzyme hydrolyzes collagen and participates in the process of wound remodeling. In the healed wound, the rates of collagen production and collagenolysis are in balance.

Maturation

As a scar matures, its physical properties change. In rat skin, 15% of preinjury bursting strength (load required to break open a wound regardless of size) is restored in a wound by 3 weeks after the injury and over 70% has re-

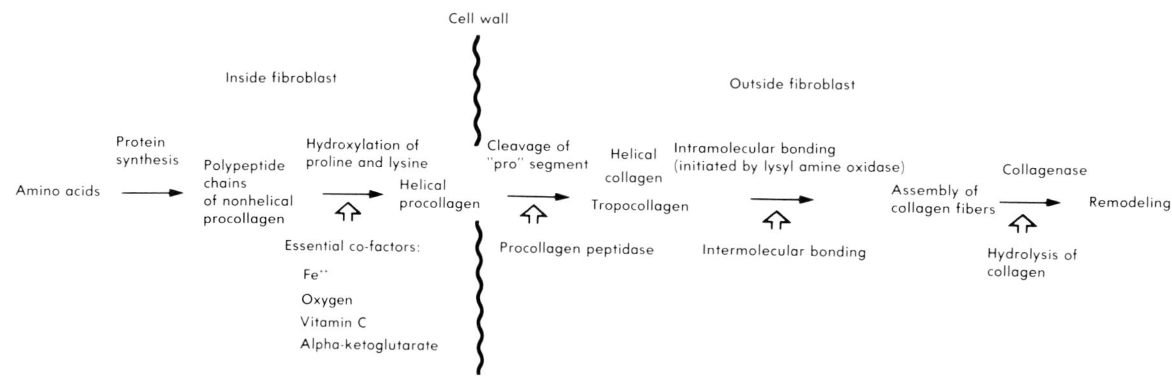

Fig. 61-3 Synthesis of collagen by fibroblast.

turned by 9 weeks.[21] An increase in wound bursting strength is observed even though there is no net increase in the scar collagen content beyond the third postinjury week. This increase in strength is explained by the development of stable intramolecular and intermolecular cross-links in the deposited collagen and by improved orientation of individual collagen fibers.[41] Type III collagen, abundant in the early scar, is gradually replaced by Type I collagen.

The immature scar is often raised, erythematous, and pruritic. As maturation progresses, the ideal scar becomes flat, white, soft, and nonirritating. A scar is usually considered mature 1 year after the injury occurred.

HEALING OF OPEN WOUNDS

Healing in the open wound progresses through stages similar to those seen in the closed wound. Wound contraction, however, assumes a more important role in the healing of an open wound. Contraction occurs by centripetal migration of the surrounding skin. This process is independent of epithelialization in the wound. The myofibroblast, a modified fibroblast, may provide the force for wound contraction.[35,36] This cell resembles a fibroblast ultrastructurally plus the addition of intracellular smooth muscle elements. Shrinkage of the wound through wound contraction and through epithelialization that progresses from the wound edges provides healing in open injuries. Wound contraction can be diminished by skin grafting; full-thickness grafts are more active than split-thickness ones in impeding contraction.[11,34]

FACTORS AFFECTING WOUND HEALING

Age

It is generally believed that advancing age adversely affects wound healing. The growth rate and multiplication of fibroblasts and the synthesis of collagen are affected by aging.[7] Wound healing does appear to be more efficient in the young. The elderly patient suffering from a wound healing problem may trace the difficulty to concurrent lung or cardiovascular disease accompanied by diminished local wound oxygen tension or circulation. Likewise, nutritional deficiencies are common in older individuals and can lead to disturbed wound healing.

Protein Nutrition

The effects of protein depletion on wound healing in animals have been previously described.[7] The incised rat wound gains strength less rapidly in the protein-depleted animal. This wound healing abnormality is probably a result of altered collagen synthesis or cross-linking in the protein-depleted rat. Adequate protein nutrition is generally believed to be important in human wound healing.[41]

Vitamins and Trace Elements

Vitamin A is an important factor in wound healing, although deficiency of this vitamin is rare. Administration of vitamin A can reverse the healing retardation caused by cortisone.[17] However, vitamin A given to an animal not deficient in the vitamin does not increase the normal healing rate.[17]

Vitamin C (ascorbic acid) has long been recognized as important in healing. Scurvy, a disease of vitamin C deficiency, is characterized by a failure in collagen synthesis. Specifically, the enzyme active in the hydroxylation of proline and lycine requires vitamin C as a cofactor.[30] Absence of ascorbic acid inhibits the action of this enzyme. Interestingly, old wounds in a scorbutic animal break down since collagenolysis proceeds normally at the same time collagen synthesis is retarded.

Zinc is necessary for the activity of DNA and RNA polymerases and transferases.[7,30] Zinc deficiency can retard epithelialization and fibroblast proliferation. A normal zinc level is essential for healing, although the administration of this element to a patient not zinc depleted does not enhance healing. In addition, ferrous iron and copper are necessary for normal collagen metabolism.

Blood Loss and Anemia

It is recognized that in animals significant blood loss and its resultant hypovolemia have a detrimental effect on wound healing. This effect may result from a decrease in tissue oxygenation during the hypovolemic state. Severe, chronic anemia is also believed to retard wound healing, although experimental data supporting this hypothesis is difficult to obtain. Mild-to-moderate normovolemic anemia does not appear to adversely effect wound healing in the otherwise healthy patient.[16]

Oxygen Tension

Oxygen is an essential element in wound healing. It is necessary for cell migration, proliferation, and protein and collagen synthesis. Although oxygen tension is low in the wound, there is little evidence that raising the normal arterial partial pressure of oxygen results in a clinically significant improvement in wound healing.[30] Nevertheless, anything that interferes with the delivery of oxygen to the wound (e.g., cardiovascular disease, diabetes, radiation) will have a detrimental effect on wound healing.

Steroids and Cytotoxic Medications

The administration of steroids can have a profound effect on wound healing.[14] The rate of protein synthesis is decreased by the administration of cortisone and glucocorticoids. Other effects of these substances include diminished capillary budding, inhibition of fibroblast proliferation, and reduction in the rate of epithelialization. The normal inflammatory reaction that occurs after wounding is inhibited by steroids. These effects on wound healing are most profound if the steroid is administered before or at the time of wounding. In this circumstance, healing does proceed to completion but at a reduced rate.

Cytotoxic drugs used in cancer chemotherapy can adversely affect wound healing.[5,10] Their action is primarily through an inhibition of cell proliferation. In general, the concentration of a cytotoxic drug in the wound, if given systemically, is insufficient to prevent wound healing; thus completion of the healing process is delayed but not prevented.

HYPERTROPHIC SCARS AND KELOIDS

Under ideal circumstances, a wound develops into a narrow, flat, white scar causing no functional or significant aesthetic problem. This ideal scar is the product of a balance between collagen deposit and its subsequent maturation and collagenolysis. An alteration in the desired process of maturation may represent itself as a *hypertrophic scar* or a *keloid*. The hypertrophic scar is characterized by the deposition of excess collagen that remains within the borders of the scar bed. The hypertrophic scar may be seen anywhere on the body and is more common in dark-skinned people and in the young. The natural course of a hypertrophic scar is spontaneous decrease in volume. A keloid scar also contains excess collagen; however, that collagen extends beyond the original lesion. The keloid is also more common in darkly-pigmented and younger individuals (Fig. 61-4). Continued growth without regression is characteristic of the keloid.[32]

Numerous techniques have been used in the treatment of hypertrophic scars and keloids. They include surgical excision, pressure, irradiation, and the administration of corticosteroids. Performance of a surgical excision alone is usually followed by recurrence of the hypertrophic scar or keloid. Irradiation and cortocosteroids both act to inhibit collagen synthesis. However, many physicians are reluctant to suggest irradiation since it is irreversible and the long-term effects of even small doses are unknown. On the other hand, the combination of surgical excision and steroid injection has proven useful in managing keloids and hypertrophic scars.[8,9,18,26,31] Pressure in the form of elastic garments prevents the formation of hypertrophic burn scars and causes regression of established lesions.[3]

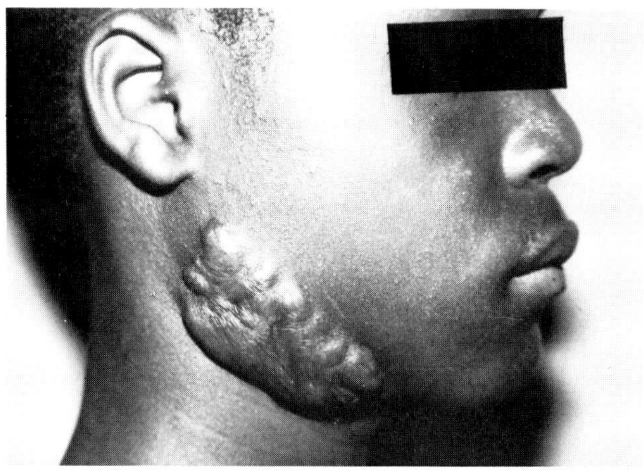

Fig. 61-4 Keloid scar that developed following a minor laceration.

Many chemical compounds have been used in an attempt to control excess scarring.[9,18] Beta-aminoproprionitrile irreversibly inhibits lysyl oxidase, preventing aldehyde formation and subsequent collagen cross-linking.[29] Penicillamine inhibits collagen cross-linking by chelating copper and interfering with the formation of aldehyde groups. Neither of these compounds has been proven safe or effective enough for broad clinical application.

SKIN GRAFTS AND FLAPS

Performing successful skin grafting is based on the observation that skin can be transplanted to a well-vascularized bed at a distant site and survive. Skin grafts are classified as either split-thickness or full-thickness (Fig. 61-5). The split-thickness graft ranges from 10/1000 inch ("thin" graft) to 15/1000 inch ("thick" graft) and is composed of the entire epidermis and a portion of the dermis. A full-thickness skin graft includes the epidermis and all of the dermis.

Once transferred, the skin graft depends on the recipient bed for survival. During the first 24 hours, the graft receives nutrients by passive diffusion from the bed. Revascularization of the graft occurs primarily by ingrowth of

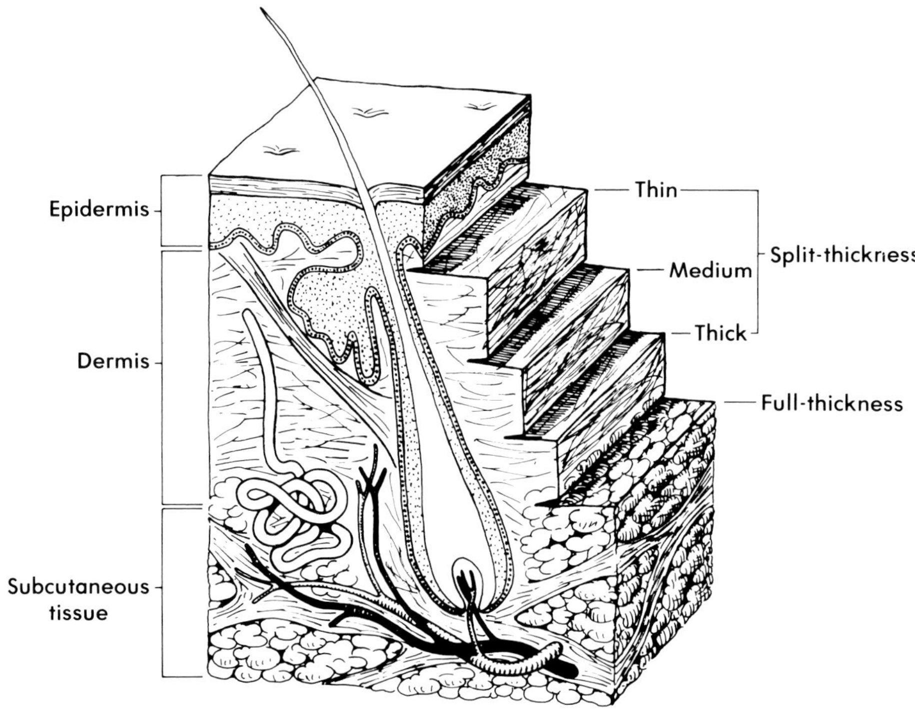

Fig. 61-5 Split-thickness and full-thickness skin grafts.

capillaries and venules from the underlying tissues. Evidence of circulation in the skin graft appears 24 to 48 hours after the transfer.

The donor site of a split-thickness skin graft heals by re-epithelialization. Keratinocytes grow from the dermal appendages (hair follicles and sweat glands) and cover the exposed dermis. A moist, sterile, and occlusive dressing promotes this process. The donor site is usually healed after 2 to 3 weeks.

Three conditions must be met for successful skin grafting. First, the bed to be grafted must be well-vascularized. A skin graft will not "take" (survive) over bone denuded of its periosteum, tendon stripped of its peritenon, or cartilage without its perichondrium. Second, the graft must be in stable contact with the vascularized bed. Motion at the wound site dislodges the graft and prevents revascularization. Similarly, a seroma or hematoma that develops between the graft and the bed can preclude survival. The use of immobilization and a bolster dressing protects against motion and fluid collection beneath the graft. Third, bacterial contamination must be minimized. A skin graft will not survive over an infected or grossly contaminated (greater than 10^5 bacteria per gram of tissue) bed.

The primary indication for skin grafting is treatment of a wound that cannot be closed by direct suturing. A large burn area, massive skin avulsion, and wide local excision of a skin tumor are examples of such wounds. Use of a skin graft can provide closure more quickly than can healing by secondary intention. Split-thickness skin grafts are selected over full-thickness ones when the area to be covered is large because they become vascularized more readily and survive transplantation more reliably. On the other hand, the full-thickness graft contracts less during healing than the split-thickness graft, making it more suitable for hand and eyelid reconstruction.

In contrast to the skin graft, a skin flap is used with its intrinsic blood supply left intact or, in the case of free-tissue transfer, with its blood supply restored immediately at the time of surgery. The skin receives its blood supply from the subdermal plexus. This plexus is in turn fed by perforating vessels from the underlying muscles. In certain anatomic areas, identifiable direct cutaneous (axial) vessels give off small arteries and veins that supply the subdermal plexus of the overlying skin. Flaps are classified as random, axial pattern, or musculocutaneous depending on their blood supply. The random skin flap is raised just to the subdermal plexus (Fig. 61-6). It is limited in size because of its reduced vascularity. An axial pattern skin flap contains an axial artery and can be larger than its random counterpart (Fig. 61-7). The musculocutaneous flap is comprised of skin and the underlying muscle and can be moved as a single vascularized unit (Fig. 61-8). In appro-

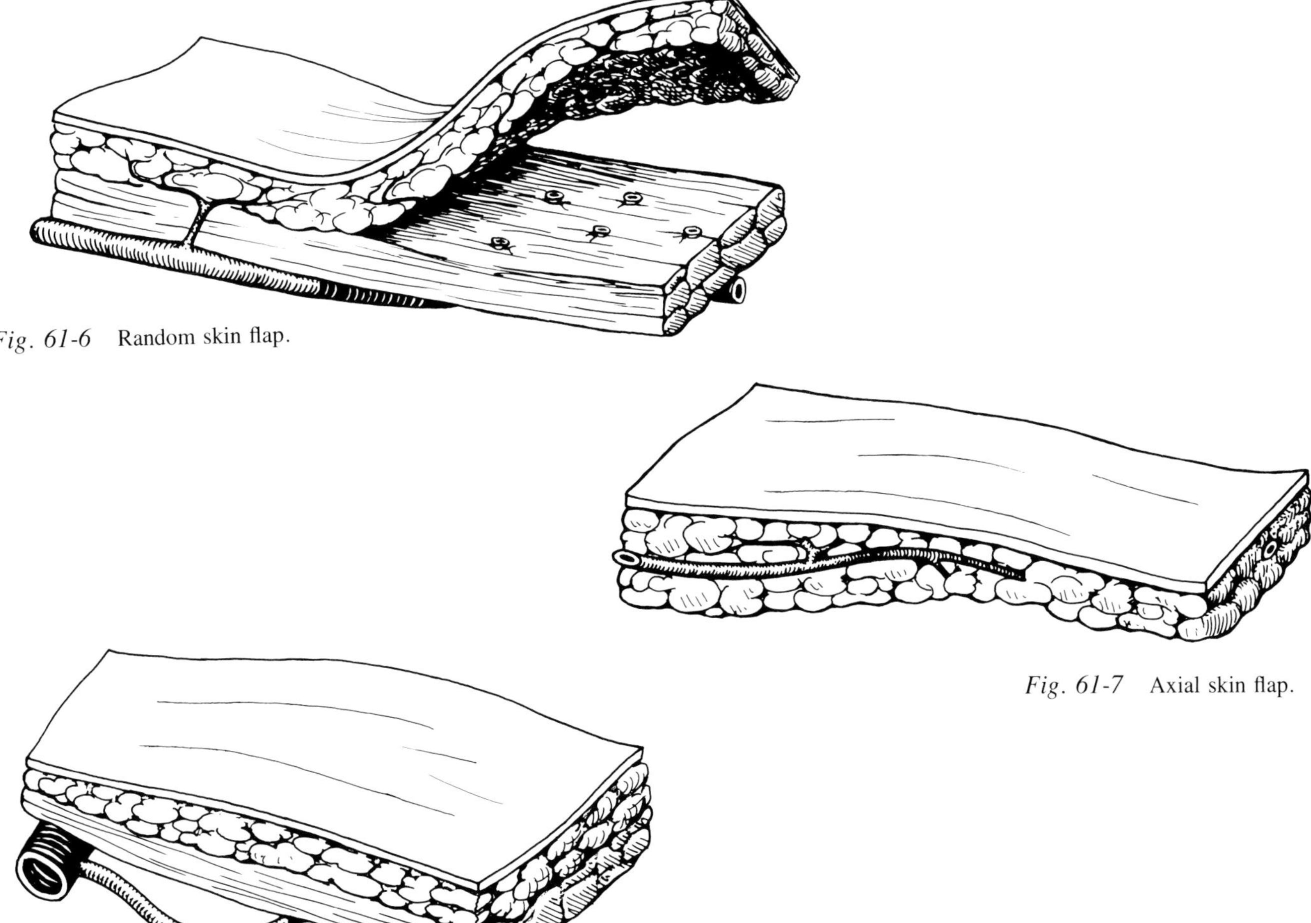

Fig. 61-6 Random skin flap.

Fig. 61-7 Axial skin flap.

Fig. 61-8 Musculocutaneous flap.

priate cases the muscle alone can be transferred, and a skin graft can then be applied. Flaps have their own blood supply and are helpful in the treatment of poorly vascularized or extensive wounds.

WOUND INFECTION

Etiology of Wound Infection

A wound infection arises when the body's defense mechanisms are inadequate to irradicate the bacteria contaminating the wound and to prevent their proliferation. Three elements predispose a patient to the development of a wound infection: (1) a compromised wound; (2) an infectious organism; and (3) a susceptible host.

A compromised wound is one that contains devitalized tissue that is separated from the circulation and the antibacterial defenses. Dead tissue, foreign bodies, and a hematoma retained in a wound can promote bacterial growth. A severely traumatized and poorly debrided wound that is repaired by suturing represents a closed space that is hypoxic, hypercarbic, acidic, and thus conducive to bacterial proliferation.

Many different organisms are capable of initiating a wound infection. A bacterial strain's ability to survive in tissue is related to its absolute numbers as well as to its capacity to damage tissue with toxins, to propagate, and to spread (i.e., its virulence). Streptococci enter through even minor wounds and may cause cellulitis. Skin and subcutaneous abscesses are often related to staphylococcal infection. Wounds associated with contamination by gastrointestinal flora may become infected by gram-negative aerobic (*E. coli*) and anaerobic *(Bacteroides fragilis)* species.

A susceptible host has some local or systemic impairment of resistance to bacterial invasion. Radiation changes and ischemia resulting from vascular disease are local factors that reduce resistance to infection. Systemic conditions (e.g., diabetes mellitus, adminstration of steroid therapy, shock burns, renal disease, cancer, and the use of immunosuppressive agents) impair host resistance. The three final common pathways of host resistance that are usually impaired are the mediation of the acute inflammatory response, phagocytic mechanisms, and opsonization.[15]

When viewed in the clinical or operating room setting, a wound can be classified as clean, clean-contaminated, contaminated, or dirty and infected.[1,6] Knowledge of these wound types helps the surgeon understand and anticipate a subsequent wound infection (see the boxed material at right). The clean wound is nontraumatic and free of inflammation. If it is created in the operating room, no break in surgical technique is recorded, and the respiratory, alimentary, and genitourinary tracts are not violated. A clean-contaminated wound is likewise nontraumatic but is characterized by a minor break in surgical technique or the involvement of the gastrointestinal, genitourinary, or respiratory tracts without significant spillage of contents. The contaminated wound classification includes all traumatic wounds caused by a dirty source, fecal contamination, a foreign body, or devitalized tissue or those receiving delayed treatment. A surgical wound in which a major break has occurred in surgical technique, gross spillage has occurred from the gastrointestinal tract, or there has been an invasion of the genitourinary or biliary tracts in the presence of infection is a contaminated wound. The rate of postoperative wound infection ranges from 1% in clean wounds to over 25% in dirty and infected ones.[15]

CLASSIFICATION OF OPERATIVE WOUNDS*

Clean
- Nontraumatic
- No inflammation
- Respiratory, gastrointestinal, and genitourinary tracts not entered
- No break in surgical technique

Clean-Contaminated
- Nontraumatic
- Involvement of respiratory, gastrointestinal, biliary, or genitourinary tracts without significant spillage
- Appendectomy without perforation or cloudy peritoneal exudate
- Prepared oropharynx or vagina entered
- Minor break in surgical technique

Contaminated
- Traumatic wound, recent
- Gross spillage from gastrointestinal tract
- Opening genitourinary or biliary tracts with infected urine or bile
- Major break in surgical technique

Dirty and Infected
- Traumatic wound with devitalized tissue, foreign bodies, fecal contamination, or delayed treatment
- Acute bacterial inflammation without pus
- Incision for drainage of pus
- Perforated viscus found during surgery

*From Burke, J.F.: Fundamentals of wound management in surgery: infection, New York, 1977, Appleton-Century-Crofts.

Prevention and Treatment of Wound Infection

Wound infection can be minimized in the operating room by shielding the surgical wound from bacterial contamination. Preoperative skin preparation, sterile draping, mechanical and antibiotic bowel preparation, systemic antibiotics administered preoperatively, and careful aseptic technique minimize contamination. Careful surgical technique and gentle handling of tissues minimizes injury and discourages bacterial proliferation.

Proper management of the traumatic wound decreases the likelihood of subsequent infection. High-pressure irrigation with physiologic saline can remove bacteria and foreign bodies from the traumatic wound. Debridement further reduces contamination because foreign bodies and devitalized tissue are removed from the site of injury. Subsequent wound closure with minimum tension maintains good vascularity of the tissues.

A wound infection is suspected if signs of inflammation (warmth, erythema, induration, and pain) or drainage appear at the operative or injured site within the first month after surgery or injury. Cellulitis is characterized by all the signs of inflammation but without a collection of pus. Beta-hemolytic streptococci typically spread through tissues without stimulating a purulent exudate. Abscess in a wound is initially seen in a purulent collection and is usually accompanied by acute inflammation.

The treatment of a wound infection must be both prompt and appropriate.[28] A sample of any wound discharge is submitted for Gram's staining, aerobic and anaerobic culture, and determination of bacterial sensitivity. Broad-spectrum antibiotic coverage is initiated before obtaining culture results. The most important aspect of early management is adequate wound drainage. A suspicious wound should be aspirated using a large bore needle. If pus is returned or if the wound remains questionable, it should be opened and drainage begun. Any abscess discovered is drained as thoroughly as possible and the wound is packed with saline-soaked dressings that are changed every 4 to 8 hours.

In a severely traumatized or contaminated wound, primary closure may risk subsequent wound infection. Delayed primary closure (within 3 days of injury) or secondary closure (3 to 7 days after injury) produces satisfactory healing and reduces the incidence of infection. Initially the wound is covered or packed lightly with saline-soaked fine mesh gauze. Whether or not healing is occurring without infection is determined through daily wound inspection. If no infection occurs, the wound is closed by suturing either with or without excision of the margins.

WOUND MANAGEMENT

Suture Material

Suture materials are classified as either absorbable or nonabsorbable.[39] They may consist of a single strand (monofilament) or of multiple strands (multifilament). The multifilament sutures are twisted or braided for strength. Nonabsorbable sutures remain in place indefinitely, and absorbable sutures are gradually removed by physiologic processes.

Absorbable sutures are useful in providing early strength to a closed wound. They are most frequently placed in an intradermal or subcutaneous position. Catgut suture is produced from bovine intestinal serosa. Chromicization of the suture prolongs absorption and strength. Absorption occurs 2 to 6 weeks postoperatively. Newer absorbable sutures (Dexon, Vicryl) are synthesized by polymerization of glycolic acid. They incite less inflammatory response than do the catgut sutures. However, the glycolic acid sutures are more difficult to tie than are the catgut ones.

Nonabsorbable sutures are most often used for skin closure and in internal sites that require prolonged tissue strength. Examples of nonabsorbable suture materials include silk, nylon, cotton, Prolene, Dacron, and stainless steel. When placed in the skin, a monofilament (Prolene, nylon, and stainless steel) suture invokes a less severe inflammatory reaction than does a multifilament (silk and cotton) suture. Skin staples allow rapid skin wound closure but leave less satisfactory skin marks if applied too tightly or if allowed to remain in the skin longer than 1 week.

The duration that a suture is left in place varies with the wound location.[42] The longer a suture remains in the skin, the more severe the tissue reaction will be to the suture. An unsightly scar may be produced at the site of each suture. In the face, skin sutures are usually removed within 3 to 5 days. Skin sutures in wounds of the extremities and trunk are generally left in position for 7 days. Skin sutures placed in a buried (intradermal) position can remain for several weeks without compromising the resultant scar.

Dressings

A dressing applied to a closed wound serves several purposes. It is absorbent and thereby removes any drainage that occurs. The dressing also serves to protect the wound against bacterial contamination. The dressing should be constructed securely enough to prevent pain from any subsequent minor trauma. The deepest layer of dressing should be nonadherent, thus assuring a pain-free removal. Some dressings, particularly those of the hand and the extremities, hold the injured part in a functional or desired position. A compressive dressing can aid in the prevention of edema at the wound site.

The duration of wound coverage by a dressing is variable. A simple skin incision closed primarily is epithelialized within 24 to 48 hours and, as such, is protected against bacterial invasion. With such a simple wound, the dressing can be removed permanently after 48 hours. Dressings may be left in place on the extremities for many days or weeks.

SUMMARY

The body's response to wounding allows survival in a harsh, pathogen-contaminated environment. When closed primarily, a wound heals by the simultaneous and interrelated processes of inflammation, epithelialization, cellular production of collagen, and maturation. A wound left open diminishes in size by contraction while undergoing the same healing phases as its closed counterpart. The speed and adequacy of healing are dependent on the patient's adequate nutrition and local vascularity. Advanced age, associated illness, and various medications have a deleterious effect on healing. Individual response to wounding determines the appearance of the mature scar, with some patients prone to develop scar hypertrophy or keloids.

The nature and extent of a wound dictates the physician's management of it. After cleansing and debridement, wounds are closed primarily, are covered with a skin graft or flap, or are allowed to heal by secondary intention. Wound infection, should it occur, is treated by incision or reopening of the wound, drainage, administration of appropriate antibiotic(s), and dressing changes. Adherence to the principles of wound care usually results in healing by primary intention and development of a scar that is satisfactory to both the patient and physician.

REFERENCES

1. Altemeier, W.A., et al.: Manual on control of infection in surgical patients, Philadelphia, 1976, J.B. Lippincott Co.
2. Arturson, G.: Pathophysiology of the burn wound, Ann. Chir. Gynaecol. **69**:178, 1980.
3. Baur, P.S., Parks, D.H., and Larson, D.L.: The healing of burn wounds, Clin. Plast. Surg. **4**:389, 1977.
4. Becker, E.L., and Stossel, T.:P.: Chemotaxis, Fed. Proc. **39**:2949, 1980.
5. Boucek, R.J.: Factors affecting wound healing, Otolaryngol. Clin. North Am. **17**:243, 1984.
6. Burke, J.F.: Fundamentals of wound management in surgery: infection, New York, 1977, Appleton-Century-Crofts.

7. Chvapil, M., and Koopmann, C.F., Jr.: Age and other factors regulating wound healing, Otolaryngol. Clin. North Am. **15:**259, 1982.
8. Cohen, I.K., and Diegelmann, R.F.: The biology of keloid and hypertrophic scar and the influence of corticosteroids, Clin. Plast. Surg. **4:**297, 1977.
9. Cohen, I.K., and McCoy, B.J.: The biology and control of surface overhealing, World J, Surg. **4:**289, 1980.
10. Cohen, S.C., et al.: Effects of antineoplastic agents on wound healing in mice, Surgery **78:**238, 1975.
11. Corps, B.V.M.: The effect of graft thickness, donor site, and graft bed on graft shrinkage in the wounded rat, Br. J. Plast. Surg. **22:**125, 1969.
12. Cuono, C.B.: Prostaglandin inhibitors and wound healing (letter to the editor), Plast. Reconstr. Surg. **70:**514, 1982.
13. Diegelmann, R.F., Cohen, I.K., and Kaplan, A.M.: The role of macrophages in wound repair: a review, Plast. Reconstr. Surg. **68:**107, 1981.
14. Ehrlich, H.P., and Hunt, T.K.: Effects of cortisone and vitamin A on wound healing, Ann. Surg. **167:**324, 1968.
15. Goodenough, R.D., Molnar, J.A., and Burke, J.F.: Surgical infections, In Hardy, J.D., editor: Hardy's Textbook of surgery, Philadelphia, 1983, J.B. Lippincott Co.
16. Heughan, C., Grislis, G., and Hunt, T.K.: The effect of anemia on wound healing, Ann. Surg. **179:**163, 1974.
17. Hunt, T.K., et al.: Effect of vitamin A on reversing the inhibitory effect of cortisone on healing of open wounds in animals and man, Ann. Surg. **170:**633, 1969.
18. Ketchum, L.D., Cohen, I.K., and Masters, F.W.: Hypertrophic scars and keloids: a collective review, Plast. Reconstr. Surg. **53:**140, 1974.
19. Kleinman, H.K., Klebe, R.J., and Martin, G.R.: Role of collagenous matrices in the adhesion and growth of cells, J. Cell Biol. **88:**473, 1981.
20. Leibovich, S.J., and Ross, R.: The role of the macrophage in wound repair, Am. J. Pathol. **78:**71, 1975.
21. Levenson, S.M., et al.: the healing of rat skin wounds, Ann. Surg. **161:**293, 1965.
22. Lord, J.T., et al.: Prostaglandin in wound healing: possible regulation of granulation. In Samuelson B., Ramwell, P.W., and Paoletti, R., editors: Advances in prostaglandin and thromboxane research, vol. 7, New York, 1980, Raven Press.
23. Lupulescu, A.: Effect of prostaglandins on protein, RNA, DNA, and collagen synthesis in experimental wounds, Prostaglandins **10:**573, 1975.
24. Majno, G., Gilmore V., and Leventhal, M.: On the mechanism of vascular leakage caused by histamine-type mediators, Circ. Res. **21:**833, 1967.
25. McGrath, M.H.: The effect of prostaglandin inhibitors on wound contraction and the myofibroblast, Plast. Reconstr. Surg. **69:**74, 1982.
26. Murray, J.C., Pollack. S.V., and Pinnell, S.R.: Keloids: a review, J. Am. Acad. Dermatol **4:**461, 1981.
27. Odland, G., and Ross, R.: Human wound repair. I. Epidermal regeneration, J. Cell. Biol. **39:**135, 1968.
28. Olson, M., O'Connor, M., and Schwartz, M.L.: Surgical wound infections, Ann. Surg. **199:**253, 1984.
29. Peacock, E.E., Jr.: Pharmacologic control of surface scarring, Ann. Surg. **193:**592, 1981.
30. Peacock, E.E., Jr.: Wound repair, ed. 3, Philadelphia, 1984, W.B. Saunders Co.
31. Pollack, S.V., and Goslen, J.B.: The surgical treatment of keloids, J. Dermatol. Surg. Oncol. **8:**1045, 1982.
32. Riley, W.B., and Peacock, E.E., Jr.: The identification, distribution, and significance of collagenolytic enzyme in human tissues, Proc. Soc. Exp. Biol. Med. **124:**207, 1967.
33. Ross, R., Everett, N.B., and Tyler, R.: Wound healing and collagen formation. VI. The origin of the wound fibroblast studied in parabiosis, J. Cell Biol. **44:**645, 1970.
34. Rudolph, R.: Inhibition of myofibroblasts by skin grafts, Plast. Reconstr. Surg. **63:**473, 1979.
35. Rudolph, R.: Location of the force of wound contraction, Surg. Gynecol. Obstet. **148:**547, 1979.
36. Ryan, G.B., et al.: Myofibroblasts in human granulation tissue, Hum. Pathol. **5:**55, 1974.
37. Samuelson, B., et al.: Prostaglandins and thromboxanes: biochemical and physiological consideration. In Coceani, F., and Olley, P.M., editors: Advances in prostaglandin and thromboxane research, vol. 4. New York, 1978, Raven Press.
38. Stewart, R.J., et al.: The wound fibroblast and macrophage. II: Their origin studied in a human after bone marrow transplantation, Br. J. Surg. **68:**129, 1981.
39. Swanson, N.A., and Tromovitch, T.O.: Suture materials, 1980s: properties, uses and abuses, Int. J. Dermatol. **21:**373, 1982.
40. Thakral, K.K., Goodson, W.H., III, and Hunt, T.K.: Stimulation of wound blood vessel growth by wound macrophages, J. Surg. Res. **26:**430, 1979.
41. Van Winkle, W.: The tensile strength of wounds and factors that influence it, Surg. Gynecol. Obstet. **129:**819, 1969.
42. Van Winkle, W., and Hastings, J.C.: Considerations in the choice of suture material for various tissues, Surg. Gynecol. Obstet. **135:**113, 1972.
43. Weissman, G., Simolen, J.E., and Korchak, H.M.: Release of inflammatory mediators from stimulated neutrophils, N. Engl. J. Med. **303:**27, 1980.

62 *Kirby I. Bland and Edward M. Copeland, III*

Breast: Physiologic Considerations in Normal, Benign, and Neoplastic States

The breast is a modified sweat gland that is embryologically unique to the mammalian species—thus the term *mammary gland*. Although variable in number among the different mammalian species, single pairs of mammary glands are observed only in human beings, apes, and monkeys (except for marmosets). The breast represents a functional part of the reproductive system, with perturbations in physiologic function that reflect similar neuroendocrine stimuli and control. These remarkable fluctuations in physiologic stimuli with metabolic and morphologic consequences are evident from prepubertal adolescence to the postmenopausal era. A comprehensive knowledge of the physiologic alterations expected in the normal breast, as well as specific deviations in the pathologic processes that are evident in the premenopausal and postmenopausal female, is essential to the diagnosis and appropriate therapy of breast disease.

RELEVANT ANATOMY

Developmental Anatomy of Mammary Gland

The mammary gland is initially recognized in the human embryo as a "milk streak" in the sixth week of embryologic development. The milk bud develops in the pectoral portion of the ectodermal thickening and extends bilaterally from the axilla to the vulva. These distinct linear elevations are called *milk lines* or the *mammary ridge*. By the ninth week intrauterine, the milk line has atrophied, except in its pectoral region, and a nipple bud appears with the formation of a proliferating mass of basaloid cells that represents the breast primordium. By month 3 of embryologic development the nipple bud is invaded by squamous cells from the ectoderm. At month 5, connective tissue of mesenchymal origin develops beneath the breast primordium into 15 to 20 solid cords. From these embryologic remnants the mammary ducts develop as ventral ingrowths that branch into primary milk ducts and terminate in lobular buds, which proliferate into acini following ovarian estrogenic stimuli. By the seventh to eighth month, these ducts are cannulated to form lumina. Thus, by termination of pregnancy, the nipple bud is penetrated by primary milk ducts to terminate at its recessed opening and shortly becomes everted and surrounded by the ectodermal thickening of the nipple (areola).

Adult Anatomic Considerations

Because the adult mammary gland represents a modification of an ectodermal vestige of a sweat gland, it is confined entirely within the superficial and deep layers of the superficial fascia of the anterior chest wall. The delicate layers of superficial fascia serve as an anatomic guide for the elevation of skin flaps of appropriate thickness of fatty and areolar tissue when performing a mastectomy. The thickness of the skin flap depends on the patient's habitus and may be only 2 to 3 mm in thin individuals, in contrast to a greater thickness in obese subjects.

The deep layer of superficial fascia crosses the retromammary space to fuse with the pectoral (deep) fascia. A distinct space is observed on the posterior aspect of the breast between the deep layer of superficial fascia and the investing fascia of the pectoralis major and contiguous muscles of the chest wall (Fig. 62-1). This retromammary bursa contributes to the mobility of the breast on the chest wall as a result of its loose areolar connections. The deep pectoral fascia is attached to the sternum and superolaterally to the axillary and clavicular fascia. This fascial envelope is contiguous inferiorly with the rectus abdominus tendon of the abdominal wall. The posterior surface of the pectoralis major muscle is continuous with the clavipectoral fascia, which also encases the pectoralis minor musculature.[6] The broad condensation of clavipectoral fascia (Halsted's ligament), which is superior and superficial to the pectoralis minor muscle, is penetrated by the anterior thoracic neurovascular bundles and the cephalic vein. A vascular sheath envelops the axillary vessels as this fascial plate continues from the roof of the axillary space to fuse with the deep fascial contributions of the anterior surface of the pectoralis major muscle.

The mammary parenchyma is interdigitated by septalike connections of fibrous processes, which extend from the posterior superficial fascia layer to the superficial layer of fascia of the skin. These suspensory Cooper's ligaments insert perpendicularly to the delicate superficial fascial layers of the corium (see Fig. 62-1). Cooper's ligaments permit remarkable mobility of the breast while providing support of the lobular and parenchymal structure.

Topographic Mammary Anatomy

With its fibrous and fatty components, the breast occupies the interval between the third and seventh ribs and extends in breadth from the parasternal to the midaxillary lines. The glandular portion of the breast rests largely on the pectoral fascia and the serratus anterior musculature. Mammary tissue typically extends in the anterior axillary fold (tail of Spence) and is often visible as a definite mass.

The anterior and lateral projections of the breast vary with the patient's age, habitus, and ovarian functional status. Thus the glandular aspects of the breast remain undeveloped and rudimentary in the male. In this circumstance

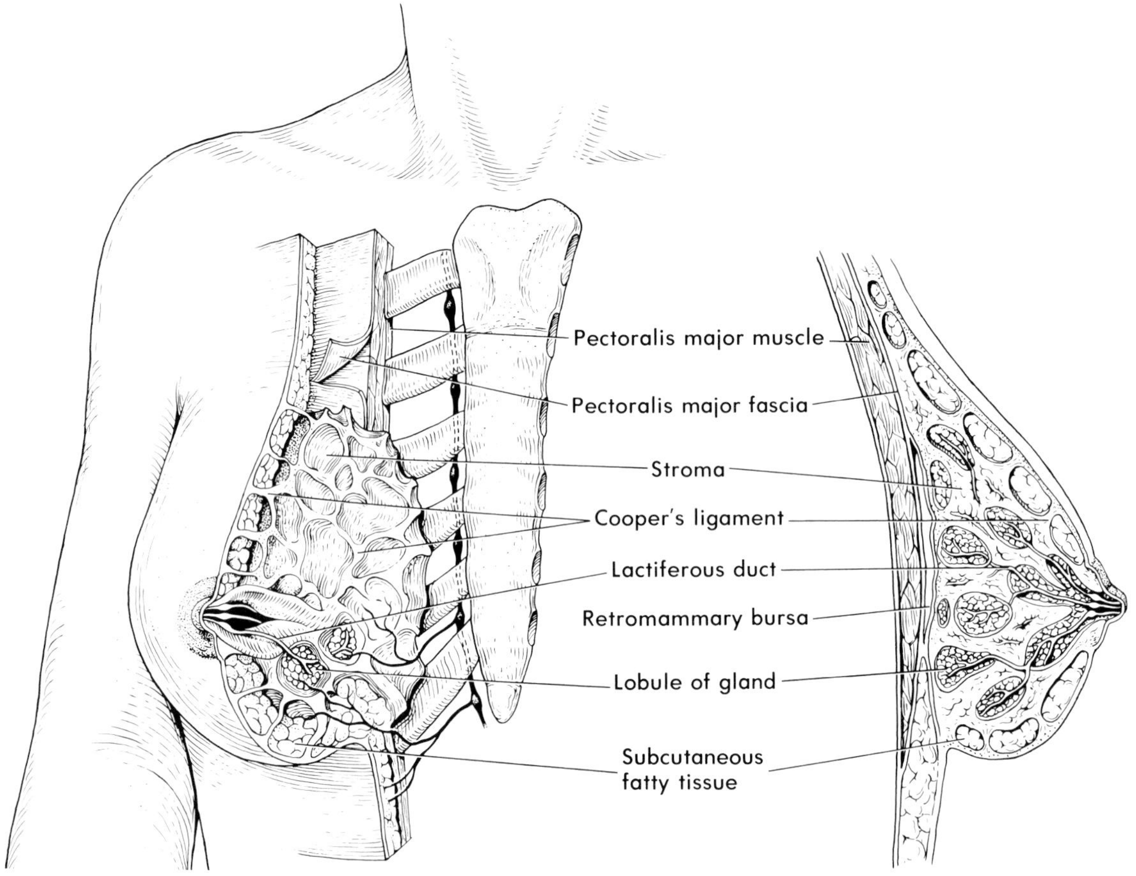

Fig. 62-1 Cross section (sagittal and tangential) view of mammary gland. The breast is invested by superficial and deep fascia. Retromammary bursa contributes to mobility of the gland. Diffuse lactiferous ductal network converges in subareolar space from glandular lobules to empty into sinus beneath nipple. Interposed fibroseptae (Cooper's ligaments) provide stromal support of breast parenchyma. Diffuse lymphatic system is interposed and parallels the extensive ductal network in periductal or perilobular position and drains 15 to 20 glandular lobules.

short ducts with poorly developed acini are evident. A deficiency of parenchymal fat and nipple-areola development are apparent and contribute to the flat appearance of the male breast.

In the female the virginal breast is hemispheric and is somewhat flattened above the nipple. In contrast, the multiparous breast is lax and large and rarely regains its initial configuration until menopause, when atrophy of glandular tissue is initiated. The postmenopausal breast consistently reveals a disappearance of parenchymal fat with loss of the active (proliferative) glandular portion as a result of cessation of ovarian function. The nonlactating breast weighs between 150 to 225 g, whereas the lactating breast may be as large as 500 g.[130]

Anomalous Developments of Breast

Anomalies of the nipples or the breast in human beings of either sex are a result of imperfect or complete suppression of the breast anlagen in embryogenesis. Further, an accessory breast represents a regression to a more primitive type of mammary arrangement in which more than a single pair of these anlagen persist.

Supernumerary (accessory) nipples or breasts may thus occur as a result of this latter embryologic event and are observed in approximately 1% to 2% of white individuals. *Accessory* breast tissue appears to occur more frequently in the female than in the male by a ratio of 2:1.[65] The anomaly is considered hereditary with autosomal dominant penetrance. Supernumerary mammary development can occur in combination or as singular components of the breast and thus involves the glandular parenchyma, nipple, or areola. In many cases only a diminutive nipple is evident, whereas the most frequent combination is a small nipple and areola bud. Classically, these anomalous structures are observed along the embryologic "milk streak" and are therefore anatomically confined to sites between the groin and axilla. These embryologic remnants are most often seen in the axilla or in the milk line just below the normal breast. The anomaly occurs more frequently in Orientals.

Conversely, *amastia,* with complete absence of one or both breasts, is a remarkably rare breast anomaly. In circumstances in which amastia occurs, it is usually unilateral, with persistence of a rudimentary breast structure, and is associated with underdevelopment and/or absence of structures of the anterior and lateral chest wall, arm, or shoulder girdle.[65]

Lymphatic Drainage of Mammary Gland and Routes for Metastases

A thorough conceptualization of breast lymphatic drainage is important to the student of this organ's pathophysiology. Metastatic dissemination occurs predominantly by lymphatic routes, which are rich and extensive and arborize in multiple directions through skin and intraparenchymal lymph ducts. These delicate lymph vessels of the corium are valveless; flow encompasses the lobular parenchyma and thereafter parallels major venous channels to enter the regional lymph nodes. The unidirectional lymphatic flow is pulsatile as a result of the wavelike contractions of the lymphatics to allow rapid transit and emptying of the lymphatic vascular spaces that interdigitate the extensive periductal and perilobular network. When obstruction to lymph flow is impeded by inflammatory or neoplastic states, a reversal in flow by way of these rich lymphatic networks is evident and accounts for the neoplastic growth in local and regional sites remote from the primary tumor.

Unlike blood circulation, lymph flow is unidirectional, except in the pathologic state just mentioned, and has preferential flow from the periphery toward the right side of the heart. Lymphatic capillaries end blindly in tissues from which lymph is collected; throughout their course these capillaries anastomose and fuse to form fewer lymph channels, which terminate in the large left thoracic duct or the smaller right lymphatic duct (Fig. 62-2). The thoracic duct empties into the left subclavian vein, whereas the right lymphatic duct drains preferentially into the right subclavian vein at the point of entry for the internal jugular vein.

Haagensen[65] emphasizes that lymphatics of the dermis are intimately related to the deep lymphatics of the underlying fascial planes, which explains the multidirection potential for drainage of superficial breast neoplasms. Preferential flow of lymph toward the axilla is observed in lesions of the upper anterolateral chest. However, at the level of the umbilicus, tributaries diverge such that chest and upper anterior and lateral abdominal wall lymph enters channels of the axilla.[6] Thus carcinomatous involvement of skin, even of the inframammary region, has preferential flow to the axilla rather than to the groin.

Haagensen[65] and Anson and McVay[6] acknowledge two accessory directions for lymphatic drainage from the breast to nodes of the apex of the axilla: the *transpectoral* and *retropectoral* routes. Lymph nodes of the transpectoral route, i.e., interpectoral nodes, lie between the pectoralis major and minor muscles and are referred to as *Rotter's nodes*. This drainage pathway begins in the loose areolar tissue of the retromammary plexus and interdigitates between the pectoral fascia and breast to perforate the pectoralis major muscle and follow the course of the thoracoacromial artery and terminate in the subclavicular (apical) group of nodes.

The retropectoral lymphatic pathway drains the superior and internal portions of the breast and arborizes on the lateral and posterior surface of the pectoralis major or under the pectoralis minor muscle to terminate at the apex of the axilla in the subclavicular (Level III) group. This route of lymphatic drainage occurs in approximately one third of patients and is a more direct mechanism of lymphatic flow to the subclavicular group. This is also the major lymphatic drainage by way of the external mammary and central axillary nodal groups (Levels I and II, respectively).

To assess the possibility of axillary nodal involvement appropriately, an appreciation of the major nodal groups is essential. Mornard[103] identified five principal axillary lymph node groups that lie on or inferior to the axillary vein and are invested by costocoracoid fascia contiguous with the axillary artery, brachial plexus, areola, and connective tissue. The five primary axillary nodal groups (see Fig. 62-2) are:

1. The *external mammary group* (Level I), which occupies the lateral margin of the pectoralis major muscle and the medial side of the axillary space and parallels the course of the lateral thoracic artery of the chest wall from the sixth rib to the axillary vein
2. The *subscapular (scapular) group* (Level I), which is closely applied to the thoracodorsal branches of the subscapular vessels and extends from the lateral thoracic wall to the axillary vein
3. The *axillary vein group* (Level I), which represents the most laterally placed and numerous group of lymph nodes of the axilla and occupies the ventral and caudal aspects of the vein
4. The *central nodal group* (Level II), which is often superficial beneath the skin and fascia of the middle axilla and is centrally located between the posterior and anterior axillary fold; the nodal group most often palpated and the one on which the clinical estimation of nodal disease is based[6, 65]
5. The *subclavicular (apical) node group* (Level III), which is the most medial and highest nodal group and is situated at the juncture of the axillary vein and its entry beneath the subclavian muscle to form the subclavian vein at the level of the clivopectoral fascia (i.e., Halsted's ligament).

The recognition of metastatic spread of breast carcinoma into internal mammary nodes as a primary route of systemic dissemination is credited to the British surgeon, W.S. Handley. Extensive investigation confirmed that median and central breast lymphatics progressed medially and paralleled the course of major blood vessels to perforate the pectoralis major muscle and empty into the internal mammary nodal chain. This major lymphatic route (see Fig. 62-2) is anatomically situated in the interspaces between the costal cartilages, approximately 2 to 3 cm within the sternal margin. These nodal groups traverse and parallel the internal mammary vessels and are invested by endothoracic fascia. Internal mammary lymphatic trunks eventually terminate in subclavicular nodal groups. The right internal mammary group enters the right lymphatic duct, and the left group enters the main thoracic duct. The presence of supraclavicular nodes (Stage IV disease) is a result of lymphatic permeation and subsequent obstruction of the inferior deep cervical group or nodes of the jugular/subclavian confluence. The supraclavicular nodal group represents the termination of efferent trunks from subclavian node(s) of the internal mammary nodal group. The nodes are situated beneath the lateral margin of the inferior

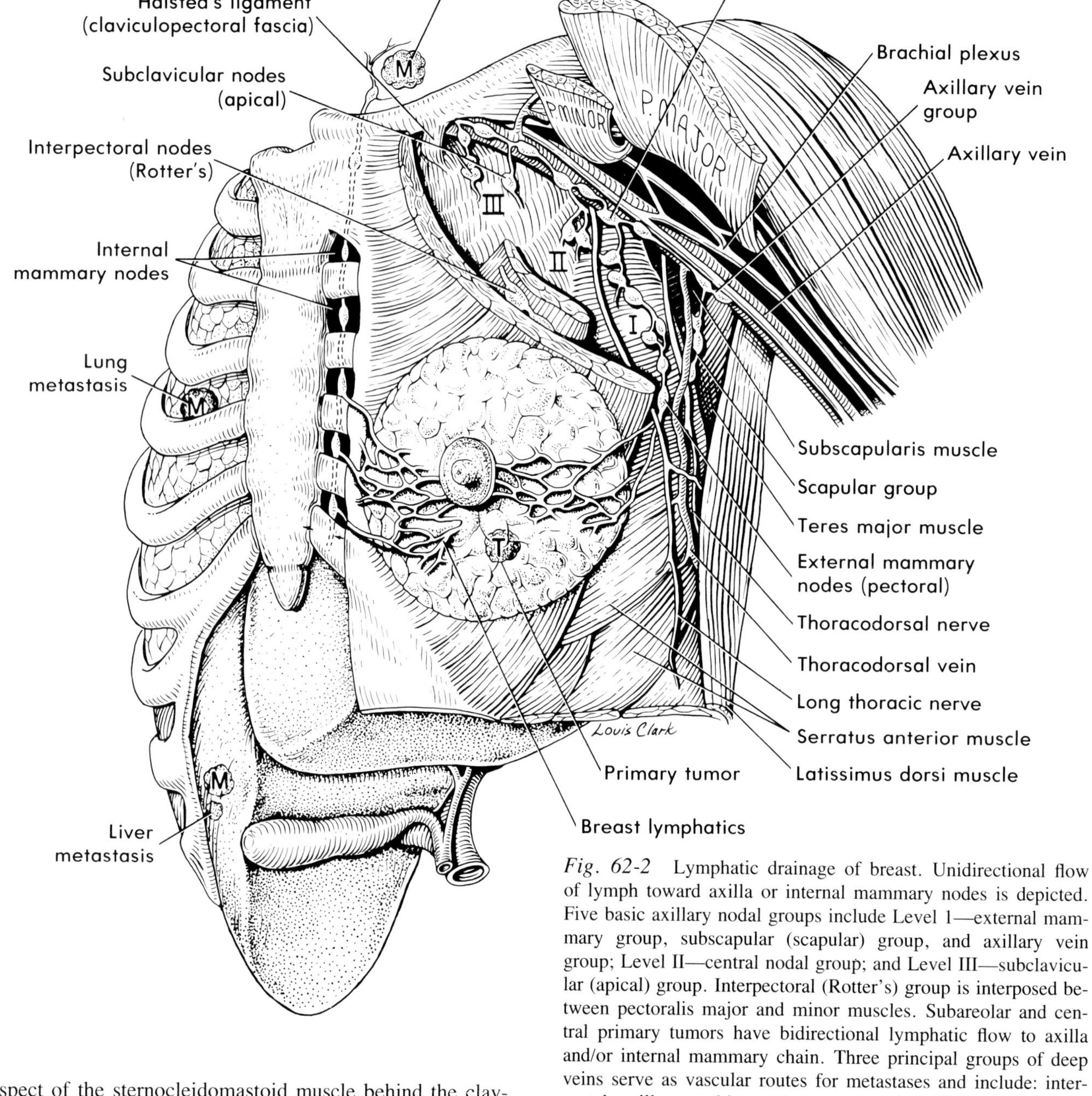

Fig. 62-2 Lymphatic drainage of breast. Unidirectional flow of lymph toward axilla or internal mammary nodes is depicted. Five basic axillary nodal groups include Level I—external mammary group, subscapular (scapular) group, and axillary vein group; Level II—central nodal group; and Level III—subclavicular (apical) group. Interpectoral (Rotter's) group is interposed between pectoralis major and minor muscles. Subareolar and central primary tumors have bidirectional lymphatic flow to axilla and/or internal mammary chain. Three principal groups of deep veins serve as vascular routes for metastases and include: intercostal, axillary, and internal mammary veins. Visceral metastases to lung or liver are possible through lymphatic or primary vascular drainage routes of breast and communicate with major venous trunks.

aspect of the sternocleidomastoid muscle behind the clavicle and represent common sites of distant metastases from breast cancer.

Cross-connections of lymphatic drainage from the breast to the opposite axilla often occur. This observation of communicating dermal lymphatics to the contralateral side explains occasional metastatic involvement of the opposite axilla and breast. Structures of the chest wall, including the external and internal intercostal musculature, have extensive lymphatic drainage, which parallels the course of their major intercostal blood supply. Thus invasive neoplasms of the lateral breast that involve deep musculature have preferential drainage toward the axillae. Conversely, invasion of medial musculature has preferential drainage toward the internal mammary nodal groups, whereas bidirectional metastases can be evident with invasive subareolar or central neoplasms.

Venous Drainage of Mammary Gland

Lymphatic drainage of the breast is the primary route for metastatic dissemination, although the vascular route for tumor emboli has a major role for dissemination of neoplasms to the lungs (see Fig. 62-2). The three groups of deep veins to the breast that serve as vascular routes are:

1. The *intercostal veins,* which traverse the posterior aspect of the breast from the second through the sixth intercostal spaces and enter the vertebral veins pos-

teriorly and the azygos vein centrally to terminate in the superior vena cava

2. The *axillary vein*, which may have many variable tributaries that drain the chest wall and the pectoral muscles and breast
3. The *internal mammary vein* perforators, which represent the largest venous network that drains the breast; this venous plexus traverses the rib interspaces to terminate in the innominate vein and thus represents a direct embolic route to the pulmonary capillary network.[6,65]

PHYSIOLOGY OF NORMAL BREAST DEVELOPMENT AND FUNCTION

The phases of breast development, growth, and involution follow alveoli and myoepithelial alterations of breast parenchyma, which result from the mammotropic effects of anterior pituitary and ovarian hormonal secretion. Breast growth and development is isometric and parallels that of body habitus before the onset of menses. The major determinant of breast development and maturation is related to the presence of ovarian estrogen and progesterone secretion. Thus, in the absence of endogenous estrogens, the amenorrheic (premenstrual) female will not develop breasts of normal size or consistency.

Hormonal Control of Breast Development and Function

Breast development in the female remains under neuroendocrine control of the anterior pituitary gland and the ovary. The gonadotropic luteinizing hormone (LH) and the gonadotropic follicle-stimulating hormone (FSH) of the female are both secreted from basophile cells of the anterior pituitary. The luteotropic lactogenic hormone prolactin (LTH) is produced by the pituitary acidophile cell. Neurohumoral pathways from the hypothalamus have a role in the production and/or release of these gonadotropic hormones.

The functions of the gonadotropic hormones of this basophilic group from the anterior pituitary are qualitatively identical in both sexes. FSH stimulates the mature ovarian graafian follicle to develop and synthesize estrogen in the presence of minute quantities of LH. When release of the basophilic LH is inhibited or impaired, the stimulated ovarian follicle will synthesize a product that, although not estrogenic, has the effect of inhibiting FSH. The presence of circulating estrogen initiates the production of LH and further inhibits basophilic cell production of FSH. Thus the presence of an augmented LH secretion with simultaneous diminution in the amount of FSH initiates ovulation and the formation of a nonfunctional corpus luteum. Prolactin hormone (LTH) initiates the release and secretion of progestogen and estrogen from the corpus luteum. Estrogen production from the ovary is initiated following FSH stimulation of the follicle in the presence of trace amounts of LH (Fig. 62-3). Both the production and release of LH, and perhaps LTH, from basophilic and acidophilic cells of the anterior pituitary are inhibited by progestogen and by estrogens in high circulating concentrations.[26]

Ovarian function in the female cannot be initiated until FSH is released, because LTH and LH have little or no effect on ovarian function in the absence of FSH. Thus menarche cannot appear until activation of FSH release from the basophilic cells of the pituitary. Further, ovulation and estrogen production, with its ultimate influence as a mammotropic hormone, cannot occur before the synthesis and release of LH from the gonadotropic basophile cell. The evacuation of the gravid uterus with the simultaneous cessation of secretion of hormones produced by the placenta initiates increased synthesis and/or release of the lactogenic (prolactin) hormone (LTH) of the anterior pituitary. Synthesis and/or release of the LTH can thus be inhibited by therapeutic doses of estrogens, androgens, or progestogens.

The previous discussion relates the biofeedback mechanism apparent for the gonadotropic hormones of the anterior pituitary with the ovary. The secretion of these hormones, which is under the purveyance of receptors of the hypothalamus, provides neurohumoral pathways to the pituitary. The feedback control of these glycoprotein gonadotropins allows the ovarian follicle to produce and release estrogen (estrone, estradiol), whereas the corpus luteum synthesizes and/or releases progesterone and estrogens. The presence of human chorionic gonadotropin (HCG) in pregnancy also initiates maintenance and production of progesterone and estrogens from the corpus luteum. The effects of estradiol in circulating levels from the ovarian follicles has numerous actions that are beyond the scope of this discussion. However, the effects to inhibit FSH and stimulate the production of LH have indirect consequences for breast development, maintenance, and function. In the prepubertal adolescent breast, estrogen induces development from the epidermal portion of the breast bud with growth of lactiferous ducts and myoepithelial cells and, to a lesser degree, of the alveoli of breast parenchyma (Fig. 62-4, *A*). Progesterone has many effects on the female reproductive system and its neuroendocrine control and promotes development of the acinar (secretory) tissues of the breast. Thus sudden loss of secretion of the gonadotropic pituitary hormones or the target organ hormones (estradiol and progesterone) will have detrimental consequences for growth, development, and maintenance of the ductal, acinar, or stromal parenchymal elements of the mammary gland.

With the onset of puberty and cyclic ovarian function resulting from the gonadotropic effects of the anterior pituitary, the mammotropic effects of estrogen are recognized (see Fig. 62-4, *B*). The lactiferous ducts and sinuses of the breast elongate with a recognizably enhanced cellular replication of columnar epithelium of the duct. Epithelial proliferation continues at the termination of the mammary tubules and initiates the formation of distinct lobules. Simultaneously, the stromal components of breast parenchyma enlarge to parallel the ingrowth and replication of ductal epithelium. This latter circumstance is responsible for the enlargement and texture of the female adolescent breast. Isometric growth with enlargement and pigmentation of the nipple and the areola occur as a result of the estrogen and progesterone effects.

The postadolescent female breast is established in cyclic ovulation, and the progesterone-secreting corpora lutae are maintained in this period. Thus the mature mammary gland has completed formation of the lobular and acinar structures following the additive effects of estrogen and progesterone (see Fig. 62-4, *C*). The characteristic lobular development evident in this phase of breast maintenance is completed approximately 12 to 18 months following menarche. Progressive development and enlargement of lactiferous ducts and acini result from the intense hormonal stimuli and secretion with each menstrual cycle or with pregnancy. Proportional enlargement of breast contour and size varies with habitus and body fat content, which are initiated in the adolescent period and maintained into the early postmenopausal era.

Data are sparse concerning the in vivo hormonal requirements in women for breast growth and differentiation in the pregnant state (see Fig. 62-4, *D*). Nonetheless, pituitary and ovarian hormones appear to be essential to growth and synthesis of milk in the mouse mammary gland. Provided the pituitary and adrenal glands are intact, growth of lactiferous ducts and alveoli to mid-pregnancy

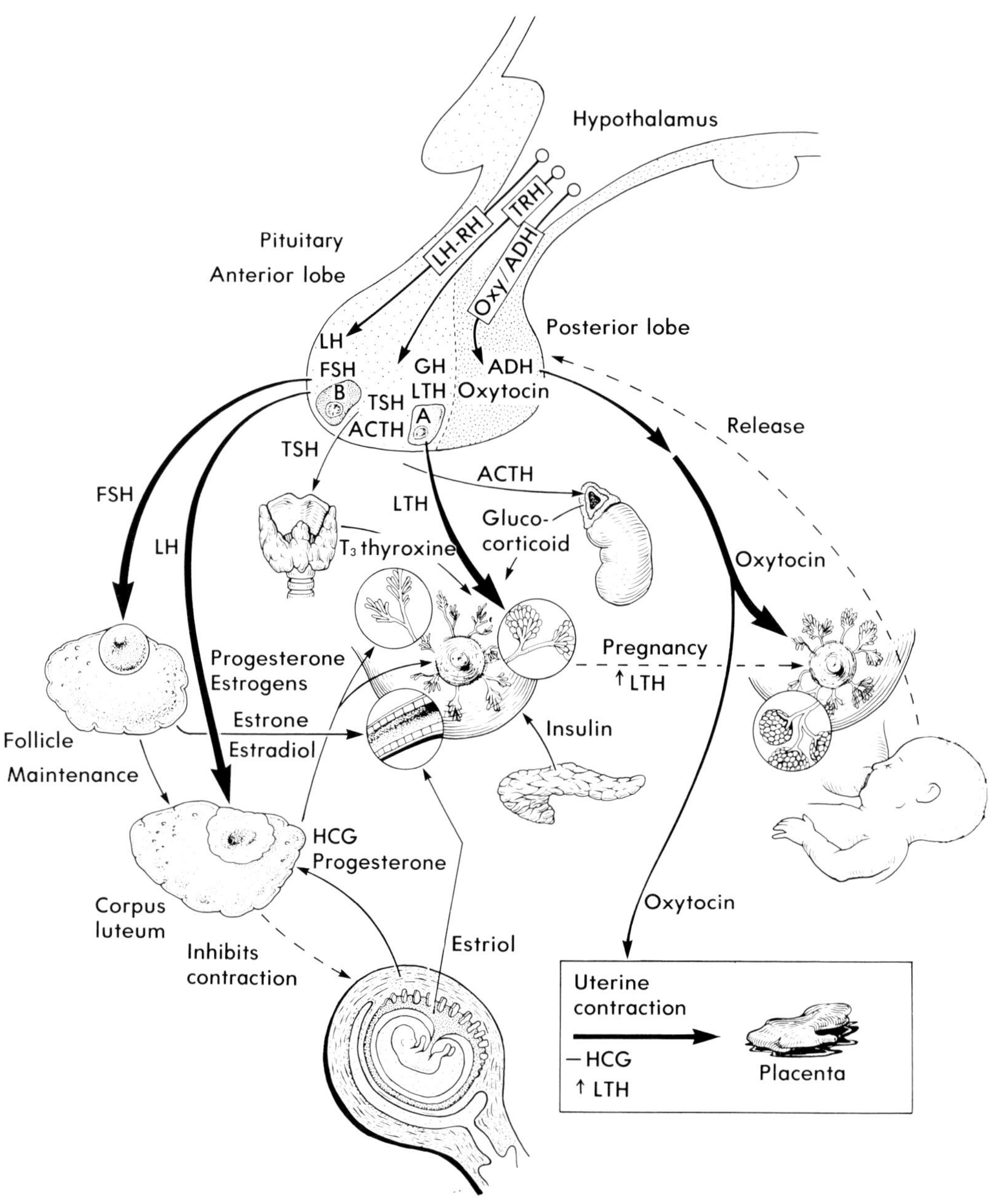

Fig. 62-3 Neuroendocrine control of breast development and function with relationships to gonadotropic hormones of anterior pituitary and ovary. Basophile secretion of LH and FSH is responsible for ovarian synthesis and release of progesterone and estrogen, respectively. Mammotropic effects of estrogen and progestin initiate myoepithelial and alveoli development. Acidophile cell secretion of LTH is initiated following evacuation of gravid uterus and is mammotropic to lobular alveoli. Suckling reflex initiates oxytocin release from posterior pituitary and is stimulatory to alveoli myeopithelial cells to initiate milk release. Neuroendocrine organs other than the pituitary and ovary provide hormones (glucocorticoid, GH, insulin, thyroxine) that are tropic to ductal and glandular maintenance and growth. (From Copeland, E.M., III, and Bland, K.I.: The breast. In Sabiston, D.C., Jr., editor: Essentials of surgery, Philadelphia, 1987, W.B. Saunders Co.)

can be achieved by administration of estrogen and progesterone to rodents. Neuroendocrine organs other than the ovary apparently provide hormones (growth hormone [GH], insulin, glucocorticoid) that are tropic to mammary ductal and glandular growth and maintenance. Milk synthesis and release begins about the fifth month of pregnancy, whereas the initiation of lactation is an event of delivery following intense LTH release of the anterior pituitary acidophile cell (see Fig. 62-4, *E*). The actual release of milk ("let down") at the time of the suckling reflex is a consequence of the action of oxytocin on the myoepithelial cells of the alveoli (see Fig. 62-3). The synthesis of oxytocin is continued in the hypothalamus and is released from the neurohypophysis following stimulation.

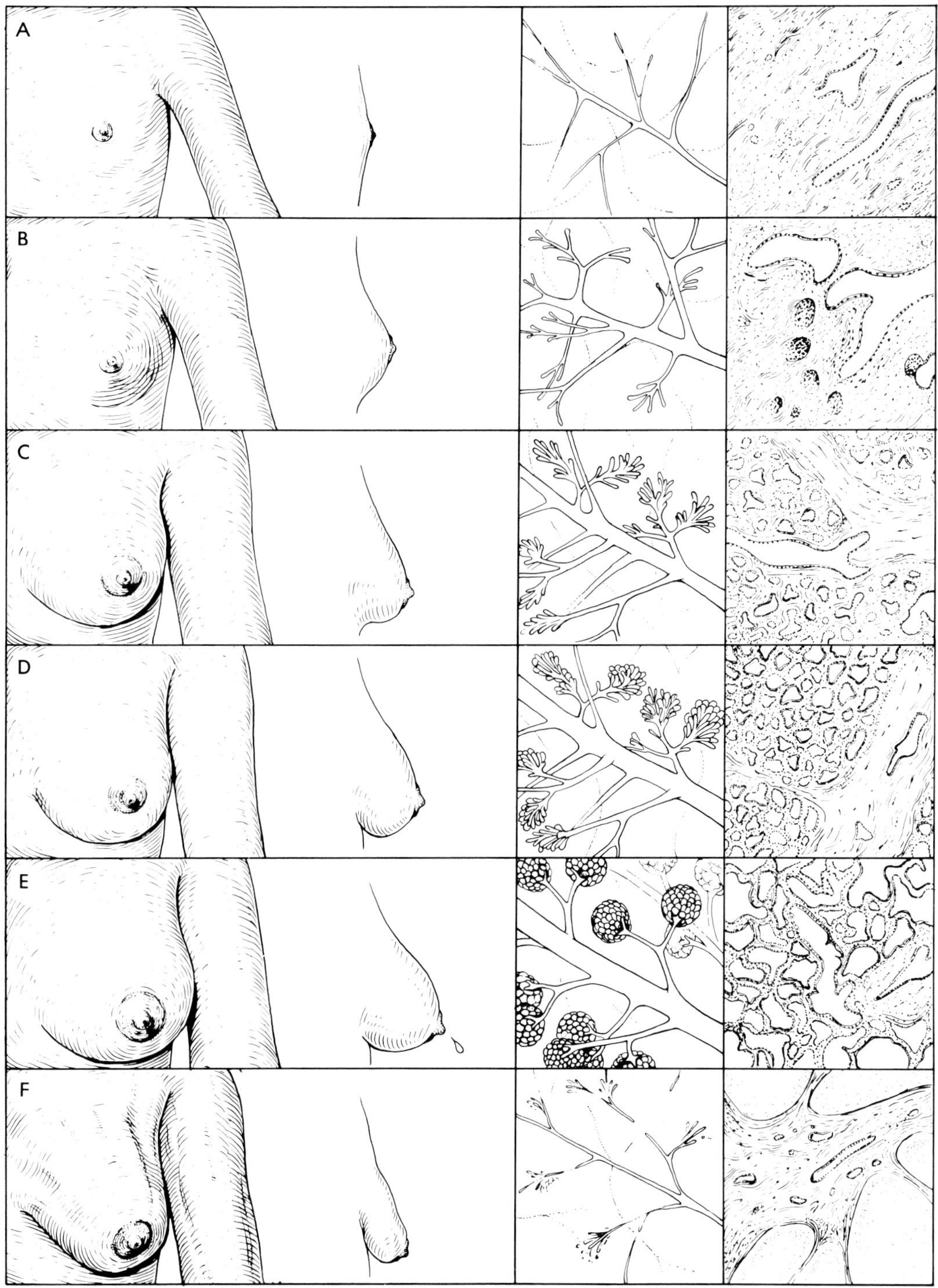

Fig. 62-4 Phases of mammary gland development, anterior and lateral view. Microscopic appearance of ducts and lobules in phases of development, growth, and maintenance. **A,** Prepubertal (childhood). **B,** Puberty. **C,** Mature (reproductive). **D,** Pregnancy. **E,** Lactation. **F,** Postmenopausal (senescent) state. (From Copeland, E.M., III, and Bland, K.I.: The breast. In Sabiston, D.C., Jr., editor: Essentials of surgery, Philadelphia, 1987, W.B. Saunders Co.)

Glandular tissue of the breast parenchyma eventually replaces the fatty elements between breast lobules as the latter proliferate with pregnancy. The primary stimuli for hyperplasia of breast glandular tissue in the pregnant state is the placental hormone, estriol. Following pregnancy and lactation, involution is incomplete, and the hypertropic and hyperplastic glandular tissues remain until menopause.

Cyclic changes of breast structure occur as a result of the gonadotropic and ovarian hormone concentrations, which may fluctuate with each menstrual cycle. Before the onset of menses, the lobules, stroma, and ducts become engorged; thereafter ducts shrink with the onset of menses, and epithelial cells desquamate and are then maintained to initiate proliferation by the second week of the cycle. The connective stroma and ductal epithelial cells increase in size and number. Remarkable variations and alterations of the hormonal milieu can be observed with the resultant effects of hypoplastic and hyperplastic dilation of ducts, connective tissue stroma, and lobules. The senile or postmenopausal breast undergoes progressive involution as a result of cessation of estrogenic and progestational effects of ovarian secretion. With menopause, regression to an atropic or hypoplastic epithelium of the lobules and ducts is apparent, whereas periductal fibrous tissue becomes dense (see Fig. 62-4, *F*). Dilation of the lactiferous duct network is noted in isolated lobules. Macrocystic formation (fibrocystic disease) occurs following enlargement of the lobular acini depleted of their columnar epithelium. On examination, the postmenopausal breast is often asymmetric with lobular irregularity and variations of cyst size. With progressive loss of fat content and the supporting periductal fibrous stroma, the senescent breast will shrink and the parenchymal and stromal tissue will blend into a homogenous, pendulous mass with loss of the original lobular structure.

CLINICAL EVALUATION OF BREAST DISEASE

General Considerations

Before visual inspection and palpation of the breast, a comprehensive personal medical history of the patient should be obtained. Detailed inquiry into associative risk factors is necessary and should include age, parity, and menstrual and nursing history. The age at menarche and cyclic alterations of breast masses that occur with menses are significant correlates of benign and malignant disease. Previous surgical procedures, especially oophorectomy, hysterectomy, adrenalectomy, or other pelvic surgery, are important to ascertain potential ablative procedures that initiate cessation of endogenous estrogen secretion. Prior use of hormonal therapy, including exogenous estrogens or oral contraceptives, may influence maintenance of mammary parenchyma. Also, the presence and nature of a nipple discharge should be ascertained. The precipitating events of such a discharge and its association with cyclic ovulation often provide distinguishing features of its etiology.

More than 80% of breast lesions are recognized by the patient before seeking medical attention. The physician should inquire about the dominant features of the presenting mass, its growth characteristics, and reproducibility of physical examination at menses. Hormonally sensitive breast lesions may present with mastodynia together with breast fullness and swelling in immediate premenstrual and postmenstrual periods. Breast cancer risk determinants are closely related to the patient's cultural background, and this may contribute to breast cancer aggregations within families. Thus a detailed inquiry of family history is necessary to determine if *hereditary breast cancer* or simple family aggregation of carcinoma exists. Breast cancer not fulfilling genetic criteria of the hereditary variant is classified as *sporadic*. Also, constitutional symptoms should be elicited and carefully recorded. The presence of progressive weight loss, hemoptysis, fever, chest pain, anorexia, and skeletal pain are important determinants of advanced local, regional, and systemic disease.

Visual Inspection

Before palpation, the physician visually inspects the patient's breasts in anteroposterior and lateral views to observe symmetry, skin changes, retraction, elevation, and color alterations. The examination is conducted with the patient's arms at her sides and then on the hips with contraction of pectoral muscles to accentuate breast contour.

Bacterial cellulitis is easily recognized by the presence of focal areas of skin involvement and associated diffuse edema of the ipsilateral breast. These findings often accompany superficial and deep *abscesses*. Regional endolymphatic permeation of the ipsilateral breast and dermal lymphatics with tumor emboli from inflammatory breast carcinoma may be confused with bacterial cellulitis. With progression of the inflammatory neoplasm, segmental entrapment of Cooper's ligaments may initiate skin retraction and dimpling. This latter finding also may be associated with common variants of infiltrating breast neoplasms. The skin may have focal sites of diffuse edema, as seen with cellulitis, and *peau d'orange* (orange peel) *edema* may occur as a result of lymphatic obstruction.

With radial growth of the tumor, an intense desmoplastic response initiates tethering with retraction of the skin secondary to contraction of Cooper's ligaments. Retraction of the skin and associated dimpling is best visualized with the patient in the sitting position, contracting the pectoral muscles to accentuate the breast profile. These maneuvers accentuate deep involvement of structures in the large breast. Similar findings are observed with benign lesions such as fat necrosis; thus physical examination alone is often insufficient to distinguish malignant tumors.

Breast Palpation

A systematic palpation of the regional sites common to metastatic involvement by breast neoplasms is conducted before initiating breast examination. Evaluation of the axillary and supraclavicular fossae requires both superficial and deep palpation to identify nodal metastases. Examination of the axillae should be done with the patient in a sitting position with the ipsilateral arm supported by the examiner. Complete relaxation of the shoulder girdle musculature is essential to allow comprehensive palpation of the five regional nodal groups. Gentle fingertip pressure best identifies small nodal deposits. Large, bulky, extramammary metastases in both these regional sites may be obvious to patient and physician. Precise documentation of location and size of nodes is important to allow accurate clinical staging. At the time the five nodal groups are assessed, the examiner should position the fingers in the axillary fold such that all infraclavicular structures lateral to Halsted's ligaments are evaluated.

A systematic evaluation of all breast quadrants is completed with the patient relaxed in the supine position with full extension of the arm and the shoulder in external rotation. A flattened sheet provides support to the ipsilateral hemithorax to accentuate breast detail. The object of the evaluation is to detect small lesions that are separate from surrounding breast fat and parenchyma. Well-circumscribed, painful lesions that are totally separable from adjacent tissues usually represent benign masses. Painless, firm, nonballottable lesions with indistinct borders should be considered malignant until proven otherwise. As noted, however, the distinction between malignancy and benignity on the basis of a physical examination is often impossible.

Following superficial and deep palpation of all quadrants of the breast, the nipple-areolar complex is carefully evaluated. The presence of associated nipple inversion should be documented, and, if unilateral, carcinoma should be suspected. If normal, an inverted nipple can usually be everted to its correct anatomic position; the inability to perform this maneuver often necessitates biopsy to disprove a malignancy. Eczema and inflammatory states of the nipple-areolar complex are often observed in the postpartum era and with lactation. In contrast, a crusty, scaly, eczematoid eruption of the areola is pathognomonic of Paget's disease of the nipple. These lesions, which are unilateral and distinct from the contralateral nipple, often bleed or weep on contact. Biopsy of the subareolar parenchyma will confirm a primary infiltrating ductal carcinoma that invades the nipple and skin of the areolar to produce the associated clinical findings.

Special Considerations

Gynecomastia

The development of gynecomastia in the pubertal male is a consequence of the estrogenic hormonal milieu and typically occurs between the ages of 13 and 17 years. Although the hormonal mechanism responsible is poorly understood, it appears that a predominant estrogenic effect in relation to androgen secretion is operative and perhaps is secondary to a delay in the reversal of the androstenedione/testosterone ratio that is normally an event of puberty.[62,65] A slight hypertropic abnormality is present and may occasionally persist either unilaterally or bilaterally. When unilateral, any relationship to hormonal dysfunction rarely exists; however, the presence of persistent bilateral gynecomastia requires a search for systemic etiology. Gynecomastia is also seen in situations where high levels of circulating estrogens are present, such as in the prepubertal child of either sex, in hepatic cirrhosis, and following use of exogenous estrogens or drugs with estrogenic properties (e.g., digoxin, dilantin) in males. In the absence of an abnormal endocrine secretory state and other abnormalities, the hypertropic breast tissue can be removed with a circumareolar incision to restore the breast contour. Biopsy typically reveals an absence of acinar growth with a background of proliferative breast stroma and lactiferous ducts.

Rapid and extensive enlargement of the female breast at puberty sometimes continues unabated. Estrogen and its target-organ effect on breast stroma and lobular hypertrophy may initiate breast enlargement to as great as 40 to 50 pounds and may represent a significant cosmetic and functional impairment. Progression in size may continue into young adulthood. Because spontaneous regression is unlikely, these hypertropic, pendulous breasts are best managed by bilateral reduction mammoplasty.

Nipple Discharge

Discharge from the nipple, although not a frequent symptom, is estimated to occur in approximately 3% to 9% of patients.[35,65,99,105] Nipple discharge has been reported in 8.8% of 10,365 women in six groups attending breast clinics and in 6.5% of 8640 women in five series subjected to breast surgery.[105] Nipple secretion represents an alteration in the normal physiologic consequences of duct epithelial secretion and may indicate an inflammatory, proliferative, or neoplastic process. Discharges of pathologic significance typically empty spontaneously from the ductal sinus/recess of the nipple ampullae. Conversely, discharges that are elicited by squeezing breast parenchyma or the nipple-areola complex are usually inconsequential.

The type of nipple discharge is the pathognomonic feature that determines its etiology. The frequently observed watery, puslike, or thick discharge of ductal ectasia may be elicited by milking or squeezing multiple lobes of the breast or the nipple. This physiologic and harmless secretion requires only patient reassurance of its benignity. Four additional types of discharge are recognized.

Bloody Discharge. This form of ductal discharge may vary from bright red to brown and represents the most common type in many series (50% to 75%). The most frequent etiologic mechanism is hyperplastic and proliferative growth of intraductal epithelium. The majority of these discharges represent benign epithelial proliferation as a component of fibrocystic disease, and an intraductal papilloma is often etiologic. On occasion, bloody discharge is secondary to a malignant epithelial proliferation such as intraductal papillary carcinoma.

The presence of a solitary mass in a postmenopausal patient is highly suggestive of a malignant process and necessitates confirmation by biopsy and/or Papanicolaou smear. The Pap smear is of value only if it is positive and should be confirmed as malignant before definitive surgical therapy. The presence of a malignancy with the finding of a bloody nipple discharge occurs in approximately 9% to 14% of patients.[55,130] Haagensen[65] observed 11.5% of spontaneous nipple discharges to be of malignant origin, 55% of which were bloody types (Table 62-1). When a palpable lesion is not identifiable clinically or mammographically, surgical exploration of the subareola is indicated. Often, milking specific quadrants and emptying the involved duct will allow identification of a papilloma. Precise localization of the offending lesion may be possible.

Table 62-1 **BREAST CONDITIONS PRODUCING SPONTANEOUS NIPPLE DISCHARGE**

Condition	Type of Nipple Discharge			Total Patients (No.)	Total Patients (%)
	Serous	Bloody	Watery		
Pregnancy	—	10	—	10	6
Menstruation	—	1	—	1	—
Cystic disease	3	—	—	3	—
Duct ectasia	3	2	—	5	3
Intraductal papilloma	53	55	—	108	69
Accessory subareolar gland papilloma	3	—	—	3	—
Papilloma of nipple ducts	9	—	—	9	5.8
Carcinoma of breast	7	10	1	18	11.5
TOTAL				157	

From Haagensen, C.D.: Physician's role in the detection of breast disease. In Haagensen, C.D., editor: Diseases of the breast, Philadelphia, 1971, W.B. Saunders Co.

Probing the duct with bimanual palpation may provide identification of the responsible tumor to allow definitive surgical resection. Radiographic imaging with contrast ductography will sometimes permit precise preoperative localization.

Chaudary and associates,[32] in an analysis of 270 patients undergoing microdochectomy for hemoglobin-positive nipple discharge, with and without an associated lump, observed a cancer incidence of 5.9%. In order of frequency, intraductal papilloma, duct ectasia, fibrocystic disease, and carcinoma accounted for over 90% of the cases.

SEROUS DISCHARGE. This thin, translucent, colorless to straw-colored discharge may occur spontaneously. It most often occurs with normal menstrual cycles, in early pregnancy, or in individuals taking oral contraceptives. This discharge is secondary to estrogen effects on duct epithelium with resultant hyperplasia and proliferation to enhance secretion. The palpation of a solitary subareolar mass is highly suggestive of an intraductal papilloma and can often be confirmed by contrast radiography or probing of the responsible duct mechanism. Simple excision of the intraductal papilloma is curative.

MILKY DISCHARGE. The discharge of fluid with the consistency and chemical composition of milk is evident many months postpartum and after cessation of breast-feeding. The production and the release of LTH can be inhibited by appropriate doses of estrogen, androgen, and progestogens. The most satisfactory normal control for secondary (delayed) breast manifestations with mastalgia, milky discharge, and engorgement is a single, intramuscular injection of testosterone enanthate and estradiol valerate (Deladumone) in the desired ratio. On occasion, acromegaly can produce a milky discharge because of the somatotropic effect of GH on breast acini and lobular secretion.

YELLOW DISCHARGE. The proliferative response of breast ductal structures and acini to excessive estrogen production in the presence of deficient corpus luteum activity is responsible for this presentation. The ductal structure with its retained fluid sometimes will spontaneously discharge a dark, yellow fluid that can also be obtained by percutaneous breast aspiration. Fluid cytology, although desirable, rarely reveals neoplastic cells unless the cyst wall has undergone the rare event of malignant transformation. The cost-effectiveness of cytology for hemoglobin-negative nipple discharge must be questioned, and, in the absence of high-risk patient factors for cancer, cytology on such fluid is not justified.

RARE CONDITIONS THAT INITIATE NIPPLE DISCHARGE. The breast represents a target organ without a physiologic feedback mechanism to inhibit multiple hormonal stimuli that may initiate prolonged secretory phases. The acidophilic lactogenic cell (LTH) from the anterior pituitary may initiate unrecognized surges in circulating serum prolactin (LTH) levels. Newman and colleagues[105] observed that serum prolactin levels were above normal in 25% of 587 patients with nipple secretion of various etiologic types. The most common physiologic factors that augmented the serum prolactin in women were nursing and breast stimulation, sexual intercourse, pregnancy, and stress.[105] Any of these etiologic mechanisms may potentiate other subliminal causes (e.g., minute doses of oral contraceptives, psychotropic drugs, antihypertensive medication).

The effect of hyperprolactinemia on depressing ovarian function and initiating secondary amenorrhea and galactorrhea is controversial. Approximately one third of patients with secondary amenorrhea and one fourth with galactorrhea will have elevated serum prolactin values.[27,105,127] Several syndromes that embrace these symptoms include Forbes-Albright[53] (pituitary adenoma), Chiari-Frommel[33,54] (postpregnancy amenorrhea and galactorrhea), and Ahumada-Argonz del Castillo[1,7] (unrelated to pregnancy symptoms). The physiologic implications of hyperprolactinemia with the shared clinical symptoms of breast secretion and amenorrhea may represent a continuum of pathologic disorder of multiple endocrine stigmata, which also include anovulatory syndromes, sterility hirsutism, obesity, acne, and loss of libido.

Kleinberg[79] observed that most (60%) pituitary tumors initiating production of prolactin are composed of specific lactomorphs. As the pituitary neoplasm enlarges, it may distort the pituitary stalk and impair the secretion and delivery of prolactin-inhibitory hormone from the hypothalamus. Thus the expansion of this neoplasm with the initiation of neurologic deficits of the optic chiasm and pyramidal tracts requires prompt surgical intervention and excision of the sella neoplasm. The differentiation between a microadenoma that may initiate amenorrhea and breast secretion and hyperprolactinemia of other causes (hypothalamic neoplasms or disease, lactomorph hyperplasia) may be impossible and only of academic interest. Indeed, in the asymptomatic patient the probability of a pituitary adenoma approximates 0.1% and is even less if the patient uses oral contraceptives or has persistent lactation.[105] Prolactin values greater than 300 ng/ml are diagnostic of tumor, whereas values between 100 and 300 ng/ml represent adenomas in approximately 50% of cases.[16]

Anovulatory syndromes associated with galactorrhea may resolve spontaneously following the inhibition of prolactin secretion with bromocriptine (Parlodel) or clomiphene (Serophene) therapy. Follow-up will allow the diagnosis of pituitary neoplasms after years of observation. The diagnosis of the triad of hyperprolactinemia, amenorrhea, and breast secretion in the absence of an associated computed tomography (CT) scan or plain-film sella abnormality deserves follow-up (serial) plasma prolactin values. Bromocriptine will control the growth of these pituitary microprolactinomas and their symptoms, but the ultimate result of chronic therapy and its potential side effects are uncertain.

DISEASE PROCESSES INVOLVING THE BREAST

Inflammatory Conditions

Acute inflammatory states of the breast are most often secondary to retrograde bacterial infections that result from disruption of the epithelial interface of the nipple-areola complex. Staphylococcal or streptococcal bacteria represent the organisms on Gram's stain and culture most frequently recovered from the nipple discharge in an active breast abscess. These infections are often related to lactation and typically occur within the first weeks of breastfeeding.[19] Progression of the inflammatory process can result in diffuse breast cellulitis with loculated subareolar or central abscesses (Fig. 62-5). Through the diffuse network of the lactiferous ducts, multilocular abscesses may form with the presentation of diffuse cellulitis and a systemically ill patient. Classically, streptococcal infections produce diffuse cellulitis without localization until an advanced course of the disease when the patient has systemic manifestations. *Staphylococcus aureus* abscesses tend to have a more localized, suppurative, and deeply invasive presentation with acute and chronic abscess formation. The multilocular abscess is seen more often in staphylococcal infections that initiate loculated suppuration between the fibroseptae of Cooper's ligaments.

The presentation of an advanced abscess requires immediate surgical attention. Lymphatic involvement secondary to streptococcal cellulitis usually requires local nursing care with the application of focal heat compresses and appropriate antibiotics such as penicillin derivatives. Focal abscess with overgrowth of any bacterial organism requires immediate and adequate surgical drainage of fluctuant areas. Thorough debridement of the abscess through a circumareolar incision or multiple incisions placed in the direction of Langer's lines is recommended (see Fig. 62-5). Open drainage of the wound with strict attention to

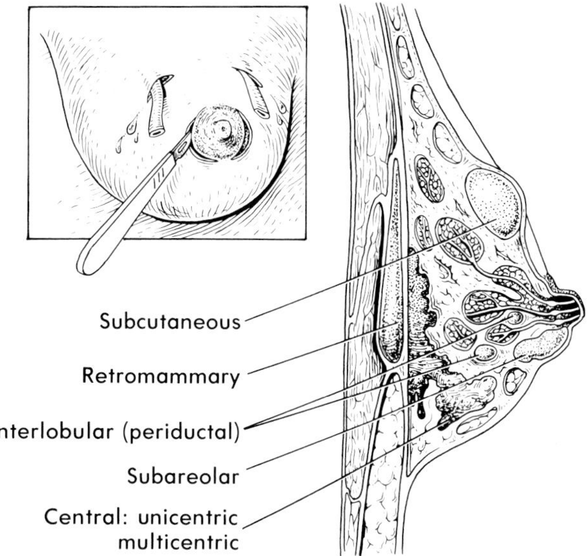

Fig. 62-5 Sagittal section of breast with potential abscess sites. Typical central abscess may be multicentric or focal. Retromammary abscess may be seen in chronic infectious or neoplastic processes (e.g., tuberculosis, carcinoma). Extensive, deep abscess may be multilocular and may communicate with subcutaneous or subareolar sites. Painful subcutaneous, interlobular, or subareolar abscess may appear with diffuse cellulitis. Thorough drainage and evacuation of breast abscesses through incisions that parallel Langer's lines are recommended treatment.

hygienic evacuation of the abscess and the nipple-areola complex are essential to avoid skin and subcutaneous necrosis.

Discontinuance of suckling in the postpartum state is recommended to prevent stasis and progressive growth of bacteria in the lactiferous ducts. The use of a breast suction pump occasionally may be advantageous to empty stagnant milk ducts and central abscess collections. The continuance of lactation following removal of the suckling reflex may necessitate the use of intramuscular injections of testosterone enanthate/estradiol valerate (Deladumone).

The presentation of *chronic* inflammatory states of the breast with abscess formation is unusual, and the differential diagnosis must include chronic infectious or neoplastic processes (e.g., tuberculosis, carcinoma). Although occurring much less frequently than two decades ago, the ubiquitous tuberculous organism remains the most common etiology of chronic bacterial mastitis.[65] Today, this diagnosis, as the coexistent finding of multiple granulomatous processes (fungi and sarcoidosis), may produce a bacteriologic and physiologic presentation similar to pulmonary tuberculosis. Classically, the breast tuberculoma is nontender and may have multiple sinus tracts extending from the anterior thorax to sites of central or subcutaneous cavitation with intervening cellulitis. The demonstration of acid-fast tubercle bacilli in the lesion or on culture is diagnostic. Adequate drainage identical to that for acute bacterial abscess and initiation of antituberculous therapy are the prerequisites of therapy. Biopsy of the drainage site is mandatory for chronic abscesses of any etiology to exclude the possibility of invasive carcinoma. Local drainage and systemic antibiotic therapy are rarely necessary before cyclic chemotherapy and mastectomy to provide control of the carcinomatous process with superimposed infection.

Mondor's Disease: Thrombophlebitis of Superficial Thoracoepigastric Vein

The presentation of acute pain in the superficial distribution of the thoracodorsal vein along its course to the hypochondrium is diagnostic of this benign state. The classic finding in Mondor's disease of a palpable, cordlike thickening that extends across the superolateral breast toward the axilla may be related to local trauma of the breast and/or axilla. This self-limiting process requires no definitive therapy. The clinical importance of this inflammatory condition is essentially its recognition and differentiation from carcinoma or other breast disease.

Hormonal Induction and Pathophysiology of Benign Breast Disease

Sir Astley Cooper is credited with the first description of benign cystic disease of the breast and subsequently classified its various forms as adenosis, cystic disease, and mastodynia. Initial opinion suggested that these forms were interrelated and together constituted the most common breast abnormalities of sexual maturity. The subsequent descriptions by Schimmelbusch (1890) of the microscopic features of cyst adenoma (Geschickter's adenosis) suggested proliferation of epithelial elements with the formation of cysts and a loss of normal interacinous connective tissues.[37] Although considerable controversy exists with regard to the variants of this entity, for purposes of discussion, mastopathy of the cystic type should be considered synonymous with "fibrocystic" disease of the breast (FCDB), chronic cystic mastitis, mammary dysplasia, benign mastopathy, and cystic disease of the breast.

Proliferative and nonproliferative diseases (gross and microscopic) are the most frequently diagnosed lesion of the mamma. As gross cystic disease does not become clinically evident until establishment of active ovarian function, the observation of its regression following menopause suggests that estrogens and progestins are operative in the etiology. The absolute prevalence of the process is unknown, but previous reports of elderly women dying of causes other than breast cancer noted histopathologic changes of benign mastopathy in 100% of the breasts studied. Kramer and Rush[81] observed that this elderly population had cystic changes in 89% of cases, apocrine metaplasia in 80%, and intraductal hyperplasia in 69%. Thus the changes of fibrosis and epithelial proliferation, which invariably occur as a result of physiologic consequences of ovarian stimulation, may represent progression to a "disease state" with macrocysts. The epithelial changes, ranging from duct adenosis to cystic alterations and from ductal epithelial proliferation to atypia and carcinoma, have been reproduced in the rodent by numerous investigators.[14,15,138] Although difficult to reproduce in mice, stromal fibrosis can be initiated following ovarian stimulation in monkeys.[61]

As already noted, the interplay and synchrony of prolactin and progesterone is necessary for estrogen to exert its active mammatropic role in breast physiology. Although synergism exists between both sex steroids, with estrogen promoting growth and development of ducts and progesterone affecting inductive growth of the alveolar system, the presence of prolactin is also necessary. In the hypothesized animal, parenteral administration of estrogen will not promote mammary development. Conversely, breast development will occur when an excess of pituitary hormones exists in the absence of estrogen. It appears that other essential endocrine factors, which are less clearly delineated but include thyroxine (T_4), insulin, adrenocorticoids, and GH, are important to allow full differentiation of the lactiferous and lobular components of the mamma.[116] The initial induction of mammary epithelial stem cell division by estrogen depends on prolactin, GH, and insulin. Also, the exposure to therapeutic levels of endogenous cortisol and insulin provides prolactin with an appropriate hormonal milieu to initiate final differentiation of alveolar epithelial cells into mature milk cells. The interregulation of pituitary hormones that interact with ovarian gonadotropins is subsequently orchestrated in synchrony with T_4 and triiodothyronine (T_3) to stimulate the end organ (breast) for metabolic regulatory control (see Fig. 62-3).

Cystic and epithelial lesions of mice produced by various regimes that augment an absolute or relative increase in serum estrogens have been observed to closely resemble the gross and microcystic lesions of human beings.[62] In species other than rodents, well-documented responses to estrogen stimulation are evident in fibrous tissue and smooth muscle of certain organs.[135] Investigators have suggested that estrogen increases stromal ground substance that has the propensity to fibrous reorganization. These data suggest that the epithelial and stromal elements of breast parenchyma may be target organs of ovarian and pituitary hormonal secretion. Further, the duration of active stimulation of the hormonally sensitive components of breast structure accounts for the peak incidence for disease and regression of symptomatic macrocystic changes following cessation of the estrogen/progesterone milieu with menopause.

The etiology of gross and microcystic breast disease appears to be multifactorial; the essential factor is relative hyperestrinism, which initiates epithelial hyperplasia. Genetic factors, mammotropic pituitary hormones, and other circulating nongonadotropin hormones (insulin, T_4, GH) also are involved. Early investigators[22] were impressed that women with FCDB had decreased fertility and often had slightly abnormal menstrual cycles. These early studies, however, did not confirm that estrogen levels in the serum of affected subjects were elevated. The hypothesis of relative estrogen excess secondary to a deficient luteal phase was thus initiated in the etiology of the entity.[62] Until recently, this hypothesis could not be tested because it required the serial measurement of estrogen/progestin hormone in various phases of the menses. The potential for abnormal end-organ metabolism as the etiology of this disease process is under investigation.

Examination of the breast of women with FCDB typically reveals diffuse fullness and fibronodularity. These multiple or solitary cystic lesions are observed to be well-demarcated, mobile, smooth masses. Following recognition of the symptomatic cystic lesion, appropriate therapy consists of needle aspiration. Typically, cystic fluid is clear or straw-colored; however, chronic cysts may be bloody or contain gray-green turbid contents. The cyst fluid should be forwarded for cytologic examination, although it is rarely of diagnostic value. The occasional finding of a positive Pap smear has profound significance and necessitates immediate biopsy. Aspiration of bloody cytologic fluid indicates frequent follow-up and warrants biopsy if a residual mass is palpable following aspiration. The presence of a solid lesion may denote a cyst cancer or a primary neoplasm coexistent with proliferative breast lesion.[17]

History of FCDB (Previous Biopsies) as Risk Indicator

As noted previously, similar mechanisms of FCDB and neoplasia relate to active ovarian hormonal stimuli. Although histologic identification of the presence of both diseases is common, circumstantial evidence for the relationship between these two entities remains controversial. The patient with advanced fibronodular breast disease marked by diffuse solid or cystic masses and with an active reproductive status should be closely scrutinized in follow-up. A positive history of familial breast cancer has added significance. Clearly, the solid-mass lesion found on clinical or xeromammographic (XMM) examination that remains unchanged throughout the menses should be considered suspicious and requires biopsy and histologic evaluation. At least one fourth of patients subjected to biopsy should have confirmation of a neoplasm, or the case selection has not been discriminating. This cancer/biopsy ratio is much higher (≅1:6 to 8) following the screening of asymptomatic women.[21]

The evaluation of prospective studies, in which women with benign biopsy specimens were followed to determine the subsequent incidence of cancer, poses several issues. Problems with statistical analyses include inconsistent intervals of follow-up and unspecified distributions of age. The clinical decision to biopsy a breast mass is subjective and is often made on clinical indications and the relative risk of cancer. Therefore patients having biopsies are considered a select, high-risk population subset. Love, Gelman, and Silen[87] compared five prospective studies for patients with biopsies who subsequently were determined to have carcinoma. For 6511 patients, an increased risk for cancer of 1.98 was evident if the breast had previously been biopsied. This relative risk was similar to the recalculated incidence of the 1970 and 1976 NCI surveys (2.13 vs. 1.86, respectively).

Histologic identification of the presence of *both* FCDB and breast neoplasia is common. Love, Gelman, and Silen[87] observed that FCDB was noted in 58% of autopsied *noncancerous* breasts but in only 26% of *cancerous* breasts. Haagensen[65] observed a 4.1-fold increase in incidence of carcinoma for patients treated previously for FCDB. The association of the two diseases is probably inevitable and coincidental because the hormonal milieu of hyperestrinism supports the genesis of both FCDB and carcinoma. Black and Chabon[14] have recommended the term *precancerous mastopathy* for the lesion with duct epithelial hyperplasia with atypia and aporcine metaplasia with atypia. These investigators report that the asymptomatic patient with ductal atypia and hyperplasia in a benign lesion is subject to developing breast carcinoma at a risk that exceeds fivefold that of the woman without these histologic findings. This risk appears to be reduced for that patient if apocrine metaplasia with atypia was included. Love, Gelman, and Silen[87] considered epithelial hyperplasia to be at least as common in noncancerous breasts as in cancerous ones (32% vs. 23%, respectively) (Table 62-2).

Table 62-2 **REPORTED INCIDENCE OF MICROSCOPIC FIBROCYSTIC DISEASE IN BREASTS REMOVED FOR CANCER AND IN NONCANCEROUS BREASTS STUDIED AT AUTOPSY**

Study	Patients (No.)	Age Range	Fibrocystic Disease (General)		Epithelial Hyperplasia (General)		Atypia	
			No.	%	No.	%	No.	%
NONCANCEROUS BREASTS STUDIED AT AUTOPSY								
Frantz*	225	13-85	117	52	32	14		
Sloss*	100	20-99			33	33		
Davis	725	13-99	360	58	210	31		
Kramer	70	70	—	—	48	69	7	10
TOTAL			360	58	258	32		
BREASTS REMOVED FOR CANCER								
Davis	327		128	40	38	12		
Kern	100	30-90	71	71	27	27	24	24
Karpas	226	20≥80			52	23	32	14
Fischerman	411	20-80	54	13	10	2		
Silverberg	398	20-99	157	40	30	8		
Bonser	220	20-80			123	56		
Fisher	1000		206	21	349	35		
Devitt	594	15-80	133	22	—	—		
TOTAL			749	26	629	23		

From Love, S.M., et al.: Reprinted, by permission of N. Engl. J. Med. **307**(16):1012, 1982.
*Studies done before 1964; these totals are included in the totals given for Davis.

Monson and co-workers[102] evaluated the cancer risk associated with "benign breast disease" (i.e., FCDB, chronic cystic mastitis) and concluded that the excess risk for dying of breast carcinoma in individuals with this diagnosis persists for approximately 30 years or longer following the diagnosis of chronic mastitis. Their data suggest that women with chronic mastitis have an escalated risk for developing carcinoma 2.5 times that of normal women. Davis, Simons, and Davis[38] concluded that proliferative histologic changes increased the risk for subsequent carcinoma 2.6 times that of the control population, whereas the neoplastic risk for women without associated proliferative changes was only 1.2 times that of the general population.

These observations have been substantiated by other investigators[41,51,80,139] with variance in the range of increasing risk. All agree with the concept that more severe degrees of epithelial proliferation and atypical changes augment the probability of cancer risk over lesser variations of atypia. Fisher and associates[51] suggest that proliferative forms occur more frequently in younger women, whereas the nonproliferative lesion is more often observed in the older age group. Carcinoma developed more frequently when epithelial proliferative lesions were present.

Page and associates[107] also observed that atypical lobular hyperplasia provides a greater predictive value than other epithelial lesions and is associated with an increased cancer risk sixfold of that expected before age 35 years, with a tripling of risk beyond this age. They noted that ductal hyperplastic lesions are associated with a twofold risk if lesions were identified at biopsy after age 45 years. These investigators suggested no increased risk for subsequent carcinoma over the control population for women with sclerosing adenosis, fibrosis, cysts, and other nonhyperplastic changes. Atypical duct neoplasms, which are typically described as having features consonant with in situ carcinoma, did not appear to have an associated elevation of cancer risk above ductal lesions that are unassociated with such severe atypia. This conclusion appears to disagree with the studies of Black and co-workers[14,15] and Kodlin and associates.[80]

The hypothesis that strong prognostic importance can be evaluated in biopsies that harbor epithelial hyperplasia of lobular and ductal patterns was reviewed by Rogers and Page.[118] This study describes a risk of fourfold to sixfold that of the general population if atypical lobular hyperplasia is present. The risk was two to three times that of the general population if ductal hyperplasia was evident in patients over age 45 years. No increased risk was evident, however, for ductal hyperplasia in patients less than 45 years of age or if sclerosing adenosis was described in the specimen.

Dupont and Page[43] recently evaluated women with benign *proliferative* breast lesions. Women having *proliferative* disease *without* atypical hyperplasia had a risk of cancer 1.9 times that of women with *nonproliferative* lesions (95% confidence interval, 1.2 to 2.9). However, the risk for women with atypical hyperplasia (atypia) was 5.3 times that in women with nonproliferative lesions (95% confidence interval, 3.1 to 8.8). The proportional hazards—the relative risks shown in Table 62-3—are useful to compare the relative risks for different subgroups within the same study. A *family history* of breast cancer had little effect on the risk for women with nonproliferative lesions. However, the risk for women with *atypia and a family history* of breast cancer was elevenfold that for women

Table 62-3 **EFFECT OF HYPERPLASIA, AGE, FAMILY HISTORY, AND CALCIFICATION ON THE RISK OF BREAST CANCER***

Numerator of Relative Risk	Denominator of Relative Risk	Relative Risk†	95% Confidence Interval	*p* Value
PDWA, age 20-45	Non-PD, age 20-45	1.9	1.2-3.2	0.012
PDWA, age 46-55	Non-PD, age 46-55	1.4	0.57-3.3	0.49
PDWA, age >55	Non-PD, age >55	5.6	0.69-46	0.11
PDWA with CAL	Non-PD without CAL	2.3	1.2-4.3	0.008
AH with CAL	Non-PD with CAL	8.6	2.5-29	0.0006
AH with CAL	Non-PD without CAL	8.3	3.5-19	<0.0001
Cysts without FH	Neither cysts nor FH	1.3	0.88-2	0.19
Cysts with FH	No cysts but FH	2.1	0.78-5.5	0.14
Cysts with FH	Neither cysts nor FH	2.7	1.5-4.6	0.0004
PDWA	Non-PD	1.9	1.2-2.9	0.003
AH	Non-PD	5.3	3.1-8.8	<0.0001
CAL	No CAL	1.3	0.87-2	0.19
PDWA without FH	Non-PD without FH	1.9	1.2-3	0.007
PDWA with FH	Non-PD with FH	2	0.63-6.1	0.25
PDWA with FH	Non-PD without FH	2.7	1.4-5.3	0.004
AH without FH	Non-PD without FH	4.3	2.4-7.8	<0.0001
AH with FH	Non-PD with FH	8.4	2.6-27	0.0003
AH with FH	Non-PD without FH	11	5.5-24	<0.0001

From Dupont, W.D., and Page, D.L.: Reprinted, by permission of N. Engl. J. Med. **312**(3):146, 1985.

*PDWA, Proliferative disease without atypia; AH, atypical hyperplasia; CAL, calcification; FH, family history of breast cancer (mother, sister, or daughter); age, age at time of entry biopsy.

†As compared with the risk in women from Atlanta (Third National Cancer Survey).

who had nonproliferative lesions without a family history (95% confidence interval, 5.5 to 24). The authors observed that calcification elevated the cancer risk if the biopsy confirmed proliferative disease. The presence of cysts and a family history of breast cancer enhanced the risk 2.7 times that for women without either of these risk factors (95% confidence interval, 1.5 to 4.6). These authors conclude that most women (70%) having breast biopsy for benign disease are not at increased risk for cancer. These data do corroborate the findings of an increased cancer risk on the basis of atypical hyperplasia and a family history of breast cancer. Fig. 62-6 denotes the proportion of patients free of invasive cancer as a function of time since biopsy. A twofold or threefold increase may have little clinical importance if the risk in the reference population is small. The adverse effect of positive family history for the patient with atypical hyperplasia becomes appreciable at approximately 20 years after biopsy.

The aforementioned clinicopathologic studies reflect the opinion that *proliferative* lesions of epithelial duct origin provide circumstantial and objective data as prognostic markers for increased cancer risk in certain age groups. A differentiation of proliferative pathologic elements in tissue sampling appears important to maximize prognostic accuracy and to enhance end-result reporting. These data further support the use of the breast biopsy report for pathologic indicators that may optimize identification of the high-risk patient with and without other commonly recognized clinical risk factors for breast carcinogenesis.

Reproductive Breast

Premenstrual fullness and tenderness of the breast parenchyma is evident during the ovulatory cycle. In this interval mammary blood flow is increased by 15 to 30 ml/cm^3. Breast parenchymal density thereafter is increased by water retention in connective tissues and is enhanced by neogrowth of the ductal and acinar cells. Breast edema may result from estrogen-induced histamine effect on the microcirculation with fluid entry into the breast interstitium. These changes have been labeled a result of the luteal phase of steroid action, although recent reports suggest that prolactin may play an essential role.

In the reproductive years the breasts undergo cyclic changes in preparation for gestation. In the proliferative phase, parenchymal proliferation with epithelial sprouts and stimulation of cellular ribonucleic acid (RNA) is evident following induction by estrogen.[116] Dilation of the ductal system and differentiation of alveoli into secretory cells follow the appearance of progesterone in the luteal phase.

These premenstrual phenomena must be differentiated from the pathologic alterations of FCDB. Thus palpation of the breast for examination purposes is most informative when performed in the early cycle phase because mammary volume is at a minimum. With termination of the menstrual cycle, the breast undergoes regressive changes characterized by cellular regression of the alveoli and reduction in the size of lumina of the lactiferous ducts.

Exogenous Hormones and Environmental Factors Etiologic in Benign Breast Disease

Endometrial abnormalities, which result from the administration of progesterone in the absence of estrogens, stimulated interest in the use of such a combined preparation for the treatment of fibrocystic mastopathy. The combination of norethynodrel and mestranol (Enovid) was reported by Ariel[8] to have good-to-excellent objective responses in 64% of subjects with FCDB. Subsequently,

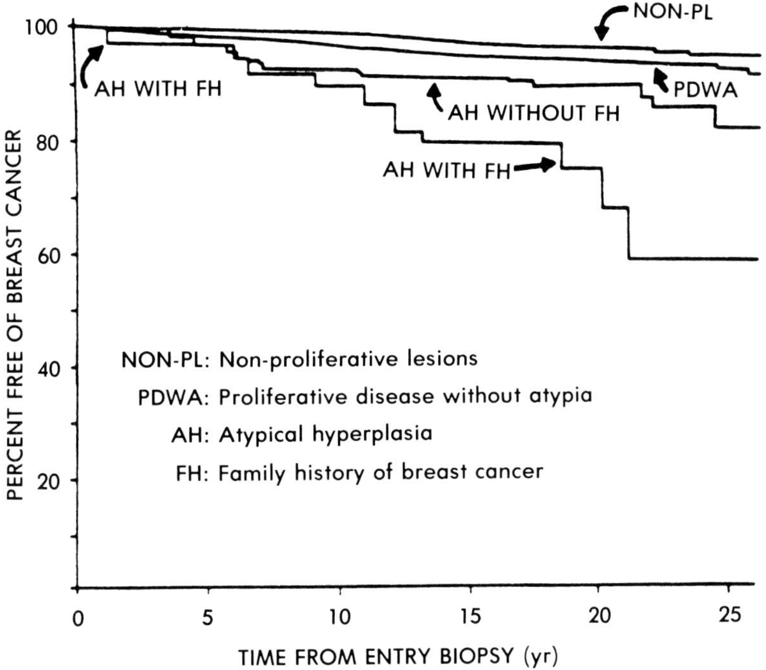

Fig. 62-6 Proportion of patients free of invasive breast carcinoma as a function of time since entry biopsy. (From Dupont, W.D., and Page, D.L.: Reprinted, by permission of N. Engl. J. Med. **312**(3):146, 1985.)

combined therapy using high-dose progesterone initiated an objective sustained response that was much improved compared with untreated patients serving as controls.[62]

Pastides and associates[109] reported that women who used oral contraceptives (OC) for 2 to 4 years or more had a decreased risk of FCDB. The findings partly agree with those of LiVolsi and co-workers[86] when cases are considered according to the degree of epithelial atypia, in that patients with FCDB exhibiting marked atypia generally had similar patterns of OC use when compared to controls. Patients with absent, low, and intermediate atypia had less OC use than controls. A negative association between OC use and FCDB-exhibiting cysts (gross and microscopic) or papillomatosis is notable. These findings suggest that a spectrum of FCDB exists and that long-term use of OC protects against the forms of FCDB that are not firmly associated with an increased risk of cancer but does not protect against the premalignant variants of FCDB.

Asch and Greenblatt[9] noted that a synthetic-impeded androgen (Danazol) may diminish secretion of LH, initiating reduction of ovarian estrogen. Their data suggest that Danazol provides competition with estrogen for receptor sites and has a direct target-organ effect on breast parenchyma through its mildly androgenic properties. The high incidence of amenorrhea (50%), acne, edema, flashes, and muscle cramps have diminished the initial enthusiasm for the use of this compound. However, a reduction of the therapeutic dose suggested for endometriosis is of value for control of mastalgia in certain subjects. The occasional involution of mastopathy to an asymptomatic state with objective regression of cyst size represents an advantage of danazol therapy.

Application of androgens, HCG, and estrogen antagonists have met with varying success in the treatment of FCDB. The disappearance of fibrocystic mastopathy during the course of pregnancy or with lactation is a common observation. Thus there is reason to speculate that lactation represents the most normal state in which the mamma can exist. In contradistinction, lactogenic factors can induce mammary epithelium and lobules to undergo a spectrum of evolution from florid or involutional FCDB to the extreme of active lactation.

More recently the effects of caffeine, cyclic nucleotides, and saturated dietary fats as mechanistic etiologic factors for benign and malignant breast disease have been suggested.[101] The role of these foodstuffs as a causation theory remains plausible, but to date their etiologic role in breast disease remains circumstantial.

Breast Neoplasia

Natural History

The attempt to characterize the preclinical stages of breast neoplasia have centered almost exclusively on proliferative lesions of the mammary epithelium or lobules. The physiologic effects of gonadal and pituitary hormones on breast parenchyma initiate proliferation and regression of the epithelium and therefore are able to induce preneoplastic lesions with unrestrained growth and metastases to a detectable clinical stage. Morphologically the effort to identify these preneoplastic states necessitates the differentiation of atypical hyperplastic lobules from lobular carcinoma in situ or the atypical proliferation of duct epithelium from an intraductal carcinoma. Despite the stringent criteria and guidelines employed, morphologic distinction is often difficult and is subject to interpretative error.

A conceptual diagram of the natural history of breast cancer is seen in Fig. 62-7. Epithelial hyperplasia is regarded as a preneoplastic lesion, in the context that it will invariably precede carcinoma, although it may have extension into other pathologic processes. The mechanism of induction and transformation from a normal epithelial cell to a preinvasive stage requires multifactorial mechanisms of dietetic, genetic, and environmental origin operating in an appropriate hormonal milieu. Sources suggest that the temporal duration for the preinvasive stage of mammary carcinoma is prolonged and may be a matter of many months to several years.[56] Further, the epithelial alterations observed in the vincinity of recognizable carcinoma may exist in multiple sites of the ipsilateral or perhaps the contralateral breast. The periductal connective tissue will show extensive changes, not only in the vicinity of invasive carcinoma, but throughout the whole breast; these changes may occur when only a single focus of carcinoma is identifiable. De Ome[40] observed that the earliest change in the duct of murine mammary carcinoma was thickening of the epithelial layer secondary to an increase in the number of cells present. These primary morphologic events occur at irregular intervals along the duct, with the observation that normal duct membrane cells intervene.

Poorly defined mechanisms initiate the duct lining to increase in cell number, with varying degrees of aberration, disarrangement, and anaplasia that range from ductal hyperplasia to intraductal carcinoma. Although these changes may occur in single or multiple duct systems, they appear to be more pronounced near invasive carcinoma. It is often possible to recognize multiple sites where disruption of the basement layer has occurred with variable amounts of periductal extension of tumor. As the carcinogenic transformation occurs within the lactiferous duct, the surrounding connective tissues become juxtaposed or have immediate contact with lymphatic vessels that traverse the periductal position.

Thus subsequent metastatic growth can occur through three mechanisms: (1) intraductal extension or change in the character of duct epithelium, (2) direct invasion of the breast connective tissues, and (3) direct embolization and extension through the intramammary peripheral lymphatics.[22]

Whole-organ studies confirm that invasive carcinoma is surrounded by nodules of hyperplastic duct epithelium foci and intraductal carcinoma.[57] Thus a tumor represents a coalescence of several "link sites" of disease, which may constitute a unicentric site of origin. Lymphatic invasion with subsequent dissemination is likely to occur early and most probably in a microscopic stage of disease (Stage 0). Thereafter, histologic and clinical changes take place in the contralateral breast, which can be recognized and confirmed as bilateral breast carcinoma. The frequency of this entity depends on the effort for which the multicentricity and bilateral probability are sought.[133]

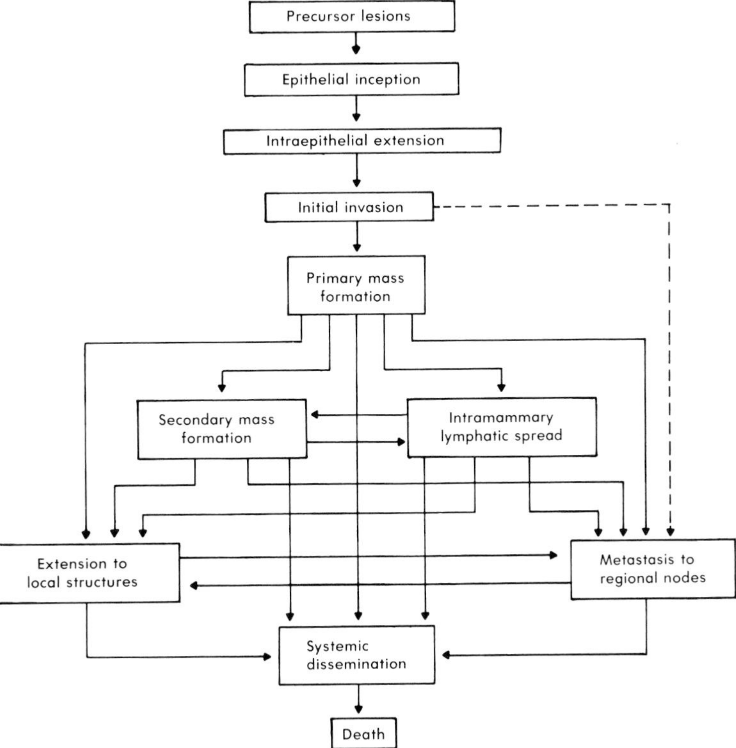

Fig. 62-7 Conceptual diagram to indicate natural history of breast carcinoma. Predictability and linear progression is evident only in early stages. (From Gallager, H.S.: Minimal breast cancer: concepts and treatment. In Burghardt, E., and Holzer, E., editors: Minimal invasive cancer [microcarcinoma]: clinics in oncology, Philadelphia, 1982, W.B. Saunders Co.)

Lobular Carcinoma and Multicentricity

Although 85% of breast carcinomas have lactiferous ductal origin, carcinogenic transformation of the alveoli is observed as the second most frequent site. Foote and Stewart[52] originally described in situ lobular carcinoma of the breast, which is regarded as a pure entity seen in association with intraductal and infiltrating carcinomas. This represents a form of breast carcinoma in which the terminal ducts and lobules are characteristically involved in neoplastic transformation following induction by a poorly understood mechanism of carcinogenesis.[74] This represented the most common bilateral carcinoma reported by Urban[133] in a series of 505 bilateral neoplasms. Further, carcinomas observed at synchronous or metachronous intervals were histologically similar to the dominant lesion and of a similar developmental stage when of the in situ lobular type. Urban noted that, when the dominant lesions were infiltrating, half the carcinomas of the other organ were also of a similar histologic type. The probability that more than half (64%) of these neoplasms will appear in the contralateral breast necessitates scrupulous follow-up and biopsy to corroborate or disprove the existence of synchronous carcinoma.[26]

Clinical Staging of Breast Cancer

The clinical staging for cancer of the breast reflects the anatomic extent of the neoplasm determined at the time of diagnosis and before therapy. Staging concepts are based on diagnostic, clinical, and biopsy information or at intervals in the postsurgical resection when all pathologic information obtained or studied from the resected specimen are used. In addition, a comprehensive evaluation by the clinician of the ipsilateral axillary and supraclavicular lymphatics and of the contralateral breast and axilla are necessary.

Over the past four decades, consistent classifications have been developed that are essential to allow comparison of treatment end-results for different investigators and among the various institutions reporting clinical trials. Three basic clinical staging systems have evolved: (1) the Manchester, (2) the Columbia Clinical Classification, and (3) the TNM (tumor, nodes, metastasis) systems.

The first system was initially developed in 1940 at the Christie Hospital and Holt Radium Institute of Manchester, England. The Manchester system was used until introduction of the more comprehensive Columbia Clinical Classification developed by Haagensen and Stout provided better clinical determinants for evaluation of the extent of involvement of the breast by the neoplastic process (e.g., edema, ulceration, fixation). The recommendation of the American Joint Committee on Cancer (AJCC) together with the TNM Committee of the International Union Against Cancer (UICC) established the TNM System, which was adopted in São Paulo, Brazil, in 1954. Since the initial development of the TNM classification, slight modifications have subsequently been formulated. The

STAGING OF CANCER: BREAST ICD-O 174

Histologic Type of Cancer

Cancer, not otherwise specified (NOS)

Ductal

- [ ]Intraductual (in situ)
- [ ]Invasive with predominant intraductal component
- [ ]Invasive, NOS
- [ ]Comedo
- [ ]Inflammatory
- [ ]Medullary with lymphocytic infiltrate
- [ ]Mucinous (colloid)
- [ ]Papillary
- [ ]Scirrhous
- [ ]Tubular
- [ ]Other:

Lobular

- [ ]In situ
- [ ]Invasive with predominant in situ component
- [ ]Invasive

Nipple

- [ ]Paget's disease, NOS
- [ ]Paget's disease with intraductal carcinoma
- [ ]Paget's disease with invasive ductal carcinoma

Other:

Definitions of Primary Tumor

[ ]T_X Minimum requirements to assess the primary tumor cannot be met

[ ]T_0 No evidence of primary tumor

[ ]TIS (Carcinoma in situ) Paget's disease of the nipple with no demonstrable tumor

[ ]T_1 Tumor 2 cm or less in greatest dimension

[ ]T_{1a} No fixation to underlying pectoral fascia or muscle

[ ]T_{1b} Fixation to underlying pectoral fascia or muscle

- [ ]I Tumor ≤ 0.5 cm
- [ ]II Tumor $> 0.5 \leq 1$ cm
- [ ]III Tumor $> 1 \leq 2$ cm

[ ]T_2 Tumor more than 2 cm but not more than 5 cm in its greatest dimension

[ ]T_{2a} No fixation to underlying pectoral fascia or muscle

[ ]T_{2b} Fixation to underlying pectoral fascia or muscle

[ ]T_3 Tumor more than 5 cm in greatest dimension

[ ]T_{3a} No fixation to underlying pectoral fascia or muscle

[ ]T_{3b} Fixation to underlying pectoral fascia or muscle

[ ]T_4 Tumor of any size with the direct extension to chest wall or skin

[ ]T_{4a} Fixation to chest wall

[ ]T_{4b} Edema (including peau d'orange), ulceration of the skin of the breast, or satellite skin nodules confined to the same breast

[ ]T_{4c} Both 4a and 4b

Lymph Nodes

Definitions for clinical-diagnostic stage

[ ]N_X Minimum requirements to assess the regional nodes cannot be met

[ ]N_O Ipsilateral axillary lymph nodes not considered to contain growth

[ ]N_1 Movable ipsilateral axillary nodes considered to contain growth

Lymph Nodes—cont'd

Definitions for clinical-diagnostic stage—cont'd

[ ]N_2 Ipsilateral axillary nodes considered to contain growth and fixed to one another or to other structures

[ ]N_3 Ipsilateral supraclavicular or infraclavicular nodes considered to contain growth, or edema of the arm

Definitions for postsurgical resection–pathologic stages

[ ]N_X Minimum requirements to assess the presence of distant metastasis cannot be met

[ ]N_0 No evidence of ipsilateral axillary lymph node metastasis

[ ]N_1 Metastasis to movable ipsilateral axillary nodes not fixed to one another or to other structures

[ ]N_{1a} Micrometastasis 0.2 cm in lymph nodes

[ ]N_{1b} Gross metastasis in lymph nodes

- [ ] i Metastasis more than 0.2 cm, but less than 2 cm, in one to three lymph nodes
- [ ] ii Metastasis more than 0.2 cm, but less than 2 cm, in four or more lymph nodes
- [ ]iii Extension of metastasis beyond the lymph node capsule (less than 2 cm in total dimension)
- [ ]iv Metastasis in lymph node 2 cm or more in dimension

[ ]N_2 Metastases to ipsilateral axillary lymph nodes that are fixed to one another or to other structures

[ ]N_3 Metastasis to ipsilateral supraclavicular or infraclavicular lymph nodes

Stage grouping

[ ]Clinical-diagnostic (cTNM)

[ ]Surgical-evaluative (sTNM)

[ ]Postsurgical resection–pathologic (pTNM)

- [ ]Stage TIS (in situ)
- [ ]Stage X (cannot stage)
- [ ]Stage I
  - [ ]T_{1ai}, N_O,M_O
  - [ ]T_{1aii}, N_O, M_O
  - [ ]T_{1aiii}, N_O, M_O
  - [ ]T_{1bi}, N_O, M_O
  - [ ]T_{1bii}, N_O, M_O
  - [ ]T_{1biii}, N_O, M_O

[ ]Clinical-diagnostic (cTNM)

[ ]Surgical-evaluative (sTNM)

[ ]Postsurgical resection–pathologic (pTNM)

- [ ]Stage II
  - [ ]T_0, N_{1a}, N_{1b}; M_0
  - [ ]T_{1a}, T_{1b}; N_{1a}, N_{1b}; M_0
  - [ ]T_{2a}, T_{2b}; N_0; M_0
  - [ ]T_{2a}, T_{2b}; N_{1a}, N_{1b}; M_0
- [ ]Stage IIIa
  - [ ]T_0, N_2, M_0
  - [ ]T_{1a}, T_{1b}; N_2, N_{1b}; M_0
  - [ ]T_{2a}, T_{2b}; N_2; M_0
  - [ ]T_{3a}, T_{3b}; N_0; M_0
  - [ ]T_{3a}, T_{3b}; N_1; M_0
  - [ ]T_{3a}, T_{3b}; N_2; M_0
- [ ]Stage IIIb
  - [ ]Any T, N_3, M_0
  - [ ]Any T_4, any N, M_0
- [ ]Stage IV
  - [ ]Any T, any N, M_1

AJCC recommended tumor staging as indicated in the boxed material on p. 1036.

These staging principles provide definition of the primary tumor with regard to size, presence or absence of lymphatic involvement, fixation, and regional or distant dissemination of the tumor. The comprehensive formulation of such principles allows one to group with regard to Stages TIS, Stage X, or Stages I to IV, depending on the advancing clinical presentation of the primary neoplasm. The diagnosis of cancer must be established by histologic study of the tumor, and the cellular type of the lesion is recorded.[11] Because the biologic behavior varies from one histologic variant of cancer to another, only similar types should be compared for reporting purposes.

The essentials of the initial examination should also include:

1. Physical examination
2. Evaluation of both breasts preoperatively using validated techniques, i.e., mammography
3. Preadmission clinical pathology examinations, including hepatic enzyme profile
4. Chest roentgenogram
5. Skeletal roentgenographic survey in select patients (when symptomatic)

Selected examinations include:

1. Technetium radionuclide, hepatic scintigraphy, or abdominal CT and/or magnetic resonance imaging (MRI) in the presence of hepatomegaly or abnormal liver profile at chemical analysis
2. Radionuclide bone scan for the following advanced stages of disease:
   a. Primary lesion T_3, T_4
   b. Evidence of regional nodal metastasis (N_1, N_2, N_3)
   c. Distant metastatic spread (M_1)

Prevailing medical opinion accepts bone scintigraphy as being too sensitive to be of cost-benefit value in the preoperative staging for patients with early breast cancers (T_1, T_2, T_1N_1). For these patients, a skeletal roentgenographic survey should be correlated with the bone scan to identify associated benign disorders that may appear as false-positive images (arthritis, healed fractures, bone islands). Burkett and associates[28] reported that 8% of 162 screening bone scans (Stages I to III) were positive, whereas the yield of scans for asymptomatic patients was only two of 150 patients (1.3%). Hayward and Frazier[66] recently reported an enhancement of sensitivity and specificity with technetium-99 bone scans employing serum alkaline phosphatase (AP) and lactate dehydrogenase (LDH) values. When *either* the AP or LDH value was abnormal, 51.7% of the scans were positive. When *both* values were abnormal, 66.7% of patients had positive bone scans.

These results suggest that breast cancer screening can be selectively enhanced with AP and LDH determinations, and that isotopic scanning should be reserved for patients with abnormal values or symptoms that suggest metastatic disease. Isotopic bone scanning remains valuable in the symptomatic patient and in the patient with chemical determination of bone involvement, but it has its greatest application in postoperative follow-up because it remains a sensitive indicator of evolving metastatic disease. Patients with suspicious findings on skeletal roentgenographic survey who have clinically palpable disease at supraclavicular or axillary sites should receive isotopic scanning in the preoperative period to serve as a baseline for future evaluations.

Currently, breast imaging may be recorded by five modalities: (1) roentgenographic (mammography), (2) heat (thermography), (3) sound (ultrasonography), (4) light (diaphanography), and (5) magnetism (MRI).[76]

To date, the primacy of *xeromammography* for mass screening of breast carcinoma is unchallenged by the other diagnostic modalities. Nonetheless, when used as an adjunct to clinical evaluation and xeromammography, these diagnostic parameters may augment the evaluation process to enhance diagnosis.

Thermography displays an intricate detail of the internal anatomy of the breast, employing invisible infrared irradiation from the skin to a thermal map. An abnormal thermogram is not of sufficient specificity to unequivocally allow diagnosis of a neoplastic disease; comparable findings may be observed in nonmalignant processes such as acute inflammatory states of the breast with heightened metabolic activity (abscess, cellulitis, fat necrosis). This technique did not enhance the diagnostic accuracy when used for mass screening in the National Breast Cancer Detection Demonstration Projects.[18]

Significant advances have been made in the instrumentation of *medical ultrasonography*. Ultrasonography uses special transducers that introduce pulsed high-frequency sound waves into breast tissues, and the reflected transmitted waves are electronically converted for display as images. This technique appears to have an advantage over xeromammography in that it can better define and precisely recognize lesions in dense (dysplastic) xeromammographic breast images where radiographic shadows may be obscured. This technique has great value in evaluating benign cysts that resemble solid masses on mammography. Its disadvantage is that of recognition and diagnosis of benign and malignant solid tumors. Distinguishing a fibroadenoma from an infiltrating carcinoma may be impossible, because differentiation of inflammatory states from diffuse neoplastic processes is not uniformly possible.

The application of *diaphanography* with visualization of mammary parenchyma by transilluminated intense light beams is not a new concept. However, the recent technologic advances by the Scandinavians to enhance imaging with this technique has great promise. Breast imaging depends on such factors as size, the composition and optical density of mammary tissues, inflammatory changes, cysts, and neoplasia, all of which affect light transmission and absorption. Clinical trials with these techniques and MRI imaging are being conducted to evaluate their diagnostic capability.

Sites for metastatic involvement with breast carcinoma in order of decreasing frequency are: bone, liver, lung, skin, extraregional lymphatics, and brain. The ipsilateral axillary lymph node basin represents the major regional drainage site for carcinoma of the breast. Approximately 40% to 50% of patients will have clinical and/or histologic involvement of this site at initial presentation. However, the detection of axillary nodal involvement at physical examination is fraught with diagnostic inaccuracies. Approximately 20% to 25% of examinations are incorrectly reported following clinical assessment. The pathologic stage of the axillary lymphatics correlates significantly with survival. For these reasons, adequate sampling of axillary lymph nodes (approximately five to 10 lymph nodes) is required to determine the future status of the patient and may indicate the necessity for adjuvant chemotherapy, radiation, or hormonal therapy. Clinical staging of the primary tumor dictates the type of surgical procedure. However, pathologic staging is the most important determinant for the necessity of adjuvant multimodal or single-agent therapy.

Options for Surgical Management

The choice of the operative procedure for breast carcinoma depends on the size of the primary lesion, the presence or absence of tumor fixation, the presence of regional adenopathy, evidence of distant disease, and the physiologic status of the patient. Carcinomas less than or equal to 5 cm in diameter that are limited to the lateral quadrants of the breast without fixation (T_{1a}, T_{2a}) are best managed by surgery alone. For regional metastatic involvement with central or medially located lesions, the combination of surgery with postoperative radiation may be appropriate to ensure chest wall control. For Stage I and Stage II diseases, the type of procedure performed and the areas receiving irradiation depend on location of the primary tumor, the presence or absence of lymphatic disease, and the pathologic findings within the operative specimen.

Neoplasms of the lateral aspect of the breast drain primarily through the axillary lymphatics, and disease can be eliminated by *modified radical mastectomy*. This procedure includes dissection of the lateral border of the sternum medically, the latissimus dorsi muscle laterally, the clavicle superiorly, and the superior border of the rectus muscle inferiorly. All breast parenchyma is extirpated from the chest wall through flaps created within the superficial investing fascia of the dermis. Dissection should be guided by principles of ablative surgery, which include an en bloc resection. To ensure that Level I, II, and III nodes are resected, the pectoralis minor muscle should be divided at its insertion on the coracoid process and origin from the ribs (Patey procedure). The final dissected specimen includes the breast, the nipple-areolar complex with associated skin, axillary contents, and the pectoralis minor muscle.

Medially located neoplasms principally drain into internal mammary lymphatics and may be associated with nodal involvement in 10% to 30% of patients. If axillary metastases are present in medial lesions, the probability may exceed 50% that the internal nodes are pathologically involved. In the absence of clinically involved axillary metastasis, medial carcinomas are treated by modified radical mastectomy. Postoperative radiation therapy has not been shown to improve survival or decrease chest wall recurrence and is no longer recommended. When metastases are identified in more than 20% of the removed nodes of the axilla, adjuvant postoperative chest wall irradiation may be used to sterilize *intransit* metastatic disease, which may exist in the endolymphatic spaces of the skin flaps. Likewise, the internal mammary and supraclavicular nodes (peripheral lymphatics) should be included in radiation portals.

Cancers that are *laterally located* with axillary nodal involvement may also have metastatic involvement of supraclavicular or internal mammary sites in as many as 25% to 30% of patients. In these cases adjuvant irradiation is also advisable for treatment of these regional nodal sites.

Radical mastectomy is reserved for medially located lesions with associated palpable axillary lymphatic metastases in patients who are not candidates for radiation therapy and for centrally located lesions that are fixed to the pectoralis major fascia. These neoplasms are likely to metastasize by way of transpectoral and retropectoral routes (Rotter's nodes). Radical mastectomy ablates the neurovascular bundle that innervates the pectoralis major muscle and through which lymphatics course medial to the pectoralis minor muscle. This procedure is technically simpler than the modified radical mastectomy, which necessitates preservation of the pectoralis major muscle and its neural innervation. The axillary dissections of both the radical and the modified radical procedures are identical and include resection of Level I, II, and III nodes.

In 1948 the *extended radical mastectomy* (supraradical mastectomy) was designed as an extension of the radical mastectomy to enhance control of regional metastatic disease with a therapeutic dissection of the internal mammary nodes. Although original reports by Margottini, Jacobelli, and Cau[93] and Lacour and asssociates[82] supported this more radical approach, most surgeons have abandoned its use and employ irradiation to achieve sterilization of internal nodal disease for control of this regional site.

An increasing interest in conservative breast surgery is apparent. These procedures have been variously labeled as *lumpectomy*, *tylectomy*, or *segmental resection*. Sine qua non to the use of breast preservation procedures is the concept that adequate removal of all primary breast cancer can be accomplished without incision into neoplastic tissue. Thus the goal is maintenance of adequate cosmetic appearance while achieving control and cure rates that equal those obtained with modified radical mastectomy. Therefore breast size and size of the primary neoplasm often dictate the prudent exercise of the more radical operative approach to facilitate adequate control of local and regional disease. Frozen-section analysis of the resected margins should always be performed to ensure that breast cancer has been removed *en bloc* with the specimen. Inadequate surgical margins that contain neoplastic disease require reexcision and, if inadequately performed, may necessitate mastectomy.

When adjuvant chemotherapy or radiation therapy is to be used, the status of the axillary nodes must be determined. *Axillary sampling* procedures are done through curvilinear incisions placed between the lateral border of the pectoralis major and latissmus dorsi muscles 4 to 6 cm below the apex of the axilla. Adequate sampling of the lateral contents of the axilla (Level I) is completed, and 10 to 15 lymph nodes are submitted for analysis.

Indications for tylectomy, axillary sampling, and comprehensive radiation to the breast, axilla, and internal mammary and supraclavicular nodes include: (1) primary neoplasm less than or equal to 4 cm, (2) clinically negative axillary lymphatics, (3) a breast of adequate size to achieve primary closure with an acceptable cosmetic result and one in which a uniform dose of radiation therapy can be delivered, and (4) a radiation therapist experienced with this modality of therapy. If these stipulations cannot be ensured, the results of segmental resection and primary irradiation may be both therapeutically and cosmetically unsatisfactory. The importance of removal of all the primary breast cancer is to be emphasized. Should viable cancer cells remain within the breast, they may be incorporated into the scar of the healing wound which is uniformly poorly oxygenated. The biologic observation that maximal irradiation effect will not be achieved for marginally oxygenated and anoxic cancer cells within scar tissue suggests that recurrence of carcinoma in the incision would be anticipated. When the initial biopsy confirms invasive carcinoma, the practice of many surgeons is to reexcise the scar and complete an axillary sampling procedure (Levels I and II), especially when the limits of the excision cannot be assessed. Approximately 50% of patients who have had their tylectomy scars reexcised have viable cancer cells present in the wound after what was initially determined to be an adequate excisional biopsy. Centers that do not advocate reexcision of the biopsy site usually boost the external beam irradiation dose by the implantation of iridium-192 needles in the area of the scar.

Veronesi, Zucali, and del Vecchio[136] of Milan, Italy, reported the results of a randomized, prospective clinical trial comparing radical mastectomy with quadrantectomy, axillary node dissection, and breast irradiation (QU.A.RT.) Between 1973 and 1980, 701 women with lesions less than or equal to 2 cm and clinically negative axillae ($T_1N_0M_0$) were evaluated. Mean time on study was 8 years. The investigators reported no significant differences between the two groups for local/regional recurrence, relapse-free survival, or overall survival. Two percent of patients in each group developed a local recurrence, and an additional 2% demonstrated a regional treatment failure. At 8 years, relapse-free survival was 79% for the mastectomy group and 80% for patients managed by the QU.A.RT. protocol; the proportion of patients surviving was 82.5% and 85%, respectively. For node-positive patients (Stage II), prolonged survival favored the QU.A.RT. group (82% vs. 79%), although the survival advantage was not statistically significant. These authors conclude that eligible patients with small breast lesions treated by QU.A.RT. protocol have no demonstrable disadvantage with regard to disease-free survival or overall survival compared to similar patient groups managed by radical mastectomy.

The results of the prospectively randomized trial for segmental mastectomy with or without comprehensive irradiation to the breast and peripheral lymphatics vs. modified radical mastectomy have been recently published by Fisher and associates[48,51] of the National Surgical Adjuvant Breast and Bowel Project (NSABP). This multi-institutional trial of the NSABP evaluated breast conservation and tumor control by segmental mastectomy in the treatment of Stage I and II breast tumors less than or equal to 4 cm in size. All patients had axillary dissections, and patients with histologically positive nodes received adjuvant chemotherapy (melphalan and 5-fluorouracil).

Life table estimates based on data from 1843 women accrued in the B-06 study indicate that treatment by segmental mastectomy, with or without breast irradiation, provides local disease-free, distant disease-free, and actuarial survival at 5 years, which equates to patients treated by total mastectomy. For women treated by segmental mastectomy with irradiation, 92.3% remained free of tumor at 5 years vs. 72.1% of those receiving no radiation ($p < 0.001$). Mean follow-up at the time of the report was 39 months, and definitive end-results must await 10-year analysis. Local recurrence in the operated breast was 8% for patients who had segmental mastectomy and breast irradiation whereas local recurrence was 28% for those women who had segmental mastectomy without radiation therapy. The study, therefore, established the importance of radiation therapy in controlling recurrence of breast cancer in the ipsilateral breast for patients with negative axillary lymph nodes. Also of note was the local recurrence in the breasts of patients with positive lymph nodes, all of whom received adjuvant chemotherapy. For node-positive patients with and without treatment with radiation therapy, local breast recurrence rates after segmental mastectomy were 2% and 37%, respectively. The 2% figure is significantly lower than the corresponding 8% recurrence rate in women with Stage I disease (negative axillary nodes) and thus suggests that irradiation may sensitize the breast neoplasm to the cytotoxic effects of chemotherapy.

For management of Stage III disease in which axillary metastases exceed 2.5 cm and are fixed or matted, the surgical procedure is designed to ablate the primary neoplasm and lymphatics, which are at a reduced probability for sterilization by irradiation alone. Control of regional nodal disease by any modality is inversely related to size of the nodes to be treated. Thus centrally located lymphatics with small deposits of cancer contiguous with axillary structures that are not resectable may be adequately controlled by radiation therapy. In these circumstances the breast tissue and Level I lymphatics are resected in what is termed an *extended simple mastectomy*. In the latter procedure, Level II and III lymphatics are left intact in the axilla to be controlled with irradiation. In this instance lymphedema of the arm is uncommon because collateral lymphatic vessels that enter the apical axilla are not ablated by the surgical procedure.

Breast carcinomas greater than 5 cm in diameter associated with minimum clinical disease in the axilla (Stage IIIA), which are biologically favorable lesions, may be treated by preoperative irradiation and/or chemotherapy followed by radical or modified radical mastectomy. Chemotherapeutic induction of the neoplasm by cytotoxic agents (cytoxan, doxorubicin [Adriamycin], fluorouracil) is highly successful to allow cytoreduction of the tumor. These therapeutic techniques may enhance locoregional control and increase the disease-free interval. Therapeutic choice of radiotherapy or chemotherapy depends on the location and site of the tumor and the total dose of irradiation necessary to be delivered to the apex of the axilla that is considered essential to provide tumor control.

Patients with Stage IV disease (distant metastasis), including supraclavicular metastases, are best treated primarily with cytotoxic chemotherapeutic agents. However, control of local chest wall disease is best achieved with limited surgical procedures that ensure skin closure and are often used with radiation therapy. The timing of these procedures must be individualized; this is often directed by the medical oncologist because the principal dilemma is control of distant disease.

RADIOLOGIC EVALUATION OF BREAST DISEASE

Mammographic Imaging of Normal Breast Parenchyma and Benign Disease

The current application of conventional mammographic techniques and xeroradiograms remains the major modality to detect occult nonpalpable breast lesions. For purposes of discussion, the xeromammogram (XMM) and the conventional biplane mammogram should be considered to have equivalent diagnostic potential.

XMMs are obtained as cephalocaudal and mediolateral x-ray images reproduced on a selenium plate with impressions in a positive or negative mode to accentuate tissue densities. Ultrasound mammography represents a noninvasive method of reproducing high-resolution tomographic sections through the breast. Development of gray-scale units has greatly improved the quality of ultrasonic images. Thermography represents a more insensitive detection method for breast cancer.[10,18] The true-positive rate for thermography was 60% to 85% in early trials of the Breast Cancer Detection Demonstration Project (BCDDP). Thermography is particularly insensitive to Stage 0 minimum cancers and Stage I invasive cancers. In contrast, the newer gray-scale diagnostic accuracy of ultrasound is approximately 79% to 87%, with a low false-negative rate (7.6%) and a false-positive rate of 18% to 20%.[36] Wolfe[142] has previously reported a false-negative rate for XMM of only 4.7%, which is much lower than most series. It appears that combined XMM-sonographic evaluation exceeds the accuracy of either method used alone.

The XMM radiographic beam consists of electromagnetic waves of energy of extremely short wavelength, such that matter is penetrated to variable degrees as a function of density. Thus the penetration of air, tissue, and water or mineral (bone) densities depends on the energy and wavelengths of the x-ray beam and the constitution of the matter being imaged. The most radiopenetrable breast substance is fat, whereas the most radiodense (radiopaque) are calcium salts, which are deposited in approximately 35% to 45% of malignant and premalignant lesions in the perilobular or periductal tissues. Microcalcification is not specific to breast cancer and may be present in epithelial hyperplasia and noninvasive and invasive cancers. The extent of calcification is a function of replication activity of epithelial cells. Microcalcification is a product of increased cellular activity in the lobuloductal complex and occurs following extrusion of calcium salts into surrounding parenchymal interstitial tissues.

The intermediate penetrability of connective tissue, blood, cyst fluid, epithelium, and duct structures accounts for the remarkable heterogeneity of breast parenchymal XMM patients. Among siblings and offspring, great variation in XMM parenchymal patterns has been observed, reflecting modification of radiopenetrability of the three variants of imaging projections. It has been suggested that certain types of proliferative disorders or dysplasias are associated with a higher incidence of breast carcinoma. Wolfe[143,144] has made attempts to identify the dysplastic breast on XMM to determine which "benign" XMM patterns on routine screening or follow-up examinations are associated with the higher risk of developing cancer. On the basis of the XMM pattern, Wolfe assigned four risk groups:

1. N_1, *Lowest risk* (Fig. 62-8, *A*)—parenchyma composed primarily of fat with small amounts of "dysplasia"; no ducts visible
2. P_1, *Low risk* (see Fig. 62-8, *B*)—parenchyma, chiefly fat, with prominent ducts in the anterior portion up to one fourth of volume of breast; may have coexisting ducts extending as bands into a quadrant
3. P_2, *High risk* (see Fig. 62-8, *C*)—severe involvement with prominent ductal pattern that occupies greater than one fourth of volume of breast
4. *DY*, *Highest risk* (see Fig. 62-8, *D*)—severe involvement with dysplasia; may obscure underlying prominent duct pattern

In the first effort to develop his thesis into a clinical application, Wolfe suggested that the DY pattern increased the risk of cancer 37-fold over the N_1 group.[142,143] This was reaffirmed by a 21-fold increase over the N_1 group in a second study.[144] Subsequently, this group was co-divided into a low-risk group (N_1/P_1) and a high-risk group (P_2/DY). Follow-up has revealed that the DY pattern will decrease with age following removal of the estrone and estradiol stimuli of ovarian secretion. Over 5 to 15 years a "shift down" occurs in more than one half of the DY patterns, with one third becoming P_2, 11% becoming P_1, and 8% becoming N_1. Although studies have confirmed the contention for increased risk in the P_2/DY pattern, Bland and associates[21] recognized the distribution of the P_2/DY XMM pattern in 83% to 87% of women aged 35 to 49 years. Analysis of 1759 histologic characteristics in biopsies of 863 patients aged 35 to 74 years with FCDB revealed ductal and lobular hyperplastic lesions, sclerosing adenosis, and epithelial cysts to be the major components of 64% to 69% of the high-risk (P_2) images ($p < 0.001$).

These data suggest that XMM parenchymal patterns observed in asymptomatic screenees incompletely correlate with known pathologic variables of proliferative and nonproliferative FCDB. The clinical integration of the XMM risk patterns apparently may allow preselection of patients who deserve frequent follow-up for breast cancer; however, they do not appear to be absolute predictors for screening strategies, nor do they decisively enhance patient management.

Recent unpublished data[121] suggest that XMM patterns are markers of high risk for breast cancer for women with a positive family history of breast cancer. Among women with a P_2/DY pattern and a positive family history, an odds ratio of 7.37 was evident compared to the N_1 pattern. A positive family history of breast cancer did not affect the odds risk among women with the N_1 pattern. In addition, for women with no family history of cancer, the

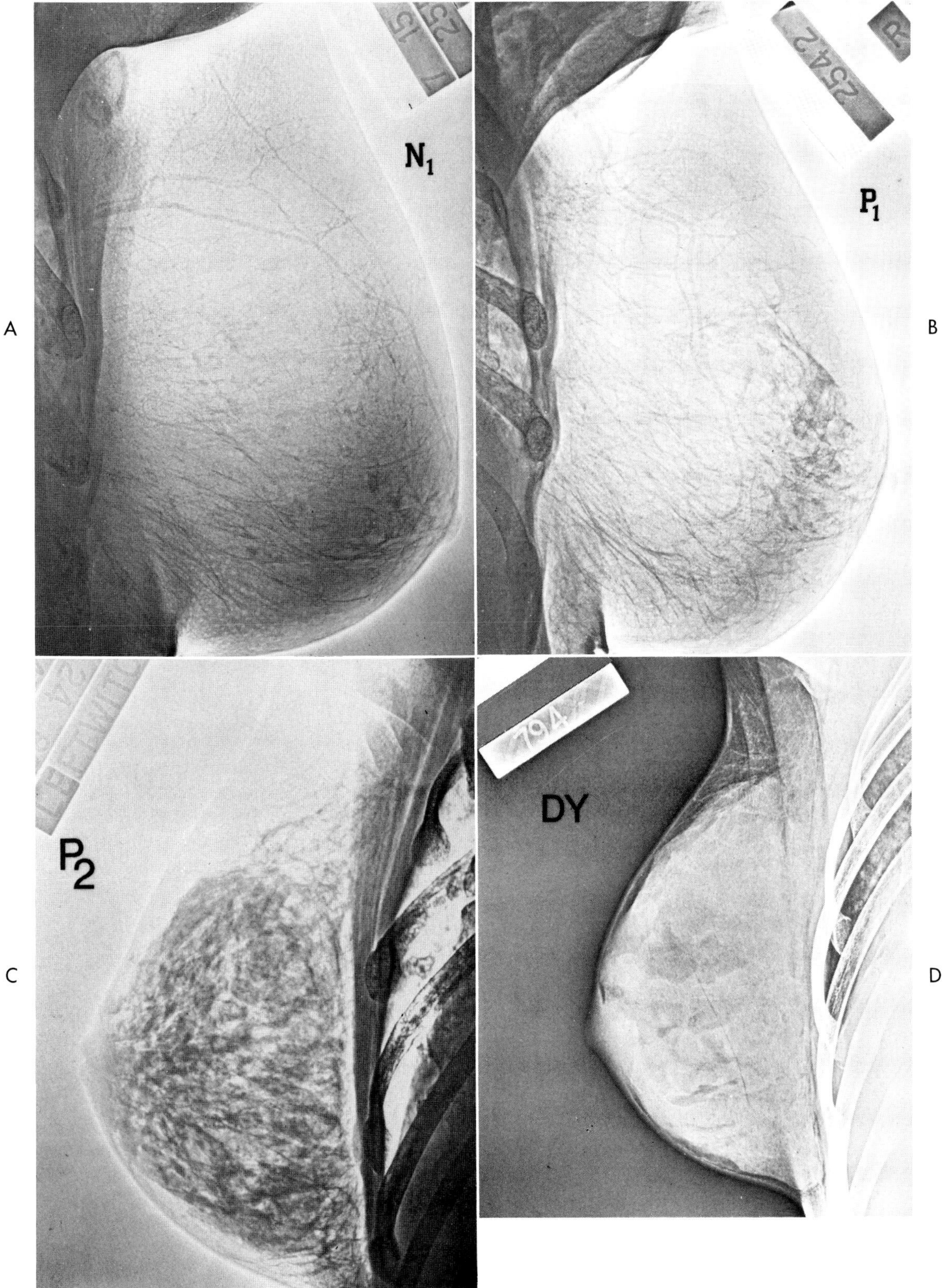

Fig. 62-8 Wolfe mammographic parenchymal patterns. **A,** N_1, Lowest risk. Breast composed predominantly of fatty tissue with no duct response. **B,** P_1, Low risk. Residual epithelial components in immediate subareolar aspects of breast, which compose 25% or less of entire breast. **C,** P_2, High risk. Severe involvement with prominent ductal pattern that occupies greater than 25 of breast volume. **D,** *DY,* Highest risk. Breast parenchyma is remarkably dense with obscure ductal response and an overall homogeneous density. (Courtesy Dr. Jerry B. Buchanan, Department of Radiology, University of Louisville, Louisville, Ky.)

P_2/DY XMM had an odds ratio of 2.42 compared with the N_1 pattern. An elevated breast cancer odds ratio of 3.68 was associated with the P_2/DY pattern in postmenopausal women; premenopausal women were unaffected. For women 50 to 64 years of age, the P_2/DY pattern had a sixfold elevation in breast cancer risks, whereas those less than 50 and 65 years or older had no significant elevation in risk.

Radiographic Imaging of Benign Disease

Proliferative breast disease, or cystic hyperplasia, denotes changes in glandular hyperplasia that primarily involve ducts, adenosis, fibrosis, duct ectasia, and multiple cyst formation. Thus the term *fibrocystic disease* has become the capricious name for a variety of histologic changes in the breast that result from uninhibited estrogen, progestogen, and prolactin stimuli on this target organ in the absence of feedback inhibition. Each of these pathologic descriptions occur in the presence of endogenous estrogens and rarely occur separately, although each is quite difficult to distinguish on a clinical or radiographic basis.[42]

The wide spectrum of XMM images relates to the proliferation that occurs in periductal fibrosis and appears as a prominent duct pattern. Often the presentation of multiple nodules or adenosis as a result of lobular proliferation is identifiable. The clinical and radiographic presentation of large cysts of proliferative origin occur because of obstruction and dilation of the lactiferous ducts. Commonly recognized benign XMM findings include:

1. *Adenosis*. Dysplastic nodules involve the entire breast or segments of a quadrant and appear as small, noncalcified multiple XMM images. A stellate appearance may be observed radiographically when associated with fibrosis and is difficult to distinguish from neoplasms. Infrequently, scattered round calcifications may be identified that resemble the microcalcifications of carcinoma.
2. *Cysts*. The use of ultrasound to differentiate cystic from solid masses has great promise in breast cysts. These palpable semisolid masses appear as oval, uncalcified lesions with sharp, smooth, well-delineated borders.
3. *Fibroadenoma*. These solitary (85%), solid, mobile, rounded or lobulated masses have sharp borders. The presence of a halo of lucency is a typical radiographic feature. On occasion, the differentiation from cysts or medullary-carcinoma is difficult. In the postmenopausal state, large, coarse calcifications may develop following mucoid degeneration with hyalinization and involution.
4. *Cystosarcoma phyllodes (giant fibroadenoma)*. The progressive growth of large variants of solitary fibroadenomas give rise to this entity. Radiographically the neoplasm appears as an uncalcified, lobulated, solid mass with sharp delineation. Differentiation from an invasive carcinoma or sarcoma can be confirmed only by excisional biopsy.
5. *Papilloma*. These intraductal neoplasms originate from the lactiferous ducts and frequently appear as bloody nipple discharge. They may present as oval masses in the subareola and are often not identifiable with biplane XMM views. The injection of water-soluble contrast into the involved duct mechanism (galactogram) often allows identification of an intraluminal filling defect.
6. *Fat necrosis*. The XMM image of fat necrosis has great variability and depends on the age of the patient and the extent of involvement of necrotic fatty substance. Smaller cysts may calcify and give rise to characteristic ringlike calcifications, whereas masses of necrotic fat may stimulate carcinoma with spiculated borders. Angular microcalcifications can occur and also stimulate carcinoma. Excisional biopsy is usually necessary to confirm the benignity of this process.
7. *Abscess*. The presentation of an inflammatory process can usually be confirmed clinically. On occasion, a central, deep, ill-defined mass, which appears with overlying skin thickening, increased vascularity, and absence of pain, may mimic carcinoma both clinically and radiographically. Thorough exploration, culture, and biopsy with drainage are indicated to confirm an inflammatory process of nonmalignant origin.

Radiographic Imaging of Malignant Disease

Gershon-Cohen and Colcher[60] and Egan[44,45] confirmed that radiographic imaging (mammography) closely reflects the pathologic changes of malignant states of the breast. These clinicopathologic correlations have been subsequently confirmed through whole-organ studies and specimen radiography. Typically the first XMM manifestation

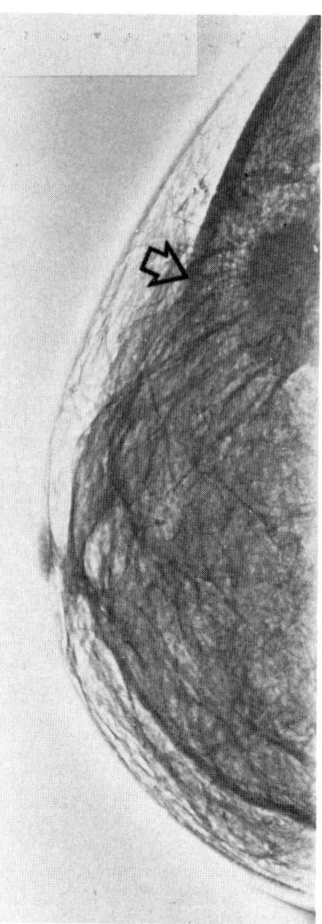

Fig. 62-9 Xeromammographic appearance of typical invasive ductal carcinoma with productive fibrosis. Distortions of normal parenchyma adjacent to dense tumor mass *(arrow)* appear as spiculated projections that radiate from neoplasm. Retraction of adjacent tissues with entrapment of Cooper's ligaments to produce peau d'orange edema was clinically evident. (Courtesy Dr. Jerry B. Buchanan, Department of Radiology, University of Louisville, Louisville, Ky.)

of breast carcinoma is a soft-tissue mass that requires differentiation from the aforementioned benign lesions of the breast. These soft tissue densities may occur in the presence or absence of microcalcification. The differentiation of the benign soft tissue mass from medullary carcinoma sometimes may be difficult because of sharp definition of both.

Characteristically, distortions of the normal parenchyma adjacent to malignant tumors occur as a spicule, i.e., long or short, fine and straight strands of tissue that radiate from the tumor site (Fig. 62-9). Retraction of tissues in the direction of the tumor occurs with loss of the margins of the malignant mass because of infiltration of tumor and subsequent reactive sclerosis. The latter characteristic adds to the XMM a spiculated or stellate appearance. The entrapment of Cooper's ligaments into the tumor mass will subsequently initiate retraction of overlying skin or nipple as the tumor extends into adjacent tissues. As the blockage of lymphatics progresses, overlying skin edema (peau d'orange) occurs, which is typically seen on XMM as heightening or thickening of skin. The presentation of inflammatory breast cancer as a lethal and aggressive clinicopathologic variant is strongly suggestive on XMM. In this case the increase of skin thickness is generalized with involvement of the entire surface of the breast and enhancement of tissue density. Asymmetric widening of the subcutaneous space with prominent subcutaneous lymphatics is evident (Fig. 62-10). Lymphatic vessels engorged by tumor are identified as fine streaks perpendicular to the skin surface.

Microcalcifications represent the early XMM findings of some cancers (e.g., comedocarcinoma, minimum). Typically, microcalcifications are irregular in shape and size and occur in linear configurations or in small clusters (Fig. 62-11). These calcifications are present histologically within areas of tumor and fat necrosis. The presence of microcalcifications in the absence of a mass may be the first sign of an intraductal or lobular carcinoma (in situ), which appears clinically as the tumor mass expands. These irregular, scattered microcalcifications must be differentiated from the benign calcifications of FCDB, which are tyically larger, oval, and more diffuse. Regardless of the circumstance, XMM identification of a site of suspicious microcalcification necessitates histologic confirmation that employs radiographically assisted biopsy techniques. Use of the Kopan needle for XMM localization followed by biopsy with a counter-incision (Fig. 62-12) allows histologic evaluation following specimen radiography.

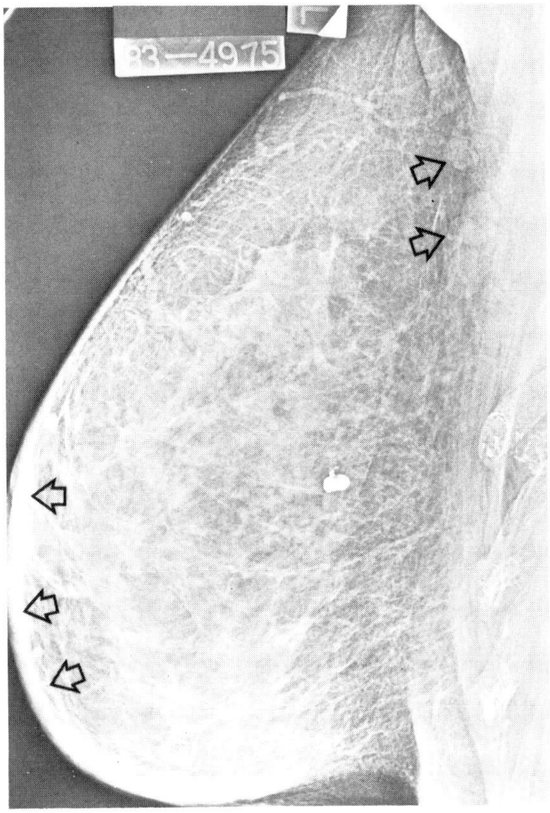

Fig. 62-10 Xeromammographic appearance of inflammatory breast carcinoma. Lymphatic vessels replaced with tumor emboli are identified as fine streaks that radiate perpendicular to skin surface. Asymmetric widening of subcutaneous space with prominent lymphatics is demonstrated *(arrows)*. Enlarged axillary lymph nodes are evident radiographically *(arrows)*. (Courtesy Dr. Jerry B. Buchanan, Department of Radiology, University of Louisville, Louisville, Ky.)

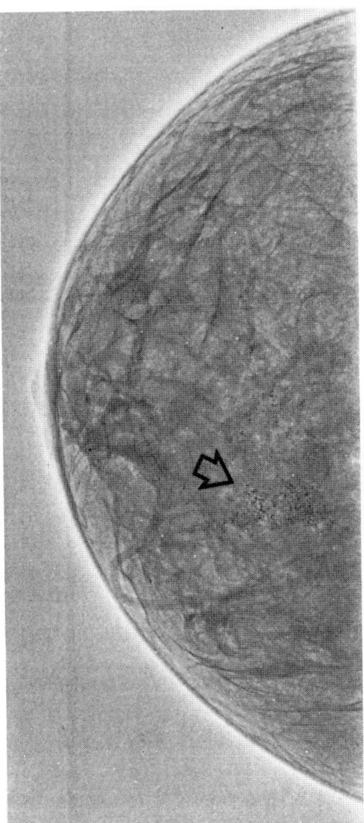

Fig. 62-11 Typical appearance of stipled microcalcifications in breast carcinoma. These calcifications *(arrow)* are typically irregular in size and shape and occur in small clusters or in linear configurations. (Courtesy Dr. Jerry B. Buchanan, Department of Radiology, University of Louisville, Louisville, Ky.)

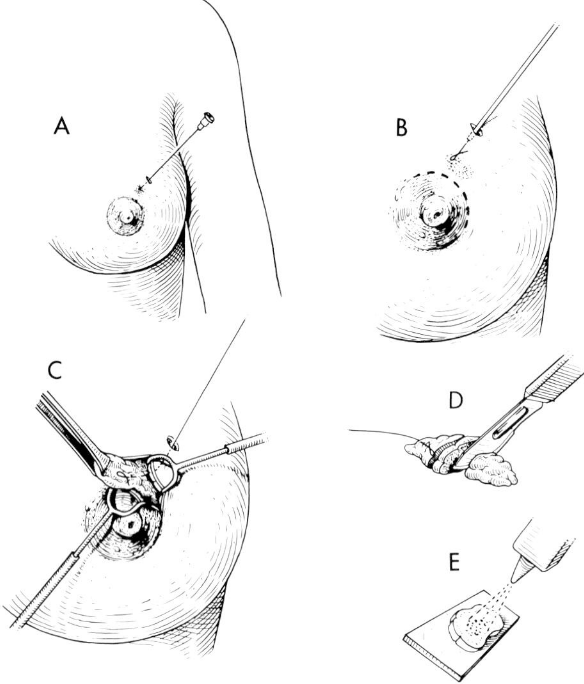

Fig. 62-12 **A** and **B,** Radiographic-assisted biopsy techniques using Kopan needle for xeromammographic localization. **C,** Circumareolar counter-incision with retrieval of hook of Kopan needle in radiographically imaged microcalcifications. **D,** Bread-loafing of biopsy specimen to identify tumor with microcalcifications employing specimen radiography **(E).** (From Bland, K.I., and Buchanan, J.B.: Preoperative localization of nonpalpable (occult) lesions of the breast. In O'Leary, J.P., editor: Techniques for surgeons, New York, Copyright © 1984, Reprinted by permission of John Wiley & Sons, Inc.)

Radiographic Imaging of Physiologically Normal and Abnormal Masses

The identification of physiologic abnormalities of breast parenchyma for asymptomatic subjects in the absence of palpable masses is possible with the use of standard XMM techniques. Currently, radiographic imaging employs standard roentgenograms or xerographic techniques with two views of each breast in a craniocaudal and mediolateral projection.

The use of XMM has been studied extensively as a screening device to detect breast cancer in an early and more favorable stage of presentation. Studies of the Health Insurance Plan (HIP) of Greater New York suggested that breast cancer could be detected mammographically in a preclinical (nonpalpable) stage. The benefit of screening in the HIP study was restricted to women over 50 years of age. The recent report of the National Cancer Institute (NCI) and the American Cancer Society (ACS) multi-insitutional study of mammography (BCDDP) supported the findings of the HIP study with regard to early detection and suggested benefit with screening for younger and elderly categories.

Bland and associates[18] confirmed minimum breast cancer (MBC) to be more prevalent in the screened population (29%) than the unscreened population (<5%). MBC lesions appeared with similar frequencies in screenees under and over age 50 years. Baker,[10] in a recent review of the final report of the NCI-ACS BCDDP results, revealed that among 3557 cases of proven breast cancer detected in the project's screening clinics, 41.6% were detected by XMM alone, 47.3% by physical examination and XMM, 8.7% by physical examination alone, and 2.4% by unknown measures. Approximately one third (32.4%) of the 3557 neoplasms were classified as MBC. Moreover, greater than 80% of all detected cancers had no evidence of regional nodal involvement.

The widespread acceptance of XMM and standard radiographic mammography to screen asymptomatic subjects and to diagnose subtle clinical breast abnormalities has occurred in the past two decades. Egan[44,45] established the value of this radiographic technique with the observation of mammographic abnormalities in 10% of the screened community patients who had clinically undetectable neoplasms, the majority (92%) of whom had absence of axillary nodal metastases. The probability of a false-negative study (clinically negative, XMM negative) exceeds 10% in most breast clinics. Conversely, the false-positive diagnosis of cancer occurs much less frequently (<5%), with diagnostic accuracy increasing as a correlate of experience of the mammographer and the radiographic technique. However, the incidence of a false-negative XMM or an equivocal report is too great to rely on mammography for exclusion of the diagnosis of cancer in the presence of a solitary mass or suspicious lesion. Further, the dysplastic (dense) multinodular, fibrocystic, and small breast may obscure or invalidate interpretation of occult neoplasms poorly imaged on XMM. *In no circumstance should mammography be considered a uniformly reliable technique for exclusion of the diagnosis of cancer, because histologic confirmation of clinically suspicious lesions by biopsy is mandatory.*

METASTASIS IN BREAST CANCER

Physiologic and Biologic Concepts

The physiologic process of tumor metastasis is a complex biologic event that is influenced by (1) the tumor-host relationship, (2) the metabolic and growth characteristics of the primary neoplasm, and (3) the physical and morphologic factors operative within the vicinity of the neoplasm. Most data that quantitate the degree and probability of metastatic spread as an aid to prognosis and treatment have thus far met with little success. These observations attest to the broad spectrum and variability for interrelationships of human breast tumors and the host-defense mechanism. The physiologic mechanism by which a primary tumor gives rise to a metastatic clone of tumor cells remains a significant factor.

Enzymatic Activity and Metastatic Potential

The role of lysosomal enzymes to initiate cellular breakdown with loss of intracellular substance may be key to initiation of tumor invasion. This local, invasive process of host tissues by malignant cells invariably follows destruction of normal tissue components juxtaposed to invading neoplastic cells. This event is concomitant with growth of neoplastic cells following infiltration into the subject tissues. A growing body of evidence suggests that neoplastic clones grow and enzymatically destroy adjacent normal cells without themselves being injured. Data suggest that tumor cell surfaces are endowed with different composition and structure such as glycoproteins, which provide innate protection against the hydrolytic effect of lysosomal enzymes. Variations of the concentration of lysosomal enzymes within invading and regressing tumors is perhaps explained by the fact that both tumor cell lines are simultaneously being destroyed by autolysis.

Immunologic Surveillance and Control of Enzymatic Activity

Berg,[13] in elaborate animal experimentation, noted that neoplastic cells are capable of initiating specific immune reactions in proven isogenic systems. In most animal models studied and in certain human cancers, tumor-specific antigens are recognizable in selective assays. However, not all tumors possess much specific immunogenicity. Mathé[95] suggested the possibility for early control of breast cancer metastases using immunologic methods to augment clinical responses. The application of these methods using monoclonal assay techniques to link active cytotoxic drugs to tumor-specific antibodies may have clinical applicability. Also, these tumor-specific antibody carriers may reduce the myelosuppression and toxicity that ensue following immunosuppression with systemic therapy. Rowland, O'Neill, and Davies[120] have used intermediate-carrier polyglutamic acid with substituted cytotoxic drugs linked to immunoglobulins to reduce active antibody activity and neoplastic growth in a rodent tumor model. However, the role of cytotoxic immunotherapy for breast cancer in clinical practice is not clearly established.

Lymphatic Metastases and Modulation of Metastases by Tumor-Host Mechanisms

Classic physiologic concepts taught by Handley suggested that breast cancer metastases represent centrifugal dissemination into and through the lymphatics to establish regional and systemic disease. This hypothesis did not recognize that neoplastic invasion facilitates entry into venulae, as well as the regional lymphatics. Although primary tumors do not contain lymphatic connections, the entry into endolymph is initiated by an invasive mechanism. Thereafter, the interstitial fluid convection currents drain and transport neoplastic cells to regional nodes by the method suggested by Butler and Gullino.[30] The presence of widely patent junctions of intercellular bridges in the lymphatics represent primary routes to transport neoplastic cells into systemic lymph.[90]

Investigators have also confirmed that cytoplasmic processes of tumor cells probe the endothelial surface to initiate and provide the best route for transport.[31] Following cellular entrapment, the neoplastic clone is transported to afferent lymph vessels to the peripheral subcapsular sinusoids of the nodes. Metabolic, morphologic, and cell-type characteristics determine the temporal duration of "nodal arrest" and the probability of subsequent entrapment. Following nodal deposition, cellular proliferation is initiated in the peripheral sinusoids and, following progressive cell division, the medullary regions of the gland are replaced. Thereafter, cells are shed into the efferent lymphatic vessels and may subsequently embolize to more distal nodes of the regional basin.

Ultimately, cells swept into endolymph are transported to systemic sites (lung, liver, brain).[131] Carr, McGinty, and Norris[31] used an anaplastic carcinogen-induced tumor to demonstrate that regional lymph nodes represent an immunologically privileged site for tumor growth. These data recapitulate Handley's concept that regional axillary nodes represent a drainage barrier that may or may not be responsive to immunostimulatory events impairing or retarding tumor dissemination. This classic teaching ignored the probability that tumor cells have additional routes to the systemic circulation by way of lymphaticovenous anastomoses.[47,91]

Although lymph node arrest may be transient, neoplastic cells traversing the sinusoids and medullary portion of the nodes retain the capacity for metastases to numerous organs. Few cells that lodge in the medullary portion of the nodes develop into subsequent metastases. This concept has been reaffirmed by Hewitt and Blake,[68] who concluded that nodes retain a constant "holding capacity" of a specific cell fraction and volume. When this threshold is exceeded, additional emboli pass through the efferent channels to directly enter the systemic venous and lymphatic circulation.

Salsbury[122] observed viable circulating neoplastic cells in peripheral human venous blood. In this and other studies,[63,64,122] malignant cells of breast and colon cancer have been readily detected in effluent venous blood, and active deoxyribonucleic acid (DNA) synthesis has been confirmed in vitro. In many experiments the threshold for "tumor-take" is higher following intravenous injection than when the subcutaneous or intramuscular routes are used. Sugarbaker[131] observed that poor clonogeneity of tumor cells cannot explain the small ratio of successful metastases to cells injected. Blood circulation apparently represents a hostile immunologic environment for nonhematogenous tumor cells.[46] Furthermore, the study by Vaage[134] suggests that immune modulation and destruction of neoplastic cells is more effective when cells are injected intravenously, although the specific dose-response effect is tumor dependent, and in many solid tumor systems only a small percentage of viable cells will survive to become metastases following injection into venous blood.

Despite the small fraction of viable cells that survive in circulation to initiate metastatic growth, the immunobiologic events occurring in distant capillary bed sites will allow growth of selective cell populations. Following cellular implantation and neogrowth, the host responds to neoplastic stimulation with a reaction that varies with the clinical stage of neoplastic growth. These host interactions vary chronobiologically and, with increasing cell populations, are influenced by metabolic and nutritional factors. In most breast neoplasms a long preclinical (occult) and prediagnostic period occurs in which tumor or host factors can modulate metastasis formation. Many human and experimental tumor cells are shown to possess tumor-associated antigens that can initiate host reactions lethal for the offending neoplastic cell.

The immune system is also known to have morphologic functional components with counterproductive capabilities that are often balanced by a large number of interrelating polypeptides akin to the endocrine system.[131] Within the lymphocytic population are thymus-dependent lymphocytes (T lymphocytes) and antibody-producing cells (B lymphocytes). An additional arm of "suppressor cells" is represented by lymphocytic cells that suppress the cytotoxic reactions of lymphoid populations. These cells have been shown to enhance tumor proliferation, whereas macrophage populations "eat" foreign cells in their confirmed role as scavengers. These phylogenetically primitive activators or suppressors of the actions of lymphocytes can kill neoplastic cells through the afferent arc of the immune surveillance system. The activity of these immune cellular subpopulations have stimulated extensive clinical trials of nonspecifc immunostimulation as adjuncts to surgical resection for breast neoplasms.

PROGNOSTIC VARIABLES CONSIDERED TO INCREASE PROBABILITY FOR RELAPSE IN BREAST CANCER

1. Histologic confirmation of metastasis to axillary lymph nodes
2. Tumor size (e.g., T_2 ($\geq$ 5 cm) vs. T_1)
3. Absence of estrogen and progesterone receptors
4. Evidence of rapid growth rate of tumor (high-thymidine labeling index or S-phase fraction).
5. High nuclear or histological grade
6. Antibody detection of occult bone marrow metastases

Modified from Lippman, M.E., and Chabner, B.A.: Editorial overview: proceedings of the NIH Consensus Development Conference on Adjuvant Chemotherapy and Endocrine Therapy for Breast Cancer, Natl. Cancer Inst. **1**:5, 1986.

Prognostic Variables for Breast Carcinoma

To justify the risk-benefit ratio of potentially toxic systemic adjuvant therapy of breast cancer, the ability to identify patients at high risk for relapse is a key consideration. The recognition by early pathologists and surgeons of the importance of quantitative axillary lymph node involvement by metastatic breast cancer is legend. The justification for this risk is that approximately one third of patients without apparent axillary lymph node involvement or recurrence die of their disease within 5 to 10 years.[84] Further, some breast carcinomas with as many as 10+ positive axillary nodes will not have recurrence within a 10-year interval. Thus the importance of reliable prognostic variables is apparent. Data presented at the NIH Consensus Development Conference on Adjuvant Chemotherapy and Endocrine Therapy for Breast Carcinoma in 1985 suggest the potential usefulness of the prognostic variables listed in the boxed material at right as important to predict risk and subsequent relapse, disease-free survival, and actuarial survival.

Clearly, estrogen and progesterone hormone receptor analyses can augment the identification of individuals at higher risk of relapse. There is an increased probability that tumors that contain no receptor proteins recur earlier than neoplasms that contain either or both of the receptors. Such data have been demonstrated conclusively from numerous retrospective and prospective trials and apply to both premenopausal and postmenopausal patients with and without nodal involvement. Although the explanation of these observations is unclear, a plausible reason is the fundamental changes in either the tumor growth rate or metastatic potential of the breast tumor that lacks these receptor proteins.

The Adjuvant Systemic Chemotherapy of Operable Breast Cancer

With revitalization of the interest in adjuvant chemotherapy during the early 1970s, the crucial indicator of success was the ability of available cytotoxic agents to exert a significant and consistent antitumor effect when administered for prolonged periods of time following standard surgical procedures. Use of this approach is scientifically justified because of the aforementioned potential of lymphatic metastasis and to modulate metastasis by tumor-host mechanisms. Even though in 90% of women with breast cancer the disease is limited to the breast and lymphatics, in many series approximately one third of these patients die of breast cancer within 5 to 10 years. Table 62-4 summarizes the essential features obtained from research protocols whose case series were studied a minimum of 5 years. All randomized studies report a significant increase in the relapse-free survival rate of chemotherapy-treated patients vs. the control population. This advantage occurred at least in the given subsets and predominantly in premenopausal women. However, in the study of the arm of the protocol testing phenylalanine mustard vs. controls, the Guy's-Manchester study[114] failed to confirm the significant superiority of the treated group observed by the National Surgical Adjuvant Breast Project (NSABP). Significant overall survival advantage has been reported thus far in given subsets. This was limited in the NSABP experience reported by Fisher and associates[50] to women $\leq$ 49 years of age with one to three nodes, to premenopausal women receiving cytoxan, methotrexate, and 5-fluorouracil (CMF) chemotherapy in Milan,[23] and to both menopausal groups treated in the Royal Infirmary (Glasgow) with radiation plus CMF.[129]

Bonadonna and Valagussa[25] note that for most published series the significant advantage achieved in relapse-free survival has not translated into a significant overall survival and thus has created a degree of skepticism of the actual value of adjuvant chemotherapy. A major criticism concerns the type and intensity of salvage therapies for which an accurate description has been omitted in almost all reports. Thus, at the time of primary failure, physicians are often forced to apply appropriate therapy by the status of the recurrent neoplasm. Therefore the subset undergoing therapy is neither selected nor comparable to control and chemotherapy-treated patients with regard to performance and receptor status, stage, and growth of the metastasis.

Bonadonna, Rossi, and Valagussa[24] recently reported the 10-year results of a trial testing radical mastectomy with and without adjuvant CMF for 386 women with Stage II breast carcinoma. Long-term analysis confirms that adjuvant CMF was able to produce a significant relapse-free survival improvement (43.4%) vs. control (31.4%, p <

Table 62-4 **ADJUVANT CHEMOTHERAPY STUDIES WITH A CONCOMITANT CONTROL GROUP WITH LOCAL-REGIONAL TREATMENT ALONE IN NODE-POSITIVE PATIENTS**

Authors	Patients (No.)	Adjuvant Treatment*	Median Follow-up (Months)	Essential Findings in Treated Groups†
Fisher[50]	370	P	82	Increased RFS and OS in premenopause, 1 to 3 nodes
Bonadonna[23]	386	CMF	92	Increased RFS and OS in premenopause
Senn[126]	118	LMF + BCG	82	Increased RFS in postmenopause; no OS difference
Wheeler[140]	227	CVFM	60	Increased RFS (mainly in postmenopause); no OS difference
Reubens[115]	312	P	48	No significant difference after P
Reubens[114]	316	CMF	48	CMF superior in premenopause; no OS difference
Morrison[104]	512	AVCMF	45	Increased RFS in premenopause; no OS difference
Smith[129]	322	CMF vs. CMF with RT	42	Increased RFS in premenopause and postmenopause after RT with CMF and CMF vs. RT alone; increased OS after RT with CMF vs. RT alone

Modified from Bonadonna, G., and Valagussa, P.: Adjuvant systemic therapy for resectable breast cancer, J. Clin. Oncol. **3**:259, 1985.
**P*, phenylalanine mustard; *C*, cyclophosphamide; *M*, methotrexate; *F*, 5-fluorouracil; *L*, leukeran; *V*, vincristine; *A*, doxorubicin (Adriamycin).
†RFS, Relapse-free survival; *OS*, overall survival; *RT*, postoperative radiation.

0.001) and a trend in total survival (55.2% vs. 47.3%) that was not statistically significant. Both relapse-free and total survival were significant for premenopausal women. Relapse-free survival was not influenced by drug-induced amenorrhea. Further, for both treatment groups results were inversely related to the number of histologically involved axillary nodes. At relapse, salvage treatment applied in the control group failed to produce superior results compared to those achieved in the CMF group and yielded a similar median survival from first relapse between control (37 months) and CMF (32 months) patients. It was concluded that CMF was able to improve the course of premenopausal women with high-risk breast cancer during the first decade following radical mastectomy.

Results of adjuvant therapies conducted over the past decade provide evidence that tumor heterogeneity represents the major determinant for success or failure in the treatment of minimal residual disease, as well as for advanced disease. Lippman and Chabner[84] note that, with examination of the summary data, adjuvant chemotherapy results in a statistically significant but small reduction in mortality for women over age 50 compared to results in younger women. Because this reduction is small (≤ 10%), many physicians have concluded that tamoxifen may be a superior therapy for this older subset when its effect on mortality and its notably reduced toxicity are considered. The overall impact of chemotherapy data for all trials using an untreated control has been considered by Peto. Using a data base of nearly 14,000 prospectively randomized women participating in trials, this author predicted a highly significant 25% reduction in mortality during the period for which follow-up is available. Thus there is unquestionably an improvement in survival with adjuvant chemotherapy. Lippman and Chabner[84] also suggest that the effectiveness of chemotherapy depends on choice of the active cytotoxic agents, scheduling and sequencing, overall dosage rate and dosage intensity, and interactions with other therapy such as irradiation or endocrine therapy. A variety of prospectively randomized trials have investigated whether chemotherapy of longer and shorter duration yields equivalent results. Trials comparing 1 vs. 2 years of therapy and 6 vs. 12 months of therapy have reached the general consensus that short, intensive courses of chemotherapy for approximately 6 months' duration are likely to be as effective as prolonged periods of chemotherapy. Further trials suggest that equivalent amounts of drug can be administered to patients receiving aggressive irradiation for the management of the primary tumor as an alternative to mastectomy in early-stage breast cancer. It appears that irradiation therapy is unlikely to have a substantial impact on the ability to deliver full-dose chemotherapy.

Hormonal Sensitivity of Metastatic Breast Cells

Breast cancers consist of heterogeneous cellular populations that have varying metabolic demands and growth fractions. The opportunity to control the metastatic tendency of the malignant breast cell during the process of tumor implantation is a correlate of steroid sensitivity of the cell clone.[141] Usually, these neoplastic cells that normally depend on the hormonal milieu for growth and function are similarly dependent when they function as a metastatic unit. Loss of response to the hormonal milieu occurs by the dedifferentiation process and appears to be a typical aspect of malignant metastatic growth. Thus cellular populations that retain this steroid sensitivity in secondary growth will respond to hormonal therapy, which will modify, enhance, or diminish cellular transport and implantation.

Progression of heterogeneous growth may revert to autonomous function of the metastatic clone, in which case hormonal sensitivity is lost. Considerable experimental evidence confirms that secondary growth, with variable hormonal sensitivities, can coexist in the same species and even in the same animal.[59] Thus secondary tumors consist of mixed cellular populations, varying fractions of which are hormone sensitive and insensitive. The mechanism by which sex steroids stimulate protein and nucleic acid synthesis in developing populations of cells appears to be mediated through a system of enzyme induction and repression.[141]

APPLICATION OF STEROID HORMONE RECEPTORS IN BREAST CANCER

Following the demonstration of hormonal dependence of breast carcinoma by Beatson[12] in 1896, observations confirmed that approximately one third of breast malignancies respond to removal of the endocrine hormonal milieu (adrenal, pituitary, ovary), as well as to additive hormonal therapy (e.g., estrogens, antiestrogens, androgens, progestins, glucocorticoids). In many institutions oophorectomy alone remains the initial method of therapy in a premenopausal patient who has recurrent breast carcinoma. In 1951, Huggins[72] and Huggins and Bergenstal[73] introduced oophorectomy combined with bilateral adrenalectomy for control of metastatic breast cancer on the assumption that carcinoma derived from hormonally dependent tissues is nonautonomous and thus may depend on this hormonal milieu for viability and growth. This concept was subsequently extended by Luft, Olivecrona, and Sjögren,[89] who also demonstrated regression of metastatic breast carcinoma after hypophysectomy, implicating a pituitary-adreno-ovarian axis with tumor regression following removal of the tropic stimuli.

The heterogeneity of the clones of breast cells correctly predicted in early investigative work suggested that carcinoma of the breast may involve two categories regarding hormonal influence. The *hormone-dependent* variant is observed to respond to one or a combination of the previously mentioned forms of endocrine ablation. Conversely, the *hormone-independent* type recapitulates the heterogenous variants of the neoplasm because clones of cells are not influenced by the modes of therapy just listed, and these autonomous cells are unaffected by steroidal, hormonal, ablative, and perhaps chemotherapeutic measures.

The proper selection of the appropriate method of sequential endocrine manipulation for the management of advanced breast carcinoma has been debated extensively. Hormonal ablation has included oophorectomy alone; oophorectomy combined with adrenalectomy; hypophysectomy; and estrogen, androgen, or adrenocortical hormone therapy. The more ancient method of endocrine manipulation, oophorectomy, remains in controversy as to its efficacy in delaying recurrence when used alone. Indeed, salutary remissions are evident when disease-free interval exceeds 12 to 18 months, and the addition of adrenalectomy often provides objective regression of metastatic lesions. A restricted use of oophoroadrenalectomy as a palliative or "therapeutic" measure for patients with disseminated breast carcinoma was adopted because surgeons were reluctant to submit patients to a radical and often nonbeneficial (60% to 70%) procedure to achieve a desired goal not possible with other modalities. In large control series of patients with Stage IV disease, irrespective of age or menstrual status, irrefutable statistical evidence suggests the equality of responses (31% to 42%) following either of the adrenal ablative methods performed without the benefit of estrogen- or progestin-receptor analyses of the metastatic lesions. Other investigators have noted similar objective remissions after therapeutic hypophysectomy (31% to 42%) and oophoroadrenalectomy (32% to 35%).[113]

The comparative retrospective analysis by Kennedy, Mielke, and Fortuny[78] for immediate castration and "late" therapeutic castration evaluated Stage I and II disease. These investigators concluded that immediate castration lengthens the disease-free interval from mastectomy to appearance of metastatic disease; however, a significant prolongation of the interval from recurrent disease to death was also noted in the therapeutic castration group. The total survival times, however, were not different in the two groups according to the statistical methods employed. These investigators extended this series to include the effects of other forms of therapy in patients with advanced disease (Stages III and IV). The additional modalities of therapy included hypophysectomy or adrenalectomy with inclusive analysis of the effects of estrogens, androgens, adrenocortical hormones, and cytotoxic agents. One third of the patients treated with immediate oophorectomy received one of these additional forms of therapy; 50% of those with therapeutic castration received adjunctive therapy. In the combined series, the proportion of improvement for the prophylactic group (17.7%) was similar to that of the therapeutic series (19.8%). The investigators concluded that for both groups of patients with prophylactic or therapeutic castration, similar objective responses are apparent following adjunctive therapy.

Thereafter, a report by the National Surgical Adjuvant Breast Project[112] failed to demonstrate that immediate oophorectomy alone either deferred the recurrence of metastatic carcinoma or prolonged survival. The subsequent application of estradiol cytosol binding of the breast cancer and its application to endocrine manipulation is legend.

A comparison of the percentage of patients who respond to the various endocrine therapies in uncontrolled studies suggests a slight advantage for ablative procedures; however, Henderson and Canellos[67] note that randomized trials fail to demonstrate a clear advantage for one form of endocrine manipulation over the other. Randomized trials that compare response and survival rates of patients treated with major ablative procedures (adrenalectomy, hypophysectomy) vs. those treated initially with additive therapy (estrogens, androgens, or possibly adrenalectomy with further disease progession) reveal no significant survival advantage of either group.[67] Randomized trials that compare additive estrogen therapy vs. antiestrogens (tamoxifen), antiestrogens vs. hypophysectomy, and aminoglutethimide vs. adrenalectomy have each failed to show significant differences in objective responses, response duration, or survival advantage.[75,123,124]

Thus the choice of endocrine manipulation depends on the available alternatives and the relative toxicities induced by the various therapies. Also, patients who respond to one type of endocrine therapy are often likely to respond to additional variants that have traditionally been administered in a sequence or cascade. Premenopausal women were first treated with oophorectomy, and, if a sustained disease-free interval was obtained, adrenalectomy would be offered following progression of disease. If these forms of therapy failed, without the *predictive* response of the estradiol-binding protein, patients would then be treated with nonendocrine therapy. Postmenopausal patients were conventionally treated with diethylstilbesterol (DES) as the initial method of therapy, because it is minimally toxic and did not portend the morbidity and mortality of adrenalectomy. If patients responded to DES and subsequently progressed, a trial of DES withdrawal would often result in a subsequent response in almost one third of patients so treated. Nonendocrine therapies were often reserved for the postmenopausal patient who had previously failed one of the forms of endocrine therapy.

Clinical trials established that patients who respond to these endocrine therapies are afforded palliation of their metastatic disease and in some circumstances have increased survival. Conversly, clinical experience suggested that approximately one third of patients with metastatic (Stage IV) breast carcinoma will respond to endocrine therapy when their menopausal status is ignored. Therefore, the nonselective application for therapy replacement or ablative endocrine therapy portends potential morbidity for therapy in approximately two thirds of subjects. Further, this additional morbidity is recognized in the absence of benefit for disease remission. For these reasons, objective parameters to predict patient selection for probability of response following endocrine therapy are desirable in the management of breast cancer patients.

The hormonally sensitive primary and metastatic breast cancer cell, as already described, can be identified at the time of breast biopsy or resection of the tumor and its regional lymphatics (mastectomy). These steroid hormone receptor analyses should be performed routinely on all patients with primary and metastatic breast cancer.

With the demonstration of estrogen receptor protein (estrophilin, ER) in hormonally responsive breast cancers by Jensen, De Sombre and Jungblut,[77] appropriate selection of subjects for endocrine ablation was remarkably enhanced. Current methods in widespread use require biochemical analysis of homogenized breast tumor tissue fractions with radioactively labeled steroid ligands. Accurate assays are now being reported for increasingly smaller quantities of tumor tissue.

The ER has thus become a marker of hormone-dependent breast cancer and has greatly simplified the approach to oncologic treatment protocols for Stages I to IV disease. The ER represents a protein located in the cytoplasm of breast neoplasms and is found in approximately 55% of breast cancers, with increasing positivity as a function of age. A negative correlate appears to exist between ER-positive tumors and (1) size of the primary tumor, (2) location of the primary tumor, (3) extent of disease, and (4) type of tissue assayed (primary vs. skin vs. nodes vs. soft tissue vs. visceral).[2] A weak correlation does exist between the frequency of reactivity of ER and the status of the axillary nodes at the time of mastectomy. However, the ER- positive tumor groups appear to contain a higher proportion of node-negative patients. The differentiation of patients with regard to the probability of response to endocrine manipulation or replacement does not appear to correlate with the site of disease, disease-free interval, menopausal status, or age.

STEROID RECEPTORS AND DISEASE-FREE INTERVAL

A correlation exists between the tumor differentiation characteristics and the reactivity of ER.[128] The observation of an inverse correlation between thymidine-labeling indices and ER status initiated a study for the relationship between ER and disease-free interval by Allegra and others[2,85] and Silva and associates.[128] Allegra[2] confirmed the relationship between disease-free interval and ER status in 182 patients with mammary cancer, of whom 79 exhibited ER-negative primary tumors (30%) that were observed to have recurrent disease. Only eight of 103 (8%) ER-positive patients were observed to have relapse. In this series 91% of the ER-positive patients were free of disease at 24 months, compared with 62% of the ER-negative patients.

Table 62-5 **RELATIONSHIP BETWEEN ESTROGEN RECEPTOR (ER) STATUS, PROGNOSTIC VARIABLES, AND RECURRENCE RATE IN BREAST CANCER**

Factor	ER Positive	ER Negative	p Value
Axillary node status			
0	5/52	8/30	≤0.02
1-3	0/13	6/23	0.08
≥4	2/20	7/21	0.05
Tumor size			
≥2 cm	4/36	7/30	≤0.04
≤2 cm	1/40	10/28	≤0.001
Menopausal status			
Premenopausal	1/20	14/32	≤0.01
Postmenopausal	4/76	7/37	≤0.01
Adjuvant chemotherapy			
No	5/67	13/41	≤0.001
Yes or unknown	3/36	11/38	
TOTAL	8/103	24/79	≤0.001

From Allegra, J.C.: The use of steroid hormone receptors in breast cancer. In Margolese, R., editor: Contemporary issues in clinical oncology: breast cancer, New York, 1983, Churchill Livingstone. By permission.

Other prognostic variables have been thought possibly to explain the difference in recurrence rates according to ER reactivity. In one study investigators compared differences in prognostic variables between ER-positive and ER-negative patients.[2] This study confirmed that neither age, tumor size, menopausal status, number of axillary nodes, nor proportion who receive adjuvant chemotherapy were different; however, younger patients were observed to have trends toward positive nodes and greater need for adjuvant chemotherapy in the ER-negative groups (Table 62-5). Thus stratification of patients with regard to their ER status appears warranted and perhaps desirable in prospective clinical trials to identify selectively patients who would gain greatest benefit with intensive cytotoxic chemotherapy.

McGuire[97] reported a correlation for level of ER in fentomoles per milligram of cytosol protein in breast neoplasms with the response rate to endocrine therapy. An 80% objective remission was observed in patients whose ER was greater than or equal to 100 fmol/mg cytosol of ER protein. A response rate of 46% was observed in women with lesser values. This objective response rate to endocrine therapy as a function of content of ER has been confirmed by others.[39,58,125]

The application of additional cytoplasmic markers of

hormonally dependent breast cancer is a more recent development, although its role in routine therapeutic management has not been firmly established.[4] The use of progesterone receptors (PR) appears to have value in augmenting selection of the endocrine-dependent breast cell.[70,98] Horwitz and McGuire[70] observed that synthesis of PR is strictly estrogen dependent and represents the end product of estradiol-stimulated pathways in breast cancer tissues. Bland, Fuchs, and Wittliff[19] established previously that premenopausal patients with nondetectable ER have a threefold increase in PR when compared to postmenopausal groups. Since high endogenous estrogens in premenopausal patients mask ER in tumor biopsies, it appears advantageous to perform PR determinations to identify an additional 15% of women with metastatic breast cancer who may benefit from endocrine therapy.

Previous studies[94,96] have correlated the trend toward higher quantitative values of ER and PR in tumors that are histologically well differentiated. These correlations have been reaffirmed by Silva and associates,[128] who observed higher mean ER and PR values and greater numbers of tissues harboring low-grade (Grade I) neoplasms when both receptors were positive.

Table 62-6 **PROPOSED THERAPEUTIC OPTIONS AND FREQUENCY OF STEROID RECEPTOR* FOR PREMENOPAUSAL AND POSTMENOPAUSAL PATIENTS WITH BREAST CANCER**

	Premenopausal		Postmenopausal	
Receptor Status	**No. (%)**	**Proposed Therapy**	**No. (%)**	**Proposed Therapy**
ER+/PR+	222 (45)	O,A,H,T T + CT Horm	520 (63)	T,A,H,CT Horm
ER+/PR−	58 (12)	O,A,H T → T + CT Horm	128 (15)	T,A,H T + CT Horm
ER−/PR−	136 (28)	CT	137 (17)	CT
ER−/PR+	72 (15)	O,A,H,T ?T + CT ?Horm	41 (5)	CT,T + CT Horm

Adapted from Bland, K.I., et al.: Surg. Forum **32**:410, 1981.

**O*, Oophorectomy; *T*, tamoxifen; *A*, adrenalectomy; *H*, hypophysectomy; *ER*, estrogen receptor; *PR*, progestin receptor; *Horm*, hormonal (estrogen, progestin, androgen); *CT*, cytotoxic chemotherapy; +, ≥10 fmol/mg of cytosol protein; −, <10 fmol/mg of cytosol protein.

THERAPEUTIC APPLICATIONS OF BIOLOGIC MARKERS FOR NEUROENDOCRINE THERAPY

Presently, quantitative ERs represent important determinants for management of recurrent breast carcinoma. Use of the PR appears most advantageous in identifying the premenopausal ER-negative patient who may benefit from endocrine ablation or additive therapy. Table 62-6 represents potential therapeutic options and the expectant frequency distribution of ER/PR reactivity in premenopausal and postmenopausal women with breast cancer.

Currently the use of the antiestrogen tamoxifen (Nolvadex) to bind cytoplasmic estrogen appears advisable in ER-positive patients. Manni and associates[92] reported an objective response rate for metastatic ER-positive cancers that is essentially identical to that of adrenalectomy. The duration of these remissions is being evaluated. Pritchard and colleagues[111] observed that tamoxifen has a higher response rate in the ER-positive premenopausal patient and may replace oophorectomy as the treatment of choice for this endocrine status. These investigators noted that response duration and rate were equal to oophorectomy and would appear predictive of subsequent response to surgical ablation of the ovaries. Future prospective trials clearly are necessary to clarify objectively the role of tamoxifen in the premenopausal patient.

Newer sequences of endocrine therapy are evolving (Fig. 62-13). Currently, many investigators consider tamoxifen to be the endocrine therapy of choice for both premenopausal and postmenopausal women. Although many methods have been proposed for the sequence of therapies to be applied in these women, current methods have avoided the sustained morbidity incurred with varying surgical procedures in favor of endocrine manipulation with pharmacologic approaches. The order in which these endocrine therapies are adminstered also depends on the relative toxicity of each approach, and data suggest that tamoxifen may not be as effective following aminoglutethimide therapy.[123,124] Finally, Ward and co-workers[137] observed that a failure to respond to estrogens does not conclusively rule out the possibility of a response to antiestrogen therapy with tamoxifen.

The report by Gapinski and Donegan[58] confirmed the aforementioned receptor data but could find no correlation between ER status and responsiveness to chemotherapy. Compared to patients with primary neoplasms poor in ER (≤300 fmol/g of tissue), those with ER-rich tumors were observed to have a longer disease-free interval, a lower incidence of recurrence following mastectomy, and a more favorable disease-free survival.

A significant role for the use of antiestrogen therapy in Stage II (node-positive) breast cancer is emerging. Hubay, Pearson, and Marshall,[71] in a prospective, randomized trial, found that CMF, when used in combination with tamoxifen, were more effective in ER-positive patients in delaying recurrence than CMF alone ($p = 0.0176$). This effect was observed to occur in both premenopausal and postmenopausal women. In premenopausal women treated with CMF alone, however, ER-poor patients were observed to recur more rapidly than ER-positive patients ($p = 0.0313$). The addition of the adjuvant immunostimulant BCG provided no therapeutic benefit over the combination of CMF and tamoxifen.

Depending on the receptor status, ER-positive postmenopausal patients with metastatic breast carcinoma should have tamoxifen as additive therapy; it apparently has a response rate and duration of response equal to all forms of endocrine therapy. Also, its side effects occur infrequently, and drug discontinuance is rare on the basis of side effects.

The application of aminoglutethimide (Cytadren) as an inhibitor of adrenocorticoid steroid synthesis for conversion of androstenedione to estrogen appears to have merit

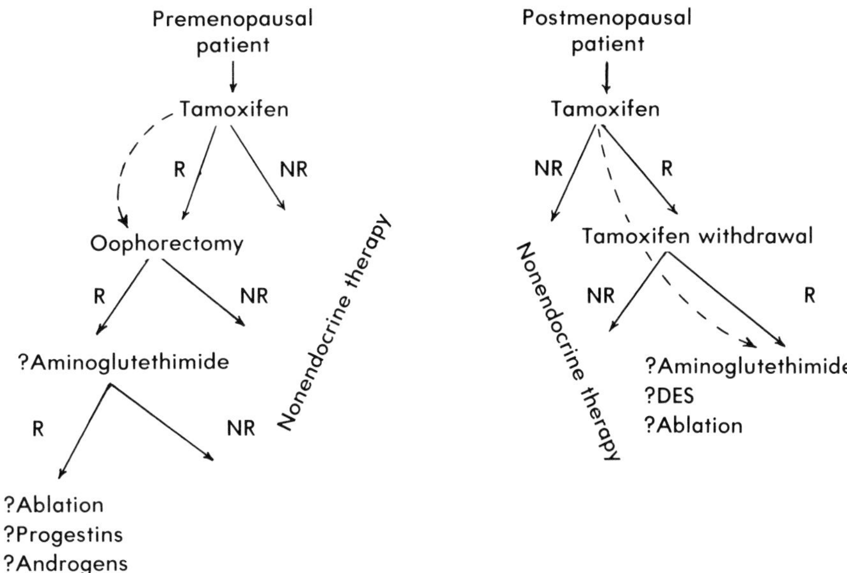

Fig. 62-13 New and future sequences for administering endocrine therapy in patients with advanced breast cancer. (From Henderson, I.C.: Breast cancer management progress and prospects [educational publication], Wayne, N.J., 1982, Lederle Laboratories, American Cyanamid Co.)

in initiating adrenal suppression. Initial trials suggest that the application of aminoglutethimide inhibition of adrenocortical function may be an accurate predictor of response to endocrine ablation with adrenalectomy and hypophysectomy.

As of 1986, seven prospective randomized clinical trials using tamoxifen as adjuvant therapy have been reported.[85,106] For six of these trials, definitive improvement in the disease-free interval was observed. The Nolvadex Adjuvant Trial Organization (NATO)[106] confirmed an improved disease-free interval and overall survival. In addition, these survival rates were enhanced, regardless of the ER status of the neoplasm. However, it should be noted that only 46% of patients in the NATO study had their tumor assayed for ER content.

The initial studies for adjuvant endocrine therapy failed to demonstrate a 5-year overall survival advantage with adjuvant castration alone, and castration plus long-term prednisone prolonged survival only in small subsets of premenopausal women over 45 years of age.[100] More recently, emphasis has been placed on the use of adjuvant endocrine therapy either alone or in combination with chemotherapy. Table 62-7 summarizes the effect of postoperative tamoxifen administered alone or in conjunction with cytotoxic agents. The largest experience thus far has been achieved by the NSABP Group that has randomly tested L-Pam-5-FU alone vs. this combination with tamoxifen in women with positive axillary nodes. The 3-year analysis confirmed that the addition of tamoxifen yielded comparatively superior relapse-free survival rates only for women 50 years of age or older. More recently, Wolmark and Fisher[145] confirmed that the effect is not uniform and depends on patient age and tumor receptor content. However, this effect is still apparent 4 years later. Patients 49 years of age or younger failed to demonstrate a prolongation in disease-free survival with tamoxifen even when the tumor estrogen receptor content was $\geq$ 100 fmol. Further, for patients $\leq$ 49 years, if the tumor progesterone receptors were less than 10 fmol, there was a significant diminution in disease-free survival and survival. Thus the overall response of the addition of tamoxifen to L-Pam-5-FU is heterogeneous, and only specific patient subsets demonstrated a salutary effect.

The recent Eastern Cooperative Oncology Group (ECOG) report on premenopausal women confirmed that 52% with ER-positive tumors had no difference in terms of disease-free survival or overall survival among the three groups receiving CMF, CMF with prednisone, or CMF with prednisone and tamoxifen for 1 year.[132] In particular, the addition of tamoxifen to CMF with prednisone was not detrimental. Two trials in postmenopausal women had been analyzed at a median follow-up of 36 months by the Ludwig group.[88] Local-regional therapy included total mastectomy and axillary dissection. CMF with additive prednisone and tamoxifen was significantly superior to prednisone and tamoxifen for women 65 years of age or younger, and both were superior to the control group in regard to disease-free survival. The addition of chemotherapy to endocrine therapy significantly improved results in ER-negative tumors, whereas in ER-positive tumors results were comparable. For patients 66 to 80 years old, randomization between prednisone plus tamoxifen vs. observation, the advantage in disease-free survival was greatest for patients with ER-positive tumors, and endocrine therapy reduced local and regional recurrence only. For the Ludwig Group,[88] in both age subsets there was no indication of a difference in overall survival. The Canadian Study by Pritchard and associates[111] was analyzed at a median fol-

Table 62-7 **EFFECT OF TAMOXIFEN ON RELAPSE-FREE SURVIVAL**

Author	Patients (No.)	Therapy*	Median Follow-up (months)	Essential Findings
Wolmark and Fisher[145]	1891	PF vs. PFT	50	PFT superior in post, PR$^+$
Tormey et al.[132]	662	CMF vs. CMFP vs. CMFPT†	36	No difference
	265	CMF vs. CMFP vs. CMFPT‡	42	CMFP ± T superior in ER$^-$
Clark et al.[34]	318	CMF vs. CMFT ± BCG	48	CMFT superior in PR$^+$
Ludwig Group[88]	463	CTR vs. CMFPT vs. PT (≤65 yr)	36	CMFPT and PT superior to control
	320	CTR vs. PT (>65 yr)	36	PT superior to control
Pritchard et al.[110]	366	CTR vs. T‡	36	T superior to control in the surgical series
NATO[106]	1124	CTR vs. T	21	T superior in post menopause with N$^+$§
Palshof[108]	284	CTR vs. T	44	T superior in postmenopause
Rose et al.[119]	1641	CTR vs. T‡	18	T superior in patients 50 to 59 years and with more than three nodes
Ribeiro and Palmer[117]	552	CTR vs. T‡	36	Survival: T superior to control in more than three nodes

Modified from Bonadonna, G., and Valagussa, P.: Review article: adjuvant systemic therapy for resectable breast cancer, J. Clin. Oncol. **3**:259, 1985.
*CTR, control; *P*, L-PAM or l-phenylalanine mustard; *T*, tamoxifen; *F*, 5-fluorouracil; *M*, methotrexate; *C*, cyclophosphamide.
†In premenopausal patients.
‡In postmenopausal patients.
§N$^+$, node-positive.

low-up of 3.1 years. Total relapse-free survival rates were significantly improved in the 1 to 3 and greater than 4 node subsets for tamoxifen (30 mg/day for 2 years) compared with controls. In an irradiated group, disease-free survival rates were no different for the tamoxifen-treated patients than for controls. Improvement in relapse-free survival rates with tamoxifen administration was strongly correlated with receptor positivity, particularly when PR was positive. In contrast, when receptors were negative or unknown there was no difference between tamoxifen-treated patients and control. For the two treatment groups, however, overall survival rates were identical, even in the presence of receptor positivity.

Considering these prospective trials and the fact that not all trials have included a homogeneous patient population base or hormone-receptor values, it is not possible at present to draw meaningful conclusions for the role of surgical adjuvant endocrine therapy.

The tumor heterogeneity of breast cancer, coupled with the probability that the predominant forms of endocrine therapy and ablation provide fractional reduction of only the ER-positive cells, suggests a predominance of refractory ER-negative cells following various endocrine therapy modalities. A previous Phase II trial by Allegra and coworkers[5] suggests the application of combination chemohormonal therapy using tamoxifen suppression for 10 days and premarin induction for 4 days, followed with methotrexate, 5-fluorouracil, and leucovorin. This combination represented an effective method to induce remission in 72% of patients with metastatic breast carcinoma. The physiologic application of chemohormonal induction represented a model of transition from basic laboratory observations to the design of a treatment regimen. Future prospective trials providing active cytotoxic therapy following hormonal induction are presently in progress. Although combinations to provide biochemical manipulation of the hormonally sensitive breast cells have met with increasing success, it is to be emphasized that therapeutic modalities for Stage IV disease rarely induce complete and sustained remissions.

THE NIH CONSENSUS DEVELOPMENT PANEL ON ADJUVANT CHEMOTHERAPY AND ENDOCRINE THERAPY FOR BREAST CANCER

The goal of the adjuvant therapy of breast carcinoma is to enhance survival while ensuring an acceptable quality of life. In September 1985 the NCI and the NIH jointly sponsored the Consensus Development Conference on Adjuvant Chemotherapy and Endocrine Therapy for Breast Cancer. The Consensus panel came to six important conclusions on the basis of their analysis of current achievements for the therapy of breast cancer and are incorporated in boxed material on p. 1053. In the future it is quite possible that a subgroup of node-negative patients with poor prognostic features will be identified who will benefit from adjuvant chemotherapy. A future consideration has been the role of adjuvant biologic response modifiers (BRMs) and their effects on breast cancer survival. Polyadenylic-polyuridylic acid has been evaluated in a randomized trial by Lacour and associates[83] for operable breast carcinoma. This group reported significant improvement in the disease-free survival, and independent verification is warranted. It is very possible that future studies that incorporate BRMs with chemoendocrine therapy as adjuvants will be initiated now that interest has been focused on this potential modality of therapy.

RECOMMENDATIONS OF NATIONAL INSTITUTES OF HEALTH CONSENSUS DEVELOPMENT CONFERENCE ON ADJUVANT CHEMOTHERAPY AND ENDOCRINE THERAPY FOR BREAST CANCER

1. Although significant changes have been made in the past five years, optimal therapy has not been defined for any subset of patients. For this reason, all patients and their physicians are strongly encouraged to participate in controlled clinical trials.
2. For premenopausal women with positive lymph nodes, treatment with established chemotherapy is recommended as standard care, regardless of hormone receptor status.
3. For premenopausal women with negative nodes, adjuvant chemotherapy is not generally recommended, but for certain high-risk patients, chemotherapy should be considered.
4. For postmenopausal women with positive nodes and positive hormone receptor levels, tamoxifen is the treatment of choice.
5. For postmenopausal women with positive nodes and negative hormone receptor levels, chemotherapy should be considered but could not, at the present time, be recommended as standard practice.
6. For postmenopausal women with negative nodes, regardless of hormone receptor levels, there is no indication for routine adjuvant therapy.

From National Institutes of Health Consensus Development Panel on Adjuvant Chemotherapy and Endocrine Therapy for Breast Cancer. Natl. Cancer Inst. Monogr. **1**:1, 1986.

SUMMARY

The heterogeneity of human mammary carcinoma appears to be a cumulative interrelationship of environmental, developmental, and genetic factors that may be identifiable with a high risk for carcinogenesis. Thus a comprehensive knowledge of the physiologic derangements and tropic events expected in normal breast development and maintenance, as well as specific variations that occur with the pathologic processes, are essential to the diagnostician in initiating appropriate therapy for breast diseases.

Breast development, growth, and involution occur as a result of the mammotropic effects of anterior pituitary and ovarian hormonal secretion. The breast should be considered an end-organ receptor that cannot initiate hormonal regulation through feedback inhibitor physiologic mechanisms. Thus the tropic effects of these target hormones on alveoli and myoepithelial components of mammary parenchyma may have uninhibited stimulatory growth with the subsequent development of benign (proliferative and nonproliferative mastopathy, fibroadenoma) or neoplastic states.

A thorough conceptualization of the natural history of benign and malignant diseases and the role of endogenous and exogenous hormones has partly clarified the therapeutic applications currently employed for diseases of this organ. Also, the identification of genetic and biochemical markers and their application for target surveillance of high-risk patients holds promise to allow identification of breast disease in a preinvasive and favorable stage of disease. The additional applications of biologic principles that govern the complex biologic events of the tumor-host relationship, metabolic and growth characteristics, and tumor metastases are being defined. The student of breast disease must retain a working knowledge of the anatomic, physiologic, and biologic events that govern deviations and neoplastic changes occurring in the ductoglandular components of this organ.

REFERENCES

1. Ahumada, J., and del Castillo, E.B.: Amenorrhea y galactorrhea, Bol. Soc. Gin Obst. **11**:64, 1932.
2. Allegra, J.C.: The use of steroid hormone receptors in breast cancer. In Margolese, R., editor: Contemporary issues in clinical oncology: breast cancer, New York, 1983, Churchill Livingstone, Inc.
3. Allegra, J.C., et al.: Steroid hormone receptors in human breast cancer, Proc. Am. Soc. Cancer Res. Am. Soc. Clin. Oncol. **19**:336, 1978.
4. Allegra, J.C., et al.: Distribution, frequency, and quantitative analysis of estrogen, progesterone, androgen, and glucocorticoid receptors in human breast cancer, Cancer Res. **39**:1447, 1979.
5. Allegra, J.C., et al.: A Phase II trial of tamoxifen, premarin, methotrexate and 5-fluorouracil in metastatic breast cancer, Breast Cancer Res. Treat. **2**:93, 1982.
6. Anson, B.J., and McVay, C.B.: Breast or mammary region. In Surgical anatomy, vol. 1, Philadelphia, 1971, W.B. Saunders Co.
7. Argonz, J., and del Castillo, E.B.: A syndrome characterized by estrogenic insufficiency, galactorrhea, and decreased urinary gonadotrophin, J. Clin. Endocrinol. Metab. **13**:79, 1953.
8. Ariel, I.M.: Enovid therapy for fibrocystic disease, Am. J. Obstet. Gynecol. **117**:453, 1973.
9. Asch, R.H., and Greenblatt, R.B.: Use of an impeded androgen—Danazol—in the management of benign breast disorders, Am. J. Obstet. Gynecol. **127**:130, 1977.
10. Baker, L.H.: Breast cancer detection demonstration project: five-year summary report, CA **32**:194, 1982.
11. Beahrs, O.H.: Staging of cancer of the breast as a guide to therapy, Cancer **53**:592, 1984.
12. Beatson, G.T.: On the treatment of inoperable cases of carcinoma of the mamma: suggestions for a new method of treatment with illustrative cases, Lancet **2**:104, 1896.
13. Berg, J.W.: Morphological evidence for immune response to breast cancer: a historical review, Cancer **28**:1453, 1971.
14. Black, M.M., and Chabon, A.B.: In situ carcinoma of the breast, Pathol. Annu. **4**:185, 1969.
15. Black, M.M., et al.: Association of atypical characteristics of benign breast lesions with subsequent risk of breast cancer, Cancer **29**:338, 1972.
16. Blackwell, R.E., et al.: Assessment of pituitary function in patients with serum prolactin levels greater than 100 ng/ml, Fertil. Steril. **32**:177, 1979.
17. Bland, K.I.: Breast carcinoma. Part I. Major risk determinants seen in asymptomatic women, Consultant: J. Medical Consultation **26**(4):65, 1986.
18. Bland, K.I., and Copeland, E.M., III: Differentiating among common breast masses, Diagnosis **7**(5):45, 1985.
19. Bland, K.I., Fuchs, A., and Wittliff, J.L.: Menopausal status as a factor in the distribution of estrogen and progestin receptors in breast cancer, Surg. Forum **32**:410, 1981.
20. Bland, K.I., et al.: Analysis of breast cancer screening in women younger than 50 years, JAMA **245**:1037, 1981.
21. Bland, K.I., et al.: A clinicopathologic correlation of mammographic parenchymal patterns and associated risk factors for human mammary carcinoma, Ann. Surg. **195**:582, 1982.
22. Bloodgood, J.C.: The pathology of chronic cystic mastitis of the female breast with special consideration of the blue-domed cyst, Arch. Surg. **3**:445, 1921.
23. Bonadonna, G., et al.: Adjuvant chemotherapy trials in resectable breast cancer with positive axillary nodes: experience of the Milan Cancer Institute. In Jones, S.E., and Salmon, S.E., editors: Adju-

vant therapy of cancer IV, Orlando, Fla. 1984, Grune & Stratton, Inc.
24. Bonadonna, G., Rossi, A., and Valagussa, P.: Adjuvant CMF chemotherapy in operable breast cancer: ten years later, World J. Surg. **9:**707, 1985.
25. Bonadonna, G., and Valagussa, P.: Editorial. Adjuvant systemic therapy for resectable breast cancer, J. Clin. Oncol. **3:**259, 1985.
26. Bond, W.H.: Natural history of breast cancer. In Stoll, B.A., editor: Host defence in breast cancer, Chicago, 1975, Year Book Medical Publishers, Inc.
27. Buchman, M.T., and Peake, G.T.: Incidence of galactorrhea, JAMA **236:**2747, 1976.
28. Burkett, F.E., et al.: The value of bone scans in the management of patients with carcinoma of the breast, Surg. Gynecol. Obstet. **149:**523, 1979.
29. Burns, T.W.: Endocrinology, In Sodeman, W.A., Jr., and Sodeman, W.A., editors: Pathologic physiology: mechanisms of disease, Philadelphia, 1974, W.B. Saunders Co.
30. Butler, T.P., and Gullino, P.M.: Quantitation of cell shedding into efferent blood of mammary adenocarcinoma, Cancer Res. **35:**512, 1975.
31. Carr, I., McGinty, F., and Norris, P.: The fine structure of neoplastic invasion: invasion of liver, skeletal muscle and lymphatic vessels by the Rd/3 tumour, J. Pathol. **118:**91, 1976.
32. Chaudary, M.A., et al.: Nipple discharge: the diagnostic value of testing for occult blood, Ann. Surg. **196:**651, 1982.
33. Chiari, J.B.V.L., Braun, C., and Spaeth, S.: In Enke and Erlinger, editors: Klinik der geburtshilfe and gynalkologie, Berlin, 1855.
34. Clark, G.M., et al.: Progesterone receptor as a prognostic factor in stage II breast cancer, N. Engl. J. Med. **309:**1343, 1983.
35. Copeland, M.M., and Higgins, T.G.: Significance of discharge from the nipple in nonpuerperal mammary conditions, Ann. Surg. **151:**638, 1960.
36. Crymes, J.E.: Current status of mammography, CRC Crit. Rev. Diagn. Imaging **11:**297, 1979.
37. Dalton, M.D.: Curt Schimmelbusch and Schimmelbusch's disease, Surgery **63:**859, 1968.
38. Davis, H.H., Simons, M., and Davis, J.B.: Cystic disease of the breast: relationship to carcinoma, Cancer **17:**957, 1964.
39. Degenshein, G.A., et al.: Hormone relationships in breast cancer: the role of receptor-binding proteins, Curr. Probl. Surg. **16:**1, 1979.
40. De Ome, K.B.: Formal discussion of multiple factors in mouse tumorigenesis, Cancer Res. **25:**1348, 1965.
41. Donnelly, P.K., et al.: Benign breast lesions and subsequent breast carcinoma in Rochester, Minnesota, Mayo Clin. Proc. **50:**650, 1975.
42. D'Orsi, C.J., et al.: Correlation of xeroradiology and histology of breast disease, CRC Crit. Rev. Diagn. Imaging **11:**75, 1978.
43. Dupont, W.D., and Page, D.L.: Risk factors for breast cancer in women with proliferative breast disease, N. Engl. J. Med. **312:**146, 1985.
44. Egan, R.L.: Mammography, an aid to early diagnosis of breast carcinoma, JAMA **182:**839, 1962.
45. Egan, R.L.: Roles of mammography in the early detection of breast cancer, Cancer **24:**1197, 1969.
46. Fidler, I.J.: Metastasis: quantitative analysis of distribution and fate of tumor emboli labeled with ^{125}I-5-iodo-2′-deoxyuridine, JNCI **45:**775, 1970.
47. Fisher, B., and Fisher, E.R.: Barrier function of lymph node to tumor cells and erythrocytes, Cancer **20:**1907, 1967.
48. Fisher, B., and Wolmark, N.: Limited surgical management for primary breast cancer: a commentary on the NSABP reports, World J. Surg. **9:**682, 1985.
49. Fisher, E.R., et al.: The pathology of invasive breast cancer: a syllabus derived from findings of the National Surgical Adjuvant Breast Project (protocol no. 4), Cancer **36:**1, 1975.
50. Fisher, B., et al.: A summary of findings from NSABP trials of adjuvant therapy. In Jones, S.E., and Salmon S.E., editors: Adjuvant therapy of cancer IV, Orlando, Fla., 1984, Grune & Stratton, Inc.
51. Fisher, B., et al.: Five-year results of a randomized clinical trial comparing total mastectomy and segmental mastectomy with or without radiation in the treatment of breast cancer, N. Engl. J. Med. **312:**665, 1985.
52. Foote, F., and Stewart, F.: Lobular carcinoma in situ, a rare form of mammary cancer, Am. J. Pathol. **17:**491, 1941.
53. Forbes, A.P., et al.: Syndrome characterized by galactorrhea, amenorrhea and low urinary FSH: comparison with acromegaly and normal lactation, J. Clin. Endocrinol. Metab. **14:**265, 1954.
54. Frommel, J.: Veber puerperale atrophie des uterus, Ztsch, Geburtsch. u Gynalkal. **7:**305, 1881.
55. Funderburk, W.W., and Syphax, B.: Evaluation of nipple discharge in benign and malignant diseases, Cancer **24:**1290, 1969.
56. Gallagher, H.S.: Minimal breast cancer: concepts and results of treatment in minimal invasive cancer (microcarcinoma), Clin. Oncol. **1:**389, 1982.
57. Gallagher, H.S., and Martin, J.E.: The study of mammary carcinoma by mammography and whole organ sectioning, Cancer **23:**855, 1968.
58. Gapinski, P.V., and Donegan, W.L.: Estrogen receptors and breast cancer: prognostic and therapeutic implications, Surgery **88:**386, 1980.
59. Gardner, W.U.: Endocrine dependence in experimental testicular tumorigenesis and tumor growth. In Brennan, J., and Simpson, W.L., editors: Biological interactions in normal and neoplastic growth; a contribution to the host-tumor problem, Boston, 1962, Little, Brown & Co.
60. Gershon-Cohen, J., and Colcher, A.E.: Evaluation of roentgen diagnosis of early carcinoma of the breast, JAMA **108:**867, 1937.
61. Geschickter, C.F., and Hartman, C.G.: Mammary response to prolonged estrogenic stimulation in the monkey, Cancer **12:**767, 1959.
62. Golinger, R.C.: Collective review: hormones and the pathophysiology of the fibrocystic mastopathy, Surg. Gynecol. Obstet. **146:**273, 1978.
63. Golinger, R.C., Gregorio, R.M., and Fisher, E.R.: Tumor cells in venous blood draining mammary carcinomas, Arch. Surg. **112:**707, 1977.
64. Griffiths, J.D., et al.: Carcinoma of the colon and rectum: circulating malignant cells and 5-year survival, Cancer **31:**226, 1973.
65. Haagensen, C.D.: Anatomy of the mammary gland. In Haagensen, C.D., editor: Diseases of the breast, ed. 2, Philadelphia, 1971, W.B. Saunders Co.
66. Hayward, R.B., and Frazier, T.G.: A reevaluation of bone scans in breast cancer, J. Surg. Oncol. **28:**11, 1985.
67. Henderson, I.C., and Canellos, G.P.: Cancer of the breast: the past decade, N. Engl. J. Med. **302:**17, 1980.
68. Hewitt, H.B., and Blake, E.: Quantitative studies of translymphoidal passage of tumour cells naturally disseminated from a nonimmunogenic murine squamous carcinoma, Br. J. Cancer **31:**25, 1975.
69. Howell, A., et al.: A controlled trial of adjuvant chemotherapy with melphalan versus cyclophosphamide, nethotrexate, and fluorouracil in breast cancer, Recent Results Cancer Res. **96:**74, 1984.
70. Horwitz, K.B., and McGuire, W.L.: Estrogen and progesterone: their relationship in hormone-dependent breast cancer. In McGuire, W.L., Raynaud, P., and Baulieu, E.E., editors: Progesterone receptors in normal and neoplastic tissues, New York, 1977, Raven Press.
71. Hubay, C.A., Pearson, O.H., and Marshall, J.S.: Antiestrogen, cytotoxic chemotherapy, and bacillus Calmette-Guerin vaccination in Stage II breast cancer: a preliminary report, Surgery **87:**494, 1980.
72. Huggins, C.B.: Control of cancers of man by endocrinology methods: review, Cancer Res. **16:**825, 1956.
73. Huggins, C.B., and Bergenstal, D.M.: Surgery of adrenals, JAMA **147:**101, 1951.
74. Hutter, R.V.P., Foote, F.W., Jr., and Farrow, J.H.: In situ lobular carcinoma of the female breast, 1939-1968. In Breast cancer, early and late, proceedings of the Thirteenth Annual Clinical Conference on Cancer, 1968, University of Texas M.D. Anderson Hospital and Tumor Institute at Houston, Chicago, 1970, Year Book Medical Publishers, Inc.
75. Ingle, J.N., et al.: Randomized clinical trial of diethylstibestrol versus tamoxifen in postmenopausal women with advanced breast cancer, N. Engl. J. Med. **304:**16, 1981.
76. Isard, H.J.: Other imaging techniques, Cancer **53:**658, 1984.

77. Jensen, E.V., De Sombre, E.R., and Jungblut, P.W.: Estrogen receptors in hormone-responsive tissues and tumors. In Wissler, R.W., Dao, T.L., and Wood, S., Jr., editors: Endogenous factors influencing host-tumor balance, Chicago, 1967, University of Chicago Press.
78. Kennedy, B.J., Mielke, P.W., Jr., and Fortuny, I.E.: Therapeutic castration versus prophylactic castration in breast cancer, Surg. Gynecol. Obstet. **118:**524, 1964.
79. Kleinberg, D.L.: Lactation and galactorrhea. In Gold, J., and Josimovich, J.B., editors: Gynecologic endocrinology, ed. 3, New York, 1980, Harper & Row, Publishers, Inc.
80. Kodlin, D., et al.: Chronic mastopathy and breast cancer: a follow-up study, Cancer **39:**2603, 1977.
81. Kramer, W.M., and Rush, B.F., Jr.: Mammary duct proliferation in the elderly: a histopathologic study, Cancer **31:**130, 1973.
82. Lacour, J., et al.: Radical mastectomy *versus* radical mastectomy plus interval node dissection, Cancer **37:**206, 1976.
83. Lacour, J., et al.: Adjuvant treatment with polyadenylic-polyuridylic acid in operable breast cancer: updated results of a randomised trial, Br. Med. J. **288:** 589, 1984.
84. Lippman, M.E., and Chabner, B.A.: Editorial Overview: Proceedings of the NIH Consensus Development Conference on Adjuvant Chemotherapy and Endocrine Therapy in Breast Cancer. NCI Monographs **1:**5-10, 1986.
85. Lippman, M.E., et al.: The relation between estrogen receptors and response rate to cytotoxic chemotherapy in metastatic breast cancer, N. Engl. J. Med. **298:**1223, 1978.
86. LiVolsi, V.A., et al.: Fibrocystic breast disease in oral-contraceptive users: a histopathological evaluation of epithelial atypia, N. Engl. J. Med. **299:**381, 1978.
87. Love, S.M., Gelman, R.S., and Silen, W.: Sounding board: fibrocystic "disease" of the breast—a nondisease? N. Engl. J. Med. **307:**1010, 1982.
88. Ludwig Breast Cancer Study Group: Randomized trial of chemo-endocrine therapy, endocrine therapy and mastectomy alone in postmenopausal patients with operable breast cancer and axillary node metastasis, Lancet **1:**1256, 1984.
89. Luft, R., Olivecrona, H., and Sjögren, B.: Hypophysectomy in man, Nord. Med. **47:**351, 1952.
90. Lunscken, C., and Strauli, P.: Penetration of an ascitic reticulum cell sarcoma of the golden hamster into the body wall and through the diaphragm, Virchows Arch. (Cell. Pathol.) **17:**247, 1975.
91. Madden, R.E., and Gyure, L.: Translymphonodal passage of tumor cells, Oncology **22:**281, 1968.
92. Manni, A., et al.: Antihormone treatment of Stage IV breast cancer, Cancer **43:**444, 1979.
93. Margottini, M., Jacobelli, G., and Cau, M.: The end results of enlarged radical mastectomy, Acta Unio Int. Contra Cancrum **19:**1555, 1963.
94. Martin, P.M., et al.: Multiple steroid receptors in human breast cancer. III. Relationship between steroid receptors and the state of differentiation and the activity of carcinomas throughout the pathologic features, Cancer Chemother. Pharmacol. **2:**115, 1979.
95. Mathé, G.: Current status of immunotherapy of human cancer: leukaemias, lymphomas, solid tumours, Drugs **8:**411, 1974.
96. McCarty, K.S., Jr., et al.: Correlation of estrogen and progesterone receptors with histologic differentiation in mammary carcinoma, Cancer **46:**2851, 1980.
97. McGuire, W.L.: Steroid receptors in human breast cancer, Cancer Res. **38:**4289, 1978.
98. McGuire, W.L., and Horwitz, K.B.: Progesterone receptors in breast cancer. In McGuire, W.L., editor: Hormones, receptors, and breast cancer, New York, 1978, Raven Press.
99. McLaughlin, C.W., Jr., and Coe, J.D.: A study of nipple discharge in the nonlactating breast, Ann. Surg. **157:**810, 1963.
100. Meakin J.W., et al.: Ovarian irradiation and prednisone following surgery and radiotherapy for carcinoma of the breast, Breast Cancer Res. Treat. **3:**45, 1983.
101. Minton, J.P., et al.: Caffeine, cyclic nucleotides, and breast disease, Surgery **86:**105, 1979.
102. Monson, R.R., et al.: Chronic mastitis and carcinoma of the breast, Lancet **2:**224, 1976.
103. Mornard, P.: Sur deux cas de tumeurs malignes des mammelles axillaires aberrantes, Bull et ném Soc. Nat. de chir. de Paris **21:**487, 1929.
104. Morrison, J.M., et al.: The West Midlands trial of adjuvant chemotherapy for axillary node positive breast cancer: a controlled clinical trial. In Jones, S.E., and Salmon, S.E., editors: Adjuvant therapy of cancer IV, Orlando, Fla., 1984, Grune & Stratton, Inc.
105. Newman, H.F., et al.: Nipple discharge: frequency and pathogenesis in an ambulatory population, NY State J. Med. **83:**928, June 1983.
106. Nolvadex Adjuvant Trial Organization: controlled trial of tamoxifen as an adjuvant agent in management of early breast cancer: interim analysis at four years by Nolvadex Adjuvant Trial Organization, Lancet **1:**257, 1983.
107. Page, D.L., et al.: Relationship between component parts of fibrocystic disease complex and breast cancer, JNCI **61:**1055, 1978.
108. Palshof, T.: Adjuvant endocrine therapy of primary operable breast cancer: a clinical trial of antiestrogen, oestrogen and placebo to pre and postmenopausal patients. Five years' results including rate of recurrence, survival and correlation to estrogen receptor status. Proceedings of the Third EORTC Breast Cancer Working Conference, (abstr.) Amsterdam, 1983.
109. Pastides, H., et al.: Oral contraceptive use and fibrocystic breast disease with special reference to its histopathology, JNCI **71:**5, 1983.
110. Pritchard, K.I., et al.: The role of tamoxifen in premenopausal women with metastatic carcinoma of the breast: an update, proceedings of the American Society of Clinical Oncology, abstract C-405, Toronto, 1981, The University of Toronto.
111. Pritchard, K.I., et al.: A prospective randomized controlled trial of adjuvant tamoxifen in postmenopausal women with axillary node positive breast cancer. In Jones, S.E., and Salmon, S.E., editors: Adjuvant therapy of cancer IV, Orlando, Fla. 1984, Grune & Stratton, Inc.
112. Ravdin, R.G., et al.: Results of a clinical trial concerning the worth of prophylactic oophorectomy for breast carcinoma, Surg. Gynecol. Obstet. **131:**1055, 1970.
113. Ray, B.S.: Carcinoma of the breast—hypophysectomy as palliative treatment, JAMA **200:**974, 1967.
114. Reubens, R.D.: Personal communication.
115. Reubens, R.D., et al.: Controlled trial of adjuvant chemotherapy with melphalan for breast cancer, Lancet **1:**839, 1983.
116. Reyniak, J.V.: Endocrine physiology of the breast, J. Reprod. Med. **22:**303, 1979.
117. Ribeiro, G., and Palmer, M.K.: Adjuvant tamoxifen for operable carcinoma of the breast: report of clinical trial by the Christie Hospital and Holt Radium Institute, Br. Med. J. **286:**827, 1983.
118. Rogers, L.W., and Page, D.L.: Epithelial proliferative disease of the breast—a marker of increased cancer risk in certain age groups, Breast Dis. Breast **5:**2, 1979.
119. Rose, C., et al.: Antiestrogen treatment of postmenopausal women with primary high risk breast cancer: 36 months of life-table analysis and steroid hormone receptor status, Breast Cancer Res. Treat. **3:**77, 1983.
120. Rowland, G.E., O'Neill, G.J., and Davies, D.A.L.: Suppression of tumour growth in mice by a drug-antibody conjugate using a normal approach to linkage, Nature **255:**487, 1975.
121. Saftlas, A.F., and Hoover, R.N.: Mammography patterns show breast cancer risk markers, Oncology Times **9:**2, 1987.
122. Salsbury, A.J.: The significance of the circulating cancer cell, Cancer Treat. Rev. **2:**55, 1975.
123. Santen, R., et al.: Aminoglutethimide scientific profile. In Santen, R., and Henderson, I.C., editors: Pharmanual: a comprehensive guide to the therapeutic use of aminoglutethimide, ed. 2, Basel, 1982, Karger Publishers.
124. Santen, R., et al.: A randomized trial comparing surgical adrenalectomy with aminoglutethimide pluse hydrocortisone in women with advanced breast cancer, N. Engl. J. Med. **305:**181.
125. Savlov, E.D., Witliff, J.L., and Hilf, R.: Further studies of biochemical predictive tests in breast cancer, Cancer **39:**539, 1977.
126. Senn, H.J., et al.: Results of adjuvant LMF/BCG in N^- and N^+ breast cancer. In Jones, S.E., and Salmon, S.E.,: Adjuvant therapy of cancer IV, Orlando, Fla., 1984, Grune & Stratton, Inc.

127. Seppala, M., Lehto Virta, P., and Ranta, T.: Discordant patterns of hyperprolactinaemia and galactorrhea in secondary amenorrhea, Acta Endocrinol. **86:**456, 1976.
128. Silva, J.S., et al.: Biochemical correlates of morphologic differentiation in human breast cancer, Surgery **92:**443, 1982.
129. Smith, D.C., et al.: Adjuvant radiotherapy/chemotherapy in breast cancer. In Jones, S.E., and Salmon, S.E., editors: Adjuvant therapy of cancer IV, Orlando, Fla., 1984, Grune & Stratton, Inc.
130. Spratt, J.S., Jr., and Donegan, W.L.: Anatomy of the breast. In Donegan, W.L., and Spratt, J.S., Jr., editors: Cancer of the breast, ed. 3, Philadelphia, 1979, W.B. Saunders Co.
131. Sugarbaker, E.V.: Cancer metastasis: a product of tumor-host interactions, Curr. Probl. Cancer **111**(7):23, 1979.
132. Tormey, C.D., et al.: Adjuvant systemic therapy in premenopausal (CMF, CMFP, CMFPT) and postmenopausal (observation, CMFP, CMFPT) women with node positive breast cancer. In Jones, S.E., and Salmon, S.E., editors: Adjuvant therapy of cancer IV, Orlando, Fla., 1984, Grune & Stratton, Inc.
133. Urban, J.A.: Bilaterality of cancer of the breast, Cancer **20:**1867, 1967.
134. Vaage, J.: Host serum factors in immune resistance to metastases. In Day, S.B., et al., editors: Biologic mechanisms and therapy, New York, 1977, Raven Press.
135. Vassar, P.S., and Culling, C.F.A.: Fibrosis of the breast, Arch. Pathol. **67:**128, 1959.
136. Veronesi, U., Zucali, R., and Del Vecchio, M.: Conservative treatment of breast cancer with the QU.A.RT. technique, World J. Surg. **9:**676, 1985.
137. Ward, H.W.C., et al.: Anti-oestrogen therapy for breast cancer—a report on 300 patients treated with tamoxifen, Clin. Oncol. **4:**11, 1978.
138. Wellings, S.R.: Development of human breast cancer, Adv. Cancer Res. **31:**287, 1980.
139. Wellings, S.R., and Jensen, H.M.: On the origin and progression of ductal carcinoma in the human breast, JNCI **50:**1111, 1973.
140. Wheeler, T.K.: Four drug combination chemotherapy following surgery for breast cancer. In Jones, S.E., and Salmon, S.E., editors: Adjuvant therapy of cancer II, Orlando, Fla., 1979, Grune & Stratton, Inc.
141. Williams, D.C.: Biological mechanisms in metastasis. In Stoll, B.A., editor: Secondary spread in breast cancer, vol. 3, London, 1977, William Heinemann Medical Books LTD.
142. Wolfe, J.N.: Analysis of 462 breast carcinomas, Am. J. Roentgenol. **121:**846, 1974.
143. Wolfe, J.N.: Breast patterns as an index of risk for developing breast cancer, Am. J. Roentgenol. **126:**1130, 1976.
144. Wolfe, J.N.: Risk for breast cancer development determined by mammographic parenchymal pattern, Cancer **37:**2486, 1976.
145. Wolmark, N., and Fisher, B.: Adjuvant tamoxifen and chemotherapy in Stage II breast cancer: interim findings from NSABP Protocol B-09, World J. Surg. **9:**750, 1985.

63 Abdominal Wall Hernias

Philip E. Donahue

The word hernia is derived from a Latin term meaning rupture of a portion of a structure. When used in the context of the abdominal wall, a hernia is a protrusion of abdominal cavity contents through an abnormal opening or defect in the fascial and muscular layers designed to contain them. Our current understanding of the abdominal wall as a site of opposing physical forces that remain in balance according to established mechanical principles or result in the appearance of a hernia when this balance is disrupted is both accurate and productive. It is accurate because the mechanical factors are considered to be the dominant explanation for the emergence of hernias; it is productive because hernias generally will not heal or resolve themselves spontaneously (an exception being the umbilical hernia), but will require surgical repair, and any such repair performed without regard to these factors is at an increased risk of failure.

No matter how many hernia repairs an experienced surgeon has performed, the clinical presentation in a given patient and the anatomic findings observed at the time of herniorrhaphy can vary considerably. This is true with respect to the patient's symptoms, the particular tissue relationships in and around the hernia itself, and the postoperative course following repair. Although the overwhelming majority of patients have an uneventful convalescence after repair of their hernias and a prompt return to gainful employment, an unfortunate few will be plagued by a complication of the procedure or by a recurrence of the hernia after its original repair. Thus hernia repair should still be considered a major surgical event demanding both technical awareness and precise skill in performance.

This chapter will highlight the important developments that have occurred during the past several decades in our understanding of the pathophysiology of hernia formation and how this knowledge is used in the modern practice of herniorrhaphy.[23]

DEFINITIONS

For an abdominal wall hernia to occur, a defect (congenital or acquired) in the musculofascial tissues supporting the abdominal cavity must exist, through which a pouch of peritoneum (the hernia sac) pushes. In evaluating the status of the hernial sac contents, the nomenclature currently used to classify different types of hernias needs to be defined. In the examination of a patient with a hernia, it is important to determine whether the contents of the hernial sac can be returned to the abdominal cavity. If this can be accomplished without difficulty, the hernia is said to be *reducible*. Occasionally the hernial contents cannot be reduced with surgical intervention. In this situation the hernia is termed an *irreducible* hernia. The word *incarcerated* is often used synonymously with the word irreducible; both terms imply that vascular compromise has not occurred. In the event that the blood supply to the hernial contents is impaired, the hernia is defined as being *strangulated*. If surgical intervention is not carried out promptly, this situation designates a surgical emergency and often results in the infarction of the viscus involved.

A *sliding hernia* indicates that a portion of the lining of the hernial sac is composed of an intraabdominal structure. This situation is especially common with groin hernias in which the cecum, appendix, or sigmoid colon may make up a portion of the sac. Although sliding hernias cannot be diagnosed before surgery, it is important to recognize the possibility of this circumstance at the time of surgery, since removal of the hernial sac as commonly performed would injure the particular viscus involved. A *Richter's hernia* indicates that a portion of the circumference of the bowel has become incarcerated in the fascial defect. If the segment of bowel wall involved becomes strangulated, localized gangrene often results. This complication can be especially life-threatening, since the segment of bowel involved is generally not obstructed as usually occurs when a portion of bowel becomes incarcerated in the hernial defect. Richter's hernias may present in a number of anatomic locations, but are particularly common with femoral hernias. A variant of the Richter's hernia is *Littre's hernia,* which occurs when an intestinal diverticulum is trapped in the fascial defect. This term is usually restricted to the herniation of a Meckel's diverticulum.

The term *ventral hernia* is a generic designation that refers to any hernia developing in the ventral abdominal wall. It usually includes umbilical, epigastric, and incisional hernias, but may also be applied to a spigelian hernia. *Groin hernias* are hernias that develop in the inguinofemoral region. Such hernias include both direct and indirect inguinal hernias, as well as femoral hernias. An *internal hernia* is the designation given to the herniation of a loop of intestine through a congenital or acquired aperture within the abdominal cavity. This may result from a defect in the intestinal mesentery or a herniation through the foramen of Winslow into the lesser sac. Occasionally an adhesion from a previously performed operation may develop between the abdominal wall and a segment of intestine, creating an aperture through which an adjacent loop of bowel may herniate. Although the hernia results from a connection with the abdominal wall, it is not technically considered an abdominal wall hernia. Internal hernias are generally not diagnosed before surgery; rather they are usually recognized when exploratory surgery is performed for a bowel obstruction, the cause of which has not been determined.

ETIOLOGIC CONSIDERATIONS IN THE DEVELOPMENT OF HERNIAS

Hernias may develop in any of the structures supporting or surrounding the abdominal cavity. They may be encountered where a previous fatal communication existed between the abdominal cavity and some distant site, when an embryologic canal fails to obliterate, when maldevelopment of a supporting structure occurs, when dilation of a normally situated hiatus results, and when the mesenchymal supporting structures constituting a portion of the body wall become attenuated, for whatever reason. Common sites where abdominal wall hernias are likely to occur include the groin, the umbilicus, the linea alba, various parts of the diaphragm, the lumbar region, along adjacent foramina in the pelvis where blood vessels and nerves exit, and within previously performed surgical incisions.

That various anatomic abnormalities play a role in the development of hernia is attested by the existence of certain types of hernia at the time of birth or their clinical presentation shortly thereafter.[2] For example, umbilical hernias occur where the umbilical ring has failed to obliterate the embryologic opening of the allantoic duct, which is ordinarily prevented by growth of the contiguous fascia of the linea alba. As many as 20% of Negro infants and 5% of Caucasian infants may present with umbilical hernias at the time of birth. A similar circumstance exists for the indirect inguinal hernia (also called the oblique hernia). This hernia arises because of an unobliterated processus vaginalis, the peritoneal connection between the abdominal cavity and the scrotum in the male and the canal of Nuck in the female. The peak incidence of the indirect inguinal hernia occurs during infancy when about 50% of males have a patent vaginal process. Congenital factors also appear to play a role in the development of direct inguinal hernias that occur between the pubic ramus and the arching border of the transversus abdominus muscle medial to the deep inferior epigastric vessels. In studies investigating the anatomic basis of this type of hernia, it has been shown that individuals who possess a transversus abdominus aponeurosis with a high arching lower border are at an increased risk for the development of this type of hernial defect. Certain types of diaphragmatic hernias and hernias involving the linea alba also appear to be related to anatomic defects as discussed elsewhere in this chapter.

Although an anatomic abnormality is certainly a predisposing factor that often plays a role in hernia development, other etiologic factors are clearly operational. For example, although structural defects may be responsible for the development of direct inguinal hernias in some patients, such defects do not explain the increased incidence of this type of hernia in advanced age groups or the tendency of elderly patients to have attenuated fascial structures of the groin. In addition, in autopsy studies as many as 20% of individuals have been noted to have a patent processus vaginalis without any clinical evidence of a hernia before death.[16] Similarly, the incidence of contralateral patency of the processus vaginalis in patients who have undergone repair of an inguinal hernia indicates that patency of this structure does not necessarily lead to inguinal herniation.[18] Similarly, the observation that 5% of young women subjected to incidental herniography (vide infra) performed after hysterosalpingography had an open processus vaginalis (diverticulum of Nuck) that was asymptomatic and without clinical evidence of a hernia further emphasizes that a patent vaginal process alone does not necessarily lead to a clinically apparent hernia.[14] It would appear therefore that equally important causes of hernia development that cannot be easily described are related to the "wear and tear" of living itself such as repetitive local trauma, degenerative changes associated with increased abdominal pressure, and altered collagen synthesis; all are possible etiologic factors in patients developing hernias in middle and older age.[1,28]

Renewed interest in the biochemical and structural aspects of herniology have followed the description of some of the molecular and cellular elements of the protective fascia and collagenous tissues that normally prevent the formation of hernia. Collagen, the major constituent of the various aponeuroses and fascial structures of the body wall, has been studied intensively. Interestingly, collagen, like all other tissues in the body, is in a state of dynamic equilibrium in which there appears to be a constant synthesis of this substance that is matched by a parallel and constant rate of degradation. When Peacock and Madden[25] studied the transversalis fascia medial to the contralateral internal inguinal ring in patients with unilateral hernia, they compared rates of collagen synthesis and collagenolysis in both inguinal regions and found that the rates of both processes were increased markedly. These findings were thought to support the concept that an abnormality of local collagen metabolism might be a factor in the eventual appearance of a hernia.[24]

Further support for the view that abnormal collagen underlies hernia formation is provided by studies of hydroxyproline (the major amino acid constituent of collagen) content in the rectus muscle aponeurosis of patients with and without groin hernia. There was a frank decrease in the concentration of this substance in patients with groin hernias that did not relate to age or muscle mass. Fibroblasts cultured from the anterior rectus sheath of these patients proliferated poorly, incorporating labeled precursors at a much lower rate than control specimens.[26] In addition, ultrastructural studies of rectus sheath collagen from patients with direct inguinal hernias were found to contain irregular microfibrils, supporting the concept of both a structural and a biochemical abnormality in adult patients who develop herniations.[26]

The specific effects of malnutrition on the evolution of hernias of the groin or other parts of the abdominal wall are as yet undefined. If the collagenous structures that guard the abdominal wall are vital living structures that constantly experience remolding and resynthesis, there is a balance between synthesis and destruction of these supporting structures that could conceivably be altered by one's nutritional status. In the surgical clinic of any large public hospital, many individuals with adult-onset hernias and malnutrition are encountered. A number of clinical and experimental observations would suggest that a correlation exists between the two conditions.

One of the first insights into this possible relationship was provided on sailing ships of a century or more ago, the crews of which suffered "scurvy." In addition to bleeding gums, periosteal pain, and weakness associated with this disease, these hapless individuals were reported to develop hernias or ruptures of healed scars. Later, a specific effect of vitamin C on collagen maturation was described, allowing a reasonable explanation of the observed effects in these patients. Another condition providing insights into the nature of acquired hernias is lathyrism, a disease resulting from ingestion of the flowering sweet pea. The active agent in the pea, beta-amino-proprionitrile, prevents the maturation of collagen and is capable of causing the appearance of groin hernias in young rats and mice.[9] Interestingly, groin hernias developed in animals less than a month old who were given sweet pea seeds in their diet in contrast to older rats who did not develop hernias when fed with a similar diet.

These examples of how nutrition may influence the formation of hernias are of particular importance because they illustrate how environmental factors affect that natural balance between collagen synthesis and lysis, eventually leading to the appearance of herniation. It may ultimately be shown that similar defects in nutrition exist in patients who seem to develop excessive numbers of hernias or have more than their share of recurrent herniations following primary repair. Of course, the relationship of hernia wound healing to one's overall nutritional status must be viewed in a multifactoral context. The hernia wound, for example, exists in the patient who may or may not have latent vitamin or mineral deficiencies, altered immunity or resistance to infection, or underlying systemic disease. In addition, such individuals may have impaired ability to generate the proteinaceous constituents of collagen and the various components of a repaired/healed defect, factors that may predispose the patient to a subsequent recurrence.

The recent description of altered levels of circulating enzymes in patients with emphysema adds another dimension to the possible role of biologic factors in hernia formation. In a provocative article by Cannon and Read,[5] serum elastolytic and antiproteolytic activity in smokers and nonsmokers was measured. It was found that smokers had the potentially undesirable combination of increases in proteolytic activity combined with reductions in alpha$_1$-antitrypsin, the major naturally occurring circulating antiprotease. This combination could possibly set the stage for the evolution of hernia formation by affecting the synthesis:degradation equilibrium of groin collagen and thereby set in motion a pathologic sequence favoring collagen degradation.

Other factors also appear to be involved in hernia formation. Patients with Laënnec's cirrhosis who develop ascites illustrate how individuals predisposed to hernias eventually develop clinically apparent hernias when subjected to stress, specifically to a hydrostatic pressure challenge. Both groin and umbilical hernias frequently appear for the first time in this group of patients. Individuals who perform repeated strenuous physical activities offer another example of hernias produced by a combination of predisposed anatomy in situational stress. In a report by Gullmo[13] in Sweden who used herniography to define the cause of obscure groin pains in a group of young athletes, a number of hernias were found, including those involving the obturator canal and incipient hernial defects at the inguinal ring that could not be diagnosed by other means. These young athletes were examined because many of them had severe pain that prevented their usual physical activity; yet they had an unremarkable initial examination.

Finally, a number of iatrogenic factors may result in the subsequent development of a hernia. Evidence exists suggesting that previous appendectomy may predispose to the later development of an ipsilateral oblique (indirect) inguinal hernia. The presumptive mechanism underlying this circumstance is damage to the innervation of the muscular constrictors of the internal ring shutter mechanism during appendectomy that later allows herniation of abdominal contents through a patent processus vaginalis. In one study laparoscopic views of the internal inguinal ring shortly after acute appendicitis and subsequent appendectomy demonstrated poor-to-absent contraction of the internal ring during coughing or straining.[33] The possibility of a temporary neuropraxia related to surgical trauma could explain these findings, but it must be kept in mind that other evidence supports the association with appendectomy. A statistically significant correlation between the appendectomy and the later development of ipsilateral hernias was shown by Arnbjornsson,[3] who described a threefold greater incidence of right inguinal hernia in men who had had appendectomy vs. the incidence of hernia formation without previous surgery.

During surgical exposure of the common femoral artery and the distal external iliac artery for various types of vascular procedures (e.g., aortofemoral bypass), the inguinal ligament and the musculoaponeurotic borders of the inguinal ring must be divided. I have noted that groin hernias occasionally occur in these individuals in the first few months after surgery, suggesting a definite relation to the first operation. The most plausible explanation for these hernias is that closure of the abdominal wall was made without attention to the principles of primary herniorrhaphy. The importance of reconstruction of the specific layers of the abdominal wall, including the internal ring, after any surgical transection of the internal inguinal ring is emphasized by these observations. Patients with a patent processus vaginalis are most susceptible to this complication, but any individual can develop it. For example, some individuals with severe groin pain after vascular access operations have no discrete hernia sac, but instead possess a lax internal ring that allows preperitoneal fat to bulge (herniate) through it. Such individuals do extremely well with surgical closure of the ring that adheres to the principles underlying hernia repair (see pp. 1062 and 1063), whether an anterior or posterior approach is used.

There is also evidence that the increased hydrostatic intraabdominal pressure associated with chronic ambulatory peritoneal dialysis (CAPD) frequently results in hernia development.[10] The reported incidence varies between 1% and 30%, with most of the hernias occurring in the groin and umbilicus and occasionally in the diaphragm, spigelian area, or the exit site of the dialysis catheter. Since the groin is the most frequent site, there is chance that congenital factors have set the stage for the appearance of the hernia in this area. However, since renal failure per se has a deleterious effect on collagen metabolism, a multifactorial pathogenesis is also possible.[6,17,29] The problem encountered in patients with CAPD is similar to that noted in patients with advanced cirrhosis and ascites, i.e., a high risk for the evolution of hernia defects caused by increased abdominal pressure, aggravated by nutritional or metabolic factors that result in poor wound healing and defective or suboptimal collagen synthesis.

Hernias appearing at the site of large latex rubber drain tracts are infrequent and are caused by the enthusiastic creation of a drainage tract by the surgeon. Some surgeons believe that a "two-finger" aperture is required for optimal drain function and that any drain tract of smaller dimension is both ineffectual and imprudent. I disagree; and, in fact, I believe the two-finger aperture is a likely cause of iatrogenic hernias. Furthermore, there is good evidence that most drains routinely placed after common surgical procedures (e.g., cholecystectomy) are unnecessary and are therapeutic only for the surgeon. On the other hand, there are certainly other situations that require generous drainage, but these are usually best handled by suction drains rather than multiple latex rubber drains and do not require extremely large abdominal wall openings. Finally, there are occasional instances in which surgeons elect to perform open drainage of either part or all of the peritoneal or retroperitoneal surfaces. The situations most commonly treated by this means are cases of hemorrhagic or necrotizing pancreatitis. When open drainage is used, it is done with full awareness that hernias of the abdominal wall are created, and usually the repair of these hernias would be planned at a later date.

TYPES OF ABDOMINAL WALL HERNIAS

Groin Hernias

Hernias may develop in any structure supporting the intraabdominal contents. Most of these involve the anterior abdominal wall, and the vast majority occur in the inguinofemoral region. Of hernias occurring in the groin, the indirect inguinal variety is most frequently encountered (50% to 60%), with direct inguinal hernias representing 25% to 35% and femoral hernias comprising approximately 5% to 10%. Because of the frequency of groin hernias, an understanding of their anatomy, clinical presentation, and surgical management is important for any student of surgery.

Anatomy

The *indirect inguinal hernia* represents a fascial defect that lies lateral to the deep epigastric artery and originates in the internal inguinal ring (Fig. 63-1, *A*). It is at least 20 times as common in males as in females; and, when it occurs in the male sex, it represents a retention or incomplete obliteration of the embryologic outpocketing of peritoneum, known as the processus vaginalis, that accompanies the testicle in its descent into the scrotum. Normally the processus vaginalis obliterates postnatally except for the portion that covers the testicle, i.e., the tunica vaginalis. If this obliterative process fails, an indirect inguinal hernia will be evident at birth or in the months thereafter. Depending on the extent of this obliterative process, the resultant hernial sac will track along varying lengths of the inguinal canal; if it extends completely into the scrotum, it is designated a *complete* indirect inguinal hernia. If the unobliterated processus vaginalis is not large enough to admit bowel, but does allow peritoneal fluid to collect, a hydrocele may develop. In view of these considerations, it is not surprising that the peak incidence of indirect inguinal hernia recurrence is at birth or shortly thereafter. A second peak occurs in the teen years and in early adulthood. As previously discussed, stress from muscular activity and the accompanying increase in intraabdominal pressure may give rise to an indirect inguinal hernia in this age group by forcing open a previously incompletely obliterated processus vaginalis. The role that congenital factors play in the pathogenesis of this hernia is further emphasized by the fact that it seldom develops after the age of 35 years. A patent processus vaginalis is probably responsible for the development of indirect inguinal hernias in females as well. In this circumstance, however, it occurs from the incomplete obliteration of the peritoneum as it descends through the canal of Nuck.

A *direct inguinal hernia* arises medial to the deep epigastric artery and somewhat inferior to the internal inguinal ring and represents a diffuse weakening of the transversalis fascia in a triangular space known as Hesselbach's triangle (see Fig. 63-1, *B*). This area is bounded laterally by the deep epigastric artery, medially by the lateral border of the rectus sheath, and inferiorly by the inguinal ligament. This type of hernia almost always occurs after the age of 35. In contrast to an indirect inguinal hernia in which the neck of the hernia may be narrow and incarceration always a potential problem, the neck with direct hernias is wide; thus incarceration is usually not encountered. Further, direct hernias are almost exclusively seen in males.

A femoral hernia develops as a peritoneal outpouching that occurs through an enlarged femoral ring (see Fig. 63-1, *C*). This space represents the medialmost compartment of the femoral canal that is bounded below by the inguinal ligament, above by the pubic bone, and medially by the lacunar ligament. The sac of a femoral hernia is always medial to the femoral vein and may progress to the level of the foramen ovale. Because the neck of a femoral hernia is narrow, incarceration and strangulation are often prone to occur. Further, the incidence of femoral hernias in the female population is much more common than with males. The specific explanation for this remains to be defined.

Clinical Presentation

The usual complaint that brings a patient to the physician's attention when a groin hernia is present is a bulge or a problem with pain, either of which may be persistent or intermittent. The pain associated with simple herniations depends on the contiguous structures that are either compressed or irritated by the presence of the hernia. The pain is usually localized, sharp, aggravated by change in position or straining, and relieved by cessation of the physical activity that precipitated it. When a hernia contains incarcerated or strangulated structures, the pain becomes persistent and is often associated with systemic signs or symptoms such as elevated temperature, tachycar-

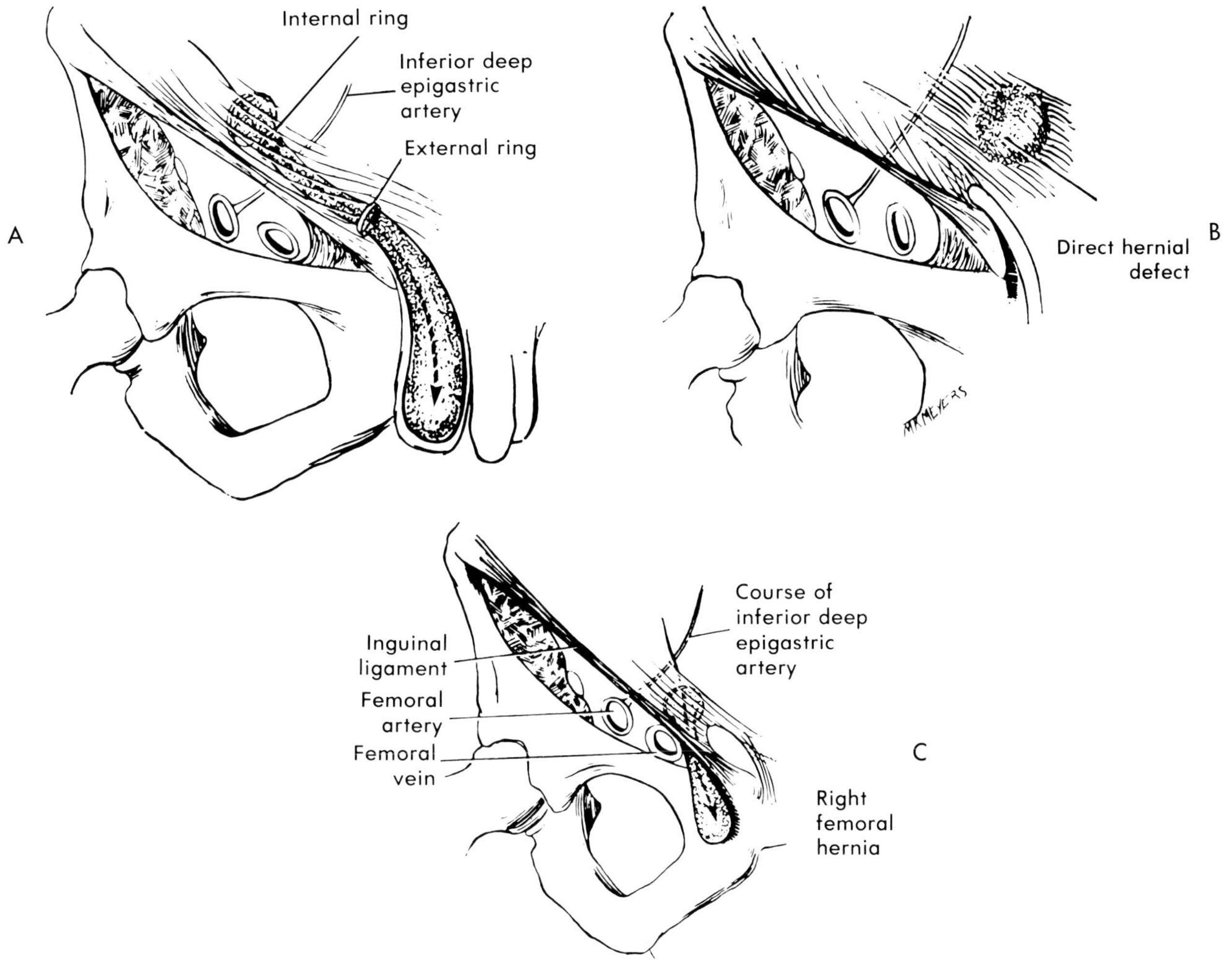

Fig. 63-1 **A,** Right indirect inguinal hernia. Hernial sac begins at the internal inguinal ring lateral to the inferior deep epigastric artery and exits from the inguinal canal at the external ring to descend into the scrotum. The sac lies anteromedial to the cord structures. **B,** Right direct inguinal hernia. Hernial sac arises in Hesselbach's triangle medial to the inferior deep epigastric artery and just above the pubic tubercle. It does not descend into the scrotum. **C,** Right femoral hernia. Hernial sac arises below the inguinal ligament and medial to the femoral vein. (From Soper, R.T.: Abdominal hernia. In Liechty, R.D., and Soper, R.T., editors: Synopsis of surgery, ed. 3, St. Louis, 1976, The C.V. Mosby Co.)

dia, vomiting, and abdominal distention. If a segment of bowel is trapped in the hernia sac, the clinical presentation may be one of bowel obstruction. Occasionally the hernia may be entirely asymptomatic and first noticed on a routine physical examination.

Groin hernias are sometimes extremely difficult to diagnose and at other times quite apparent. The standard maneuver to diagnose a groin hernia is based on digital palpation of the floor of the inguinal canal. The patient should initially stand while visual inspection of the groin is conducted. The physician examines the external genitalia to check for any localized swellings along the spermatic cord on either side, or for abnormalities in the testicle or scrotal contents. In a female there may be palpable swelling noted on the side of the patient's complaints. In any case, ipsilateral swelling in a groin in which pain is apparent requires definite explanation, and the inference that a hernia is present becomes quite tenable.

When examining the floor of the inguinal canal in the male, there are three prerequisites for a complete examination: first, following invagination of the scrotal skin along the axis of the canal, the examiner palpates the fascial border or the external inguinal ring to direct the examining finger to the floor of the canal where all inguinal hernias occur. The external ring is only a landmark to guide the examination in the appropriate region; its size or consistency has nothing to do with the hernia itself. On identification of this ring, digital palpation of the floor of the canal and the overlying spermatic cord are next performed to ascertain any apparent weakness. A weakness or mass in the region of the external ring is usually indicative of a direct hernia. Finally, examination of the internal ring itself is performed. The area of the internal ring is first palpated, and then the examiner asks the patient to strain for 5 to 10 seconds to increase intraabdominal pressure while at the same time the examining finger is withdrawn 1 cm. The patient is asked to give a gentle cough. A positive response is a palpable "tap" against the fingertip (suggestive of an indirect hernia) or along the medial side of the finger (indicative of a direct hernia), caused as the distended hernia sac transmits the cough-induced increase in pressure; alternatively, a "gurgle" of peritoneal fluid may be appreciated passing beneath the examining finger. At times, the positive response will be a reproduction of the patient's pain; this latter situation, however, demands careful interpretation to exclude other possibilities as discussed later in this chapter.

If the patient has had a previous inguinal hernia repair, the same principles of examination are followed. When such a patient complains of pain during the examination, the differential diagnosis may include ilioinguinal nerve entrapment or neuroma of a branch of the nerve severed previously. In situations in which the patient complains of a typical pain syndrome, but the physical examination is negative, I recommend a waiting period during which the patient is reexamined at monthly intervals. If the pain persists despite exclusion of other causes, surgical exploration of the groin can be justified even when the examiner has no absolute evidence that a hernia exists. A patient must have realistic expectations of results after such surgical intervention, however, and be informed that, although most patients do well following surgery, some will have persistent postoperative discomfort. In my experience there have been occasional patients, usually one every year or two (0.1% to 0.3% of groin hernias), who report a typical pain syndrome but have no definite hernia on physical examination. After several negative examinations the patient comes with an ultimatum from his employer that he return to work immediately or face the loss of his job and accrued benefits. Often the possibility of malingering or latent personality disorder is considered more likely than occult hernia, and the patient is inappropriately consigned to such a diagnosis. Following the principles described, I have been gratified by the response of such individuals to surgical exploration and have *always* found a definite explanation for the complaint when a localized area of tenderness in the groin was present; either a small indirect hernia or a patulous internal ring has been the usual explanation for the pain.

In contrast to most inguinal hernias that can be diagnosed with a minimum of difficulty, the femoral hernia is often a diagnostic challenge and usually appears as a subtle mass lesion in the inguinal crease, somewhat medial to the femoral artery. It is extremely important that the examiner realizes that the mass lesion may be quite small ($\leq$ 1 cm in diameter) and that in obese individuals or those patients with edematous overlying skin the hernia may be clinically occult. In such situations the general condition of the patient will have to serve as a guide for the specific management plan undertaken. Patients who experience an unexplained acute onset of local pain in the femoral region and/or an unexplained mass or tenderness suggestive of an increased hernia should have prompt surgical exploration. Inattention of such findings could put the patient at extreme risk for incarceration of ischemic bowel and the devastating complications arising therefrom.

The only laboratory test worth consideration in the diagnosis of inguinofemoral hernias is peritoneography (herniography). This test involves the intraperitoneal injection of contrast material and trapping of that material in an inguinal defect. In performing this technique, I have used Gullmo's approach, which consists of the intraperitoneal injection of 50 to 60 ml of renographin after instillation of diluted xylocaine.[13] There is no question that this procedure has great potential for the discovery and definition of hernias that may not be clearly identifiable clinically, but it cannot be performed casually and will require the expertise of an interested and committed radiologist experienced in the subtleties of interpretation for it to give useful information. But this test is used so infrequently that decisions to operate are usually not greatly influenced by it.

Surgical Management

Once present, hernias in the groin will not resolve spontaneously, and therefore with few exceptions (e.g., terminal malignant disease) they should be repaired surgically to prevent complications such as incarceration and strangulation. The illuminating work of Condon[7,8] has defined several important aspects of the anatomy of the groin that are germane to repair of hernias in this area of the abdominal wall (Fig. 63-2). The precise definition of the term "fascia and aponeurosis" is especially applicable in this context as is the precise use of the designation "ligament." A fascia is a condensation of connective tissue into a definable, homogenous layer that may vary from a thin layer to an easily observed stout structure. An aponeurosis is a tendinous insertion of a major muscle composed of strong individual collagenous fiber bundles. Ligament is a term applied to any definable tissue "banding" two or more structures, whether bony or visceral, and may refer to structures of either areolar or aponeurotic consistency.

When referring to a groin hernia, one must be careful not to confuse the transversus abdominus aponeurosis and transversalis fascia. The latter term is incorrectly applied at times to the transversus abdominus muscle and the transversus abdominus aponeurosis. The transversalis fascia of and by itself is of varying density and possesses little intrinsic strength. It usually represents the first anatomic boundary to visceral structures as they herniate through the abdominal wall but by itself cannot form the basis of groin hernia repairs. Instead, all herniated structures must first be restored to their anatomic position behind and deep to the transversalis fascia, and repair of the hernia defect performed by suturing neighboring tendinous aponeuroses and ligaments that can hold sutures properly.[7,8]

The repair of all common groin hernias is designed to permanently eliminate the defect in the abdominal wall by means of sutures placed into the solid structures that line the defect. The aponeurosis of the external oblique muscle inserts at the pubic tubercle and has a flattened medial portion that is recurved beneath the floor of the inguinal canal.

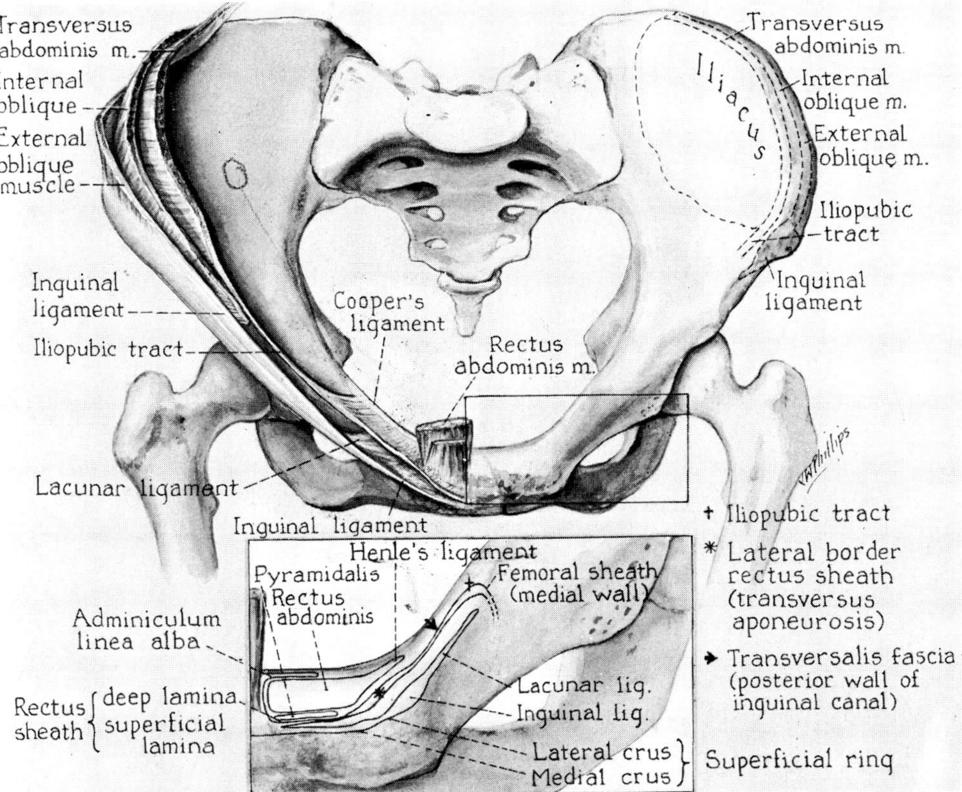

Fig. 63-2 Left pelvis: Origins of the three flat muscles are shown. The oblique and transversus muscles arise from the iliacus fascia and iliopectineal arch (not shown). Inset shows the insertions of the muscle layers of the groin into the pubis. Right pelvis: Internal oblique is not shown, but would arch above the spermatic cord to insert into the rectus sheath. (From Condon, R.E.: Anatomy of the inguinal region and its relation to groin hernia. In Nyhus, L.M., and Condon, R.E., editors: Hernia, ed. 2, Philadelphia, 1978, J.B. Lippincott Co.)

The relationship of the inguinal ligament to the fascia of the tranversus abdominus muscle is that of contiguous, but quite separate, structures. The lacunar ligament, a structure that extends from the posterior border of the inguinal ligament to the pectineal fascia (1 cm below the pectin) is separate and superficial to the ileopubic tract. One must be aware of this relationship, since the rationale for modern hernia repair involves the reconstruction of separate layers of the abdominal wall, with an attempt to preserve the "shutter" mechanism effected by the different layers of the abdominal wall. This shutter mechanism consists of structures moving simultaneously in different planes and is analogous to the shutter on a camera: the planes of motion occur within the internal oblique and transversus abdominus layers of the abdominal wall.[19] Conventional herniorrhaphy does not result in a functional shutter mechanism unless the principles of anatomic repair of the hernia are followed; i.e., the dynamic components of the shutter are compression of the potential hernial defect by traction of the superior and inferior crus of the internal inguinal ring. This contraction of the transversus muscle results in narrowing of the internal ring and lateral traction on the spermatic cord. The shutter mechanism thus affords continuous protection for the two most vulnerable areas of the groin—the area where direct hernias exit through Hesselbach's triangle and the inguinal canal through which "oblique" herniation occurs, beginning at the internal inguinal ring.

The components of adequate groin herniorrhaphy are knowledge of the anatomic structures involved, precise identification of these structures by surgical dissection, meticulous repair of the defect in the transversus/transversalis plane, and measures to reduce tension on suture lines where appropriate. These principles are true for direct or indirect inguinal hernias or for femoral hernias.

Anterior Repair

Inguinal hernias. Although multiple procedures (e.g., Bassini, Halstead, McVay, Shouldice) have been recommended to repair inguinal hernias (each with its advocates), the details of which can be obtained in standard textbooks of hernia repair,[23] I am a "regionalist," preferring to view the entire transversus/transversalis area as a single entity and therefore using the same basic approach to repair any hernial defect in this most important layer. The most essential technical aspect of repair is the creation of a tension-free union between the arching transversalis abdominus aponeurosis and its adherent transversalis fascia above and the ileopubic tract below. This repair is readily achieved if meticulous dissection has defined the floor of the inguinal canal and the structures in question. For both direct and indirect inguinal hernias, the repair is carried out through a transverse skin incision positioned above (approximately 2 cm) and parallel to the inguinal ligament to prevent injury to the iliohypogastric and ilioinguinal nerves (Fig. 63-3).

For hernias lateral to the inferior epigastric vessels (i.e., indirect inguinal hernias), repair primarily involves obliteration of the communication that exists between the peritoneal cavity and the hernial sac. Thus the sac is carefully dissected free from its fibroareolar connections, ligated at its base so that such ligation is flush with the internal inguinal ring, and any sac distal to this ligation resected (Fig. 63-4). In infants and children high ligation of the sac

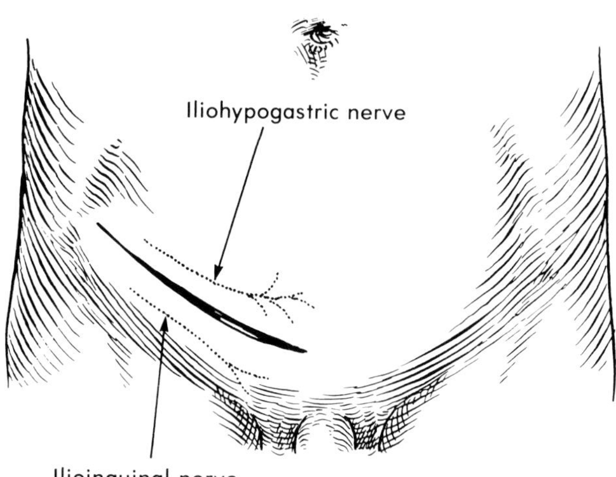

Fig. 63-3 Skin incision is made approximately 2 cm above the inguinal ligament in a gentle curve following Langer's lines. (From Ponka, J.L.: Hernias of the abdominal wall, Philadelphia, 1980, W.B. Saunders Co.)

is usually all that is required; in older children and adults some reconstruction of the musculoaponeurotic structures is generally needed, in addition to sac division and ligation to tighten the internal inguinal ring around the cord structures. Occasionally an indirect inguinal hernia will be encountered that has been present for many years and has enlarged to such an extent that a good portion of the supporting structures medial to the internal ring have been destroyed. In this situation a more extensive aponeurotic fascial repair will be required following the principles described below for the repair of a direct inguinal hernia.

In the repair of a direct inguinal hernia or of a deficient posterior wall of the inguinal canal in a patient with a large indirect inguinal hernia, the cremaster fibers surrounding the spermatic cord must be circumferentially removed at the internal inguinal ring.[11] When this has been accomplished, fatty and areolar tissues are excised from the inferior aspect of the canal to bare the shelving portion of the inguinal ligament and the iliopubic tract. Through careful dissection, the attentuated floor of the inguinal canal is excised, the hernial sac is simply reduced (no need for resection as with the indirect inguinal hernia), and the defect in the floor is repaired by suturing the transversus/transversalis complex above to the ileopubic tract below (Fig. 63-5), using interrupted nonabsorbable suture material. If only a direct hernial defect is present, the internal ring is not completely displayed. However, in all instances the cremaster muscle is completely excised from the posterior inguinal wall, and the spermatic cord dissected to identify the obliterated vaginal process at the internal ring. Only by so doing is the risk of a "missed" indirect hernia eliminated.

Because the suture repair of any large defect in the pos-

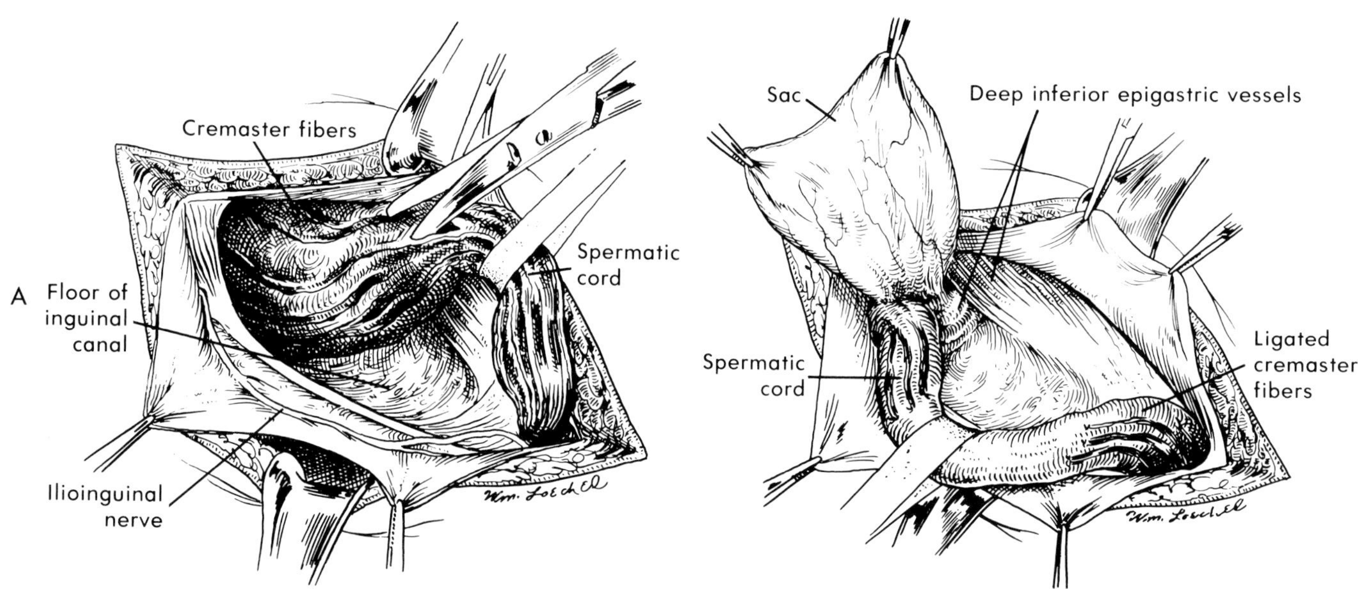

Fig. 63-4 **A,** Steps in the repair of a right indirect inguinal hernia. The external oblique aponeurosis has been opened. The cord is freed from the inguinal floor. The freed ilioinguinal nerve is seen overlying the retracted lower leaflet of the external oblique aponeurosis. The cremaster muscle is being dissected free of the cord. **B,** Peritoneal sac must be dissected free of the cord and the abdominal wall at the internal abdominal ring. (**A** to **F** from Ponka, J.L.: Hernias of the abdominal wall, Philadelphia, 1980, W.B. Saunders Co.)

terior inguinal wall places undue tension on the superior portion of the repair, there has been a long interest in maneuvers to reduce the abnormal stress resulting from such surgery. The Tanner "slide" procedure is one of the best known early attempts at relieving this stress through the creation of a relaxing incision.[32] Tanner rightfully recognized that an incision along the internal oblique portion of the anterior rectus sheath would allow the lateral portion of this sheath and its attached transversus arch to "slide" inferolaterally to close a large inguinal hernial defect. The necessity for such a relaxing incision is fully recognized and accepted in modern hernia surgery and forms an integral part of all direct and large indirect inguinal hernia repairs (Fig. 63-6). McVay[20] has beautifully illustrated the importance of the relaxing incision and has further shown that the pyramidalis muscle can conceal aponeurotic transversus fibers, which if unrecognized would lead to failure of the relaxing incision to relax. Usually the relaxing incision is made before tying the sutures that have been placed to effect the hernial repair.

Occasionally the size of a direct inguinal hernia will prohibit effective repair with a patient's own tissue and

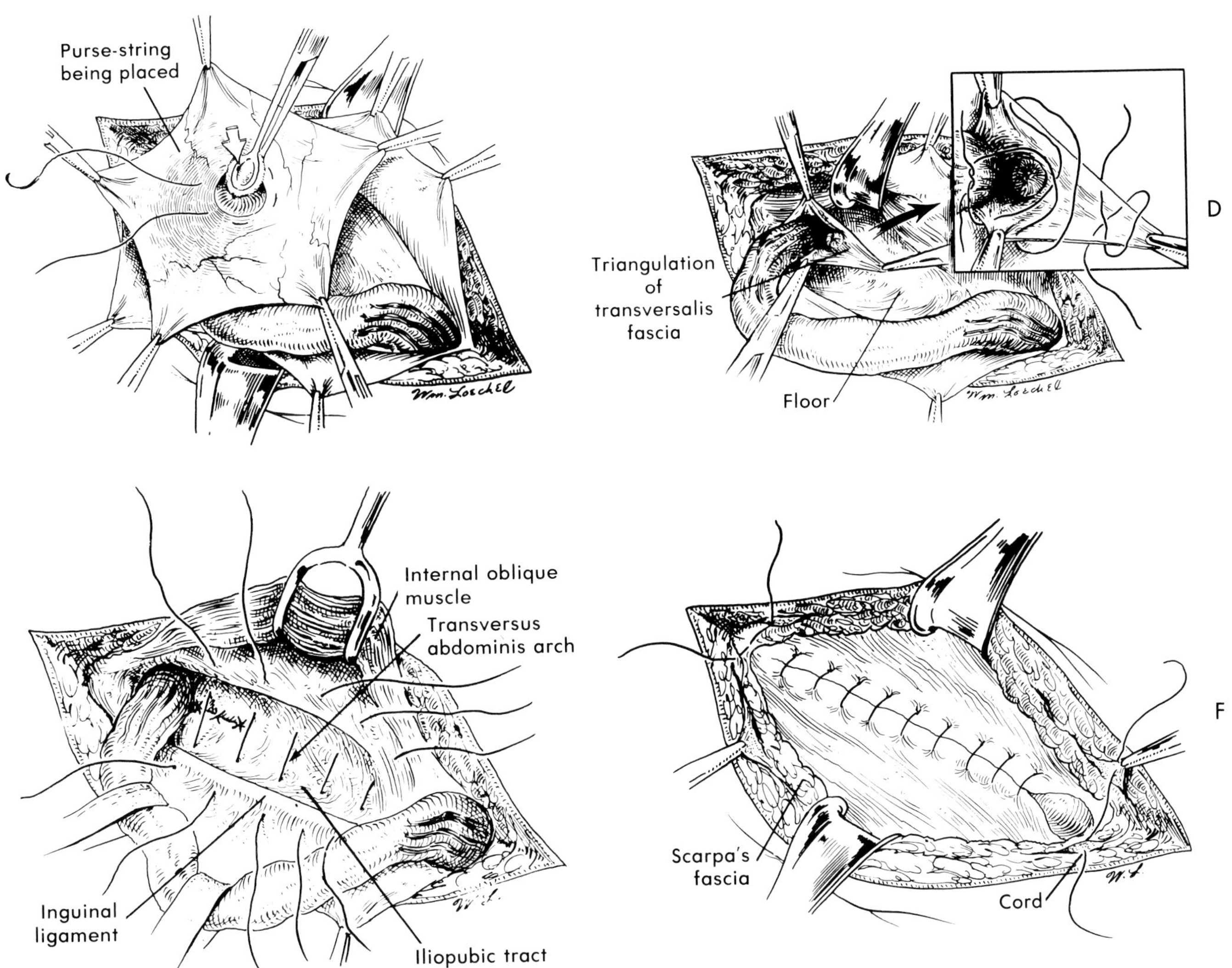

Fig. 63-4, cont'd. **C,** Technical detail of high ligation of the sac is important in an orderly repair. The peritoneum must be freed of omentum, and adherent viscera must be detached. Appendices epiploicae or omentum must not be caught in the closure. **D,** Components of the transversus abdominis lamina must be accurately identified and closed at the internal ring. Triangulation of the transversalis fascia (shown here) is a useful detail to help achieve accurate closure at the internal ring. **E,** Transversus abdominis arch is sutured to the iliopubic tract and inguinal ligament. **F,** External oblique aponeurosis is closed over the spermatic cord. Slight imbrication of this structure gives an excellent closure. Scarpa's fascia is then closed with interrupted sutures of No. 3-0 plain catgut, and the skin edges approximated with sutures or steri strips.

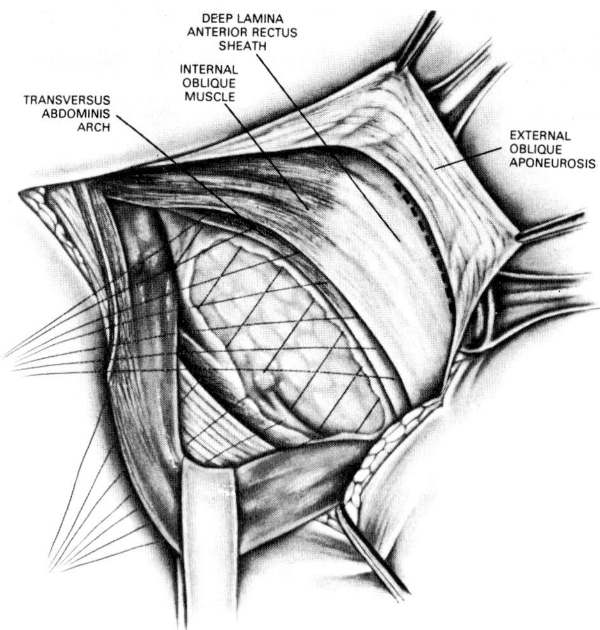

Fig. 63-5 External oblique aponeurosis (superficial lamina of the rectus sheath) has been dissected medially and superiorly to its line of fusion with the rectus sheath. The placement of a relaxing incision in the deep lamina of the rectus sheath (transversus abdominis and internal oblique aponeurosis) is indicated by the dotted line. (From Condon, R.E.: Anterior iliopubic tract repair. In Nyhus, L.M., and Condon, R.E., editors: Hernia, ed. 2, Philadelphia, 1978, J.B. Lippincott Co.)

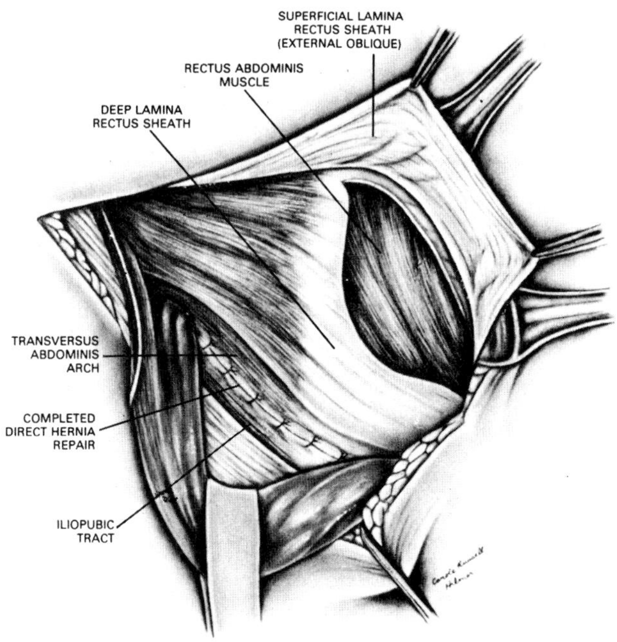

Fig. 63-6 Completed direct hernia repair demonstrates that the relaxing incision allows the transversus abdominis to slide inferiorly. As the relaxing incision opens, the rectus muscle is exposed, but the overlying intact superficial lamina (external oblique aponeurosis) of the rectus sheath supports the muscle externally while the intact fascia posteriorly shields the potential hernial defect. (From Condon, R.E.: Anterior iliopubic tract repair. In Nyhus, L.M., and Condon, R.E., editors: Hernia, ed. 2, Philadelphia, 1978, J.B. Lippincott Co.)

necessitate the use of some biologic or synthetic substance. Of the biologic substances available, fascia lata grafts have been most popular. Of the synthetic materials, polypropylene (Marlex) and dacron mesh grafts have been most extensively used.[27,31,34] These materials have been used either to bridge the hernial defect itself by suturing the substance to the fascia lining the hernial ring or as a buttress to enhance a primary repair. Some surgeons have even used synethetic meshes to repair all hernias; however, most authorities believe this is unnecessary and that primary repair using the patient's own tissues is most appropriate when it can be successfully accomplished.

Femoral hernias. Although femoral hernias are less commonly encountered than inguinal hernias, surgical repair is also the treatment of choice. The principles underlying inguinal hernia repair also apply to femoral hernias. Usually the same type of skin incision is used; the sac, once identified, is reduced of its hernial contents, divided and ligated at its neck; and the entrance into the femoral canal giving rise to this entity is obliterated. This can be accomplished by attaching the transversus/transversalis complex to Cooper's ligament to close off the empty space in the femoral canal.

POSTERIOR REPAIR. The idea of approaching the transversalis/transversus layer posteriorly (Fig. 63-7) has been suggested as an adequate means of repairing some types of groin hernias over the past 60 years but has been particu-

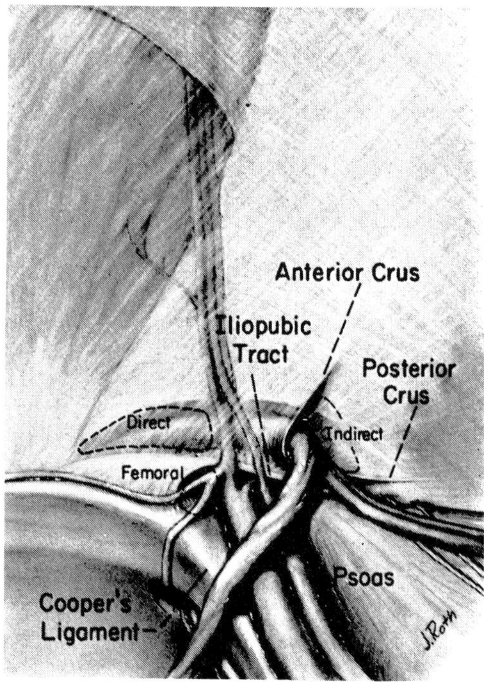

Fig. 63-7 The preperitoneal exposure of the posterior inguinal wall displays the important structures that form the boundaries of groin hernias. Repair of hernial defect(s) is readily accomplished by suture after preliminary reduction of the hernia. If an indirect hernia sac extends into the scrotum, it is not necessary that the entire distal sac be removed. Note that application of mesh is quite easy, since the posterior wall is completely exposed. (From Nyhus, L.M.: The preperitoneal approach and iliopubic tract repair of inguinal hernia. In Nyhus, L.M., and Condon, R.E., editors: Hernia, ed. 2, Philadelphia, 1978, J.B. Lippincott Co.)

larly strongly advocated by Nyhus[22] in recent years. This technique, when properly applied, is extremely useful in the repair of three major types of hernia: (1) the recurrent inguinal hernia, (2) the primary femoral hernia, and (3) incarcerated hernias of all types.

It is not surprising that surgeons who are unfamiliar with the posterior approach sometimes have difficulty in achieving effortless exposure of the proper tissue planes. For this reason it is imperative that anyone interested in gaining technical expertise with this approach should first watch an experienced surgeon perform this type of repair, also referred to as the preperitoneal repair. In this operation there is no substitute for experience in defining the sometimes subtle transversalis fascia layer.

As with anterior approaches to groin hernia repair, the skin incision should be placed transversally above and parallel to the internal inguinal ligament. After the incision to the level of the rectus sheath is deepened, the anterior fascia layer of this sheath is incised, and the rectus muscle retracted toward the midline. The exposed transversalis fascia is then incised to gain access to the preperitoneal space; this space always has a variable amount of fat present. The appearance of fatty tissue is the signal that the proper plane has been entered; at this point the incision through the abdominal musculature is widened toward the anterior iliac spine to pass about 2 cm above the internal inguinal ring. When this has been accomplished, the posterior inguinal wall is bared of fatty and areolar tissue from the line of incision to the superior pubic ramus. If the deep epigastric vessels obscure proper exposure, they can be ligated and divided as needed.

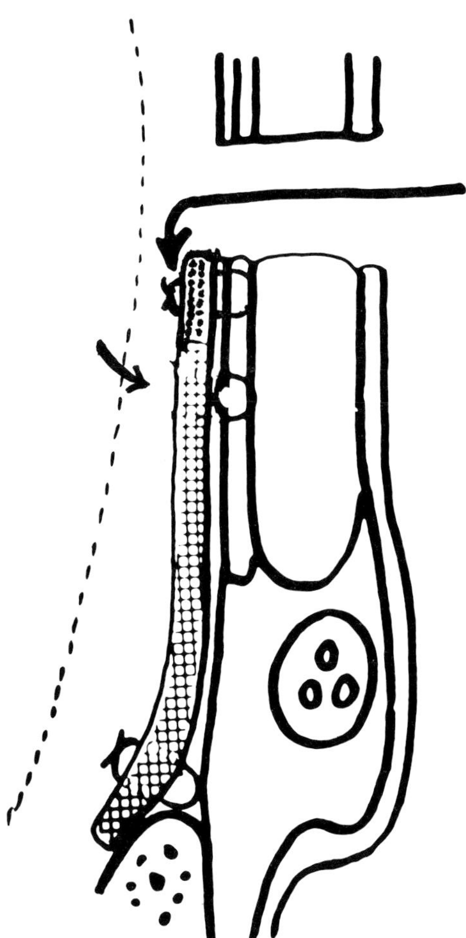

Fig. 63-8 Large arrow illustrates the approach to the preperitoneal space, above the inguinal canal. Small arrow shows the preliminary repair of the hernia defect before insertion of the "regional" prosthetic reinforcement that extends from the primary incision to the pubic ramus and from the midline to lateral of the internal ring.

After the posterior inguinal wall has been exposed, the herniated structures are identified and reduced. If there is an incarcerated hernia, it is prudent (and easy) to inspect all portions of incarcerated bowel for signs of ischemia or infarction. If there is any doubt concerning these possibilities, the surgeon can easily observe the tissues in question until the decision as to whether or not to resect has been made. After the walls of the hernial defect have been identified, the repair is fashioned to approximate the margins of the defect with interrupted sutures of permanent material. As with the anterior approach to hernia repair, the spermatic cord must also be examined to ensure that an additional oblique hernia is not present.

The posterior approach is strongly recommended for the repair of a recurrent hernia because it provides an opportunity to perform the operation in virgin tissue, which is clearly a distinct advantage over any anterior approach. The only difference between repairing a recurrent hernia posteriorly and other types of hernias is that a synthetic mesh buttress should be sutured to the posterior wall following repair of the hernia defect to prevent the possibility of another recurrence (Fig. 63-8).

Complications

There are many possible problems that may develop following inguinofemoral herniorrhaphy. The boxed material on p. 1068 lists the local or regional complications that can occur. In addition, the surgeon must always be aware of the systemic complications that may attend a groin herniorrhaphy such as those arising from the anesthetic technique used or secondary to an underlying associated disease such as that involving the heart or lungs. As with any operation, fatalities do at times occur, but these are quite rare and usually associated with an underlying cardiovascular problem.

Several complications related to the hernia repair itself need to be considered. One problem that is not uncommonly encountered in male patients undergoing groin hernia repair is that of a postoperative swollen testis. It may arise from venous engorgement or lymphatic congestion secondary to the repair itself, compromise to the arterial blood flow as a result of intraoperative trauma, a subfascial hematoma, or a missed hernia (such as an indirect inguinal hernia when a direct hernia was being repaired). In these troubling cases the management is usually guided by evaluating the overall clinical picture over a period of time. It will usually resolve over a period of 4 to 12 weeks, and the patient will only need the mature guidance of the surgeon during this interval to allay any fears that he may have. In those situations in which the blood supply to the testicle has been compromised, late atrophy of the testis will be noted; this complication is not rare, yet the true

LOCAL OR REGIONAL COMPLICATIONS FOLLOWING REPAIR OF GROIN HERNIAS

Acute

Wound infection/hematoma
Ilioinguinal/iliohypogastric nerve injury
Preperitoneal hemorrhage
Femoral vein/artery laceration or trauma
Thrombosis femoral vein/pulmonary embolus
Transection of vas deferens
Ligation of spermatic artery
Perforation of viscus (sliding hernia)
Nonclosure of internal ring
Loss of domain of erstwhile incarcerated structures
Scrotal ecchymosis/hematoma
Swollen testis
Missed hernia
Urinary retention

Chronic

Recurrent hernia
Hernia in a contiguous area
Late wound/suture sepsis (>5 to 10 years later)
Neuroma
Testicular atrophy
Hydrocele
Pseudoaneurysm of femoral artery
Groin pain
Loss of cremasteric reflex
Periostitis of pubis
Sexual dysfunction

incidence is hard to determine because of limited follow-up studies in most reported series of patients undergoing groin herniorrhaphy. Occasionally an acute infarction of the testicle will develop postoperatively that will require immediate surgical intervention and orchiectomy.

Occasionally a patient will develop a persistent pain following groin herniorrhaphy (see the boxed material at right). The great majority of patients have a rapidly subsiding pain that is usually manageable by the second postoperative week. After 3 to 4 weeks postoperatively, there is only a residual tenderness to deep palpation, and by 3 to 4 months there are no symptoms referable to the operation. Occasional patients have persistent complaints that can be quite troublesome and that can prove difficult to assess and treat successfully. The physical examination is very useful because it gives precise information about the possible sources of pain. For example, if the testicle is swollen or inflamed or if the epididymis is quite tender, a genitourinary infection might be suspected. Alternatively, the floor of the inguinal canal may be painless, whereas the pubic tubercle area is exquisitely tender, indicating periostitis of the pubic bone where a suture was placed to effect adequate repair. In all cases I avoid any specific intervention until at least 3 to 4 months have passed to allow the acute perioperative reaction to subside because most subjective complaints disappear during this interval. In patients with persistent pain, point tenderness along the floor of the inguinal canal (but not at the internal ring)

GROIN PAIN AFTER HERNIORRHAPHY

Wound infection
Stitch abscess
Epididymitis/urinary infection
Recurrent hernia/femoral hernia
Missed hernia
Neuroma
Desmoplastic scar
Thrombophlebitis
Hidradentis
Sebaceous cyst
Pubic periostitis

suggests the possibility of a neuroma. In this circumstance an injection of 2 to 3 ml of 1% xylocaine can be made at the point of tenderness to determine whether the groin discomfort disappears. If such a response occurs, the site can be reinjected with a mixture of cortisone and xylocaine into the "trigger" point. Most patients will respond to this type of treatment with a clear decrease in symptoms and not require any further treatment. If such management is unsuccessful, surgical excision of the superficial scar tissue and nerve tissue is indicated, with care to include cut nerve endings within the ligated tissue. When neuromas occur during groin hernia surgery, they are usually a consequence of injury to the ilioinguinal or iliohypogastric nerves.

The most important complication directly relating to the repair itself is that of hernia recurrence. Because of the mobility of our society and the consequent difficulty of following patients over the long term, the actual incidence of recurrence is probably not known. Most series would suggest that this incidence is somewhere between 2% and 10%. In a 22-year analysis of inguinal and femoral hernias repaired by Halverson and McVay[15] and McVay and Chapp,[21] a 3.2% recurrence rate in over 1200 cases was noted. Almost 40% of the recurrences occurred after 5 years following the initial operation, illustrating the constraints of short evaluation periods. The best results ever reported in terms of recurrence rates are those from the Shouldice Clinic.[11,12] The Shouldice repair is performed through an anterior incision and includes maneuvers to ensure adequate exposure of the internal inguinal ring followed by an overlapping repair of the floor of the inguinal canal. The principles of this repair are narrowing of the internal ring and a multilayer reinforcement of the transversalis fascial layer. This repair is made without relaxing incisions and without the need for prosthetic mesh insertion. Several authors have reported less than a 1% recurrence rate with this technique, whether primary or recurrent hernias were being treated. Whether other surgeons using this technique but not reporting their results are having the same degree of success remains unknown. Thus, when results from different clinics are evaluated, apparent differences may not be borne out when subjected to critical statistical analysis. For this reason it is difficult to be sure which operation is "the best."

Umbilical Hernia

Umbilical hernias occur where the umbilical ring has failed to obliterate the opening of the allantoic duct. The majority of these hernias are congenital in origin and are particularly common in Negro infants. Most of these hernias close spontaneously by the ages of 4 to 6 and almost never become incarcerated or strangulated. For this reason infant congenital umbilical hernias rarely require surgical closure. Exceptions to this stance include hernias that are symptomatic, those in which the umbilical ring is excessively large so that external trauma poses a threat, and those that have demonstrated no significant closure by 6 years of age.

Umbilical hernias may also develop in adults. When they occur in this population, a number of predisposing factors appear to give rise to their development, including abdominal distention secondary to massive ascites from underlying disease such as Laënnec's cirrhosis; induced ascites as occurs in patients undergoing chronic ambulatory peritoneal dialysis, pregnancy, and obesity; and in certain situations where there may be abnormal or defective collagen synthesis secondary to nutritional deficiencies or advancing age. Because many of these hernias have a small neck, the risk of incarceration and strangulation remains a continuing threat. Thus most of these hernias should be surgically repaired, which can be easily accomplished through an infraumbilical or supraumbilical skin incision in which the sac is removed and the fascial edges surrounding the hernial defect directly approximated with nonabsorbable sutures.

Hernias of the Linea Alba

In addition to the umbilical hernia, a number of other hernial defects may involve the linea alba. These hernias usually occur between the xiphoid process and the umbilicus, in which case they are termed *epigastric hernias;* occasionally they may appear below the umbilicus. Hernias of the linea alba are usually small, often multiple, and typically contain preperitoneal fat. Their presentation clinically is often deceptive and may be apparent only as pinpoint convexities overlying the erect patient's linea alba. If the physical examination is negative but the patient's complaint is persistent pain in this region anatomically, surgical exploration may be required to provide a definite diagnosis. The most cogent explanation at present for the development of these hernias is provided by anatomic studies of the linea alba. This structure is a complex network of three musculoaponeurotic components of the rectus sheath[4] and varies considerably in its inherent strength. There are at least three recognizable patterns of decussation of these fibers in the midline, all of which may be aggravated by marked distention of the abdominal wall. In addition, there are discreet areas midway between the xiphoid process and umbilicus that are subjected to repetitive stresses by phrenic aponeurotic bands that insert in the midline fascia; perhaps these latter structures eventually weaken the midline fascia and therefore help explain the location of most hernias in this area.[4] Like umbilical hernias, repair of hernias involving the linea alba consist of excision and closure of the hernial sac and direct approximation of the edges of the defect in the fascia with nonabsorbable sutures.

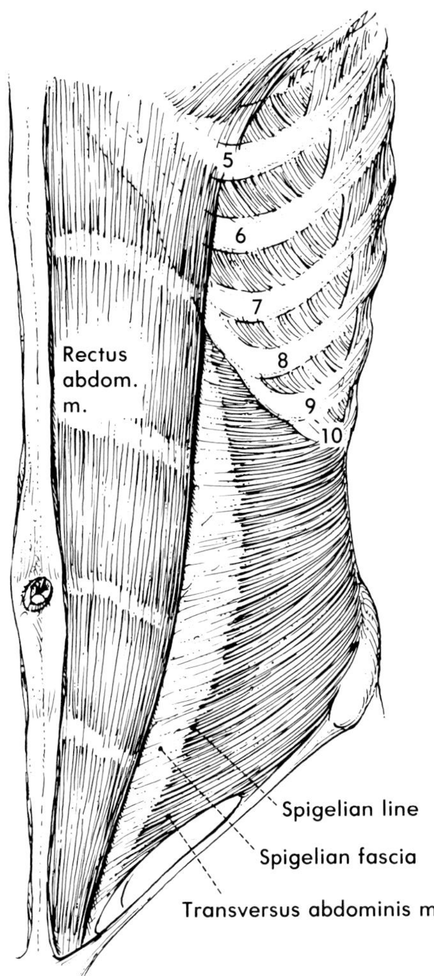

Fig. 63-9 The rectus muscle aponeurosis extends from the fourth, fifth, and six ribs. The hernias along the lateral border of the rectus muscle do not penetrate the external oblique layer.

Spigelian Hernia

The spigelian hernia develops through a defect in the spigelian fascia (named after the Flemish anatomist Spieghel who described it in the 1600s), which is that site where the semilunar and semicircular lines just lateral to the lower one third of the rectus muscle join (Fig. 63-9). The development of a hernia in this area is often subtle and frequently presents a diagnostic challenge.[30] Presenting findings include pain and tenderness and occasionally an abdominal mass along the rectus muscle just inferior to the umbilicus. Most of the difficulty in diagnosis results from the fact that these hernias are usually intramural so that they may track from their site of origin in almost any direction being covered by the external oblique muscle. Consequently, they are not obvious as hernial defects traversing the abdominal wall. Recently the use of ultrasonography has been demonstrated to be of value in the diagnosis of spigelian hernia. Spangen reported that B-mode scans were of particular value in discovering spigelian hernias in a relatively large number of individuals in his clinic.[12] The author has also had some success with ultrasonic diagnosis of spigelian hernias and believes that it is a useful adjunct in the diagnosis of patients with unexplained abdominal wall pain, particularly if the clinical finding strongly suggests this type of hernia despite negative physical findings.

Because incarceration and strangulation may occur with spigelian hernias, they should be surgically repaired when diagnosed. Such repair is accomplished through a transverse incision over the site of origin, with division of the external oblique fascia for proper exposure of the hernial defect. Since the defect involves the aponeurosis of the transverse abdominus and internal oblique muscles, repair involves approximation of these two fascial layers and subsequent closure of the divided external oblique fascia.

Lumbar Hernia

Hernias arising in the lumbar region through the posterior abdominal wall are called *lumbar* or *dorsal hernias*. One of two sites is generally involved. The superior lumbar triangle, also called Grynfeltt's triangle, is the most common site of origin; the inferior lumbar triangle (also called Petit's triangle) is less frequently involved. The common clinical presentation is usually a mass in the flank that may or may not be associated with pain. On palpation this mass is generally reducible, and incarceration and strangulation are usually not problems. Most lumbar hernias represent incisional hernias occurring in old nephrectomy incisions, but they may on occasion occur spontaneously. Surgical repair with approximation of the fascial edges of the hernia defect is the treatment of choice.

Pelvic Hernias

A variety of rare hernias may occur through the various foramina in the pelvic floor through which nerves and blood vessels pass into the buttocks or out of the pelvis. Various intraabdominal structures may make up the hernial contents, small bowel being particularly frequent. The two common types of pelvic hernias include those that pass through the greater sciatic foramen and the obturator foramen. The diagnosis of these types of hernia is often first made at the time of surgery when a portion of intestine becomes incarcerated, necessitating abdominal exploration. Occasionally an obturator hernia will be diagnosed as a swelling in the upper and medial aspect of the thigh associated with pain radiating to the medial aspect of the knee in the distribution of the obturator nerve (i.e., Howship-Romberg sign). In a patient in whom a sciatic or obturator hernia is suspected, herniography provides confirmation. Both types of hernias are usually repaired through an abdominal approach in which the hernial sac and its contents are reduced (with resection of necrotic bowel if indicated) and primary closure of the fascial defect.

Another type of pelvic hernia may occur when there is a defect in the levator sling in the floor of the pelvis. A protrusion through this defect is called a *perineal hernia* and usually appears as a bulge just lateral to the midline perineal raphe. These hernias are usually secondary to a previous surgical procedure such as an abdominoperineal resection or a prostatectomy. Repair involves fascial closure of the perineal defect, usually through a combined abdominal and perineal approach. Perineal hernias are often asymptomatic, but depending on their location they may be associated with pain on sitting or a variety of urinary complaints, predominantly dysuria.

Incisional Hernia

An incisional hernia is one that develops through a surgical incision in the abdominal wall. These hernias most commonly involve incisions of the anterior abdominal wall, although they may be responsible for other types of hernias such as those occurring in the lumbar region (from a previous nephrectomy incision) and in the perineal region (from a previous abdominoperineal resection). The hernia may appear clinically shortly following the placement of the initial incision or develop many years thereafter. When arising in the anterior abdominal wall, incisional hernias are more commonly encountered in vertical than in transverse incisions.

A variety of etiologic factors are involved in the development of incisional hernias that can generally be grouped under the two broad headings of poor postoperative wound healing or postoperative wound infection. Any factor related to poor surgical technique can result in inadequate wound healing. Thus, if sutures are placed too close to the edges of the wound being apposed or they are tied too tightly so as to necrose the involved tissues, poor wound healing may result. Other contributing factors relating to surgical technique include knots becoming untied, use of the wrong type of suture material for a particular incision, the development of wound hematomas from poor hemostasis, and the placement of drains through the incision itself, all of which may adversely affect healing. Further, if the incision has not been closed properly and the patient develops a problem with increased intraabdominal pressure (secondary to such factors as hiccuping, abdominal distention, and postoperative coughing), undue strain may be placed on the suture line that ultimately may give way. Finally, wound infections are known to be directly related to the subsequent development of an incisional hernia, particularly if the infection extends to the level of the fascia. Thus any factor contributing to the development of a wound infection will also influence the likelihood of recurrent incisional hernia.

The treatment of most incisional hernias is not dissimilar to that of other hernias. Thus for small or moderate-sized hernias the hernial sac is excised, and the defect closed with interrupted sutures. For larger hernias such closure may not be possible without placing undue tension on the repair. In this circumstance either a fascia lata graft or a synthetic mesh material such as Marlex should be used to bridge the hernial defect.

A variant of the incisional hernia is that which occurs through the same fascial opening created for a colostomy or ileostomy. This type of hernia is termed a *parastomal hernia* and usually occurs when the stomal opening is placed lateral to the rectus muscle. Often this type of hernia can be managed by tightening the fascial defect around the stoma with interrupted sutures. When this is not possible, the colostomy or ileostomy should be taken down and moved to a new site, preferably through the rectus muscle. The remaining fascial defect from the previously placed ostomy is then closed from within the peritoneal cavity.

Diaphragmatic Hernias

A number of hernias may occur within the diaphragm that separates the thoracic from the abdominal cavity. These hernias may be congenital, in which case they arise through defects or apertures resulting from developmental abnormalities; or they may be acquired through enlargement of preexistent apertures or disruption of points of weakness.

A congenital diaphragmatic hernia represents an arrest in the development of some portion of the diaphragm (Fig. 63-10). When it occurs posterolaterally (which is the most common site), it is called a foramen of Bochdalek's hernia and involves the left hemidiaphragm 70% to 85% of the time. This type of hernia, which allows abdominal viscera to readily migrate into the left thorax, is one of the surgical emergencies of the newborn period and is associated with a substantial mortality rate as a result of the accompanying respiratory distress and ventilatory impairment. The clinical presentation of this type of hernia and the physiologic principles underlying its management are discussed in detail in Chapter 65. Another type of congenital hernia is that which results from failure of fusion anteriorly of the sternal and costal portions of the diaphragm. The resulting midline defect creates a hiatus, known as Morgagni's foramen, through which a hernia may occur. When normal fusion results, only the internal mammary vessels pass through this area and continue into the abdomen as the superior epigastric vessels. When the defect remains, however, various portions of bowel (usually small bowel) or omentum may herniate through this abnormal hiatus. In contrast to the Bochdalek hernia, which clinically presents at birth, most hernias protruding through Morgagni's foramen do not become symptomatic until middle age or later. Often the first demonstration of their presence is a mechanical bowel obstruction that may result in strangulation of the involved bowel and can develop into a severe mediastinitis if not emergently treated. When diagnosed, they should be repaired surgically, usually by a transabdominal approach.

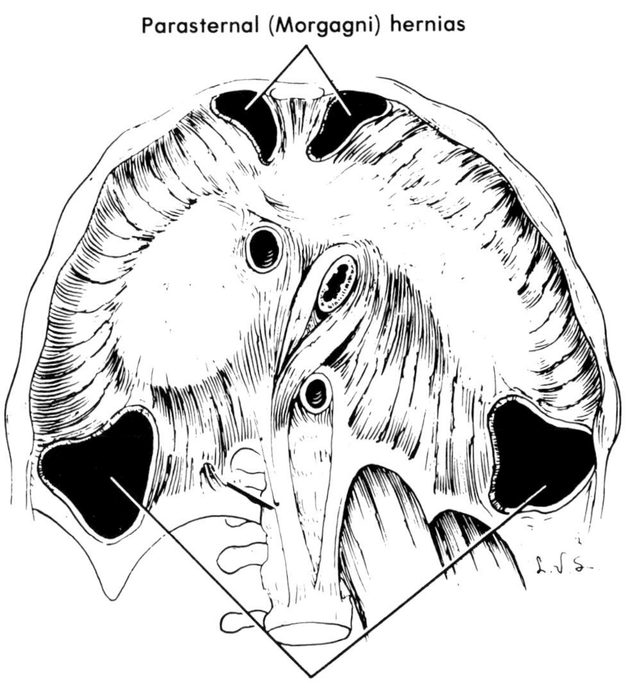

Fig. 63-10 Sites of congenital diaphragmatic herniation. (From Grimes, O.F., and Way, L.W.: Esophagus and diaphragm. In Way, L.W., editor: Current surgical diagnosis and treatment, ed. 7, Los Altos, Calif., 1985, Lange Medical Publications.)

Of the acquired types of hernias that may affect the diaphragm, the most common is the sliding hiatus hernia, which may or may not be associated with esophagitis. This type of hernia is discussed in detail in Chapter 14. Less commonly encountered clinically is the parahiatal hernia, also called the paraesophageal hernia (Fig. 63-11). Since the esophagogastric junction is not disturbed in this condition, esophagitis is not a problem. Usually the presenting symptoms are vague epigastric and lower chest pain that may be aggravated on recumbency. With this type of hernia, all or part of the stomach may herniate into the thorax adjacent and to the left of the gastroesophageal junction. Radiologically this type of hernia may give the appearance of an upside-down stomach on barium contrast study. Paraesophageal hernias are often associated with the complications of ulceration and bleeding and not uncommonly become incarcerated and at times even strangulated. For this reason the most prudent method of management is to return the herniated stomach to the abdomen and surgically repair the aperture in the diaphragm.

One additional type of acquired hernia of importance is

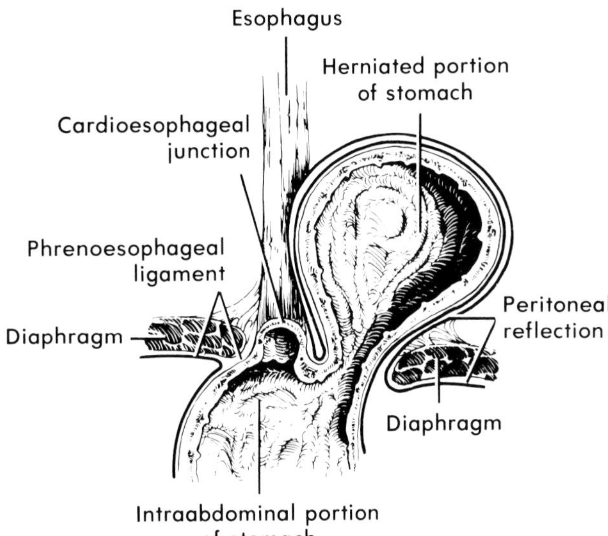

Fig. 63-11 Paraesophageal hernia. (From Grimes, O.F., and Way, L.W.: Esophagus and diaphragm. In Way, L.W., editor: Current surgical diagnosis and treatment, ed. 7, Los Altos, Calif., 1985, Lange Medical Publications.)

that produced by rents in the diaphragm that may result from penetrating or blunt trauma.

Because of the protective effects of the liver on the right, these traumatic hernias almost always occur on the left side and can result in considerable respiratory embarrassment from herniation of abdominal viscera into the left chest if they are of sufficient size. Surgical repair of the diaphragmatic tear with reduction of the herniated viscera into the abdomen is the treatment of choice.

SUMMARY

Hernias of the abdominal wall are commonly encountered in the practice of surgery and may arise in any structure surrounding or supporting the contents of the abdominal cavity. These hernias are particularly common anteriorly, with the vast majority arising in the groin. Other sites of relatively frequent occurrence include the umbilicus and previous incisions. The clinical presentation of a hernia is usually obvious and exhibits a bulge at the site of the hernial defect, often in association with pain. Less commonly, an unexplained intestinal obstruction may be the presenting finding in which a segment of bowel has become trapped in the hernial defect. Because hernias generally do not resolve spontaneously (an exception being the congenital umbilical hernia), surgical repair is the treatment of choice once the diagnosis has been established. This includes careful identification of the hernial ring, reduction of any contents that may be within the hernial sac, and in most circumstances excision of the sac itself. When these maneuvers have been accomplished, the defect is then repaired by approximating its edges and interrupted nonabsorbable sutures. Occasionally the hernial defect will be sufficiently large that primary closure is not possible without creating undue stress and tension. In this circumstance, as may occur with large groin hernias, umbilical hernias, and some incisional hernias, fascia lata or some type of synthetic material (such as Marlex) may be used to bridge and/or buttress the hernial defect to ensure an adequate repair and reduce the possibility of recurrence. The key to any successful hernia repair is an understanding of the underlying anatomy and its restoration to normalcy. With this principle in mind, most hernias can be repaired without difficulty and a good-to-excellent result can be expected.

REFERENCES

1. Andrews, E.: A method of herniotomy utilizing only white fascia, Ann. Surg. **80:**185, 1984.
2. Anson, B.J., Morgan E.H., and McVay, C.B.: Surgical anatomy of the inguinal region based upon a study of 500 body-halves, Surg. Gynecol. Obstet. **111:**707, 1960.
3. Arnbjornsson, E.: Development of right inguinal hernia after appendectomy, Am. J. Surg. **143:**174, 1982.
4. Askar O.: Surgical anatomy of the aponeurotic expansions of the anterior abdominal wall, Ann. R. Coll. Surg. Engl. **59:**313, 1977.
5. Cannon, D.J., and Read, R.C.: Metastatic emphysema, a mechanism for acquiring inguinal herniation, Ann. Surg. **194:**270, 1981.
6. Colin, J.F., Elliot, P., and Ellis, H.: The effect of uraemia upon wound healing: an experimental study, Br. J. Surg. **66:**793, 1979.
7. Condon, R.E.: Surgical anatomy of the transversus abdominis and transversalis fascia, Ann. Surg. **173:**1, 1971.
8. Condon, R.E.: The anatomy of the inguinal region and its relationship to groin hernia. In Nyhus, L.M., and Condon, R.E., editors: Hernia, ed. 2, Philadelphia, 1978, J.B. Lippincott Co.
9. Conner, W.T., and Peacock, E.E., Jr.: Some studies on the etiology of inguinal hernia, Am. J. Surg. **126:**732, 1973.
10. Engeset, J., and Youngson, G.G.: Ambulatory peritoneal dialysis and hernia complications, Surg. Clin. North Am. **64:**385, 1984.
11. Glassow, F.: Recurrent inguinal and femoral hernia, Br. Med. J. **1:**215, 1970.
12. Glassow, F.: The Shouldice repair of inguinal hernia. In Nyhus, L.M., and Condon, R.E., editors: Hernia, ed. 2, Philadelphia, 1978, J.B. Lippincott Co.
13. Gullmo, A.: Herniography: the diagnosis of hernia in the groin and incompetence of the pouch of Douglas and pelvic floor, Acta Radiol. **36:**1, 1980.
14. Gullmo, A., Broome, A., and Smedberg, S.: Herniography, Surg. Clin. North Am. **64:**229, 1984.
15. Halverson, K., and McVay, C.B.: Inguinal and femoral hernioplasty: a 22-year study of the author's methods, Arch. Surg. **101:**127, 1970.
16. Hughson, W.: The persistent or preformed sac in relation to oblique inguinal hernia, Surg. Gynecol. Obstet. **41:**610, 1925.
17. Jorkasky, D., and Goldfarb, S.: Abdominal wall hernia complicating chronic ambulatory peritoneal dialysis, Am. J. Nephrol. **2:**323, 1982.
18. Keith, A.: On the origin and nature of hernia, Br. J. Surg. **11:**455, 1924.
19. Lytle, W.J.: Internal inguinal ring, Br. J. Surg. **32:**441, 1945.
20. McVay, C.B.: Groin hernioplasty: Cooper's ligament repair. In Nyhus, L.M., and Condon, R.E., editors: Hernia, ed. 2, Philadelphia, 1978, J.B. Lippincott Co.
21. McVay, C.B., and Chapp, J.D.: Inguinal and femoral hernioplasty—the evaluation of a basic concept, Ann. Surg. **148:**499, 1958.
22. Nyhus, L.M.: The preperitoneal approach and iliopubic tract repair of inguinal and femoral hernia. In Nyhus, L.M., and Condon, R.E., editors: Hernia, ed. 2, Philadelphia, 1978, J.B. Lippincott Co.
23. Nyhus, L.M., and Condon, R.E., editors: Hernia, ed. 2, Philadelphia, 1978, J.B. Lippincott Co.
24. Peacock, E.E., Jr.: Biology of hernia. In Nyhus, L.M., and Condon, R.E., editors: Hernia, ed. 2, Philadelphia, 1978, J.B. Lippincott Co.
25. Peacock, E.E., Jr. and Madden, J.W.: Studies on the biology and treatment of recurrent inguinal hernia. II. Morphological changes, Ann. Surg. **179:**567, 1974.
26. Read, R.C.: Attenuation of rectus sheath in inguinal herniation, Am. J. Surg. **120:**610, 1970.
27. Read, R.C.: Bilaterality and the prosthetic repair of large recurrent inguinal hernias, Am. J. Surg. **138:**788, 1979.
28. Read, R.C.: The development of inguinal herniorrhaphy, Surg. Clin. North Am. **64:**185, 1984.
29. Robinson, R.R., et al.: Surgical considerations of continuous ambulatory peritoneal dialysis, Surgery **96:**723, 1984.
30. Spangen L.: Spigelian hernia, Surg. Clin. North Am. **64:**351, 1984.
31. Stoppa, R.E., et al.: The use of dacron in the repair of hernias in the groin, Surg. Clin. North Am. **64:**269, 1984.
32. Tanner, N.C.: A "slide" operation for inguinal and femoral hernia, Br. J. Surg. **29:**285, 1942.
33. Tobin, G.R., Clark, D.S., and Peacock, E.E., Jr.: A neuromuscular basis for development of indirect inguinal hernia, Arch. Surg. **11:**464, 1976.
34. Usher, F.C.: Hernia repair with Marlex mesh. In Nyhus, L.M., and Condon, R.E.,, editors: Hernia, ed. 2, Philadelphia, 1978, J.B. Lippincott Co.

64 Pathophysiology of Thermal Injury

Donald H. Parks, Harold R. Mancusi-Ungaro, and David J. Wainwright

Thermal injury elicits major pathophysiologic alterations beyond the obvious cutaneous manifestation. Although the burn wound itself can present unique challenges in terms of therapeutic management and is responsible for the high incidence of infection that occurs in thermally injured patients, a number of metabolic aberrations and associated dysfunction of various organs are also commonly encountered that directly contribute to morbidity and mortality. The magnitude of these latter derangements has led to the proposal that the burn patient is the universal trauma model.[101] Major progress has recently been achieved in understanding many of the pathophysiologic mechanisms that occur in burn injury and has facilitated patient management and improved survival. Such progress has been attributed to the development of specialized burn centers, increased investigative efforts in burn research, and the development of the team concept in patient management.[51]

THE BURN WOUND

Biophysics of Thermal Injury

When the skin is heated, damage occurs from the transfer of thermal energy. The magnitude of this tissue destruction is a function of both the quantity of heat transferred and the speed at which it dissipates. These factors are determined by the physical properties of the burning agent, the recipient tissue that is burned, and the incipient environment.

Burning Agent

The temperature and duration of exposure to the burning agent are the most important determinants of the degree of injury. For a specific level of injury, there is an inverse relationship between these two parameters[75,85] (Fig. 64-1). As the temperature is reduced, a progressively longer exposure time is required to inflict the same injury. At a theoretic "threshold temperature," the heat source would have to be applied for an infinite time. Temperatures below this "threshold" do not result in tissue damage, regardless of the duration of application. The exposure interval is related not only to the actual removal of the offending agent, but also to the rate at which the heat source loses its energy to the environment. For example, at lower temperatures at which duration is important, a different degree of injury will result when a metallic object

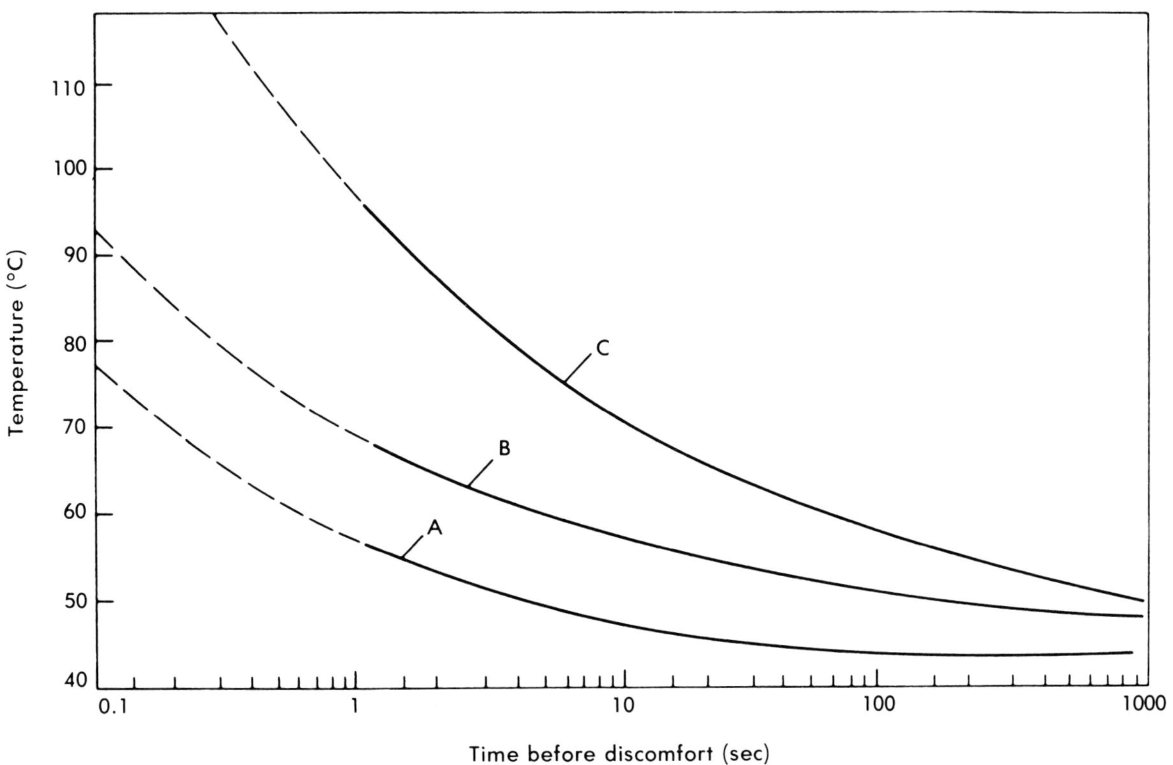

Fig. 64-1 Relationship between temperature and the duration of contact for first-degree *(A)*, second-degree *(B)*, and third-degree *(C)* injuries. (Reprinted by permission of the Council of the Institution of Mechanical Engineers from Lawrence, J.C., and Bull, J.P.: Thermal conditions which cause skin burns, Eng. Med. **5**:61, 1976.)

and liquid are exposed to the same temperature. The liquid will lose its heat more slowly.

Recipient Tissue

Certain physical properties of the heated object are also important in determining the extent of damage. These parameters reflect how much energy must be expended to raise the temperature of the object and how efficiently and quickly the heat is transferred. Skin, because of its high water content, has a high specific heat and a low thermal conductivity. Thus slow overheating of the tissues and delayed dispersion of the energy result. This is illustrated by measuring the temperature 1 mm below the skin surface after a 10-second scald burn (Fig. 64-2). There is an initial rapid, but not immediate rise in temperature as the heat is applied. Even more dramatic is the length of time required for the temperature to return to baseline values. In this way heat damage may continue after the offending agent is removed. Heat energy is lost primarily by conduction to the surrounding tissues, with removal by the circulating blood making only a small contribution.[76]

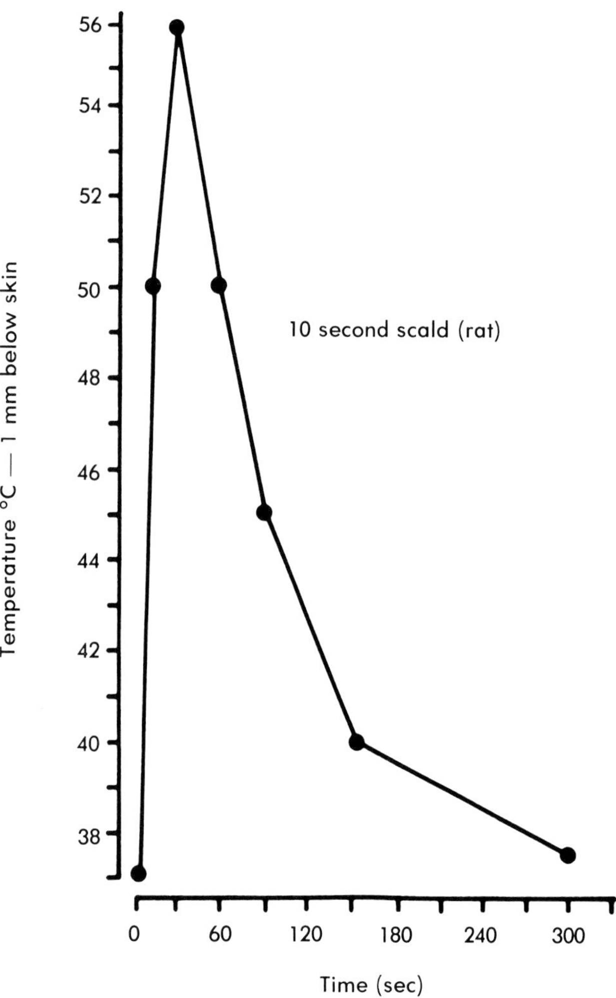

Fig. 64-2 Temperature curve measured by a thermocouple 1 mm below the skin surface during a 10-second scald. The skin's low thermal conductivity results in a slow dispersion of the energy, leading to additional tissue injury subsequent to the removal of the offending agent. (From Moncrief, J.A.: The body's response to heat. In Artz, C.P., et al., editors: Burns: a team approach, Philadelphia, 1979, W.B. Saunders Co.)

Environment

Heat dissipation occurs not only through adjacent tissues, but also into the surrounding environment. Heat loss is therefore maximized in a cooler environment. For example, the rapid application of cold water to burned skin has been shown to decrease the severity of the injury by rapidly reducing the elevated tissue temperature.[131] There is also evidence that cooling the burn wound will minimize edema[49,52] by decreasing the amount of histamine released[27] through stabilization of the mast cell membrane.[48] Preservation of the dermal microcirculation has likewise been demonstrated by immediate cooling of the thermally injured tissues,[49,105] presumably through a reduction in thromboxane production.[69]

Histopathology of the Burn Wound

The severity of a burn injury is determined by the anatomic surface area involved and the pathologic depth. A *first-degree burn* is characterized by painful, erythematous, and edematous skin. Histologically vasodilation is present in the dermal microvasculature, and there is an increase in the interstitial fluid volume secondary to increased permeability. If the insult is more severe, necrosis of the epidermis occurs, and blistering of the skin is found clinically. A hyperemic response is again observed in the vessels within the dermis accompanied by extravasation of fluid. In this instance the fluid accumulates not only within the connective tissue of the dermis, but also at the dermal-epidermal junction leading to vesicle formation. The composition of the blister fluid has been extensively examined by a number of investigators.[9,67,90,114] Compounds with a relatively low molecular weight (i.e., electrolytes, urea, glucose, antibiotics) diffuse freely into the tissues and are found in the same concentrations in the serum, interstitial fluid, and blister fluid. On the other hand, low-molecular-weight proteins that are generally found only in small concentrations in tissue fluid have been shown to attain up to 80% of their plasma concentration within the vesicles. Significant quantities of intracellular enzymes and purine/pyrimidine compounds are also found, reflecting the extent of cellular damage. Elevated concentrations of several chemical mediators (i.e., prostaglandins) have also been reported in the blister fluid.

In this *partial-thickness injury* or *second-degree burn* the epidermal appendages are preserved and are responsible for resurfacing the wound. The epithelium in the surviving sweat glands and hair follicles multiplies and begins to migrate across the wound, coverage being complete within 7 to 14 days. This injury is typically painful because of direct nerve-ending damage coupled with the release of irritant chemical mediators into the wound.

An even greater thermal insult leads to additional dermal necrosis. The cellular components are irreversibly damaged, and the connective tissue is sufficiently disrupted that it is unable to fulfill its function of support and protection. If this extends to a depth below the level of the epidermal appendages, a *full-thickness* or *third-degree burn* has occurred. Reepithelialization is only possible from the wound edge, a process that would take a considerable length of time for even small defects. A dry, leathery appearance is seen clinically since the tissues have lost their ability to hold water. This wound is painless because the nerve endings have been destroyed.

Pathophysiology of the Burn Wound

Progressive Ischemia

An important conceptual model of the burn wound is that proposed by Jackson.[73] He described three zones of graded thermal trauma (Fig. 64-3). Centrally the "zone of coagulation" is an area of irreversible tissue destruction. Temperatures in this region are extreme and lead to immediate cell death, the depth of necrosis dependent on the quantity of heat transferred. On the periphery, a "zone of hyperemia" exists where vasodilation and permeability changes are present. Here the tissues are viable and generally heal uneventfully. The "zone of stasis" lies between these two areas. In this zone the flow through the microvasculature is sluggish or has ceased, leading to progressive ischemia and cell death.[29] Jackson[73] conceived that these changes were a direct effect of the heat energy on the tissues and that eventual tissue necrosis within the zone of stasis within 24 to 48 hours was inevitable. However, other investigators believe that the tissues in this region have not been permanently damaged and thus have the potential for a full recovery.[135] Any deterioration is the result of a combination of physical factors and local inflammatory processes leading to persistent stasis and ischemia with conversion to a "zone of coagulation."

Systemic Factors. The progressive nature of the dermal ischemia occurs secondary to the influence of both systemic and local factors as outlined in the boxed material at right. Depletion of the intravascular volume from fluid leaking into the injured tissues diminishes the filling pressure of the left ventricle and in turn the perfusion pressure within the micro-circulation. Stroke volume is also reduced secondary to compromised myocardial contractility. A so-called "myocardial depressant factor" liberated from the heat-damaged tissues has been implicated as being responsible for these adverse effects on the function of the cardiac musculature,[19,81,103] but its existence remains disputed. Constricting eschar in circumferential burns of the extremities can also lead to reduced perfusion pressures in distally burned tissues.[38]

Local Factors. Local factors can be categorized into intraluminal, extraluminal, and those associated with changes in the vessel wall itself. Within the lumen of blood vessels, cellular debris may accumulate, leading to

FACTORS CONTRIBUTING TO PROGRESSIVE ISCHEMIA

Systemic Factors
1. Diminished circulating volume
2. Myocardial depression
3. Constricting eschar

Local Factors
1. Intraluminal
   a. WBC margination
   b. Platelet microthrombi/microemboli
   c. Erythrocyte agglutination
2. Vessel wall changes
   a. Endothelial cell shape
   b. Vasoconstriction
      (1) Direct
      (2) Through chemical mediators
3. Extraluminal
   a. Interstitial edema

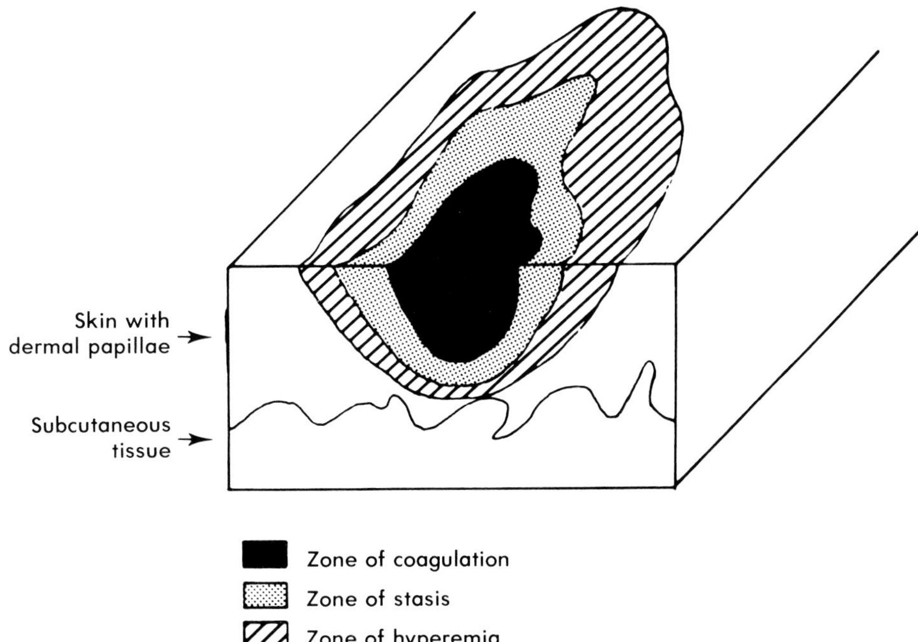

Fig. 64-3 Jackson's three zones of graded thermal injury. (From Moncrief, J.A.: The body's response to heat. In Artz, C.P., et al., editors: Burns: a team approach, Philadelphia, 1979, W.B. Saunders Co.)

a reduction in the functional diameter for flow. White blood cells respond to the thermal injury with increased margination along the vessel wall. As fluid leaks out of the intravascular space, hemoconcentration occurs that may encourage erythrocyte aggregation and agglutination, further diminishing local blood circulation. Platelet microthrombi and microemboli have also been observed to block the microvasculature within the injured area.[28] Release of tissue thromboplastin from the injured tissues and the platelet aggregating properties of certain members of the prostaglandin family are both believed to contribute to the generation of these products of coagulation. Despite these observations, the use of anticoagulants has been unsuccessful in reducing the extent of tissue damage.[111] Outside the vessel wall, the interstitial tissue pressure slowly increases as the lymphatics are unable to contend with the continual fluid extravasation. This leads to compression of the microvasculature within this region and a reduction in flow.

The vessel wall itself contributes to the reduction of nutrient flow by structural changes in the endothelial cells and vasoconstriction. As a response to direct damage or ischemia, the endothelial cells are less able to regulate their internal electrolyte balance. Water therefore enters the cells, and their normally hexagonal shape assumes a more spherical form.[95] In this way the thickness of the vessel wall increases and impinges on the diameter of the lumen. The vasoconstriction is likely the result of a multitude of factors. Increased sympathetic tone and eicosanoid release (especially thromboxane) appear to be the most important causes. Since the changes in the caliber of the lumen secondary to vessel wall alterations are often transient,[28] the other pathophysiologic changes detailed above probably play a more important role in reducing blood flow.

In order for the cells within the zone of stasis to survive, nutrient flow within the microvasculature must be maintained. By preserving these tissues, one may prevent a partial-thickness injury from becoming full thickness and therefore requiring grafting. Clinically this is achieved by maintaining the vascular volume and in turn the perfusion pressure through adequate resuscitation with intravenous fluids at the time of initial treatment. Similarly, wound care is important to prevent dehydration and infection, which can contribute to increasing the depth of injury. There is evidence that, by preserving an intact blister or covering the denuded partial-thickness injury with a skin substitute, dehydration of the exposed dermis is minimized and maximal tissue preservation is achieved.[80,135] More recently, attempts at pharmacologic manipulation of the offending chemical mediators have been made to preserve and/or reestablish the flow in this vascular bed.[108,110] In particular, promising results have been obtained using specific inhibitors of thromboxane production (e.g., imidazole, dipyridamole, methimazole). In a guinea pig burn model, India ink perfusion[50] and xenon 133 washout studies[112] have demonstrated a significant reduction in dermal ischemia following the administration of these compounds. The selective effect on thromboxane production was confirmed with the use of specific antiprostaglandin antibodies.

Cellular Alterations

In areas of irreparable damage, cell membranes are disrupted with the escape of intracellular contents. The connective tissue proteins undergo denaturation, and the water content is lost, leaving a solid amorphous substance. This fusion of the dermal and epidermal heat-damaged tissue is referred to as coagulation necrosis. As a reaction to the presence of this damaged and necrotic tissue, a marked inflammatory response characterizes the early phase of the burn wound. In locations where destruction is less extensive, cellular ultrastructure remains intact; however, function is often compromised. Resting membrane potentials are found to be above normal (> -90 mv) in this region, and cellular swelling is observed histologically.[17] This is likely the result of decreased adenosine triphosphate production from tissue ischemia.[34,71] The function of the ATP-dependent sodium pump is impaired, permitting a shift of sodium and water into the cell, further compounding the loss of intravascular volume. A specific example of this is the altered function of the endothelial cells, the shape of which has been changed in response to a local thermal insult,[95] as discussed above.

Fluid Shifts in the Wound

The inflammatory response typical of heat-damaged tissues is characterized by tremendous edema formation. Although various physical and chemically mediated factors are responsible, the fluid efflux depends on the restoration of adequate blood flow to the injured area. Perfusion is maintained by a combination of fluid resuscitation and local vasodilation, the latter following an initial period of transient sympathetic vasoconstriction. The magnitude and time course of the tissue edema is therefore subject to the timing and volume of fluid resuscitation.[54]

The cause of the increased fluid extravasation is multifactorial, with a tremendous amount of synergism between the responsible mechanisms. These can be broadly grouped into two major categories: (1) those that affect the permeability or ''leakiness'' of the vessel wall, and (2) those whose effect is mediated through alteration of the Starling forces (see boxed material below).

CAUSES OF EDEMA FORMATION

VESSEL WALL CHANGES

Vasodilation
Heat-induced damage
Vasoactive substances

ALTERED STARLING FORCES

Increased capillary hydrostatic pressure
- Vasoconstriction
- Partial blockage (platelets, white blood cells, red blood cells)

Decreased intraluminal colloid osmotic pressure
Increased interstitial colloid osmotic pressure
Lymphatic obstruction

Permeability Changes

Physical factors. The ease by which fluid, solutes, and macromolecules can exit the vessel lumen is influenced directly by architectural changes in the vessel wall and indirectly by a variety of chemical mediators. Vasodilation opens the endothelial gaps, promoting the efflux of fluid. The damaged endothelial cells exhibit an increase in both the number of intracellular vacuoles and the number of open intercellular junctions,[40] the latter secondary to these cells and assuming a more spherical shape.[95] These findings are first observed in the venules and later in the capillary bed. Since more channels are open along the vessel wall than exist normally, the outflow of fluid will naturally increase.

Humoral correlates. The release of vasoactive substances is perhaps the most important cause of the increased permeability seen in the early burn wound. The effect of these agents is primarily on the endothelial cells of the microvasculature where they cause both an increase in the number and size of the channels. This results in an increase in the amount of fluid escaping from the vessel lumen and more importantly allows a greater number of macromolecules to enter the interstitial compartment. Proteins of up to 150 Å have been shown to escape into the interstitial compartment, resulting in a decreased intravascular oncotic pressure.[6,10] Studies have demonstrated that the integrity of the microvasculature to macromolecular leak is restored by 8 to 12 hours following thermal injury. Hence, this is the time period during which some clinicians initiate colloid infusions in their resuscitation regimen.[36]

A variety of mediators have been implicated in the generation of these permeability changes (Fig. 64-4), but the most important appear to be histamine and the prostaglandins.[4,68,108] Kinins[5] and serotonin[20] have been shown to play only a minor role. Recently, much interest has been generated by the leukotrienes and the oxygen-free radicals[25] liberated by neutrophils.

The permeability changes seen within the burn wound take on a biphasic pattern[66] (Fig. 64-5). The initial increase is primarily caused by the action of histamine[72] and the direct thermal damage to the microvasculature. The specific cause of the second, more prolonged phase is less clear but is likely the result of activated components of the kallikrein-kinin system or prostaglandin release, primarily those of the E_1, E_2, and F_2 types. Although the prostaglandins themselves do not directly initiate fluid extravasation, they do have an enhancing effect on other responsible agents.

The use of specific histamine H_2-receptor blockers (e.g., cimetidine) in reducing the early phase of edema formation has been successful in animals[30,134]; however, their clinical use seems to be ineffective in this regard[31] and is occasionally associated with undesirable side effects.[123] These findings are consistent with the fact that histamine is not responsible for the longer, more pronounced phase of increased permeability; therefore its inhibition is unlikely to make an appreciable effect.

It is as yet unknown why certain subgroups of prostaglandins are released in thermally injured tissue. A variety of prostaglandin end products have been identified in the

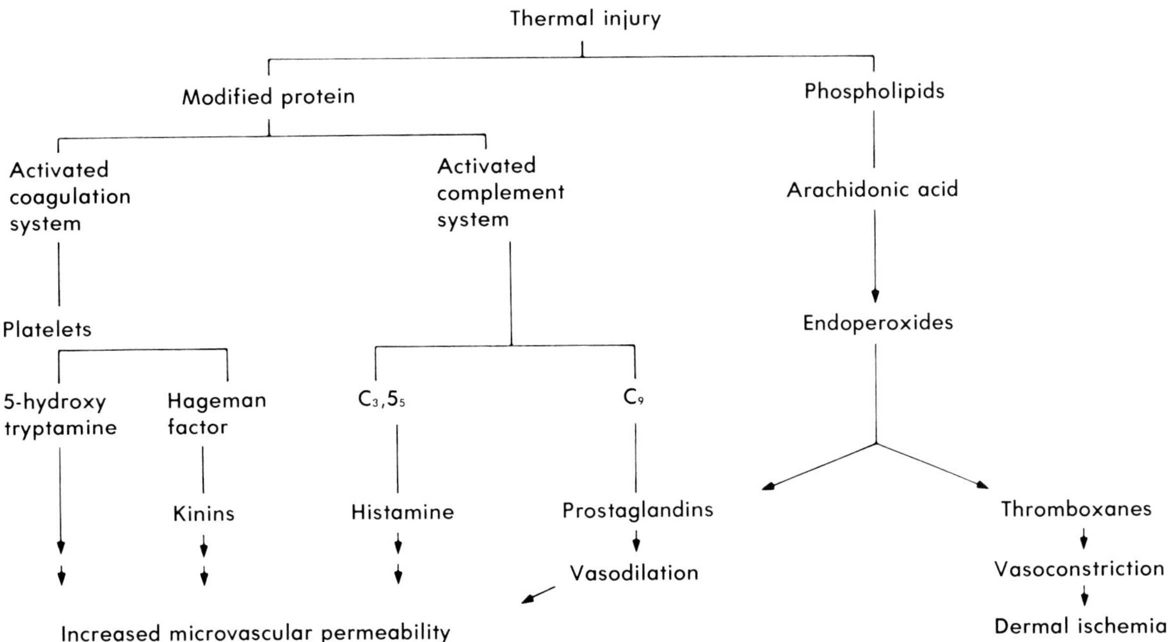

Fig. 64-4 Agents responsible for the generation of the permeability changes and progressive dermal ischemia in the burn wound. Superoxide radicals may also play a role in the increased permeability by both a direct effect and an augmentation of prostaglandin production. (From Davies, J.W.L.: Physiological responses to burning injury, London, 1982, Academic Press Inc.)

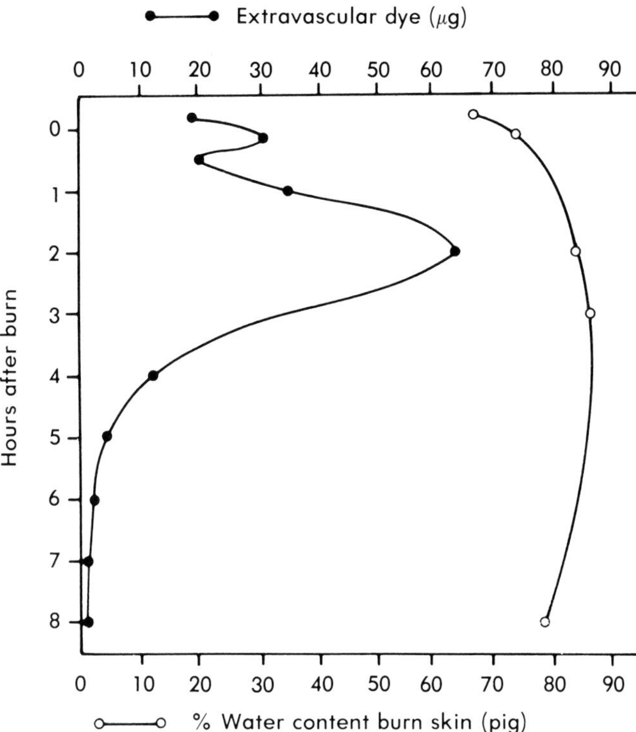

Fig. 64-5 Biphasic pattern of capillary permeability. (From Moncrief, J.A.: The body's response to heat. In Artz, C.P., et al., editors: Burns: a team approach, Philadelphia, 1979, W.B. Saunders Co.)

burn wound, many having completely opposite effects.[117] For example, prostaglandin E_2 (PGE_2) and prostacyclin (PGI_2) are vasodilators and inhibit platelet aggregation, whereas prostaglandin F_2(PGF_2) and the thromboxanes are potent vasoconstrictors and promote platelet aggregation. A steady-state relationship exists between these pairs of oppositely functioning prostanoids (e.g., PGE_2-PGF_2; prostacyclin-thromboxane) in uninjured tissues. However, a traumatic stimulus may disrupt this balance and initiate increased production of a particular group of prostanoids. Several studies have demonstrated that thromboxane is the responsible agent for many of the progressive ischemic changes seen in the dermal microcirculation and that inhibiting its production can prevent necrosis.[50,112] Further definition of the stimuli responsible for this preferential synthesis of certain prostaglandins and their specific inhibition is presently a very active area of research. Interest in the effect of prostaglandins on the progression of the injury is also evident in frostbite[104] and electrical injuries.[109] The final common pathway of the prostanoids' influence on cellular function appears to be their effect on intracellular cAMP levels.

The stimulus for the mediator response is the connective tissue protein that has been modified by thermal injury. Its effect on activating the complement and clotting mechanisms leads to the generation of the various mediator compounds (see Fig. 64-5). Specifically the C-3 and C-5 components of complement are responsible for mast cell histamine release, whereas the C-9 component initiates prostaglandin release from platelets.[7] The other minor factors are generated through activation of the clotting cascade.

In addition to vasoactive chemical release, a number of compounds are liberated that are chemotactic and result in a brisk cellular response to the injury. The polymorphonuclear leukocytes and macrophages are primarily responsible for the phagocytosis of the necrotic tissue. In the phagosome of the neutrophil, superoxide anion radicals and hydrogen peroxide are produced in large quantities to break down the ingested debris. These free radical substances are normally rendered harmless by the action of superoxide dismutases and catalases that convert them to oxygen and water. It has been postulated that a sufficient quantity of these substances may escape into the interstitial fluid where the necessary enzymes for their reduction are present only in small amounts.[7] These radicals not only can increase capillary permeability directly and cause additional tissue damage, but can also result in further prostaglandin release by their action on the phospholipid layer of the cell membrane.[120] To compound the local tissue injury, several lysosomal hydrolases (collagenase, elastase, cathepsin G) are also released from the phagosome, leading to further connective tissue destruction.

Starling Forces. In normal tissues the balance of the Starling Forces results in a slight efflux of fluid from the intravascular to the extravascular compartment (Fig. 64-6). A steady state is maintained by resorption of this fluid through the lymphatic channels. The lymphatic route is also the only avenue by which proteins can be returned to the vascular space to maintain the oncotic pressure gradient between the interstitial and intravascular compartments. In the burn wound these forces are altered so that this extravasation of fluid is greatly enhanced. Within the capillary lumen hydrostatic forces are increased above normal. The opening of the precapillary sphincters allows the arterial pressure to be transmitted directly to this vascular bed. In addition, intraluminal pressures rise proximal to a partial obstruction to flow caused by platelet microthrombi/microemboli, white blood cell margination, and red blood cell debris. In contrast, capillary intravascular osmotic pressure is decreased by the loss of colloid molecules into the interstitial space (especially albumin), whereas the extravascular osmotic activity rises, which tends to pull fluid out of the vessels.[9] The heat-denatured collagen is thought to be responsible for this effect. This denatured protein tends to hold the fluid within the interstitial space, thereby delaying resorption. Initially the lymphatics increase their flow to compensate for this additional interstitial volume; however, the maximum effect of this flow is achieved within an hour following thermal injury. Not infrequently, blockage or destruction of the lymphatic channels delays resorption of the increased interstitial volume, further compounding this problem. Although tissue pressures rise as the quantity of edema fluid increases,[74] this alteration is not sufficient to counteract the forces responsible for flow out of the vessels.

Nonburn Wound Edema. In large burns (i.e., over 40% body surface area), edema is observed in both burned and nonburned tissues. Increased capillary permeability of distant vascular beds may be caused by the systemic effect of chemical mediators released from the damaged tissue.[10,41,65] Excessive white blood cell margination in the nonburned microcirculation has also been considered as a

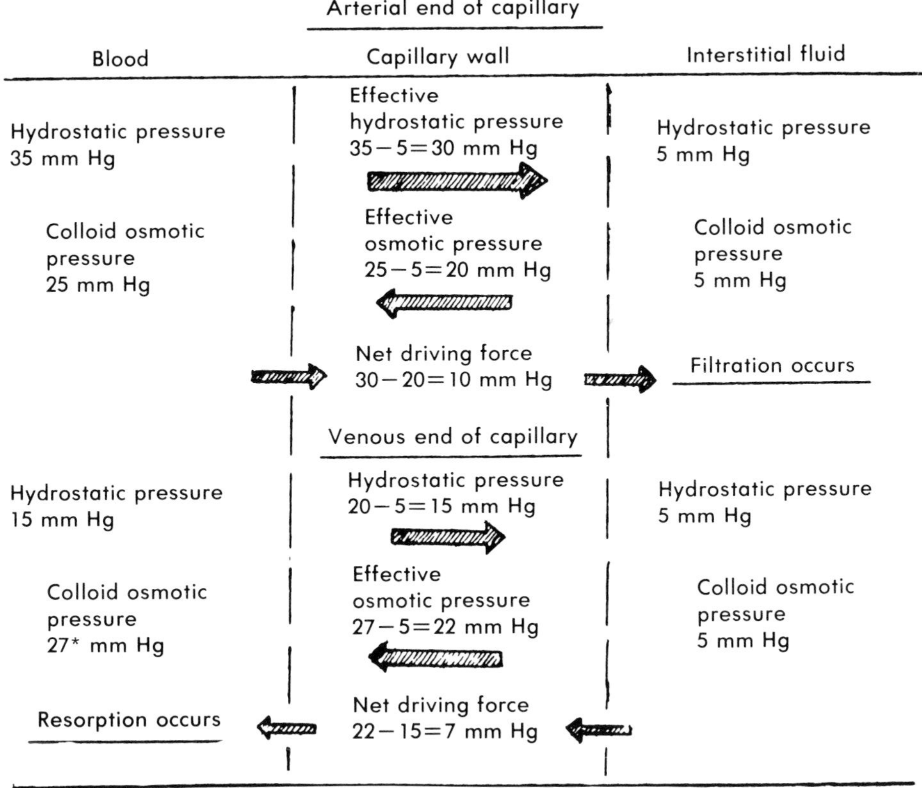

Fig. 64-6 Starling forces.

possible cause.[61] Recently, Demling, Kramer, and Harmes[53] and Demling[55] have proposed that intravascular hypoproteinemia may be responsible for this effect. They suggested that the plasma oncotic pressure is lowered not only by protein loss through the burn wound but also by dilution from the crystalloid solutions used in burn resuscitation. By administering colloid during the resuscitative period, he observed that the edema in nonburned tissues was significantly diminished.

METABOLIC ALTERATIONS

Hypermetabolic Response

The insult of a major burn results in a greater elevation of the metabolic rate than is observed in all other forms of trauma (Fig. 64-7). This phenomenon of hypermetabolism generally begins within 48 hours after the injury. It includes an elevated resting consumption of oxygen, coupled with increased nitrogen losses and protein catabolism.[8]

The hypermetabolic response to thermal injury appears to be associated with an intrinsic elevation in body core temperature as a result of a direct resetting of the hypothalamic temperature-regulating mechanism. Evidence supporting this contention relates to the observations that unburned skin remains vasoconstricted even when ambient temperatures are increased and evaporative losses are minimized.[33,129] On the other hand, although the hypermetabolic state does not depend on changes in ambient room temperature, it does appear to be sensitive to such alterations, since heat production and the energy cost of healing a large surface area can be reduced by keeping patients in a warm environment.[100,127]

The magnitude of the hypermetabolic response reflects the extent of the thermal injury. It increases over the first week following injury and decreases in response to wound healing and the diminishing size of the burn wound. During this time, a protein catabolic state is produced that is characterized by increased urinary nitrogen losses that are associated with protein degradation proportional to the severity of the burn. The hypermetabolic state generates a net caloric deficit. Although much of that deficit could be met through the use of fat deposits, the oxidation of fat requires simultaneous oxidation of carbohydrates. Once glycogen stores are exhausted, protein breakdown becomes the obligatory source of the carbohydrate.[77] In the process of gluconeogenesis, muscle protein is expended to liberate alanine and glutamine.[77,81] Without exogenous nutritional support, skeletal muscle becomes the target organ of the catabolic process.[128]

The factors mediating postburn hypermetabolism remain to be defined. Because denervation of a burned extremity does not affect the systemic metabolic rate nor the febrile state, it seems unlikely that neural factors are involved. In contrast, the increased flux of amino acids from muscle together with the febrile response may be attributed to a leukocytic endogenous mediator (LEM).[62] The infusion of isolated LEM caused a similar hypermetabolic state in normal animals. In terms of identifying such a humoral mediator, it has been suggested that LEM may be interleukin I.[77] If such is the case, the result of tissue injury and/or the burn wound itself becomes the cause of the hypermetabolic state.

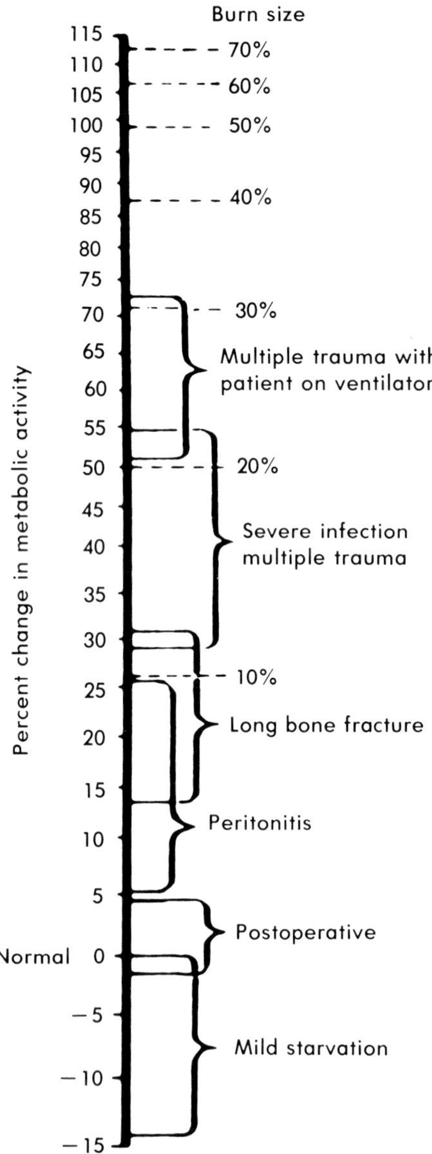

Fig. 64-7 Relative metabolic rates for various forms of trauma. (From Goodwin, C.W.: Crit. Care Clin. **1**:97, 1985.)

Postinjury Catabolism

The postinjury period is characterized by prolonged protein catabolism (particularly in muscle), negative nitrogen balance, and weight loss, all of which vary according to the extent of thermal injury. Although it remains a nonsteady state for weeks, the catabolic state ultimately reaches a plateau and does not change in response to caloric replacement.[16,133] For a 50% total body surface area burn, the magnitude of catabolism may be twice that which normally occurs following an injury. Weight loss develops because of a breakdown of lean body mass. The loss of 300 to 600 g of body weight per day can be equated to a daily loss of 75 to 150 g of protein.[92] Although treatment with calories and nitrogenous sources does not affect breakdown of muscle protein, it can increase its synthesis.

This apparent metabolic paradox can be appreciated by briefly reviewing the cycle through which carbohydrates are produced and used. Gluconeogenesis uses amino acids, principally alanine and glutamine. The source of these two gluconeogenic amino acids is skeletal muscle. Although that source appears to be obligatory, exogenous amino acids can either decrease muscle efflux or contribute to increased muscle synthesis.[63] The increase in conversion of alanine to glucose is accompanied by a reduction in the incorporation of exogenous alanine into protein and an increase in the release and synthesis of alanine by muscle.[13] At the same time, a reduction in circulating branched chain amino acids suggests that the administration of exogenous amino acids, especially those of the branched chain variety, may stimulate de novo synthesis of alanine and glutamine by skeletal muscle.[26]

The process of gluconeogenesis from skeletal muscle requires energy. In this process skeletal muscle uses fatty acid substrates.[91] Meanwhile, glucose from the liver's new stores is only partially used in the periphery, being converted to a three-carbon precursor, which in turn must return to the liver for reconversion into new glucose. The process of reconversion, the Cori cycle, also requires fatty acid substrates.[125] Although increased lipolysis and lipid mobilization occur in the burn patient, exogenous administration of fatty acids appears to be of little nutritional value and may be related to variation in the body's ability to clear lipids when in a state of stress.[78] Following thermal injury, it has been noted that a diet consisting of 5% to 15% of the nonprotein calories as fat was optimal and that a diet consisting of more was deleterious.[82] In man the inhibition of triglyceride lipase by insulin may lead to a futile cycle of triglyceride metabolism.[77] Immediately after a burn, for example, there is increased lipoprotein lipase activity and clearance of triglycerides as insulin levels fall and glucagon and glucose levels rise. In response to plasma triglycerides, lipase activity increases. However, the resulting free fatty acids cannot be used without carbohydrates and eventually must be reesterified to triglycerides. For a more detailed discussion of these considerations, see Chapter 1.

Therapeutic Implications

The dramatically increased metabolic expenditure following thermal injury must be compensated by increased nutritional support to avoid the plethora of potential complications associated with nutritional deficiency. Energy requirements in terms of caloric needs can be calculated according to the formula below proposed by Curreri and associates[45]:

25 kcal/kg of body weight + 40 kcal/percent of body surface burn

Carbohydrate is the major source of calories and contributes to nitrogen sparing. The major carbohydrate form is glucose, and it must be administered with nitrogen-containing nutrients to improve nitrogen balance and allow more calories to be used for the restoration of nitrogen balance. Approximately 20% of caloric requirements should be protein or amino acid equivalents; improved survivals have been demonstrated with a 100:1 calorie to nitrogen ratio diet.[3] Essential fatty acids must also be provided, and 2% to 4% of daily calorie requirements should consist of linoleic acid.[64] In addition to preventing a fatty acid deficiency state, fat also provides extra calories. In patients with large burns, enteral tube feeding is almost always necessary to achieve nutritional goals. Most patients, when left to their own dietary habits, do not consume adequate nutrients orally. Generally a high-calorie, high-protein diet should be administered in addition to the calculated tube requirement. Further, vitamin and mineral requirements must be provided in all nutritional programs. Rarely is total parenteral nutrition indicated because it is fraught with a number of complications as discussed in Chapter 2.

Daily weight gain is the most effective single index for assessing the adequacy of nutritional support and must be continually monitored. Nitrogen balance studies generally are very inaccurate when large open wounds exist, and indices of immunologic status and visceral protein pool have not been shown to accurately predict specific nutritional deficiencies.[64]

ORGAN SYSTEM ALTERATIONS

Cardiovascular Responses

The initial cardiovascular response to extensive thermal injury is a fall in cardiac output of 50% of normal or greater. Hypovolemia and circulating serum factors probably derived from the burn wound have been cited as causes. As previously indicated, an unidentified circulating factor called myocardial depressant factor has been implicated in eliciting reduced cardiac contractility,[19,81,103] even though its existence has never been firmly established. There is usually an early transient rise in blood pressure; however, central venous pressure and pulmonary artery wedge pressures are generally low initially. All of these alterations are accompanied by an initial cutaneous vasoconstriction in unburned areas.

Most of these responses tend to normalize as plasma volume is restored through resuscitative efforts, although the cardiac output generally returns to normal and may actually exceed normal values before complete restoration of plasma volume. This resultant hyperdynamic circulatory response appears to complement the hypermetabolic response previously discussed, and both appear to reflect an effort of the body to heal the injured wound.

The increased cardiac output is associated with a major shift of blood flow to the burn wound. Blood flow studies in burned extremities have demonstrated that flow increases in the surface of the injured extremities, but not in injured extremities where the unburned skin remains vasoconstricted.[13,14] In contrast, perfusion in muscle remains the same in both burned and unburned extremities.[91] Therefore this increased blood flow in response to an increased cardiac output is a direct contributor to the metabolic and physiologic demands of the wound itself.

Renal Responses

The burn patient is initially in a state of antidiuresis. In the presence of a hyperdynamic circulatory response, oliguria occurs as a result of increased and inappropriate ADH secretion. It has also been shown that glomerular vessels become constricted, prolonging transit time through the kidney and decreasing urinary output. Metabolism within the kidney appears to increase as evidenced by a consistent uptake of glucose, whereas renal plasma flow remains essentially unaltered.[15,130]

Despite the glomerular vascular changes, renal complications are relatively uncommon in thermally injured patients with the improved knowledge of resuscitation over the past 10 to 15 years. The initial renal lesion following burn injury appears to be a biphasic proteinuria. The initial phase includes a mild, transient albuminuria followed in 4 to 7 days by a proteinuria with a relatively low albumin composition.[115] Any relationship between the proteinuria and the subsequent development of renal failure remains unclear. When renal failure does ensue, it proceeds characteristically with polyuria in the face of a rising serum creatinine.

Oliguric renal failure is quite rare. When it occurs, it develops early and appears to be related to inadequate resuscitation. In contrast, the more common polyuric renal failure generally arises in the second or third week following the burn injury and does not seem to be caused by hypovolemia. The findings of low urinary sodium and high urinary potassium indicate intact distal tubular function. These observations indicate that burn-related dysfunction in the glomerulus and proximal tubule presents the distal nephron with a solute load, producing a "downstream" diuresis.[98] The cause of this form of renal failure remains unknown and it is unique to the burn patient.

Endocrine Responses

A complex endocrine response is elicited by thermal injury that probably is related to peripheral nervous stimulation of the hypophyseal-hypothalamic axis of the brain that then in turn intricately interacts with metabolic, immune, and other body systems.[57] Sustained, elevated levels of adrenocorticotropic hormone (ACTH) from the anterior pituitary gland have been reported throughout the acute phase of thermal injury and only decrease to normal as the burn wound heals.[99] If one uses measurements of plasma cortisol as an index of ACTH secretion, however, no consistent patterns have been noted in burn patients.[121] Generally thyroid-stimulating hormone is suppressed or normal in burn injury. When suppressed, though, there is no evidence of clinical hypothyroidism in burn patients, and in fact many patients have signs suggestive of hyperthyroidism.

Growth hormone secretion is inconsistent in burn patients but often is elevated following thermal injury. Normally, growth hormone increases nitrogen storage and protein synthesis, but it appears that in the catabolic phase of thermal injury increased growth hormone secretion produces effects that are deleterious and characterized by increased urinary nitrogen losses and body weight loss. Gluconeogenesis appears to be enhanced, using amino acid substrate and producing urea. Follicle-stimulating hormone and luteinizing hormone secretion are depressed in burn patients, whereas prolactin secretion may be suppressed in children but elevated in adults.[83] The significance of these observations remains unknown.

Antidiuretic hormone (ADH) measurements reveal high levels in both blood and urine of adults and children during the first week after burn. Oversecretion is apparently independent of plasma and urine osmolality and volume but related closely to the severity of the thermal injury.[47]

Glucocorticoids, mineralocorticoids and 17-ketosteroids are the major hormonal groups secreted by the adrenal cortex. Cortisol is high in burn patients with loss of the normal circadian rhythm, particularly in the first week following thermal injury. This elevation is believed to be essentially unrelated to ACTH hypersecretion but does relate closely to the size of the burn.[47] Aldosterone is secreted in markedly increased amounts and produces sodium retention and increased potassium loss, which persists for many weeks in adults with major burns.[47] The 17-ketosteroids are also elevated in burn patients as measured in the urine, but the significance of this finding is unknown.

Adrenalin and nonadrenalin synthesis are dramatically increased in thermal injury as detected in the serum and urine of burn patients. Catecholamine elevation is indicative of increased adrenergic activity, which has been related to the extent of the burn and the increased oxygen consumption resulting therefrom. These findings suggest that catecholamines are major mediators of the hypermetabolic response.[124]

Immunoreactive insulin is elevated following thermal injury, and this elevation persists until healing of the burn wound. Insulin hypersecretion is usually accompanied by elevated glucose in the blood, implying a relative insulin resistance.[132] Plasma glucagon levels are also elevated and appear to play a key role in the hypermetabolic response.[23] It is thought that glucagon released from alpha cells of the pancreas is more influential in producing postburn hyperglycemia than the so-called insulin resistance.[24]

T4 and T3 blood levels are generally low in burn injury, although a less pronounced decrease in T4 and a transitory increase in reverse T3 have been identified.[22] The significance of these observed hormonal alterations is uncertain, since as, previously noted, there is no evidence of hypothyroidism in burn patients and in fact some patients have signs of hyperthyroidism. In addition, evidence exists suggesting that the thyroid may play a partial role in burn hypermetabolism.[97]

RESISTANCE TO INFECTION

Infection remains the most common cause of death in hospitalized burn patients. Resistance is impaired in these patients through disruption of the skin's mechanical barrier and defects in the body's immune system. Fauci[59] has conveniently classified the body's defense capabilities into the categories of nonspecific immune system and specific immune system. Although many defects in the capacity to resist infection have been defined in thermally injured patients, direct relationships between burning and immunologic alterations are complex and unclear and have eluded successful therapeutic intervention.

Disruption of the Skin's Mechanical Barrier

Loss of the morphologic and physiologic integrity of the skin as a result of thermal injury allows access of microorganisms to deeper tissues and the systemic circulation. Not only is devitalized tissue a nutritious medium for the growth of bacteria, but thermally injured skin may be a source of circulating substances or toxins that can contribute to multi-faceted, systemic alterations, including impairment in the synthesis of secretory immunoglobulins, bone marrow depression, and myocardial depression.[12,19,47,113]

Impairment of the Nonspecific Immune System

Phagocytic cell activity and accumulation are enhanced in response to tissue injury through an inflammatory reaction characterized by increased vascular permeability. This appears to be mediated by vasoactive amines, prostaglandins, C-reactive proteins, and other components of inflammation.[46] In addition, the release of chemotactic substances from injured tissues or through the influence of gram-negative organisms enhances the attraction of phagocytes to intruding microorganisms. Should bacteria not be contained at the site of invasion, the fixed macrophages, particularly in the regional lymph nodes, may prove effective in killing invading bacteria.

Opsonins are antibodies that enhance the phagocytic process by rendering the microorganisms more susceptible to phagocytosis. Complement and fibronectin are characterized opsonins. Complement is a system of serum proteins that participates in inflammation and phagocytosis and in neutralizing viruses, enhancing leukocyte chemotaxis and killing bacteria. Fibronectin is a glycoprotein existing in a soluble circulating form in the plasma and a relatively insoluble form in connective tissue. Fibronectin enhances macrophage phagocytosis and may prevent organ failure through inhibition of fibrin aggregation among other functions. Other undefined regional defense mechanisms also participate in protecting the host from hostile microorganisms.

The presence of major thermal injury adversely affects this nonspecific inflammatory protective system. Both circulating and fixed phagocytic cells, with or without the help of opsonizing factors, are functionally impaired following a major burn. Not only is phagocytic activity decreased in burn injury, but bacteriocidal activity is also decreased and chemotaxis is impaired through decreased complement activation.[2,88,122]

Impairment of the Specific Immune System

The specific immune system includes both humoral and cellular components and their respective products. The production of specific antibody requires a complex interaction of many cell types. Once an antigen is recognized, it is processed by macrophages and presented to "thymic-dependent" lymphocytes (T cells). T cells proliferate and in turn activate bursal-dependent lymphocytes (B cells) that ultimately produce a specific antibody to the antigen. Stimulated T lymphocytes have other important functions such as antigen memory storage, direct cytotoxic effects, and production of mediators of immune reactivity regulating both the specific and nonspecific immune responses and including such mediators as macrophage inhibition factor.

Antibody formation is influenced by a specific subset of T cells known as T helper cells and a second subset known as T suppressor cells. T suppressor cells generally modulate responses preventing uncontrolled immune reactions by inhibiting T cell stimulation of antibody production. Interleukin I is produced by macrophages and is active in antigen processing; interleukin II is produced by T cells and is effective in subsequent functions. Other factors involved in a specific immune response include interferon, B cell–activating factor and various growth factors.[88]

In patients with burns on more than 20% of their total body surface area, essentially all immune functions are affected. This is especially true of the T cells.[88] Following burning, T cell concentrations are decreased in peripheral blood, whereas the B cell population is relatively normal.[93] T suppressor cell activity is increased, whereas helper activity decreases. This depresses T cell–generated responses, including production of cytotoxic cells, B cell activation, and recruitment of uncommitted lymphoid cells to an immune function. Immunoglobulin synthesis is also decreased, particularly IgG production, in contrast to IgM and IgA, which are altered very little. Factors that may be responsible for these specific immune system alterations include prostaglandins, leukotrienes, endotoxin, and so-called "burn toxins."[94] Various anesthetic agents used during debridement and grafting of burn wounds are also thought to play a role in immunosuppression in burn victims.[94]

PULMONARY CONSEQUENCES OF THERMAL INJURY

Pulmonary alterations as a result of thermal injury occur in response to direct pulmonary injury caused by the inhalation of the products of combustion and indirectly as a response to cutaneous burns alone.

Inhalation of the Products of Combustion

Inhalation injury accounts for the vast majority of deaths in fires and is responsible for the high mortality in patients who survive to be admitted to hospitals. The following classification has proven useful in categorizing the various disorders related to inhalation injury and is based on mechanisms of disease[118]:

1. Carbon monoxide poisoning
2. Smoke toxicity
   a. Direct injury caused by
      (1) Hot gases
      (2) Super-heated particulate matter
      (3) Conversion of gases to acid and alkali
   b. Smoke poisoning caused by thermodegradation of
      (1) Natural substances
      (2) Synthetic substances

Carbon Monoxide Poisoning

Carbon monoxide is a clear, colorless, odorless gas produced by the incomplete combustion of organic fuels. Carbon monoxide has an affinity for hemoglobin that is approximately 250 times that of oxygen and shifts the oxyhemoglobin dissociation curve to the left. Thus the oxygen that remains bound to hemoglobin is not readily available to cells, resulting in a decreased tissue oxygen tension that is considerably lower than that seen with simple hypoxia (Fig. 64-8). The toxic effect of carbon monoxide may be the result of this hypoxia alone or binding to heme-containing proteins at the cellular level.[56] Carbon

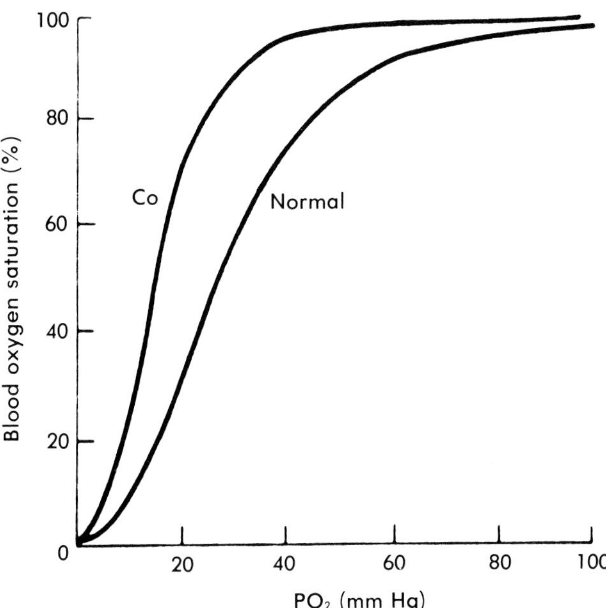

Fig. 64-8 Oxygen-hemoglobin dissociation curve. Note the shift to the left in the presence of carbon monoxide (CO), indicating that oxygen is more tightly bound to the hemoglobin molecule.

monoxide impairs the cytochrome chain through competition with oxygen for cytochrome a_3 and has been observed to have a direct toxic effect on mammalian lung tissue.[107] Carbon monoxide also binds to cardiac and skeletal muscle, producing carboxymyoglobin that dissociates slower than carboxyhemoglobin. This circumstance may become apparent during initial treatment as a rebound type of response. Pure carbon monoxide poisoning produces no grossly detectable lung pathologic alteration although, histologically, alveolar Type II cellular organelles are physically altered.[70]

The clinical symptoms of carbon monoxide poisoning range from dyspnea and headache at levels of 10% to 20% to coma and death when inspired air contains levels in excess of 60%. Cherry red skin discoloration is usually not apparent because of facial burning, but a high index of suspicion based on the history of burning in an enclosed space, orofacial burns, and nasal hair singeing suggests the diagnosis. A laboratory carboxyhemoglobin determination confirms the diagnosis, and treatment consists of rapid evacuation from the toxic source and the administration of 100% oxygen, preferably by endotracheal tube, in symptomatic poisoning. The half-life of carboxyhemoglobin in room air is approximately 210 minutes, but on 100% oxygen it can be reduced to 40 to 60 minutes. Hyperbaric oxygen has been proposed as a treatment modality in severe poisoning on the basis of a rapid decrease in the half-life of carboxyhemoglobin and clinical evidence of improved neurologic recovery.[89]

Smoke Toxicity

Direct Injury. Direct heat injury as a result of inhalation of hot gases is extremely rare below the vocal cords because of the efficiency of heat dissipatory reflexes.[86] However, more proximally, oropharyngeal burns causing local edema may occur, and single-dose steroids have been recommended for the control of such edema. Direct parenchymal injury to the epithelium in distal air passages, however, may be observed by the inhalation of superheated steam that has 4000 times the heat capacity of air. Superheated particulate matter and soot that is not filtered out in the proximal airways may produce local thermal burns in the alveoli.[42]

Corrosive acids and alkalis resulting from the reaction of sulfur and nitrogen oxides adherent to soot particles with lung surface water also produce direct, local parenchymal injury, although the pathophysiology is uncertain and the extent of such injury is difficult to define.[118]

Smoke Poisoning. The incomplete combustion of both natural and synthetic products in smoke produces noxious gases that are inhaled and elicit both local and systemic effects. The magnitude of injury depends on the type of noxious gas inhaled, its concentration and solubility, and the duration of exposure. Water-soluble chemicals such as ammonia, sulfur dioxide, chlorine, and hydrogen chloride tend to dissolve in the upper respiratory tract, whereas lipid-soluble gases such as the aldehydes, phosgene, and nitric oxide tend to reach more distal lung radicals.[43] Cyanide, a product of the combustion of synthetic materials such as polyurethane, produces its effects through systemic absorption and cellular poisoning.

The effect of inhaled toxic products includes direct epithelial destruction, mucosal edema, ciliary paralysis, and surfactant deficiency, the latter resulting from injury to Type II alveolar epithelial cells.[21,102] Pulmonary alveolar macrophages secrete chemotaxins producing leukocyte sequestration, which in turn releases proteolytic enzymes and oxygen-free radicals that potentiate pulmonary injury from the microvascular side.[70] Subsequent pathologic alterations depend on the severity and character of the inhalation and include a fulminant adult respiratory distress syndrome (ARDS), pulmonary edema, bronchial pneumonia, and sepsis, all of which contribute to the high mortality rate observed in patients with inhalation injury.

The diagnosis of smoke inhalation is based primarily on history, blood gas analysis, carboxyhemoglobin, and cyanide determinations, as well as on special procedures, including bronchoscopy, xenon clearance, and pulmonary function tests. Physical examination and chest x-ray films, although essential, may be misleading, particularly under acute conditions when a paucity of physical signs tends to be the rule even in severe inhalation injury.

Careful monitoring of patients suspected of sustaining smoke poisoning is essential. In less severe injuries, treatment consists of the use of humidified air, vigorous pulmonary toilet, and the judicious use of bronchodilators. In severe poisoning intubation with a soft cuff nasotracheal tube and the use of a volume-cycled ventilator with carefully controlled positive end expiratory pressure is indicated. Invasive monitoring to include pulmonary wedge pressure and thermodilution cardiac output parameters is often essential, particularly when positive end-expiratory pressure is used. Although evidence suggests that steroids are not indicated in the management of smoke toxicity,[87] the high incidence of pulmonary infection in these patients dictates the use of broad-spectrum antibiotics.

Indirect Pulmonary Injury

Pulmonary edema following pure cutaneous burning without inhalation injury relates to alterations in the pulmonary microvasculature. Hemodynamic alterations related to resuscitation, increased capillary permeability, and alterations in blood flow characteristics as a result of cutaneous thermal injury may contribute to indirect lung damage. Recently, patients with major thermal injury and noninhalation pulmonary dysfunction have been shown to have consistently high concentrations of fragment D resulting from fibrinogen degradation. This phenomenon is associated with systemic complement depletion and platelet aggregation with release of platelet products that may cause increased translocation of water and protein from the pulmonary microcirculation contributing to the development of an ARDS picture.[44] In addition, activated complement may stimulate leukocyte aggregation, resulting in trapping of these aggregates in the pulmonary microcirculation. These leukocytes may then produce extremely toxic oxygen metabolites that may also contribute to the development of ARDS. Later pulmonary alterations generally relate to the onset of sepsis and may also manifest themselves as ARDs or bronchial pneumonia. Current therapies are primarily directed toward supportive intervention, but mortality from the pulmonary manifestations of burns remains high. For a more detailed discussion of these considerations, see Chapter 35.

PHYSIOLOGIC CONSIDERATIONS IN MANAGING THE BURN PATIENT

Fluid Resuscitation

The most important priority in the initial management of the burn patient is fluid resuscitation. The pathophysiologic alterations caused by the fluid losses in acutely burned patients requires volume replacement to preserve vital functions and to prevent hypovolemic shock. Fluid losses as a result of increased capillary permeability in injured and noninjured tissues are greatest in the first 24 hours following burning and diminish thereafter. Accompanying intravascular deficits also need to be corrected but generally are less responsive to resuscitative efforts until the volume losses from "capillary leaking" are adequately controlled.

The optimum approach to fluid resuscitation remains controversial in terms of both the volume of fluid to be administered and its composition. A wide variety of fluid replacement formulas have been proposed over the years,* each with its advocates, differing primarily from one another with respect to salt and colloid content. Virtually all fluid formulas are based on patient weight and the extent of skin surface burned. Only burns reaching a depth of second degree or greater are considered in these calculations. The fluid formulas provide guidelines for the resuscitation of burn patients and are altered according to the response to treatment.

The effectiveness of administered fluid in early burn resuscitation with regard to its colloidal or noncolloidal content remains unresolved. Advocates of colloid-containing fluids recognize their potential use in maintaining plasma

*References 18, 39, 58, 84, 96, and 106.

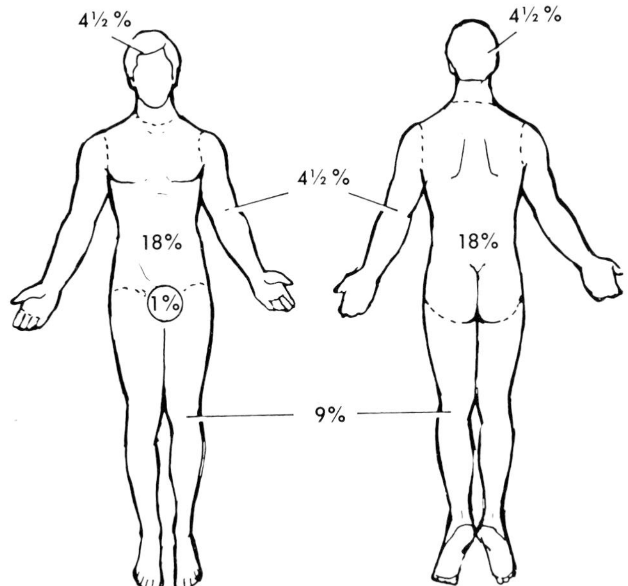

Fig. 64-9 "Rule of Nines" for adults. Rapid estimation of extent of burn injury can be accomplished by using the "Rule of Nines" as an approximation of body surface areas involved. (From Parks, D.H., Carvajal, H.F., and Larson, D.L.: Surg. Clin. North Am. **57:**875, 1977.)

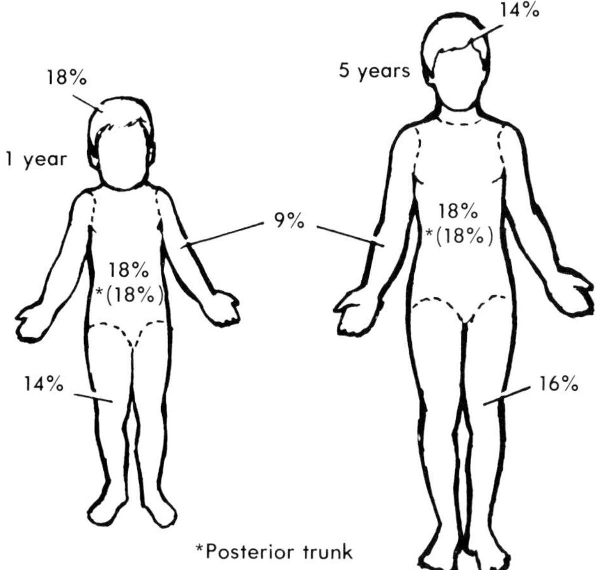

Fig. 64-10 Modified "Rule of Nines" for ages 1 and 5. Adult proportions assumed at age 15. (From Parks, D.H., Carvajal, H.F., and Larson, D.L.: Surg. Clin. North Am. **57:**875, 1977.)

oncotic pressure and intravascular volume. Those opposed to such solutions emphasize the increased capillary permeability in the first 24 hours after thermal injury that results in leakage of plasma protein, particularly albumin, into the interstitium. It is argued that adding exogenous protein (i.e., colloid) to the extravascular protein pool raises this interstitial oncotic pressure further and thereby prevents restoration of an adequate circulating blood volume. There is general agreement, however, that the administration of colloid-containing fluids during the second 24 hours following burn and thereafter is associated with intravascular colloid retention and thus decreased fluid requirements.

In contrast to the colloid controversy, sodium ion administration appears to be essential to successful resuscitation. Balanced salt solutions are quite popular and effective, although the use of hypertonic saline solutions has been recommended.[84] The decreased volume loading with hypertonic solutions may be particularly useful in the elderly patient or in patients with cardiovascular compromise in whom excessive volume may be detrimental.

Body surface charts are available for the determination of surface area burned and are based on delineating body surface components (e.g., head, back, extremity) as a percentage of the whole body surface[35,79,96] (Figs. 64-9 and 64-10). This method improves the accuracy of the determination and provides the basis for the use of the various formulas. Patients with second- and third-degree burns involving greater than 15% of their body surface area should receive parenteral fluids, and the effectiveness of resuscitation should be monitored precisely.

An Approach to Resuscitation

The replacement program that we used has proven to be convenient and successful over many years of application and will be described. In this program, losses of fluid and daily maintenance requirements are related to the total body surface area and the surface area burned (in square meters) as calculated from a standard height-weight nomogram. This approach has proven to be highly accurate and allows standardization of fluid therapy in managing both adults and children. During the first 24 hours following burning, fluid requirements are calculated as follows:

2000 ml/m^2 of body surface per 24 hours
(maintenance requirements)
+
5000 ml/m^2 of body surface burned per 24 hours
(fluid losses)

One half of the calculated volume is infused in the first 8 hours following burning, and the remainder in the subsequent 16 hours. During this first 24-hour period the patient should not receive oral fluids except for the administration of antacids, which are given hourly by a nasogastric tube to prevent the development of Curling's ulcers (see Chapter 16).

For such resuscitation, a single, standard solution for intravenous therapy is used with adaptation to the patient's needs as necessary. This solution consists of:

Lactated Ringer's solution in 5% dextrose and water
+
12.5 g of salt-poor albumin per liter

We have found such a solution to be ideal. This isotonic protein-containing fluid ensures the provision of lactate to combat any systemic acidosis and an adequate carbohydrate load to ensure protein-sparing. Because of the hyperkalemia associated with tissue injury, addition of potassium to this solution during the first 48 hours after burning is inappropriate and may be detrimental.

During the second 24 hours following burning, fluid requirements generally decrease, and oral fluid administration is begun. The fluid requirements during this second 24-hour period are calculated on the basis of the following formula:

1500 ml/m^2 of body surface area per 24 hours
(maintenance requirements)
+
4000 ml/m^2 of burned body surface area per 24 hours
(fluid losses)

Such requirements are administered in equal hourly aliquots over this 24-hour period. Assuming that oral alimentation can be initiated, oral fluid in the form of homogenized milk is given, and the intravenous fluid needs decreased proportionately. When the milk intake increases sufficiently, the antacid therapy begun during the first 24 hours is decreased. In most cases oral fluid administration will completely replace intravenous therapy at the end of 48 hours following burning, allowing removal of the intravenous catheter.

Daily fluid requirements after the initial 48 hours of fluid resuscitation generally remain the same as those for the second 24 hours; but, as the burn wounds are covered and healing commences, requirements are generally diminished, and fluid therapy revised accordingly. As already indicated, initial oral alimentation is usually administered through a nasogastric feeding tube that is retained for several days thereafter to ensure adequate oral nutrition. Until the convalescent phase is well underway, milk should continue to be given on an hourly basis to protect the stomach from the development of a Curling's ulcer. In those patients who have a lactate deficiency, a soy-based formula should be substituted. Patients should be started on regular meals in addition to this milk diet as soon as such alimentation can be adequately tolerated.

As indicated in an earlier section of this chapter, the burn patient remains in a hypermetabolic state requiring high caloric support until wound coverage has been achieved. It has been estimated that evaporative losses alone may amount to 4 L/m^2 of the burn area, which results in an expenditure of 576 kcal/L of water evaporated. Thus, to ensure adequate caloric intake in the burn patient, the following formula has been used by the authors:

1800 calories per m^2 of body surface per 24 hours
+
2200 calories per m^2 of body surface burned per 24 hours

Milk by itself provides approximately 0.66 calories per milliliter of fluid administered. With the additional calories provided by a regular diet, most caloric requirements can be adequately met. If there is any problem in ensuring this possibility, nutritional needs should be guaranteed by the administration of appropriate feeding regimens through a nasogastric feeding tube.

Monitoring Fluid Resuscitation

The effectiveness of the resuscitation program must be constantly monitored and altered if deviations from the expected course are noted. Among the most useful physical signs to determine the adequacy of resuscitation are the general appearance and state of alertness of the patient and the stability of pulse and blood pressure, including peripheral perfusion characteristics. The urine output (by means of an indwelling urinary catheter) is the most readily obtained measure of effectiveness of resuscitation, and a urine volume of 30 to 50 ml/hour in the adult and 20 to 40 ml/m^2 of total body surface area per hour in children is expected. A significantly higher urine output may indicate overhydration or other complications (e.g., poluric renal failure, excessive glucose loading), since in the acutely burned patient an antidiuretic state caused by multiple factors, including ADH secretion, is present.

Baseline laboratory studies should be obtained at the time of admission and repeated in 12 and 24 hours or more frequently as needed. Among the values to be obtained initially are a complete blood cell count; serum levels of sodium, potassium, chloride and bicarbonate; a blood urea nitrogen and creatinine, urine protein, and serum protein electrophoresis; and arterial blood gases. An initial hemoconcentration is expected, regardless of the resuscitation program instituted; and therefore an elevated hematocrit and slight elevation of other parameters may be identified. Metabolic acidosis is particularly significant in children and may indicate inadequacy of resuscitation.

A chest x-ray film, electrocardiogram, and complete urinalysis are usually performed on admission and repeated only as indicated during the subsequent course. Invasive monitoring with Swan-Ganz catheters or central venous lines is not routinely performed except in elderly patients, patients with cardiovascular compromise, or patients with inhalation injury requiring machine ventilation.

The timely administration of carefully monitored parenteral fluids to the acutely and extensively burned patient facilitating the body's own compensatory physiologic alterations will prevent early complications, minimize physiologic disturbances, and provide a basis on which future care of the acutely burned patient depends.

Management of the Burn Wound

After fluid resuscitation has been successfully ensured, attention is next directed to the burn wound itself. The wound is cleansed with a suitable antiseptic solution such as povidone-iodine (Betadine) and debrided of foreign matter, necrotic tissue, and any blebs or vesicles that may be present. Since hypothermia may be a problem during this debridement period, overhead radiant energy sources are usually used to minimize the loss of body heat.

Because the burn wound is essentially an extensive area of coagulation necrosis with accompanying ischemia from the underlying thrombosis of the local microcirculation, this avascular dead tissue is an excellent bacterial culture medium that can rapidly become a source of bacterial growth and the development of sepsis from hematologic dissemination of microorganisms. For this reason topical antimicrobial agents are applied directly on the burn wound during the early period after the burn. In the historical development of burn management over the past several decades, a variety of agents have been developed for this purpose, each with its particular advantages and disadvantages. Presently four such agents are in use at burn centers across the United States as summarized in Table 64-1. Each of these agents, in varying degrees, sat-

Table 64-1 **TOPICAL ANTIMICROBIAL AGENTS**

Characteristics	(0.5%) Silver Nitrate	Mafenide	Silver Sulfadiazine	Organic Iodine
Type of preparation	Aqueous solution	Cream	Cream	Foam
Method of wound care	Closed	Open or closed	Open or closed	Open or closed
Allergic reactions	None	10%	10%	5%
Pain on application	None	Severe	None	Moderate
Amount absorbed	None	5%	1%	Variable
Associated complications	Significant losses of Na and K into wet dressings, methemoglobinemia	Acidosis, hyperventilation caused by renal carbonic anhydase inhibition	None	None
Fungal overgrowth	—	Often	Often	Often
Bacterial resistance	Bacteriostatic	Rare	Rare	Occasional
Cost	Inexpensive	Moderate	Moderate	Moderate

Modified from Curreri, P.W.: Burns. In H.C. Polk, Stone, H.H., and Gardner, B., editors: Basic surgery, ed. 3., Norwalk, Conn., 1987, Appleton-Century-Crofts.

isfies the characteristics of an ideal topical agent, which include: (1) anti-bacterial activity that is both broad spectrum in nature and nontoxic locally or on absorption, (2) resistance to the development of strains of bacteria that would not be covered, (3) adequate permeation and the maintenance of continuing activity in the burn eschar, (4) absence of pain on application, and (5) absence of adverse effects on the behavior of the wound, including its healing properties. Of the agents currently available, 1% silver sulfadiazine is the most popular among burn specialists and is our choice. This drug is essentially nontoxic, is easy to apply and soothing to the patient, and has a broad spectrum of antimicrobial activity and minimal problems with the development of resistant strains. Its only major disadvantage is its limited penetration through the eschar and its relative ineffectiveness when deep eschar colonization with microorganisms has already occurred. When the latter circumstance exists, a gentamycin cream is usually substituted if the cultured organisms are sensitive. Silver sulfadiazine is applied in a thin layer (usually 1 mm thick) two or three times daily, using a sterile glove or tongue depressor. Although some specialists leave the treated burn wound open to the air, we generally apply a thin layer of fine mesh gauze impregnated with the cream over the treated burn area and further retain it with a netlike dressing.[96] This approach allows patients to move about freely and guarantees contact of the cream with the burn wound at all times. At the present time, all first-degree and superficial second-degree burns are managed in this fashion, enabling spontaneous reepithelialization to occur.

For deep-second degree burns and all third-degree burns, early surgical excision is now considered the procedure of choice.[96] For deep partial-thickness burn wounds, a technique called *tangential excision* is used. This technique involves the excision of the necrotic surface of a burn by removing shavings of eschar until a pattern of pin-point deep dermal bleeding is reached and then immediately autografting the excised surface. The rationale underlying this approach is that the removal of the zone of coagulation protects the viable elements in the zone of stasis and thereby exposes a surface that readily accepts an autograft. As much as 20% of the body surface may be excised at one time. The major problem with this technique is that considerable blood loss may occur, necessitating the need for substantial blood replacement (particularly in major burns in which such excision may need to be repeated several times within a period of days) and the careful monitoring of anesthesia to prevent other problems such as shock with its attendant complications. For full-thickness burns, excision is carried down to the level of the fascia, and an autograft is then placed on the exposed base. These aggressive surgical approaches to burn management have demonstrated several advantages to the more traditional methods of debridement using various proteolytic enzymes, the most popular of which has been sutilains (Travase). Such advantages have included improved function of extremities (particularly hands), a better cosmetic result, a definite decrease in the incidence of hypertrophic scarring after the burn, and a considerable reduction in hospitalization time.

In the event that a patient may have extensive body burns limiting the amount of nonburn areas that can be used for the acquisition of skin grafts, temporary coverage of the surgically debrided burn may be obtained with various biologic dressings, including amnion or procine xenografts. A more recent innovative approach has been the use of artificial skin. Several types of synthetic skin have been evaluated investigationally. Of these, the bilaminate membrane appears to be the most useful.[32] This substance consists of reconstituted collagen with a silicon synthetic epidermis. Application of this substance to the debrided burn surface results in vascularization of the collagen layer with the production of an underlying neodermis. When donor sites become available, the silicon synthetic epidermis is stripped from the underlying collagen, and an autograft placed on the neodermis. Initial results with such an approach have proven quite gratifying and open up exciting possibilities in the management of burn wounds in the future.

A unique problem that occasionally develops with deep second-degree or third-degree circumferential burns, especially when involving the extremities or trunk, is the resulting tourniquet effect. This occurs because the elastic membrane of the dermis is destroyed with these types of burns and no longer allows the skin to stretch, which is necessary to accommodate the underlying edema formation. In the chest such circumferential eschar formation may prevent normal respiration. If not corrected, the rapid development of respiratory acidosis may ensue. When this problem exists, incision through the eschar should be carried out and deepened into the subcutaneous fat to effect adequate release of the constricted tissue. This can be accomplished by making vertical anterior axillary line incisions that are curved medially to the level of the suprasternal notch. In addition, transverse incisions at the level of the diaphragm will effect further release of the constricted tissue. In the extremities eschar constriction often results in a decreased venous outflow from the affected part and in time jeopardizes the arterial inflow. Ischemia then results, which may be manifest by decreased capillary refill of the nail beds, severe pain within the involved muscle compartment of the extremity, or the development of motor and/or sensory deficits. Often, elevation of the affected extremity may allay the need for escharotomy, but continuous monitoring of the peripheral pulse, usually with an ultrasound detector, must be assured. If this cannot be guaranteed, lateral longitudinal incisions through the burn eschar should be made to the level of the subcutaneous fat to release the pressure in the constricted muscle compartments. Both extremity escharotomies and those involving the chest can generally be performed without the assistance of anesthesia, since the burn wound is usually insensitive to painful stimuli.

SUMMARY

The disruption of the physiologic equilibrium of the human organism by thermal injury varies with the extent and depth of the burn. The burn wound is characterized by a central irreversible zone of coagulation necrosis surrounded by reversibly altered tissues that may be irreversibly compromised by progressive ischemia as a result of systemic factors such as hypoperfusion and local factors such as prostaglandin derivatives. Major fluid shifts caused by permeability alterations occur as a result of physical changes in the microcirculatory ultrastructure and local release of vasoactive substances. Such alterations disrupt normal Starling forces and potentiate these fluid losses. Additional fluid extravasation in unburned tissues contributes to the hypovolemic state and may relate to increased capillary permeability and plasma oncotic pressure alterations.

Thermal injury induces a state of marked hypermetabolism mediated by catecholamines and requires an intense nutritional replacement program to overcome the potentially disastrous consequences of malnutrition. The initial fall in cardiac output observed in burn patients that is possibly related to an unidentified myocardial depressant serum factor released from the burn wound is followed by an intense hyperdynamic circulatory response. A state of antidiuresis is induced, and the hormonal milieu of the body is dramatically altered in concert with the metabolic and immune alterations.

Resistance to infection is severely compromised in thermally injured patients through alterations in both nonspecific and specific immune systems. Thermally altered tissue allows access of microorganisms and provides a medium for bacterial growth. Phagocytic activity is decreased along with bacteriocidal activity within the phagocytes. T cell populations are decreased in peripheral blood, and T suppressor cell activity is increased, whereas T helper cell activity and other beneficial responses are depressed.

Smoke inhalation is responsible for the majority of deaths in fires. Carbon monoxide poisoning is the most common mechanism of injury, and, if treated quickly enough with oxygen, a successful outcome can be realized. Smoke toxicity as a result of direct injury to the airways or smoke poisoning caused by inhalation of thermodegradation of natural and synthetic substances is less well understood. Therapy has been primarily directed toward supportive care. Until the pathophysiology of this pulmonary injury is better understood, the prognosis for these patients will remain poor.

Understanding the pathophysiologic events that occur in response to a burn has significantly improved care of the burned patient over the past several decades not only by decreasing morbidity but also by enhancing survival. Particularly germane in this regard has been the recognition of the need for aggressive fluid resuscitation in the first 24 hours following burning and the importance of controlling bacterial colonization of the burn wound with its potentially deleterious effects should infection and sepsis supervene.

REFERENCES

1. Alberti K.G., et al.: Relative roles of various hormones in mediating the metabolic response to injury, J. Parent. Enteral Nutr. **4:**141, 1980.
2. Alexander, J.W., and Wixson, D.: Neutrophil dysfunction of polymorphonuclear leukocytes in patients with burns and other trauma, Surg. Gynecol. Obstet. **130:**431, 1970.
3. Alexander, J.W., McMillan, B., and Stinnett, J.: Beneficial effects of aggressive protein feeding in severely burned children, Ann. Surg. **192:**505, 1980.
4. Anggard, E., Arturson, G., and Jonsson, C.E.: Effect of prostaglandins in lymph from scalded tissues, Acta Physiol. Scand. **80:**46, 1970.
5. Arturson, G.: The plasma kinins in thermal injury, Scand. J. Clin. Lab. Invest. (suppl.) **24**(107):153, 1969.
6. Arturson, G.: Microvascular permeability to macromolecules in thermal injury, Acta Physiol. Scand. (suppl.) **463:**111, 1979.
7. Arturson, G.: Pathophysiology of the burn wound, Ann. Chir. Gynecol. **69:**178, 1980.
8. Arturson, G.: The pathophysiology of severe thermal injury, J. Burn Care Rehab. **6:**129, 1985.
9. Arturson, G., and Mellander, S.: Acute changes in capillary filtration and diffusion in experimental burn injury, Acta Physiol. Scand. **62:**457, 1964.
10. Arturson G., and Jonsson, C.E.: Transcapillary transport after thermal injury, Scand. J. Plast. Reconstr. Surg. **13:**29, 1979.
11. Arturson, G., Hamberg, M., and Jonsson, C.E.: Prostaglandins in human burn blister fluid, Acta Physiol. Scand. **82:**270, 1973.
12. Asko-Seljavaara, S., Sundell, B., and Rytomaa, T.: The effect of early excision on bone-marrow cell growth in burned mice, Burns **2,3:**140, 1976.
13. Aulick, L.H., and Wilmore, D.W.: Leg amino acid turnover in burn patients, Fed. Proc. **37:**536, 1978.
14. Aulick, L.H., et al.: Influence of the burn wound on peripheral circulation in thermally injured patients, Am. J. Physiol. **237:**901, 1977.
15. Aulick, L.H., et al.: Visceral blood flow following thermal injury, Ann. Surg. **193:**112, 1981.

16. Bartlett, R.H., et al.: Nutritional therapy based on positive caloric balance in burn patients, Arch. Surg. **112**:974, 1977.
17. Baxter, C.R.: Fluid volume and electrolyte changes in the early post-burn period, Clin. Plast. Surg. **1**:693, 1974.
18. Baxter, C.R., and Shires, G.T.: Physiologic response to crystaloid resuscitation of severe burns, Ann. N.Y. Acad. Sci. **150**:874, 1968.
19. Baxter, C.R., Cook, W.A., and Shires, G.T.: Serum myocardial depressant factor of burn shock, Surg. Forum **17**:1, 1966.
20. Baxter, C.R., et al.: Excretion of serotinin metabolites following thermal injury, Surg. Forum **14**:61, 1963.
21. Beal, D.D., Lambeth, J.R., and Conner, G.H.: Follow-up studies on patients treated with steroids following pulmonary thermal and acrid smoke injury, Laryngoscope **78**:396, 1967.
22. Becker R.A., Wilmore D.W., and Goodwin C.W.: Free T4, free T3 and reverse T3 in critically ill, thermally injured patients, J. Trauma **20**:713, 1980.
23. Becker, R.A., et al.: Relation of glucagon and other non-thyroidal hormones to resting hypermetabolism after burn injury, abstracted from The Seventh International Congress of Endocrinology, Quebec, 1984.
24. Bingham, H.G., et al.: Burn diabetes: a review, J. Burn Care Rehab. **33**:179, 1982.
25. Bjork, J., et al.: The possible involvement of free radicals in acute edema formation after mild thermal injury, Microvasc. Res. **17**:S104, 1979.
26. Blackburn, G.L., et al.: Branched chain amino acid administration and metabolism during starvation, injury, and infection, Surgery **86**:307, 1979.
27. Boykin J.V., and Crute, S.L.: Mechanisms of burn shock protection after severe scald injury by cold-water treatment, J. Trauma **22**:859, 1982.
28. Boykin, J.V., Eriksson, E., and Pittman, R.N.: Microcirculation of a scald burn: an "in vivo" experimental study of the hairless mouse ear, Burns **7**:335, 1981.
29. Branemark, P-I., et al.: Microvascular pathophysiology of burned tissue, Ann. N. Y. Acad. Sci. **150**:474, 1968.
30. Brimblecombe, R.W., et al.: Histamine H2 receptor antagonists and thermal injury in rats, Burns **3**:8, 1976.
31. Burge, P.D., and Gilbert, S.J.: Effect of a histamine H2 receptor antagonist on the swelling of the burned hand, Burns **6**:30, 1979.
32. Burke, J.F., et al.: Successful use of a physiologically acceptable artificial skin in the treatment of extensive burn injury, Ann. Surg. **194**:413, 1981.
33. Caldwell, F.T.: Energy metabolism following thermal burns, Arch. Surg. **111**:181, 1976.
34. Carney, S.A., Hall, M., and Ricketts, C.R.: The adenosine triphosphate content and lactic acid production of guinea pig skin after mild heat damage, Br. J. Dermatol. **94**:291, 1976.
35. Carvajal, H.F.: A physiologic approach to fluid therapy in severely burned children, Surg. Gynecol. Obstet. **150**:379, 1980.
36. Carvajal, H.F., and Linares, H.A.: Effect of burn depth upon oedema formation and albumin extravasation in rats, Burns **7**:79, 1980.
37. Carvajal, H.F., Reinhart, J.A., and Traber, D.L.: Renal and cardiovascular functional response to thermal injury in dogs subjected to sympathetic blockade, Circ. Shock **3**:287, 1976.
38. Clayton, J.M., et al.: Sequential circulatory changes in the circumferentially burned limb, Ann. Surg. **185**:391, 1977.
39. Cope, O., and Moore, F.D.: The redistribution of body water in the fluid therapy of the burned patient, Ann. Surg. **126**:1013 (footnote), 1947.
40. Cotran, R.S., and Majno, G.: The delayed and prolonged vascular leakage in inflammation. I. Topography of the leaking vessels after thermal injury, Am. J. Pathol **45**:261, 1964.
41. Cottam, G.L., Mitchell, M.D., and Baxter, C.R.: Measurement of 13,14-dihydro-keto-Prostaglandin F and 11-deoxy-13,14-dihydro-keto-11,16-cyclo Prostaglandin E2 in human plasma following thermal injury, J. Burn Care Rehab. **5**:324, 1984.
42. Cox M.E., et al.: The Dellwood Fire, Br. Med. J. **1**:942, 1955.
43. Crapo R.O.: Smoke inhalation injuries. JAMA **264**:1694, 1981.
44. Curreri, P.W.: Supportive therapy in burn care, J. Trauma **21**(suppl):724, 1981.
45. Curreri, P.W., et al.: Dietary requirements of patients with major burns, J. Am. Diet. Assoc. **65**:415, 1974.
46. Daniels J.C., et al.: Serum protein profiles in thermal burns: II. Protease inhibitors, complement factors, and C-reactive protein, J. Trauma **14**:153, 1972.
47. Davies, J.W.L.: Physiological responses to burning injury, 1982, Academic Press, Inc.
48. deCamara, D.L., Heggers, J.P., and Robson, M.C.: Response of mast cell granules to thermal injury, Surg. Forum **32**:560, 1981.
49. deCamara, D.L., Raine, T., and Robson, M.C.: Ultrastructural aspects of cooled thermal injury, J. Trauma **21**:911, 1981.
50. DelBeccaro, E.J., et al.: The use of specific thromboxane inhibitors to preserve the dermal microcirculation after burning, Surgery **87**:137, 1980.
51. Demling R.H.: Burns, N. Engl. J. Med. **313**:1389, 1985.
52. Demling, R.H., Mazess, R.B., and Woldberg, W.H.: The effect of immediate and delayed cold immersion on burn edema formation and resorption, J. Trauma **19**:56, 1979.
53. Demling, R.H., Kramer, G.C., and Harms, B.: Role of thermal injury-induced hypoproteinemia on edema formation in burned and nonburned tissue, Surgery **95**:136, 1984.
54. Demling, R.H., et al.: The study of burn wound edema using dichromatic absorptionmetry, J. Trauma **18**:124, 1978.
55. Demling, R.H., et al.: Effect of nonprotein colloid on postburn edema formation in soft tissues and lung, Surgery **95**:593, 1984.
56. Dolan M.C.: Carbon monoxide poisoning. CMAT **133**:392, 1985.
57. Dolovek, R.: The endocrine response after burns: its possible correlations with the immunology of burns, J. Burn Care Rehab. **6**:281, 1985.
58. Evans, E.I., et al.: Fluid and electrolyte requirements in severe burns, Ann. Surg. **135**:804, 1952.
59. Fauci, A.: Host defense mechanisms against infection, Current concepts/scope publication, Kalamazoo, Mich. 1978, Upjohn Co.
60. Felig, P.: The glucose-alanine cycle, Metabolism **22**:179, 1973.
61. Ferguson, M., Eriksson, E., and Robson, M.C.: Effect of methylprednisolone on oedema formation after a major burn, Burns, **5**:293, 1979.
62. Fiser, R.H., Denniston, J.C., and Beisel, W.R.: Infection with Diplococcus pneumoniae and Salmonella typhimurium in monkeys: changes in plasma lipids and lipid proteins, J. Infect. Dis. **125**:54, 1972.
63. Freund, H., et al.: The role of the branched-chain amino acids in decreasing muscle catabolism in vivo, Surgery **83**:611, 1978.
64. Goodwin, C.W.: Metabolism and nutrition, Crit. Care Clin. **1**:97, 1985.
65. Harms, B.A., et al.: Prostaglandin release and altered microvascular integrity after burn injury, J. Surg. Res. **31**:274, 1981.
66. Hayashi, H., et al.: Endogenous permeability factors and their inhibitors affecting vascular permeability in cutaneous Arthus reactions and thermal injury, Br. J. Exp. Path. **45**:419, 1964.
67. Heggers, J.P., et al.: Evaluation of burn blister fluid, Plast. Reconstr. Surg. **65**:798, 1980.
68. Heggers, J.P., et al.: Histological demonstration of prostaglandins and thromboxanes in burned tissues, J. Surg. Res. **28**:110, 1980.
69. Heggers, J.P., et al.: Cooling and the prostaglandin effect in the thermal injury, J. Burn Care Rehab. **3**:350, 1982.
70. Herndon, D.N., Thompson, P.B., and Traber, D.L.: Pulmonary injury in burned patients, Crit. Care Clin. **1**:79, 1985.
71. Hershey, F.B., et al.: Effect of ATP on glucose metabolism of thermally injured skin in vitro, J. Trauma **11**:931, 1971.
72. Horakova, Z., and Beaven, M.A.: Time course of histamine release and edema formation in the rat paw after thermal injury, Eur. J. Pharmacol. **27**:305, 1974.
73. Jackson, D.M.: The diagnosis of the depth of burning, Br. J. Surg. **40**:588, 1953.
74. Kingsley, N.W., Stein, J.M., and Levenson, S.M.: Measuring tissue pressure to assess the severity of burn induced ischemia, Plast. Reconstr. Surg. **63**:404, 1979.
75. Lawrence, J.C., and Bull, J.P.: Thermal conditions which cause skin burns, J. Inst. Mech. Eng. **5**:61, 1976.
76. Lepenye, G., Novak, J., and Nemeth, L.: The biophysics of thermal injury, Acta Chir. Plast. **20**:77, 1978.
77. Long, C.L.: A response to trauma and infection: metabolic changes and immunologic consequences, J. Burn Care Rehab. **6**:188, 1985.

78. Long, J.M., III, et al.: Effect of carbohydrate and fat intake on nitrogen excretion during total intravenous feeding, Ann. Surg. **185:**417, 1977.
79. Lund, C.C., and Browder, W.L.: Healing of second-degree burns: comparison of effects of early application of homografts and coverage with tape, Plast. Reconstr. Surg. **49:**552, 1972.
80. Miller, T.A., and White, W.L.: Healing of second degree burns. Comparison of effects of early application of homografts and coverage with tape, Plast. Reconstr. Surg. **49:**552, 1972.
81. Moati, F., et al.: Biochemical and pharmacological properties of a cardiotoxic factor isolated from the blood serum of burned patients, J. Pathol. **127:**147, 1979.
82. Mochizuki, H., et al.: Optimal lipid content for enteral diets following thermal injury, J. Parent. Enteral Nutr. **8:**638, 1984.
83. Molteni L.B., et al.: Prolactin, corticotropin, and gonadotropin concentrations following thermal injury in adults, J. Trauma **24:**1, 1984.
84. Monafo, W.W.: The treatment of burn shock by the intravenous and oral administration of hypertonic lactated saline solution, J. Trauma **10:**575, 1970.
85. Moritz, A.R., and Henriques, F.C.: Studies of thermal injury. II. The relative importance of time and surface temperature in the causation of cutaneous burns, Am. J. Pathol. **23:**695, 1947.
86. Moritz A.R., Henriques F.C., Jr., and McLean, R.: The effects of inhaled heat on lungs: an experimental investigation, Am. J. Pathol. **21:**311, 1945.
87. Moylan J.A., Jr., and Chan, C.K.: Inhalation injury—an increasing problem, Surgery **188:**34, 1978.
88. Munster, A.M., and Winchurch, R.A.: Infection and immunology, Crit. Care Clin. **1:**119, 1985.
89. Myers, R.A.M., et al.: Value of hyperbaric oxygen in suspected carbon monoxide poisoning, JAMA **246:**2478, 1981.
90. Nanto, V., and Viljanto, J.: Observations on the chemical composition of the blister fluid of burned patients, Acta Chir. Scand. **124:**19, 1962.
91. Newman, J.J., et al.: Altered muscle metabolism in rats after thermal injuries, Metabolism **31:**1229, 1982.
92. Newsom, T.W., Mason, A.D., Jr., and Pruitt, B.A., Jr.: Weight loss following thermal injury, Ann. Surg. **178:**215, 1973.
93. Ninneman, J.L.: Suppression of lymphocyte response following thermal injury. In Ninneman, J.L., editor: The immune consequences of thermal injury, Baltimore, 1981, The Williams and Wilkins Co.
94. Ninneman, J.L.: Immune depression in burn and trauma patients: the role of circulating suppressors. In Ninneman, J.L., editor: Traumatic injury: infection and other immunologic sequelae, Baltimore, 1983, University Park Press.
95. Nozaki, M., et al.: Permeability of blood vessels after thermal injury, Burns **6:**213, 1980.
96. Parks, D.H., Carvajal, H.F., and Larson, D.L.: Management of burns, Surg. Clin. North Am. **57:**5, 1977.
97. Pinky, T.W., and McCloud, C.G., editors: Pathology of thermal injury, a practical approach, Orlando, Fla., 1985, Grune & Stratton, Inc.
98. Planas, M., et al.: Characterization of acute renal failure in the burned patient, Arch. Intern. Med. **142:**2087, 1982.
99. Popp, M.B., et al.: Anterior pituitary functioning thermally injured male children and young adults, Surg. Gynerol. Obstet. **145:**517, 1977.
100. Pruitt, B.A., Jr.: The burn patient. II. Later care and complications of thermal injury, Curr. Probl. Surg. **16:**1, 1979.
101. Pruitt, B.A., Jr.: The Scudder oration on trauma, Bull. Am. Coll. Surg. **70:**2, 1985.
102. Pruitt, B.A., Jr., Erickson, M.D., and Morris, A.: Progressive pulmonary insufficiency and other pulmonary complications of thermal injury, J. Trauma **15:**369, 1975.
103. Raffe, J., and Trunkey, D.D.: Myocardial depression in acute thermal injury, J. Trauma **18:**90, 1978.
104. Raine, T.J., et al.: Antiprostaglandins and antithromboxanes for treatment of frostbite, Surg. Forum **31:**557, 1980.
105. Raine, T.J., et al.: Cooling the burn wound to maintain microcirculation, J. Trauma **21:**394, 1981.
106. Reiss, E., et al.: Fluid and electrolyte balances in burns, JAMA **152:**1309, 1953.
107. Rhodes, M.L.: The effect of carbon monoxide on mitochondrial enzymes in pulmonary tissue, Am. Rev. Respir. Dis. **103:**906, 1971.
108. Robson, M.C., DelBeccaro, E.J., and Heggers, J.P.: The effect of prostaglandins in the dermal microcirculation after burning and the inhibition of the effect by specific pharmacological agents, Plast. Reconstr. Surg. **63:**781, 1979.
109. Robson, M.C., Murphy, R.C., and Heggers, J.P.: A new explanation for the progressive tissue loss in electrical injuries, Plast. Reconstr. Surg. **73:**431, 1984.
110. Robson, M.C., et al.: Prevention of dermal ischemia following thermal injury, Arch. Surg. **113:**621, 1978.
111. Robson, M.C., et al.: The effect of heparin on dermal ischemia after burning, Burns **5:**260, 1979.
112. Robson, M.C., et al.: Increasing dermal perfusion after burning by decreasing thromboxane production, J. Trauma **20:**722, 1980.
113. Schoenenberger, G.A.: Burn toxins isolated from mouse and human skin their characterization and immunotherapy effects, Monogr. Allergy **9:**72, 1975.
114. Shakespeare, P.G., Levick, P.L., and Vaitheespara, R.B.: Proteins in blister fluid, Burns **4:**254, 1978.
115. Shakespeare, P.G., et al.: Proteinuria after burn injury, Ann. Clin. Biochem. **18:**353, 1981.
116. Till G.O., et al.: Oxygen radical dependent lung damage following thermal injury of rat skin, J. Trauma **23:**269, 1983.
117. Trang, L.E.: Prostaglandins and inflammation, Semin. Arthritis Rheum. **9:**153, 1980.
118. Trunkey, D.D.: Inhalation injury. Surg. Clin. North Am. **58:**1133, 1978.
119. Turner, R., Carvajal, H.F., and Traber, D.L.: Effects of ganglionic blockade on renal and cardiovascular dysfunction induced by thermal injury, Circ. Shock **4:**103, 1977.
120. Uriuhara, T., and Movat, H.Z.: Role of PMN leukocyte lysosomes in tissue injury, inflammation and hypersensitivity. V. Partial suppression in leukopenic rabbits of vascular hyperpermeability due to thermal injury, Proc. Soc. Exp. Biol. Med. **124:**279, 1967.
121. Vaughn, G.M., Mason, A.D., Jr., and Shirani, K.Z.: Hormonal changes following burns: an overview with consideration of the pineal gland, J. Burn Care Rehab. **6:**275, 1985.
122. Warden, G.D., Mason, A.D., and Pruitt, B.A., Jr.: Evaluation of leukocyte chemotaxis in vitro in thermally injured patients, J. Clin. Invest. **54:**1001, 1974.
123. Watson W.C., Kutty, P.K., and Colcleugh, R.G.: Does cimetidine cause ileus in the burned patient? Lancet **2:**720, 1977.
124. Wilmore, D.W.: Nutrition and metabolism following thermal injury, Clin. Plast. Surg. **1:**603, 1974.
125. Wilmore, D.W.: Carbohydrate metabolism in trauma, Clin. Endocrinol. Metabol. **5:**731, 1976.
126. Wilmore, D.W.: Hormonal responses and their effects on metabolism, Surg. Clin. North Am. **56:**999, 1976.
127. Wilmore, D.W., and Aulick, L.H.: Metabolic changes in burned patients, Surg. Clin. North Am. **58:**1173, 1978.
128. Wilmore, D.W., et al.: Catecholamines: mediator of the hypermetabolic response to thermal injury, Ann. Surg. **180:**653, 1974.
129. Wilmore, D.W., et al.: Alterations in hypothalamic function following thermal injury, J. Trauma **15:**697, 1975.
130. Wilmore, D.W., et al.: Effect of injury and infection on visceral metabolism and circulation, Ann. Surg. **192:**491, 1980.
131. Wilson, C.E., et al.: Cold water treatment of burns, J. Trauma **3:**477, 1963.
132. Wolfe, R.R.: Glucose metabolism in burn injury: a review. J. Burn Care Rehab. **6:**408, 1985.
133. Wolfe, R.R., et al.: Response of proteins and urea kinetics in burn patients to different levels of protein intake, Ann. Surg. **197:**163, 1983.
134. Yoshioka, T., et al.: Cimetidine inhibits burn edema formation. Am. J. Surg. **136:**681, 1978.
135. Zawacki, B.E.: Reversal of capillary stasis and prevention of necrosis in burns, Ann. Surg. **180:**98, 1974.

65

Thomas R. Weber

Physiologic Problems in the Pediatric Surgical Patient

Surgeons caring for the pediatric patient are presented with challenges that are unique and in most instances significantly different from those involved in caring for the adult patient. These differences become most obvious in the surgical neonate, and, as a consequence, surgery in neonates and small infants has provided the springboard for the speciality of pediatric surgery. Among the factors that make the neonate and infant a challenging surgical patient are the dynamic adjustment of the newborn to extrauterine life, increased energy and nutritional demands produced by rapid growth, continued organ development and maturation in function, small physical size, rapid metabolic rates that can change the physiologic status of the child almost within minutes, and anatomic defects that are usually congenital rather than acquired in origin. These factors, combined with the fact that the pediatric patient cannot give a history or list complaints or symptoms, make care of the pediatric surgical patient demanding and leave little room for error.

This chapter will describe the unique characteristics of the pediatric patient, present the physiologic principles that can guide the management of the patient in this age group, and apply these physiologic principles to the most common defects seen. The diagnosis and management of various common congenital and acquired diseases of infancy and childhood will also be briefly discussed.

CIRCULATION, FLUIDS, AND ELECTROLYTES

Circulation

A complete discussion of the normal circulation of the fetus and newborn is beyond the scope of this chapter, but certain salient points that seem to contribute to some neonatal disorders discussed later will be emphasized.

The circulation just before birth consists of parallel circuits with both right and left ventricles pumping blood that eventually goes through the descending aorta either to the capillary bed or through the umbilical arteries and then to the placenta where oxygenation takes place. The oxygenated blood returns to the heart through the umbilical vein, ductus venosus, and inferior vena cava. Because of extremely high pulmonary artery resistance, only about 7% of the cardiac output flows through the lungs, with the remainder of the right ventricle output traversing the ductus arteriosus to enter the descending aorta. Because of the exclusion of the lungs during fetal life, intrauterine congestive heart failure initially appears as generalized edema (anasarca).

Immediately after birth, the state of the circulation is best described as transitional[14] and continues in that state for the first week or two of life. With the newborn's first breath the pulmonary artery resistance falls rapidly, resulting in reversal of flow through the ductus arteriosus, temporarily becoming left-to-right. The ductus venosus functionally closes, followed by the foramen ovale. Toward the end of the first day of life, as systemic and pulmonary pressures stabilize, the ductus arteriosus closes as a result of the poorly understood influences of prostaglandins, blood oxygen, carbon dioxide, and pH. Anatomic closure of the ductus arteriosus is complete at 10 to 14 days, whereas foramen ovale may remain anatomically patent for months or years.

Although shortly after birth the neonatal circulation abruptly changes from a parallel to a series arrangement, many fetal characteristics remain, and the possibility of returning to a fetal pattern of circulation exists. This becomes critically important in disorders such as meconium aspiration and congenital diaphragmatic hernia, discussed later, in which persistent pulmonary hypertension and fetal circulation patterns cause hypoxemia, which is extremely difficult to treat. Shortly after birth the right and left ventricles are equal in muscular thickness, and the pulmonary vasculature has increased muscularity, making the muscle extremely reactive to stimuli. Hypoxia, acidosis, and hypercarbia have all been shown experimentally and clinically to cause variable degrees of pulmonary vasoconstriction.[6,12,15] Gradually, over a period of weeks the muscular wall of the pulmonary arteriole becomes thinned and much less reactive to stimuli.

The circulatory development of the premature infant is entirely different from that of the term baby. The pulmonary arteriole muscle develops late in gestation. Thus the more premature the infant, the less vasoactive the pulmonary vasculature, making the pulmonary vascular pressure lower. This allows more left-to-right shunting through the ductus arteriosus, resulting in increased pulmonary vascular congestion and decreased peripheral perfusion. Hy-

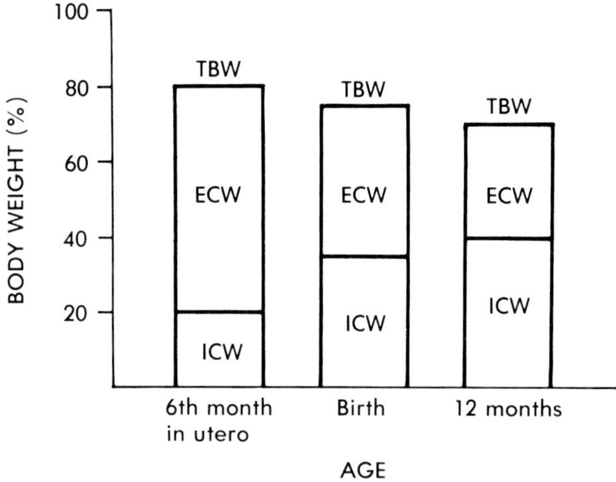

Fig. 65-1 Change in body water content with age. Note gradual decrease in total body water *(TBW)* and extracellular water *(ECW)* and associated expansion of intracellular water *(ICW)* as age increases.

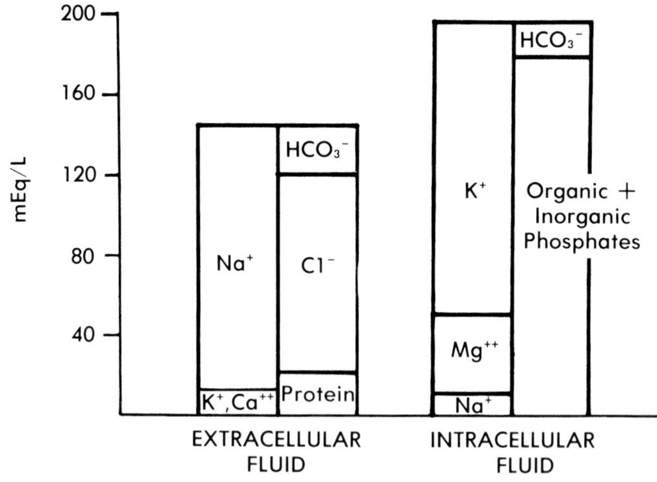

Fig. 65-2 Electrolyte composition of intracellular and extracellular compartments in the newborn.

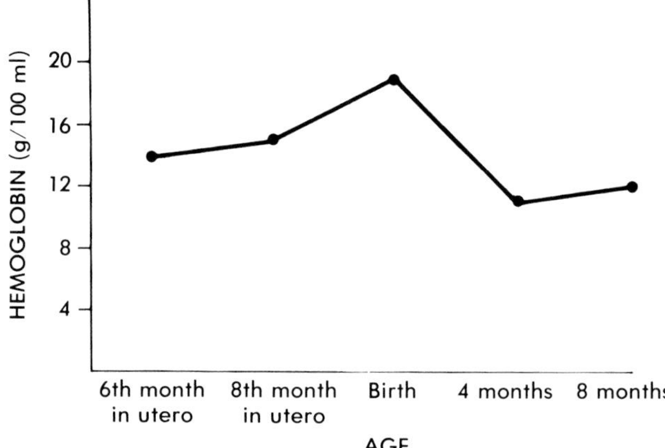

Fig. 65-3 Changes in blood hemoglobin concentrations with age. Hemoglobin is highest at birth and falls to adult levels at age 8 months.

poxia, often present in premature infants for a variety of reasons, tends to delay closure of the ductus, resulting in more shunting. The increased work required of the left ventricle and pulmonary vascular congestion added to already marginal pulmonary reserve from lung immaturity make closure of the ductus by either pharmacologic (indomethacin) or surgical means an important factor in the overall management of circulatory disorders in premature infants.

Body Fluids

The blood volume, red cell mass, extracellular water content, and electrolyte profile of a newborn infant (Figs. 65-1 to 65-3) are significantly different than at any other time throughout life. The blood volume for a term infant ranges from 78 ml/kg to 98 ml/kg of body weight, depending on how quickly the cord is clamped after birth and the resultant amount of placental transfusion needed. The premature infant tends to have a slightly higher blood volume at birth (89 m/kg to 105 ml/kg of body weight), primarily because of increased plasma volume and extracellular water. By the third day of life, the blood volumes have fallen to approximately 80 ml/kg for term babies and 92 ml/kg for prematures, gradually decreasing with time to the adult value of 60 ml/kg of body weight at age 2 years.

The total body water is conveniently divided into intracellular and extracellular compartments. At approximately the sixth month of gestation, the total body water comprises 80% of body weight, three fourths of which is located in the extracellular intravascular and interstitial spaces (see Fig. 65-1). At birth the total body water has fallen slightly to 78% of body weight, but marked changes have occurred in the distribution of water, with the intracellular and extracellular components essentially equal. Further contraction of extracellular water occurs after birth so that, by 1 year of age, intracellular water has become 40% of body weight, whereas the extracellular component is only 30%. The decrease in extracellular water fraction corresponds to improvement in renal function and increasing urine output.

Premature infants have body composition, (i.e., increased extracellular water and plasma volume and smaller intracellular water content) consistent with their gestational age. These factors must be taken into account when calculating parenteral fluid replacement for premature infants. In addition, the transition from fetal to newborn body composition must be preserved in all babies receiving intravenous fluids. Overzealous intravenous fluid replacement may result in chronically expanded extracellular volume, resulting in undesirable complications such as patent ductus arteriosus with congestive heart failure and necrotizing enterocolitis.

The daily maintenance fluid requirements consist of insensible water loss, urine and stool losses, and loss of water for tissue growth. The insensible water loss has been studied extensively by numerous investigators. The ideal method of calculating the insensible fluid loss in newborns is somewhat controversial, giving rise to variations in technique and study design that result in normal values that vary between 0.7 to 1.6 ml/kg/hour. Theoretically the most accurate reference unit for insensible water loss uses caloric expenditure of evaporative heat loss through the skin and respiratory tree. However, since there is no simple means of measuring energy expenditure, attempts have been made to use either surface area or body weight to calculate fluid losses. Although these latter techniques have drawbacks, they are the most widely used methods of calculating fluid therapy in the newborn and infant.

Several factors alter insensible fluid losses in newborns. Insensible water loss is inversely proportional to birth weight and gestational age. Small infants have a relatively large heat-losing surface area in relation to body weight when compared with larger infants. Also, preterm infants have higher respiratory rates in contrast to term infants, further aggravating insensible losses. Finally, hyperthermia (increasing ambient temperature with a radiant warmer) significantly increases insensible fluid loss, as does the use of phototherapy for hyperbilirubinemia. The use of these therapeutic modalities has been shown to increase insensible fluid losses by as much as three times.[11] Factors reducing insensible water loss include (1) use of a heat shield, (2) a high ambient humidity, and (3) the use of humidified gas during ventilation. The savings in insensible water loss from these factors vary from 30% to 90% and must be taken into account when calculating fluid replacements.

The endocrine control of fluid balance, although immature in early infancy, has important functions. The pituitary gland (antidiuretic hormone) and adrenal cortex (mineralocorticoids) both function within certain physiologic limits to aid in the maintenance of fluid homeostasis. Renal tubular–concentrating mechanisms in the newborn can produce a urine of 800 mOsm/L, whereas the adult can achieve 1200 mOsm/L. Both decreased antidiuretic hormone and renal tubular function may be involved in limiting the ability of the neonate to concentrate urine. In contrast, during water loading, only infants older than 5 days can excrete normally. Aldosterone levels are quite high in newborns and young infants, but appropriate feedback mechanisms exist between sodium intake and excretion and aldosterone levels.

Renal function in newborns and infants has been assumed to be immature and incapable of responding to fluid changes that differ significantly from intrauterine life. However, recent evidence suggests that the newborn glomerular and tubular functions are capable of withstanding all but an overwhelming fluid and electrolyte load or deprivation.[11] This seems to be related to gestational age as well, with preterm infants less able to respond to abnormal physiologic conditions.

When these various factors are taken into account, an appropriate figure of 80 to 100 ml/kg/day can be used as a starting point for the calculation of maintenance fluid requirements. This starting point is based on the assumption that losses through stool, urine, and insensible routes are normal but it does not adequately reflect replacement of abnormal losses such as diarrhea, nasogastric suction, or emesis. In addition, a child who is already dehydrated when initially seen must have extra fluid administered on the basis of a calculation of the percent of dehydration. An estimate with the use of sequential body weights is the most accurate means of estimating acute fluid loss. However, it should be remembered that a weight loss of 5% to 10% is normal during the first week of life as a result of contraction of the extravascular space. If accurate body weights are unavailable, the presence of dry skin and slightly sunken fontanels are indicative of 5% dehydration; loose skin turgor, sunken eyes, and severely sunken fontanels suggest 10% dehydration; and circulatory collapse, shock, and a moribund appearance indicate dehydration of 15% or more.

Electrolyte loss can be ascertained by the nature of abnormal fluid losses and by measuring serum and urine electrolytes. Severe diarrhea usually causes an isotonic dehydration (serum sodium near normal), whereas a prolonged febrile course in addition to diarrhea frequently results in the loss of more water than sodium, giving a high serum sodium level (hypertonic dehydration). A very low serum sodium level might result from inappropriate fluid administration or antidiurectic hormone secretion.

The electrolyte losses from prolonged vomiting (i.e., pyloric stenosis) have a rather characteristic pattern. Because of the large amount of chloride ion present in gastric juice (100 to 150 mEq/L), hypochloremic and hypokalemic alkalosis result, and serum bicarbonate levels in the range of 35 to 45 mEq/L are not unusual. Intravenous replacement fluids for these deficits must include normal saline and potassium chloride at 1½ to two times maintenance infusion until serum bicarbonate levels return to normal.

Fluid and electrolyte therapy in critically ill patients of any age must be monitored very closely; this is especially true for the neonate and young infant. The minimum amount of information needed includes accurate records of all intake (enteral and parenteral), daily body weights, daily or twice daily serum electrolytes, urine volume, osmolarity and specific gravity, and abnormal fluid and electrolyte losses through such factors as diarrhea, vomiting, and nasogastric drainage. The goal in fluid management of the critically ill patient should be maintenance of normal serum electrolytes and urine output of 0.5 to 1 ml/kg/hour. Frequent readjustment of rate and content of intravenous fluid may be necessary on the basis of the clinical and biochemical parameters listed previously.

Electrolyte Composition

The electrolyte composition of the newborn infant depends on gestational age and maternal factors. Premature infants tend to have a higher extracellular solute load, primarily because of the expanded extracellular water space. Because fetal fluid and electrolyte balance depend on maternal and placental exchange, abnormal electrolyte conditions such as hyponatremia in the mother can produce similar electrolyte imbalances in the fetus and newborn.

As demonstrated in Fig. 65-2, the primary extracellular cation is sodium, whereas the major anions are chloride and bicarbonate. In contrast, the intracellular space has potassium and magnesium as the prinicipal cations, whereas phosphorus and, to a minor degree, bicarbonate make up the majority of the anion load.

Circulatory Collapse and Shock

Although the cause of shock in the pediatric surgical patient can conveniently be categorized as hypovolemic, septic, and cardiogenic, these various causes of shock share may pathophysiologic pathways, and the therapies overlap these divisions. It seems much more useful to discuss the unique features of shock in young patients in a unified approach. This might be further emphasized by a single definition of shock, which is "a severe pathophysiologic syndrome associated with abnormal cellular metabolism and a fall in energy production, usually caused by poor tissue perfusion." The overall goal in shock resuscitation and therapy is improvement in tissue perfusion by normalizing intravascular volume, cardiac output, and vascular tone.

The most common cause of shock in infants and children is hypovolemia, resulting either from salt and water loss (caused by diarrhea or vomiting) or blood loss (caused by conditions such as trauma and gastrointestinal hemorrhage). Septic shock from pneumonia, meningitis, necrotizing enterocolitis, appendicitis, and infections in the urinary tract is not rare in the young child. Cardiogenic shock associated with congenital heart defects is less common but can be rapidly lethal, sometimes requiring immediate definitive repair. Congenital heart defects are discussed in Chapter 39; the bulk of the discussion here will concern hypovolemia and sepsis.

The initial response of the human to acute hypovolemia is sympathicoadrenal, resulting in tachycardia and increased cardiac output. A newborn's ability to respond in this fashion is limited, and bradycardia from acidosis and myocardial dysfunction is more common in this age group. Venous constriction increases the volume of blood returning to the heart for distribution to vital organs (e.g., heart, brain), whereas arteriolar constriction in nonvital circulatory beds (e.g., skin, muscle, viscera) causes further redistribution of blood flow to other organs. This results in insufficient oxygen delivery to these peripheral tissues, forcing the cellular metabolism to anaerobic glycolysis. This is an extremely inefficient method of energy production, since only two molecules of adenosine triphosphate are manufactured from a molecule of glucose anaerobically, in contrast to 36 molecules of adenosine triphosphate produced from a molecule of glucose in aerobic glycolysis. The sodium-potassium pump suffers from decreased energy availability, and further abnormal cellular metabolism ensues. This simplified overview emphasizes that restoration of intravascular volume by transfusion and crystalloid diffusion is necessary to restore cellular metabolism to a normal state.

One of the more common shock-producing lesions that pediatric surgeons must deal with is peritonitis caused by a perforated viscus as in appendicitis, necrotizing enterocolitis, midgut volvulus, and Hirschsprung's disease. This causes rapid shifts of fluid from intravascular to peritoneal spaces ("third space loss"), followed soon afterwards by a septic course from the absorption of bacteria, toxins, and vasoactive substances from the peritoneal cavity. Since the intravascular volume of an infant is very limited (70 to 80 ml/kg of body weight), a loss of only a small amount of fluid into the peritoneal cavity can result in rapid intravascular depletion and hypovolemia. In these situations both hypovolemia and sepsis are present and must be treated rapidly.

Sepsis in itself has numerous cellular and organ function implications, a complete discussion of which is beyond the scope of this chapter. Briefly, sepsis produces abnormal cellular metabolism by affecting functions such as oxygen uptake and use, mitochondrial function, gluconeogenesis, and energy production to name only a few. The ability of young infants to deal effectively with infection and sepsis is severely limited, making the frequent combination of hypovolemia and sepsis rapidly fatal in this age group. Myocardial failure is common in infant sepsis,[18] but whether it is the result of inadequate oxygen and energy substrate delivery, direct myocardial depression by toxic substances, or severe hypovolemia with irreversible cellular damage is unclear. Survival in these instances thus depends on improvement in myocardial performance and cardiac output.

The initial therapy of shock in the child has as a short-term goal, the normalization of physiologic parameters, followed by correction of the original process that caused shock. Since almost all forms of shock include hypovolemia, a rapid infusin (20 ml/kg of body weight over 30 to 60 minutes) of 5% dextrose in Ringer's lactate will begin to correct deficits. The use of colloid-containing fluids (plasma or albumin) remains controversial, although they are probably beneficial as a one-time infusion. If hypovolemia is the result of blood loss, the measures described above should be used only until blood is available for transfusion. The use of massive doses of corticosteroids, thought to have a role in adult septic shock, has not been extensively investigated in the pediatric age group.

Inotropic agents that have been found to be effective in pediatric patients include isoproterenol, epinephrine, and dopamine. The use of such agents in septic infants seems justified on the basis of experimental data that show rather profound cardiac depression, with low cardiac outputs in neonatal shock models,[18] The efficacy of isoproterenol and epinephrine has been confirmed by numerous studies, but the newborn and young infant response to dopamine is questionable, on the basis of both experimental and clinical studies.[13,17] The lack of dopaminergic receptors in neonates has been suggested as an explanation for this apparent lack of response. Further studies are clearly needed to clarify the role of these agents for circulatory support in pediatric patients.

RESPIRATORY PHYSIOLOGY

The newborn and infant lung presents unique challenges to physicians involved in the management of patients in these age groups. This is especially true for premature infants who require ventilatory support. Although the anatomy of the fetal and newborn lung has been extensively investigated and seems well understood, only recently have the biochemical and physiologic differentiation and functions of lungs in these age groups been elucidated. Pulmonary physiology in the pediatric surgical patient becomes important in such disorders as diaphragmatic hernia and in complications associated with such pulmonary diseases as cystic fibrosis. For these reasons, a brief review of lung development and physiology is useful.

The developing lung bud first appears as an outpouching from the primitive foregut at 3 to 4 weeks of gestation. Branching continues until 10 weeks at which time cartilage appears; complete bronchial formation is complete at 16 weeks of fetal life. Pulmonary arteries arising from the sixth pharyngeal arch branch within the lung buds parallel to the developing airways and end in a vast capillary bed that has anastomoses with the developing bronchial arteries. The pulmonary vein forms as an outpouching from the left atrium at 4 to 5 weeks of gestation, developing in a dorsal direction to join the forming vascular endothelial channels within the lung bed.

The developing lung airway is solid until 18 to 20 weeks, at which time differentiation and canalization begin. The cells lining the primitive airways are rich in glycogen and appear to differentiate into two types of cells as further branching occurs: (1) Type I pneumocytes, which are flat cells with scant cytoplasm and no glycogen that line the alveolar spaces and serve in the regulation of diffusin of gas between alveolus and capillary bed; and (2) Type II pneumocytes with microvilla and inclusions that appear to be responsible for the manufacture and secretion of surface-active phospholipids (surfactants) that maintain the alveolar integrity. Very little of this cellular differentiation has occurred, however, before week 28 of gestation; this explains in part the difficulties in maintaining adequate ventilation in infants born before this time.

The period of 28 to 32 weeks is one of rapid maturation and differentiation of developing lungs; and toward the end of this period numerous Type I and Type II cells are seen lining alveolar spaces, and the pulmonary capillary vasculature becomes normal in appearance histologically. Type II pneumocytes contain lamellar inclusions, which are typical for surfactants. The lungs at this stage are much better able to provide respiratory function—hence the marked improvement in survival of neonates born with gestation over 32 weeks.

The biochemical maturation of the lung consists primarily of the formation of surface-active phospholipids to act as surfactants. The principal surfactants are thought to be phosphatidyl choline and phosphatidyl glycerol, both lecithin. They are formed primarily from a pathway that includes the combination of cytidine diphosphate choline and D-alpha, beta-diglyceride, resulting in desaturated phosphatidyl choline, which later becomes saturated. These changes are occurring simultaneously with the appearance of Type II pneumocytes within the lung, as outlined above. The level of lecithin (phosphatidyl choline) in the amniotic fluid which can be measured, seems to correlate well with the maturation of the lung; whereas the level of another phospholipid (sphingomyelin) remains constant in amniotic fluid throughout gestation. The lecithin level increases as more of the compound is manufactured and excreted by Type II pneumocytes. A ratio of lecithin to sphyingomyelin (L/S ratio) of 2:1 is considered indicative of relatively mature lung function.

It has been found experimentally that administration of glucocorticoids to fetuses in utero will result in advanced lung maturation; thus acceleration of the maturation of biochemical and histologic aspects of lung function have been attempted.[8] Extending these data to the human, controlled trials of the administration of steroids to women in premature labor have shown acceleration in lung maturation with these compounds,[9] provided the steroid is given in 27 to 32 week pregnancies and at least 48 hours before delivery. The numerous theoretic side effects of steroid therapy in a newborn have tempered enthusiasm for this approach, but nonetheless these exciting data demonstrate that increased survival in infants with very immature lungs may be forthcoming, with new methods of accelerating maturation of lung function.

The implications of developing neonatal pulmonary function in the pediatric surgery patient are numerous. Disorders such as diaphragmatic hernia and congenital cystic lung lesions occur frequently in the period of most active growth of the lung (10- to 20-weeks' gestation). Impairment of lung growth and/or maturity can occur with such space-occupying lesions, giving rise to pulmonary insufficiency shortly after birth. More details concerning the pathophysiology of diaphragmatic hernia will be given later.

ABDOMINAL WALL DEFECTS

Omphalocele

The incidence of omphalocele is approximately 1:4000 live births, and numerous familial occurrences of omphalocele have been noted. Increased incidence with advanced maternal age has been observed, and a high rate of spontaneous abortion has been seen among women giving birth to infants with omphalocele, suggesting placental dysfunction.

The anomaly is a covered defect within the umbilical cord, through which intra-abdominal contents herniate. Unless it is ruptured during birth, there is always a sac covering the herniated gut, composed of amnion externally and peritoneum internally. The defect is 2 to 10 cm in diameter and may contain small and large bowel and liver. The most widely accepted theory of embryogenesis of omphalocele is that of Duhamel,[5] who believed the omphalocele was a failure that occurs early in gestation (3 to 4 weeks) of embryonal formation of the cephalic, caudal, and especially the two lateral embryonic folds that fuse at the umbilicus. Other authors consider an omphalocele a result of faulty migration of myotomes, caused by failure of the return of the bowel from the yolk sac into the developing abdominal cavity.

Omphalocele is associated with a significant (greater than 50%) incidence of associated anomalies and syndromes, including malformations in the alimentary tract, genitourinary, musculoskeletal, cardiac, and nervous systems. It is also seen commonly in the Beckwith-Wiedemann syndrome (gigantism, macroglossia, hypoglycemia) and trisomy 13-15 and 16-18. Two other syndromes in which an omphalocele is present but away from the umbilical cord include Pentalogy of Cantrell (upper midline omphalocele, diaphragmatic defect, sternal cleft, free pericardio-peritoneal communication, and intracardiac defects); and the lower midline syndrome (low-lying omphalocele, cloacal exstrophy, imperforate anus with colonic atresia, and vesicointestinal fissure separating the two halves of the bladder). Colonic or appendiceal duplications are commonly seen, and sacral or vertebral anomalies may be present with associated myelomeningocele.

The physiologic considerations in the infant with omphalocele include the preoperative evaluation and resuscitation, intraoperative management, and postoperative recovery period. Before surgery the management of the infant includes attention to the prevention of hypothermia, maintenance of a sterile environment, and fluid resuscitation. Hypothermia is related to excessive radiant heat losses from the surface of the omphalocele sac. Placing the infant to the level of his axillae in an impermeable plastic bag with drawstrings ("bowel-bag") will decrease radiant heat loss and, in addition, will effectively limit evaporative heat and water loss from the exposed surface. This is particularly important in the premature infant, in whom high transepithelial water loss is possible.

Rapid fluid shifts caused by "third space" losses from the surface of the omphalocele can deplete the intravascular volume at an alarming rate in these newborns. The neonate has a limited capacity to respond to abnormal fluid losses because of a low plasma oncotic pressure, poor renal concentrating mechanisms, relative hyponatremia, and immature sympathicoadrenal responses. In addition, limited energy stores (a paucity of fat and glycogen) put demands on a gluconeogenic mechanism that may not be fully developed or functional in the hypovolemic state of the preterm or term infant. This set of circumstances may lead to metabolic acidosis from poor tissue perfusion and anaerobic metabolism that can lead to adverse cardiac and pulmonary vascular responses. The resultant hemoconcentration (hematocrit frequently in the 65 to 75 g/100 ml range) may result in increased blood viscosity and further decrease in tissue perfusion. Thus in these infants an intravenous line must be established immediately, preferably in a vein above the diaphragm, with a bolus of 20 ml/kg of 5% dextrose in lactated Ringer's solution over 1 hour. This can be safely administered even if a cardiac anomaly is suspected. This should be followed by maintenance fluids of 5% or 10% dextrose in 0.45% normal saline at a rate of 150 to 175 ml/kg/day until urine output is obtained. Potassium chloride, 2 to 3 mEq/kg/day, can be added after urine output is established. If the omphalocele sac has ruptured, significant blood loss may occur, and this should be replaced with transfusion as soon as possible.

Because of limited host defense mechanisms, these babies are at high risk for infectious complications. Intravenous ampicillin (100 mg/kg/day) and gentamycin (5 mg/kg/day) are given in divided doses (every 12 hours for the first week of life). In addition, providing a sterile environment as outlined above is an important adjunct.

After the resuscitation period, attention is directed toward complete work-up to assess for other anomalies or syndromes. In most pediatric centers this includes consultation with a cardiologist, geneticist, neurologist, neonatologist, and others. In cases of cloacal exstrophy and ambiguous genitalia, a gender assignment committee may also become involved. Chromosome analysis is frequently necessary to assess the possibility of trisomy syndromes.

The actual treatment of the omphalocele defect should be individualized. The recommended methods of management include nonoperative treatment with escharotics, primary repair, skin flap closures with later ventral hernia repair and use of prosthetic sheeting with staged reduction. The factors that determine the optimal method of treatment include the size of the defect, the overall condition of the patient, presence of other anomalies (especially those that are potentially lethal), and whether the sac is intact or ruptured. If the sac is intact, the choice can be made on a less urgent basis, and all of the above factors can be taken into consideration.

Nonoperative therapy with escharotic agents has been practiced since 1899, when alcohol application was used successfully. This caused granulation tissue, and then epithelium to form over the sac. Later aqueous mercurichrome was used, but mercury poisoning has been observed, and its use has largely been abandoned. The use of silver nitrate (0.25%) and silver sulfadiazene creme, agents frequently used on burn wounds, has been suggested recently. Silver nitrate has the disadvantage of being hypotonic, causing sodium depletion, which must be monitored and replaced intravenously. Because of the need for prolonged hospitalization, the resulting large ventral hernia that requires later repair, and the inability to inspect the intra-abdominal viscera for other anomalies, nonoperative therapy is reserved primarily for specific patients. These might include a premature infant with an extremely large defect, infants with severe hyaline membrane disease or other life-threatening condition, newborns with chromosomal (trisomy) syndromes in whom prolonged survival is not expected, and the infant with potentially lethal cardiac defects such as hypoplastic left ventricle.

Primary closure of the defect is obviously the most efficacious surgical approach in dealing with omphalocele. Most small and medium-sized defects can be dealt with in this manner. After the sac has been carefully excised and the umbilical vessels ligated the contents are inspected for evidence of intestinal atresia or vitelline duct remnant and reduced. Removal of portions of the gastrointestinal tract, liver, and spleen have been reported to facilitate reduction, but these techniques are unnecessary.

For large defects in which full reduction of intra-abdominal contents is not possible, placement of a prosthetic "silo" is an excellent alternative to nonoperative therapy. This allows staged reduction over a 7 to 10 day period, at which time the baby is returned to the operating room for removal of the prosthetic and abdominal wall repair. This technique is more fully described in the section on gastroschisis, where it has had more widespread application. Yet another alternative for large defects, especially those involving liver, includes the use of an internal polyethylene or silastic sheet placed directly over the viscera, with application of a polypropylene or Marlex mesh superficially, with skin flap coverage of the entire prosthesis. Staged repair by reopening the skin, resecting the central portion of the prosthesis, and resuturing the prosthesis in the midline will gradually result in an enlarged abdominal cavity and eventual removal of the entire prosthesis. This may require 4 to 5 operations over a several year period.

The postoperative management of these infants is usually straightforward. Intravenous fluids (120 to 150 ml/kg/day) and antibiotics are continued, the latter for 5 to 7 days or until all external prostheses are removed. Bowel function usually returns within several days after surgery, and oral feeding is begun. The associated anomalies are managed appropriately. Current survival in infants with omphalocele is 65% to 75%; the high mortality rate is the result of associated anomalies (especially cardiac) rather than factors directly related to repair of the defect.

Gastroschisis

Gastroschisis (Greek for "belly cleft") is characterized by a full-thickness abdominal wall defect, usually to the right of the umbilicus, through which antenatal evisceration of bowel occurs. Unlike omphalocele, there is no sac present, allowing the herniated gut to be exposed to the amniotic fluid (pH 7). This results in a chemical peritonitis, with thickened, edematous, inflamed, and foreshortened bowel. If the defect is very small, the blood supply to the eviscerated gut can be compromised, leading to frank necrosis or intestinal atresia (10% of cases). The incidence of other anomalies is very low in contrast to omphalocele, although 40% to 60% of infants with gastroschisis are either premature or small for gestational age, making their management exacting and frequently complicated.

The true incidence of gastroschisis is difficult to ascertain, although many authors think that the number of infants born with gastroschisis is increasing.[7] The mean maternal age is younger for gastroschisis than omphalocele, and a significant number (50%) are born to teenage or primigravida mothers. Familial occurrences are extremely rare.

Much controversy surrounds the cause of gastroschisis. Various authors have proposed a defect in differentiation of somatopleuric mesenchyme lateral to the umbilicus, whereas others consider gastroschisis to be a consequence of rupture of the amniotic membrane at the base of a hernia of the umbilical cord. This latter circumstance may occur when involution of the primitive right umbilical vein leaves a weakened area on the abdominal wall. Most authors agree that gastroschisis does not represent a ruptured omphalocele but rather is a distinct entity. The fact that omphalocele is so often associated with chromosome abnormalities and other anomalies, whereas gastroschisis is not, lends support to the concept that omphalocele and gastroschisis are different entities.

As with omphalocele, the physiologic considerations in the newborn with gastroschisis include immediate attention to life-threatening problems and preoperative preparation, intraoperative therapy, and postoperative management. Immediately after birth a sterile, warm environment must be provided for the child. Placing the lower two thirds of the baby in a "bowel bag" as outlined for omphalocele will help conserve heat, provide a sterile and impervious barrier, and limit evaporative fluid loss by allowing water vapor to accumulate within the confines of the bag. The use of extremely wet dressings may lead to rapid hypothermia even within a plastic bag and should be avoided.

An intravenous line should be established as quickly as possible, and a fluid bolus (20 ml/kg) of 5% dextrose in lactated Ringer's solution given over the first hour. Metabolic acidosis because of poor peripheral perfusion is common but usually responds rapidly to increased intravascular volume. The administration of colloid in the form of plasma or albumin is also advisable since the composition of the fluid "leaking" from the exposed surface of eviscerated bowel is rich in plasma proteins. Intravenous antibiotics (ampicillin and gentamicin) are given after the intravenous line is established.

After preoperative preparation the patient is taken to the operating room for repair. Unlike omphalocele, nonoperative therapy is not an option in infants with gastroschisis. Maintenance of a warm environment and close attention to replacement of fluid and blood loss are critical factors in successful surgical management of these infants. The decision for the most appropriate surgical approach is made at the operating table. Primary reduction of all viscera with closure of the abdominal wall is highly desirable but only successful in 40% to 50% of cases for the following reasons: (1) the eviscerated gut can be extremely thick, edematous, and enlarged and may not be reducible into the small abdominal cavity; (2) vascular compromise to bowel may develop if forceful reduction is attempted; (3) compression of the inferior vena cava by increased intra-abdominal pressure may decrease cardiac output; and (4) upward pressure on the diaphragms by the same mechanism may cause respiratory distress, prompting the use of increased ventilatory pressures that can be harmful to the newborn lung. If any of the above complications arise during primary reduction, staged reduction with the use of a silastic "silo" is an excellent alternative. With the use of a sheet of reinforced silastic, an envelope is constructed around the bowel that cannot be reduced and sutured to the skin and fascia of the defect. An occlusive dressing is applied around the silastic with topical antibiotic cream (povidone-iodine) application. The gut can be gradually reduced by gently squeezing the top of the silo daily or every other day, using umbilical tape to ligate the distal sac to maintain reduction. When the gut has been fully reduced (usually 7 to 10 days), the infant is returned to the operating room for removal of the silo and abdominal wall repair.

The fluid requirements for infants immediately after repair of gastroschisis are significantly higher than maintenance rate. The fluid deficits after surgery are related to the amount of fluid given before surgery and intraoperatively, the extent of exposure of gut to the amniotic fluid, and the degree of chemical peritonitis present. Lymphatic and venous obstruction of exteriorized bowel may increase "third-space" losses into either the silo or the peritoneal cavity. Vascular dilation, hyperemia, and increased capillary permeability may also be present in the bowel wall, resulting in an outpouring of interstitial fluid that is not available for reabsorption into the intravascular space. Taking these factors into account, volumes of 175 to 300 ml/kg/day have been used intravenously for the first 24 to 48 hours after reduction, usually in the form of 5% dextrose in lactated Ringer's solution. Maintenance fluids can be used after 48 hours, when mobilization of extravascular fluid usually begins.

Depending on the degree of thickening and inflammation present within the bowel wall, a period of adynamic, ineffective intestinal peristalsis can be expected for as long as 30 days, occasionally longer. Because of the increased caloric demands, the placement of a central venous catheter and administration of intravenous total parenteral nutrition is a valuable adjunct and is probably responsible for most of the improvement in survival in gastroschisis over the past 15 years. The catheter is usually placed after the removal of the silastic prosthesis, at which time the risk of sepsis and bacteremia is reduced. Total parenteral nutrition must be used until relatively normal bowel movements begin, but even then elemental diets might be necessary when commencing feedings since malabsorption of fats, protein, and sugar is not uncommon in these infants.[7] In addition, gastrointestinal transit time remains prolonged for up to 6 months after reduction. Fortunately, by 12 to 18 months of age most infants demonstrate normal growth, development, and gastrointestinal function.

Improvements in preoperative and postoperative care, the availability of the silastic prosthesis for management of the irreducible gut, and total parenteral nutrition have all played important roles in increasing survival rate to 85% to 90% in most series of gastroschisis. Prenatal diagnosis of gastroschisis with ultrasound should allow better preparation for delivery, immediate resuscitation, and repair of this common abdominal wall defect.

HYPERTROPHIC PYLORIC STENOSIS

Hypertrophic pyloric stenosis is an obstructing lesion of the pyloric canal that seems to be unique to the young infant. This disorder was first described in the 1700s, but a complete description awaited the astute observations of Hirschsprung in 1887. The latter report included autopsy results in two children. The first suggestion that the ideal treatment of these infants might be surgical was made by Schwyzer in 1896, who thought either pyloric dilation or gastroenterostomy would be effective. Gastroenterostomy was used as the early therapy, but as of 1910 a 61% mortality rate was recorded. Early attempts by Fredet to perform pyloroplasty by resuturing the muscle transversely after the muscle had been split longitudinally (the lumen of the stomach was not entered) proved extremely difficult, and Fredet himself remained convinced that muscle-splitting procedures were superior to gastroenterostomy for this disease. The operation performed today was first described by Ramstedt in 1912.

The cause of pyloric stenosis remains unknown. Interestingly, both environmental and hereditary factors seem to influence the development of this lesion in infants. The symptoms of pyloric stenosis develop later in infants born in hospitals when compared to those born at home. Maternal-fetal-neonatal hypergastrinemia has been implicated in the development of pyloric stenosis. In addition, in a series of monozygotic twins with one twin affected, the other twin developed pyloric stenosis only 67% of the time. It is well recognized that first-born children are more frequently affected, and sporadic ''epidemics'' of pyloric stenosis within a community have been reported.

There also seems to be a genetic predisposition to the development of pyloric stenosis. Boys are affected five times more frequently than girls. In addition, 10% to 15% of sons and 3% to 7% of daughters of affected patients develop pyloric stenosis, with the higher incidence present if the mother has had the disease. Twins, triplets, and multiple siblings with pyloric stenosis have all been reported.

The presenting symptom is vomiting, which is nonbilious in color and frequently consists of the feeding given shortly before. The vomiting typically begins within 1 to 2 weeks after birth and rapidly progresses to projectile emesis as the pylorus becomes essentially completely obstructed. This results in dehydration and loss of hydrogen, potassium, and chloride ions. Stimulation of the renin-aldosterone mechanisms results in increased urinary potassium loss to conserve sodium, perpetuating the metabolic alkalosis. Thus a typical serum electrolyte pattern might include a relatively normal level of sodium (135 to 140 mEq/L), depressed levels of potasium (3 to 4 mEq/L) and chloride (75 to 90 mEq/L), and a greatly elevated serum bicarbonate level (30 to 45 mEq/L). The urine is usually acidic.

Taking these electrolyte deficits into account, the ideal fluid for resuscitation in these infants is 5% dextrose in normal saline with 20 to 40 mEq of calcium chloride per liter added at a rate of 150 to 200 ml/kg/day. A bolus of 5% dextrose in normal saline (20 ml/kg) over an hour is sometimes necessary in severe dehydration. Even though the serum sodium level is usually normal, these infants have isotonic dehydration and benefit by replacement with sodium. As the hypochloremia resolves, the serum bicarbonate level falls. Most clinicians feel that general anesthesia can be safely administered when the serum bicarbonate level is below 30 mEq/L, but this may take 48 hours of vigorous intravenous therapy or more. There is no role for attempts at oral hydration in these seriously ill neonates.

After adequate preparation the operation for pyloric stenosis is one of the safest, most straightforward, and curative procedures performed in pediatric surgery. A small right upper quadrant incision is made, and the peritoneal cavity entered without dividing the rectus muscle. The pylorus is delivered into the wound, and a longitudinal incision made in the anterior wall of the hypertrophied pylorus from the duodenopyloric junction proximally for the extent of the muscular thickening. With a blunt instrument or a ''spreader'' the muscle fibers are divided to the submucosa, allowing the mucosa to bulge into the defect. If the mucosa is injured and the lumen entered, several fine silk sutures can be used to repair the defect, but these must be placed so the stenosis is not recreated. A nasogastric tube is not routinely left in place after surgery unless the lumen has been entered.

Following surgery intravenous fluids are continued until a diet is tolerated. Because the lower esophageal sphincter pressure is abnormally low in these infants for a time after repair, gastroesophageal reflux is common and may result in continued vomiting. An upright position and thickened feedings may be necessary for several weeks after surgery to decrease the risk of reflux and its sequelae.

NECROTIZING ENTEROCOLITIS

Neonatal necrotizing enterocolitis (NEC) is an intriguing disease that seems to affect only newborns and very young infants, primarily those who are born prematurely. An increase in the incidence of NEC over the past 15 years par-

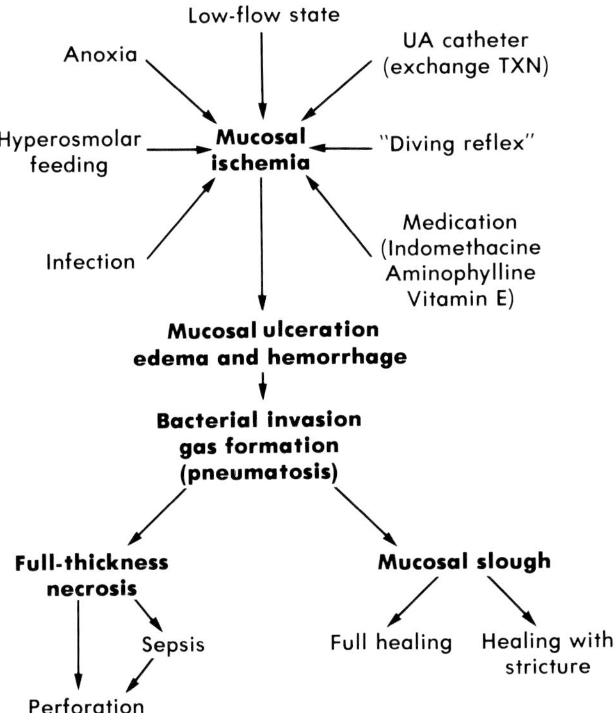

Fig. 65-4 Causes and natural history of newborns with necrotizing enterocolitis. Multiple factors result in mucosal ischemia, which may lead to bacterial invasion. Full healing, healing with stricture, or full-thickness necrosis are possible outcomes. *TXN*, transfusion; *UA*, umbilical artery.

allels the emergence of neonatal intensive care units and the improved survival of premature infants. Although the disease has certainly been present for many years, its pathology was explored only after numerous cases were recognized and managed. Although the exact cause remains obscure, recent experimental and clinical studies have increased the understanding, prevention, and management of NEC.

The basic disorder responsible for bowel necrosis present in NEC is ischemia. Several factors may contribute to the abnormal oxygen delivery to the mucosa and other bowel wall layers (Fig. 65-4). A mesenteric vasospastic reflex after an hypoxic episode, similar to that present in diving mammals, may be responsible for a decrease in mesenteric blood flow from arterial vasoconstriction. This mechanism allows shunting of blood to the brain and heart, providing protection for those vital organs at the expense of others. This is a normal physiologic defense mechanism in many animal species, but its presence in humans has never been proven. Umbilical artery catheterization with positioning of the catheter tip in the descending aorta may also produce vasospasm in the superior mesenteric artery. The infusion of certain substances (e.g., calcium) may contribute to the occurrence of this complication.

Microemboli and thrombi have also been found in instances of NEC, which may be a result of substances infused through an umbilical artery catheter, especially exchange transfusion. Hyperviscosity and platelet aggregates have also been found in some babies with NEC, but these findings may be a secondary process rather than an inciting one.

Low flow states as a result of congenital heart disease or patent ductus arteriosus have been implicated in NEC. Severe dehydration and shock from any cause may also be an inciting event in NEC.

Bacteria appear to be vital to the development of NEC. The gas present within the bowel wall is derived from bacterial action on a carbohydrate substrate, documented by the predominance of hydrogen in gas bubble analysis. Several bacteria and viruses have been implicated in "epidemics" of NEC, but no one organism predominates. Invasion of bowel wall by enteric flora or pathogens may be a primary factor in the development of NEC or may occur secondarily after the ischemic insult. Prophylactic administration of oral broad-spectrum antibiotics in infants at risk has been attempted in several prospective, randomized studies, with inconclusive results. The fear of emergence of resistant organisms has decreased the enthusiasm for this technique.

It has been recognized for several years that babies fed milk-based formulas, especially those that are hyperosmolar, are at risk for the development of NEC. In contrast, breast milk seems to be protective against NEC. The difference may be because of the presence of secretory IgA and macrophages within breast milk. However, since NEC has been seen both in breast-fed infants and in babies who have never been fed, obviously other factors must be implicated.

Several medications given to newborns as therapy for a variety of disorders have recently been found to increase the incidence and severity of NEC in both experimental and clinical studies. Indomethacin, a prostaglandin synthetase inhibitor used for nonsurgical closure of a patent ductus arteriosus, has been associated clinically with an increase in the number of cases of NEC.[10] Vitamin E given to prevent retrolental fibroplasia and aminophylline used as a respiratory stimulant have been found experimentally to increase the severity of bowel necrosis in a rat model of NEC.[4] These studies suggest that extreme care must be exercised in using medications of any kind in the newborn infant.

The most common early signs and symptoms in NEC are presented in Fig. 65-5. The onset is usually insidious, although fulminant cases are occasionally seen. The physical examination of the abdomen in the infant with NEC, although difficult, can nonetheless frequently be valuable. Abdominal wall erythema and edema (especially in the periumbilical region), localized tenderness or crepitance, abdominal mass (edematous, thickened loop of bowel), and splinting of the abdomen by the use of chest wall accessory muscles of respiration are all valuable physical signs in the infant with NEC. In fulminant cases grossly bloody stools and rapid deterioration to a moribund state within a several-hour period usually signifies the presence of a large amount of necrotic bowel.

The roentgenographic signs of necrotizing enterocolitis have been described in numerous publications and include pneumatosis intestinalis, localized bowel distention, portal vein gas, free intraperitoneal air, thickened bowel wall, and a "gasless" appearance, signifying fluid-filled loops

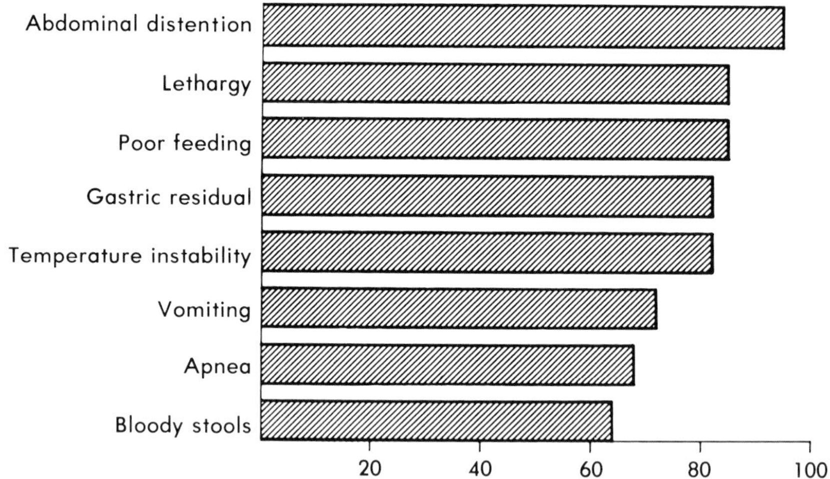

Fig. 65-5 Percent frequency of signs and symptoms associated with necrotizing enterocolitis in newborn infants.

of bowel. The use of metrizamide, a water-soluble contrast agent to aid in the diagnosis of NEC, has proven to be a valuable adjunct in recent studies.[2] Free intraperitoneal air and portal vein gas seem to be the most ominous x-ray signs of NEC, suggestive of perforation and/or extensive necrosis. The laboratory evaluation of the infant with suspected or confirmed NEC should include a white blood cell count; hematocrit; platelet count, blood gas and pH analysis; and a study of renal and liver functions. A very low white blood cell count suggests overwhelming sepsis. A low platelet count has been observed in cases of gangrenous bowel, thought to be caused by disseminated intravascular coagulation, sequestration into the area of necrotic bowel, or binding to endotoxin with removal by the spleen. Although it is useful for following the baby, a very low platelet count is not considered to be an absolute indication for surgery by most neonatal surgeons. Persistent metabolic acidosis or blood gas analysis is a reliable indicator of poor perfusion, is suggestive of bowel necrosis, and is useful when combined with physical and radiologic findings.

The principles of nonoperative management include restoration of intravascular volume to improve gut circulation, prevention of infection, and bowel rest. Candidates for this form of treatment include those infants without perforation; with stable or improving clinical status, including laboratory data; and without massive gastrointestinal hemorrhage. Most neonatologists will institute medical therapy in any infant suspected of having NEC, even if there is little firm evidence that the baby has the disorder. Frequent reexamination by abdominal palpation, x-ray films, and laboratory data (white blood cell count, platelet count, blood gas and pH analysis) are necessary in infants receiving such nonoperative therapy. Since perforation is not detected by x-ray film in as many as 50% of cases, total reliance on radiologic procedures is risky and may result in high mortality because of late diagnosis of peritonitis.

An infant suspected or confirmed of having NEC should have an orogastric or nasogastric tube placed. Intravenous antibiotics (gentamicin and ampicillin) should be given. Poorly absorbed oral antibiotics have not been shown to be efficacious in controlled studies. Intravenous fluids, both crystalloid (0.45% NaCl in 5% dextrose) and colloid (albumin 1 g/kg or fresh-frozen plasma 10 ml/kg), are used at rates necessary to obtain normal renal output. This may require unexpectedly high volumes (200 to 250 ml/kg/day). Cardiac failure from sepsis or vigorous intravascular volume replacement may necessitate the use of inotropic agents (dopamine, isoproteronal, epinephrine) until the clinical status stabilizes. After the onset of resolution (usually 2 to 3 days), the use of intravenous alimentation should be considered. However, the septic premature infant seems to be most susceptible to cholestasis from total parenteral nutrition, and thus liver functions must be monitored carefully.

The timing for the resumption of oral feedings remains controversial since recurrence of NEC has been reported after beginning oral formulas. Most neonatologists would wait 3 to 4 days after resolution of ileus, pneumatosis, and hematochezia before resuming an oral diet.

The timing for surgical intervention in NEC is important since a negative exploration may be dangerous in these critically ill neonates. Pneumoperitoneum, failure of medical therapy as judged by clinical deterioration, persistent acidosis, and thrombocytopenia have been used in various combinations as surgical indications. Of these, pneumoperitoneum seems to be the most reliable, although unfortunately it also signifies a poorer prognosis.

A laparotomy is performed, usually through an upper abdominal transverse incision. All bowel is exteriorized and examined carefully for sites of necrosis and/or perforation, most commonly found in the terminal ileum, ascending colon, transverse and left colon, and proximal small bowel in decreasing order of frequency. Areas of frank bowel necrosis or perforation are resected, even if several separate segmental resections are necessary. Bowel that appears marginally viable is not resected but returned to the abdomen with the possibility of second-look laparotomy 24 to 36 hours later. Although a few investigators have advocated primary anastomosis of bowel, most neonatal surgeons prefer to exteriorize the ends of the bowel as ostomies, either through the wound or through separate incisions, to be closed at a later date. Usually culture-positive purulent fluid or stool is found within the peritoneal cavity, and this should be copiously irrigated.

The postoperative care is directed toward optimizing the circulatory status; correcting shock, acidosis, and sepsis; maintaining hematologic homeostasis; and providing nutrition. This is accomplished by the administration of fluid (colloid and crystalloid), blood and platelets, antibiotics, and later parenteral nutrition. An oral elemental diet can be started 7 to 10 days after surgery, but rarely can sufficient calories be given by the enteral route, and total parenteral nutrition is a valuable adjunct in the management of these infants.

Since the majority of patients with NEC are premature infants, they are suceptible to the disorders that are common to that age group (e.g., hyaline membrane disease, jaundice, meningitis, and intracerebral hemorrhage). Exacting care is necessary to achieve survival in these seriously ill neonates.

ESOPHAGEAL ATRESIA AND TRACHEOESOPHAGEAL FISTULA

Infants with esophageal atresia frequently have early symptoms of severe respiratory distress and excess salivation. Choking, coughing, and cyanosis are frequently encountered on the first attempted feeding. Infants with an associated tracheoesophageal fistula will often develop acute gastric dilation because of air entering the distal esophagus and stomach with each inspired breath. As most neonates have an incompetent lower esophageal sphincter, this ultimately leads to reflux of gastric acid through the fistula into the lungs, resulting in aspiration and chemical pneumonitis. There are five recognized anatomic variants of esphageal atresia. These include atresia of the esophagus without a fistula, esophageal atresia with a proximal tracheoesophageal fistula, esophageal atresia with a "double" tracheoesophageal fistula (from both proximal and distal segments), proximal atresia with a distal tracheoesophageal fistula (most common form—88%), and "H" type tracheoesophageal fistula without esophageal atresia. The incidence of this anomaly is approximately 1:1500 births, with boys and girls equally affected. The ultimate survival of these infants usually depends on prompt recognition and expeditious transfer to institutions fully equipped and staffed with experienced personnel familiar with the often complicated care required. Approximately one third of the infants will be of low birth weight. Associated anomalies are common (70%), particularly those of the cardiovascular system, gastrointestinal tract (imperforate anus and duodenal atresia), genitourinary tract, and musculoskeletal system. Tracheoesophageal fistula has also been observed in patients with Down's syndrome and Trisomy 18. In addition, many may have the VATER association (*V*, vertebral or vascular defects; *A*, anal anomalies; *T*, tracheoesophageal fistula; *E*, esophageal atresia; and *R*, radial limb or renal anomalies).[19]

The defect may be anticipated if maternal polyhydramnios is noted before the baby's delivery. Most infants with esophageal atresia without a fistula will have polyhydramniotic mothers (greater than 90%), whereas in only (approximately) 20% of infants with a distal tracheoesophageal fistula will this be observed. In the latter cases the fetus will swallow amniotic fluid, which overflows the blind esophageal pouch only to pass through the tracheoesophageal fistula into the gastrointestinal tract and will be absorbed normally in utero. The diagnosis of esophageal atresia is not difficult to confirm—attempted passage of a firm red rubber or synthetic catheter through the nose into the esophagus will demonstrate obstruction at the level of atresia. A frontal and lateral x-ray film of the chest and abdomen should be obtained with the catheter in place, showing the tip of the catheter at the end of the atretic proximal esophageal pouch. If gas is present in the gastrointestinal tract, a tracheoesophageal fistula must therefore also be present. If no gas pattern is observed below the diaphragm, a fistula is unlikely. These simple observations will allow a diagnosis in at least 95% of cases of esophageal atresia. Occasionally contrast studies are required for the diagnosis of the more rare forms of proximal esophageal fistula or a double fistula from both the proximal and distal esophageal segments and the "H" type fistula without atresia. The "H" type fistula may be suspected in infants with severe respiratory distress who have a dilated, air-filled esophagus on plain x-ray films. Endoscopy with updated telescopic Storz infant bronchoscopes can usually directly observe the "H" type fistula.

Emergency care of the infant involves aspiration of the oral pharynx to clear secretions. This may be accomplished by insertion of a Replogle sump catheter into the blind pouch. The catheter is maintained on continuous suction to keep the pouch dry. The secretions should be cultured, and the infant started on antibiotic therapy. The truly emergent aspect in the care of this anomaly concerns the occurrence of potentially lethal aspiration pneumonia caused by reflux of gastric juice from the dilated stomach through the tracheoesophageal fistula. The deleterious chemical effects of gastric juice on the tracheobronchial tree and pulmonary parenchyma are well known. The infant should be maintained in semi-Fowler's position to keep the gastric fluid meniscus low in the stomach, reducing reflux. An emergency gastrostomy is performed, usually under local anesthesia, to decompress the stomach; this eliminates the problem of reflux in 95% of the cases. The gastrostomy is maintained on straight drainage. If the infant is full term and shows no evidence of associated anomalies, sepsis, or pneumonitis, a definitive extrapleural thoracotomy is then undertaken, using general endotracheal anesthesia. The fistula is divided, the tracheal side oversewn, and an end-to-end anastomosis is attempted between the dilated thickened proximal pouch and the small distal esophagus. Tension and poor blood supply (particularly to the distal segment) are two problems encountered during this anastomosis and are directly related to the incidence of anastomotic leaks that may occur in as many as 15% of patients. An extrapleural leak, however, will drain to the outside, much like an incision and drainage of an abscess, with little or no effect on the infant's condition; in fact, many infants do not even demonstrate an elevation in temperature when this occurs. However, if a transpleural operation is performed, a leak would result in empyema, which is associated with a significant morbidity and mortality in the neonatal age group. Thus there is probably no role for the transpleural approach in the initial thoracic exploration of an infant with esophageal atresia. This concept is supported by a 20% higher survival rate in infants undergoing extrapleural operations. In patients of low birth weight (premature or small for gestational age) or those with evidence of associated congenital anomalies, sepsis, or severe pneumonia, the thoracic operation is delayed following gastrostomy. Improved pulmonary toilet, hydration, and antibiotic therapy are initiated with suction on the proximal pouch, and the gastrostomy set to straight drainage. The definitive procedure is delayed until the infant is better able to withstand a general endotracheal anesthetic and thoracotomy. This "staging" period often lasts only from 1 to 4 days and significantly improves the baby's general condition and chances for survival. At the time of thoracotomy, if the ends of the esophagus are too far apart for a "safe" anastomosis (even under tension), a number of alternatives may be considered. First, closure of the distal end and approximation of the muscular segments without opening the proximal pouch may be attempted, allowing the two ends of the esophagus to spontaneously stretch with reoperation at 4 to 6 weeks. Others have used manual or electromagnetic bougienage of the blind proximal pouch over a 6- to 8-week period with subsequent reexploration to achieve the same goal. An additional technique is that of circular esophagomyotomy that allows distal descent of the end of proximal atretic pouch and primary anastomosis to be performed at the initial operation. In general, the goal has been to avoid esophageal replacement by interposition of colon or a gastric tube whenever possible. Neither of these replacement organs functions as well as the infant's own esophagus. These procedures, however, are sometimes required when the two ends of the esophagus are much too far apart or if any of the previously mentioned surgical adjuncts fail (particularly in instances of atresia without an associated fistula). In these cases, a cervical esophagostomy is performed, and the infant is maintained on gastrostomy feedings until an appropriate time for interposition procedures (usually at age 18 months). Sham oral feedings are also given in the interim so that the infant does not forget how to swallow.

The care of infants with variants of esophageal atresia is exacting and demanding. However, when it takes place at skilled neonatal centers particularly designed and equipped with personnel skilled in the management of these critically ill patients, good survival rates can be obtained.

Many of these survivors will require periodic dilation of the esophageal anastomosis. In addition, long-term follow-up is essential since some of the patients will need additional surgical procedures to repair associated cardiac, renal, and other gastrointestinal anomalies.

In recent years a high incidence of gastroesophageal reflux has been noted in these patients. Gastroesophageal reflux has been incriminated in the many chronic pulmonary problems seen in these children (aspiration pneumonia, "asthmatic" condition), and some may require an antireflux operation (Nissen fundoplication).

CONGENITAL DIAPHRAGMATIC HERNIA

Congenital posterolateral diaphragmatic hernia, through the foramen of Bochdalek, is the most common surgically correctable cause of severe respiratory distress in the newborn. Occurring in 1/2200 births, the defect is on the left side in 85% of cases, on the right side in 13%, and bilateral in 1% to 2%. Most infants with diaphragmatic hernia are term babies, and therefore any "large" baby with severe respiratory distress should be suspected as having congenital defect.

This anomaly forms as the gut makes its normal return to the abdominal cavity from the yolk sac simultaneously with the formation of the diaphragm and the development of lung buds. Failure of the pleuroperitoneal foramen of Bochdalek to close before return of the gut allows the viscera to herniate into the hemithorax, preventing the full development of the ipsilateral lung. If the mediastinum is shifted, compression of the contralateral lung takes place, interfering with its development as well. The result is moderate-to-severe respiratory distress, usually present immediately at birth or shortly thereafter. The degree of distress tends to worsen rapidly as swallowed air distends the gut within the chest, causing further lung compression and mediastinal shift. Cyanosis, tachypnea, pallor, gasping respirations, retractions, or complete cardiorespiratory arrest are the usual findings as the baby struggles to expand his lungs. Breath sounds are usually absent on the side of the hernia, and heart sounds are shifted to the opposite hemithorax. The typical appearance of a barrel chest and scaphoid abdomen is frequently present.

The differential diagnosis on the basis of clinical examinaton will be that of pneumothorax, chylothorax, meconium, or other aspiration syndromes and congenital cystic lung lesions (lobar emphysema or cystic adenomatoid malformation). If possible, a chest x-ray film should be obtained at the first sign of respiratory distress, before the institution of invasive resuscitative procedures such as tube thoracostomy. Occasionally the x-ray film will show an opacified hemithorax if the infant has not swallowed sufficient air to fill the gastrointestinal tract. If confusion exists in the interpretation of the x-ray film, a repeat x-ray film should be performed to further define the problem. Frequently, this will demonstrate the gut within the chest.

The therapy for newborns with diaphragmatic hernia consists of preoperative stabilization and preparation, operative reduction of the hernia and repair of the defect, and postoperative care and support. It is well accepted that most infants with diaphragmatic hernia benefit from a brief period of preoperative stabilization, which should include direct endotracheal intubation with ventilator assistance. Assisted ventilation by mask and bag should be avoided since this technique may introduce excessive amounts of air into the portion of the gastrointestinal tract herniated into the chest, causing further lung compression. After intubation the child should be rapidly ventilated with 100% oxygen, and a blood gas determination made to assess the effectiveness of ventilation (P_{CO_2} level and oxygenation (P_{O_2} level). High pressures should be avoided during ventilation since the development of pneumothorax from lung "blow-out" can be rapidly fatal in these infants with marginal pulmonary reserve. A nasogastric tube should be placed early in resuscitation to empty the gastrointestinal tract. Maintenance of a warm environment for preservation of body temperature is critically important. An intravenous line should be inserted as quickly as possible, and sodium bicarbonate given to correct metabolic acidosis, if present. Using several minutes to stabilize and improve the metabolic status in this way makes the baby a much better candidate for surgical repair and optimizes his chances for survival.

The surgical approach for these infants is usually straightforward. A transverse or upper vertical incision is used. The viscera are gently reduced from the chest, and an assessment is made regarding primary closure of the diaphragm defect (usually possible) or, if the defect is very large, the use of a prosthesis or muscle flap for defect closure. A tube thoracostomy is inserted through the fifth intercostal space and placed on a low level of suction (5 to 8 cm of water). Occasionally, after the defect is repaired, the abdominal cavity is too small to accommodate the viscera. In these instances creation of a ventral hernia by closing only skin and subcutaneous tissues, followed later (3 to 6 months) by ventral hernia repair, is an acceptable alternative. In cases where prolonged ventilatory support is anticipated, particularly with high peak inspiratory pressures, a chest tube is placed prophylactically in the contralateral chest to prevent development of an unsuspected tension pneumothorax if that lung should rupture.

The postoperative management of these infants is demanding and frequently frustrating. Arterial blood gas monitoring should be performed frequently, and appropriate changes in ventilator settings made immediately. The development of pulmonary hypertension, which can become apparent immediately or after a so-called ''honeymoon'' period of 6 to 12 hours is the most serious complication following surgery. This condition, leading to a fetal circulatory pattern with right-to-left shunting at the atrial (foramen ovale) and ductus arteriosus levels, has proven very difficult to treat and leads to mortality in the majority of infants who develop it.[3]

The cause of pulmonary hypertension in these infants is unclear. Histologically, an increase in musculature within the pulmonary arteriole has been found in the lungs of nonsurvivors vs. age-matched controls, suggesting increased pulmonary vascular resistance by lumen narrowing.[16] An exaggerated response of the pulmonary vasculature to factors known to cause pulmonary artery vasospasm might lead to suprasystemic pressures in the right ventricle, leading to right-to-left shunting. Shunting in these infants has been confirmed by simultaneous arterial Po_2 measurements from above (right radial artery) and below (foot artery) the level of the ductus arteriosus.

The circumstances that have been shown to cause pulmonary artery vasoconstriction are alveolar hypoxia, hypoxemia, hypercarbia, and acidosis. Other factors that result in pulmonary artery vasospasm include epinephrine and norepinephrine, serotonin, propanalol, and hypothermia. Respiratory factors shown to reverse vasospasm include high inspired oxygen concentrations, often combined with hyperventilation to lower Pco_2 levels and thus to resolve respiratory acidosis, even to the point of alkalosis (arterial pH 7.5 or greater). The medications that lower pulmonary artery resistance include tolazoline, prostaglandin E, chlorpromazine, acetylcholine, and nitroprusside.

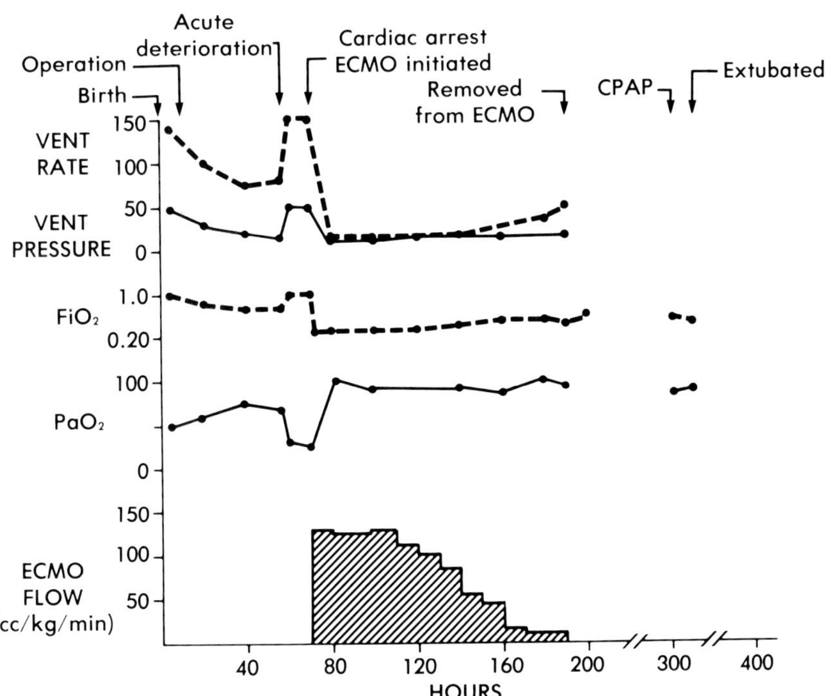

Fig. 65-6 Typical clinical course of an infant after repair of congenital diaphragmatic hernia. After a ''honeymoon'' period of relative stability, acute deterioration occurred in blood gases, probably related to pulmonary hypertension and right-to-left shunting. Extracorporeal membrane oxygenation *(ECMO)* was then used for approximately 100 hours, until the pulmonary hypertension resolved. *FIo_2*, fraction of inspired oxygen; *Pao_2*, partial pressure of oxygen in arterial blood; *CPAP*, continuous positive airway pressure.

The postoperative management of these infants is thus directed toward creating a situation favorable to limiting or reversing pulmonary artery vasoconstriction. Hyperventilation with 100% oxygen at rapid rates (120 to 150/minute) to keep the arterial Po_2 above 80 mm Hg and reduce Pco_2 to 30 mm Hg or lower, combined with continuous infusion of tolazoline (1 to 2 mg/kg/hour), is generally used to attempt to prevent or reverse a cycle of hypoxia–hypercarbia–pulmonary–vasoconstriction–right-to-left shunting–increased hypoxia. Unfortunately, these maneuvers have been shown to be only marginally effective, at best.

The use of extracorporeal membrane oxygenation has recently been described in newborns with severe respiratory distress, including several with diaphragmatic hernia.[1] Cannulae are placed in the right atrium through the jugular vein for venous outflow and in the aortic arch through the right carotid artery for return of oxygenated blood. The blood is circulated through a membrane oxygenator and heat exchange with a variable speed roller pump before return to the patient. By varying the oxygen delivery to the membrane oxygenator, Po_2 levels of 300 to 400 mm Hg and Pco_2 levels of 15 to 25 mm Hg can easily be obtained. Fig. 65-6 shows a typical clinical course for a baby treated with extracorporeal membrane oxygenation after diaphragmatic hernia repair who was unresponsive to conventional medical management. This technique can rapidly reverse pulmonary vasospasm, which allows weaning from the apparatus and resumption of routine pulmonary care. Although the long-term effects of carotid artery and internal jugular vein ligation, which are necessary components of this therapy, remain to be determined, extracorporeal membrane oxygenation holds great promise for saving many of these infants who would otherwise die.

ALIMENTARY TRACT OBSTRUCTION

Congenital lesions resulting in alimentary tract obstruction constitute a major group of anomalies. These lesions formerly were thought to be associated with significant morbidity and mortality, but early recognition and prompt appropriate therapy now results in excellent survival rates in most pediatric centers.

The presence of intestinal obstruction may be anticipated by carefully obtaining a family history to record instances of cystic fibrosis, aganglionosis, pyloric atresia, and rare cases of multiple gastrointestinal atresia, all of which may be inherited disorders. Prenatal ultrasound may detect alimentary tract obstruction in utero, allowing for predelivery preparation and timely transfer to a pediatric surgical center, if appropriate.

There are four cardinal signs of alimentary tract obstruction in the newborn: maternal polyhydramnios, bilious vomiting, abdominal distention, and failure to pass normal amounts of meconium spontaneously in the first 24 hours of life. Although none is pathognomonic, the presence of two or more strongly suggests intestinal obstruction and mandates further work-up.

Amniotic fluid in excess of 1500 to 2000 ml is considered to be polyhydramnios. A 25% to 40% amount of amniotic fluid is swallowed by the fetus and usually reabsorbed in the first 20 to 25 cm of jejunum. A high alimentary tract obstruction (e.g., esophageal atresia without tracheoesophageal fistula, pyloric atresia, duodenal atresia, or high jejunal atresia) may be associated with maternal polyhydramnios. Other causes of polyhydramnios include fetal swallowing problems, particularly in infants with central nervous system abnormality (i.e., anencephaly). Maternal conditions resulting in poly-hydramnios include toxemia and cardiac, renal, or hepatic disease. Idiopathic polyhydramnios is also observed. Current evaluation of the polyhydramniotic female should include ultrasound of the fetus to attempt to detect upper alimentary tract obstruction.

Bilious vomiting in a newborn or young infant is always pathologic and must be investigated. The newborn's stomach normally contains less than 15 ml of clear gastric juice at birth. More than 20 ml of clear gastric secretions or gastric juice containing bile suggests alimentary tract obstruction. Bilious vomiting may also be seen in septic infants with adynamic ileus. If alimentary tract obstruction is suggested by a large amount of gastric juice, the stomach should be gently emptied by an orogastric tube, which should be left in place and connected to either low suction or gravity drainage. Fluid and electrolyte losses from the stomach can be considerable and should be replaced with 5% dextrose in normal saline, with added potassium (20 to 50 mEq/L).

The normal contour of the newborn's abdomen is round, unlike the usual spheroid appearance of the adult abdomen. However, a grossly distended abdomen in the neonate is pathologic. Physical findings associated with distention include visible veins on the abdomen wall caused by attenuation, "bowel patterning" (visible intestinal loops with or without peristalsis) and occasionally respiratory distress caused by elevation of the diaphragms. In each case it is essential to obtain a supine and decubitus or cross-table x-ray film of the abdomen to evaluate the nature of the distention. Distention may be the result of free air (perforated viscous), fluid (hemoperitoneum, chyloperitoneum), or distended bowel caused by mechanical obstruction or adynamic ileus. In general, only lower intestinal obstruction (ileal or colonic) gives significant abdominal distention.

Normal meconium is composed of amniotic fluid, squames, lanugo hairs, succus entericus, and intestinal mucus. It is dark green or black in color and sticky in consistency. As much as 250 mg of meconium may be passed, and failure to pass normal amounts in the first 24 hours of life may be pathologic. Infants with low small bowel obstruction, colon atresia, Hirschsprung's disease, meconium plug syndrome, or small left colon syndrome may fit this category. Other diseases that may be associated with failure of meconium passage include prematurity, hypothyroidism, sepsis with adynamic ileus, and maternal narcotic addiction.

Pyloric Atresia

Pyloric atresia accounts for 1% of all alimentary tract obstruction in neonates. Occasionally there is a familial tendency to pyloric atresia, and cases have been noted in siblings. Infants with this malformation present with nonbilious vomiting. Maternal polyhydramnios is found in two thirds of cases. In some infants epidermolysis bullosa is associated with pyloric atresia.

Plain x-ray film of the abdomen shows a single large gastric bubble with no evidence of air beyond the pylorus. Contrast studies are usually unnecessary. The infant may initially have hypochloremic alkalosis as a result of the loss of hydrochloric acid from vomiting. An orogastric tube should be placed to prevent vomiting and minimize the risk of aspiration. Intravenous fluids are required to prevent dehydration and to replete electrolyte losses (10% dextrose in 0.45% saline).

When the electrolyte pattern stabilizes, the infant should be taken to the operating room for the relief of obstruction. The atretic lesion is usually mucosal in nature. Excision of the prepyloric atretic web and pyloroplasty is an effective treatment, with a temporary Stamm gastrostomy usually performed as a complementary procedure.

Duodenal Obstruction

Congenital obstruction of the duodenum, whether complete (atresia) or incomplete (stenosis) represents a significant cause of neonatal alimentary tract obstruction. Duodenal atresia develops early in intrauterine life. A mucosal web is the most frequent type of atretic lesion noted. Eighty-five percent of duodenal atresias are located just distal to the ampulla of Vater, thus making bilious vomiting the presenting symptom in a majority of cases.

Polyhydramnios is observed in 33% to 50% of cases. Of these infants 40% are premature, and one third have Down's syndrome. Hyperbilirubinemia is also often observed. Between 50% and 75% of babies have associated anomalies, including cardiac, genitourinary, musculoskeletal, and other gastrointestinal defects (i.e., esophageal atresia, imperforate anus). As a result, these infants are very high–risk patients and should be managed in a sophisticated neonatal intensive care facility.

Plain x-ray film of the abdomen demonstrates the classic ''double-bubble'' sign of duodenal obstruction. There is no evidence of air in the gastrointestinal tract beyond the obstruction in atretic cases. An orogastric tube should be placed on drainage. Fluid and electrolyte disturbances may be seen as a result of losses related to bilious vomiting, and thus appropriate intravenous therapy is a prerequiste in the preparation of the infant for surgical therapy of the obstruction. This condition does not represent a true surgical emergency, and a period of time as long as 48 hours may be necessary to completely stabilize the infant.

The surgical treatment of choice is a duodenoduodenostomy to bypass the obstruction. In instances of duodenal web, duodenotomy and excision of the web may be possible, but care must be taken to not injure the ampulla of Vater, which is frequently located immediately adjacent to the web. The greatly dilated duodenum proximal to the obstruction frequently results in delayed (7 to 10 days) anastomotic function. Tapering of the dilated antimesenteric border of the proximal duodenum has also been recommended.

Duodenal stenosis may be associated with annular pancreas, malrotation with Ladd's bands (incomplete rotation and fixation), an anterior (preduodenal) portal vein, or an intrinsic web with a small diaphragm. Plain x-ray film shows a ''double-bubble'' with a small amount of intestinal air distal to the duodenum. The preparation and treatment of infants with stenosis are similar to that outlined for infants with duodenal atresia.

Intestinal Atresia

Four types of small bowel atresia (exclusive of duodenal atresia) are recognized. Type I represents a mucosal web or diaphragm and is probably caused by epithelial plugging. In Type II an atretic cord exists between two blind ends, and the mesentery is intact. In Type IIIa there is complete separation of the blind ends by a U-shaped mesenteric gap. Type IIIb represents instances of atresia with an ''apple-peel'' deformity, in which the bowel distal to the atresia receives a retrograde blood supply from the ileocolic or right colic artery. Type IV represents cases of multiple atresias.

Types II, III, and IV atresias result from late intrauterine mesenteric vascular accidents. The possible causes of these episodes include instances of intrauterine emboli, volvulus, internal hernia, intussusception, or gastroschisis. Most cases of small bowel atresia are solitary; however, in 10% multiple atresias (Type IV) are observed. Since 10% of atresias, especially ileal, occur in infants with cystic fibrosis, appropriate work up (sweat chloride determination) should be performed on each child before discharge.

Infants with high jejunal atresia are usually products of polyhydramniotic pregnancy and initially have bilious vomiting. The plain abdominal x-ray film demonstrates several dilated loops of small bowel with no air distal to the atresia. Jaundice is a frequent finding in newborns with jejunal atresia.

The preoperative clinical management should include placement of an orogastric tube combined with rehydration and electrolyte stabilization with appropriate intravenous fluids. At laparotomy, bowel proximal to the atresia is greatly dilated and atonic with poor peristalsis. This dilated bowel is usually resected back to the ligament of Treitz, where an end-to-end anastomosis is performed. The disparity in size between the large proximal bowel and the smaller distal gut may be alleviated by an end (90-degree) to oblique (45-degree) approximation, generally using a single layer of nonabsorbable suture. When short bowel length is present, as is frequently the case in Types IIIb and IV, the proximal dilated segment can be used rather than resected by a tapering jejunoplasty.[20] This is accomplished by an antimesenteric resection of the dilated gut for a length of 4 to 8 cm, which then allows an end-to-end anastomosis. When the diameter of the gut is reduced in this way, normal peristalsis is restored, and valuable gut length is maintained. A 7- to 10-day delay in the onset of anastomosis function is not unusual, and a gastrostomy provides excellent gastric drainage in these circumstances. Postoperative nutritional support is provided by intravenous solutions of amino acids, glucose, and lipids, occasionally administered through a central venous catheter if a prolonged period of parenteral nutrition is anticipated.

Infants with low small bowel obstruction initially have bilious vomiting and significant abdominal distention. Abdominal x-ray films demonstrate numerous loops of dilated bowel, usually associated with air-fluid levels. Since the infant colon does not show haustral markings on x-ray film, a barium enema can be performed in cases of low intestinal obstruction and should be the first enema that the baby receives. The barium enema differentiates between small and large bowel distention, determines whether the colon is used or unused (microcolon) and therefore identifies the level of obstruction (small or large bowel), and evaluates the position of the cecum with regard to intestinal rotation and fixation (i.e., malrotation).

Occasionally the abdominal x-ray film demonstrates calcification within the abdominal cavity. This signifies either the presence of meconium peritonitis from intrauterine bowel perforation or bowel wall necrosis resulting in "mummification." In either case, barium enema is as unnecessary as laparotomy is imperative.

Ileal Atresia

Infants with ileal atresia present with abdominal distention and bilious vomiting and may fail to pass meconium. Abdominal x-ray film multiple loops of distended small bowel with many air-fluid levels (with one loop larger than the others). The barium enema shows an unused microcolon, delineating the obstruction to the distal small bowel.

These cases are usually managed by resection of the proximal dilated segment with end-to-end anastomosis. Tapering ileoplasty may be used in cases with short gut to preserve bowel length. In the presence of peritonitis or in instances of questionable bowel viability, a temporary enterostomy may be required.

Meconium Ileus

Meconium ileus is a unique form of congential intestinal obstruction that occurs in 10% to 15% of newborns with cystic fibrosis. A deficiency of pancreatic enzymes and an abnormality in the composition of meconium are factors responsible for the solid intraluminal concretions that produce an obturation form of obstruction in this disorder. A careful family history should be sought when this hereditary disease is suspected. The presence of low small bowel obstruction occurring in identical twins is almost always caused by meconium ileus. These infants present with abdominal distention and bilious vomiting and fail to pass meconium.

Certain x-ray film findings may help distinguish between ileal atresia and meconium ileus. In infants with meconium ileus, the x-ray film often demonstrates significant dilation of similar-sized loops with few, if any, air fluid levels. A ground glass appearance in the right lower quadrant (Neuhauser's sign) may be observed and represents viscid meconium mixed with air. The contrast enema shows an unused colon similar to ileal atresia, but reflux of contrast into the distal ileum may demonstrate the unusual obstructive concretions. Treatment of meconium ileus depends on whether it is uncomplicated (simple obstruction with concretions) or complicated by atresia, volvulus, meconium peritonitis, or giant cystic meconium peritonitis.

The initial treatment for uncomplicated meconium ileus is nonoperative, using hypertonic contrast enema (Hypaque or Gastrograffin). These substances allow fluoroscopic visualization of the gut, whereas their hypertonic character draws fluid into the thick, meconium pellets from the bowel wall, resulting in relief of obstruction. This therapy may cause significant fluid shifts with intravascular depletion, reducing cardiac output by as much as 35%, thus making an intravenous line mandatory during the procedure. Careful attention to fluid balance, blood pressure, pulse rate, and urine output during the enema and for several hours afterwards is essential. Occasionally the enema must be repeated to relieve the obstruction.

Unsuccessful nonoperative attempts in uncomplicated instances of meconium ileus and all cases with complications require surgical intervention. Contemporary surgical management consists of intraoperative irrigation of the viscid meconium and obstructive pellets by means of an enterotomy. The bowel is irrigated with saline and dilute Hypaque or Gastrograffin to lower the viscosity of the meconium and relieve the obstruction. This procedure obviates the need for resection and/or enterostomy in most cases, thus avoiding the risks of later enterostomy closure. For cases complicated by volvulus or gangrene, bowel resection with anastomosis or enterostomy may be required.

Careful family counseling and parental instruction regarding diet, enzyme replacement, and pulmonary toilet are important components of the overall care of these patients.

Colonic Obstruction

Causes of colonic obstruction in the newborn include meconium plug syndrome, aganglionic megacolon (Hirschsprung's disease), colon atresia, small left colon syndrome, and the various types of imperforate anus. The two most common causes, meconium plug and Hirschsprung's disease, will be discussed.

Meconium plug syndrome was first described by Clatworthy in 1956. Although a few cases may be associated with Hirschsprung's disease, the majority have no known cause. Meconium plug syndrome is not equivalent to meconium ileus and therefore has no relationship to cystic fibrosis. The infant initially has distention and fails to pass meconium. Plain x-ray films of the abdomen show numerous dilated loops of bowel with air-fluid levels. Contrast enema shows a small, unused left colon with a dilated transverse colon containing copious intraluminal meconium. The enema is both diagnostic and therapeutic since the thick meconium can frequently be irrigated and expelled. Occasionally a second enema is required to completely evacuate all of the inspissated material, after which the infants usually have no further obstruction.

Hirschsprung's disease is a neurogenic form of obstruction characterized by an absence of ganglion cells in the myenteric (Auerbach's) and submucosal (Meissner's) plexus. Hypertrophic nerve fibers are frequently observed. This absence of parasympathetic innervation causes an uninhibited sympathetic tone in the gut musculature, resulting in failure of relaxation of the internal sphincter. The failure of internal sphincter relaxation with anal dilation is the basis for manometric diagnosis of this disorder. A lack of craniocaudal migration of ganglion cell precursers is believed to be responsible for the disorder, perhaps related to ischemia of the gut in utero.

The aganglionosis always begins at the anorectal line and extends proximally to the sigmoid in 80% of cases. In

10% of patients, the aganglionic segment extends to the splenic flexure, whereas in an additional 10% the entire colon and, in some cases, portions of ileum are involved. Total aganglionsis of the entire gastrointestinal tract has also been reported. The disease has a definite familial tendency, with children of one affected parent having a 5% to 15% risk of having Hirschsprung's disease.

Most patients with this disease will become symptomatic shortly after birth, and 95% will fail to pass meconium in the first 24 hours of life. Abdominal distention, bilious vomiting, and severe constipation are the signs that should lead one to suspect aganglionosis. Plain x-ray films may show many dilated loops of bowel, a large amount of stool above the level of aganglionosis, and air-fluid levels. Barium enema might look normal in the newborn, but a normal infant will expel the barium within 6 to 12 hours, whereas an infant with Hirschsprung's disease will retain the contrast for over 24 hours. Older infants and children will have a "transition zone" visible on contrast enema, with dilated bowel narrowing to a narrow spastic segment.

An occasional infant will present with abdominal distention and alternating constipation and diarrhea. Diarrhea associated with Hirschsprung's disease is known as enterocolitis and has been the subject of investigation for many years. Bacterial overgrowth, passive diffusion of fluid into the bowel with static contents, poor lymphatic flow caused by lack of peristalsis, and abnormalities in prostaglandin metabolism have been postulated as causes for this disorder, but a combination of these is the most likely cause of this complication.

A rectal biopsy demonstrating the absence of ganglion cells confirms the diagnosis. A submucosal aspiration biopsy is 90% accurate, whereas a full-thickness biopsy showing no ganglion cells is pathognomonic but must be performed using general anesthesia. Once the diagnosis is made, the therapy of choice is a colostomy or enterostomy at the lowest point of normal ganglion cell distribution, as judged by frozen section control. When the infant reaches 1 year of age, a definitive pull-through procedure of the classic Swenson, Duhamel (retrorectal), or Soave (endorectal) is undertaken, depending on which method is best used by the surgeon involved. Long-term results are excellent with the use of any one of these techniques.

SUMMARY

The pediatric patient, especially in the first month of life, presents unique challenges in management for the surgeon should an operation become necessary. These challenges relate to the dynamic adjustment to extrauterine life with which the newborn infant must cope, the energy and nutritional demands invoked by this period of rapid growth, the relative immaturity of the infant's organ systems, the rapid metabolic and physiologic changes that are occurring during this time, and the infant's small physical size. Coupled with these features is the inability of these young patients, and frequently their parents, to provide an adequate history of complaints or symptoms, making diagnosis of disease often tedious and demanding and allowing little room for error in management. Notwithstanding these potential difficulties in defining the cause of a given patient's problem, the most common signs and symptoms encountered in this age group include respiratory distress, vomiting, failure to pass meconium, diarrhea, abdominal distention, sepsis, and abdominal wall defects. A number of well-defined clinical abnormalities are generally responsible for these findings and include such disorders as omphalocele, gastroschisis, hypertrophic pyloric stenosis, necrotizing enterocolitis, various forms of esophageal atresia, congenital diaphragmatic hernia, intestinal obstruction secondary to atresia, malrotation or meconium ileus, and Hirschsprung's disease. An understanding of the physiologic derangements coincident with each of these disease processes and their accompanying clinical presentations will ensure early diagnosis and expeditious treatment. These considerations coupled with a knowledge of the fluid dynamics and respiratory physiology unique to this age group will guarantee the optimum in clinical care and the minimum in morbidity and mortality.

REFERENCES

1. Bartlett, R.H., et al.: Extracorporeal membrane oxygenation for newborn respiratory failure: forty-five cases, Surgery **92:**425, 1982.
2. Cohen, M., et al.: A new look at the neonatal bowel: contrast studies with metrizamide (Amipaque), J. Pediatr. Surg. **18:**442, 1983.
3. Collins, D.L., et al.: A new approach to congenital posterolateral diaphragmatic hernia, J. Pediatr. Surg. **12:**149, 1977.
4. Dalsing, M., et al.: The relationship of aminophilline and caffeine in the treatment of neonatal apnea and necrotizing enterocolitis (NEC), Surg. Forum **23:**202, 1982.
5. Duhamel, B.: Embryology of exomphalos and allied malformations, Arch. Dis. Child. **38:**138, 1963.
6. Fishman, A.P.: Hypoxia on the pulmonary circulation: how and where it acts, Circ. Res. **38:**221, 1976.
7. Grosfeld, J.L., and Weber, T.R.: Congenital abdominal wall defects: gastroschisis and omphalocele, Curr. Probl. Surg. **19:**158, 1982.
8. Liggins, G.C.: Premature parturitian after infusion of corticotrophin or cortisol into fetal lambs, J. Endocrinol. **45:**515, 1969.
9. Liggins, G.C., and Howie, R.N.: A controlled trial of antepartum glucocorticoid treatment for prevention of the respiratory distress syndrome in premature infants, Pediatrics **50:**515, 1972.
10. Nagaraj, H.S., et al.: Gastrointestinal perforation following indomethacin therapy in very low birthweight infants, J. Pediatr. Surg. **16:**1003, 1981.
11. Oh, W.: Fluid and electrolyte management. In Avery, G., editor: Neonatology: pathophysiology and management of the newborn, Philadelphia, 1981, J.B. Lippincott Co.
12. Peacham, G.J., and Fox, W.W.: Physiologic factors affecting pulmonary artery pressure in infants with persistent pulmonary hypertension, J. Pediatr. **93:**1005, 1978.
13. Perkin, R.M., et al.: Dobutamine: a hemodynamic evaluation in children with shock, J. Pediatr. **100:**977, 1982.
14. Riemenschneider, T.A., et al.: Disturbances of the transitional circulation: spectrum of pulmonary hypertension and myocardial dysfunction, J. Pediatr. **89:**662, 1976.
15. Rudolph, A.M., and Yuan, S.: Response of the pulmonary vasculature to hypoxia and H^+ ion concentration changes, J. Clin. Invest. **45:**399, 1966.
16. Shochat, S.J., et al.: Congenital diaphragmatic hernia: new concept in management, Ann. Surg. **190:**332, 1979.
17. Vane, D.W., et al.: Systemic and renal effects of dopamine in the infant pig, J. Surg. Res. **32:**477, 1982.
18. Vane, D.W., et al.: Peritonitis: failure of hemodynamic response with dopamine, J. Pediatr. Surg. **18:**426, 1983.
19. Weber, T.R., Smith, E., and Grosfeld, J.L.: Surgical experience in infants with the VATER association, J. Pediatr. Surg. **15:**849, 1980.
20. Weber, T.R., Vane, D.W., and Grosfeld, J.L.: Experience with tapering enteroplasty in infants with bowel atresia and short gut, Arch. Surg. **117:**684, 1982.

66

Ronald Fairman and John L. Rombeau

Physiologic Problems in the Elderly Surgical Patient

In 1982 the White House Conference on Aging estimated that 25 million people in the United States were 65 years of age or older. In 1900 this subset constituted 4% of the population, whereas now the figure is 11%. Today approximately 2 million people are age 85 and older, about 1% of the U.S. population; it is expected that this number will grow to 5.4 million by the year 2000. At that time, one in 20 Americans will be older than 85. At present, 75% of those born can be expected to reach age 65, and 50% of those who survive to 65 can expect to live 80 years. Because of both medical and social progress, it is clear that we are moving at an accelerating rate toward a more elderly society.

Because of the increase in life expectancy, the number of aged patients who require major surgical procedures for correction or palliation of disease has also increased. Powers[44] noted that a peak incidence of operative procedures occurred in the seventh decade of life; the highest incidence of coexisting diseases was also found in this decade. Surgical mortality was highest in patients with the largest number of coexisting diseases, especially cardiovascular diseases. He further noted that a steadily increasing incidence of intercurrent disease began in the fifth decade of life. Also, elective surgery performed in patients over age 60 was associated with a 5% increase in mortality risk, and emergency surgery carried a 20% increase in risk compared with a younger population. In this subset of the population older than 60 years of age, complications were more frequent postoperatively and convalescence was generally longer, especially if associated intercurrent diseases were present.

These data lend support to the need for a specific physiologic approach to the management of surgical disease in the elderly high-risk patient. Only through precise attention to primary as well as intercurrent pathology will surgical therapy be successful in this population.

CELLULAR DYNAMICS OF AGING PROCESS

Aging is a biologic process of deterioration in structure and function over time. Although the precise etiology is unclear, the process is unavoidable and constantly present. Fig. 66-1 illustrates the decline in major functional capacities in the aged patient. The changes leading to functional impairment are multifactorial. It is difficult to separate the physiologic or primary causes of aging from pathologic or secondary causes that are acquired and accelerate the process. Environmental forces also play a role in this process. A decreasing ability to survive stress and impairment of the mechanism(s) of internal homeostasis are characteristic of aging.

Such observations fit with Kohn's characterization[32] of the aged population as having (1) diseases that are progressive, (2) increased incidence of coexisting diseases, and (3) a diminished reaction to stress with increased mortality from injuries and various insults. Reaction to stress is delayed in the elderly individual. It takes longer for the blood glucose level to return to baseline during a standard glucose tolerance test in this patient population. The heart rate likewise takes longer to return to the resting level after physical activity.

Kohn[32] has shown that the mortality from most diseases increases with aging. The explanation for this is uncertain. It is known that the aging process involves decreasing immunologic efficiency, and consequently an increased incidence of infections, cancer, and autoimmune disorders occurs in the elderly patient. Increasing age brings a progressive loss of lymphoid tissue from the thymus, spleen, bone marrow, and lymph nodes. The decline in function is most pronounced in the T-cell population and is apparent in a test of delayed skin reactivity.[29] Burnett[6] has proposed that the thymus is central to all the changes in the aging immune system. Changes in the B cells, or the humoral response, are smaller and appear to be secondary to changes in the T-cell population. Whether this decline in immunologic surveillance is the etiology of the aging process or a result of it is still unclear.

On a cellular level much has been learned about the process of aging in recent years. In the aging cell the nucleus shows clumping of chromatin, with an increased number of nucleoli.[53] The nuclear membrane becomes invaginated, and the amount of endoplasmic reticulum is reduced, perhaps accounting for the reduced synthetic capability of the cell. The cytoplasm undergoes both regressive and degenerative changes, leading to altered cellular metabolism. Water is lost from the cytoplasm so that it becomes gel-like in consistency, causing a reduction in biologically active surfaces. These changes produce a depression of basic cellular biochemical functions which affects the energy pathways of the cell. With the loss of both smooth and rough endoplasmic reticula, the decreased protein synthesis accounts for the reduced presence of cytoplasmic protein and reduced production of mucopolysaccharides by the Golgi apparatus. The process of glycolysis continues, but at a reduced rate.[53]

Researchers have also noted reduced efficiency of fatty acid utilization in aged cells, especially acetoacetic acid and beta-hydroxybutyric acid.[46] These reductions seem to be related to changes in mitochondrial metabolism. Aged mitochondria appear to have increased fragility. Since 90% of the oxidative reactions in mammalian tissues occur

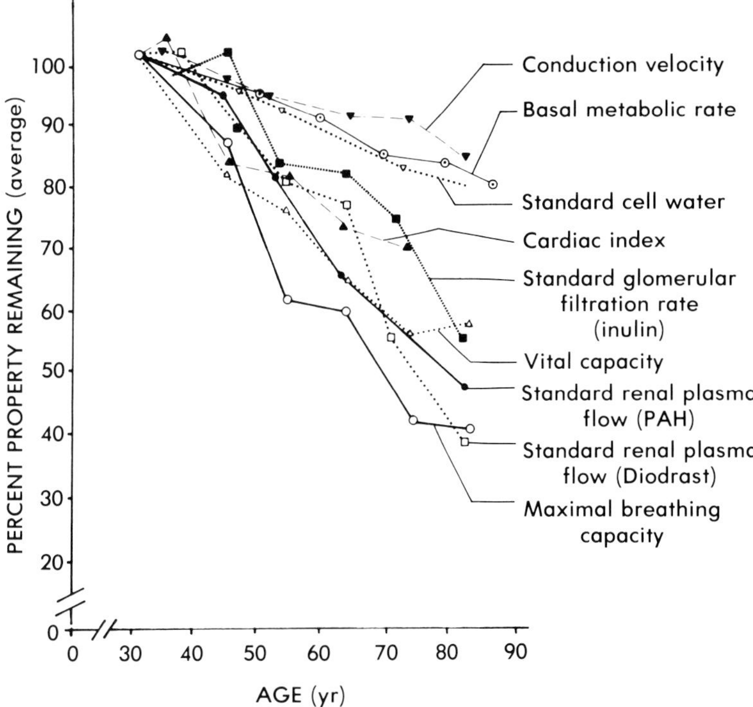

Fig. 66-1 Decline in major functional capacities in the aged patient. (From Timiras, P.S.: Developmental physiology and aging, New York, 1972, Macmillan Publishing Co., Inc. With permission.)

in the mitochondria, the major changes induced by senescence apparently originate within the mitochondria. Harman[20] has theorized that the life span of a species may be related to the rate of oxygen consumption in the mitochondria, which is known to increase as cells become senescent. Andrew[1] has observed a reduction in the number of mitochondria in aged cells but an increase in their volume. The finding of a reduced level of the enzyme succinate dehydrogenase has suggested an impairment of the Krebs cycle in the aged cell. Furthermore, oxidative phosphorylation appears to be less efficient, and phosphate utilization by the mitochondria is reduced.

Evidence from tissue culture has shown that the enzyme 5′-nucleotidase increases with each cell doubling and may have increased by as much as 10 times at senescence.[54] This higher concentration may inhibit the reconversion of adenosine monophosphate (AMP) to adenosine triphosphate (ATP), thereby decreasing the efficiency of energy pathways in the aged cell. Decreased production of ATP results in reduced protein synthesis, reduced immunoprotein synthesis required to combat sepsis, and diminished collagen formation needed for wound healing. Such derangements in protein synthesis during collagen formation alter cross-linking within this substance, leading to the stiff, brittle, wounds typically observed in elderly patients after a traumatic insult or surgical incision.

The aging cell also undergoes changes in membrane function, resulting in increased permeability of the cellular membrane. The sodium-potassium pump becomes less efficient, and other cations such as calcium begin to accumulate intracellularly. The red blood cell becomes more permeable to water reducing osmotic resistance.[49] The extracellular space increases because of a shift of water out of cells. A gain in total extracellular sodium occurs, with a decrease in intracellular sodium. Total potassium is also reduced in the intracellular compartment.[19]

Rockstein and Brandt[46] have noted reduced activity of magnesium-activated ATPase in the muscle of the aged rat, suggesting a lack of metabolic enzyme reserve in the elderly. Furthermore, gluconeogenesis as a major source for substrate during the stress response is inhibited in the senescent cell.[50] A cycle of energy depletion caused by the lack of enzymes and substrate transport mechanisms then follows.

All these observations emphasize the delicate homeostatic balance that exists in the aged organism. In short, the senile cell has difficulty responding to stressful situations. Changes in total sodium and potassium cause a brittleness following fluid administration. A therapeutic need exists for glucose, amino acids, insulin, and vitamins, as well as a need to prevent catabolism of endogenous proteins from muscle. Successful treatment of disease in the elderly patient requires recognition of these limitations and therapeutic needs.

THEORIES OF AGING

On a cellular level several theories have been proposed to account for the primary physiologic process of aging. According to the *programmed theory* of aging, all cells carry specific genes that are programmed to turn off, in sequential fashion, various intracellular processes, which in turn account for the signs of aging. Thus, according to this theory, the end point of cellular differentiation is cellular senescence.[29]

Cowdry[11] proposed a *wear-and tear theory* of aging based on the limited ability of "postmitotic" cells such as muscle and nerve fibers to divide. Since these cells cannot be replaced by new ones, they are substituted with "intermitotic cells" such as connective tissue. These intermitotic cells continue to duplicate and accumulate in the aging individual, filling in spaces formerly occupied by postmitotic cells. The cross-linking of collagen and the accumulation of the aging pigment lipofuscin are sequelae of this process.

According to the *somatic mutation theory*, mitotic errors may play an important role in aging. Curtis[12] proposed that frequently dividing cells replace themselves and have a minor role in aging. Cells that rarely divide, such as muscle cells, have no opportunity for spontaneous or induced mutation and are responsible for the aging process. On the other hand, Jarvik,[27] working with long-term tissue cultures, has noted frequent mitotic errors, particularly chromosomal losses. If such errors occur in the organism, then aging may represent the accumulation of mitotic errors and inappropriate molecules that are unable to support the cell's metabolism. This theory has been used to support the species' life span being inversely related to basal metabolic rate. The faster the metabolic rate, the faster is the rate of cellular turnover and the greater chance for mitotic error.

Other theories have suggested that aging results from the failure to repair errors in the transcription of deoxyribonucleic acid (DNA) or from the exhausted supply of redundant genes and the inevitable expression of gene errors.[29]

Walford[59] has proposed that the aging process is rooted in an autoimmune disorder resulting from the increased circulating levels of gamma globulin and autoantibodies in elderly persons. If this is a factor, immunosuppressive drugs may have a role in prolonging the life span.

Denckla[15] has suggested that the secretion of a pituitary "killer" hormone diminishes the response of peripheral cells to thyroid hormone. Both the cardiovascular and the immune systems depend on adequate thyroid activity. Depression of the effects of thyroid hormone certainly could contribute to the demise of these systems and the organism.

A final notable theory comes from Harman.[20] He proposed that free radicals, which are chemical intermediates containing an unpaired electron, are the agents responsible for the changes seen in aging cells. Free radical reactions occur normally in metabolic processes, but diffusible free radicals may cause molecular instability and interference with the cellular oxidative reactions that produce energy. These free radicals may accumulate from materials in the diet or in the atmosphere or from irradiation by ultraviolet light. The older the organism is, the more likely the accumulation of such substances from these potentially inciting causes.

BODY COMPOSITION CHANGES

In addition to these cellular alterations with aging, several compositional changes are also known to occur within the body as a whole and within specific organs. One example is the decrease in height that occurs with age. This begins at about 30 years of age and progresses at a rate of 1 cm each decade thereafter. This loss of height is equally divided between trunk length and extremity length. Other changes with age include a decrease in shoulder width, partly from loss of muscle mass in the deltoids, and an increase in the pelvic diameter. Loss of elasticity of the lungs and thorax with age leads to an increase in the anteroposterior diameter of the chest. Likewise, the abdominal cavity increases in depth with age.

Changes in body weight also occur with age. Generally, body weight increases and peaks in the middle fifties; weight then tends to decline in the sixties and seventies.[47] A variety of factors may influence these weight changes, including alterations in fat content, total body water, and the body cell mass. In general, total body water constitutes 60% of the body weight of the average young male and slightly less in the young female. In the elderly person, however, this value drops to approximately 54% in the male and 46% in the female.[29] If one uses total body water as an index of fat content, the change in weight in older people represents a change in the ratio of lean body weight to fat and is associated with a decreased specific gravity of the body. Thus the contribution of fat to total body weight increases in the elderly, whereas fluid volume is reduced, primarily in the intracellular space.

This reduction in the intracellular space can also be demonstrated by measuring the body cell mass with a marker such as exchangeable potassium or whole body counting of the naturally occurring potassium-40 isotope (^{40}K). Such measurements demonstrate a reduction in lean body mass relative to body weight in older patients, the loss primarily being from muscle mass.[41] Using exchangeable sodium (Na^+) as an extracellular marker, a shift of this ion toward the extracellular space appears to occur with aging, along with its reduction in the intracellular compartment (K^+). This further emphasizes a reduction in the body cell mass with aging.[36]

Understanding these body conformation and composition changes is necessary to ensure the appropriate use of fluids and drugs in the elderly patient.

WOUND HEALING

In general, surgeons believe that wound healing diminishes with age. Many systemic factors do affect wound healing, and the presence of intercurrent disease renders the elderly patient more susceptible to complications such as sepsis, wound dehiscence, and pathologic scar formation. As a general principle, wounds in the elderly heal more slowly than in the young. As far back as 1916, Du Nouy[17] observed that in epithelial wounds of equal size, the rate of healing varied inversely with age. More rapid healing was noted in the young, and aging constantly diminished the velocity of healing. It is easy to criticize this work since the study comprised a small number of patients ranging in age from 20 to 39 years of age. Nonetheless, as early as the 1920s, Carrel and Ebeling[10] proposed the existence of a growth-retarding substance in older individuals and demonstrated inhibition of cell multiplication by adult serum.

Howes and Harvey[24] in the 1930s showed that wound healing was accompanied by a short lag period in the young rat that tended to lengthen with age. Although the rate of cell proliferation was no greater in the young rats, fibroplasia began 1 day earlier in the young rat and lasted longer. Of equal interest, Billingham and Russell[3] noted that the rate of healing of open skin wounds depended on the wound's rate of contraction. They found that wounds contracted sooner in younger rabbits than in older ones. Other investigators have demonstrated delayed rates of cicatrization when healing by secondary intention.[16]

Sandbloom, Petersen and Muren[48] determined the breaking strength of 5-day-old experimental surgical skin incisions in 13 patients aged 22 to 87 years of age. They noted that the wounds of the patients older than 70 years were substantially weaker than those of the younger patients. Efimov[18] found that the healing of full-thickness skin wounds occurred 10 times as fast in newborn rats compared to young adult rats. When completely healed, the scar had a mean area of 8% of the removed skin section in newborn rats, compared with 42% in young adult rats. This further supports the theory that wound closure proceeds faster in younger animals and that epithelialization is more complete in the young.

Other investigators have noted similar differences in sutured incisions. Holm-Pedersen and Viidik[22] noted that healing in skin incisions of wounds in young rats (3 months of age) had better mechanical properties (i.e., greater strength and elasticity) than those of older rats (up to 23 months of age). Microscopically, at 3 weeks postoperatively, collagen fiber meshwork was more complex and organized in the wounds of the younger rats. Sussman[55] was unable to demonstrate a difference in the tensile strength of healing skin incisions 2 to 13 weeks postoperatively in rats 8 and 20 months of age; however, the younger rats produced an increased amount of connective tissue as well as reparative tissue with different mechanical properties than did the older rats.

Further work by Holm-Pedersen, Nilsson, and Branemark[23] demonstrated that vascular proliferation and microvascular function in healing skin incisions was faster in young rats. Wounds in young rats contained more coiled and tortuous vessels of variable diameter, whereas in older animals the blood vessels were straighter and more uniform in size. Viidik, Holm-Pedersen, and Rundgren[58] demonstrated that collagen matured at a faster rate (increased cross-linking) in the wounds of old rats compared to young ones. This gradual increase in cross-linking of collagen is one of the characteristics of the normal aging process.

Several conclusions can be drawn from these studies regarding the influence of aging on wound healing. Although there have been problems with study design and analysis, a primary delay of fibroplasia seems to occur with advancing age. The rate of collagen synthesis is affected directly by aging, leading to a decreased rate and quality of wound healing and longer convalescence. Secondary factors in the aged, both local and systemic, also adversely affect the healing of wounds. The rate of cross-linking of reparative collagen in the wounds of the elderly appears increased. On the other hand, the rate of collagen formation and its reorganization proceed at a faster rate in younger animals. The morphology of the vascular network differs in wounds of the young and old. The net result is a healing wound of increased strength in the young.

A discussion of the secondary factors affecting wound healing is also important. Several factors other than the age of the organism influence wound healing. These variables assume particular importance, however, in the elderly. Nutritional status has been shown to correlate with ability to heal wounds. Protein-calorie malnutrition and deficiencies of ascorbic acid, vitamin A, and trace elements, which often occur in aged individuals, all negatively affect wound healing. Hormonal influences also play a role. Excess corticoids, which many older patients take for arthritis, diminish the inflammatory response and inhibit fibroplastic proliferation and collagen synthesis. Furthermore, the clinical impression is that anemia adversely affects wound healing. Whether this is true remains to be clarified, but decreased serum albumin levels have a negative influence on wound healing.[45] Degenerative metabolic processes such as diabetic microangiopathy and atherosclerosis diminish blood flow in the area of a peripheral wound and also adversely affect healing. Tissue hypoxia, from whatever cause, negatively affects the healing wound as well.[25] Both local and systemic sepsis impair wound healing, and evidence suggests that systemic infection may have a more deleterious effect on wound healing in the elderly.[2]

These secondary factors, which may further compromise wound healing in the elderly patient give rise to several important principles that must be followed in the management of wounds in this population. First, wounds in older persons require meticulous attention to systemic as well as local care. Underlying conditions that may adversely affect the healing process should be corrected preoperatively when possible. These include acute and chronic nutritional deficiencies, hypoproteinemia, serious anemia, and respiratory and cardiovascular metabolic and physiologic derangements. Moreover, minimizing tissue injury at surgery is of fundamental importance in the elderly patient. Prevention or early treatment of shock, sepsis, and acidosis is vital to avoid delayed wound healing. Finally, early ambulation and physical therapy are essential in elderly patients to preserve their ability to handle daily activities. The key to the management of wounds in the elderly is total care.

FLUIDS, ELECTROLYTES, AND NUTRITIONAL SUPPORT

To provide effective and precise fluid therapy for the elderly patient, one must recall the alterations in body composition that accompany senescence. The reduction in the body cell mass is accompanied by a reduction in intracellular water and total body potassium. The extracellular space expands so that plasma volume and exchangeable sodium (Na^+) increase. With the reduction in estrogen and androgen production with age, a shift toward catabolism occurs leading to further reductions in the muscle mass, red cell mass, and metabolic expenditure.

Since physical activity is generally reduced in the elderly, caloric requirements are also reduced. Despite the diminished caloric needs in older patients, protein requirements are unchanged. This is important to remember since malnutrition is not uncommon in the elderly, and because of the expanded extracellular space, weight loss may not be present. Patients with advanced cardiac or renal disease may have significant vitamin and nutritional deficiencies in the absence of weight loss.

Thus preoperative management of elderly patients must include recognition and correction of deficits in nutrition, plasma volume, and electrolyte imbalances. The negative impact of hypoproteinemia on wound healing is discussed in the previous section.

The metabolic response to surgery does not differ from younger to elderly patients; however, intercurrent disease acts to compound this effect. Patients who suffer from cardiac, hepatic, and renal insufficiency have an acquired state of hyperaldosteronism. This aggravates the expansion of the extracellular space, which is a normal response to surgery and part of the normal aging process. This circumstance further accentuates alkalosis and hypokalemia.[42] Significant alkalosis results in cardiac irregularities and decreased cerebral blood flow, accentuates hypokalemia, and shifts the dissociation of oxygen to the left. Lactic acidosis and tissue ischemia result. Hypokalemia also may result in cardiac arrhythmias, as well as disturbances in muscle contractility and intestinal motility.

Hyponatremia frequently occurs in the elderly patient and is usually a consequence of dilution resulting from the expanded extracellular volume and hyperaldosteronism. Measurement of body weight as well as urinary sodium losses can help reveal the etiology of hyponatremia. The presence of gross edema or ascites supports a dilutional process, which can be appropriately treated by restriction of water, promoting gentle, free water diuresis.

Elderly patients tolerate hypovolemia poorly and develop a low cardiac output. Likewise, with chronic cardiopulmonary disease, overhydration is also poorly tolerated. Thus both intraoperative and postoperative fluid management must be carefully balanced between overhydration and maintenance of adequate cardiac out. Large volumes of crystalloid added to an already expanded extracellular space are not well tolerated. One must remember that the elderly patient with associated cardiac or pulmonary dysfunction is maintaining a precarious homeostasis. Recognition of the body compositional changes associated with the aging process, as well as of the normal metabolic response to surgery, should enable appropriate management of fluids and electrolytes and correction of nutritional deficits.

IMPACT OF AGING ON ORGAN SYSTEMS AND ASSESSMENT OF SURGICAL RISK

The loss of elasticity and distensibility that accompanies aging has significant impact on the heart and circulatory system. The aged myocardium becomes stiff, and the amount of collagen in the myocardium itself increases with the aging process. Elastic tissue is also reduced in arteries, whereas the collagen and smooth muscle content increases. The deposition of calcium and the increased cross-linking of collagen leads to further reductions in compliance with age and an increased load on the left ventricle. The loss in elasticity in both the heart and the arterial vessels results in an increase in the velocity of pulse-wave transmission and a decrease in amplification of the arterial pulse between the aorta and the femoral artery.[29] Loss of elastic tissue also affects the veins, causing varicosities in the lower extremities. On a capillary level the basement membrane is thickened, and diffusion capability is adversely affected.

Functionally, changes in the myocardium occur with advancing age, resulting in a reduction in the cardiac output and cardiac index with a corresponding increase in peripheral resistance (Fig. 66-2). These functional changes are secondary to the anatomic changes listed previously. The increase in vascular resistance (about 1% per year) causes some reduction in cellular perfusion. Cardiac output reportedly decreases 1% each year, starting at age 20, and the stroke volume decreases 0.7% per year.[29] Although resting heart rate appears unchanged, maximum heart rate is reduced linearly with age. Systolic and diastolic pressures both increase with age.

Changes in the respiratory system also contribute to older patients' decreased ability to acquire and deliver oxygen to actively metabolizing tissues. Although the number of alveoli remains constant despite aging, they become smaller as ducts enlarge, thereby reducing total alveolar surface area. Total lung capacity does not change throughout life, but the vital capacity falls linearly with age (Fig. 66-3). The lung also loses it elastic properties, and the anteroposterior diameter of the chest expands. The functional residual capacity increases about 10% by age 60.[9] Calcification also contributes to reduced chest wall compliance. Diaphragmatic breathing assumes greater importance in the elderly because of this reduced compliance. Furthermore, timed ventilatory functions, such as expiratory flow velocity and maximum breathing capacity, are reduced in elderly patients even when they are free of lung

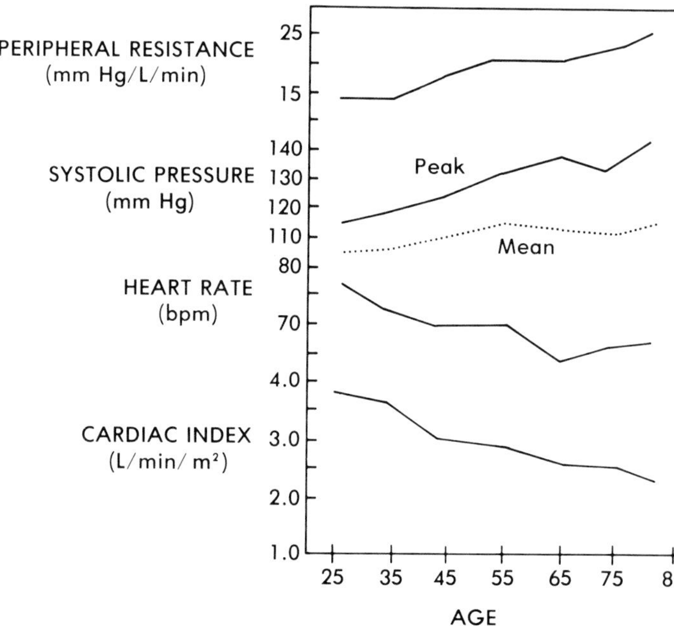

Fig. 66-2 Age-related changes in the cardiovascular system. (Reproduced with permission from Kenney, R.A.: Physiology of aging: a synopsis. Copyright © 1982 by Year Book Medical Publishers, Inc., Chicago.)

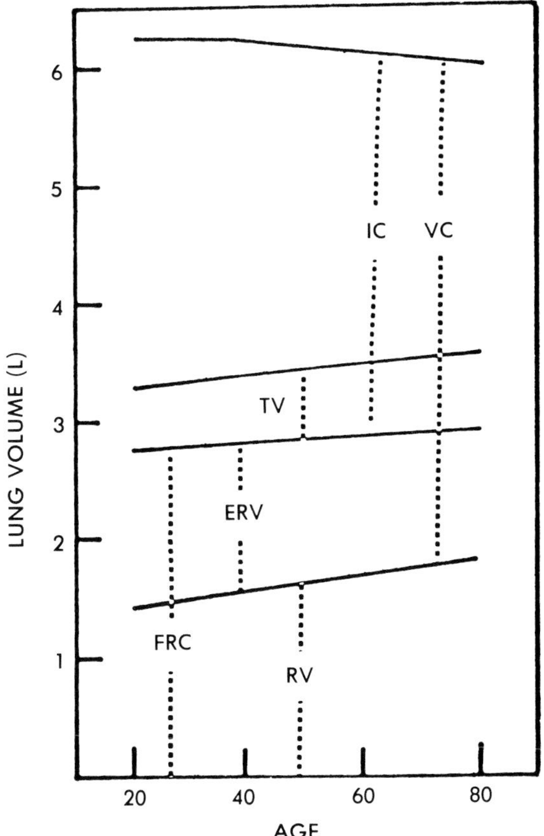

Fig. 66-3 Age-related changes in lung volume. (Reproduced with permission from Kenney, R.A.: Physiology of aging: a synopsis. Copyright © 1982 by Year Book Medical Publishers, Inc., Chicago.)

disease.[29] The closing volume in older patients is increased so that ventilation is not uniform during the breathing cycle. Other changes in respiratory dynamics include an increased alveolar-arterial oxygen difference and a decreased concentration of 2,3-diphosphoglycerate (DPG), causing a left-sided shift in the oxygen dissociation curve.[13,35] Also, mechanical barrier defenses within the tracheobronchial tree against particulate matter are adversely affected by decreased numbers of functioning cilia.

The impact of these alterations is obvious. Cardiovascular disease is the most prevalent abnormality in elderly patients, with pulmonary defects the second most common.[38,63] Powers[44] noted a 6% incidence of cardiovascular disease in the fifth decade of life, which increased to 23% in the sixth decade, 45% in the seventh decade, and was present in all patients in the eighth decade. Nachlas, Abrams, and Goldberg[39] reported on the influence of cardiovascular disease on surgical mortality in older patients. In a large controlled series the average mortality of 2.4% increased to 6.6% in patients with associated cardiovascular disease. Mortality climbed to 7.2% in patients older than 60 years and to 14.3% in those over 70 years.

Skinner and Pearce[51] noted that with preexistent heart disease, the surgical mortality for routine cholecystectomy, subtotal gastrectomy, and bowel resection all doubled in older patients (Fig. 66-4). Significant increases in mortality were also noted with major orthopedic procedures and whenever a body cavity such as the pleural space or peritoneum was violated. The operative mortality in elderly patients also doubled for emergency abdominal procedures in the presence of preexistent cardiac disease (Table 66-1).

Studies have determined that specific features of cardiac disease may be used as predictors of surgical mortality. Topkins and Artusio[57] found the most ominous feature to be a documented history of an acute myocardial infarction

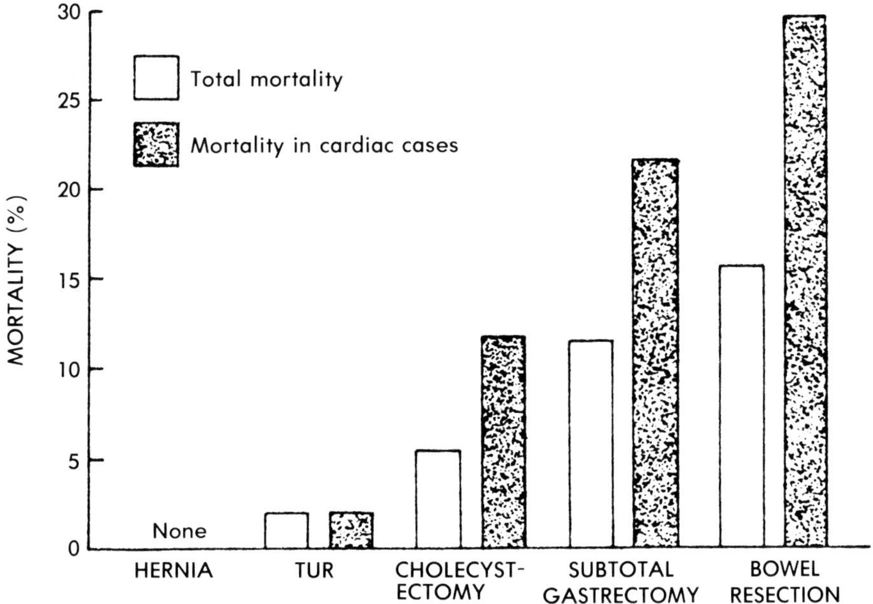

Fig. 66-4 Influence of preexistent heart disease on surgical mortality. (From Siegel, J.H., and Chodoff, P., editors: The aged and high risk surgical patient: medical, surgical, and anesthetic management, New York, 1976, Grune & Stratton, Inc.)

Table 66-1 **EFFECT OF ARTERIOSCLEROTIC AND HYPERTENSIVE HEART DISEASE ON SURGICAL MORTALITY**

			Intrathoracic or Intraabdominal Surgery	
Disease	**Total No. of Patients**	**Mortality (%)**	**No. of Patients**	**Mortality (%)**
Angina pectoris (all cases)	192	11	64	27
Angina with possible or definite hypertensive heart disease	70	9	20	25
Healed myocardial infarction (all cases)	170	14	70	23
Healed myocardial infarction with possible or definite hypertensive heart disease	45	18	13	31
Possible and definite hypertensive heart disease (all cases)	293	13	92	26
Angina and healed myocardial infarction	61	16	22	27
Unstable angina	20	10	6	33
Acute myocardial infarction less than 3 months before surgery	10	40	4	25

Table 66-2 **INCIDENCE OF POSTOPERATIVE MYOCARDIAL INFARCTION (MI) ACCORDING TO DURATION SINCE PREOPERATIVE MI**

Duration Since Preoperative MI	No. of Patients with MI	Incidence of Postoperative MI (%)
< 6 months	22	54.5
> 6 months, < 1 year	36	25.0
> 1 year, < 2 years	49	22.4
> 2 years, < 3 years	51	5.9
> 3 years	493	1.0
TOTAL	651	

(MI) within 6 months of surgery (Table 66-2); i.e., the reinfarction rate was 6.6% postoperatively, and the operative mortality was 54%.[56] In the absence of a previous MI, the postoperative infarction rate was less than 1%, with a 26% operative mortality. Tarhan and associates[56] noted the highest reinfarction rates after intrathoracic, intraabdominal, and major orthopedic procedures.

Skinner and Pearce[51] also noted that angina pectoris and uncontrolled hypertension were associated with an increased surgical risk. Mortality associated with major surgery was considerably enhanced when systolic blood pressure was elevated over 200 mm Hg or diastolic was elevated over 100. Other risk factors included preoperative atrial fibrillation, atrial premature contractions, or incomplete heart block. Left bundle branch block was a particularly serious preoperative finding. Using the New York Heart Association Functional Classification, Skinner and Pearce found a close relationship between operative mortality and the severity of cardiac disease (Table 66-3). Following elective intra-abdominal or intrathoracic surgery, functional Class I patients had an 11% mortality, which increased to 21% for Class II, 42% for Class III, and 100% for Class IV patients.

Pulmonary disease is the second most important major organ system abnormality in the elderly patient contributing to surgical morbidity and mortality. In the absence of any unusual occupational history that may affect the lung, pulmonary abnormalities first become important factors possibly influencing operative outcome in the fifth decade of life. The peak incidence of pulmonary dysfunction related to aging occurs between 60 and 70 years; emphysema, chronic bronchitis, and atelectasis are the most common preoperative abnormalities noted in this age group. Powers[44] found that operative mortality was a direct function of the severity of pulmonary dysfunction in patients with symptoms of overt pulmonary disease. Lewin and associates[33] have stressed the need for quantitative physiologic studies of the lung preoperatively to obtain a valid estimate of surgical risk in those patients older than 60 years.

Although definite changes in renal hemodynamics and tubular function are associated with the normal aging process, enormous functional reserve of the kidneys remains. With intercurrent disease or injudicious management of fluid and electrolyte replacement, unusual demands may be placed on renal function, resulting in deterioration. For this reason and because renal disease is a common intercurrent disorder of senescence, the next paragraph briefly reviews the changes in renal physiology that accompany the aging process.

The kidney continues to grow in size until early adulthood and loses mass somewhat rapidly after age 50 years. This age-related loss of mass involves entire nephron units.[8,37] Wesson[60] has reported a gradual decrease in glomerular filtration rate (GRF) in males from ages 20 to 60 years. Beyond 60 years the falloff in GRF is quite abrupt. In association with a cardiac index that drops by 2.6% each decade of life, the effective renal plasma flow (ERPF)

Table 66-3 **RELATIONSHIP OF FUNCTIONAL HEART CLASSIFICATION TO MORTALITY**

Functional Classification	Total No. of Patients	Mortality (%)	Intrathoracic or Intra-abdominal Surgery: No. of Patients	Intrathoracic or Intra-abdominal Surgery: Mortality (%)
Class I	46	4	9	11
Class II	569	11	199	21
Class III	145	25	59	42
Class IV	6	67	1	100

drops by 10% per decade.[14] The filtration fraction (FF), or that portion of the ERPF that is filtered by the glomeruli, increases linearly with age, probably because of autoregulatory processes. Morphologic vascular changes appear to result in reductions in the pattern of perfusion. The result is that kidneys of elderly patients receive a lower percentage of the cardiac output than those of younger patients. Alterations in medullary structure and perfusion cause a significant loss of concentrating ability in the older kidney.[34] Further, the aged kidney loses the ability to buffer an acid or base load because of associated tubular effects. At normal metabolic loads, however, acid-base homeostasis is maintained. Thus fluid and electrolyte management and acid-base balance must be meticulously maintained in this special subset of patients.

RESULTS OF SURGERY

The surgical literature is replete with reports of successful treatment of surgical disease in the elderly; age alone no longer represents a contraindication to surgery. Recognizing that intraopertative complications are not well tolerated in elderly patients and that postoperative complications will threaten survival, the surgeon must seriously consider the risk/benefit ratio of a procedure. In the absence of an acute surgical problem requiring emergency intervention, careful preoperative attention to nutrition, fluid and electrolytes, and cardiopulmonary status will favorably influence the outcome. The goals of surgery are not the same in the elderly high-risk patient as in the young adult. The ambition to cure should be tempered by a realization of the limitations imposed by aging, such that palliation of disease assumes greater importance.

As mortality rates for all surgical procedures have declined, surgeons have taken a more aggressive approach to surgical problems in the elderly. The key to success in the elderly population is the avoidance of postoperative complications. Wilder and Fishbein[62] noted that postoperative complications resulted in a 62% mortality rate in patients older than 80 years compared with a 13% mortality in patients whose postoperative course was uneventful.

Ziffren and Hartford[64] performed a comprehensive review of mortality rates for abdominal procedures in elderly patients (Table 66-4). They noted the highest mortality rates in association with an exploratory laparotomy for an inoperable lesion, closure of a wound dehiscence, and cholecystostomy. Most elective abdominal procedures had comparable mortality rates among all age groups. However, emergency procedures for patients older than 80 years carried a significantly increased risk. Burnett and McCaffrey[7] reported similar results and noted that pulmonary complications were most frequent, with bronchopneumonia being the most common cause of death.

Boyd, Bradford, and Watne [5] studied operative risk factors in elderly patients undergoing colon resection and found that mortality rates were correlated with the number of associated illnesses and not with age as an isolated factor. Both mortality rate and rate of infectious complications increased in the group requiring emergency procedures. Similarly, the mortality from acute appendicitis in the elderly is higher than in younger patients, and perforation is a more frequent finding.[43]

Nehme[40] reported a 10-year experience with 1755 groin hernias in patients aged 65 years and older. The mortality rate for emergency procedures was 7.5% compared with 1.3% for elective cases. The postoperative morbidity rate was 56% in emergency cases in contrast to 20% in elective cases. The presence of intercurrent cardiovascular and pulmonary disease carried the worst prognosis. Procedures performed under local anesthesia had the least sequelae. These data support the repair of groin hernias in the elderly under elective conditions.

Pulmonary resection also appears to be well tolerated in the elderly patient provided that the results of pulmonary function testing are within normal ranges.[28] In general the mortality rate for a pulmonary resection is higher than for procedures performed transabdominally. Also, the mortality rate for esophagectomy rises significantly with age: 4% in the sixties, 26% in the seventies, and 33% in the eighties, as shown in the data of Ziffren and Hartford.[64]

Stephenson, MacVaugh, and Edmunds[52] reported experience with 89 patients from 70 to 82 years of age who underwent cardiac procedures using cardiopulmonary bypass. Coronary artery bypass grafting and aortic valve replacement performed together carried a mortality rate of 10%, whereas and 0% rate was reported for the coronary grafting alone. Eighty-four percent of the hospital survivors were symptomatically improved by at least one class rating using the New York Heart Association Classification of Heart Disease. Mitral valve replacement was associated with a mortality rate 7.3 times greater in the age 70 to 82 group than in patients less than 70. Other authors have reported similar data.[26]

Herbsman and associates[21] investigated survival following breast cancer surgery in the elderly and found it com-

Table 66-4 **MORTALITY FOR ABDOMINAL PROCEDURES**

Procedure	Mortality (%) by Age Groups			
	Under 60 Years	60-69	70-79	80 or Over
Repair of incisional hernia	0.5	1.1	1.9	0.0
Repair of umbilical hernia	2.8	7.3	0.0	3.3
Closure of wound dehiscence	17.7	15.7	36.3	66.6
Repair of femoral hernia	1.3	0.0	2.7	6.6
Repair of inguinal hernia	0.1	0.2	1.6	3.3
Exploratory laparotomy for inoperable lesion	6.9	9.0	16.6	31.6
Aortic graft	7.5	9.2	16.4	22.2
Splenectomy	6.2	17.3	9.0	—
Repair of hiatal hernia	10.0	0.0	0.0	0.0
Cholecystostomy	6.6	16.6	18.1	17.2
Cholecystectomy	0.8	2.8	5.5	5.4
Choledochostomy	0.0	2.2	13.2	5.5
Suture of perforated duodenal ulcer	16.1	22.2	23.0	40.0
Partial gastrectomy	3.9	5.0	11.2	19.8
Pyloroplasty or gastrojejunostomy with vagotomy	5.6	7.4	10.8	15.3
Freeing of adhesions in intestinal obstruction	6.7	10.0	17.6	14.2
Resection and anastomosis of small intestine in obstruction	14.2	13.9	24.3	35.7
Partial colectomy	6.4	6.8	5.4	9.0
Abdominoperineal resection	0.7	4.3	7.6	11.5
Colostomy	5.6	8.1	8.3	14.2
Closure of colostomy	0.1	0.0	0.0	0.0
Appendectomy	0.1	3.3	2.7	16.6

Reprinted with permission from the American Geriatric Society. From Ziffren, S.E., and Hartford, C.E.: Comparative mortality for various surgical operations in older versus younger age groups, J. Am. Geriatr. Soc. **20**:485, 1972.

parable to that of younger patients regardless of race, type of surgery, histology, or tumor size. They concluded that comventional surgical treatment of elderly patients with breast cancer should not be avoided solely on the basis of advanced age.

Renal transplantation has also been successfully performed in selected elderly patients. Kock and associates[31] reported a series of 39 patients over age 60 years with mortality rates comparable to those of younger groups. Graft survival was also comparable. Finally, both vascular and orthopedic reconstructive procedures are characteristically performed in elderly patients, and aggressive rehabilitative and psychosocial support yields satisfactory results.[4,30,61]

SUMMARY

The successful management of elderly surgical patients demands a comprehensive physiologic approach. Not only must the primary surgical disorder be addressed, but an understanding of the cellular dysfunction is essential. At the cellular level the stress response is blunted, and both fluid resuscitation and administration of substrates are associated with brittle responses. Several important changes in body composition occur in the elderly. The reduction in lean body mass and the expansion of the extracellular compartment are typical findings. Recognition of these body composition changes will ensure appropriate use of drugs and fluids. Aging is associated with decreased rate and quality of wound healing, which leads to a lingering convalescence. Secondary systemic factors play a key role in clinical outcome. Recognition of the cardiac, pulmonary, and renal changes associated with aging will enable appropriate risk assessment preoperatively. Finally, with the advancing age of our population and the trend toward aggressive surgery, the key to success appears to be avoidance of postoperative complications since these are poorly tolerated among elderly patients. An aggressive surgical approach in the older patient will be quite rewarding when total care, including social, emotional, and physiologic needs, are addressed. Although postoperative recovery and rehabilitation may be prolonged, returning elderly patients to function in society is an achievable goal.

REFERENCES

1. Andrew, W.: The fine structural and histochemical changes in aging. In Bittar, E.E., and Bittar, N., editors: The biological basis of medicine, vol. I, New York, 1968, Academic Press.
2. Baer, P.N., Garrington, G.E., and Kilham, L.: Effect of age and H-1 virus on healing fractures in hamsters, J. Geronol. **26**:373, 1971.
3. Billingham, R.E., and Russell, P.S.: Studies on wound healing with special reference to the phenomenon of contracture in experimental wounds in rabbit's skin, Ann. Surg. **144**:961, 1956.
4. Bouhoutsos, J., and Martin, P.: The influence of age on prognosis after arterial surgery for atherosclerosis of the lower limbs, Surgery **74**:637, 1973.
5. Boyd, J.B., Bradford, B., Jr., and Watne, A.L.: Operative risk factors of colon resection in the elderly, Ann. Surg. **116**(2):153, 1981.
6. Burnett, F.M.: An immunological approach to aging, Lancet **2**:358, 1970.
7. Burnett, W., and McCaffrey, J.: Surgical procedures in the elderly, Surg. Gynecol. Obstet. **134**:221, 1972.
8. Calloway, N.O., Foley, C.F., and Lagerbloo, P.J.: Uncertainties in geriatric data. II. Organ size, Am. Geriatr. Soc. **13**:20, 1965.
9. Campbell, E.J., and Lefrak, S.S.: How aging affects the structure and function of the respiratory system, Geriatrics **33**(6):68, 1978.

10. Carrel, A., and Ebeling, A.H.: Age and multiplication of fibroblasts, J. Exp. Med. **34:**599, 1921.
11. Cowdry, E.V.: Cowdry's problems of aging, Baltimore, 1952, Williams & Wilkins.
12. Curtis, H.J.: Biologic mechanisms underlying the aging process, Science **141:**686, 1963.
13. Davies, C.T.M.: The oxygen transporting system in relation to age, Clin. Sci. **42:**1, 1973.
14. Davies, D.F., and Shock, N.W.: Age changes in GFR, ERPF, and tubular excretory capacity in adult males, J. Clin. Invest. **29:**496, 1950.
15. Denckla, W.D.: A time to die, Life Sci. **16:**31, 1975.
16. Doberauer, W.: Effect of age on wound healing process, Geronol. Clin. **4:**112, 1962.
17. Du Nouy, P.L.: Cicatrization of wounds. III. The relation between the age of the patient, the area of the wound, and the index of cicatrization, J. Exp. Med. **24:**461, 1916.
18. Efimov, E.A.: Comparison of healing of full thickness wounds in newborn and sexually mature rats, Bull. Eksp. Biol. Med. **65:**75, 1968.
19. Friedman, S.M., Sreter, F.A., and Friedman, C.L.: The distribution of water, sodium, and potassium in the aged rat: a pattern of adrenal preponderance, Gerontologia **7:**44, 1963.
20. Harman, D.: Free radical theory of aging: effect of free radical inhibitors on the mortality rate of LAF mice, Gerontology **23:**476, 1968
21. Herbsman, H., et al.: Survival following breast cancer surgery in the elderly, Cancer **47**(10):2358, 1981.
22. Holm-Pedersen, P., and Viidik, A.: Tensile properties and morphology of healing wounds in young and old rats, Scand. J. Plast. Reconstr. Surg. **6:**24, 1972.
23. Holm-Pedersen, P., Nilsson, K., and Branemark, P.I.: The microvascular system of healing wounds in young and old rats, Adv. Microcirc. **5:**50, 1973.
24. Howes, E.L., and Harvey, S.C.: Age factor in velocity of growth of fibroblasts in the healing wound, J. Exp. Med. **55:**577, 1932.
25. Hunt, T.K., and Pai, M.P.: The effect of varying ambient oxygen tensions in wound metabolism and collagen synthesis, Surg. Gynecol. Obstet. **135:**561, 1972.
26. Jamieson, W.R., Thompson, D.M., and Munro, A.I.: Cardiac valve replacement in elderly patients, Can. Med. Assoc. J. **123**(7):628, 1980.
27. Jarvik, L.: Quote. In Benes, A.M., and Sacher, G.A., editors: Aging and levels of biological organization, Chicago, 1965, University of Chicago Press.
28. Jezek, V., et al.: Cardiopulmonary function in lung resection performed for bronchiogenic cancer in patients above 65 years of age, Respiration **27:**42, 1970.
29. Kenney, R.A.: Physiology of aging, Chicago, 1982, Year Book Medical Publishers, Inc.
30. Kihn, R.B., Warren, R., and Beebe, G.W.: The "geriatric" amputee, Ann. Surg. **176:**305, 1972.
31. Kock, B., et al.: Kidney transplantation in patients over 60 years of age, Scand. J. Urol. Nephrol. (Suppl). **54:**103, 1980.
32. Kohn, R.R.: Principles of mammalian aging, Englewood Cliffs, N.J., 1971, Prenctice-Hall, Inc.
33. Lewin, I., et al.: Physical class and physiologic status in prediction of operative mortality in the aged sick, Ann. Surg. **174:**217, 1971.
34. Lindeman, R.D.: Age changes in renal function. In Goldman, R., and Rochester, M., editors: Physiology and pathology of human aging, New York, 1975, Academic Press.
35. Lynne-Davies, P.: Influence of age on the respiratory system, Geriatrics **32**(8):57, 1977.
36. MacGillioray, I., Buchanan, T.J., and Billewicz, W.Z.: Values for total exchangeable sodium and potassium in normal females based on wieght, height, and age, Clin. Sci. **19:**17, 1960.
37. Miller, J.H., McDonald, R.K., and Shock, N.W.: Age changes in maximal rate of renal tubular reabsorption of glucose, J. Gerontol. **7:**196, 1952.
38. Monroe, R.T.: Diseases in old age: a clinical and pathologic study of 7941 individuals over 61 years of age, Cambridge, 1951, Harvard University Press.
39. Nachlas, M.M., Abrams, S.J., and Goldberg, M.M.: The influence of arteriosclerotic heart diseases on surgical risk, Am. J. Surg. **101:**447, 1961.
40. Nehme, A.E.: Groin hernias in elderly patients: management and prognosis, Am. J. Surg. **146**(2):257, 1983.
41. Novak, L.P.: Aging, total body potassium, fat free mass and cell mass in males and females between ages 18 and 85 years, Gerontology **27:**438, 1972.
42. Olson, J.E., and Moore, F.D.: Metabolic management of elderly surgical patients. In Powers, J.E., editor: Surgery of the aged and debilitated patient, Philadelphia, 1968, W.B. Saunders Co.
43. Peltokallio, P., and Tykka, H.: Evolution of the age distribution and mortality of acute appendicitis, Arch. Surg. **116**(2):153, 1981.
44. Powers, J.H.: Coexisting debilitating and degenerative diseases: preoperative investigation and management of elderly patients. In Powers, J.H., editor: Surgery of the aged and debilitated patient, Philadelphia, 1968, W.B. Saunders Co.
45. Rhoads, J.E., and Alexander, C.E.: Nutritional problems in surgical patients, Ann. NY Acad. Sci. **63:**268, 1955.
46. Rockstein, M., and Brandt, K.: Muscle enzyme activity and changes in weight in aging white rats, Nature **196:**142, 1962.
47. Rossman, I.: Anatomic and body composition changes with aging. In Finch, C.E., and Hayflick, L., editors: Handbook of the biology of aging, New York, 1977, Van Nostrand Reinhold Co.
48. Sandbloom, P., Petersen, P., and Muren, A.: Determination of the tensile strength of the healing wound as a clinical test, Acta Chir. Scand. **105:**252, 1953.
49. Schumer, W.: Metabolic mechanisms of the aging cell. In Siegel, J.H., and Chodoff, P., editors: The aged and high risk surgical patient, New York, 1976, Grune & Stratton, Inc.
50. Singhal, R.L.: Effect of age on the induction of glucose-6-phosphatase and fructose-1,6-diphosphatase in rat liver, J. Gerontol. **22:**77, 1967.
51. Skinner, J.F., and Pearce, M.L.: Surgical risk in the cardiac patient, J. Chronic Dis. **17:**57, 1964.
52. Stephenson, L.W., MacVaugh, H., III, and Edmunds, L.H., Jr.: Surgery using cardiopulmonary bypass in the elderly, Circulation **58**(2), 1978.
53. Strehler, B.L.: Aging at the cellular level. In Rossman, I., editor: Clinical geriatrics, Philadelphia, 1971, J.B. Lippincott Co.
54. Sun, A.S., Aggarival, B.B., and Packer, L.: Enzyme levels of normal human cells: aging in culture, Arch. Biochem. Biophys. **170:**1, 1975.
55. Sussman, M.D.: Aging of connective tissue: physical properties of healing wounds in young and old rats, Am. J. Physiol. **224:**1167, 1973.
56. Tarhan, S., et al.: Myocardial infarction after general anesthesia, JAMA **220:**1451, 1972.
57. Topkins, M.J., and Artusio, J.F.: Myocardial infarction and surgery, Anesth. Anag. **43:**716, 1964.
58. Viidik, A., Holm-Pedersen, P., and Rundgren, A.: Some observations on the distant collagen response to healing wounds in young and old rats, Scand. J. Plast. Reconstr. Surg. **6:**114, 1972.
59. Walford, R.L.: Immunologic theory of aging, Baltimore, 1970, Williams & Wilkins.
60. Wesson, L.G., Jr.: Physiology of the human kidney, New York, 1969, Grune & Stratton, Inc.
61. Wilcock, G.K.: A comparison of total hip replacement in patients aged 69 years or less and 70 years or over, Gerontology **27**(1-2):85, 1981.
62. Wilder, R.J., and Fishbein, R.H.: Operative experience with patients over 80 years of age, Surg. Gynecol. Obstet. **113:**205, 1961.
63. Wilson, L.A., Lawson, I.R., and Brass, W.: Multiple disorders in the elderly, Lancet **2:**841, 1962.
64. Ziffren, S.E., and Hartford, C.E.: Comparative mortality for various surgical operations in older versus younger age groups, J. Am. Geriatr. Soc. **20:**485, 1972.

67 *Harvey J. Sugerman*

Morbid Obesity

A number of definitions have been developed over the years in an attempt to standardize the description of morbid obesity.[8] Indices of obesity include the Body Mass Index (BMI) in which weight (W) in kilograms is divided by the height (H) in square meters ($BMI = W/H^2$), the Ponderal Index (PI) in which the height of an individual in centimeters is divided by the cube root of the weight in kilograms ($PI = H/\sqrt[3]{W}$, the Broca Index (BI) that equals the weight in kilograms minus the height in centimeters minus 100 ($BI = W - H - 100$), and the Adipocity Index that includes a measurement of triceps skinfold thickness in its formula. More commonly used criteria are based on deviation from a standard or desirable weight for a given body build and height. The most frequently used ideal weight standards are those that were developed in 1959 by the Metropolitan Life Insurance Co. for men and women of small, medium, and large frames. These data were modified in 1983 with a new set of tables that increased ideal weight standards by approximately 10% to 15%.[25] A morbidly obese person has been arbitrarily defined by some investigators as anyone with a weight of 100 pounds above ideal body weight and by others as twice ideal body weight. In a United States survey in the early 1970s, severe obesity (>244 pounds for men or >225 pounds for women) was estimated to be present in 4.9% (≈2.8 million) of men and 7.2% (≈4.5 million) of women.[8]

ETIOLOGY

Obesity is secondary to a positive energy balance in which there is an excess of caloric intake relative to caloric expenditure. The causes of morbid obesity are unknown but could include inherited errors of metabolism, abnormalities of the neural and/or humoral transmitters to the hypothalamic hunger and/or satiety centers, derangements in the hypothalamic centers themselves, acquired psychologic oral dependency drives learned in a pathologic family environment, or an inappropriate response to stress.[47] It is conceivable that most of these factors are involved, singly or in various combinations, in each patient with morbid obesity. Clinical studies have shown that some morbidly obese patients have low basal caloric energy expenditure, whereas others appear to consume normal or even large amounts of calories while at rest.[11] Some investigators have suggested that each patient has a weight level that is dictated by the number of fat cells developed before birth and during infancy and that there is a "body weight set point" where a patient's weight tends to stabilize.[45] These considerations have been offered as possible reasons why some patients do well and others do poorly following surgery for morbid obesity.

Of interest experimentally, several strains of obese mice have been developed (ob/ob, ad/ad, fa/fa) in which various defects have been identified that may be important in the pathogenesis of their obesity. The defects include derangements in the normal balance between satiety and hunger mechanisms mediated by the hypothalamus, deficiencies in various enzymes (e.g., liproprotein lipase and glycerokinase, which are necessary for the appropriate use and metabolism of fat and glucose), and defects in endogenous opioid metabolism, which appears to be involved in maintaining normal feeding behavior by regulating a hyperphagic or anorexic response to feeding.[12,46,60] Whether any of these experimental observations is pertinent in explaining the etiology of morbid obesity in human beings remains to be determined. The observation that many morbidly obese patients are delighted with the early satiety that follows surgical procedures for obesity suggests a nonpsychologic cause for this problem.

MORTALITY AND MORBIDITY

Morbid obesity, like alcoholism, is a disease of addiction that produces a large number of associated illnesses that lead to significant morbidity and early mortality. The cost of obesity in terms of lost jobs, psychologic impairment, and number of days requiring hospitalization must be enormous. Drenick and associates [9] noted a 12-fold increase in mortality in a group of morbidly obese men in the 25- to 34-year age group compared to the total population of men in this age range (Fig. 67-1). A study of the association between body build and blood pressure by the Society of Actuaries in 1959 noted only a 168% mortality ratio of obese patients over what was expected in the general population.[52] It must be noted, however, that this study was performed in an insured population group that was, therefore, probably a better underwriting risk with a lower mortality rate than a standard obese population. In a study of 750,000 men and women by the American Cancer Society from 1959 to 1972, a 50% increase in mortality was noted in individuals 30% to 40% above average weight for their height and age; this mortality rate was 90% higher in individuals who were more than 40% over average weight.[28]

Severe obesity is associated with a large number of problems that give rise to the term "morbid" obesity:

- Hypertension
- Coronary artery disease
- Heart failure (right-sided and/or left-sided)
- Diabetes mellitus
- Obesity hypoventilation syndrome
- Obstructive sleep apnea syndrome
- Pseudomotor cerebri

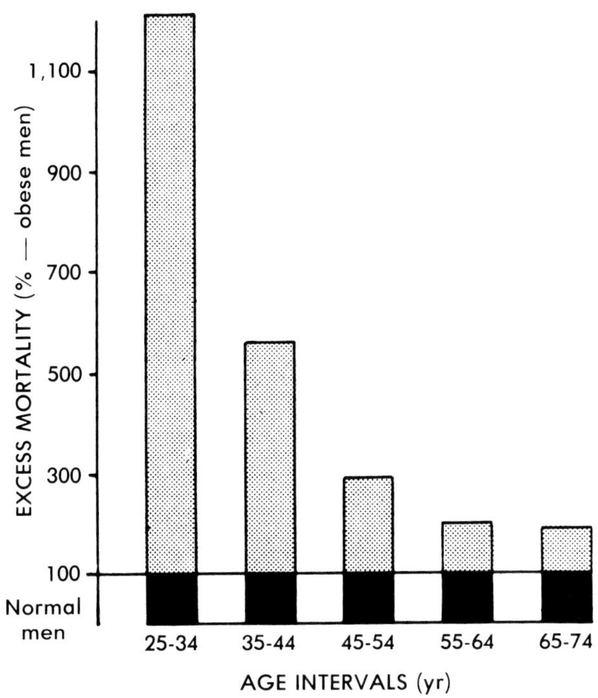

Fig. 67-1 As computed for decades, percent of excess probability of dying among morbidly obese men relative to mortality of United States men as a whole. (From Drenick, E.J., et al.: JAMA **243:**443, Copyright 1980, American Medical Association.)

Degenerative osteoarthritis
Cholelithiasis
Thrombophlebitis
Stasis ulcers
Pulmonary emboli
Necrotizing subcutaneous infections
Wound infections/dehiscence
Gastroesophageal reflux
Stress overflow urinary incontinence
Sexual hormone imbalance
Dysmenorrhea
Infertility
Uterine carcinoma
Stein-Leventhal syndrome
Psychosocial impairment

Several of these problems are the underlying causes of the earlier mortality associated with obesity; they include coronary artery disease, systemic hypertension, impaired left-ventricular function, adult onset diabetes mellitus, obesity hypoventilation syndrome, sleep apnea syndrome, hypercoagulability leading to an increased risk of pulmonary embolus, and necrotizing panniculitis. Morbidly obese patients can also die from peritonitis as a result of difficulties in recognizing its signs and symptoms in a very heavy individual.

A number of other obesity-related problems are not associated with death but can lead to significant physical disability. They include degenerative arthritis, pseudotumor cerebri, cholecystitis, and various infections. Many morbidly obese patients suffer from severe psychologic and social disability. Although most individuals with this problem are typically pictured as "the jolly fat man or woman," the majority have a very negative self-image, problems in relating to the opposite sex, and difficulty obtaining jobs or occupational advancement.

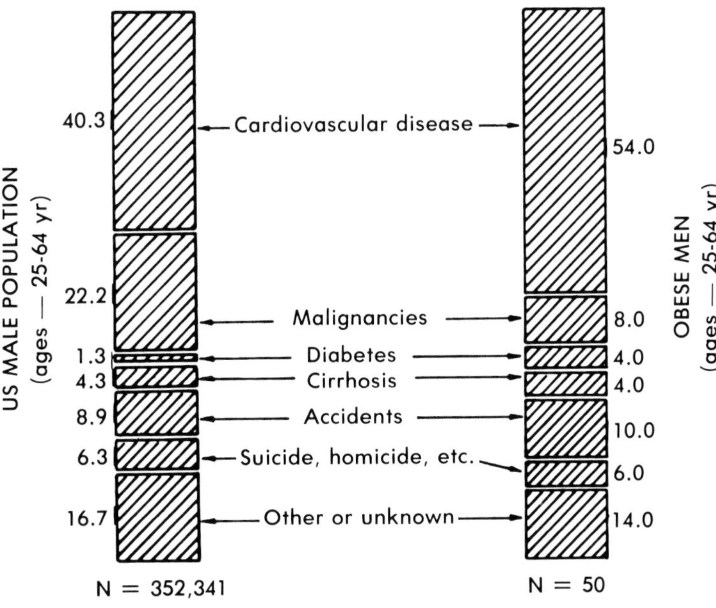

Fig. 67-2 Frequency of common causes of death in morbidly obese men vs. United States male population in same age range. (From Drenick, E.J., et al.: JAMA **243:**443, Copyright 1980, American Medical Association.)

Cardiac Disease

The primary cause of mortality in the morbidly obese patient is cardiovascular in origin (Fig. 67-2). It relates to the cardiomegaly and impaired left-ventricular function so commonly observed in these patients.[7,9] Although obesity is also associated with hypertension, the impaired cardiac function is not necessarily related to (but may be aggravated by) systemic hypertension. The cause for this impairment is unknown, but it probably relates to the increased demand for blood flow through the miles of capillaries in fatty tissue. Some investigators believe that correction of morbid obesity may improve cardiac function in these patients, although data supporting this contention is far from conclusive.

Morbid obesity is also associated with an accelerated rate of coronary atherosclerosis.[8,24,52] Patients with this disease often have hypercholesterolemia and an elevated ratio of high density to low-density lipoproteins in their blood.[8] This situation may be related to the high intake of simple carbohydrates, cholesterol, and polyunsaturated fats, which have been clearly demonstrated to increase the risk of heart attack, consumed by these patients. The abnormal lipoprotein ratio reverts toward normal following either the jejunoileal bypass or gastric procedures performed for morbid obesity.[14]

Respiratory insufficiency associated with morbid obesity can result in hypoxemic pulmonary arterial vasoconstriction, which in severe cases may lead to right-sided heart failure.[20] In my experience, correction of the respiratory insufficiency after surgically induced weight loss also corrects the pulmonary artery hypertension within 3 months to 1 year.

Pulmonary Disease

The respiratory insufficiency of morbid obesity is associated with either the obesity hypoventilation syndrome,[40] obstructive sleep apnea syndrome,[17] or a combination of these two entities. In the classic description of this problem, the term Pickwickian syndrome was coined by Burwell and associates[4] to describe a 54-year-old morbidly obese man who fell asleep in a poker game holding a hand containing three aces and two kings.

The obesity hypoventilation syndrome results from the increased weight placed on the chest wall and diaphragm.[40] As a result, the lungs are squeezed. Patients initially seen with this syndrome have a markedly decreased expiratory reserve volume and reductions in other lung volumes. They have hypoxemia and hypercarbia while awake and a blunted ventilatory response to carbon dioxide. The hypercarbia leads to carbon dioxide narcosis and daytime somnolence. The chronic hypoxemia leads to pulmonary artery vasoconstriction and right-sided heart failure. These patients also have increased risk of developing fatal arrhythmias and pulmonary embolism.

The obstructive sleep apnea syndrome, also associated with severe obesity, is caused by depression of the normal genioglossus reflex and by deposition of fat within the hypopharynx resulting in a narrowing of the airway.[17] The genioglossus muscle is normally activated during inspiration, bringing the tongue forward. The cause for the depressed function of this reflex in obese patients is unknown but may be related to fat deposition within the muscle and the increased weight of the tongue. These patients are notorious snorers and suffer from severe daytime somnolence with tendencies to fall asleep while driving or at work. Two of my patients were fired from their jobs for falling asleep on the job; one was a state prison guard. Another patient fell asleep while shaving and woke up when his head hit the mirror. This daytime somnolence is probably secondary to impaired rapid eye movement (REM) sleep. On occasion, this syndrome has been associated with sudden death.

The diagnosis of obstructive sleep apnea is suggested by a history similar to the patients described previously and the performance of screening capnography in which expired carbon dioxide is measured during sleep. In this test, a mask with a carbon-dioxide–sensitive electrode is placed over the patient's mouth and nose. During inspiration the carbon dioxide tension falls abruptly and then rises sharply during expiration (Fig. 67-3). If the patient has an apneic episode, the carbon dioxide tension, which has risen during end-expiration, gradually falls as carbon dioxide washes out of the face mask.

Although the findings enumerated through the use of capnography suggest the presence of obstructive sleep apnea, this test is not able to differentiate the obstructive type from the central type of sleep apnea. To confirm the diagnosis of the obstructive type requires the use of polysomnography. This procedure includes the use of electroencephalography and of electromyography of the genioglossus muscle, the measurement of esophageal pressure, the determination of nasal and oral temperatures (which documents air flow), and chest wall excursion (Fig. 67-4). Performance of polysomnography documents the cessation of airflow during sleep that is associated with the persistence of respiratory efforts. Patient arousal as demonstrated by the electroencephalogram is associated with the return of air flow.

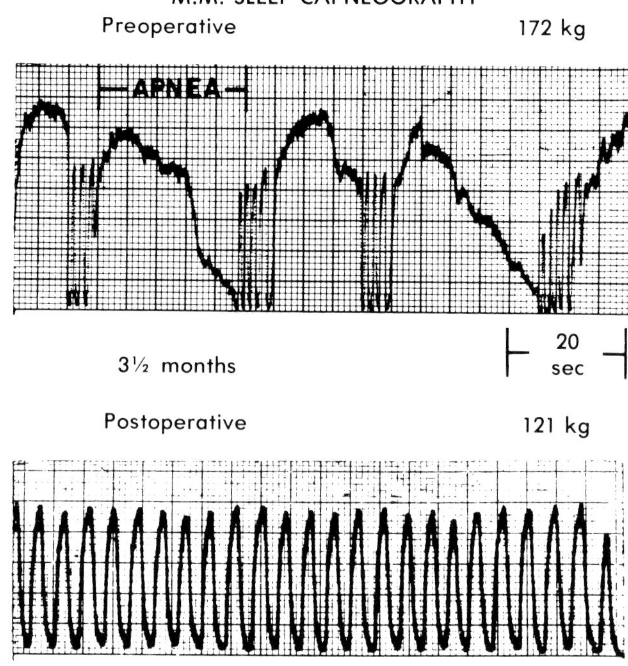

Fig. 67-3 Sleep capnography in patient; vertical axis is qualitative measurement of expired carbon dioxide. Frequent apneic episodes were noted before gastroplasty and 51-kg weight loss, and absence of apnea was noted afterward. (From Sugerman, H.J., et al.: Ann. Surg. **193:**677, 1981.)

Some patients, such as the man with the Pickwickian syndrome described by Burwell and associates,[4] have both the obesity hypoventilation and obstructive sleep apnea syndromes. In my experience, 12% of patients who have undergone gastric surgery for morbid obesity have had respiratory insufficiency.[48] Of the 38 patients with this problem, 10 had sleep apnea syndrome, nine had obesity hypoventilation syndrome, and 19 had both syndromes. Obesity is not the only factor, however, for respiratory dysfunction since many of our markedly obese patients had few or no significant pulmonary problems. Other contributing factors to pulmonary dysfunction in these patients included sarcoidosis, heavy cigarette abuse, and myotonic dystrophy.

Both the obesity hypoventilation and obstructive sleep apnea syndrome are associated with high mortality and serious morbidity.[30] Weight reduction will cure both of them (Figs. 67-3 and 67-5).[48] However, there appears to be a critical weight associated with respiratory insufficiency since loss of relatively small amounts of excess weight results in its correction in some patients. As stated previously, it has been our experience that hypoxemic pulmonary artery vasoconstriction and right-sided heart failure will respond to weight loss and correction of the respiratory insufficiency.

Hypertension

There is little doubt that obesity increases the incidence of systemic hypertension.[8,24,52] However, determining

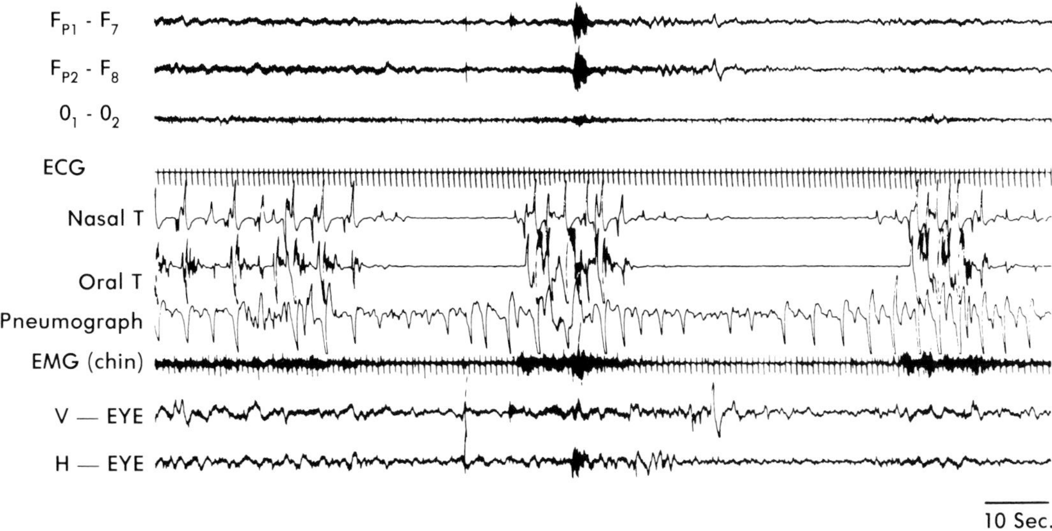

Fig. 67-4 Polysomnography in patient with obstructive sleep apnea syndrome. Readings represent a simultaneous electroencephalogram (EEG) using leads F_{P1}-F_7, F_{P2}-F_8, and O_1-O_2, an electrocardiogram *(ECG)*, nasal and oral airway temperature *(T)*, a pneumogram using a circumferential chest belt, and an electromyogram *(EMG)* of submental muscle and random eye movements *(V* and *H)* showing cessation of airflow with persistence of respiratory efforts. Patient aroused (note EEG and EMG) after 25- and 45-second apneic episodes with return of air flow. (From Sugerman, H.J., et al.: Ann. Surg. **193:**677, 1981.)

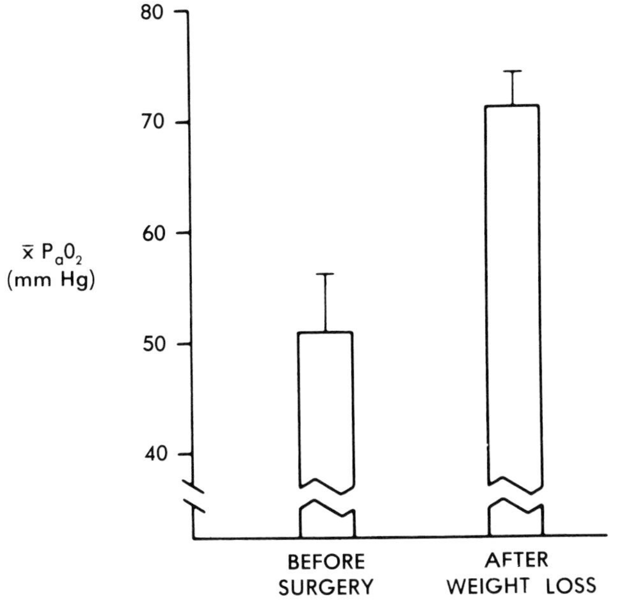

Fig. 67-5 Increase in arterial oxygen tension (Pa_{O_2}) following gastric surgery–induced weight loss in four patients with obesity hypoventilation syndrome. (From Sugerman, H.J., et al.: Ann. Surg. **193:**677, 1981.)

which patients are hypertensive may be difficult since there is a question regarding the validity of blood pressure measurements in morbidly obese patients. The use of standard blood pressure cuffs yields spuriously elevated pressures. Thus it is necessary to use a thigh cuff for these patients. Hypertension has been proven to be associated with a decreased life expectancy. Weight reduction will lower mean arterial pressure in many, but not all, obese patients.

Diabetes

Obesity is a frequent cause in the development of adult onset diabetes mellitus. However, only 5% of morbidly obese patients in my personal experience required insulin or oral hypoglycemic agents for blood sugar control. It has been suggested that 20 to 25 years of gross obesity will produce diabetes in one half of the morbidly obese population.[8,52] Morbidly obese patients can be very resistant to insulin because of the marked down-regulation of insulin receptors. Following weight reduction after gastric surgery for morbid obesity, all but two of twenty patients in our experience who had previously required 30 to 200 U of NPH insulin daily no longer needed this drug. The tendency toward hyperglycemia manifested by obese patients is another probable risk factor for atherosclerosis and coronary artery disease. Diabetes also increases the risk of fatal, severe subcutaneous infections, but since diabetes in these patients is of the adult onset variety, ketoacidosis or severe renal disease is rarely encountered.

Hypercoagulability

Morbidly obese patients are also at increased risk for thrombophlebitis, venous stasis ulcers, and pulmonary embolism.[21] They have low levels of antithrombin III, which may increase their risk to form blood clots.[2] The increased weight within the abdomen may increase inferior vena cava pressure with an accompanying resistance to venous return, which could increase the tendency toward clot formation. A similar mechanism may be responsible for the increased risk of pulmonary emboli in patients with pulmonary hypertension secondary to respiratory insufficiency and hypoxemic pulmonary artery vasoconstriction. Starvation, particularly in the postoperative period, may be associated with high levels of free fatty acids that may pre-

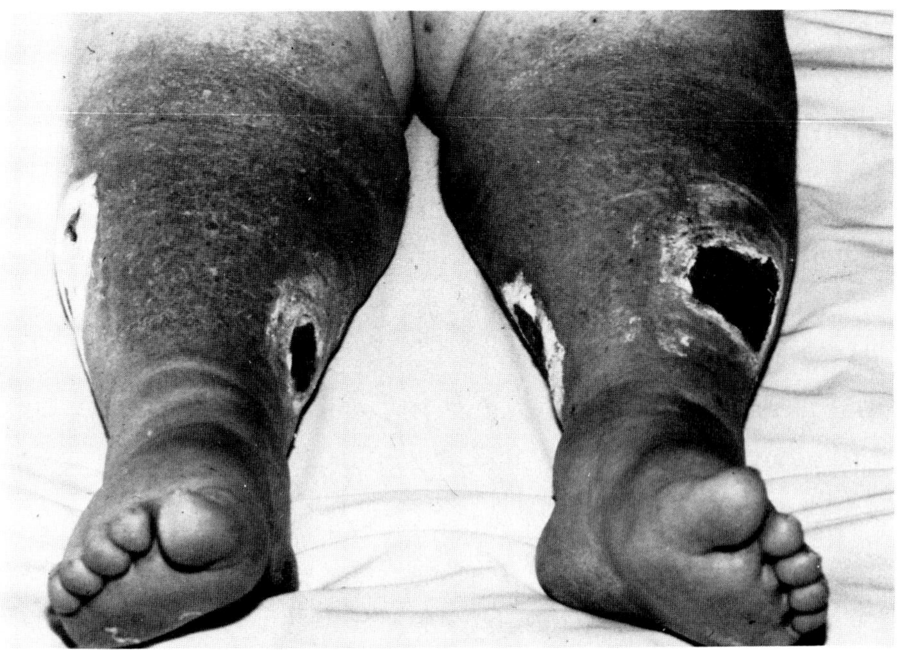

Fig. 67-6 Stasis ulcers in patient with morbid obesity. They resolved only after gastric surgery induced weight loss.

dispose to perioperative thrombotic complications. The stasis ulcers (Fig. 67-6) that may develop in these patients can be incapacitating and extremely difficult to treat. Weight reduction may be the critical factor in treatment since pressure stockings and wound care are usually ineffective.

Necrotizing Subcutaneous Infections

An increased risk of overwhelming necrotizing subcutaneous infections has also been noted in morbidly obese patients.[41] These infections often occur in association with adult onset diabetes and usually involve both aerobic and anaerobic organisms. Fat is notoriously susceptible to rapidly spreading infections. These infections usually begin in the perineum or in a massive abdominal panniculus. Treatment requires broad-spectrum antibiotics for both aerobic and anaerobic organisms and early, aggressive, and radical surgical debridement that may necessitate surgical resection of the offending fat tissue.[41] Despite this approach, these infections are often fatal. In my personal experience, all but one of eight patients with a severe necrotizing subcutaneous infection, who also suffered from diabetes and morbid obesity, died.

Cholelithiasis

Thirty percent of morbidly obese patients have already had a cholecystectomy for gallstones or have gallstones identifiable when the patients are initially seen for obesity surgery.[8] This percentage is in contrast to the 10% of patients with cholelithiasis in the average population. The cause for the increased lithogenesis in obesity is unknown but is probably related to the diet that these patients eat. The intestinal bypass operation for obesity is lithogenic,[58] which may be the result of a diminished bile acid pool secondary to the loss of bile salts from the enterohepatic circulation. Gastric operations for obesity are also lithogenic,[56] probably as a result of an increased prehepatic cholesterol load caused by its mobilization from fat stores. These stores may resolve spontaneously or respond rapidly to oral chenodeoxycholic acid.[56] The increased prehepatic load may also contribute to the increased lithogenicity of the intestinal bypass procedure.

Degenerative Joint Disease

The increased weight in the morbidly obese patient leads to early degenerative arthritic changes of the weight-bearing joints including the knees, hips, and spine. Efforts to replace these joints with prosthetic devices are fraught with considerable difficulty. Generally patients undergoing such joint replacement do poorly because of the inability of the prosthesis to withstand the enormous pressures to which it is subjected.[38] The problem encountered is primarily one of the prosthetic material loosening from the glue within its bony housing. Orthopedic surgeons at the Medical College of Virginia refuse to insert total hip or knee prosthetics in patients weighting over 250 pounds because of the unacceptable incidence of early failure. Obviously degenerative arthritis leads to a great deal of patient disability and unemployment.

Pseudotumor Cerebri

Occasionally morbidly obese patients suffer from frequent, daily, incapacitating headaches which are associated with papilledema and elevated cerebrospinal fluid (CSF) pressures, known as pseudotumor cerebri. The cause for this phenomenon in the morbidly obese patient is unknown but may be related to a mechanical impairment of CSF absorption. An association with hypervitaminosis

A has also been observed in nonobese patients. It is possible that the increased adiposity in obese patients may lead to an increased store of vitamin A, which could be responsible for the syndrome. Treatment includes periodic spinal taps with CSF fluid drainage and the use of diuretics. One study questioned the relationship of obesity to pseudomotor cerebri[6]; however, in my experience, weight reduction lowered the CSF pressure and cured the syndrome in four morbidly obese patients. One patient, 4 feet 11 inches tall, had an opening CSF pressure of 370 mm of water that was associated with incapacitating headaches when she weighed 235 pounds. Weight loss following gastric surgery for obesity cured her headaches. At a weight of 110 pounds following surgery, her CSF opening pressure was 130 mm of water.

Nephrotic Syndrome

Rarely patients with morbid obesity develop the nephrotic syndrome.[57] This syndrome is secondary to increased right atrial, vena caval, and renal vein pressures and may occasionally be associated with renal vein thrombosis. Kidney biopsy reveals a mesangial glomerulopathy. In the absence of renal vein thrombosis, the proteinuria with morbid obesity must be quite uncommon since I was unable to find more than trace protein in the urine of more than 50 patients undergoing obesity surgery.

Psychosocial Incapacity

Many morbidly obese individuals have very low self-esteem. Although typically pictured as jolly, they are often severely depressed. Guilt feelings associated with this low self-esteem coupled with their inability to ambulate without difficulty tends to make them reclusive. This behavior increases their sedentary habits and decreases their caloric expenditure, producing a vicious cycle that leads to further weight gain.

Morbidly obese patients have difficulty in obtaining good jobs, especially if the job requires "exposure" to the public. In addition, obesity hypoventilation and sleep apnea syndromes, degenerative arthritis, pseudotumor cerebri, and other complications of morbid obesity all reduce employability. If the morbidly obese patients are successful in gaining employment, they frequently encounter difficulty obtaining job advancement. Following surgically induced weight loss, there is generally a significant improvement in emotional feeling and self-image.[42] Several of my patients have obtained jobs or promotions that they are convinced were unobtainable had they not lost weight.

Obese patients have difficulty in attracting members of the opposite sex because of their unappealing appearance. Those patients who do marry often have pathologic relationships that can be jarred when the obese partner loses weight and becomes more attractive to the opposite sex. Because of problems with estrogen and androgen metabolism in obese women, they tend to be hirsute and have problems with menstrual regularity and fertility. In fact, pregnancy may be a "complication" of weight loss. Morbidly obese patients often have problems with personal hygiene (e.g., wiping themselves after a bowel movement or washing areas under a large abdominal panniculus) and often suffer from stress overflow urinary incontinence. They often have an offensive body odor that makes them even more unattractive.

SURGICAL MORBIDITY AND MORTALITY IN MORBIDLY OBESE PATIENTS

Difficulties in Recognizing Peritonitis

Extremely obese patients may demonstrate very few clinical signs of peritonitis. Although they may complain of severe abdominal pain, there may be no guarding, rigidity, or rebound tenderness. This circumstance has been well documented in patients who have developed a gastric leak following surgery for morbid obesity.[35] Signs of gastric perforation include fever, tachycardia, and tachypnea. Symptoms of peritonitis include shoulder pain, back pain, scrotal pain, pelvic discomfort, tenesmus, urinary frequency, and of particular importance, marked anxiety. I have recently had a morbidly obese patient with a known history of duodenal ulcer disease appear in the emergency room with severe epigastric pain, absent "peritoneal signs" during physical examination, and normal upright chest and abdominal radiograms. She was discharged only to return 2 days later with free air demonstrable on a chest radiogram indicating a perforated viscus. Exploratory laparotomy revealed a perforated duodenal ulcer with severe peritoneal soilage that suggested that the perforation was at least 24 hours old. The lack of physical signs in this morbidly obese lady understated the severity of her problem when she was first evaluated.

Two of my other patients appeared to have had a massive pulmonary embolus the third day following gastroplasty. One patient suffered a cardiac arrest in the nuclear medicine department while undergoing a ventilation-perfusion lung scan. Both patients had, in fact, developed a gastric leak and peritonitis. Autopsy failed to reveal any evidence of pulmonary embolus in either patient. Thus peritonitis should be seriously considered in any patient who has abdominal surgery and develops sudden air hunger and hypoxemia postoperatively. Mason and associates[35] have reported similar findings in patients initially thought to have had a pulmonary embolism only to find later that the clinical course was secondary to peritonitis from a gastric leak. A high index for suspicion of peritonitis is required in any postoperative morbidly obese patient whose clinical course appears to be deteriorating. Obtaining radiologic contrast studies may be indicated for patients with few clinical signs, and performing an exploratory laparotomy may be necessary in spite of negative barium studies to substantiate the presence or absence of a perforated viscus.

Thrombosis and Pulmonary Embolism

As previously noted, morbidly obese patients, especially those with respiratory insufficiency, have an increased tendency toward venous thrombosis and pulmonary embolism.[21,30] Of 565 patients who have undergone obesity surgery at the Medical College of Virginia, there have only been three patients with thrombophlebitis and four patients with nonfatal pulmonary embolism—in contrast to the reported incidence of these problems. My findings are almost certainly related to the routine use of intermittent venous compression boots in morbidly obese patients during surgery and for the first 2 to 3 postoperative days. The use of intermittent venous compression boots has, in random trials in nonobese patients, decreased the incidence of deep vein thrombosis.[5] Equally important, every attempt should be made to ambulate morbidly obese patients early, beginning the evening of their surgery. The need to use prophylactic subcutaneous heparin in these patients is uncertain, and I have not routinely used it. With these precautions, pulmonary embolism should be an uncommon event following surgery in the morbidly obese. If symptoms do arise that suggest pulmonary embolus (e.g., acute air hunger, tachypnea, and hypoxemia), it cannot be emphasized too strongly that in this patient population such clinical manifestations suggest an equal likelihood of peritonitis with septic-induced adult respiratory distress syndrome.[35]

Pulmonary Problems

In addition to the well-recognized association of the obesity hypoventilation and sleep apnea syndromes with morbid obesity, anesthetic induction may also be difficult and dangerous in patients with this disease. To minimize anesthesia-related problems, an arterial blood gas analysis should be obtained before surgery in all morbidly obese patients. Because of a high incidence of hypoxemic pulmonary arterial vasoconstriction and left-ventricular dysfunction, it is my policy to insert a Swan-Ganz catheter in all patients with an arterial oxygen tension (PaO_2) less than 60 mm Hg or arterial carbon dioxide tension ($PaCO_2$) greater than 45 mm Hg. Efforts should also be used to optimize cardiac function, possibly requiring digitalization, diuresis, and supplemental oxygen therapy. An arterial catheter has also been helpful for ventilator management during and after surgery.

Induction of anesthesia is accomplished with thiopental (Pentothal) and succinylcholine. Ventilation with 100% oxygen is achieved by using an oral airway with a tight-fitting mask over the mouth and nose and the neck hyperextended. This procedure may require one person to hold the mask and jaw and another to compress the ventilation bag. Oral-tracheal intubation is then attempted. If difficulties are encountered with this procedure, the attempt is abandoned after 1 minute, the oral airway is reinserted, and the patient again is ventilated with a mask. This procedure is repeated as necessary until the patient is successfully intubated. A fiberoptic bronchoscope placed through the endotracheal tube may further facilitate intubation.

Patients with symptoms suggestive of the obstructive sleep apnea syndrome (i.e., daytime somnolence and loud snoring) should undergo screening sleep capnography (see Fig. 67-3) or polysomnography (see Fig. 67-4). If more than 25% of their sleep is apneic (an amount obtained by dividing the duration of all apneas by the duration of sleep), they should be given a trial of nocturnal continuous positive airway pressure (cPAP). If nocturnal cPAP is ineffective or the patient cannot tolerate it, a tracheostomy should be performed after tracheal intubation. The increase in pharyngeal edema following oral-tracheal intubation (especially a traumatic intubation) may place the patient in jeopardy of postoperative upper-airway obstruction and possible respiratory arrest.

Following surgery, morbidly obese patients have better gas exchange if they are placed in the reverse Trendelenburg position since this posture permits increased diaphragmatic excursion.[53] This position places increased pressure on the leg veins and further supports the need for use of intermittent venous compression boots. Patients with obesity hypoventilation syndrome require postoperative mechanical ventilation using a volume ventilator. Positive end-expiratory pressure is rarely necessary and can even impair oxygenaton by impeding blood flow to well-ventilated alveoli. As the abdominal pain subsides and more effective breathing is obtained, the patient can be weaned from the ventilator when the arterial blood gas measurement returns to its preoperative value while the patient breathes room air even though this value would not normally be acceptable in nonobese patients.

Wound Complications

Morbidly obese patients have a greater risk of wound infection and fascial dehiscence. I have recently completed a randomized, prospective study comparing running No. 2 Dexon sutures (54 patients) with interrupted No. 28 stainless steel wire sutures (51 patients) used for abdominal wall closure. One dehiscence occurred in the wire closure group, and four incisional hernias occurred in each of the two groups. Performing running Dexon closure was significantly faster than performing the interrupted wire closure. Since there was no obvious difference in morbidity between the two methods of closure, it is currently my practice to use running No. 2 Dexon to close the fascia of the abdominal wall because this technique is faster, easier, and distributes tension more evenly than with an interrupted suture closure approach.

My patients have experienced only nine wound infections in the last 340 procedures for morbid obesity operations with which I have been associated, an incidence of 2.6%. Eight of these infections were small collections, which were easily managed on an outpatient basis. I believe that this low incidence is a result of the technique used for wound closure, which included irrigation with 1% neomycin, using no subcutaneous sutures (which have been shown to increase the frequency of wound infection), using a large suction drain, and using stainless steel skin staples.

DIETARY MANAGEMENT OF MORBID OBESITY

A number of dietary programs are available for weight reduction. They include hospital supervised programs, psychiatric behavioral modification programs, commercial approaches (e.g., Weight Watchers, Inc. and American Weight Loss Clinic), fad diets (e.g., Stillman Diet, Watkins Revolutionary Diet), and diet pills provided by unscrupulous physicians. Using these various approaches, many patients have lost considerable weight only to gain it back after an expenditure of thousands of dollars.

Unfortunately, none of these dietary approaches has achieved uniform long-term success. Although many individuals can lose weight successfully through dietary manipulation, the incidence of recidivism with a return to the predietary weight (or more) approaches 100% (Fig. 67-

MEAN WEIGHT CHANGES IN THREE GROUPS FASTING FOR VARYING PERIODS

Group	N	Duration of fast (days	Baseline weight (kg)	Baseline weight excess (%)	Weight loss with fast (kg)	% of subjects fasting to < 30% excess	Minimum weight after fasting plus dieting (kg)	Weight excess after fasting plus dieting (%)
1	49	<30	138.6	78.4	14.1	22.4	120.0	53.6
2	101	30-60	140.0	89.9	28.6	36.6	105.1‡	41.8
3	57	>60	150.0*,†	96.7	41.4	54.4	105.0‡	35.9
TOTAL	207	47	143.0	89.0	28.2	38.2	108.4	43.1

*Difference from group 1 is significant at $P < 0.05$
†Difference from group 2 is significant at $P < 0.01$
‡Difference from group 1 is significant at $P < 0.001$

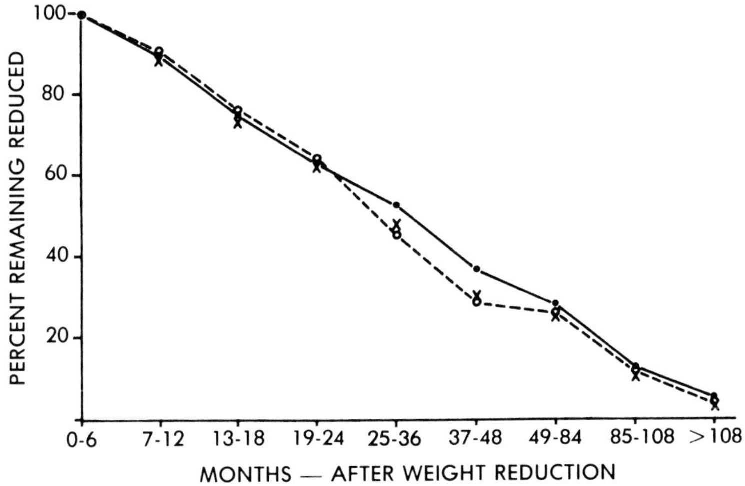

Fig. 67-7 Percent of patients maintaining reduced weights at various time intervals after they accomplished diet-induced weight loss. Solid line represents 60 patients with onset of obesity before age 21; broken line represents 42 patients with onset of obesity after age 21. (*X*, mean experience.) (From Johnson, D., and Drenick, F.J.: Arch. Intern. Med. **137:**1381, 1977.)

7).[23] In my experience, candidates for surgery have made multiple attempts at nonsurgical weight reduction. Particularly popular among these patients have been the various liquid protein diets, which became available in the late 1970s and provided 300 to 400 kcal per day in the form of a collagen hydrolysate. Unfortunately, by 1977 60 deaths, presumably secondary to ventricular arrhythmias, had been reported to the Center for Disease Control in Atlanta in individuals who were using these diets. More recently, very low-caloric diets containing high-quality protein and mineral supplements (e.g., Cambridge Diet) have also been used and have been associated with a mortality that may be similar to the liquid-protein diets (0.6%).[55] These diets have been distributed by lay people without adequate nutritional training and with inadequate patient follow-up.

SURGICAL MANAGEMENT OF MORBID OBESITY

Surgical Eligibility

Patients are only considered candidates for surgery to treat morbid obesity if they are at least 100 pounds overweight based on the ideal body weight tables published by the Metropolitan Life Insurance Co.[25] and if they have repeatedly tried for a minimum of 5 years to lose weight using various dietary regimens but without success. If a patient is just a little more than 100 pounds over ideal body weight and does not have an associated weight-related medical problem (e.g., diabetes, respiratory insufficiency, or pseudotumor cerebri), an attempt is made to talk that patient out of surgery since the attendant risks associated with surgery may exceed its potential benefits. In heavier patients (i.e., ones 200 pounds or more over ideal body weight), the potential benefits to be derived from surgery, despite the operative risks, far outweigh the risks associated with the morbidly obese state itself. Thus I am much more enthusiastic about offering surgery to this group of patients than ones with less excessive weight problems. In any case, the patient is fully appraised of the potential surgical complications and the chances of success. In addition, patients are routinely given the Hopkins Symptom Checklist to screen for significant psychopathology. If answers to questions on this checklist suggest a severe emotional problem, patients are referred to a psychiatrist for full psychologic assessment. If the patient is considered emotionally unstable, operative treatment of morbid obesity may be denied. However, several patients have been referred to me by psychiatrists for surgical treatment, and these patients have had a marked improvement in emotional stability associated with the improved self-image that accompanied weight reduction following surgery. Most insurance carriers have recognized the medical risk of morbid obesity and have underwritten the cost that these patients encounter when undergoing surgery.

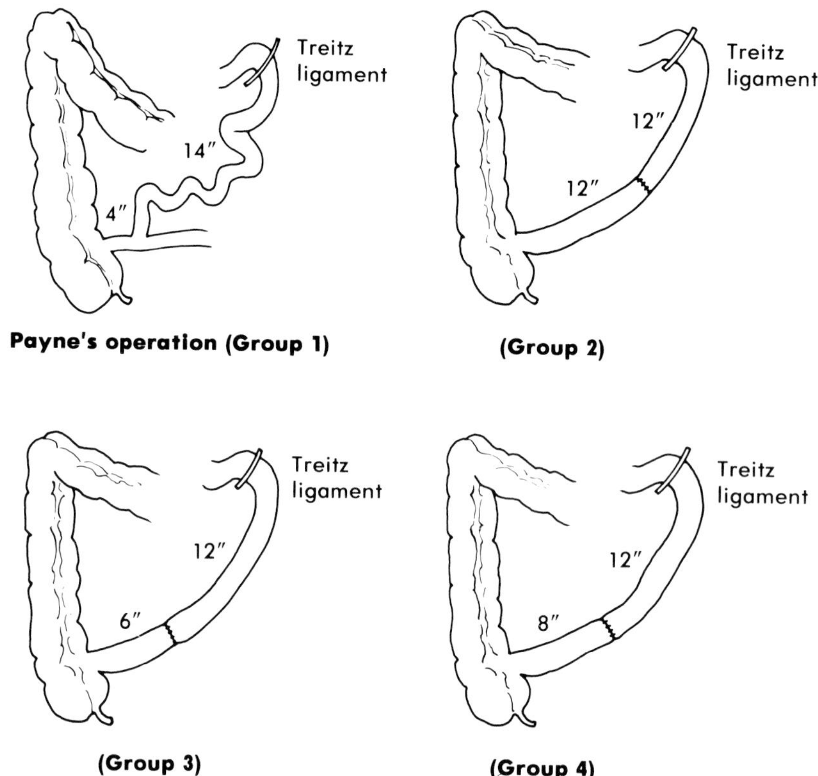

Fig. 67-8 End-to-side and various types of end-to-end jejunoileal bypass procedures. (From Scott, H.W., Jr., et al.: Surg. Gynecol. Obstet. **145**:661, 1977.)

Surgical Options

Jejunoileal Bypass

The first popular surgical procedure for the treatment of morbid obesity was the jejunioleal bypass, initially introduce by Payne and associates[37] and later modified by Scott and associates.[44] This operation produces an obligatory short-bowel syndrome that results in a malabsorptive state by short-circuiting the small intestine. The procedure connects various lengths of jejunum (8 to 14 inches) to the distal ileum (4 to 12 inches) as an end-to-end or end-to-side anastomosis (Fig. 67-8). The end-to-end procedures, which were associated with a greater weight loss, required decompression of the bypassed small intestine into the large bowel. In any of its forms, the jejunoileal bypass is distinct from the partial intestinal bypass for control of Type I hyperlipidemia in which only the distal 40 cm of ileum are bypassed.

Experience with the jejunoileal bypass has demonstrated a number of significant early and late complications[18,22].

- Liver failure
- Interstitial nephritis
- Rheumatoid-like arthritis
- Oxalate nephrolithiasis
- Gallstones
- Hypocalcemia
- Hypokalemia
- Hypomagnesemia
- Metabolic acidosis
- Hypoalbuminemia
- Diarrhea
- Bypass enteritis
- Pneumatosis cystoides intestinalis
- Intussusception
- Blind loop syndrome
- Small bowel obstruction

Liver failure, caused by either protein-calorie malnutrition or absorption of degradation products from bacterial overgrowth in the bypassed intestine, is associated with a 50% mortality rate. A rheumatoid-like arthritis may also occur and is a result of the absorption of bacterial products from the bypassed intestine since antibodies to the bacterial cell walls have been found in the joint fluids of patients with this problem. Malabsorption of bile salts increases the risk of cholelithiasis because of the decrease in cholesterol solubility, of hypocalcemia as a result of chelation of calcium with bile salts, and oxalate nephrolithiasis because of increased oxalate absorption across the colon where it is normally bound to calcium and unavailable for absorption. Intractable, malodorous diarrhea with associated potassium and magnesium depletion, metabolic acidosis, and severe malnutrition can occur. Vitamin B_{12} deficiency is relatively common following jejunoileal bypass. Bacterial overgrowth in the bypassed intestine can also lead to vitamin K deficiency, pneumatosis cystoides intestinalis, and a bypass enteritis associated with occult blood in the stools and iron-deficiency anemia. Since many of the problems enumerated previously are associated with anaerobic bacterial overgrowth in the bypassed intestine, they may be ameliorated with the antibiotic metronidazole. Mechanical complications can also occur following jejunoileal bypass and include small bowel obstruction and intussusception of the bypassed intestine.

Randomized, prospective studies have shown that the gastric bypass operation is associated with a weight loss comparable to and a complication rate lower than that of the jejunoileal bypass.[3,16] Furthermore, in some patients, the complications associated with jejunoileal bypass have necessitated its dismantling with the reestablishment of

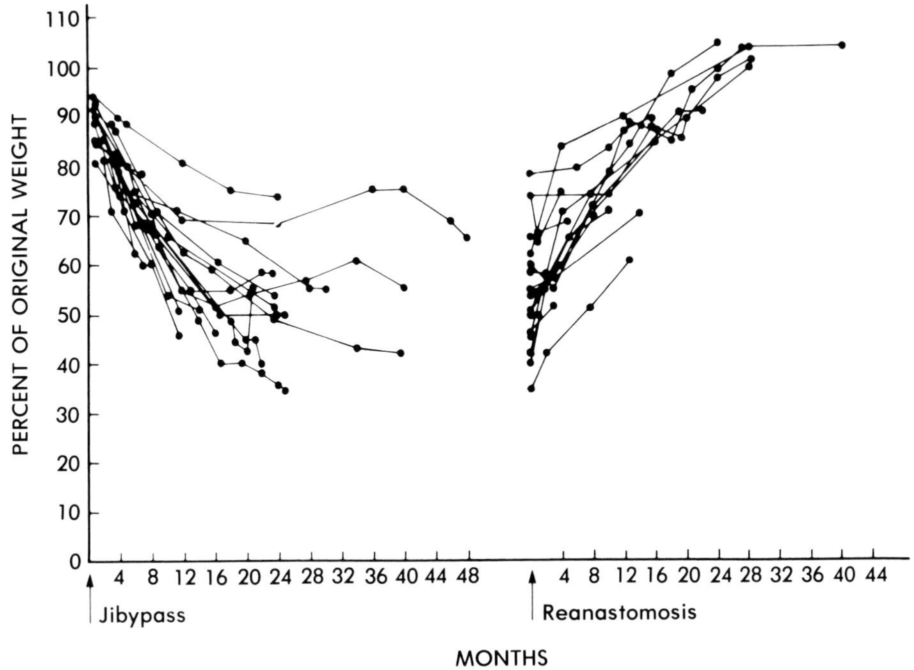

Fig. 67-9 Weight loss after jejunoileal bypass and weight gain after reanastomosis. (From Halverson, J.D., et al.: Surgery **84:**241, 1978.)

normal gastrointestinal continuity. Although reversal of the jejunoileal bypass is invariably associated with regaining lost weight (Fig. 67-9), this problem can be prevented by conversion to a gastric bypass during the same operation. In view of these studies, investigators at most academic centers now believe that the jejunoileal bypass should no longer be performed.

Recently a modification of the jejunoileal bypass, known as the partial biliopancreatic bypass, has been proposed as an alternative operative approach for the management of morbid obesity.[43] This operation includes a high subtotal gastrectomy and an anastomosis between the stomach and the distal 200 cm of the small intestine with an end-to-side anastomosis of the proximal small intestine 50 cm from the ligament of Treitz (Fig. 67-10). This procedure is apparently devoid of most of the jejunoileal bypass complications since there is no ''blind loop.'' Despite its potential ability to control morbid obesity surgically, it is a formidable operation when compared to the gastric procedures currently available. Randomized, prospective trials have not yet been performed to evaluate the safety and efficacy of partial biliopancreatic bypass for the treatment of morbid obesity.

Gastric Procedures for Treating Morbid Obesity

In 1966 Mason and Ito[33] reported weight loss results following division of the stomach into a small proximal pouch (approximately 10% of the total capacity of the stomach) that was anastomosed to a loop of jejunum and bypassed the distal 90% of the stomach and duodenum. The rationale for this procedure was based on the weight loss that followed subtotal gastrectomy for the treatment of duodenal ulcer disease, and the procedure was designed to interfere with food intake rather than with digestion and absorption such as occurs with the jejunoileal bypass. Although there was initial concern that peptic ulcers could

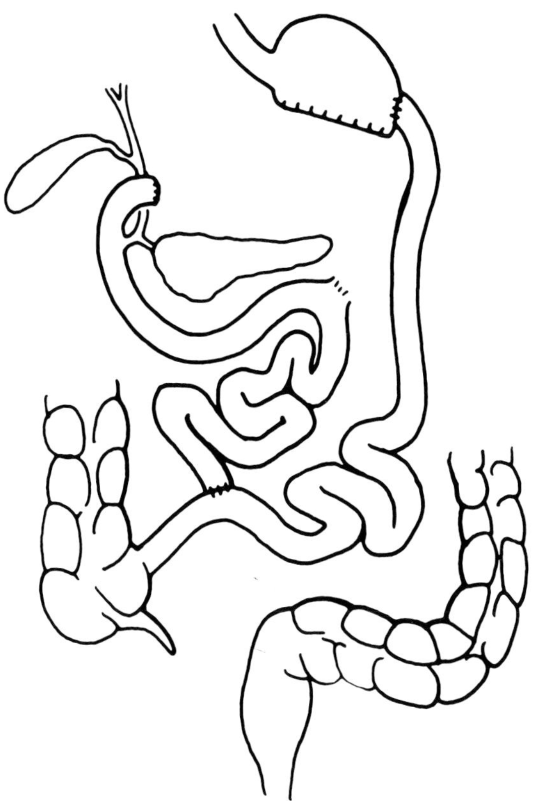

Fig. 67-10 Biliopancreatic bypass that requires a distal two-thirds gastrectomy and a gastroenterostomy to distal one half of the small intestine. Proximal one half of small intestine is anastomosed to ileum 50 cm proximal to the ileocecal valve. (From Griffen, W.O., and Bell, R.M.: Contemp. Surg. **23:**15, 1983.)

develop in the bypassed stomach or duodenum, experience with this procedure has indicated that the incidence of this complication is low. Serum gastrin levels have been normal in these patients, probably as a result of the preservation of an intact acid inhibitory mechanism for antral gastrin release.[34] Since this initial report, other modifications for gastric bypass have been developed. In addition, the technique has been greatly simplified with the use of stapling instruments. Furthermore, newer procedures have been developed that compartmentalize the stomach through a precisely measured opening, avoiding the need entirely for bypass into a loop of intestine. This latter approach is called "gastroplasty."

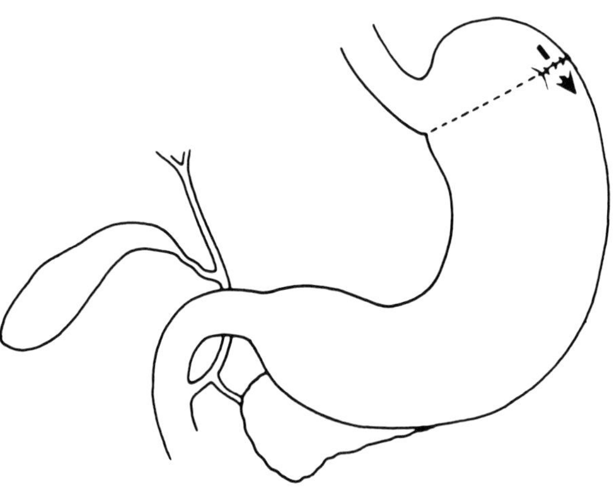

Fig. 67-11 Horizontal gastroplasty with stoma on greater curvature. (From Griffen, W.O., and Bell, R.M.: Contemp. Surg. **23:**15, 1983.)

Gastroplasty Procedures

Gastroplasties can be performed with the placement of sutures either horizontally (Fig. 67-11) or vertically (Fig. 67-12). The former approach requires ligation and division of most of the short gastric vessels between the stomach and the spleen and carries with it the risk of devascularization of the gastric pouch and possible splenic injury. Types of horizontal gastroplasties include a single application of the 90-cm stapling device without suture reinforcement of the stoma between the upper- and lower-gastric pouches[36] or a double application of staples with either a central or a lateral polyproylene-reinforced stoma (Gomez).[15] Using these three horizontal procedures, our failure rate was 71%, 46%, and 42% respectively (Fig. 67-13).[49] Failure was defined as the loss of less than 40% of excess weight, loss of early satiety following surgery with increased ability and desire to eat, and radiologic or endoscopic evidence of suture-line disruption or stomal enlargement. Complete stapling of the stomach with a 1-cm gastrogastrostomy constructed anterior to the staple line has also been recommended. With all of these procedures, other investigators [26,27,29,39] and I[49] have had an unacceptably high incidence of patients who fail to lose weight or who regain it once it has been lost.

Recently Mason[32] has proposed a vertical banded gastroplasty in which, with the end-to-end stapling device, a stapled opening is made in the stomach 5 cm from the cardio-esophageal junction (see Fig. 67-12). Two or three applications of a 90-mm stapling device are made between the opening and the angle of His, and a 1.5- × 5-cm strip of polypropylene mesh is wrapped around the "stoma" on the lesser curvature and is sutured to itself and not to the stom-

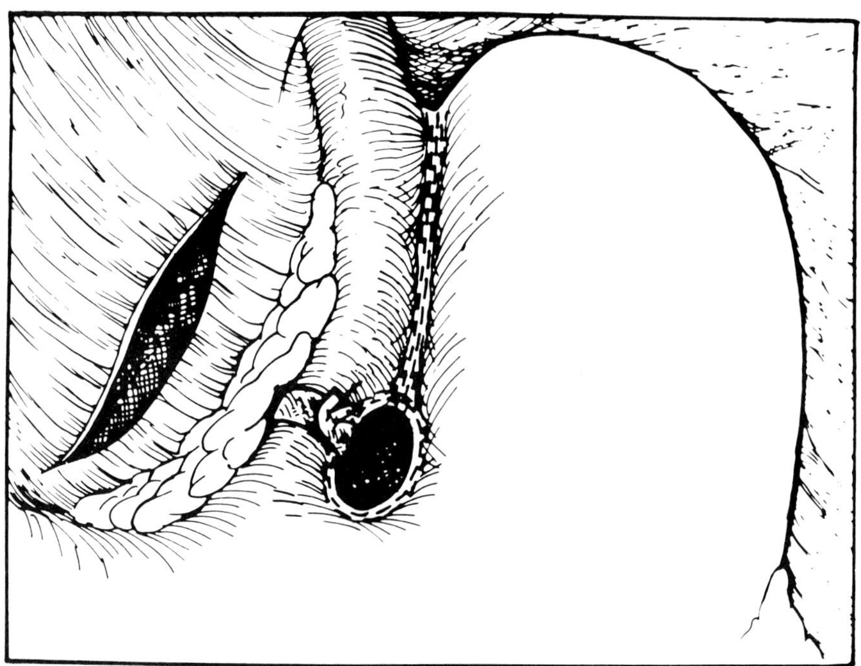

Fig. 67-12 Vertical banded gastroplasty with measured pouch volume of 50 ml or less at pressure of 50 cm. Two sets of staples and 5-cm polypropylene mesh collar reinforced outlet. (From Mason, E.E.: Arch. Surg. **117:**701, Copyright 1983, American Medical Association.)

ach. Erosion of the mesh into the stomach has been a very rare complication with this procedure. This approach presently is the best of the gastroplasty procedures available.

Gastric Bypass Procedures

The gastric bypass can also be performed with placement of staples in a vertical or a horizontal direction. In my experience, the vertical approach (Fig. 67-14) is preferred since there is less risk of gastric pouch devascularization or splenic injury. With either approach, however, there is no need to transect the stomach. The gastrojejunostomy can be a loop, a loop with a jejunojejunostomy constructed below the gastrojejunostomy, or a Roux-en-Y. The latter two procedures prevent bile reflux into the gastric pouch. I prefer the Roux-en-Y approach (see Fig. 67-14) since it would theoretically limit food intake should stomal dilation occur. In any case, the gastric pouch should be restricted to a 30-ml volume and the stoma to a 1-cm opening to produce early satiety and to impede rapid gastric emptying. The gastric pouch has limited acid secretory capacity and has been associated with a low incidence of marginal ulcer (7% in my series) in the absence of vagotomy.

Gastroplasty vs. Gastric Bypass

There have been several randomized, prospective studies comparing the gastric bypass procedure to unbanded gastroplasty procedures, including the gastrogastrostomy and Gomez techniques.[26,27,29,39] Each of these studies has shown a significantly greater weight loss using the gastric bypass procedure (Fig. 67-15). I have recently compared a vertical Roux-en-Y gastric bypass to the newer vertical banded gastroplasty and have also found a significantly greater weight loss with the gastric bypass procedure.[50] When patients were divided according to different categories of pathologic eating behavior based on a preoperative dietary interview, it was found that "sweets eaters" had a significantly more pronounced weight loss following a vertical banded gastroplasty than after gastric bypass when compared with individuals not addicted to sweets. Sweets eaters were defined as individuals who ate more than 300 calories of simple carbohydrates (e.g., candy, sodas, and Kool-Aid) a minimum of three times per week. There was no significant difference in weight loss between sweets eaters and nonsweets eaters in the gastric bypass group itself. The more favorable weight loss in sweets eaters following gastric bypass when compared to vertical banded gastroplasty was probably a result of the development of the dumping syndrome following gastric bypass. Many, but not all, of my gastric bypass patients claimed that sweets produced one or more of the following symptoms—nausea, light-headedness, flushing, and diarrhea; most of these patients stated that they had lost their taste for sweets. Unfortunately, the group of patients undergoing gastric bypass also had a higher incidence of stomal ulcer, stomal stenosis, vitamin B_{12} deficiency, and iron deficiency anemia.[51] Other postoperative complications were comparable between vertical banded gastroplasty and gastric bypass. On the basis of these observations, I currently favor Roux-en-Y gastric bypass for sweets eaters and vertical banded gastroplasty for nonsweets eaters.

The mechanism(s) of weight loss following gastric re-

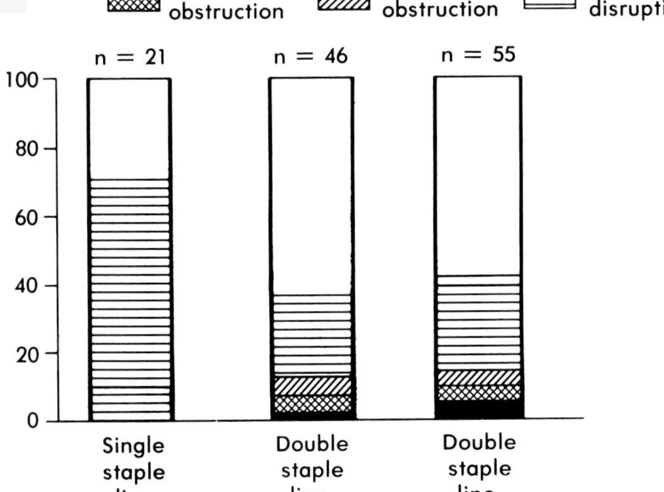

Fig. 67-13 High incidence of stomal disruption, stomal stenosis requiring dilation or repeat surgery for obstruction, or leaking following single staple line, double staple line with central stoma, or Gomez gastroplasties. (From Sugerman, H.J., and Wolper, J.L.: Am. J. Surg. **148**:331, 1984.)

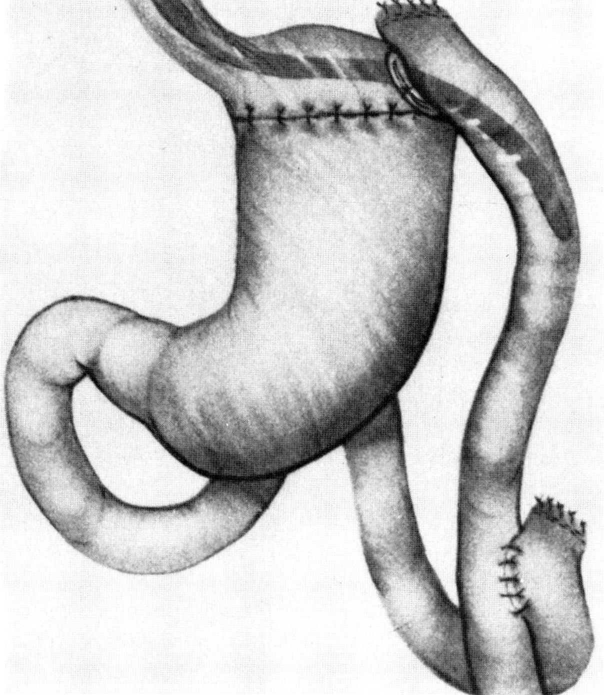

Fig. 67-14 Roux-en-Y gastric bypass with anterior gastric pouch. (From Linner, J.H., and Drew, R.L.: Contemp. Surg. **26**:46, 1985.)

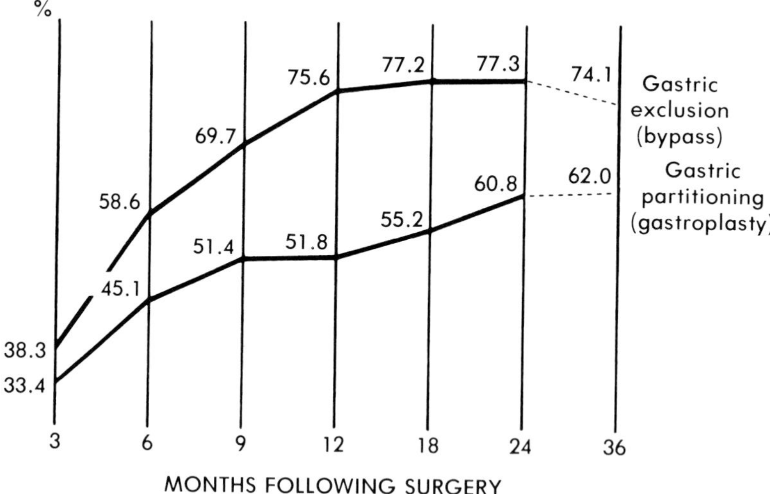

Fig. 67-15 Percentage of mean excess weight loss by patients with gastric exclusion compared with patients with gastric partitioning. (From Lechner, G.W., and Elliott, D.W.: Arch. Surg. **118:**685, Copyright 1983, American Medical Association.)

strictive surgery is unknown. Most patients claim that they lose their appetites following such surgery and that small amounts of food make them feel full. Dilation of the gastroplasty stoma is usually associated with the return of insatiable hunger and a regain of weight. Possible mechanisms for feeling full include stimulation of the hypothalamic satiety center or inhibition of the hunger center by afferent vagal impulses or release of hormones such as cholecystokinin.[46] The hormonal mechanism is probably the more important of these two possibilities since three patients of mine who had undergone a truncal vagotomy for duodenal ulcer disease still had early satiety following gastric bypass. A direct effect on gastric motility and inhibition of "hunger pains" may also be involved through the effect of pouch distention on the gastric pacemaker.[54]

Complications of Gastric Surgery for Morbid Obesity

The most feared complication of gastric surgery for morbid obesity is a postoperative gastric leak with the development of peritonitis. This leak can occur at the staple line of the proximal gastric pouch or in the distal bypassed stomach. A leak from the pouch is probably secondary to ischemic necrosis since this has occurred more often in our experience with either horizontal gastroplasty or gastric bypass procedures with "take-down" of the short gastric vessels. Blowout of the distal stomach occurs most often in gastric bypass procedures, possibly as a result of edema at the ligament of Treitz, in the afferent limb of the loop gastrojejunostomy, or at the jejunojejunostomy of a Roux-en-Y procedure with the development of a closed loop obstruction. For this reason, most surgeons who operate on morbidly obese patients believe that gastric-bypass patients should have a gastrostomy tube placed in the distal gastric pouch. The gastrostomy tube is clamped progressively as tolerated and generally is removed several weeks after surgery. In patients undergoing conversion from a jejunoileal bypass to a gastric bypass, the gastrostomy tube can be used for feeding until oral intake permits weight stabilization.

The most dangerous aspect of a gastric leak is the difficulty in recognizing the symptoms of peritonitis.[35] I have had personal experience with 18 leaks in 565 patients, with six occurring after conversion of a failed gastroplasty to gastric bypass.[49] Delayed recognition of the symptoms of leak following Gomez gastroplasties led to the death of two of these patients. Other series have reported similar results.[13,35] All of the leaks encountered in my experience have occurred within the first 4 postoperative days. None has arisen after hospital discharge.

Sudden death has been observed following gastric surgery for obesity. I have had five cases of sudden death, which occurred 3 days, 5 weeks, 3 months, 12 months, and 18 months following surgery, in a total of 565 patients. The three patients on whom autopsies were performed had unrevealing findings. Before obesity surgery, however, each of these patients had underlying heart disease, including myotonic dystrophy in one patient who had a pacemaker for complete heart block (a functioning pacemaker was noted at autopsy), hypertrophic subaortic stenosis in another patient, and combined right-sided and left-sided severe ventricular dysfunction in a third patient, which was associated with the respiratory insufficiency of obesity. In the two patients who were not autopsied, a pulmonary embolus could have been responsible for death.

An incidence of marginal ulcer has been noted in 7% of our gastric bypass patients. Such ulcers have responded to histamine-receptor blockade in all but three patients. Two of these patients had been converted from a failed gastroplasty to a Roux-en-Y gastrojejunostomy; they subsequently developed large ulcers, which failed to respond to either cimetidine or ranitidine, on both the gastric and jejunal sides of their gastrojejunostomies. Both patients subsequently required total proximal gastrectomy and esophagojejunostomy. Gastrin levels were normal in both patients. The etiology of the ulcers is uncertain but was probably secondary to ischemia.

Stomal stenosis developed in 15% of my patients following Roux-en-Y gastric bypass. This problem was effectively treated with endoscopic balloon stomal dilation that could almost always be done as an outpatient procedure and usually required only one dilation.[59] On occasion, hospitalization and multiple dilations were necessary.

A rare syndrome of polyneuropathy has been noted following gastric surgery for morbid obesity. This problem has usually occurred in association with severe protein-calorie malnutrition and the patient's failure to take multivitamins.[10] Acute thiamine deficiency has been thought by some to be responsible for this condition. Vitamin B_{12} deficiency has been observed following gastric bypass and mandates long-term follow-up of these patients with vitamin measurements.[19,31] B_{12} deficiency is probably caused by the failure of the coupling of B_{12} to the intrinsic factor, which occurs in the presence of acid in the body of the stomach. This deficiency can be corrected with large doses (500 μg/day) of oral B_{12}. In contrast to these findings, deficiencies in vitamin C, thiamine, or folic acid are generally not a problem in gastroplasty or gastric bypass patients. Iron deficiency anemia can occasionally be seen in menstruating women following gastric bypass. This deficiency can be refractory to supplemental ferrous sulfate tablets since iron absorption requires acid and takes place primarily in the duodenum and upper jejunum. Iron-dextran injections may be necessary to manage this problem, although I have recently noted improved absorption with ferrous sulfate elixir. Deficiencies in zinc, calcium, or magnesium have not been observed in these patients following surgery.

Cholecystitis is seen in approximately one third of morbidly obese patients. Gastric surgery for obesity significantly increases the risk of developing cholelithiasis.[56] Of 92 patients I managed with normal preoperative sonography, 14% developed cholecystitis and 2% developed asymptomatic cholelithiasis 6 months to 2 years following gastric surgery for obesity. Since bile salt absorption is probably normal in these patients, it is my hypothesis that the increased bile lithogenicity is a result of cholesterol mobilization from storage areas with an increased prehepatic cholesterol load. Because of the high incidence of gall bladder disease following surgery, one group of investigators has recommended prophylactic cholecystectomy.[56]

Other complications, which are observed with any type of surgery in obese patients, have already been discussed and include wound infection, wound dehiscence, incisional hernia, thrombophlebitis, and pulmonary embolus.

Failed Gastroplasty

Attempts to revise a failed gastroplasty are fraught with problems.[49] They include recurrence of stomal dilation and difficulties with postoperative gastric emptying, which are probably secondary to damage to the nerves of Latarget. Repeat surgery in these patients is extremely difficult because of the extensive adhesions to the liver and spleen. Thus it is not surprising that these nerves can be damaged during the repeat surgery. Results are generally better when the failed gastroplasty is converted to a Roux-en-Y gastric bypass. Nonetheless, because of technical difficulties, patients with this problem must be adequately informed that the risk of serious complications is far more pronounced after a secondary than after a primary gastric bypass.[49] Such informed consent may play a role in whether a patient chooses to undergo surgery for morbid obesity.

SUMMARY

Selectively applied gastric procedures can yield a very satisfactory weight reduction in the morbidly obese patient, with an average loss of 68% of excess weight within 1 to 1½ years after surgery. Weight becomes stable at this level in most patients when caloric intake meets caloric expenditure. Following surgery, these patients may have difficulty eating chicken or red meats but usually tolerate fish, seafood, and vegetables well. They must be followed carefully to ensure an adequate protein intake, a deficiency of which may be responsible for the occasional sudden deaths observed secondary to acute cardiac arrhythmias. Rarely a patient may request that the procedure be reversed because of dissatisfaction with the operative results. If such a procedure becomes necessary, a large gastrogastrostomy is usually required above the staple line and may be associated with a gastric emptying problem postoperatively because of injury of the nerves of Laterget.

The weight loss following surgery for morbid obesity will completely correct insulin-dependent diabetes and the headaches associated with cerebral spinal fluid pressure elevation in pseudotumor cerebri in almost all patients. The obstructive sleep apnea syndrome will resolve completely with the weight loss. Hypoxemia and hypercarbia seen in the obesity hypoventilation syndrome and the associated right-sided and left-sided cardiac pressure abnormalities will return toward normal with the accompanying weight loss. Furthermore, the loss in weight will permit healing of chronic venous stasis ulcers associated with venous insufficiency and improve low back pain as well as joint related pain; in fact, weight loss may permit successful total artificial joint replacement. Patient self-image is markedly improved following gastric obesity surgery, although this change can cause serious marital difficulties. Patients report being able to do things that most of us consider routine but that they could not do before weight loss such as washing their feet, wiping themselves after a bowel movement, or cleaning their homes. Some patients have been able to gain excellent employment, which they are certain would not have become available had they not lost weight.

A recent study has shown results from an intensive physician-supervised dietary program were equivalent to results from Gomez gastroplasty for weight reduction.[1] However, the amount of weight regained was significantly less for patients receiving the Gomez gastroplasty than for patients who tried diet control so that the total weight loss was significantly better in patients undergoing surgery. Since the Gomez gastroplasty is inferior to either gastric bypass or the newer vertical banded gastroplasty, it can be presumed that these operations would be even better than diet alone in enhancing weight loss and preventing its regain.

Although current surgical procedures have provided an effective means of enhancing weight loss in the morbidly obese patient, the ultimate goal of the surgeon should be the replacement of surgical procedures with less invasive, less dangerous, and more effective nonsurgical approaches. Hopefully, understanding the physiology responsible for the satiety provided by gastric surgical intervention will yield clues to the pathophysiology of morbid obesity and will enable more effective medical management of this common, incapacitating, and potentially life-threatening disease.

SUGGESTED READINGS

Mason, E.E.: Surgical treatment of obesity, vol. 26, Major problems in clinical surgery, Philadelphia, 1981, W.B. Saunders Co.

Stunkard, A.J.: Obesity, Philadelphia, 1981, W.B. Saunders Co.

REFERENCES

1. Andersen, T., et al.: Randomized trial of diet and gastroplasty compared with diet alone in morbid obesity, N. Engl. J. Med. **310**:352, 1984.
2. Batist, G., et al.: Low antithrombin III in morbid obesity: return to normal with weight reduction, J.P.E.N. **7**:447, 1983.
3. Buckwalter, J.A.: A prospective comparison of the jejunoileal and gastric bypass operations for morbid obesity, World J. Surg. **1**:757, 1977.
4. Burwell, C.S., et al.: Extreme obesity associated with alveolar hypoventilation: a Pickwickian syndrome, Am. J. Med. **21**:811, 1956.
5. Coe, N.P., et al.: Prevention of deep vein thrombosis in urological patients: a controlled, randomized trial of low-dose heparin and external pneumatic compression boots, Surgery **83**:230, 1978.
6. Corbitt, J.J., and Mehta, M.P.: Cerebrospinal fluid pressure in normal obese subjects and patients with pseudomotor cerebri, Neurology **33**:1386, 1983.
7. DeDivitis, O., et al.: Obesity and cardiac function, Circulation **64**:477, 1981.
8. Drenick, E.J.: Definition and health consequences of morbid obesity, Surg. Clin. North Am. **59**:963, 1979.
9. Drenick, E.J., et al.: Excessive mortality and causes of death in morbidly obese men, JAMA **243**:443, 1980.
10. Feit, H., et al.: Peripheral neuropathy and starvation after gastric partitioning for morbid obesity, Ann. Intern. Med. **96**:453, 1982.
11. Feurer, I.D., et al.: Resting energy expenditure in morbid obesity, Ann. Surg. **197**:17, 1983.
12. Foch, T.T., and McClearn, G.E.: Genetics, body weight, and obesity. In Stunkard, A.J., editor: Obesity, Philadelphia, 1980, W.B. Saunders Co.
13. Freeman, J.B., and Burchett, H.J.: A comparison of gastric bypass and gastroplasty for morbid obesity, Surgery **88**:433, 1980.
14. Gleysteen, J.J., and Barboriak, J.J.: Improvement in heart disease risk factors after gastric bypass, Arch. Surg. **118**:681, 1983.
15. Gomez, C.A.: Gastroplasty in morbid obesity, Surg. Clin. North Am. **59**:1113, 1979.
16. Griffen, W.O., Young, V.L., and Stevenson, C.C.: A prospective comparison of gastric and jejunoileal bypass for morbid obesity, Ann. Surg. **186**:500, 1977.
17. Guilleminault, C., and Delment, W.G., editors: Sleep apnea syndromes, New York, 1978, Alan R. Liss, Inc.
18. Halverson, J.D., et al.: Jejunoileal bypass for morbid obesity: a critical appraisal, Am. J. Med. **64**:461, 1978.
19. Halverson, J.D., et al.: Gastric bypass for morbid obesity: a medical-surgical assessment, Ann. Surg. **194**:152, 1981.
20. Harvey, R.M., and Enson, Y.: Pulmonary vascular resistance, Adv. Intern. Med. **15**:73, 1969.
21. Hassan, F.M., Auchincloss, J.H., Jr., and Gilbert, R.: Thromboembolic disease and cardiorespiratory syndrome of obesity, N.Y. State J. Med. **76**:272, 1976.
22. Hocking, M.P., et al.: Jejunoileal bypass for morbid obesity. Late follow-up in 100 cases, N. Engl. J. Med. **308**:995, 1983.
23. Johnson, D., and Drenick, E.J.: Therapeutic fasting in morbid obesity, Arch. Intern. Med. **137**:1381, 1977.
24. Keys, A., et al.: Coronary heart disease: overweight and obesity as risk factors, Ann. Intern. Med. **77**:15, 1972.
25. Knapp, T.R.: A methodological critique of the "Ideal Weight" concept, JAMA **250**:506, 1983.
26. Laws, H.L., and Piantadosi, S.: Superior gastric reduction procedure for morbid obesity: a prospective, randomized trial, Ann. Surg. **193**:334, 1981.
27. Lechner, G.W., and Callender, A.K.: Subtotal gastric exclusion and gastric partitioning: a randomized prospective comparison of one hundred patients, Surgery **90**:637, 1981.
28. Lew, E.A., and Garfinkel, L.: Variations in mortality by weight among 750,000 men and women, J. Chronic Dis. **32**:563, 1979.
29. Linner, J.H.: Comparative effectiveness of gastric bypass and gastroplasty, Arch. Surg. **117**:695, 1982.
30. MacGregor, M.I., Block, A.J., and Ball, W.C., Jr.: Serious complications and sudden death in the Pickwickian syndrome, Johns Hopkins Med. J. **126**:279, 1970.
31. MacLean, L.D., Rhode, B.M., and Shizgal, H.M.: Nutrition following gastric operations for morbid obesity, Ann. Surg. **198**:347, 1983.
32. Mason, E.E.: Vertical banded gastroplasty for obesity, Arch. Surg. **117**:701, 1982.
33. Mason, E.E., and Ito, C.: Gastric bypass in obesity, Surg. Clin. North Am. **47**:1345, 1967.
34. Mason, E.E., et al.: Effect of gastric bypass on gastric secretion, Am. J. Surg. **131**:162, 1976.
35. Mason, E.E., et al.: Risk reduction in gastric operations for obesity, Ann. Surg. **190**:158, 1979.
36. Pace, W.G., et al.: Gastric partitioning for morbid obesity, Ann. Surg. **190**:392, 1979.
37. Payne, J.H., et al.: Surgical treatment of morbid obesity: sixteen years of experience, Arch. Surg. **106**:432, 1973.
38. Pellicci, P.M., Salvati, E.A., and Robinson, H.J.: Mechanical failures in total hip replacement requiring re-operation, J. Bone Joint Surg. **61A**:28, 1979.
39. Pories, W.J., et al.: The effectiveness of gastric bypass over gastric partition in morbid obesity: consequence of distal gastric and duodenal exclusion, Ann. Surg. **196**:389, 1982.
40. Rochester, D.R., and Enson, Y.: Current concepts in the pathogenesis of the obesity hyperventilation syndrome, Am. J. Med. **57**:402, 1972.
41. Rouse, T.M., Malangon, M.A., and Schulte, W.J.: Necrotizing fascitis: a preventable disaster, Surgery **92**:769, 1982.
42. Saltzstein, E.C., and Guttmann, M.C.: Gastric bypass for morbid obesity: preoperative and postoperative psychological evaluation of patients, Arch. Surg. **115**:21, 1980.
43. Scopinaro, N., et al: Two years of clinical experience with biliopancreatic bypass for obesity, Am. J. Clin. Nutr. **33**:506, 1980.
44. Scott, H.W., et al.: New considerations in use of jejunoileal bypass in patients with morbid obesity, Ann. Surg. **177**:723, 1973.
45. Sims, E.A.H., and Horton, E.S.: Endocrine and metabolic adaptation to obesity and starvation, Am. J. Clin. Nutr. **21**:1455, 1968.
46. Smith, G.P., and Gibbs, J.: Gut peptides and postprandial satiety, Fed. Proc. **43**:2889, 1984.
47. Stunkard, A.J.: Obesity, Philadelphia, 1980, W.B. Saunders Co.
48. Sugerman, H.J., et al.: Gastric surgery for respiratory insufficiency of obesity, Chest **89**:81, 1986.
49. Sugerman, H.J., and Wolper, J.L.: Failed gastroplasty for morbid obesity: revised gastroplasty versus Roux-en-Y gastric bypass, Am. J. Surg. **148**:331, 1984.
50. Sugerman, H.J., Birkenhauer, R., and Starkey, J.V.: A randomized prospective trial of gastric bypass versus vertical bonded gastroplasty for morbid obesity and their effects on sweets or nonsweets eaters, Ann. Surg. (In press.)
51. Thompson, W.P., et al.: Complications and weight loss in 150 consecutive gastric exclusion patients, Am. J. Surg. **146**:602, 1983.
52. Van Itallie, T.B.: Obesity: adverse effects on health and longevity, Am. J. Clin. Nutr. **32**:2723, 1979.
53. Vaughan, R.W., Bauer, S., and Wise, L.: Effect of position (semirecumbent versus supine) on postoperative oxygenation in morbidly obese subjects, Anesth. Analg. **55**:37, 1976.

54. Villar, H.V., et al.: Mechanisms of satiety and gastric emptying after gastric partitioning and bypass, Surgery **90:**229, 1981.
55. Wadden, T.A., et al.: The Cambridge diet: more mayhem? JAMA **250:**2833, 1983.
56. Wattchow, D.A., et al.: Prevalence and treatment of gall stones after gastric bypass surgery for morbid obesity, Br. Med. J. **286:**763, 1983.
57. Weisinger, J.R., et al.: The nephrotic syndrome: a complication of massive obesity, Ann. Intern. Med. **81:**440, 1974.
58. Wise, L., and Stein, T.: The effect of jejunoileal bypass on bile composition and the formation of biliary calculi, Ann. Surg. **187:**57, 1978.
59. Wolper, J.C. et al.: Endoscopic dilatation of late stomal stenosis following gastric surgery for morbid obesity, Arch. Surg. **119:**836, 1984.
60. Yim, G.K.W., and Lony, M.T.: Opioids, feeding, and anorexias, Fed. Proc. **43:**2893, 1984.

INDEX

C

G

I

N

S

W

X